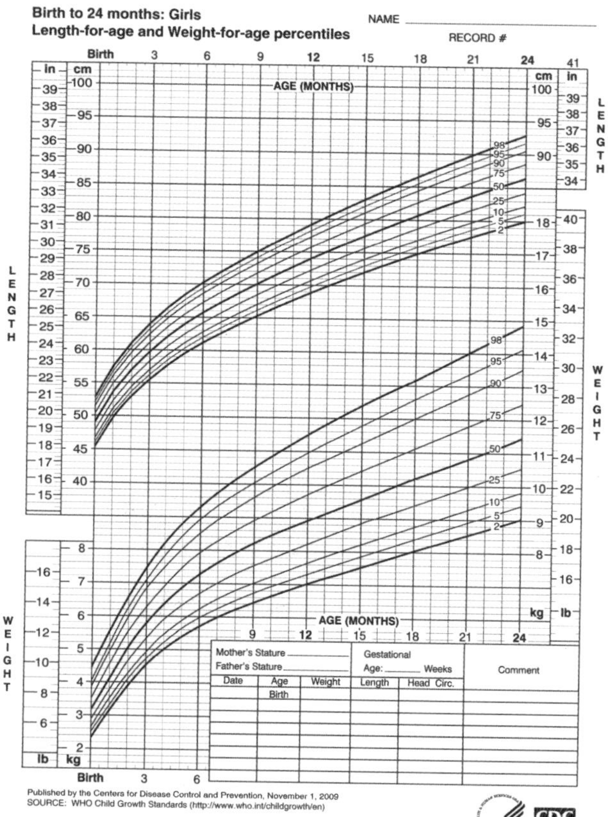

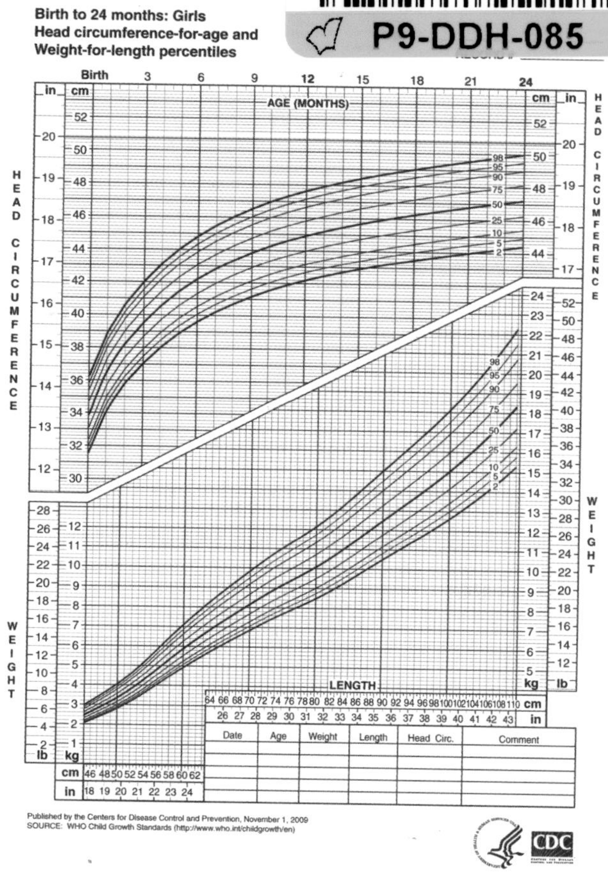

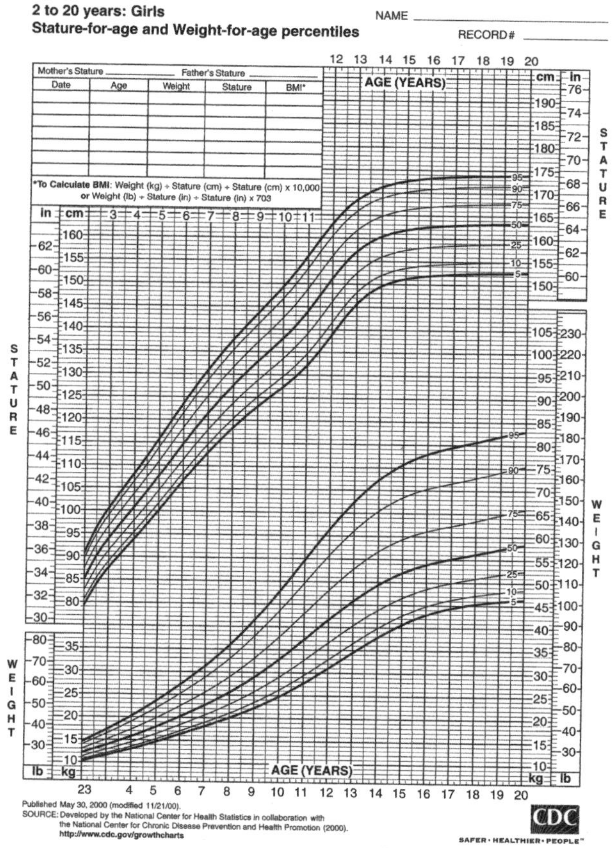

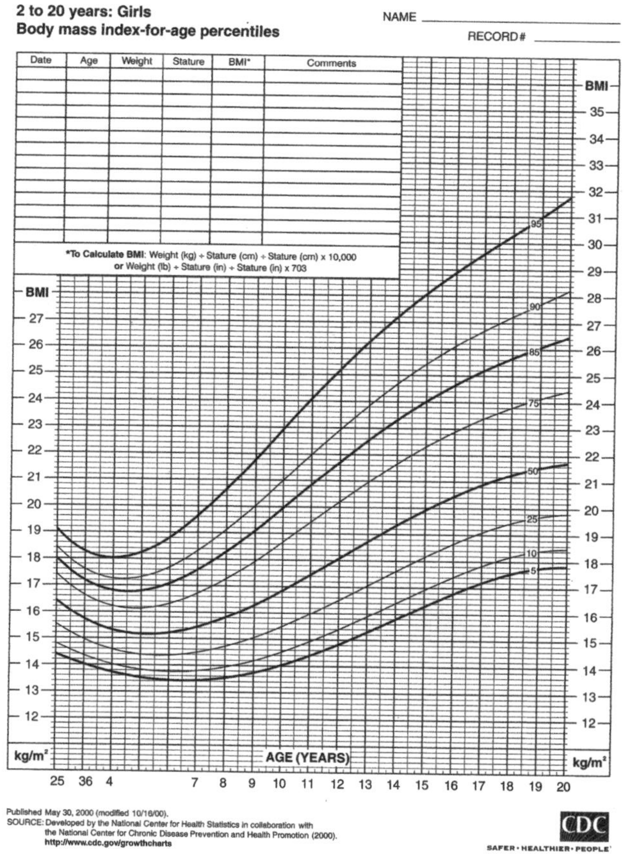

• **Figure 2** (1) Birth to 24 months: girls' length-for-age and weight-for-age percentiles. (2) Birth to 24 months: girls' head circumference-for-age and weight-for-length percentiles. (Published by the Centers for Disease Control and Prevention, November 1, 2009. From WHO Child Growth Standards. Available at www.cdc.gov/growthcharts.) (3) 2 to 20 years old: girls' stature-for-age and weight-for-age percentiles. (4) 2 to 20 years old: girls' body mass index-for-age percentiles. (From the National Center for Health Statistics in collaboration with the National Center for Chronic Disease Prevention and Health Promotion, 2000.)

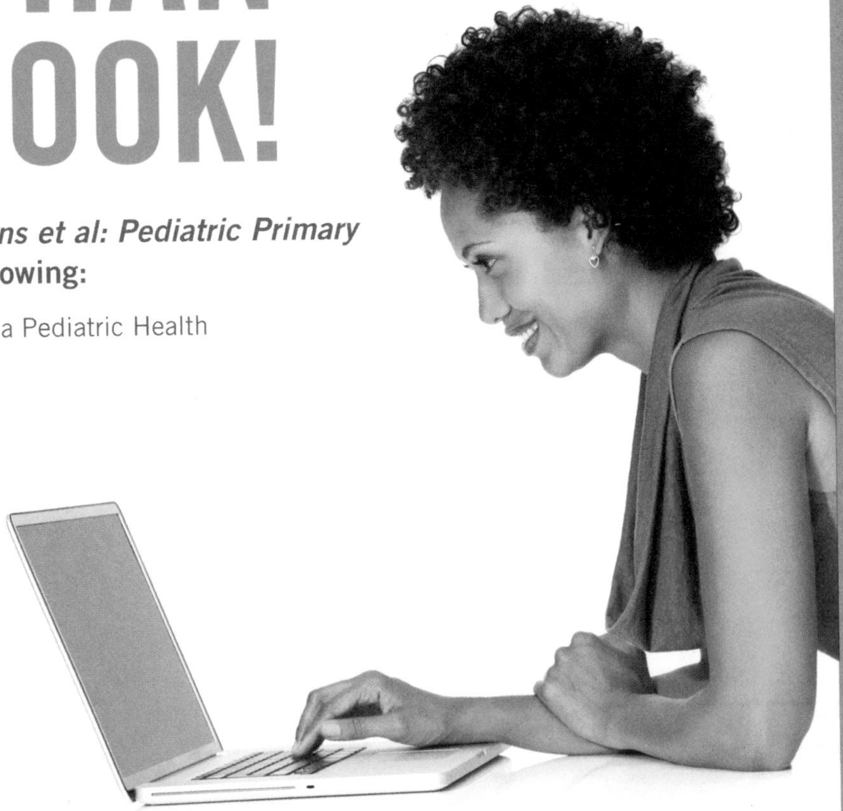

Pediatric Primary Care

Sixth Edition

Editors

Catherine E. Burns, PhD, RN, CPNP-PC, FAAN

Professor Emeritus
Primary Health Care Nurse Practitioner Specialty
School of Nursing
Oregon Health & Science University
Portland, Oregon

Ardys M. Dunn, PhD, RN, PNP

Associate Professor Emeritus
University of Portland School of Nursing
Portland, Oregon;
Professor, Retired
School of Nursing
Samuel Merritt College
Oakland, California

Margaret A. Brady, PhD, RN, CPNP-PC

Professor
School of Nursing
California State University Long Beach
Long Beach, California;
Co-Director, PNP Program
School of Nursing
Azusa Pacific University
Azusa, California

Nancy Barber Starr, MS, APRN-BC (PNP), CPNP-PC

Pediatric Nurse Practitioner
Advanced Pediatric Associates
Centennial, Colorado

Catherine G. Blosser, MPA:HA, RN, PNP

Pediatric Nurse Practitioner, Retired
Oak Grove, Oregon

Dawn Lee Garzon, PhD, PNP-BC, CPNP-PC, PMHS, FAANP

Clinical Professor
Washington State University
Vancouver, Washington

Associate Editor

Nan M. Gaylord, PhD, RN, CPNP-PC

Associate Professor
College of Nursing
University of Tennessee
Knoxville, Tennessee

ELSEVIER

ELSEVIER

3251 Riverport Lane
St. Louis, Missouri 63043

PEDIATRIC PRIMARY CARE, SIXTH EDITION ISBN: 978-0-323-24338-4

Previous editions copyrighted 2013, 2009, 2004, 2000, 1996.

Library of Congress Cataloging-in-Publication Data

Names: Burns, Catherine E., editor.
Title: Pediatric primary care / editors, Catherine E. Burns [and 6 others].
Other titles: Pediatric primary care (Burns)
Description: Sixth edition. | St. Louis, Missouri : Elsevier, [2017] |
Includes bibliographical references and index.
Identifiers: LCCN 2015045933 | ISBN 9780323243384 (hardcover : alk. paper)
Subjects: | MESH: Pediatrics | Primary Health Care | United States
Classification: LCC RB145 | NLM WS 100 | DDC 618.92–dc23 LC record available at
http://lccn.loc.gov/2015045933

Executive Content Strategist: Lee Henderson
Content Development Manager: Billie Sharp
Content Development Specialist: Charlene Ketchum
Publishing Services Manager: Catherine Jackson
Senior Project Manager: Rachel E. McMullen
Design Direction: Brian Salisbury

Printed in Canada

Last digit is the print number: 9 8 7 6 5 4 3

Contributors

Michele E. Acker, MN, ARNP
Pediatric Nurse Practitioner
Seattle Children's Hospital
Seattle, Washington

Jan Bazner-Chandler, RN, MSN, CNS, CPNP
Assistant Professor, Nurse Practitioner
Azusa Pacific University
Azusa, California

Anita D. Berry, MSN, CNP, APN, PMHS
Director, Healthy Steps for Young Children Program
Advocate Children's Hospital
Downers Grove, Illinois

Jennifer Bevacqua, RN, MS, CPNP-AC, CPNP-PC
Pediatric Nurse Practitioner
Oregon Health & Science University (OHSU)
Portland, Oregon

Crisann Bowman-Harvey, CPNP, AC, PC, MSN
Instructor
University of Colorado
Aurora, Colorado

Donald L. Chi, DDS, PhD
Associate Professor
University of Washington, School of Dentistry, Department of Oral Health
Seattle, Washington

Cynthia Marie Claytor, MSN, PNP, FNP
Graduate Nursing Faculty
Azusa Pacific University
Azusa California

Sara D. DeGolier, RN, MS, CPNP
Pediatric Nurse Practitioner
Department of Emergency Medicine
The Children's Hospital Colorado and University of Colorado Denver
Aurora, Colorado

Joy S. Diamond, MS, CPNP
Pediatric Nurse Practitioner
Advanced Pediatric Associates
Children's Hospital Colorado
Aurora, Colorado

Mary Ann Draye, MPH, APRN
Assistant Professor, Emerita
DNP FNP Program
School of Nursing
University of Washington
Seattle, Washington

Martha Driessnack, PhD, PPCNP-BC
Associate Professor
Pediatric Nurse Practitioner Program
Oregon Health & Science University (OHSU) School of Nursing
Portland, Oregon

Karen G. Duderstadt, PhD, RN, CPNP
Clinical Professor
Coordinator PNP Specialty
Academic Coordinator of International Student Programs and Special Studies
University of California San Francisco
School of Nursing
Department of Family Health Care Nursing
San Francisco, California

Susan Filkins, MS, RD
Nutrition Consultant
Oregon Center for Children & Youth with Special Health Needs
Oregon Health & Sciences University
Portland, Oregon

Leah G. Fitch, MSN, RN, CPNP
Pediatric Nurse Practitioner
Providence Pediatrics, Carolinas HealthCare System
Charlotte, North Carolina

Maxine Fookson, RN, MN, PNP
Pediatric Nurse Practioner, School Based Health Program
Multnomah County Health Department
Portland, Oregon

Lauren Bell Gaylord, MSN, CPNP-PC
Pediatric Nurse Practitioner
Etowah Pediatrics
Rainbow City, Alabama

Teral Gerlt, MS, RN, WHCNP-E, PNP-R
Instructor
Oregon Health & Science University
School of Nursing
Portland, Oregon

Terea Giannetta, DNP, RN, CPNP, FAANP
Associate Professor/Chief Nurse Practitioner
California State University, Fresno/Valley Children's Hospital
Fresno, California/Madera, California

Denise A. Hall, BS, CMPE
Practice Administrator
Advanced Pediatrics Associates
Aurora, Colorado

Anna Marie Hefner, PhD, RN, CPNP
Associate Professor
Azusa Pacific University
Upland, California

Pamela J. Hellings, RN, PhD, CPNP-R
Professor Emeritis
Oregon Health & Science University
Portland, Oregon

Susan Hines, RN, MSN, CPNP
Pediatric Nurse Practitioner
Sleep Medicine
Children's Hospital Colorado
Aurora, Colorado

Sandra Daack-Hirsch, PhD, RN
Associate Professor
The University of Iowa, College of Nursing
Iowa City, Iowa

Belinda James-Petersen, DNP, RN, CPNP
Pediatric Nurse Practitioner-Gastroenterology
Children's Specialty Group
Children's Hospital of the Kings Daughters
Norfolk, Virginia

Rita Marie John, EdD, DNP, CPNP, PMHS
Associate Professor of Nursing at CUMC
PNP Program Director
Columbia University School of Nursing
New York, New York

Veronica Kane, PhD, RN, MSN, CPNP
Clinical Assistant Professor, Coordinator—Pediatric Nursing Specialty
MGH Institute of Health Professions, School of Nursing
Boston, Massachusetts;
Pediatric Nurse Practioner, Pediatrics, Urgent Care
Harvard Vangard Medical Associates
Braintree, Massachusetts

Julie Martchenke, RN, MSN, CPNP
Pediatric Cardiology Nurse Practitioner
Oregon Health & Science University
Portland, Oregon

MiChelle McGarry, MSN, RN, CPNP, CUNP
Certified Pediatric and Urology Nurse Practitioner/ Program Director/Owner
Pediatric Effective Elimination Program Clinic & Consulting, PC
Highlands Ranch, Colorado

Peter M. Milgrom, DDS
Professor of Oral Health Sciences and Pediatric Dentistry,
Adjunct Professor of Health Services,
Director, Northwest Center to Reduce Oral Health Disparities
University of Washington
Seattle, Washington

Carole R. Myers, PhD, RN
Associate Professor-College of Nursing
University of Tennessee
Knoxville, Tennessee

Jennifer Newcombe, MSN, PCNS-BC, CPNP-PC/AC
Nurse Practitioner, Pediatric Cardiothoracic Surgery
Loma Linda Children's Hospital
Loma Linda, California

Noelle Nurre, RN, MN, CPNP
Suspected Child Abuse and Neglect (SCAN) Nurse Practitioner
Oregon Health and Science University Doernbecher Children's Hospital and CARES Northwest
Portland, Oregon

Catherine O'Keefe, DNP, CPNP-PC
Associate Professor/NP Curriculum Coordinator
Creighton University, College of Nursing
Omaha, Nebraska

Gabrielle M. Petersen, MSN, CPNP
Medical Examiner
Children's Center
Oregon City, Oregon

Ann M. Petersen-Smith, PhD, APRN, CPNP-PC, CPNP-AC
Assistant Professor
University of Colorado Anschutz Medical Campus
College of Nursing;
Associate Clinical Professor
University of Colorado Anschutz Medical Campus
School of Medicine
Section of Pediatric Emergency Medicine
Aurora, Colorado

Michele L. Polfuss, PhD, RN, CPNP-AC/PC
Assistant Professor
University of Wisconsin–Milwaukee;
Nurse Researcher
Children's Hospital of Wisconsin
Milwaukee, Wisconsin

Ruth K. Rosenblum, DNP, RN, PNP-BC
Assistant Professor, DNP Program Coordinator
San Jose State University
San Jose, California

Mary Rummell, MN, RN, CNS, CPNP, FAHA
Clinical Nurse Specialist
The Knight Cardiovascular Institute, Cardiac Services
Oregon Health & Science University
Portland, Oregon

Susan K. Sanderson, DNP, APRN, FNP-BC
Pediatric Infectious Diseases Nurse Practitioner; Instructor
Department of Pediatrics
Division of Infectious Diseases
University of Utah School Of Medicine
Salt Lake City, Utah

Arlene Smaldone, PhD, CPNP, CDE
Associate Professor of Nursing at CUMC
Associate Professor of Dental Behavioral Sciences (in Dental Medicine) at CUMC
Assistant Dean, Scholarship and Research (School of Nursing)
Columbia University
New York, New York

Isabelle Soulé, PhD, RN
Human Resources for Health Rwanda
University of Maryland
Baltimore, Maryland

Robert D. Steiner, MD
Executive Director
Marshfield Clinic Research Foundation;
Professor of Pediatrics
University of Wisconsin
Marshfield, Wisconsin

Ohnmar K. Tut, BDS, MPhil
Adjunct Senior Research Fellow
Griffith University;
Program Consultant Investigator
HRSA Oral Health Workforce Activities—FSM
Brisbane, Queensland, Australia;
Affiliate Instructor
University of Washington
Seattle, Washington

Becky J. Whittemore, MPH, MN, FNP-BC
Nurse Practitioner
Institute on Development and Disability
Oregon Health & Sciences University
Portland, Oregon

Elizabeth E. Willer, RN, MSN, CPNP
Pediatric Nurse Practitioner
Kaiser Permanente
Walnut Creek, California

Teri Moser Woo, PhD, RN, ARNP, CNL, CPNP, FAANP
Associate Professor
Associate Dean for Graduate Nursing Programs
Pacific Lutheran University
Tacoma, Washington

Robert J. Yetman, MD
Professor of Pediatrics
Director, Division of Community and General Pediatrics
University of Texas–Houston Medical School
UT Physicians Pediatrics—The Kid's Place
Houston, Texas

Yvonne K. Yousey, RN, CPNP, PhD
Pediatric Nurse Practitioner
Kids First Health Care
Commerce City, Colorado

Reviewers

Jennifer P. D'Auria, PhD, RN, CPNP
Associate Professor
The University of North Carolina–Chapel Hill School of Nursing
Chapel Hill, North Carolina

Martha Driessnack, PhD, PPCNP-BC
Associate Professor
Pediatric Nurse Practitioner Program
Oregon Health & Science University (OHSU) School of Nursing
Portland, Oregon

Melissa J. Geist, EdD, PPCNP-BC, CNE
Associate Professor of Nursing
Whitson-Hester School of Nursing
Tennessee Technological University
Cookeville, Tennessee

Beverly P. Giordano, MS, RN, CPNP, PPCMHS
Pediatric Nurse Practitioner
Child Development/ADHD Clinic
University of Florida
Gainesville, Florida

Sunny Hallowell, PhD, PPCNP-BC, IBCLC
Pediatric Nurse Practitioner & Lactation Consultant
Research Fellow
Center for Health Outcomes and Policy Research
University of Pennsylvania School of Nursing
Philadelphia, Pennsylvania

Judith W. Leonard, PNP-BC, MSN
Pediatric Nurse Practioner-Board Certified
Southern Orange County Pediatric Associates
Lake Forest, California

Ann Parsons, MN, PPCNP
Nurse Practitioner
TEDI EAR Children's Advocacy Center at East Carolina University
Greenville, North Carolina

Debra P. Shockey, DNP, APRN-BC, CPNP
Assistant Professor
Family and Community Health Nursing
Virginia Commonwealth University School of Nursing
Richmond, Virginia

Leigh Small, PhD, RN, CPNP-PC, FNAP, FAANP, FAAN
Associate Professor and Chair
Department of Family and Community Health Nursing
Virginia Commonwealth University
School of Nursing
Richmond, Virginia

Preface

We are delighted to introduce the sixth edition of *Pediatric Primary Care*. This book was first developed 20 years ago as a resource for advanced practice nurses serving the primary health care needs of infants, children, and adolescents. Pediatric nurse practitioners (PNPs) and family nurse practitioners (FNPs) are our primary audience. However, physicians, physician assistants, and nurses who care for children in a variety of settings also find the book to be a valuable resource. The field of pediatric primary care has also grown and changed since the first edition of this book. The interdisciplinary Institute of Medicine (IOM) and the Affordable Care Act have explicitly recognized the critical role of nurse practitioners and nurses in providing health care to the population in the United States (IOM Report, 2010).

The book emphasizes prevention and management of problems from the primary care provider's point of view. Each chapter is organized to introduce key concepts and foundations for care in a narrative format followed by a discussion of the identification and management of diagnoses using an outline format. Experienced clinicians can simply jump to the topic or diagnosis in question while the student can read the chapter for immersion into the topic. Additional resources for each chapter include websites to access organizations and printed materials that may be useful for clinicians, their patients, and families. Our contributing authors are experts in their fields.

Special Features of the Sixth Edition

Some features of the sixth edition about which we are particularly excited include the following:

- **Updated content** reflects the latest developments in our understanding of disease processes, disease management in children, and current trends in pediatric health care
- **NEW Pediatric Pharmacology chapter**
- **NEW Specialist Referral highlights** to alert busy practitioners to cues that signal the need for urgent referral
- **NEW graduate-level Quality and Safety Education for Nurses (QSEN) integration** (Cronenwett et al, 2009): The Safety, Informatics, Teamwork and Collaboration, and Evidence–based competencies
- **NEW full-color design and illustration format** to improve usability and teaching/learning value
- **NEW focus on diversity among cultures** in Chapter 3 provides greater emphasis on the need for providers to approach differences between themselves and their clients with humility and competence
- **Reorganized application of Gordon's Functional Health Patterns** to provide a more conceptually consistent flow of content (Gordon, 1987, 2010)
- **Expanded coverage of health literacy**—obtaining, reading, understanding, and using health care information to make appropriate health decisions
- **Expanded, updated coverage of growth and development** for greater consistency with contemporary theories of development
- **Unique chapter on integrative/complementary therapies** promotes the primary care provider's knowledge about many of the less conventional health care strategies that families may be inquiring about or using
- **Refocused Practice Management chapter (Chapter 44) is now available to readers on the Evolve website.** This chapter focuses on content more specific to pediatric practice management, including the various settings for pediatric primary care, such as school-based clinics and the health care home. This refocused chapter also addresses informatics and other essential topics influenced by the Affordable Care Act, as well as National Patient Safety Goals and the growing trend of interprofessional collaboration.
- **Discussion questions and NEW PowerPoint slides** are available on the Evolve site for educators. These are written by nurse practitioner educators to assist students to think about the implications of the material for their clinical practice.

Organization of the Book

We recognize that children are a special population and that providing health care to them must be approached using several unique perspectives: their developmental changes over time, their dependency on their parents, the differential epidemiology of child health, the different demographic patterns of children and their families, and the individuality of their genetic makeup. These themes are carried throughout the text.

The book is organized into four major sections—Pediatric Primary Care Foundations, Management of Development, Approaches to Health Management in Pediatric Primary Care, and Approaches to Disease Management. Each chapter follows the same format. Standards and guidelines for care are highlighted, the physiologic and assessment parameters are discussed, management strategies are identified, and management of common problems is presented in a problem-oriented format. The scope of practice of the primary care provider is always kept in mind with appropriate referral and consultation points identified.

We hope this text will continue to promote the very best evidence-based care possible for children and families in primary care settings by all the providers with whom they come in contact.

Editors
Catherine E. Burns, PhD, RN, CPNP-PC, FAAN
Ardys M. Dunn, PhD, RN, PNP
Margaret A. Brady, PhD, RN, CPNP-PC
Nancy Barber Starr, MS, APRN-BC (PNP), CPNP-PC
Catherine G. Blosser, MPA:HA, RN, PNP
Dawn Lee Garzon, PhD, PNP-BC, CPNP-PC, PMHS, FAANP

Associate Editor
Nan M. Gaylord, PhD, RN, CPNP-PC

References

Cronenwett L, Sherwood G, Pohl J, et al: Quality and safety education for advanced nursing practice, *Nurs Outlook* 5(6):338–348, 2009.

Gordon M: *Nursing diagnosis: process and application*, New York, 1987, McGraw-Hill.

Gordon M: *Manual of nursing diagnosis*, ed 12, Sudbury, MA, 2010, Jones and Bartlett.

Institute of Medicine (IOM) of the National Academies: *The future of nursing: leading change, advancing health*, 2010. Available at: http://www.iom.edu/Reports/2010/The-Future-of-Nursing-Leading-Change-Advancing-Health (accessed October 28, 2014).

Acknowledgments

A book of this size and complexity cannot be completed without considerable help—the work of the contributors who researched, wrote, and revised content; the consultation and review of experts in various specialties who critiqued drafts and provided important perspectives and guidance; and the essential technical support from those who managed the production of the manuscript and the final product. Lee Henderson and Charlene Ketchum have provided consistent Elsevier support through the past two editions.

Contributors to the Fifth Edition

These people were instrumental in helping us develop the fifth edition of the book. Although they are not authors in this edition, their ideas and work have contributed greatly to our work, and we are deeply indebted to them: Barbara Deloian, Mary Murphy, Maxine Fookson, Lynn Frost, Denise Abdoo, Roberta Bentson Royal, Veronica Kane, Martha K. Swartz, Anne Albers, Melissa Reider-Demer, Shirley Becton McKenzie, Peggy Vernon, Jan Bazner-Chandler, and Constance Brehm.

Our Thanks to Family and Friends

- To my husband, Jerry Burns: Thanks so very much for giving me the time and support to work on this text one more time; to my loving daughters Jennifer and Jill and their families; other family and friends; and to the many PNPs, FNPs, and NP faculty who have expressed their appreciation for this text and encouraged us to continue the project. *Catherine E. Burns*
- To Marvin Dunn; Malcolm and Megan Dunn; Philip Dunn and Liz Flynn, grandchildren Miles, Claire, Simon, and Eleanor Dunn (from "the craziest Nana in the whole wide world!")—thanks for being my joy and inspiration; and to so many other family and friends, you are the spice of a well-flavored life. *Ardys M. Dunn*
- With deep appreciation for the circle of love and support from my dear family and friends who are always there surrounding me with warmth, laughter, and joy. *Margaret A. Brady*
- Aloha and mahalo to my Jon, Jonah, and AnnaMei. I am ever grateful for the joy you bring to my life as well as your support of my time with "the book." Likewise, I am ever thankful for Denise and my APA colleagues who give me the flexibility and challenge to work hand in hand to provide model pediatric care. *Nancy Barber Starr*
- To my husband, Terry, for his continued love and support and my admiration for all the littlest Blosser offspring for their years of sharing their humor, strides, and challenges—they are amazing examples of the wonder of growth and development. *Catherine G. Blosser*
- My thanks to the students, parents, and families who make me a better person; to Rachel and Elizabeth Garzon who give my life meaning; and to Amy DiMaggio, friends, and family for loving me and giving me wings. *Dawn Lee Garzon*
- To my parents who first loved, supported, and encouraged me. To my husband, Mark, who loved me second and continues to love, support, and encourage me in all my professional endeavors. To my children, Curtis and Leah, who make life fun and will continue to do so with their own children. *Nan Gaylord*

Contents

Resources on the Evolve Website

UNIT 1

Pediatric Primary Care Foundations

1 Health Status of Children: Global and National Perspectives

KAREN G. DUDERSTADT

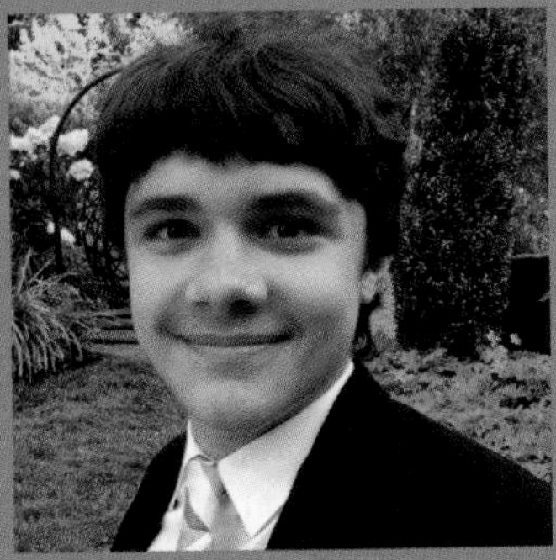

The health status of all children must be viewed with a global lens. Whether considering pandemic infectious diseases or the global emigration of populations between continents, the health of all children is interconnected worldwide. Inequalities in the health status of children globally and nationally are largely determined by common biosocial factors affecting health, which include where they are born, live, are educated, their work, and their age (World Health Organization [WHO], 2014a). The biosocial factors also include the systems in place to address health and illness in children and families.

The biosocial circumstances or social determinants of child health are shaped by economics, social policies, and politics in each region and country. In order to impact health outcomes, scaling up the efforts nationally and globally to build better health systems is required. Significant progress has been made in reducing childhood morbidity and mortality using this approach. The framework of the United Nations Millennium Development Goals 2014 (United Nations, 2015) and the Healthy People 2020 (U.S. Department of Health and Human Services [HHS] Office of Disease Prevention and Health Promotion, 2015a) goals set the mark for improving child health status. It is for societies to embrace and prioritize these goals on behalf of children.

This chapter presents an overview of the global health status of children, including the issue of global food insecurity, child health status in the United States and current health inequalities, the progress toward achieving the Millennium Development Goals and Healthy People 2020 targets, the effect of health care reform in the United States on access to care for children and adolescents, and the important role pediatric health care providers have in advocating for polices that foster health equity and access to quality health care services for all children and families. The final section addresses the health frameworks and tools available to pediatric health care providers to assess and monitor the health and well-being of children from infancy to young adulthood.

Global Health Status of Children

Thirty-five million children younger than 20 years old are part of the international migration of populations across continents (UNICEF, 2014). Emigrant children have increased health and educational needs that impact the health and well-being of communities; many of these communities have fragile health care systems. The United Nations Convention on the Rights of Children (UNCRC) charter was established 25 years ago and declares the minimum entitlements and freedoms for children globally, including the right to the best possible health (United Nations International Children's Fund, 2009). Emigrant children have the right to be protected under this charter (Box 1-1). Governments are advised to provide good quality health care, clean water, nutritious foods, and clean environments so that children can stay healthy. The charter is founded on the principle of respect for the dignity and worth of each individual, regardless of race, color, gender, language, religion, opinions, origins, wealth, birth status, or ability. The UNCRC continues to work on ensuring that all children have these basic human rights and freedoms. Special emphasis is placed on the responsibility and strength of families and the vital role of the international community to protect and secure the rights of children, including access to health care and primary health care services.

Health equity is the absence of unfair or remediable differences in health services and health outcomes among populations (WHO, 2014b). Although the rate of child mortality globally remains high, there have been significant

• BOX 1-1 UNICEF* Summary of the United Nations Convention on the Rights of Children

The UNICEF conventions include 42 articles that are summarized in the following list. They represent the worldwide standards for the rights of children. The conventions apply to *all* children younger than 18 years old. The best interests of children must be a top priority in all actions concerning children.

- Every child has the right to:
  - Life and best possible health
  - Time for relaxation, play, and opportunities for a variety of cultural and artistic activities
  - A legally registered name and nationality
  - Knowledge of and care by his or her parents, as far as possible, and prompt efforts to restore the child-parent relationship if they have been separated
  - Protection from dangerous work
  - Protection from use of dangerous drugs
  - Protection from sale and social abuse, exploitation, physical and sexual abuse, neglect and special care to help them recover their health if they have experienced such toxic life events
  - No incarceration with adults and opportunities to maintain contact with parents
  - Care with respect for religion, culture, and language if not provided by the parents
  - A full and decent life in conditions that promote dignity, independence, and an active role in the community, even if disabled
  - Access to reliable information from mass media, television, radio, newspapers, as well as protection from information that might harm them
- Governments must do all that they can to fulfill the rights of children as listed above.

*UNICEF stands for the full name United Nations International Children's Emergency Fund. In 1953, its name was shortened to the United Nations Children's Fund. However, the original acronym was retained.

reductions in the rate over the past few decades. Since 1990, child mortality in children younger than 5 years old has decreased by 47% due to targeted policies to reduce childhood pneumonia, diarrhea, and malaria and also to reduce the number of preterm births and perinatal complications. Despite these efforts, 6.3 million children younger than 5 years old die each year worldwide (Wang et al, 2014). To reach the World Health Organization (WHO) target of two-thirds reduction in mortality for children younger than 5 years old, more rapid progress is needed, particularly in sub-Saharan Africa, where the highest rate of infant mortality occurs. Currently, sub-Saharan Africa and Southern Asia account for 81% of the infant mortality globally (United Nations, 2015).

Diarrhea and pneumonia remain the leading infectious causes of childhood morbidity and mortality globally. The highest proportion of deaths due to these two conditions is in children younger than 2 years old; undernutrition, suboptimum breastfeeding, and zinc deficiency contribute significantly to the mortality rate from these diseases. (Zinc reduces the duration and severity of diarrhea and likelihood of reinfections for 2 to 3 months. As a micronutrient, it is essential for protein supplementation, cell growth, immune function, and intestinal transport of water and electrolytes [Khan and Sellen, 2015].) Rotavirus is the most common cause of diarrhea globally and *Streptococcus pneumoniae* is the leading cause of pneumonia (Walker et al, 2013). Both of these are vaccine-preventable infectious diseases.

Successful vaccination programs have markedly reduced the mortality caused by some infectious diseases, particularly measles and tetanus. Cambodia serves as a noteworthy example. To reduce childhood mortality in children younger than 5 years old, Cambodia targeted measles vaccination due to the high mortality associated with the disease. Within a decade, health workers were able to increase the rate of measles immunization by 71% in children younger than 1 year old (United Nations, 2015). To achieve complete eradication of measles, WHO helped the Cambodian national immunization program to identify and reach communities at high risk for low rates of immunizations. A national immunization program also began providing a booster dose of a measles-containing vaccine after 18 months old. The result was measles eradication in Cambodia since 2012. Such sustained immunization programs by partnerships between communities, governments, and international aid organizations can markedly improve global child health status. However, emerging viral and bacterial infectious diseases present complex challenges to public health infrastructure and threaten the global progress made on reducing childhood mortality (see Chapter 24).

The majority of the extremely poor live in five countries—India, China, Nigeria, Bangladesh, and the Democratic Republic of Congo. The risk of maternal death from pregnancy-related complications and childbirth in developing regions is 230 deaths per 100,000 births; this rate is 14 times higher than in developed countries (United Nations, 2015).

Global Food Insecurity and Effect on Children's Health

Hunger and undernutrition are often referred to as *food insecurity,* which is the condition that exists when populations do not have physical and economic access to sufficient, safe, nutritious, and culturally acceptable food to meet nutritional needs. Food insecurity occurs in impoverished populations in developing countries and in industrialized nations, particularly among migrant populations. Children affected by migration and family separation are at risk for food insecurity and are vulnerable to further health consequences, including exposure to exploitation and child trafficking. Growing evidence on climate change indicates the dramatic effect on food crops that lead to food distribution issues, which is one of the primary contributors to food insecurity (Fig. 1-1).

Globally, undernutrition is an important determinant of maternal and child health and accounts for 45% of all child

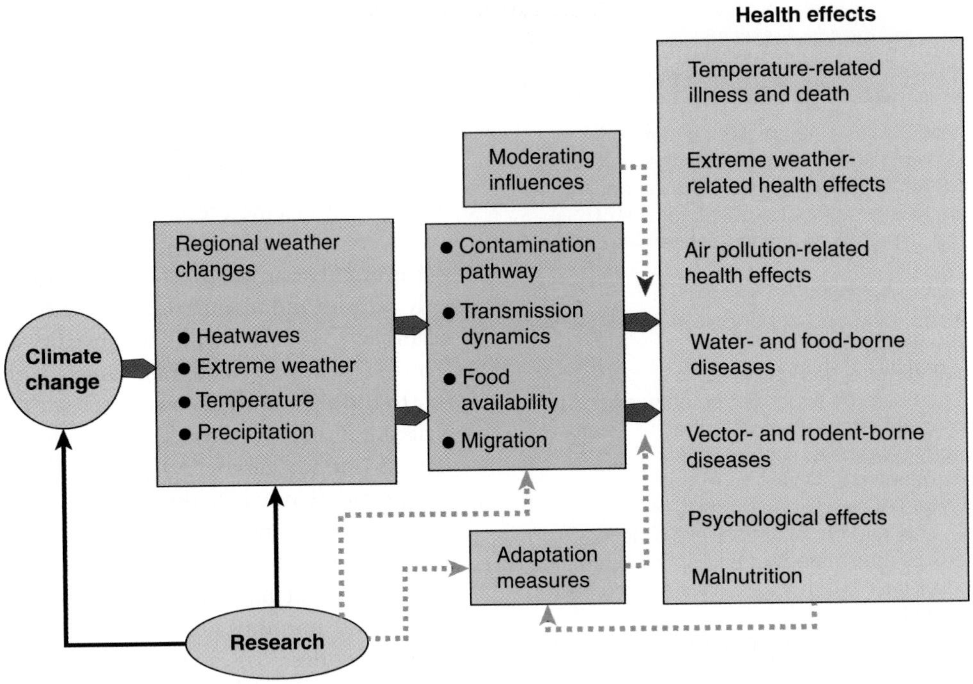

• **Figure 1-1** Health effects of climate change.

deaths in children younger than 5 years old (United Nations, 2015). Suboptimal breastfeeding remains a problem in developed and developing nations. Children who are exclusively breastfed for the first 6 months of life are 14 times more likely to survive than non-breastfed infants (United Nations, 2015). Vitamin A and zinc deficiencies also contribute to the disease burden in mortality for children younger than 5 years old. In developing countries, 55 million women are stunted from undernutrition and lack of micronutrients, including iron, folic acid, vitamin A, and zinc (Save the Children, 2015). Preventable nutritional deficiencies are a compelling case for further implementation of the Millennium Development Goals and increased support for micronutrient supplementation for children in developing regions.

United Nations Millennium Development Goals: Project Goals

The Millennium Project, a global health project of research and study to improve prospects for a better future for humanity, publishes a framework (Millennium Development Goals) annually to address the challenges, both local and global, facing the world populations. Health and access to health care in the context of social determinants are covered in the document. Figures 1-2 and 1-3 and Box 1-2 illustrate the collaborative action required among governments, international organizations, corporations, universities, and individuals and societies to address the issue of health equity from a global perspective (The Millennium Project, 2014).

One of the main goals of the Millennium Development Goals framework is to reduce infant mortality by at least two-thirds by 2016 in 27 countries. Eight goals consist of 21 quantifiable targets measured by 60 health indicators (see Fig. 1-3). They provide a framework for the international community to ensure socioeconomic development reaches all children.

Progress on the Millennium Development Goals

Significant progress has been made in many areas, including reductions in child mortality and preterm birth. In 30 developing countries, progress toward achieving reductions in child mortality has been faster than predicted due to income, education, and secular shifts in living and work environments (Wang et al, 2014). However, increased assistance in improving economic status and levels of maternal education is required to sustain the effort.

Since 1990, progress has been made by reducing world poverty by half, access to clean drinking water has improved for 2.3 billion people, chronic undernutrition in children causing stunting has decreased by 40%, and 90% of children in developing regions are attending primary school (United Nations, 2015). The achievements are the result of the collaborations between governments, international communities, civil societies, and private corporations. To make further sustained progress, expansion and acceleration of the interventions by the WHO are required to target the leading causes of death in the target countries.

The economic growth potential remains strong in many of the developing regions, and partnerships between

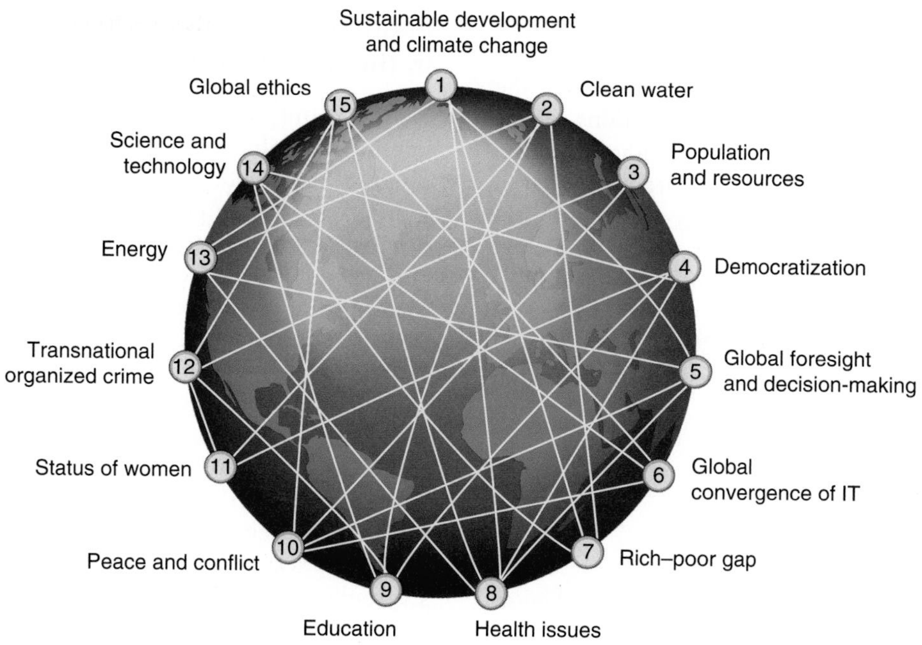

• **Figure 1-2** Fifteen global challenges facing humanity. *IT,* Information technology.

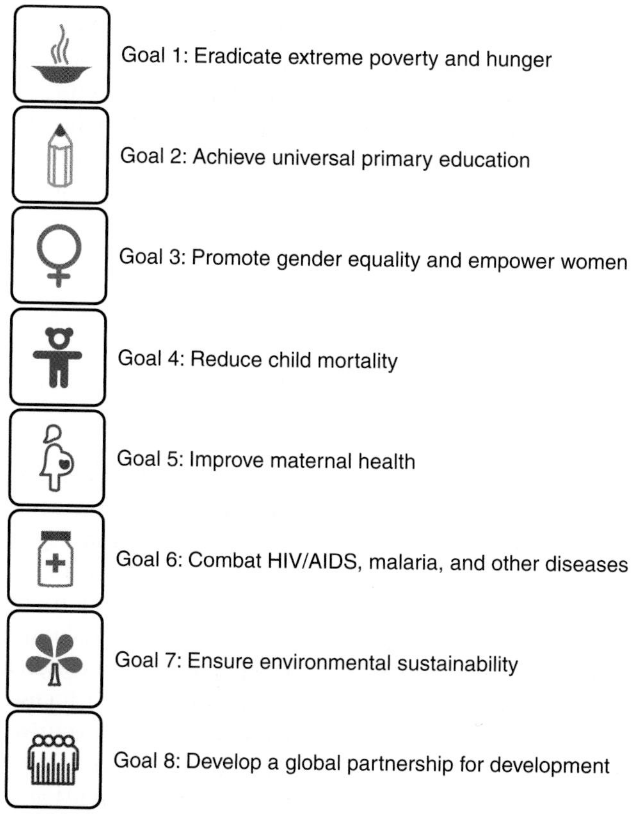
Goal 1: Eradicate extreme poverty and hunger
Goal 2: Achieve universal primary education
Goal 3: Promote gender equality and empower women
Goal 4: Reduce child mortality
Goal 5: Improve maternal health
Goal 6: Combat HIV/AIDS, malaria, and other diseases
Goal 7: Ensure environmental sustainability
Goal 8: Develop a global partnership for development

• **Figure 1-3** List of eight Millennium Development Goals. *AIDS,* Acquired immune deficiency syndrome; *HIV,* human immunodeficiency virus.

• BOX 1-2 Preterm Birth Rate by Race and Ethnicity

Births before 37 weeks' gestation can result in lifelong disabilities, and children born preterm are at higher risk of death during their first few days of life.

Race and Ethnicity	Preterm Birth Rate
African American, non-Hispanic mothers	16.5%
American Indian or Alaska Native mothers	13.3%
Hispanic mothers	11.6%
White, non-Hispanic mothers	10.3%
Asian or Pacific Islander mothers	10.2%

The African American preterm birth rate is more than 1.5 times higher than that experienced by Asians or Pacific Islanders.

HHS Office of Disease Prevention and Health Promotion: LHI infographic gallery: maternal, infant, and child health (April 2014): preterm births and infant deaths, HealthyPeople.gov (website): www.healthypeople.gov/2020/leading-health-indicators/LHI-Infographic-Gallery#Apr-2014. Accessed August 13, 2015.

developing countries and nongovernmental organizations (NGOs) continue to provide significant sources of developmental assistance. Official development assistance is at the highest level ever recorded by the United Nations agency partners (United Nations, 2015). Developing countries require further debt relief, reduced trade barriers, improved access to technologies for renewable energy production, and enhanced protection from and response to environmental disasters to sustain current advances. Further, global political efforts are required to support achievement of the Millennium Development Goals beyond 2015 and a renewed commitment to the future health and well-being of children everywhere.

Health Status of Children in the United States

Globalism will increasingly affect child health in the United States. The demographic mix of children and families cared for by pediatric health care providers in the United States has become increasingly complex, with a greater number of children living in poverty who are at increased risk for chronic physical and mental health conditions and exposure to intimate partner violence (IPV), gun violence, and abuse (American Academy of Pediatrics [AAP], 2014). Child poverty rates in the United States remain higher than in other economically developed nations. One in five children (out of 16.3 million) in the United States live in families with incomes below the federal poverty level (FPL) (Annie E. Casey Foundation, 2015). The rate of household poverty is higher (one in three) for Latino and African American children.

Most concerning among the child health indicators is the percentage of overweight and obese children. Seventeen percent of youth are "obese" as defined as a body mass index (BMI) greater than the 95th percentile for age on the BMI age and gender–specific growth charts. For infants and children younger than 2 years old, the rate of obesity is 8.1% as determined by weight for recumbent length charts. Although rates of obesity among children and youth remain high, surveillance studies show that the rate of increase in overweight and obesity has stabilized. The obesity rate among 2- to 5-year-olds showed a significant decrease of 5.5% between 2004 and 2013 (Ogden et al, 2014).

Obese and overweight children and youth are more at risk for developing adult health problems, including heart disease, type 2 diabetes, stroke, and osteoarthritis. Poor eating patterns are a major factor in the high rate of obesity among children and adolescents. Children's diets have been out of balance over the past two decades with too much added sugar and saturated fats, and limited fruits, vegetables, and whole grains. Of all the child health indicators, overweight and obesity will significantly affect the cost of providing health care services in the United States in the coming years. Chapter 10 discusses childhood obesity, the comorbidities, and the related cost of health care.

Food Insecurity in Children in the United States

Despite many government food assistance programs, nearly one in five children in the United States lives in a food-insecure household. Children who are food insecure are more likely to have poorer general health, higher rates of hospitalization, increased incidence of overweight, asthma, anemia, and experience behavioral problems. Factors other than income do impact whether a household is food insecure. Maternal education, single-parent households, intimate-partner violence, and parental substance abuse also contribute to food insecurity in households. Children living in households where the mother is moderately-to-severely depressed have a 50% to 80% increased risk of food insecurity (Gundersen and Ziliak, 2015).

Three-quarters of children spend some portion of the preschool years being cared for outside of the home. Depending on child care arrangements, the care can contribute to or ameliorate the effects of food insecurity for children. Young children who attend a preschool or child care center have lower food insecurity, whereas children cared for at home by an unrelated adult are at higher risk for food insecurity (Gundersen and Ziliak, 2015). The Supplemental Nutritional Assistance Program (SNAP), the Special Supplemental Nutrition Program for Women, Infants, and Children (WIC) and the School Breakfast Program (SBP) are federally funded programs with the purpose to combat childhood hunger. In 2013, 11.2 million children participated in the SBP for a free or reduced price, and WIC served 8.7 million women and children at a cost of $6.45 billion (Gundersen and Ziliak, 2015). The average monthly WIC benefit for families is $43.

Addressing Children's Health in the United States

Healthy People 2020

The Healthy People 2020 goals for children include foci specific to early and middle childhood and adolescents, social determinants of health in childhood, health-related quality of life for children, and on specific disparities in child health to improve health care services and health outcomes (HHS Office of Disease Prevention and Health Promotion, 2015a). With increased proportions of children with developmental delays, Healthy People 2020 focuses on objectives to increase the percentage of children younger than 2 years old who receive early intervention services for developmental disabilities and to increase the proportion of children entering kindergarten with school readiness in all five domains of healthy development—physical well-being and motor development, social emotional development, approaches to learning, language development, and cognition, and general development. The objectives also address the increase in maladaptive behaviors in the pediatric population and set benchmarks to increase the percentage of young children who are screened for autism and other developmental delays at 18 and 24 months old (Annie E. Casey Foundation, 2015; National Center on Birth Defects and Developmental Disabilities, Centers for Disease Control and Prevention [CDC], 2015).

Healthy People 2020 objectives also address the need for increasing the proportion of practicing primary care providers, including nurse practitioners, to improve access to quality health care services. The demand for primary care services will increase as more children, adolescents, and young adults qualify for health insurance plans through the Affordable Care Act of 2010 (ACA) and seek preventive health care. An integrated workforce can provide appropriate evidence-based clinical preventive services to reduce overall health care costs, as well as improve access and facilitate communication and continuity of care for children and families. Approaches to health care must be interprofessional and must consider the biosocial factors in the delivery of health care to achieve child health outcomes far beyond the biomedical dynamics of disease (Holmes et al, 2014).

Social Determinants of Health and Health Equity

The social determinants of health result in unequal and unavoidable differences in health status within communities and between communities (HHS Office of Disease Prevention and Health Promotion, 2015b). Individuals are affected by economic, social, and environmental factors in their communities. Social determinants of health recognize the impact of home, school, workplace, neighborhoods, and access to health care as significant contributors to child health outcomes. Many of the Healthy People 2020 leading health indicators address social determinants of health, but the specific objective targeted for this objective is the number of students who graduate in 4 years of high school with a regular diploma. The target is 82.4% for the on-time graduation rate. Progress has been made toward the goal with a rate of 78.2% over the past 4 years (HHS Office of Disease Prevention and Health Promotion, 2015b). However, the target falls significantly below what is required to decrease the economic inequalities between communities and neighborhoods.

The United States has the highest rate of death in the first day of life among the 27 industrialized nations (Save the Children, 2015). Healthy People 2020 sets targets for reductions of infant deaths and the rate of preterm births (infants born at or before 37 weeks' gestation). Significant inequalities exist in communities in the rate of preterm births—particularly in the Southeastern states (see Box 1-2). The overall rate of preterm births in the United States has only decreased 0.6% since 2002 despite interventions to decrease the incidence. One out of nine preterm births results in complications, including greater risk of breathing problems, developmental delays, and vision and hearing problems. All of these complications increase the cost of health care. The Centers for Disease Control and Prevention (CDC) is collaborating with state health departments, university researchers, and private foundations to understand and reduce preterm births and implement evidence-based interventions to improve prenatal care in those communities and hospitals with high rates of preterm births.

Adverse Childhood Events and Impact on Child Health Outcomes

There is growing evidence on the disruptive impact of toxic stress on biologic mechanisms that impact childhood development. Exposure to chronic stress and high levels of elevated cortisol are believed to play a role in the encoding of memory and other bodily functions. The structural development of the brain in childhood is guided by environmental cues; optimum development of the neuroendocrine system is dependent upon the absence of early toxic stress and toxins (e.g., lead, mercury, alcohol, and drugs) and adequate nutrition (AAP, 2015).

Early adverse stress is linked to later impairments in learning, behavior, and physical and mental well-being (AAP, 2015; Shonkoff et al, 2012). Toxic stress results from strong or frequent and prolonged activation of the body's stress response systems in the absence of the protection of a supportive, adult relationship (Shonkoff et al, 2012). The adversity can occur as single, acute, or chronic events in the child's environment, such as emotional or physical abuse or neglect, IPV, war, maternal depression, parental separation or divorce, and parental incarceration (Box 1-3). Although discussed here as a problem in the United States, adverse childhood events is a significant worldwide problem.

Toxic stress in childhood has implications that carry over into adulthood. Evidence suggests that the results of the prolonged and altered biologic mechanisms lead to chronic health conditions in adulthood, including obesity, heart disease, alcoholism, and substance abuse (Shonkoff et al, 2012). A child who has experienced adverse childhood events is also more likely to engage in high-risk behavior, such as the initiation of early sexual activity and adolescent pregnancy. Limiting the impact of adverse childhood events through effective interventions that strengthen the capacity of nations, communities, and families to protect young children from the disruptive effects of toxic stress improves

• BOX 1-3 Adverse Life Experiences of Children

- Emotional abuse or neglect
- Physical abuse or neglect
- Sexual abuse
- Mother treated violently
- Household substance abuse
- Household mental illness
- Parental separation of divorce
- Incarcerated household member

child health outcomes and decreases financial costs to individuals and societies (Shonkoff et al, 2012).

Child Health and Quality Improvement Measures

As part of the effort in the United States to reform health care, quality and performance measures have gained significant importance in the national dialogue. Many measures relevant to the overall health of children are tracked annually in the National Healthcare Disparities Report (NHDR). The report focuses on four components of pediatric health care: (1) prevention, (2) treatment, (3) management, and (4) access to care.

Lack of health care insurance is the single strongest predictor of quality of care for children in the United States—greater than the effects of race, ethnicity, family income, or education (HHS Office of Disease Prevention and Health Promotion, 2015a). Quality of care is measured by the timeliness and effectiveness of care, as well as the safety of the care delivered. Measures of access to care include health insurance coverage, utilization of health care services, and barriers to care. Both access and quality are required to eliminate the impact of disparities in health.

Understanding the changing demographics of the pediatric population is critical to shaping the health care workforce and health care services for future generations of children. Further, the debate on whether to expand health care to immigrant children needs to become part of the dialogue in order to further decrease health disparities.

The Role of Advanced Practice Nurses for Improving Child Health

Advanced practice nurses (APNs) have a key role in advocating for child health locally, nationally, and globally. A growing body of evidence demonstrates that APNs deliver high-value primary care services (Naylor and Kurtzman, 2010). APNs provide continuity of care in the ambulatory care setting for underserved children with health conditions, such as asthma, pneumonia, and vaccine-preventable conditions that might otherwise lead to greater utilization of costly emergency departments and hospitalizations. Increasing access to APNs who deliver primary care services would reduce health care costs, improve health outcomes, and produce health care savings—all steps toward allowing the United States to lead rather than trail the other economically developed countries in child health indicators. Additionally, APNs have the potential to influence economic and political decisions to ameliorate health disparities and increase health equality among populations and communities in order to build a healthier generation of adults.

Health care reform places a greater emphasis on primary care infrastructure, including identifying a pediatric health care/medical home in order to coordinate the care of children and youth across settings and providers. The concept is supported by the American Academy of Pediatrics, the Institute of Medicine, and the Patient-centered Primary Care Collagorative (PCPCC). The model promotes holistic care of children and their families through a collaborative relationship with qualified pediatric health care providers inclusive of nurse practitioners (National Association of Pediatric Nurse Practitioners [NAPNAP], 2009). Exemplary innovative models in pediatric health care/medical home services delivered by nurse practitioners are being implemented in several states. Interventions in successful models must address the concepts of family-centered partnerships, community-based systems, and transitional care from pediatric to adult services.

Health Promotion and Evidence-Based Clinical Preventive Services

Many children are not receiving the recommended preventive services and developmental surveillance required for health promotion. There are many barriers to effective well child care, including time constraints; low level of reimbursement for preventive care and developmental screening services; lack of provider education in current strategies to identify child development, emotional, and behavioral problems; and lack of community referral sources to assist children, adolescents, and families. These issues have led to inconsistent quality of preventive health care services affecting children and families.

Much of the basis for primary care practice is not yet evidence based. Primary care would benefit from strong scientific clinical research that would strengthen primary care principles and prevention. Lack of funding and infrastructure to support such primary care clinical research stands in sharp contrast to the organized commitment and emphasis on advancing knowledge in disease entities and treatment options. This gap provides an area of research open to pediatric nurse researchers and other pediatric health care providers trained in clinical research. Increased evidence in the primary health care domain would help to move the public dialogue toward a greater focus on primary prevention and away from a disease-focused health care system.

Health Supervision Guidelines

American Academy of Pediatrics Guidelines

The AAP publishes the *Recommendations for Preventive Pediatric Health Care* annually. However, it became clear that the number of recommended health directives for well child care had far surpassed the time available to pediatric health care providers (Schor, 2004). Recent recommendations from the AAP to improve the efficiency and effectiveness of health promotion and preventive pediatric care have placed a greater emphasis on behavioral and developmental issues. Their recommendations suggest uncoupling the periodicity of well child visits with the required immunizations and providing greater emphasis on healthy growth and developmental surveillance (Tanner et al, 2009). Part of the revision includes basing well child care on the evidence-based research available on child and family development rather than the periodicity of required immunizations. This necessitates a revision of the current recommendations that guide practice, which can be found in the Bright Futures publication.

Bright Futures

Bright Futures is a national health promotion initiative dedicated to the principle that "every child deserves to be healthy and that optimal health involves a trusting relationship between the health professional, the child, the family, and the community as partners in health practice" (Hagan et al, 2008, p 1). Bright Futures helps providers deliver prevention-based, developmentally oriented care in a family-focused manner and fosters the aforementioned relationships. The parent tools included in Bright Futures empower families with greater skills and knowledge to be active partners in their child's healthy growth and development. Bright Futures is available to health care providers and parents at www.brightfutures.org.

For a complete list of references, please visit http://evolve.elsevier.com/Burns/pediatric/.

2

Child and Family Health Assessment

CATHERINE E. BURNS AND KAREN G. DUDERSTADT

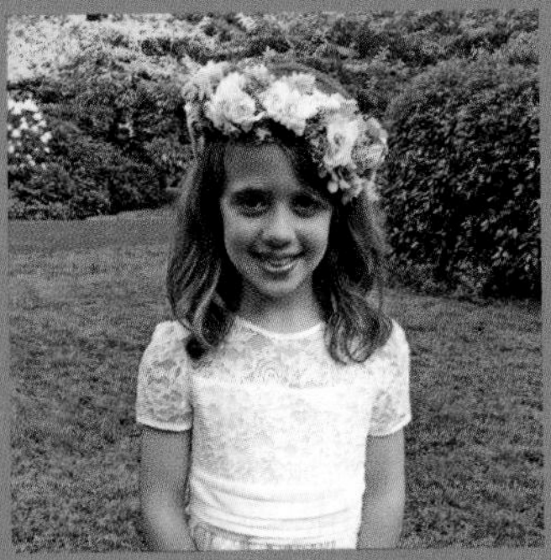

Patient/family-centered community-based primary care for children is recognized as the best possible practice model for providing health care services to children and their families (American Academy of Pediatrics [AAP], 2014a). The family is the most influential factor in a child's life, and its functioning is totally intertwined with the child's health and well-being. Providing family-centered care demands the highest level of primary care—considering both child and family as the units of care.

Delivery of family-centered care for children requires the provider to shift focus from "child as the unit of analysis" to "family as the unit of analysis," depending on the problem at hand. Although the child's welfare is ultimately the goal, the family is so integral to a child's well-being that unless the family is healthy, the child cannot achieve true physical, developmental, and psychological health. Moving from child to family and back again during the assessment process is a complex task, but it is an essential one for providing excellent care.

This chapter presents a child assessment model that integrates some family issues and a family assessment model that is useful when greater focus on the family is needed. The outline for assessment of children in this chapter is consistent with the organization of the entire textbook in which development, functional health issues, and diseases are the three domains for pediatric practice and are the major units of this book. Throughout this book, family is considered integral to the child's life and care. This chapter provides foundations for an integrated assessment of the child, using a family-centered community-based approach.

Foundations for Child and Family Assessment

Child Health Assessment Foundations

A careful, complete, and thoughtful assessment of the child's health status is absolutely essential to provide excellent primary health care. This assessment is based on knowledge of child development, family structure and functions, culture, anatomy and physiology, pathophysiology, pharmacology, health care delivery systems, communities, and standards of primary health care for children. The assessment must also be viewed through the lens of the provider's experience to allow the provider to modify perceptions and validate data on the basis of previous work. When providers analyze patient care situations, they are engaged in critical thinking. This chapter cannot teach critical thinking nor does it teach physical assessment. Rather, it provides frameworks for gathering data to facilitate expert decision-making in areas of pediatric practice.

Nursing has declared a set of Essentials of Master's Education in Nursing (American Association of Colleges of Nursing [AACN], 2011):

- *Essential I: Background for practice from science and humanities*: The child health assessment process must integrate scientific findings from nursing, biologic, psychological, social, genetic, and public health fields to comprehensively understand the health care issues.
- *Essential IV: Translating and integrating scholarship into practice:* The assessment process changes over time as new knowledge informs practice. Hopefully the experienced clinician uses strategies for assessment beyond those learned as a student and the student will learn strategies recently informed by scholarship as well as the wisdom of clinician mentors.
- *Essential V: Informatics and health care technologies*: In order to be comprehensive yet efficient, the primary care provider (nurse or other) needs to use appropriate health care and information technologies within the practice setting, not only as record-keeping and communication tools among providers over time, but also incorporating the patient and family into the technology network. Health teaching and monitoring are examples of new uses. A new term, health-enabling technologies (HET), more broadly encompasses the uses of the information-accessing opportunities available in the world today (Knight and Shea, 2014).

- *Essential VII: Interprofessional collaboration for improving patient and population health outcomes:* Comprehensive assessment requires several levels of data gathering, validation of data, and decisions about the appropriate data to be collected. No one provider is expected to be "all knowing." Rather, the clinician should understand the value of collaboration with other professionals to make appropriate clinical decisions and provide the best care possible. Knowing when and how to collaborate is essential.
- *Essential VIII: Clinical prevention and population health for improving health:* Sometimes the primary care provider focuses on the individual child and family as the target for services, both preventive and restorative. However, sometimes the appropriate target for services is the community or a population at risk. Assessment concepts addressed in this chapter focus on the child and family as the basic units of care. However, throughout the text, there are many opportunities for care strategies to be translated into care for communities. The clinician is expected to be able to shift focus as needed to meet the needs of those with health risks. Care may be direct or indirect.

These are broadly written for graduates in diverse areas of practice. The advanced pediatric assessment process described in this chapter is consistent with several of these tenets.

• BOX 2-1 The Classic Health History

I. Patient-identifying information: name, birth date, gender, address, record number, and name of historian, along with relationship to the patient stated
II. Chief complaint (CC)
III. History of present illness (HPI)
IV. Past medical history (PMH)
  A. Prenatal, natal, postnatal
  B. Past illnesses
  C. Allergies
  D. Accidents
  E. Hospitalizations
  F. Immunization history
  G. Nutrition history
  H. Growth
  I. Development
V. Review of systems (ROS)
  A. Physical—body systems
  B. Psychological—Adjustment to home, school, neighborhood Temperament Sleep—amount, habits, problems
VI. Family history (FH)
VII. Socioeconomic (SE)
  A. Occupations of father and mother
  B. Time spent with child by parents, activities together
  C. Finances—adequacy
  D. Persons in the home
  E. House or apartment living arrangements
  F. General relationship of family members
  G. Community support systems—friends, church, agencies involved with family
  H. Safety precautions

Domains of Health Care Problems

When analyzing patient problems, most providers use medical/disease diagnoses for organizing data collection, analysis, management, and recording. The classic health history format drives diagnostic decisions into these categories. Box 2-1 shows this classic health history format.

The classic medical history is written to expand on the chief complaint, which is generally a physical problem. Issues such as nutrition, development, and activities of daily living are included, primarily as they relate to various diseases. This classification system works well and has generally been taught to physicians, nurse practitioners (NPs), and other providers. The system fails, however, to provide a framework for integrating the daily living (also called *functional health patterns*) and developmental issues of children into the problem lists and management plans. Without that framework, primary care providers, especially NPs who emphasize developmental and functional health areas of practice, may fail to clearly identify and document many of the unique contributions they make to child health care. Without that identification, the special aspects of their work with children and families remain invisible.

An alternate model is offered in this chapter that integrates the nursing and medical aspects of primary care work conceptually and clinically. This assessment model (Burns, 1991, 1992, 1993) is based on the assumption that patient problems can be grouped into three distinct domains: developmental problems, functional health problems, and diseases (Box 2-2 and Fig. 2-1). Although it was originally developed for NPs, the framework is useful to all pediatric health care providers.

Developmental Problems

The developmental domain includes the long-term issues of development and maturation over the lifespan. In pediatrics, developmental issues are prominent. The National Survey of Children's Health estimates that 15% of children are at moderate risk for developmental, behavioral, or social delays and another 11% are at high risk for similar delays (National Survey of Children's Health, 2011/12). Failing to identify a developmental problem or to plan for its management is as serious as missing type 2 diabetes mellitus or a dislocated hip. Physical as well as developmental problems can affect a child's entire future if not remedied or managed to minimize their effects. Clinicians assess for developmental problems in the areas of gross motor, fine motor, speech and language, cognitive, social/emotional, and adaptive behaviors.

Zero to Three (2005) has developed a taxonomy of developmental diagnoses, *DC:0-3R: Diagnostic Classification of Mental Health and Developmental Disorders of Infancy and Early Childhood, revised edition,* which may be a useful resource for developmental problem diagnoses. It is currently being revised.

• BOX 2-2 Suggested Integrated Classification System of Diagnoses for Use by Primary Care Providers: Domains and Examples of Diagnoses

Domain I: Examples of Developmental Diagnoses

Cognitive development
- Cognitive delay
- Learning disorder

Language development
- Language delay
- Speech delay

Motor development
- Gross motor delay
- Fine motor delay

Social development
- Social developmental delay
- Attachment failure

Domain II: Examples of Functional Health Diagnoses

Health perception and health management pattern
- Decisional conflict
- Home-care resources inadequate
- Home-maintenance management impaired
- Risk of injury—suffocation, poisoning, trauma, aspiration
- Self-care deficits—dressing, toileting, hygiene

Nutritional—metabolic pattern
- Anorexia or bulimia
- Breastfeeding ineffective, interrupted, or effective
- Infant-feeding pattern ineffective
- Nutrition alterations less than or more than body requirements
- Swallowing impaired

Elimination pattern
- Constipation
- Encopresis or enuresis

Activity and exercise pattern
- Activity intolerance
- Fatigue
- Physical mobility impaired

Sleep pattern
- Sleep pattern disturbance
- Obstructive sleep apnea

Cognitive and perceptual pattern
- Attention-deficit disorder
- Sensory-perceptual alteration—visual or auditory deficits

Self-perception and self-concept pattern
- Body image disturbance
- Personal identity disturbance
- Self-esteem disturbance—chronic or situational

Role relationships pattern
- Abuse/neglect/family violence
- Caregiver role strain
- Communication impaired—verbal
- Parenting alteration
- Risk of alteration in parent-infant-child attachment
- Social interaction impaired
- Social isolation

Sexuality pattern
- Sexual pattern alteration

Coping and stress tolerance pattern
- Anxiety
- Depression
- Grieving—anticipatory, dysfunctional
- Hopelessness
- Pain, chronic
- Post-trauma response
- Substance misuse
- Violence potential, self or others

Values and beliefs pattern
- Spiritual distress

Domain III: Examples of Pediatric Disease Categories for Diagnoses

Infectious diseases
Endocrine, nutritional, metabolic, and immune diseases
Diseases of blood and blood-forming organs
Neurologic and sense organ diseases
Circulatory system diseases
Respiratory system diseases
Digestive system diseases
Dental disorders
Genitourinary system disorders
Gynecologic disorders
Skin diseases
Musculoskeletal diseases
Symptoms, signs, ill-defined conditions
Injury and poisoning
Environmental: Exposure to toxin (specify)

Functional Health Problems

Functional health problems are derived from Gordon's functional health patterns (Gordon 1987, 2010) and are incorporated into the international taxonomy of nursing diagnoses (NANDA International, 2014). These patterns provide a framework for thinking about the problems that nurses have always managed independently. Other primary care providers are also asked to manage functional health problems of children. These patterns represent the universal health behavior patterns of all humans, regardless of culture, sex, age, or economic status. Gordon's 11 patterns include health beliefs and behavior, nutrition, elimination, activity, sleep, role relationships, coping, self-perception, cognition and perception, sexuality, and values and beliefs. All functional health problems involve the family, because the family really is the primary caregiver for infants and children. NPs and other providers become involved when the family's knowledge and experience are insufficient to meet the needs of the child or when the family directly contributes to the child's problems, such as with the role-relationship problem of child abuse.

Labels for many problems in the functional health domain are found in the NANDA taxonomy terms (NANDA International, 2014), which is expanded and updated every 2 years. Many terms are also found in the *International Classification of Diseases, Tenth Revision, Clinical Modification* (ICD-10-CM) (World Health Organization [WHO], 2015) and other taxonomies, such as the *International Classification of Sleep Disorders, third edition* (ICSD-3) (2014).

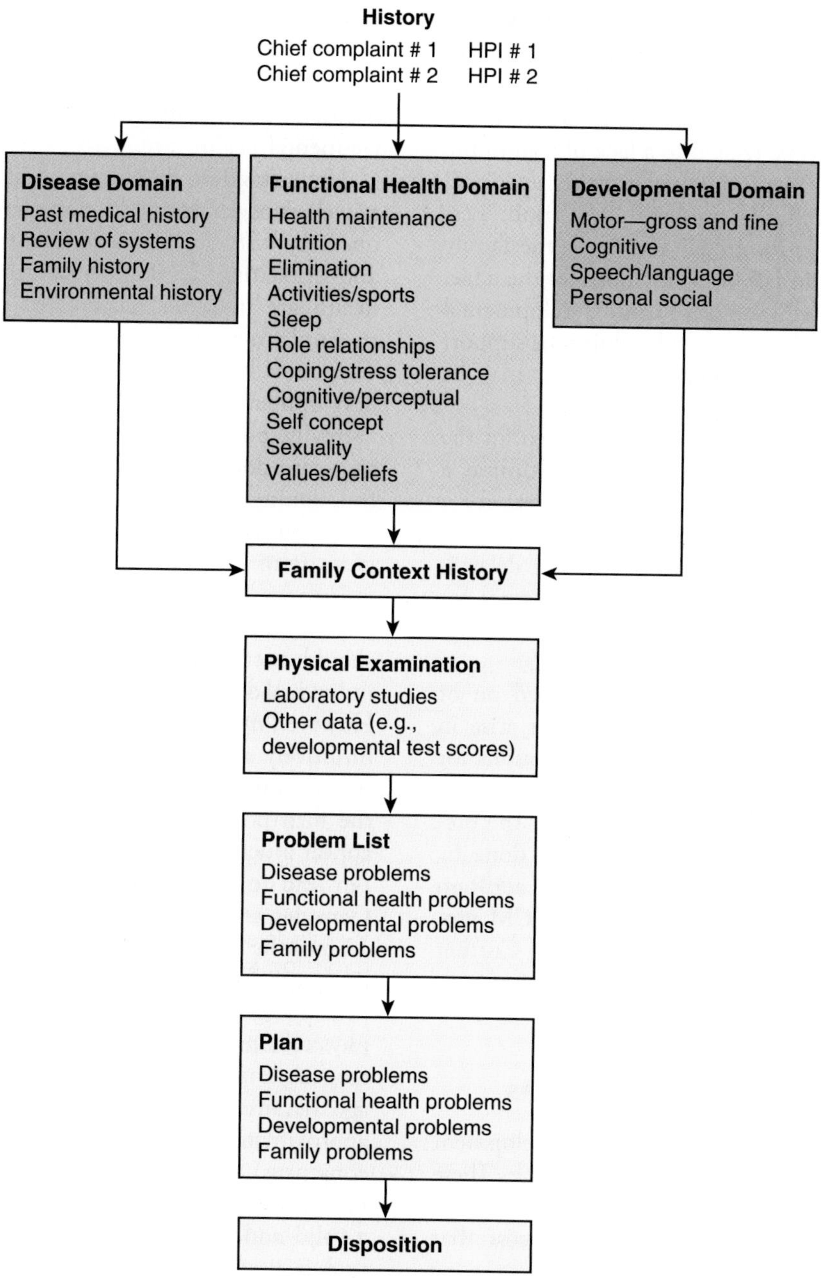

• **Figure 2-1** Model for data collection using the disease, functional health, and development domains. *HPI,* History of present illness.

Diseases

Diseases are conditions assessed and managed at the tissue or organ level of analysis. The diagnoses found in the disease domain generally comes from the ICD-10-CM. Otitis media, streptococcal pharyngitis, and appendicitis are examples of disease diagnoses. Providers should use the diagnosis that best guides understanding of etiology and management.

The ICD-10-CM is designed to represent the primary phenomena of concern to physicians. It is broad and mature in scope. It represents physiologic problems extremely well but includes few labels, or rubrics, for the behavioral, social, and developmental problems that NPs also manage. The ICD-10-CM listings are recognized by many insurance carriers for billing purposes and, as such, have become the "currency" for much health care delivery in the United States, whereas the NANDA nursing diagnoses have not yet achieved that recognition. Fortunately, a variety of diagnoses similar to those in the NANDA classification can be found among the medical listings, thus facilitating reimbursement for management of functional health patterns.

Problem Interactions

The concept of interactions of problems across domains is important to understand. For instance, iron deficiency anemia can be considered a disease if looked at from the effects of lack of iron on heme production, red blood cells, oxygen transport, and cellular metabolism. The clinician can diagnose this disease and prescribe an iron supplement to manage the problem at this physiologic level. However, if the problem is found to be related to a lack of iron in the diet, the provider can choose to intervene at the functional health-nutrition level, call the problem "Nutrition: Less Than Body Requirements for Iron," and teach the family how to increase the selection of iron-rich foods for the table. Iron deficiency has also been shown to cause developmental delays. If a goal for the visit is to provide additional support in the school setting, a developmental problem may be diagnosed.

A particular domain can also serve as the context for the problem in another area. For instance, Down syndrome, a chromosomal disorder, can be the cause or context for a cognitive development problem. If the intervention is for cognition, a developmental problem of cognitive delay is listed—not simply "Down syndrome." Content issues for which the clinician is planning interventions are the diagnoses. The contextual issues are not the diagnoses.

Most importantly, interventions must be based on or derived from diagnoses. A situation should never arise in which the provider intervenes without explicit reasons for doing so. The reasons are stated as diagnoses, either actual or potential, and enumerated in the problem list. The preventive work (i.e., to avoid potential problems) done by clinicians also needs to be identified. Diagnoses, in addition to interventions, must be recorded. The ICD-10-CM provides the lists of reimbursable diagnoses, and the Current Procedural Terminology (CPT) codes provide the therapeutic intervention codes.

Developmental Assessment Foundations

Several assumptions underlie the concept of development in children and are threaded throughout this book. These include the following:

- Development is a self-fueling, ongoing process that requires physical and emotional energy.
- Development occurs in stages and is dynamic and interactional.
- Development is influenced by the child and his or her environment.
- Development occurs in "spurts and lulls." Periods of disorganization, disharmony, and turbulence are usually followed by periods of harmony, balance, and organization because all areas of development are interrelated.

Children are generally healthy and have adaptive capabilities. Therefore, the goal of the provider is to maximize health and development and a child's overall potential, rather than solely to resolve problems. Although development is judged in terms of milestones, individual differences among children are reflected in developmental variations that reflect the unique characteristics of families, cultures, and social circumstances. Individual developmental variations and positive adaptations should be appreciated and facilitated. Further, children and families have the capacity to learn from and grow beyond their limitations when interventions are based on their abilities. Finally, preventive health care for children includes developmentally supportive mental health care.

Understanding development, incorporating the physical as well as psychosocial developmental stages for every child on every visit into the assessment and management plan, and evaluating developmental outcomes as a measure of health are the core concepts of pediatric health care. It cannot be overemphasized that *children are not little adults.* They must be cared for within the parameters of their own development. Because children change so quickly developmentally, one cannot be lax about including development as a core domain for assessment. The 6-month-old infant functioning at a 3-month level is 50% behind!

Monitoring children's developmental progress brings pleasure in watching them master expected developmental milestones. With time, many providers develop an intuitive sense about the general ages at which particular milestones should occur. Experience also brings an appreciation of individual differences in infants, families, and ethnic groups. However, many variables can make it difficult to appreciate intuitively all the various developmental skills of any particular child. For example, a premature infant at or below the fifth percentile for height and weight may physically appear much younger. The discrepancy between size and age can lead to an inaccurate estimate of the child's abilities. Consider an infant who is 15 months old chronologically, 12 months old adjusted age, but physically at the 9 month level and developmentally at the 8-month-old level. If the provider evaluated this infant developmentally based on physical size, the development level might appear appropriate (size and development at 9 months old). Adjusting for age because of the infant's prematurity (adjustment to approximately 2 to 3 years though this is an area of poor consensus), the infant might still appear normal, and the need for intervention and referral might be missed. When a valid and reliable standardized developmental screening tool is used, it is more readily apparent that the infant requires referral and intervention services. Competent developmental care requires three strategies: (1) monitoring (surveillance), (2) screening, and (3) assessment. Success using these strategies begins when the health care provider builds rapport and a trusting relationship with parent and child. Gaining the parents' and child's trust and engagement in the interview process are critical to obtaining accurate and reliable information. The parent interview requires the provider to encourage parents to share sensitive information, ask questions, and express concerns about their child's development. The child interview requires an understanding of child development and ages. The provider must be skilled in the use of age-appropriate strategies, both verbal and nonverbal, to engage the child and be sensitive to the unique needs of each child. One example is to sit at the same level as the child in order to establish eye contact. Targeted questions around daily routines often provide

TABLE 2-1 Areas for Developmental Assessment

Developmental Area	Definition
Physical development	Physical stability, growth, sexually
Regulatory skills	State control and modulation, ability to manage sensory input (e.g., light, noise, touch, movement) from the external internal environment; self-regulation and control
Adaptive skills and fine motor skills	Self-care skills that are involved in daily routines (e.g., feeding, bathing, dressing, brushing teeth)
Motor skills	Skills that facilitate overall movement and locomotion
Communication and language	Verbal and nonverbal communication skills, including behaviors, gestures, signs
Social-emotional development and parent-child interaction	Ability to interact with others and the environment and overall affect; the reciprocal relationship between the child and his or her caregivers
Cognitive and intellectual development	Cognitive and intellectual skills, including problem-solving, decision-making, and goal-setting

insight into a child's daily activities and parents' areas of concern. Observation of the child and the child's attention, activities, verbalization, connection with the parent, processing of information, quality of movements, cooperation, and ability to follow requests are all components of developmental screening and assessment. See Table 2-1 for areas of development to assess.

Developmental Monitoring (Surveillance)

The American Academy of Pediatrics (AAP) Council on Children with Disabilities recommends that developmental monitoring be incorporated into each well-child preventive visit (Council on Children with Disabilities et al, 2006). Monitoring encompasses all primary care activities related to the development of children, including:

- Eliciting and attending to parental concerns
- Obtaining a relevant developmental history
- Making accurate and informative observations of children

Emphasis is placed on monitoring development over time within the context of the child's overall well-being rather than viewing development during an isolated testing session.

One focus of developmental monitoring is to build parental competence and confidence, which in turn enhances the child's overall well-being. When providers share their observations of a child's unique developmental strengths and skills, parents increase their knowledge of development and create their own parenting style. When parents feel success in their current parenting role, they do a better job meeting their child's future needs.

Developmental Screening and Assessment

Because developmental monitoring was found to be insufficient to identify children with developmental problems—in some cases lower than a 54% identification rate (Sheldrick et al, 2011)—developmental screening and assessment strategies must also be used.

Screening

Screening is considered a first-level contact with an individual to identify potential and actual developmental concerns. Developmental screening is a brief, inexpensive method to identify children who may need a more comprehensive assessment and diagnostic evaluation. It allows the practitioner to document a child's progress over time and objectively identify and reinforce a child's developmental strengths. It may also serve as a tool to stimulate parent questions about development and facilitate parent education.

Typical areas of developmental screening and assessment include language, motor, social-emotional, and cognitive skills. Regulatory and sensory systems as a part of the child's overall development and functioning should also be assessed. Regulation refers to infants' daily patterns of sleep-wake cycles, which include sleeping, eating, moving, responding, and reacting to their internal and external environments. Sensory system evaluation includes assessment of the child's ability to receive, process, and respond to both internal and external stimuli. Finally, although it is conceptually a part of the child's social skill set, it is important to review parent-child interactions and the family and environmental context in which the child is living. A comprehensive approach to developmental screening and assessment that includes the areas of regulation and adaptive skills in daily routines is presented for each age group in Chapters 4 through 8. Table 2-1 provides examples of information to gather within each of these areas.

Strategies Specific to Developmental Screening

A standardized screening test is recommended for children at a minimum of 9 months old, 18 months old, and 24 to

30 months old (AAP, 2014a). A parent self-report screening tool can be completed in the waiting room or examination room, scored by a nurse or medical assistant, and then reviewed by the provider with the parent. Aspects of the screening should be incorporated into the physical examination. By doing this, the provider not only sees the child "in action" but also has an opportunity to demonstrate to parents the infant's or child's current or emerging skills. After completion of developmental screening, the provider should review the findings with the parents. This discussion helps families focus on concerns that they may have, provides opportunities to answer specific parent questions, addresses parenting issues, and is conducive to providing anticipatory guidance.

When developmental screening is omitted or delegated to medical assistants but not reviewed by the primary provider, the significance of subtle variations of normal behavior or behavior that is very near the abnormal range may be overlooked. Use of standardized developmental screening tools enhances the efficiency and quality of the practice. Such tools provide a consistent, reliable, and efficient method of documentation of care provided and set standards for referral. Use of developmental screening tools involves engaging other providers and office staff with some minimal training and imparting knowledge of community resources for referral of children identified with developmental problems. Implementing this standard of practice increases parent satisfaction and engagement as experts on their child and recognizes the provider-parent partnership in the care of the child (Halfon et al, 2011).

Developmental screening tools should have well-established psychometric qualities, including sensitivity, specificity, validity, and reliability that have been standardized on diverse populations. A variety of standardized screening tools are available and recommended for developmental screening. Many of these tools have been developed to meet the demands of a busy, efficient office practice. Chapter 4-8 on the management of the development domain provide suggested developmental screening or assessment tools that are age-appropriate. Some recommended tools include the following (Berry et al, 2014):

- Ages & Stages Questionnaires, Third Edition (ASQ-3)
- Ages & Stages Questionnaires: Social-Emotional (ASQ:SE)
- Parents' Evaluation of Developmental Status (PEDS)
- Modified Checklist for Autism in Toddlers (M-CHAT)
- Edinburgh Postnatal Depression Scale (EPDS)
- Pediatric Symptom Checklist (PSC)
- Patient Health Questionnaire-9 (PHQ-9)
- CRAFFT and Patient Health Questionnaire-2 (PHQ-2) are recommended for teens (see Boxes 2-3 and 2-4)

See Chapter 6 and 19 for guides to these resources.

Developmental screening strategies are appropriate for all children, although culture and life experiences may affect some outcomes and need to be taken into consideration. Screening is conducted with the assumption that some children's developmental skills will fall outside the normal limits identified by the screening tool, thus requiring a referral for a more in-depth developmental assessment. In addition, parent education to facilitate the "next steps" of development for the child may also be needed.

Developmental Assessment

A developmental assessment, more in-depth than a developmental screening, is conducted when a definitive diagnosis and a more individualized approach to guide the plan of care and manage the child's problems are required. Assessment is a second level of analysis, focusing on a narrower, often complicated problem. Generally, assessments confirm a developmental problem, identify the type of problem, describe the level of functioning in one or more developmental domains, and provide parents with anticipatory guidance and referrals to appropriate therapy, early intervention services, or community resources.

Strategies Specific to Developmental Assessment

Developmental assessment tools are significantly different from screening tools and are appropriate when concerns require more in-depth developmental or diagnostic evaluation. Assessment tools for developmental and behavioral diagnosis, home assessment, family assessment, parent-child interaction assessment, parent stress, and parental competency are most frequently used in research but may also be of value in the clinical setting. These tools can be used for a thorough assessment of the child within the family context, to look at the parent-child interaction, and to develop a substantiated diagnosis for the child. The information also improves the practitioner's ability to structure individualized interventions for both the child and the parents, and it can be used to evaluate the effectiveness of recommended interventions. Tools used for overall development can include the Bayley Scales of Infant Development (Aylward, 1995), the Child Developmental Inventory (Ireton, 1992), and the Mullen Scales of Early Learning (Mullen, 1989). Tools used to evaluate specific behaviors or characteristics may include the Autism Diagnostic Observation Scale-Generic (ADOS-G) (Lord et al, 1994) or the Childhood Autism Rating Scale (CARS) (Schopler et al, 1986). Because of the complexity of issues that might need evaluation, developmental assessment tools require more knowledge, practice, and skill to perform reliably, interpret the findings, and plan appropriate interventions. These tools generally require special training or credentials to administer accurately. Often they are completed by specialists after referral from the primary care setting.

Family Assessment Foundations

The Family's Role in Health Care of Children

Understanding family health promotion begins with understanding family dynamics. Research has provided definitive evidence that children, from birth through adolescence, need nurturing and attention from the significant adults in their lives. These adults most often are the child's birth or adoptive parents, but they may also be grandparents,

• BOX 2-3 Adolescent Health History

The adolescent history should be adapted depending upon the teen's developmental level: Early (11-14 years old), middle (15-17 years old), or late (18-21 years old)

I. Contextual and Family Information Database
   A. With whom do you live?
   B. In the past year have there been any changes in your immediate family, such as marriage, separation, divorce; serious illness or injury; loss of job; moves; change of school; births or deaths?
   C. What languages are spoken in your home?

II. Disease Database
   A. Chief complaint
      1. *Teen:* Since your last visit, how have you been? What health problems, concerns, or questions have you had? How are things going with your family, friends, school, and work?
      2. *Parent:* Do you have any questions or concerns about your child's physical well-being, growth, or pubertal development? Emotional well-being, feelings, behavior, learning?
   B. Physical health
      1. In the past year, have you had any injury or illness that made you miss school or cut down on activities, or that required medical care?
      2. Have you been hospitalized or gone to an emergency department in the past year?
      3. Do you have any illnesses or medical conditions?
      4. Are you taking any medications?
   C. Review of systems
      1. Focus on the issues of physical development for teens such growth in height and weight, pubertal changes, acne, sports injuries,

III. Development Database
   Chapter 8 is especially useful in elaborating on developmental assessment of teens. Throughout the history, listen for data that allow you to assess the following areas:
   A. Motor development
      1. All teens should be active in a variety of physical activities and sports.
      2. Fine motor development should also be mature.
      3. Special arts or crafts or occupational activities may be learned.
   B. Cognitive development
      1. *Early adolescents* are still concrete and generally present oriented rather than future oriented. Questions can be answered quite literally.
      2. *Middle adolescents* can use and understand "if then" statements. They are able to understand long-term consequences and think of the future. They might challenge many ideas and rules with their newfound skills in logic and reasoning.
      3. *Late adolescents* are able to consider options before making decisions, engage in sophisticated moral reasoning, and use principles to guide their decisions.
   C. Social development
      1. *Early adolescents* are egocentric in thinking. They can vacillate between childish and mature behavior, especially around their parents. Their peers are usually of the same sex. Group activities are the norm.
      2. *Middle adolescents* are concerned with their identity within society and less concerned with their sexual identity unless they are struggling with recognizing their homosexuality. They tend to distance themselves from parents, spend less time at home, and increasingly challenge parental control. Cliques or friends prevail, with only a few close friends. Physical intimacy can occur during this stage, and romantic partners are common.
      3. *Late adolescents* have distanced themselves from parents and then reestablished relationships with family on a new basis of independence. Romantic and emotional intimacy appears.
   D. School and vocational development
      1. *Early adolescents* are usually adjusting to the expectations of middle school or early high school. Setting priorities and completing homework independently can be a challenge. Future goals are often unrealistic and change frequently.
      2. *Middle adolescents* are entering high school and beginning to develop an awareness that their performance in school will affect their future options for work or college. They do not usually have specific ideas about future vocations in mind.
      3. *Late adolescents* are making decisions about vocations, college, working, or entering the military.

IV. Functional Health Database
   A. Health maintenance and health perception—safety issues
      1. Do you always wear a helmet and protective gear when you participate in physical activities, such as biking, skateboarding, team sports, or water sports? Do you always wear a seat belt when riding in a vehicle?
      2. In the past year, have you been in a car when the driver has been drinking or using drugs? What do you do to stay safe?
   B. Nutrition—diet/eating behaviors
      1. How do you feel about the way you look? Do you feel you are underweight or overweight? How much would you like to weigh? Are you doing anything to change your weight?
      2. Which meals do you usually eat each day? Do you skip meals? If so, how many times a week?
      3. How many servings of dairy products did you eat yesterday? Other calcium-containing foods? Fruits? Vegetables?
      4. Does your family ever not have enough food?
      5. Are there foods you won't eat?
      6. How often do you drink juice or soft drinks?
   C. Activities
      1. Do you participate in any physical activities? (Listen for variety, frequency, duration of activity.)
      2. What do you do after school?
      3. What are your interests outside of school?
      4. How much time do you spend watching TV, videos, or DVDs each day? How many hours a day do you spend on the computer outside of study time?
      5. Do you participate in any physical activities with your parents?
      6. Do you have physical problems that limit your exercise?
      7. Do you have questions or concerns about exercise or physical activity?
   D. Sleep
      1. How many hours do you sleep on weekdays? Weekends?
      2. Do you have trouble sleeping? Tiredness?
   E. Role relationships
      1. How do you get along with your friends? Do you have at least one friend that you really like and feel you can talk to?

Continued

• BOX 2-3 Adolescent Health History—cont'd

2. Who are the important adults in your life? Is there someone outside your family that you can talk to?
3. How are you getting along as a family? Do your parents listen to you? What do you do together?
4. How connected do you feel to your family in terms of your family's cultural or family life?
5. Do you have some responsibilities or chores? What rules does your family have for you?

F. Drug and alcohol use, emotions, violence
   1. Drugs and tobacco use
      a. Use the CRAFFT screening for drugs and alcohol (see Box 2-5)
      b. Have you ever used steroids or drugs to enhance your sports performance without a physician telling you to do so?
      c. Do you or your friends ever smoke cigarettes, e-cigarettes, or use smokeless tobacco? Does anyone you live with smoke or use smokeless tobacco?
      d. Do you ever sniff, huff, or breathe in substances to get high?
   2. Emotions/depression
      a. Use the two-question Patient Health Questionnaire-2 (PHQ-2) (see Box 2-6)
      b. Do you worry a lot or feel overly stressed out? How do you cope when you are stressed?
      c. Do you ever feel so sad that you wish you weren't alive or that you wanted to die?
      d. Do you keep remembering something bad that happened, such as an accident or being hurt by someone?
      e. Do you think counseling would help you or someone in your family?
      f. Do you have any questions or concerns about physical, sexual, or emotional abuse? Has anyone ever hurt you? Has anyone been bullying you directly or on the computer?
   3. Weapons and violence
      a. Is there a gun in your house? A friend's house? A relative' house? Is it locked and ammunition stored and locked separately?
      b. In the past year, have you ever carried a gun, knife, razor blade, or other weapon (even for self-protection)?
      c. Have you been in a physical fight during the past 6 months?
      d. Are guns or violence a problem in your neighborhood? Have you ever witnessed a violent act? Do you know anyone in a gang?
      e. When you are angry, what do you do?
      f. Have you and your friends done anything that could have gotten them into trouble?

G. Cognitive and learning issues
   1. In general do you like school? Why?
   2. Are your grades this year better or worse than the year before? What are your usual grades?
      a. Areas to explore if school is a problem: Have you ever had to repeat a grade in school? Cutting classes? On time to school? Days missed this year? Suspension or dropped out? Supports for school success tried?
   3. What do you plan to do after high school?
   4. Do you have any questions or concerns about school or your learning?

H. Self-perception and self-concept
   1. What do you like about yourself?
   2. What do you do best?
   3. If you could, what would you change about your life or yourself?

I. Sexual and menstrual
   1. Early teen:
      a. Have you and your parents discussed the physical changes that occur during puberty?
      b. Have you talked with your parents about dating and sex?
      c. Have you had sexual intercourse or oral or anal sex?
   2. Sexually active teens:
      a. Was your sexual experience wanted or unwanted? Have you been forced to do something you didn't want to do sexually?
      b. How many partners have you had this past year? Male, female, or both? Younger, older, or the same age? Do you think you might be gay, lesbian, bisexual, or transsexual?
      c. Have you ever been told that you have a sexually transmitted disease?
      d. Do you practice abstinence or use a birth control method? If so, which one(s)? Girls: Are you worried about getting pregnant? Boys: Do you worry about getting someone pregnant?
      e. Do you want information or supplies to prevent pregnancy or sexually transmitted diseases, including human immunodeficiency virus (HIV)?
      f. If you are in a relationship, are you making good choices to avoid emotional hurt to yourself or your partner?

J. Values and beliefs and religious orientation
   1. Are you involved with any religious groups or activities on regular basis?
   2. Do you have any strong ethical, moral, or religious beliefs?

Adapted from Hagan JF, Shaw JS, Duncan PM, editors: *Bright Futures: guidelines for health supervision of infants, children, and adolescents*, ed 3, Elk Grove Village, IL, 2008, American Academy of Pediatrics and other sources.

extended family members, or foster parents. Factors such as a mother's level of education, her beliefs and attitudes about health, and her own health practices have significant influences on the health status of her children. Parental stress and mental health problems, such as depression, affect health care for children (Earls, 2013; Raphael et al, 2010). Maternal depression in the first year of her infant's life has been associated with poorer caregiving that results in poorer language development at 3 years old (Paulson et al, 2009; Stein et al, 2008). Maternal depressive symptoms were also predictive of asthma symptoms in inner-city African American families (Otsuki et al, 2010). Similarly, paternal depression also affects a child's health (Ramchandani et al, 2011).

BOX 2-4 Symptom Analysis

1. Onset—initial and episodic; date and time, sudden or gradual, setting
2. Location of pain—local, radiation, generalized, superficial, or deep
3. Duration—how long, has it eased, gotten worse?
4. Characteristics and course:
   - Symptom quality: Nature of symptoms
   - Symptom quantity: Severity, frequency, volume, number, size or extent, degree of functional impairment
   - Course: Continuous or intermittent, pattern of variation
5. Activating (precipitating) and aggravating factors
6. Relieving factors
7. Tests and treatment, including complementary therapies: What, when, where, who, and results, including complications and sequelae
8. The meaning of the symptoms to patient and family and patient's reactions to symptoms

Evidence is strong that when children are raised without consistent, affectionate attention and without sensitive interactions with a caring adult, the results can be devastating for both child and society (Kazak et al, 2010). For example, family cohesion, beyond dyadic family relationships, is a protective factor for adolescent violence against authority (parent abuse and student-to-teacher violence) (Ibabe et al, 2013).

Although inadequate or poor parenting is linked to factors such as poverty, substance abuse, and minimal education, research suggests that a poor "fit" between a child and a significant adult can occur in any family, including those in which the adults are well educated, socially competent, and economically successful. In contrast, when a parent or another significant adult responds consistently and sensitively to a child's needs, such as a need to play, to eat, to sleep, to be comforted, or to be left alone, the child is likely to grow up competent to initiate and build strong, nurturing relationships. Issues of family relationships and family disruption are discussed more fully in Chapter 17.

Family Assessment Basic Elements

Family assessment begins with the assumption that families are central to and inseparable from the health of children. It is based on a family health promotion framework that assumes that the vast majority of family members are competent, want to do what is best for their children, and desire to be active participants in their children's health care. Family assessment in a primary care practice with children requires attention to family structure, family life cycle stage, family functioning, and social network. In other words, a basic family assessment addresses characteristics of the family, transitions that the family is experiencing, how family members interact and accomplish tasks, what they believe and value, and how they interact with the community.

It is important to recognize that providers' own definitions of family and healthy family functioning are culturally and temporally bound, determine who is and who is not family, and can profoundly affect assessment, treatment, and outcomes. Providers might find it useful to periodically examine their own assumptions and beliefs regarding families and use the knowledge gained to foster increased sensitivity and openness to the rich diversity that their families present.

Legal definitions of family usually address bonds of blood, marriage, and adoption. A significant number of contemporary families do not fit such restrictive definitions. To address this reality, Whall defined family as "a self-identified group of two or more individuals whose association is characterized by special terms, who may or may not be related by bloodlines or law, but who function in such a way that they consider themselves to be a family" (Whall, 1986, p 240). Wherever practitioners' personal definitions might fall on a continuum of inclusiveness, it is imperative that they know and understand the implications of that definition in practice.

Family Structure and Roles

Assessment of a family's structure and roles includes the composition of the family or household, demographic data, intergenerational data, and information about family roles. Implicit in the data is the way the family defines itself and how the family gets its work done.

Family Life Cycle

Family life cycle assessment includes data on the present family life cycle stage (such as, a family with young children), family life cycle transitions or developmental crises (such as, serious illness of a frail, elderly grandparent), and family life cycle events that are untimely or "out of sync" (such as, the terminal illness of a young wife and mother).

Family Functioning

Healthy family functioning should result in what Terkelsen (1980), in his classic paper, called the "good-enough family." Families have both strengths and limitations, but the majority of families are able to meet most of their members' needs most of the time. This is a hopeful stance, one that allows for the less than perfect family to feel successful and empowered.

Family resilience is a helpful concept referring to healthy family functioning (Benzies and Mychasiuk, 2009). On a broad definition, family resilience is the ability of the family to rebound from adversity stronger and more resourceful than before. Walsh (2006) sees nine keys to resilience in three different areas: (1) family belief systems, (2) family organization and resources, and (3) family communication. Within the belief systems, resilient families view crisis as a shared challenge, something that can be manageable and meaningful when family members work together. Such families maintain a positive outlook and find meaning in moral and spiritual values. Within the family organization and resources area, resilient families are flexible, connected with one another, and supported by social and economic resources. Finally, resilient families share clear consistent messages, express their emotions openly, and work together to solve problems. Protective factors for family resilience include individual, family, and community supports. Some individual factors include internal locus of control, emotional regulation, and effective coping skills. Some family factors include structure, stable partner relations, cohesion, social support, and adequate income, whereas some supportive community characteristics include community involvement, peer acceptance, supportive mentors, a safe neighborhood, and access to a quality school, day care, and health care (Benzies and Mychasiuk, 2009).

Characteristics of healthy family functioning have been identified by a number of researchers. Open communication, mutual respect and support, differentiation, shared problem-solving, shared decision-making, flexibility, enhancement of members' personal growth, sense of play and humor, and a shared value of service to others are some of these assets. The AAP states that a child will thrive best when cared for by two mutually committed parents who respect and support each other, who have adequate social and financial resources, and who both are actively engaged in the child's upbringing. Characteristics of the successful family are described by the AAP as being cohesive, enduring, and mutually appreciative. Such families communicate effectively and often, adapt to changing circumstances, spend time together, are committed to the family, and embrace a common religious or spiritual orientation (Schor and AAP Task Force on the Family, 2003). "Family members share their lives emotionally and together fulfill the multiple responsibilities of family life" (AAP, 2014b).

Family Social Network

Positive social support exists when the family feels emotional support, has tangible help, and is informed (Benzies and Mychasiuk, 2009). The family's social network includes those individuals, activities, agencies, and institutions that have the potential to support, harm, or drain energy from the family. Assessing the family's relationships with extended family, friends, and the community provides information on which to base recommendations and further assessment.

Genograms

A genogram is an approach to developing a family database. It does not require the purchase of standardized assessment tools, and it can be updated over time, which is a characteristic making it valuable to pediatric providers in understanding patterns in the lives of children and families. Genograms provide graphic representations of complex family data; they allow the providers to map the family structure and roles, life cycle transitions, family functioning, and social networks clearly and to update the picture as it emerges. Further, genograms provide efficient clinical summary, making it easier for providers to keep in mind family members, patterns, and events that may have recurring significance in a family's ongoing care. They provide a means for interacting with children and their family members in a focused, nonthreatening way around potentially complex and difficult issues. The genogram is inherently appealing to families, because it helps them see themselves in new ways and provides a way for families to be partners in their own diagnosis and management. Even if not explicitly constructed during a visit, conceptually, the genogram assists the provider to organize family data for analysis and identification of problems. It is a subjective, interpretive tool to help generate tentative hypotheses for further systematic evaluation.

Providers who use genograms in their practice frequently come to the conclusion that the tools are as useful for intervention as they are for assessment. In addition, those working with children find that including the children in the construction and updating of genograms helps children be active in their own care and provides data on family interactions. Although the genogram looks similar to a genetic pedigree, its purpose is to understand the family's structure and function—not the family's genetic risk factors.

Genogram Construction

Genograms are sociometric paper-and-pencil tools used to depict a family's composition and history across generations (Fig. 2-2). Although not essential, computer programs to facilitate genogram data management are available and can be easily included in computerized patient records. These programs have made updating genogram data easy and efficient (e.g., Genopro).

Priorities for organizing genogram data for clinical use rely less on formal blood and legal links and more on repetitive symptoms in members and relationships or patterns of functioning seen across the family or over generations. They are most effective when constructed during an initial visit with children and their families and then revised as new information becomes available.

The provider begins by drawing a basic family tree, with the present family members guiding identification of family members. It is clinically useful to identify members of the current household in which children live. In fact, it can be more informative and useful to learn who is living in a household than who is related by blood or birth. This objective can be met by drawing a circle around the members of the genogram who currently live together (e.g., the circle may include parents and three children, or it may include one of two parents, two of three children, and a grandparent). It is also useful to include at least three generations of the family. Standardized symbols and a sample can be found at www.genogram.org/gmm_sample_win.html.

Health history information, including serious medical, behavioral, and emotional problems, can be noted on the genogram (e.g., drug or alcohol problems, serious problems with the law, and causes of death). Likewise, family information that is significant to the health of the child can be included, such as ethnic background, language spoken in the home, education of parents, occupations, religious affiliation, major family moves, and current location of family members. Significant others who live with or are important to the family should be included (for example, family

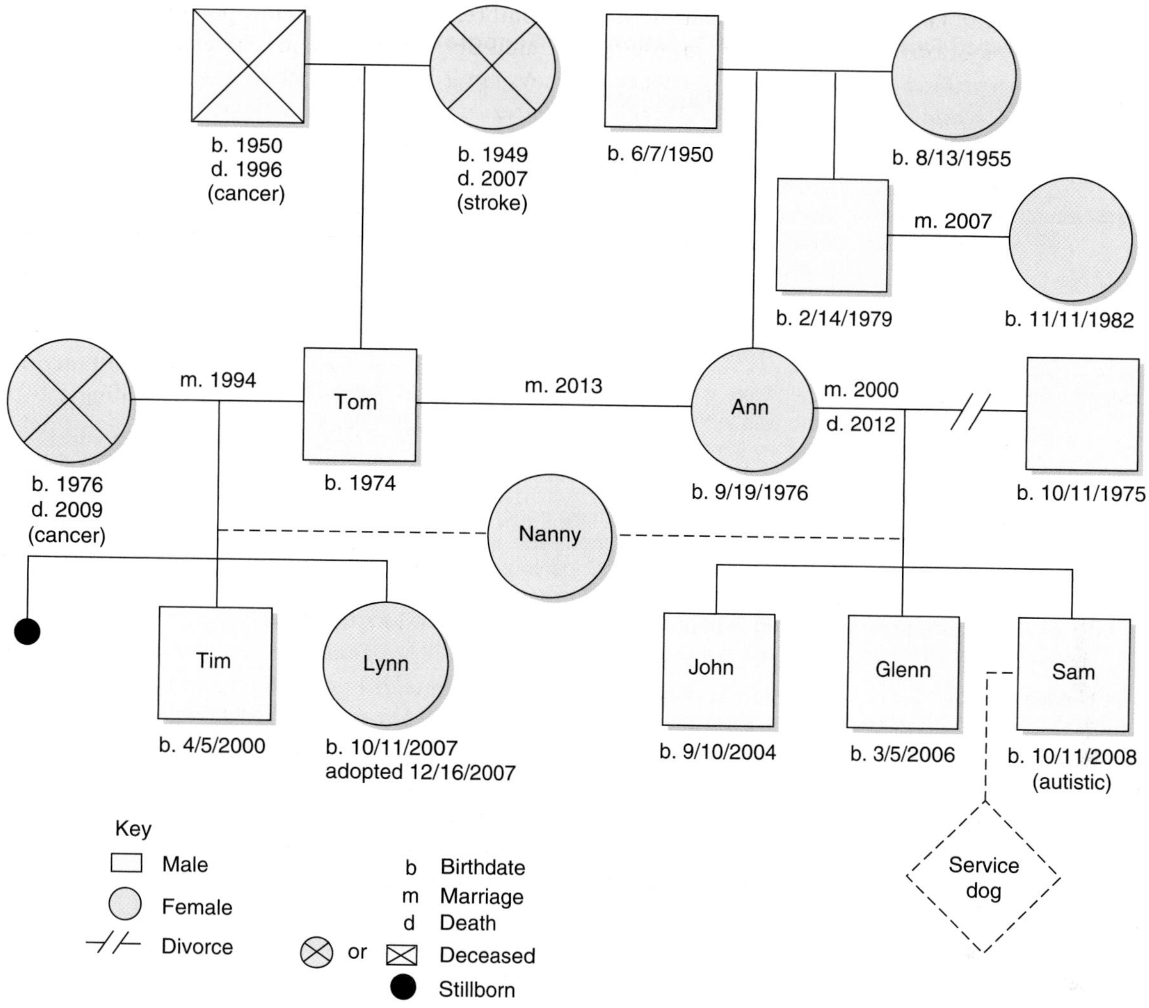

• **Figure 2-2** A three-generational genogram of a blended family.

friends, foster children, and babysitters). In some cases, the significant other is a family pet.

Practical pointers include using pencil instead of pen, unless there are legal or institutional requirements to use a pen; leaving space at the bottom of the page for notes; and including a key to notations or unusual symbols. It also is useful to provide children with their own paper and pencils or crayons to use while conducting the interview; ask them to draw a picture of their family for you.

The genogram interview can begin with an open question, such as, "Tell me about your family." It can be addressed to children, parents, or both. As the genogram is being constructed, questions can be used to elicit information about family functioning. Some examples of questions that may help to understand the functioning of various family forms are found in Table 2-2. They are examples only and should not be viewed as exhaustive.

The Ecomap is a similar tool that is used to construct a picture of the family structure and relationships within the family and in the community that are supportive or harmful. For those interested in pursuing how individual family members work together or against one another and use outside resources to support themselves as a family that may or may not be successful, the genogram is a highly recommended tool.

The Environment for Data Collection

Setting up the Assessment Environment

Health care is a family event in pediatrics, and pediatric primary health care is delivered in many settings, not just examination rooms in outpatient clinics. Wherever the child and the family are to be cared for, privacy must be ensured. People should have places to sit down, and the room in which the examination is conducted should be well lit and allow the patient to lie down comfortably. The examiner must be able to work comfortably, too. The health care provider should sit down during the history to make data collection a conversation, to equalize the status of patient and examiner, and to help the children and their families feel that they have time to talk. Sitting also helps the provider conserve energy for a busy day. The environment must be safe, given the developmental ages of the children to be cared for, and should present an atmosphere of warmth and welcome.

TABLE 2-2 Some Suggested Family Assessment Questions for Genogram

Family History Topic	Suggested Questions
Family composition and structure	Who is in your family? Broadly define *family*—not just blood relatives but those living together in a supportive, committed relationship.
Current family situation	Who currently lives with you and your child? If the relationships are not clear: How are you related to the members of your household? If divorce or separation is involved: Where does the child's other parent live? How often does the child see or hear from the other parent? Have there been any changes in your family since your last visit? What, if any, changes do you anticipate in the near future?
Extended family situation	When were your parents born? Where? Who were their parents? Who was in their families while they were growing up? Are they living? If yes, where do they live now? How often do you have contact with them? If no, when did they die? What was the cause of death?
Family relationships and roles	How do you generally make important decisions in your family? Who in your family is responsible for monitoring your children's health? What are some of the things you do together as a family? How often? To whom does your child tend to tell problems and concerns? How do family members show their support for one another? How well do you think your family adapts to change?
Two-parent families	How do you decide who does what at home? Who has primary responsibility for daily child care? How is that working? How many hours do you work outside the home in a typical week? How does that affect your family life? What tensions do you anticipate (or are you experiencing) to be associated with balancing work and home? What child care arrangements have you made? How satisfactory are they? What would you change if you could?
Families with a child with a chronic illness	How are things going on a day-to-day basis with your child's care? How is the child's illness affecting your child's relationships with other children? How is the child's illness affecting family life? How is school going? What do you need most right now to better care for your whole family?
Blended families	Have things gone as you expected they would in your new family? How is each child coping with the new family? How has their child care or school situation changed, and how have they responded? What do the parents identify as the most significant loss for each child in the blended family? The most significant benefit? How are the relationships between parents (including stepparent) and children? Among the children?
Single-parent families	What is the best thing about being your child's only parent? What is most challenging for you about being a single parent? How do you get the support that you need as a parent? What would most help you raise your child at this point in time?

Communication with Children and Families

"Communication is the most common 'procedure' in medicine" (Levetown and AAP Committee on Bioethics, 2008, p 1441) and is identified as critical to the provision of health care. It must be responsive to the needs of the child and family within the context of their own dynamics. It is essential to diagnosis and successful treatment planning and results in better patient outcomes, including physical and psychosocial benefits, increased patient satisfaction, patient knowledge, adherence, functional status, and adaptation to challenging situations. "Poor communication, on the other hand, can prompt lifelong anger and regret, can result in compromised outcomes for the patient and family, and can have medicolegal consequences for the practitioner" (Levetown and AAP Committee on Bioethics, 2008, p 1441).

The three elements they identify as essential to excellent communication are as follows:

- Communication needs to provide information.
- Communication should be sensitive interpersonally, with affective behaviors indicating the provider's attention

to and interest in the parents' and child's feelings and concerns.

- Communication should help to build a partnership among the three parties, allowing discussion of concerns, perspectives, and suggestions from all.

Health care communication is different from normal discourse because very personal issues are discussed—hopes and fears; sexuality; mental health issues; painful issues such as abuse, drug use, school and personal failure; and serious or terminal illness. Communication involves both cognitive and affective elements. When drug use, alcohol consumption, and smoking were addressed with mothers, parent-provider relationships were positively affected (Garg et al, 2010). Similarly, discussion of maternal stress also results in greater maternal satisfaction with care (Brown and Wissow, 2008).

The pediatric health history has several unique aspects. First, the participants in the conversation may include the child, caregiver, or both, and provider—more than just the patient and provider as in the adult care model. Second, the topics emphasized vary significantly depending on the child's developmental stage. Third, the process of communication with the child and the extent to which he or she is involved with health care decisions vary with age. The provider should introduce himself or herself at the start of the interview. Families typically want to be addressed by their last names and to shake hands with the provider (Amer, Fischer, 2009). For young children, the conversation time gives them the opportunity to become familiar with the examiner and setting, which is essential for cooperation when needed. Remember that young children are learning the "script" for health care visits. The visit should help them learn a script that is understandable and not too stressful. When the script is to be varied (e.g., no immunizations this visit), alert them to the change with cues and explanations for the new experiences of this visit and the likelihood that the new script will be repeated at future visits.

The provider is also observing parent-child interactions during the visit. For example, are the parents responding to their baby? Do the parents contribute to the school-age child's self-esteem? Cues to mental health problems in any family member or the child should be addressed.

For adolescents, the history can be started with the parents and teen together; however, they then need to separate, with the provider getting information from the parents and the teen independently. Interviewing teens requires patience, because they are learning to take responsibility for their own health care. Interactions will change as teens mature developmentally or as the situation is modified.

Data can be collected verbally, through record review, via written forms completed by the family, or through a combination of these methods. It might not be practical for data to be fully collected on the first visit; rather, the collection can be staged according to the visit priorities. When time with patients is limited, it is common to ask new families to come early for their first appointment to complete a written history before meeting the clinician. Notation of any missing data should be made so that further baseline data can be collected at the next visit.

Interpreter services must be available if the clinician and family are not fluent in each other's languages. These services are mandated by law. Use of family members as interpreters is never recommended. Family members may try to protect the patient or themselves by hiding important information. Legally, the provider may be at risk if information was not transmitted correctly or completely either to or from the clinician.

Redesigning Primary Care to Achieve Assessment Goals

Although the data that needs to be collected during a first-time primary care health care visit is extensive, many well child visits are of very short duration—11 to 20 minutes (47%). Longer visits are associated with more anticipatory guidance, more psychosocial risk assessment, and stronger family-centered care ratings (Halfon et al, 2011). Receiving a developmental assessment, having enough time to ask questions, and satisfaction with the provider are all associated with longer visits. Some efforts are being made to redesign clinical practices to provide for developmental-behavioral promotion and family-oriented services (Glascoe and Trimm, 2014). For example, health educators may do more anticipatory guidance and developmental/behavioral/psychosocial surveillance and screening (Coker et al, 2014).

Health literacy is a concept discussed in several chapters of this text. If the family or child does not have the skills to understand, read, write, and discuss health issues in the language required, communication may be broken with possible, including jeopardized, quality of care outcomes and misunderstandings.

The Database

The Child Health History

It is a common saying in medicine that 80% of diagnoses are made on the basis of the history. The physical examination only provides a partial view of the situation as it is at the moment. It is often a cloudy picture because the body frequently responds similarly to different assaults. It is the history of the problem—its onset, duration, progress, associated symptoms, meaning, and effects on daily living—that brings the health care provider to an understanding in sufficient depth to choose appropriate management. Functional health and developmental problems present the same issues for the provider. A thorough, thoughtful history is essential.

The database described in this chapter summarizes the child health history and physical examination and the family assessment. The model presented uses a basic problem-oriented format that begins with subjective data (the history), moves to objective data (the physical examination, laboratory, and test data), then lists the problems by domain (identified through the subjective and objective data), and finally, outlines plans of care, problem by problem. The items listed under each topic are suggestions; they are not required data to obtain from every patient. As children age, the emphasis will change (e.g., less time spent on birth and infancy histories). The history needs to be individualized, considering family, culture, health status, and environment. The complete format should be mastered so that it becomes core to the provider's approach to all patient situations. If data are omitted, the omissions should be by choice, not by an error committed through haste, distraction, ignorance, or habit. The adolescent history needs special modification because adolescents' health care needs, risks, and developmental characteristics are so different from those of infants and young children and because adolescents are interviewed directly. Box 2-3 shows a modification of the initial health history for adolescents.

The Initial (Complete) Health History

Patient-Identifying Information

Data here are standard to medical records: date, name, medical record number, birth date, gender, address, phone number, and names of other family members. Data about the informant are designed to give the reader a sense of the probability that the history is accurate, complete, and from a knowledgeable source. Health literacy can be determined with "the newest vital sign," which is a single question, "How many children's books are in your home?" An answer of less than 10 is a meaningful indicator of inadequate household health literacy (Driessnack et al, 2014)

The Database: Subjective Information

Chief Complaint and History of Present Problem

- *Concerns:* The health care visit should begin with open-ended questions to allow the child and family to voice their concerns. What brings the child to the clinic today? The chief complaint is a brief statement of the problem and its duration. Remember that new concerns can arise at any point during the visit. Agendas can be hidden or unconscious. The chief complaint or complaints can involve disease, the functional health pattern, or development, and the problem may lie primarily with either the child or family.
- *Present problem history:* For each concern, a chronologic description should be made that includes a symptom analysis (i.e., onset, duration, characteristics or symptoms, exposure to illnesses or other causative factors, similar problems in other family members or neighbors, previous episodes of similar illnesses or symptoms, previous diagnostic measures, pertinent negative data, things that have been tried in attempts to manage the concern and their success, and the meaning of the concern for the family and child). Box 2-4 shows symptom analysis.

Even though the child comes in for a specific problem, always ask some screening questions that tap into the other domains of the history—disease, functional health, and developmental. At visits for minor illnesses, health promotion and disease prevention issues should be considered in addition to the problem at hand. An immunization history, if appropriate, should be completed at every visit.

Disease Domain Database

Past Medical History

- *Prenatal:* Planned pregnancy? When did prenatal care begin? What was the mother's health during pregnancy? Drug, alcohol, and tobacco use? Illnesses and medications? Weight gain? Accidents? (With age and history of a healthy baby, these sections may become less significant.)
- *Perinatal:* Where was the baby born and who delivered the infant? Duration and process of labor? Vaginal or cesarean delivery and process? Infant response to labor and delivery (breathing, crying)? Resuscitation needed? Apgar scores? Birth weight, length, and head circumference? Gestational age? Neonatal course: infections or other health problems, physiologic stabilization, feeding, responsiveness? Jaundice? Weight at discharge? Hospital duration? Neonatal follow-up over the first few weeks? (Again, with age and health, this section is given less attention.)
- *Past disease profile:* What health problems has the child experienced, and what have the outcomes been? Who has provided care? Infectious diseases?
- *Other current health problems (not related to the chief complaint):* What problems does the child have now? What was the date of onset? Who is the principal health care provider for each problem, and what is the current status (e.g., medications, awaiting surgery, problem in remission)?
- *Operations, hospitalizations, emergency department visits:* Has the child been hospitalized for any reason? Why, when, where, outcomes? Response to hospitalization? Problems resolved? Emergency department visits? Why, when, and outcomes?
- *Injuries:* What significant injuries has the child experienced? What care was needed, was care sought at emergency department(s), and does the child have any sequelae?
- *Allergies:* Allergies to foods, medications, or environmental factors? How are the allergies manifested? When did the allergies develop? What care is given?
- *Growth:* What has the child's growth pattern for height, weight, and head circumference been? (Always plot growth data and body mass index [BMI] on a growth grid to assess progress.) Is the child similar in size to peers? Are clothing sizes changing? Has growth been a worry for the child or family?
- *Immunizations and laboratory tests:* Obtain a record with dates for all immunizations received in the past. Reactions? Blood tests and screening tests?
- *Medications:* Is the child taking any medications (prescription drugs, over-the-counter agents, or folk remedies)? What? Why? How much? Responses to the medication?

Review of Systems. Remember that this section documents the history of body system functioning, not the physical assessment findings. The goal is to seek information about all the body systems that may be related to the present problem or the child's general health status.

- *General:* Is the child considered to be well, happy, and developing normally?
- *Skin:* History of birthmarks, lesions, or skin conditions, including hair and nails?
- *Head:* Head trauma? Head growth—microcephaly, macrocephaly? Headaches?
- *Eyes, ears, nose, throat:* Vision and eye problems? Hearing and ear problems? Nose—discharge or bleeding episodes, breathing interference? Throat problems or infections?
- *Respiratory:* Breathing problems? Respiratory infections? Blue spells? Cough? Snoring at night or obstructive sleep apnea?
- *Cardiovascular:* Heart murmur history? Cyanosis? Blood pressure problems? Activity intolerance? Syncope?
- *Gastrointestinal:* Infections, diarrhea, constipation, vomiting, or reflux? Structural problems? Anal itching or fissures? Stomachaches? Weight loss?
- *Genitourinary:* Infections, discharges? Structural problems? Stream appearance? Frequency or burning?
- *Gynecologic:* Menarche and menstrual history including length of menses, frequency of cycle, cramps, and clots? Vaginal discharge or bleeding? Itching?
- *Musculoskeletal:* Movement or structural problems? Broken bones or joint sprains? Joint inflammation?
- *Neurologic:* Seizures? Movement disorders? Tremors? Tics? Loss-of-consciousness episodes? Headaches?
- *Endocrine:* Problems with growth or pubescence?
- *Hematologic:* Anemia history or symptoms? Blood transfusions? Bleeding disorders?
- *Dentition:* Number of teeth and eruption pattern? Dental trauma? Dental care? Use of fluoride? Teeth brushing and flossing? Toothaches? Use of appliances?

Family History of Diseases. Classically the three-generation pedigree is used to map out risks for genetic diseases in families, but can be used more broadly to detect conditions with modifiable risk factors. The family history is a good proxy for the genetic, environmental, and behavioral risks to health (Doerr and Teng, 2012). It can be helpful to individualize preventive care for a variety of conditions, such as obesity and diabetes. It requires patients to report reliably and is somewhat time-consuming though it is a reimbursable process (CPT code 99202 for a new patient and one return visit [99213]). Families can use checklists to note conditions or construct a pedigree online (www.familyhistory.hhs.gov) although they need access to the Internet and the record may not work well with the electronic medical record in use (Doerr and Teng, 2012). Health literacy is essential. It is discussed in greater depth in Chapter 9.

Now that the human genome has been mapped out, genetic diseases are receiving more attention, making the three-generation pedigree an important component of the health history.

- *Mother and father:* Ages and health history.
- *Mother's pregnancy history:* Number of pregnancies, births, status of offspring.
- *Familial diseases:* Age, sex, and health status of each family member. Familial and communicable diseases, such as diabetes, epilepsy, tuberculosis, hypertension or heart disease, cancer, sickle cell anemia, birth defects, known genetic disorders.
- *Genogram and/or pedigree:* Draw out a genogram of the family members, including sex, age, and health status of each member. (See Chapter 41 for pedigree notations.)

Environmental History. This section is used to consider toxic exposures. What foods does the child eat and how are they prepared? What is the quality of the child's living environment(s)—water and air quality? Pesticides used? Are chemicals or heavy metals stored in or near the home? Has the child been exposed to tobacco smoke or lead? Exposure to other toxins? What are the noise levels in the child's environment?

Functional Health Domain Database. The questions in this section are organized by functional health patterns.

Health Maintenance and Health Perceptions. All people take steps to influence and protect their health. These choices include selection of health care providers, use of safety devices, learning how to take care of oneself, and daily care of the body. Problems identified might include health-seeking behavior, altered health maintenance, or noncompliance with a preventive or adaptive health care regimen. Usual data include the following:

- Usual primary care provider: Last visit?
- Dentist: Last visit?
- Child's self-care or caregiver needs for more knowledge of caregiving?
- Health care recommendations that the family chooses not to follow or is unable to follow?
- Safety measures used: Car seats or seat belts? Smoke and carbon monoxide alarms? Window screens? Home safety measures? Pools? Firearms in the home? Helmet use?
- Routine health promotion regimens?
- Home and health management resource issues for the chronically ill or handicapped child? Home nursing? Equipment needs? Transportation needs?

Nutrition. Quality and quantity of the daily diet and the processes of feeding and swallowing, in addition to data to support diagnoses, such as nutrition, less than or greater than body requirements; anorexia; bulimia; impaired swallowing; and breastfeeding issues would be found in this section.

- Daily diet: Breakfast, lunch, snacks, and dinner? Aversions and preferences?
- Cultural patterns related to nutritional preferences and eating?
- Supplements and vitamins?
- Feeding patterns: Mealtimes and snack times? Feeding strategies? Self-feeding skills?

- Breastfeeding and bottle-feeding issues?
- Nutritional restrictions or special needs: Calories? Other?
- Satisfaction with weight?
- Difficulties chewing or swallowing? Reflux?

Elimination. Problems of elimination can be analyzed at the physiologic level of the genitourinary or gastrointestinal systems or in terms of daily living patterns. Enuresis and encopresis are daily living problems (bowel and bladder habits) that fall into this area. Physiologically, the child is well, but the elimination habits are problematic.

- Urinary patterns: Bed-wetting? Toilet training? Voiding schedule?
- Bowel patterns: Constipation or soiling? Stooling patterns? Toilet training?

Activities. Physical mobility and the diversional and occupational activities of daily life should be described here.

- Amount, timing, and types of physical activities? Other play opportunities and activities?
- Television and computer or electronic games time?
- Reading time?
- Sports, organized activities, and hobbies of older children and adolescents?
- Activity limitations caused by health problems?
- Special equipment used or needed to support mobility?

Sleep. Sleep and rest patterns are described here.

- Hours?
- Disturbances for the child or family?
- Sleep aids?
- Sleep position for infants?
- Signs of sleepiness?

Sexuality. All people have sexuality issues that affect their lives. Within their sexual preferences and habits, problems are identified when these patterns are interrupted or viewed as problematic by the client or family. Pregnancy, viewed from the psychosocial perspective, is also a sexual issue that should be explored.

- Sexual habits?
- Sexual relationships?
- Development of sexual identity?

Values and Beliefs. This section explores spiritual patterns and personal values and beliefs that affect the child's health.

- Involvement with church?
- Religious rituals?
- Sense of alienation?
- Sense of spiritual meaning in one's life?
- Values the family wants to impart to their children?

Role Relationships. Role relationships include family relationships and relationships with peers and friends in the community. Both family and individual diagnoses need to be considered here. Family coping, family process alteration, parenting alteration, abuse, and social interaction or isolation can be addressed. This section assesses family functioning in greater depth than the introductory family functioning section of the history.

- Family interactions: Between parents? Parents and children? With other family members?
- Parenting style and activities?
- Peers and social supports for the child and family? Special adults in the child's life?
- Communication with and by the child: Verbal? Nonverbal?
- School performance for school-age children and teens?
- Concerns that anyone has abused the child?

Self-Perception or Self-Concept. Personal role identity, body image, and self-esteem are issues identified in this functional health domain.

- Satisfaction with self?
- Feelings of depression?

Coping and Temperament, Mental Health, and Discipline Issues. People select and use a variety of coping strategies in their daily lives. Temperament is also important to understand child behavior and likely responses to the environment. Discipline strategies used in families are important to identify. Anxiety, fear, hopelessness, grief, powerlessness, substance abuse, pain, and potential for violence might be identified diagnoses.

- Stressors for the child and family? Losses?
- Coping strategies of the child and caregivers?
- Use of alcohol or drugs? (Use CRAFFT; Box 2-5)
- Temperament characteristics of the child and the "fit" with other family members?
- Problem behavior, discipline strategies used and their outcomes?
- Indications of depression, suicide, violent behavior, anxiety? (Use PHQ-2; Box 2-6)

Cognitive and Perceptual. Cognitive or perceptual problems are identified here. Attention-deficit disorder is an example.

- Hearing or vision problems?
- Learning disorders or attention problems?
- Adaptations made at home and school to assist the child, especially for problems of comprehension?

Development Domain Database. The levels of different aspects of development are assessed and documented in this area. Both past milestones and current functioning are important. Developmental surveillance is expected at all visits, and screening tests should be administered periodically to infants and young children (AAP, 2014a).

- *Motor landmarks*—gross and fine motor: sitting, standing, walking, use of hands and arms
- *Language landmarks*—words, sentences, intelligibility, comprehension
- *Personal and social*—play, attachment, self-care, peer and family relationships
- *Scholastic grade and progress*
- *Developmental and psychological test scores*—need to be recorded and considered when problems are being identified

Family Database. The intent of this section is to identify basic family, day care, school, work, or community agency factors that form the context of the child's life and need to be considered in planning care. The provider also needs to shift to the "family as unit of care" here to identify family

• BOX 2-5 CRAFFT Screening Interview for Drug and Alcohol Risks

Begin: "I'm going to ask you a few questions that I ask all my patients. Please be honest. I will keep your answers confidential."

Part A

During the PAST 12 MONTHS, did you:

	No	Yes
1. Drink any alcohol (more than a few sips)? (Do not count sips of alcohol taken during family or religious events.)	☐	☐
2. Smoke any marijuana or hashish?	☐	☐
3. Use anything else to get high? ("anything else" includes illegal drugs, over the counter and prescription drugs, and things that you sniff or "huff")	☐	☐

For clinic use only: Did the patient answer "yes" to any questions in Part A?

No ☐ → **Ask CAR question only, then stop**

Yes ☐ → **Ask all six CRAFFT questions**

Part B

	No	Yes
1. Have you ever ridden in a **CAR** driven by someone (including yourself) who was "high" or had been using alcohol or drugs?	☐	☐
2. Do you ever use alcohol or drugs to **RELAX**, feel better about yourself, or fit in?	☐	☐
3. Do you ever use alcohol or drugs while you are by yourself, or **ALONE**?	☐	☐
4. Do you ever **FORGET** things you did while using alcohol or drugs?	☐	☐
5. Do your **FAMILY** or **FRIENDS** ever tell you that you should cut down on your drinking or drug use?	☐	☐
6. Have you ever gotten into **TROUBLE** while you were using alcohol or drugs?	☐	☐

SCORING INSTRUCTIONS: FOR CLINIC STAFF USE ONLY

CRAFFT scoring: Each "yes" response in **Part B** scores 1 point.
A total score of two or higher is a positive screen, indicating a need for additional assessment.

Probability of Substance Abuse/Dependence Diagnosis Based on CRAFFT Score[1,2]

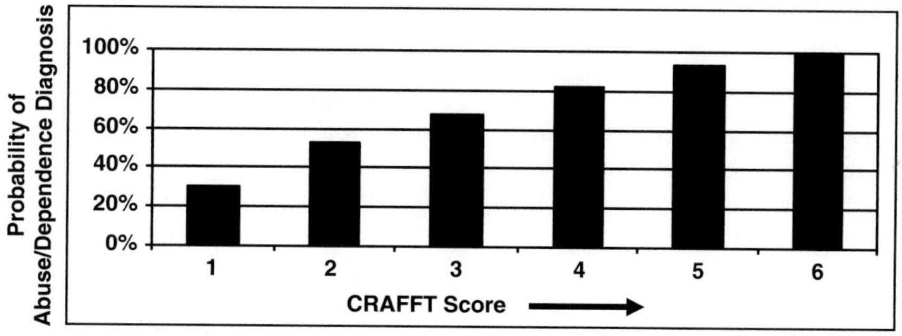

DSM-IV Diagnostic Criteria[3] (Abbreviated)

Substance Abuse (one or more of the following):

- Use causes failure to fulfill obligations at work, school, or home
- Recurrent use in hazardous situations (e.g., driving)
- Recurrent legal problems
- Continued use despite recurrent problems

Substance Dependence (three or more of the following):

- Tolerance
- Withdrawal
- Substance taken in larger amount or over longer period of time than planned
- Unsuccessful efforts to cut down or quit
- Great deal of time spent to obtain substance or recover from effect
- Important activities given up because of substance
- Continued use despite harmful consequences

References:

1. Knight JR, Shrier LA, Bravender TD, et al: A new brief screen for adolescent substance abuse, *Arch Pediatr Adolesc Med* 153(6):591–596, 1999.
2. Knight JR, Sherritt L, Shrier LA, et al: Validity of the CRAFFT substance abuse screening test among adolescent clinic patients, *Arch Pediatr Adolesc Med* 156(6):607–614, 2002.
3. American Psychiatric Association: *Diagostic and statistical manual of mental disorders,* ed 4, Washington DC, 2000, American Psychiatric Association.

• BOX 2-6 Patient Health Questionnaire-2 for Depression

The Patient Health Questionnaire-2 (PHQ-2)

Patient Name_______________ Date of Visit_______________

Over the past 2 weeks, how often have you been bothered by any of the following problems?	Not At All	Several Days	More Than Half the Days	Nearly Every Day
1. Little interest or pleasure in doing things	0	1	2	3
2. Feeling down, depressed or hopeless	0	1	2	3

The Patient Health Questionnaire-2 (PHQ-2)—Overview

The PHQ-2 inquires about the frequency of depressed mood and anhedonia over the past 2 weeks. The PHQ-2 includes the first two items of the PHQ-9.

- The purpose of the PHQ-2 is not to establish a final diagnosis or to monitor depression severity, but rather to screen for depression in a "first step" approach.
- Patients who screen positive should be further evaluated with the PHQ-9 to determine whether they meet criteria for a depressive disorder.

Clinical Utility

Reducing depression evaluation to two screening questions enhances routine inquiry about the most prevalent and treatable mental disorder in primary care.

Scoring

A PHQ-2 score ranges from 0-6. The authors* identified a PHQ-2 cutoff score of 3 as the optimal cutoff point for screening purposes and stated that a cutoff point of 2 would enhance sensitivity, whereas a cutoff point of 4 would improve specificity.

Psychometric Properties*

MAJOR DEPRESSIVE DISORDER (7% PREVALENCE)				ANY DEPRESSIVE DISORDER (18% PREVALENCE)			
PHQ-2 Score	Sensitivity	Specificity	Positive Predictive Value (PPV†)	PHQ-2 Score	Sensitivity	Specificity	Positive Predictive Value (PPV†)
1	97.6	59.2	15.4	1	90.6	65.4	36.9
2	92.7	73.7	21.1	2	82.1	80.4	48.3
3	**82.9**	**90.0**	**38.4**	**3**	**62.3**	**95.4**	**75.0**
4	73.2	93.3	45.5	4	50.9	97.9	81.2
5	53.7	96.8	56.4	5	31.1	98.7	84.6
6	26.8	99.4	78.6	6	12.3	99.8	92.9

†Because the PPV varies with the prevalence of depression, the PPV will be higher in settings with a higher prevalence of depression and lower in settings with a lower prevalence.

*Kroenke K, Spitzer RL, Williams JB: The Patient Health Questionnaire-2: Validity of a Two-Item Depression Screener, *Med Care* 41:1284–1294, 2003.

problems—another level of issues. Family problems might include impaired communication among family members, social isolation, family violence, impaired parents, alterations in parenting, caregiver role strain, and others. In general, families appreciate concerns and inquiries related to the health of their family. For some topics, such as domestic violence, mothers may prefer to discuss the issues away from the children. Providers should not hesitate to ask questions about the family.

Family Composition and Structure. Who lives in the home—family and others? How are they related? What is the meaning of the family structure to the child? In other words, does the child feel like a member of the family—cared for and supported? Does the family feel whole or is it missing members from the child's or another's point of view?

Current Family Situation. An understanding of the current family situation is helpful, especially if a significant period has elapsed since the child and family were last seen. Understanding changes that the family is facing and where they are in the family life cycle is also important. Are there family problems that put the family at risk—"out of sync" issues, such as a seriously ill parent, young teen parent, or grandparenting by an ill elder?

Extended Family Context. Data about the extended family may not seem relevant to parents or children, but patterns that can have an effect on children's health often do not become evident until this kind of intergenerational mapping is done. This more extensive mapping of a family may be used when the clinical picture includes conflicting information or when the effectiveness of a prevention activity is a concern. For example, knowing that both the mother and grandmother of the young adolescent in your office became pregnant at 14 years old and dropped out of high school may be helpful in deciding how to best use a brief visit. "It would help me to help your child if I knew more about your child's grandparents, aunts, uncles, and other relatives. Let's begin with your mother's family..." Knowledge of the timing and repetition of significant family events or behavior may be helpful. For example, adolescent pregnancy, alcohol abuse, dropping out of high school, and suicide may be patterns of behavior in a family's intergenerational history.

Genogram Data. Demographic data include dates of birth, death, adoption, marriage, separation, divorce, significant illness, and major family events; culture and ethnicity; religion; education; and occupations. The provider can probe for more information about specific data as they appear to be significant in a given situation. For example, faith and strength of adherence to a specific religion may have an unexpected effect on care decisions for a child. Disagreement about adherence within a family may result in mixed messages and uneven follow-through with a treatment plan.

If gaps in data become evident, they need to be explored. It is also helpful to keep in mind events external to the family that may have influenced family choices. For example, the years of conflict in Iraq and Afghanistan have interrupted many life plans. Immigration, voluntary or forced, can have an effect on family health status. Natural disasters (such as, floods, hurricanes, and droughts) have changed family histories and the health status of family members.

Family Relationships and Roles

- Primary caregiver? Who helps? Stresses of caregiver: Is the caregiver well both physically and emotionally?
- Does anyone require more attention from the primary caregiver than the child?
- How much time do parents and child spend in the home together?
- How are family decisions made? How are arguments worked out?
- What is the relationship between caregiver and partner?

Family Social and Community Network

- What community resources and family support systems are used?
- What agencies work with this child and family?
- Where does the child go for day care, school, work (teens), and is each setting safe?

Family Environment and Resources

- What is the home environment: Apartment, home, or farm?
- Fenced yard or perceived unsafe neighborhood?
- Family financial resources: Health insurance? Money for necessities?
- What are the sources of money for the family? Jobs or government assistance?
- Family stresses over resources and home environment?

Adolescent Health History Adaptations

For adolescents, the SSHADESS (**S**trengths, **S**chool, **H**ome, **A**ctivities, **D**rugs/substance abuse, **E**motions/depression, **S**exuality, **S**afety) is recommended as a psychosocial screening test (Ginsburg and Carlson, 2011). The CRAFFT screening tool (see Box 2-5) consists of six questions that screen for adolescent substance abuse (Center for Adolescent Substance Abuse Research [CeASAR], 2014). It is recommended by the AAP in *Bright Futures: Guidelines for Health Supervision of Infants, Children, and Adolescents* (Hagan et al, 2008). The PHQ-2 is a rapid screen for depression in adolescents (see Box 2-6). The Rapid Assessment for Adolescent Preventive Services (RAAPS) is a 21-item questionnaire that assesses the risk behaviors contributing most to morbidity, mortality, and social problems of teens. It has been positively evaluated by primary care providers (Darling-Fisher et al, 2014; Yi et al, 2009). It is available as a proprietary product via the website www.raaps.org.

The Interval History

The complete history usually needs to be completed only once for new patients. After that for routine scheduled health maintenance visits, the history is updated only from the last contact to the present. The format remains the same as for the complete history; however, questions are modified to verify that the situations are as they were in the past or to add new information. All areas of the history should be assessed.

The Episodic History

Families often bring their children in for help with specific problems. The history includes the chief complaint with symptom analysis and history of present illness sections of the complete history. The other areas of the history should be updated since data were last collected. Always listen for emerging problems and developmental progress. The symptom analysis assists with organization of presenting problem data (see Box 2-4).

The Psychosocial Problem History

Psychosocial or behavioral problems also must be assessed. Some considerations are summarized in Box 2-7. Much of the data related to psychosocial concerns will be collected in the functional health pattern domain database.

The Physical Examination

The physical examination is conducted following the history, although younger children might do better with developmental testing preceding the physical examination. Height, weight, head circumference, BMI, and vital signs, including a pain assessment, are recorded. A list of principal findings that the provider is expected to identify is presented in Box 2-8. Screening tests for hearing and vision, in addition to laboratory data and data from other disciplines, are included as other types of objective information. More experienced providers collect some of the history while conducting the physical examination. Content of the examination varies depending on the child's age and the various problems under consideration. Further discussion of physical examination techniques and findings are found in specific disease chapters.

Other Data

Laboratory and Radiographic Data

Record hearing, vision, hematocrit or other blood tests, lead, urinalysis, newborn screening tests, and tuberculosis screening.

Data from Other Disciplines

Summarize social work, nutrition, physical therapy, occupational therapy, medical specialist, speech pathology, education, and other reports.

Creating the Problem List

The problem list is derived from analysis of the subjective and objective data collected. Differential diagnosis is the clinical decision-making process used to derive the problems listed (Fig. 2-3). To use this process, the provider considers all the possible diagnoses for the problems presented by the child. Then the factors that support or rule out each of the various options considered are analyzed. Identification of the best fit of the subjective and objective data with the possible diagnoses is the goal. If further data are needed to confirm a diagnosis, collection of these data is incorporated into the plan. For example, the differential diagnoses for coryza (a runny nose) include, among others, allergic rhinitis, upper respiratory infection, and a foreign body in the nose. The clinician uses data about related symptoms (e.g., itchy eyes, a sore throat, systemic symptoms, or bilateral or unilateral drainage from the nostrils) to choose which diagnosis best fits the child's picture. That analysis for fit is the diagnostic reasoning process.

Functional health problems and developmental problems are also subject to the notion of differential diagnosis. For example, a child who is not sleeping well might be fearful, a trained night feeder, or might experience episodes of obstructive sleep apnea. The interventions for each problem are different. Thus the provider must use the differential diagnosis process to identify the problem or problems at hand. A problem should never be included on the problem list that is not supported by subjective and objective data found and recorded in the database. "Rule out" should not be listed as a diagnosis. (It may be considered part of a plan.) The diagnosis would be the unexplained symptom (e.g., "dysuria").

• BOX 2-7 Suggestions for the Psychosocial Complaint History

1. Use good communication skills—listen. Nonjudgmental approach. Seek a balanced give and take of information.
2. Interview the child or adolescent alone and with parents. Time alone with the preschooler may be used for play or drawing.
3. Have questionnaires or checklists from parents, teachers, and child care workers available. Use the information in the interview.
4. Be alert to emotional tone and interactions among family members.
5. Review the context for the concern:
   - Information about parents and family members: Illnesses, mental health problems, poverty, employment, violence, social isolation
   - Information about the child: School, peer relationships, temperament, neglect or abuse history, foster home placements, losses
   - Information about child-parent relationships: Attachment unrealistic expectations, poor family communication, lack of knowledge of child development and appropriate parenting
6. The history of present illness becomes an amalgam of information from the multiple sources—child, parents, others. Do not assume that both parents have the same views of the issues.
7. Remember that the interview itself may be therapeutic.

Avoiding Diagnostic Errors

Data collection for clinical practice, just as for research, must be as reliable and valid as possible. To assist with reliability, consider the following techniques:

- *Test-retest:* Ask the question again later. Take a blood pressure or a head circumference reading twice. Look for the physical finding a second time a bit later.
- *Interrater reliability:* Ask someone else to listen, palpate, and so on for the same finding. Does someone else get the same answer to the same question you asked?

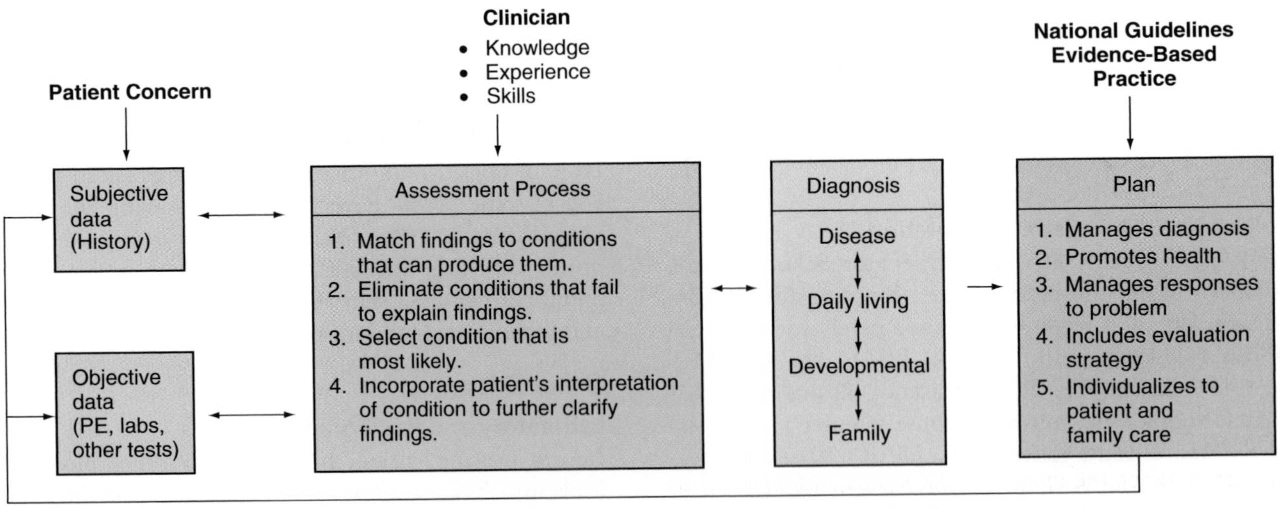

• Figure 2-3 Model for clinical decision-making. *PE,* Physical examination.

• BOX 2-8 Essential Physical Examination Data to Collect

General appearance: Ill or well, distressed, alert, cooperative, body build; reaction to parents; characteristic position, movements, nutrition, developmental appearance as contrasted with the stated age
Skin: Color—pigmentation, cyanosis, jaundice, carotenemia, erythema, pallor; vascular—visible veins, arteries; eruptions, petechiae, ecchymosis, hives, rashes; lesions; texture, scaling, striae, scars; sweat, edema, turgor; subcutaneous tissue; distribution and color of hair; nail appearance
Lymph nodes: Occipital, postauricular, preauricular, cervical, parotid, submaxillary, sublingual, axillary, epitrochlear, inguinal; size, mobility, tenderness, heat
Head: Position, shape, sutures, fontanelles; size—circumference, microcephaly, macrocephaly, hydrocephaly; facial paralysis, twitching
Eyes: Vision, visual fields, cover test; blinking; position—exophthalmos, enophthalmos, hypertelorism, hypotelorism; movements—strabismus, extraocular movements, nystagmus; ptosis—eyelids, sclera, conjunctivae; lesions—styes, chalazion; corneas—corneal reflex; discharge; pupils—accommodation, iris; retina—red reflex, fundus
Ears: Anomalies; position; discharge; tenderness; canals; tympanic membranes—redness, light reflex, landmarks, bulging or retraction, perforation, mobility; mastoid; hearing; vestibular function
Nose: Shape; alae nasi, flaring; mucosa, secretions, bleeding, airway; septum; polyps, tumors
Mouth: Odor; teeth—number, edges, occlusion, caries, formation, color; gums—discoloration, bleeding; buccal mucosa; tongue—coating, protrusion, color, tremor, lesions; palate—cleft, arch; tonsils—size, color, exudate; pharynx—appearance, color, lesions
Neck: Size; anomalies—webbing, edema, nodes, masses; sternocleidomastoid; trachea; thyroid; vessels; motion—head drop, tilting, nodding, range of motion
Chest: Shape—circumference, symmetry, Harrison groove; movement—flaring, expansion, abdominal or thoracic breathing, intercostal retractions
Breasts: Tanner stage of development, symmetry, redness, heat, tenderness, lumps; gynecomastia
Lungs: Respiration—type, rate, dyspnea; exercise tolerance; cough, hemoptysis, sputum; palpation—masses, tenderness, fremitus; percussion—dullness, hyperresonance, diaphragm location; auscultation—breath sounds, crackles (rales), rubs, rhonchi, wheezes, vocal resonance
Cardiovascular and heart: Blood pressure and pulse rate; inspection—vascularity, bulging, impulse; distress, cyanosis, edema, clubbing, pulsations, venous distention; palpation—femoral pulses, point of maximal impulse, thrill; auscultation—first and second heart sounds, rhythm, split, third heart sound, gallop, friction rub, venous hum, murmurs
Abdomen: Inspection—shape, distention, transillumination; umbilicus, diastasis rectus, veins; peristaltic, gastric waves; auscultation—bowel sounds, bruits; palpation—superficial or deep tenderness, rebound; spleen, liver, masses, kidneys, bladder, uterus; percussion—masses, fluid, flatus
Genitalia: Discharge, foreign body; *male and female*—Tanner staging; *female*—tags; labia, adhesions, vagina, clitoris; vaginal, bimanual examination for teenage girls (pelvic examination observations are discussed further in Chapter 35); *male*—penis—hypospadias, epispadias, phimosis, meatus; scrotum, testes, hydrocele, hernia; cremasteric reflex
Anus and rectum: Buttocks, fistula, fissure, prolapse, polyps, hemorrhoids, rashes; rectal—rectum, fistula, megacolon, masses, prostate, tenderness; sensation
Musculoskeletal: Anomalies, length, clubbing, pain, tenderness, temperature, swelling, shape, symmetry; gait—stance, balance, limp; foot position; spine—tufts of hair, dimples, masses, spina bifida, tenderness, mobility, scoliosis; posture—lordosis, kyphosis; joints—heat, tenderness, mobility, swelling, effusion; muscles—development, pain, tone, spasm, paralysis, rigidity, contractures, atrophy
Nervous system: General impression, abilities, responsiveness, position, spontaneous movements, play activity; development—consistent with age or current level; state of consciousness, irritability, seizure activity; gait, stance, limp, ataxia; coordination, Romberg sign; tremors, twitching, choreiform movements, athetosis, spasticity, paralysis, flaccidity; reflexes—superficial, deep tendon, clonus, Chvostek sign; primitive reflexes for infants and children with neurologic impairments—Moro, tonic neck, Babinski, grasp, suck; thumb position; sensation—hyperesthesia, paresthesia, temperature, touch; stereognosis; cranial nerves I to XII; hearing and vision.

- *Internal consistency:* Look for a logical consistency to the findings obtained. If something is "out of sync," question it. For example, do the height or head circumference points on the graph line up, or is one significantly off the trajectory? If there is significant variation, consider a measuring error before looking for a health problem that has altered growth. Does the history support the physical findings? Does the story keep changing?

Algorithms, computer algorithms, protocols, and flow sheets can improve the consistency and reliability of the data collected, especially when several staff members are involved with the data for a given patient.

To assess the validity, or meaning, of data collected, the provider should consider sources of error:

- Do the cumulative data fit and support a given diagnosis? If not, perhaps the diagnosis was inadequate or an error in data collection, sequencing, or interpretation occurred. Providers constantly need to attend to age, gender, race, culture, and other issues when they consider data. Is it likely for a Caucasian child to have sickle cell disease? What diagnoses should one consider when a teenage girl has abdominal pain, as opposed to the diagnoses possible for a boy of the same age?
- Was the diagnosis made on the basis of one isolated finding or a cluster? For instance, diagnosing pneumonia after hearing a cough or diagnosing failure to thrive with one growth measurement are mono-operation bias errors.
- Sometimes two problems occur with overlapping findings. One problem might be missed, whereas the other is pursued.
- The teen might change the data provided because of stress or worry about the outcomes of the visit. Both findings and their meaning to teens need to be explored

with the adolescent without the family and then with the family present.

- Provider expectations can also influence accurate diagnosing.
- Were cues missed or questions unasked?
- Data are often compared with specific criteria (e.g., heights and weights for age are known, developmental milestones are established, and laboratory norms are set for children of different ages). Which test has been used? What is its specificity and sensitivity? Is the right criterion being used?
- Were all data (such as, laboratory studies) reviewed promptly?

Creating the Management Plan

A plan must be developed for every identified problem. It is helpful to consider diagnostic, therapeutic, and educational interventions for every problem listed. Of course, not every problem requires work in all three areas, but they should be considered. The management activities are listed in the record. The plan should always include a recommendation for the next visit and what is to be done at that visit in an attempt to move the child into a health maintenance pattern rather than being seen only episodically. Just as the problem list must be consistent with the data at hand, plans must address diagnoses that are included in the problem list. In other words, the plan is internally consistent with the data and diagnoses.

Shared Decision-Making with Child and Family

Using newer models of family collaborative decision-making, plans for care should be communicated to the family with a discussion of alternatives for management of issues with risks and benefits for each option. Active parent-child involvement with creation of the plan of care is the most desirable. Shared decision-making involves a provider and patient's family working together to find a health care decision that is acceptable to both parties (Légaré and Thompson-Leduc, 2014). Four key characteristics need to be present in a shared decision: (1) both patient and providers participate in the phases of shared decision, (2) information is shared between parties, (3) the expressed treatment preference is shared between the parties, and (4) agreement is reached. Patients who feel that they have been an active participant in the shared decision-making process have improved health outcomes (Shay and Lafata, 2014). A recent study found that a provider's positive attitude toward shared decision-making can help a patient to engage in the process (Légaré et al, 2011).

Again, health literacy is a prerequisite to good decision-making.

Communicating Assessment Data

An important corollary to health assessment is the skill to communicate information obtained in both oral and written forms. A record of the care given must always be written to communicate the provider's logical thinking based on data obtained. This record is important because it provides information for later care, serves as a communication link with other providers, documents the quality of care provided, may be used for research purposes, and serves as a legal and billing document. Verbal communication of health care information is also essential. The words must paint a picture of the child and family for the reader or listener (e.g., a consultant). Knowledge of the classic format used by other health care providers is important. Using that same format or one that is closely related facilitates efficient communication about patient problems.

Informatics and Child Health Care

Communities of pediatric health care providers are addressing the needs to bring data collection and management systems for pediatric health care forward. There are many areas for utilization of technology to make caregiving more efficient, effective, and safe. However, systems must be tailored to the issues of infants and children, attending to the developmental, family, and differences in the everyday living experiences of youth. Core pediatric data must be managed across systems. Maternal and newborn health information, tracking immunization information, monitoring and tracking growth and development, providing age-appropriate medication dosing and laboratory test result interpretation, protecting patient privacy, and identifying patient data accurately and precisely (e.g., names for newborns, gender when it has yet to be determined), and providing selective data for clinical research and quality improvements are all areas of concern (Lehmann et al, 2011). Creating special systems for children with special needs, adolescents, and care for children in special situations (such as, child abuse assessments for forensic documentation) increase the complexities of data management system creation, utilization, and evaluation. Further, there are significant problems yet to be solved regarding the interface of computer systems across agencies. Evidence-based care, clinical guidelines, and decision-making trees can support pediatric health care decisions, but how and by whom will they be incorporated and updated in information systems? Telemedicine is another area where informatics can be supportive. Patients do not need to be in the same room to receive excellent care. Rural care, as well as regional specialty care, can be provided via telemedicine. Finally, health care education can make use of information technologies—education both for providers and children and their families. Videos, interactive methods, the Internet, texting, and group conferences among professionals or patients and families can all be used to enhance health care.

For a complete list of references, please visit http://evolve.elsevier.com/Burns/pediatric/.

3 Cultural Considerations for Pediatric Primary Care

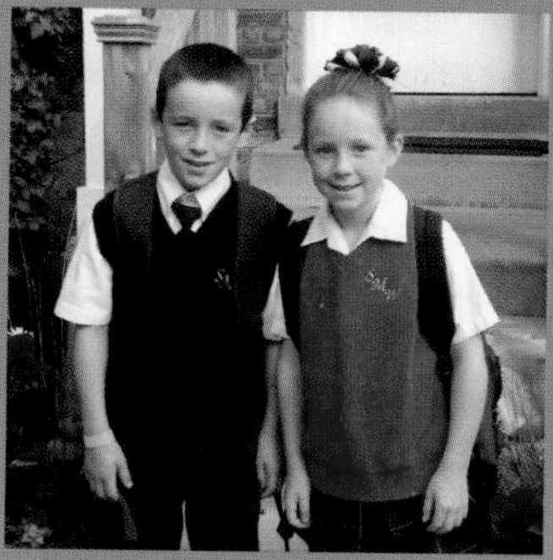

ARDYS M. DUNN AND ISABELLE SOULÉ

Recent political and economic crises have resulted in a marked increase in the migration of people across international borders, increasing contact among groups with widely varying backgrounds and worldviews. According to the 2010 United States census, about 36% of the population belongs to a minority racial or ethnic group—a number expected to reach more than 50% by 2050. Nearly 13% of United States residents are foreign-born and, depending on the state, the range of foreign-born residents is between 2% and 27% (U.S. Census Bureau, 2013). Latinos from Mexico, the Caribbean, and South and Central America have been the fastest growing population group in the United States for the past 20 years. This phenomenon has generated an increased awareness of the impact of dissimilar worldviews, values, and customs on the lived experiences of health and illness. Unfortunately, these differences often manifest themselves in health inequities and poor health status, even though health professionals strive to eliminate health care disparities and achieve positive health status among all populations. Achieving a goal of health equity requires valuing everyone equally, using ongoing efforts to address preventable inequalities, and working to correct historical and contemporary injustices. This requires attention to population diversity and to how the social determinants of health affect diverse groups (see Chapter 1). Health professionals and health care systems are being called upon to not just increase their knowledge of other cultures but to alter traditional ways of working with clients, families, and communities and to change the way in which they perceive the world and their place in it (Pernell-Arnold et al, 2012). Understanding the influence of culture and its effect on interpretive meaning is essential for health care providers in contemporary practice.

This chapter reviews some foundational concepts related to culture and its relationship to health care. It presents a model of ways health care providers can learn to improve care given to diverse groups. It also includes a section on immigrant, refugee, and asylee health. A more comprehensive discussion of this important topic can be found in the following books: *Immigrant Medicine* (Walker and Barnett, 2007) and *When People Come First: Critical Studies in Global Health* (Biehl and Petryna, 2013).

Culture

Culture is a complex, dynamic, learned pattern of behavior that is integral to the being of individuals and communities. Culture structures how people view the world, including ways of thinking and living—beliefs, attitudes, values, norms, customs, and expectations. An individual's cultural reality is created within a specific context of experiences. One's ethnicity; gender; age; sexual orientation; spiritual practices; social, educational, and economic status; and geographic location help shape one's cultural worldview. The degree to which one experiences discrimination or persecution also influences beliefs and behaviors. No one belongs to only one culture. Each individual, family, and community represents a unique blend of overlapping and nested cultures that influence perception, attitudes, and behavior.

Essentialist and Constructivist Concepts of Culture

An essentialist view of culture dominates in the health care literature today, often portraying an ethnic minority group as having a static set of traits. Although members of a culturally defined group may share values, attitudes, or behaviors, an essentialist perspective tends to oversimplify cultural information, applying these traits to all members of the group, unwittingly creating an artificial "package" that minimizes the complexities present in all cultures. Failure to address the diversity that exists within a cultural group results in ethnic groups being considered as homogeneous when, in fact, the variations within the group may be greater than the differences between cultural groups. Providers with essentialist assumptions about cultural differences may have a false sense of competence and instead of demonstrating respect as they intend, may stereotype the client, family, and community (Leung et al, 2013; Stith, 2011).

• BOX 3-1 Essentialist and Constructivist Views of Culture

Essentialist

Simplistic
Static
Known
Single culture (e.g., ethnic) identity
Resides in client, family, and community
Predictable response to health and illness
Mindlessness (unconscious)

Constructivist

Complex
Dynamic
Unknowable
Multiple cultural identities
Influences all individuals, including providers
Unique response to health and illness
Mindfulness (conscious)

In contrast, a constructivist view, which this text uses, recognizes culture as a complex, dynamic process, evolving and changing as individuals and communities move in and out of numerous cultures over time, thus generating a unique cultural mosaic. This view acknowledges that individuals belong to multiple cultures simultaneously, directs attention to social and political as well as individual factors, and validates the multidimensional nature of human experience within any given group. From a constructivist perspective, a health professional does not have to be an expert in cultural minutia but rather focuses on resource-sharing, alliance-building, cross-disciplinary collaboration, and the individuality and uniqueness of each client and his or her life story. Health professionals also recognize the limits of their knowledge when confronted with the mystical nature of health and illness, and they acknowledge the accumulated wisdom and resilience of clients, families, and communities (Box 3-1).

Individualism and Collectivism

Individualism, rooted in a belief in the separation and autonomy of individuals, underpins the United States health care system. This understanding is so pervasive and deeply ingrained that it is seldom recognized, let alone questioned. Individualism recognizes the individual, not the group, as the basic unit of survival. In contrast, many clients residing in the United States come from cultures that are based on a collectivist viewpoint. Collectivists perceive themselves as intrinsically part of a group and emphasize interdependence over independence, affiliation over confrontation, and cooperation over competition. Both individualism and collectivism have merits. However, it is important to understand that each relies on different mechanisms and values in decision-making, that behaviors may differ as a result, and that those behaviors may be in conflict with mainstream United States medical expectations. For example, a client may wish to integrate the extended family into the clinic visit, yet the examination room only accommodates several people; or a provider may want to tell the client that she has a terminal illness, but the family believes that such information-sharing is inappropriate (Segal and Hodges, 2012).

Culture, Privilege, and Health Care

Frequently, culture is implicitly and explicitly addressed as problematic in health care, a risk factor rather than an asset or a source of strength and resilience. In fact, ethnicity, spirituality, sexuality, age, ability, and other dimensions of difference are *not* intrinsically problems; they are simply differences. However, prejudice, discrimination, and cultural conflict *are* problems. Recent social-psychological research has recognized the detrimental effects of unconscious bias that contribute to health and health care disparities. *Institutionalized racism* is used to describe the invisible, but presumed neutral, Eurocentric values and assumptions (including an individualistic, essentialist perspective) that underlie the United States health care system and whose authority defines knowledge, membership, and language within the system. However, these values are not neutral. They have power to define expectations, often at the expense of marginalized groups within the same system. This power is expressed in the form of "white privilege," reflecting a system that creates political, economic, and institutional suffering for non-dominant members of the same community (Cook et al, 2012).

Privilege has been described as an advantage that an individual or group has over, and often at the expense of, other individuals or groups. Health care providers share unique privilege as a result of their educational level, professional and socioeconomic status, and even national citizenship. Because it is a part of the "natural" socialization process, members of privileged groups may not recognize their privilege nor understand that it is the source of the distance between them and less privileged groups. When biases, prejudices, and privilege are not understood and appreciated for the impact they have on the delivery of health care, providers may inadvertently contribute to disparities (Hannah and Carpenter-Song, 2013). Scholars have noted that health care interactions, behaviors, and clinical judgments are influenced to a greater extent by the providers' own expectations, assumptions, reactions, and worldview than the data at hand (Willen, 2013). Even well-meaning, culturally sensitive, fair-minded individuals can unwittingly activate and rely on unconscious biases, and stereotypes and prejudices can be invisible to those who use them (DeLilly and Flaskerud, 2012; Stone and Moskowitz, 2011).

Taken broadly, biases are not rooted initially in individual choice but are a part of the cultural socialization process, naturally occurring within the larger cultural context. All humans innocently acquire bias and prejudice as a result of their sociohistorical setting, social position, and personal experiences. Using this broad perspective to examine the development of prejudice and bias can help health care providers move beyond the guilt often associated with undesirable attitudes to a deeper understanding of the influences that initiate and reinforce those ways of thinking. It can also highlight the fact that attitudes, biases, and prejudices can be changed.

Biomedicine and the Culture of Client, Family, and Community

Beliefs, values, and explanatory models of health and illness differ markedly across cultural groups. Biomedicine, a newcomer to the healing professions, is a system based on a belief in the power of science and technology, personal autonomy, and the capacity to overcome disease. It springs from a Western professional culture, embedded in individualism, competition, and cognitive knowing. From a biomedical perspective, the more ancient healing traditions, whose underlying frameworks are intrinsically holistic, are often referred to as complementary and alternative medicine (CAM). The values that underlie biomedicine may be at odds with these more traditional models, and biomedical providers may think of them as nonrational, even superstitious. Providers may distrust or disparage the mystical or metaphorical aspects of ancient traditions and reduce them to appendages of the main body of "real" or biomedicine. As a result, a client's choice to use complementary and alternative healing practices, spiritual healers, or community-based support mechanisms as primary sources for healing or health maintenance may conflict with the beliefs and practices of the provider. For much of the world, however, biomedicine is the alternative model, conceptualizing health as an individual phenomenon that separates the physical, mental, and spiritual aspects of individuals from the family and community in which they are embedded.

The challenge is to find ways to reach a mutual understanding of these differences within the client-provider interaction. By eliciting a client's ideas about his or her illness, the health care provider will have a framework from which to begin negotiating an acceptable plan of care. Kleinman and colleagues (1978) developed a set of questions as a basic tool to facilitate cross-cultural health communication (Box 3-2). These questions focus on specific areas related to health and illness in which cultural differences are expressed: (1) how health and illness are perceived and manifested; (2) what is thought of as the cause of illness; (3) the roles of health professional, client, family, and community in the caregiving process; and (4) how treatment is negotiated, implemented, and evaluated.

• BOX 3-2 Questions to Elicit Cultural Perspective of Clients

- What do you think has caused your problem?
- Why do you think it started when it did?
- What do you think your sickness does to you? How does it work?
- How severe is your illness? Will it have a long or short course?
- What kind of treatment do you think you should receive?
- What are the most important results you hope to receive from this treatment?
- What are the chief problems your sickness has caused you?
- What do you fear most about your sickness?

Cultural Humility and Cultural Competence

As health care provision moves from medical authority and privilege to client-centered care, two concepts have emerged for working effectively across diverse cultures: cultural humility and cultural competence. Although these concepts are interconnected, they also have unique and distinguishing features.

Cultural Humility

Cultural humility is defined as the lifelong commitment to self-evaluation and self-critique, and to developing mutually beneficial, nonpaternalistic partnerships (Guskin, 1991; Tervalon and Murray-Garcia, 1998). Cultural humility is based on a model of passive volition, receptivity, and being open to learn from others. It means interacting in a non-judgmental way with people who have different ways of looking at things; asking questions rather than giving answers, for example, in an effort to have a clearer understanding of another's perspective. From a cultural humility perspective, difference is legitimate and all worldviews are valued. To be humble is not self-depreciatory nor does one have a low self-opinion. Rather, one who demonstrates humility is self-aware, has an accurate opinion of the self, acknowledges limitations, stays "curious," and is willing to be influenced and changed by alternate values and worldviews.

In a multiethnic, multiclass society, providers interact with coworkers and clients from every subgroup and identity imaginable, and it is not possible to become competent in the many permutations of "culture" that exist in all individuals and communities. In a model of cultural humility, the most serious barrier to culturally appropriate care is not a lack of knowledge of the details of any given cultural orientation, but the providers' failure to develop self-awareness and a respectful, open attitude toward diverse points of view. Arrogance, an exaggeration of one's own importance, narrows the health care provider's thinking and creates distance between provider and client, making it difficult if not impossible to negotiate a collaborative plan of care. Interacting from a starting point of humility rather than professional expertise generates a different, more positive, type of health care encounter.

Cultural Competence

Cultural competence, the prominent cultural paradigm in United States health care today, assumes an inclusive approach to health care practice; this enables a health care provider or system to provide meaningful, supportive care that preserves the human rights and dignity of all. Cultural competence implies active volition in acquiring cultural knowledge, becoming proficient, competent, and skillful. Sensitivity to the culture of the client, family, and community is considered the cornerstone in culturally competent practice. However, health care education and professional systems that primarily emphasize competence vis-à-vis empiric and cognitive understanding can lead to a false sense of security in *knowing*. Representing an essentialist perspective (see earlier discussion), this can generate a climate of arrogance and exclusivity in which new inquiry and discovery and the capacity to understand and accept the worldview of another are blocked. In addition, a narrow focus on cultural traits can obscure the interlocking systems and oppressive relations that establish and maintain power imbalances and health disparities among groups in the United States and worldwide. Cultural competence education has not addressed this issue well. In fact, it has been criticized for overly focusing on the culture of clients without concomitantly exploring how the culture of health care systems and individual providers contribute to health disparities (Hannah and Carpenter-Song, 2013).

As the concept of cultural competence has evolved, it has moved from rather simplistic attempts to educate health professionals about minority groups, their cultural norms, and cultural peculiarities regarding health and health care into something more akin to client-centered care. This more complex and dynamic understanding of cultural competence includes the integration of the cognitive, relational, emotional, practical, aesthetic, and spiritual aspects of human experience (Soulé, 2014). There is also a physical aspect to this awareness and understanding. A distinction between cognitive and embodied knowing of culture can be made; the first is a traditional external knowing "about" culture; the latter, an internal, physical sense "of" culture, an *embodiment* of what culture means. In one's own culture, this embodiment is for the most part, unconscious; things simply *feel right*. This *feeling right* can be considered the physical manifestation of ethnocentrism in which one's own culture is experienced as central to reality. As one becomes more self-aware, sensitivity to the *feeling* of appropriateness (multisensory awareness) increases. An argument has been made that values create a context that influences sensory perceptions and that the body can become an instrument to effectively gather information about culture (Bennett and Castiglioni, 2003; Soulé, 2014). An exclusive emphasis on the cognitive aspects of cultural competence can mask the deeper phenomenon of the embodiment of culture, and without a *feeling* for another culture, one's depth of understanding and ability to adapt and build rapport with others can be limited. Because health care providers are in a practice that relies on developing perceptual acuities in order to notice, see, hear, and feel events and signs that they could not recognize before their education, they are well suited to understand the physical nature of cultural awareness and to develop the ability to work skillfully across diverse groups.

Best Practices for Developing Cultural Humility and Cultural Competence

Cultural humility and cultural competence share the pivotal understanding that every encounter is a cultural encounter. Both of these perspectives challenge providers to develop intellectual, attitudinal, and behavioral flexibility, including a lifelong commitment to reflective self-scrutiny. Implementing them in the health care encounter is a first step toward redressing the power imbalances between provider and client.

Broadly speaking, in order to work effectively with diversity, individuals must be interested in other cultures, be sensitive enough to notice cultural differences, and then be willing to modify their attitudes and behavior as an indication of respect for the people of diverse cultures. This can prove very challenging, particularly for health professionals whose values and practices differ sharply from those of many clients. Integrating a foreign perspective is fundamentally unnatural, and discomfort, apprehension, resistance, and fear of being perceived as either discriminatory or giving preferential treatment are likely responses. Mental anxiety, which is often present in the face of significant cultural difference, is consistently accompanied by physical tension. Physiologically, this stricture of mind and body can lead to limited thinking and a skewing of perceptions, which may include withdrawal, defensiveness, and/or hostility (LeBlanc, 2009; Swartz, 2012). For example, a nurse may check on a hospitalized client only when it is essential, rather than comfortably visiting from time to time, because she is not at ease in her interactions with the client and uncertain how she will be received.

In health care education cultural competence is taught alongside the concept of professionalism. Topics such as spirituality and humility, which are not often discussed in professional circles, may not be simply overlooked but may be perceived as antithetical to competence, professionalism, and professional practice. Because many health professionals are educated to think in these terms, they may be quick to misunderstand or reject teachings that offer an unrecognized worldview or alternate set of truths. Moreover, building partnerships where health professionals respect the expertise of the client and family in their own health care decisions runs contrary to how professionalism is taught and role modeled in our schools and professions today.

A new model that can be used in health education to help providers work toward cultural humility and cultural competence identifies three interconnected themes (awareness, engagement, and application) that cross four domains (intrapersonal, interpersonal, system/organization, and global) (Soulé, 2014). The following sections describe

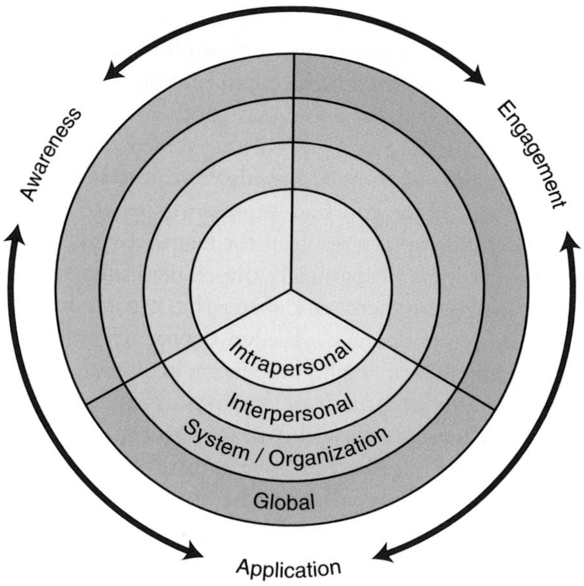

• **Figure 3-1** Components of a model for cultural humility and cultural competence. (From Soulé I: Cultural competence in health care: an emerging theory, *Adv Nurs Sci* 37(1):48–60, 2014; with permission from Advances in Nursing Science.)

and clarify the intersection of these themes and domains (Fig. 3-1).

Awareness

Awareness includes simultaneous discernment of self and others including the larger context in which individuals live and interpret their worlds. There is a continuum of awareness that ranges from a lack of awareness (mindlessness, reactivity, interference or impediment of a specific mindset, and "entrenchment") on one end to self-awareness (mindfulness, openness to new information, and ability to imagine from multiple perspectives) on the other.

Engagement

Engagement represents thoughtful consideration, active involvement, and reflection occurring in synchrony. Results of successful engagement include empathy, connectivity, and high-quality relationships.

Application

Application denotes moving beyond cultural knowledge toward action, such as intervention or operationalization, requiring different thinking at different levels. Application spirals back to awareness, engagement, and additional reflection, thus allowing for meaningful change. Although awareness, engagement, and application are interwoven, awareness is a precursor to both engagement and application across all domains. These three overarching concepts are expressed in intrapersonal, interpersonal, system/organization, and global domains.

Intrapersonal Domain

Intrapersonal refers to understanding ourselves as unique cultural beings, including our distinctive blend of attitudes, beliefs, values, and stereotypes, and the larger context of sociohistorical and personal experiences from which they have been shaped.

Awareness

Health care providers are encouraged to understand the genesis of their own values, beliefs, and bias. They must examine the social and historical context in which they have been raised and educated in order to gain insight into how that context helped create their values, beliefs, and biases. Specifically, they are encouraged to explore how they are privileged and to reflect on how their position can both enhance and inhibit optimal health and health care for clients, families, and communities. This self-awareness is considered the cornerstone of a culturally competent encounter and an effective cross-cultural relationship.

Engagement and Application

Health care providers must be flexible in order to understand the self. Flexibility includes being open and available to learn, conceive of alternate sets of values, appreciate how mindsets develop, and understand that all behaviors make sense in context. The truly flexible individual is able to see oneself in the perceptual world of another and understand the world through another's specific viewpoint and life experience. Flexibility stands in contrast to being entrenched in a fixed set of values, singular mindset, or set of actions. Examination of the self, one's limitations, biases, prejudices, and so forth, can be difficult, even frightening. Self-reflection requires a personal commitment to deeply explore one's underlying motivations; look at the questions one asks or doesn't ask, the things one "sees" or "doesn't see." There is an uncertainty to what may be found that can produce anxiety. One must be healthy—physically, emotionally, intellectually, and spiritually—to engage fully in the process. This personal well-being is an essential precursor to building the emotional and intellectual capacity for self-examination and reflection. Strategies such as sensitivity training, consciousness-raising, group discussions, and counseling can be used to reflect on the self and increase self-awareness.

Interpersonal Domain

Interpersonal refers to how cultural competence is manifested between and among individuals. Although commonly thought of in the context of a provider-client encounter, the interpersonal domain applies to all relationships within the health care setting.

Awareness

In the interpersonal domain, health care providers must be aware of, acknowledge, and accept alternate viewpoints as valid. By reflecting on how their own viewpoints differ from those of others, providers may see how their own are incomplete or limited. Understanding these limitations can provide an incentive to be open to worldviews of others—a key skill in the development of trust and empathy.

Engagement and Application

Interpersonal engagement and application require skillful communication, leading to empathy and strong relationships. Use of interpreters and conflict negotiation are two specific strategies discussed here.

Communication

Communication across cultures is challenging. Different languages may be spoken, but much communication happens below the level of language. Nonverbal messages, style, tone, unspoken meanings, and explanatory models are also operating. In order to build rapport, it becomes necessary to engage all the senses, not just auditory, when communicating with clients of diversity. One must note visual cues, discern meaning, and make oneself "present" (i.e., actively engage, or "bear witness"). Multiple sensory pathways are at work, and the whole body becomes a tool in the communication process. When it works, there is synchrony of energies between client and provider, a feeling of connection. On the provider's part, noticing, mirroring, listening, and asking questions are strategies that can facilitate this process.

Noticing. Interpersonal noticing requires bidirectional conscious attention. First, noticing is directed outward toward how the client and/or family communicate. This includes style, tone, pace, use of language (e.g., specific terms), and nonverbal cues, such as gesturing, body posture, personal space, and degree of eye contact. Second, noticing is directed inward to one's own style, tone, pace, use of terms, and nonverbal cues. Providers must be highly attuned to the style clients and families use to communicate and flexible enough to adjust their own style to ensure mutual understanding.

Mirroring. Mirroring is best thought of as technique in which the provider subtly reflects both verbal and nonverbal communication of another, including behaviors, actions, and body language. Mirroring and noticing are closely related and when skilled communication happens, they occur in synchrony.

Listening. One must "listen to understand." This involves active listening, allowing the client to tell his or her story and responding appropriately without trying to inform, fix, or advise. Listening to understand is a strategy that respects the client as an individual, gains clarity on client priorities and concerns, and creates a collaborative environment for negotiating a plan of care. It is similar to the process used in motivational interviewing (see Chapter 9) where the roles of expert and learner are blended and where provider and client work together to reach mutual understanding.

Asking Questions. Asking questions can focus thinking and generate new information. Although it can be uncomfortable, providers can ask the client questions about his or her lived cultural experience; this sends the message that client differences are recognized and valued, and that the provider intends to prevent negative encounters from happening (e.g., "Have you had experiences where you have been treated poorly as a result of the fact that you have dark skin color or look Hispanic? Is that something that you're afraid of happening here? And if so, what can we do to keep that from happening?"). Asking deeper questions and engaging in deeper dialogue with clients and families enhances the development of empathy on the part of the provider. Empathy is the ability to understand and share the feelings of others, to be receptive to others and effectively enter into the perceptual experience of another, including intellectual, attitudinal, and behavioral aspects. Empathy involves a deep connection between individuals in a relationship, and it is evident in the way people act and treat others. This connectivity creates trust where children and families feel seen, heard, understood, and accepted.

In a complex health care system, time constraints, technology, and other demands make establishing deep relationships between clients and providers difficult. Skillful communication and empathy make it easier to build high-quality relationships between and among individuals, and it is ultimately relationships upon which trust and collaboration depend.

Use of Interpreters

The use of interpreters represents a distinctive aspect of communication. Providers are encouraged to become "linguistically appropriate." As a part of this effort, federal standards relating to linguistic competence have been developed—Culturally and Linguistically Appropriate Services (CLAS) (HHS Office of Minority Health, 2001). It is helpful to speak the client's language; although sharing a common language can enhance rapport, that ability alone is not sufficient and may not always be possible or necessary to be linguistically appropriate. Interpreters can be used very effectively and the importance of using a qualified interpreter cannot be overemphasized (Perez-Stable and Karliner, 2012). Federally funded managed care networks and community health centers are required to have interpreters accessible for all clients with limited English proficiency (LEP).

Interpreters who are familiar with the culture and the language are especially helpful because they are likely to be more sensitive to the nonverbal cues patients give. The term *cultural broker* is used to describe an individual who bridges two or more cultures and can translate both linguistic and cultural meaning.

In some immigrant communities, especially those that are small, there may be few qualified interpreters. Also, as members of a small, closely knit community, both interpreter and client may find it awkward to discuss sensitive personal information in a clinical setting and then return to their culturally prescribed social roles in the community. In larger immigrant communities, several languages or dialects may be spoken; language barriers may arise even among people who speak the same language because communication patterns differ among classes, subcultures, and regions of the country of origin. Also, there may be a wide range of literacy levels in all language groups. Some health care facilities do not have adequate interpreter services and providers rely on family members or unqualified facility staff to translate. In all these cases, patient confidentiality, provider/family understanding, and quality of care can be jeopardized. Contracting with a commercial telephone interpreter service may be a possibility in these instances and has been shown to be as effective as an "in-person" interpreter in many cases (Napoles et al, 2010).

Interpreters and providers may experience conflict related to control of the clinical situation. Providers may not be sure that the interpreter is accurately conveying their (the providers') message or completely relaying the client's comments. Providers may see the interpreter as a tool to be used, not as a part of the team, whereas interpreters may take on a "co-diagnostician" role in which they make decisions that can affect care without consulting the provider. Something as "minor" as neglecting to fully disclose what the client has said because the interpreter did not think it important, or the interpreter offering the client advice beyond that given by the provider can compromise care. The provider must be sensitive to the relationship between the client and the interpreter, and a working relationship based on trust between the provider and interpreter and a clear understanding of the role of each are necessary and must be actively negotiated (Hsieh, 2010; Hsieh and Kramer, 2012; McCarthy et al, 2013).

The qualified interpreter stands or sits behind the provider so that he or she will not interfere with eye contact between the child, the parent, and the provider. If privacy is an issue, the interpreter can stand or sit behind a screen. If topics related to sexuality are to be discussed, clarify with the patient which gender he or she perfers the interpreter to be; generally, patients prefer interpreters of the same gender.

The interpreter should make an effort to translate the dialogue as closely and accurately as possible for both parties. This does not necessarily mean a "word-for-word" translation, especially since some English words have no translation into some other languages, and vice versa. But, when a provider's yes-or-no question results in a lengthy response, for example, the interpreter must ensure that the provider is apprised of what the whole statement means, including any seemingly unrelated data. It is especially difficult to convey emotion through verbal translation, and this component of communication may be lost or diminished when interpreters are used. This should not be perceived as lack of concern on the part of the client or family, and the clinician should be alert for nonverbal cues. Nonverbal cues may have their own cultural connotative meaning, however, so clarification should be sought (e.g., "You seem very upset; I noticed your face changed when we talked about _____. Are you worried about _____?"). Regarding instructions for home management, it may be helpful if the interpreter can write instructions (having assessed for literacy) for the family in the family's language and review them again before the family leaves.

Interpreters should work toward the following goals:

- Make the client's description and understanding of the problem clear to the provider.
- Communicate accurately the provider's interpretation and explanation of a health problem (e.g., pathophysiology) to the client.
- Facilitate the discussion to develop a management plan.
- Assess the child's and parents' level of knowledge and understanding of what is being said.

Conflict Negotiation

Conflict is a natural outcome of working with others, particularly when there are significant differences, in complex organizational systems, and when difficult decisions are required. Poor working relationships, aggression, and bullying are commonly found among provider groups (Steen, 2011) and between providers and clients, families, and communities. Conflict can generate poor health outcomes, as well as decrease provider satisfaction with work. Practitioners with creative conflict negotiation skills will be more able to resolve tensions that arise than those who avoid or "give in" to conflict.

System/Organization Domain

The *system/organization* domain refers to institutions of health care delivery. This domain has two aspects: intra-organizational and extra-organizational. The intra-organizational aspect refers to internal processes, such as mission statements, strategic plans, policies and procedures, hiring practices, employee behavior expectations, and performance appraisals. The extra-organizational aspect includes a system's or organization's relationship to the surrounding community.

Awareness

Just as individual reflection is necessary to develop self-awareness, an examination of the underlying assumptions of the United States health care system and health care facilities is essential to develop system/organization awareness. Complex issues (such as, power, privilege, racism, and institutional racism) create and sustain health disparities; they cannot be changed unless they are clearly identified and understood.

Engagement and Application

Three central themes relate to engagement and application in the system/organization domain: (1) infrastructure of the organization, including intra-organizational standards; (2) client-centered care; and (3) collaborative relationships with the community.

Intra-Organizational Standards

The way a system operates reflects its commitment to cultural diversity, and institutional standards can serve to create an environment where humility and culturally competent behavior are the expected norms. Some of the issues addressed by culturally sensitive standards include:

- Level of cultural humility and competence among caregivers: Are expectations clear that *all* members of the organization will be held accountable to demonstrate attitudes and behaviors aligned with principles of cultural humility and competence? Is evidence of such behaviors a part of employee performance reviews?
- Use of the organization's resources to develop a staff that exemplifies cultural humility and competence: Are training programs available? Do staff members have opportunities to interact with diverse communities? Is there support to work abroad? Are culturally sensitive client educational materials created? Does the organization hire and consistently use professional interpreters? Does the environment support the practice of cultural humility and competence? For example, are providers able to interact with clients in a way that strengthens their relationship? Or are they under constant pressure to produce and required to use technology (e.g., cell phones, beepers, electronic charting, and email) that competes for their time with clients?
- Dedication of leadership to cultural humility and competence: Do administrators, nurses, physicians, supervisors, and others in leadership positions actively support efforts toward cultural humility and competence? Cultural humility and competence are not just limited to client-provider interaction; they are important concepts for building strong relations among a workforce that often includes large rank, ethnic, and class differences. The infrastructure of standards, behaviors, and performance appraisals can be a mechanism to ensure institutional accountability for culturally humble and competent practice. If an organization has a "critical mass" of employees who function from a base of cultural humility and competence, culturally appropriate care for all becomes the norm, and those who are less skilled find support in dealing with a variety of cultural backgrounds.

Client-Centered Care

Client-centeredness in the system/organization domain requires altered provider, client, and family roles. In the more traditional relationship, clients are expected to conform to a system in which health care providers give "care" and clients adhere to the advice and regimen prescribed. Traditionally, clients are expected to change their behavior (or, if they do not, are labeled "noncompliant"), while the provider and system remain the same. In a client-centered approach, there is reciprocal relationship and the system, as well as clients and families, will change. This approach requires different skill sets from providers and systems. In clinical rotations, for example, students need to learn how to communicate with clients, understand the client's perspective, understand their own biases, be compassionate, be aware of issues that impact clients' health (such as, social determinants of health and health literacy), and adapt interventions to meet the needs, abilities, and desires of clients.

Building Collaborative Relationships with Communities

Organizations and systems need to establish collaborative relationships with the communities in which they are engaged. There is no "one-size-fits-all" solution in developing these relationships, but they take time and require a high level of resolve on the part of the organization. Many health care institutions have a history of conflict with the communities in which they function (e.g., due to acquisition of land for expansion, incidents of abuse or neglect of patients from minority neighborhoods, and so on), so their task is complicated by a negative history that must be overcome. In this process, organizations must give up some of their power and resources, shift their focus to include needs as identified by the community, and enthusiastically incorporate the opinions and expertise of the community as essential for making organizational decisions. A true partnership includes the community as active decision-makers in the life of the organization. In a service organization such as a health care facility, this means overcoming the traditional relationship of dependence in which the provider "gives" care and the community "receives" care on the provider's terms. Instead, the goal is an interdependent partnership in which the community and organization identify mutual priorities and create common ground to achieve them. Organizations must work closely with the community to identify its unique qualities (including strengths and needs); establish mechanisms to ensure ongoing communication; share information and resources; and receive and provide feedback, evaluation, and support for needed and desired change (Purnell et al, 2011; Soulé, 2014).

Collaborative relationships between health care organizations and communities can be fostered through community-based participatory research (CBPR). CBPR is transformative research that bridges the gap between science and practice by actively engaging communities with formally trained researchers. It is based on partnerships that respect the diverse expertise of community members and researchers; power, resources, credit, results, and knowledge are equally shared. CBPR differs from traditional research in significant ways. In CBPR projects, the community fully participates in all aspects of the research process, including identifying priority issues of concern, gathering and interpreting data, and disseminating information most useful to the community. Instead of creating knowledge for the advancement of an academic field, CBPR incorporates research, reflection, and action with the goal of improving health for the community as they define it (Minkler and Wallerstein, 2008).

Because the CBPR model blends the accumulated wisdom of community members with the skill of formally trained researchers, the quantity and quality of data are strengthened, making the findings more relevant to the community it affects the most. In addition, informing the entire community of findings in culturally appropriate ways is a priority of this model. As a result, findings are more relevant to the groups that can benefit most, the applicability of the research is validated, and importantly, trust between the community and researchers is enhanced. This foundational trust can pave the way for future research collaboration; it also can lead to findings being translated more quickly into policy and practice, which increases the possibility of priority issues being addressed promptly, resulting in better health outcomes for the community.

Global Domain

The *global* domain recognizes the worldwide movement toward integration and interconnection of the world's people functioning together economically, politically, technologically, and socioculturally. In the context of world population growth and migration, this area of study includes concepts such as global citizenship and local, national, and international diversity.

Awareness

It is essential that practitioners in contemporary practice have a basic understanding of the major diseases that affect humans worldwide and the social, political, economic, even geologic factors that contribute to them. The World Health Report (World Health Organization [WHO], 2013) is one key resource of global health epidemiology. By learning, for example, that when war broke out in Syria in 2014 polio reappeared (it had been eradicated 14 years earlier), health care providers can appreciate how health care systems, politics, and conflict between countries can impede the delivery of cost-effective vaccination services (Coutts and Fouad, 2014). As another example, surveys in 22 African countries showed that when households owned at least one insecticide-treated mosquito net there was a 13% to 31% reduction in the mortality of children younger than 5 years old. In addition, environmental factors (such as, climate change and natural disasters) must be understood for the impact that they have on the health of communities (Bell, 2011).

Engagement and Application

Successful engagement with diverse global communities can help providers learn how to work collaboratively at the regional, national, or international level. In addition to clinical work in the United States, many international volunteer opportunities for students and experienced providers are available (for example, the American Medical Association [AMA] has an Office of International Medicine. See www.ama-assn.org/). Application of a global perspective includes demonstrating social accountability to a global society; examining issues of paternalism and institutional racism; and having a willingness and ability to adjust to the needs of clients, families, and communities both nationally and globally (Lindgren and Karle, 2011; Soulé, 2014). Care must be taken that providers who participate in international experiences work collaboratively with on-site personnel to ensure that skilled care is given and follow-up happens. There is a movement toward these competencies in graduate programs focused on clinical practice, research, scholarship, and policy development; but this field of study is still in its infancy, and more work is needed to integrate and evaluate essential global health curriculum (Clark et al, 2011; Frenk et al, 2011; Veras et al, 2013).

Health Care for Immigrant and Refugee Populations

Immigrants, Refugees, and Settlement Processes

Immigrants to the United States come from many countries and have a wide range of motivations for leaving their country of origin. They may be authorized or unauthorized, and some engage in circular migration, moving back and forth between their country of origin and the United States. Many immigrants come to the United States seeking a better life with economic, educational, or social advantages. Refugees and asylum seekers, in contrast, have been displaced by hardship, trauma, or war, or they seek protection through the justice system in a third country due to risk of life, safety, or well-being in their country of origin. It appears that the majority of refugees and asylees ultimately return to their country of origin. According to the United Nations High Commissioner for Refugees (UNHCR), only about 1% of refugees with which the UNHCR works is resettled in a third country (UNHCR, n.d.).

Once in the United States, refugees face many challenges. They are assisted in settlement in a number of ways. Currently, 10 private voluntary agencies (VolAgs) and one state agency work with the U.S. Department of State, Bureau of Population, Refugees, and Migration to provide "initial reception and placement" of new refugees (see Additional Resources). Refugees may be "anchored" (i.e., have a family member or friend who assumes some responsibility for their placement) or "free" (i.e., without a community of support in the United States). In early 2008, for example, all refugees from Burma and Bhutan were designated as "free," because this population was so new to the United States that no well-established community was available to support new immigration. "Free" refugees usually have no role in deciding where they will be placed. However, if a "free" refugee does have a family member or friend in the United States, the individual may request placement and be designated "free with geographic preference" or "free-o," even though the family or friend (who also may be a recent immigrant) has limited responsibility for resettlement; the VolAg assumes primary responsibility. Not all states are able to accept "free" refugees.

VolAgs assist new arrivals to settle into the community. Each refugee family is assigned a VolAg caseworker who ideally meets the refugees at the airport; arranges housing and basic household supplies; provides an orientation to the community; assists in application for Social Security cards, draft status (if applicable), public assistance (if necessary), school and English class (English as a second language [ESL]) enrollment, and employment; arranges for medical care and refugee screening; facilitates travel for family reunification; and gives special care to separated or unaccompanied minors.

In response to large refugee populations, some states and municipalities work with VolAgs to develop coordinated, integrated programs of service, support, and information for both clients (i.e., immigrants) and providers (e.g., the Minnesota Refugee Health Program can be accessed at www.health.state.mn.us/divs/idepc/refugee), and many volunteer groups provide services both in countries of origin and in the United States (e.g., American Refugee Committee International [see Additional Resources]). In contrast, immigrants applying for resident status who are not refugees or are not seeking asylum are not assigned caseworkers or considered for service under refugee programs.

Prearrival Health Requirements

When applying for permanent resident status in the United States, all foreign-born persons, whatever their history or circumstance, have the same health requirements. These requirements serve to identify health problems and necessary care for incoming individuals and to protect the United States population from diseases that may be introduced by new arrivals. Applicants for permanent resident status *must* present a health assessment. Individuals who apply for a temporary visitor status are not required to have a health assessment. Nor would unauthorized immigrants have an assessment but, as with temporary visitors, they could require medical care and/or represent a health risk to the United States population.

Health assessments are done by physicians in the applicant's country of origin (panel of physicians appointed by the U.S. Department of State Consulates) or by physicians in the United States (civil surgeons appointed by the U.S. Citizenship and Immigration Service) (Centers for Disease Control and Prevention [CDC], 2014b). If applicants are found to have an inadmissible health condition (Box 3-3) or are underimmunized, treatment may be given or vaccines administered to help them meet the requirement for admission. Because a vaccine series can take months to complete, applicants become eligible for immigration when the series is begun. The applicant may also request a waiver for an inadmissible condition. The United States embassy or consulate in the individual's country of origin decides to grant or deny an immigrant visa; the ultimate decision to admit an applicant to the United States rests with the U.S. Citizenship and Immigration Service. This decision is based in part on the health findings. Applicants who present at a port of entry to the United States with an inadmissible condition or who have been exposed to such a condition (e.g., Ebola or severe acute respiratory syndrome [SARS]) may be placed in isolation or quarantine. There are 20 quarantine stations at United States borders, staffed by the Centers for Disease Control and Prevention (CDC) and managed by CDC's Division of Global Migration and Quarantine (CDC, 2014a).

• BOX 3-3 Inadmissible Conditions for United States Immigration Purposes

- Communicable diseases of public health significance
  - Active, infectious tuberculosis
  - Active syphilis
  - Other sexually transmitted diseases (chancroid, gonorrhea, granuloma inguinale, lymphogranuloma venereum)
  - Hansen disease (leprosy)
- No documentation of vaccination against vaccine-preventable diseases (see Box 3-6)
- Physical or mental disorders with associated harmful behaviors
- Substance-related disorders (drug abuse or addiction)

Postarrival Health Care

Medical care and screening with a primary care provider are to be arranged for refugees within 90 days of entry into the community—ideally within 30 days. If an applicant has a medical waiver for entry, health care should be arranged sooner than the 90 days. The CDC Division of Global Migration and Quarantine is responsible for notifying state and local health departments of new arrivals who need medical treatment and/or follow-up.

Refugees may qualify for Medicaid coverage for this care; for those who do not, the Office of Refugee Resettlement, Refugee Medical Assistance program may pay for up to 8 months of health care from the date of their arrival in the United States (Walker et al, 2014) (see Additional Resources). Nonrefugee immigrants, depending on their resources, may enter the health care system as any resident client would do; they may pay "out of pocket," have insurance through a job, or apply directly for public assistance and Medicaid. They may also access public health resources in their community.

Initial Health Visit, Screening, and Assessment

In addition to identifying health status and needs and beginning appropriate interventions, a major goal of the refugee or immigrant's initial visit with the primary care provider is to establish trust. It is hoped that such trust will encourage clients to engage in an ongoing relationship with the health care provider, creating a medical home for needed care in the future.

• BOX 3-4 Immigrant Health Needs: Considerations for Primary Care Providers

- Acute conditions: Infectious diseases (tuberculosis [TB], hepatitis B), dental caries, diseases of malnutrition
- Chronic conditions: Diabetes, malaria, parasites, others (e.g., thalassemia, sickle cell)
- Mental health conditions: Both acute and chronic, and related to both circumstances of immigration and intrinsic variables (i.e., the condition would have manifested without immigration)
- Conditions related to the social circumstances of immigration:
  - Stress of transition, particularly a move from rural to urban environment
  - Posttraumatic stress disorders: Although children suffer psychologic trauma of war, dislocation, and violence, there are many factors (e.g., family attachment, peer support, and extended social networks) that serve to help the child cope and demonstrate resilience
  - Exposure to environmental and safety hazards in new location (e.g., traffic and population density; farmworkers' occupational health)
  - Malnutrition secondary to poverty and lack of access to high-quality nutrients

Assessment

Care given at the initial visit includes a thorough history, physical examination, mental health assessment (see Chapter 2; Boxes 3-4 and 3-5), and assessment for both acute and chronic conditions (Walker et al, 2014). Although the evaluation is standard, there are some special considerations to keep in mind when working with new arrivals, including:

- Emphasize that the examination is aimed at benefiting the client and will not affect the client's immigrant status. Confidentiality should be explained to the client.
- Explain that the provider is interested in learning more about the client's culture; explanations from the client are welcome, and the provider will ask questions related to culture.
- Understand that the recent history of the client (e.g., displacement, trauma, refugee camp experience, loss) may set a context that exacerbates difficulties adjusting to life in United States culture.
- It may be extremely difficult or impossible to get a complete and accurate history.
- Include traditional, herbal, or other complementary medications when soliciting medication history.
- Include use of substances (e.g., betel nut in Thailand and khat in East Africa) when soliciting alcohol, tobacco, or drug use history.
- Ask about education level and literacy.
- Attend especially to mental health and nutrition concerns.
- Provide for same-gender examiners when conducting examinations of genitalia or asking questions related to personal or intimate matters.
- Get a thorough vaccination history; ask to see any documentation the client has from other providers (e.g., the panel physician who conducted the admission examination overseas; vaccine card given to parents in the country of origin). Remember that new arrivals may not have received all vaccinations prior to arrival. Box 3-6 lists vaccination requirements for United States immigration.
- Anticipate the need for referral, and assist the client to make contact with referral sources as needed. Work closely with caseworkers and public health nurses assigned to clients.

• BOX 3-5 Components of the Initial Screening and Assessment Visit

- Review all available records, including chest radiograph. (Ask for overseas records.)
- Complete a history and physical examination, including vision, hearing, and dental evaluation.
- Conduct mental health screening and, when clinically indicated, a more detailed social history, including any history of trauma/torture or rape.
- Evaluate for infectious disease, including tuberculosis, human immunodeficiency virus (HIV), and other sexually transmitted infections, and malaria and other parasitic infections (schistosomiasis and intestinal nematodes, including *Strongyloides*), depending on local epidemiology.
- Review overseas records for presumptive therapy for strongyloidiasis, schistosomiasis, or malaria, depending on point of departure.
- Evaluate for chronic diseases, including obesity, hypertension, diabetes, and nutritional deficiencies, such as vitamin B_{12} deficiency in select populations.
- Perform age-appropriate cancer screening, such as mammography, colonoscopy, or Papanicolaou test.
- Update immunizations as needed.
- Complete laboratory testing (hematologic testing, urinalysis, lead [as appropriate], HIV testing, hepatitis B serology for those arriving from countries with prevalence greater than 2%, specific sexually transmitted infection testing, or other screening, such as basic metabolic panel and liver function testing, when clinically appropriate).

From Walker PF, Stauffer WM, Barnett ED: *Arrival in the United States: health status & screening of refugees, immigrants, & international adoptees*. In Centers for Disease Control and Prevention (CDC): *Health information for international travel 2014*, New York, 2014, Oxford University Press.

Management

Primary care providers face heightened challenges when working with immigrants and refugees. The same cultural barriers discussed earlier operate: differences in language, worldviews, cultural norms, and perceptions and interpretations of the meaning of health and illness. In addition, immigrants experience restricted access to and discrimination in the health care system (Clough et al, 2013). Added to these barriers are the unique experiences of refugees and asylees: dislocations, major shifts from rural to urban living, violence, physical and emotional trauma, extreme poverty, marginalization, and fear. In the dislocation process, families face changes in gender roles, social expectations, and responsibilities. All of the rules change: Children may be lost,

• BOX 3-6 Vaccination Requirements for Immigration to the United States

Under the immigration laws of the United States, a foreign national who applies for an immigrant visa abroad, or who seeks to adjust status to a permanent resident while in the United States, is required to receive vaccinations to prevent the following diseases:

- Mumps
- Measles
- Rubella
- Polio
- Tetanus and diphtheria toxoids
- Pertussis
- Haemophilus influenzae type B
- Hepatitis B
- Any other vaccine-preventable diseases recommended by the Advisory Committee for Immunization Practices (ACIP)

The vaccine must be an age-appropriate vaccine as recommended by the ACIP for the general United States population, and at least one of the following:

- The vaccine must protect against a disease that has the potential to cause an outbreak; or
- The vaccine must protect against a disease eliminated in the United States, or is in the process of being eliminated in the United States

From U.S. Citizenship and Immigration Services (USCIS): *Vaccination requirements, USCIS* (website): www.uscis.gov/news/questions-and-answers/vaccination-requirements. Accessed August 21, 2014.

orphaned, or abandoned; women may take a more visible public role; and adolescents may be unsupervised, largely operating in peer groups. The ability to cope that derives from a strong social support network is jeopardized as families are uprooted and disoriented. As a part of the skill set of cultural humility and competence discussed previously, providers of care to refugees need to develop a knowledge base related to the following (Suurmond et al, 2010):

- Political situation and experience of clients in the country of origin
- Transition time experienced by clients: Were they in refugee camps? Where? For how long? What were conditions there?
- Diseases common in the country of origin and in transition sites
- Effects on health that result from being a refugee (e.g., stress, malnutrition)
- Legal context for refugees in the United States
- Effective management of trauma: physical, psychological, and emotional

The experience of inequality, marginalization, and stress can create lasting changes that lead to acute and chronic physical and mental health concerns (Morin and Schupbach, 2014). However, because of compromised coping, refugees may not use health care services and following health care recommendations may be low on their list of survival needs. Immigrants use health services far less than do native-born United States residents (Tarraf et al, 2012); unauthorized immigrants, in particular, may make efforts to avoid public scrutiny and remain isolated from services and agencies.

For a variety of reasons, the health status of immigrants deteriorates the longer that they are in the United States (Lee et al, 2013) and health care providers need to find ways to ensure that health needs will be met. Communicating effectively on the initial health visit can set the stage. Clearly explaining the United States health care system to clients is essential. The use of community-based participatory action to meet refugee health needs has been shown to be effective—where immigrant clients are involved in planning systems, and primary care providers have support from a larger system, including public health nurses, interpreters, social workers, and voluntary community agencies (Culhane-Pera et al, 2010).

Finally, providers must be alert to the fact that care of second-, third-, and older-generation immigrants will differ from that of first-generation or new arrivals. As they acculturate into the United States lifestyle, immigrants begin to look and act more like others in their community; adolescents take on behaviors of their peer group, for example, and may seem like "typical" United States teenagers. But they do not have the same historical cultural context as their peers, and as a result, providers may make incorrect assumptions about them or use cultural references in health education that make no sense to the client.

Providing care to clients of diversity is a challenge to both health care workers and the system as a whole. High-quality care requires significant changes in beliefs, attitudes, and practices on the part of providers. It also requires changes in the ways health care systems deliver care. By working sensitively with these clients, sharing ideas and information, learning from and about each other, and celebrating differences and similarities, clients and clinicians can become full participants in creating a new cultural context for the health and illness experience.

For a complete list of references, please visit http://evolve.elsevier.com/Burns/pediatric/.

UNIT 2

Management of Development

4

Developmental Management in Pediatric Primary Care

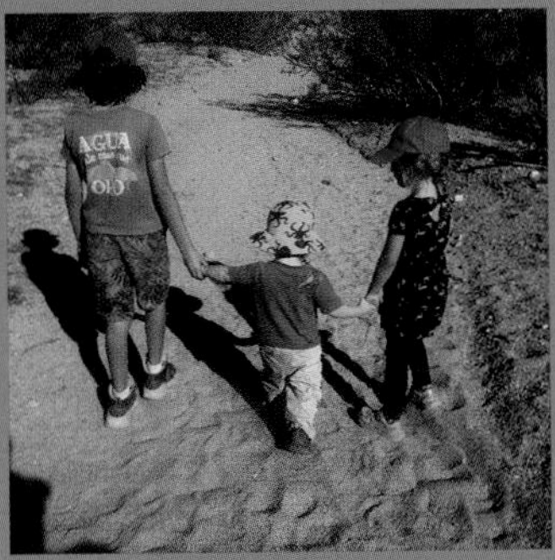

DAWN LEE GARZON

Modern approaches to managing children's well-being differ dramatically from those that prevailed at the turn of the past century when health supervision often consisted of a brief examination to detect communicable or contagious diseases. In the twenty-first century significant social, economic, and demographic changes influence the American family and affect children's health. Children's health supervision uses a broader approach than one necessary for disease detection. Pediatric primary care providers (PCPs) have a responsibility to monitor children's overall physical, cognitive, and psychosocial development and to provide anticipatory guidance to families as children grow. PCPs are key players who help parents and families adjust to the life changes that occur throughout childhood. This requires a strong background in child development, knowledge of strategies that help parents understand and respond to their child's development, and an ability to establish effective relationships with children and their parents.

Pediatric providers offer parents support and suggest diverse approaches to childrearing. They help parents understand the challenges that growth and developement and new accomplishments create, and how to best handle these challenges. Providers who develop a close relationship with parents and their children share in the parents' pride as their child grows. Research indicates that parents value receiving reassurance about their child and their parenting and desire opportunities to discuss concerns with health care providers who respect their parental role and with whom they have an ongoing relationship (Radecki et al, 2009). The opportunity to provide parental support is not limited to periodic wellness visits. All pediatric office visits provide rich opportunities for parents to discuss their concerns, to validate information received from other sources, and to learn about their child's growth and development. Studies indicate parents believe the most desirable anticipatory guidance topics include developmental and behavioral issues, how to reach health care providers with concerns when episodic visits are less frequent (e.g., when visits become annual), how to best communicate with their child, and the best way to keep a child healthy (Combs-Orme et al, 2011). Unfortunately, only 74% of parents are able to recall at least one anticipatory guidance item, and 65% report having at least one unmet need after their child's last well visit (Combs-Orme et al, 2011; Radecki et al, 2009).

This chapter presents an introduction to principles of development, developmental theories, methods of developmental assessment, and identification and management of developmental problems. Chapters 5 through 8 review how developmental theories are applied by age group, describe normal patterns of development, identify "red flags" related to development, and recommend anticipatory guidance for families of infants, toddlers and preschoolers, school-age children, and adolescents.

Developmental Principles

Development is a lifelong, dynamic process. Achievement of milestones in one phase sets the stage for the next phase. Development is a dynamic and reciprocal process that is influenced by the child's internal and external environments. Key principles provide a contextual understanding of developmental concepts. Exactly how these principles manifest in a particular child depends on the child's genetic background, personality or temperament, and intrauterine and extrauterine environmental factors.

Principle 1. Growth and development are orderly and sequential. Although children differ in rates and timing of developmental changes, they generally follow certain predictable stages or phases. Specific examples include the rapid growth during the first year of life, progress toward independence throughout childhood, and the development of secondary sex characteristics during adolescence.

Principle 2. The pace of growth and development is specific for each child. Developmental changes vary considerably for each child. Some children demonstrate early skill in motor coordination, and others demonstrate early skill in language acquisition. These changes are unique to each child.

Principle 3. Development occurs in a cephalocaudal and proximodistal direction. An example of this principle is seen as infants develop increasing motor coordination, gaining head control before sitting and walking. Similarly, developmental progress is seen in controlled movements that occur first near the midline of the body, such as rolling over, progressing to distal coordination of the hands, such as mastery of the pincer grasp.

Principle 4. Growth and development become increasingly integrated. Behavior that is taken for granted, such as self-feeding, occurs as a result of numerous small changes and skills acquired by the child. Simple skills and behaviors are integrated into more complex behaviors as the child grows and develops.

Principle 5. Developmental abilities increasingly organize and differentiate. As a result of increasing maturation and experience, children's behaviors and responses to internal and external cues become more regulated, organized, and differentiated. The infant who cries and moves because of hunger is different from the hungry toddler who walks to the refrigerator and points.

Principle 6. The child's internal and external environments affect growth and development. Opportunities for play, societal norms, cultural values, family traditions, and family beliefs all influence child development. Similarly, children influence their environment to achieve desired experiences and opportunities.

Principle 7. Certain periods are critical during growth and development. Critical periods are points of time when developmental advances occur and are particularly susceptible to alterations due to internal and external influences. For example, fetal exposure to certain viruses during the first trimester of pregnancy increases the risk of congenital abnormalities.

Principle 8. Development is a continual process, often without smooth transitions. Developmental phases are marked by periods of change, growth, and stability plateaus.

Theories of Child Development

Developmental theories include an array of ideas about how children progress from infancy through adolescence and provide many perspectives on children's growth and development. Health care providers need to stay abreast of changing ideas regarding child development and appreciate new developmental theories relating to children. Developmental theories are based on various cultures, personalities, environmental issues, philosophical beliefs, and investigative methods. When using a developmental perspective in practice, the provider should understand how the theory was developed and how it may relate to a particular family and child. Developmental theories provide guidelines for understanding the child's emerging behavior, personality, and physical abilities. It is usually necessary to combine several theories to holistically view the child.

Ethology: Animal Studies

The study of animal behavior, looking at the concepts of bonding, altruism, social intelligence, and dominant and submissive behavior, led to theoretic assumptions that frame the study of child development. Bowlby (1969) first generalized theories developed about animal behavior to bonding for humans, articulating the concept of attachment theory. Ainsworth and colleagues (1971) examined the elements of early attachment and separation in child development and personality. This was followed by Klaus and Kennel's work (1976), which emphasized the importance of early mother-infant contact. Their work later became the basis for changes in hospital rooming-in care.

Maturational Theories: Developmental Milestones

Early theories about human behavior set the stage for studies of child development. Rousseau's (1762) descriptions of the natural, innately good growth of the child, if not misled by a "corrupt social environment," provided the foundation for maturational theories. Gesell (1940) is credited with the term *maturation* in reference to the orderly, sequential developmental changes that occur over time. He described behavior cycles that correspond to certain chronologic ages. His work resulted in the chronologic growth and development norms for motor, affective, linguistic, and social domains that are now used to assess developmental progress.

Lewin (1936) identified growth principles and defined the stages of infancy, early childhood, and adolescence. He provided an understanding of how a child's play and decision-making change as he or she develops.

Havighurst's work (1953), a summation of ideas from many theorists, popularized the concept of developmental tasks. He theorized that when individuals successfully master skills, this fosters happiness and sets the stage for successful attainment of future skills. Failure, on the other hand, leads to feelings of unhappiness, societal disapproval, and difficulty attaining future skills.

Cognitive-Structural Theories: Language and Thought

Cognitive-structural theories examine the ways in which children think, reason, and use language. They are based on assumptions about central nervous system maturation and children's interactions with their environment. Individual differences are ascribed to genetic endowment and environmental influences.

Jean Piaget's observations, many of which were of his own children, provide an understanding of children's cognitive development and their perception and interaction with the world around them. Piaget (1969) described how children actively use their life experiences, incorporating them into their own mental and physical being over time. He emphasized how children modify themselves depending on their environmental experiences and their stage-related competency level. Piaget described four stages of cognitive development (Table 4-1).

Sensorimotor Stage (Birth to 2 Years)

At the sensorimotor stage, children learn about the world through their actions and sensory and motor movements. Key concepts during this period include object permanence, spatial relationships, causality, use of instruments, and combination of objects. The child's framework for learning is the self, and there is little cognitive connection to objects outside the self.

Preoperational Stage (2 to 7 Years)

Children next attempt to make sense of the world and reality. In this stage, children are egocentric and are only able to reason when there are connections to concrete objects. They learn cause and effect, and their reasoning is often flawed. Children begin to use semiotic functioning, or the use of one thing to represent another. Intuitive reasoning emerges toward the end of this stage, but reasoning remains connected to the concrete reality of the here and now.

Concrete Operational Stage (7 to 12 Years)

Children use symbols to represent concrete objects and to perform mental tasks. This requires cognitive skill to organize experiences and classify increasingly complex information. Most schoolwork requires functioning at this level. This stage is characterized by flexibility of thought, declining egocentrism, logical reasoning, and greater social cognition.

Formal Operational Stage (13 Years through Adulthood)

At this stage, children begin to think abstractly and imagine different solutions and outcomes to problems. Adolescents begin to develop increased awareness of health and illness and recognize how their behaviors can impact health. Renewed egocentrism may be noted early in this stage as a result of a lack of differentiation between what others are thinking and one's own thoughts. This egocentric thinking eventually gives way to an appreciation of the differences in judgment between the adolescent and other individuals, societies, and cultures. This is the basis of an adolescent's ability to think about politics, law, and society in terms of abstract principles and benefits rather than focusing only on the punitive aspects of societal laws.

Piaget's work was expanded by theorists, such as Flavell (1977) and Siegler and colleagues (1973), who looked at specific intellectual capabilities via the information processing model. This model included concepts of attention, perception, memory, and making inferences and provided an initial understanding of how mental activity leads progressively to more sophisticated ways of handling information.

Kohlberg (1969) focused on theories of moral development and socialization, emphasizing the process by which children learn the expectations and norms of their society and culture (see Table 4-1). Kohlberg's work primarily involved male participants. Gilligan (1982) suggested that female thoughts and actions involve significantly different objectives and goals; specifically that girls tend to think more in terms of caring and relationships, basing their moral judgments on complexities that they perceive in human interactions.

Fowler's theory (1981) described the spiritual dimension of human life, or the development of faith. This theory addressed the process by which humans develop meaning for daily life. Faith is described as the structure that people use to build their lives. Fowler emphasized that achieving the stages is not due to intelligence but rather occurs through valuing, thinking, and interacting with others.

The Role of Social Interaction in Cognitive Development

Vygotsky's theory of child learning (1978) states that as children interact with others, they develop as individuals within cultural contexts. They simultaneously develop memory, problem-solving skills, attention, and concept formation. Core to Vygotsky's theory is the "zone of proximal development," which is the difference between what a child can do on his or her own and what he or she can do with help from others.

Vygotsky believes that children learn by watching adults and other children, and that children learn best when their parents and caregivers provide them with opportunities in the child's zone of proximal development. This theory holds that cognitive development occurs in a social, historical, and cultural context and that adults guide children to learn. Development depends on the use of language, play, and extensive social interaction. One of Vygotsky's examples is the process of the child learning to point his or her finger. Initially, the infant points his or her finger without meaning; however, as people, and especially caregivers, respond to the finger pointing, the infant learns there is meaning to the movement. What starts as a muscle movement becomes a means of interpersonal connection between two people. This theory further holds that play and learning should be constructed to take into consideration the child's needs, inclination, and incentives. This theory supports the benefit of adult social learning opportunities via group interaction and observation.

Psychoanalytic Theories

Personality and Emotions

Psychodynamic theorists study factors that influence the emotional and psychological behavior of individuals. Personality includes the characteristics of temperament and motivation, in addition to concepts related to self-esteem and self-concept. Sigmund Freud (1938) was one of the most influential theorists in this area. Freud sought to find

TABLE 4-1 Comparison of Early Developmental Theorists

		Kohlberg		Piaget		Erikson	
Age	Freud	Stages		Stages/ Substages	Characteristics	Psychological Crisis	Themes
0-12 mo	Oral stage	Stage 1 "premoral" preconventional level	1: Punishment avoidance and obedience	Sensorimotor stage: Reflexive stage: 0-1 mo Primary circular stage: 1-4 mo Secondary circular stage: 4-8 mo Coordination of secondary circular stage: 8-12 mo	Innate infant reflexes Repetitive responses Outward-directed behaviors Object permanence and goal-directed behaviors	Trust vs. mistrust	To get; to give in return
12-18 mo				Tertiary circular reactions stage: 2-18 mo	Causality and object permanence through several steps	Autonomy vs. shame	To hold on; to let go
18-36 mo	Anal stage	Stages 1-2 preconventional level	2: Instrumental realistic orientation—recognizes needs in others as long as own needs are met	Mental combinations stage: 18-24 mo	Memory used for problem-solving		
3-6 yr	Oedipal stage	Stages 1-2 preconventional level		Preoperational stage: Preconceptual stage: 2-4 yr Intuitive stage: 4-7 yr	Increased use of symbols, especially language; representational thought, egocentrism, assimilation, and symbolic play Increased symbolic functioning, language, decreasing egocentricity, imitation of reality	Initiative vs. guilt	To make things; to play

Continued

TABLE 4-1 Comparison of Early Developmental Theorists—cont'd

		Kohlberg		Piaget		Erikson	
Age	Freud	Stages		Stages/ Substages	Characteristics	Psychological Crisis	Themes
6-11 yr	Latency stage	Preconventional (stage 2): Up to 7 yrs Conventional (stages 3 and 4): 7-10 yrs Post-conventional (stage 5): 10-11 yrs	3: Interpersonal acceptance of "nice" girl and "good" boy social concept—does not want relationships with others harmed 4: The "law and order" orientation—rules are not flexible or changeable 5: Social contract and utilitarian orientation—rules can change on social needs	Concrete operational stage	Flexible thought: Understands rules of reversibility and deconcentration, conservation, and identity Declining egocentrism: Ability to understand another's perspective Local reasoning: Understands concepts of relation, ordering, conservation; able to classify objects Social cognition: Improved sense of equality and justice	Industry vs. inferiority	To make things; to complete
12-17 yr	Adolescence (Oedipus complex)	Stages 5-6 post-conventional level	6: Universal ethical orientation principles are source of rules; inner conscience present	Formal operational stage	Development of logical thinking, able to work with abstract ideas; able to synthesize and integrate concepts into larger schemes	Identity vs. role confusion	To be oneself; to share being oneself or not being oneself
17-30 yr	Young adult	Stages 5-6		Formal operational stage		Intimacy vs. isolation	To lose and find oneself in another

links between the conscious mind and the body through the unconscious mind (see Table 4-1). Some of his most significant contributions were his descriptions of the interactions of id, ego, and superego.

Anna Freud continued the work of her father, focusing particularly on children. It was through her studies that the implications of psychoanalysis for raising normal children were developed. She believed that psychoanalytic theory could help parents gain "insight into the potential harm done to young children during the critical years of their development by the manner in which their needs, drives, wishes, and emotional dependencies are met" (Freud, 1974).

Erikson (1964) expanded Freud's theories, describing the stages of the individual throughout the lifespan (see Table 4-1). Each stage presents problems that the individual seeks to master. Erikson believed that if problems were not resolved, they would be revisited again at future stages.

Sullivan (1964) emphasized the importance of self-concept and the environmental influences that modulate it. He defined the parents and home as the most crucial cultural environment. Sullivan posited that progression toward mature relationships is based on communication skills and the integration of social experiences inhibited or enhanced by the parents' relationship between themselves.

Mahler and colleagues (1975) analyzed the development of an infant's evolving independence through study of the mother-infant dyad. Three phases of development were proposed: autism, symbiosis, and separation-individuation. They posited that these phases account for the infant's gradually increasing awareness of self and others. In the autistic phase (3 to 5 weeks old), the infant has no concept of self but works, physiologically, to achieve homeostasis in the extrauterine world. The second phase, symbiosis, refers to a period of undifferentiation or fusion with the mother in which infant and mother form a dual unity. Separation-individuation (from about 4 to 5 months old onward) is characterized by a steady increase in awareness of the separateness of the self and the other.

Infant attachment within the context of separation and connectedness has been explored by Stern (1985), Emde and Buchsbaum (1990), and Rogoff (1990). They propose that the quality and consistency of infant-caregiver relationships help the infant develop an affective, or emotional, sense of self. The early beginnings of the sense of self are based on three biologic principles: self-regulation, social fittedness, and affective monitoring (Emde, 1988). Infants with attachment security and a sense of connectedness are more likely to explore and be autonomous; they also have what is called an *internal working model* to guide them in later attachments.

The concept of *intersubjectivity*, or mutual understanding of meaning and mutual engagement in social interactions, underlies attachment theory. Observing that even very young infants demonstrate an ability to interact beyond an instinctive or reflexive manner with a sympathetic individual, Trevarthen and Aitken (2001) conducted an extensive review of the literature on the topic of infant intersubjectivity. They concluded that the infant's capacity for self-regulation may be based in the operation of an intrinsic motive formation (IMF) developed in the parieto-temporal region of the prenatal brain. Studies of the brain and infant behavior suggest that this IMF guides the newborn's ability to integrate sensory-motor coordination, orient to preferred stimuli (e.g., mother's voice), sustain mutual attention with an affectionate other, and anticipate what to expect in the environment. Successful development of the infant's "purposive consciousness" and the ability to cooperate with and learn from another depends on the neurologic functioning and the presence of a supportive environment. The parent guides the infant to connect with others and experience mutuality. Social interactions and infant engagement with their parents and objects in their world are major developmental influences.

These theories help the provider assist parents to understand why, for example, 12-month-old infants (who now understand object permanence) look over the side of the highchair for food or a toy that has fallen to the floor and smile and laugh when they spot it, because they knew it would be there. These same infants may call a parent to their room in the middle of the night; they now have "person permanence." They picture their parent in their mind and, perhaps experiencing normal separation anxiety, they want the parent to come to them. The PCP can use the concepts of attachment theory and intersubjectivity to explain that this behavior is that of a normal developing infant trying to have his or her needs met. The behavior reflects an infant who is attached and who uses the parent as a secure base from which to explore the world. It is not a problem, nor is the child being "bad."

Behavioral Theories: Human

Actions and Interactions

Behaviorism, the study of the general laws of human behavior, focuses on the present and ways that the environment influences human behavior. Skinner's view of child development (1953) examined learning that was controlled through classic operant conditioning. Behavior modification therapy is largely based on Skinner's work. Bandura's social learning theory (1962) looks at imitation and modeling as a means of learning, emphasizing the social variables involved. Bijou and Baer (1965) responded to critics of behaviorism's view of the child as a passive object and argued that children's responses to environmental stimuli are dependent on their genetic structure and personal history.

Humanistic Theories

Innermost Self

Maslow (1971), Buhler and Allen (1972), and Mahrer (1978) are among the most well-known humanistic theorists and examined development throughout the lifespan. Maslow's hierarchy of needs included physiologic, safety, belongingness and love, esteem, and self-actualization needs. He differentiated deficiency needs from growth or self-actualization needs. Rather than proposing stages through which children or adults mature, the humanists believe that individuals and those around them are responsible for any movement they make from one plateau of needs to another; intrinsic forces do not move them along.

Ecologic Theories

The key concepts of human ecology theory (Bronfenbrenner, 1979) emphasize the interdependence between environmental settings (roles, interpersonal relations, and activities) and the developing child. Development is described as the growing capacity to discover, sustain, or alter the self or the environment. Children are viewed as dynamic entities who increasingly restructure the settings where they live. Environments influence children, leading to mutual accommodation and reciprocity. Children's perceptions of the environment influence their behavior and development more than objective reality does.

Children are influenced by the home and family, child care settings, schools, entertainment and recreational activities, their parents' work, and broad economic opportunities in society. Recognition is given to ecologic transitions or changes in an individual's role or setting, such as the birth of a sibling or changes in family structure. Family routines and rituals can powerfully mediate children's development. The quality of the parents' relationship with each other and each parent's individual development strongly impacts parent-child interaction. When parents successfully complete their own developmental tasks and they experience positive mutual feelings, the parent-child relationship is strengthened. Alternatively, when parents experience mutual antagonism or interference, the parent-child relationship may be impaired (Pridham et al, 2010). These theories are especially useful to assist PCPs to understand how interpersonal violence and unhealthy relationships impact child development.

Temperament

The work of Chess and Thomas (1995) explains the role that temperament plays in child behavior. They identified characteristics or qualities of temperament and introduced the concept of "goodness of fit" to describe the degree to which the child's environment and parents' characteristics, including the parents' temperament, are congruous with the child's natural temperamental characteristics. Understanding the child's unique temperament prepares the health care provider to help parents and other caregivers to better understand the child's behavior, especially when the behaviors are confusing or problematic for the parents. The provider can discuss with parents their view of their child's temperament, how it "fits" with the parents' temperament or that of other family members, and what parent-child strategies can be used if conflicts emerge between the child's temperament and the caregivers' personal style. The intent is to alleviate guilt and frustration, to support the parenting role, and to assist parents to develop skills that enhance positive behaviors rather than exaggerate difficult temperamental characteristics. Supporting both the parents' and child's needs can prevent significant problems later on. Table 4-2 further defines characteristics of temperament.

TABLE 4-2 Temperament Characteristics

Temperament Characteristic	Description
Activity	What is the child's activity level? Is the child moving all the time he or she is awake, some of the time, or rarely?
Rhythmicity	How predictable is the child's sleep-wake pattern, feeding schedule, and elimination pattern?
Approach or withdrawal	What is the child's response when presented with something new, such as a new toy, a new experience, or a new person? Does he or she immediately approach or turn away?
Adaptability	How quickly does the child get used to new things? Quickly or not at all?
Threshold of response	How much stimulation does the child require for calming? A quiet voice and touch or more intense, loud voice or firm grasp?
Intensity of reaction	Are the child's responses (crying or laughing) very subtle or extremely intense?
Quality of mood	Is the child's mood usually outgoing, happy, joyful, pleasant or unfriendly, withdrawn, or quiet?
Distractibility	How easily is the child distracted by outside disturbances, such as a phone ringing, TV, and siblings?
Attention span and persistence	How long will the child continue to play with a particular toy or engage in a certain activity? Does this continue even when there are distractions?

Self-Regulation

Self-regulation involves a transition from reflexive responses in the newborn period to the ability to recognize and control one's thoughts and actions. Both genetics and environment influence the development of self-regulation (Vohs and Baumeister, 2011). Examples of self-regulation are early infant sleep patterns and the ability to self-soothe, the toddler's ability to manage emerging emotions, the preschooler's ability to transition from home to school, the school-age child's ability to focus attention on important tasks, and the adolescent's sense of confidence and competence. Learning self-regulation is influenced by differences in an individual child's abilities (e.g., attention, cognition, and impulsivity), temperament, genetics, and characteristics of the child's environment. Children best learn to self-regulate when they experience loving and nurturing parenting, consistent discipline, and when they are provided opportunities to learn without fear of negative outcomes if failure occurs (Vohs and Baumeister, 2011). The prefrontal cortex controls memory, attention, planning, and behavioral inhibition and is considered to be critical to the ability self-regulate. However, further work is needed to understand how neurobiologic development and environmental influences combine to influence individual children's abilities.

Early Brain Development

The understanding of early brain development has grown considerably in the past few decades. Landmark work done in the 1990s changed the understanding of early child development and revealed the critical brain growth that occurs in the first few years of life. By 8 months old, brain synapses have increased from 50 trillion to 1000 trillion and remain at this level throughout early childhood. During the rest of childhood and adolescence, the efficiency of the neuronal networks, especially the prefrontal cortex that is responsible for judgment and impulse control, is refined.

Research on the developing brain confirms a number of key points, including:

- Some physical brain characteristics are genetically determined, and most neurons are present at birth.
- The capacity to build the brain structures that support social, emotional, and mental development is greatest in early childhood and decreases over time.
- Failure to prune synapses hinders some learning in later life (Stephan et al, 2012).
- Early stimulation is necessary for optimal brain development.
- The brain grows rapidly in early childhood; by 6 years old, the brain is about 95% of its adult size.
- Ongoing stress, including child abuse, neglect, maternal depression, substance abuse, or family violence, can damage the growing brain (McCrory et al, 2010).
- Normal brain development requires good nutrition.

Studies confirm the fact that early experiences affect the brain development and lay the foundation for intelligence, emotional health, and moral development (Institute of Medicine [IOM] and National Research Council [NRC], 2012). Positive early experiences have a positive effect on brain cell formation. The IOM and NRC report emphasizes the following developmental concepts:

- Healthy early development depends on nurturing and dependable relationships.
- How young children feel is as important as how they think, particularly with regard to school readiness.
- Although society is changing, the needs of young children are not being met in the process.

The PCP plays an important role in helping parents understand how daily experiences (such as, feeding, playing, diapering, calming, and sleep) influence infants' brain development. Specifically, providers can teach parents that providing predictable, consistent, and loving care helps the infant learn trust, which is the first stage of psychosocial development according to Erikson.

Theories of Family and Parenting Development

PCPs recognize that pediatric care occurs within the context of the family. Just as an infant is not born fully developed, families and parents grow and change over time. Parents and families are influenced by a wide variety of stimuli including sociocultural norms, changes in family members, learned behaviors from past experiences, and internalized individual expectations and desires. Family function and parental comfort and capability in their parenting role have profound impacts on child development and child well-being. Thus, PCPs should be familiar with theories on how parents develop in their roles and how families develop as units.

Family Theories

Family systems theory provides a framework to help PCPs understand how family dynamics influence adult and child behaviors. Originally described by Bowen in the 1960s, this theory holds that an individual's emotional dysfunction has a profound impact on overall family health (Bowen, 1966). Differentiation of self and emotional fusion are key concepts in this theory. *Differentiation of self* refers to the individual's ability to recognize that he or she is a unique individual, with characteristics and traits different from those of other family members, who can function as a distinct person while developing and maintaining emotional connections to others. *Emotional fusion* reflects the ability to emotionally react to and communicate with others without conscious thought or speaking. Highly-fused relationships can cause stress and anxiety because of fear of rejection and/or emotional distance. Anxious family members, those with highly-fused relationships or those with poor self-differentiation, express their anxiety in ways that result in family dysfunction. This can cause parental discord, parent or child health or emotional problems or triangulation, a process where anxiety and/or tension between two family members is passed on to a third family member (Haefner, 2014). This theory helps explain how parental relationship problems can result in child behavior difficulties or how an enmeshed parent-child relationship can result in inappropriate worries about child health and/or strain in the parents' relationship. PCPs aid families by helping them recognize triangulation and other signs of unhealthy self-differentiation and emotional fusion, by helping families modify unhealthy behaviors, and by referring to mental health specialists when significant concerns and dysfunctions occur.

Evolutionary life history theories explain how the family environment affects family conflict and child development (Gillette and Gudmunson, 2014). Core to these theories is the belief that just as physical evolution occurs in nature, families evolve over time and learned family behaviors are inherited. These theories hold that behaviors are intrinsic and the genetic influences of behavior are largely driven by the biologic imperative to reproduce. Family behaviors affect parenting practice and child development because children learn how to interact with others and social skills are developed via interactions with and mimicking of family members. Innate, unconscious thought processes that are driven by the neuroendocrine system shape parenting behaviors. According to this approach, some parents focus on long-term pair bond outcomes and selective interpersonal relationships and tend to be highly invested in their parenting role and the long-term success of their offspring. Other parents focus more on short-term gains and may be more focused on forming pair bonds and less focused on parenting (Gillette and Gudmunson, 2014). This can result in cool parent-child relationships, early onset sexual expression, and inappropriate relationship expectations, especially in adolescent females.

Parent Development Theory

The parent development theory asserts that the parenting role begins in childhood, evolves over time, and is influenced by personal experience, social norms, the health of the parent-child relationship, family dynamics, and the child's own characteristics (Mowder, 2005; Sperling and Mowder, 2006). Parent development theory defines the parent as the individual who assumes the responsibility of caring for and raising a child. It identifies six characteristics of parenting that vary in their importance based on the child's developmental needs (Table 4-3). These behaviors occur as part of the parent-child relationship, are dynamic, and occur within a social context. Parenting evolves as a child ages. For example, a parent of a toddler who is just learning to walk has a very different role from the parent of an adolescent who is a senior in high school and preparing to leave for college.

Expectations for parental behaviors are also shaped by societal norms and personal beliefs (Mowder, 2005). If parents view their role as primarily that of a disciplinarian, they may have very specific and defined ways they expect their child to behave, and many of the interactions they have with their child will focus on the child's behavior within the context of the parent's rules. On the other hand, parents who view their primary role as a nurturer and comforter may spend more time expressing love and affection for the child. There is no single approach to parenting, and parenting differs from family to family. Parenting roles are not fixed, parents may move from one role to another depending on the situational context.

It is important for PCPs to recognize that one parenting style does not "fit all." The PCP serves to provide information and act as a support for the knowledge and skills parents need to develop a healthy parent-child relationship.

TABLE 4-3 Parent Role Characteristics in the Parent Development Theory

Role Characteristic	Signs of Healthy Role Development
Bonding	Parents feel and express love and affection for the child. They positively regard the child.
Discipline	Parents set limits for the child's behavior and make sure the rules are understood and followed. They give consistent parental responses.
Education	Parents share information with their child to help them understand the world around them. They teach and guide their child, and they model good behaviors.
General welfare and protection	Parents make sure their child is safe and has physical needs met. They provide a safe, healthy environment with adequate food, water, clothing, and shelter.
Responsivity	Parents pay attention to their child and are responsive to cues from the child, addressing needs beyond those of general welfare and protection. They help, encourage, and support the child.
Sensitivity	Parents listen to the verbal and nonverbal communication of the child and are able to accurately interpret the child's needs. They respect, empathize with and comfort the child, and give appropriate responses to the child's needs.

From BA: Parent development theory: understanding parents, parenting perceptions and parenting behaviors, *J Early Child Infant Psychol* 1:45–64, 2005.

Concerns develop when there is a mismatch of parent role and child development or when strife in the parent-child relationship occurs.

Cultural Influences on Development

Cultural and ethnic traditions shape the development of infants, children, adolescents, parents, and families. Some cultural groups manifest childhood developmental milestones differently from others. Health care providers should understand that these differences are normal. Early milestones, such as eating solid food, weaning from the breast or bottle, sleeping through the night, and toilet training, may occur at different ages and be considered normal. Parental responses to their children's needs also vary by culture. Group differences, however, may be less important when providing individualized care for a particular child and family. More accurate assessments of families and children come from understanding the specific culture of a family and community. To understand family culture, additional assessment is needed beyond the traditional health history and physical examination.

Tools such as the genogram, ecomap, and family functioning model (Minuchin, 1974) can help identify family structure, strengths, resources, and health responses, beliefs, and practices. The Childhood Health Assessment Questionnaire (CHAQ) and Child Health Questionnaire (CHQ) have been adapted to a number of cultural groups (Ruperto et al, 2001), and cross-cultural tools to be used with specific illnesses (e.g., lupus erythematosus, rheumatoid arthritis) are available (Moorthy et al, 2010). The interview process clarifies families' unique qualities and resources, and it serves as an avenue for communicating interest in, and understanding of, individual families and their ethnic or cultural values, differences, and commonalities (see Chapters 2 and 3). Using a validated screening tool with high sensitivity, specificity, and reliability helps the provider to better determine which children need referrals. Once the child reaches kindergarten, children from all cultural backgrounds should have similar development (Hagan et al, 2008).

Providers need to recognize their own cultural biases and how their culture and ethnic traditions affect approaches to certain aspects of the well-child visit. By gaining this awareness and understanding, they more effectively work with others (see Chapter 3).

Management Strategies in Child Development

Promoting Parent Development and Parent-Child Interaction: Anticipatory Guidance

Parents need clear information about expectations for child development, and providers must educate parents and families about normative development and best practices for managing development. The broadly defined goal of anticipatory guidance is to help parents plan for and cope with anticipated changes and to increase parenting skills, confidence, and competence in problem solving so that children can reach their maximum potential for health and wellness. Anticipatory guidance is intended to assist parents to adapt parenting styles and strategies to their child's temperament, growth, and development and should include the following:

- Assessment of the child's development.
- Determination of the parents' knowledge of child development.
- Determination of the parents' knowledge of, and comfort and experience with, the parent role.
- Assessment of the parents' problem-solving and coping skills.
- Information about normative child development, including common developmental variations. Include age-appropriate written educational materials as well as referrals to additional sources (i.e., online resources, community and professional organizations, and support networks).
- Assisting parents to develop realistic expectations of their child's development.
- Education about parenting strategies and concepts.
- Continuous process evaluation and reinforcement of healthy parental role development.

Promoting parent development through anticipatory guidance may be more challenging than providing physical care, especially in primary care practices in which time is limited. The standard of care in pediatric practices should include opportunities for providers to address parenting issues or concerns. Quick, pat answers to complex parenting issues do not facilitate parental growth. To achieve this standard, creative strategies can be used to structure prenatal visits, hospital discharge rounds, early discharge newborn follow-up, breastfeeding consultations, well-child visits, and referrals. An organized parent support program in practice settings, for example, can help providers listen, hear, and act on parents' concerns. Without an organized plan that connects the child's developmental needs, parents' concerns and educational needs, providers' abilities and resources, and community resources, it is easy to overlook, delay, or deny important parenting issues.

The interview and counseling conducted during anticipatory guidance should be based on a consistent framework. Programs such as Touchpoints (Brazelton and Sparrow, 2006), Bright Futures (Hagan et al, 2008), Healthy Steps for Young Children (Minkovitz et al, 2007), and The Incredible Years (Webster-Stratton, 2005) can be used. Specific questions are suggested to elicit responses from parents and guide the visit and to provide anticipatory guidance and counseling. No matter what framework is selected, anticipatory guidance should include information that helps reinforce positive health behaviors, minimizes or eliminates health risks, and facilitates optimal family functioning—all grounded in an understanding of the child's developmental stage and individual developmental needs.

• BOX 4-1 Parenting Red Flags

Moderate Concern

Disinclination to separate from child or prematurely hastening separation
Signs of despondency, apathy, or hostility
Fearful, dependent, apprehensive
Disinterested in or rejecting of infant or child
Overly critical, mocking, and censuring of child; tendency to undermine child's confidence
Inconsistent in discipline or control; erratic in behavior
Highly restrictive and overly moralistic environment
Turning away from eye-to-eye contact

Extreme Concern

Extreme depression and withdrawal; rejection of child
Intense hostility; aggression toward child
Uncontrollable fears, anxieties, guilt
Complete inability to function in family role
Severe moralistic prohibition of child's independent strivings
Domestic abuse or violence in the home
Self-destructive behaviors—alcohol or drug abuse
Untreated mental health issues (e.g., parent with diagnosis of bipolar disorder, schizophrenia, or delusional disorder)

There is a wealth of popular literature available to guide parents as they raise their children. The PCP can be an invaluable resource for parents by accurately assessing and competently caring for the child's needs; by supporting positive parent behaviors or actions; and by providing the information, suggestions, strategies, and guidance needed to be good parents. PCPs should be familiar with popular parenting books, television shows and parenting "experts" so they can help parents to better evaluate the parenting advice they contain. Giving parents positive feedback, being open to teaching, and listening to parents' concerns build parent confidence, create a trusting relationship, and establish comfort for bringing forth more difficult concerns if such discussion is necessary. The provider-family relationship can be a powerful tool to guide family members' management of their child's temperament, behavior, and development. The benefit of establishing a long-term, continuous relationship with a child and family cannot be overestimated.

Certain "red flags" related to parent-child interactions indicate that further assessment of the home environment, parent-child interaction, and child's development is indicated. Box 4-1 identifies some of these parental red flags.

Discipline

Children do not always behave the way their parents would wish. The question of how parents should deal with children's misbehavior has led to a wealth of books on parenting and discipline, strategies for child management, and many frustrated parents. Parents often use a combination of strategies—spanking, yelling, timeout, taking away a favorite toy, or reasoning with the child—and ideally they will tailor their response to the age and situation. Although families have differing temperaments, styles, and beliefs, there are some basic principles and guidelines about discipline that providers can discuss with parents to help them handle discipline. The American Academy of Pediatrics (AAP), in its 1998 policy statement (reaffirmed in 2014), stated that "effective discipline requires three essential components: (1) a positive, supportive, loving relationship between the parent(s) and child; (2) use of positive reinforcement strategies to increase desired behaviors; and (3) removing reinforcement or applying punishment to reduce or eliminate undesired behaviors" (AAP, 1998, p 723). All three of these components guide the principles discussed here:

- Parents should talk with each other to come to agreement on how they will handle discipline and their child's misbehavior.
- They should distinguish between discipline and punishment.
  - Discipline is training or education that molds the behavior, mental capacities, or moral character of an individual. Discipline is used by the parent to teach the child appropriate behavior and to keep the child safe.
  - Punishment, on the other hand, is loss, pain, or suffering that is administered in response to behavior; it is a form of retribution.
- Parents should focus their interactions with children on discipline, rather than punishment. As with the food pyramid in which wholesome grains, proteins, fruits, and vegetables form the base for good nutrition, a "parenting pyramid" describes teaching, play, guidance, role modeling, and thoughtful correction of a child's behavior as the broad base for parent-child interactions (Fig. 4-1; Webster-Stratton, 2005). Like nutrient-empty foods, punishment should be used as little as possible.
- Misbehavior can often be prevented. When a child appears willful, bored, or out-of-sorts, distraction and active engagement with the parent (e.g., giving the child something to do; talking to, playing with, or dancing with the child) can be used to stop misbehavior before it starts.
- Parents need to be alert to when children reach their limits (i.e., are nearing "meltdown" because they are tired, hungry, or overstimulated) and intervene to prevent problems from occurring.
- Children who are at a "meltdown" stage are not able to relate rationally to a parent's reasoned explanation or request; the underlying problem—hunger, lack of sleep, and so on—must be dealt with first. Conversely, parents may need a "timeout" from the child to cool down and regain self-control. Parents should have a plan for help when they need respite.
- All children need rules, limits, and expectations that should be reasonable and appropriate to the age and developmental capabilities of the child. A 3-month-old,

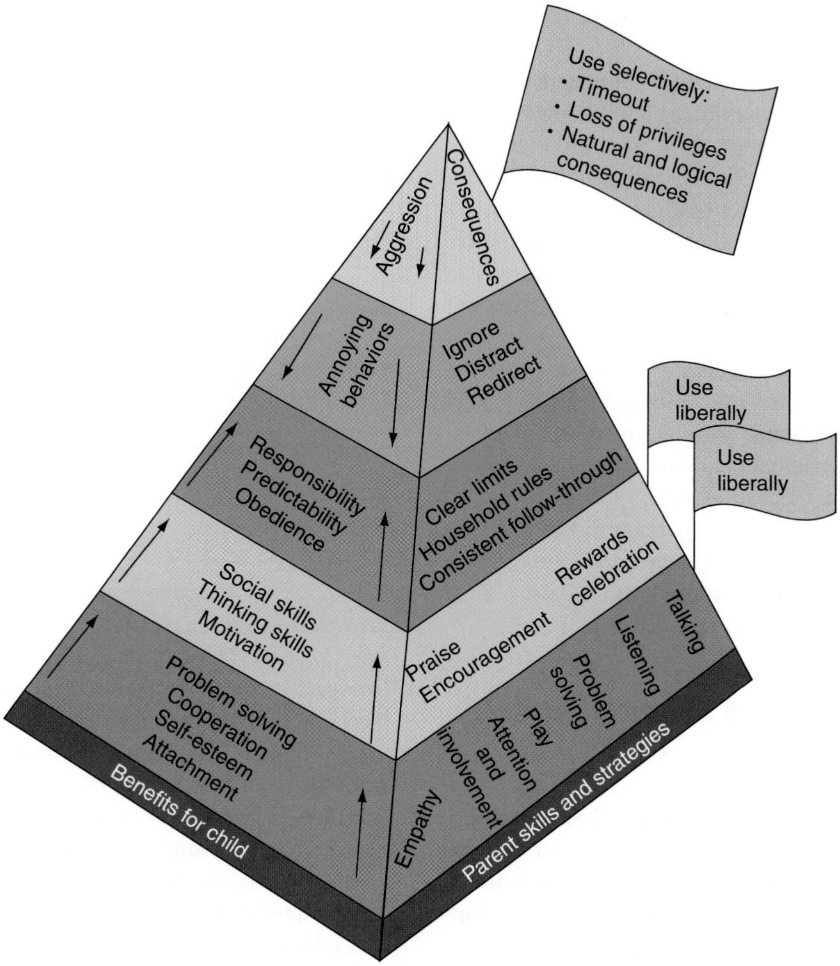

• **Figure 4-1** Parenting pyramid. (From Webster-Stratton C: *The incredible years: a trouble shooting guide for parents of children aged 2-8*, Seattle, 2005, Incredible Years Press.)

for example, cannot be expected to stop crying when her parents tell her to. As children grow, they should negotiate with their parents to help set the rules. This parent-child interaction helps children learn how to be active, valued family members and builds their social skills.

- Parents should be sure that the rules are clear and specific and should strive for consistency in adhering to them. Even young children benefit when the parent explains what the rules are and why they are necessary.
- Be flexible when responding to a child's behavior. Parents should agree about what issues are important to stand firm on. A wise parent learns to not sweat the small stuff, and chooses to ignore very minor infractions while rewarding positive behaviors.
- Parents should role model expected behaviors.
- Adhering to rules should be rewarded. Parents should be encouraged to catch their children "being good" and give praise, encouragement, or rewards. Praise and encouragement are powerful reinforcements for good behavior. Some parents find a 4:1 ratio to be a good rule of thumb (that is, four positive reinforcements for every negative).
- Praise and rewards for following the rules are different from "bribes" for being good (e.g., "If you stop crying, I'll get you an ice cream cone."), which should be discouraged.
- Children should be treated with respect and empathy, even when being reprimanded for misbehavior.
- Breaking rules should lead to natural and logical consequences.
- Consequences should be given immediately, be fair, and should relate to the rule broken.
- Consequences should be appropriate to the age and developmental capabilities of the child. Timeout, being sent to the child's room, restricting a favorite activity, and turning off the television or video games are all examples of consequences that have been successfully used. For example, if a 6-year-old child refuses to share, he can be sent to his room for "alone time." If a 4-year-old pushes or punches her sibling, she can be given a timeout or not be allowed to play with a friend. If a 10-year-old breaks the neighbor's window with her baseball, she can be expected to apologize, help clean up the mess, and work to pay for the new window. As

children grow, they should help determine the consequences for misbehavior.

- Parents should follow through on limits. Frequent threats (e.g., "If you do that one more time, I'll send you to your room!") without follow-through teach the child that they can continue their misbehavior without consequence and may lead to a parent's belief that their children won't listen to them. Learning early that they are accountable for their behavior is an invaluable lesson for children.
- Punishment should never be a withdrawal of the parent's love or affection.
- Corporal punishment is unnecessary and has the potential to cause physical and/or psychologic damage.

No parent is perfect, and parents bring their own upbringing to the role. Parental behavior may reflect efforts to "be like my parents were" or, as seems more often the case, "not do things wrong, like my parents did with me." Providers should acknowledge that parents are trying to do the best that they can and encourage them to relax and discover how they and their child can best interact.

Concerns about Delayed Development

Developmental Red Flags

Child development is exceptionally varied. A 2-year-old girl may use full complex sentences, whereas her 3-year-old neighbor relies on three-word directives (e.g., "Want milk, peeze.") to get what he desires. Both can be normal, but the differences may be striking, and parents may express concern that their child is "delayed." Prevalence estimates of developmental and behavioral disorders in the United States range from 12% to 16% (Berry et al, 2014). Health care providers should keep in mind certain red flags related to normal child development when seeing infants and children for well-child care or minor acute illnesses. These red flags are highlighted in each of the following chapters in this unit.

A standardized developmental screening is needed at every well visit and any time a concern is noted, with a follow-up developmental assessment as appropriate. A decision must be made as to whether the child is progressing appropriately or whether intervention is indicated. Information from the history, physical examination, developmental screening and assessment, hearing and vision screening, and other indicated tests are essential in making this decision. It is also important to consider the cause of developmental delays when making a judgment whether to intervene directly or to refer (Box 4-2).

Children with screening findings that are very near normal may be mildly delayed but not eligible for early intervention services (criteria for early intervention vary from state to state, and a child may need to be between 25% and 50% delayed to be eligible in some states). Children with a mild delay and/or those who are at risk may benefit from activities, such as encouraging "tummy time" when awake (e.g., for an infant who is not yet rolling over).

• BOX 4-2 Etiologies of Developmental Delays

- Central nervous system dysfunction
- Mental health problem
- Chronic disease affecting either functional abilities or activity tolerance (e.g., cardiovascular, visual, auditory)
- Child abuse and neglect
- Maternal or paternal stress
- Developmentally inappropriate animate or inanimate environment, or both
- Lack of parental knowledge of development
- Genetic syndromes
- Depression
- Attention-deficit hyperactivity disorder
- Autism spectrum
- Regulatory or sensory dysfunctions
- Unknown causes

Providers can use a manual such as the *Hawaii Early Learning Program (HELP) at Home Manual* (see Additional Resources) to assist them with suggestions for parents who have children with mild delays in various domains. They can also make referrals to early intervention programs, such as Early Head Start and YMCA classes. These opportunities can also allow parents to begin working on an area while waiting for early intervention services to begin.

Understanding possible causes helps the provider plan appropriate developmental care, including parent counseling, educational programs, and referral choices (e.g., Which developmental specialist is most appropriate to further assess the child? Which treatment modality, such as speech or physical therapy, would be most effective?). The discussion in Chapter 28 of the management of cerebral palsy illustrates the decision-making process used in cases of developmental delay. The PCP should not assume that waiting will remedy a problem when parents express a concern or when developmental delays are noted; even though developmental progress may occur, the rate and quality can be abnormal. In addition, parents' stress and anxiety about their child can cause further problems. Neither can the PCP assume that all developmental problems can be fixed with home remedies (e.g., changing parenting or environmental factors), sometimes developmental problems are indicators of serious systemic, particularly neurologic, dysfunctions.

Vulnerability and resilience are two characteristics that have been shown to significantly impact health and wellness. *Vulnerability* refers to a person's sensitivity and inclination to decompensate in the face of life stressors. *Resilience* (sometimes called *hardiness*), in contrast, is a person's capacity to survive intact, both psychologically and physically, despite adversity. In children, these characteristics affect outcomes as stressors come and go in the child's life experiences. Many children demonstrate remarkable resilience despite significant risks; others are less capable of coping. Any child who fails to move ahead as expected, or begins to deteriorate developmentally requires an immediate developmental assessment and diagnostic evaluation.

Talking with Parents about Developmental Delays

Talking with parents on a routine, ongoing basis about their child's development usually makes it easier should a specific developmental problem appear, although it can be a challenging process. It is essential for the PCP to listen and be sensitive to parental concerns. Typically, parents notice differences in the child first and seek reassurance or confirmation of problems from their health care provider. Parents have reported that they have expressed their concerns to their health care provider only to be reassured or told let's "wait and see." Later on, as problems become more obvious and a referral is finally made, they are understandably frustrated that they were not listened to initially and that services to their child have been delayed.

When a problem is found, a strength-based approach can help soothe the experience of receiving "bad news." Each infant and child has areas in which development is progressing, even if the progress is not consistent with usual development. Discussing these areas in addition to the parents' concerns is important. Focusing on strengths *first* provides parents with a framework for understanding their child's unique strengths along with any particular developmental challenges.

Parents may be overwhelmed with the news that their child has a developmental problem. To determine whether parents understand what they have been told, the provider can ask the parent how they are going to explain what has been discussed to others at home. To increase parents' follow-through, providers need to be very familiar with referral resources. They should walk the parent through the next steps in the process, and after allotting time for the family to complete the referral visit, follow up with a phone call or office or home visit with the family.

Above all, it is important to be honest, positive, and realistic. Most often, the long-term prognosis for developmental delays is unknown because of continuing brain development. Parents want to know what they can do and, specifically, how they can assist their child. They also need support and time to cope with their own feelings. Different families have different expectations for their children, so a child with mild delay may be more devastating to one family than a child with severe developmental delays may be to another.

Implementing Individualized Interventions

Early Intervention Programs

Children with developmental delays should receive appropriate referral or more frequent visits, or both, particularly during the first year of life (see Chapter 21 for a discussion of issues related to children with chronic illnesses). Many difficulties with parent-child interaction and/or learning, behavioral, and attachment problems can be avoided or more effectively managed by offering parental counseling or referral to appropriate community services (e.g., a social worker, community health nurse, or mental health specialist) during the first year of life. The longer the problem lasts, the more difficult it is to resolve. Most communities have early infant education programs for infants and young children (birth to 3 years old) provided for under Public Law 108-466. This law, the Individuals with Disabilities Education Improvement Act of 2004, is a reauthorization of Public Law 99-457 that was enacted at the federal level in 1986. This law requires developmental screening and early intervention programs for infants and young children at risk for developmental delay. The individualized family service plan (IFSP) is a process that includes the family in planning services for children. PCPs may be asked to participate in the meetings in which the IFSP is developed with the family. Often, however, PCPs are not involved in IFSP development, but they should be aware of the plan. These plans can be established through school systems, health departments, or developmental programs and vary significantly in quality and comprehensiveness from one community to another. The importance of structured plans that stimulate growth of all children cannot be overestimated. Providers need to be familiar with community resources and educate community leaders and legislators about the developmental and health needs of children and families.

There are a number of comorbidities associated with developmental disorders that occur because of the functional impairment or secondary to the medical management of these conditions. Common complications of developmental disorders include alterations in gastrointestinal motility, malnutrition, urinary tract infections, impaired airway clearance, frequent upper respiratory tract infections, and altered neuromuscular tone (Garzon et al, 2010). Children with developmental delays may require special attention in many areas, including assessment of medical and dental needs, feeding, sleep, elimination, activity, temperament, and behavior. Interventions, such as education regarding medications, modifications of therapies as a result of the child's health status, referrals to parent groups, and assistance regarding organization of the child's health records, are greatly appreciated by the family.

School Intervention Resources

Public Law 94-142, enacted in 1975, addresses the needs of children older than 3 years. Under this legislation, schools are mandated to provide appropriate education to all children with developmental delays, including opportunities for mainstreaming children with developmental delays or handicaps into regular classrooms. Special education services assist in this process through the development of an individualized education plan (IEP).

Planning sessions for IFSPs or IEPs determine the developmental or school services offered during a designated period of time for a particular child, usually each calendar year or each school year. If a child's or family's needs are not identified, services are not made available. Often health care

TABLE 4-4 Comparison of Child-Centered and Family-Centered Care

Child-Centered Care	Family-Centered Care
Goal: Focus on child's care.	*Goal:* Parental empowerment and child advocacy for the life of the child.
Child's needs are primary focus.	Family needs to assist the child are the focus.
Professionals decide on the plan of care.	Family and professionals decide on the plan of care.
Parents' opinions are not consistently requested or valued.	Parents' ideas are requested and valued.
Families are considered part of a particular group.	Families are all considered to be unique.
Parents participate as observers.	Parents are considered to be equal members at whatever level they are comfortable.
Parental differences are judged as not being in the best interest of the child.	Family culture, language, ethnicity, and structure are respected.
Test results of the child are the most important factor used to plan care.	Focus is on addressing parental concerns, issues, questions, and their need for assistance in problem-solving.
One-way communication is used—professional to parent.	Two-way communication is used with parents encouraged to have input into the child's care plan.

needs are not considered in these planning sessions. Primary health care providers should advocate for families and children. In this role, they help clarify children's health needs and ensure that parental concerns, health care services, and educational services are appropriately coordinated (Jackson Allen et al, 2010).

Family-Centered Care

The National Association of Pediatric Nurse Practitioners (NAPNAP) (2009), Public Law 99-457, and the AAP (AAP and Duby, 2007) all emphasize the importance of pediatric health care providers working with the family when addressing children's health. A partnership with the family is crucial in order for families to become comfortable and engaged in creating the plan of care for their child. Each family's cultural values, learning styles, and health beliefs and practices must be respected. The shift from child-centered to family-centered care is represented in Table 4-4.

Care Coordination

The Maternal and Child Health Bureau (MCHB) and the AAP define children with special health care needs as "those who have or are at increased risk for chronic physical, developmental, behavioral, or emotional conditions and who also require health and related services of a type or amount beyond that required by children generally" (McPherson et al, 1998, p 138). Care coordination is one of the key elements for children with special needs, and the PCP is ideally suited to direct the health care home. Because of their nursing background and appreciation for the complex needs of this population, nurse practitioners (NPs) have the unique skills to function as care coordinators. In order to help families access parent and community resources to sustain the long-term care of their child, PCPs must become "community-wise" through professional networks, parent groups, and educational connections. It is essential to develop a system with up-to-date referral agencies and contact information (see Chapter 9). Children with special health care needs are best served when they receive tailored, family-focused, culturally appropriate care from a health care home that supports shared decision-making and individualized care (Lindeke et al, 2010).

There are public and private entities that provide support services for children with special health care needs, and it is critical that PCPs be aware of which services are available in their area. However, it is not enough simply to give a family a name and phone number of a referral source. All too often, parents' phone calls lead to busy signals, disconnected numbers, or the wrong agency for their needs. These deterrents can discourage even the most willing family from pursuing needed resources for their child. Parents may hesitate to seek resources because of apprehension about the outcome of the referral, costs, time constraints, or lack of understanding about the need for timely follow-up. When the provider intervenes to guide families through the referral process and coordinate services, parents have greater confidence in the new health care or educational resource and are more likely to achieve appropriate follow-up for their child.

For a complete list of references, please visit http://evolve.elsevier.com/Burns/pediatric/.

5 Developmental Management of Infants

JOY S. DIAMOND AND ANITA D. BERRY

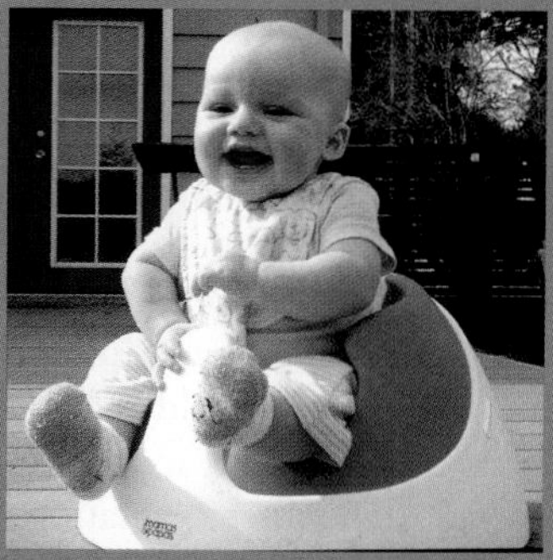

Infancy is an exciting time for everyone involved—the infant, his or her immediate family, extended family members, and others in the infant's immediate community. Pediatric health care providers are privileged to be able to work with families during this period of rapid, predictable (yet individually unique), and challenging change. As part of the routine care of infants and their families, primary care providers assess and monitor growth and development; educate parents about child development; collaborate with other health professionals; offer guidance about ways to foster healthy growth and development; identify and manage health problems; and guide, counsel, and support parents dealing with their infant's health or illness.

During pregnancy and early life, internal physiologic and neurologic factors and external factors (such as, light, sound, touch, position, taste, and movement) affect the infant. In the first year, physical growth, brain development, the infant's environment, and particularly the actions of the infant's caregivers influence an infant's ability to develop consistent and predictable responses to internal and external stimuli. General learning and skills acquisition for later reading and writing begin at birth, not in kindergarten or first grade. Language and literacy skills grow with everyday loving interactions—sharing books, telling stories, singing songs, and talking to one another. Adults play a very important role in preparing young children for future school success and becoming self-confident and motivated learners. Responsive, nurturing relationships between infants and their adult caregivers help build positive attachments, support healthy social-emotional development, and are the foundation of mental health for infants, toddlers, and preschoolers. Such relationships strengthen all aspects of an infant's development.

Birth Rates and Infant Mortality

National trends in birth rates and infant mortality are important measures of population-based infant health. The number of live births in the United States was slightly higher in 2013 than 2012. The general fertility rate was 62.9 births per 1,000 women aged 15 to 44, which was down slightly from 2012, and a record low. The birth rate for teens 15 to 19 years old declined by 10% in 2013, which was another historic low for the nation, with rates declining for both younger and older teenagers. The birth rate for women in their early 20s declined to a record low of 81.2 births per 1,000, and birth rates for women in their 30s and 40s rose. The preterm birth rate fell for the seventh year in a row to 11.38% in 2013 (Hamilton et al, 2014). In all age groups, the populations with the highest birth rates are Hispanics and non-Hispanic African Americans, whereas Asians and non-Hispanic whites have the lowest birth rates (Hamilton et al, 2013).

Infant mortality rates in the United States vary greatly by race and ethnicity. From 2009 to 2010, the infant mortality rate declined by 3% for non-Hispanic white women and 8% for non-Hispanic black women. The highest rate of infant mortality was that of infants of non-Hispanic black mothers. The leading causes of infant mortality are congenital malformations, low birth weight, prematurity, maternal delivery complications, multiple gestations, sudden infant death syndrome (SIDS), and unintentional injuries. Of the 3.98 million babies born in the United States every year, approximately 4,200 infants die for no obvious reason. SIDS is the third leading cause of overall infant mortality in the United States and is estimated to cause half of the cases of unexplained infant death (Mathews and MacDorman, 2013). The SIDS rate declined significantly since 1992 when the American Academy of Pediatrics (AAP) began its "Back to Sleep" campaign (Task Force on Sudden Infant Death Syndrome and Moon, 2011).

Development of Infants

Birth to One Month Old

Physical Development

Newborn assessment begins with gestational age determination using the Dubowitz/Ballard examination or similar gestational age scale (see Chapter 39). It is important to document significant prematurity, intrauterine growth restriction (IUGR), and size for gestational age (i.e., either large for gestational age [LGA] or small for gestational age [SGA]). Compare the reported gestational age with the infant's birth weight, length, and head circumference.

The infant may initially lose up to 5% to 8% of birth weight but should regain it within 10 to 14 days. Weight loss of 10% or more requires close monitoring and may require further evaluation. Weight gain after the initial loss averages 0.5 or 1 ounce (14 to 28 g) per day, or about 2 pounds (nearly 1 kg) per month. Nutritional needs to promote growth are approximately 110 kcal/kg/day (see Chapter 10).

Term newborns have cyclical arousal states, which are equivalent to the level of consciousness in older children and adults. Normal newborns move from state to state in smooth transitions. There are two sleep states: quiet sleep and active sleep. Quiet sleep occurs when the infant is in deep sleep, shows little movement, and is difficult to arouse even when touched or stimulated by sound. Active sleep, the most common type of sleep, involves rapid eye movement (REM), smiling, sucking, and brief fussing or crying. Babies who fuss during active sleep are not in distress or hungry. They wake when cold, hungry, and so on; and they typically respond to touch, rocking, or voices. There are four common awake states:

- Drowsy: Infants in this state are quiet and appear sleepy but can become fussy or active if stimulated. They respond to stimuli slower than those in an alert state. Blinking and yawning are common.
- Quiet but alert: Infants in this state frequently look around and quietly observe their environment; they brighten with stimulation from caregivers or other sources. Infants who are quiet but alert are often described as being happy. It is common for infants to transition from quiet but alert to sleep states or the alert and active state.
- Crying: Infants in this state have bursts of crying that last at least 15 seconds. Hunger, cold, fatigue, and other noxious stimuli make this phase more pronounced. Infants typically transition from crying to sleep or alert and active phases.
- Alert and active: Infants in this state keep their eyes open but are likely to fuss if hungry, soiled, tired, or overstimulated. They may wiggle and make faces during this time. When consoled by caregivers, they can calm and either fall asleep or go into a quiet but alert state.

The infant's autonomic nervous system stability is evaluated through heart rate, respiratory rate, temperature control, and color changes. The infant should demonstrate some degree of arousal state regulation and transition easily from deep sleep through quiet alert to active alert and crying. A variety of techniques can be used to arouse the newborn for feedings. The newborn sleeps about 16 out of 24 hours and, if encouraged to breastfeed every 2 to 3 hours, may have one longer stretch of four hours at night. It is important to assess for a normal-pitched cry because problems, such as hypothyroidism and genetic disorders (e.g., cri du chat syndrome), can cause voice alterations.

Motor Skills Development

The newborn's flexed posture allows the infant to self-console when positioned so that the hands reach the face and mouth. Primary reflexes, such as sucking, rooting, asymmetric tonic neck, Moro, and grasp, should be present and symmetric. Passive muscle tone is not normal in term newborns and is observed on the gestational age scales by assessing shoulder (scarf sign) and knee flexibility (popliteal angle). Arm and leg recoil provide information about the infant's active movements, particularly symmetry and coordination. Jerkiness and tremors may be noted. The neonatal period begins a remarkable series of fine and gross motor skill milestones for the infant (Table 5-1).

Communication and Language Development

The newborn gives clear signals of distress, such as crying, arching, or gagging. These help the caregiver respond to the infant's needs. The newborn should orient to sound and light. Newborns use self-consoling or self-calming behaviors such as sucking, moving hand to mouth, or grasping clothing. Articulation begins at birth with the infant's first cry. In the first few weeks of life, infants make sounds of comfort and discomfort.

Social and Emotional Development

Social skills are evident as the newborn quiets and turns to the parent's voice. The caregiver can foster social and emotional development by making eye contact; speaking, crooning, or singing in a soft voice; and touching, caressing, and holding the baby. Reading to newborns can be soothing for both parent and the baby.

Cognitive-Sensory Development

Vision is limited, but the newborn has the ability to focus briefly on a face or bright object when it is brought into visual range (about 8 to 12 inches from the infant's face). Newborns visually track objects to midline. Of all the senses, the sense of smell is most acute in newborns. Hearing is also fairly well developed.

One through Three Months Old

Physical Development

During the first 3 months the infant experiences many physical and developmental changes. Length increases about 1.4 inches (3.5 cm) per month, and head circumference increases about 0.8 inch (2 cm) per month, with more rapid growth for the younger infant. The infant typically gains 0.5 to 1 ounce (14 to 28 g) per day and has 8 to 10 feedings in 24 hours, each lasting 20 to 30 minutes. Feedings lasting longer than 40 minutes and shorter than 20 minutes need to be evaluated. At about 6 to 8 weeks, the infant may experience a growth spurt and fuss to eat more frequently. Mothers who are breastfeeding need extra encouragement during this time because they may believe

TABLE 5-1 **Fine Motor and Gross Motor Development Milestones for Infants**

Age	Fine Motor Movement	Oral Movement	Motor Movement
Birth	Flexion	Suckling tongue movements, extension-retraction of tongue, up-and-down jaw movements, low approximation of lips	Momentary head control when held sitting
1 month old	Extension, nondirected hand swipes	Rooting	Turns head when prone
4 months old	Directed swipes, corralling, reaching		Sits with support, begins to roll over, head steady in sitting
4-5 months old	Ulnar-palmar grasp		"Swims" in prone position, no head lag
6-7 months old	Radial-palmar grasp, raking	Sucking with negative oral cavity pressure, rhythmic jaw movements, firm approximation of lips	Sits independently, rolls over, rocks on hands and knees, free head lift in prone position
7-8 months old	Radial-digital grasp	Phasic bite reflex, rhythmic bite and release pattern	Supports weight standing, bounces when held
7-9 months old	Scissors grasp	Munching, early chewing	Sits alone well, may crawl
9-10 months old	Voluntary release		Cruises, pivots while seated, pulls to stand
12 months old	Picks up pellet with pincer grasp	Chewing with spreading and rolling tongue movements, tongue lateralization, rotary jaw movements, controlled sustained bite	Walks with one hand held, stands alone momentarily

that they do not have enough milk for their baby. Provider reassurance can be backed up by an interval infant weight check if the mother is overly concerned. Providers should instruct mothers to follow their infant's cues for feeding; pointing out that the extra suckling will increase the milk supply sufficiently to meet their growing infant's needs (see Chapter 11). Elimination patterns become more regular. Infants go from defecating with each feeding to having one or two bowel movements daily or every other day if formula fed, and bowel movements that range from once or twice daily to once every 3 to 5 days or longer if breastfed. Wet diapers typically occur after each feeding.

Sleep cycles become more regular, about 15 to 16 hours per day, with defined sleep-wake patterns. Regular nap or nighttime routines help keep infants calmer. The infant may need more organized play periods when sleep periods consolidate into more consistent naps. Many infants have fussy periods in the late evening that may last 1 to 3 hours. Infant crying tends to peak at this age, but fortunately this fussiness usually lasts only a few weeks. The provider should discuss with parents plans to cope with crying before this time is upon them. This is a good time to explain "shaken baby syndrome" and the period of PURPLE crying to parents (see Crying section later in this chapter and Additional Resources). It is important to talk with parents about how to respond when they feel frustrated or overwhelmed by their baby. Encourage them to take a parental "time out," to allow the infant to cry in the crib, and to encourage identifying a back-up helper for when they are overstressed or overtired. Encourage them and others who care for the infant to have a repertoire of coping skills.

Motor Skills Development

Fine motor skills begin to emerge as primitive reflexes become integrated. Infants attempt to grasp rattles, fingers, and clothing. They demonstrate visible head control, lifting the head off the bed about 45 degrees when in the prone position and showing little head droop when held in suspension. All normal body movements are symmetric (see Table 5-1).

Communication and Language Development

Parents should be encouraged to observe how their infant looks at them when they are talking and how intently the infant looks at faces, especially during the quiet alert state, which is the time when the infant is most interactive. Infants "connect" with parents, even if only for a few moments. Parents encourage early language development when they talk to their infant during caregiving activities. Infants start to make cooing and babbling sounds, much to the delight of their parents. Table 5-2 lists receptive and expressive language skills for the first year of life. However, body movements (e.g., snuggling, turning the head, arching the body) are the primary form of communication, and

TABLE 5-2 Speech and Language Milestones: Areas for Surveillance

Age	Receptive Language	Expressive Language
0-3 months old	Attends to voice, turns head or eyes Startles to loud sounds Quiets in response to voice Smiles, coos, gurgles to voice	Undifferentiated but strong cry Coos and gurgles Single-syllable repetition *g, k, h,* and *ng* appear
3-6 months old	Actively seeks sound source May look in response to name Responses may vary to angry or happy voice	Increased babbling, vocal play Increased repetitive babbling (gaga) Laughs Vocalizes to toys Spontaneous smile to verbal play Increased intensity and nasal tone Vocalizes to removal of toy Experiments with own voice
6-9 months old	May look at family member when named Inhibits to "no" Begins interest in pictures when named Individual words begin to take on meaning	Babbles tunefully Increased sound combinations Uses *m, n, b, d, t* Initiates sounds, such as click or kiss Uses nonspecific "mama" and "dada"
9-12 months old	Gives toy on request Understands simple commands Turns head to own name Understands "hot," "where's ...?" Responds with gestures to "bye-bye"	Increased imitating efforts Has one word with specific reference Accompanies vocalizations with gestures Jargon increases Imitates animal sounds

providers can help parents identify and become more skilled at interpreting their infant's cues.

Social and Emotional Development

At this age, the infant becomes highly social, imitating the parent's expressions and visually following the parent. Infants are more responsive to sounds in their environment, attending to sounds by quieting body movements or demonstrating visual responses. By 3 months old, infants demonstrate a social smile and will usually smile in response to their parent's voice. As infants become more active, alert, and responsive, parents may mistakenly assume that the infant can handle more activity and stimulation. It is important for caregivers to develop sensitivity to infant cues for the need to rest or to have decreased stimulation.

Cognitive Development

By 4 to 8 weeks old, infants readily begin to take in more of their environment. The infant visually tracks faces or toys past midline, vertically, and horizontally. Even very young infants demonstrate various facial expressions, respond to sounds, and attempt to imitate mouthing movements. By 3 months old, infants begin to enjoy toys and may wave their arms when a toy is brought into sight.

Four through Five Months Old

Physical Development

Infants 4 through 5 months old have regular patterns of eating, sleeping, and playing. They sleep 12 to 15 hours a day with five feedings during the day and one during the night. By this age, infants begin to sleep through the night without feeding. Somewhere between 4 and 6 months old, infants double their birth weight, and growth slows to a gain of about 5 ounces (140 g) a week. The infant's length increases about 0.8 inch (2 cm) per month, and head circumference about 0.4 inch (1 cm) per month. Growth may appear in spurts, although the overall growth chart will show a steady upward curve. Weight gain can be influenced by the amount of play activity and the sleep schedule.

Motor Skills Development

Fine motor skills are demonstrated as infants play with their hands and begin to reach for and pull at clothing or other objects that are close, such as the parent's hair, earrings, or eyeglasses. They grasp toys and start to place their hands on the breast or the bottle in an attempt to hold or pat it.

Motor skills progress (see Table 5-1) as the Moro and asymmetric tonic neck reflexes are integrated and infants no longer reflexively extend their arm when their head turns. The Landau reflex emerges. Infants at this age begin to roll. Those who spend sufficient time in a prone position generally roll first front to back and then from back to front. Head control becomes stronger and more sustained, and there should be no head lag when the baby is pulled to sit. When in the prone position, infants hold their head up at 45 degrees, gradually progressing to 90 degrees for sustained periods of time. The infant learns to sit, first in the tripod stance, and then unassisted with the head held erect. When lying supine, infants can lift their legs and bring their feet to their mouth. They bear full weight when standing and enjoy bouncing up and down in a parent's lap. All their body movements should be symmetric.

Communication and Language Development

Infants' social skills increase and verbal skills become more evident (see Table 5-2). They begin babbling, using vowel sounds, cooing, laughing quietly, and experimenting with variations in tone and pitch, such as low-pitched chuckles and deeper belly laughs. Eventually they laugh out loud, much to the enjoyment of those around them. Infants' responses to sounds gradually become more localized, and they search for the sound of a bell or rattle.

Oral-motor development is a prerequisite for speech. Throughout infancy oral development progresses from sucking and rooting to rhythmic biting and chewing. Beginning at about 6 months old and continuing through 2 years old, the child learns to chew by moving the jaw up and down while flattening and spreading the tongue, and to control biting by using rotary jaw movements with lateralization of tongue placement. These motor skills, essential for the production of speech, are among the most complex movements that the young child must master.

Social and Emotional Development

At this age, infants' social skills become more evident, and parents often find their baby to be engaging and entertaining. Usual behavior includes spontaneous smiling at parents and others while visually following the caregiver around the environment and turning the head a full 180 degrees. They promptly look at an object when it is placed in front of them; they notice things. The infant's increasing awareness of the environment facilitates more complex social interactions. Infants begin to recognize that their parents are responding to their needs. They notice, for example, as the parent prepares to offer the breast or get a bottle ready for feeding. Because infants notice other things, parents can often distract them from demanding immediate gratification by talking, playing, or using other social interactions, such as reciprocal vocalizations and eye contact. As a result, infants learn that their hunger needs will be met, but that there are other satisfying interactions they can have with their caregiver. Infants at this age begin to more actively reciprocate their parents' attention and enjoy playing with their parents. Crying may reflect tiredness or a need for social interaction, not just hunger. Parents should acknowledge their child's unique personality, because this reciprocal recognition is an important aspect of infant-parent attachment.

Cognitive Development

Visual exploration increases during this age as infants seek out objects in the environment, such as mobiles, mirrors, their hands, and the toys they are holding. They prefer to look at their parents' or another person's face. Chewing and mouthing are means of exploration used to differentiate textures, tastes, and shapes. As their muscle control improves, they are able to bring a toy to their mouth, first when lying on their back and then when sitting.

Six through Eight Months Old

Physical Development

As infants reduce their breast milk or formula intake and add solids to their diet, growth velocity changes. Weight gain slows to 3 to 4 ounces (85 to 110 g) a week, or about 1 pound (0.5 kg) a month; length gains are about 0.5 to 0.6 inch (1.2 to 1.5 cm) per month; and head circumference increases about 0.2 inch (0.5 cm) per month. Teething symptoms can begin at about 6 months as the central incisors emerge and at 8 months when the lateral incisors emerge. The first childhood illness might occur at the same time as teething behaviors start and these events can disrupt the infant's previous sleep routine (see Chapter 34 for a discussion of teething).

Motor Skills Development

Infants at this age love to explore their environment, an activity that fosters motor skills development. Infants sit erect for longer periods of time and may scoot while in a sitting position. Crawling begins with the infant pushing up to the hands and knees and rocking in place, then eventually mastering the rhythm of hands and knees working together. Many infants will pull themselves along on the floor with their arms and use one foot or toe to push while their stomachs remain on the floor, prior to beginning to use hands and knees to crawl. Infants may stand, fully supporting their weight, when their hands are held at shoulder height.

Fine motor skills continue to be honed, and babies are more adept at using their palm and all of their fingers to pick up objects. Initially they rake at small objects and are able to hold a small cube, lifting it off the table. Gradually they use fingers and thumb to pick up objects. They reach for and grasp toys, can hold a toy in each hand at the same time, and can transfer objects from one hand to another. Some families introduce solid food to infants using the "infant-led-weaning" method with all foods being manipulated by the infant (see Chapter 10).

Communication and Language Development

Vocalizations increase in pitch and tone, and specific sound imitation begins. Infants articulate single-sound units that may be vowels, consonants, or blends, such as "ah," "ba," "da," "ga," "ch," and "bl." Gradually, they progress to double-consonant sounds (e.g., "dada") and occasionally will vocalize using three or more different syllables. They use "mama" and "dada," but they do not understand the meaning behind these sounds. Infants delight their parents as they respond to verbal cues and play at making sounds and noises when alone. They enjoy imitating oral sounds, such as "raspberries" and coughing.

Although infants' expressive language skills are limited, their receptive language is evident when they listen and respond to their parents' talking. Infants distinguish facial expressions and gestures, may stop or quiet when their parent uses "no" or a different tone of voice, and turn toward their parents' voices and other sounds, localizing directly to the sound.

Instruct parents to begin daily reading to their child by 6 months old if they have not already done so. This can be introduced as part of the bedtime routine. Parents should focus on simple board books and use books as a way to talk to their infants, because they do not have the attention span to sit through a whole book. Infants should not watch TV or videos (both are passive media), because they are more positively stimulated and learn language best when interacting with another person, listening to parents' or caregivers' voices, and looking at a face that responds to them.

Social and Emotional Development

Infants at this age greatly enjoy social play, and their individual personality and temperament continue to be expressed. Infants may express frustration or do things like reject a spoon during feeding, preferring instead to feed themselves. Small issues with give-and-take and control may arise even if parents understand their infant's cues and engage with the infant responsively. Infants use gestures such as pointing, reaching with outstretched arms, tugging, vocalizing, and throwing things to get their parent's attention and communicate their needs. As infants' abilities and desires become more complex, and they expand their repertoire of communication cues, parents need to learn new parenting skills (e.g., how to handle a determined child) to meet their infant's social development needs. Stranger and separation anxiety may appear at this time.

Cognitive Development

Infant cognitive development grows significantly between 5 and 8 months old. The infant understands cause-and-effect relationships in activities like ringing a bell; pulling on a string to retrieve a ring, train, or phone; and dropping a toy from the crib or highchair. They visually follow a toy if it falls and remains within their visual field. For some older infants, beginning object permanence is evident, because they will look for partially hidden objects and play peek-a-boo. The infant is increasingly aware of surroundings and begins to express individual preferences more clearly. This is often a time when resistance to bedtime, feeding, and parental separation occurs.

Nine through Twelve Months Old

Physical Development

At 9 to 10 months old, the infant's growth may follow a different growth curve than the one established early in infancy. Growth spurts become more apparent to parents as the infant seems to outgrow clothes "overnight." At the same time, illnesses, decreased solid food intake caused by teething, and the infant's increased activity level can slow the growth rate. It is important to estimate the infant's total caloric intake if there is a significant decrease in the infant's growth or if feeding problems are present. Early intervention for feeding problems at this time can result in a much easier resolution (see Chapter 10).

Infants at this age show regular bowel and bladder elimination patterns. Some parents inaccurately interpret their ability to predict their infant's bowel movements as readiness for toilet training. Sleep problems, if managed with consistency, begin to resolve, although there might still be struggles with bedtime.

Between 11 and 12 months old, infants gain about 1 pound (0.5 kg) per month. Growth in length continues to occur in spurts. Older infants usually eat solids well, want to feed themselves, and are able to recognize their own hunger or satiation needs. They usually do not eat the same amount at each meal and often demonstrate specific food preferences. They typically eat breakfast, lunch, and dinner, with midmorning and afternoon snacks.

Motor Skills Development

Fine motor development allows older infants to entertain themselves for sustained periods of time. They hold objects of different sizes and pick up small objects using the sides of the fingers and eventually a fine pincer grasp, most often transferring the object directly to their mouth. Infants at this age enjoy putting objects into containers and taking them out again and, by 11 or 12 months old, can stack blocks one on top of the other. They often begin to hold a cup with two hands, but may still have difficulty sealing their lips around the edge of the cup to take sips.

At 9 to 10 months old, most infants sit for long periods and crawl on hands and knees. They "cruise," walking around furniture holding on with both hands, and pull themselves off the floor to a standing position. They begin to let themselves down from furniture with fairly good control and take steps if someone holds both their hands, although they quickly transition to standing with one hand held. Eventually they take a few steps from one object or person to another. Some may momentarily stand alone, and others may walk independently.

Communication and Language Development

Receptive language skills improve, and infants participate in games, such as pat-a-cake and peek-a-boo. Babies at this age momentarily stop activity when they hear "no," but they do not truly understand what "no" means. They are still very focused on observing activities in their environment and attend well to the new information when given names of things. They enjoy songs and rhymes and may participate by "singing" along.

By 12 months old, infants' expressive language expands to three or four words. Words such as "dada," "mama," or "ba-ba" (for bottle) can be recognized. They are able to name a picture in a book, visually look for an object when named, and follow simple one-step requests.

Social and Emotional Development

Stranger anxiety persists at this age and some demonstrate fear of new situations or experiences. As a result, they look to their parent for reassurance and attempt to engage the parent in eye contact while watching their parent's expression. Emotions, such as affection, anger, jealousy, and anxiety, become more evident in late infancy. However, once familiar with new people, particularly if introduced by their parents, babies enjoy initiating interactive games and social interchanges. Overall, 11- to 12-month-olds appear to be in love with the world, love to explore, and have little understanding of those things that can cause them harm. They help with dressing by extending an arm or leg and retrieve an object if it is dropped. Most take great pride in mastering new skills or overcoming their fears, and they look to others around them to take notice as well.

Cognitive Development

Cognitively, older infants complete more complicated tasks, such as stacking and container play. They master object permanence and easily locate a toy placed out of sight or under a cloth. This skill allows them to take a more active role in playing hide-and-seek or peek-a-boo. They hold a crayon or pencil with their whole hand and make dots on a piece of paper, imitating a drawn line.

Infants' curiosity blossoms as they explore visually, with mouthing and chewing, grasping, poking, shaking, pushing, pulling, and stacking. They develop their own games or explore different ways of playing with familiar toys or objects. Play and other activities become more spontaneous and self-directed. Parents can foster ongoing development by following the infant's lead during play, imitating the child's interest, and modeling newer activities related to the same toy or game (e.g., playing pat-a-cake and then adding a song).

Developmental Assessment of Infants

Monitoring the overall growth and development of infants is critical because of the rapid changes during this time. If a delay or concern is detected early, prompt treatment improves the likelihood of positive outcomes. Effective assessment occurs with consistent visits with the same provider. Seeing the same provider on a regular basis also strengthens the parent-child-provider relationship and makes it easier to pursue follow-up questions and concerns, provides anticipatory guidance, validates parental efforts, and reinforces parental successes.

Screening Strategies for Infants

Every well-child visit should include developmental surveillance that assesses parents' concerns, includes a relevant developmental history, and completes a thorough and accurate examination, looking particularly at the infant's development over time. Developmental screening with a standardized, valid, and reliable instrument should be conducted at the 2-, 4-, 6-, 9-, and 12-month well-child visit and whenever there is a parent or provider concern (Council on Children with Disabilities et al, 2006) (Table 5-3). The Ages & Stages Questionnaires (ASQ) or the Parents' Evaluation of Developmental Status (PEDS) is recommended for infants and young children and can be completed by parents while waiting to see the provider. Other tools may be used for specific areas of concern, such as speech and language, and social and emotional behavior. Simply completing a checklist of developmental milestones or asking about specific milestones is not adequate to assess an infant's developmental status, especially for those born prematurely. When developmental screening indicates an infant is not progressing at the expected rate, additional testing to determine the degree of delay or to refer to another health professional for further assessment and management is necessary.

Anticipatory Guidance for Infants

Many of the issues of infancy can be addressed through educating and providing anticipatory guidance to parents. New parents can be bombarded by their own parents, neighbors, friends, the media, and others with more information and opinions than they can manage. When confronted with a question as common as, "When do I begin to feed my baby solid foods?" parents, especially first-time parents, can be confused by all the options. Health care providers help parents sort through the information, understand what it means, and decide what is best for their family. There are several goals to keep in mind when working with new parents of infants. These include helping parents:

- Identify and develop a set of skills that they can use as their child grows
- Understand infant development and capabilities
- Understand and appreciate their own child's abilities
- Interact with their child in a way that strengthens the child-parent bond, nurtures and cherishes the child, and increases their self-confidence as parents

To achieve these goals, providers must listen carefully to parents, especially to their perception of any problems or concerns they have about their baby. Discussion can then directly address specific concerns. Too much information, or information that the parent feels is irrelevant; however, can be overwhelming, so providers must be sensitive to the parents' learning needs. Frequently, time limitations in a clinic or office setting lead to use of a "laundry list" of topics for anticipatory guidance rather than information individualized to the infant and family being seen. Alternative approaches, such as parent groups or classes that focus on commonly shared parenting issues, are good additions to visit-based education.

It is important that providers validate parents' efforts to do their job as parents. Parents should always be asked what they have tried that has worked, and their successes should be reinforced. When providers acknowledge specific positive aspects of the parents' skills before offering anticipatory

TABLE 5-3 Standardized Screening Tools for Infants

Screening Tool	Use	Website
Ages & Stages Questionnaires, edition 3 (ASQ-3) (2009)	Screening and surveillance of developmental milestones. Measures communication, gross motor, fine motor, problem solving, personal-social, and overall development. For use with 1-month-olds to 5½-year-olds. Parents report on 30 items plus overall concerns. Written at the 4th- to 6th-grade level. Manual includes activity handouts for parents. Available in English and Spanish. The ASQ-2 available in French and Korean.	www.brookespublishing.com
Ages & Stages Questionnaire: Social-Emotional (ASQ:SE)	Screening of social-emotional development. For use with 3- to 60-month-olds. Parents report on 32 items. Takes 10 to 20 minutes or less to administer.	www.brookespublishing.com
Infant-Toddler and Family Instrument (ITFI)	Assesses infant, family, and home environment. Includes gross and fine motor, social and emotional development, language, coping, and self-help. For use in 6- to 36-month-olds. Parent interview: Takes two 45- to 60-minute interviews.	www.brookespublishing.com
Battelle Developmental Inventory, edition 2 (BDI-2)	Screening for early childhood developmental milestones. Measures personal-social, adaptive, motor, communication, and cognitive ability. For use from birth to 8 years old. Parents report on 100 items. Takes 10 to 30 minutes; complete test in 1 to 2 hours.	www.riversidepublishing.com/products/bdi2/
Parents' Evaluations of Developmental Status (PEDS)	Screening/surveillance of development/social-emotional/behavior/mental health. For use from birth to 8 years old. Parents complete 10 questions. Test takes 2 minutes to administer. Available in English, Spanish, Vietnamese, and many other languages.	www.pedstest.com
Temperament and Atypical Behavior Scale (TABS)	Screening for behavioral concerns. Measures detached, hypersensitive and hyperactive, under-reactive, and dysregulated behaviors. For use from birth to 6 years old. Parent interview with 55 questions. Takes 15 to 20 minutes to complete.	www.brookespublishing.com
Child Development Inventories (CDI)	Measures gross and fine motor, language, social, and comprehension skills. For use from 3 to 72 months. Parents complete 60 yes/no questions. Takes less than 10 minutes to complete.	www.childdevrev.com/page15/page17/cdi.html
Short Sensory Profile (SSP)	Screens for sensory processing patterns. Measures tactile sensitive, taste-smell sensitivity, movement, underresponsiveness, auditory filtering, low energy and weakness, visual and auditory processing. For use from birth to adult. Parents complete 25 items. Takes 15 to 20 minutes to complete.	www.pearsonclinical.com

guidance, the parent's confidence is strengthened, and parents are more likely to be open to new ideas and suggestions.

Providers should be alert for developmentally appropriate parent-child interactions in the office, and reinforce the parents' behavior with immediate positive feedback. Observing and commenting on aspects of the child's development during the office visit is also a "teachable moment" that allows the provider to initiate discussions with parents about concerns or anticipatory guidance topics. Providers can model developmentally appropriate activities during the well-child examination. They can show parents ways to interact with their infant that stimulate, comfort, or soothe the baby. During these demonstrations, parents can be asked to give examples of things they do at home as they care for their infant. If a problem was discussed at a previous well-child care visit and a plan made to try certain activities (e.g., creating a nighttime ritual to manage a 10-month-old who refuses to go to sleep in her own bed), providers should review the outcome and provide positive feedback and encouragement for the efforts made and successful results.

Health education and anticipatory guidance help parents gain the skill to become their child's advocates and to maximize their child's potential. The following sections cover specific topics of anticipatory guidance that practitioners can provide to help parents through the remarkable, fast-moving first year of their child's life.

The Prenatal Visit

The prenatal visit is an opportunity to form a relationship between provider and family and to assess parents' knowledge and receptiveness to anticipatory guidance. These meetings provide a foundation for later visits and establish the provider as a resource for the parents. It is especially important for first-time parents, parents unknown to the provider, single parents, and those with certain high-risk characteristics (e.g., families with high-risk pregnancies, parents of multiples, those experiencing pregnancy complications, and those who have experienced the loss of a child) (Cohen and Committee on Psychological Aspects of Child and Family Health, 2009; Simon et al, 2014). The prenatal visit should include discussions of the benefits of breastfeeding, the need for immunizations, family wishes regarding circumcision, and injury prevention with focus on safe sleep, common causes of newborn injury, and car seats. This is an ideal time to explore parental expectations for health preventive services, including well-child visits, and to discuss situations that may affect the way the family will adjust to the new baby's arrival (e.g., a toddler who may become jealous, an upcoming move, a recent job loss, or economic stressors). Providers can use this visit to conduct a family history, including genetic risk factors, and to screen for risk factors for perinatal depression (e.g., previous history of depression or previous postpartum depression or lack of social support).

The Neonatal Visit

The newborn visit in the hospital should focus on family readiness, infant behaviors, feeding, safety, and routine baby care. Parents should leave the hospital knowing how to interpret their infant's hunger and discomfort signs and what signs and symptoms related to feeding (breast milk or formula), jaundice, and infant care (e.g., umbilical cord) are of concern and warrant a call to the provider. Guidelines for newborn care during the immediate postnatal period should be provided in writing. The hospital visit is the least opportune time to discuss infant care because of the mother's physiologic state, which can diminish her ability to absorb new information. Written information should include the phone numbers of the practice and specifics about how to reach the provider after hours and on weekends. A follow-up visit in the office should be scheduled within 48 to 72 hours of discharge to screen for feeding problems and jaundice.

Birth to One Month Old

Regulation and Sleep-Wake Patterns

- Normal neonates require an average of 16 hours of sleep every 24 hours, but some will require more (Dewar, 2013). (For additional discussion regarding the sleep cycle, see Chapter 14.) Breastfed infants may need to eat more frequently than babies who are formula-fed and may wake more frequently in the night.
- Infants need assistance to develop day-night cycles because they do not distinguish between days and nights. Using a consistent daily routine helps the infant establish a good sleep-wake cycle.
- Placing the infant in a bassinet or crib for naps during the day assists with nighttime sleep.
- Infants need a variety of movement, voice, or touch to move them from sleep to wake states. Rhythmicity of voice, movement, or touch calms infants or lowers their state, and a parent's slow, easy movements during caregiving will lessen the infant's startle or Moro reflex.
- Some infants benefit from external stimuli, such as music, voice, or movement to help calm them and support their self-regulation. Gentle massage or swaddling helps some infants adjust to state changes.

Strength and Motor Coordination

- Infants' gradual increase in strength makes it possible for them to lift their heads. Parents should place their infants in the supine position for sleep, but they should give their babies "tummy time" when awake and alert as soon as the newborn comes home from the hospital. Tummy time consists of supervised time spent playing with the baby in a prone position. It is best to start with sessions less than 4 minutes, two or three times a day, but time intervals should gradually increase until the infant spends a total of 1 hour daily while prone. Time spent prone allows infants to develop strong neck muscles and decreases the likelihood of positional plagiocephaly.

Feeding and Self-Care

- A primary developmental activity of the newborn is organizing feeding responses. The first step is bringing the infant slowly to an awake state for feeding. If the infant is overstimulated or disorganized, it may be necessary to reduce external stimuli (e.g., lights and noise), increase the infant's flexion of arms and legs, or bundle the infant to assist with central nervous system control and improve feeding responses.

- Infants need regular suck-swallow and breathing rhythms for feeding. If milk flows through the breast or bottle too rapidly or too slowly, adjustments are needed to help the baby manage the feeding. Feedings that are longer than 40 minutes or shorter than 20 minutes should be evaluated.
- Infants are good at regulating how much they need to eat. It may not always be consistent from one meal to the next. Understanding and respecting an infant's hunger and satiation cues help protect against later feeding and nutritional problems, such as obesity. Burping techniques may also be different for each infant. Burping is an important time for a rest during feeding and provides social interaction.
- Urinary output is one indicator of adequate intake, but it is not the only one. Weight gain, feeding type (breast milk or formula), frequency and duration, frequency of spit-ups, and infant activity level must be evaluated to determine adequate nutrition.
- The face-to-face feeding position is important because it encourages eye contact and parent-child communication and interaction.
- The infant's reach for breast or bottle represents beginning exploratory learning and should be encouraged. Parents also can encourage the grasp reflex while the baby is feeding through finger play or finger holding.
- Evidence indicates that the use of a pacifier during sleep decreases the risk of SIDS (Task Force on Sudden Infant Death Syndrome and Moon, 2011). Randomized control studies show no significant relationship between pacifier use and decreased breastfeeding. Thus, the AAP recommends that all infants be provided a pacifier to decrease SIDS risk, but it should be delayed in breastfed infants until breastfeeding is well established (Task Force on Sudden Infant Death Syndrome and Moon, 2011). Pacifiers may be given when parents place their infant to sleep, but pacifiers should not be inserted or reinserted after the infant is asleep. If the infant refuses the pacifier, he or she should not be forced to take it. Pacifiers should not be coated with sweet solutions or placed in the parent's mouth prior to giving it to their infant, and they need to be cleaned frequently and replaced regularly (Nelson, 2012).
- Support and guidance for breastfeeding mothers may require additional counseling, observation of feedings, and referral to a lactation consultant, in addition to guidance on strategies for returning to work while breastfeeding (see Chapter 11).

Communication and Language

- Newborn's communication skills are seen during arousal state transitions as they experience periods of alertness, feeding, and sleep routines. Parents must be alert to nonverbal infant communication (e.g., fussiness, turning the head away) to understand their infant's needs.
- Attending promptly to infant crying helps the infant to develop a sense of trust.
- Imitating infant sounds encourages an infant to vocalize and experiment with different types of sounds.

Social and Emotional Growth

- Newborns benefit from brief periods of social interaction when they are in an alert state. Orienting to visual stimuli (e.g., a parent's smiling face) helps the infant keep a stable alert state. Parents need to learn how to help the infant achieve this alert state and how to avoid overstimulating a newborn. These are discussed more fully later.
- It is important for newborns to be gently touched and held. Encourage parents to hold their infant and assure them that holding does not spoil a baby but meets the infant's need for emotional support and tactile contact, and it fosters infant-parent bonding.
- Facilitating overall family development and emotional growth is important, especially for siblings. Based on the sibling's age, parents may need ideas of appropriate ways for the older child to interact with the newborn.
- Two-parent families may need the opportunity to discuss how to delegate and share parental roles and responsibilities.

Parental development is fostered by pointing out concrete ways that parents are meeting their infant's needs (more than just "You are doing a good job"). Parents' concerns should be followed up closely with support, guidance, and reassurance when appropriate.

Cognitive and Environmental Stimulation

- Parents should encourage opportunities for the infant to look at things and to hear sounds in their environment. As infants develop, a variety of objects placed within their field of vision encourages them to visually explore their surroundings and move their heads from side to side. It is also helpful to periodically place infants at different ends of the bed. Placing mobiles at the side of the bassinet or crib helps prevent overstimulation. Softly played music enriches the infant's auditory experience. Including infants in family activities during their awake times exposes them to many sounds and visual images.

One through Three Months Old

Regulation and Sleep-Wake Patterns

- Structuring an infant's day (e.g., regular feeding schedules and nap times) helps meet the infant's ongoing need for external routines and helps the infant transition through the arousal states.
- The infant's immature nervous system (e.g., continuation of Moro or asymmetric tonic neck reflex) creates a need for swaddling and sensitive movements.
- Sleep location, safety, position ("back to sleep"), and the establishment of a naptime and nighttime ritual all influence later sleep habits for the infant. Helping infants learn to go to sleep on their own can begin with parents placing drowsy, but still awake, infants in the bassinet or crib instead of holding them until they fall asleep.

- The capacity of an infant to self-soothe develops in the first 3 months of life.
- Factors such as the parents' work schedule, child day care attendance, breastfeeding patterns, and infant and parental temperaments influence family decisions about sleep schedules and nighttime interactions between the parent and infant.

Strength and Motor Coordination

- Placing the infant in different positions for playtime and when awake, especially the prone position, encourages upper body strength, and neck, arm, and head control. Family members can help stimulate the infant by encouraging the infant to look up at faces during tummy time.
- The supine position stimulates movement of the fingers, hands, feet, and legs, and makes it easier to hold toys.

Feeding and Self-Care

- Feedings become more consistent, and the infant continues to have a strong need for sucking, especially for nonnutritive sucking, such as sucking on fingers, pacifiers, and toys.
- Feedings continue to be important to meet both nutritional and developmental needs. This is a time for close, affectionate communication between parent and baby.
- Infants demonstrate cues for readiness to eat and satiation. For example, they may vocalize and increase their movements as they see the parents prepare for a feeding, and seal their lips, turn their head, or slow or stop sucking when they are satiated. Overfeeding can occur if parents do not recognize and respond to the infant's cues that he or she has eaten enough.
- Positive reinforcement for continued breastfeeding is essential and strategies for the mother who is returning to work are beneficial (see Chapter 11).

Communication and Language

- Talking and singing to infants during routine daily activities should be encouraged. The value of hearing the parent's voice is great, even if the infant does not understand the words.
- Helping parents understand and respond to their infant's cues and sleep-wake states supports communication between parent and infant.
- Reading as part of daily or evening routine should be encouraged.

Social and Emotional Growth

- An infant's hands are often described as an infant's "first toy." In addition, they are used for self-consoling and hand-to-mouth exploration.
- Responding to infants' cries as soon as possible reassures them that their needs will be met and decreases the chances of crying later on.
- Infant temperaments are increasingly expressed in the child's behavior. Parents' perception of their infant's temperament plays an important role in how they respond to their infant. They may describe their infant as easy, average, or challenging, and they will compare their infant with other babies, siblings, or with themselves.
- Infants have an increasing social need and desire to play with the caregiver. Often fussing or crying is misinterpreted for hunger. Parents may need assistance to set up "play stations" (different play activities) so that the infant can be moved easily from one activity to another. As a result of the infant's short attention span, approximately 10 to 15 minutes at each station for a total of 1 hour will usually lead to a tired, happy baby.
- Parents need to develop strategies to have time together as a couple. Providers can help them identify criteria for child care resources and how to locate those resources.

Cognitive and Environmental Stimulation

- The infant's visual acuity is increasing and visual diversity is needed, such as changes in position and location and the use of stimulating objects like a mobile or mirror.
- Toy and equipment selection should include assessment of safety and developmental appropriateness. Toys should be semi-rigid, unpainted, and have varying textures. Special care is needed to avoid toys that pose choking hazards (e.g., those with small pieces or are smaller than the size of the infant's fist). Toys that rattle and make sounds are entertaining and encourage waving arms and kicking legs.

Four through Five Months Old

Regulation and Sleep-Wake Patterns

- Infants need to be allowed to self-soothe when they awaken at night. Infants who are placed in their crib while drowsy but not yet asleep are more likely to go back to sleep without comforting from the parent when they wake.
- Nighttime rituals are an important aspect of helping the infant anticipate what is going to happen next, which builds a sense of security.
- The infant's emerging temperament and the parents' perceptions of the infant's behaviors may lead to conflicts that will need to be resolved.
- Parents need varied approaches to infants of different temperaments (e.g., patterns of eating and sleeping), and individualizing their activities to their baby's style makes parenting much easier.

Strength and Motor Coordination

- As the infant becomes more mobile, safety measures become more critical; parental supervision and childproofing the home, relatives' homes, and child care or day care settings are essential for safety (e.g., locks on cabinets and gates for stairs).
- Floor-time play encourages motor strength and coordination. Playpens can be limiting, but can be effectively used as a safety measure. Movable walkers are unsafe and have not been commercially available for some time;

however, they can be purchased at resale and garage sales. Only nonmobile, sitting/reclining devices are recommended and use should be limited to brief periods (e.g., 10 to 15 minutes).

Feeding and Self-Care

- Drooling can be due to teething but primarily occurs because of salivary gland maturation. The infant gradually develops the ability to swallow excessive saliva.
- It is important for parents to respond appropriately to the infant's hunger and satiety cues.
- Infants are ready for solids as they and their gastrointestinal tract mature. Specifically, they should have good head control, be able to sit alone, and have diminished tongue thrust reflex before solids are introduced. Listen closely to parents' questions and beliefs and the influence of others on the introduction of solids. Exclusive breastfeeding is best until 6 months old, but solid food can be introduced after 17 weeks old, although timing for solid food introduction should be individualized (Grimshaw et al, 2013).
- Spoon-feeding helps the infant develop new oral-motor skills. Infant-led feeding, in which the child picks up pieces of food and self-feeds, also strengthens fine and gross motor skills (see Chapter 10). Cereal should not be given in a bottle or cup. Infants learning to eat solids should have constant supervision during feedings.
- Interacting with the infant during feeding fosters the parent-child relationship and makes feeding time fun rather than just a routine
- Allowing infants to pat the breast or bottle and place their hands on the bottle promotes self-feeding. Bottles should not be propped because the infant can aspirate.

Communication and Language

- Parents' use of reciprocal or "back-and-forth talking" with their infant, especially using changes in voice inflection and intonation, is important in developing communication skills.
- Parents' talking to their infant during caregiving activities holds the infant's attention, especially when the infant is fussy. Talking to the infant makes it easier to change diapers, prepare meals, and attend to the infant's needs in other ways. It also stimulates the infant's language skills.
- Reading to an infant, looking at picture books and describing the pictures, colors, and actions in them, is beneficial even at this early age, and can be a first step in developing habits of quiet time, reading time, and parent-child together time. Providers may want to participate in Reach Out and Read, the national early literacy program for children 6 months through 5 years old.

Social and Emotional Growth

- The infant continues to need nonnutritive sucking as a means of self-regulation. Sucking on fingers or toys requires different oral-motor movements from those needed to suck on a pacifier.
- Discipline can be discussed and differentiated from punishment. The important role of "parents as teachers" may be a new concept to some parents. Helping parents understand the importance of modeling desired behaviors and redirecting behavior should be discussed before it is needed (see Chapters 4 and 17).
- Information about infant development and strategies to deal with difficult behaviors is important. Referral to parenting classes that provide information on developmental milestones and anticipated changes may be helpful. Although parents may have books on development, a one-page handout given at the clinic visit that addresses a particular subject of immediate concern is likely to be more useful. Such handouts are available through Healthy Steps and Bright Futures (see Additional Resources).
- Both parents need to be involved in ongoing communication about their roles, responsibilities, and expectations. Differences between parental expectations need to be discussed (e.g., to allow an infant to cry at bedtime or not).
- Reinforce that parents need to be encouraged to find time for themselves because their emotional well-being and availability is an important aspect of their infant's overall care. Infant behaviors often mirror the emotional state of their caregivers.
- Also important is counseling about how to select safe and appropriate child care (Chapter 6) and toys.

Cognitive and Environmental Stimulation

- With the infant's increasing activity and awake time, parents need strategies to provide more attention and play activities. The infant will attempt to obtain the parents' attention by smiling, making sounds, or crying. Suggest using a variety of activities and toys, such as soft stuffed toys, rattles, a crib gym or busy box, and toys of different sizes, weights, shapes, materials, and colors. Home objects that infants see every day (like plastic containers and pots) can be used as "toys" for stacking, shaking, and rolling.
- Infants may enjoy looking at themselves in a mirror, and placing a mirror next to the changing table is a good diversion.
- Activities such as walks to the park, visiting neighbors, or trips to the grocery store are all part of an infant's learning experiences.

Six through Eight Months Old

Regulation and Sleep-Wake Patterns

- By 6 months old, most babies can go for a 6- to 12-hour period without being fed. This extended period coincides with the longest sleep period. Thus after 6 months old, feeding in the night can be considered a learned behavior. There is no scientific evidence to support the myth that feeding cereal to infants helps them sleep through the night.
- Infants may have settled into a good sleep routine through the night, only to have it interrupted by teething

or illness. They may need assistance to resume their regular sleep-wake patterns. Parents may need to go to the infants to assure them they are safe, but they should not feed infants for comfort or to help them return to sleep.
- An increased need for consistency of nighttime rituals to help the infant transition from playtime to sleep time (e.g., bath time and a story) may be evident.
- Teaching infants to sleep in their own crib can be a struggle for some parents. Begin by putting them to bed while they are drowsy but still awake. If the infant wakes in the night, parents should help them return to sleep with the least amount of intrusion (e.g., use voice, face, touch, and then holding).
- Infants are now more capable of waiting for gratification, and parents can use talking and tone of voice to distract, calm, and reassure infants that their needs will be met.

Strength and Motor Coordination

- Floor time is essential for the infant to learn to crawl and walk. Parents must provide for infant safety.
- Childproofing the home becomes increasingly important. Stress topics that decrease risk of falls, burns, and poisonings, such as putting gates at the top and bottom of stairs, padding sharp corners, covering electrical outlets, removing small objects and balloons from the infant's reach, and keeping curtain or iron cords safely out of the way. Make sure that parents and other caregivers have the telephone number for a poison control center handy (1-800-222-1222). Some parents find it helpful to lie on the floor where the infant plays to find hazards visible to the infant.
- Bath-water temperature must be checked (should not be above 100° F [37.8° C]), and infants should never be left alone even for a few seconds in the tub. Parents should be encouraged to set the water temperature on their hot water heater to 120° F to 125° F (48.9° C to 51.7° C).
- Active supervision is the best way to prevent injuries as an infant becomes more mobile; it requires parents to be within reach and free of distractions while watching their infant.

Feeding and Self-Care

- If not already started, solids should be introduced at 6 months old. Breastfed infants need iron-fortified foods. Parents often need specific information about types of foods to start with, quantity, and feeding positions (see Chapter 10). Parents should be given information to use an infant seat or a highchair (properly seated high enough that the infant's back and sides are supported and arms are at the level of the tray).
- Structured mealtimes are important to help the family maintain regular infant routines.
- Allowing the child to hold a spoon or cup encourages self-feeding and begins preparing the infant for later weaning from bottle or breast. With infant-led feeding, the child is given "finger foods" that can be picked up, held, and "gummed" (e.g., cooked vegetables, slices of soft fruit [no raw apples] or bread). Often parents are uncomfortable with the messiness of infant feeding. Discuss ways they can minimize the mess (e.g., sheet or plastic tablecloth on the floor, small portions of food) and still allow the infant to explore, look at, touch, smell, and taste the new foods. Assure the parents that there will always be some mess.
- Introducing solid foods and infant teething often occur simultaneously. Cleansing the teeth (use a soft cloth or soft toothbrush) and providing fluoride supplements, if the water supply is not fluoridated, are important at this time (see Chapter 34).

Communication and Language

- Using the names of objects, encouraging gestures, talking about everyday activities, and responding to the infant's increasing vocalizations are important.
- Early lessons in "reading to an infant" include showing the infant picture books and magazines and talking about the pictures.
- Naming body parts while changing diapers and during bath time is an enjoyable activity for parents. To demonstrate the infant's responsiveness, the provider can model this behavior during the physical examination.

Social and Emotional Growth

- Identifying and encouraging the child to have a "transitional object" (e.g., a favorite toy or blanket) can ease the coming developmental phase of separation anxiety.
- It is important to discuss parents' feelings regarding limit setting, consistency of care, and parental consensus about discipline.
- Positive parental responsiveness and attention supports infant social and emotional growth.

Cognitive and Environmental Stimulation

- Toys that involve cause-and-effect reactions, stacking, and container play are important. Most often, favorite toys are common household objects, such as wooden spoons, plastic bowls, pull toys, or a telephone. Especially popular is any object that the parents use. Continue to stress the risk of choking caused by small objects.
- Interactive games are important, and infants should be encouraged to initiate actions and guide play.

Nine through Twelve Months Old

Regulation and Sleep-Wake Patterns

- A "transitional object" can ease the infant's experience in new situations and provide a sense of comfort or familiarity.
- Predictability in the daily schedule allows the infant to gain mastery over new situations. Efforts to establish and maintain regular mealtimes, a nighttime routine, and consistent caregivers increase the infant's sense of security during transitions.

- The infant's temperament becomes more evident in activity level, curiosity level, and ease in adjusting to new situations. Inquiring about the infant's temperament and discussing positive parenting strategies can generate creative solutions.

Strength and Motor Coordination

- The parents' natural tendency to "cheer" their infants on as they refine old and achieve new motor skills is an example of positive reinforcement for the child in other areas of development.
- Childproofing the environment is critical because the infant is increasingly mobile and curious. Parents need help to anticipate their infant's next major developmental achievement and prepare for the child's natural curiosity. Babies at this age are able to get into trouble but not get themselves out (e.g., falling in a slippery bathtub).
- Safe storage of purses or personal item bags, medicines, cleaning agents, matches, and hazardous objects (e.g., kitchen knives should not be left lying on counters; firearms should be in locked cabinets, not just out of reach, with the ammunition separated from the gun) are essential precautions for mobile older infants with increased fine motor skills and unbounded curiosity.
- Bath-water temperature must be checked, and infants should never be left alone even for a few seconds in the tub.
- Plastic bags, balloons, and small objects must be kept away from the curious, exploring infant.
- As fine motor skills improve, oral exploration is still one of an infant's primary learning methods, so almost everything ends up in the mouth. Having the 24-hour poison control telephone number available and posted for caregivers is critical.
- Active supervision, with the parent within reach and without distractions, is the best way to prevent injuries as an infant becomes more mobile. Once the infant can pull to stand in the crib, the crib mattress should be lowered to the lowest rung.
- Outings for both parents and child help relieve stress and provide wonderful learning opportunities for the infant.

Feeding and Self-Care

- The division of responsibility in feeding becomes more obvious during this time. Parents are responsible for providing healthy foods in an environment that is pleasant and conducive to eating. Children are responsible for determining how much of the healthful foods they will eat. Nine- to 12-month-old infants refine their ability to self-feed and demonstrate clear preferences and dislikes. Discussing the division of responsibilities and the control issues that may arise at this time can help families establish healthy eating patterns for a lifetime.
- Dental hygiene and caries prevention include use of a soft cloth or soft toothbrush to cleanse teeth and gums. Toothpaste is not necessary, but when used should not contain fluoride. Fluoride supplements should be given if the family's water supply is not fluoridated (see Chapter 34).
- Some infants will transition from purees to blended foods, finger foods, and soft solids; some will continue an infant-led process, eating a wider range of table foods. Both involve major changes for infant and parents. Remind parents that it can take 10 to 20 exposures for infants to accept a new food into their diet.
- Practicing with spoons and cups during play and at mealtime helps develop the infant's dexterity skills and promotes self-feeding. Infants should be weaned from the bottle and pacifier at 12 months old.
- Establishing consistent mealtimes and snack times and avoiding the habit of "grazing" (i.e., having food constantly available, including juices or milk) will encourage appropriate intake of foods. Because hunger is inconsistent for infants, three meals and two or three snacks will ensure adequate nutrition. Having the infant sit in a highchair to eat sets a pattern and expectation for eating at the table.
- It is important for infants to eat with their family at least once a day. The likelihood that infants will try new foods increases as they observe others eat. Eating with others keeps the infant focused on meals. Distractions, such as toys and television, should be avoided. Mealtime conversation should be pleasant, helping all family members enjoy their time together.

Communication and Language

- Encourage parents to reinforce the infant's effort to communicate through gestures, pointing, and ambiguous vocalizations. Parents should not try to anticipate exactly what the child needs but rather encourage the child to "ask" for what he or she wants. This "practice" with language provides the groundwork for future speech skills.
- Naming utensils and the color, smell, taste, and texture of foods builds language skills and keeps the infant engaged during mealtime.
- Naming body parts and pointing to them provides distraction during diaper changes and bath time.
- Reading is more interactive as the infant points to pictures in a book, imitates animal sounds, and assists in turning pages. Encourage parents to read to their infant often.

Social and Emotional Growth

- As infants reach 12 months old, their emerging will, desire for autonomy, need for control, and sense of initiative become more evident. They begin to distinguish themselves from their parents.
- It is important to help parents understand that discipline is a guidance process used to teach positive behaviors (as compared with punishment in which constraints are applied to negative behaviors).
- Distraction is very effective when guiding an infant's curiosity by redirecting behavior to desirable activities.

- The infant's stranger anxiety may be difficult for parents to handle. Parents may need help establishing a separation ritual that helps the infant understand the parent is leaving but will return. The parents may need to express their feelings of concern or even disappointment when their infant enjoys the time away from them.
- Parents may have difficulty finding the energy needed to deal with busy, mobile infants and appreciate suggestions on how to cope when exhaustion occurs.
- Parents need positive reinforcement for their continually developing skills, just as their children do.

Cognitive and Environmental Stimulation

- Playing with the child strengthens the parent-child bond and stimulates the infant's cognitive development.
- Allowing the child to take the lead in play activities is important, but parents can use play to model new activities and skills.
- Interactive games such as peek-a-boo, pat-a-cake, and rolling a ball back and forth encourage reciprocal social play. Interaction with the caregiver is still the most important activity for the infant.
- Books, music, blocks, stacking toys, container toys, and pull toys allow self-initiated activities.
- Many 12-month-old children have a box of toys that they enjoy dumping out for play. An infant's curiosity and interest can be sustained if toys are "cycled" (some put away and brought out at a later date).
- Bath time, water tables, and sandboxes provide safe opportunities to engage in messy play that most infants enjoy. Infants need this type of tactile stimulation.

Common Developmental Issues for Infants and Families

Parents' concerns during the infant's first year of life are often related to inexperience or lack of knowledge about infant growth and development. Few infants have developmental delays. Having a "normal" baby does not make the parents' concern any less compelling, and the health care provider has a responsibility to answer parents' questions, provide essential information about development, make accurate assessments to rule out problems, treat or refer problems appropriately, and provide follow-up care and support. Some of the more common developmental issues that trouble parents are discussed in this section. When parents understand the complexity of infant growth and development, they are better able to make healthy decisions for their infants and family.

Sleep

Infant sleep varies widely from birth to 12 months old. Infants who don't sleep well often disrupt the sleep of other family members. Thus concerns about sleep and promoting healthy sleep patterns are important topics in primary care. Chapter 14 includes detailed information about pediatric sleep.

Feeding

Guidelines for nutrition and breastfeeding are found in Chapters 10 and 11. Infant feeding concerns or problems (particularly a less than expected weight gain or decrease in weight) should be assessed through an observation of a feeding in the clinic (or at home, if resources allow). A detailed feeding history, a minimum 3-day diet history, and calorie analysis are needed. The infant's oral motor skills and general development should be assessed because early feeding issues may indicate other subtle developmental delays that can benefit from early intervention. A standardized feeding assessment, using a tool such as the NCAST Feeding Scale, provides information about the parent-child relationship and assists in the development of individualized recommendations for the parents.

Crying

Infant crying and irritability can cause parents to worry that something is wrong. It can disrupt the family and create a strained parent-child relationship. Often, people interpret a newborn's tears as a sign of pain or distress when it is a normal developmental phenomenon. Labeling the crying as "colic" may or may not console stressed parents and may result in reinforcing the parent's belief that something is wrong with their baby (see Chapter 33). Parental education about normal infant crying patterns and effective soothing strategies can empower parents and help decrease parental stress.

Normal crying varies from "fussing" to strong crying where babies pull up their legs, their faces become red, and they cry out in forceful screams. Crying can indicate an infant is tired, soiled, chilled, or it may have no identifiable cause. Normal infants cry as many as up to 5 hours a day, especially in the first few months of life.

The Period of PURPLE Crying Initiative (www.purplecrying.info) is a resource to assist parents during the developmentally normal fussy period that typically starts at about 2 weeks old, peaks between 3 and 5 weeks old, and lasts until 3 to 5 months old. The term *PURPLE crying* is an acronym (Fig. 5-1) to help explain normal crying patterns for young infants.

It is important to assess the infant's crying patterns and frequency and to ascertain the success of soothing caregivers have used. Providers can best plan education about crying when they understand the caregiver's concerns and beliefs about crying. Caregiver education about crying focuses on:

- Identifying the reason why the infant is crying (e.g., wet diaper, hungry, a hair wrapped around a finger or toe) if possible. Remove the source of the discomfort (when possible).
- Removing noxious stimulation, such as excessive noise, light, or movement.

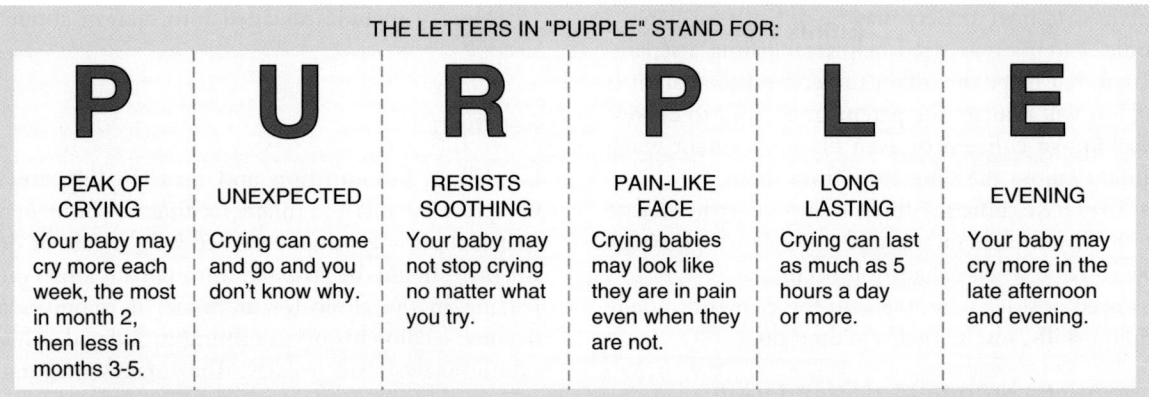

THE LETTERS IN "PURPLE" STAND FOR:

P	U	R	P	L	E
PEAK OF CRYING	UNEXPECTED	RESISTS SOOTHING	PAIN-LIKE FACE	LONG LASTING	EVENING
Your baby may cry more each week, the most in month 2, then less in months 3-5.	Crying can come and go and you don't know why.	Your baby may not stop crying no matter what you try.	Crying babies may look like they are in pain even when they are not.	Crying can last as much as 5 hours a day or more.	Your baby may cry more in the late afternoon and evening.

• **Figure 5-1** The PURPLE acronym for the period (meaning the crying has a beginning and an end) of PURPLE infant crying. (Available online at http://purplecrying.info/what-is-the-period-of-purple-crying.php.)

- Using comfort measures, such as swaddling, white noise, holding the baby while making eye contact and making soothing sounds, taking the baby on a car ride, and providing a pacifier.
- Allowing the infant to cry in the crib, especially if the caregiver feels overwhelmed.
- Instructing to never shake a baby because of the risk of accidentally harming the infant's developing brain.

Postpartum Depression

Infant social and emotional development is closely linked to the mother's emotional state—60% to 80% of mothers experience "baby blues" in the first 2 weeks postpartum; 10% to 15% have postpartum depression during the first year of the infant's life; and 0.1% to 0.2% present with postpartum psychosis (National Institute of Mental Health [NIMH], n.d.).

"Baby blues" are normal and often result in maternal feelings of inadequacy, worry, unhappiness, and fatigue that typically do not cause significant impairment and will resolve spontaneously within a few weeks after birth. Postpartum depression usually starts between a week and a month after delivery but can occur anytime during the first year. It is characterized by the mother's periods of sadness, anxiety, loss of interest in activities, and impaired ability to care for herself and her infant. Postpartum psychosis generally presents in the first weeks after delivery and is much more significant as it may result in maternal thoughts of harming herself and/or her newborn. The rate of postpartum psychosis is significantly higher if there is maternal schizophrenia or bipolar disease, or when the mother's history is positive for previous postpartum psychosis (Spinelli, 2009).

Pediatric health care providers are critical to the early detection of this significant disorder. Infants' well-child visits should be used as opportunities to screen mothers and families for factors that can affect the infant's growth and development, including depression and intimate partner violence.

The parenting role is stressful, even if all goes well. Fatigue and maternal depression resulting from hormonal shifts are common. Encourage parents to identify and make use of supportive people, arrange time for rest and time alone, and keep their expectations reasonable. When a mother seems to be having significant difficulty adjusting to her new infant, it is imperative that the provider keep in mind the possibility of postpartum depression and be ready to intervene on the behalf of the infant, the mother, and the family. The 10-question Edinburgh Postnatal Depression Scale (EPDS) is an easy-to-administer tool and a valuable and efficient way to identify mothers at risk for perinatal depression (Fig. 5-2). Women with postpartum depression need not feel alone; intervention should be individualized, with possible referral for mothers whose score indicates a depressive illness.

Red Flags for Infant Development

Developmental delay in infants involves disorders that manifest as motor problems (e.g., cerebral palsy), communication problems (e.g., receptive or expressive communication and behavior), and/or cognitive problems (e.g., problem solving, mental retardation, specific deficits in processing information). Processing disorders include peripheral problems, such as deafness and blindness; central processing that results in motor, language, and perceptual dysfunction; and behavioral problems. Disorders may be degenerative (e.g., muscular dystrophy) or static (e.g., brachial plexus injury), and they may have clear signs in infancy or have delayed presentations. Signs and symptoms of developmental delay may also be a function of the disorder itself (e.g., progressive neurological loss) or secondary to the disorder (e.g., contractures with cerebral palsy).

Infant developmental problems can be difficult to identify, but the provider must be alert to "red flags" that place the infant at risk or indicate a potential problem. Providers should also listen carefully to parents' concerns about their child's development. Often it is the parent who first notices

TABLE 6-3 Language Development of Toddlerhood

Age	Receptive Language	Expressive Language
12 to 18 months	Follows one-step commands Each week understands new words Increased interest in naming pictures Differentiates environmental sounds Points to familiar objects and body parts when named Understands simple questions Begins to distinguish "you" from "me"	Uses all vowels, many consonants Increased use of real words Jargon is sentence-like Likes to use negatives (i.e., says "no" often) Names a few pictures By 18 months old, articulates 15 to 20 words and understands 50 Imitates non-speech sounds (e.g., cough, tongue click) Names some body parts
18 to 24 months	Follows two-step commands Vocabulary increases rapidly Enjoys simple stories and songs Recognizes pronouns	Imitates two-word combinations Dramatic increase in vocabulary Speech combines jargon and words Names self Answers some questions Begins to combine words Begins to use pronouns
24 to 30 months	Understands prepositions *in* and *on* Seems to understand most of what is said Understands more reasoning ("when you are finished, then ...") Identifies object when given function (wear on feet, cook on)	Babbles less Two- to three-word sentences Repeats two numbers Increased use of pronouns Asks simple questions Joins in songs and nursery rhymes Can repeat simple phrases and sentences
30 to 36 months	Listens to adult conversations Understands preposition *under* Can categorize items by function Begins to recognize colors Begins to take turns Understands "big" and "little," "boy" and "girl"	Answers questions ("wear on feet," "to bed") Repeats three numbers Uses regular plurals Can help tell simple story
36 to 42 months	Understands *fast* Understands prepositions *behind* and *in front* Responds to simple three-part commands Increasing understanding of adjectives and plurals Understands "just one"	Understands and answers ("cold," "tired," "hungry") Mostly three- to four-word sentences Gives full name Begins rote counting Begins to relate events Lots of questions, some beginning prepositions (on, in)
42 to 48 months	Recognizes coins Begins to understand future and past tenses Understands number concepts—more than one	Uses prepositions Tells stories Can give function of objects Repeats longer than six-word sentences Repeats four numbers Gives age Good intelligibility
48 to 60 months	Responds to three-step commands	Asks "how" questions Answers verbally to questions, such as "How are you?" Uses past and future tenses Can use conjunctions to combine words and phrases

The intelligibility rate jumps to about 66% between 24 and 36 months, with 90% intelligibility by 3 years old. By 4 years old, speech should be completely intelligible with the exception of particularly difficult consonants. By 5 years old, the tongue-contact sounds of "n," "t," "d," "k," "g," "y," and "ng" are more intelligible. Some sounds, such as the "zh" sound, are not added until the child is 6 to 8 years old. Figure 6-1 identifies sounds articulated by children at specific ages.

During the second year, the child practices playful changes in pitch and loudness. Three- and 4-year-olds show normal hesitance in speech or stuttering. They "stutter" by repeating words, especially those at the start of a sentence, or when excited, such as when they want to convey an important message (e.g., "Mommy, I… Mommy, I… Mommy, I want to tell you I hear the ice cream truck"). This normal speech variant does not include syllable repetition or cause undue stress for the child. These dysfluencies

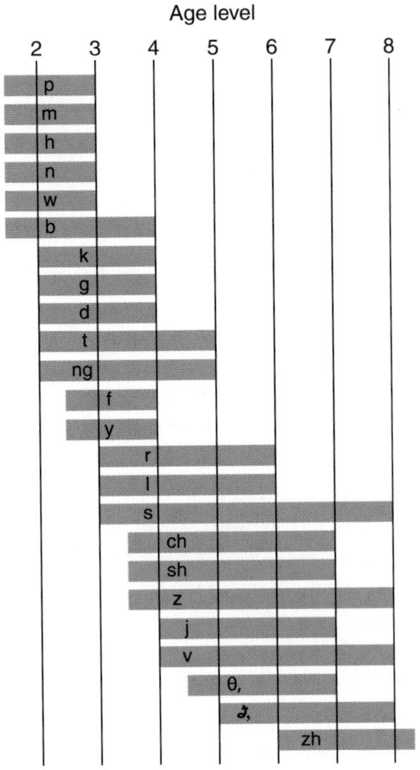

• **Figure 6-1** Norms for development of speech sounds. *θ, th* as in *thin*; ð as in *this*. (From Van Riper C, Erickson RL: *Speech correction: an introduction to speech pathology and audiology*, ed 9, Needham Heights, MA, 1996, Allyn & Bacon, p 98. Reprinted by permission.)

are usually temporary; they are considered abnormal if they cause significant stress for the child, if they occur in children over 5 years old, or if they involve syllable instead of word repetition.

Children usually progress through a regular sequence of mispronunciations as they learn new articulation skills. At first, they simply omit the new sound, and then they try to substitute a more familiar sound for the new one (e.g., the "w" for "r" substitution, as in "wabbit" for "rabbit"). Distortion is followed by "addition" as the child adds an extra sound (e.g., "gulad" for "glad"). Knowing each of these steps allows the examiner to assure the parent whether the child is developing normally or needs monitoring.

Lexicon

Lexicon refers to vocabulary. Vocabulary size is influenced by many factors, including environment, stimulation, intelligence, multilingualism, culture, and personality. Children usually understand more words than they are able to express, and addition of words to their expressive vocabulary comes with continued practice. Girls typically say their first word between 8 and 11 months, boys by about 14 months. Most 2-year-olds have more than 200 words in their vocabulary, and most 4- to 5-year-olds add approximately 50 words a month to their vocabulary. Five-year-olds should be able to define some words with other words (e.g., "cup" is "you drink with it," or "chair" is "to sit on").

Syntax

Syntax, or grammar, refers to the structure of words in sentences or phrases. The ability to construct sentences that convey meaning is a complex skill, proceeding through several stages in children: receptive, holophrastic, and telegraphic speech. Much of this skill is developed between 8 months and 3½ years. By 8 months, children develop receptive language (i.e., they understand others who use a new word or structure before they are able to use it themselves). When asked "Where is the ball?" an 8-month-old searches for the ball. Between 12 and 18 months, children begin to use holophrases or single words to express whole ideas. The child says "milk," perhaps to mean the whole sentence, "I want a glass of milk." A complex idea is expressed in one succinct word. Holophrastic sentences are denominative (labeling) or imperative (commanding).

Around 18 months, children begin using telegraphic speech, phrases that have many words omitted and sound like a telegram, to convey their message (e.g., "get milk," "go bye-bye"). At around 2 years old, children begin to expand their vocabulary and to form short sentences like "my big ball" and "the yummy cookie." This is the age when toddlers begin to mimic phrases and gestures used by caregivers like "Oh, my goodness." Sentence structure becomes more complex as children move from active sentences, to questions, to passive and negative construction, and then add plurals (at 3 years old) and past tenses (at 4 years old) to their grammar. Three- or four-word sentences should be evident by 3 years; and by 5 years old, the child's syntax is close to adult style, including use of future tense and complete sentences of five or six words in length.

Semantics

Semantic development, the understanding that words have specific meaning and the child's use of words to convey specific meaning, is an ongoing process extending into adulthood. This development occurs in stages from global to more specific and requires interaction through conversation, listening, and reading. Words used in any language have both denotative (the specific, concrete referent of the word) and connotative (a broader range of feelings aroused by the word) meanings. Even though children may be quite adept at using words correctly, they may have only a vague, diffuse connotative understanding of these words. For example, the 3-year-old who drops a toy and uses an expletive that she heard when her father dropped a dish does not understand the connotative meaning of what she has said. As language progresses from simple to more complex, meaning and cognitive understanding evolve.

Each child develops speech at different rates. Hearing is vital to speech development. Table 6-3 lists common speech and language milestones.

Bilingualism

Raising children to be bilingual can help preserve the family culture and heritage, and studies suggest that fluent bilingual children have greater mental flexibility and enhanced employment and lifestyle opportunities. Initially, normal toddlers from bilingual homes may show mild delays in initial spoken words and mixing of the words and phrases from the two languages.

Parents often ask primary care providers and educators how best to introduce two languages to children. Often they are told to use the one-parent-one-language approach. Many bilingual preschoolers meet language milestones at the predicted time in their primary language, but skill attainment in the second language may lag behind (MacLeod et al, 2013). Most are proficient in sorting one language from the other, although they may "code switch" to the other language for clarity as they talk. They switch languages depending on the person with whom they are speaking and the circumstances. Some even translate for others, seeming to understand that not everyone speaks or understands both languages. Ultimately, whether a second, third, or even more languages are learned simultaneously or sequentially, most children have one dominant language. Bilingual children with significant vocabulary delays require the same evaluation as delayed monolingual children.

Social and Emotional Development

Psychosocial changes in early childhood are remarkable. Emotions and cognition are interconnected so that assessment of any one area of development is somewhat arbitrary. Toddlers spend most of their time up, running about, verbalizing, and demanding to join in family activities. These are years of intense learning about and managing feelings (such as, love, happiness, anger, frustration, aggression, and jealousy) and social skills (such as, sharing, giving, and receiving affection). They learn the words that go with their feelings and, with guidance, the appropriate behaviors. A major developmental milestone for this age is the achievement of a sense of independence and autonomy. The road from depending on parents for everything to doing some things for themselves, however, can be rocky and uneven.

During early childhood a child's ability to achieve independence is influenced, in part, by the strengths in his or her social environment. In particular, maternal depression (chronic and postpartum) has a significantly negative effect on the development of normal infant engagement behaviors that can persist into the toddler and preschool years and affects the child's social, emotional, and language development (Goodman et al, 2011). Maternal depression is related to infant avoidant and disorganized attachment patterns and negative mother-infant interactions, which are linked to externalizing behavior problems during toddlerhood, higher levels of internalizing and externalizing behavior problems in preschoolers, and conduct problems in adolescents (Bagner et al, 2010). Maternal depression is one of the most potent risk factors for child and adolescent depression.

Toddlers need a great deal of love, warmth, and comfort, primarily from their parents and caregivers. Toddlers learn to give love and find satisfaction in pleasing their parents. They learn to respond to kisses, hugs, and cuddles that they have received by giving kisses, hugs, and cuddles in return. Toddlers who make these early attempts at giving love and are rejected or ignored soon stop trying and begin to find pleasure elsewhere. Toddlers with sensory issues learn to avoid some gestures unless they are in control and decide that they can handle the tactile or sensory feelings. Some toddlers find that thumb sucking, rhythmic body movements, and body manipulation are more pleasurable and reliable than person-to-person contacts.

Preschoolers develop more sophisticated ideas about feeling, giving, and sharing. Four- and 5-year-olds move away from the self-centered attitude of earlier toddlerhood. At this stage, parents are the epitome of wisdom, power, integrity, and goodness. If early stages of the love relationship are not satisfied, preschoolers show more fears, inhibitions, explosive behavior, and demands for attention.

Toddlers and preschool-age children gradually increase their ability to follow commands consistently as they work to gain and maintain approval of adults and to behave the way "good" children are expected to. By the preschool years, children begin to show interest in table manners, being polite, saying "thank you" without a reminder, sharing, saying (and meaning) "I'm sorry," and taking turns. These social skills are learned through daily interactions at home, school, and church, from parents, peers, relatives, and neighbors. Children learn to read others' social cues (e.g., the voice tone, slight facial expression, posture) and to correct their own behavior. Some children, frequently boys, find these cues vague and difficult to learn, and parents can help by modeling, explaining, and discussing them.

Children at this age vacillate between being a big boy or big girl and mommy's or daddy's baby. They take great pride in doing as many things as possible for themselves, yet they need to feel totally secure in their parents' care. On some days, toddlers cling to their parents' side, not letting their parents out of sight; on other days, the child can play for short periods in the next room, trotting back every so often to see, touch, and hear the parent and be reassured by the parent's presence. The child who is securely attached uses the parent as a base from which to go out and safely explore the world. Gradually the periods of separation lengthen, and the child needs only to hear the parent's voice or to check occasionally for security. Separation anxiety is frequent during these years and can be traumatic for both parents and child.

Preschool children are much less dependent on their parents and frequently tolerate physical separation for several hours. As this sense of separateness increases, children are more aware that they are different from their surroundings, their families, and their friends. They begin to realize that other persons also have feelings, fears, and doubts. Peer dependence and learning about how to have and be friends begin to be important.

Toddlers like to have a choice in matters and quickly learn the power of the word "no." They can become extremely negative, practicing the power of "no" every day for months, even when their answer is actually "yes." As toddlers practice making choices, they are clumsy, awkward, and frequently wrong. This can be very frustrating for them, and their outraged responses can be equally annoying for their parents. Toddlers discover the delights of control over others and themselves. This increases their sense of power but can also lead to misunderstandings and hurt feelings if their parents do not read their moods properly. With time, they become more skilled, make better choices, have more successes, and feel more powerful. They no longer have to work so hard to show others their power, and the negative stage passes.

Preschool-age children are more verbal than toddlers and are able to perform many more self-care tasks (e.g., feed themselves using appropriate utensils, blow their own noses, and go to the bathroom unassisted). Interactions become easier and more enjoyable as the child learns to verbally express needs and feelings.

Morality

Morality, or the ability to know right from wrong, is based on external control during the toddler years and stems from children's love of their parents and a desire to please them (see Chapter 16). Parent teaching generally focuses more on helping the child to make safe decisions rather than moral ones. Toddlers cannot be expected to make correct choices if left alone in potentially dangerous situations because their internal sense of conscience is rudimentary and judgment is absent. Any room with electrical sockets, knobs for technical equipment, guns, open windows, unsecured television and furniture, or hot food represents a risk. As toddlers gain language skills, they begin to echo the parent's firm "no," but they do not understand the full meaning of the term. By 24 months, many toddlers show beginning internalization by saying "no" to themselves and stopping the act; they may then continue with the act as they talk to themselves, still saying "no."

Preschoolers form a foundation for their moral development as they develop socioemotionally and cognitively. For the 4- to 5-year-old, morality is more internally controlled. Instead of basing all decisions on the knowledge of the consequences of the act (e.g., "If I take a cookie, I will be sent to my room"), older children show an elementary understanding of what is right and wrong, fair or unfair. They recognize others' needs and may express a desire to help or comfort others. They begin to think ahead and are able to plan and control their urges, thus avoiding punishment. Four-year-olds can internalize some demands from their parents, and feelings of guilt can be elicited after some transgressions.

Peer Relationships

Toddlers may be fascinated by children their own age and demonstrate curiosity by physically examining the other child closely, poking and probing. However, they generally do not engage with their peers in an interactive way. Parallel play is the norm. Preschoolers learn to interact with peers as their social world grows. As symbolic language develops, play becomes more interactive, cooperative, and shared. Play offers more than cherished memories of growing up; it allows children to develop creativity and imagination while developing physical, cognitive, and emotional strengths (Milteer et al, 2012). Fantasy and make-believe are very important during these years. Imaginary play leads to "pretend play," role-playing, and creation of imaginary friends. Play is the major mechanism through which toddlers and preschoolers practice social roles, such as housekeeping, caring for baby dolls, "fixing" household items, going to work or school, cooking, and doing garden and yard work. Children need both structured and free play. Shared or cooperative play makes simple games of hide-and-seek and tag possible. Games with complicated rules can be frustrating to the preschooler, who prefers simple games with the option of making up the rules as the game proceeds. Cheating is common because the boundaries of acceptable play are not yet clear, and the earliest stages of moral behavior are only beginning to emerge.

Children today spend less time playing outside than previous generations, and they are more likely to play in their yard than any other location. Neighborhood environments may play an important role in children's planned and incidental physical activity. Parents report that when they live closer to play areas, children are more active overall and more likely to engage in moderate-to-vigorous activity. When there are fewer connecting streets and more visually appealing play areas, children are more active in their neighborhood; and children are more likely to use public recreation spaces that are free from crime and have walk and cycle facilities. Creating communities where children are closer to safe play areas may be the best way to improve children's physical activity and, in turn, reduce their risk of obesity and associated chronic disease (Tappe et al, 2013).

Body Image

Toddlers are often highly concerned about bodies. They realize that they are separate persons and begin to take notice of their own bodies. They may become fascinated with the different body parts and how they work. Bodily injury becomes a concern, and cuts and bruises elicit much discussion. Toward the end of the second year, children may notice the inner feelings of their bodies (e.g., the urge and tension to move the bowels, the release and relaxation resulting from going to the bathroom, the discomfort of hunger, and the pleasure of eating). These are abstract feelings that toddlers cannot put into words but can show with actions.

Preschoolers are equally curious about their bodies but are more capable of understanding and expressing themselves. They reexamine themselves frequently, and worries over a lost tooth or a skinned knee are common. Curiosity about their bodies and those of others generates a wealth of innocent questions that generally require only a simple answer. They learn that genital manipulation brings pleasure, and masturbation peaks around 3 to 4 years old.

Cognitive Development

Cognitively, toddler thinking is highly concrete. According to Piaget, 18- to 24-month-old children use mental imagery and infer causality when they can see only the effect. For example, if they see a puddle of milk on the floor, they might say "uh-oh" because they recognize it was spilled by someone. By the end of the second year, children enter the preoperational stage with preconceptual and intuitive thinking. Primitive conceptualization processes begin with the development of symbolic thinking. A block becomes a car; words become symbols for ideas. The 3-year-old continues to develop symbolic thinking, and this manifests through drawing and acting out elaborate play scenarios. However, children at this age generally are unable to take another's perspective but view the world egocentrically. Attending to one characteristic at a time is another feature of preschool thinking. For example, the child will try to fit a jigsaw puzzle piece using either color or shape but not both.

Parents may have difficulty understanding the thoughts of preschool children. On the surface, preoperational thinking has many characteristics that resemble adult thinking, and parents are often deceived into believing that children are able to think as adults do. Preschool children, for example, are developing the use of language and the ability to symbolize concepts mentally. Some of their verbalizations appear quite precocious, as evidenced by the 3-year-old who stares out the window and then states, "Look, Mommy, the trees are saying yes and no." Preschool children continue to be concrete and egocentric in their thinking, and their logic is the source of many communication problems between parents and children. Table 6-4 identifies major characteristic of preschool thinking and gives examples of each.

Language development through the toddler and preschool years remains one of the most sensitive indicators of cognitive development, and assessment tools plot language ability as a way of measuring cognitive levels. Social development and adaptive skills are also major indicators of

TABLE 6-4 Examples of Preschool Children's Thinking Using Piaget's Preoperational Stage

Characteristic	Example
Egocentrism	"It's snowing so I can go play in it."
Unable to see another's viewpoint	If John is holding a doll with its face toward Ann, Ann thinks John can also see the doll's face.
Mental symbolization of the environment	"The wind is crying." "The (flushing) toilet is an angry animal."
Incomplete understanding of sequence of time	Knows names of time components (today, tomorrow, yesterday, minutes, days, weeks, and so on), but uses them inconsistently: "I'm not going to take a nap yesterday." Yesterday means any time before now; tomorrow means any time in the future. Historical events are conceptualized in terms of the present: "Mommy, do you know George Washington?"
Developing sense of space: From experiencing space as a part of their activity to moving through it to understanding space in terms of detail and direction	Frequently used words: *in, on, up, down, at, under.*
Evolving ability to categorize or order objects and phenomena	*Early preschooler:* No understanding of concept of class or groups; undisturbed to see a new Santa Claus on every corner. *Cluster phenomena:* When asked to sort a series of blocks, the child may cluster a small, medium, and large block as a "baby," "mommy," and "daddy" block. By 4 to 5 years, child is able to consistently use one or two categories to arrange objects in some order (color, number, form, or size).
Developing ability to establish causality (e.g., realism, animism, artificialism)	*Realism:* Intellectual (dreams are actually real) and nominal (a horse can only be called a horse, not a stallion or filly). *Animism:* Two- to 3-year-olds think objects possess innate person-like qualities that cause results: "The chair made me fall down." *Artificialism:* Three- to 4-year-olds think things are caused by some controlling force that controls the world.
Transductive reasoning: from particular to particular	If the child does not like one particular vegetable, he or she will not like another particular fruit: "I can't eat my banana because my potatoes are burned."
Developing sense of conservation of quantity, weight, mass	Preschoolers are usually unable to conceptualize that change in shape does not affect quantity, weight, or mass of an object. Generally, 50% of 5-year-olds have mastered conservation of quantity, and 50% of 6-year-olds have mastered conservation of weight or mass.
Rigidity	Generally, children in the preoperational stage are very rigid in their thinking.

cognitive abilities. Differentiation of the self from others, with increasing sensitivity not only to the rules and norms for social interaction but also to the perception of the perspectives and feelings of others, requires ever increasing cognitive capability. Finally, play quality is an indicator of cognitive development. Through play, children manipulate and learn to control their environment in safe, yet stimulating ways.

Developmental Assessment of Early Childhood

Developmental assessment is an essential part of each health maintenance visit and includes both surveillance and screening using validated tools. Its goal is to monitor the child's growth and development and to determine at an early stage if problems or concerns exist. The process begins by building rapport with the parents, encouraging them to share developmental concerns and complete parent report tools, and listening to their comments with care and attention. Data are collected through parent interviews, screening tools, observation of the interactions between the child and parents, physical examination, and laboratory or other diagnostic measures. If there are questions about the child's development or if a child is identified through screening as having a possible problem, a thorough diagnostic assessment is needed. Referral to an appropriate specialist should be made to determine the degree of developmental delay and to identify management priorities.

Screening Strategies During Early Childhood

Toddlers and preschoolers need screening for physical and motor skills, communication and language, and social, emotional, and cognitive development. This can be done at well-child visits and at visits for episodic illnesses. Validated screening tools provide a quick, inexpensive method of identifying potential delays or concerns. These tools are generally appropriate for all children, although culture and experience can affect outcomes and must be taken into consideration. Parents can complete a screening tool in the waiting room, or providers can directly ask the parent questions. Providers should make sure they understand the parents' responses and follow up with more probing questions to clarify any concerns. Table 6-5 lists a variety of developmental screening tools. Tables 6-6, 6-7, 6-8, and 6-9 list questions that can be used to assess behavior and include the purpose or rationale for these questions.

Physical Development

Annually, toddlers and preschool children need anthropometric measurement, including blood pressure for 3-year-olds and at-risk children. Hearing and vision assessment is recommended at 4 and 5 years old (Hagan et al, 2008). The American Academy of Pediatric Dentistry (AAPD)

TABLE 6-5 Screening Tools for Toddler and Preschoolers

Screening Tool	Use	Website
Ages & Stages Questionnaires, ed 3 (ASQ-3) (2009)	Screening and surveillance of developmental milestones. Measures communication, gross motor, fine motor, problem solving, personal-social, and overall development. For use with 1-month-olds to 5½-year-olds. Parents report on 30 items plus overall concerns. Written at the 4th- to 6th-grade level. Manual includes activity handouts for parents. Available in English and Spanish. The ASQ-2 is available in French and Korean.	www.brookespublishing.com
Ages & Stages Questionnaire: Social-Emotional (ASQ: SE)	Screening of social-emotional development. Parents report on 32 items. For use with 3- to 60-month-olds. Takes 10 to 20 min or less to administer.	www.brookespublishing.com
Battelle Developmental Inventory, ed 2 (BDI-2)	Screening for early childhood developmental milestones. Measures personal-social, adaptive, motor, communication, and cognitive abilities. Parents report on 100 items. For use from birth to 8 years old. Takes 10 to 30 min; complete test 1 to 2 hours.	www.riversidepublishing.com/products/bdi2/
Child Development Inventory (CDI)	Screening for development milestones. Measures fine motor, gross motor, social skills, expressive language, language comprehension, self-help, letters, and numbers. Parents report on 300 items. For use with 15-month-olds to 6-year-olds. Test takes 30 to 40 min to administer.	www.childdevrev.com/index.html

TABLE 6-5 Screening Tools for Toddler and Preschoolers—cont'd

Screening Tool	Use	Website
Parents' Evaluations of Developmental Status (PEDS)	Screening/surveillance of development/social-emotional/behavior/mental health. Parents complete 10 questions. For use from birth to 8 years old. Test takes 2 min to administer. Available in English, Spanish, Vietnamese, and many other languages.	www.pedstest.com
Pediatric Symptom Checklist (PSC)	Psychosocial screen designed to recognize cognitive, emotional, and behavioral problems. Parents complete 35 items. For use with 4- to 11-year-olds. Test takes 5 to 10 min to complete. Available in English and dozens of other languages.	www.massgeneral.org/psychiatry/services/psc_forms.aspx
Temperament and Atypical Behavior Scale (TABS)	Screening for behavioral concerns. Measures detached, hypersensitive and hyperactive, underreactive, and dysregulated behaviors. Parent interview with 55 questions. For use from birth to 6 years old. Takes 15 to 20 min to complete.	www.brookespublishing.com
Short Sensory Profile (SSP)	Screens for sensory processing patterns. Measures tactile sensitive, taste-smell sensitivity, movement, underresponsive, auditory filtering, low energy and weakness, visual and auditory processing. Parents complete 25 items. For use from birth to adult. Takes 15 to 20 min to complete.	www.pearsonclinical.com
Modified Checklist for Autism in Toddlers, Revised with Follow-Up (M-CHAT-R/F) (2013)	Screening for symptoms of autism spectrum disorders. Parents complete 20 items. For use from 16 to 30 months. Takes 5 min to complete. Available in multiple languages.	www.mchatscreen.com/Official_M-CHAT_Website.html

TABLE 6-6 Surveillance of Physical Development and Motor Skills: Questions and Rationales

Question	Rationale for Question
Tell me about your child's health.	Invites discussion of somatic issues and complaints.
Does your child appear to be developing in a way similar to other children of the same age?	Assesses parent perceptions of physical development; developmental milestones.
Has any illness affected your child's daily activities?	Assesses possible chronic medical problem and effects on development.
Tell me about your child's daily habits: elimination, toilet training, sleeping, eating.	Assesses parent understanding of readiness, child's cues, changing behaviors, and current status.
How does your child get from place to place?	Assesses gross motor skills (e.g., walks, climbs, runs, pedals tricycle), and activity level.
How does your child feed himself or herself (e.g., cup, bottle, utensils)?	Assesses fine motor skills.
Tell me about your child's play activities.	Assesses gross and fine motor skills.

developed guidelines for preventive oral health interventions, including anticipatory guidance and preventive counseling for infants, children, and adolescents. The guidelines recommend the first examination occur at the time of the eruption of the first tooth and no later than 12 months old. Health professions should support the identification of a dental home for all infants by 12 months old (AAPD Clinical Affairs Committee, 2013).

Motor Skills Development

Toddlers and preschoolers develop and refine their motor skills, driven by curiosity, desire for independence, and

TABLE 6-7 Surveillance of Communication and Speech Development: Questions and Rationales

Question	Rationale for Question
How does your child communicate needs and desires?	Assesses verbal and nonverbal communication strategies, vocabulary, and expressive language.
How much do you think your child understands?	Evaluates cognitive level and receptive language.
How does your child respond to one-step commands? To two- or three-step commands?	Evaluates receptive language; evaluates short-term memory and auditory sequencing.
Does your child use plurals, pronouns, phrases, and sentences?	Indicates increased understanding of more complex structures.
How well can you understand your child's speech? How well can others?	Indicates increased articulation ability.

TABLE 6-8 Surveillance of Psychosocial and Emotional Development: Questions and Rationales

Question	Rationale for Question
Is your child able to feed himself/herself, dress, and take care of his or her own toileting?	Assesses adaptive skills, comfort with own abilities.
How does your child behave with family members he or she lives with? How does he or she behave with other family members?	Assesses child's development of roles within the family system; attachment should be evident.
How do you guide or discipline your child without always saying "no"?	Evaluates adaptability, creativity, repertoire of parent's skills in response to child's behaviors.
How does your child respond when you set limits?	Assesses child's understanding of limits of appropriate behavior, social rules, and self-control.
How does your child react to strangers or new situations?	Evaluates child's ability to deal with increasingly complex social situations.
Tell me about any tantrums your child has. What causes them? How does he or she behave? How do you respond?	Evaluates responses to stress, development of independence, and social control.
What does your child do for play?	Indicates social and emotional well-being.
How does your child behave around other children?	Considers social development with peers and development of appropriate play.
What is your child's best friend's name? Does he or she have shared activities with peers?	Indicates child is developing a social circle and increasing opportunities for practicing new social skills.
Does your child seem to understand the feelings of others?	Assesses empathy.
Is your child afraid of anything in particular? How do you handle that fear?	Evaluates parent's responses to child's emotional stresses and understanding of child's view and feelings.
Does your child have imaginary friends? Does she or he have a fantasy play time?	Allows child to explore emotions and developing roles in a safe way.

endless energy. Asking parents about the child's development is an important part of developmental surveillance. Gross and fine motor skills are best assessed using standardized, validated screening tools, such as the Ages & Stages Questionnaire-3 (ASQ-3).

Fine motor development is evaluated by assessing finger, hand, and oral movements. Gross motor skills are evaluated by assessing the child's large muscle skills, such as the ability to crawl, sit, walk, run, hop, skip, and climb. The quality of the child's movements during these activities is important to note as well.

Communication and Language Development

Communication is a vital part of being a happy, functioning human being, and language assessment is important during early childhood. A careful history of the child's abilities and pattern of learning (e.g., when did the child first articulate words?) provides much of the essential information. Listening to children and talking with their parents are essential, but the provider should also remember that parents may not be fully sensitive to speech problems because they are accustomed to hearing the child's current speech. Physical examination helps to determine if physical

TABLE 6-9 Surveillance of Cognitive Development: Questions and Rationales

Questions	Rationale for Questions
Questions Asked of 1- to 3-Year-Olds	
Tell me about a typical day. What sorts of things does your child do? With whom does she or he play? (Ask parent.)	Assesses complexity of manipulation of objects, parallel and cooperative play, and role-playing.
Can your child follow simple instructions? (Ask parent.)	Assesses ability to retain and process instructions and respond to input.
Does your child speak clearly? How much do you understand when your child speaks to you? Can your child understand what you say to him or her? (Ask parent.)	Assesses progress in decoding, encoding, and using a language system effectively.
How does your child behave in the family and with other children? (Ask parent.)	Indicates understanding of social systems and norms.
What is your name? Are you a boy or girl? How old are you? (Ask child.)	Three-year-olds should know these facts.
Questions Asked of 4- to 5-Year-Olds	
Ask child general information questions (e.g., colors, numbering, objects).	Assesses general fund of knowledge.
Ask child what makes the sun come up.	Illustrates child's belief about causality.
Ask child about concepts of time (e.g., What time do you have lunch? What time do you go to bed?).	Assesses understanding of a relatively sophisticated concept.
Ask child about spontaneous play (e.g., with puppets or dolls), imaginative use of play materials (e.g., clay, crayons, other toys).	Assesses imagination and magical thinking.
Ask child to draw a person.	50% of 4-year-olds draw a three-part person; by 5 years old, child can draw an eight-part person.
How does the child behave in preschool or child care setting? (Ask parent.)	Assesses language, social, and play development in relation to peers in a setting where expectations differ from those at home.

structures necessary for speech are intact (e.g., a cleft uvula may indicate an occult cleft palate that could interfere with the child's ability to shape words). Finally, using tools like the Early Language Milestone (ELM) brief screening for speech intelligibility (at 3 to 4 years old) may be necessary to refine the assessment (Table 6-10).

Language screening evaluates expressive and receptive language skills. Because language and cognitive skills are intricately interwoven, most intelligence tests have language sections that can be useful in assessing the total child. Expressive language screening places emphasis on articulation and vocabulary. Receptive language looks at comprehension, repetition, and follow-up of language heard (e.g., child's ability to follow directions).

Social and Emotional Development

Assessment of psychosocial and emotional development addresses children's roles in the family, success in making friends and working with peers, self-esteem, and feelings of contentment and security. This area of development should be assessed at each visit. The social emotional section of the ASQ assesses these behaviors but a more complete screening can be done by using the specific Ages & Stages Questionnaire: Social-Emotional (ASQ: SE) for children 3 months to 5 years old. The Pediatric Symptom Checklist (PSC) is a validated screening tool that can be used beginning at 4 years old to screen for psychosocial issues or concerns.

Cognitive Development

After 2 years old, as thinking moves into the preconceptual stages, cognitive development is increasingly expressed through symbol systems and language. Toddlers begin to enjoy make-believe, and preschoolers love stories and become masters at games of pretend and fantasy.

Anticipatory Guidance for Early Childhood

Anticipatory guidance for toddlers and preschoolers helps parents and children transition from a highly dependent relationship to one in which the child has an established sense of autonomy with an evolving understanding of the self as a separate, creative, and powerful being. During the process, parents learn new communication and interaction skills with their children. Although the toddler and preschool years can be frustrating at times, the ultimate outcome of good communication and relationships that support the potential of both child and parent is worth the

TABLE 6-10 Speech and Language Evaluation Tools

Evaluation Tool	Age Assessed and Test Characteristics	Source
The Capute Scales: Cognitive Adaptive Test and Clinical Linguistic and Auditory Milestone Scale (CAT/CLAMS)	Use from birth to 36 months. Interview. Tests language and problem-solving skills to help clearly identify between the two.	Paul H Brookes Publishing www.brookespublishing.com
Clinical Evaluation of Language Fundamentals—Preschool (CELF-P)	Use from 3 to 6 years. Assesses receptive and expressive language.	Pearson Assessment www.pearsonclinical.com/language/products/100000316/celf-preschool-2-celf-preschool-2.html
Early Language Milestone Scale (ELM Scale-2)	Use from birth to 36 months. Tests visual and auditory receptive, auditory expressive abilities. History, testing, and observation completed in 3 to 10 min.	Pro-Ed www.proedinc.com
Goldman-Fristoe Test of Articulation	Use from 2 to 22 years old. Assesses articulation skills.	Pearson Assessments www.ags.pearsonassessments.com
Peabody Picture Vocabulary Test	Use from 2½ to 90+ years old. Screens for receptive vocabulary.	Pearson Assessments www.pearsonclinical.com
Receptive-Expressive Emergent Language Test, ed 3 (REEL 3)	Use from birth to 36 months. Interview or direct observation of expressive and receptive language.	Pearson Assessments www.linguisystems.com

effort. According to the AAP recommendations for preventive pediatric health care and the *Bright Futures Guidelines,* providers should offer anticipatory guidance in all of the following areas: family support, child development, mental health, healthy weight, healthy nutrition, physical activity, oral health, healthy sexual development and sexuality, safety and injury prevention, community relationships, and resources; they should also provide educational counseling and support services (Hagan et al, 2008).

Regulation and Sleep-Wake Patterns

- Discuss the need to assist toddlers and preschoolers to transition from one state to another. Consistent sleep and naptime schedules are essential. Use of a comfort object (e.g., teddy bear) and bedtime rituals help.
- Explain how children at this age process information and control themselves. They can be overwhelmed if they have too much stimulation.
- Explain that some children may have sensory integration issues that require structuring and modulation of their environment.
- Discuss how to help children identify and name their feelings. This ability will help them to more successfully organize and integrate the sensations they experience and respond appropriately (Brazelton and Sparrow, 2006).
- Encourage parents to provide opportunities for children to have some control and choice in daily activities (e.g., can select the story to be read at bedtime), while maintaining important rituals.
- Discuss sleep problems that may appear at this time, including sleep resistance, bruxism, nightmares, and somnambulism (see Chapter 14).
- Encourage parents to offer naps and opportunities for rest but not to force them on children. It is the parents' job to make sure the child has ample rest time.
- Encourage parents to form good sleep routines for the child, to provide positive reinforcement of healthy sleep behavior, and to use firm, loving, and consistent discipline when dealing with sleep refusal and other behavioral sleep problems.

Strength and Motor Coordination

- Encourage parents to provide a wide range of safe play opportunities that use both fine and gross motor skills.
- Urge parents to allow children to take the lead during play and to follow and expand on whatever the child is interested in.
- Encourage parents to provide their children with a variety of play activities that expose children to nature, such as the following:
  - Take children to a park or playground to run, throw balls, swing, and slide.
  - Encourage children to play with natural materials, water, sand, grass, and leaves.
- Provide children with age-appropriate play materials: stickers, pencils, crayons, paper, paints, utensils, blocks, cardboard boxes, and building toys.

- Explain how parents can incorporate motor skills practice as part of daily routines (e.g., have child help pour the milk, hold the cup, or squeeze the toothpaste; encourage child to do own buttons, snaps, and zippers).
- Emphasize the need for constant adult supervision of children's activities.
- Discuss how parents can make the environment safer for their child: securing doors and using window guards; removing toxic substances and dangerous objects; providing toys that are developmentally appropriate and safely constructed.
- Reinforce teaching about car seat use and explain the need for larger car seats and booster seats as the child grows. Explain to parents the importance of modeling for the child by using their own seat restraint.

Feeding and Self-Care

- Provide parents with information about healthy foods and nutritional needs of their child (see Chapter 10). Three meals and two nutritious snacks per day are encouraged.
- Discuss the parents' responsibility to provide children with healthy foods and to allow children to make choices from healthy food options; it is the parents' job to provide the child with nutritious foods, and it is the child's job to decide how much they will eat. Starting with very small portions of food will help the child choose a variety of foods. Discourage parents from making separate meals for their young children.
- Young children may go on "food jags," refusing some foods or requesting the same food day after day. Parents need to make sure the food eaten is nutritious.
- Explain how changes in toddlers' eating habits are caused by developmental changes (e.g., child has a decrease in appetite, is easily distracted, demonstrates more curiosity about what is going on around him or her than in eating, is more interested in using gross motor skills than in sitting still).
- Explain nonnutritive value of food and eating (e.g., finger foods stimulate fine motor and cognitive development, in addition to fostering a child's sense of control and independence; eating together as a family can strengthen relationships and develop social skills).
- Encourage self-feeding to help the child gain new skills.
- Encourage parents to structure family mealtimes that are pleasant and interactive; this may mean offering the toddler foods that can be eaten in short periods of sitting. Avoid making meals a power struggle.
- Discuss plans for weaning (if the child has not already weaned).
- Explain the importance of the child gaining mastery of self-care (e.g., toileting, bathing, dressing, eating) and the valuable role the parent plays as teacher in the process. Assist parents to cope with the frustration or tensions generated by toddlers and preschoolers wanting to "do it myself." Ask the parents how they handle these situations.
- Ask if parents are concerned about the child becoming overweight.

Communication and Language

Children learn and refine communication and language skills best through their interactions with others. When parents and caregivers listen to them, talk interactively with them, and read to them, children's language blossoms (Hammer et al, 2010). Encourage parents to stimulate their child's language skills by doing the following:

- Read to children daily, using short, simple stories or picture books.
- Model appropriate language.
- Talk to the child, explaining in clear, simple language what is happening around the child; this helps increase vocabulary and the child's understanding of the world.
- Listen with care and respond actively to the child's verbalizations.
- Provide the child with opportunities to interact verbally with other children and adults.
- Do not allow children younger than 2 years old to watch television, and limit television viewing, smartphone, tablet and videos to 1 to 2 hours or less of appropriate programs per day for older children. Remove televisions from children's bedrooms (Hagan et al, 2008; National Association of Pediatric Nurse Practitioners [NAPNAP], 2009).
- When young children watch something on television, the parents should watch with them and talk about what is happening.

Providers should give parents the following anticipatory guidance:

- Explain that children need constant reinforcement of their speech and language efforts, but that nonverbal language, especially touch, continues to be crucial.
- Give parents an opportunity to explain their expectations for their child; discourage parental pressure on the child to perform (e.g., use of flash cards, requirement that child articulate sounds correctly) but point out that daily activities provide a wealth of opportunities to practice language skills.
- Reassure parents that language errors of young children usually disappear as children grow.
- Inform parents that children learn receptive language first, then expressive, and that they may not fully understand the meaning, especially connotative meaning, of what they hear or say (e.g., a 4-year-old may innocently ask a stranger about their private body parts). Parents should explain clearly, simply, and unemotionally which words are appropriate and in which settings.

Social and Emotional Growth

The emotional development of toddlers is an area in which parents may need a great deal of anticipatory guidance and support. The balance between dependence and independence is constantly in flux for young children and their parents, and conflict can develop as a result of inconsistent or extreme behavior. Toddlers and preschoolers need to master multiple social tasks during these years. They need to learn how to identify, control, and manage their feelings and emotions around anger, joy, love, and frustration. They learn about making and keeping friends, sharing, cooperative play, and living socially within a family. They learn to handle separation from parents, home, and neighborhood. To help families with this process, providers should do the following:

- Reemphasize the role of parents as guides of their child's social and emotional growth. Parents must actively engage with their children, showing interest in their activities and giving them guidance on appropriate behavior.
- Encourage parents to give their children opportunities to expand social skills and form important attachments outside the immediate family by doing the following:
  - Provide toys that children can use creatively.
  - Allow children to explore, guiding them to activities that are fun and stimulate their curiosity.
  - Structure time for children to play in natural settings. "Nature play" enhances physical, mental, and emotional health of children (McCurdy et al, 2010).
  - Allow children to make choices when possible; do not give children a "choice" when there really is none (e.g., "Do you want to go to bed?"). Instead, use "toddler's choices" that allow the child to have a say and yet still get toward the final objective (e.g., "Do you want to put your pants on or your shirt on first? Do you want to take the bunny or the bear with you during your nap?").
  - Discuss differences among people openly and positively.
  - Help children identify, name, and express feelings, both positive and negative.
  - Teach children to manage anger and resolve conflicts without violence.
  - Discuss television programs and movies to help children distinguish fantasy from reality.
  - Take children on trips to places of interest in the community.
  - Arrange play times with other children; encourage cooperative play (e.g., tag, hide-and-seek).
  - Reinforce positive child behavior ("catch the child being good").
  - Make the limits of what is expected of children clear, consistent, and achievable.
- Differentiate discipline and teaching from punishment.
- Discuss parenting and discipline (see Chapters 4 and 17).
- Clarify each parent's expectations of the child's behavior.
- Discuss how parents plan to resolve differences in expectations.
- Provide information to parents related to child development and what parents can expect their child to be able to do.
- Recommend parenting classes that provide information on developmental milestones, anticipated changes, and management strategies as children grow.
- Encourage parents to show affection in the family.
- Explain to parents that myths or fables can be important ways of teaching children abstract concepts, such as love, sharing, and giving.
- Inform parents of the need to provide children a feeling of safety and security. Parents can do the following:
  - Support use of comfort or transitional objects to allay fears (e.g., blanket).
  - Consider use of a nightlight.
  - Provide reassurance if nightmares or fears occur and respond to the child's fears.
  - Explain about "good" and "bad" touch.
  - Reinforce that the child can always come to the parent for comfort.

Cognitive and Environmental Stimulation

- Explain to parents that toddlers and preschoolers are concrete and preoperational in their thinking. As a result, parents need to be ready to explain things over and over patiently, without expecting the child to understand the adult's interpretation clearly. Also, children may use words to convey thoughts and feelings, but many responses are repetitive, and trial-and-error problem solving is usually crude. They frequently attend to only one aspect of a problem, giving partial answers.
- Emphasize that parents should avoid putting their own meaning on the child's behavior or statements. For example, the child's statement, "What if you just bought a new house, and I was allergic to something in the house? I guess you'd have to get rid of me," should not be interpreted to mean the parents have somehow failed to show the child how much they love him or her. Rather the child can be exploring the concepts of place, ownership, belonging, size, or importance. In the child's mind, a house is much bigger than he or she is and may be more important. An appropriate response from the parent might be, "No, we'd probably have to get a new house or take out whatever you are allergic to. Even if we just bought it, you are more important than any house, and we wouldn't want to lose you."
- Reassure parents that "Why?" will not continue to be the child's most frequent question. Toddlers and preschoolers are actively exploring meaning in their world and have learned that asking "Why?" brings them more information—and attention. As parents answer them, children begin to show threads of symbolic and more abstract thought.

Common Developmental Issues in Early Childhood

Sibling Rivalry

Interaction patterns between siblings vary and are affected by factors, such as gender, age, temperament, degree of attachment, nature of family interactions, types of discipline used in the family, and children's perceptions of how equally parents treat each child. Many toddlers or preschoolers regress when a new baby arrives, whereas older children may experience excitement, love, and enhanced self-esteem with a new sibling. Parents need to promptly limit any aggression expressed by the older child, provide love and attention, and talk about feelings. When older children fight, parents need to describe the situation and provide even-handed control. Blaming a child, except in a clear-cut instance of misbehavior, is usually unproductive. Promoting support, loyalty, and friendship is important for sibling interactions.

The birth or adoption of a sibling is a life-changing experience for the older sibling. Many parents voice concerns about the potential challenges with the older siblings, especially transient behavioral regressions that occur after a new infant is brought home. The developmental stage of the older sibling at the time of the new sibling's arrival is an important consideration in helping parents prepare their older child for the new sibling and in dealing with rivalry behaviors. For example, the 2-year-old working on developing autonomy often feels highly vulnerable with the appearance of a new sibling.

Additionally, many school-age children experience feelings of sibling rivalry, which may continue in varying degrees as the children grow and develop. Sibling rivalry involves the realization by the child that he or she must share his or her parents' attention and affection. The child may feel threatened or displaced.

Assessment

To assess sibling rivalry after the arrival of a new infant, ask the parent whether the older child has:

- Manifested regressive behaviors since the new sibling arrived (e.g., bed-wetting, return to the bottle, temper tantrums, separation issues)
- Made negative comments about the new sibling or has demonstrated verbal or physical aggression toward the parents or new sibling
- Voiced psychosomatic complaints

To assess sibling rivalry at any point, ask parents to:

- Describe sibling behaviors that concern them—fighting, verbal abuse, bickering.
- Identify any precipitating events or situations that seem to elicit negative behaviors between the siblings.
- Identify how rivalry behaviors between siblings were handled in the past and encourage the siblings to resolve the issues between them rather than the parents.

The provider should also ask parents to describe how they reacted to the behaviors or verbal comments and if and how they have disciplined the child.

Management

The cornerstone of the management of sibling rivalry is anticipatory and preventive. The provider needs to prepare parents before the arrival of the new sibling for the possibility of sibling rivalry and guide them in managing this situation. Before delivery or adoption:

- Explain to parents that at the time of the arrival of the new baby the other sibling(s) may exhibit regressive behaviors.
- Encourage parents to do the following:
  - Tell the child about the pregnancy or adoption of the new baby, using a time frame and language appropriate to child's developmental stage.
  - Investigate the possibility of sibling preparation classes for older siblings.
  - Prepare the child for a change in daily routines and change in the amount of time he or she will have with the parents.
  - Give children realistic expectations of their interactions with the baby.
  - Include an older child in preparations for the new baby and in the excitement of the event (e.g., have the child visit the mother and baby in the hospital if possible).

After the infant or child comes home:

- Encourage parents to consistently spend "alone time" each day with the older sibling.
- Have parents include the older sibling in the care of the new baby as appropriate (e.g., the toddler can help by bringing Mommy a diaper).
- Reinforce the older sibling's efforts to be a "big brother or sister;" praise the child for helping.
- Explain the need for tolerance when a child exhibits regressive behaviors, knowing the behaviors are not permanent.
- Educate parents about teaching children to distinguish between acceptable and unacceptable behaviors as well as accountability for negative behaviors.

As siblings grow, parents should avoid intervening for minor squabbles; rather they should encourage child-centered articulation of more significant arguments, and intervene if physical or verbal abuse occurs. Box 6-1 has other strategies to help siblings develop healthy relationships.

Temper Tantrums

Parents struggle with how to handle temper tantrums, which are episodes in which the child is frustrated and angry and loses control of his or her feelings (see Chapter 19).

Child Care and Preschools

Child Care

Many parents return to work during the first year of their child's life and must make arrangements for child care. In 2011, 12.5 million (61%) of the 20.4 million children under 5 years old attended regular child care (Laughlin, 2013). In 2014, nearly 64% of mothers with preschool-aged children (younger than 6 years old) were employed, and 75% of women with children between 6 and 17 years old were employed (Bureau of Labor Statistics, 2013). Child care issues affect millions of people and can be a

• BOX 6-1 Managing Sibling Rivalry

Do

Allow children to vent negative feelings.
Encourage children to develop solutions for problems with siblings.
Anticipate problem situations.
Foster individuality in each child.
Spend time with children individually.
Compliment children when they are playing together.
Tell children about the conflict you had with your siblings when you were a child.
Define acceptable and unacceptable behaviors for sibling interactions.

Do Not

Take sides.
Serve as a referee.
Foster rivalry by comparing siblings or their accomplishments.
Use derogatory names.
Permit physical or verbal abuse between siblings.

source of significant parental concern. Parents are challenged with evaluating and selecting a qualified child care provider whom they are sure provides a safe, nurturing, and developmentally appropriate setting. The individual needs of the child together with parental needs for work coverage and flexibility must be matched with the philosophy and constraints of the child care setting. The primary care provider is often called on to advise parents about how to select a suitable provider (Box 6-2).

Preschool

Entering preschool can be stressful for both the young children attending the school and their families. Some children have difficulty adapting to the more structured school environment, whereas others may be comfortable with limits and rules. Parents may find their child compared with other children, and a child with developmental delays (e.g., speech, motor, physical) may be singled out as different, not fitting in, or as having a behavior problem. Preschool and kindergarten were originally intended to help children learn separation, sharing, listening, paying attention, and simple social skills. Now, kindergarten students are often expected to show pre-academic skills, such as writing, counting, and letter and word recognition in addition to the preschool social skills of paying attention and sitting still. In making their preschool selection, parents should select a play-based learning curriculum, because this is the most comfortable way for young children to learn. Chapter 7 includes an in-depth discussion of school readiness.

When selecting a preschool, it is important to consider the following child characteristics:

- Social skills (e.g., ability to separate from parent for several hours)
- Language skills, both expressive and receptive
- Physical size
- Energy level (e.g., ability to actively participate)

• BOX 6-2 A Five-Step Approach to Help Parents Select a Child Care Provider

Step 1

You should begin searching for child care as early as possible. Deciding whether to use a child care center or an individual home is a very personal decision. It can take a while to find the right setting to fit your child and family.

Step 2

The search for a child care also means familiarizing yourself with local child care rules and regulations. Local and state child care licensing boards can provide referrals to accredited child care facilities and can give you information about the rules and regulations in your area. They also can provide information about formal child care complaints and violations.

Step 3

Visit potential child care sites. Drop in at different times and pay attention to the environment and how the staff responds to the children in their care.

- Ask what the adult-to-child ratio is. Older children do not need the same level of attention as infants, so ratios tend to increase as the child ages. Make sure you know what the minimum state ratios are for your area.
- Ask how many children are in each class/group. Think about your child's personality and needs and try to match the group size to what is best for your child. Large groups with multiple adults are very different from smaller groups with fewer adults.
- Ask how child care providers are selected and what training and education they require. Child cares that have caregivers with degrees in early child education or who have special training have skills that will foster your child's learning. It is also important to know what kinds of continuing education is provided for the caregivers.
- Ask how often children change caregivers and ask about staff turnover. Children do best with consistent care and with regular caregivers. Just like they crave routine at home, children desire routines and consistent caregivers in child care.
- Ask if the child care provider has accreditation from a national organization. Accredited providers have demonstrated they meet standards that are usually higher than state standards. National accreditation can be verified by visiting the accrediting agency's website.

Step 4

When you make your decision about which child care provider to use, start by thinking about your child's and family's needs. Take into account all the information you received during your search.

Step 5

Stay involved with your child's child care. Talk to your child's caregivers. Don't be afraid to ask questions about your child's day and how he/she is doing during the day. Tell your child's caregiver about how your child is doing at home. For example, if your child is having trouble napping at home, asking about how naps are going at the child care can give you important information. Try to attend special events like field trips or holiday parties. You are your child's most important caregiver, and children do best when parents and child care caregivers work together as a team.

Child Care Aware: *Five steps to choosing care* (website). http://childcareaware.org/parents-and-guardians/child-care-101/5-steps-to-choosing-care. Accessed December 12, 2014.

- Neurologic maturation required for fine and gross motor activities (e.g., writing, cutting, coloring, climbing, running, walking)
- Neurologic maturation of sensory and cognitive function (e.g., visuospatial perception, tactile maturation, auditory processing, attending skills, memory)

Toileting

Toileting skills and training are major milestones for a child and the parents. It is a complex developmental skill that many children master effortlessly, but some children and families need guidance and support along the way (see Chapter 12).

Safety

Parents should safety proof any environments their children spend time in but also need to know that safety proofing is not enough; toddlers and preschool children need to have adult supervision at all times (see Chapter 40 for more information).

Early Childhood Developmental Red Flags

Although a wide range of normal development may be seen when assessing children, the provider needs to be alert to developmental red flags—signs of delayed or abnormal development. In addition to obvious abnormalities, minor problems that are left untreated can develop into major concerns; minor signs and symptoms that persist can indicate a more serious underlying problem, or a major problem can occur as a one-time event (e.g., a child who sets a fire). Some children and families are at high risk and need careful monitoring and guidance to detect problems at an early stage or to prevent their occurrence (e.g., very early premature infants, families with history of violence, families with chronic medical or mental health problems, some single-parent families). The warning signs, or red flags, can be found in Table 6-11. Children who demonstrate these behaviors should be referred. Immediate referral is required for children who stop eating, demonstrate cruelty to animals or other people, are self-harmful, start fires, or talk of harming themselves, their peers, or others.

Physical Disorders

Children should be monitored for physical growth milestones. Further investigation, screening, and referral may be appropriate when children fall outside normal growth parameters or when children follow a normal growth pattern and begin to level off or fall below that range. If children have symptoms—they stop eating, complain of tiredness, are not as active as usual, or the parents state that the child has regressed—it is time to investigate.

Cognitive Disorders

Mental and cognitive delays are more difficult to recognize and categorize without the help of a screening tool or more in-depth assessment. These tools rank children on the basis of a standardized score or against standardized criteria (e.g., word definition). Children with scores below 85 on intelligence scales, for example, predictably have more difficulty in school. Significant discrepancies between test scores taken over time also suggest problems. The causes of delay must be carefully assessed as well because some children may have a neurologic limitation, whereas others may be delayed as a result of material or environmental deprivation. Identifying the causes is necessary to plan effective interventions. In any case, when delays are suspected, prompt referral to developmental specialists or early childhood intervention programs for more detailed assessment is essential.

Language Disorders

Language delays or disorders are problems in learning communication systems and, when present, affect other areas of development, especially cognitive, social, and emotional development. Because language development is the best indicator of cognitive development, language delays may indicate serious issues that require developmental and educational intervention.

Children with language delays experience problems in either receptive or expressive language, or both. They may start talking late, talk very little as toddlers, or have prolonged stages of normal stuttering, distortion, and substitution.

Cognitive, familial, environmental, physical, psychological, or cultural factors can cause language delays. Language delays or disorders may occur if the child does not hear, is not immersed in a language-rich environment, or has a disorder, such as severe deprivation or autism. Speech disorders (i.e., problems producing sounds) are associated with physical problems (e.g., cleft lip, cleft palate, cerebral palsy, hearing impairments) or they can be idiopathic.

Language evaluation involves assessment of the child's physical, cognitive, social, emotional, and perceptual characteristics. Expressive and receptive language needs to be evaluated. The inability to use the symbols of language may be characterized by the following:

- Improper use of words and their meanings
- Inappropriate grammatical patterns
- Improper use of speech sounds

Speech disorders involve problems producing correct speech sounds and may be characterized by difficulty in the following:

- Producing speech sounds (articulation)
- Maintaining speech rhythm (fluent speech)
- Controlling vocal production (voice)

Management of children with language disorders requires a clear understanding of the nature of the problem. Referral to a specialist (e.g., pediatric speech pathologist) to make

TABLE 6-11 Red Flags of Early Childhood Development

Age	Growth, Rhythmicity, Sleep, and Temperament	Psychosocial and Emotional Skills	Cognitive Abilities	Gross Motor, Language, and Hearing	Fine Motor, Feeding, and Self-Care	Strength and Coordination
12 months		No big smiles or joyful expressions		No babbling No recognizing name when called	Is not pointing or using sounds to get desired object; may just cry	
15 months	No nighttime ritual Difficulty with transitions Parents express concern about temperament or control issues	Problems with attachment to caregiver	Lack of object permanence	No words Only single words by 16 months Lack of consonant production, uses mostly vowel sounds Consistent and frequent omission of initial consonants Does not imitate words No gestures or pointing	No self-feeding	No attempts at walking
18 months	Poor sleep schedule Problems with control and behavior	Does not pull person to show something	Primary play: mouthing of toys No finger exploration of objects Lack of imitation Not using toys as they were intended	Unable to follow simple directions (e.g., "no," "jump") Excessive, indiscriminate, irrelevant verbalizing	Does not try to scribble spontaneously Unable to use spoon	Not yet walking or frequently falls when walking
24 months	Falling off growth curve Poor sleep schedule Awakens at night; unable to put self back to sleep	Absent symbolic play No evidence of parallel play Displays destructive behaviors Always clings to mother	No pretend play	No meaningful two-word phrases Use of noncommunicative speech (echolalia, rote phrases) Unable to identify five pictures Unable to name body parts No jargon History of greater than 10 episodes of otitis media	Unable to stack four or five blocks Still eating pureed foods Unable to imitate scribbles on paper Unable to dump pellet from bottle	Unable to walk downstairs holding a rail Persistent waddle walk Persistent toe walking

30 months	Resistance to regular bedtime Beginning behavior issues	Problems with biting, hitting playmates, parents Not able to play with others	Cannot follow two-step commands	Cannot name self Does not use pronouns	Unable to feed self Unable to build a tower of six blocks Unable to imitate circle shape Unable to imitate vertical stroke	Unable to jump in place Unable to kick ball on request
36 months	Problems with toilet training Unable to calm self	Not able to dress self Does not understand taking turns No expanded pretend play	Cannot name familiar colors Does not understand "same" and "different" Unable to recognize common objects Unable to recall parts of a story	Unable to give full name Unable to match two colors Does not use plurals Does not know two or three prepositions Unable to tell a story Unclear consonants Unintelligible speech Unable to construct a sentence	Unable to build a tower of 10 blocks Holds crayon with fist Unable to draw circle	Unable to balance on one foot for 1 second Toeing-in causes tripping with running
48 months	Lack of bedtime ritual Behavior concerns: withdrawn or acting out Stool holding Problems with toilet training	Unable to play games, follow rules Unable to follow limits or rules at home (e.g., put toys away) Cruelty to animals, friends Interest in fires, fire starting Persistent fears or severe shyness Inability to separate from mother	Unable to count three objects Unable to recall four numbers Unable to identify what to do in danger, fire, with a stranger Consistently poor judgment	Difficulty understanding language Problems understanding prepositions Limited vocabulary Unclear speech	Lack of self-care skills—dressing feeding, Unable to button clothes Unable to copy square	Unable to balance on one foot for 4 seconds Unable to alternate steps when climbing stairs
60 months	Continued sleep problems Concerns with night terrors Hair pulling—scalp or eyelashes	Difficulty making and keeping friends; no friends Difficulty understanding sharing, school rules, organization of daily activities Cruelty to animals, friends Interest in fires, fire starting Bullying or being bullied Prolonged fighting, hitting, hurting Withdrawal, sadness, extreme rituals	Unable to count to 10 Unable to identify colors Unable to follow three-step commands	Speech pattern not 100% understandable Cannot identify a penny, nickel, or dime Abnormal rate or rhythm of speech	Unable to copy triangle Unable to draw a person with a body	Difficulty hopping, jumping

that determination is often the first step. Deficits identified in Table 6-11 are cause for referral for additional testing. Other criteria that warrant referral include the following:

- There are unusual confusions, reversals, or telescoping in connected speech.
- There is a loss of previously acquired language skills.
- The child stops talking.
- The child reacts to his or her own speech with embarrassment or withdrawal.
- The child's voice is monotone, extremely loud, largely inaudible, or of poor quality.
- Pitch is not appropriate to the child's age and gender.
- Hypernasality or lack of nasal resonance occurs.

For a complete list of references, please visit http://evolve.elsevier.com/Burns/pediatric/.

7 Developmental Management of School-Age Children

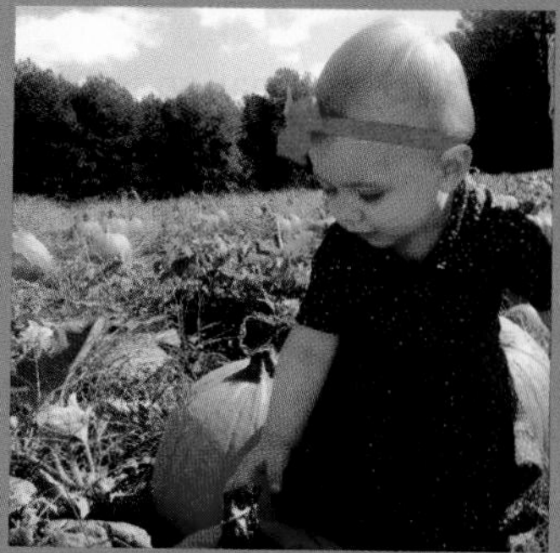

YVONNE K. YOUSEY

School-age children are busy, active, curious, and creative. With guidance and encouragement, they eagerly apply the skills they learned as toddlers and preschoolers as they move into more structured school environments, home schooling, or community settings. Their physical abilities advance, they engage in casual play with friends or siblings, and they may choose to play organized sports. Cognitively and emotionally, school-age children face daunting challenges. They must master the intellectual skills of reading, writing, mathematics, science, and other academic work. They become skilled socially, separating from home and family, establishing friendships, negotiating with siblings and other family members, and working on developing a sound sense of who they are as unique members of the community.

School-age children pass through several phases from preschool innocence to adolescent complexity. The school-age years can be divided into early childhood (5 to 7 years old), middle childhood (8 to 10 years old), and late childhood (11 to 12 years old). Children in each of these phases demonstrate different developmental goals and achievements. Each school-age child is unique, and patterns of "normal" development have broad parameters. The developmental goals of school-age children include laying the groundwork for lifelong learning, creating a sense of self-worth, developing the ability to contribute to the world around them, and, ultimately, gaining satisfaction with life.

Primary health care providers must be familiar with theoretic models of psychosocial development and physical growth for this age group. Parents often turn to their health care provider for understanding and guidance. Some authors characterize the school-age period as one of quiescence, but a remarkable amount of growth takes place, and the route is not always smooth. Providers can support children and their families to be successful in their achievements during these important years.

Development of School-Age Children

Physical Development

School-age children gain strength and coordination and become more physically capable, setting the stage for participation in sports, dance, gymnastics, and other activities. Success and enjoyment of these physical activities establish healthy patterns for a lifetime. Social status among children is often based on physical competence; therefore the child's feelings about physical development can be as important as the physical growth itself.

The growth rate of school-age children increases significantly from that of the toddler and preschooler and occurs in "spurts" where the child literally "grows out" of his or her clothes in a matter of weeks. The best way to evaluate an individual child's growth is to monitor his or her progress for height, weight, and body mass index (BMI) on a growth chart. Head circumference increases slowly but is no longer routinely measured. By middle childhood, the brain is about 90% of its adult size with full adult size reached by approximately 12 years old. Myelination of the brain, which is necessary for information processing, is not complete until early adulthood. The cerebral cortex (responsible for intelligence) and the frontal lobe (responsible for problem-solving and decision-making) are the last to fully develop. The increasing maturation of the brain allows children to complete increasingly complex motor and cognitive skills and to have greater control over their bodies. Organ development is complete. Most school-age children sleep about 10 hours per night (range 8 to 14 hours) without naps, particularly during the school

TABLE 7-1 Physical Development of School-Age Children

Body System	Developmental Change
Skin and lymph	At about 6 years old, tonsils and adenoids reach thier largest size. Prepubescence is characterized by more active sebaceous glands and vasomotor instability that can lead to uncontrolled blushing.
Head, eyes, ears, nose, and mouth	Head size becomes smaller in proportion to body size. Undeveloped sinus cavities contribute to increased susceptibility to upper respiratory infections, sinus irritation, and sinus headaches. By 6 to 7 years old, the retina is fully developed, and visual acuity is 20/20. By middle childhood, the Eustachian tube grows longer, narrower, and more slanted. By 5 to 6 years old, first primary teeth are shed, and the first permanent teeth erupt, usually the central incisors. Each year after 6 years old, approximately four teeth are replaced—one set in the upper jaw, and one set in the lower jaw.
Pulmonary	Through childhood, the lungs gradually descend into the thoracic cavity. By 8 years old, alveolar development is complete. During middle childhood, tidal volume increases; normal adult respiratory rate is achieved (18 to 30 breaths per minute). Increased maturation of the macrophagocytic activity of mucus and ciliary function in lungs makes the child more resistant to respiratory infections.
Cardiovascular	By 5 years old, the heart is four times larger than at birth. By 7 years old, the left ventricle thickens; it is two to three times greater in size than right; blood pressure increases to 90 to 108/60; cardiac volume increases; heart rate declines to 60 to 100 bpm. Atherosclerosis begins in childhood.
Gastrointestinal	By middle childhood, the GI system is of adult size and function.
Genitourinary	By 6 years old, elimination patterns are established; greater than 90% of children are toilet trained. Bladder capacity continues to expand. Between 10 and 14 years old, puberty begins but can be normal in any child after 8 years old for females and 9 years old for males. Delayed puberty is diagnosed if no secondary sex changes (e.g., breast budding; penis or testicle growth) are noted at 13 years old in girls and 14 years old in boys.
Musculoskeletal	Long bones grow, leading to the taller, thinner school-age child. Spine becomes straighter; legs become straighter. Facial bones are actively changing as nasal accessory sinuses grow.
Immune system	Rapid maturation of the immune system during middle childhood. Allergic conditions may appear.

bpm, Beats per minute; *GI*, gastrointestinal.

year. Night terrors or sleepwalking may emerge (see Chapter 14). Table 7-1 lists the normal physical development for school-age children.

Motor Skills Development

In middle childhood, gross motor skills continue to be refined, allowing children to run, jump, climb, hop, skip, tandem walk, alternate their foot patterns, and use an overhand motion. Activities that require balance and coordination (such as, riding a bicycle, swimming, and roller skating) demonstrate children's expanding skills. In late childhood, gross motor skills become more controlled and purposeful. Skills are perfected with much practice. A sense of competition is high as children try to outlast or outperform one another. Consequently, school-age children enjoy participating in competitive sports.

Mastery of fine motor skills includes improved dexterity and better control of scissors and writing tools, such as crayons and pencils. In early childhood, children become adept at dressing themselves, including being able to tie knots and manage buttons and zippers. Their drawings become more recognizable, showing details of eyes, ears, and other body parts. Self-care skills (e.g., combing hair, brushing teeth) are improved. In late childhood, hand-eye coordination improves, and the child is able to use each hand independently with speed and smoothness. During this time, skill in playing musical instruments emerges.

Communication and Language Development

The child's language patterns provide insight into the status of the neurologic system because the maturing brain is capable of increasingly complex language skills. Both receptive and expressive language skills improve. Six-year-olds have a well-developed vocabulary and are able to retrieve words quickly. They have basic syntactic abilities and can follow simple directions. The language demands of school can be challenging for 6-year-olds. First, they may not be accustomed to attending to total auditory stimuli, which occurs in the classroom environment. Second, they are still mastering connotative and semantic rules, such as understanding the concepts "before" and "after," relative clauses (e.g., "the cat was chased by the dog"), and the structures of sentences. These factors can make it difficult for them to follow complicated directions or cope with the increased demand to recall information within a specific time frame. Narrative skills can be poor, and reading may be difficult. The expressive language of 6-year-olds should be fully intelligible. Stuttering has usually resolved by school age but may be seen if young children are overly eager to express themselves. Developmentally normal stuttering that does not cause the child distress should be ignored at this age.

Seven-year-olds' receptive language is strong; they generally have language decoding mastered and are working on encoding information. They organize previous knowledge and express it verbally or in writing. They can solve word problems. Articulation mastery may not be achieved until 7 or 8 years old with the sounds of "l" and "th."

Eight- to 9-year-old children demonstrate significant syntactic growth with better use of pronouns, allowing them to understand convoluted sentences. Comparatives are learned, and the child is able to distinguish qualities, such as more or less, near or far, and heavy or light. By 8 years old, children follow complex directions. They begin to tell jokes because they understand different meanings of words. In their expressive language, children have better narrative abilities and significantly improved storytelling and the summarization skills needed for such activities as explaining a task to other children. Vocabulary grows, and there are gradual improvements in grammar (e.g., noted by the use of past and future tenses and plural forms of nouns, particularly irregular nouns and verbs).

At 10 years old, children are able to discuss ideas and understand inflections and metaphors. Their ability to understand the ambiguities of sentence structure, word meaning, and language contributes to their increasing ability to enjoy jokes and riddles. They use concrete operational thinking to analyze and interpret language and are more aware of the inconsistency in spoken languages. Children in late childhood understand that words can mean more than their literal definition. By 12 years old, children normally answer questions involving sophisticated concepts. Their sentences should be grammatically correct, and they have more detail in their verbal skills. The ability to express emotions also develops. Language becomes a means of socializing, and fewer gestures are used. Language can become a game as children make up words and participate in storytelling using proper sequence and pronouns.

Speech and language problems are among the most common developmental disorders among children in early childhood affecting from 4% to 10% of children; motor dysfunction is associated with language impairment in 40% to 90% of these children. Language delays and hearing impairment have been linked with motor coordination, behavior, and psychiatric comorbidities, such as attention-deficit/hyperactivity disorder (ADHD) (Stevenson et al, 2010). Although it is important that language delays and motor impairment be identified at a younger age, interventions and therapy for these conditions extend into school-age years. The perceptual difficulties experienced by these children require continued intervention to ensure learning success. Physical, occupational, and speech therapy are necessary interventions through school years (Müürsepp et al, 2012).

Social and Emotional Development

The psychosocial development of school-age children puts to rest the notion that childhood is a "quiescent" period. Challenges that school-age children face are especially difficult because the child's skill and ultimate success are dependent on evolving abilities. Gaining social acceptance from one's peers, for example, depends on skills such as being socially responsive, understanding the group "rules," using the group jargon, being appropriately assertive, and being empathetic. Children who do not have those skills can experience a sense of failure when they are compared with their peers who do. Erikson posited that school-age children are eager to learn and internally motivated to achieve mastery and recognition. They need experiences in an environment that recognizes, adjusts for, and supports their maturing set of skills, where they can explore creatively, learn actively, and be recognized for their successes.

The stages through which children progress as they become more socially and emotionally mature are sequential and are built on since birth, with each being a prerequisite for the next (Table 7-2) (see Table 4-1 and discussion in Chapter 4 on theoretic models of development). In particular, school-age children must develop social interaction skills including how to:

- Understand meaning in social situations and interpret others' social cues
- Initiate interactions
- Terminate interactions positively
- Gain impulse control and manage emotions
- Resolve conflicts

Mastery of these skills enables children to:

- Refine their role within the family system
- Separate self from family
- Develop and maintain peer friendships
- Develop positive relationships with adults outside the family
- Achieve social acceptance
- Strengthen a sense of self

The earliest school-age psychosocial milestone occurs when children learn to separate easily from family, allowing them to go to school. As they move into the community,

TABLE 7-2 **Developmental Characteristics of the School-Age Child**

Approximate Stages and Ages	Psychosexual Development	Social and Emotional Development	Cognitive and Problem-Solving Development	Moral Development
Early childhood (5 to 7 years old) (carried over from the toddler and preschool years to about 6 years old)	*Phallic stage (Freud):* Attaches to the parent of the opposite sex. Usually sexual identity occurs at the end of this phase, and sexual urges are quiescent.	*Initiative vs. guilt (Erikson):* Moving into a larger social environment and thus able to initiate activities on their own. Begins to learn to modulate their own behaviors through development of a consciousness as to what is appropriate for parents and society.	*Preoperational period (Piaget):* Representative language and early reasoning. Problem-solving is intuitive rather than logical. Thought process involves magical thinking, egocentrism, centration, syncretism, juxtaposition, animism, artificialism, participation, and irreversibility.	*Preconventional stage (Kohlberg):* Stage 1: Reasoning is based on rewards and punishment or the consequences of behavior. Stage 2: Begins to base behaviors on own needs and at times the needs of others. Reciprocity is concrete. Others' feelings are secondary.
Middle childhood (7 to 10 years old)	*Latency stage (Freud):* The superego or conscious is internalized. Energy is put into acquiring cultural and social skills. Guidelines established by the family are followed.	*Industry vs. inferiority (Erikson):* Begins to appreciate individual interests and skills, and seeks to become a successful member of a group. Internal motivation to achieve, compete, and obtain recognition. If unsuccessful, learning motivation is lost.	*Early concrete operational (Piaget):* Begins to use logic and becomes more objective using an external point of view. Thinking becomes dynamic, decentralized, using conservation, transitivity, seriation, classification, and reversibility. Learns to understand size, shape when the physical properties can be manipulated.	*Conventional stage (Kohlberg):* Stage 3: Begins to act to please others. Stage 4: Begins to conform to rules.
Late childhood (10 to 12 years old) (carried into adolescence)	*Genital stage (Freud):* Reemergence of sexual impulses.	*Industry vs. inferiority (Erikson):* Continuation of socialization with other children and groups. Development of hobbies and interests outside of school allows recognition of individual worth.	*Late concrete operational (Piaget):* Able to conceptualize size, shape, quantity, space, and thus able to problem-solve using abstract thought. Able to classify items into a hierarchical system. *Formal operational (Piaget):* Distinguished by the ability to use abstract thinking, complex reasoning, thinking, flexibility, and hypothesis formation. Becomes more aware of contradictions, falsehoods, and shortcomings in previous beliefs. Becomes aware of how others think of them.	*Postconventional stage (Kohlberg):* Stage 5: Begins to appreciate that their behaviors benefit society. Stage 6: Begins to form principles from conscience, even if they differ from what is generally acceptable in society. Looks for rationale in rules. Respect for authority and maintaining social order.

children maintain their role and feelings of belonging to a family, but also develop secondary attachments with other adults outside the home. Having good relationships with adults outside the home is especially important when the family is not wholly functional or not responsive to and supportive of the child.

Peer Relationships

A major task of school-age children is to develop competence in social relationships. The ability of children to form friendships depends on development of their social cognition, a direct result of parent-child relationship during the developing years (Fenning et al, 2011). Social acceptance is especially important at this age. Friends are generally chosen because of shared skills, interests, personality, and loyalty. Children often see themselves through the eyes of their friends. As early as 7 years old, some children are more concerned about a friend's opinion than about adults' opinions. They develop "best friends" and dress and talk like their peers. A special-friend phase should occur at around 10 years old. This is an intense attachment to a same-gender child. With that friend, the child expands the self, learns altruism, shares feelings, and learns how others manage problems. Talking on the telephone, texting or emailing friends, and sleepovers become more common. These early friendships are the basis for later relationships. Family conflicts can arise when peer activities and expectations conflict with family rules and values.

Children's temperaments affect the way they interact with peers, teachers, family, and others in their environment. Adverse environments create stress in the lives of children that alters their development. Emotional problems during these years often follow frustrations, losses, and situations in which the child's self-esteem is threatened or the child is faced with adversity. Relationships are crucial in normalizing biologic and behavioral systems in at-risk children. These supportive, responsive relationships foster healthy child behavioral and biologic development (Thompson, 2014).

Morality

Although there is variability in moral development, moral reasoning in early childhood is usually determined by the consequences of behavior: to avoid punishment, receive rewards, or meet one's needs. There is some consideration of the feelings of others, but only as it serves one's needs. By 7 years old, most children can name a site for their conscience (heart or brain), and school-age children tend to be rather rigid in their views of right and wrong, which is consistent with concrete thinking. They understand the relationships between responsibility and privileges and realize that choices between right and wrong behaviors are within their control. Some children at this age act appropriately to get a direct reward, whereas others do their duty, viewing moral behavior as following the rules of higher authority. In late childhood, children begin to move into Kohlberg's (1981) postconventional stage where respect for authority and social norms develops.

The ability to reason through difficult situations with a variety of factors operating is heavily dependent on cognitive development; however, school-age children do not have the cognitive maturity to cope with all situations. The school environment, where rules and values may differ from those of the immediate family, must be confronted and negotiated daily. This presents a challenge to the child's concepts of right and wrong. Social pressures may make it difficult to choose actions that the child believes are right. The pressures of gangs, drugs, and peers push many children to make decisions about their activities and behaviors before they are developmentally ready. Furthermore, the values of the family are challenged as the child learns that other families make decisions and have beliefs that differ from their own.

Body Image

School-age children may appear to be totally unaware of their bodies (e.g., the 9-year-old boy who does not change his shirt for 3 days) perhaps because they are so busy with their daily lives. In fact, children at this age are extremely curious about changes happening to them as they grow, and they are sensitive to others around them. Highly literal in their thinking, they can be very frank with questions to people they trust (e.g., "Grandma, why are you growing a moustache?"). At the same time, they are learning the importance of social politeness (e.g., what is appropriate in certain situations and how to behave themselves), so they may be uncomfortable or shy about new or unusual situations. Modesty is characteristic of school-age children.

Sexual exploration, including masturbation, is common. Children in early childhood, 5 to 7 years old, often play "doctor," and in middle childhood, children will compare their bodies with friends of the same gender.

Physical growth and neurologic maturation give children the ability to master many new skills. Young swimmers, runners, skateboard enthusiasts, and soccer players all emerge at this time. Their achievements and failures help them define who they are and are the basis for their evolving self-image. Their body images come from the experiences they have and the feedback from family, peers, teachers, and others in the community. This feedback can help clarify their understandings and allow the child to gain in self-confidence and feelings of worth.

Coping Skills

As a part of the process of developing relationships with others, school-age children refine their ability to identify, label, and manage their feelings. However, their experiences are limited, and their cognitive abilities are still expanding. They continue to need help labeling complex emotions, such as sadness, depression, worry, and envy. They also need help to consciously manage those and other feelings in acceptable ways.

Impulse control is an important coping skill learned by school age. Without impulse control, random behavior occurs; on the other hand, overly controlled children appear hostile, uncreative, or both. By 7 years old, children should have developed sufficiently to function in a variety of settings (e.g., home, school, and playground) with increasing competence.

School-age children face a variety of stressors in society today, including violence, bullying, parental divorce, substance abuse in the family, early responsibilities, and lack of support in school. Violence is a constant problem for many, not only in neighborhoods where children live and play but also within their families and in the schools where they go to learn. Anxiety is the most common mood disorder of middle childhood, with most cases diagnosed before 12 years old (Beesdo et al, 2009).

Some children are given heavy responsibility at a young age. Many children care for themselves after school while their caregivers work. Latchkey children remain alone, housebound, and unsupervised until adults return at the end of the day. Some also have responsibility for caring for younger siblings.

Many schools lack resources to maintain small class sizes or offer special programs for children with learning difficulties. Children with these issues are at risk for passing from grade to grade without remediation of their fundamental learning problems and with the stigma of failure.

Children with chronic illnesses or disabilities may have trouble adapting to their conditions during the school-age years and may need special help to foster independence and a sense of self-esteem. Latchkey children with chronic illnesses are especially vulnerable, because they may need to make decisions about their health care without adult advice, such as whether to take more medication or complete a treatment. Affected children need to understand their illness, medications, where to go for emergency care, how to write down instructions or messages, and how to follow important rules. Children vary in their ability to manage their self-care. A child's capacity for self-care of chronic illnesses depends on the illness, its stability, and the child's age and cognitive skills. Children's coping abilities are significantly affected by the availability of social supports from caregivers (Thompson, 2014).

Cognitive Development

In early childhood, children transition from preoperational thinking that uses intuitive problem-solving to early concrete operational thinking. At this stage, they are capable of the logical thought processes described in Box 7-1. Children are more likely to be ready for school when they make this transition. Magical thinking and egocentric logic fade, and concepts of conservation, transformation, reversibility, decentration, seriation, and classification emerge. Children's ability to mentally manipulate the world, relationships, and viewpoints of others is facilitated when they have the opportunity to physically manipulate concrete materials (e.g., using paints, paper, and glue; building things; making dams and forts of mud, sand, snow, or rocks).

By middle childhood, children need to understand relationships of mass and length and multiple variables relating to objects. School-age children should be able to classify or group materials in relation to other information. By late childhood, children should have well-developed concrete operational thinking. They should be able to focus on more than one aspect of a problem and use logical thinking. For effective cognitive work, young people must process information, recognize salient cues in the environment, organize their thoughts, consider relationships with other information, use short- and long-term memory retrieval and storage skills, make decisions based on the analysis of information, take action, and use feedback to further their learning.

Concrete operational abilities allow children to read, write, and communicate thoughts effectively. Learning about the world, its people, and the views and values of others becomes possible. Logical thinking and new social skills appear with the ability to understand the viewpoints of others and the decline of egocentricity. Empathy, or the ability to share and understand another's feelings, emerges—and with it the capacity to make deep friendships. School success fosters the development of a personal sense of competence. This is further facilitated by caregiver support.

• BOX 7-1 Piaget's Concrete Operational Stage: Characteristics of Thought Process

Decentration: Can focus on more than one aspect of a situation at a time (e.g., keeping track of both color and shape when working on a jigsaw puzzle)

Conservation: Can understand that some aspects of things, such as weight and mass, remain the same despite changes in appearance (e.g., one cookie, though broken into two pieces is still one cookie)

Transitivity: Can deduce new relationships from sets of earlier ones (e.g., if a first-grade rule is to sit still when the teacher talks, and if all grades have the same rules, then children in the second grade should sit still when the teacher talks)

Seriation: Can sequence in order (e.g., ordering triangle shapes from smallest to largest)

Classification: Can group objects on the basis of common features (e.g., separating out all the triangles from circles, squares, and stars)

Reversibility: Can mentally reverse a process or action (e.g., ice can melt to water and then refreeze)

Developmental Assessment of School-Age Children

Preventive health visits include monitoring, screening, and anticipatory guidance related to developmental, behavioral, and emotional issues. By reviewing the child's progress, offering suggestions, and validating parents' efforts, providers can best assist school-age children and families. Table 7-3 summarizes key points to discuss with children and their caregivers.

Developmental surveillance (see Chapter 2) is an essential aspect of each contact with the school-age child because

TABLE 7-3 Topics for Preventive Health Visit

5 to 7 Years Old	8 to 10 Years Old	11 to 12 Years Old
Adaptation to school	Progress at school	Progress in school
After-school activities	After-school activities	After-school activities
Development of peer relationships Family relationships	Peer relationships: Friendships, bullying, or victimization Family relationships	Peer relationships Family relationships Bullying or victimization
Activities that support positive self-esteem	Activities that support positive self-esteem	Activities that support positive self-esteem
Problem-solving away from home, without parents immediately available	Community safety; joining gangs Problem-solving away from home Handling emotions—sadness, anger, worries	Community safety; membership in gangs Problem-solving away from home—avoiding drugs, alcohol, and smoking Handling emotions—sadness, anger, and worries
Nutrition and physical activity at each visit Routine dental care	Initiating sexual education Nutrition and physical activity Routine dental care	Completion of basic sexuality and reproductive health education Nutrition and physical activity Routine dental care
Safe Internet and technology use	Safe Internet and technology use	Safe Internet and technology use

visits are less frequent during the school years. Although annual wellness visits are recommended, most visits are for minor acute illnesses rather than health maintenance. Data must be collected on the child's physical, nutritional, neurodevelopmental, psychosocial, behavioral, and emotional status during all visits. As with all children, assessment of the family system is crucial; for the school-age child, it is particularly important to evaluate how well the family is nurturing the child while supporting the child's efforts to separate, become more independent, and create a unique self in the community.

The assessment process begins by building rapport with the parents and the child. Direct questions are asked first to the child, encouraging him or her to share aspects of daily routines, family experiences, school activities, and sensitive developmental concerns. Parents can then be invited to expand on data collected, providing information not only about the child's abilities but also about interactions between child and parents.

Screening Strategies for School-Age Children

Formal developmental screening tools and/or questionnaires should be used with all children (Table 7-4). These tools allow the child, parent, and teachers to provide specific information about a child's development, behaviors, and emotional status. They also document a baseline status, highlight potential need for referrals, and evaluate the effectiveness of intervention strategies. Parent, teacher, and child perceptions about specific issues may differ. Parental reports of skills and concerns about language, fine motor, cognitive, and emotional-behavioral development have been shown to be highly predictive of true problems. This information gives the provider insights into areas needing further investigation and those that may require counseling, therapy, or other intervention strategies (see Additional Resources for links to various developmental and behavioral screening tools).

Physical Development

A traditional history should be obtained and a physical examination conducted with findings documented. Growth measurements (weight, height, and BMI) and blood pressure should be evaluated and compared with gender- and age-appropriate norms at each visit. Immunization status should be checked each time the child is seen. Hearing and vision should be screened at routine health visits. Hemoglobin or hematocrit is done for at-risk children between the age of 5 years; girls should be screened again after beginning menstruation. Perform fasting glucose, insulin, and lipid levels; total cholesterol; and liver function tests to assess for diabetes mellitus, hyperlipidemia, and metabolic syndrome in children 4 years old or older with a BMI equal to or greater than 95% or if BMI is greater than 85% and other risk factors are present, such as family history of diabetes or cardiovascular disease. Lead screening should be conducted if no previous screen has been done, there is a past positive lead screen, or there has been a change in risk factors (see Chapter 42). Likewise, a tuberculin testing should be performed if there is a positive on the risk screening questions or a change in risk. Tanner staging should be a part of the physical examination because pubertal changes can begin as early as 8 years old, and some endocrine problems may emerge in the school years. Also evaluation for specific conditions listed in Box 7-2 can provide direction for the provider in the

TABLE 7-4 Screening and Assessment Tools for the School-Age Child

Screening Tool	Appropriate Age and Screening Time	Characteristics
Pediatric Symptom Checklist (PSC) PSC-17 Youth Self-Report Pediatric Symptom Checklist (Y-PSC)	6 to 16 years old 35 items 17 items—shorter version of PSC Self-administered or completed by parent Y-PSC—For 11-year-olds and older	Psychosocial screening tool to identify cognitive, emotional and behavioral problems
Patient Health Questionnaire (PHQ) (2001) PHQ-9 and PHQ-2 are modified versions	Children and adults	Psychosocial screening tool for depression and suicide
Columbia Impairment Scale (CIS) (1993) Parent and youth versions	Children and adolescents 13 items Scored using Likert scale	Psychosocial screening tool for impairment—interpersonal relationships, psychopathological domains, school or job functioning, and use of leisure time
Parent's Evaluation of Developmental Status (PEDS) (2002) Available online with M-CHAT Parent interview with open-ended questions	Birth to 8 years old; 2 min 10 questions	Identifies children at low, moderate, high risk for disabilities and delays
Short Sensory Profile (SSP) (1999)	Birth to adult; 15 to 20 min	Parental questions in seven areas: tactile sensitive, taste-smell sensitivity, movement, underresponsive, auditory filtering, low energy and weakness, and visual and auditory
Vanderbilt Assessment Scale (2002) Teacher Rating Scale Parent Rating Scale	School-age children and adolescents 55 items 10 min	Evaluates inattention, hyperactivity, conduct disorders, and anxiety or depression
Conners 3—Parent and Teacher Rating Scale (2004) ADHD Index Global Index	6 to18 years old Parent: 48 items 6 to 18 min Teacher: 28 items 6 to 18 min Youth: 8 to 18 years old Written at 6th- to 9th-grade level depending on version The long forms correspond to the DSM-IV diagnostic criteria for ADHD	ADHD and mental health Full length and short versions available Online version available Norm-referenced screening and assessment forms to identify symptoms of ADHD and other problem behavior Evaluates general psychopathology, inattention, hyperactivity/impulsivity, learning problems, executive functioning, aggression, peer relations, family relations, ADHD inattentive, ADHD hyperactive-impulsive, ADHD combined, oppositional defiant disorder, conduct disorder
Behavioral Assessment for Children—ed 2 (BASC-2)	2 to 21 years old 25 to 30 items Teacher version Parent version Child version (6+ years old)	Social, emotional, mental health Parent/child relationship Used to further assess children who have positive findings on BESS-2

TABLE 7-4 Screening and Assessment Tools for the School-Age Child—cont'd

Screening Tool	Appropriate Age and Screening Time	Characteristics
Behavioral and Emotional Screening System for Children (BESS-2)	36 months to 17 years old 100 items Parent report, teacher report, and self-report, depending on child's age Approximately 10 min to administer; must be scored by a qualified professional	Norm-referenced behavioral questionnaire comprised of items from BASC-2 Social emotional and mental health Scales assess hyperactivity, aggressive behavior, anxiety, depression, communication and social skills, attention, learning
Eyberg Child Inventory	2 to 16 years old 36 to 38 items with Likert scale Parent report 10 min Two scales: (1) Intensity (severity of disruptive behavior) and (2) Problem (parent perception of child's behavior) Three-factor structure: Inattentive, oppositional defiant, and conduct problem behavior	Norm-referenced screener for indicators of disruptive behavior problems at home and school Measures the frequency of specific problematic behaviors Has a scale that reflects the impact of the problem (tolerance, stress) on the parent and/or teacher The items reflect the behaviors most frequently reported as problem by parents and teachers

ADHD, Attention-deficit/hyperactivity disorder; *DSM-IV, Diagnostic and Statistical Manual of Mental Disorders,* ed 4.

BOX 7-2 More Common Physical Conditions Associated with the School-Age Child

- Congenital heart disease
- Encopresis
- Enuresis
- Genetic syndromes
- Lymphadenopathy
- Obesity
- Scoliosis

physical examination. Oral health screening is indicated and referral to a dental home if the child does not have a regular dentist.

Motor Skills Development

Strength and coordination can be evaluated using a systematic musculoskeletal and neurologic examination as identified in Table 7-5. Concerns about balance, coordination, strength, and mobility should be followed up depending on attention, school performance, and overall developmental function. Problems in this area may account for school performance or learning difficulties.

Communication and Language Development

Assessment of communication and language development is ongoing during the health care visit as the provider talks directly with the child, probing for the child's level of understanding (e.g., Can child follow directions? Does the child understand explanations given by the provider?); listening to the child's articulation, vocabulary, sentence structure, and grammar; and noting the child's ability to interact socially with the examiner, the parent, and others in the setting. The child can be asked to write something on a sheet of paper to screen writing skills. Assessment is also based on reports from the parent and/or teachers.

Social and Emotional Development

Assessment of social and emotional development is an important aspect of the well child examination because 20% to 25% of children in the United States are affected by mental health, psychosocial problems, and risk-taking behaviors. It is especially important to assess for life stress, anxiety, depression, self-esteem issues, and parent-child relationships. The biologic effects of stress undermine the child's ability to concentrate, remember things, and control and focus his or her own thinking (Thompson, 2014). It is also important to observe the interaction between parents and child during the examination and examine the child's role in the family. The child's success in making friends and working with peers, and his or her feelings of contentment and security are to be explored (see Chapter 19 for mental health screening guidelines).

Cognitive Development

Assessment of cognitive development is difficult in school-age children. Generally, standardized paper-and-pencil tests are more accurate than clinical judgments. Knowledge about the child's performance compared with that of peers in the classroom, the child's grades, and information from parent-teacher conferences provide data. Referral to a psychologist is recommended if more definitive information is needed.

Diagnostic Studies

If problems are suspected, additional testing can be performed (e.g., bone age can be determined by using x-rays

TABLE 7-5 Guidelines for Neurodevelopmental Assessment of the School-Age Child

Assessment Area	Findings
Overall impression	Behavior, attentional skills and distractibility, motor activity level, impulsivity, degree of cooperativeness, strategies for and persistence in task completion, problem-solving, organizational skills, ability to follow directions and ask for assistance.
Cerebral	State control, attention, behavior, orientation, cooperation, participation, and separation from parents. Are judgment, orientation, memory (short- and long-term ability to remember eight familiar objects in "memory box"), affect, and calculation age appropriate or immature?
Cranial nerves	Note any asymmetries or oral-motor dyspraxia.
Cerebellar functioning	*Fine motor movements:* Evaluate for dysfunctions, including problems with balance, fine motor control (rapid alternating movements), and pincer or pencil grasp. *Coordination:* Evaluate coordination, including balance (Romberg, balance on one foot), tandem walk (heel-toe walk), duck walk, and coordination while throwing and catching a ball (use a small ball with older children).
Sensory functioning	Evaluate problems recognizing body parts or body position, sensitivity to touch, asymmetric or poor graphesthesia (letters or numbers) or stereognosis (objects).
Gross motor function	Evaluate overall gait, coordination for age while skipping, running, and walking on a balance beam; appropriateness for age; note posture, ability to sit in chair straight vs. leaning on desk; and ability to stand for periods of time without leaning on something.
Extraneous movement, tremors	Evaluate for synkinesis (motor overflow), dyskinesis (incomplete or fragmented movements), mild dyspraxic movements, dysdiadochokinesia (inability to perform rapid movements), and motor impersistence.
Auditory perceptual abilities	Evaluate discrimination, processing, integration, memory, and comprehension of auditory information. Evaluate ability to follow twofold and fivefold directions. Note directionality and consistent or inconsistent use of right or left eye, hand or foot. Note the ability to remember series of spoken words and numbers forward and backward, and the ability to understand or comprehend a written paragraph. Note expressive language ability (word retrieval, formulation, and articulation). Evaluate conversation spoken spontaneously through story or history. Evaluate ability to define words appropriate for age.
Visual perceptual	Identify memory recall (short- and long-term), visual discrimination, visuospatial perception, visual abilities, memory for objects, visual discrimination of subtle differences in words (e.g., ten and tin), object assembly, and decoding.
Visual motor integration	Note ability to copy a design (+, 0, square, or triangle) and handwriting. Evaluate picture of a person and coordination drawn by the child for age appropriateness.
Organization	Observe problem-solving of math problems.
Learning style	Evaluate concrete and abstract thinking, sequential or stimulus processing, thought integration, perseveration, ritual and routine; control; adaptation to changes; modulation of behaviors; exaggeration (overdo or underdo) activities.

of the left hand and wrist to determine epiphyseal fusion; intelligence testing can establish cognitive abilities). Further endocrine, nutrition, genetic, or other assessments may be necessary if the child does not meet the norms for physical growth.

Anticipatory Guidance for School-Age Children

Anticipatory guidance should be an individualized discussion with parents to help them understand, respond to, and guide their child's behavior and development (see Table 7-3). Because children assume more responsibility for self-care as they grow, anticipatory guidance should be discussed with them in an age-appropriate manner. The list of anticipatory guidance topics discussed in this chapter is not intended to be exhaustive, but it is provided to illustrate how developmental concepts can be applied to everyday living. Further information about assessment management of specific problems is found in later chapters (e.g., sleep problems are discussed in Chapter 14).

Parent Development

The role of parents is central in preparing and supporting their child's transition during the school-age years. Often families are constrained by social and economic conditions as they raise their children, and parents need help to fulfill their responsibilities. They typically welcome the support,

suggestions, and connection to resources that providers can give them. Parent and caregiver support is essential to the child's adjustment and his or her ability to manage stressful life events.

A child's entry into school can be emotionally stressful for parents because they must adjust to a new social situation, routine, and a changing relationship with their child. Some parents feel that they have "lost" their child, watching him or her move from dependence on the family to participation in a new world of which the parent is not a part. Other parents anticipate the new opportunities facing the child and family and are ready to help their child cope with challenges that emerge in the school environment. Parents also have a responsibility to provide an environment that reinforces their child's educational efforts. School performance can be damaged by excessive media and technology use and by parents' failure to monitor their child's exposure to age-inappropriate material.

The Internet also introduces new risks for school-age children. With the widespread availability of social networking websites, Internet safety is becoming a growing concern for school-age youth. Research suggests that the greatest risk factors for victimization that occurs via the Internet are family conflict, depression, conversing with unknown people about sex, and sending personal information to strangers. Victims of child maltreatment (physical, sexual abuse, or neglect) are at particular risk (Noll et al, 2009). Further information about safe use of social media is found in Chapter 8.

As children grow from 6 to 12 years old, parents will continue to extend freedoms and give them new responsibilities. They need to provide opportunities that allow children to experience and master new challenges and adjust family patterns of nutrition, sleep, activities, health maintenance, safety, and communication to fit with the child's needs and emerging skills. Parents need to be available to children to ensure the child has both the social and emotional skills essential to move into and succeed in school environments. Supportive parents should know their child's whereabouts after school and know their child's friends. Children who participate in after-school activities have higher self-esteem, better school grades, and higher academic performance. At the same time, activity participation is associated with a reduction in withdrawal behaviors, depression, fighting, substance use, and engaging in other risky behaviors (Robl et al, 2012).

Regulation and Sleep-Wake Patterns

Family routines provide a support to the daily life of the child and help the child self-regulate. If children have routines that they can rely on, they are more comfortable exploring new areas and trying new skills. Family routines strengthen the relationship between parent and child, provide family stability and continuity, and serve as a buffer during times of change and transition. Stronger family relationships also serve as protection against risk factors, such as divorce, alcoholism, substance abuse, or violence. Suggestions the provider can make to parents include the following:

- Encourage the family to establish and recognize traditions or family activities that are special (e.g., birthday celebrations, Sunday afternoon walks, and videos and popcorn on Saturday night).
- Help parents explore ways to adapt the child's new schedule in an effort to maintain previous routines or readjust routines to meet the new schedule (e.g., if the child must meet a school bus at an early hour, making a school lunch the night before can become part of a new evening routine).

Strength and Motor Coordination

Because of the maturity of the central nervous system and cognitive advances, most children are physically capable. Most enjoy playing hard and developing physical skills, strength, and coordination. Parents can support this growth if they do the following:

- Encourage children's participation in daily exercise.
- Provide for activities that are fun, involve family or peers, and require cognitive or social skills, including rules, strategies, and skills.
- Include children's friends in family activities (e.g., hiking, skiing, and swimming).
- Support children's interest in physical activities that are healthful; personal achievement in an activity can be crucial to children's self-image.
- Encourage hobbies and activities that foster fitness and increased motor skills.
- Encourage activities that require training, commitment, and effort, especially for older children.
- Help children prevent the stress of overscheduling.
- Limit activities that include TV, video games, or computer time.
- Let the children "own" the activity (e.g., Little League baseball games should be fun for the children, not a contest among parents over whose child is the best).
- Explore ways children with physical limitations can participate in preferred activities and with their peers (see Chapter 14 regarding Special Olympic sports activities for families and children with physical challenges).

Nutrition, Self-Care, and Safety

Nutrition

Careful attention to nutrition is important because 31% of school-age children are overweight or obese. Diets can be deficient in iron or vitamin C, and high-fat snack foods can become a habit. Choosing nutritious foods while away from home and learning to eat new foods are areas for learning. Eating well at breakfast and dinner becomes especially important, because food is not readily available all day at school. High-calorie snacks and other high-calorie foods contribute to obesity in school-age children, and monitoring and weight control programs are needed at earlier ages

(see Chapter 10). Parents should be advised to do the following:

- Ensure that the child has three nutritious meals and two nutritious snacks daily.
- Know that food jags are common.
- Establish an eating routine, with at least one daily meal together as a family. Maintain family meals as much as possible to preserve family time and share interests and experiences from the day's activities.
- Monitor food choices and opportunities to determine best foods.
- Teach children to understand the importance of eating healthy foods.
- Encourage participation in meal planning, food shopping and selection, and meal preparation.
- Discuss making nutritious choices for quick meals, school lunches, and when eating out.

Self-Care

For school-age children, learning to take responsibility for their own health begins with simple goals and moves to more complex decision-making strategies. For example, children may begin by deciding to have a fruit or vegetable at each meal and then progress to helping plan some meals and participate in their preparation. Other areas in which children take increasing responsibility are dental health, hygiene and grooming, snacking, and exercise. Children at this age see health in positive terms and equate it with being able to participate in desired activities. Parents can do the following to assist the child's achievement in self-care:

- Explain the relationship between good health and self-care.
- Supervise personal hygiene, such as brushing teeth, combing hair, and doing nail care; for older school children, supervision is minimal, with an occasional reminder.
- Set clear limits on expectations for cleanliness, healthy exercise, hours of sleep, and other health promotion behaviors.
- Recognize that children may be "noncompliant" as a means of exerting independence; a discussion about decision-making and healthy choices may be needed to resolve the issue.
- Be flexible.
- Provide children with opportunities to experiment with appropriate healthy behaviors that allow them to develop self-expression (e.g., school-age children can enjoy new hair styles or temporary tattoos).
- Encourage shared decision-making and self-care during illnesses and for chronic disease management.
- Give children an opportunity to ask questions about sexuality, drugs, alcohol, and tobacco; encourage discussion about these topics as a family; teach about puberty changes.
- Model healthy behaviors related to nutrition, physical activity, and other healthy self-care behaviors.

Safety

Unintentional injuries are common among school-age children. Often their growing bodies allow them to get into situations that they cannot get out of without help. They need guidance and direction to be safe and make safe choices. Although parents do not provide the constant supervision they did for toddlers and preschoolers, they should work with their school-age child to ensure safety. The health care provider can give guidance to parents and encourage them to do the following:

- Help children learn "survival skills" (e.g., name, telephone number, address, use of 911, how to ask adults for help, and what to do if lost).
- Require use of protective gear when riding bicycles, skateboards, or scooters and as appropriate in sports activities.
- Use booster seats or wear seatbelts as appropriate.
- Use sunscreen (sun protection factor [SPF] 15 or higher) before prolonged sun exposure.
- Teach children to swim; supervise their activities near water.
- Educate children about hazards, both physical and social (e.g., pedestrian traffic on busy streets; facts about pregnancy, intercourse, and sexually transmitted infections; what to do if they find a weapon or syringe).
- Monitor Internet, TV, app, video, and social media use. Use security tools to prevent children from instant messages from strangers. Use parental controls to limit access on phones, tablets, computers, and TVs.
- Educate children that Internet and technology use is an opportunity—not a right.
- Get rid of firearms or ensure that they are unloaded and locked, with ammunition in a different location and the key is accessible only to the parent.
- Help children to think about safety aspects of activities; talk about safety.

Communication and Language

Mastering the ability to read, comprehend, and write is essential for the school-age child's academic success. Parents can help children learn these skills by doing the following:

- Provide structured time and space for children to complete school writing and reading assignments.
- Read stories to children; even older children enjoy listening to stories that are exciting or relevant to them.
- Listen to the child read aloud.
- Role model by reading and writing often.
- Encourage the child to make notes, keep a journal, and write letters to friends and family members. Skill with writing supports reading and vice versa.
- Play word games with the child (e.g., finding all the things that "start with B" while on a road trip can entertain a 6-year-old; Junior Scrabble or Boggle is fun for older children). Let the child lead the play; the parent

should not be "out to win," and the child should not be made to feel inadequate for not knowing everything.
- Talk with the child and actively listen as the child talks.
- Enroll the child in structured, voluntary after-school programs that offer an opportunity to engage in active conversation with other children and adults.
- Never punish a child by removing books or writing materials.
- Limit television, computer activities, and video games to 1 to 2 hours per day; do not have a television in the child's bedroom.

Social and Emotional Growth

The hallmark of successful school-age social and emotional growth is finding family and peer support while establishing individuality and independence. Providers can help foster that growth by encouraging parents to do the following:
- Enhance goal setting with charts, calendars, and tally sheets. Care should be taken not to reward children too much because this can decrease motivation. Let children set goals while parents monitor activities and point out options.
- Appreciate the products of the child's work at home and at school; encourage activities in which the child can have success or excel.
- Provide positive expressions of love, concern, and pride to promote a sense of family belonging.
- Share family history and encourage visits with relatives to help children be proud of their heritage.
- Help children feel that the home base is secure to increase their confidence as they move into other domains.
- Make home rules and expectations clear and use consistency in applying them.
- Discuss family values and rules and explain the differences that the child may face when away from home.
- Play and work together as a family to teach children how to work together with their classmates and to function as a team; children should maintain their responsibilities to the family (e.g., jobs or chores around the house).
- Provide opportunities for children to make and develop friendships with a variety of children, teaching them how to initiate, sustain, and terminate relationships with friends.
- Include the child's friends in some family activities and outings.
- Teach children how to read social cues.
- Provide social skills training and supervise experiences in which child can practice new skills successfully.
- Help children learn to communicate well with other adults.
- Teach respect for authority and rules away from home.
- Help children identify and appropriately express their emotions.
- Provide fantasy play opportunities to allow children to deal safely with their emotions and concerns and to develop their creativity.
- Provide guidance about how to appropriately express feelings of aggression, anger, and emerging sexuality; discuss sexual values.
- Help children with decision-making and accepting consequences of actions.
- Model positive conflict resolution and good communication.
- Teach anger-management and conflict-resolution skills.
- Help children learn delayed gratification and increase their frustration tolerance, while still remaining sympathetic.
- Provide children with opportunities for appropriate behavior when values are challenged (e.g., "You can say, 'No, my mom won't let me do that,' and then walk away").
- Recognize that parents are role models and that children internalize parental values as they begin to form a conscience.
- Recognize that children may identify with a special person, such as a movie star or athlete.
- Recognize that having a strong sense of self-esteem helps "inoculate" children against some of the negative peer pressures children may experience.
- Monitor communication activities on social networking sites.
- Set and adhere to rules for Internet use and social networking sites both inside and outside the home.

Cognitive and Environmental Stimulation

School is a major source of intellectual stimulation and an arena where the children experience cognitive growth. Expectations for performance increase over the school years with examinations, graded papers, projects, and homework assignments. Reading becomes a tool to attain and master knowledge rather than being an end in itself. Thus poor readers begin to experience broader academic failure and can become increasingly frustrated. Unless these children are provided with social and remedial support, they may see school as an unpleasant burden, develop feelings of failure, and look for validation through nonacademic experiences. Social supports can help children cope with this stress, and interacting with healthy, interested, and caring adults is the strongest support children can have.

The family also provides the child with stimulation for cognitive growth. Parents can be counseled to do the following:
- Read to the child and have the child read to the parent.
- Establish and build trust with children through joint use of computers and online activities.
- Stimulate the younger child's thinking about comparisons and differences (e.g., changes in shape, volume, directions to and from school) to facilitate cognition at the concrete operations level.
- Discuss variables in objects or situations as experienced, seen on television, or read about to help move the child's thinking away from the earlier egocentric style.

- Provide opportunities to gain knowledge through books, outings, classes, and family discussions.
- Engage children in experiences with other languages, music, and cultural groups.
- Explore and explain the environment and community to the child to promote broader understanding of the world.
- Establish a regular homework time and place to help the child maximize time for cognitive practice.
- Establish an environment that encourages children to focus and complete tasks with limits clearly defined.
- Provide help early if children experience school problems to lessen secondary problems with emotions and conflict; seek the teacher's assistance in securing needed educational resources and services to assist the child at school (e.g., request an individual education plan [IEP]).
- Volunteer at the child's school or participate in school activities for parents.
- Recognize academic achievement because success motivates further work.
- Stay involved with school assignments and evaluate progress to support the child's work.
- Encourage problem-solving efforts.
- Provide more complex opportunities to plan and complete projects that use skills learned at school, such as planning and cooking meals, planning family outings, and managing money and a budget.

Common Developmental Issues for School-Age Children

School Readiness

School entrance is based on chronologic rather than developmental age. What children bring with them from other life experiences to school either enhances or inhibits their capacity to learn. School entry is stressful for all children, but immature children have increased stress because the expectations for performance are beyond their abilities, and they may not have adequate coping resources. Children who lack necessary skills to meet school demands and expectations may be unsuccessful, and early school failure can result in significant negative consequences. Health care providers have a responsibility to work with parents and their communities to promote optimal development and school readiness for children.

School participation requires skills to perform self-care, interact with a variety of new people, act with a sense of responsibility, and emotionally separate from the family and home base. Children need to meet school standards, which may be different from those at home. There is a social expectation to gain an awareness of "the group"—an ability to go along with the group while meeting some personal needs through the group's achievements.

An estimated 30% of 5-year-olds are not ready for school, a number that increases to almost 50% for socioeconomically disadvantaged children (Isaacs and Brookings Institute, 2012). Causes for failed school readiness include language deficiencies, emotional immaturity, poor socialization, presence of problem behaviors, lack of early math and reading skills, and poor physical health. Parents may have ambivalent attitudes toward their child's school and may distrust the school's capacity to meet children's educational needs. Socially and economically disadvantaged children are at greatest risk for difficulties. Head Start or comparable early childhood education experiences have been shown to improve school readiness in these high-risk populations (Bierman et al, 2008). Attention to social and emotional factors and to nurturing relationships in the life of a child will facilitate healthy development in preparation for success in school.

Clinical Findings

History

- *Child experiences:* Evaluate opportunities for participating in activities away from home, following directions, playing with other children, habits, and interest in school.
- *Parents and family:* Assess the parents' feelings about their child entering school. What do they think their child will experience at school (e.g., racism, bullying, teachers who do not recognize or appreciate their child's unique strengths)? What do they think the school will expect of their child (e.g., to be appropriately sociable, to sit still, to learn quickly)? Do they think their child will be able to handle the demands of school? Do they think that the chosen school can meet the child's needs? Reluctance on the parents' part may be communicated to their child. Ask what parents have done to prepare their child for school. Ask about family activities, sibling school experiences, traumatic events, or separation on the part of the child or parents. Communicate to parents that parent expectation is the strongest predictor of school success.
- *Home environment:* Inquire about daily routines, family activities together, parent- versus child-initiated activities for learning.
- *Developmental progress:* Ask about the child's developmental opportunities and skills in communicating needs, fine motor and gross motor activities, behaviors, fears, separation from parents, play with other children.
- *Other issues:* Ask about other concerns (e.g., chronic illness, economic issues, homelessness, and family stressors) that might compromise regular school attendance or school success.

Physical Examination

The child should have a complete physical examination with special focus on the following:

- Neurologic development, including sensory, cognitive, and language
- Height, weight, BMI, blood pressure
- Dental health
- Immunization status
- Evaluation of the normative skills listed in Table 7-6

Diagnostic Studies

All children should have hearing and vision screening prior to beginning kindergarten. Screening tests to evaluate school readiness have established norms and are generally reliable in predicting developmental outcomes (Table 7-7). They should be used to consider all areas of readiness (social, behavioral, and cognitive) and to provide an explanation of readiness for parents. Test results should be evaluated in conjunction with history, observation, family situation, and previous experiences. Children can be referred to local Head Start programs and school districts if more in-depth testing is required.

TABLE 7-6 Basic First-Grade School Readiness Skills

Language skills	Counts 10 or more objects Uses complete sentences of at least five words Uses future tense Gives first and last name Recognizes four colors Defines five to seven words Communicates needs Recalls parts of a story Follows three-part commands Understands number concepts
Personal and social skills	Separates easily from parent Dresses without supervision Plays interactively with other children Has toilet skills Follows instructions Feels support from other adults
Fine motor and adaptive skills	Copies geometric shapes (circle, square, triangle) Draws a person (six parts with distinct body) Prints some letters Classifies similar objects
Gross motor skills	Hops on one foot Catches bounced ball Walks backward heel to toe Balances on each foot for 6 seconds

Management

Preventive strategies for high-risk children begin before the school-age years and include enrollment in preschool, interactive reading with the child from an early age to promote language mastery, increased time for young children to play with peers and engage in creative play activities, and interaction with caring adults.

Ensuring school readiness involves sharing data with school counselors and teachers, parents, and primary care providers and offering anticipatory guidance in the following areas:

- Teach and encourage parents to assist their child with skills that will be needed for school (e.g., knowing colors and numbers, behavioral expectations).
- Encourage parents to visit the school, meet the teacher, and discuss their child's characteristics with the teacher.
- Instruct parents to rehearse school activities with their child before school begins (e.g., getting to school, finding class, eating meals, going to the bathroom, asking for help, getting home, and following the rules).
- Help parents deal with their own stress of separation. Review their expectations of the child and identify what will be new and different.
- Provide parents with available community and school resources that they may need to access to meet the developmental needs of their child.
- Encourage children to start school with their developmental-appropriate group. Children who are not ready often need extra support at school and would benefit by spending another year at home or in preschool.
- Be an advocate for parents and children with identified deficits to ensure that the school adequately assesses both strengths and weaknesses of children and develops a program of study (e.g., an IEP) that maximizes children's strengths).

TABLE 7-7 Screening Tests to Evaluate School Readiness

Test	Source	Content
Beery Visual-Motor Integration, ed 5 (VMI-5)	Pro-Ed Inc. www.proedinc.com	Test of visual motor integration
Denver Developmental Screening Test II	Denver Developmental Materials, Inc. www.denverii.com	Divided into four areas: Gross motor Language Fine motor Personal and social
Pediatric Examination of Educational Readiness (PEER) and Pediatric Examination of Educational Readiness at Middle Childhood (PEERAMID)	Educators Publishing Service, Inc. www.epsbooks.com	Combined neurodevelopmental, behavioral, and health assessment

- Counsel parents that deficits in a child's readiness may occur even with the best of parenting.
- Develop a "catch-up" or "tutorial plan" with parents to address deficits in a comprehensive way while preserving the child's self-esteem.
- Monitor the child's progress through the year, advocating as necessary.

Learning Problems

Learning problems can be a hidden handicap that presents during the school-age years. Ability to manage school learning expectations requires growth in four areas: basic processing of information, memorization, increased attention span and recall of important events, and beginning problem-solving skills.

Knowledge (the sum of what children know) rapidly expands as a result of schoolwork, experiences at home, and activities with friends. The organization of knowledge improves as school-age children grow older and integrate knowledge into existing concepts. Self-awareness, reflected by children's ability to predict performance, develops slowly and in areas in which children have the most knowledge (Table 7-8). Although children with learning problems generally have difficulties with basic thinking skills, they may have specific problems in linguistic skills, attention, and organizational skills; higher cognitive functions, such as memory and sensory function; motor capacities; visuospatial analysis and neuromotor function; and social awareness and behavior.

Clinical Findings

History

A complete, in-depth history is needed to examine underlying or related issues because learning difficulties are attributed to many different causes. The history often provides the most information about how a child's learning affects aspects of the child's life. It should also identify areas of strength on which the child and family can build strategies for managing the child's learning difficulties. The history includes the following:

- *Medical history:* Prenatal history, including in utero exposure to drugs, toxins, and alcohol; neonatal history; recurrent or chronic medical conditions; allergies; medications; hospitalizations; syndromes; congenital, neurologic, metabolic, or endocrine conditions; current illnesses; vision and hearing problems; fetal alcohol spectrum disorder (FASD); history of accidents, concussions, or other brain injury
- *Developmental history:* Achievement or regression of developmental milestones, especially in language; experiences for achieving developmental skills at home or in preschool; daily routines and preferred play activities; temperament; behavioral concerns of the parents; ability of the child to handle transitions and change; child's initiation of activities versus parent-guided activities; repetitive behaviors
- *Family medical history:* Family history of difficulties in school or school dropout, learning difficulties, ADHD or attention-deficit disorder (ADD), mental retardation, or genetic disorders; overall family members' functioning; substance abuse
- *Family social history:* Problem-solving and decision-making skills, use of community resources, financial resources, family stressors, substance abuse, homelessness, violence, criminal behavior

Physical Examination

A complete physical examination, with special attention to the neurodevelopmental assessment (see Table 7-5), should be performed.

Diagnostic Studies

- *School records:* Information needs to be obtained from the school system to evaluate the child's school performance and to review any educational testing that has

TABLE 7-8 Developmental Changes in Thinking Skills

Component	Developmental Changes	Examples
Basic skills	Improvements in the speed and efficiency of memory, attention, language processing, motor implementation	Ability to work for longer stretches of time Use of adult-like logical principles Development of reading skills
Strategies	Use of active, complex strategies to improve basic skills	Greater spontaneous use of strategies Wider repertoire of strategies Greater likelihood of generalization to new areas
Knowledge	Expansion of what is known and greater organization of knowledge	Development of hobbies and special areas of interest More complex network of concepts
Metacognitive awareness	Development of explicit self-conscious knowledge about how to think	Ability to predict success or failure Ability to plan and to modify strategies

From Feldman H: Development of thinking skills in school-aged children, *Pediatr Ann* 18(6):358, 1989.

been done. Testing identifies the child's strengths and weaknesses, revealing the cognitive styles that teachers and parents will be most successful in tapping.
- *Psychological testing:* The school may or may not have the capacity for psychological evaluations. Often parents must ask for this, and they may need to seek outside evaluations. Schools are required, under Public Law 94-142, to provide appropriate education to all children identified with developmental delays.
- *Cognitive testing:* The school's ability to provide cognitive and learning evaluations may be limited, and some school districts cannot provide testing for a dyslexia diagnosis because it is not a recognized educational diagnosis. An evaluation for a learning disorder is not complete without cognitive testing (see Additional Resources, International Dyslexia Association).
- *Developmental assessment:* A multidisciplinary developmental evaluation through a developmental program may be needed to provide the most appropriate plan of care for an individual child. Additional testing may be recommended, such as genetic testing with chromosome studies, brain scans, or endocrine and metabolic testing.

Differential Diagnosis

The following diagnoses need to be considered in children with learning problems:
- Vision problems
- Hearing problems
- Mental retardation—genetic syndrome, neurologic insult, or malformation
- Cognitive developmental delay
- Speech or language delay
- Depression
- ADHD
- Autism spectrum disorder
- Toxin-related delay (e.g., lead, FASD, other intrauterine substance exposure)
- Medication-related delay (e.g., anticonvulsant, psychotropics, antihistamine)
- Neurologic problems
- Traumatic brain injury
- Dyslexia

Management

Providers can encourage parents to obtain an early diagnosis and identify and access appropriate school programs. Some children qualify for special educational support through IEPs (see Chapter 4). Parents need to review educational plans, provide an environment rich with experiences for children, and set realistic goals. They also need to act as advocates for their children during every school year because classrooms and teachers change. Parents should work to correct secondary problems, such as poor self-esteem, hopelessness, or depression. Finally, providers can encourage parents to avoid the use of the many unsubstantiated cures for learning disabilities (see Chapter 20 for further discussion of ADHD and other cognitive-perceptual problems).

School Refusal (Phobia)

Description

School refusal is a term that was introduced in the 1970s to describe the heterogeneity of its causes. The prevalence ranges from 0.4% to 18% of all school-age children. Ninety percent of children who experience school refusal, commonly called *school phobia,* have a psychiatric diagnosis (Ek and Eriksson, 2013). The disorder includes, but is not limited to, separation anxiety disorder, simple and social phobias, and depression. The criteria for a diagnosis include the following: (1) severe difficulty attending school or refusal to attend school; (2) severe emotional upset when attempting to go to school; (3) absence of significant antisocial disorders; and (4) staying at home with the parent's knowledge. Children may request to stay home from school with a variety of physical complaints, including stomachaches, headaches, dizziness, fatigue, or a combination of these. The symptoms gradually improve as the day progresses and often disappear on weekends. Unexcused school absences peak with the beginning of school attendance and again at 11 to 12 years old.

Clinical Findings

History

Because child, parent, family, and school environmental factors may all play into the causes of school refusal, an in-depth history exploring these areas is needed. Specific areas include the following:
- Frequent somatic complaints or sleep difficulties
- Parents' ambivalent feelings about children's attendance at school, evidence of overindulgence or overprotection
- Difficult home situation (e.g., children may try to stay at home to care for a chronically ill parent or may have a substance abusing parent who is not attending to the child's academic needs)
- Recent or anticipated loss or separation
- School environment and evidence of bullying, violence, humiliation, lack of privacy (in bathroom especially), mismatch with teacher

Physical Examination

A complete physical examination and any indicated laboratory testing should be done to rule out specific indications of organic disease.

Diagnostic Studies

Laboratory testing that is symptom specific, noninvasive, and cost effective to rule out organic disease is appropriate to assure child and parents that the problem is taken seriously. Both parent and child may then be more willing to accept the lack of organic disease and work toward addressing the underlying psychological issues and cooperating in the development of a treatment plan.
- Depression and anxiety questionnaires (see Chapter 19)
- ADHD evaluation tools (see Chapter 20)

Differential Diagnosis

Anxiety disorders are the most common reason for school refusal, usually manifesting as an inability to cope with anxiety, especially anxiety stemming from separation.

- Somatic illness or overresponse to minor illness: Avoid provider overresponse with excessive diagnostic testing.
- Depression: Isolation from peers, withdrawal from activities, sleep disturbances, erratic moods, poor self-esteem, and decreased activity level.
- ADHD and conduct disorder: Children who are unsuccessful in school, either academically or socially, may try to withdraw from the school environment.
- Sexual or physical abuse: Children who are being abused or who experience violence either at home or at school can feel intimidated to the point that they refuse to attend school.
- Chronic physical illness with poor adaptation.
- Learning disability with poor adaptation.
- Substance abuse in the family.
- Parental criminal activity.
- Pregnancy.
- Family dysfunction.
- Truancy.

Management

Intervention is generally successful when behavioral measures are combined with supportive counseling of parents. The physical complaints must be reasonably evaluated to rule out organic disease without excessive medical attention or diagnostic testing. Once the possibility of organic disease is set aside (or a plan is established to evaluate somatic problems), children must go to school. Generally, once they are at school, symptoms resolve.

- Support parents in getting children to school and insist on full attendance.
- Notify school personnel and encourage them to support and expect child's attendance and intervene to improve any situation related to children's anxiety.
- Assess home situation and identify issues that must be handled. Provide referrals as needed for family and parent problems for counseling, social services, or other resources. Notify child protection services in the case of threat of harm from parental inability to provide for adequate supervision and needs.
- Refer for psychiatric care if no improvement occurs within 2 weeks.
- Criteria for mental health referral include the following:
  - Unresponsive to pediatric management
  - Out of school for 2 months
  - Psychosis
  - Depression
  - Panic reactions
  - Parental inability to cooperate with plan

Recurrent Physical Symptoms

Complaints of recurrent symptoms, such as headaches, abdominal pain, and limb pain are frequent in school-age children. There is no validated medical explanation for these symptoms, but the frequency of complaints in school-age children suggests a correlation with developmental factors. Children with recurrent symptoms may have parents with increased psychosocial problems and preoccupation with somatic complaints, but many times the cause is not clear. Often children receive a great deal of attention for these symptoms (see Chapter 33 for evaluation and management of recurrent abdominal pain).

Clinical Findings

History

- Vague and intermittent complaints of abdominal pain, headaches, nausea, or malaise, but absence of significant findings on physical examination
- Normal function between episodes
- No episodes of vomiting, diarrhea, or constipation
- Possible family member with similar symptoms
- Stress in school or home environment (e.g., new social situation, new sibling, new school, change in teacher, examination, peer group conflict, moving, family illness or loss, parental or self-initiated pressure for achievement or perfection)

Physical Examination

No evidence of organic disease.

Differential Diagnosis

- Chronic, recurrent abdominal pain (see Chapter 33): Consider irritable bowel syndrome, food intolerance, acid peptic disease, inflammatory bowel disease, sickle cell anemia, porphyria, hereditary angioedema, systemic lupus erythematosus, and dysmenorrhea in adolescent females (see Chapter 36)
- Neurologic conditions (see Chapter 28 for discussion of headaches)
- School refusal

Management

The following are keys to the management of recurrent symptoms:

- Do not "medicalize" the problem with a barrage of tests if the initial history and physical examination do not indicate systemic symptoms.
- Encourage the child to keep a food or pain diary.
- Reassure the child and expect normal participation in activities.
- Refer for mental health counseling if symptoms persist.
- Discuss coping strategies to deal with stressors.
- Discuss family strategies that are supportive, but do not reinforce the illness behavior.

Red Flags for School-Age Children

The school-age child may present with more serious problems. Table 7-9 outlines "red flags" that may be found in five specific areas: (1) psychosocial and emotional,

TABLE 7-9 Developmental Red Flags: School-Age Child

Age	Psychosocial and Emotional Skill	Cognitive and Visual Abilities	Language and Hearing	Fine Motor	Gross Motor
6 years old	Problems with peer relationships Latchkey: Stays home alone Unable to state special quality about self Flat affect, depression, withdrawn Cruelty to animals, friends Interest in fires or fire setting	School problems with grades, behavior, interest in school Unable to sit still in class Unable to give age Watching television and play video games more Unable to name interests	Language partially unintelligible	Unable to copy "+" Picture of self includes less than eight parts	Unable to catch a ball
8 years old	Lack of hobbies Lack of best friend Cruelty to animals, friends Interest in fires or fire setting Flat affect, depression, withdrawn Defiant attitude	Unable to state days of the week Unable to add and subtract Unable to identify right and left	Unable to read simple phrases Unable to relate simple story	Unable to copy a diamond and square Unable to print name Unable to tie shoes Picture of self includes less than 12 to 16 parts	Unable to walk a straight line Poor coordination, endurance, strength
10 years old	Lack of team sports or extracurricular activities at school Lacks understanding of rules Poor peer influence, interest in gangs Cruelty to animals, friends Interest in fires or fire setting Flat affect, depression, withdrawn	Lack of operational thinking: Cause and effect, relationships of whole and parts, non-egocentric thinking	Problems with reading and math	Difficulty holding pencil with penmanship or cursive writing	Problems throwing or catching
12 years old	Risk-taking behaviors: Smoking, alcohol, sex Inappropriate for age sexual behavior Cruelty to animals, friends Interest in fires or fire setting Flat affect, depression, withdrawn Defiant, rebellious attitude	Difficulty with school work Lack of organizational skills for homework	Problems understanding, following through with verbal instructions Problems with reading comprehension	Problems getting written homework done because of difficulties holding pencil or doing paper-and-pencil tasks	Unable to list strengths and physical things he or she likes to do

(2) cognitive and verbal abilities, (3) language and hearing, (4) fine motor, and (5) gross motor for children 6 to 12 years old. Providers must be alert for indications that something is amiss and, if needed, assess the child and family more thoroughly. This assessment involves consideration of the child's developmental processes, risk-taking behaviors, and school success.

The wide variation in the growth and development of school-age children necessitates looking at problems based on age, developmental tasks of each age, and family functioning. The family status significantly impacts the child's ability to move through developmental stages during school years. Because most children who have a chronic condition that impacts development have been identified by the time they reach school age, red flags may be related to issues that arise from these chronic conditions.

Assessment of risk behaviors in school-age children requires looking at both the child's interest in engaging in risk-taking behaviors and the specific behaviors themselves. It is unclear if risk-taking behaviors in school-age children are indicators of risky behavior in adolescence. Child temperament plays a role in risk-taking behaviors, and boys are more likely to engage in risk behaviors than girls. The family maintains an influential role, but increasingly, peers and influences outside the family during school years impact children's decisions related to risk-taking behaviors.

In addition to identifying high-risk behaviors, the health care provider must be alert to "red flags" that jeopardize children's school success and be ready to intervene with families and school professionals to obtain necessary evaluations and resources to address these problems. Learning problems may not surface until the child is in school, and early identification is important to ensure that children are able to access resources that result in a positive school experience.

The well-child history provides the foundation for identifying developmental issues, behavioral risk factors, and problems the child may have at school. For school-age children, it includes the following:

- Presence of chronic illness
- Accidents and injuries (number and severity)
- Vision and hearing problems
- Progress, interest, and success in school
- Identification of learning problems with appropriate school plans and placement based on needs and abilities
- Sudden changes in school performance
- Changes in vocabulary and receptive language
- Cognitive processes: Logical reasoning and ability to problem-solve
- Socialization: Friends, involvement with peer group, community
- Antisocial behavior and/or destructive acts
- Participation in group sports
- Development of self-concept and self-identity
- Socialization away from family to peer or community groups
- Family circumstances, such as death of a family member, divorce, or changes in parents' health

Primary care providers have skills to address risk factors with families to prevent further problems. In situations where the child has been referred, the primary care provider has a crucial role in working with other professionals to ensure that children and families receive timely and appropriate services.

For a complete list of references, please visit http://evolve.elsevier.com/Burns/pediatric/.

8 Developmental Management of Adolescents

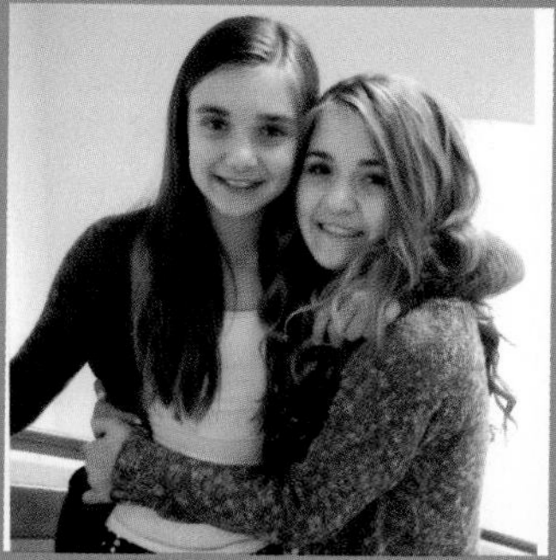

DAWN LEE GARZON AND ARDYS M. DUNN

The changes a young person experiences during the transition from childhood to young adulthood are dramatic. The extent of physiologic growth and maturation during this time rivals that occurring during infancy. Social and psychological changes are also extreme and can create a tenuous sense of balance during this phase of development. The common question on the minds of most adolescents is "Am I normal?" Reassurance and information during well-child care about what to expect as they grow are among the most valuable services a health care provider can offer the adolescent. This chapter focuses on the normal physical and psychosocial growth and development of adolescents and provides practitioners with a framework for structuring care of the adolescent client.

Adolescent Development

Puberty is the term for the biologic process that ultimately leads to fertility. The hormonal regulatory systems in the hypothalamus, pituitary, gonads, and adrenal glands undergo major changes between the prepubertal and adult states. Accompanying these changes are rapid growth in height and weight, development of secondary sex characteristics, and onset of fertility (Fig. 8-1) (see Chapters 26 and 36). Normal development can be difficult to define and is, at best, an approximation rather than a precise parameter. However, even though the timing (tempo) of adolescent development is variable, the sequence of events is orderly (Fig. 8-2).

Adolescence refers to the psychosocial and emotional transition from childhood to adulthood. The physical changes of puberty are accompanied by significant cognitive and psychosocial development that affects how adolescents view themselves and how the world views adolescents. Successful development in adolescence culminates in achievement of goals that can provide the basis for a healthy and productive adult life.

Physical Development

Tanner Stages

Pubertal growth and maturation can be divided into five stages ranging from prepubertal (sexual maturity rating [SMR] 1) to adult (SMR 5). These divisions are termed *Tanner stages* (Tanner, 1962) (Figs. 8-3, 8-4, and 8-5). Pubertal changes occur on a continuum, with individual differences in timing or tempo.

Female Stages

Females enter puberty earlier than males do, and their puberty usually progresses sequentially in the following pattern:

- Ovaries increase in size; no visible body changes occur.
- Breast budding (thelarche) traditionally occurs between 9 and 10 years old, with 97% of girls having initial breast development by 12 years old (Cabrera et al, 2014) (Fig. 8-3). Evidence indicates that adolescent girls are entering and completing puberty younger than girls did 50 years ago, with the average age decreasing by 1 year in the past few decades (Biro et al, 2012; Cabrera et al, 2014). Most girls (85%) experience the development of breast buds approximately 6 months before the appearance of pubic hair. African American girls, on average, reach thelarche and onset of menstruation (menarche) approximately 6 months prior to their Caucasian peers (Cabrera et al, 2014). The timing of the onset of breast development in females has no relationship to breast size at the completion of puberty.
- Rapid linear growth usually begins shortly after the onset of breast budding and reaches its peak about 1 year later. Ninety-five percent of females reach peak height velocity (PHV) between the ages of 10 and 14 years, and most girls experience PHV about 6 to 12 months before menarche, generally between 11 and 12 years old (Busscher et al, 2012). Early developers may experience a height

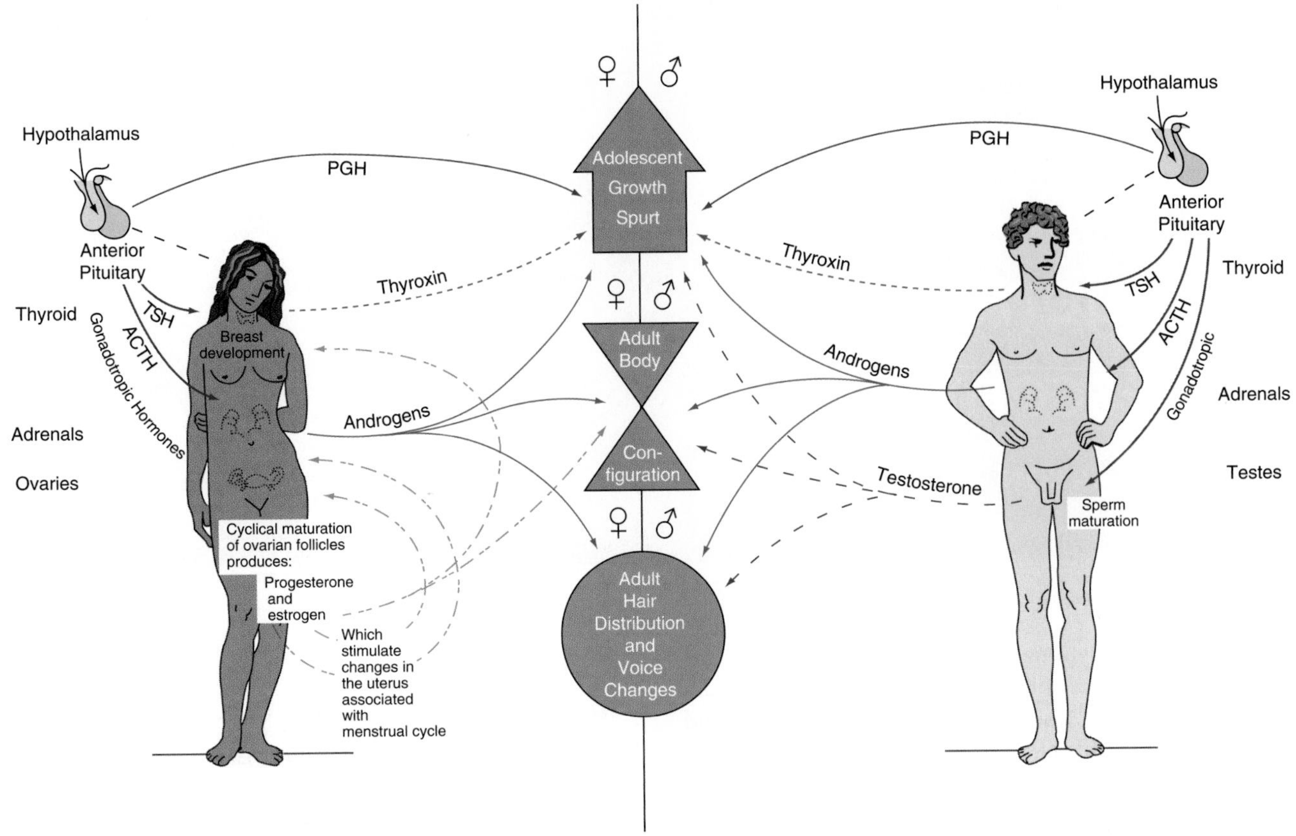

• **Figure 8-1** The endocrine system at puberty. *ACTH,* Adrenocorticotropic hormone; *PGH,* pituitary growth hormone; *TSH,* thyroid-stimulating hormone. (From Valadian I, Porter D: *Physical growth and development from conception to maturity*, Boston, 1977, Little, Brown.)

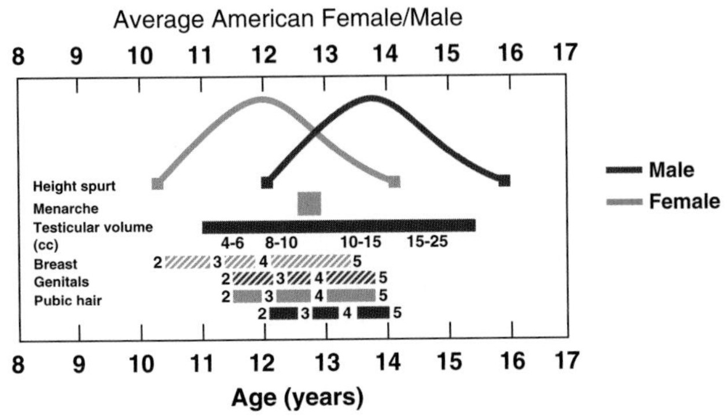

• **Figure 8-2** Sequence of pubertal events. Breast, genital, and pubic hair development indicate Tanner stages 2 to 5. (Adapted from Division of Adolescent Medicine, Children's Hospital Medical Center, Cincinnati, OH, 1995.)

spurt between 9 and 10 years old, whereas late developers may not experience a height spurt until between 13 and 14 years old. Final height is determined by the amount of bone growth at the epiphyses of the long bones. Growth stops when hormonal factors shut down the epiphyseal plates.

- Appearance of pubic hair (adrenarche or pubarche) commences at about 11½ years old and is related to adrenal rather than gonadal development, not to thelarche; therefore, it is less valid than other secondary sex characteristics in assessing sexual maturation (Fig. 8-4).
- The first menstrual period (menarche) occurs, on average, at 12½ years old. More than 95% of girls experience menarche between 10½ and 14½ years old. The mean age of menarche is highly dependent on ethnic, socioeconomic, and nutritional factors. Menarche generally occurs approximately 2½ years after thelarche (Cabrera et al, 2014). It may be 18 to 24 months after menarche before females establish regular ovulatory cycles. To some degree, menstrual cycles can be affected by athletic activity. The American Academy of Pediatrics (AAP) and the American Congress of Obstetricians and Gynecologists (AGOG) recommend that health care providers recognize the menstrual cycle as a "vital sign" because of the need for education regarding normal timing and characteristics of menstruation and other pubertal signs (ACOG Committee on Adolescent Health Care, 2006; Hagan et al, 2008).

Changes in the body composition of females occur during puberty, and adolescent girls benefit from the primary health care provider's reassurance that these changes are normal. Initial breast development usually begins as a unilateral disk-like subareolar swelling, and many adolescents and parents may initially present with concerns about breast tumors. Girls often have asymmetric breasts and need

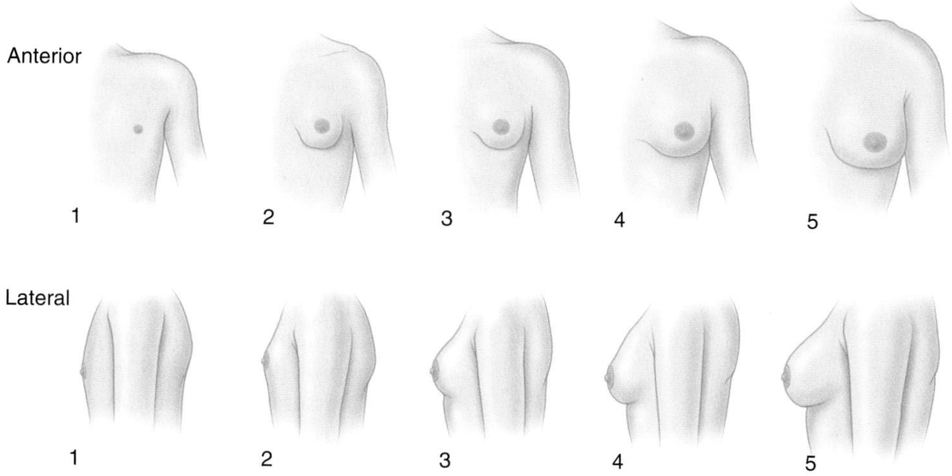

• **Figure 8-3** Normal female breast development, Tanner stages 1 to 5. (From Duderstadt K: *Pediatric physical examination: an illustrated handbook*, ed 2, St. Louis, 2014, Elsevier/Mosby, p 235.) (Original source Herring JA: *Tachdjian's pediatric orthopaedics*, ed 4, Philadelphia, 2008, Saunders/Elsevier.)

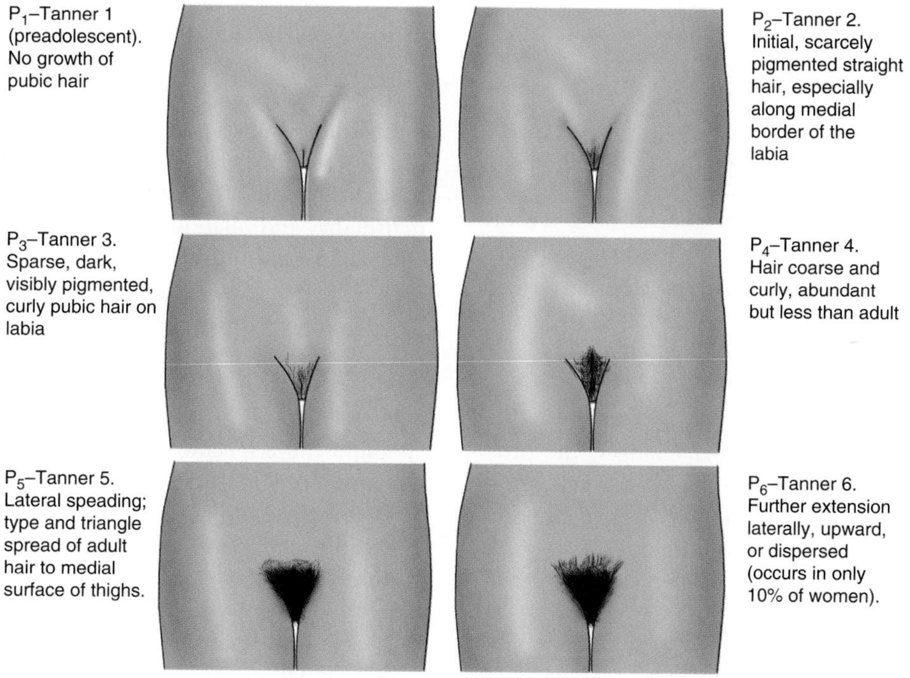

P1–Tanner 1 (preadolescent). No growth of pubic hair
P2–Tanner 2. Initial, scarcely pigmented straight hair, especially along medial border of the labia
P3–Tanner 3. Sparse, dark, visibly pigmented, curly pubic hair on labia
P4–Tanner 4. Hair coarse and curly, abundant but less than adult
P5–Tanner 5. Lateral speading; type and triangle spread of adult hair to medial surface of thighs.
P6–Tanner 6. Further extension laterally, upward, or dispersed (occurs in only 10% of women).

• **Figure 8-4** Normal female genitalia development, Tanner stages 1 to 6. (From Duderstadt K: *Pediatric physical examination: an illustrated handbook*, ed 2, St. Louis, 2014, Elsevier/Mosby, p 245.)

assurance that breasts become more or less the same size within a few years after the onset of breast budding. The female body shape changes as girls progress through puberty, with broadening of the shoulders, hips, and thighs. Girls experience a continuous increase in proportion of fat to total body mass during puberty. They enter puberty with approximately 80% lean body weight and 20% body fat. By the time puberty ends, lean body mass drops to about 75%. Body fat is an important mediator for the onset of menstruation and regular ovulatory cycles. An average of 17% of body fat is needed for menarche, and about 22% is needed to initiate and maintain regular ovulatory cycles.

Male Stages

Physical body changes of puberty generally occur sequentially in males as follows:

- The initial sign of male puberty is testicular enlargement, on average at 11 years old (Hagan et al, 2008). Growth of the testes occurs approximately 6 months before the development of pubic hair in most males. If testicular

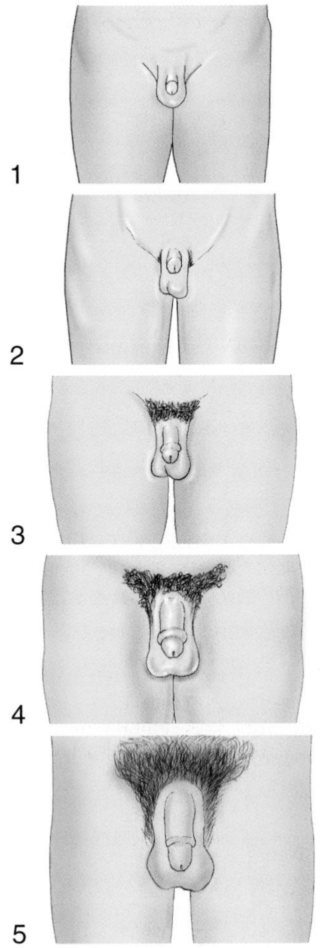

• **Figure 8-5** Normal male genitalia development, Tanner stages 1 to 5. (From Duderstadt K: *Pediatric physical examination: an illustrated handbook*, ed 2, St. Louis, 2014, Elsevier/Mosby, p 216.)

enlargement does not precede other changes, the provider should consider whether the boy is taking exogenous anabolic steroids. Once puberty begins, the left testis generally hangs lower than the right.

- Pubic hair development follows a pattern similar to that of girls (Fig. 8-5).
- First release of spermatozoa (spermarche) generally occurs in mid puberty at a mean age of 13½ to 14½ years. However, it can occur at any stage of development from SMR 2 to 5.
- Elongation and widening of the penis usually begin in SMR 3 and continue through SMR 5 (see Fig. 8-5).
- Rapid growth in height occurs. The PHV for males tends to occur late in mid puberty to early in late puberty. Boys generally lag about 2 years behind girls, but 95% have their growth spurt between 12 and 16 years old. Males typically have a higher peak growth velocity than females. Males can continue to grow, although minimally, well beyond their teenage years.
- Change in the male voice coincides with the PHV.
- Development of axillary, facial, and body hair occurs. Axillary hair generally does not appear before SMR 4 pubic hair. Facial hair appears only after SMR 4 pubic hair and does so in an ordered sequence. It starts at the outer corners of the upper lip and moves inward, then appears on the upper parts of the cheeks and middle of the lower lip, and finally grows along the sides and lower border of the chin. The extent of body hair is determined to a large extent by genetic factors. Body hair develops gradually after facial hair. Body hair changes should not, however, be used to assess pubertal maturation related to changes in the endocrine system.

As with girls, the body composition of adolescent boys changes, sometimes causing great concern for the adolescent. The provider can be an invaluable source of information and reassurance. In contrast to females, males generally increase muscle mass and lose body fat during puberty.

Some changes associated with puberty may be unwelcome. Up to 65% of males experience *gynecomastia,* a transient enlargement of breast tissue, typically within a year of achieving PHV (Limony et al, 2013). Gynecomastia generally lasts 12 to 18 months and resolves completely in nearly all cases by late puberty. In a small percentage of males, however, some palpable breast tissue may persist. Acne starts in early puberty, and by mid puberty many males have moderate to severe acne, which becomes somewhat worse by the end of puberty. Although generally benign, gynecomastia can occur secondary to anabolic steroid or illicit drug use. In cases of persistent gynecomastia or severe acne, the provider should ask questions about the use of alcohol, marijuana, and anabolic steroids, all of which can exacerbate these conditions.

Psychosocial, Emotional, and Cognitive Development

Adolescents transitioning from childhood to adulthood should achieve specific cognitive, emotional, and psychosocial developmental milestones that help them:

- Feel a sense of belonging in a valued group
- Acquire skills and master tasks that are important to the valued group
- Develop a sense of self-worth
- Develop at least one reliable relationship with another individual
- Demonstrate cognitive potential

Influences on Psychosocial, Emotional, and Cognitive Development

The adolescent's ability to achieve these goals depends in part on brain functioning. Although full sized, the adolescent brain continues to develop functional ability. In particular the prefrontal cortex (PFC), which coordinates executive functions of abstract thinking, reasoning, judgment, self-discipline, ethical behavior, personality, and behavioral modification and emotions, experiences rapid growth. As with the infant brain, a process of pruning and reinforcement occurs, based on the stimuli, activities, and experiences of the teenager.

The brain is subject to chemical, hormonal, physical, and biologic changes. Dopaminergic and noradrenergic receptors become more active and neurotransmitter levels increase during adolescence. Neuroimaging studies indicate the cortical and limbic structures, including the midbrain, amygdala, and hippocampus, change in size and are particularly affected by puberty. The communication between the amygdala (the center for emotional response and perception) and the PFC diminishes during adolescence and is stronger from the amygdala to the PFC (Gee et al, 2013). This explains many of the socioemotional responses of adolescence. The adolescent brain is particularly vulnerable to toxic stress from life events, abuse/maltreatment, mental illness, altered social interaction, and chronic illness. It is hypothesized that chronic stress affects the limbic and cortical brain structures and may predispose affected adolescents to developing chronic mental illness, risky adult behaviors, and decreased satisfaction with interpersonal relationships (Eliand and Romeo, 2013; Whittle et al, 2013). See Chapter 19 for an in-depth discussion of mental health and illness.

Drugs and alcohol have a significant negative effect on the adolescent brain, damaging the neural circuitry in the "reward" or motivation pathways and shutting down the body's ability to respond to stimuli that normally generate feelings of pleasure. In essence the drug becomes the only thing that leads to pleasurable feelings, and a craving for the drug is "etched" into the brain—the individual becomes addicted. In addition to contributing to addiction, brain changes resulting from exposure to alcohol, especially binge drinking, can lead to loss of memory and cognitive function. It is theorized these occur because of neurotoxicity and damage to the myelin sheath in the prefrontal cortex (Coleman et al, 2014; Pascual et al, 2014). Genetic structures of individuals vary, however, and not all brains respond to drugs in this way, but the adolescent brain is highly vulnerable.

Principles of Behavior Changes

A wide variety of normal behavior characterizes the process of psychosocial, emotional, and cognitive development in adolescents (Table 8-1). Three general principles may be used to understand these changes:

- Transition is continual and generally smooth.
- Disruptive family conflict is not the norm.
- The quality of thinking changes from concrete to formal operational thinking.

Smooth Transition

The first principle of adolescent psychosocial development is that the transition from adolescence to adulthood is continuous and generally smooth. A commonly held myth is that adolescence is a period of "storm and stress." This view was originally described by G. Stanley Hall in 1908. Although his argument was not based on research, this myth continues to be widely believed. It is important to remember that adolescence is only one of many transitional phases in life; and although some experience significant challenges during these years, others pass through this critical time with relative ease.

Family Relationships Change

The second principle of adolescent psychosocial development is that the biologic, cognitive, and emotional changes experienced by adolescents require a reworking of family relationships. Some degree of adolescent-parent conflict is to be expected because of this reworking of relationships, but disruptive family conflict is not the norm. Mundane, everyday issues (such as, which clothes to wear, hairstyles, household chores, curfew, and friends) continue to be the usual sources of parent-adolescent conflict, and negotiation between parent and child is essential. Inexperienced in negotiation, adolescents will often argue a point to excess. It may help to remind parents that this verbal debate, or "arguing," is a normal behavior of teens that reflects their use of more abstract thinking skills. It is a way of practicing abstract thinking and engaging parents. However, the parent should not become too deeply engaged because the adolescent rarely is, and the "arguments" tend to blow over fairly quickly (Box 8-1).

Families should not experience one crisis after another. It is a cause for concern if family crises are the norm. When

• BOX 8-1 Tips for Parents: Adolescent Survival Guide

Start with clear rules and expectations before children are teenagers. Work on developing good communication with children early and continue through adolescence. State expectations and future consequences before trouble has occurred (e.g., identify curfew expectations before the dance, not when the teen comes home late).

Be firm and follow through.

Try to be flexible and allow teenagers to negotiate. Discussing principles and negotiating solutions are valuable life skills for the future. Do not negotiate rules that are nonnegotiable.

Fighting and arguing are typical, often used by teens as they practice their developing reasoning skills. Often teens are engaged more recreationally than emotionally. Therefore, when the parent is tired, disengage and walk away. Try not to take what they say personally.

Teenagers want parents to be involved, concerned, and ask questions. They just may not know it or know how to express their desire.

Know who their friends are and call those parents from time to time. Compare household rules if possible.

Be involved at their school if possible. Try to meet their teachers and stay in contact with them.

Continue to involve teenagers in family activities, even when they no longer want to. Bringing friends along will help.

Keep promises made to teens. This builds trust and respect and makes you a role model.

Model good behavior. Adolescents recognize the hypocrisy of saying one thing and doing another.

Don't forget that teenagers still need adult supervision at times.

Keep communication lines open and don't be afraid to start conversations. Adolescents sometimes want to talk to adults but are nervous about speaking first.

TABLE 8-1 Central Issues in Early, Middle, and Late Adolescence

Variable	Early Adolescence	Middle Adolescence	Late Adolescence
Sexual maturity rating (SMR)	1 to 2	3 to 5	5
Somatic	Secondary sex characteristics Beginning of rapid growth Awkward appearance	Height growth peaks Body shape and composition change Acne and odor Menarche/spermarche	Physically mature Slower growth
Cognitive and moral	Concrete operations Unable to perceive long-term outcome of current decision-making Conventional morality	Emergence of abstract thought (formal operations) May perceive future implications, but may not apply in decision-making Questioning social mores	Future-oriented with sense of perspective idealism; absolutism Able to think things through independently
Self-concept/ identity formation	Preoccupied with changing body Self-conscious about appearance and attractiveness Fantasy and present-oriented	Concern with attractiveness Increasing introspection "Stereotypical adolescent"	More stable body image Attractiveness may still be of concern Emancipation complete Firmer identity
Family	Increased need for privacy Increased bid for independence	Conflicts over control and independence Struggle for acceptance of greater authority	Emotional and physical separation from family Increased autonomy
Peers	Seeks same-sex peer affiliation to counter instability	Intense peer group involvement Preoccupation with peer culture Peers provide behavioral example	Peer group and values recede in importance Intimacy/possible commitment takes precedence
Sexual	Increased interest in sexual anatomy Anxieties and questions about genital changes, size Limited dating and intimacy	Testing ability to attract partner Initiation of relationships and sexual activity Questions of sexual orientation	Consolidation of sexual identity Focus on intimacy and formation of stable relationships Planning for future and commitment
Relationship to society	Middle school adjustment	Gauging skills and opportunities	Career decisions (e.g., college, work)

(From Kleigman RM, Stanton BF, St. Geme JW, et al: *Nelson textbook of pediatrics*, Philadelphia, 2011, Elsevier, p 650.)

true turmoil exists, it usually represents psychopathology and will not be simply "outgrown." Careful assessment and treatment are required. Behavior that results in negative consequences is especially worrisome. For example, fights over hair color may not be worthwhile because hair color will grow out, but behavior that results in school and/or work difficulties should be addressed.

Cognitive Changes

The third principle of adolescent psychosocial development is about change in cognitive abilities. Adolescents develop what Piaget referred to as *formal operational thinking,* characterized by the use of propositional thinking and abstract reasoning. The principal difference between concrete and formal operational thinking is the ability to reason using verbal manipulation rather than in terms of concrete objects. In early adolescence, thinking tends to be very concrete. The classic example is an adolescent who when asked, "Are you sexually active?" responds, "No, I just lie there," or when asked, "What brought you here to see me today?" answers, "The bus." Most teenagers acquire increasing sophistication in abstract thought after they are 14 years old. They learn to conceptualize about past and future events and to relate actions to consequences. During this process, adolescents begin to:

- Consider values: The ones they challenge most are those with which they are most familiar, ones they have grown up with.
- Understand concepts of good and evil and understand human nature (e.g., not all authority figures are good people).
- Be aware of contradictions between what is said and what is done (e.g., adolescents are acutely aware when parents tell their children not to smoke or drink even though they do, or when they tell them to wear their seat belts although the parent does not).
- Understand the significance of their place within the construct of time (past, present, and future) and

begin thinking about what they will be doing in the future (e.g., college, technical school, job, marriage, and family).

Although most teenagers develop the ability to translate experiences into abstract ideas and think about the consequences of actions, approximately one third do not achieve more fully sophisticated thinking abilities, even as adults. Neurologic changes underlie the development of executive function, memory, social inhibition, intelligence, and cognition in adolescence. Emerging scientific evidence indicates that a combination of environmental influences (e.g., drugs, alcohol, noise, and so on) and genetic susceptibility can have long-term effects on cognitive ability and higher executive function (Erus et al, 2015; Luna et al, 2010).

Emotional Changes of Adolescence

Hormones present during puberty cause emotional and physical changes. As with physical growth and development, emotional changes appear differently in males than in females. Some males may experience an association between an increase in testosterone and sad or anxious feelings, acting out, aggressive behavior, or interest in sexual activity.

Some emotional changes that occur are not directly associated with hormonal changes. Research shows that boys with adult-like physiques are given more leadership roles, are more proficient in sports, are perceived as more attractive and smarter than their peers, and are more popular than others in their age group. In general, they demonstrate higher self-esteem in early adolescence. Late-maturing boys who are short and child-like in appearance until 15 years or older tend to show more personal and social maladjustment over the entire course of adolescence. They can be insecure, suggestible, vulnerable to peer pressure, and subjects of bullying or seen as weak, immature, and less competent than average. Males, as they progress through puberty, typically develop a more positive self-image and mood, whereas females may feel a diminished sense of attractiveness as their bodies mature. Boys tend to be more satisfied with their body image and, depending on their current size, may want to either gain or lose weight, whereas girls are more likely to express a desire to lose weight. Dieting and disordered eating is unfortunately common in adolescence. Studies indicate that within the previous year almost half (45.8%) of females and 31.1% of males dieted, 50.2% of females and 38.1% of males had unhealthy weight control behaviors, and 6.8% of females and 3.9% of males engaged in extreme weight control measures (Neumark-Sztainer et al, 2012).

The emotional affect and behavior of pubescent females differ in other ways from those of boys. Both early-maturing boys and girls demonstrate more risky behaviors than do adolescents who are late maturing, but girls are at greater risk as a result of romantic liaisons. Often these early bloomers get "bumped up" to an older group of peers and become the objects of sexual attention from older males. The developing body of early-maturing females may not match their chronologic age or emotional maturity. This difference can influence their behavior and place them at risk for early sexual activity, delinquency, and substance abuse (Stattin et al, 2011).

Egocentrism of Adolescents

Changes in the quality of adolescent thinking coupled with physical and emotional changes give rise to a form of egocentrism. This change may result in a rather self-centered, but not necessarily selfish, view of the world. This may survive into later adolescence and adulthood and is generally recognized to encompass four major types of egocentrism first described by Elkind (1984):

- *Imaginary audience:* Everyone is thinking about them.
- *Personal fable:* They are special.
- *Overthinking:* They make things more complicated than they are.
- *Apparent hypocrisy:* Rules apply differently to them than to others.

Imaginary Audience. Abstract thinking allows teenagers to wonder what others are thinking about. At the same time, adolescents are obsessed by the physical changes brought about by puberty. These changes and their new thinking abilities create the notion that everyone is thinking about the same thing that they are (i.e., them). Teenagers may believe that one can read minds and know what others are thinking. For example, a boy who goes to the pharmacy to purchase a condom may feel that he is "on stage," the object of everyone's scrutiny. An adolescent with orthodontic braces may think that everyone is staring at him. A young girl who has a pimple on her nose may feel that it is the first thing others see when they look at her.

Personal Fable. If everyone is watching you and thinking about you (thanks to the imaginary audience), you must be someone special. The personal fable is the concept that the laws of nature do not apply to oneself and that one's thoughts and feelings are totally unique. The personal fable has a very positive aspect in that it provides adolescents with a sense of importance, purpose, and hope; it helps them to imagine possibilities and opportunities in their lives and futures. Personal fables can also have a negative effect (e.g., when adolescents believe that they will never grow old, cannot get pregnant [especially the first time], cannot get a sexually transmitted infection [STI] despite engaging in unprotected intercourse, or will not suffer long-term consequences from substance use).

Overthinking. Overthinking involves making things more complicated than they need to be. An example is an adolescent who attributes complicated motives to simple oversights (e.g., an adolescent boy who thinks that his parents would not have divorced if only he had helped more with the chores around the house or an adolescent girl who breaks up with her boyfriend because she assumes that he does not like her because he did not compliment her on her new red dress).

Apparent Hypocrisy. Apparent hypocrisy is the notion that rules apply differently to adolescents than they do to others. For example, an adolescent girl may believe that she should have free access to her parent's clothes and electronic equipment (such as, a tablet or music player), whereas her parents entering her room to borrow something constitutes an invasion of privacy.

Developmental Screening and Assessment

Principles and Approaches to Assessment

Throughout infancy and the preschool and school years, the focus of the health care visit is the parent or caregiver and the child as a unit. This dyad changes with adolescence. Teenagers must be evaluated independently of their parents, and developmental issues must be discussed privately with the adolescents themselves. Nonetheless, parents remain concerned, and it is ideal that they be involved in their child's health care. Adolescents continue to be part of the family system, and providers should work with adolescents to maximize communication with parents around health issues. Some providers believe that involving parents or other significant adults in the adolescent's care is essential. However, that decision is not always the provider's to make, and it may not always be in the best interest of the adolescent. Adolescents must be actively included in decisions about sharing information with others. For many sensitive health issues, providers need to help the teenager understand and evaluate the risks and benefits of involving family members. They must also provide guidance and support on how to best inform the family, if that is the final choice. This approach can help protect a teen from the parent who may be abusive or unsafe. It can also reduce the problem of parents who are upset if they feel they are denied information about the child they love and for whom they feel responsible.

Effective interviews with adolescent clients are based on the use of good general interviewing techniques: demonstrating respect for the client; establishing parameters of what can be accomplished during the visit; using appropriate body language, active listening, and communication techniques; and working with the client to develop a realistic, individualized treatment plan. The provider gives the message that the teenager and his or her concerns are important, that no judgments will be made, and that the provider and teenager are a team, working together to achieve the healthiest outcome possible.

Preserving confidentiality with the teenager is essential. Adolescents should be reassured that the provider will not share information with the child's parent or caregiver (general confidentiality) unless the adolescent agrees, or unless the health of the child or others may be compromised (e.g., threat of potential suicide, violence, evidence of an eating disorder). Providers must inform the teenager that there are limits to confidentiality (limited confidentiality). As "mandatory reporters," primary health care providers are required by law to report information that puts the child or others in danger (e.g., physical or sexual abuse; some states require reporting teen sexual activity, even if consensual, if an age difference of 3 or more years exists between the couple). If adolescents perceive that their provider will maintain confidentiality, they are more likely to disclose more sensitive, relevant information (Gilbert et al, 2014), and it has been found that even when providers tell adolescents that there are limits to their confidentiality, teens continue to disclose. For teenagers who are hesitant to discuss sensitive issues, a questionnaire or checklist may be an effective way to collect information. Questionnaires used to identify adolescent strengths have been created by the Search Institute and have been used by communities to enhance adolescent self-concept, whereas programs like the Rapid Assessment for Adolescent Preventative Services (RAAPS) can help PCPs identify risky adolescent behaviors (see Resources, Chapters 2 and 18).

Focus of Assessment

Physical Development

Adolescents should have height, weight, body mass index (BMI), and blood pressure measured at each health maintenance visit. The growth trajectory should be evaluated, using growth grids to identify norms. The Tanner stage (SMR) should be recorded at each visit to evaluate progression of pubertal changes initiated by the endocrine system. Testicular growth can be directly assessed by palpation of the testes in the scrotum and comparison of their size with a standardized orchidometer. Self-assessment is generally reliable, and adolescent males can be asked to evaluate their own level of development if provided with standards against which to compare themselves. Varicocele, or enlarged veins palpable in the scrotum, may develop at sexual maturity and are not cause for alarm unless a discrepancy in testicular size is noted on examination. Gynecomastia in boys should be noted. Scoliosis may develop rapidly at this age, and assessment should be done annually. The thyroid gland should be palpated because goiter may appear in this age group. Additionally, the teen should be questioned about attitudes regarding physical growth and development. Dissatisfaction with body appearance might warrant further probing to elicit unhealthy behavior (e.g., bingeing and purging, steroid use) (see Chapter 19 for information about eating disorders).

Cognitive Development

Assessment should include questions about school attendance, school performance, and educational or career goals. Connectedness to school has been found to be a significant predictor of adolescent well-being; the extent to which a child connects to school depends on characteristics of both the child and the school (Saab and Klinger, 2010; Waters et al, 2010). Children who are behind a grade have a much greater risk of dropping out of school, thus leading some to consider school failure as a form of adolescent failure to thrive. Chronic absenteeism, class skipping, and other types of school avoidance indicate a problem that may be related to cognitive ability and should be assessed in depth. Objective assessment of cognitive development, as with school-age children, requires formal psychological testing, which is best done through schools.

Social and Emotional Development

Key areas to assess in relation to social and emotional development include adolescents' emerging independence from family, relationships with peers, and goals for the future (an area that older teenagers should address more specifically than younger adolescents).

Adolescents should be interviewed about school, family, and peer relationships; safety (e.g., use of seat belts); exposure to violence, abuse, or weapons in their home or community; mental health issues, such as mood, depression, anger problems, or suicidal ideation; sexuality, sexual activity, and sexual orientation; and involvement in risk behaviors, such as tobacco, alcohol, and prescription or street drug use and eating disorders.

Parent Assessment

Parents change in response to the adolescent's influence on the family. Parents, too, need advice, support, and encouragement. The normal mood swings of adolescence can trigger strain on family relationships and result in arguments. Parents with balanced approaches that include unconditional love, clear boundaries, and consistent discipline are more likely to have adolescents with less depression and risk-taking and better academic success than parents who are authoritarians. It is important to assess parental concerns about their adolescent's health at each of the episodic wellness visits because these concerns can give insight into the teen's physical, socioemotional and mental health, and they provide a glimpse into the family functioning and the health of the parent-child dyad. If problems exist in the parent's view or a discrepancy and potential conflict emerge in the interviews, the provider should bring the teen and parent together to clarify the concern and offer counseling.

Anticipatory Guidance During Adolescence

Anticipatory guidance should be an individualized discussion with teenagers that helps them understand, respond to, and take responsibility for their own behavior and development (Table 8-2). Separate discussions need to be conducted with parents to help them understand and support their child's maturation and need for independence. In these discussions, the provider should clarify what values and expectations parents have for their child and how the teenager perceives those expectations. Some discussion points are outlined in each of the adolescent phases discussed later. They should be incorporated into the health supervision visit, but they are not all-inclusive, and they should not be covered exhaustively at each visit. Ideas for assessment and management of problems that emerge from these discussions can be found in subsequent chapters (e.g., sexuality issues are discussed in Chapter 15).

Phases of Adolescence

One simple way to understand adolescence is to divide it into three psychosocial developmental phases: (1) early, 11 to 14 years old or junior high school; (2) middle, 15 to 17 years old or high school; and (3) late, 18 to 21 years old or college, work, or vocational-technical school.

Each phase is characterized by certain behavior. Understanding such behavior assists in the evaluation of areas of concern to the adolescent or family. Within each developmental phase, adolescents deal with issues of autonomy, body image, identity development, and peer group involvement.

Early Adolescence (11 to 14 Years Old)

Early adolescence is the most difficult adjustment period for young people. Rapid changes occur simultaneously in all parts of the adolescent's life; cognitive skills may not keep pace with physical changes; emotional reactions may overwhelm the child's ability to understand and cope. Early adolescents are often confused, even frightened, by the changes they are experiencing. They can be difficult people to be around, and the responses their behavior elicits from parents and other adults may be exactly the opposite of the support, caring, and understanding they desperately need.

Physical Development

Physical changes in early adolescence vary widely, with some young people achieving Tanner stage 3 or even 4, whereas others are still at SMR-2 by age 14 (see previous discussion of physical development).

Cognitive Development

As their thinking abilities develop, teenagers daydream frequently. Parents and teachers need to be reminded that daydreaming is cognitive work for adolescents and that they need time to participate in this activity. At the same time, early adolescents should be given the opportunity to use their growing reasoning skills to actively solve problems, explore values, and examine principles on which they make decisions. Early adolescents set idealistic goals that change frequently. One day they want to be an engineer and the next day a pilot or a parent who stays home to raise children. Some adolescents at this age experience a drop in academic performance in junior high school, which is related to motivation rather than ability.

Social and Emotional Development

Young adolescents begin to renegotiate relationships with parents and other significant adults and develop more intimate contacts with their peers. Because they lack experience and social skills, early adolescents may not yet be a part of an adolescent subculture and can be very lonely. At this stage, teenagers can appear to be anti-adult, preferring to spend more time with friends than with family, and suddenly finding their parents to be an

TABLE 8-2 Adolescent Development and Related Anticipatory Guidance

Area of Development	Anticipatory Guidance
Physical	
Experience growth from prepubescence to sexual maturity	Teach child about body functions (e.g., menstruation, nocturnal emissions) of both genders. Teach about the timing and descriptions of primary and secondary sexual characteristics of both genders (e.g., changes in breasts, genitals, and hair). Discuss masturbation. Discuss sexual orientation, sexual feelings.
Reach adult parameters of height and physical growth by late adolescence	Provide counseling regarding substance abuse, safety, and unintentional injuries. Teach and encourage correct and consistent use of helmets, seat belts, and proper sports equipment. Emphasize safety and responsibility regarding access to and use of guns and other weapons.
Become comfortable with one's body	Offer reassurance that physical findings are normal; explain what to expect; listen to adolescents' concerns; encourage exercise, sports participation, and body fitness; encourage healthy nutrition and sleep patterns.
Cognitive	
Move from concrete thinking to ability to reason abstractly	Emphasize value of successful completion of school. Discuss how meeting academic responsibilities is a priority and needs to be integrated with other activities. Explain how changes in cognitive abilities may contribute to "overthinking" or a sense of confusion; encourage teen to do "reality checks" with a trusted adult. Engage adolescent in conversation, explain procedures, and answer questions; listen.
Develop personal value system and moral integrity	Encourage discussion of what the adolescent believes is important and what the adolescent finds valuable. Help the adolescent develop skills in conflict resolution and prevention. Discuss how learning to identify feelings is the first step in understanding how "feelings" influence mental and physical processes. Discuss respect for rights, needs, and opinions of others. Teach that maturation involves understanding and appreciating multicultural differences.
Move from dependence on others to self for risk reduction	Provide information about how to resist peer pressure to engage in risky behavior. Discuss injury prevention strategies at home, work, and school. Emphasize dangers of weapons.
Psychosocial	
Establish independence from parents	Explain to parents an adolescent's need for privacy and that not joining in all family activities is not a sign of rejection of the family. Some privacy within the home should be expected.
Develop sense of self-identity	Encourage adolescents to take responsibility for their own health care. Encourage adolescents to take on new challenges; discuss plans for the future (e.g., school, work, and family). Help adolescents identify their own personal strengths and joys.
Create new relationships with peers and other adults	Discuss importance of activities with peers; identify healthy ways to be part of a group. Provide counseling on: • Avoiding gang involvement • Bullying, which may be physical, emotional, or sexual • Preventing the use of drugs, cigarettes, and alcohol • Stopping substance use for those who are using Discuss the notion that maturation includes increased independence *and* increased responsibility at home, school, and in the community. Encourage the adolescent to participate in community activities. Provide information and opportunity to discuss questions regarding sexuality, how to differentiate between "love" and "infatuation," how to be sexually responsible, and how to protect against pregnancy and STIs. Discuss dating relationships. Emphasize that healthy relationships are based on mutual respect. Discuss how to prevent date rape or other abusive relationships. Advocate for safe social media usage.

STI, Sexually transmitted infection.

embarrassment. This behavior is a normal and healthy step toward maturity and a first step toward independence. One way of demonstrating independence is to challenge parental authority. The adolescent may become more argumentative and disobedient, refuse to do chores, and want to renegotiate rules (e.g., curfews, allowance, household responsibilities).

Wide mood swings—from euphoria to sadness—can occur within a matter of minutes. Normative fluctuations of mood are linked to adolescent developmental processes and are characterized by their transient nature, commonly measured in hours or days. These emotional fluctuations can and should be distinguished from the unremitting, long-standing mood and behavior changes of serious depressive disorders.

During this period adolescents become extremely conscious of their bodies as they adjust to the physical changes they are experiencing. They begin to spend more time in front of the mirror combing their hair, checking their skin, and putting on makeup. Clothes and appearance become more important for all teenagers, including those with a developmental delay or chronic handicap. The onset of secondary sex characteristics increases anxieties about menstruation, wet dreams, masturbation, and size of the breasts or penis. This is an opportune time to dispel myths (e.g., masturbation causes blindness and acne) and to provide anticipatory guidance (e.g., a premenarcheal girl often has vaginal leukorrhea, which is generally a clear, mucoid discharge).

Early adolescents have a desire for greater privacy. They often spend more time in their room alone listening to music, using social media, texting, or talking on the phone. They magnify their problems and believe that no one could possibly understand what they are feeling. Much of the adolescents' time is used in the development of new friendships as a greater number of opportunities become possible. Same-sex friendships occur, usually with one best friend. These strong friendships may lead to fleeting same-sex experimentation as sexual feelings emerge and adolescents begin developing their sexual identity. Contact with the opposite sex is usually in groups (e.g., middle school dances with boys on one side of the gym and girls on the opposite side). Other sexual behavior of the early adolescent includes masturbating, telling dirty jokes, making lewd remarks to others, demonstrating interest in watching explicit sexual scenes in the media, or looking at magazines of nude individuals. The type of sexual experimentation may vary greatly, depending on the adolescent's subculture. For example, by this age, some teenagers have already experienced sexual intercourse or pregnancy, whereas others have not even held hands.

Early adolescents begin developing their own value system. They may try value systems other than the one that they have learned from their family, often leaving family members befuddled or even threatened. The peer group serves the purpose of aiding continued identity development.

Health Supervision

Annual health supervision visits are recommended. Critical components of the visit include developmental surveillance; assessing social and academic progress, including quality of interpersonal relationships and school performance; identifying emotional wellness (e.g., mood, mental health, sexuality); and risk reduction, including injury prevention, substance use prevention, and healthy sexuality. Immunization for human papillomavirus (HPV), diphtheria and tetanus toxoids and acellular pertussis vaccine (DTaP), influenza, hepatitis A, and meningococcal meningitis is recommended. Serum lipoprotein analysis should be done if not done earlier in childhood.

Anticipatory Guidance

Anticipatory guidance for the early adolescent focuses on explaining the rapid changes that are occurring; helping the adolescent in the early process of developing self-concept, autonomy, and independence; and providing reassurance that he or she is "normal." Specifically discuss:

- What physical changes to expect as puberty progresses.
- How the adolescent can best manage the rapid physical changes (e.g., engage in physical activity or sports; focus on injury prevention [e.g., bike helmets]; identify strategies to deal with onset of menstruation while at school; eat a well-balanced diet; get enough sleep).
- Nutritional needs: Increased iron and calcium intake is needed as menstruation begins and during periods of rapid growth.
- What emotional and psychological changes are occurring, and what coping strategies do the child and family have to manage them.
- What does it mean to be sexually responsible, both physically and emotionally; include abstinence counseling.
- Transition to adult health care: Initial conversations regarding transitioning to adult health care should begin between 12 and 13 years of age. This consists of informing the teen and family about the practice's transition policies. Those with chronic health care needs should begin to learn about their condition and the management regime. By age 14 to 15, a transition plan should be developed with the adolescent and parent (AAP et al, 2011).

Middle Adolescence (15 to 17 Years Old)

Middle adolescence is the essence of adolescence and its subculture. Picture in your mind's eye what typical adolescents look like and how they behave. What are they wearing? How do they act? What language are they using to communicate to adults and to one another? The picture that probably comes to mind is that of a middle adolescent. Middle adolescents stand out for their unique appearance.

Physical Development

Physical development is nearing completion. Middle adolescents have less concern about body changes, but increased interest in making themselves more attractive. As body attractiveness increases in importance, teenagers spend more time with hairstyles, clothes, and, for some, dieting or activities to build muscle mass. Teenagers with apparent handicaps are equally concerned about their body image and participate in the same activities to improve their appearance. Middle adolescents defy the limits of their bodies, and many have periods of excessive physical activity followed by periods of lethargy.

Cognitive Development

Intellectual sophistication and creativity increase in middle adolescents. Practicing the skills of reasoning, logic, and decision-making strengthens the adolescent's ability to establish healthy patterns as an adult. School and extracurricular activities are often the focus of the middle adolescent's life. Middle adolescents demonstrate increased concern with neighborhood and societal issues, such as poverty, peace and the environment.

Social and Emotional Development

Peer group involvement is intense and includes the establishment of a dress code, communication style, and code of conduct. Middle adolescents tend to be more non-adult than anti-adult, a characteristic of early adolescents. They spend twice the time with peers than adults. The need for peer contact is important for all middle adolescents, but it is especially important for teenagers with developmental disabilities, chronic handicaps, or both. However, peer involvement may be more limited for this group for any number of reasons (e.g., ostracism by the peer group, parental overprotectiveness, lack of social skills, and physical constraints).

Sexual drive emerges, and middle adolescents begin to explore their ability to attract a partner. National trends demonstrate that the mean age for initiating dating, sexual experimentation, and intercourse is in mid to late adolescence (Kann et al, 2014). Frequently, physical urges precede emotional maturity, and societal pressure to experiment with sex is great. Further discussion about adolescent sexuality is found in Chapter 15.

Because of the developing egocentrism and the concept of personal fable with feelings of omnipotence, invulnerability, and immortality, risk-taking and behavioral experimentation intensify. This may include smoking, alcohol use, sexual activity, general risk-taking behavior, or drinking and driving. Parental conflict peaks as middle adolescents continue to argue and renegotiate issues, such as curfew, allowance, going to parties or movies, and dating. Rules and expectations must be clear by this stage.

Health Supervision

Annual health supervision visits are recommended, including annual influenza immunization; developmental surveillance; and assessment of social and academic progress, quality of interpersonal relationships, school performance, and emotional wellness (e.g., mood, mental health). Screening for STIs is needed if the adolescent is sexually active. Papanicolaou (Pap) smears are no longer recommended until after age 21 years regardless of sexual activity. Tuberculosis and lipid screening is needed if risk factors are identified. If a plan for transition to adult health care is not already in place, one needs to be developed. These plans must be based on an assessment of the adolescent's ability to provide self-care and the needs and desires of the teen and his or her family. Plans, once in place, should be reevaluated annually (AAP et al, 2011).

Anticipatory Guidance

Anticipatory guidance for the middle adolescent focuses on the teen's expanding physical, cognitive, and socioemotional capabilities; consolidating self-concept; and identifying areas for continued growth and development. The provider should reinforce healthy behaviors and acknowledge and validate the adolescent's physical, intellectual, and social growth. Specifically discuss:

- Physical changes that allow for increasing skills; recommend regular, vigorous physical activity, fitness, and engagement in a wide range of activities.
- Dangers in use of drugs, cigarettes, performance-enhancing drugs, diet pills, and alcohol.
- Injury prevention (e.g., use seat belts, bike helmets; no texting when driving; emphasize safety and responsibility if using weapons [e.g., for hunting]).
- Involvement in extracurricular activities (e.g., clubs, hobbies, volunteer work, and community activities).
- Nutrition and the relationship between good nutrition, health, and a positive body image. Emphasize limiting sugary and caffeinated beverages and not skipping meals.
- Healthy sleep habits (see Chapter 14).
- Importance of completing school and making plans for the future.
- Sexuality. Emphasize:
    - Responsible sexual behaviors
    - Implications of sexual intercourse
    - Preventing date rape and other forms of intimate partner violence
    - Importance of remaining abstinent or returning to abstinence
    - Prevention of STIs
    - Birth control, including emergency methods
    - Sexual orientation
    - Breast or testicular self-examination (Note: Although the U.S. Preventive Services Task Force [USPSTF] guidelines do not recommend self-examination [USPSTF 2011, 2011], this is common practice and is included in the *Bright Futures* recommendations; the USPSTF recommendations are challenged by many (Hendrick and Helvie, 2011).
- Nature of peer relationships: based on mutual respect and caring? Gang involvement? Bullying?
- Nature of relationship with parents: reasonable limits set? Parents show interest and concern for teenager?

- Emotional maturity: how does adolescent resolve conflicts? Manage feelings of anger? Reduce stress?
- Potential for self-harm (e.g., cutting, bingeing, and purging).

Late Adolescence (18 to 21 Years Old)

Late adolescence is a time when the individual has a clearer self-concept, life choices are made, and decisions about how to contribute to society as a responsible adult are implemented. These are all examples of normal behavioral autonomy.

Physical Development

Physical development is typically complete, although the late adolescent may continue to add stature into his or her early 20s.

Cognitive Development

Late adolescents have an adult level of reasoning skills. They are generally capable of understanding the consequences of their actions and behavior and can make complex and sophisticated judgments about human relationships. They no longer base their judgments about people on overt behavior, but they have a good understanding of inner motivations, including multiple determinants of an action. Of course, neither teenagers nor adults consistently use this mature level of thinking, and some never reach this level of cognitive maturity.

Social and Emotional Development

By now, adolescents usually relate to the family as adults. Relationships with parents and family are gradually renegotiated to a more adult-adult basis. The role of the parent during late adolescence should be one of support. By the end of late adolescence, this status has optimally progressed to autonomy for adolescents in the context of continuing strong ties of affection to the family. Once adolescence is complete, young adults often have a modified value system very similar to the one with which they grew up.

Much of the final shaping of identity centers on adolescents' perceptions of their future options as adults. Many late adolescents are preparing for high school graduation or entry to college. They work, enter the military, marry, or participate in a vocational or technical training program. Approximately 68% of U.S. 2014 high school graduates went on to study in colleges or universities, and 73% of those not attending postsecondary institutions were in the workforce (U.S. Bureau of Labor Statistics, 2013). In many significant ways, the years in college offer a "moratorium," or a prolonged adolescence, a time to further clarify one's self-image. College life offers both maximal autonomy and a structured, supportive environment in which to complete developmental tasks. Those adolescents who enter the workforce and leave home immediately out of high school have quite different tasks and experiences. Their identity may be formed earlier, because they do not have the added time and supportive structures of the college experience. They cannot delay facing the issues of earning a living, forming a family, and accepting other adult responsibilities. Adolescents who are unsuccessful in the educational system or the workplace (underemployed or unemployed) may establish an identity by joining peers in gangs or by becoming socially isolated. Some late adolescents opt to join the military and, especially in times of war, face demands that force them to take on adult responsibilities for which they may not be psychologically or emotionally prepared. Individuals in the military and those affected by violence and other traumatic events can experience years of stress that jeopardize their sense of self.

A substantial number of late adolescents have established their sexuality and entered into an intimate, committed partner relationship, including marriage. Selection of a partner is based more on individual preferences and less on the peer group's values.

Health Supervision

Annual health supervision visits are recommended, including an annual influenza immunization. Screening for STIs is needed if the adolescent is sexually active, and Pap smears should begin at age 21 regardless of sexual activity. Tuberculosis screening is needed if risk factors are identified. A fasting lipoprotein analysis is recommended once during late adolescence.

Providers should assist the adolescent to learn about health insurance, how to enter and use the health care system, and to take responsibility for self-care. A plan for transition to adult care should be clearly developed by this time. Transition involves providing medical records and referring the adolescent to an adult health care provider. Many teens may benefit from a pretransfer visit with an adult provider (AAP et al, 2011).

Anticipatory Guidance

Anticipatory guidance for the late adolescent centers on the transition from being a teenager to taking on the responsibility and role of an adult. Specifically discuss:

- How physical exercise, good nutrition, sleep, and rest are incorporated into the late adolescent's lifestyle.
- Strategies to balance responsibilities of school, family, and job.
- Conflict resolution and stress management strategies.
- Choices made to achieve positive future goals and plan for the future—college, vocational training, military, and job or career.
- Ways the late adolescent is clarifying values and beliefs; identifying talents and interests to be pursued, and taking on challenges that increase self-confidence.
- Relationships with family, parents, siblings, friends, significant others, and community.
- Strategies to prevent injuries.
- Sexuality. Emphasize:
  - Responsible sexual behaviors; abstinence, a return to abstinence, or safe sex for those who are sexually active.

- Continued clarification of sexual orientation and how the late adolescent manages sexual feelings.
- Prevention of STIs.
- Prevention of date rape and other intimate partner abuse.
- Birth control, including emergency methods. Childbearing may be a decision for some late adolescents.
- Breast or testicular self-examination (see controversy discussed in middle adolescence)

Common Developmental Issues for Adolescents

Risk Behavior: General

Description

Risk behavior consists of actions that jeopardize adolescents' physical, psychological, or emotional health. Although health-risk behaviors among adolescents have decreased in the past few years, they continue to be the major cause of morbidity and mortality for adolescents (Kann et al, 2014). It is a paradox of adolescence that developmental tasks (i.e., gaining independence, developing one's own values, becoming comfortable with one's body, and establishing meaningful relationships) may be achieved (albeit in negative ways) through risk-taking behavior. Adolescents needing peer affiliation and striving for increased autonomy are likely to explore, experiment, and otherwise push the limits of their personal experience—often in ways that put them at risk for health-compromising outcomes. Many adolescents engage in risk behaviors without apparent negative outcomes. Other behaviors may appear risky at first glance, but do not pose significant risk to the adolescent. Is an adolescent who is sexually active but uses condoms on a regular basis engaged in risk behavior? Is an adolescent who goes to a party on the weekend and has a beer at risk? It is also important to recognize that some teenagers who seem at high risk do not engage in risk behaviors. Primary care providers should recognize factors that are protective for and those that increase risk of risky behavior.

Factors that Contribute to Risk-Taking

Although it is normal for behavioral experimentation to occur during this time, adolescents vary tremendously in their ability to think abstractly about the consequences of risky behavior. Their thinking is often characterized by the notion that "it can't happen to me" (personal fable). Although adolescents have an increase in abstract cognitive skills, thinking related to emotionally charged topics (e.g., substance use, sex, school performance, and peer pressure) is often less sophisticated. An adolescent who is drinking may be doing so in part to be accepted by friends or to feel a sense of independence and maturity. Because the behavior meets important developmental needs, it may be difficult for the adolescent to look at it objectively and give it up. In addition, the effect of alcohol on brain function further limits the adolescent's reasoning ability.

Environmental factors, both social and physical, can also influence adolescents' decisions to take risks. Factors that contribute to the adolescent engaging in risk behaviors include, but are not limited to, the following (McKnight-Eily et al, 2011):

- Poor academic performance or low intellectual function
- Impulsivity or attention deficit-hyperactivity disorder
- Role models for deviant behavior (e.g., parents with mental health disorders or who abuse drugs or engage in criminal behavior)
- Lack of constructive support or encouragement from others in social environment
- Low self-esteem
- Sense of hopelessness or helplessness
- Child abuse or other types of early emotional trauma
- Depression or other mental-emotional disorders
- Illiteracy or lack of job skills
- Poverty
- Insufficient sleep

Protective Factors

Protective forces may help counter the effects of risk factors and help adolescents make healthier lifestyle choices. It is important for adolescents to have active parental influence during these critical years, and these relationships serve as strong protective factors for adolescents. Also, community support of positive adolescent behavior appears to minimize risk-taking (see Chapter 17). Examples of adolescent protective factors (Hagan et al, 2008) are:

- High self-esteem
- Sense of future
- Academic success
- Parental engagement
- Positive family environment
- Relationships with caring adults
- Community involvement (e.g., school, religious institutions, volunteering)
- Access to recreation

Adolescents with multiple risk factors and few protective factors are more likely to engage in risk behavior, with potential health- and life-threatening results. These adolescents need prompt attention and assessment to determine the likelihood of negative outcomes. Conversely, resilient adolescents who are doing well, despite multiple risk factors, should be acknowledged and applauded.

Assessment

All adolescents should be assessed for their level of risk-taking behavior. The provider's approach to a discussion of sensitive issues should include ensuring confidentiality, providing privacy, using constructive communication strategies, and establishing rapport.

The HEEADSSS technique is a method of assessing risk behavior. Areas for assessment include **H**ome, **E**ducation and employment, **E**ating, **A**ctivities, **D**rugs, **S**exuality,

• BOX 8-2 Questions for HEEADSSS Assessment

Questions focus on relationships with others, function in school and work, self-efficacy, resilience, and independent decision-making.

Home: Who lives with you? How are your relationships with the other people with whom you live? Have there been any changes at home? Do you feel safe at home?

Education/employment: What do you like/dislike about school? How is school going? How are your grades? Have you ever had trouble at school? Do you work? How many hours do you work? Where do you work? Do you have friends at school? At work?

Eating: Are you comfortable with your body? Are you interested in gaining/losing weight? How do you manage your weight? Tell me about how often you exercise. Tell me about what you normally eat every day.

Activities: What do you do for fun? What types of things do you like to do with your friends? What types of things do you like to do with your family? Do you play sports? Are you in clubs or other organizations? How much time do you watch TV? Use the computer? Text? Listen to music? What types of activities do you like to do online? On your phone?

Drugs: Do you, anyone in your family, or your friends use drugs/tobacco/drink alcohol? Have you ever used performance-enhancing drugs?

Sexuality: Do you date? Have you ever had a romantic relationship? What do you consider to be sex? Have you ever had sex? How many partners have you had? Are you interested in males/females or both? Have you ever had someone hurt or threaten you sexually? Do you use birth control/condoms? How often?

Suicide/depression: Do you ever feel like you are all alone or no one cares? Do you feel sad most of the time? Have you ever thought of actually hurting yourself? Do you ever need to use drugs (alcohol, tobacco, street drugs) to make you feel better? Have you lost interest in being with friends or doing things you previously liked to do?

Safety: Have you ever been hurt by or threatened by someone (who)? Have you ever been seriously injured? Do you use sports safety equipment? Do you use seat belts? Do you text/talk when you drive? Do you ever feel unsafe (where)? Have you ever been bullied? Have you ever met (or do you plan on meeting) someone you first met online?

Suicide/Depression, and **S**afety (Box 8-2) (Klein et al, 2014). Providers should also be alert for red flags at each developmental stage, because delays in development may contribute to negative behavior (Table 8-3).

The following are considered examples of risk behavior:

- Tobacco use (discussed later)
- Substance use or abuse, including alcohol
- Poor academic performance
- Risky sexual activity (including multiple partners, unprotected sexual intercourse)
- Drinking and driving
- Body dysmorphism or eating disorders (see Chapter 19)
- Behaviors that result in injury or violence.
- Delinquency or involvement with gangs
- Violence-related behavior, such as carrying weapons or making threats of violence
- Mood disorders or signs of mental disorders
- Signs of physical, mental, sexual, or emotional abuse
- Poor nutrition and physical inactivity

The consequences of such behavior can be addiction, school failure, pregnancy, and STIs (nearly half of all cases of STIs in the United States occur in 15- to 24-year-olds [CDC, 2012]), accidents, conviction for driving under the influence, incarceration, or death. Engaging in chronic risk-taking behavior often arrests developmental progress toward adult emotional maturity.

Management

Interventions should be considered when the adolescent's behavior threatens the accomplishment of developmental tasks or the adolescent's health, safety, and well-being. Generally, when adolescents' behavior supports the achievement of developmental tasks, such behavior should be encouraged. Adolescents who pierce their noses, shave half of their heads, and spend evenings with friends, for example, may be irritating to parents, but their behavior can help them establish their autonomy, identity, and ability to relate to others. On the other hand, such behavior may be an indicator of more serious problems. Tattoos and body piercings, especially among younger adolescents, have been shown to have a strong correlation with risk-taking behaviors (Jennings et al, 2014). It is important to understand the meaning of the behavior for the adolescent before making decisions about intervention.

The approach used when providing care to teenagers differs from that used with younger children. Earlier, parents were central to the success of interventions. Although parents are still critical to successful intervention, health care providers must recognize that the teenager makes the decisions, and mediation between parent and teen may be necessary at times. The provider's role is to give the adolescent information and guidance to make the best decisions possible. Such information can have a big effect.

Generally, high-risk teenagers require numerous services. Health care providers need to know their state laws regarding adolescent health issues, how to access community resources, and how to use other professionals collaboratively. The following list identifies basic services that at-risk teenagers may need:

- Food resources for teenage parents and their offspring
- Temporary shelters for teenagers
- Counseling and mental health services for teenagers and their families
- Foster care services for teenage parents and their offspring
- Local medical and social work services
- Local juvenile justice system and protective services
- Drug rehabilitation programs for teenagers
- Alternative school and vocational education programs
- Sports, fitness, and community activities for teenagers, including after school programs
- Support programs for teenagers, such as Big Brothers or Big Sisters

TABLE 8-3 Developmental Red Flags: Adolescent

Age	Physical and Sexual Development	Psychosocial Development	Cognitive Development
All phases of adolescence	*Physical development:* Poor vision close or distant Female kyphosis or scoliosis Poor nutrition, poor oral health, caries, malocclusion Loss of appetite/ underweight Chronic disease, such as heart disease, hypertension, dyslipidemia, diabetes, or a family member with a chronic or lifelong illness No physical activity; overweight Sleep disturbance	*Social habits:* Drug or alcohol abuse; blackouts *Relationships:* Permissive or authoritarian parental style No participation in home chores History of family violence School fights No close or "best" friend No identified peer group Friends or siblings in gangs Cruelty to animals *Sexuality:* Sexual orientation worries *Mood:* Pervasive sad mood, feelings of hopelessness, suicidal thoughts or gestures, history of previous suicide attempt Flattened affect without expressions of joy, sorrow, or excitement Excessive worrying or rumination *Self-concept:* Believes self to be "ugly" or "fat"; is dieting despite normal body size and shape Negative feelings of self-worth	Low IQ Behind in grade or failing classes Chronic absenteeism or class skipping Attention problems Lack of organizational skills for homework Disruptive behavior Lack of impulse control Unable to control own behavior (e.g., anger, impulsivity)
Early adolescence (11-14 years old)	Less than Tanner stage 2 Female short stature or lack of height spurt *Sexuality:* Early sexual experimentation	*Sexuality:* Fears about emerging sexuality/sexual orientation *Self-concept:* Does not fantasize or dream about adult career	Unable to identify feelings
Middle adolescence (15-17 years old)	Male kyphosis or scoliosis Less than Tanner stage 4 Male short stature or lack of height spurt Male muscular growth without testicular maturation Male persistent gynecomastia and acne Female primary or secondary amenorrhea Risky sexual activity, including unprotected sexual intercourse and multiple sexual partners	*Social habits:* Drinking and driving *Relationships:* Excessively oppositional, defiant of all authority Abusive dating relationships *Sexuality:* Sexual orientation worries	Unable to differentiate emotional states from physical states Poor judgment
Late adolescence (18-21 years old)	Less than Tanner stage 4 or 5 Risky sexual activity, including unprotected sexual intercourse and multiple sexual partners	No life goals Does not fantasize or dream about adult career *Social habits:* Drinking and driving *Relationships:* Lacks intimate relationships Abusive dating relationships Unable to separate from peer groups Unable to separate from parents Unable to keep a job *Sexuality:* Sexual orientation worries	School dropout Persistent egocentrism Unable to reason or plan based on future and abstract concepts Poor judgment Chronic health care seeking for psychosomatic complaints

IQ, Intelligence quotient.

Advocating for children and adolescents at risk; involving their families, communities, and schools; and helping young people identify an individual who cares for them and trusts them are important actions all health care providers can take.

Risk Behavior: Tobacco Use

Description

Tobacco use, primarily smoking, appears within a cluster of risk-taking behaviors, and adolescent smokers are more likely than their nonsmoking peers to use marijuana and hard drugs, sell drugs, have multiple drug problems, drop out of school, and experience early pregnancy and parenthood. These adolescents are also at higher risk for low academic achievement and behavioral problems at school, stealing and other delinquent behaviors, and use of predatory and relational violence (Ellickson et al, 2008). More in-depth discussions of sexuality and substance abuse are found in Chapters 15 and 19.

Many adolescents experiment with tobacco use but may stop after a short period before becoming addicted to nicotine. Tobacco dependence (addiction) varies from one individual to another and can appear at any time after initiating tobacco use, so prevention and early intervention are essential. As previously discussed, the adolescent brain is particularly susceptible to the influence of substances (like nicotine), and there is a resulting higher rate of dependence in teenagers than in adults.

Current data indicate that 41% of adolescents have tried cigarette smoking and 22% are current tobacco users (defined as use within the past 30 days). Sixteen percent of adolescents report current cigarette use and the highest smoking rates occur in males, Caucasians, and Hispanics, with a peak occurring in 11th grade (21.1%). Current smokeless tobacco use is 8.8%, with highest rates among males and Caucasians (Kann et al, 2014).

Of growing concern is the use of hookahs and electronic cigarettes. Many adolescents consider these vehicles to be a "safe" form of tobacco use. Rates of hookah and e-cigarette use have doubled in the past few years and increasing evidence indicates that e-cigarette use is a significant risk factor for future marijuana and other substance use (CDC, 2014; Kandel and Kandel, 2014). Because nicotine is used in both of these delivery systems, risk of dependence and addiction remains the same as for traditional cigarette and smokeless tobacco use.

Assessment

Direct questioning is the best way to assess adolescents' smoking patterns. At every visit, children should be asked whether they or their friends smoke or use other forms of tobacco. Biochemical tests to measure tobacco by-products (e.g., carbon monoxide in serum or expired alveolar air; urine cotinine, a primary metabolite of nicotine; and thiocyanate, a detoxification product of hydrogen cyanide in tobacco smoke) are used primarily in the research setting and are not appropriate diagnostic studies in primary care. Exposure to cigarette smoke, directly or indirectly, causes increased incidence of respiratory problems, including asthma (see Chapter 42 for a discussion of environmental tobacco smoke).

Management

Adolescent tobacco management includes primary prevention, with a goal of keeping the child from starting to use and secondary prevention, with a goal of cessation (Table 8-4). The use of behavioral interventions in pediatric primary care for tobacco use is controversial in that a meta-analysis indicates that effects of such programs are small and mostly effective for young non-users (Patnode et al, 2013). Educating young people about tobacco use in their age group may be a means of preventing them from initiating tobacco use. This approach is based on the social norms theory, which states that the perceptions an individual has of group norms of behavior will influence one's own behavior. The social norms approach has effectively reduced

TABLE 8-4 Primary and Secondary Prevention and Tobacco Use Cessation Strategies for Adolescents

Primary Prevention	Secondary Prevention
Provide multimedia, multisite health information, not limited to schools Use social norms theory to encourage adolescent to forgo tobacco use Emphasize skills to avoid peer pressure Focus on adolescents' developmental need to belong to a social group	Ask at every visit whether adolescent or friends use tobacco Inform adolescent of health risks of tobacco use and process by which one becomes addicted to nicotine; emphasize that it is easier to stop early Develop mutual understanding of problem Determine realistic stop-use date Help adolescent identify barriers to stopping and ways to overcome those barriers Provide information about self-help and support groups; encourage adolescent to try to stop smoking with a friend Provide nicotine patch protocol if adolescent feels this will help Schedule follow-up visits to monitor progress; reinforce positive efforts Assess parents' tobacco use patterns; provide information and support to stop use

alcohol misuse on college campuses and appears to reduce violence against women (Moreira et al, 2009). The social norms approach suggests that if young people believe that "everyone is smoking" or even a majority of youth are smoking, they are more likely to begin smoking as well. Informing the child that nearly 98% of very young adolescents and 80% of older adolescents do not smoke can support a personal decision to not smoke.

Other effective tobacco prevention strategies include making tobacco products more expensive, creating smoke-free zones in schools and buildings, using school-based programs, and supporting anti-smoking messages from parents (Butt et al, 2009). Intervention by dental providers can also prevent initiation or support smoking cessation.

Many children are exposed to nicotine in utero or to secondhand smoke of parents or other caregivers. This puts them at risk for cognitive deficits, low test scores, and decreased school performance (Herrmann et al, 2008); also, children who live in a family with smokers are more likely to become smokers themselves. Although pediatric providers are not the parents' primary caregivers, they can intervene with parents in several ways. Parents can be encouraged to talk to their children about the dangers of smoking; there is evidence that when parents teach their children that smoking is bad, children are less likely to begin, even if the parent continues to smoke (Jackson and Dickinson, 2006). Parents should also be encouraged to stop smoking.

Another strategy shown to be effective is the implementation of population-based interventions to help clients stop tobacco use. These include tracking and monitoring smokers, providing insurance coverage for tobacco-cessation services, educating employees not to use tobacco, and lobbying for public anti-smoking campaigns and increased taxes on tobacco products.

Risk Behavior: Self-Injurious Behaviors

Description

Self-injurious behaviors (SIBs) are repetitive behaviors with the intent of intentionally causing physical harm to oneself for nonsocially sanctioned and nonsuicidal reasons. Symptoms must have occurred at least five times and be associated with at least two of the following:

- Previous negative emotions
- Preoccupation with activity and a repetitive desire to engage in activity
- Feelings of relief from negative emotions or a sensation of positive feelings with activity
- Impaired interpersonal relationships (American Psychiatric Association [APA], 2013)

Excluded from this diagnosis are behaviors like piercings and tattoos, because these are seen as socially acceptable. SIBs vary widely and include cutting (the most common mechanism); scraping; hitting; burning or ripping of skin, subdermal tissue, or hair; hindering wound healing (e.g., picking at scabs); swallowing toxic substances; breaking bones; and bruising oneself (Kameg et al, 2013). The common factor among SIBs is that they are used as a coping strategy to relieve distress, anger, and stress and to create a sense of calm. Patients often report that the physical pain associated with these acts helps relieve emotional pain. These are not suicide attempts, but it is important to note that individuals who engage in SIB are more likely to attempt suicide or to have an eating disorder, a history of abuse or trauma, a mood disorder, or psychological distress than those in the general population and should be assessed for suicide risk (Brickell and Jellinek, 2014; Kameg et al, 2013).

SIB typically begins in mid to late adolescence and declines in early adulthood (APA, 2013). Many believe the prevalence of SIB is increasing, but there are no historical data for comparison, and many studies do not differentiate SIB from suicidal SIB. Data indicate that 13% to 25% of adolescents and young adults report engaging in SIB at least once, with as many as 80% having experimental or mild SIB (Kameg et al, 2013; Williams et al, 2010). Females, Caucasians, and those who identify themselves as homosexual or bisexual are more likely to report SIB. Recent evidence indicates that males and females have similar rates of SIB, although females are more likely to report symptoms (Brickell and Jellinek, 2014). Approximately half of adolescents and young adults who engage in SIB have a history of physical, sexual, and/or emotional abuse.

Assessment

History should include focused questions about present and past experiences with self-injury, description of the frequency of these behaviors, and what emotional or mental responses the adolescent gets from self-injury. Given the association of SIB with abuse, adolescents should be assessed for physical and emotional signs of abuse (see Chapter 17). Although these self-injuries can cause a decrease in emotional pain, they often result in guilt. Therefore, adolescents who engage in SIB often hide evidence of their activities, intentionally mask physical marks, and deny or will not disclose their SIBs, thus making diagnosis difficult. Suspicion should be raised if adolescents present with hoodies or heavy clothing on hot days, or when there is resistance to allow skin examination. The most common locations for SIB injuries are the arms, legs, and front of the torso. There may be scratches or cuts in various stages of healing or that appear to be in patterns or that form words (Williams et al, 2010). Traction alopecia may be present.

Management

Suicide and mental health assessment is needed when adolescents present with suspected SIB. Self-injurers will often accept help during acute phases but lose motivation for help when symptoms are not as acute. The presence of any wounds should be recognized as a call for help. Appropriate therapeutic interventions range from cognitive behavioral, dialectical and family therapy, to antidepressant and psychotropic medications (although none are U.S. Food and

Drug Administration [FDA] approved), and even hospitalization (Kameg et al, 2013). Therapeutic response is usually contingent on the self-injurer feeling recognized by the provider and is achieved when positive emotional coping skills are learned. Prompt referral to a mental health professional is needed if symptoms of psychosis or suicide ideation are present. However, not all adolescents who use SIB need psychiatric referral. Those who have no other signs of mental illness and who are experimenting with self-injury, or who have engaged in SIB because of peer pressure may not require immediate intervention but should have close follow-up (Williams et al, 2010).

Risk Behavior: Social Media Use

Description

Technology allows for ever-increasing connectivity and social interaction, and social media can be a positive influence when used appropriately. Adolescents are drawn to social media because they allow them to connect with friends, families, and classmates and give them a platform to express their thoughts, feelings, and points of view to a broad audience. These websites and apps provide opportunities for positive interactions, but not all websites and apps are good for adolescents. A spur-of-the-moment online interaction can have profound implications beyond the developmental ability of many teens. Half of all adolescents report using social media on a daily basis, whereas one in five accesses online websites and applications 10 or more times daily (O'Keeffe et al, 2011).

Assessment

Parents and primary care providers should have open discussions with adolescents regarding their social media use. Risky social media usage includes:

- Bullying and harassment
- Sexting: Sending nude or provocative photos, and/or sexual messages
- Depression and social withdrawal (O'Keeffe et al, 2011)
- Signs of media addiction: Obsessing about social media use, avoiding interactions with others in order to engage online, getting in trouble because of social media use
- Meeting strangers through online profiles

Management

It is important for primary care providers to approach teens nonjudgmentally, because there is often a technology gap between adolescents who grew up with the usage of computers, tablets and smartphones and adults who begin technology use later in life. It is common for teens to state that adults don't understand how "everyone" uses social media and how not using technology can have a negative social impact. Providers should remind adolescents that electronic images and communications can be accessed and used by others even after being deleted. Therefore, the teen needs to understand that any posting can, and possibly will be, shared with others and that digital footprints can be accessed years later and negatively impact their future (e.g., university admission and/or employment). Many adolescents do not realize that possession of nude or suggestive photos can be considered child pornography, although enforcement of this varies from state to state (O'Keeffe et al, 2011). Counsel teens to not post when they are emotionally upset (e.g., angry, sad, scared), because spur-of-the-moment expression can cause long-standing problems. Educate them that online profiles can be real but may also be complete fabrications designed to meet others under false pretense.

An important part of managing social media usage involves parental education and encouraging supervision of social media usage. Ask parents to preview and approve websites and applications that the adolescent is interested in and to block those that are inappropriate for teens. Parents need to educate themselves about adolescent technology use and risks. Lastly, active supervision and communication are more effective than software tracking and remote monitoring (O'Keeffe et al, 2011).

For a complete list of references, please visit http://evolve.elsevier.com/Burns/pediatric/.

UNIT 3

Approaches to Health Management in Pediatric Primary Care

9

Introduction to Functional Health Patterns and Health Promotion

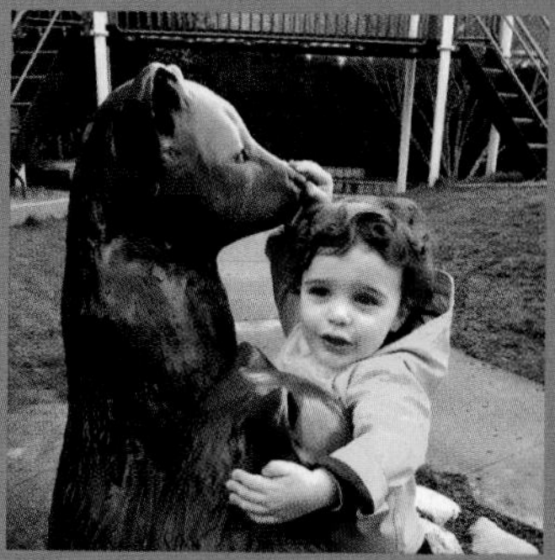

ARDYS M. DUNN

Health is a dynamic and complex phenomenon. The World Health Organization (WHO) defines health as "a state of complete physical, mental and social well-being and not merely the absence of disease or infirmity" (WHO, 2015). WHO further affirms that health is a universal human right. These principles reflect the thinking that health is not just a function of biomedical factors, either in terms of cause or choice of treatment and management. Interrelated biomedical, social/cultural, economic, and political circumstances all influence health policy, interventions, and outcomes. This understanding that health is influenced by factors other than biomedical phenomena is not new; it finds its roots in the discipline of social medicine that has existed since the late 19th century (Porter, 2006; Rosen, 1947). Skilled health care providers have a clear understanding of the nature of these social determinants of health and their relationship to health status (see Chapter 1). Currently, the notion of global health is gaining prominence in health care literature and practice. For example, *Healthy People 2020* goals retain many traditional health indicators from *Healthy People 2010* (Box 9-1), but new areas of focus include issues specifically related to early and middle childhood, adolescents, social determinants of health, global health, and health-related quality of life and well-being (U.S. Department of Health and Human Services [HHS], 2014). Holmes and colleagues (2014) contend that, although global health broadens "the scope of biomedicine," the field to date lacks integration and will only realize its potential as it draws from the tradition of social medicine and truly becomes "global *social* health" (emphasis added).

Healthy individual lifestyle behaviors promote children's health. Appropriate nutrition, exercise, stimulation, rest, and emotional and social nurturance are all critically important. Also, prevention and management of illness and injury are essential to children's growth and development. Teaching and modeling healthy behaviors help children learn to promote their own health and, because many health problems of children are carried into adulthood, educating children has long-term health effects on the whole population. Family, community, and global health are also important. Children cannot thrive in unhealthy, unsafe, or insecure families and communities; and the impact of global phenomena on health (e.g., physical displacement, psychological trauma, infectious disease outbreaks related to wars) is significant.

Approaches to managing health care must be interdisciplinary and must consider social factors far beyond biomedical dynamics of disease. A broad array of professionals and citizens must be involved. Nurses, physicians, teachers, health educators, city planners, legislators, the industrial and business community, volunteers, and others from all levels of society need to guide the development of an infrastructure that supports health. Interdisciplinary intervention at the individual, family, community, health care systems, and policy levels often makes more of a difference in children's health than working with individual patients alone (Braveman et al, 2011; Holmes et al, 2014; Institute of Medicine [IOM], 2001; Phelan et al, 2010). Although this text focuses primarily on management of individual children within families, a broader perspective on community and global intervention and support for health needs to be maintained.

This chapter introduces the functional health patterns unit of the book and examines the first of those patterns: health perception and health management. Topics presented in the health perception and health management pattern include the components of health perception, children's conceptualization of health, models that predict health behavior, factors that influence health behaviors, assessment methods, and specific management strategies for use with children and families. These topics serve as a

• BOX 9-1 *Healthy People 2010* Goals that Continue to 2020

- Physical activity
- Overweight and obesity
- Tobacco use
- Substance abuse
- Responsible sexual behavior
- Mental health
- Injury and violence
- Environmental quality
- Immunization and infectious diseases
- Access to health care

foundation for the subsequent chapters of this unit, where the remaining functional health patterns and their relationship to health are discussed. This chapter's goal is to give the reader tools to help families create environments in which children will thrive physically, mentally, emotionally, and developmentally.

Functional Health Patterns—The Behaviors of Health

The functional health patterns construct, which is unique to nursing (Gordon, 1987, 2010), is a model appropriate to the practice of all pediatric primary care providers. The use of functional health patterns emphasizes health promotion and focuses the provider's attention directly on lifestyle behaviors that affect children's health, such as nutrition, activity, coping and stress tolerance, tobacco and drug use, and accident prevention.

The 11 functional health patterns that Gordon (1987, 2010) used to describe the domain of nursing practice serve as the framework for the chapters in this unit. The patterns describe the health-related behaviors in which people engage. These functional health patterns are universal, applying to all humans regardless of age, sex, culture, health status, or other factors. All people need to eat, sleep, and eliminate, for example. Each pattern is described as follows:

- *Health perception–health management pattern:* Describes client perceptions of personal health and health care behaviors and one's ability to control or influence health. Health management includes the actions taken to deal with these experiences. Health management is based on health perceptions and reflects the judgments of individuals and families, the ways they solve problems, and the decisions or choices they make. Positive health management assumes that wise decisions are made and that resources are available for families to implement those decisions.
- *Nutrition-metabolic pattern:* Describes patterns of food and fluid intake. Includes choice of foods and food supplements, eating habits, and schedules.
- *Elimination pattern:* Describes patterns of bowel and bladder excretion. Includes schedule and habit patterns and use of healthful foods or other methods to facilitate excretory functions.
- *Activity-exercise pattern:* Describes patterns of activity and exercise, including type of activity, schedule of participation, vigor, effect on leisure, physical state, and meaning of activity to the child.
- *Sleep-rest pattern:* Describes patterns of sleep and rest, including schedule, habits, aids to sleep, and perceived feelings of renewal, fatigue, or exhaustion.
- *Cognitive-perceptual pattern:* Describes sensory-perceptual and cognitive patterns, including adaptations to hearing, vision, or other perceptual losses; includes pain perception and the process of finding meaning from environmental stimuli and the effectiveness of efforts to compensate for deficits.
- *Self-perception–self-concept pattern:* Describes patterns of perception and valuing of the self, in addition to evaluation of strengths and weaknesses and sense of self-worth.
- *Role-relationships pattern:* Describes pattern of roles and responsibilities of the client and patterns of relationships with family and others.
- *Sexuality-reproductive pattern:* Describes patterns of satisfaction or dissatisfaction with sexuality and sexual relationships. Involves perception and development of sexual identity, in addition to reproductive expectations, behaviors, and outcomes.
- *Coping-stress tolerance pattern:* Describes patterns of coping with the range of stresses experienced. Includes strategies used, effectiveness, support systems, and perceived ability to control and manage difficult situations.
- *Values-beliefs pattern:* Describes patterns of values and beliefs that influence daily living activities, guide decision-making, and provide meaning to life. Involves religious and spiritual activities and personal values and beliefs.

Health Perception and Health Management Functional Health Pattern

Health Perception

Components of Health Perception

All people in all cultures make decisions that affect their health and well-being. Chapter 3 discusses cultural dynamics that influence these decisions. Providers, by exploring health perceptions of individuals and families, can begin to see reasons behind health decisions. Components of health perception include (1) the beliefs and feelings individuals have about their general state of health (past, present, and future), and (2) the belief that there is a relationship between health status and health practices—specifically, that individual behaviors can affect one's health status (i.e., self-efficacy).

The first of these components, beliefs and feelings about children's health status (i.e., the *meaning* parents, caregivers, and children themselves give to health), are shaped by several interrelated variables, including:

- Susceptibility to the condition
- Severity of the condition
- Extent to which the condition has an effect on the child's and family's ability to function
- Knowledge about the condition
- Experience with the condition
- Developmental stage of the child
- Knowledge about how a child's developmental stage affects his or her responses to illness
- Cultural or social cues about the condition and about health and illness in general (see Chapter 3)

The second component of health perception, the degree to which parents and children believe that they can influence their health status, varies. Individuals with an "internal locus of control" believe that they can take actions that will make a difference in health outcomes. They are motivated to make change, are active problem-solvers, and are able to more effectively cope with health problems. Those who believe that health outcomes are beyond their control are more likely to be passive and dependent, and they may fail to follow through with recommended treatments. Success with past experiences, external support, and cues to action reinforce a sense of self-efficacy.

Children's Conceptualizations of Health and Illness

Children's concepts of health and illness must be considered within a developmental framework. One model for understanding how children process health information is Piaget's theory of cognitive development (see Chapter 4). Koopman and colleagues (2004) found support for this theory in their study of 158 Swedish children, 80 children with diabetes mellitus and 78 healthy children. They also found that the child's development of illness concepts is congruent with Piaget's concept of physical causality. For very young children, in Piaget's sensorimotor stage, causes are invisible, they simply are, and the child is not aware of them. As they move into the preconceptual stage, children have little understanding of their internal bodies. They lack understanding of time and transformations, so the process of healing, for example, is not clearly understood. They see illness from a distance perspective, caused by external activities, in some cases, magically. Also in the preconceptual stage, children later add the notion of proximity—one must be close to people, objects, and events for illness to occur. In the concrete-operational stage of thinking, children do not yet distinguish between body and mind, and they may believe that illness can be caused by bad thoughts or behavior as well as contact or contamination. Later in this stage, children begin to conceptualize the cause of illness as being within the body: an external element (e.g., germs) or an unhealthy condition (e.g., obesity) may damage something within the body. This is a process of internalization. In this stage, children generally need overt signs of illness or health to recognize the health status of a person. In the formal stage of thinking, children can describe and explain how the body works and how illness may be related to the body and its environment (body processes). Adolescents understand the difficulties of defining health (e.g., a person who may look well but has a cancerous tumor inside vs. a person with limited mobility who is actually healthy). A final stage occurs with sophisticated thinking in which the child conceptualizes the mind and body interactions of illness, is sensitive to feeling states, and differentiates between mental and physical health. With more experience and knowledge, children can incorporate more elaborate concepts into theories of how the body works, contagion, and differences between physical and mental well-being (Myant and Williams, 2008).

A model of how scientific reasoning develops in children supports this developmental approach to children's perceptions of illness (Piekny and Maehler, 2013). Piekny and Maehler (2013) examined differences in children's ability to evaluate evidence, experiment with data, and generate hypotheses, and found that preschool-age children can evaluate information that does and does not match; that, by primary school age, children understand that evidence can be manipulated or experimented with; and that older children are able to generate hypotheses based on evidence given. In all children, greater ambiguity in the information given requires more sophisticated cognitive abilities to understand and coordinate reasoning.

Children's understandings of mental illness also become more refined with age and development. Fox and colleagues (2010) used Leventhal's model of how adults frame illness (i.e., description, cause, timeline, consequences, and curability) to examine children's understanding of mental illness (Leventhal et al, 1984). They found that younger children rely on what they already know about physical illness to explain mental illness. Younger children tend to conceptualize physical and mental conditions similarly; they often cite contagion (e.g., "she caught it [dementia]") as a cause of mental illness and medicalize the consequence (e.g., she needs "to see a doctor" vs. needing support of family, friends, and community). By the end of middle childhood, children are able to understand that there is a clear difference between physical and mental illness and that the interaction between the mind and body as well as external factors are important in explaining mental illness.

Unfortunately, many children develop an attitude stigmatizing mental illness at an early age. Longitudinal research conducted in 1986 and 1994 found that, by kindergarten, most children have a negative attitude toward mental illness, and this attitude largely endures into childhood. Children reinterviewed in 1994 did demonstrate more acceptance of and willingness to relate to individuals with mental retardation, but continued to stigmatize other forms of mental illness (Weiss, 1994). Little current research has been done on children's attitudes toward mental health, but there is evidence that attitudes of adults *toward* children with emotional and behavioral problems may reflect a negative bias. Hirsch (2013) developed a scale to identify biases toward children with psychological and behavioral disorders and found that mental health professionals were less biased than teachers, who, in turn, were less biased than the general public. The question of whether this bias translates into discrimination against children was not examined in this project (Hirsch, 2013). Nonetheless, advocates for children believe that significant public health steps can be taken to improve accessibility and utilization of child mental health services for those who may avoid it because of the stigma attached (Adelsheim, 2014).

Providers can also educate children about their bodies, health, and illness in order to increase understanding and foster abilities to take action. In particular, children living with parents or siblings with a mental disability need clear explanations about the condition in order to decrease anxiety and fear and help them cope in a positive way (Mordoch, 2010; Unal and Baran, 2011). Research indicates that clinicians must tailor health information to the child's current knowledge and experience and base it on developmental abilities, not solely on age.

Assessment Foundations: Health Behavior Prediction Models

Health perceptions and prediction of health behaviors can be assessed using a number of different models. Several models are discussed here: the health belief model, the self-efficacy model, the transtheoretical (stages of change) model of behavior change (Prochaska, 1995; Prochaska et al, 1992, 1994), and the health promotion model (Pender et al, 2011).

Health Belief and Self-Efficacy Models

The health belief model originally explained behavior used to prevent disease rather than behavior to promote health. According to this model, individuals believe that:

- They are vulnerable or susceptible to the disease or health problem.
- The disease will have negative consequences for them if they are affected.
- Taking some action will reduce their risk.
- The benefits of action outweigh the costs.

A determination of cost to benefit in this model takes into consideration:

- Perceived barriers to action: What needs to be overcome?
- Perceived ability to make a change: Am I strong enough, capable enough, to make a change?
- Activity-related effects or subjective feelings that will occur: What changes will I undergo, and how will those changes make me feel?
- Interpersonal influences such as social norms or personal sources of influence: What messages of support (or not) am I getting from people around me, what cues to action? What behaviors do people who matter to me expect of me?
- Situational influences: Will the social structure I live/work/play in support or hinder the change I want to make? For example, working in a smoke-free environment would support someone who is trying to stop smoking.

In 1988, the health belief model more fully incorporated the concept of self-efficacy (Bandura, 2004). Bandura explained that one's sense of personal efficacy, in conjunction with goals, expected outcomes, and the perception of whether social variables will hinder or facilitate change, determines whether behavior change will be initiated, how much effort will be expended, and whether that change will be maintained. One's self-efficacy is based on past accomplishments, observing the results of other's efforts, positive verbal feedback, and emotional arousal. The individual needs to believe that if he or she performs as well as expected, the outcome will be favorable.

This model can be illustrated by assessing the motivation for toothbrushing behavior: clients must believe that they could have caries; that dental treatment, pain and expenses, or tooth loss or disfigurement could result from caries; that brushing teeth can prevent caries; and that the benefits of brushing outweigh the inconvenience, time, and costs of maintaining a supply of toothbrushes and toothpaste. If individuals are able to afford supplies, have access to a bathroom, and interact with others who value good dental hygiene, they are likely to find "costs" more easily overcome.

Based on this model, the provider's role is to help clients understand unhealthy conditions, the effects if the client does nothing, actions that can be taken to prevent problems, and the improved outcomes possible if they take action. Providers also strive to reinforce clients' beliefs that they can initiate coping behaviors that will benefit their health. Finally, providers help clients master the skills to take effective action or provide necessary resources to clients.

Stages of Change (Transtheoretical) Model

The transtheoretical model is in wide use. It incorporates elements from health belief and self-efficacy theories to describe the stages of change that individuals go through as they initiate behaviors to promote health. The model describes five stages of change (precontemplation, contemplation, preparation, action, and maintenance), 10 processes that facilitate movement from one stage to another, and two patterns that individuals use to progress through the various stages (relapse and recycling) (Fig. 9-1) (Prochaska et al, 1992).

Stages of Change. Shifts in attitudes and behaviors occur at each stage, and the time spent in each stage depends on the individual and the task to be attempted.

- *Precontemplation:* At this stage, the individual does not acknowledge that a serious problem exists, although a wish to change may be expressed. Resistance to change is the hallmark of this stage, and the reasons not to change are clear.
- *Contemplation:* The individual is aware that the problem exists and struggles with the costs and energy required for change. Many individuals remain stuck in this phase.

Transtheoretical Model of Behavior Change

Stages of Change and Associated Processes of Change

STAGES: Precontemplation | Contemplation | Preparation | Action | Maintenance

PROCESSES*:
- Consciousness raising
- Dramatic relief
- Environmental reevaluation
- Self-reevaluation
- Self-liberation
    - Reinforcement management
    - Helping relationships
    - Counter-conditioning
    - Stimulus control
- Social-liberation

PATTERNS:

Relapse

Recycling

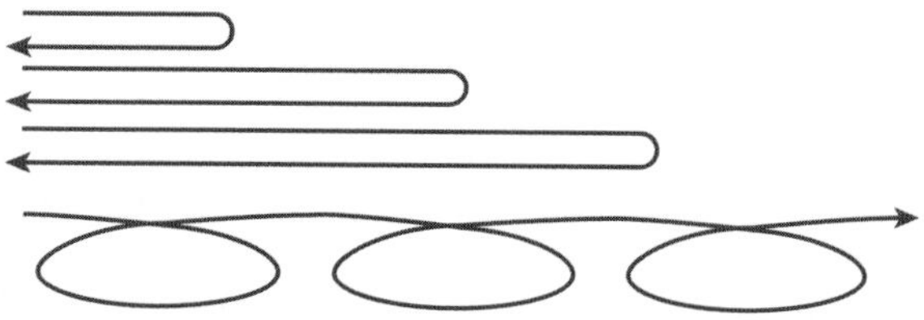

DECISIONAL BALANCE: "cons" outweigh "pros" | "pros" outweigh "cons"

Explanations of Processes of Change	Associated Interventions
Consciousness raising: gathering information about self and problem†	Observation of others, confrontations Classes, bibliotherapy, interpretations
Dramatic relief: feeling and expressing feelings related to problem	Role play, psychodrama, grief work
Environmental reevaluation: assessing one's behavior on environment	Documentary information, empathy training
Self-reevaluation: exploring one's feelings about self and the problem	Value clarification, imagery Corrective emotional experience
Self-liberation: choosing to act, changing belief in ability to change‡	Decision-making training Making resolutions, commitment-enhancing techniques
Social liberation: increasing alternatives and support for health behaviors	Empowerment and advocacy activities, policy interventions
Reinforcement management: establishing a reward system	Overt and covert reinforcement, contingency contracts
Helping relationships: trusting and sharing problem with a caring person*	Therapeutic alliance, buddy system, self-help/support groups
Counter-conditioning: substituting alternatives for problem behavior	Relaxation, desensitization, assertive skills, self-affirmations
Stimulus control: avoiding triggers of problem behavior	Restructuring environment, avoidance techniques, cue identification

*Most frequently used. Used more frequently for psychologically distressing problems.
†Second most frequently used.
‡Third most frequently used. Used more frequently for weight control.

• **Figure 9-1** Transtheoretical (stages of change) model. (Adapted from Prochaska JO, DiClemente CC, Norcross JC: In search of how people change: applications to addictive behaviors, *Am Psychol* 47(9):1102–1114, 1992.)

- *Preparation:* Planning begins in this stage. Small behavior changes may occur in preparation for commitment to the actual plan.
- *Action:* Behaviors to eliminate the problem occur in this stage. These may include initiating new behaviors, accessing resources, modifying the environment, and mitigating barriers.
- *Maintenance:* Plans occur here to prevent relapse, consolidate gains, and establish new behaviors as long-term changes. Maintenance occurs after at least 6 months in the action stage.

Patterns of Change. Most people do not proceed through all five stages in a linear way. Environmental barriers, external pressures to change beyond the individual's own desires, or problems with maintenance can contribute to relapses. Recycling is a regression from the action stage to the contemplation or preparation stages. The person spirals through small increments of change, recycling and moving forward again. Success with the change increases with effort, action, and mastery of the tasks of each stage.

Decisional Balance. Another component of the transtheoretical model is the cognitive exercise of weighing the pros and cons of change, or balancing the decision to change against the decision to remain the same. In the precontemplation stage, change is seen as more negative than no change (e.g., "If I stop smoking, I'll gain weight"). To initiate and sustain behavior in the action stage and move to the maintenance stage, the reasons to change must outweigh the reasons to return to old ways (e.g., "Not smoking is less expensive than smoking").

Providers who understand the stages of change can facilitate movement from resistance to action for many health behaviors. Interventions need to be designed to help clients assess the benefits and barriers to change and identify how they can successfully cause change. Providers must reinforce the sense of self-efficacy clients demonstrate. Motivational interviewing, discussed later in this chapter, is a strategy based on the stages of change that appears to have excellent success rates for many health-related behaviors; it helps individuals identify their own strengths and take responsibility for their own change.

Health Promotion Model

Pender and colleagues (2011) developed a broad model with a focus on health promotion rather than on disease prevention. The model consists of two main domains—*cognitive-perceptual factors* and *modifying factors*—that explain participation in health promotion behaviors (Fig. 9-2). The cognitive-perceptual factors include all the concepts in the health belief and self-efficacy models, locus of control notions, and individuals' definitions of health and their own health status estimates, as previously discussed. Modifying factors include demographic, biologic, behavioral, and situational factors; interpersonal influences; social support structures; the emotional competence of family members; past experience; education and knowledge level (health literacy); and values and cultural perspectives. Cognitive-perceptual and modifying factors interact as a person decides whether and when to engage in health promotion behaviors. The model can be applied to any health behavior.

Health Management

Health management is the process of making decisions and taking action to restore, maintain, and/or promote health and to prevent disease. A major component of health management is the effective use of resources, both in the family and in the community. Health management reflects the underlying beliefs and perceptions that families, parents, and children have about health, as discussed previously. Also, as previously noted, the way children's health is managed is strongly influenced by social determinants of health (see Chapter 1).

Assessment of Health Management Pattern

Assessment of the functional health patterns—sleep, nutrition, elimination, exercise, use of primary care services, and others—needs to be part of the general health assessment as much as possible (see Chapter 2). Specific conditions are present within each functional health pattern however (e.g., a child may present with night terrors, a condition discussed in the sleep functional health pattern), and these conditions require more focused assessment. The following chapters in this unit examine these specific conditions in more detail, discussing assessment, clinical findings, and management.

Assessment of health perception and health management patterns is broad in scope, and can give providers a better understanding of the family's health decisions and actions and areas of concern. It can also help providers find ways to work with families to generate appropriate interventions. Table 9-1 provides helpful, practical assessment questions. These fall into the domains of general perceptions of health in the family, strategies used to maintain health of the family members, decision-making about health issues, use of health care resources, health of the family environment, and managing the child with special needs.

Clinical Findings Indicating Health Perception and Health Management Functional Health Pattern Problems

Families with a positive health management pattern identify, access, and use appropriate social, community, family, and health-related resources effectively and efficiently. When that is not the case, children's health status can be compromised. Some of the clinical findings that indicate problems in this area include:

- No regular health care provider for the child
- History of lack of continuity or fragmented care
- Use of emergency department for nonemergent conditions
- Lack of follow-up care for the child seen in the emergency department

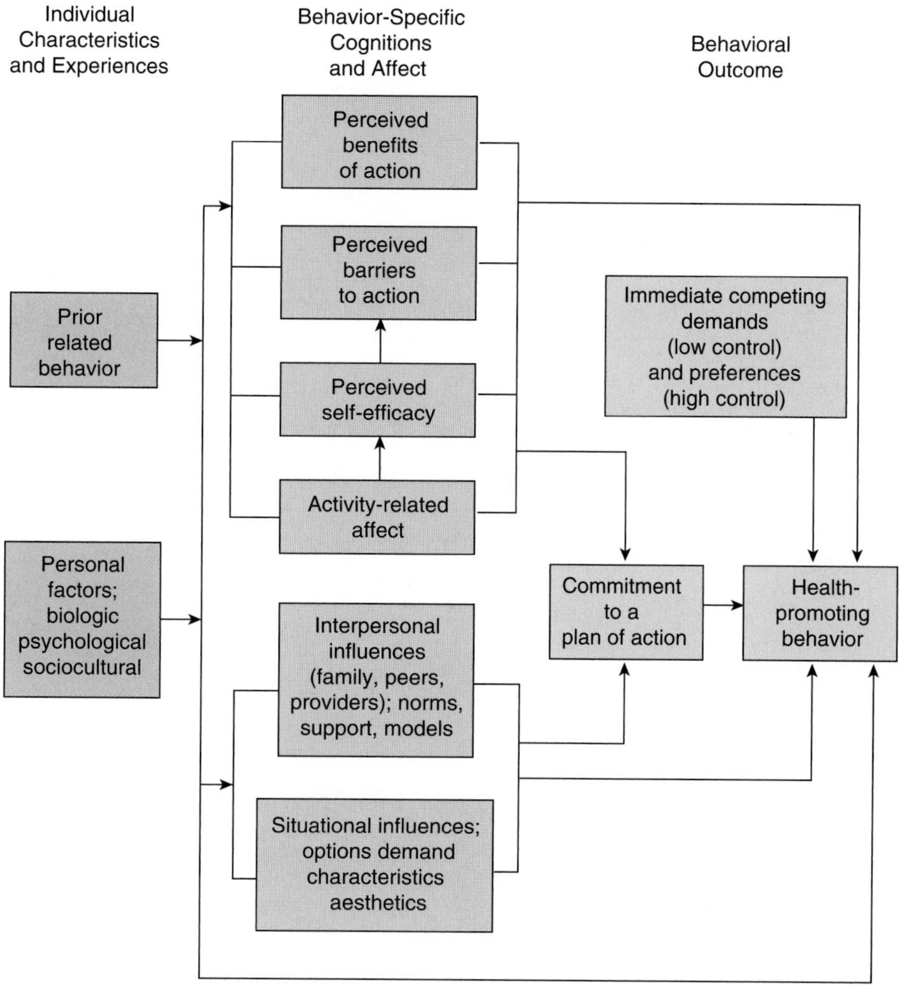

• **Figure 9-2** Health promotion model. (From Pender N, Murdaugh CL, Parsons MA: *Health promotion in nursing practice*, ed 6, Upper Saddle River, NJ, 2011, Prentice-Hall).

TABLE 9-1 Health Perception/Health Management Pattern Screening Questions

Topic	Questions
General assessment	How would you describe your child's health right now? Compared with other children, how healthy would you say your child is? What does it mean for you to say that your child is "healthy"? How do you describe good health in your family? Do you have any questions or concerns about your child's health, growth, or development? How important is it to you to have a regular health care provider?
Belief that health practices affect health status	What do you know about this current condition? What caused it? What can you do about it? What can you do to prevent it? Has your child had a problem like this before? How do you expect your child to respond when sick? To this particular sickness? What have you done for it in the past? What do you do or have you done that you believe makes a difference in how your child responds to illness? What things can you do to help your child cope with being sick? What kinds of feelings do you have when confronted with sudden changes in plans or a disruption of normal routine caused by illness in the family? How do you deal with those feelings? How do you think those feelings affect the way you handle your child's health and illness?

Continued

TABLE 9-1 Health Perception/Health Management Pattern Screening Questions—cont'd

Topic	Questions
Decision-making	What do you do when your child has health problems? What makes you decide to call your health care provider or take your child in for an examination? Who makes decisions about health care in your family? How do you make those decisions? Do you talk things over? Do you get advice from others? Why do you think that you make decisions in that way? What are the most important things that you consider when making a decision about your child's health care? What is most difficult for you when you have to make decisions related to your child's health?
Health behaviors and use of resources	Do you have a regular health care provider for your child? When did you see that person last? What health care resources are available to you? Is there a primary care provider you can get to conveniently? Clinics? Pharmacies? What immunizations has your child received? What have you done to protect your child from injuries? There has been much focus on healthy lifestyles, such as eating right and exercising. What does your family do regularly to stay healthy? Does anyone in your family (adolescents, you) smoke, drink, or use drugs? How often? What kind? Are there other things that your family does that you think are bad for your children's health? Who cares for your child when you are not at home and the child is not in school? What helps you learn about health problems and how to take care of them—talking to others, reading, using the Internet, watching videos? For this illness: How are you managing household, work, school, and other child care responsibilities? What is most difficult for you? Having sick children can create a financial strain on families. Is this a problem for your family? What is the most difficult part? How comfortable do you feel managing this illness? Have you had experience in the past that helps you manage?
Environment	Do you use booster seats, seatbelts, or child restraints for your child when riding in a car? Where does your child play? Do you believe it is safe? Have you gone over personal safety with your child (e.g., "saying no")? Is your home childproof? If you have firearms, are they unloaded and locked? Is ammunition locked separately? Are pools fenced and gated? How do you heat or cool your home? Is it comfortable? Is there any danger of falls? Is your child dressed warmly for cold weather? Do you have a working smoke alarm? What would you do if your child had a health emergency? Do you have a car, or is there a friend, family member, or neighbor close by who could help you? What other conditions in your child's environment do you think could be a health risk?
Children with special needs	What does it mean for you to say that your child is "healthy"? How did you feel when your child's problem was diagnosed? What did you do? What coping strategies do you use as you care for your child? How has managing a chronic illness changed your family functioning? How does your family function? Who is providing specialty care to your child? Do you believe this is adequate? What other special needs do you believe your child has that require care? How comfortable are you in providing home care? What would you need to be more comfortable? How are your child's regular health needs met (i.e., those not directly related to the chronic illness, such as immunizations)? What resources do you know about that can help you understand and manage your child's illness? What special physical arrangements have you made to accommodate your child's illness? At home? In the car? At school or day care?

- Failure to adhere to prescribed medical treatment or standards for well-child health supervision after having adequate information for decision-making
- Child at risk for delayed or ineffective treatment, or both
- Poor health status of children as a result of untreated illness or other health problem
- Lack of appropriate immunizations
- Barriers to health care services
- Knowledge deficit about children
- Knowledge deficit related to illness
- Parents' dissatisfaction with health care providers
- Risk-taking behaviors

Management Strategies for Functional Health Patterns

Pediatric primary care providers work with children and families to help them make sound decisions, access necessary resources, and achieve and maintain healthy behavior changes. Providers also give information, guidance, prescriptions, and referrals that can strengthen a family's ability in these areas. The process of fostering behavior that promotes health is broad in scope, encompassing actions in the examination room, the primary care practice, the family, and the community (Fig. 9-3). This section discusses some general strategies for promoting effective health management. As will be seen in subsequent chapters, these strategies can also be applied to management of other functional health pattern problems.

The Provider-Child-Family Triad: Family-Centered Collaborative Negotiations

Developing a relationship of trust and respect is the first basic step to any intervention, and an environment in which the family is comfortable and welcome facilitates the working relationship. This is particularly evident when providers work with clients of diverse cultures, but it is true of *all* clients. Parents bring their perspectives, questions, and priorities to the health care visit. They also bring an expertise based on knowledge and experience with their child. Providers have skill and expertise in their clinical area. The goal and challenge is how to integrate the two in a process of collaborative negotiation that maximizes health. Providers can foster collaborative negotiation when they:

- Provide opportunities for parents and children (as appropriate) to discuss concerns
- Acknowledge ambivalence, disorganization, and stress faced by parents and the family
- Solicit parents' and children's thoughts and beliefs
- Acknowledge and value parents' expertise, strengths, and desire to help their child
- Validate parents' efforts at parenting; provide support and guidance
- Work closely with families to develop intervention strategies appropriate to the skills, needs, and desires of parents and children
- Demonstrate knowledge and skill in which families can place their trust

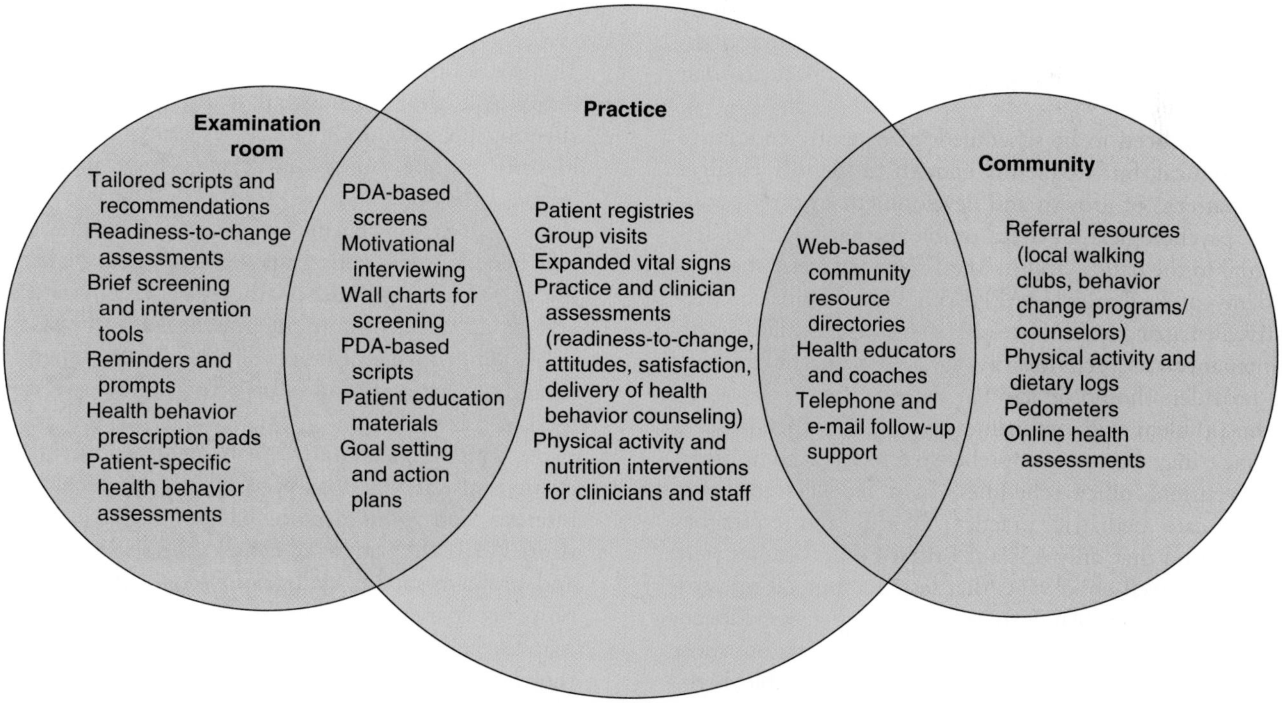

• **Figure 9-3** Integration of health behavior change strategies in primary care. *PDA,* Personal digital assistant (handheld computer). (From Cifuentes M, Fernal DH, Green LA, et al: Prescription for health: changing the health care practice to foster healthy behaviors, *Ann Fam Med* 3(Suppl 2):S8, 2005.)

- Be willing to discuss issues beyond the provider's traditional role
- Demonstrate positive affect and body language
- Recognize the biases and perspectives the provider brings to the interaction

This collaborative approach cannot be overemphasized and is increasingly the model expected by parents and families (Glascoe and Trimm, 2014). Children should be encouraged to participate in the process consistent with their developmental abilities. Adolescents, especially, are at a stage at which they can make many decisions independently of their parents.

Health Promotion Care

The use of functional health patterns emphasizes health promotion, and the regular clinical visit, timed to offer periodic screening opportunities, is an essential management strategy. The purpose of the health supervision visit is to assess strengths and weaknesses in health and to intervene to promote the best health possible. Health supervision includes the clinical interview, developmental and educational surveillance, observation of parent-child interaction, physical examination, and screening procedures, such as measuring height, weight, head circumference, body mass index (BMI), vision, hearing, blood pressure, and diagnostic tests like hemoglobin or hematocrit.

Visits with the provider also allow assessment of home, family, culture, and social life, teaching about growth and development, and problem-solving related to issues that affect children's health status. The visits can be used to enhance children's sense of independence and positive self-concept and to encourage children to make healthy lifestyle decisions. As children mature, they should be actively involved in the visit, with the provider asking them questions directly and providing appropriate feedback to their responses.

The visits need to be scheduled infrequently enough to be economical, but frequently enough to identify changes in the patterns of growth and development or early physiologic, psychological, or social problems that might be detrimental to the child's health. The Bright Futures/American Academy of Pediatrics' (AAP) Recommendations for Preventive Pediatric Health Care (2014) lists appropriate health maintenance care activities by age. All pediatric primary care providers should be familiar with its use.

The problem with guidelines for health supervision is that they may be too comprehensive to be accomplished within current office schedules. In a recent study of a primary care pediatric practice, Norlin and colleagues (2011) found that only 42% of Bright Futures topics were addressed in well-child visits that lasted about 20 minutes each. An alternative plan is to determine, using an evidence-based approach, which topics and interventions are most essential (i.e., are most likely to have measureable high-quality outcomes). If efforts were directed toward the most effective interventions, time and costs could be saved without sacrificing quality (Mangione-Smith et al, 2011). Much work needs to be done in this area, and providers need to be alert to research that supports or refutes some of the standard interventions recommended in well-child care. Although providers are given a comprehensive framework for provision of quality care, they need to select and prioritize the guidelines to make care realistic and meaningful.

Behavioral Counseling Interventions

The term "counseling" implies a cooperative mode of interaction between client and provider rather than a more directive teacher-learner model; behavioral counseling is usually directed at complex behaviors. The goal of behavioral counseling is self-management of the problem behavior by the client in order to change and sustain healthy patterns of living. Many behavioral counseling interventions are based on the health beliefs, self-efficacy, and transtheoretical models discussed earlier. Certain attributes of clients predispose them to successful behavior change:

- There is a desire to change for clear, personal reasons.
- Few obstacles to behavior change are perceived.
- The client has the skills and self-confidence for the needed changes.
- The client feels that there will be benefits to the change.
- The changes are viewed as congruent with the client's self-image and norms of his or her social or cultural group.
- Reminders, encouragement, and social support at key times and from persons and the community whom the client values will support the behavior changes.

The Five As

Originally developed by the American Cancer Institute for use in smoking cessation interventions, the construct of "the five As" can be an effective behavioral counseling strategy.

The five As are as follows:

- *Assess:* Ask about behavioral health risks and factors affecting behavioral choices, goals, and methods used. Identify unique family and client circumstances that impact behavior.
- *Advise:* Give clear, specific information, including harms and benefits of various behavioral options. Personalize the information to address the patient's circumstances and experience. Minimize judgment, using phrases, such as "As your provider, I must tell you…" rather than "You should…" Various models of patient education can be used in this step.
- *Agree:* Find a collaborative plan that the provider and client can agree on that is based on the client's goals, interests, and willingness to change.
- *Assist:* Assist the patient to achieve the self-management and problem-solving skills, confidence, and social supports necessary to make and maintain changes. Providers may use behavior change techniques with the individual; they may also assist in overcoming barriers and connecting the patient to needed resources.
- *Arrange:* Schedule follow-up contacts with the client to provide further guidance, support, and encouragement

to continue with the plan or make adjustments as needed. This step might also involve referral to special sources of help.

Motivational Interviewing

Motivational interviewing (MI) is a specific behavioral counseling method to help patients recognize and change risky behaviors. MI effectively supports change in a variety of behaviors, including smoking, drug addiction, inactivity, obesity, diabetic care, and asthma. While working with clients with problem drinking behaviors, Miller and Rollnick (1991) discovered that eliciting the client's own intrinsic motivation to change, using persuasion rather than coercion, and using support rather than argument were more effective in helping clients change their behaviors. MI is effective in brief encounters of only 15 minutes, although more than one encounter will increase the likelihood of success. The technique is particularly helpful with clients who are reluctant to change or ambivalent about the need to change. It works particularly well with adolescents, because developmentally they are trying to make their own decisions.

In a meta-analysis of studies comparing MI with other strategies, MI outperformed traditional advice-giving in approximately 80% of studies. No studies reported it to be harmful (Rubak et al, 2005). Suarez and Mullins (2008) completed an extensive review of MI in pediatric practice and found it to be an effective strategy for decreasing adolescent substance abuse, decreasing health risk behaviors, and increasing adherence to regimens for treatment of various conditions. It also works with parents.

MI has 10 basic components, none of which are unique to MI, but which, when used together, comprise the technique. Motivational interviewing:

1. Is a conversation about change, often behavioral change
2. Uses a method of collaborative partnership between the client and counselor
3. Honors autonomy and self-determination, allowing people to make their own decisions
4. Seeks to evoke and strengthen one's personal motivation for change
5. Draws out the individual's motivation for change
6. Uses specific interviewing skills (OARS):
   - Elaborate: Using **O**pen-ended questions
   - **A**ffirm: Using statements that acknowledge the client's perspective
   - **R**eflect: Listening and responding to client's meanings
   - **S**ummarize: Asking questions and making statements to summarize provider's understanding and consolidate client's message.
7. Works to clarify and resolve ambivalence in the direction of change; may generate ambivalence during the conversation
8. Is guided by the client's forms of speech as they discuss issues (i.e., "change talk")
9. Responds to client's change talk in specific ways (i.e., OARS)
10. Responds to resistance by being nonconfrontational and avoiding argument

A four-step process is involved in the motivational interview approach. When using a motivational interview approach, pediatric providers should:

1. Develop rapport with the child and family. In this first step, the client and provider engage in establishing a relationship based on trust and respect. Studies support the ideas of active listening, forming a working alliance, and clarifying the patient's views with reflective comments.
2. Set an agenda. The second step in the process is to guide the conversation in a way that clarifies the issue and finds a focus ("What is it that you think is going on?"). At this stage, the provider can share information and advice as requested by the client.
3. Once the agenda is set, ask scaling questions to assess the patient's confidence and abilities in making a behavior change, perceptions about barriers, and so forth. "Why do you feel you are at 4 out of 10 in terms of confidence in yourself to be able to quit smoking? What would help raise your score? " Respond and summarize selectively to further guide the client to identify what it is he or she hopes to accomplish.
4. Collaborate with the client to identify a plan. At this step, the provider uses MI skills to reinforce the client's commitment to change, encouraging and assisting as requested.

See Box 9-2 for some essential features of MI. Skilled MI is best learned through short training sessions, followed by several days of supervised practice with real patients.

Reframing

Reframing is a counseling strategy in which one changes the context of an experience to give it a new meaning (i.e., to

• BOX 9-2 Essential Features of Motivational Interviewing

- Motivation to change comes from within the patient and is not externally imposed by the provider or others.
- Provider guides patient to identify discrepancy between current behavior and goals for change.
- Ambivalence must be articulated and resolved by the patient, not the provider. The provider can help facilitate the patient's expressions of both sides of the issue and guide the patient toward a resolution that triggers a desire for change.
- Direct persuasion by the provider will not resolve ambivalence. Unsolicited advice is not given.
- An intervention style that is quiet and eliciting works best.
- Readiness for change is not a patient trait, but a changing product of interpersonal interaction.
- The provider allows the patient to resist change, while encouraging self-efficacy and articulation of ambivalence.
- The provider-patient relationship must develop as a partnership rather than an expert-novice or teacher-student relationship.

refocus interpretation of an experience). The goal is to create a frame of reference that focuses on a desired outcome rather than a current problem. For example, a teenager may experience pain with braces on his teeth and can complain and be miserable, making the entire family miserable; or he can reframe the experience to understand that pain indicates the braces are working as they should and will lead to a healthy smile. As another example, a child may be labeled "stubborn," but reframing changes the label to "determined," a positive trait that will be helpful as the child grows. One needs to be careful, however, not to use reframing to discount, deny, or ignore real problems faced by families. For example, the child who is setting fires should not be described as "demonstrating scientific curiosity." Support groups can help people reframe their current condition, and patients who find positive meaning in their condition may become more invested in self-care.

Health Education

Education about health and illness is a mainstay of primary care pediatric practice. It is a dynamic process that requires contributions from both family and provider to achieve its end goal—arriving at mutual understanding of the problem or concern and creating a shared plan for dealing with that problem. Providers typically offer parents anticipatory guidance about what to expect as their child grows, ways to prevent illness and injury and to reduce health risks, strategies to implement positive lifestyle changes, and steps to maintain a healthy environment. The educational interventions of providers are most useful when the patient and family are motivated and self-sufficient and when families are given an opportunity to explore options for action. In pediatrics, the learner may be the parent, caregiver, or a child or teen who is able to manage some of his or her own health behaviors. Many strategies can be applied in the educational process, and the way in which information is given may be as important as the information itself, but there are some guiding principles to consider no matter which technique is used. This section discusses some of the principles and approaches to health education, focusing particularly on adults, parents, and caregivers of children. Teaching children, especially adolescents, can include many of the same steps but is based on a careful assessment of the child's developmental level. Children have often been described as "little sponges," soaking up information and learning from a wide range of experiences. The Management of Development unit of this textbook (Chapters 4 through 8) extensively discusses children at different ages and stages of development, looking specifically at their learning capabilities, health-related issues (e.g., anticipatory guidance topics), and educational strategies and interventions that are most appropriate at each stage.

Assessing and Fostering Health Literacy

For the educational process to function well, clients must be "health literate." Literacy is the ability to comprehend and interpret prose (narrative), documents (charts, tables, and so on), and numeracy (numbers within the context of written information). Barriers to literacy include limited language, especially English, proficiency; sensory, neurologic, or cognitive impairment; and economic, social, and physical limitations.

Health literacy is defined as the ability to read and communicate, evaluate and interpret health information, understand health concepts, apply information to make informed health care decisions, accurately manage medications and treatments, and know how to access and use resources properly (IOM, 2001). More recently the definition has been expanded to include the skills needed to navigate the health care system and the need for clear communication between providers and patients. Verbal skill as a component of health literacy has not been extensively researched but may be a way to mitigate the effect of low health literacy in reading, writing, and numeracy (Berkman et al, 2011). An additional element that affects the outcome of health literacy is that the individual must be able to act on the informed decisions made; this is not always the case when poverty, absence of health services, lack of access, or other social variables are present.

Low health literacy impacts health status. In a review of research on the relationship between health literacy and health status, Berkman and colleagues (2011) found that adults with low health literacy are more likely to use emergency room care; have greater risk of hospitalization; are less likely to take preventive measures (mammograms and influenza immunizations); have poorer skills in managing medications; are less likely to understand or accurately interpret health information; have greater incidence of depression; and, in the elderly, have higher morbidity and mortality rates (Berkman et al, 2011). Although Berkman's group did not find strong evidence for it, Sanders and colleagues (2009) noted that adults with low health literacy are 1.2 to 4 times more likely to exhibit negative health behaviors that affect child health. Teens with low general literacy are twice as likely to exhibit aggressive or antisocial behavior. And chronically ill children who have caregivers with low general literacy are twice as likely to use more health services (Sanders et al, 2009). See Figure 9-4 for a model of the relationship between individual characteristics, external and social variables, health literacy, health behaviors, and health management.

It is difficult to accurately state the prevalence of low health literacy in the population, because it is mediated by many variables, and different literacy screening tests can arrive at different numbers for the same population. A study conducted by Dunn-Navarra and colleagues (2012), for example, found that inadequate health literacy was seen in 83.8% of Latino respondents using the Newest Vital Sign (NVS) screening tool but only 35.7% when respondents were tested with the Short-Test of Functional Health Literacy in Adults (S-TOFHLA). For both screening tools, different variables (e.g., college education, length of residency in the United States, having a regular care provider,

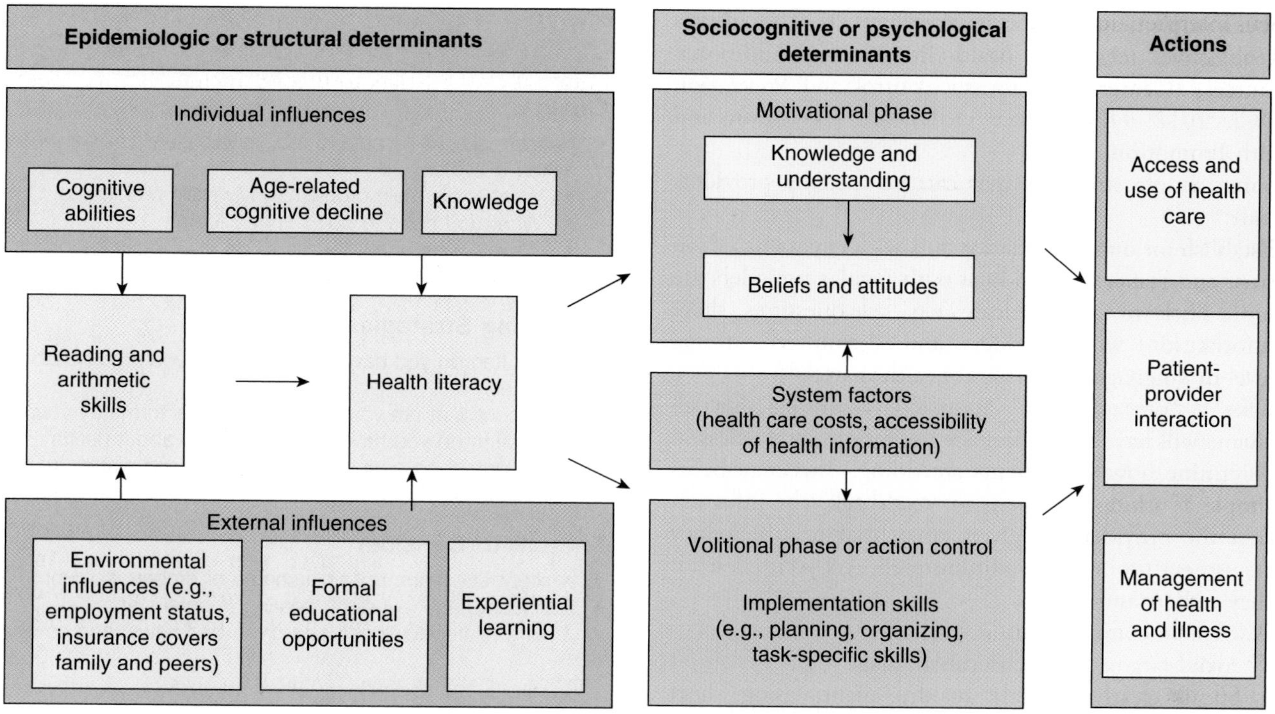

• **Figure 9-4** Health literacy and health actions. (From von Wagner C, Steptoe A, Wolf M, et al: Health literacy and health actions: a review and a framework from health psychology, *Health Educ Behav* 36(5):863, 2009. Used with permission.)

whether born in the United States or not) influenced the responses of subjects.

Nonetheless, many individuals demonstrate poor health literacy. A 2009 review article determined that one third of adolescents and young adults had low health literacy. More than 28% of parents had below basic to basic health literacy. Sixty-eight percent were unable to enter names and birthdates correctly on a health information sheet, and 46% were unable to perform at least half of medication-related tasks. Those with low health literacy reported difficulty understanding over-the-counter medication labels and nutrition labels (Yin et al, 2009).

A variety of tools to screen for health literacy are available to clinicians, and more are being developed in an effort to find one that accurately measures as many parameters of literacy as possible, in as many populations, and for as many clinical conditions as possible—and does so quickly with minimal inconvenience to client and provider. Most screening tools currently being used provide only a moderately accurate assessment of literacy. The traditional method of using level of education as a measure of health literacy does not adequately evaluate reading, comprehension, and analytic ability. Also, as noted previously, different tools can generate different results in the same population (Dunn-Navarra et al, 2012); this is probably due to the different focus, scope, and structure of the instrument being used (Al Sayah et al, 2013). However, despite any limitations, screening tools can be used to identify clients who may need more assessment and/or assistance to manage health information. The NVS is an orally administered tool that takes about 3 minutes to administer and assesses ability to understand and interpret the provider (Weiss et al, 2005) (see Additional Resources). Several different tools assess reading level and ease of readability of material, such as a patient handout (e.g., Fog Index, SMOG, Flesch-Kincaid Readability Tests) (see Additional Resources). The best tool to estimate reading level is the SMOG, and a level no higher than fifth grade is best for patient materials (Wilson, 2009). In their review of tools appropriate for adult patients with diabetes, Al Sayah and colleagues (2013) outline the type and scope, characteristics (number of items, time to administer, and so on), scoring, and reliability and validity of 12 different instruments. Some providers are developing their own tools (Cawthon et al, 2014). In addition, a Rapid Estimate of Adolescent Literacy in Medicine (REALM-Teen) is available to screen teens in middle school and high school and takes less than 3 minutes to administer (Davis et al, 2006). Also, a recent study indicated that findings from use of a "home literacy environment single-item screening question" (i.e., How many children's books are in the home?) confirmed findings found when the NVS literacy assessment tool was used. Homes with 10 or fewer children's books tended to have lower health literacy levels (Driessnack et al, 2014).

Improving health literacy is an international goal, being approached in a variety of ways. For example, recent U.S. legislation (The Plain Writing Act of 2010) requires that written material from the federal government have multiple headings with short sentences using verbs in the active tense; a National Action Plan to Improve Health Literacy has been implemented, and *Healthy People 2020* has identified objectives related to health literacy (see Additional Resources) (Centers for Disease Control and Prevention [CDC], 2012; HHS Office of Disease Prevention and Health Promotion, 2010).

Some simple strategies that can be used by providers include:

- Establish an ongoing relationship with clients based on trust and respect. Individuals with regular providers are more likely to communicate (e.g., ask questions, share information) with providers, and, despite educational level or language, understand health materials.
- Take a "precautionary" approach, assuming that all clients will have health literacy limitations, and assess to determine how well clients are doing. This may be as simple as asking the client to "read-back" the information the provider has given; or a brief health literacy assessment tool may be administered. Ask your clients if they understand you.
- Be clear in communication with clients:
  - Avoid jargon and technical language
  - Speak clearly, directly to the client, using short sentences
  - Use multiple forms of educational materials (e.g., visual images, video, written words)
  - Use written materials presented at a fifth-grade level
  - Limit lists to seven items or less
- Identify target groups and solicit their specific issues and communication patterns (e.g., a client population that is predominately Somali, Spanish-speaking, or teens). For children, health care providers must consider the developmental level and provide materials that are understandable to them—more pictures for younger children, written materials at the appropriate grade level, and use of social support to "scaffold" learning in new areas for the child (Borzekowski, 2009). Improved written materials with brief counseling have been shown to improve adherence (DeWalt and Hink, 2009) (Box 9-3).

BOX 9-3 Goals, Screening, and Interventions for Low Health Care Literacy

Goals

- Patients should be able to articulate a clear answer when asked to state:
  - What is my main problem? ("My main problem is…")
  - What do I need to do? ("I need to…")
  - Why is it important for me to do this? ("It is important for me to do this because…")

Screening Strategies

- How often do you have someone help you read health materials?
- How confident are you to fill out medical forms by yourself?
- How often do you have trouble learning about health conditions because it is hard to understand written information?

Factors to Consider

- Anxiety, stressors, possible shame or embarrassment
- Language, age, eyesight, hearing, mental status
- Timing related to illness, just given bad news, and so on

BOX 9-4 The Patient Education Process

- Set the climate for learning—make introductions, provide comfortable environment.
- Assess the learner's style of learning, level of knowledge and competency, readiness, physical and developmental capabilities, attitudes, and feelings.
- Plan—identify the parent and/or child's learning goals and objectives, specifying behaviors that the learner will exhibit to demonstrate learning.
- Manage the learning intervention—use methods and resources for instruction with the patient or family (or both) to implement the plan. Provide information, role modeling, practice, and opportunity for discussion. Use various aids that facilitate teaching—books, pamphlets, diagrams, videos, and models.
- Evaluate the outcomes—judge achievement of objectives and then reformulate the plan to move the learner to the next level.

Patient Education Process

The traditional core methodology for patient education for individuals and groups is reviewed here and summarized in Box 9-4.

1. *Set the climate for learning:* Patients, families, or groups need to be in an environment that is comfortable, free of distractions, and provides cues that learning activities will occur. Introductions and a mutually agreed-on time limit are helpful. For example, mothers who are worried about being home when the school bus drops off their children attend poorly to teaching, no matter how skilled the provider.
2. *Identify mutual goals of learner and provider:* Learner and provider must reach agreement on what is to be achieved. Clients do not always come to the provider with preestablished goals or needs, yet if learning is to be successful, the client must recognize a need for new knowledge. The MI process discussed previously can be used to help clients express questions, concerns, and, ultimately, identify health goals; this process also allows the provider to give information that will assist individuals to clarify their thinking and arrive at a mutual understanding of the learning goal that they have defined.
3. *Assess the learner:* A health literacy assessment tool can be used in the assessment process (Al Sayah et al, 2013). Providers can also assess learners' capacity with questions in the following areas:
   - Readiness
     - Does the individual ask questions?
     - Does the individual have multiple stresses in his or her life that inhibit learning?

- Is the individual coping with survival issues (e.g., chronic poverty, debilitating chronic illness, unemployment, or rehabilitation from substance abuse) that inhibit learning? When is the best time to meet, given other daily expectations?
- Attitudes and feelings
  - Does the individual demonstrate self-efficacy? Do statements indicate that the individual believes the problem could be managed through personal actions?
- Style of learning
  - What are the preferred learning modalities for this individual?
- Level of knowledge
  - What does the individual already know about the subject?
- Physical and developmental capabilities
  - Does the individual have any limitations to consider (e.g., limited English proficiency, caregiver is a grandparent who is hard of hearing)?
  - Judging from the individual's developmental level, how abstract can the teaching be?

4. *Plan:* The plan begins by stating learning objectives. As with goals, objectives should be developed through negotiation and mutually agreed upon by client and provider. Objectives identify specific behaviors that will be seen if learning has occurred. They must be realistic, achievable, and relevant to the client's goals (e.g., Goal: Safe and accurate administration of medication; Objective: The parent will demonstrate correctly measuring prescribed amount of oral medication using device provided by pharmacist). Both short-term and long-term objectives are written if the goals will not be achieved in one teaching session. Using both types of objectives helps the client and provider set priorities and stage education in achievable steps. In routine pediatric visits, objectives are often verbally stated, not written.
5. *Advise:* Manage the learning intervention. The process of implementing the teaching plan is carefully orchestrated so that the client is actively engaged. Progress is constantly monitored, new information added, success reinforced, feedback assessed, the pace adjusted, and outcomes and achievement of objectives evaluated.
6. *Evaluate the outcomes:* Judge achievement of objectives (e.g., Were the desired behaviors achieved?) and then reformulate the plan to move the client to the next level. Evaluate learning using a variety of methods, such as asking questions that require use of new knowledge to answer, watching for new behaviors, and looking for expressions of new understanding and feelings of achievement.

Patient Education Strategies

A number of strategies or interventions can be used effectively in health education.

Provide Data and Verbal Advice. Providing data about a child's health status to the parents or adolescent can be a powerful yet easy intervention. Describing and interpreting information from the height and weight grid and developmental screening or laboratory test scores can significantly reinforce the work that parents have been doing. Interpreting information is important so that the parents know how their child compares with appropriate norms. Data provided should include both normal outcomes and areas of concern.

Verbal advice is used in 99% of client-pediatric provider encounters and also can be a simple, powerful intervention (e.g., "Bicycle helmets reduce head injuries in children, so make sure your child wears his whenever he's on his bike"), yet it is limited by the client's health literacy or ability to focus or recall, especially when clients are stressed or depressed (Glascoe and Trimm, 2014).

Role Model. Social learning theory suggests that role modeling is an effective way for people to learn. Modeling appropriate parenting techniques can be useful, especially when the parent rehearses the desired behaviors with positive reinforcement. The provider must be careful to create a situation in which parents feel competent—that they are doing a fine job rather than that someone else could do it better. Parents need to feel new confidence as they try out new behaviors. Parenting classes and support groups often provide more time for role modeling and new behavior practice. Parents may need several sessions to learn new responses to their children's behavior, and part of the process requires that parents make decisions about when to use the new responses they are learning. Providers can serve as reflective listeners, reinforcing success, as parents discuss their efforts.

Bibliotherapy. Providing reading material can be an excellent primary care intervention. Books or pamphlets are helpful if information is well organized and presented in a manner that facilitates retention. Written materials allow patients or families to self-pace their learning and can serve as a familiar future reference if needed. The reading level of patients must be assessed to make sure appropriate materials are shared. Good readers use reading materials efficiently, scanning for important words, stopping to summarize the material learned, and using illustrations to enhance the meanings derived from the text. Unskilled readers may either spend an inordinate amount of time trying to master the material or simply set the task aside, usually without letting the provider know. Some parents with low health literacy may ask a family member or friend who is more literate to help them with written material.

Reading provides vicarious role models for children and parents, acts as a support by acknowledging the feelings and problems encountered by others with similar problems, and expands perspectives on various health-related issues. Stories help children, especially adolescents, explore new ideas, clarify their own feelings and perceptions, and serve as an impetus for change. Many providers participate in the Reach Out and Read program, offering age-appropriate reading materials to children and families.

Multimedia Instruction. Learning is often facilitated with exposure to a variety of media. Such a multimedia approach can include videos, DVDs, interactive technology using CD-ROM, smartphone applications, office-based kiosks with touchscreens, and Internet-accessed programs (e.g., Play Nicely, a teaching model for how to manage aggressive behavior in toddlers and preschool children) among others. Not all families have easy access to the Internet and, for those who do, many must be educated as to how best to interpret the information they are able to find. Providers have a responsibility to help families distinguish reliable information from biased sources. Having a list of "approved websites including social media and smartphone applications with appropriate content" can help families in this challenging process (Glascoe and Trimm, 2014).

Health System Interventions

Families with children have many complex needs that could often be met by resources other than the primary care provider's practice. These include governmental agencies; other health care services, including clinics, screening programs, health promotion programs, and hospitals; and community volunteer programs. A problem in the health management pattern occurs when families do not gain access to needed resources. Providers can intervene to (1) give parents the skills and assistance to more easily and appropriately gain access and (2) remove barriers to access.

Skills to Access Resources: Referrals, Email, and Telephone Communication

Referrals are made when specialty care or special types of intervention, such as a support group, class, or practice opportunities, are needed. Referrals may also be made if treating the child and working with parents requires more time for intervention than is available in the current setting. Managed care settings, in most cases, make internal referrals and seem to discourage referrals outside the system, but that option may be in the best interest of the patient at times.

Identifying, locating, and using resources may require knowledge and skills that some families do not have. Providers can serve as advocates by helping families locate local, regional, or national health care resources to meet their health needs. It is important that providers develop and maintain a resource list relevant to their practice. Using a resource list facilitates making referrals and recommendations to parents; it gives the clear message that the family is not alone with their concern, that help is available, and that the primary care provider is a knowledgeable ally in the family's effort to maintain good health. It is helpful to discuss with the family what they can expect from the referral; for example, what the process for entering the system will be; what transportation or financial accommodations will need to be made; and what services can be anticipated.

As advocates, providers make every effort to encourage independent action and decision-making by families, but if the family's coping abilities are compromised, it is not enough simply to give the name of a resource or contact to the family. In these situations, providers may need to contact the resource themselves or assist the family to make the contact. For some families in crisis, it is appropriate to refer them to a community or mental health professional for help to establish and maintain contact with a supportive network.

Increasingly, health care practices use email to communicate with clients, get information from them, and assess and give clinical advice. This trend is increasing, but there is no clear evidence to evaluate the effectiveness of such communication (Atherton et al, 2012). As with any form of communication, providers who use email should clearly establish with the parent how the technology is to be used (e.g., which types of questions, how quickly can a response be expected, and security measures to protect confidentiality).

Telephone interaction between parent and provider can be a critical factor in accurately interpreting a child's condition, deciding on appropriate measures of care, and establishing confidence and trust. See Chapter 21 for a discussion of how pediatric care providers can work with parents to use the telephone in the management of illnesses. The same strategies can be applied to the management of health promotion.

Remove Barriers to Care

Financial and insurance issues are key barriers to health care. Since the passage of the Patient Protection and Affordable Health Care Act (2010), many of these barriers have been removed. Insurance companies are now required to provide coverage to children with preexisting conditions; Medicaid programs, providing care to low-income children and families, have been expanded in most states; state-based health insurance exchanges offer health insurance to everyone—most often with lower premiums than previous plans. As a result, a significant number of Americans who were previously uninsured have access to health care insurance.

Providers can also find ways to help parents decrease costs while maximizing a practice's resources; for example, scheduling fewer visits and performing only necessary diagnostic tests. Providers who offer clinical services outside normal working hours (i.e., evening and weekend clinics) help many families access care without losing pay or having to use limited "sick time" hours. Some providers are offering home visits for their patients. Other barriers to health care access are geography and lack of essential infrastructure services, such as transportation and child care. The lack of primary care resources in rural and isolated areas can prevent families from obtaining regular care. If a family does not have adequate transportation or child care services, the cost of seeking well-child care or treating minor acute problems that can worsen without medical intervention often outweighs the perceived benefits.

Providers can consult with parents and social workers to identify resources in the community that help overcome some of these barriers. For example, transportation may be available through some managed-care plans or local volunteer organizations (e.g., churches), or a relative may have time to care for other children while the parent takes one child to the clinic. For other barriers, however, the solution lies in making changes in the way health care services are organized and financed. This task goes far beyond the primary care setting, but it is nonetheless the responsibility of all pediatric primary care providers to be aware of and to participate in the process of restructuring and reorganizing the health care system to ensure necessary care is given.

Management Strategies for Children with Special Needs

Health management of children with special needs is challenging. Children with chronic illness receive expert illness care from a number of specialists, but their primary care needs may often be neglected. Primary care providers can serve to coordinate health maintenance care with ongoing specialty illness management. Communication and collaboration with the child's specialty physician or care team are essential, as well as clear communication with the parents about the role of each provider in the child's care. Providers also need to adapt normal intervention techniques when providing primary care to children with chronic illness. The regular immunization schedule may need to be adjusted, for example, or special techniques for obtaining height and weight or vital signs might be necessary. Parents and children should be assisted to develop ways to meet daily living needs consistent with the child's ability. Children with physical handicaps, for example, require special intervention to meet activity and exercise needs for growth and development.

Evaluating Health Promotion Interventions

The care that many health care providers deliver is rarely evaluated, except in larger organizations; yet as Pender and colleagues (2011) suggest, evaluation is essential to ensure quality care. The health care team should build evaluation into health delivery services. This begins with identification of goals, program objectives and indicators of success—short-term, midterm, and long-term outcomes.

Evaluations may be quantitative or qualitative or both. The type of program determines the type of evaluation method used. Although a randomized control trial is considered the best form of outcome evaluation, mixed methods of data collection are often used. Measures should consider program effectiveness, efficiency, efficacy, and equity. Evaluations assess *outcomes;* for example, how many children were up to date on immunizations? How many children lost weight? What was the decrease in use of emergency department services for treatment of asthma? Program evaluation also assesses the *process* of delivering care; for example, efficiency and time use, or satisfaction with care by staff, parents, and child.

Program evaluation includes the following questions:

- What knowledge, behavior changes, or outcomes are expected?
- Is the intervention practical and effective in clinical practice?
- How long does it take to become effective?
- How long do the intervention effects last?
- Are there unintended consequences?
- Are families satisfied?
- What could be done to improve the intervention?
- How much did the intervention cost?

Data should be collected and analyzed as part of clinic management routines, on an ongoing basis. With the use of automated systems and records in many institutions, the job should be more manageable than in the past. Ultimately the goal is to demonstrate that attention to health promotion and health maintenance activities has benefits for multiple stakeholders: patients, providers, and payers.

The functional health patterns of children need continual reassessment in light of their developmental change. Parents also need continuing information and new skills, such as teaching behaviors, to manage their children's evolving health care needs adequately. In addition, a multitude of factors—the social determinants of health—shape children's health behaviors. In some ways, health promotion care for children can be more difficult than managing an illness. Although it is no easy task, developing the skills to manage health promotion for children and their families is worth all the effort.

For a complete list of references, please visit http://evolve.elsevier.com/Burns/pediatric/.

10 Nutrition

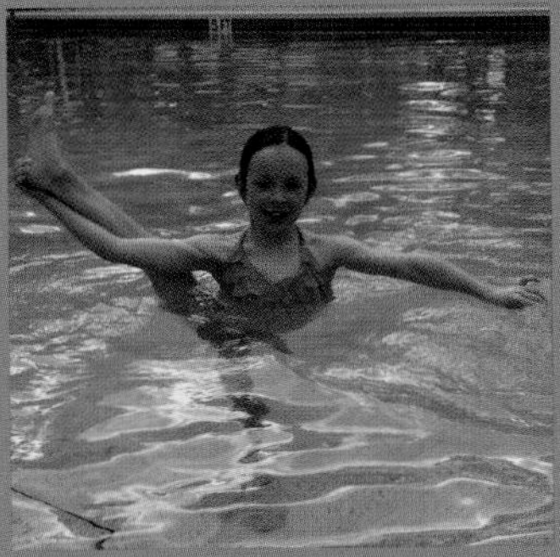

SUSAN FILKINS AND ARDYS M. DUNN

Optimal nutrition is the foundation for healthy physical and mental growth and development. Without adequate nutrients to achieve a high level of health, children's ability to interact with their environment, to be curious, to explore and learn, and to have sufficient energy for exercise can be compromised. For children with acute or chronic illness, appropriate nutrition can be essential to healing and/or successful management of their condition.

The pediatric primary health care provider's goals are to assess whether children are meeting their nutritional requirements and prevent any problems related to poor nutrition. To accomplish this, providers must conduct thorough assessments, provide relevant education, develop clear and appropriate treatment plans, and refer the child and family to nutritional specialists as needed. Interventions are based on certain assumptions, including the following:

- Children's nutritional needs vary as they grow and are influenced by their state of health.
- A wide range of food choices and feeding behaviors are used to meet nutritional needs.
- Dietary reference intakes (DRIs) are *guidelines* only.
- Parents and other caregivers are responsible for providing food choices that are nutritionally adequate and for establishing healthy eating patterns; to do so, they must be well informed.
- Family patterns of nutrition and eating are based on social, economic, cultural, and psychological dynamics. Patterns are not related to nutrients alone.
- The primary care provider is a source of information regarding nutrition, feeding patterns, and health.
- The primary care provider works with a network of specialists (e.g., registered dietitian nutritionists) to manage children's nutrition status.

This chapter looks at the nutritional requirements of children and the ways providers can use nutrition to help children be their healthiest. It begins with the nutritional standards for preventive care recommended by certain professional groups, followed by a review of the functions of specific nutrients in the body and the DRIs for these nutrients. It must be emphasized that these recommendations are just that—recommendations, not requirements—and the fact that they are often given as a range (e.g., 25% to 35% of energy intake in the form of fat) reinforces the concept that there is latitude in healthy nutritional intake.

Approaches to general assessment, diagnosis, and management of nutritional status are then presented. The chapter concludes with sections on "normal" and "altered" patterns of nutrition. The section on "normal" nutrition outlines age-specific considerations related to food intake and includes discussions of vegetarian diets and nutrition for the pregnant teenager. In the section on altered patterns of nutrition, several tables summarize nutritional considerations of specific conditions (e.g., diabetes mellitus). It would be impossible within the scope of a general text to discuss nutritional needs of all acute and chronic conditions, so general categories are outlined: conditions that require increased caloric intake, those that require decreased caloric intake, and so on. The epidemiology, etiology, assessment, and management of obesity, which has become an epidemic in the United States and other developed countries, is also discussed.

Standards for Preventive Care

Nutrition standards for children emphasize that:

- Breast milk is the best food for infants.
- Children's diets should include a wide variety of foods predominantly from plants, especially whole grains, fruits, vegetables, legumes, and nuts.
- Iron-rich foods are essential, especially for infants and adolescents.
- Fat intake, particularly saturated fats, should be limited. Trans fats should be eliminated from the diet.
- Simple carbohydrates (e.g., refined grains, white bread, sugar, high-fructose corn syrup, and sodas) should be limited.
- Extra calcium, iron, and folic acid are important nutrients in adolescent girls' diets.
- Children's diets should include adequate fiber and sodium.

The American Academy of Pediatrics (AAP) recommends exclusive breastfeeding until about 6 months old and continued breastfeeding, supplemented with appropriate foods for infants, for "1 year or longer as mutually desired by mother and infant" (AAP Section on Breastfeeding, 2012). The AAP also recommends 400 international units (IUs) of vitamin D for all breastfed infants until they are 1 year old and for all children and adolescents with diets deficient in vitamin D (Kleinman and Greer, 2013). The National Committee for Quality Assurance (NCQA) recommends assessment of body mass index (BMI) for all children 3 to 17 years old (NCQA, 2014). The U.S. Preventive Services Task Force (USPSTF) recommends interventions to promote and support breastfeeding, that children ages 6 years and older be screened for obesity, and that they be given, or referred for, comprehensive intensive behavioral interventions to improve weight (USPSTF, 2010). The Institute of Medicine (IOM) has published ways to ensure that school food programs meet current dietary recommendations (IOM Committee on Nutrition Standards for National School Lunch and Breakfast Programs et al, 2010). *Bright Futures in Practice: Nutrition* (Holt and Wooldridge, 2011) presents nutritional guidelines, discusses issues and concerns related to pediatric nutrition, and outlines tools for providers to assess and manage nutrition in children.

• BOX 10-1 Categories of Daily Reference Intakes

- Estimated average requirements (EAR): The average daily nutrient intake level that is estimated to meet the requirements of the healthy individuals in a particular life stage and gender group.*
- Recommended dietary allowance (RDA): The average daily dietary nutrient intake level that is sufficient to meet the nutrient requirements of nearly all (97% to 98%) healthy individuals in a particular life stage and gender group.
- Adequate intake (AI): The recommended average daily intake level based on observed or experimentally determined approximations or estimates of nutrient intake by a group (or groups) of apparently healthy people that are assumed to be adequate; used when an RDA cannot be determined.
- Tolerable upper intake level (UL): The average highest daily nutrient intake level that is likely to pose no risk of adverse health effects to almost all individuals in the general population. As intake increases above the UL, the potential risk of adverse effects may increase.

Otten JJ, Hellwig JP, Myers LD, editors: *Dietary Reference Intakes: the essential guide to nutrient requirements,* Washington DC, 2006, Institute of Medicine, National Academies Press, p 8.

*In the case of energy, an estimated energy requirement (EER) is required. The EER is the average daily energy intake that is predicted to maintain energy balance in a healthy adult of a defined age, gender, weight, height, and level of physical activity consistent with good health. In children and pregnant and lactating women, the EER is taken to include the needs associated with the disposition of tissues or the secretion of milk at rates consistent with good health.

Nutritional Requirements and Dietary Reference Intakes

The body requires energy, water and electrolytes, and macro- and micronutrients in order to survive. The amounts of these requirements vary greatly. The Food and Nutrition Board (FNB) of the National Academies of Science and IOM list DRIs based on diets consumed in the United States and Canada. Released in a series of reports from 1997 to 2005, the DRIs include four categories of values (Box 10-1). DRIs identify parameters of nutrient intake that will meet body needs and prevent adverse effects of excessive intake. They do not, however, set a standard below which the diet is judged inadequate to prevent pathology (basal requirement), or a standard that is sufficient for the body to maintain a healthy body reserve (normative requirement) (FNB and IOM, 2005). Based on extensive analysis of scientific evidence on diet and nutrition and referencing the DRIs developed by the FNB, the U.S. Department of Agriculture (USDA) and U.S. Department of Health and Human Services (HHS) publish Dietary Guidelines for Americans every 5 years. These guidelines address questions of nutritional adequacy, energy balance, weight management, and food safety and technology and make recommendations regarding intake of macro- and micronutrients, water, cholesterol, salt, and alcohol (USDA and HHS, 2015). They can assist families and providers to make healthful dietary decisions to meet the nutritional needs of individual children.

Energy

Three body processes require energy, which is measured in kilocalories:

- Basal metabolism, primarily regulatory functions: respiration, digestion, temperature regulation, circulation, and so on. Most of the body's energy is used for this function, measured in basal metabolic rate (BMR) or resting energy expenditure (REE).
- Growth, which is greatest in infancy and adolescence.
- Activity, exercise, and other metabolic demands, including illness.

The body meets these energy demands, or estimated energy requirement (EER), by using stored energy sources or calories consumed on a daily basis. EERs for healthy children can vary significantly by age, health status, and activity level. Tables providing a formula to calculate caloric needs of infants and toddlers and children age 2 to 18 years old can be found on the inside front cover of this text.

Macronutrients (protein, carbohydrates, and fats) and alcohol provide calories that supply energy. The body makes no distinction as to the *source* of calories; it will use whichever calories are consumed. Caloric intake for children is recommended to be distributed among the three macronutrients, with each providing a certain percentage of total daily caloric intake. These recommendations are given as an acceptable macronutrient distribution range (AMDR) and are presented in Table 10-1. They are based on age for

TABLE 10-1 Recommended Daily Allowance or Adequate Intake of Nutrient by Age for Children of Average Height, Weight, and Physical Activity Level

	Age								
Nutrient	0-6 mo	7-12 mo	1-3 yr	4-8 yr	Boys: 9-13 yr	Boys: 14-18 yr	Girls: 9-13 yr	Girls: 14-18 yr	Pregnant: <18 yr
Protein, g/day	9.1*	11	13	19	34	52	34	46	71
Protein (AMDR)	ND	ND	5-20	10-30	10-30	10-30	10-30	10-30	10-35
Carbohydrates, g/day	60*	95*	130	130	130	130	130	130	175
Carbohydrates (AMDR)	ND	ND	45-65	45-65	45-65	45-65	45-65	45-65	45-65
Fats, total, g/day	31*	30*	—	—	—	—	—	—	—
n-6 Polyunsaturated fatty acids (linoleic acid), g/day	4.4*	4.6*	7*	10*	12*	16*	10*	11*	13*
n-3 Polyunsaturated fatty acids (alpha-linolenic acid), g/day	0.5	0.5	0.7	0.9	1.2	1.6	1.0	1.1	1.4
Fats, total (AMDR)	ND	ND	30-40	25-35	25-35	25-35	25-35	25-35	20-35
Vitamin A (RAE), mcg	400*	500*	300	400	600	900	600	700	750
Thiamine (B_1), mg	0.2*	0.3*	0.5	0.6	0.9	1.2	0.9	1	1.4
Riboflavin (B_2), mg	0.3*	0.4*	0.5	0.6	0.9	1.3	0.9	1	1.4
Niacin, mg	2*	4*	6	8	12	16	12	14	18
Pyridoxine (B_6), mg	0.1*	0.3*	0.5	0.6	1	1.3	1	1.2	1.9
Folate, mcg	65*	80*	150	200	300	400	300	400	600
Vitamin B_{12}, mcg	0.4*	0.5*	0.9	1.2	1.8	2.4	1.8	2.4	2.6
Vitamin C, mg	40*	50*	15	25	45	75	45	65	80
Vitamin D, mcg	10*	10*	15*	15*	15*	15*	15*	15*	15*
Vitamin E, mg	4*	5*	6	7	11	15	11	15	15
Vitamin K, mcg	2*	2.5*	30*	55*	60*	75*	60*	75*	75*
Calcium, mg	200*	260*	700	1000	1300.0	1300	1300	1300	1300
Fluoride, mg†	0.01*	0.5*	0.7*	1*	2*	3*	2*	3*	3*
Iron, mg	0.27*	11	7	10	8	11	8	15	27
Zinc, mg	2*	3	3	5	8	11	8	9	12

Adapted from Food and Nutrition Board, Institute of Medicine: *Dietary reference intakes for energy, carbohydrate, fiber, fat, fatty acids, cholesterol, protein, and amino acids,* Washington, DC, 2005, National Academies Press; U.S. Department of Agriculture and U.S. Department of Health and Human Services: *Dietary guidelines for Americans 2010,* Washington, DC, 2010, U.S. Government Printing Office.
AMDR, Acceptable macronutrient distribution range; *ND,* no data; *RAE,* retinol activity equivalents.
*Adequate intake.
†Fluoride supplement is not necessary if the water supply contains ≥0.6 part per million fluoridation.

children who are of average height, weight, and physical activity level. If more calories than are required for energy needs are consumed, they will be converted to fat and stored. The body requires essential nutrients as well as energy for growth and health. If the food a child eats is high in calories (calorie dense) but low in nutrients (nutrient poor, which is often referred to as "empty calories"), the child will gain excess weight and still be undernourished. Data from the National Health and Nutrition Examination Survey (NHANES) from 2009 to 2010 show that 33% of American children's total energy intake came from empty calories as solid fat and added sugar (Poti et al, 2014).

Water and Electrolytes

Water

Water is the primary component of body tissue, and maintaining fluid balance is essential to good health. Because of the wide variation of healthful intake and output, there is no specific recommended daily requirement for water (Rush, 2013). Thirst is generally an adequate indicator of the need to take in more water. Children do not always appreciate the feeling of thirst, however, and may need to be offered water or foods that contain water. Infants present special concerns because they have a large skin surface per unit of body weight, their renal systems are not fully mature to process solutes, they have a high daily water turnover (up to 15% of body weight), and they are unable to express thirst. All of these factors make infants uniquely susceptible to rapid variations in water balance.

Water loss is increased by illness, activity, high altitude, high ambient temperature, and dry air. When more than 10% of body weight is lost without replacement, dehydration can become life threatening. If a child is vomiting and has diarrhea, water loss can be significant. Children who exercise strenuously, especially in a warm, dry environment, require additional water intake. After strenuous or prolonged exercise, however, high water intake without electrolyte replacement can lead to water intoxication (see Chapter 13 for a discussion regarding fluid intake during and after exercise).

Sodium

Sodium functions primarily to regulate extracellular fluid volume. It also regulates osmolarity, acid-base balance, and the membrane potential of cells and is involved in the cell membrane transport pump, exchanging with potassium in intracellular fluid. Sodium loss occurs with vomiting, diarrhea, and perspiration. Sodium requirements vary with the rate of extracellular fluid expansion, which is most rapid in infants and very young children. It is not necessary to add sodium to the diet, even for children who exercise and perspire heavily. In fact, the typical North American diet far exceeds minimum requirements for sodium intake, with most sodium coming from salt added during food processing and manufacturing. For children 1 to 3 years old, 1000 mg per day is considered an adequate intake of sodium; for children 4 to 8 years, the adequate intake is 1200 mg per day; and for children 9 to 18 years, it is 1500 mg per day (FNB and IOM, 2005).

Potassium

Potassium helps maintain intracellular homeostasis and contributes to muscle contractility and transmission of nerve impulses. Severe potassium deficit (hypokalemia) can lead to cardiac dysrhythmias and death. Excessive potassium (hyperkalemia) can cause cardiac arrest. The urinary and gastrointestinal systems regulate potassium levels, and extreme imbalances are almost always due to disease processes or medication rather than dietary factors. Potassium requirements increase as lean body mass increases and are higher during the rapid growth of infancy and adolescence than during middle childhood. Fruits, vegetables, and fresh meat have high potassium content.

Chloride

Chloride functions with sodium to maintain fluid and electrolyte balance. Loss of chloride occurs through the same routes as sodium loss: vomiting, diarrhea, and perspiration. The major source of chloride is salt (NaCl or KCl) added to foods during processing. There is no recommended daily allowance for chloride, but adequate amounts are ingested with a normal diet.

Macronutrients

Protein

Protein is a fundamental component of all body cells. Dietary protein is broken down into amino acids, which are required for the synthesis of body cell protein and nitrogen-containing compounds, some enzyme and hormone activity, cell transport, and tissue growth and development. Ten "indispensable" or essential amino acids are not synthesized by the body and must be provided in the diet (phenylalanine, leucine, methionine, lysine, isoleucine, valine, threonine, tryptophan, histidine, and arginine [arginine is required in diet for infants but not adults]). Depending on their age, children should receive approximately 5% to 30% of daily calories from proteins (see Table 10-1).

Protein and amino acid deficiencies rarely appear alone but follow other dietary deficits (such as insufficient carbohydrate intake), although young children are vulnerable to protein deficiency when cow's milk is replaced with low protein beverages, such as plant-based milk (e.g., rice, almond) (Le Louer et al, 2014). Extreme stress and disease can deplete nitrogen, a process that contributes to tissue wasting and creates an increased demand for protein. Growth needs of the premature infant require higher levels of protein intake than those of infants born at term. The demand for protein is not generally increased with normal activity except with some illnesses or to build additional muscle tissue during body conditioning.

Carbohydrates

Carbohydrates are the body's major dietary source of energy. More than half (45% to 65%) of children's body energy requirements should be supplied by carbohydrates (FNB and IOM, 2005; USDA and HHS, 2015). There are two forms of carbohydrates: simple sugars (the monosaccharides and disaccharides of sucrose, fructose, and lactose found in fruits, vegetables, milk, and prepared sweets) or complex carbohydrates (starches found in cereal grains, potatoes, legumes, and other vegetables). Most dietary carbohydrates should be in the complex form and refined food products should be limited. Because carbohydrates are essential to facilitate protein synthesis, if carbohydrates are extremely limited or absent from the diet (e.g., with a ketogenic diet used to manage intractable epileptic seizures [see Chapter 28]), the body uses stored triglycerides, oxidizes fatty acids, and breaks down dietary and tissue protein, leading to an accumulation of ketone bodies.

Fats

Lipids, fats, and fatty acids are used by the body to provide energy, to facilitate absorption of the fat-soluble vitamins (A, D, E, and K), and to maintain integrity of cell membranes and myelin. Two essential polyunsaturated fatty acids, linoleic acid (LA) and alpha-linolenic acid (ALA), are not produced by the body and must be included in the diet. These essential fatty acids are precursors of omega-6 and omega-3 fatty acids, respectively. LA is found in soy oil, corn oil, and sunflower, safflower, pumpkin, and sesame seeds. ALA is found in large quantities in flaxseed and flaxseed oil and in lesser quantities in walnuts, canola oil, and wheat germ. Adequate amounts of omega-3 and omega-6 fatty acids are produced in the body if there is adequate intake of these two essential fatty acids as well as the vitamins and minerals (vitamins B_3, B_6, and C; zinc and magnesium) necessary to facilitate their conversion.

It is recommended that fat intake for children 1 to 3 years old be 30% to 40% of total caloric intake; children more than 3 years old should gradually adopt a diet of 25% to 35% of total calories from fats. Saturated fat intake should be minimal (less than 10% of total calories in the form of saturated fat) and trans fatty acids should be excluded from the diet (FNB and IOM, 2005; USDA and HHS, 2015). Numerous studies indicate that diets with high plant fibers, limited saturated fats, low cholesterol, and zero trans fats reduce serum cholesterol and low-density lipoprotein (LDL) levels without affecting normal growth and development (Niinikoski and Ruottinen, 2012; Oranta et al, 2013). When counseling parents, providers should emphasize that a diet with less than 20% of the total energy intake from fat can put the child at nutritional risk.

Micronutrients

Vitamins

Recommendations for daily intake of fat- and water-soluble vitamins are listed in Table 10-1. Table 10-2 identifies specific metabolic functions, dietary sources, and signs of deficient or excessive intake of these vitamins.

Fat-Soluble Vitamins

Several characteristics of fat-soluble vitamins (A, D, E, and K) have implications for dietary assessment and management:

- They can be stored for long periods of time in body tissues. As a result, temporary dietary deficiencies may not affect the body's growth and development. If stores are depleted and nutritional intake is inadequate, signs of vitamin deficiency appear. If intake is excessive, which can occur when supplements are taken, toxic effects can appear.
- They are fairly stable when heated, as in cooking. Food preparation does not destroy fat-soluble vitamins as readily as water-soluble vitamins.
- They are absorbed in the intestines along with fats and lipids in foods. Low-fat diets and increased intestinal motility or malabsorption syndromes put individuals at risk for fat-soluble vitamin deficiency.
- They require bile for absorption. Conditions that compromise the hepatobiliary system put the individual at risk for decreased vitamin absorption.
- They do not contain nitrogen and do not act as coenzymes in cellular metabolism of nutrients.

Water-Soluble Vitamins

In contrast to fat-soluble vitamins, water-soluble vitamins (C and B complexes) are stored in very small amounts in the body. If water-soluble vitamin intake is more than that needed by the body, absorption (primarily in the jejunum) decreases, and excess vitamins are excreted. As a result, daily intake of water-soluble vitamins is necessary, and there is little risk of toxicity from large doses. The B vitamins contain nitrogen and serve as essential coenzymes in the body's metabolism of nutrients. Niacin (vitamin B_3) plays a significant role in increasing high-density lipoproteins (HDLs).

Minerals and Elements

Three major minerals—calcium, magnesium, and phosphorus—are present in the body in amounts greater than 5 g. DRIs have been set for boron, calcium, chromium, copper, fluoride, iodine, iron, magnesium, manganese, molybdenum, nickel, phosphorus, selenium, silicon, vanadium, and zinc. Table 10-1 identifies recommended allowances for calcium, fluoride, iron, and zinc.

Peak bone density is directly related to calcium intake during the years of bone mineralization, primarily before 20 years old. Bone calcification continues for several years more, however, so to ensure maximum peak bone density, dietary calcium needs to remain high until about 25 years old. Breastfed infants or those who are fed an approved infant formula receive sufficient calcium and should not be given a supplement. Minerals and essential trace elements, their functions, dietary sources, and signs of deficit or excess are presented in Table 10-3. Foods rich in iron are listed in Table 10-4.

Use of Vitamin and Mineral Supplements

National surveys reveal that many children in the United States have suboptimal nutrient intakes, especially a deficit of fruits and vegetables that contain many vitamins and minerals. Project EAT (Eating Among Teens) data show a trend toward eating fewer fruits and vegetables as adolescence progresses (Nielsen et al, 2014), and school-age children are at high risk for vitamin and mineral deficits (Robinson-O'Brien et al, 2010).

In light of these data and when confronted with a "picky eater," parents are justifiably concerned and often ask if

Text continued on p. 167

TABLE 10-2 Vitamins: Function, Dietary Sources, Interactions, Deficiency, and Excess

Function	Dietary Sources	Interactions Affecting Absorption or Utilization	Signs of Deficit	Signs of Excess
Fat-Soluble Vitamins				
Vitamin A				
Vision, cellular differentiation and growth, reproductive and immune system function	Liver, fish liver oils, fortified milk, eggs, red and orange vegetables, dark green leafy vegetables	Facilitated by dietary fat, protein, and vitamin E Absorption of vitamin A is hindered by lack of protein, iron, or zinc	Anorexia, dry skin, keratinization of epithelial cells of respiratory tract, night blindness, corneal lesions, increased susceptibility to infections	Headache, vomiting, double vision, hair loss, dry mucous membranes, peeling skin, liver damage Toxic at 10 times the RDA Excessive intake of carotenoids (e.g., carrots) may cause hypercarotenosis, a benign condition of yellowing of the skin
Vitamin D				
Bone growth and development; regulates intestinal absorption of calcium and phosphorus	Sunlight, artificial ultraviolet light, fortified food products, especially milk, fish	Utilization compromised in patients with renal failure Increased exposure to sunlight increases synthesis Darker skin and aging skin inhibit synthesis	Inadequate bone mineralization, rickets or skeletal malformations, delayed dentition	Anorexia, nausea, vomiting, diarrhea, weakness, hypercalcemia, hypercalciuria, calcium deposits in soft tissue, permanent renal or cardiovascular damage
Vitamin E				
Antioxidant, traps free radicals, prevents oxidation of polyunsaturated fats	Vegetable oils, margarine, nuts, seeds, wheat germ, green leafy vegetables	Low serum levels have been associated with prematurity and congenital defects of the hepatobiliary system (e.g., cystic fibrosis, biliary atresia)	Macrocytic anemia and dermatitis in infants; neurologic defects in severe malabsorption	None known in dietary doses Supplements may cause hemorrhagic effects, especially if taken long term
Vitamin K				
Forms proteins that regulate blood clotting	Green leafy vegetables, milk, dairy products, liver	Inhibited by long-term antibiotic use, hyperalimentation, chronic biliary obstruction, or lipid malabsorption syndromes	Defective coagulation of blood, hemorrhages, liver injury	Vitamin K–responsive hemorrhagic condition, especially if patient is being treated with anticoagulants
Water-Soluble Vitamins				
Vitamin C				
Essential for collagen formation and function; promotes growth and tissue repair; enhances iron absorption; improves wound healing	Vegetables and fruits, especially citrus fruits, broccoli, collard greens, spinach, tomatoes, potatoes, strawberries, peppers	Vitamin C is easily lost in food storage and preparation with exposure to heat, oxygen, and water Exposure to cigarette smoke increases vitamin C requirement	Scurvy, cracked lips, bleeding gums, slow wound healing, easy bruising	Unknown; excess vitamin is excreted in urine

Continued

TABLE 10-2 **Vitamins: Function, Dietary Sources, Interactions, Deficiency, and Excess—cont'd**

Function	Dietary Sources	Interactions Affecting Absorption or Utilization	Signs of Deficit	Signs of Excess
Thiamin (Vitamin B_1)				
Necessary for carbohydrate metabolism; promotes normal appetite and digestion	Whole grains, brewer's yeast, legumes, seeds and nuts, fortified grain products, organ meats, lean cuts of pork	Availability inhibited by presence of thiaminase (found in raw fish); alcohol contributes to thiamine deficiency Rarely, deficiency may follow gastric sleeve surgery for weight loss	Beriberi: Muscle weakness, ataxia, confusion, anorexia, tachycardia, heart failure in infants	None by oral intake; excess excreted in urine
Riboflavin (Vitamin B_2)				
Necessary for oxidation-reduction reactions; essential for function of vitamin B_6 and niacin; helps maintain integrity of skin, tongue, and lips	Dairy products, meat, poultry, fish; enriched or fortified grains, cereals, and breads; green vegetables, such as broccoli, spinach, asparagus, turnip greens	Positive nitrogen balance contributes to function of riboflavin	Oral-buccal cavity lesions, generalized seborrheic dermatitis, scrotal and vulval skin changes, normocytic anemia, dimness of vision	None known
Niacin (Vitamin B_3)				
Essential for energy metabolism, glycolysis, fatty acids; maintains nervous system, integrity of skin, mouth, tongue	Meats, fortified grains, cereals, legumes Milk, eggs, and meats contain tryptophan	Requires riboflavin for absorption and utilization Grains treated with lime have more biologically available niacin Dietary tryptophan converts to niacin	Pellagra: Dermatitis, diarrhea, inflammation of mucous membranes, indigestion	No known toxicity with dietary doses; heat rush and flushing with excessive doses
Vitamin B_6 (Pyridoxine)				
Essential for metabolism of amino acids, lipids, nucleic acids, and glycogen	Chicken, fish, kidney, liver, pork, red meat, eggs, unrefined rice, soybeans, oats, whole wheat, peanuts, walnuts, fortified cereals	Riboflavin enhances function Increased protein intake increases requirements for vitamin B_6	Seen in combination with other B-complex vitamin deficiencies; dermatitis, anemia, convulsions, neurologic symptoms, and abdominal distress in infants	Ataxia, sensory neuropathy when taken in gram quantities for months or years
Folate (Folacin)				
Essential for amino acid metabolism and nucleic acid synthesis; red blood cell formation	Liver, fortified grain products yeast, dark green leafy vegetables, green vegetables, legumes, orange juice, wheat germ	Only about 50% of folate in foods is directly bioavailable for absorption in intestine; more efficiently absorbed if serum levels are low	Megaloblastic anemia in severe cases; macrocytic anemia, glossitis, gastrointestinal disturbances; increased risk of neural tube defects and growth retardation in infants of folate-deficient mothers	None known in dietary doses; excessive folic acid supplementation may reduce serum levels of phenytoin, carbamazepine, and valproate and contribute to seizures in epilepsy controlled by these medications
Vitamin B_{12}				
Essential for neurologic function, adequate red blood cell formation, and DNA synthesis	Animal products: meat, eggs, and milk; shellfish; fortified foods	Absorbed in ileum; intrinsic factor-mediated In strict vegetarians, the vitamin excreted in the bile is reabsorbed	Megaloblastic anemia, neurologic symptoms, sore tongue, weakness	None known

DNA, Deoxyribonucleic acid; *RDA*, recommended dietary allowance.

TABLE 10-3 Minerals and Trace Elements: Function, Dietary Sources, Interactions, Deficiency, and Excess*

Function	Dietary Sources	Interactions Affecting Absorption or Utilization	Signs of Deficit	Signs of Excess
Minerals				
Calcium				
Development of bone tissue; vital role in nerve conduction, membrane permeability, blood clotting, and muscle contraction	Milk and milk products, green leafy vegetables, broccoli, kale, and collards, soft bones of fish, sardines, foods processed or fortified with calcium	Absorption enhanced in the presence of vitamin D, adequate protein intake, during periods of rapid growth, and if dietary intake of calcium is low; inhibited by excess sodium or protein	Decreased bone strength, increased risk for fractures	Constipation, increased risk for urinary stone formation; risk for decreased renal function
Phosphorus				
Essential for bone integrity and general metabolism; provides essential energy during the metabolic process	Almost all foods, especially meat, poultry, fish, milk, cereal grains; food additives in processed foods	Absorption inhibited by aluminum hydroxide in antacids and by excess iron	Bone loss, weakness, malaise, anorexia, and pain	None known
Magnesium				
Activates enzymes, facilitates cell metabolism, maintains electrical potential of cell membranes, enhances transmission of nerve impulses, assists to maintain adequate serum levels of calcium and potassium	Nuts, legumes, whole (unmilled) grains, green vegetables; bananas provide some magnesium	Absorption reduced with high-fiber diet, excess sodium, calcium, vitamin D, protein, and alcohol	Nausea, muscle weakness, irritability	None in healthy individual; with impaired renal function, excess may contribute to nausea, vomiting, hypotension, bradycardia, central nervous system depression
Iron				
Formation of the heme molecule; used in oxygen transport	Meat, eggs, vegetables, cereals, foods fortified with iron additives; Table 10-4 identifies a number of iron-rich foods	Absorption is enhanced if iron stores or daily intakes are low; presence of ascorbic acid increases absorption Heme iron in meats is more bioavailable than nonheme iron from grains, fruits, and vegetables Absorption inhibited if the iron-rich food is ingested with milk or caffeine or in presence of phytic acid, oxalic acid, or tannic acid	Anemia Children are particularly susceptible to iron deficiency during periods of rapid growth combined with low dietary iron intake: from about 6 months to 4 years old and during early adolescence; menstruation puts adolescent girls at risk	Iron poisoning can be fatal; for a 2-year-old, a fatal dose is approximately 3 g; for adolescents and adults, 200 to 250 mg/kg may be fatal
Zinc				
Cellular metabolism, growth, and repair	Meats, animal products, seafood (especially oysters), eggs	Absorption may be decreased if taken with high-fiber diet, excess iron, copper, folic acid, ascorbic acid	Anorexia, growth retardation, skin changes, immunologic abnormalities	Gastrointestinal disturbances, vomiting, acute toxicity, impaired immune response

Continued

TABLE 10-3 Minerals and Trace Elements: Function, Dietary Sources, Interactions, Deficiency, and Excess—cont'd

Function	Dietary Sources	Interactions Affecting Absorption or Utilization	Signs of Deficit	Signs of Excess
Iodine				
Production of thyroid hormones	Water, seafood, airborne water from ocean mist, iodized salt, food processing related to milk and bread	None known	Thyroid dysfunction ranging from simple goiter to cretinism and mental retardation	Thyrotoxicosis; goiter, rare and not seen in children with intake up to 1 mg/day; toxic levels not known
Trace Elements				
Selenium				
Unknown	Seafood and organ meats; may be in grains grown in soil containing selenium	Intake linked to vitamin E intake; if vitamin E is adequate, selenium is likely to be also; may need to supplement in lactating women TPN feedings contribute to deficiency	May be related to muscle weakness and pain, cardiomyopathy (Keshan disease) in young children	Nausea, abdominal pain, diarrhea, fatigue, nail and hair changes or loss; toxic levels not known
Copper				
Normal growth	Organ meats, seafood, nuts, seeds; fetus stores copper in liver during gestation	TPN feedings contribute to deficiency; high vitamin C, molybdenum, or zinc intake may reduce retention or bioavailability	Bone loss, anemia, neutropenia, growth impairment	Liver disease, gastrointestinal symptoms, diarrhea, vomiting
Manganese				
Unknown, may be related to reproductive health, normal growth	Whole grains and cereals	Increased absorption during third trimester of pregnancy	Unknown; may be related to growth retardation	Unknown; may be related to learning disabilities, anemia
Fluoride				
Prevents dental caries, enhances bone health	Fluoridated water, tea, meat and bones of marine fish, potatoes, wheat germ	Processing foods in fluoridated water or cooking with Teflon increases content; cooking foods in aluminum reduces fluoride	Dental caries; may be related to poor bone health	Mottling of teeth, kidney disease, bone disease; may affect muscle and nerve function
Chromium				
Assists in glucose metabolism	Brewer's yeast, calves' liver, American cheese, wheat germ	TPN feedings can contribute to deficiency	May be related to impairment of glucose tolerance	Unknown; requires further study
Molybdenum				
Enzyme function	Milk, beans, breads, cereals	TPN feedings can contribute to deficiency	Unknown	Related to loss of copper; may lead to gout-like symptoms

TPN, Total parenteral nutrition.
*Nearly all trace minerals are toxic in large quantities because many are metals.

TABLE 10-4 Iron-Rich Foods*

Food	High Levels (5 mg/serving)	Moderate Levels (2-4 mg/serving)	Low Levels (<2 mg/serving)
Breads, grains, cereals, seeds†	Almonds (1 cup, whole, oil roasted) Cashews (1 cup, dry roasted) Pumpkin seed kernels (¼ cup, roasted) Fortified cereals Mixed nuts (1 cup, dry roasted with peanuts) Brown glutinous rice (1 cup, cooked) Sunflower seeds (1 cup, dry roasted) Watermelon kernels (1 cup, dried) Wheat germ (1 cup, toasted)	Bagel (1, egg or plain) Bread, Indian fry (1 piece) Breadstick (10, plain, without salt) Filberts (1 cup, dried) Gingerbread (1 piece) Muffin (1 wheat) Peanuts (1 cup, dried) White rice (1 cup, enriched, regular, cooked) Waffles (2 each) Walnuts (1 cup, dried)	Biscuits (1 each) Bread (1 slice, whole wheat) Egg noodles (1 cup, cooked) English muffin (1 each) Pancakes (1 each) Peanut butter (2 Tbsp) Oatmeal (1 cup, cooked)
Fruits†	Apricot (1 cup, dried halves)	Avocado (1 whole) Currants (1 cup, dried Zante) Fig (10 each, dried) Pear (10 each, dried halves) Prune juice (1 cup) Raisins (½ cup)	Apple (1 medium, unpeeled) Apple juice (1 cup) Banana (1 medium) Dried mixed fruit (2 oz) Orange (1 medium) Orange juice (1 cup)
Vegetables†	Kidney beans (1 cup, cooked, fresh) Lentils (1 cup, cooked) Soybeans (1 cup, cooked) White beans (1 cup, cooked) Spinach (1 cup, cooked) Tofu (½ cup, cooked)	Black beans (1 cup, cooked) Garbanzo beans (1 cup, cooked) Refried beans (1 cup, canned) Beet greens (1 cup, cooked) Potatoes (1 medium, with skin, baked) Peas (1 cup, fresh, cooked) Snow peas with pods (1 cup, raw or cooked) Spinach (1 cup, raw) Molasses (2 Tbsp, blackstrap) Spinach (1 cup, frozen, cooked)	Kidney beans (1 cup, canned) Green beans (1 cup, raw or cooked) Broccoli (1 cup) Carrots (1 cup) Corn (½ cup) Lettuce (1 cup) Potato (½ cup, baked, with skin) Sweet potatoes (1 cup, fresh, boiled, mashed) Tomatoes (1 cup fresh) Tomato juice (1 cup, canned) Turnip greens (1 cup, cooked)
Meats, poultry, fish, other protein sources‡	Clams (3.5 oz, 5 each, or 1 cup = 22 mg iron) Oysters (3.5 oz) Beef heart meat (3.5 oz, cooked) Beef liver (3.5 oz, simmered) Veal liver (3 oz, simmered) Chicken liver (3.5 oz, cooked) Turkey liver (3.5 oz, cooked)	Ground beef (3 oz, cooked lean) Catfish (1 piece, floured, fried) Tuna (1 cup, canned, water packed) Lamb (3.5 oz, cooked)	Roast beef (3 oz, lean) Chicken (1 cup, dark or light meat) Egg (1, whole) Halibut (1 piece, baked or broiled) Ham (1 cup, roasted) Bacon (3 pieces, cooked) Pork (3 oz, lean shoulder roast)

Adapted from Hands ES: *Food finder: food sources of vitamins and minerals,* ed 3, Salem, OR, 1995, ESHA Research; and Hands ES: *Nutrients in food,* Philadelphia, 2000, Lippincott Williams & Wilkins.

*Cooking in cast iron pans increases iron intake, especially with high-acid foods (e.g., tomatoes).

†Iron in plant foods is better absorbed when eaten with vitamin C or meat products.

‡Iron in meat, poultry, and fish is more bioavailable than iron in other food sources.

they should be giving their child a vitamin and mineral supplement. Parents should be advised that supplements are not a substitute for food but may be appropriate in some cases. A child's intake should be assessed over a 3-day period (i.e., DRIs for all foods do not have to be met every day), and strategies to encourage the child to eat a healthful, varied diet should be put in place. If, after assessment, the provider concludes that the child is at risk for nutritional deficit, multivitamins can be given. Preterm or low-birth-weight babies and children with chronic illness may need supplements, and all pregnant teenagers should receive prenatal vitamins. The AAP recommends a vitamin

D supplement (400 IUs) in breastfed infants, beginning at discharge from the hospital (which would be in the first days of life for infants delivered at home), and children and adolescents whose diet does not include an equivalent amount. The Endocrine Society recommends vitamin D intakes of 400 to 600 IU per day to maximize bone health (Holick et al, 2011).

Assessment of Nutritional Status

Assessment of nutritional status is done to determine if there is deviation from normal growth and development, whether the child's diet is adequate, and what variables may be influencing the child's dietary intake. Much data can be collected in the intake interview or using a 3-day diet recall. Other tools available to assess diet include Bright Futures nutrition questionnaires for infants, children from 1 to 10 years old, and children to young adults from 11 to 20 years old (in the Bright Futures Tools section); the Healthy Eating Index-2010 (HEI-2010), which assesses quality of nutrient intake; as well as a variety of software programs available through the USDA National Nutrient Database (see Resources on the Evolve Website).

A review of a child's dietary intake (DRIs) is only one component of a nutritional status assessment. Ideally, intake data are combined with clinical, biochemical, and anthropometric information to provide a more complete picture of nutritional status. Also, when doing nutritional assessment, it is important to remember that eating is a social, cultural, and economic activity. The nutritional value of foods is not the only variable in a child's or family's decisions about what, how, and when to eat. In all cases, the individual's true requirement and usual intake can only be approximated. Thus, assessment of dietary adequacy for an individual is imprecise and must be interpreted cautiously in combination with other types of information about the individual.

History

Questions to elicit a history of nutritional status can be grouped into several categories:

- Nutritional status of mother during pregnancy
- Food and fluid intake of child and of family:
  - Type of feeding method used during infancy: If not exclusively breastfed, formula name and preparation. Any problems? When weaned? When solids started? Any allergies or intolerances noted?
  - Current nutritional intake of child, types and amounts of foods and fluids eaten (may use 24-hour recall, 3-day diet history, or length of time and frequency that child is at breast)
  - Additional intake (e.g., vitamin, fluoride, or iron supplements)
  - Is child's intake different from the rest of the family? How?
- Eating patterns:
  - Frequency of eating (nursing, meals, snacks)
  - Bottle feeding: Is bottle propped? Does child take bottle to bed at night or at naptime? Who feeds child?
  - Breastfeeding: On demand or scheduled? How flexible is mother to demands of infant? Is mother working? Is breast milk frozen and fed by someone other than the mother?
  - Feeding patterns or behaviors for both child and family
  - Describe mealtimes: Does family sit down together? Are meals prepared at home? Does child eat at school? How often are "fast foods" eaten? What amount of time is spent eating? How long does it take to feed child? Does the family view TV or other media during meals?
  - Does family eat out frequently? Types of restaurants? How many times per week?
- Reactions to and attitudes about foods:
  - Any reaction to particular foods (e.g., vomiting, diarrhea, abdominal pain, rash)?
  - Food preferences or dislikes? How does child demonstrate likes and dislikes?
  - Cultural factors: What beliefs or attitudes does family have about how and what child should eat or how family should eat?
  - What is child's attitude about foods and eating?
  - Feeding abilities of child: For example, does child choke, gag, vomit, have suck or swallow difficulties, or refuse certain foods, perhaps because of texture or smell?
  - Parents' and child's knowledge of foods and nutritional needs
- Management of foods in the family:
  - Who plans, purchases, and prepares food and meals for family?
  - What economic and environmental factors influence how food is managed? For example, are finances adequate to supply nutritious foods? Is there a refrigerator? Does family have a car to carry larger amounts of food from store? Is there a full-service grocery store in the neighborhood? What is the socioeconomic status of family? Is food shopping budgeted? Are food stamps or other supplemental programs used?
- Health status affected by nutrition:
  - Special considerations for children or family related to food: For example, does child have a chronic condition that requires a special diet, formula, enzymes, or device for feeding?
  - Are any medications being taken that must be given with or without food?
  - Are any medications being taken that will affect the body's ability to digest or process foods?
  - Elimination patterns
  - Dental status and care of teeth
  - Patterns of wound healing, infections, colds, and mild illnesses

- Any change in hair, nails, skin, or mucous membranes?
- Tolerance for hot or cold weather?
- Growth, activity, and exercise pattern: For example, has child been growing as parent expects? Has there been a history of unusual weight gain or loss? Does child have energy to play? Is the child engaged in strenuous activity, such as an athletic training program?
- Family history: Hypertension, diabetes, hyperlipidemia, obesity, heart disease, allergies, eating disorders?

Physical Examination

A complete physical examination with vital signs should be done with a review of all systems. Include a BMI measurement for children older than 2 years old. Plot all growth measures on appropriate growth charts (see the table on the inside front cover of this textbook for average weight and height gains expected during childhood); measure arm circumference and triceps and subscapular skinfold caliper of children at risk for obesity or malnutrition.

Diagnostic Studies

Laboratory and diagnostic studies are performed as indicated:

- Hemoglobin or hematocrit
- Iron and/or ferritin levels
- Serum levels for various elements: albumin, nitrogen balance, minerals, lipids, vitamin D
- Bone radiographs for suspected iodine, vitamins C and D, or copper deficiency or to compare bone age with height age (age at which 50% of children reach the height that the child has at the time of the examination)

Management Strategies for Optimal Nutrition

It is the parents' responsibility to provide healthful food that is adequate to meet the child's nutritional needs in an environment that makes eating enjoyable; it is the child's responsibility to decide what and how much of these healthful foods to eat (Satter, 1986). Critical to this interaction is a parent who knows which foods are healthful and which are not and who is aware of and responsive to the child's cues around feeding. Also essential is the parents' ability to provide healthful foods; this can be extremely difficult for some low-income families. Food insecurity is common among low-income multiethnic groups, even in high-income countries (Coleman-Jensen et al, 2014).

It is the providers' responsibility to counsel parents and children about making good decisions about nutrition and to facilitate families' access to healthful foods. Providers may need to refer families to public health resources for assistance to find adequate food sources (e.g., food stamps; Women, Infants, and Children [WIC] program) and/or to pediatric dietitians for access to and management of special needs diets. Providers may know what nutrients are necessary for healthy growth and development, but translating that information into day-to-day dietary intake can be complex and confusing, and counseling families can be a challenge. What advice should the provider give when there is such a wide range of "normal" intake? What does it mean, for example, that 35% or less of energy requirements should be in the form of fats? Will it be harmful if a 3-month-old is introduced to commercially prepared fruits and vegetables, or to table foods? What, if any, are the benefits of eating organic foods? Should children avoid sugar or flavored milk? The questions are endless and often without clear answers. But the basic message providers should give parents is simple (Pollan, 2008):

- Eat mostly plant-based foods (versus processed, edible food-products that contain additives, fats, and few nutrients)
- Eat appropriate portions, do not overeat
- Exercise

Developing Healthy Eating Behaviors

Parents Decide What Foods to Eat

The responsibility of parents to provide healthful foods to their children cannot be overemphasized. Children learn eating behaviors by observation and instruction, and parents are the primary teachers in the process. Often that teaching is done without conscious reflection or planning on the part of parents—both fathers and mothers—but has lifelong ramifications (Lloyd et al, 2014). Parents have a choice and a serious responsibility to their children's long-term health. They may rationalize giving their child empty calories rather than nutrient-rich food by stating, "That's all my child will eat, and I know she needs the energy." But it is the parent—not the child—who decides if an 18-month-old's "treat" is French fries or fruits. Specifically, high-sugar, high-salt, and high-fat foods should make up a very small part of the diet; however, overly restricting them, especially in children, can contribute to unhealthy attitudes toward food. If these foods are occasionally available, children learn to make better choices about how to fit them into a healthful diet. Intervention by providers in the child's first year of life to teach parents which foods are healthy and encourage them to provide those foods helps establish healthy eating patterns in older children (Vitolo et al, 2012). If children learn early that healthy, nutrient-filled foods are readily available and that their parent(s) enjoy(s) them, they are likely to enjoy them as well.

Parents Create an Environment Conducive to Healthy Eating

A positive environment related to meals, food, and eating supports healthy eating habits. Parents should be encouraged to provide the following:

- Positive examples of healthy intake; parents are the child's role model

- Limits, but not prohibitions, on consumption of non-nutritious sugars and "sometimes" foods
- Food prepared in a form that stimulates children's appetites
- Regular, structured mealtimes when the family sits down to eat together; this may occur only once a day
- A pleasant, relaxed environment for mealtimes
- Clear, developmentally appropriate expectations for children's behavior at mealtimes
- Developmentally appropriate access to and instruction in the use of utensils
- Appropriate supervision during mealtimes
- Developmentally appropriate opportunities to participate in planning, preparing, and serving meals
- Adequate exercise, sleep, and rest to stimulate appetites

Children Decide How Much of Healthful Foods to Eat

Often parents will try to decide exactly how much their child should eat (e.g., they make a child sit at the table to finish his or her vegetables). Appetite fluctuations and preferences are typical of children, and parents should be aware that children may appear to eat less than the parent thinks is sufficient or too much of one particular food to the neglect of others. If parents punish a child for not eating or force a child to eat, they have taken away the child's responsibility to choose. As a result, the child may develop an aversion to certain foods, overeat, or act-out in other ways. Mealtimes can become contests of will between parents and children, creating feelings and patterns of interacting that extend far beyond the dinner table. Parents need to find out what healthy foods their children enjoy (e.g., it is perfectly all right to eat only carrots, peas, or broccoli as one's vegetable for several weeks in a row) and make those available. If provided a nutritious variety of foods they like, children tend to select those necessary for their healthy growth, in terms of both amount of calories and other nutrients. A general principle to keep in mind when considering portions is to serve 1 tablespoon of food per year of age. For children younger than 5 years old, one serving is about one-fourth to one-third of an adult serving; for older children, one serving is about one-fourth to one-half of an adult serving. Children's appetites vary, however, and parents should be alert to cues that the child wants more or less of any particular food.

The range of nutrients available to the growing child will be greater with a wide variety of foods, but the introduction of new foods can create tension between parents and children. Parents should be informed that children may reject new foods, often because of taste or texture, as many as 15 to 20 times before they become accustomed to it and enjoy eating it. Parents should not be too concerned if a child refuses a particular food. Rather than force the child to try the new food or give in to the child's feeding demands, the food should be removed without comment, then offered again at another meal. With a well-balanced diet, not eating a vegetable prepared at one meal, for example, will not compromise the child's health. However, parents should be encouraged to avoid becoming the child's "short-order cook," preparing a special dish if the child rejects what has been fixed for the family. If a child chooses not to eat much at a particular meal, he or she will be hungrier at the next. Between meals, children should be offered age-appropriate snacks, but snacks should not be a substitute for meals; "grazing" or eating whenever food is available tends to override the child's natural sense of satiety and encourage overeating.

Strategies that can be used to increase the chances of children accepting a new food include the following:

- Offer the food when children are hungry.
- Allow children to taste a little of the food rather than eating a full portion.
- Expose children to the food by preparing and serving the food without expecting them to eat it.
- Provide an example of parents eating and enjoying the food.
- Prepare the food the way children prefer: few spices, lukewarm, and recognizable.

Finally, remind parents that individuals do not need to eat all foods. The parent may not eat some foods because of a personal dislike (e.g., anchovies, sushi, and/or cilantro); children should be accorded the same courtesy if they have been offered the food numerous times and repeatedly demonstrate dislike. There are many food options for attaining the same nutrients. As children become older, parents can help them master the social skill of politely trying new foods in new situations (e.g., visiting friends or dining in public places).

Nutritional Education

Education about nutrition should include information about children's age and developmental abilities and characteristics, nutritional requirements, foods that meet children's nutritional needs, and strategies to facilitate the development of healthy eating behaviors. Providers should explain the relationship between diet and health conditions, including obesity. Finally, providers can help parents examine their own values and patterns related to eating, identify and reinforce those they would like to foster in their children, and eliminate those they see as negative.

MyPlate, MyPlate for Kids, and SuperTracker

MyPlate, MyPlate for Kids, and the SuperTracker are useful tools for educating families and children of all ages about a healthful diet (Fig. 10-1) (see Resources on the Evolve Website, USDA). Based on DRI guidelines of the FNB and the 2010 Dietary Guidelines for Americans, these tools can be used to calculate an individual's nutrient needs by age, gender, and activity level. They illustrate proportions of a healthy diet, emphasizing a foundation of grains, fruits, vegetables (particularly beans and peas), and lean meats, fish, and poultry. These tools provide in-depth information, resources, and a wide variety of nutrition-related activities to engage individuals in assessing and planning healthy nutrition. School nutrition is also addressed.

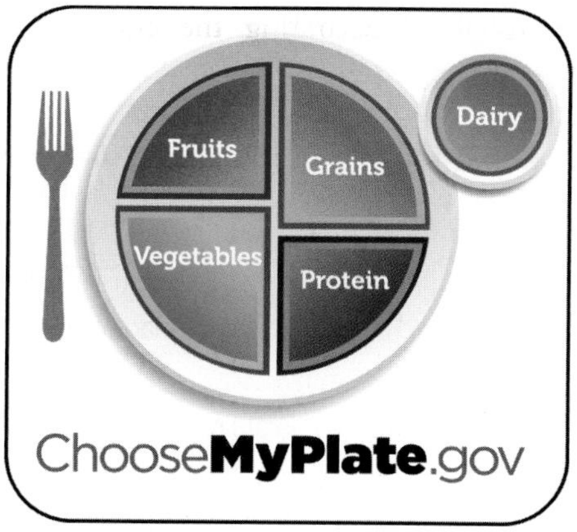

• **Figure 10-1** ChooseMyPlate. (U.S. Department of Agriculture (USDA): ChooseMyPlate (website), available at choosemyplate.gov. Accessed March 10, 2015.)

Age-Specific Considerations

Healthy eating habits are essential to good nutrition. The role that food plays in the family, the meaning it has for family members, and the way it is incorporated into family dynamics (e.g., parents may use sweets to reward children for good behavior) must be considered as providers counsel families about nutrition. Healthy eating habits begin during gestation and continue throughout the lifespan. A healthy pregnancy most often leads to a healthy term newborn, ready to learn and master the skills of eating. The toddler and preschool years are critical to establishing lifelong patterns of eating. Many eating problems, including obesity, are in part due to poor eating habits learned in infancy and early childhood that are reinforced through the school-age and adolescent years. Special considerations related to developing healthy eating habits and specific nutritional needs are presented for each of the age groups in the sections that follow.

Newborns and Infants

Energy. Rapid infant growth requires high caloric intake. The table found on the inside front cover of this textbook can be used to calculate the energy needs of infants to meet demands of metabolism and growth. Adequate intake of breast milk or infant formula meets all energy needs for infants until they are 4 to 6 months old.

Fat. For proper myelination to occur, infants must have adequate fat intake. Children younger than 2 years old can require more than 30% dietary fat for neural development. The lipids in breast milk and formulas meet infants' dietary requirements. During the second year of life, cow's milk can be included in children's diets. The AAP recommends transitioning to unflavored 2% to fat-free cow's milk for children between 12 and 24 months old. Appropriate fat content should be decided by parents and health care providers based on growth, appetite, intake of other foods, intake of other sources of fats, and potential risk for obesity and cardiovascular disease (Expert Panel on Integrated Guidelines for Cardiovascular Health and Risk Reduction in Children and Adolescents, 2011). As part of a varied diet, reduced-fat milk contributes to adequate fat intake and has no negative effect on growth or body composition (Wosje et al, 2001).

Vitamins. In general, vitamin supplements are not necessary for healthy term breastfed or formula-fed infants who eat a variety of cereal, fruits, vegetables, and proteins after 4 to 6 months old. The one exception is vitamin D (400 IUs daily) that is recommended for all breastfed infants and infants who receive an unfortified formula from birth until they are 1 year old. Infants should have an adequate source of vitamin C after they are 4 to 6 months old. A multivitamin supplement is recommended for infants at nutritional risk.

Iron. Iron deficiency is the leading cause of anemia in children, and iron supplements are necessary in some cases. Term infants who are breastfed usually have adequate iron supplies until they are 4 to 6 months old. Premature or low-birth-weight infants, infants who are exclusively breastfed beyond 4 to 6 months old, and infants who are fed cow's milk before they are 12 months old are at high risk for iron deficiency anemia. Iron-fortified cereals and iron-fortified formulas are excellent sources of dietary iron supplements for 6- to 12-month-olds. Earlier supplementation may be necessary for premature infants, especially those who are breastfed.

Fluoride. The American Dental Association (ADA) recommends fluoride treatment starting at 6 months old (Casamassimo and Holt, 2014). (See Chapter 34 for recommended fluoride dosages.) The level of fluoride in the water that is used to mix formula should be ascertained in order to ensure that infants do not receive excess fluoride. If the water supply is fluoridated, formula-fed infants younger than 6 months old can be given ready-to-feed formula, or non-fluoridated bottled water can be used to prepare formula.

Infant Formulas. Breast milk is the ideal food for newborns and infants and should be promoted unless it is medically harmful to the infant. Most iron-fortified infant formulas provide adequate nutrition and, for some families, may be an appropriate alternative to breastfeeding. Table 10-5 outlines various types of commercial formulas available.

Occasionally infants demonstrate intolerance to formula, showing irritability, weight loss or slow gain, vomiting, diarrhea, constipation, other gastrointestinal problems, or atopic dermatitis. The provider must work closely with parents to identify a formula tolerated by the infant, being careful to allow sufficient time for the baby to respond to a new formula as it is introduced. This can be a time- and energy-consuming process in which parents need support, reassurance, and encouragement. Referral to a registered dietitian can be helpful.

Introduction of Solid Foods. A number of variables converge at about 6 months that make this an appropriate time to introduce solid foods into the infant's diet:

- Infants' sucking patterns have changed sufficiently to allow mastery of chewing and swallowing.

TABLE 10-5 Specialized Infant Feeding Guidelines*: Formula Selection

	Products	Indications	Contraindications	Main Features
Breastfeeding				
	Breast milk	With very few exceptions, breastfeeding is indicated for all infants When extra fortification is required infant formula may be added to breast milk	Mother: Illegal drug use HIV-positive Infant: Galactosemia	Protein: Whey and casein, with a changing ratio over the duration of lactation Whey/casein ratios: Early lactation: 90/10 Mature lactation: 60/40
Formulas				
Routine	Enfamil Infant Similac Advance Similac Sensitive	Healthy infants born >34 weeks gestational age	Cow's milk protein allergy	Protein: Intact cow's milk proteins (casein and whey)
Partially hydrolyzed	Enfamil Gentlease Good Start Gentle Good Start Soothe Similac Total Comfort	Note: Marketed as intolerance formulas; not truly hypoallergenic Good Start Gentle: FDA approved for use in reducing risk of atopic dermatitis in high-risk infants	Cow's milk protein allergy	Protein: Cow's milk proteins partially hydrolyzed into small peptides Note: Good Start and Similac: 100% whey
Thickened	Enfamil A.R. Similac for Spit Up	Uncomplicated GERD Note: Decreased efficacy when used with proton-pump inhibitor medications (e.g. Prilosec, Prevacid)	Premature infants <38 weeks GA Do not concentrate above 24 kcal/oz	Protein: Intact cow's milk proteins Note: Contains rice starch, which thickens upon contact with stomach acid Formulation maintains appropriate nutrient composition as opposed to adding cereal to formula
Soy	Enfamil Prosobee Good Start Soy Similac Soy Isomil	Vegan diet Family preference Galactosemia (Isomil and Prosobee powder only)	Prematurity Colic Constipation Cow's milk protein-induced enteropathy	Protein: Soy protein isolates Note: All soy formulas are lactose free
Free amino acid	EleCare Infant (Abbott) Neocate Infant (Nutricia) PurAmino (Mead Johnson)	Cow's milk and soy protein allergy Multiple food protein allergies GERD Short bowel syndrome Malabsorption Eosinophilic esophagitis Galactosemia Note: Limited availability and expensive		Protein: Synthetic free amino acids Fat: EleCare and Neocate: 33% MCT oil Note: Mixing ratios differ from standard formulas; refer to manufacturer's instructions
Low mineral	Breast milk Similac PM 60/40 (Abbott)	Impaired renal function Neonatal hypoglycemia		Protein: Intact cow's milk proteins Note: Breast milk's efficient absorption rate results in a naturally low mineral content Similac PM 60/40: Iron supplementation may be needed
Post-discharge premature	EnfaCare (Mead Johnson) Neosure (Abbott)	Birthweight >2000 g (4.5 lb) and <34 weeks GA Can be used until 1 year corrected age Contraindications: Full term infants and FTT infants due to the risk of hypervitaminosis and hypercalcemia		Protein: Intact cow's milk proteins Note: Provides 22 kcal/oz at standard dilution

From Oregon Pediatric Nutrition Practice Group, 2015, available at www.eatrightoregon.org. Accessed February 24, 2015.

FDA, U.S. Food and Drug Administration; *FTT*, failure to thrive; *GA*, gestational age; *GERD*, gastroesophageal reflux disease; *HIV*, human immunodeficiency virus; *MCT*, medium-chain triglycerides.

*These are general guidelines; not intended for use in the treatment of a specific clinical condition or without medical supervision.

- Infants can sit with some support, and they are able to purposefully move their heads.
- Infants are able to grasp, pick up, and bring objects to their mouths.
- Iron stores present at birth are being depleted.
- Growth demands require nutrients other than those provided in milk alone.
- Developmental needs (cognitive, sensory, and motor) are stimulated by new foods, textures, smells, tastes, and use of utensils.

Solid foods can be introduced in whatever sequence the family desires, often based on cultural or family customs, though nonallergenic cereals are often the first infant foods. Cereals are convenient because they can be prepared in small volumes and mixed with formula or breast milk. Infants generally are able to pull the cereal from a spoon with their lips. The concept of "baby-led weaning" is gaining popularity with Western parents. Infants feed themselves soft, mashable table foods using their grasp, rather than being spoon-fed, allowing the infant more control in the feeding process. To self-feed in this fashion, an infant must have the ability to sit with little or no support and to reach and grasp for objects. Research is needed to determine if baby-led weaning is a feasible approach to infant feeding that affords protection from obesity by improving self-regulation (Cameron et al, 2012). Whether fed by spoon or finger-fed, home-prepared foods, such as grains (e.g., oatmeal, bread, crackers, and rice), soft fruits, cooked vegetables, and blenderized meats, can meet all the child's nutritional needs. Although not necessary, commercial baby foods can provide adequate nutrition, but labels should be examined to determine their content, especially for calories, fats, additives, salt, and sugar. Box 10-2 lists some principles to keep in mind when beginning solid foods.

• BOX 10-2 Principles for the Introduction of Solids into the Infant's Diet

- Introduce one food at a time, waiting a day or so before offering another to assess for adverse reaction.
- If there is a family history of allergies or atopy, consider introducing nonallergenic cereals as the first food.
- Introduce cereals, fruits, and vegetables in any sequence desired.
- Feed only iron-fortified cereals.
- Prepare food appropriate to child's developmental abilities (e.g., strained, mashed, or finger foods).
- Use home-prepared or commercially prepared foods.
- Provide a variety of foods.
- Help child develop healthy patterns of eating:
  - Be alert and responsive to child's cues when eating. Never force a child to eat.
  - Offer about 1 tablespoon per year of age as a serving for infants; for older children, offer about one-fourth to one-half an adult serving.
  - Include the child in family mealtimes.

Eating Habits. Feeding on demand in early infancy is important, and neonates should not be allowed to sleep for long periods of time without feeding. Parents should be counseled to respond promptly to a child's feeding cues and to allow the child to initiate and guide the feeding interaction. However, feeding primarily to comfort a child should be discouraged; every time a child cries, he or she is not necessarily hungry. Do not encourage the child to overeat. Bottle-fed infants, whether formula or breast milk is given in the bottle, can easily be overfed (e.g., the caregiver often urges the infant to take that extra half ounce just to empty the bottle even when the infant has indicated he or she wants to stop feeding). As a result, infants can learn to ignore feelings of satiety. Self-regulation of intake is evident in young infants, but by the early toddler years, children are influenced by social cues around feeding and can eat more than they need. Normal-weight term infants, especially those who are formula-fed, who rapidly gain weight in the first weeks and months of life appear to be at higher risk for obesity (Weng et al, 2012). Formula-fed infants introduced to solid foods before 4 months old are six times as likely to be obese at 3 years old than breastfed infants (Huh et al, 2011). Bottle feeding beyond 12 months old also appears to be a risk factor for being overweight (Bonuck et al, 2010).

A selection of varied, healthful foods gives the older infant a chance to explore textures, smells, colors, and taste. Feeding is also a time when older infants and toddlers learn physical skills of fine motor control, cognitive skills of relationships between action and consequence (e.g., the dog *will* eat whatever is dropped on the floor), and skills of social exchange among family members.

Toddlers and Preschoolers

Energy and Protein. The growth rate of toddlers and preschoolers is slower than that of infants, resulting in decreased energy needs per unit of body weight. But because of increased size and activity, these children require an increased number of total calories. Addition of muscle mass also demands a continued high protein intake.

Vitamin and Mineral Supplements. Vitamin supplements are usually not necessary for young children because many foods are fortified and, as noted, supplements should not be considered as a substitute for food. Findings from the Feeding Infants and Toddlers Study (FITS) show that most children who do not use supplements receive adequate amounts of vitamins, and adding a multivitamin supplement can actually place children at risk of excessive vitamin and mineral intake, particularly of folate, vitamin A, and zinc (Butte et al, 2010). Evaluate a child's intake over the course of a week. If children persist with *extremely* limited food choices or picky eating behavior, they might benefit from a children's multivitamin plus mineral supplement.

Eating Habits. Toddlers become more skilled in managing eating, using utensils, joining the family for regular mealtimes, and demonstrating more distinctive food likes and dislikes. They learn how and what to eat by observing adults around them and by responding to the foods adults provide for them. Older infants and toddlers may show an initial aversion to new foods and may demonstrate "food jags," eating only a few kinds of food. With time, guidance, and patience, toddlers will learn to eat a wide variety of foods (see Developing Healthy Eating Behaviors). Parents should continue to be responsive to the child's cues for hunger and satiety, providing age-appropriate portions and not insisting on the "clean-plate" approach at mealtimes.

School-Age Children

Energy and Protein. Energy and protein needs of school-age children vary greatly, depending on body size, growth patterns, and activity and exercise levels. Protein needs increase in older children as they gain more muscle mass. Active boys from 10 to 18 years old generally need between 2200 and 3200 calories a day, whereas active girls require about 1800 to 2400 calories daily; older children require the higher intake of this range (see the table on the inside front cover of this textbook).

Vitamin and Mineral Supplements. Poor eating habits place school-age children at risk for deficiencies in iron, thiamin, vitamin A, and calcium. Teaching children about specific nutrient sources and encouraging healthy eating habits can prevent many problems; supplementation with a daily multivitamin is usually not necessary—except vitamin B_{12} for the child eating a vegan diet.

Eating Habits. Food likes and dislikes carry over from the preschool years. There is great variation in appetite and intake as a result of uneven growth and activity levels. School-age children have a tendency to skip meals and are more likely to snack as they become engrossed in activities. This tendency is exacerbated in families with hectic schedules, unstructured mealtimes, and reliance on fast foods. Parents and children can identify healthful fast foods that fit a busy school-age child's schedule (e.g., homemade burritos, stir-fry chicken, peanut butter sandwiches, an apple, carrot sticks, string cheese, and a bagel on the way to soccer practice). As noted previously, high-fat, high-calorie, low-nutrient snacks (such as, chips, soda, and pizza) should be a very small part of a child's diet.

Adolescents

Energy and Protein. The growth rate of adolescents is remarkable (see the table on the inside front cover of this textbook), and the description by some parents that their children never seem to stop eating is apt. High levels of energy are needed to support adolescents' rapid growth, and if children participate in sports or other exercise programs, additional caloric intake can be needed. Adequate protein intake is essential to produce muscle mass. The average intake of protein in the American diet is significantly greater than the DRI, so additional supplementation is usually not necessary.

Vitamin and Mineral Supplements. Thiamin, riboflavin, niacin, folate, iron, zinc, and calcium needs increase during adolescence (see Table 10-1). Most adolescents who eat a well-balanced diet need no supplements, but their irregular eating habits put them at risk for deficits. Adolescent girls are at risk for iron deficiency when menstruation begins, and children who eat a vegan diet need vitamin B_{12} supplements.

Eating Habits. Eating habits of adolescents are influenced by their increasing independence and social activity, perceptions of body image, and physical growth patterns. Adolescents often have erratic eating patterns; skip meals; eat high-fat, high-calorie, low-nutrient snack foods; and consume calories late in the day. Teens who participate in sports and adolescents who eat a mainly vegetarian diet tend to have healthier eating habits than their non-sports-involved or meat-eating counterparts (Croll et al, 2006; Dunham and Kollar, 2006).

Pregnancy in Adolescence

Pregnancy presents added nutritional demands for growing adolescents. During the pubertal growth spurt, the teenager's body competes with the fetus for nutrients. This is particularly true of girls younger than 15 years old. Infants born to teenage mothers are at higher risk for prematurity, low birth weight, chronic illness, disabilities, and death. Proper nutrition and early prenatal care can increase the chance of a successful pregnancy.

The nutrition needs of pregnant teenagers also are high at a time when the typical teen is likely to have irregular eating patterns. Calcium; iron; zinc; vitamins A, D, E, and B_6; riboflavin; folic acid; and total calories—all essential to fetal growth—are often found to be inadequate in the diets of female adolescents (Baker et al, 2009).

When caring for the pregnant teenager, providers should carefully assess dietary intake and counsel the adolescent to eat a varied and healthful diet. A prenatal multivitamin and mineral supplement, including iron, calcium, and folic acid, is essential. The pregnant teenager should strive for a total of 1300 to 1500 mg of calcium through diet and supplements each day. Daily folic acid intake of 0.4 mg is recommended for all girls capable of becoming pregnant, increased to 0.6 mg during pregnancy (see Table 10-1).

Gestational weight gain in adolescents should be carefully monitored using World Health Organization (WHO) growth charts. Adolescents should not gain more than a recommended healthy gestational weight, just because they are adolescents. Healthy teens who are still growing (i.e., less than 4 years after menarche) should gain the amount they would normally gain in 9 months if they were not pregnant plus a normal gestational weight gain. For adolescents who are 4 years past menarche, gestational weight gain should be similar to that of adult women (IOM and National Research Council, 2009). Adolescents who begin pregnancy when they are overweight are at high risk for neonatal and perinatal morbidity (Todd et al, 2015). Gestational weight gains of 15 to 25 pounds in overweight and obese adult women and 15 pounds or less in morbidly obese women are associated with fewer adverse outcomes (Crane et al, 2009). There are no data on adolescents to match those of the study by Crane and colleagues, but weight gain should not be excessive, and all adolescents would benefit from comprehensive prenatal nutrition programs (Todd et al, 2015). For those adolescents who meet income guidelines, the WIC program is a valuable resource. In addition to providing nutritious foods, WIC offers nutrition education and counseling.

Physical Activity

Physical activity is integrally related to healthy nutrition. It is recommended that children and adolescents engage in 60 minutes of physical activity every day, most of which is moderate- or vigorous-intensity aerobic (exercise that makes them breathe hard); they should do vigorous activity at least 3 days a week and muscle- and bone-strengthening activity at least 3 days a week (HHS, 2009). Increased activity creates a demand for more calories and nutrients; more sedentary behavior means that the body needs fewer calories, and sedentary lifestyles combined with poor eating habits can contribute to obesity (see Fig. 13-1, Children's Activity Pyramid, for suggestions of activities).

Vegetarian Diets

Vegetarian diets are increasingly common and offer striking health benefits. If vegetarian children continue to follow a plant-based diet into adulthood, they can expect to have lower levels of obesity, high blood pressure, heart disease, diabetes, and perhaps cancer. Vegetarians tend to fall into several categories and can have extremely varied diets:

- Vegans, or strict vegetarians, eat only foods of plant origin, including fruits, vegetables, grains, nuts, seeds, tofu, and legumes (e.g., beans, peas, lentils, and peanuts). Some individuals restrict the type of plants they eat, consuming only nuts and legumes, or no fruit or some other dietary variation. Some macrobiotic diets in which whole grains form the bulk of food eaten are an extreme type of veganism; yet some macrobiotic diets include fish or meat, so they would fit in the "flexitarian" or "sometimes" category.
- Lacto vegetarians include milk and dairy products in their diet, in addition to all plant-based foods.
- Lacto-ovo vegetarians consume eggs, dairy products, and all plant-based foods in their diet.
- "Flexitarians" have a diet that consists mostly of plant-based foods, but they occasionally eat fish, chicken, or some seafood, usually avoiding or severely limiting red meat.

Vegetarian and vegan diets can meet all nutritional needs of growing children, including athletes (Van Winckel et al, 2011). For children who are lacto or lacto-ovo vegetarians, or who from time to time eat fish or other meat, it is easy to achieve adequate nutrients needed for proper growth and development. In fact, the diet of these children is often healthier and more likely to meet the Healthy People 2020 goals than that of their red meat–eating peers (Sabaté and Wien, 2010). However, strict vegan diets may be deficient in some nutrients, specifically protein, vitamin B_{12}, iron, calcium, zinc, riboflavin, and (if exposure to the sun is limited) vitamin D. Attention must also be paid to ensure adequate intake of essential fatty acids (Table 10-6).

Management

Families and children who select vegetarian diets should be supported for their healthy dietary decisions, counseled about potential deficits, educated about alternative sources of nutrients that may be lacking in the diet, and assessed regularly to ensure adequate growth and development is occurring. Nutritional assessment of the child with a vegetarian diet should include regular anthropometric measurements, diet recall and analysis, and laboratory assessment of vitamin B_{12}, zinc, iron, and vitamin D; supplementation may be necessary.

Parents and children should be counseled that some plants have less protein, or less of one kind of protein, than other plants (e.g., soy protein uses nitrogen more efficiently than wheat protein). If the diet is high in one type of protein alone, growth could be affected. Consuming a variety of plants with different configurations of protein can meet the child's needs. This combination has often been called *complementary,* one plant providing the protein lacking in another. It is not necessary that these complementary proteins be eaten in the same meal; intake throughout the day is more important (Van Winckel et al, 2011). Examples of foods that provide adequate protein intake include combinations of legumes and grains, nuts, or seeds (e.g., peanut butter on wheat bread, beans and rice, lentils and rice, lentils and sunflower seeds, peas and rye or wheat, or tofu and almonds).

Vitamin B_{12}, in the form of a supplement or fortified foods, is required for the child who is a vegan because bioavailable vitamin B_{12} is present only in animal-based foods. Most edible algae (blue-green) used in supplements contains pseudo-vitamin B_{12}, which is inactive in humans (Watanabe et al, 2014).

Iron needs of vegetarians are calculated to be 1.8 times greater than non-vegetarians because the non-heme iron in plant-based foods is less bioavailable (phytates in grains and legumes also bind with iron to decrease its absorption). Iron absorption can be enhanced by combining intake with vitamin C found in fruits and some vegetables and by processing seeds and grains (e.g., soaking, sprouting, fermenting, or making into bread). Over time, it appears that the absorption of iron from plants improves, and most vegetarians in the United States are not iron deficient (Craig and Mangels, 2009).

Phytates in grains and legumes also bind with zinc to inhibit its absorption. As with iron, eating zinc-rich foods (e.g., soy, nuts, cheese, legumes, and grains) with organic acids (e.g., citrus) and processing these foods by soaking, sprouting, or leavening with yeast increases zinc absorption. Most vegetarians in the United States do not have zinc

TABLE 10-6 Vitamins and Minerals at Risk for Deficit in Strict Vegetarian (Vegan) Diets

Vitamin and Minerals at Risk for Deficit	Usual Sources	Alternative Sources in Vegan Diet
Vitamin D	Animal products: Egg yolk, butter, liver, salmon, sardines, tuna; sunlight	Fortified cereals, milk, or margarine; sunlight (20 to 30 min/day, two or three times per week)
Vitamin B_{12}	Animal products only: Meat, fish, eggs, dairy products	Fortified soy milk, fortified soy-based meat substitutes, nutritional yeast, fortified cereals, vitamin supplements
Riboflavin	Dairy products and meat are best sources; also in eggs, dried yeast, grains, dark-green leafy vegetables, avocado, broccoli	Brewer's yeast, wheat germ, fortified cereal, beans, almonds, soybeans, tofu, dark-green leafy vegetables, avocado, broccoli, orange juice
Calcium	Dairy products are best source; also in some fruits, nuts, dark-green leafy vegetables	Fortified soy milk, dried fruits, almonds, sunflower seeds, filberts, whole sesame seeds, green leafy vegetables (at same meal, avoid eating spinach, Swiss chard, beet greens, whose oxalic acid hinders calcium absorption)
Iron	Iron in meat sources is more bioavailable than iron in plants; lentils, beans (cooked black, soy, garbanzo, lima) are good sources	All legumes, almonds, pecans, dates, prunes, raisins, fortified cereals, white or brown rice; absorption is enhanced by ascorbic acid–rich foods
Zinc	Meats, animal products, seafood (especially oysters), eggs; found in whole grains, brown rice, nuts, spinach; however, best plant sources also contain phytic acid, which inhibits zinc absorption	Whole grains, fortified cereal, brown rice, almonds, wheat germ, tofu, pecans, spinach

deficiency. Vegans are at higher risk for zinc deficiency and may need a supplement (Craig and Mangels, 2009).

Because plant-based diets tend to be high in fiber and lower in calories, the child may feel full before consuming sufficient calories and nutrients. Recent research, however, indicates that children with a high fiber intake from a wide variety of plant-based foods grow well, have adequate energy intake, and experience a reduction in total serum and low-density cholesterol levels (Niinikoski and Ruottinen, 2012). Like all children, those eating a vegetarian diet should emphasize a wide variety of nutrient-dense foods to achieve adequate energy and nutrient intake.

It is important that providers offer advice, counseling, and support within the context of the child's and family's belief system. But in extreme cases, such as highly restrictive diets resulting in growth failure or if the child is using vegetarianism as a form of eating disorder, intervention and possible referral are necessary.

Complications

A high incidence of vitamin B_{12} deficiency and suboptimal zinc status has been noted in children who eat a strict vegan diet, and children are at risk for developmental retardation without these nutrients. If girls who are vegetarian become pregnant, the fetus is also at risk for vitamin B_{12} deficiency, with potentially severe and permanent neurologic damage. Finally, some individuals with an eating disorder may choose a vegetarian diet as one way to restrict weight gain (Bardone-Cone et al, 2012).

Altered Patterns of Nutrition

Many children have chronic illnesses, developmental disabilities, developmental special needs, or handicapping conditions that affect their nutritional status. According to the 2011 to 2012 National Survey of Children with Special Health Care Needs, approximately 14.6 million (19.8%) American children 17 years old or younger have special health care needs, and some 10% of those have nutritional problems, specifically related to swallowing, digesting, or metabolizing food (HHS, Health Resources and Services Administration, Maternal and Child Health Bureau, 2013).

The number of children with chronic conditions that require specialized nutrition interventions is increasing as a result of expanded screening programs, increased survival rates, and improved prognosis for the very small (less than 1500 g) underdeveloped neonate. Nutritional management of children with special health care needs requires a multidisciplinary team and interventions directed at specifically diagnosed feeding problems. Physical, occupational, and speech therapists, particularly speech pathologists, can assess head and trunk control, positioning, body mechanics, and

• BOX 10-3 Suggested Criteria for Nutrition Referral

Markedly overweight or underweight (height or length for weight less than the 5th or more than the 95th percentile)
Mechanical feeding difficulties or neuromotor dysfunction
Feeding skills less than those anticipated for developmental level or mental age
Unusual food habits (e.g., pica or food faddism)
Inadequate or imbalanced dietary intake, according to dietary history or 24-hour recall
Nutrition treatment central to medical management (e.g., inborn errors of metabolism, diabetes, congestive heart failure, malabsorption syndromes, allergy)
Overt physical signs of nutritional deficiency (e.g., extreme underweight, overweight, anemia)
Emotional disturbances and associated feeding and nutrition problems (e.g., anorexia nervosa, autism)
At high risk for compromised nutritional status (e.g., takes stimulant or anticonvulsive drugs, family below poverty level, inadequate housing, pregnant adolescent)

oral-motor skills. Depending on the child's symptoms and diagnosis, gastroenterologists, allergists, endocrinologists, and other specialists may need to participate in the child's care; surgical and medical intervention may be necessary. For children who are socially or economically deprived, or both, public health nurses, social workers, and psychologists are central to appropriate assessment, counseling, and referral to outside services and agencies. Pediatric dietitians can be critical to success, and the family must be included as an integral component of the team. Primary care providers must carefully assess the nutritional status of children in this population and make appropriate referrals. Children who meet the criteria outlined in Box 10-3 should be referred to a registered dietitian for comprehensive nutrition assessment and further referral or treatment.

Nutrition and health problems are related in a number of ways: Some conditions require more caloric intake (e.g., athetoid cerebral palsy); others require less (e.g., Prader-Willi); some, depending on the individual, may require either more calories or fewer calories (e.g., autism). Some conditions demand special supplements or vitamins and others require special feeding strategies (e.g., the child with cleft palate). The following section outlines principles of care in these categories and highlights several specific conditions.

Disorders Requiring Increased Caloric Intake

A common nutrition problem in children with special health care needs is inadequate weight gain and delayed growth. Inadequate caloric intake should be suspected in any child with a weight-to-age ratio below the 10th percentile on standardized growth and BMI charts. For children who are genetically small or have a disabling condition that limits growth, a weight-to-length ratio or weight-to-height ratio below the 10th percentile indicates suboptimal nutrition. A number of conditions put children at risk for insufficient caloric intake, including the following:

- Conditions in which activity level is increased, either by purposeful or involuntary muscle work, such as athetoid cerebral palsy, attention-deficit/hyperactivity disorder (ADHD), or chronic lung conditions
- A hypermetabolic state (sometimes complicated by secondary malabsorption), which may be present in the child who has acquired immunodeficiency syndrome (AIDS), cancer, burns, fever, or frequent infections, or who has recently had surgery
- Chronic renal insufficiency
- Psychosocial factors, such as inadequate resources, poor feeding relationship with caregiver, and improper dilution of formula, which can lead to delayed growth and require increased calories for the child's catch-up growth
- Oral-motor impairment or chronic conditions, such as congenital heart disease (CHD), which can contribute to fatigue and poor feeding
- Low-birth-weight or premature infants
- Medical treatment (e.g., a child receiving corticosteroid treatment for Crohn disease)
- Conditions in which malabsorption occurs (e.g., cystic fibrosis)

Clinical Findings

When a child is malnourished, regardless of cause, the nutritional insult follows a predictable course. In the early stages, the child maintains or begins losing weight, then the child's linear growth slows or ceases. Finally, head circumference, indicating compromised brain development, levels off.

History

A thorough history should be taken, assessing for the following:

- Diet and eating habits:
  - Type and amount of foods and liquids consumed (e.g., nutrient content and consistency)
  - Amount of food that falls from utensils, cups, or bottles during feeding and is not ingested
  - Physical effort and time required for meal (i.e., the child can sometimes use more calories eating than he or she consumes)
  - Any impaired oral functions (e.g., poor suck and swallow, tongue thrust, drooling, difficulty chewing, choking, or aspiration)
  - Position of child during feeding
  - Family's pattern of feeding child (e.g., time, place, and utensils used)
  - Child's apparent food likes and dislikes
- Other reported concerns may include:
  - Paleness
  - Fatigue, inactivity
  - Vulnerability to infections
  - Delayed healing

BOX 10-4 Growth Charts for Children with Special Conditions

- Achondroplasia
- Cornelia de Lange syndrome
- Cri du Chat syndrome
- Down syndrome
- Marfan syndrome
- Noonan syndrome
- Prader-Willi
- Pseudoachondroplasia
- Rubinstein-Taybi syndrome
- Russell-Silver syndrome
- Trisomy 13
- Trisomy 18
- Turner syndrome
- Williams syndrome
- Myelomeningocele, male and female, 2 to 18 years old
- Sickle cell anemia

From Gripp KW, Slavotinek AM, Hall JG, et al: *Handbook of physical measurements,* ed 3, Oxford, 2013, Oxford University Press; Platt OS, Rosenstock W, Espeland MA: Influence of sickle hemoglobinopathies on growth and development, *N Engl J Med* 311(1):7–12, 1984.

- Behavior problems; irritability
- Poor academic performance, poor vocabulary
- Perceptual difficulties

Physical Examination

Anthropometric measurements are reliable indicators of a child's growth and development, especially if measured accurately and compared over time. Growth charts indicate the child's height, weight, head circumference, and BMI at a point in time, as well as whether the child is following a consistent growth curve over time. Growth charts specific to children with various chronic conditions have been developed, although there can be problems with their use and interpretation and they should be used with caution (Box 10-4). Because these charts are "descriptive" of the growth of small populations, they may overrepresent undernourished individuals, particularly if the condition is associated with oral feeding difficulties (Brooks et al, 2011). Anthropometric measurements taken at each visit include the following:

- Height, weight, weight-to-height ratio, BMI, head circumference
- Mid-upper arm circumference and triceps skinfold measurements

A feeding evaluation can be included in the physical examination, particularly for the child with oral-motor or behavioral problems associated with eating. In this type of assessment, parents or caregivers are asked to replicate the home experience, using the same types of foods, utensils, and positioning. If possible, the parents should videotape the child eating at home, and providers should review the video with them. By observing the interaction between the child and the caregiver during feeding, the health care team can more accurately assess feeding success and problems, along with emotional or psychological issues related to feeding.

Diagnostic Studies

Laboratory studies are done if indicated, including hematocrit or hemoglobin for anemia, serum ferritin and transferrin levels, and metabolic screening (chemistry screen).

Initial basic workup for failure to thrive (FTT) (see Chapter 33) includes complete blood count (CBC) with reticulocytes, chemistry screen and thyroid studies, urinalysis with culture and sensitivity, stool for ova and parasites and stool culture for enteric pathogens (e.g., *Escherichia coli*), and bone age.

Management

The management of the child with delayed growth or poor weight gain varies with the underlying cause of the problem and often requires intervention by specialists. Although the primary provider can coordinate the plan of care, a team approach to management is needed.

A child with an increased activity level, a metabolic condition that increases energy requirements, or a condition that decreases the body's ability to absorb nutrients needs to receive caloric- and nutrient-dense meals and snacks frequently, at 2- to 4-hour intervals.

A child with a chronic disease that decreases the appetite (e.g., AIDS, cancer) needs creative approaches that consider food preferences, optimal times of day for snacks and meals, and family dynamics that encourage eating. Some children may be placed on medication to stimulate their appetite.

A child with a condition that affects oral-motor control will need special equipment, specific feeding techniques, proper positioning, and use of foods and liquids with appropriate consistency to improve oral intake.

A child who is not receiving enough food because of neglect, inadequate financial resources, or other psychosocial factors requires referral to appropriate health care professionals and social services. The public health nurse can be an invaluable resource for these children.

Although feeding by the oral route is preferable from a developmental perspective, tube feedings or parenteral feedings may be necessary. Frequently, a medical crisis precipitates the use of supplemental feedings.

Premature or low-birth-weight infants (particularly those with a poor suck) frequently require supplemental feedings. Breastfeeding is both possible and desirable for these infants and ensuring that they receive higher-fat hindmilk is important; pumping may be necessary (see Chapter 11). Human milk fortifiers (i.e., adding formula to breast milk) or premature formulas that increase the caloric density from 20 to 24 kcal/oz can be used. Regular infant formulas can be mixed to increase the kilocalorie-to-ounce ratio from 20 to 24 kcal/oz or 27 kcal/oz, and nutrient-dense formulas for older infants and children are available (see Table 10-5).

Practical suggestions for increasing calories, protein, and nutrients needed for weight gain and growth are outlined

• BOX 10-5 Suggestions for Increasing Energy Intake

Establish regular times for meals and snacks, 2 to 4 hours apart. Do not allow the child to nibble continually on small amounts of food.
Keep mealtimes relaxed and pleasant. Avoid scolding, nagging, or forcing the child to eat.
Allow the infant or child to provide cues regarding hunger and satiety.
Use readily available, economic foods that are familiar to the child.
Fortify milk by adding 1 cup of nonfat dry milk powder to 1 quart of whole milk. Drink or use to prepare cooked cereals, creamed soups, pancakes, pudding, and milkshakes. (Do not use with children younger than 24 months.)
Add additional butter or cheese to potatoes, vegetables, casseroles, rice, pasta, cooked cereals, and so on.
Encourage high-calorie snacks, such as dried fruits, nuts, bananas, cheese cubes, pudding or custard, cereal with whole milk, fruit yogurt (alone or as a dip for fruit), cheese or peanut butter on crackers, olives, or sliced or mashed avocado (as a dip for vegetables or crackers).
Add instant breakfast mixes to whole milk.
Use commercially prepared formula with high calorie content.
Use commercial liquid supplements, such as PediaSure, for children with lactose intolerance.

• BOX 10-6 Estimating Catch-Up Growth Requirements*

$$\text{Catch-up growth requirement (kcal / kg / day)} = \text{Calories required for weight age (kcal / kg / day)} \times \text{Ideal weight for age (kg)} \div \text{Actual weight (kg)}$$

1. Plot the child's height and weight on the WHO or CDC growth charts.
2. Determine at what age the present weight would be at the 50th percentile (weight age).
3. Determine recommended calories for weight age (see the tables on the inside front cover of this textbook).
4. Determine the ideal weight (50th percentile) for the child's present age.
5. Multiply the value obtained in step 3 by the value obtained in step 4.
6. Divide the value obtained in step 5 by actual weight.

Estimated protein requirements during catch-up growth can be calculated similarly (see Table 10-1):

$$\text{Protein requirement} = \text{Protein required for weight age (g / kg / day)} \times \text{Ideal weight for age (kg)} \div \text{Actual weight (kg)}$$

CDC, Centers for Disease Control and Prevention; *WHO,* World Health Organization.

in Box 10-5. A "complete" multivitamin and mineral supplement is also recommended, because it contains the entire spectrum of these nutrients and can usually be chewed or crushed and mixed into soft foods. For children who are underweight or growth retarded, it is not sufficient to simply increase intake to age-specific norms. These children require excess calories and protein for "catch-up" growth until growth is normalized. A method for calculating calories and protein required for catch-up growth is presented in Box 10-6. Calculations for catch-up growth in children with chronic diseases that contribute to poor weight gain (e.g., cystic fibrosis) can be found in more detailed nutrition texts. Some chronic conditions may require more complex treatment, such as growth hormone therapy. Frequent monitoring of the child with inadequate caloric intake is necessary. Infants should be weighed at least weekly, and length and head circumference should be measured once a month. Children older than 2 years old should be measured for height and weight at least once a month.

Complications

Children with a chronic medical condition that requires increased caloric intake are at risk for frequent illness, medical complications, and impaired development, including growth delay. In some cases, restoring nutritional status does not ultimately resolve growth deficits. In the case of environmental deprivation, the success of catch-up growth depends on the timing, length, and severity of the nutritional insult.

Complications secondary to treatment must also be considered for children with caloric deficits. Providers must be alert to negative effects caused by a sudden change to a high-calorie, high-protein diet. The child on a high-protein diet should be counseled to drink adequate fluids. Care must be taken that infants do not receive excess protein in concentrated infant formulas because the breakdown and excretion of protein by the kidneys may place an excessive demand on the renal system. Diarrhea can result from an abrupt increase in carbohydrate intake. Gradually changing the child's diet can decrease these negative effects.

Disorders Requiring Decreased Caloric Intake

Health conditions that contribute to decreased metabolic activity or reduced energy output in children can require a decrease in caloric intake. If children's caloric intake exceeds their metabolic needs, they are at risk for overweight, obesity, and additional health problems.

Any disorder or disability that reduces energy output places the child at risk for overweight. Obesity is common, for example, in children with Prader-Willi syndrome, myelomeningocele, or Down syndrome. Excess weight gain occurs in 50% of children with spina bifida (Spina Bifida Association, 2014).

The child with Prader-Willi syndrome is hypotonic and may demonstrate dysphagia and FTT as an infant. By 3 to 4 years old, the child becomes hyperphagic, lacking the internal regulation responsible for satiety. Children with Prader-Willi syndrome are short in stature. Most children with Down syndrome have short stature, and before they are 3 years old, they may have a low weight-to-height ratio.

As a result of a lower resting metabolic rate or hypothyroidism, a child with Down syndrome requires fewer calories than a child without the syndrome, and overweight is common, but not inevitable; its incidence can be decreased with healthy eating and exercise habits begun in early childhood (Ivan and Cromwell, 2014).

Clinical Findings

History

The history should assess the following:

- Level of physical activity in which child engages
- Diet recall (3 days) and mealtime patterns
- Concerns and attitudes of parents and child regarding weight gain
- Previous interventions or attempts to control weight
- Risk for overweight and its complications (e.g., diabetes mellitus, limited mobility, family history of obesity)
- Use of food as a reward or incentive for desired behavior

Physical Examination

Key components of the physical examination include the following:

- Weight-to-height or weight-to-length ratio: Ratio greater than 75th percentile on growth chart indicates at risk for overweight; greater than 95th percentile indicates overweight
- Triceps skinfold measurement (greater than 85% of norm indicates overweight)
- Mid-upper arm circumference
- Body frame type; central adiposity and waist circumference (used more in adults)
- Muscle mass
- BMI in the 85th to 95th percentile indicates overweight; 95th percentile or higher is obese

A child's growth pattern is evaluated over time. A child who is consistently in the 85% weight-to-height ratio may be genetically programmed to be big, whereas a child who suddenly moves from the 60% to the 90% weight-to-height ratio can be developing a weight problem.

Diagnostic Studies

Laboratory studies include those to rule out metabolic conditions that may cause overweight (e.g., thyroxine [T_4] and thyroid-stimulating hormone [TSH] to rule out hypothyroidism). Because of complications of obesity (e.g., hyperlipidemia, hypercholesterolemia), children older than 4 years old should be monitored annually for risk factors, and tests should be done as appropriate, including blood glucose, complete lipid profile, and liver function tests.

Management

The goal of nutritional management of children with medical conditions that reduce energy expenditure is to ensure that the child receives adequate nutrients without excessive caloric intake. Families should be referred to a registered dietitian to establish an appropriate caloric level and eating plan individualized to each child's growth needs. A complete multivitamin with mineral supplement is recommended because a restrictive diet can result in nutrient deficiencies. Children should be encouraged to engage in regular physical activity. Although they may not be able to meet the recommended 60 minutes of moderate to vigorous activity each day, the goal is to increase calories used and the child's level of fitness. A team approach, involving a physical or recreational therapist or both, is advised to develop exercise strategies.

In some cases (e.g., children with brain dysfunction affecting hypothalamic control or Prader-Willi syndrome), access to food needs to be rigidly enforced and may include locks on refrigerators, cupboards, and garbage cans in the child's environment. Frequent monitoring is necessary to assess compliance and devise alternate strategies as indicated; weekly weight and monthly height measurements are recommended.

Support is essential for families and children. Despite the best efforts, many children gain excess weight. Primary care providers can model and encourage a positive, accepting attitude toward the child, independent of weight gain or loss.

Disorders Requiring Restricted or Supplemental Diets

Body metabolism requires hormone, enzyme, or cofactor activity. When there is either too much or not enough of these factors, or when absorption of nutrients is limited, nutritional status is at risk. Under these conditions, nutritional intake must be adjusted by restricting diet or adding supplements (e.g., enzymes) in order to maximize the body's ability to use foods.

A number of metabolic conditions or defects of absorption or transport affect nutritional status in children (Table 10-7), and primary care providers may be part of the team managing the care of a child with inflammatory bowel disease (Crohn disease or ulcerative colitis), short bowel syndrome, celiac disease, or other conditions that fall into this category.

Metabolic disorders may be due to inborn errors of metabolism, genetic conditions other than inborn errors of metabolism, and autoimmune diseases (see Chapter 26). Surgical intervention, drugs and medications, tumors, and infectious disease also contribute to metabolic dysfunction and problems of absorption or transport. For some individuals, a genetic predisposition to the disorder can be triggered by environmental factors, and the disorder appears later in life.

Clinical Findings

Clinical findings related to specific disorders are discussed in Unit 4. If nutrition is inadequate in children with these chronic conditions, clinical signs and symptoms worsen, pathophysiologic processes of the disorder accelerate, and health is compromised.

TABLE 10-7 Metabolic Conditions Affecting Nutrition in Children

Organ Affected	Excessive Hormone/Enzyme Production	Deficient Hormone/Enzyme Production
Pancreas	Reactive hypoglycemia Organic or fasting hypoglycemia	Diabetes mellitus Cystic fibrosis
Thyroid	Hyperthyroidism Graves disease	Hypothyroidism
Parathyroid	Hyperparathyroidism	Hypoparathyroidism
Adrenal cortex	Cushing syndrome Corticosteroid therapy	Addison disease Congenital adrenal hyperplasia
Inborn errors of metabolism		PKU (deficiency of phenylalanine hydroxylase) Maple syrup urine disease Tyrosinemia Urea cycle disorders Organic acidemias Fatty acid oxidation disorders Galactosemia Glycogen or lysosomal storage disorders

PKU, Phenylketonuria.

Management

Disorders of absorption and metabolism are usually managed with specialized diagnostic studies and treatments and require the efforts of a coordinated health care team. Although not a cure for disease, nutrition is an essential component of treatment plans and can make a critical difference in the child's outcome. The goals of nutritional intervention in these conditions are to provide for normal growth and development, maintain optimal health, prevent or delay complications related to progression of the disease (e.g., diarrhea, fistulas), and prevent or delay the need for more aggressive intervention (e.g., bowel resection).

Nutritional intervention in chronic disorders can be extremely complex. Referral to a registered dietitian is necessary, and primary providers should consult frequently with the dietitian. In some conditions, dietary restrictions are lifelong requirements, and success of dietary intervention depends on the child's and family's willingness to adhere to the plan of care. Cooperation is enhanced if the child and family are actively included in decision-making and if meal plans are developed that minimize disruption to the family's lifestyle and maximize flexibility and normalcy for the child. Families and children must be given ample opportunity to express their concerns and frustrations regarding the child's condition. Support, empathy, and encouragement from providers can be vital elements in determining how well a family copes with the child's chronic condition.

Certain principles of nutrition related to disorders of absorption and metabolism guide the dietitian, primary care provider, and family as they create diet plans. Boxes 10-7 through 10-10 outline these principles for several specific conditions.

Complications

See Unit 4 for complications of specific disorders. Additionally, fetuses of women with higher than normal phenylalanine levels are at risk for microcephaly, congenital heart defects, and other birth defects. All pregnant women should be questioned about a history of phenylketonuria (PKU) or special diets during childhood, and maternal PKU should be considered in any woman who has delivered an infant with microcephaly or has experienced spontaneous abortion, as the phenylalanine level may be high enough to damage the fetus without harming the mother.

Disorders Requiring Physical Alterations in Diet Management

Physical conditions, such as cleft lip or palate, esophageal atresia, cerebral palsy, gastroesophageal reflux, and pyloric stenosis, can create difficulty sucking, chewing, swallowing, or retaining food and liquids in the gastrointestinal tract. Most of these conditions are congenital, and a combination of environment, heredity, and behavior appears to influence their development. Stenoses, atresias, or fistulas can also be secondary to environmental trauma, such as a chemical burn.

Gastroesophageal reflux (GER) is common in normal individuals following a meal. All babies "spit up," especially directly after a feeding or when burped. A small regurgitation of undigested formula or breast milk is usually not of concern. GER in infants can occur during, immediately after, or several hours after a feeding and can be exacerbated

• BOX 10-7 Principles for Dietary Management of Diabetes Mellitus

- Individualize diet: There are many types of meal planning systems for those with diabetes; what works best for child and family, minimizes conflicts and issues of control and "normalizes" child's intake. Many programs rely on a liberal diet plan with close insulin coverage.
- Space food intake to account for type of insulin used.
- Structure diet to include foods that everyone else eats; do not be overly restrictive; use insulin coverage to allow child to eat as typical a diet as possible.
- Vary specific nutrient intakes depending on child's age, size, and activity level.
- Evidence suggests that there is no ideal percentage of calories from carbohydrate, protein, and fat for all people with diabetes; therefore, macronutrient distribution should be based on individualized assessment of current eating patterns, preferences, and metabolic goals. Once the desired amount of carbohydrate intake is determined, learn to "count carbs." Identify estimated grams of carbohydrates (carbs) in certain foods (e.g., there are about 15 g in one slice of bread or one six-inch tortilla). Learn to read food labels to find grams of carbs per serving.
- Maximize carbohydrate intake from vegetables, fruits, whole grains, legumes, and dairy products rather than from other carbohydrate sources, especially those that contain added fats, sugars, or sodium.

Vitamins and Minerals

- Same as for child without diabetes; if diabetes is poorly controlled, supplements are recommended.

Sweeteners

- Noncaloric sweeteners, such as aspartame and saccharine, may be used but are not encouraged.
- Caloric sweeteners, such as fructose, sucrose, glucose, sorbitol, and mannitol, can be used (with caution) as a substitute for carbohydrate calories.
- Excess sorbitol intake can contribute to diarrhea.

Adapted from American Diabetes Association: Executive summary: standards of medical care in diabetes—2014, *Diabetes Care* 37(Suppl 1):S5–S13, 2014.

by increased intraabdominal pressure (as with crying, coughing, defecation, or external pressure from movement or position). Children with insufficient lower esophageal sphincter tone are especially susceptible to GER. Reflux becomes symptomatic early in life, peaks at about 4 months old, and spontaneously resolves for most children by 12 to 24 months old. GER is a common problem in children with cerebral palsy. These children (and others with neurodevelopmental problems) may already have difficulty chewing or coordinating suck-swallow skills, and, if GER is present, the child may refuse food. Gastroesophageal reflux disease (GERD) is discussed in Chapter 33.

Clinical Findings

History

A thorough history of the infant's feeding patterns, incidence of gagging or vomiting, arching and crying during

• BOX 10-8 Principles for Dietary Management of Cystic Fibrosis

- Nutrients needed (high protein, high fat, high energy) may cause physical distress; work with family to help them understand the balance between comfort and adequate nutrition sought.
- Small, frequent meals, eaten slowly are better tolerated.
- Consume nutrient-dense foods; avoid "empty calories."
- Increase fluid intake to prevent dehydration and help liquefy secretions.
- Assess intake on a 3- to 5-day diet record rather than daily.

Energy

- Energy needs are increased as a result of malabsorption of nutrients, extra effort needed for respirations, and frequent pulmonary infections. At least 120% to as much as 150% of recommended dietary allowance (RDA) caloric intake is recommended.
- Vary caloric intake for each child, depending on condition, activity, and growth.

Carbohydrates

- Obtain 40% to 50% of total calories from carbohydrates. Simple sugars may be better tolerated than complex carbohydrates.
- Include extra fiber; increase fiber as complex carbohydrates are increased.

Protein

- Higher need than for children without cystic fibrosis; 15% to 20% of caloric intake should be in proteins.
- Breastfed children may need supplements (e.g., casein hydrolysates).

Fat

- Increase to level of tolerance, minimum of 35% and as much as 40% to 50% of total caloric intake.
- Use medium-chain triglyceride (MCT) oils to enhance absorption and decrease steatorrhea.
- Use corn or soy oil and include absorbable linoleic acid in diet to ensure essential fatty acid intake.

Vitamins and Minerals

- Daily multivitamin supplement and water-soluble preparation of vitamins A, D, and E are recommended; 50 to 100 mcg/day of vitamin K is recommended.
- Daily calcium supplements are necessary to prevent bone loss.
- Normal diet is usually adequate to replace sodium lost through excessive sweat; can use salt tablets (intake is more easily monitored than adding salt to diet) if exercise or fever leads to profuse sweating.

Supplements

- Pancreatic enzymes should be consumed with all meals and snacks.
- Other supplements include casein hydrolysates and powdered or liquid nutrient-dense preparations.

• BOX 10-9 Principles for Dietary Management of Phenylketonuria

- Intervene promptly. Infants who begin treatment before 3 weeks old do not suffer mental retardation secondary to phenylketonuria (PKU).
- All children require phenylalanine in their diet. Mother's milk and/or standard infant formula furnish this during infancy.
- The goal of PKU dietary therapy is to prevent excess phenylalanine accumulation in the body.
- Recommended daily intake of phenylalanine is individualized based on laboratory monitoring. Maintain serum phenylalanine levels between 2 and 6 mg/dL in children. Plasma phenylalanine levels greater than 6 mg/dL should be controlled with dietary therapy. Dietary restrictions continue for life.
- Most foods contain phenylalanine (approximately 5% of all protein is phenylalanine).
- Involve older children in preparation of nutritional supplements.
- Supplements may be more palatable if served as frozen drinks or flavored with juices or fruits.

Energy, Carbohydrate, Fat, Vitamin, and Mineral

- Basic requirements are same as for child without PKU. Restrictions on high-phenylalanine carbohydrates.
- Daily multivitamin is recommended unless needs are met with phenylalanine-free formula.
- Nutrient requirements not met by commercial formulas must be supplemented by a phenylalanine-deficient food.

Protein

- Recommendations for total protein intake exceed age- and gender-specific dietary reference intakes (DRIs), because L-amino acids found in most medical foods are absorbed and oxidized more rapidly than amino acids in intact protein of a regular diet.
- Low or minimal phenylalanine medical foods are necessary to meet protein requirements.

Adapted from Singh RH, Rohr F, Frazier D, et al: Recommendations for the nutrition management of phenylalanine hydroxylase deficiency, *Genet Med* 16(2):121–131, 2014.

• BOX 10-10 Principles for Dietary Management of Inflammatory Bowel Disease

- Restrict irritating and poorly absorbed foods (e.g., carbonated beverages, fried foods, and spicy foods).
- Decrease intake of foods that stimulate peristalsis (e.g., high-fiber foods) during inflammatory periods. High-fiber foods, especially those that retain water, can be introduced as clinical signs and symptoms decrease.
- Small, frequent meals are better tolerated.
- Vary specific nutrient intakes depending on child's age, size, activity level, and severity of disease.
- Exclusive enteral nutrition early in disease is recommended by some (Day and Burgess, 2013). Mild disease can require supplemental formulas; severe disease can require enteral elemental nutrition via tube feeding or total parenteral nutrition.
- Condition can be complicated by lactose or gluten intolerance.

Energy

- Teens need 40 to 50 kcal/kg of ideal body weight per day; younger children need up to 120 kcal/kg of ideal body weight per day.

Protein

- Greater than 1.5 g/kg of ideal body weight per day.

Fat

- Low fat (40 g/day) intake is necessary.
- Emulsified fats or medium-chain triglycerides (MCTs; commercial preparation) are better tolerated.

Vitamins and Minerals

- Take a 100% to 150% daily multivitamin with minerals supplement.
- May need additional vitamin and mineral supplements (e.g., water-soluble vitamins, vitamin B_{12} intramuscularly), folic acid, iron, zinc, copper, calcium, potassium, and magnesium.

feeding, timing of emesis in relation to feeding, character and quantity of emesis, and associated symptoms is essential. Parents also should be asked about treatments they have tried and whether they have been successful.

Physical Examination

Clinical signs can be present at birth, and a diagnosis of the underlying condition, such as cleft lip or palate, can be made in the delivery room. Roentgenography and endoscopy are used to confirm atresias or fistulas. Some conditions, such as pyloric stenosis, occur later in the neonatal period (see Chapter 33).

Management

The treatment goals related to conditions that require biomechanical or physical intervention include the following:

- Provide adequate nutrients for normal growth and development.
- Provide increased calories to add more weight if needed before surgical procedures.
- Strengthen infant's resistance to infection.
- Prepare infant to tolerate stress of surgical procedures.
- Facilitate healing processes postoperatively.
- Ensure correct development and use of oral-facial and oropharyngeal muscles and structures.
- Minimize disruption of family processes.
- Prevent development of feeding problems.

Some conditions require surgical correction of the underlying condition. In many cases (e.g., a simple cleft lip), initial surgical intervention is sufficient and the child progresses normally. In others, especially for the child with serious or multiple anomalies, long-term treatment is required. Additionally, the treatment itself can lead to problems that require further management. For example, correction of esophageal atresia, tracheoesophageal fistula, or presence of a tracheostomy can result in scarring and strictures, which in turn put the child at risk for impaired swallowing, choking, and aspiration. Table 10-8 lists strategies related to feeding children with cleft lip or palate. GER usually can be managed in the outpatient setting. Table 10-9 lists specific suggestions related to managing GER.

Providers must also support parents emotionally and psychologically as they care for their children. Parents of a child with birth anomalies can suffer shock, loss, guilt, anger, or disappointment and may find it difficult to accept their child. Difficult feeding or uncertainty about the child's long-term prognosis adds additional pressure to parents who are already facing an extremely stressful situation. Creating a positive feeding experience can facilitate a healthy parent-infant bond. Providers can intervene in the following ways:

- Encourage parents to express their feelings.
- Listen without judging, acknowledging those feelings.
- Demonstrate techniques that increase feeding success.

TABLE 10-8 Strategies for Feeding in Children With Cleft Lip or Palate

Age	Problem Presented	Management Strategies
Infants	Poor suction when nursing	Individualize position used to feed infant; semi-upright (60 to 90 degrees) position is often most effective.
	Nasal regurgitation	Breastfeed if possible; experiment with nipple position: position nipple toward side of mouth, do not put nipple into cleft.
	Swallows air	Use of longer, soft, or cross-cut nipples and squeezable bottles benefits infants with weak suck. Specialty nursing bottles require training of parents to ensure effectiveness. Use of prosthetic device may be helpful. Wean child by 12 months old. Tube or gavage feedings may be necessary in severe cleft. Burp frequently.
	Fatigue	Allow sufficient time for feeding; work toward providing adequate nutrients in 30 minutes.
Toddlers	Risk of aspiration Nasal regurgitation	Encourage use of cup, spoon, and finger foods as developmentally appropriate. Avoid small, hard, sticky foods that can lodge in palate opening; supervise feeding.
School-age children and adolescents	Malocclusion Difficulty coordinating chewing, swallowing, and breathing Aspiration Anorexia secondary to decreased sense of taste and smell	Dental referral and treatment are essential. Teach child how to chew, swallow, and breathe; not to talk and chew at the same time. Inform parents that child will chew with mouth open. Cut food into small pieces; child can take sips of water while eating. Plan diets that stimulate appetite; provide child's favorite foods.

TABLE 10-9 Strategies for Feeding in Children With Gastroesophageal Reflux

Condition	Management Strategies
Mild	Position infant in flat prone position after feeding if awake and being observed; position in flat supine position if infant will be sleeping. Semi-sitting position applies abdominal pressure and causes more reflux. Burp frequently during feeding. Thicken formula with rice cereal if formula feeding to decrease episodes of vomiting. May need to use large-hole nipple. One tablespoon of rice cereal per ounce of regular 20 kcal/oz formula increases energy density to 34 kcal/oz, so infant may be at risk for excess intake unless volume per feeding is decreased. Consider using anti-regurgitation (AR) formulas that thicken in the stomach without changing the energy composition.
Moderate to severe	Position infant in flat prone position after feeding if awake and being observed; position in flat supine position if infant will be sleeping. Prone or lateral position is not recommended for sleep due to risk of sudden infant death syndrome (SIDS) (Vandenplas et al, 2009). If formula fed, use trial of extensively hydrolyzed or amino acid–based formulas. If breastfed, try removing cow's milk from mother's diet. Reduce volume at each feeding; may need to increase caloric density of feeding to meet infant's energy needs. Consult with pediatric gastroenterologist. Medication may be indicated (see Chapter 33). Surgical referral may be necessary in cases that do not respond to medical management.

- Explain the child's condition, treatments, and prognoses, both short and long term.
- Emphasize how the parent can be involved in the child's progress.
- Encourage parents to make decisions related to their child's care; provide suggestions and guidance as the child grows, as treatment is carried out, and as needs change.
- Give positive reinforcement for parents' success.

Complications

Aspiration with damage to lung tissue, FTT, poor parent-child bond, esophagitis, and esophageal strictures are complications of difficulty in feeding.

Eating Disorders

An eating disorder is defined as "a situation where the time spent eating (or not eating) in response to an external stimulus is greater than the time spent eating in response to internal hunger cues" (Hahn, 1998, p 395). Although problems with feeding (e.g., colic, food refusal, picky eating) are common among children, anorexia nervosa, bulimia, and binge (or out of control) eating are the conditions most frequently identified as eating disorders in the pediatric population. These conditions are discussed in detail in Chapter 19.

Obesity and Overweight

Excessive adipose tissue is the hallmark of obesity and overweight, and it may be due to an increase either in the size of fat cells (hypertrophy) or in the number of fat cells (hyperplasia). Childhood-onset overweight that is hyperplastic in nature is especially difficult to control because fat cells can be reduced in size but not in number.

BMI and weight-for-height ratios are used to define parameters of overweight. In adults, normal BMI ranges from 18.5 to 24.9, and an individual is defined as obese if BMI is 30 or greater. In children, the definition of obesity and overweight is less specific, especially for infants and toddlers. Children are compared with a normative group of peers, and percentiles specific for their age and gender are considered to be a more valid indicator of underweight, normal weight, overweight, or obesity than is an absolute BMI. Children 2 to 18 years old with a BMI greater than or equal to the 95th percentile for age and gender, or those with a BMI greater than or equal to 30 (whichever is lower) are considered obese. Children with a BMI between the 85th and 95th percentiles for age and gender are overweight. This terminology avoids the confusion of "at risk for overweight or obesity" and more clearly categorizes those obese children who are likely to have health problems as a result of their weight. There are no BMI parameters for children younger than 2 years; those with a weight-to-height ratio of greater than or equal to the 95th percentile are categorized as overweight. BMI measurements must be used cautiously to assess individual children, because some children have a body weight or BMI in excess of the norm for their age, gender, and height without having excess fat. Children who have genetically larger skeletal frames, for example, or athletic adolescents with more muscle mass may weigh more and may have a higher BMI than their peers.

The rapid rise in overweight and obesity in the United States occurred between the 1960s and 2000, with about 5% of all children 2 to 19 years old being obese in the 1971–1974 NHANES study, and 13.9% in 1999–2000. NHANES data from 2012 found that nearly one third (31.8%) of American children 2 to 19 years old were overweight OR obese; approximately 17% were obese (Fryar et al, 2014). The *severity* of obesity has also worsened. In 1976 to 1980 NHANES data, 1.1% of boys and 1.3% of girls were severely obese (120% of the 95th percentile) (Wang et al, 2011). By 2012, that number had increased to 5.9% of all children 2 to 19 years old. In 2010, nearly 12% of children 2 to 19 years old had BMIs equal to or greater than the 97th percentile; and in 2012, 2.1% had BMIs equal to or greater than 140% of the 95th percentile (Skinner and Skelton, 2014). There is a significant difference in obesity prevalence by race and gender (Fryar et al, 2014): 12.6% of 2- to 19-year-old non-Hispanic white boys, 19.9% non-Hispanic black boys, 24.1% Hispanic boys, and 24.2% Mexican American boys have BMIs equal to or greater than the 95th percentile. Similar differences are found in girls: 15.6% of non-Hispanic white girls, 20.5% non-Hispanic black girls, 20.6% Hispanic girls, and 21.1% Mexican American girls are obese.

Overweight and obesity are increasingly common among infants and toddlers. Although both providers and parents seem reluctant to identify infants as obese, NHANES data from 2011 to 2012 indicate that nearly 10% of children younger than 2 years old are overweight (95th percentile or greater for weight to recumbent height), and data from the Early Childhood Longitudinal Study found 31.9% of 9-month-olds and over 34% of 2-year-olds either at risk or obese (Moss and Yeaton, 2011). Ongoing research indicates that "fat babies" will not necessarily be healthy children. Rapid weight gain in infants from birth to 8 months old and overweight and obesity in infants and toddlers are strong predictors of overweight in children and adolescents, putting them at risk for subsequent obesity and metabolic syndrome (Moss and Yeaton, 2012, 2014).

Risk Factors and Predictors for Obesity

Obesity results from a complex relationship of genetics, environment, and the body's response to environmental factors (e.g., neurohormonal regulation). Although studies show a variety of risk factors and predictors for obesity (Box 10-11), the specific moderators of excess weight gain vary and the relationship among variables is complex. New discoveries of the factors (e.g., hormones, brown fat, microbes, and brain activity) involved in the dynamics of satiety, insulin sensitivity, and weight regulation are being made daily. It may be that most obesity is a function of a genetic

• BOX 10-11 Risk Factors and Predictors of Overweight and Obesity in Children

- Maternal smoking during pregnancy
- Rapid weight gain in infancy, beginning at birth
- Bottle feeding
- Early introduction of solids
- Intake of high-glycemic foods (e.g., sugars, soda, processed bakery goods) (contributes to disruption of normal balance of hormones, proteins, and so on, leading to hyperinsulinemia and insulin resistance)
- Limited intake of high-fiber foods (e.g., whole grains, fruits, vegetables) (contributes to disruption of normal balance of hormones, proteins, and so on, leading to hyperinsulinemia and insulin resistance)
- Use of food as a reward or a "comfort" during stress
- Sedentary lifestyle (e.g., watching television, screen time with technology, limited physical exercise)
- Television in the bedroom
- Overweight or obese parents
- Family stressors
- Middle or low socioeconomic status

predisposition combined with environmental stimuli (Locke et al, 2015). The following discussion outlines what are currently believed to be major causes or predictors of obesity.

Biological Mechanisms

First, a biologic imbalance of hormones, peptides, proteins, and other factors may contribute to obesity; extensive research is being done in this area with exciting discoveries that may yield clinical application in the future. Insulin and leptin are two major hormones that normally serve to control satiety and influence weight. Resistance to insulin and to leptin, which is seen in some racial and ethnic groups and often found in obese individuals, may contribute to the body's failure to register satiety. Lustig (2006) posits that chronic hyperinsulinemia may be the source of insulin and leptin resistance. Leptin normally stimulates the ventromedial hypothalamus (VMH), sending the message that the body has adequate energy stores. Insulin and leptin share the same "signaling cascade" in the VMH, however, and if insulin levels are high, leptin is prevented from signaling its message of satiety. Hyperinsulinemia thus prevents the message that the body is satiated from getting through, and overeating to satisfy a feeling of hunger can result. Hyperinsulinemia in children has three sources: genetics, epigenetics (small- and large-for-gestational-age infants experience hyperinsulinemia and insulin resistance), and environment. Environmental dynamics contributing to hyperinsulinemia are threefold:

- Increased stress leads to increased cortisol production, which can lead to insulin resistance.
- Decreased physical activity contributes to insulin resistance.
- Diet, especially high levels of fructose and decreased fiber, leads to excess insulin secretion. "High-glycemic" foods (such as, soda, sweetened juices, processed breads, pastries, and crackers) are more quickly converted to serum glucose, and they stimulate a sharp rise in insulin production. With the high insulin level, glucose is moved quickly into cells, the extra insulin stays in the blood, and the resulting hypoglycemia stimulates hormone release that further increases appetite. The end result is overeating and increased fat storage (Lustig, 2008).

Food Addiction

A second proposed etiology for obesity is the concept that some people may be "addicted" to certain foods; animal and human research in this area is expanding to determine to what extent and by what mechanisms food may be addictive (Ziauddeen et al, 2012). Others contend that food, per se, is not addictive, but a dietary pattern of restricting and bingeing, especially fats and sweets, can lead to a behavioral (in contrast to physiological) addiction (Avena et al, 2012). Overweight children may increase their intakes of "comfort foods" when stressed (Roemmich et al, 2011) or engage in emotional or night eating (Wildermuth et al, 2013).

Physical Activity

Decreased physical activity is a third explanation for increased overweight and obesity: less physical activity results in decreased energy consumption and, logically, if dietary intake remains the same, individuals will gain weight; increased physical activity would lead to weight loss. With the obesity epidemic, it is argued that children have increased the time they spend on sedentary activities (e.g., "screen time" with television, computers, hand-held electronic devices), more schools have discontinued physical education classes (Centers for Disease Control and Prevention [CDC], 2014), many children are driven to school rather than walking or riding bicycles, and many neighborhoods are unsafe for outdoor play. These are all environmental factors that contribute to the problem of excess weight gain. The use of electronic media by children is rapidly becoming the norm. Although television is still used more frequently than other media by young children, nearly twice as many children younger than 8 years old used mobile devices in 2013 than in 2011 (72% vs. 38%), and the time spent using them tripled over those 2 years (Rideout, 2013). Thirty-six percent of children younger than 8 years old and over two thirds of all children have a television in their bedroom (Rideout, 2013; Strasburger et al, 2010). The Common Sense Media survey found that children younger than 8 years old watch about 1 hour of television per day (Rideout, 2013). Although most older children watch television, they prefer online interaction. According to a recent study, 96% of 13- to 24-year-olds watch free online video (approximately 11.3 hours per week), 71% view subscription online video (10.8 hours per week), and 57% watch free online television (6.4 hours per week). Eighty-one percent of 13- to 24-year-olds watch broadcast, cable, and satellite television (8.3 hours per week) and an additional 56% watch prerecorded television (7.5 hours per week) (DEFY Media, 2015). Excess screen time and having a bedroom TV are associated with increased risk of obesity (Wethington et al, 2013).

The relationship between a more sedentary lifestyle and obesity appears straightforward, but it may not be that simple. Although most children do not get the amount of exercise recommended by the Centers for Disease Control and Prevention (CDC), it is hard to say how much less active today's children are than those of previous generations. Although, as noted, increased physical activity contributes to weight loss, it may not be lack of physical activity alone that is at the heart of the problem. Changes in eating habits, rather than a decrease in physical activity, may be more important. Watching television replaces active play, but it also exposes children to snack-food advertising and increases the likelihood that children will overeat and eat more empty calories. This pattern of overweight and poor nutritional intake related to watching television is international in scope (Sigman, 2012).

Temperament

A fourth risk factor for obesity may be temperament; in one study, 12-month-old male infants with shorter attention spans and female infants with a greater need to be soothed or negative reaction to food were more likely than their counterparts to be overweight at 6 years old (Bergmeier et al, 2014).

Psychosocial and Environmental Factors

A number of psychosocial and environmental factors put children at risk for being overweight (see Box 10-11). Food may be used to regulate emotions or cope with stress, or individuals may overeat in response to inappropriate body image perceptions, social pressure to be thin, depression, and low self-esteem. Children who suffer neglect or abuse or have an overcontrolling parent may turn to food for comfort and solace, with overeating as a result. An association has been found between caesarean section births and obesity; it is posited that the process of vaginal delivery may affect the infant's metabolism and immune system in ways that make the child less susceptible to becoming overweight (Darmasseelane et al, 2014). Some research suggests that prenatal exposure to endocrine disruptors, such as bisphenol-A or estrogen, may predispose to overweight and obesity (Dhurandhar and Keith, 2014), but associations are inconsistent and more research is needed to more adequately assess whether such exposure is associated with childhood obesity and related conditions (metabolic syndrome, diabetes, and future cardiovascular disease) (Meeker, 2012).

Clinical Findings

Clinical assessment of obesity is the first step to effectively address the problem. Unfortunately many providers do not conduct thorough assessments or address the topic of weight in their routine well-child care. A study examining provider's perceptions of what they had done to assess weight found large discrepancies between what providers said they had done and what they documented having done. For example, 93.1% of physicians reported they had calculated BMI, but only 79% actually documented the data; and only 22% of the children found to be obese were documented as being so (Chelvakumar et al, 2014). Reviewing data from the National Hospital Ambulatory Medical Care Surveys from 1997 through 2000, Cook and colleagues (2005) found that of nearly 33,000 well-child visits for 2- to 18-year-olds, only 281 (0.78%) had a diagnosis of excess weight gain, obesity, or morbid obesity, despite the fact that approximately 15% of this population reportedly had BMIs equal to or greater than the 95th percentile.

Additionally, most parents of overweight children perceive their child as normal weight or even underweight, so they may not present a concern to the pediatric provider. A recent meta-analysis of studies worldwide found "the overall rate of parental underestimation of overweight/obese child's weight" to be 67.5% (corrected to 50.7% to allow for heterogeneity of study findings) (Lundahl et al, 2014). This analysis also found that one in seven parents underestimated their normal-weight child's weight; overweight parents were more likely to state that their normal-weight child was underweight. Another meta-analysis affirmed that 63% of parents of overweight children fail to recognize overweight of their child, and 86% of parents of overweight 2- to 6-year-olds fail to recognize it (Rietmeijer-Mentink et al, 2013).

History

The history should review patterns of eating and exercise for both the child and the family system. Also consider underlying factors and comorbid conditions, such as hypothyroidism, polycystic ovary disease, depression, diabetes, and cardiovascular disorders. The history should include the following:

- Dietary intake, including:
  - Total caloric intake and nutrient adequacy
  - Fat intake as percentage of total calories
  - Carbohydrate intake as percentage of total calories
  - Portion sizes
  - Amount of sweetened beverages, sodas, and 100% fruit juices consumed
- Eating patterns, including breakfast, eating outside home, frequency, and types of meals and snacking
- Exercise pattern and hours and type of sedentary activity
- Parental obesity
- Age at onset of excessive weight gain
- Family history of diabetes and cardiovascular disease (hypertension, CHD)
- Family or child history of hypothyroidism or other medical conditions that could contribute to overweight
- Episodes of sleep apnea
- Social adjustment, peer group, friends

TABLE 10-10 Calculation and Interpretation of Ideal Body Weight from Centers for Disease Control and Prevention Growth Charts*

Ideal Body Weight for Healthy Children	Interpretation
>120%	Overweight
90%-110%	Normal
80%-90%	Mildly underweight
70%-79%	Moderately underweight
<70%	Severely underweight

From Centers for Disease Control and Prevention (CDC): Growth charts.
*Ideal body weight percentage = Current weight ÷ Weight at 50th percentile for current stature × 100

- Family and child readiness and ability to participate in a weight management treatment program based on healthy eating and activity
- Barriers to exercise and healthy eating (e.g., environmental constraints, physical disability)

Physical Examination

A complete physical examination is necessary to determine the child's level of fitness and anthropometric status, looking especially at the following:

- Blood pressure (measured with cuff that covers 80% of arm) and vital signs
- Height and weight (height-to-weight ratio is a better indicator than BMI of overweight in infants and children younger than 2 years old)
- BMI and ideal body weight (Table 10-10)
- Skin (for acanthosis nigricans)

Diagnostic Studies

- Fasting lipid profile
- Fasting glucose tolerance test
- Thyroid screen, TSH, T_4
- Metabolic panel
- Glycated hemoglobin (HbA_{1c})

Differential Diagnosis

The differential diagnoses include medical conditions, such as hypothyroidism, polycystic ovary disease, Down syndrome, and Prader-Willi syndrome.

Management

Pediatric providers often state that they are uncomfortable managing childhood obesity (Chelvakumar et al, 2014), and they may not raise the issue with parents and their children. Only 25% of the parents of children identified on the NHANES as having an 85% or higher BMI recalled being told by the provider that their child was overweight (Perrin et al, 2012). National data from 2010 found that less than 40% of children seen by pediatric providers were counseled on healthful exercise; about 56% were counseled on healthy nutrition (HHS Agency for Healthcare Research and Quality, 2014). A review of data from 2001 through 2004 indicated that only about one quarter (24.4%) of normal-weight children 4 to 18 years old received obesity prevention counseling (i.e., diet/nutrition and exercise) during well-child visits. A concerning finding in this latter study was that Hispanic children, children on Medicaid, and children seen in hospital-based clinics (populations at high risk for obesity) were significantly less likely than Caucasian, insured children to receive counseling (Branner et al, 2008). Further, parents' misperceptions that their child is not overweight or obese may hinder treatment, especially if the intervention plan requires family lifestyle changes. These misperceptions may also put normal weight children at risk of being encouraged to overeat, which is an issue that may need to be addressed by the provider as a part of well-child care.

Prevention of overweight and assertive treatment of children who are already overweight are priorities for care, and lifestyle changes are key to successful treatment.

Lifestyle Changes

For most children who are overweight or obese, the primary goal of weight management is to normalize, not necessarily reduce, weight. Because children are growing and developing, recommendations for treating overweight focus on slowing the rate of weight gain, thereby allowing children to grow into their weight. If the child is beyond a weight into which he or she will reasonably "grow," weight reduction becomes the treatment goal.

A staged management approach with active monitoring by the primary care provider and involvement of the entire family is recommended (Barlow and Expert Committee, 2007). Both the child and family must change their lifestyle patterns, and family therapy may be necessary. If initial efforts are unsuccessful, more rigorous management may include behavior modification, highly structured monitoring and control, multidisciplinary interventions, medication, or surgery.

Providers can use motivational interviewing (described in Chapter 9) when working with adolescents and parents of overweight children to make lifestyle changes. This approach allows the provider to:

- Educate parents about:
  - Children's growth patterns and nutritional needs
  - Ways children communicate hunger and satiety
  - Strategies for developing healthy eating habits
  - Strategies to encourage physical activity in children
  - Risk factors for overweight
  - Early indicators of overweight
- Assist parents and adolescents to recognize problems related to the child being overweight and clarify goals
- Assist parents and adolescents to identify barriers to weight loss and strategies to overcome them

- Assist parents to implement behavioral change interventions, including lifestyle changes suited to the family's structure, abilities, and needs
- Provide ongoing support to families
- Monitor the child for anthropometric parameters (every 3 months)
- Identify, assess, and reward other parameters of progress with the child and family (e.g., improved dietary habits; increased physical activity, fitness, strength, and enhanced self-esteem)

Effective treatment for obesity may also need to take into consideration the "subgroups" of obese children: chronically obese (i.e., have never been normal weight), transiently obese (i.e., have significant weight gain and then spontaneous loss without treatment), children with a dual diagnosis or significant comorbidity (e.g., ADHD, depression), and obese children who are "well-functioning" (Panzer, 2010). When the entire family is involved, the overweight child has a much greater chance to normalize weight. Box 10-12 outlines suggestions for counseling overweight children and their families.

Community Changes

Individual and family interventions may not be sufficient to deal with the causes of obesity. If children cannot safely play outside, for example, it may be impossible for them to get the recommended 60 minutes of moderate-to-vigorous daily exercise they need. Community change is imperative to support individual and family efforts to lose weight. The CDC recommends community action in six different areas (CDC, 2009) (see Resources on the Evolve Website):

- Increasing access to affordable healthy foods
- Supporting healthy food choices
- Promoting breastfeeding
- Encouraging physical activity
- Providing safe communities in which to exercise
- Organizing at the grass roots to create and continue health-supportive change

Primary care providers can make the detailed recommendations presented in the CDC Guidebook that is available to community policymakers, give policymakers information about obesity as a public health problem, and support public policy that creates positive change.

Medications

Lifestyle changes should be the primary treatment for obesity in children and adolescents. Medications should only be used after an intensive, formal trial of lifestyle change has proven ineffective and the child is excessively obese (greater than 95th percentile) or overweight (greater than 85th percentile) with comorbidities present (Boland et al, 2015), and even then medications should be an adjunct to diet and exercise programs—not the only intervention used. Several medications are used to control weight in adults and adolescents, some available over the counter (OTC) or as herbal or diet supplements. Providers should inquire about whether the family or child is self-medicating

• BOX 10-12 Parental Guidelines for Managing Childhood Weight Problems

- Do not put child on a diet (unless medically indicated and supervised). Instead, gradually modify *the entire family's* eating habits. For example, serve fruit as a substitute for dessert, switch to nonfat or 1% milk, experiment with low-fat, low-sugar recipes and methods of food preparation, and use reduced-fat salad dressings and other condiments.
- Breastfeed infants if at all possible. If not breastfeeding and infant is at risk for overweight or obesity, consider providing lower-protein formula (within the range of normal protein—the infant should *not* be given an inadequate protein intake). Higher protein content in infant formula has been found to be related to higher body mass index (BMI) and higher fat mass in infants and young children (Escribano et al, 2012; Weber et al, 2014).
- Respond to cues of satiety. Do not force infants to empty the bottle or children to clean their plates. They should eat only until they are full.
- Serve age-appropriate portions (e.g., one-quarter to one-third adult portion for young children).
- Schedule and maintain regular times for meals and snacks. Do not skip meals. Do not allow children to "graze" throughout the day.
- Have a family meal at least five or six times a week, eating, sharing, and enjoying food together.
- Reduce the number of meals eaten outside the home (e.g., in restaurants, fast-food chains).
- Serve low-calorie, low-glycemic, nutritious snacks, such as fresh fruit and vegetables, air-popped popcorn, pretzels, low-fat yogurt, frozen fruit juice bars, skim milk, and low-sugar cereals. Do not have high-calorie, high-glycemic snacks (e.g., chips, cookies, cakes, pies, ice cream, candy, soda pop, and doughnuts) in the home.
- Increase fiber intake. The Institute of Medicine's (IOM's) dietary reference intake (DRI) for dietary fiber is 14 g fiber/1000 kcal consumed or between 19 and 38 g per day in children, depending on age (Kranz et al, 2012).
- Do not use food as a reward.
- Do not overly restrict children's intake. This approach can actually lead to overeating and subsequent overweight.
- Promote physical activity. Start slowly, with low-weight–bearing exercise. Set reasonable goals and celebrate achieving them. Make daily exercise a priority. Encourage family participation, individual exercise, and team sports and structured activities with peers as appropriate. Strive for 1 hour or more a day of vigorous activity.
- Limit "screen time" to 2 hours or less per day. Replace screen time with family activities, hobbies, or chores. Remove televisions from children's bedrooms (if present). Children who watch 4 or more hours of television per day are twice as likely as other children to become obese. Children are more sedentary when they watch television, and frequent food advertising is linked to increased snacking.
- Praise and reward children for the progress they make in reaching nutrition, activity, physical fitness, self-esteem, or weight goals.
- Emphasize the uniqueness of each child, pointing out special talents, abilities, and positive qualities.

and with what products. Orlistat (decreases fat absorption) is approved by the U.S. Food and Drug Administration (FDA) for children 12 years and older, and it is available OTC and by prescription; OTC preparations should not be taken by children younger than 18 years old. Several appetite suppressants (phentermine and metformin) are used to treat obesity in adults. Metformin does not have FDA approval for use in treatment of obesity, but it has been used experimentally. All these medications have potential side effects and, other than orlistat, are not recommended for use with children and adolescents (Boland et al, 2015). Orlistat is contraindicated in individuals with gallbladder disease, malabsorption syndromes, pregnancy, and sensitivity to the drug. Major side effects of orlistat are fatty stool and gastrointestinal upset; fiber supplements (e.g., glucomannan) can be used to help control side effects.

Surgery

Bariatric surgery (Roux-en-Y gastric bypass; laparoscopic adjustable gastric binding) has not been widely used as a therapy for adolescents and children, but can be effective in treating morbidly obese adolescents with comorbidities (Brandt et al, 2010). In the recent past, the use of sleeve gastrectomy has increased in all age groups, including adolescents (Pallati et al, 2012).

Adolescents selected for bariatric surgery using criteria set by the National Institutes of Health (NIH) should have a BMI of 40 or higher, be at their adult height, and have serious health problems, such as type 2 diabetes or sleep apnea, that may improve with surgery (National Institute for Diabetes and Digestive and Kidney Diseases [NIDDK], 2011).

Some providers believe that having surgery during adolescence (rather than waiting until adulthood) may be more beneficial for some individuals with childhood-onset obesity (Fitzgerald and Baur, 2014), and a recent study indicates that bariatric surgery of 277 adolescents was generally safe (8% had major complications; 15% minor complications within a 30-day postoperative period) (Inge et al, 2014). However, the surgery has potentially serious side effects, and adolescents must be carefully monitored to determine risks and benefits and to clarify exact indications for surgery (Nobili et al, 2015).

Although surgery has been used experimentally in younger children (Dan et al, 2010) and more frequently in adolescents, primary care providers are still cautious about referring patients for the procedure. Table 10-11 summarizes recommendations for both pharmacotherapy and bariatric surgery when treating adolescents.

Complications

Children who are overweight are at much higher risk for related conditions, including hypertension, impaired glucose tolerance, sleep apnea, orthopedic problems (e.g., slipped capital femoral epiphysis), social rejection, lowered self-esteem, depression, and suicide. In a child with a

TABLE 10-11 Recommendations for Pharmacotherapy or Bariatric Surgery

Expert body	Recommendations for Pharmacotherapy	Recommendations for Bariatric Surgery
American Academy of Pediatrics (AAP)	Candidates have: (a) attempted comprehensive multidisciplinary intervention; (b) maturity to understand risks; (c) willingness to maintain physical activity.	Severe obesity not responsive to behavioral interventions
Endocrine Society	Pharmacotherapy considered if formal intensive lifestyle modification has failed to limit weight gain and severe comorbidities persist after lifestyle modification; BMI must be >95th percentile or >85th percentile with significant comorbidities. Pharmacotherapy should only be offered by clinicians who are experienced in the use of antiobesity agents and are aware of the potential for adverse reactions.	Tanner stage 4 or 5 and at final or near-final adult height BMI >50 or BMI >40 and significant, severe comorbidities Severe obesity and morbidity persists in spite of formal lifestyle modification program, with or without medication trial Psychological evaluation confirms the stability and competence of the family unit Access to an experienced surgeon in a medical center capable of providing long-term follow-up, and the institution is participating in a study of bariatric surgery outcomes or sharing research data The patient demonstrates the ability to adhere to the principles of healthy diet and activity

Data from August GP, Caprio S, Fennoy I, et al: Prevention and treatment of pediatric obesity: an Endocrine Society clinical practice guideline based on expert opinion, *J Clin Endocrinol Metab* 93(12):4576–4599, 2008; Woo T: Pharmacotherapy and surgery treatment for the severely obese adolescent, *J Pediatr Health Care* 23(4):206–212, 2009.

BMI, Body mass index.

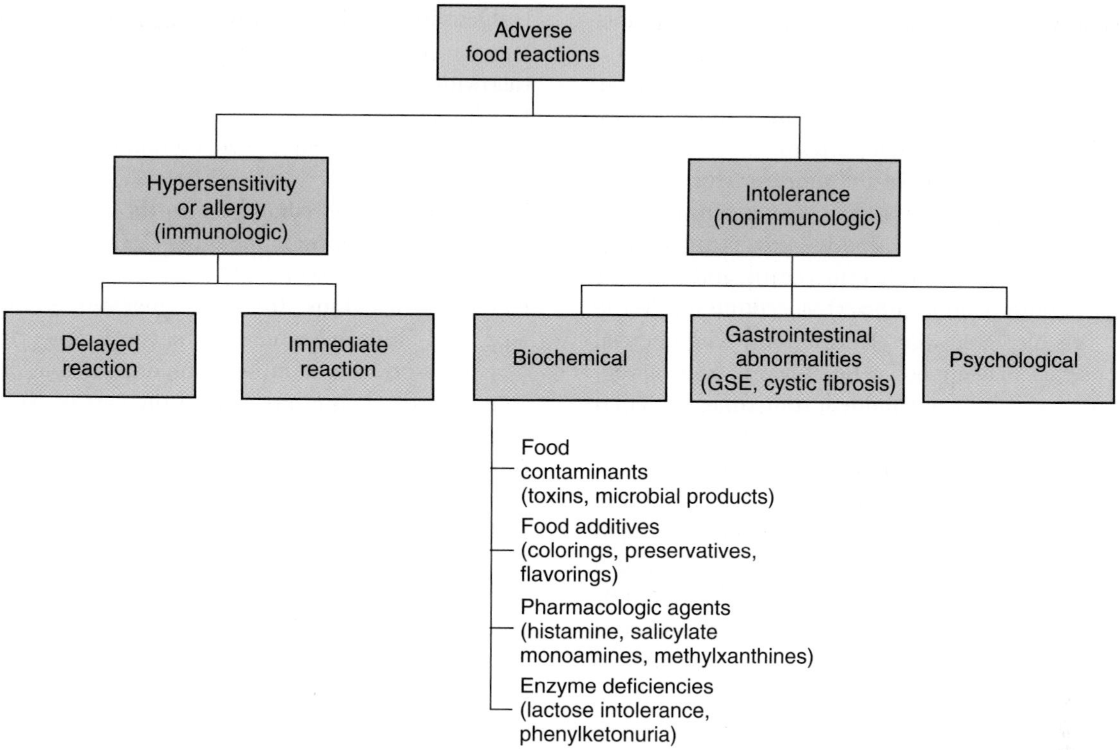

• **Figure 10-2** Adverse food reactions. (From Davis J, Sherer K: *Applied nutrition and diet therapy for nurses*, Philadelphia, 1994, Saunders.)

physical disability, overweight can further impair mobility and reduce energy expenditure.

Adverse Food Reactions

A distinction is made between *food allergy,* a hypersensitivity to a food or food additive with a reproducible immediate or delayed immune system response (e.g., anaphylactic reaction to ingestion of nuts; atopic skin reaction), and *food intolerance,* a nonimmunologic inability to process or tolerate the food product (e.g., enzyme deficiencies [lactase] or PKU secondary to the body's inability to metabolize phenylalanine) (Fig. 10-2). Food can also be toxic (e.g., food poisoning or toxins from bacteria growing in the food) or create pharmacologic effects (e.g., headaches after eating ice cream). All are considered adverse reactions to food; this section discusses food allergy and intolerance.

Many individuals believe they have a food allergy or intolerance, with up to 20% changing their diets because of this belief. Actually very few people have true food allergies, although there have been more food allergies reported in the past two decades. A 1998 study indicated that only 1% to 2% of individuals met the criteria of a severe immunoglobulin E (IgE)-mediated or anaphylactic reaction or had a positive double-blind, placebo-controlled food challenge (Hourihane, 1998). More recently, NHANES 2007–2010 data reveal that, based on serum IgE, an estimated 3.51% of the American population has food allergies to four foods (peanuts, cow's milk, eggs, and shrimp) (McGowan and Keet, 2013). In another sample of 38,480 United States households, by parents' self-report, 8% of children had food allergy and 2.4% had multiple food allergies (Gupta et al, 2011). From 1997 to 2008, peanut allergy in American children younger than 18 years old increased from 0.4% to 1.4% (Sicherer and Sampson, 2014). Although few children are allergic to foods, one study found food to be the most common cause of anaphylaxis in children seen in an emergency department over a 5-year period (Russell et al, 2010). Factors contributing to adverse food reactions include the following:

- Heredity: Children with a history of food allergy in their family are more likely to have an allergy themselves. Children born with a metabolic disorder can have adverse reactions to specific foods.
- Infant diet: Breastfeeding may be protective against allergies, though the data about this are mixed (Sicherer and Sampson, 2014). It also appears that solid foods should be introduced by 6 months of age, including foods that are considered allergenic (e.g., eggs, peanuts), because later introduction may actually increase food sensitization (Du Toit et al, 2015; O'Keefe et al, 2014).
- Immature gastrointestinal tract: Before 7 months old, the infant gastrointestinal tract is more permeable to large molecules, including most food proteins. Allergies

to milk and eggs are more common in younger infants and are often outgrown with age and maturity.
- Compromised gastrointestinal tract: As a result of injury or illness, the gastrointestinal system can be more permeable to allergens, such as large proteins.
- Type of food: Some foods are more allergenic than others, and some individuals have greater sensitivity to certain foods. Only a few foods—cow's milk, eggs, peanuts, soybeans, wheat, fish, crustaceans, and tree nuts (including almonds and cashews)—account for nearly 90% of IgE-mediated allergic reactions. Commercial baby foods that may appear to be only one fruit or vegetable can have eggs or milk added, sometimes under an unfamiliar name.
- Allergic load or tolerance level: Conditions such as, illness, stress, surgery, or trauma can place excessive metabolic demands on the body. An individual who is susceptible to food intolerance or allergy can have a reaction when these conditions are present. Additionally, individuals may be allergic to more than one food and experience a reaction if more than one allergen is present.

Clinical Findings

The goals of a thorough clinical assessment are to determine whether an allergic reaction has occurred, whether it is related to food, to which food is it related, and how serious the problem is. This process is extremely challenging and can require referral to a registered dietitian or use of a team approach with primary provider, dietitian, and allergist for a more in-depth diagnostic workup.

History

The history should assess the following:
- Age of child
- Suspected food
- Route of exposure: Ingested? Skin touched? Food dust inhaled?
- Amount of exposure
- Onset of symptoms relative to exposure
- Description of symptoms (gather data about change over the course of the reaction)
- Description of other factors that are present and may contribute to or aggravate an allergic response (e.g., stress, environment, exercise)
- Treatment given and child's response
- Does child have previous history of symptoms following exposure to this food?
- What is the child's diet history? When and what types of foods were introduced into the diet?
- Does the child have a history of symptoms frequently seen in food allergies (e.g., respiratory distress, eczema, urticaria, rashes, colic, vomiting, diarrhea) unaccompanied by other signs of illness or history of exposure to infectious agents?
- Is there a family history of allergies, especially a history of reaction to certain foods?

Describe the child's usual intake. A food diary is an excellent mechanism for obtaining these data and includes the following:
- All foods and fluids ingested for at least 3 days
- How food is prepared (e.g., commercially, at home, fried, baked)
- How food is stored and fed to the child
- All medications, including herbs and dietary supplements
- Child's reactions to foods ingested (food-symptom diary). This can become a time-consuming, cumbersome task, especially if more than one food is involved; it requires real commitment on the part of parents.

Physical Examination

Signs and symptoms of adverse food reactions vary by type and severity, from a mild local reaction to life-threatening anaphylaxis, making it often difficult to diagnose the condition definitively. Table 10-12 lists possible clinical manifestations of food allergies or intolerances by body system, and Table 10-13 relates clinical features of a reaction to the level

TABLE 10-12 Possible Clinical Manifestations of Food Allergies or Intolerances by Body System

System	Symptoms
Respiratory system	Chronic rhinitis Asthma Croup Cough Serous otitis media Bronchitis
Gastrointestinal system	Tingling and swelling of lips, mouth, throat Nausea, vomiting Diarrhea Colic Protein-losing enteropathy Bloating, flatulence Constipation Gastrointestinal blood loss Malabsorption
Integumentary system	Eczema Pruritus Atopic dermatitis Rashes Urticaria
Central nervous system	Headaches (sinus, migraine) Fatigue Drowsiness, listlessness Irritability Depression Excessive sweating
Circulatory system	Hypotension Cardiac dysrhythmias Anaphylaxis Pallor

TABLE 10-13 Severity of Allergic Reactions to Foods

Severity	Clinical Manifestations
Mild	Localized cutaneous erythema, urticaria, angioedema, oral pruritus
Mild	Generalized erythema, urticaria, angioedema
Mild	At least one or two manifestations listed above plus gastrointestinal symptoms, rhinoconjunctivitis
Moderate	Mild laryngeal edema/mild asthma
Severe	Marked dyspnea; hypotension

Adapted from Clark AT, Ewan PW: Food allergy in childhood, *Arch Dis Child* 88(1):79–81, 2003.

of severity of the child's condition. Height and weight should be monitored closely in children with food allergies, because food elimination and use of alternative foods may compromise nutrition and affect growth.

Diagnostic Studies

A double-blind, placebo-controlled food challenge is recognized as the gold standard for determining the presence of food allergy, but this is not usually practical for the clinical setting. Laboratory studies are used more commonly and include (O'Keefe et al, 2014):

- Skin tests: The skin prick test (SPT) is very sensitive. Cutaneous response may not correlate with a clinical systemic response, however. Antihistamine medications must be discontinued 3 to 20 days before the test, and the test should be avoided in children who have generalized skin lesions, dermographism, or a severe reaction to food following skin contact or inhalation.
- Serum IgE and eosinophil count (elevated serum IgE and eosinophilia greater than 400/mm^3 are usually related to allergies). This test is done if the child cannot have an SPT done, but it can be expensive, especially if more than one food is suspected. Results must be interpreted carefully by an allergist because findings can reflect exposure to other allergens.
- Atopy patch tests: The atopy patch test looks for skin reaction to food, but is not widely used in the clinical setting.
- Food elimination and challenge: When a food has been identified as a potential source of the problem, elimination and an oral food challenge can be used to confirm the diagnosis. Medical supervision during the elimination and challenge is essential (to ensure prompt treatment in case of a severe reaction), and interpretation of responses should be done by an allergist or immunologist; overall the procedure has been found to be relatively safe (O'Keefe et al, 2014). The suspected foods are completely eliminated from the child's diet for at least 3 days and up to 4 weeks and then gradually reintroduced, one at a time. The initial reintroduction dose should be small and then increased until either a reaction recurs or the amount normally eaten is given. If exercise is thought to contribute to the initial allergic reaction, exercise must be part of the challenge. An allergy or intolerance is confirmed if symptoms cease when the food is eliminated and then reappear as it is reintroduced (Koletzko et al, 2012). If there is a possibility of a severe reaction to a food (e.g., anaphylaxis), the child should be hospitalized with emergency cardiovascular support available for the challenge part of this process.

Differential Diagnosis

The differential diagnoses for food allergy and food intolerance include:

- Reactions related to other environmental allergens
- Asthma as a result of other causes
- Immunodeficiency
- Psychological reactions to feeding
- Malabsorption syndromes (e.g., celiac disease), cystic fibrosis
- Lactose intolerance
- Chronic diarrhea
- Heiner syndrome, a milk-induced pulmonary disease with infiltrates, should be suspected in infants and young children who have persistent pulmonary disease without a clear cause.

Management

The goal of managing children with adverse food reactions is to maintain nutrition levels adequate for normal growth and development, prevent nutritional deficits, avoid exposure to offending food or foods, and respond promptly and appropriately to adverse reactions after exposure. Achieving these goals requires the coordinated efforts of pediatric allergists, dietitians, the primary care provider, and teachers or child care providers, in addition to children and their families. Once a child has been assessed as to the cause and severity of the response, a treatment plan can be made. The National Institute of Allergy and Infectious Diseases (NIAID) has developed guidelines for managing food allergies (Burks et al, 2011) (see Resources on the Evolve Website).

Elimination Diet

The standard of practice is to avoid the offending food or foods. Efforts to eliminate the food from the diet raise challenging issues:

- The foods to which most individuals are allergic are very common and very nutritious. Extensive use of elimination diets can lead to malnourishment; these diets should be used for as short a time as possible.
- Sometimes the individual is allergic to the food in its raw form but can eat it in a cooked (heat-treated) form; completely eliminating it means unnecessary loss of a good source of nutrients.

- The food may contaminate other foods or be found in minute amounts in other foods (e.g., processed foods).
- Skin or inhalant contact may occur (e.g., breathing peanut dust) even if food is not eaten.
- Cross-reacting allergens may further limit diets.

Restricted foods need to be replaced with those of equivalent nutrient value in the context of a well-balanced diet. Additionally, the physical problems caused by allergies (e.g., diarrhea, vomiting, dehydration, eczema) can create a need for extra nutrients to maintain health and foster growth. Consultation with a dietitian is recommended. For formula-fed infants allergic to cow's milk, hypoallergenic formula preparations are available. Extensively hydrolyzed cow's milk–based preparations may protect against allergy but can be expensive, and the infant may not accept the taste. Elemental formulas, synthesized free amino acids with vitamin and mineral supplements, can be used. Soy-based formulas are often a first choice alternative for older infants, but many infants allergic to cow's milk are also sensitive to soy (see Chapter 33).

Immunotherapy

In some cases, the allergenic food need not be avoided and may even be therapeutic in controlling the allergy. There are many studies currently under way evaluating the use of oral, sublingual, subcutaneous, and epicutaneous immunotherapy for food allergies with some promising results. To date, however, allergic side effects are common in these trials, and long-term studies to determine whether permanent desensitization occurs have not been done. Immunotherapy for food allergies should not be used routinely in clinical practice; safety is paramount and avoidance of the food allergen is the standard of practice (O'Keefe et al, 2014).

Revisiting the Food Challenge

The child's allergic status should be reevaluated regularly. Because food allergies and intolerances are often outgrown, the child may be challenged with most offending foods every year or 2 years. Cow's milk and egg allergies are often outgrown by 2 years old (Burks et al, 2012). Some foods appear to remain allergenic for longer periods (e.g., seafood, peanuts, and tree nuts) (Gupta et al, 2013). If the child's reaction has been serious or even life threatening, the parents may decide to continue to avoid the food. Many fatalities related to food allergies occur among older children, teenagers, and young adults.

Medication

Self-administered epinephrine is prescribed for children with moderate or severe allergies. Children, their parents, and other caregivers should be educated on intramuscular injection using a prepared epinephrine injection (EpiPen). Children at risk for food-related anaphylaxis should carry two doses of epinephrine (Rudders et al, 2010). Antihistamines are prescribed for children with mild allergies, unless there is a history of a reaction to trace amounts of the allergen or the child has asthma from another cause; in these cases, epinephrine is appropriate. Children with food allergies should wear a medical-alert bracelet or necklace. School personnel should be informed of the child's allergy, and a medical plan should be implemented in the school.

Education

Education of families, children, and adults who are responsible for the child's well-being is critical. The provider can do outreach to teachers, schools, and day care centers with information about how to understand and safely manage the child's condition and be an ongoing source of suggestions, support, and advocacy for parents. Management of food intolerances secondary to metabolic disorders is discussed earlier in this chapter (see Disorders Requiring Restricted or Supplemental Diets).

Complications

Complications of adverse food reactions include anaphylaxis, asthma, convulsive coughing (leading to aspiration and choking), malnutrition, gastrointestinal dysfunction, secondary skin infections, and disruption of family processes.

Effect of Medications on Nutritional Status

Medications are designed to alter the body's biochemistry in order to produce a healing effect. These biochemical changes have implications for the individual's nutritional status. Some medications deplete essential nutrients from the body; others interfere with the body's ability to metabolize nutrients; still others have an adverse effect on the appetite or cause nausea. Although a medication can have an immediate effect on an individual, adverse changes in nutritional status are most often seen after prolonged therapy.

Drug-induced malnutrition results from drug-related alterations in the body's ability to absorb, distribute, metabolize, use, or excrete nutrients and their metabolites (Woo and Wynne, 2011). Absorption is affected by characteristics of the molecule being absorbed (size, ionization, lipid solubility), gut motility (too rapid as with diarrhea or too slow as with Hirschsprung disease), and environment of the gastrointestinal tract (e.g., gastric pH, lack of intrinsic factor). As medications change gastrointestinal motility or environment, they influence the absorption of nutrients.

Distribution of nutrients is affected by plasma protein-binding capabilities, total body water content, and relative fat content in the body. For example, if a drug that binds highly with plasma protein is taken for long periods of time or if a child has low serum albumin, nutrients have to compete for protein-binding sites.

Metabolism occurs primarily in the liver, and drugs can either inhibit or stimulate hepatic enzyme activity, thus influencing the body's ability to metabolize nutrients for use at the cellular level. The relationship of medications and nutrients in terms of excretion is less marked than with absorption, distribution, and metabolism, but drugs can have an effect on renal function, especially tubular reabsorption, which then affects nutritional status.

Clinical Findings

Diet history, anthropometric measurements, and physical examination are essential components of the clinical assessment and have been discussed previously. Specific attention should be paid to assessing nutrients in the diet for which drug therapy places the child at risk of deficiency.

Management

Management involves ongoing monitoring and anticipatory intervention to prevent nutritional problems for children on drug therapy. Table 10-14 provides dietary suggestions related to specific classes of medication. This list is limited, and a comprehensive pharmacology reference should be consulted for specific drugs. Referral to a dietitian can also be helpful. General interventions include the following:

- Alter dietary intake to include more foods containing the affected nutrients.
- Supplement diet with required vitamins or minerals, or both.
- Administer medications in a manner that minimizes their effect on nutrition.
- Consider alternative medications and treatment modalities.

Complications

Malnutrition, slowed growth, delayed healing, and drug toxicity are complications of the effects of medication on nutritional status.

Toxic Exposures in Foods

Exposure to toxins and chemicals through the food chain contribute to many health problems in children. Chapter 42 examines the relationship between toxic exposure in foods and children's health.

Controversies in Pediatric Nutrition

Effects of Sugar or Food Additives on Behavior

Food affects the body and its ability to function in complex and sometimes unclear ways. Many parents, teachers, and children believe that sugar intake causes behavior problems, primarily hyperactivity. An extensive review of controlled scientific studies failed to find evidence of a causal link between sugar and behavior or cognitive performance (Cruz and Bahna, 2006), and a recent random, double-blind, placebo-controlled test found no relationship between food additives and child behavior (Lok et al, 2013). But an association has been found between high sugar intake and poor diet quality and emotional symptoms in children as reported by parents (Kohlboeck et al, 2012). It may be that rapid change in blood sugar levels could contribute to mental and emotional lability. Additionally, sugar consumption is often related to activities (e.g., birthday parties, Halloween) that result in excited behavior among children. An elimination diet can be tried; if symptoms improve, a double-blind, placebo-controlled challenge can be used to confirm a relationship.

The role of the provider is to educate and reassure parents that low sugar consumption in healthy children rarely results in adverse behavior. High-sugar diets are to be avoided, because these foods tend to replace more nutrient-dense foods and contribute to overweight and obesity, dental caries, and other health problems. The American Heart Association (AHA) recommends that less than half of an individual's discretionary calories should come from added sugar (i.e., sugar not found naturally in fruits, milk, and so on) (AHA, 2014). For the preschooler who consumes 1200 to 1400 calories per day, this amounts to about 4 teaspoons of added sugar; for the 4- to 8-year-old with a 1600 calorie intake, it is about 3 teaspoons; and for older children and adults who consume 2000 calories daily, it is about 5 to 8 teaspoons each day. According to the Harvard School of Public Health, "the average can of sugar-sweetened soda or fruit punch provides...the equivalent of 10 teaspoons of table sugar" (Harvard T.H. Chan School of Public Health, 2015).

Gluten-Free Diets

In recent years, eating a low-gluten or gluten-free diet has become more popular in the United States. The gluten-free product market grew by 44% from 2011 to 2013 and is expected to reach $15.6 billion in sales in 2016 (Pauk, 2014). A gluten-free diet is the only known, effective treatment for celiac disease (see Chapter 33). Very few individuals, approximately 0.7% of the American population, have this chronic inflammatory disease. Other individuals may be sensitive to wheat or other grains. "Non-celiac wheat sensitivity" or "patients who avoid wheat and gluten" are terms that describe individuals with symptoms associated with wheat consumption, such as indigestion, abdominal pain, bloating, or fatigue. These symptoms may be due to dietary fermentable oligo-di-monosaccharides and polyols (FODMAPs) (e.g., fructose, lactose, fructans, galactans, polyols; disaccharides and oligosaccharides occurring in many foods, not exclusively wheat) (Aziz and Sanders, 2014). The incidence of non-celiac gluten sensitivity is unknown, but research is continuing to clarify the extent and significance of this condition (Catassi et al, 2013).

Many individuals eat gluten-free foods for reasons other than intolerance or sensitivity. According to consumer market research data, 53% of survey respondents who fit into this category state that they believe gluten-free foods are healthier and 27% believe that they will help them lose weight (Pauk, 2014). However, gluten-free grain products are often highly processed and not enriched with iron or folate. Sugar and fat may be added to enhance their flavor and improve their physical structure. Many are so low in protein that they are used for patients with metabolic diseases, like PKU, who have a severely restricted

TABLE 10-14 Nutritional Risks of Selected Drugs

Drug Category or Name	Nutritional Risk	Nutritional Intervention
Antibiotic (e.g., chloramphenicol)	Inhibits vitamin K–producing intestinal microflora Increases excretion of riboflavin Nausea, vomiting, diarrhea Decreases absorption of calcium, fat, and protein Decreases lactase activity Suppresses bone marrow (chloramphenicol) May cause aplastic anemia	Use acidophilus tablets, acidophilus milk, or yogurt to replace gastrointestinal organisms Supplement with vitamin C, B-complex vitamins, vitamin B_{12}, biotin, vitamin K, or well-balanced vitamin and mineral supplement Use lactose-reduced milk
Antihistamine (e.g., cimetidine, diphenhydramine)	Decreases gastric acid secretion, increases pH Decreases absorption of iron, folate, vitamin B_{12} May lead to hyperglycemia May disrupt vitamin D metabolism	
Barbiturate (e.g., phenobarbital)	Breaks down vitamin D May cause calcium deficiency, rickets, or osteomalacia May decrease serum folate, vitamin B_{12}, pyridoxine (vitamin B_6), magnesium May cause nausea, vomiting, constipation	May need vitamin D and calcium supplements Give drug with meals Give high-fiber and high-fluid diet If folic acid supplementation is indicated, administer cautiously
Corticosteroid	Increases protein catabolism and gluconeogenesis; decreases protein synthesis contributing to nitrogen wasting Stimulates appetite May cause stomach upset May cause hypokalemia, hyperglycemia, hypernatremia, hypocalcemia associated with osteoporosis May elevate serum lipids	If edema occurs, restrict sodium intake High doses require calcium and vitamin D supplements Supplement with vitamin B_6, vitamin C, and folic acid Monitor weight and restrict calories if there is excessive weight gain Increase dietary protein
Digoxin	May cause anorexia and nausea, weight loss May cause hypokalemia May increase urinary excretion of magnesium and calcium	Increase dietary potassium Evaluate need to increase dietary magnesium and calcium
Isoniazid	Interferes with enzyme pathway for creation of niacin Increases excretion of vitamin B_6 and folic acid May cause nausea and vomiting Decreases absorption of vitamin E Increases absorption of iron May cause hyperglycemia	Give vitamin B_6 supplement Increase foods high in folate, niacin, vitamin B_6, and magnesium Avoid foods with histamine and tyramine, such as tuna, mackerel, sardines, dry sausages and meats, imitation and hard cheeses, meat and protein extracts, and excessive amounts of caffeine
Methotrexate	Folate antagonist, contributes to folate deficiency May cause stomatitis, anorexia, diarrhea Decreases absorption of vitamins A, D, E, and K, beta-carotene	Give folate
Oral contraceptive	Increases vitamin A and calcium absorption Causes low serum vitamin C; possibly contributes to low levels of vitamins B_1, B_2, B_6, B_{12}, folate, magnesium, zinc	Increase intake of vitamins C, B_1, B_2, B_6, B_{12}, folate, magnesium, zinc
Phenothiazine hydantoin, phenytoin	Increases excretion of riboflavin May cause nausea, vomiting, constipation May cause hyperglycemia Impairs metabolism and absorption of folate; may lead to megaloblastic anemia Inactivates vitamin D; can lead to osteomalacia Decreases serum vitamin K	Supplement with vitamin D, vitamin K, folate, but excessive folate levels can decrease action of anticonvulsants Administer drug with, or immediately after, a meal
Supplements		
Calcium	If taken with iron supplement, only calcium carbonate does not affect iron absorption; if taken with fluoride, absorption of both is decreased	
Zinc	>1500 mg/day: decreases copper absorption, possibly leading to anemia-related fatigue	
Iron	Causes nausea, possibly anorexia	
Theophylline	May cause vitamin B_6 deficiency	Give pyridoxine supplements

protein allowance. A Swedish study of the dietary intakes of children and adolescents with celiac disease identified inadequate energy, fiber, magnesium, and vitamin D and higher than recommended intakes of sucrose and saturated fats in subjects who adhered to a gluten-free diet (Öhlund et al, 2010). Individuals without celiac disease may also have inadequate nutritional intake on a gluten-free diet.

For a complete list of references, please visit http://evolve.elsevier.com/Burns/pediatric/.

11 Breastfeeding

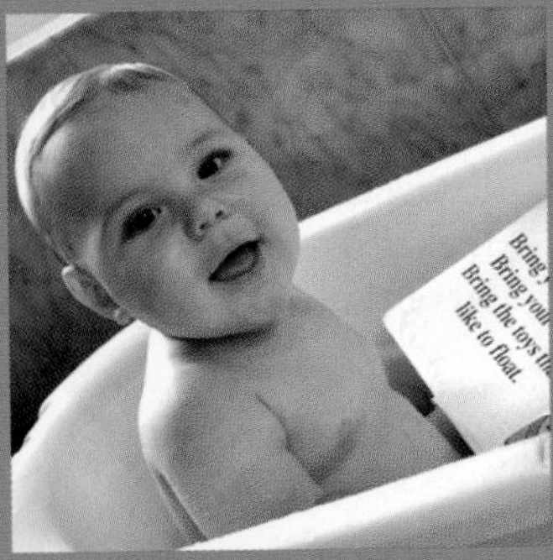

ARDYS M. DUNN, ANNA MARIE HAFNER, AND PAMELA J. HELLINGS

Breast milk is the ideal food for newborns and infants and supports infant nutrition essential for optimal growth and development. In addition to healthy nutrients, breast milk contains many immune substances that protect the newborn against infections. Breastfeeding also offers parents and infants physical, psychological, and emotional benefits that last a lifetime. Breastfeeding should be promoted and supported whenever possible.

Health care providers engage in assessment, education, support, outreach, and advocacy as they promote breastfeeding. Breastfeeding is a learned skill for both the mother and the infant; providers must assess the mother's knowledge level and provide information and guidance to increase the skills of the mother-infant dyad as the breastfeeding experience develops. Providers can educate families about the benefits of breast milk and how to recognize and prevent common problems. As a result, families can make educated choices about infant feeding and quickly find answers to questions and concerns. Breastfeeding is supported when providers take the time to determine the cause of a breastfeeding problem, develop a plan to address the problem, and guide the family through difficulties; these interventions can make all the difference in the decision to continue breastfeeding. Outreach and advocacy for breastfeeding is demonstrated when providers contribute to hospital, clinic, and community committees, advisory boards, and task forces to develop policies that promote and support breastfeeding. Providers act as advocates for breastfeeding when they advise and educate colleagues on breastfeeding issues, teach breastfeeding content to students in the health professions, and serve as expert contacts for the media on issues related to breastfeeding. In all these activities, health care providers serve an important leadership function in promoting and supporting breastfeeding.

Breastfeeding Recommendations

Major health professional organizations, including the National Association of Pediatric Nurse Practitioners (NAPNAP), the American Academy of Pediatrics (AAP), the American Academy of Family Physicians (AAFP), and the American Dietetic Association recommend breastfeeding exclusively for the first 6 months of life and then breastfeeding combined with other nutrients for at least the first year (AAFP, 2008, 2012; AAP, 2012; James et al, 2009; NAPNAP, 2013).

Breastfeeding goals for *Healthy People 2020* include the following targets:

- 81.9% of mothers will initiate breastfeeding in the neonatal period.
- 60.6% will be breastfeeding at 6 months old and 34.1% at 1 year old.

There are also efforts to remove the barriers mothers who are separated from their children (e.g., working mothers) encounter when attempting to breastfeed (U.S. Department of Health and Human Services [HHS], 2014). Although breastfeeding rates have increased in the United States (Table 11-1), they continue to be well below the Healthy People 2020 goals (Centers for Disease Control and Prevention [CDC] Division of Nutrition, Physical Activity, and Obesity [DNPAO], 2014). Much work remains to be done, and providers can make a major contribution to the success of efforts to support breastfeeding. One model that can be used to further these goals encourages providers to focus on interventions that (1) support the mother's self-efficacy to breastfeed, (2) provide lactation support to mother and family, and (3) increase lactation education for both mother and providers (Busch et al, 2014).

Hospital-Based Support

The Baby-Friendly Hospital Initiative

In 1991, the Baby-Friendly Hospital Initiative (BFHI) was developed by the World Health Organization (WHO) and the United Nations International Children's Emergency Fund (UNICEF) to recognize hospitals that provide optimal lactation support. This worldwide initiative trains providers and hospitals to promote breastfeeding internationally (UNICEF, 2009). The 10 criteria to meet a "baby-friendly hospital" standard are outlined in the original joint WHO/UNICEF statement (WHO/UNICEF, 1989) and are used

TABLE 11-1 Healthy People 2020 Objectives: Initiation and Duration of Breastfeeding for Children Born in 2011

Healthy People 2020 Objective	Actual Percentage of Total Population Breastfeeding by Age of Infant	Number of States Meeting Healthy People 2020 Objective*
81.9% of mothers will initiate breastfeeding	79.2%	17
60.6% of mothers will be breastfeeding 6-month-old infant	49.4%	7
34.1% of mothers will be breastfeeding 12-month-old infant	26.7%	8
46.2% exclusive breastfeeding through 3 months old	40.7%	20
25.5% exclusive breastfeeding through 6 months old	18.8%	6

Data from Centers for Disease Control and Prevention (CDC) Division of Nutrition, Physical Activity, and Obesity (DNPAO): Breastfeeding report card, 2014: www.cdc.gov/breastfeeding/pdf/2014breastfeedingreportcard.pdf. Accessed September 18, 2014.

*Alaska, Hawaii, Oregon, and Vermont have met all five *Healthy People 2020* breastfeeding objectives; California, Utah, and Washington have met four of the five.

to assess the quality of a lactation program. Every facility that provides maternity services and care for newborn infants should:

- Have a written breastfeeding policy that is routinely communicated to all health care staff.
- Train all health care staff in skills necessary to implement this policy (18 hours of formal training are recommended).
- Inform all pregnant women about the benefits and management of breastfeeding.
- Help mothers initiate breastfeeding within ½ hour of birth.
- Show mothers how to breastfeed and how to maintain lactation even if they are separated from their infants.
- Give newborn infants no food or drink other than breast milk, unless medically indicated.
- Practice rooming in (i.e., allow mothers and infants to remain together) 24 hours a day.
- Encourage unrestricted breastfeeding.
- Give no artificial teats or pacifiers (also called *dummies* or *soothers*) to breastfeeding infants.
- Foster the establishment of breastfeeding support groups, and refer mothers to them on discharge from the hospital or clinic.

Currently, more than 20,000 facilities in 150 countries have been designated "baby-friendly" internationally—most in developing countries (WHO, 2015). As of August 2015, 288 hospitals and birthing centers in the United States held a "baby-friendly" designation, and, statistics for 2014 show 7.9% of births in the United States were in "baby-friendly" facilities, close to the Healthy People 2020 goal of 8.1%. Still, much work remains for American health care providers (Baby-Friendly USA, 2015; CDC, 2014).

Benefits of Breastfeeding

With rare exception, breast milk is the ideal food for the human infant. Each mammalian species provides milk uniquely suited to its offspring, and milk from the human breast is no exception. It is a living fluid rich in vitamins, minerals, fat, proteins (including immunoglobulins and antibodies), and carbohydrates (especially lactose). It contains enzymes and cellular components, including macrophages and lymphocytes, in addition to many other constituents that offer ideal support for growth and maturation of the human infant. Amazingly, as the infant grows and develops, the properties of breast milk change. The sequence of colostrum, transitional milk, and mature milk meets the changing nutritional needs of the newborn and infant. Thus, the milk of a mother of a 9-month-old has different concentrations of fat, protein, and carbohydrates and different physical properties, such as pH, when compared with the milk of the mother of a newborn or 1-month-old. In addition, some of the constituent properties in the milk are different from one time of the day to another.

In addition to providing optimal nutrition for growth and development, breastfeeding confers many short- and long-term health benefits to infants. A review of studies examining the effect of breastfeeding on infant health indicates a lower risk of nonspecific gastroenteritis, necrotizing enterocolitis, acute otitis media, severe lower respiratory tract infections, asthma, atopic dermatitis, type 1 and type 2 diabetes, obesity, sudden infant death syndrome (SIDS), and childhood leukemia in breastfed infants (Ip et al, 2009; Kramer and Kakuma, 2012).

In the short term, studies show that breastfed babies have added protection against bacterial, viral, and protozoan illnesses during infancy. Human-milk glycans and immunoglobulins appear to inhibit pathogens from adhering to intestinal mucosa, replicating, and causing disease. Oligosaccharides in breast milk also support the growth of the infantis strain of *Bifidobacterium longum* in the intestine of the breastfed infant, while suppressing pathologic bacteria such as *Escherichia coli, Clostridium perfringens,* and *Enterococcus* (Marcobal et al, 2010; Zivkovic et al, 2011).

Breastfeeding also appears to reduce the incidence of fever after immunization (Pisacane et al, 2010).

The long-term benefits of breastfeeding for 6 months may include a decreased incidence of atopic diseases and an association with lower rates of asthma in young children (Dogaru et al, 2014). Breastfeeding may also be protective against obesity, has been associated with lower cholesterol in adults (Owen et al, 2008), and may be protective against type 1 and type 2 diabetes in youth (Geddes and Prescott, 2013).

Initiating breastfeeding is crucial; the infant enjoys health benefits with every day of breastfeeding. Maintaining breastfeeding is also crucial; there is evidence that infants who are exclusively breastfed for a minimum of 4 months have less risk for infection than those breastfed for less time (Duijts et al, 2010). However, exclusive, prolonged breastfeeding beyond 6 months may actually contribute to health problems. Studies have shown that infants *exclusively* breastfed for 9 months or longer have had an increased incidence of atopic dermatitis and food hypersensitivity in childhood (Pesonen et al, 2006) and prolonged breastfeeding (i.e., beyond 12 months) contributed to the incidence of atopic dermatitis in young Korean children, regardless of the family history for atopic dermatitis (Hong et al, 2014). Complementary foods should be added to the infant diet by 6 months of age (see Chapter 10); breastfeeding provides important nutritional and health-related benefits and should be continued until the child is at least 1 year old.

There are also benefits for the mother that include more rapid return to her nonpregnant state, establishment of the strong bond associated with successful nursing, decreased risk for breast cancer (De Silva et al, 2010) and ovarian cancer, especially if the lastborn child is breastfed (Feng et al, 2014; Titus-Ernstoff et al, 2010), for metabolic syndrome (Gunderson et al, 2010), type 2 diabetes (Jäger et al, 2014), postpartum depression (Ip et al, 2009), and a variety of other conditions (Stuebe and Schwarz, 2010).

Breastfeeding also provides an economic incentive as a free and plentiful source of excellent infant nutrition. The cost of formula and other necessary supplies exceeds several thousand dollars each year for a family. In addition to individual costs, it is estimated that if 90% of women complied with the recommendation to exclusively breastfeed their infant until 6 months of age, 911 infant deaths and $13 billion in care of infants would have been avoided (Bartick and Reinhold, 2010), and as much as $17.4 billion related to maternal morbidity and mortality would be saved in the United States (Bartick et al, 2013).

Contraindications to Breastfeeding

In addition to all the beneficial nutrients that are provided to the infant during breastfeeding, certain infections and many drugs or medications can be passed to the infant via breast milk. Although rare, contraindications to breastfeeding occur in some of these situations. A small number of infant conditions also preclude breastfeeding. Contraindications to breastfeeding include the following (AAP, 2012):

- Infant with classic galactosemia
- Maternal diagnosis of human T-cell lymphotrophic virus type I or II
- Maternal diagnosis of untreated brucellosis
- Maternal diagnosis of active, untreated tuberculosis (TB) (expressed breast milk can be fed to the infant)
- Maternal diagnosis of cancer and treatment
- Maternal human immunodeficiency virus (HIV) infection (except in some areas, see WHO recommendations [Box 11-1]; breastfeeding for HIV-infected mothers is not recommended in developed countries)
- Herpetic lesions on the mother's nipples, areolas, or breast (expressed breast milk can be fed to the infant)

Special Situations

Additional circumstances require special consideration regarding the advisability or management of breastfeeding. These circumstances include the following:

- Significant maternal or infant illness affecting the ability to feed

• BOX 11-1 World Health Organization Recommendations for Breastfeeding with Human Immunodeficiency Virus

The primary goal is to balance the risk of human immunodeficiency virus (HIV) infection of the infant transmitted through breast milk with protection from other causes of child mortality that breast milk provides.

For HIV-positive mothers who live in countries where breastfeeding and antiretroviral treatments (ART) are promoted, the World Health Organization (WHO) recommends exclusive breastfeeding for the first 6 months and breastfeeding with nutritional supplements until 12 months.

National or subnational health authorities should decide whether HIV-infected mothers should either:

- Breastfeed and receive ART

or

- Avoid breastfeeding completely, implementing replacement feeding

Replacement feeding should not be used unless it is:

- Acceptable (socially welcome)
- Feasible (facilities and help are available to prepare formula)
- Affordable (formula can be purchased for 6 months)
- Sustainable (feeding can be sustained for 6 months)
- Safe (formula is prepared with safe water and in hygienic conditions)

Adapted from World Health Organization (WHO): Consolidated guidelines on the use of antiretroviral drugs for treating and preventing HIV infection: recommendations for a public health approach, 2013, WHO (website): www.who.int/hiv/pub/guidelines/arv2013/download/en/. Accessed September 24, 2014; WHO: Guidelines on HIV and infant feeding 2010: principles and recommendations for infant feeding in the context of HIV and a summary of evidence, 2010, WHO (website): www.who.int/maternal_child_adolescent/documents/9789241599535/en/. Accessed September 24, 2014.

- Maternal illness, such as TB (treated), chickenpox, or hepatitis B or C
- Invasive breast surgery, in particular breast reduction in which the areola is removed and reattached
- Documented history of milk supply problems
- If mothers cannot breast feed their infants but want their baby to receive breast milk, or if the infant requires breast milk to survive, a network of breast milk banks is available to families. Although it is expensive, the Human Milk Banking Association of North America (HMBANA) provides breast milk at three centers in Canada and 17 in the United States (see Additional Resources). Nursing mothers may also donate their milk to these banks. Increasingly, it is possible to buy breast milk online; however, this could be hazardous for the infant, since many of these donors are unscreened, and many samples purchased online have been found to be contaminated or adulterated (Keim et al, 2015).

Characteristics of Human Milk

The uniqueness of human milk to support the growth and development of the human infant cannot be overestimated. Scientists continue to find new components and to clarify the purposes of known components. More than 200 constituents of milk have been identified (Lawrence and Lawrence, 2011).

Colostrum

Colostrum production begins at about 20 weeks of gestation. The pregnant woman may notice a small amount of yellow discharge on her nipple or clothing. After delivery of the baby, production of colostrum increases but is still of low quantity. This thick, rich, yellowish fluid has fewer calories than mature milk (67 vs. 75 kcal/100 mL) and is lower in fat (2% vs. 3.8%). It is rich in immunoglobulins, especially immunoglobulin A (IgA), and other antibodies. In addition, it is higher in sodium, chloride, protein, fat-soluble vitamins, and cholesterol than mature milk, and it facilitates the passage of meconium. Because of the outstanding contribution to the infant's immunologic status, colostrum is often referred to as the infant's "first immunization." Premature infants in particular benefit when receiving colostrum from their own mothers or from a donor with an infant who matches the gestational age of the preemie (Moles et al, 2015). Colostrum meets all nutritional needs of a normal term newborn in the first few days of life. No supplementation is necessary.

Transitional Milk

Transitional milk appears several days after delivery. Significant variability is seen in the constituent properties of transitional milk between mothers and within samples from the same mother. However, as a general rule, transitional milk has more lactose, calories, and fat and less total protein than colostrum.

Mature Milk

Mature milk gradually replaces transitional milk by about the second week after delivery and provides, on average, 20 kcal/oz.

Water

Approximately 90% of human milk is water. Breast milk can meet the fluid needs of the infant without any supplementation, even in tropical and desert climates.

Lipid (Fat) Content

Various lipids (fats) make up the second greatest percentage of constituents of human milk. They are also the most variable component, with differences noted within a feeding, between feedings, in feedings over time, and between different mothers. On average, the fat content is approximately 3.8% and contributes 30% to 55% of the kilocalories in human milk. During feeding, the fluid content of the mammary gland becomes mixed with droplets of fat in increasing concentration. Thus, the fat content is higher at the end of the feeding (hindmilk) than it is at the beginning (foremilk). The type and amount of fat in the maternal diet are thought to affect the type of lipid but not the total amount of fat found in the mother's breast milk.

The cholesterol content varies little in human milk and is approximately 240 mg/100 g of fat. Changes in the maternal diet do not produce changes in these cholesterol values. Breastfed infants have higher plasma cholesterol levels than do formula-fed infants. Research suggests, however, that breastfeeding may have a protective effect against cardiovascular disease, because adolescents and adults tend to have lower cholesterol levels if they were breastfed (Owen et al, 2008). Research on fatty acids, such as docosahexaenoic acid (DHA) and other long-chain polyunsaturated fatty acids (LC-PUFAs), indicates that they play an important role in brain and retinal development (Brenna and Carlson, 2014; Lassek and Gaulin, 2014). If infants are not breastfed, formula should be supplemented with DHA.

Protein

Approximately 0.9% of the content of human milk is protein. When milk is heated or exposed to enzymes as in digestion, a clot, or casein, is formed. The clear portion that remains is known as *whey.* In human milk, 60% to 70% of the protein is whey, which primarily consists of α-lactalbumin and lactoferrin, and 30% to 40% is casein. In contrast, cow's milk is 20% β-lactalbumin and 80% casein, with distinct chemical differences between the casein found in cow's milk and that found in human milk. The curds of human milk are more easily digested by the infant. Other proteins include immunoglobulins, nonimmunoglobulins, and lysozyme—a nonspecific antibacterial factor.

Carbohydrates

The primary carbohydrate of human milk is lactose, which is synthesized by the mammary gland from glucose. Lactose is highly concentrated in human milk (6.8 vs. 4.9 g/100 mL in cow's milk) and appears to be essential for growth of the human infant. In addition, lactose enhances the absorption of calcium, a potentially important role because of the relatively low level of calcium in human milk.

Vitamins and Minerals

Human milk has more than adequate amounts of vitamins A, E, K, C, B_1, B_2, and B_6. However, the level of vitamin D in breast milk may not be adequate for breastfed infants. There are two ways to address this issue: (1) nursing mothers can take vitamin D supplements to ensure adequate concentrations in breast milk, and (2) the infant can be exposed directly to sunlight. Further research is needed to determine exactly what supplemental dose of vitamin D is necessary for nursing mothers, but the recommended 400 IU/day does not appear to be enough; it may need to be up to 10 times the currently recommended dose (Thiele et al, 2013). Direct, unprotected exposure to sunlight, however, is a more effective way than diet for the body to get vitamin D and provides other benefits to the infant. A rule of thumb is to expose the infant to an "amount of sunlight that is about 50% of what it would take to cause a mild sunburn" (i.e., slight pinkness to the skin 24 hours later) followed by good sun protection (i.e., clothing, hat, and/or sunscreen) (Wacker and Holick, 2013). Sunscreen blocks vitamin D absorption. A supplement of 400 IU/day, beginning shortly after birth for all infants, including those exclusively breastfed, and 600 IU/day for children and adolescents is also recommended (Perrine et al, 2010; Wacker and Holick, 2013).

Low levels of iron are found in human milk. However, iron absorption from human milk is highly efficient, with 49% of the available iron absorbed in contrast to 4% from formula. A full-term infant who is exclusively breastfed for 4 to 6 months is not at risk for iron deficiency anemia. Zinc is readily available in human milk and has an absorption rate of 41% versus 31% from cow's milk protein formulas and 14% from soy formulas.

Anatomy and Physiology

Pregnancy brings about the final stage of mammogenesis—growth and differentiation of the mammary gland and development of the structures to support breast milk production. Estrogen, progesterone, placental lactogen, and prolactin all play a role in mammogenesis. By approximately 20 weeks, the breast is capable of milk production. The actual production of breast milk is triggered by the fall in progesterone concentration after birth of the baby. Placental retention inhibits milk production because of the influence of progesterone and other hormones.

Suckling by the infant is essential to establish and maintain lactation. The amount of milk produced depends on stimulation of the breast, removal of milk from the breast, and release of hormones. The concept of "supply and demand" is an important one for providers and parents to understand. Suckling stimulates the hypothalamus to decrease prolactin-inhibiting factor and permits release of prolactin by the anterior pituitary, which leads to a rise in the level of prolactin. Prolactin levels are directly proportional to the level of suckling by the infant and are more important to the initiation than to the maintenance of lactation. The hypothalamus also stimulates the synthesis and release of oxytocin by the posterior pituitary (Fig. 11-1). Oxytocin reacts with receptors in the myoepithelial cells of the milk ducts to initiate a contracting action that results in forcing milk down the ducts. This action increases milk pressure called the *letdown reflex* or *milk ejection reflex*. Oxytocin also aids in maternal uterine involution.

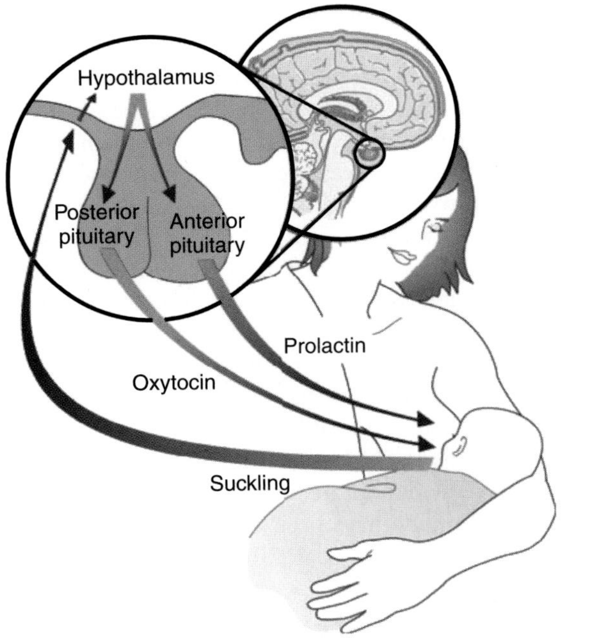

• Figure 11-1 Neuroendocrine loop.

Under the influence of the hormones mentioned previously, the mammary gland undergoes a dramatic change with an increase in size and rapid growth of the lobuloalveolar tissue. The alveoli are the site of milk production and combine in numbers of 10 to 100 to form lobuli. Twenty to 40 lobuli combine into lobes, and 15 to 25 lobes empty into a lactiferous duct. The ducts transport the milk to the nipple (Fig. 11-2).

The nipple and surrounding areola serve as a visual and tactile target to assist with latch-on. The size and shape of the woman's breast and areola vary greatly. Fortunately, the size of the breast is not a predictor of breast milk volume. Women with very small breasts can successfully breastfeed. The provider should be alert, however, for the occasional presence of insufficient glandular tissue, which is characterized by the absence of breast changes associated with pregnancy, a unilaterally underdeveloped breast, or conical-shaped breasts.

The size, shape, and position of the nipple also vary among women. The nipple may be everted (protuberant from the breast), flat, or inverted. It is not always possible to detect an inverted nipple by observation only. The "pinch test" may be needed to identify nipples that invert with tactile stimulation to the areola. To do the pinch test, place

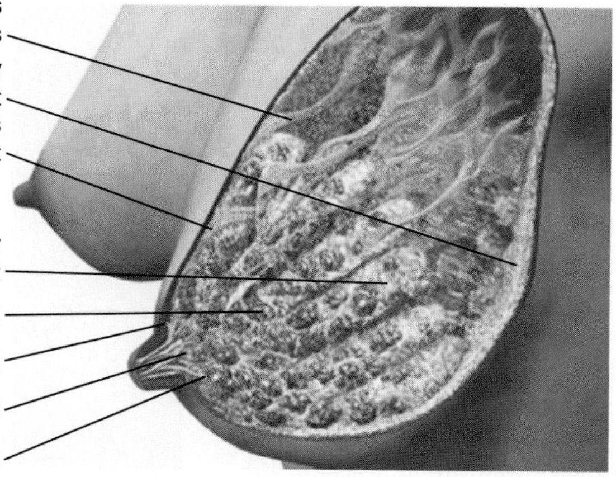

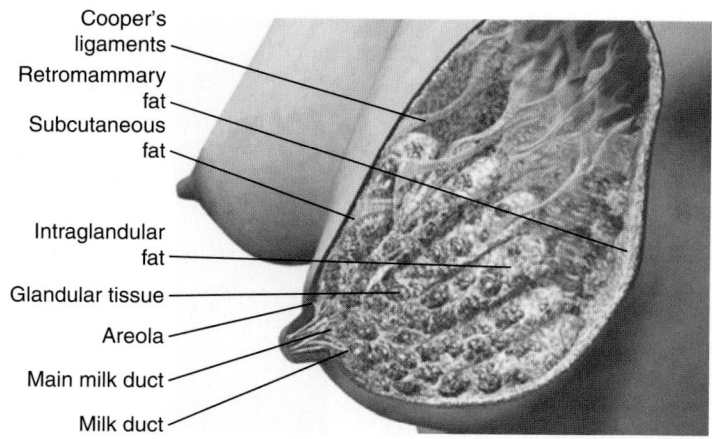

• **Figure 11-2** Anatomy of the breast. (From Ramsay DT, Kent JC, Hartmann RA, et al: Anatomy of the lactating human breast redefined with ultrasound imaging, *J Anat* 206(6):525–534, 2005.)

the thumb and forefinger on opposite sides of the areola about 1 to 1½ inches back from the nipple-areolar junction. Gently compress as though bringing the two fingers together, causing the nipple to become more everted or inverted. This assessment should be conducted prenatally on every patient (Fig. 11-3). Management of inverted nipples is discussed later in this chapter.

Despite the complexity of the anatomic and physiologic processes, the great news is that breastfeeding can proceed for the mother and the baby with little or no awareness on their part of these considerations.

Assessment of the Breastfeeding Dyad

Prenatal assessment focuses on maternal expectations for breastfeeding; knowledge about breastfeeding, especially techniques for getting off to a good start; and identification of any contraindications to breastfeeding. A nipple evaluation should be completed. All pregnant women should be assessed, not just primigravidae. In the early postpartum period, assessment focuses on the transition to breastfeeding and should include close observation of a feeding. In addition, signs of progress for successful breastfeeding should be reviewed, and the names and phone numbers of contact persons should be given to mothers for follow-up or questions.

Maternal History

In general, data should be collected about the following areas:

- Overall health, including documentation of any chronic illnesses or allergies
- Previous breastfeeding experience
- Cultural expectations about breastfeeding
- Routine use of over-the-counter, prescribed, or recreational or street drugs, including tobacco, alcohol, and herbal preparations or supplements

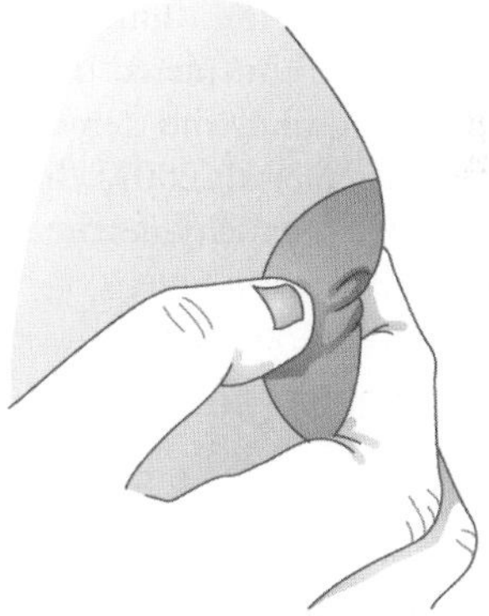

• **Figure 11-3** Pinch test.

- Surgical interventions, especially to the breast or thoracic region
- Nutritional status
- Family and community support for breastfeeding
- Pregnancy history, especially any complications or need for medications
- Labor and delivery history, including medications, procedures, or complications

Infant History

Data are gathered on the infant in the following areas:

- Overall health status
- Congenital conditions, such as cardiac, respiratory, or orofacial conditions
- Trauma or complications during delivery
- Medications received during labor and delivery or in the early postpartum period
- Activities including circumcision, use of bilirubin lights, or use of bottle, cup, or tube feeding
- Gestational age
- Early responses to feeding attempts

Maternal Examination

Examination of the mother should focus on an evaluation of the breast in the following areas:

- Type of nipples—everted, flat, or inverted
- Presence of surgical scars on the breast or thoracic area
- Any nipple bruising or bleeding

Infant Examination

Evaluation of the infant's oral-motor skills and structures is the basis for the examination. The examiner's finger should be inserted beyond the gum line nearly to the soft palate. The infant should be able to suck smoothly and evenly in a wavelike motion of the tongue as the finger is drawn in for suckling. The hard and soft palate should be intact, without palpable clefts or submucosal clefts. The infant should be able to extend the tongue over the lower gum with no evidence of a tight frenulum. Although there are no standard criteria for diagnosis of what constitutes a frenulum that is *too* tight (i.e., ankyloglossia or "tongue-tie"), a frenotomy may be considered in some infants whose tongue does fully extend and who demonstrate feeding difficulties (Ito, 2014; Segal et al, 2007). In the process of the examination, the infant's state of alertness and readiness for feeding are also observed.

Positions for Breastfeeding

Getting off to a good start begins with positioning the baby at the breast in a way that is comfortable for both the mother and baby and that allows for good latch-on. The three most common positions are the cradle, side-lying, and football-hold positions.

Principles of Correct Positioning

Several principles are common to all of the various positions for breastfeeding, including the following:

- Both the mother and the baby should be comfortable.
- The infant should be positioned "face on" at nipple height so that no head turning or tilting is required. The nipple should be directed toward the center of the infant's mouth.
- The infant should be lying on the side, not the back.
- The infant's body should be in good alignment, with a straight line from the ear to the shoulder to the hips.
- The infant's top and bottom lips should be flanged out (Fig. 11-4).
- The infant's tongue should extend forward over the lower gum line and cup around the nipple and areola.
- Good latch-on results in quiet feedings. No "clicking" or "popping" sounds should be heard from the infant. After mother's milk is in, audible swallowing, such as a "glug" or air blowing out the baby's nose, should be heard.

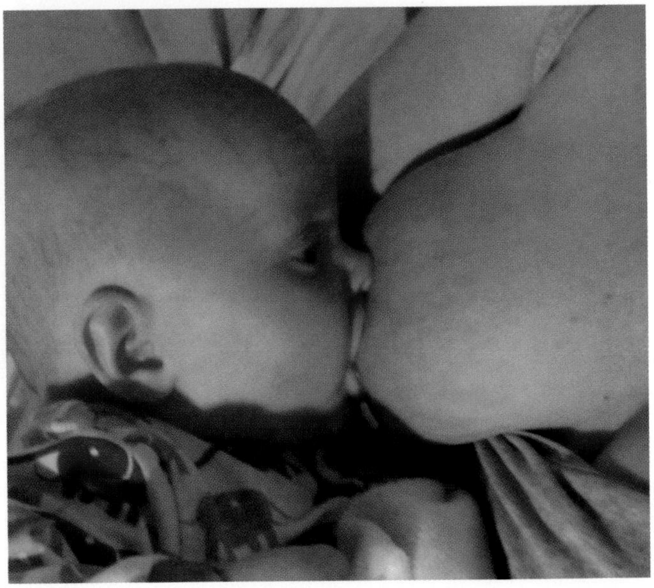

• **Figure 11-4** Lip position.

Cradle Position

The cradle position (also called the *Madonna* or *cuddle position*) and its variation, the cross-cradle position, begin with the mother sitting upright or leaning slightly forward with her feet on the floor or stool or her legs crossed in front of her. The infant is held with the mouth at nipple height, and the mother and infant are in a tummy-to-tummy arrangement. The mother uses her free hand to support the breast, if needed, while keeping her fingers well back from the areola so that she does not interfere with latch-on. The "cigarette hold," or pinching of the breast tissue, should not be used. In the regular cradle position, the baby's head is supported in the crook of the elbow on the same side as the breast being suckled (Fig. 11-5). In the cross-cradle position, the opposite hand supports the baby's head and shoulders. This position often works well for a premature infant because it provides extra support to the head and trunk.

After positioning the baby, the mother should touch the baby's lower lip with her nipple to stimulate mouth opening. As the mouth opens, the mother should bring the baby close so that the lips come up and over the nipple and back onto the areolar tissue and the nipple rests on top of the baby's tongue. Once the baby appears latched on, the mother can check the lips for a flanged, open placement. At this point, the baby is very close to the breast, with the tip of the infant's nose touching it. Mothers often need to be shown that the baby is able to breathe without a need to press down on the breast tissue. If the baby appears to be pushed into the breast, the infant's buttocks should be brought closer into the tummy-to-tummy position. As the mother looks down at her baby, she should see a straight line from the baby's ear to the shoulders to the hips. Once the baby is suckling well, the mother can usually remove the hand that was supporting her breast and use it to cradle the baby in

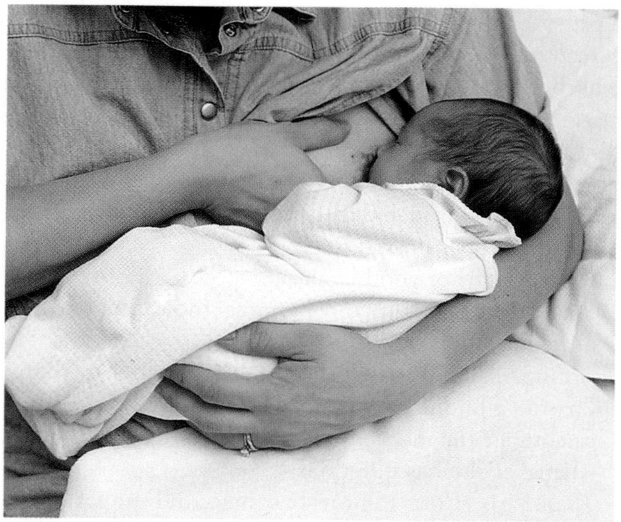

• **Figure 11-5** Cradle hold. The mother positions the infant's head at or near the antecubital space and level with her nipple with her arm supporting the infant's body. Her other hand is free to hold the breast. Once the infant is positioned, pillows or blankets can be used to support the mother's arm, which may tire from holding the baby. (From McKinney ES, James SR, Murray SS, et al: *Maternal-child nursing*, ed 4, St. Louis, 2013, Elsevier/Saunders.)

her arms. She can also relax back from the forward-leaning position that she used at the beginning.

Side-Lying Position

The side-lying or other lying-down variations are often helpful when the mother is uncomfortable sitting up or wishes to nap or sleep with her baby. In the early days of learning to achieve latch-on, the side-lying position is not easy to use because the mother cannot see her breast and nipple quite as well. In the hospital, a nurse should be available to help the mother and infant. At home and with practice, the mother and infant can achieve latch-on without assistance.

In the side-lying position, the mother lies on her side, cradles her infant in her elbow, and supports the infant's back and neck. The mother or the nurse should arrange one to two pillows under the mother's head and shoulders and a rolled towel or blanket along the infant's back to keep the infant in a side-lying position. As in the cradle position, the mother may support her breast with her upper hand (Fig. 11-6).

Football Hold

In the football hold, the infant is supported off to the side of the mother. This position is often used by a mother who has had a cesarean delivery, because it does not require that the infant be positioned along her abdomen or by a mother of multiples when she would like to feed two babies at once. Finally, mothers with flat or inverted nipples are often able to achieve latch-on more easily with this position.

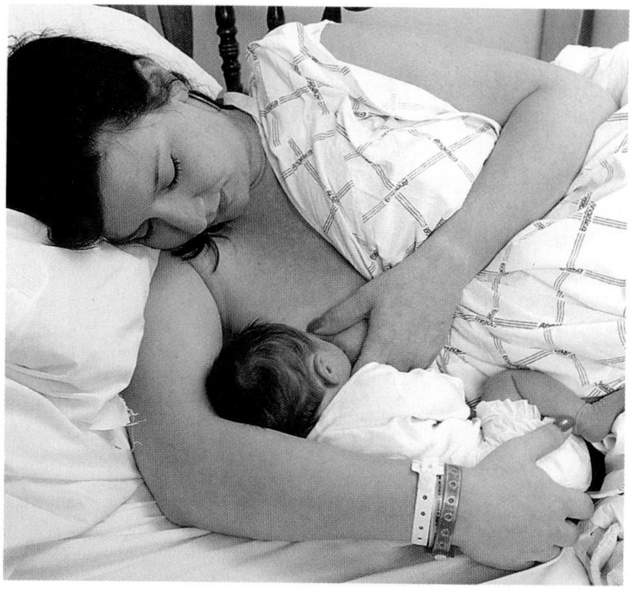

• **Figure 11-6** The side-lying position prevents pressure on episiotomy or abdominal incisions and allows the mother to rest while feeding. She lies on her side, with her lower arm supporting her head or placed around the infant. A pillow behind her back and between her legs provides comfort. Her upper hand and arm are used to position the infant on the side at nipple level and hold the breast. When the infant's mouth opens to nurse, the mother leans slightly forward or draws the infant to her to insert the nipple into the mouth. (From McKinney ES, James SR, Murray SS, et al: *Maternal-child nursing*, ed 4, St. Louis, 2013, Elsevier/Saunders.)

One or two firm pillows should be placed at the mother's side to help support the infant. The baby is in a side-lying position and flexed at the hips, with the buttocks back against the chair or couch. As in other positions, the mother may support her breast to assist with latch-on and remove her hand once the baby is suckling well (Fig. 11-7).

Dynamics of Breastfeeding

Early Feedings

The first breastfeeding should take place as soon after birth as possible. Full term neonates often have an alert period for 30 to 60 minutes after delivery that is ideal for the first feeding practice. This first feeding can take place in the delivery area, if necessary, and should be encouraged by all in attendance. It will not delay, to any significant extent, any procedures required, such as weighing and measuring the infant, instilling ointment or drops in the infant's eyes, and giving vitamin K injections. These procedures can be done one at a time in the delivery room or at the bedside after return to the room. The mother and infant should remain together as much as possible, with rooming-in preferable. The family's desire to promote close contact and initiate breastfeeding should be made clear to and supported by staff. In addition, the health care provider should advocate changes in institutional policy to support the needs of breastfeeding families.

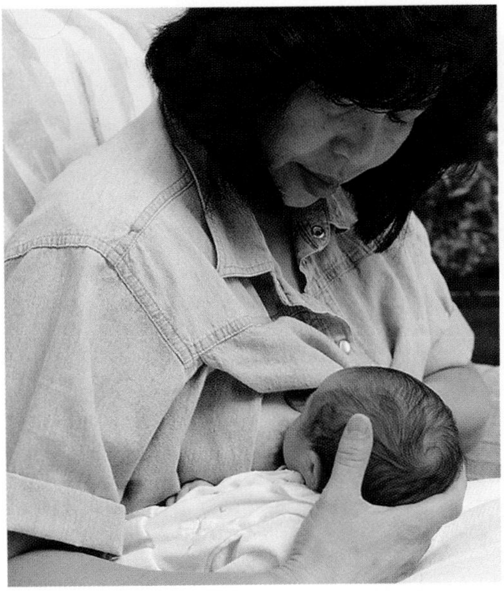

• **Figure 11-7** Football hold. The mother supports the infant's head in her hand, with the infant's body resting on pillows alongside her hip. This method allows the mother to see the position of the infant's mouth on the breast, helps her control the infant's head, and is especially helpful for mothers with heavy breasts. This hold also prevents pressure against an abdominal incision. (From McKinney ES, James SR, Murray SS, et al: *Maternal-child nursing*, ed 4, St. Louis, 2013, Elsevier/Saunders.)

The infant usually goes into a deep sleep after the initial alertness and is difficult to wake for feeding practice. Parents should be instructed to watch for any awakening behavior, such as opening eyes or movement in the bed. Many newborns will not cry at this point, so parents need to be alert for these signs of feeding readiness. Full term infants are born with stores of fluid and energy to carry them through this early transition to the non-uterine environment, a time of infrequent feeding and low volume of colostrum. The infant's stomach, liver, and kidneys are gearing up for the larger volumes of higher-fat food that will come in a few days. It is not necessary to provide any supplement, including water, to a healthy, full term neonate. In addition, feeding with a rubber or silicone nipple may lead to nipple confusion, because it does not work like the breast in delivering milk.

During this transition time, assistance and support from an individual knowledgeable in breastfeeding can be helpful to the mother and infant as they practice latch-on and suckling. The infant should be encouraged to go to each breast for at least 10 to 15 minutes of active suckling, although some infants may spend even longer—up to 20 or 30 minutes. The infant's behavior is much more important during this time than the clock. However, an infant who falls asleep in 5 minutes should be stimulated to continue active suckling. Attention to proper positioning and technique becomes important as the frequency and duration of the suckling behavior increase. A mother is unlikely to get sore or cracked nipples when her infant is latched on correctly. These early feedings are excellent "practice" sessions both for the mother, who gains confidence in her breastfeeding ability, and for the infant, who gets first colostrum and then milk for the efforts at suckling.

The goal of discharge planning is to maintain successful breastfeeding and includes the following:

- Review proper positioning.
- Review signs of good latch-on.
- Review signs of infant progress indicating adequate nutrition (Table 11-2).
- Arrange daily follow-up for 2 to 3 days after discharge.
- Provide a phone contact for questions and concerns.
- Encourage the mother to contact breastfeeding resources whenever she has questions.

These early efforts to provide contact and support during the transition to home can make all the difference in maintaining breastfeeding. Problems encountered during engorgement, sleep deprivation, and times of uncertainty or lack of confidence can be addressed quickly and directly rather than after a bottle has been introduced or the mother's nipples are cracked and bleeding.

Frequency and Duration of Feedings

After the first 24 hours, the infant should be going to the breast 8 to 12 times (or every 2 to 3 hours) in 24 hours for approximately 20 to 45 minutes at each feeding. Frequent suckling stimulates milk production and establishes a regular routine. Exclusive breastfeeding for the first month should be encouraged to ensure the establishment of adequate milk supply and prevent any nipple confusion. Parents need to be alert for an infant who sleeps for 4 to 5 hours at a time or who goes to sleep at the breast in 5 minutes. These infants must be actively wakened and stimulated for feeding.

If the mother and infant must be separated for one or more feedings or supplements are medically necessary, they may be given with a dropper, a cup, or a 5-French feeding tube placed at the breast. Proper instructions, close supervision, and follow-up are needed for each of these methods, and they should not be used routinely.

Pumping

Routine pumping is unnecessary for mothers who are available for a feeding every 2 to 4 hours. However, if the mother and infant must be separated for more than one or two feedings, pumping should be part of the plan to assist with milk production. If the mother and infant are separated right after birth, pumping should begin as soon as possible, within the first 24 hours. The mother should pump six to eight times in 24 hours for 15 minutes if she is using a double-pump setup, or 10 minutes per breast if she is using a single-pump setup. She should be encouraged to save even the smallest amounts of colostrum to give to her infant.

TABLE 11-2 Signs of Infant Progress: A Handout for Parents

	First 8 Hours	8-24 Hours	Day 2	Day 3	Day 4	Day 5	Day 6 and Beyond
Milk supply	You may be able to express a few drops of milk.		Milk should come in between the second and fourth day.			Milk should be in. Breasts may be firm or leak milk.	Breasts should feel softer after nursing.
Baby's activity	Baby is usually wide awake in first hour of life. Put to breast within ½ hour of birth.	Wake your baby. Babies may not wake on their own to feed.	Baby should be more cooperative and less sleepy.	Look for early feeding cues: rooting, lip smacking, hands to face. Note that baby swallows regularly while nursing.			Baby should appear satisfied after feeding.
Feeding routine	Baby may go into a deep sleep 2 to 4 hours after birth.	Feed your baby every 1½ to 3 hours or as often as wanted.	Feedings should be at least 8 to 10 times each day.			May go up to 5 hours between feedings (once in a 24-hour period).	
Breastfeeding	Baby will wake up and be alert and responsive for several more hours after the initial deep sleep.	Nurse at both breasts as long as baby is actively suckling and mother is comfortable.	Try to nurse on both sides at each feeding, aiming for 10-15 minutes at each side. Expect some nipple tenderness.	Consider hand expressing or pumping a few drops of milk to soften the nipple if the breast is too firm for the baby to latch-on.	Nurse at least 10-15 minutes at each side every 2 to 3 hours for the first few months of life.		Mother's nipple tenderness is decreased or gone.
Baby's urine output		Baby must have at least one wet diaper in first 24 hours.	Baby should have at least one wet diaper every 8 hours.	Wet diapers should increase to four to six in 24 hours.	Baby's urine should be light yellow.	Baby should have six to eight wet diapers per day of colorless or light yellow urine.	
Baby's stools		Baby should have a black-green stool (meconium stool).	Baby may have a second very dark (meconium) stool.	Baby's stools should be changing from black-green to yellow.		Baby should have three to four yellow seedy stools per day.	The number of stools may slowly decrease after 4 to 6 weeks.

From Thilo EH, Townsend SF: Early newborn discharge: have we gone too far? *Contemp Pediatr* 13:29–46, 1996.

Hand expression and manual pumps work well for infrequent or short-duration pumping, and some women may choose to hand express exclusively. However, a hospital-grade, piston-style pump that permits pumping both breasts at the same time is ideal for a mother who will have to pump for several weeks or months. No pump works as well as an infant in stimulating production, but frequent pumping goes a long way toward establishing a milk supply and provides the mother with a concrete, healthful contribution to her sick or preterm infant. As the volume of milk goes up over the first few days, the mother can see the success of her efforts. She should be counseled about the increase in production in contrast to the small volume of colostrum produced in the first few days.

Collection and Storage of Breast Milk

A mother who is pumping should be reminded to wash her hands well before she begins pumping and to use clean containers for collection and storage. In addition, the pump parts should be thoroughly cleaned after each use. Many of the pump parts can go through a dishwasher, but the directions that come with the pump should be consulted for specific instructions on cleaning.

Milk collected from pumping should be stored in clean plastic bottles or disposable milk bags. It is preferable to store breast milk in small amounts so that only the amount that is needed is defrosted and used. Milk that has been defrosted and not used within 24 hours should be discarded. Pumped breast milk should be refrigerated as soon after pumping as possible and can be stored there for up to 8 days. It can be stored with reusable cooler packs in a cooler for about 24 hours. If it is not going to be used in that time, it should be frozen. In a refrigerator freezer that maintains a steady temperature, breast milk can be stored for 3 months. Breast milk can be stored for up to 12 months in a freezer where 0° F is routinely maintained. The bottles or bags should be labeled with the date of collection so that the oldest milk can be used first. If the milk must be transported to the hospital or day care facility, it should be placed in ice or on a blue ice unit to minimize the amount of warming or thawing. The American Academy of Pediatrics recommends that breast milk not be saved from an unfinished bottle for use at another feeding (AAP et al, 2011), and no studies have been done to determine the safety of unfinished milk. Others suggest that an unfinished bottle can be refrigerated and reused within 4 hours without problems for the infant (Lawrence and Lawrence, 2011).

Growth Spurts

Just when parents begin to think that breastfeeding is going well, the first growth spurt occurs and they may become concerned. The term *growth spurt* is used to describe those times during breastfeeding when the baby's growth demands exceed the breast milk supply at that moment. For 2 to 4 days, the infant seems to be "hungry all the time" and demands to be fed more frequently. The best response is to feed on demand and increase the number of feedings (i.e., "cluster feedings") because increased stimulation of the breast will increase milk production to the amount needed. However, an inexperienced parent may begin supplementation that can actually lead to a decrease in breast milk production. Once the level of milk production has risen, the infant returns to the normal feeding pattern. Growth spurts tend to occur every 3 to 4 weeks, but parents seem to notice them less as time goes on. The behavior becomes an expected part of the breastfeeding experience.

Breastfeeding Toddlers

Many mothers find breastfeeding an enjoyable experience and may continue into the child's second year of life. In some cases, a second pregnancy may occur and the mother chooses to breast feed both the infant and toddler (tandem feeding). There are many benefits to breastfeeding toddlers who have a wide range of foods in their diet. Breastfeeding continues to provide immunity, strengthens the maternal-child bond, is a source of comfort to the child, and is readily available when the child needs quick nourishment and none other is available. Breastfeeding the toddler can help prevent constipation (Inan, 2009) and may reduce the prevalence of obesity in children, especially if sugar-sweetened beverages are not a part of the diet (Davis et al, 2014). One drawback to breastfeeding the toddler is the effect it may have on dental health. Research indicates that prolonged contact with sweet substances or fermentable carbohydrates (e.g., lactose) leads to demineralization of enamel and subsequent caries. Prolonged and nocturnal breastfeeding (when the natural defense of saliva is decreased), especially after the child is 12 months old, is therefore a risk factor for caries (Çolak et al, 2013). Considerations for breastfeeding toddlers include:

- Breastfeed after the child has eaten a meal, not before
- Breastfeeding should not be on demand as with the infant; mothers can establish times and places (e.g., only at home, before bedtime) when breastfeeding will occur
- If tandem feeding, always feed the infant first
- Have parent consult with the child's dentist regarding potential caries development with breastfeeding
- Have toddler brush teeth before bedtime, but *after* breastfeeding

Weaning

The decision about the time for weaning is an individual one. Breastfeeding should be encouraged for at least one year, but individual circumstances may dictate a different choice for a family. Sometimes weaning is led by the mother and other times by the infant. Typically, a natural weaning process occurs as other foods become a part of the infant's diet and the infant begins to participate in self-feeding.

When a family inquires about the ideal time to begin weaning, the provider can counsel them to consider factors, such as the following:

- Beliefs and desires of individual family members
- Developmental readiness of the infant
- Nutritional replacements for breast milk
- Social and environmental issues affecting the decision

Whether weaning occurs as a planned or unplanned activity, it is best to implement it gradually. Some mothers use a plan over a week or so of having three feedings a day, then two, then one either in the morning or at bedtime. If necessary the mother can use a breast pump to gradually decrease milk production and prevent breast engorgement, blocked ducts, and discomfort. A good approach is to pump when uncomfortable and to pump only to comfort, not to empty. In situations where weaning was not an anticipated or planned event, the health care provider may help the mother deal not only with the act of weaning but also with her feelings about it. Some mothers grieve the early loss of the breastfeeding experience.

In an effort to prevent premature weaning, providers should maintain close communication with families, especially those who are more likely to wean early. Early identification and support of these families may assist them to continue breastfeeding for a longer period. Factors associated with early weaning include the following (Wijndaele et al, 2009):

- Younger mothers
- Low socioeconomic status
- Low maternal education
- Maternal smoking
- Formula feeding or short duration of breastfeeding
- Lack of information or support from health professionals
- Early return to work, lack of support from family, advice from older female family members to wean, and being from a non-Hispanic black cultural group also influence mothers' decisions to introduce solids or wean earlier than recommended

Clinical Indications of Successful Breastfeeding

Infant Weight Gain

Normal newborn infants lose 5% to 8% of their birth weight in the first few days of life. It is helpful for parents to be aware of both the birth and discharge weights. Once the maternal milk volume increases, the infant begins to gain weight in the range of 0.5 to 1 oz/day or 4 to 7 oz/wk. Most breastfed infants have regained their birth weight by 2 weeks. One criterion for failure to thrive is lack of return to birth weight by 3 weeks. Breastfed infants usually double their birth weight by the time that they are 5 to 6 months old and triple it by 1 year old.

The CDC recommends that providers in the United States use the WHO growth standards for children up to 24 months old. WHO standards are based on growth of an international population of healthy infants of whom 100% were "breastfed for 12 months and predominantly breastfed until at least four months old" (Grummer-Strawn et al, 2010). If growth charts other than WHO charts are used, breastfed infants show an apparent decline in growth from 6 to 9 months when compared to formula-fed infants, which may lead a provider to falsely conclude that the infant is not growing well. Use of the WHO growth standards with these same breastfed infants, however, shows them to be on target for growth; in fact, when using the WHO charts, formula-fed infants have apparent excessive weight gain (van Dijk and Innis, 2009), which may "signal early signs of overweight" (Grummer-Strawn et al, 2010). It is essential to assess developmental progress and other measures of growth in all infants, as well as height, weight, and head circumference. Characteristics of a healthy breastfed infant include the following:

- Active and alert state
- Developmentally appropriate progress
- Age-appropriate height and head circumference
- Good skin turgor and color
- Sufficient output of at least six wet diapers and several stools per day
- Contented and satisfied behavior after feeding

Urine Output Guidelines

In the first 2 days of life as the volume of breast milk is increasing, the infant may urinate only one to three times in 24 hours. By day 3, the infant should have four or more wet diapers in 24 hours; and by day 4, the infant should have four to six wet diapers per 24 hours. Over time, the infant should have a minimum of six to eight wet diapers in a 24-hour period. The urine should be light yellow with no strong odor. If the parents are anxious or if they have a question about breastfeeding progress, a diary of wet diapers can be kept to aid in the accurate assessment of progress. Parents need to be alerted, however, to the difficulty of doing accurate diaper counts with disposable diapers and may elect to insert a tissue liner into the diaper or to use cloth diapers for the first few weeks. Ultra absorbent diapers should be avoided when close monitoring of output is necessary.

Stool Output Guidelines

In the first 24 hours after delivery, the baby should have at least one meconium stool followed by another on the second day of life. By the third day, stools are beginning to make the transition to the characteristic loose, yellow, seedy stools of breastfeeding, and the infant should begin having two to three stools in 24 hours. That number may continue to increase in the first few weeks of life. Some infants stool with every feeding. After the first month, the pattern may change again, because some infants begin to stool less frequently and may go several days between stools. As long as the infant is healthy and gaining weight, there is no problem. However, infrequent stooling, especially in the first month, should stimulate a feeding history and possibly a weight check to make sure that the infant is getting enough breast milk.

Maternal Nutritional Needs during Breastfeeding

Maternal nutritional needs increase during lactation. Characteristics of a good diet include the following (Lawrence and Lawrence, 2011):

- A minimum of 1800 calories—about 300 extra calories than prepregnancy (This may vary slightly depending on how much body fat the woman has and how active she is.)
- Generous intake of fruits and vegetables, whole grain breads and cereals, calcium-rich dairy products, and protein-rich fish, meats, and legumes
- Rich sources of calcium, zinc, folate, magnesium, and vitamin B_6
- Culturally appropriate foods
- Supplementation with calcium or prenatal vitamins or both only if the diet is poor

The mother should be encouraged to eat well for her own sake to keep herself healthy and to meet the energy demands of nursing. In addition, an adequate intake of fluid is necessary, but excessive use of fluids does not increase breast milk production. A good guideline for adequate fluid intake is maternal urine that is light yellow and has no strong odor. Eligible mothers and infants should be referred to the Women, Infants, and Children (WIC) special supplemental food program for nutritional counseling and for food supplements. Most WIC programs offer food supplements for the breastfeeding mother's diet, because she does not need formula for the infant. Even with a diet that is adequate in nutrients and calories, a gradual maternal weight loss of 1 to 2 pounds per month usually occurs. In fact, breastfeeding is the ideal way for a mother to return to her prepregnancy weight.

No foods need to be routinely excluded from the maternal diet, unless there is evidence that a particular food bothers the infant or the infant appears to be allergic to it. Sometimes the food does not need to be eliminated but merely decreased. For infants with colic, it can be helpful to reduce allergenic foods (e.g., cow's milk, eggs, peanuts, tree nuts, soy, fish, and wheat) in the mother's diet (Iacovou et al, 2012). When a mother has markedly decreased or eliminated cow's milk from her diet, she must add another source of calcium. Certain foods, such as onions and garlic, may change the flavor and odor of the milk, but they do not negatively affect its quality. The nutrient characteristics of breast milk are fairly stable. One positive way to look at the variety of foods in the diets of mothers from all over the world is to acknowledge that infants are getting early exposure to the foods of their culture.

Alcohol intake of an amount more than 0.5 g/kg of maternal body weight (two cans of beer, 8 oz of wine, or 2 to 2.5 oz of liquor) can impair the milk ejection reflex (Institute of Medicine Subcommittee on Lactation, 1991). Although alcohol is transmitted in breast milk, amounts are not clinically relevant, and recommendations for alcohol intake are the same for women who are breastfeeding as for those who are not (Haastrup et al, 2014).

Large amounts of caffeine from coffee, sodas, or chocolate should be discouraged, because caffeine is transmitted via breast milk to the infant, can be associated with jitteriness in the infant, and may have a negative effect on the iron content of the breast milk. However, the equivalent of one to two cups of coffee per day does not pose a problem (Santos et al, 2012).

Medications for Breastfeeding Mothers

Frequently, women question whether they can take certain medications while they are breastfeeding. Concerns relate primarily to two areas: (1) the effect of the drug on maternal milk supply and (2) the effect of the drug on the infant. General guidelines for maternal drug recommendations include the following:

- Give drugs that are normally safe for infants or have been tested in infants.
- Avoid long-acting forms of a drug.
- Schedule feeding at times when the drug level is lowest. Often breastfeeding immediately after taking the drug is the safest time.
- Observe the infant for changes in feeding pattern, fussiness, vomiting or diarrhea, or rash.
- Consider all appropriate options, and select the drug with the lowest level in breast milk.
- Avoid drugs that inhibit prolactin release, such as estrogen, antihistamines, and ergot compounds.
- Be cautious about the use of herbal preparations.

A good drug reference should be readily available for providers. Four excellent drug references are shown in Box 11-2. Not all references available to providers offer adequate up-to-date information. Two retail pharmacy databases and the Physician's Desk Reference (PDR), for example, have been found to carry recommendations that inappropriately could interfere with breastfeeding (Akus and Bartick, 2007). Decisions about drug selection are difficult, especially when contraindicated drugs are being considered, but the consequences of weaning and loss of breast milk for the infant must be included in the deliberations.

Returning to Work

Women who return to work outside the home after initiating breastfeeding should be encouraged to continue breastfeeding and be supported in their decision with

• BOX 11-2 Drug References

American Academy of Pediatrics (AAP) Committee on Drugs, Sachs HC: The transfer of drugs and therapeutics into human milk: an update on selected topics, *Pediatrics* 132(3):e796–e809, 2013.

Hale TW, Rowe HE: *Medications and mothers' milk 2014*, ed 16, Plano, TX, 2014, Hale Publishing. Updated and reprinted every other year. Order from 800-378-1317 or www.ibreastfeeding.com.

U.S. National Library of Medicine, National Institutes of Health, Health & Human Services: LactMed: a TOXNET database, TOXNET (website): www.toxnet.nlm.nih.gov/newtoxnet/lactmed.htm. Accessed September 1, 2015. Updated monthly.

Woo TM, Wynne AL: *Pharmacotherapeutics for nurse practitioner prescribers*, ed 3, Philadelphia, 2011, FA Davis.

accurate information about how to manage both work and breastfeeding. Increasingly, employers are taking responsibility to provide resources for lactating women, but women continue to need support, encouragement, and education from their health care provider. Education particularly focuses on pumping, storing, and transporting breast milk; introducing the bottle; and handling challenges of multiple demands (Box 11-3). The ideal work environment provides the following:

- A location dedicated to pumping breast milk that is private, convenient, and has access to a sink for washing up and a refrigerator for storage
- Breaks or lunchtime (or both) in which the mother can pump or go to the infant: The average time needed to set up equipment, express milk, and clean up is approximately 30 minutes (Academy of Breastfeeding Medicine Protocol Committee, 2010).
- Supportive colleagues and supervisors
- Maximum of 8 hours of work per day

In addition to providing support and information to the mother, providers can advocate for community and corporate initiatives that promote these conditions in work settings. Women are more likely to continue breastfeeding if they have workplace support (Tsai, 2013), and employers benefit from breastfeeding mothers whose infants tend to be healthier (Ball and Bennett, 2001). Employers can work with the March of Dimes to support their breastfeeding employees (see Additional Resources).

The National Conference of State Legislatures (NCSL) maintains a database on laws related to breastfeeding, including breastfeeding in public and breastfeeding in the workplace. Twenty-seven states, the District of Columbia, and Puerto Rico currently have laws specifically related to work and breastfeeding. Individual practitioners can access this website for an update on the laws in their location (www.ncsl.org/research/health/breastfeeding-state-laws.aspx) (NCSL, 2015).

• BOX 11-3 Advice for Mothers on Returning to Work

Before Delivery

Discuss plans with employer before maternity leave.
Provide employer with information to help in planning (see www.usbreastfeeding.org).
Discuss options with other employees who have continued to breastfeed after returning to work.
Gain support of coworkers.
Investigate pumps, including rental or purchase.
Identify place to pump and to store breast milk at work.

During Maternity Leave

Practice method of breast milk expression that will be used at work.
Begin freezing milk. After the baby feeds at each breast, pump each breast and freeze in disposable milk bags. Amount will be small initially, but the supply will increase with continued pumping (see Collection and Storage of Breast Milk).
Introduce bottle after breastfeeding is well established (usually around 3 to 4 weeks).

After Return to Work

If available, use on-site or nearby child care so that you can go to infant during day.
Ask employer if caregiver for child can bring infant on-site once a day to nurse.
If possible arrange work hours to maximize times to nurse infant (e.g., arrive at work at 8:30 instead of 8:00).
Have a picture of your baby at the pump.
Plan on 15 to 30 minutes to complete pumping.
Wear clothes for easy access to breasts and to hide leaks.

Feeding Breast Milk

Warm or thaw milk in warm water.
Do not use microwave, because milk heats unevenly and presents a risk for burns.
Refrigerate thawed milk for no more than 24 hours; do not refreeze.
Do not add milk to a bottle that has already been used.

Important Reminders

Wash hands before and after pumping.
Rinse pump parts with cool water, then wash with dish detergent, and rinse well after each use.

From Tully MR: Working & breastfeeding: helping moms and employers figure it out, *AWHONN Lifelines* 9(3):198–203, 2005; Marinelli KA, Moren K, Taylor JS, et al: Breastfeeding support for mothers in workplace employment or educational settings: summary statement, *Breastfeed Med* 8(1):137–142, 2013.

Common Breastfeeding Problems

Flat or Inverted Nipples

A nipple can look as though it is inverted, but a "pinch test" is necessary to determine what happens to the nipple during breastfeeding (see the previous description and Fig. 11-3 for the technique). If the nipple pulls in, it is inverted. If the nipple does not pull in, as happens most often, or everts with compression, it is considered to be flat.

Inverted nipples can make it more difficult for the infant to latch-on in the early days, because it is harder to pull the nipple into the mouth for suckling. As the baby continues to breastfeed, the nipple tissue elongates; with time, the problem usually becomes less severe, and successful breastfeeding is possible. Flat nipples do not generally change over time, but the infant develops a style to more easily latch-on successfully. Adhesions cause retraction or inversion of the nipples. Flat nipples are often found in women with larger breasts.

Differential Diagnosis

The differential diagnosis for flat or inverted nipples is dimpled, fissured, or unusually shaped nipples.

Management

Prenatal

If the patient is not at risk for preterm labor, breast shells can be used during the third trimester for inverted nipples. The obstetrician or nurse-midwife should be notified before their use. Shells are plastic, dome-shaped devices with small holes for ventilation. An opening in the portion that lies against the skin fits over the nipple, and gentle suction during use helps stretch the nipple tissue. The bra cup holds the shell comfortably in place, and the use of shells during the last trimester generally helps stretch out adhesions in preparation for breastfeeding.

Postpartum

The provider should stay with the mother during early feeding attempts; give extra praise, reassurance, and support; and emphasize the need for extra patience and persistence. Encourage use of the football-hold position during feedings and have the mother lean slightly forward as she latches the baby on.

The mother may find any of the following helpful:

- Wear breast shells between feedings.
- Manually pull or roll the nipple immediately before latch-on.
- Use a breast pump for 1 or 2 minutes before latch-on.
- Put a cold cloth or ice on the nipple for a few seconds before latch-on.
- Avoid pacifiers and bottle nipples until the infant is 4 to 6 weeks old.
- If supplementation is medically indicated, use a syringe, dropper, feeding tube, or supplemental nutrition system.

Complications

Complications of flat or inverted nipples include the following:

- Frustration
- Loss of self-confidence
- Inadequate infant nutrition and its sequelae
- Severe maternal engorgement, plugged ducts, or mastitis
- Discontinued breastfeeding

Sore Nipples

Soreness of the nipples is pain caused by irritation or trauma to the nipples and areola, often accompanied by a breakdown in skin integrity. Sore nipples have many causes, including the following:

- Improper latch-on and positioning at the breast
- Prolonged negative pressure
- Inappropriate suction release from the breast
- Use of or sensitivity to nipple creams and oils
- Incorrect use of breastfeeding supplies (e.g., pumps, shells, shields)
- Thrush (candidiasis)
- Leaking nipples that are not properly air-dried

Clinical Findings

The nipples, areolae, and breasts are tender, bruised, raw, cracked, bleeding, blistered, discolored, swollen, or traumatized.

Differential Diagnosis

The differential diagnoses for sore nipples include the following:

- Mild tenderness, which is sometimes described by new mothers as they are getting used to the infant's suckling
- Breast or nipple trauma from another cause
- Thrush (candidiasis)
- Mastitis
- Abscess
- Milk plugs at the nipple pores

Management

The following measures can be taken to manage sore nipples:

- Assess breastfeeding at an early feeding. Prevent the problem by demonstrating and reinforcing the proper latch-on technique and positioning of the infant.
- Counsel mothers to seek help early for more than mild tenderness. Nipples can be damaged by constant high negative pressure and do not "toughen up" as breastfeeding progresses. Cracking and bleeding are not normal.
- Rub a few drops of colostrum or hindmilk onto the nipple and areola after every feeding and let it air-dry.
- Expose the nipples to air for short periods several times a day.
- Use breast shells to prevent the bra or clothing from rubbing against the nipple.
- Nurse from the least sore side first.
- Use short, frequent feedings.
- Pump the affected breast if pain is too severe to allow nursing.
- Use mild analgesics, as necessary.
- Refer to a lactation specialist as appropriate.

Severe Engorgement

Severe engorgement is characterized by extremely full, sore, and swollen breasts, beyond the normal fullness experienced as the milk comes in. Engorgement is caused by milk stasis in the breast from inadequate emptying.

Clinical Findings

The following are seen in severe engorgement:

- Painful, hard, lumpy, swollen breasts
- Breasts usually warm to the touch
- Nipples flattened by the swelling
- Bruising or trauma to the nipples and areolae

Differential Diagnosis

The differential diagnosis for severe engorgement is bilateral mastitis.

Management

The following measures can be taken to manage engorgement:

- Take a hot shower or wrap the breasts with warm, wet compresses for 5 to 10 minutes before nursing. Disposable diapers can be moistened with hot water and then wrapped around each breast and "tabbed" to hold them in place. The plastic liner holds the heat in longer than an ordinary washcloth or towel does.
- Gently massage the entire breast or use an electric pump with intermittent suction on the minimal setting for several minutes after using wet heat.
- Manually express milk before feeding to soften the areola and make it easier for the infant to latch-on properly.
- Nurse frequently and make certain that latch-on and position are correct and audible swallowing is heard.
- Avoid long stretches between feedings in the early weeks as the milk supply is being established. Pump the breasts if a feeding will be missed.

Mastitis

Although rarely seen in the postpartum hospital setting, mastitis is an infection of the breast that can occur at any time during lactation. Occasionally, it has been identified during the third trimester of pregnancy. *Staphylococcus aureus*, streptococci, and corynebacteria are most commonly associated with mastitis (Arroyo et al, 2010). Predisposing factors include:

- Stress, fatigue
- Cracked nipples, plugged ducts
- Constricting, improperly fitting bra
- Inadequate emptying of the breast
- Sudden weaning or a significant decrease in the number of feedings

Clinical Findings

The following are commonly noted in mastitis:

- Malaise
- Breast tenderness or pain
- A reddened, warm lump in any quadrant, sometimes associated with red streaking
- Flu-like symptoms, including fever, chills, and body aches

An old adage is that the "flu" in a breastfeeding woman is mastitis until proved otherwise.

Management

Recommendations for treatment of mastitis include the following:

- Empty the breast. Nurse frequently, or if pain is severe, pump milk carefully from the affected breast. Breast milk is not infected and is fine for the infant.
- Use analgesics as necessary.
- Oral Lactobacillus fermentum CECT5716 or Lactobacillus salivarius CECT5713, probiotics isolated from human milk, has been found to be as effective as antibiotic therapy (Arroyo et al, 2010; Fernández et al, 2014).
- Although more studies are recommended to determine the appropriate role of antibiotics to treat mastitis (Jahanfar et al, 2013), antibiotic therapy has been a mainstay of treatment. Administer oral antibiotics such as penicillinase-resistant penicillin or a cephalosporin that covers *S. aureus*. Treatment should be maintained for 10 to 14 days. Dicloxacillin is often used, and amoxicillin-clavulanic acid and cefuroxime have been found to be effective with few adverse effects (Benyamini et al, 2005).
- Rest (extremely important).
- Do not wean abruptly because of the possibility of mastitis progressing into an abscess.
- Take warm showers or use warm wet compresses.
- Increase fluids.

Complications

Abscess and septicemia are complications of mastitis.

Nipple Confusion

Nipple confusion occurs when an infant is accustomed to nursing from a bottle and is introduced to the breast. Different oral-motor skills are used in breastfeeding and bottle feeding, and infants who have been given a bottle or pacifier sometimes attempt to breastfeed using the same sucking pattern as with a bottle. This can make it difficult to obtain adequate nourishment and may contribute to maternal sore nipples. The infant may cry, fuss, or push away with their arms during attempts to nurse.

Clinical Findings

The following are seen in nipple confusion:

- Ineffective suckling at the breast
- Breast refusal
- Sore, red, or bruised maternal nipples

Differential Diagnosis

The differential diagnoses for nipple confusion are other causes of fussiness and refusal to feed.

Management

The following are recommended to manage nipple confusion:

- Avoid all rubber bottle nipples and pacifiers for the first 4 to 6 weeks or until the infant is breastfeeding successfully, unless absolutely necessary.
- Retrain the infant to suck correctly at the breast by correct positioning, proper latch-on technique, suck training to repattern tongue movements, and supplementation via alternative methods if required.
- Consult with a lactation specialist as indicated.
- If supplements are medically indicated, give with an eyedropper, spoon, syringe, or cup or through a 5-French feeding tube (attached to a 20- or 30-mL syringe) taped to the areola or breast. The end of the tubing protrudes slightly past the end of the nipple so that the tube, nipple, and areola are in the infant's mouth.
- Using a thin silicone nipple shield may help the infant successfully latch-on and suckle, especially with the preterm infant (Eglash et al, 2010), but there is little evidence supporting the safety or effectiveness of nipple shields to ensure adequate intake; it is recommended that nipple shields be used with caution (McKechnie and Eglash, 2010). Cleansing and drying both the shields and breast after feeding are important to prevent skin breakdown and infection.

Complications

The following are complications of nipple confusion:

- Failure to thrive
- Hyperbilirubinemia
- Colic and crying
- Prolonged feedings
- Sore and cracked nipples
- Plugged ducts
- Mastitis
- Frustration

Breast Milk Jaundice

Breast milk (late onset) jaundice is an elevated serum indirect bilirubin concentration with the peak level occurring on or after day 7 to 10 of life in an infant drinking an adequate amount of breast milk with no other signs of liver abnormality. The exact cause of breast milk jaundice is unknown; however, an enzyme may be present in some mothers' milk that inhibits the action of glucuronyl transferase and increases intestinal absorption of bilirubin. Breast milk jaundice is more common in Asian and North American Indian infants. Siblings with the same mother are often affected. True breast milk jaundice is uncommon and estimated to occur in less than 1 in 200 births (Clark, 2013; Preer and Philipp, 2011).

Clinical Findings

Physical Examination

The following are seen with breast milk jaundice:

- Healthy and thriving infant
- Adequate stooling and voiding
- Appropriate weight gain
- Appearance of elevated bilirubin levels between day 7 and 10 of life
- Bilirubin peaks around day 10 to 15
- Persistence into the third month of life

Diagnostic Tests

The following tests are usually indicated:

- Serum bilirubin
- Urine and other cultures, which are sometimes necessary to rule out infection

Differential Diagnosis

The differential diagnosis for breast milk jaundice is pathologic jaundice.

Management

Continue breastfeeding unless clinical signs of pathologic jaundice are observed. See Chapter 39 for a discussion of pathologic jaundice. The family should be reassured that breast milk jaundice is not harmful.

Thrush

When oral candidiasis is diagnosed in the infant or found on the nipple or areolae of the nursing mother, both members of the dyad should be treated. See Chapter 37 for a discussion of candidiasis.

Poor Weight Gain

Problems associated with poor weight gain occur at two different times and represent different challenges for management. During the newborn period, initiation of breastfeeding may not proceed normally, and the infant may actually continue to lose weight or, at best, gain very slowly. After the newborn period, infants may gain weight more slowly than expected given normal parameters for their age.

Poor weight gain has a number of contributing factors, including the following:

- Infrequent or inadequate feeding because of poorly managed breastfeeding or environmental or social circumstances in the family system
- Inadequate milk production
- Genetic predisposition
- Infection
- Organic disease
- Physical anomaly that prevents good suckling or swallowing

Clinical Findings

The following may be seen in poor weight gain:

Infant Factors

- Continued weight loss after 5 to 7 days old
- Failure to regain birth weight by 2 to 3 weeks old
- Failure to maintain an ongoing weight gain of 0.5 to 1 oz/day
- Weight below the third percentile for age (This finding can be a pattern over time or a sudden change.)
- Lethargic, sleepy, inactive, unresponsive infant
- Newborn or young infant sleeping longer than 4 hours between feedings
- Dry mucous membranes
- Poor skin turgor

Technique Factors

- Ineffective latch-on or sucking
- Short time at the breast (The infant is removed before nursing is finished, thus reducing access to hindmilk and total consumption.)
- Infant kept on a preset schedule despite cues for more feeding
- Infant given water between feedings to "get through" to the next feeding
- Infant encouraged or allowed to sleep through the night before 8 to 12 weeks old
- Fewer than eight feedings in 24 hours
- Infant fed in a distracting environment
- In older infants, breastfeeding offered after solids are given
- Infant in a day care setting that does not facilitate breastfeeding

Maternal Factors

- Does not initially respond to infant's cues for feeding or does not recognize that waking is needed to establish feeding
- Hectic schedule with limited time for breastfeeding
- Recent illness or significant weight loss
- Uses oral contraceptives or other hormones

Differential Diagnosis

The differential diagnoses for poor weight gain are a pattern of slower but normal weight gain in healthy breastfed infants and failure to thrive.

Management

The following measures should be taken to manage poor weight gain:

- Complete a thorough history to elicit information regarding infant and maternal factors.
- Conduct a thorough assessment of breastfeeding techniques to accurately determine the extent to which mismanagement is a cause.
- Provide instruction, encouragement, and reinforcement for correct breastfeeding techniques.
- Refer for treatment of physical or organic causes.
- Be alert for any infant who has lost too much weight and is unable to feed with vigor at the breast; such infants require an immediate infusion of calories for energy.
- Use a supplemental system at the breast if supplementation is required.
- Encourage and reassure the parents.

Complications

Complications of poor weight gain include developmental delay, poor bonding, and severe dehydration. In situations of early failure to establish breastfeeding, some infants may appear to be in a septic state and require hospitalization for rehydration and further evaluation.

For a complete list of references, please visit http://evolve.elsevier.com/Burns/pediatric/.

12

Elimination Patterns

ARDYS M. DUNN AND MICHELLE MCGARRY

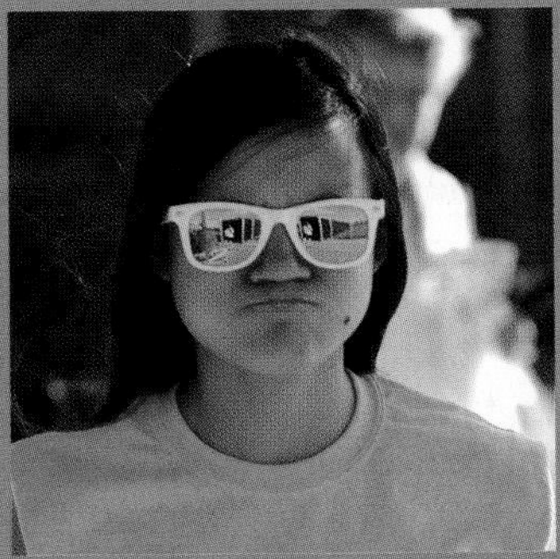

Gastrointestinal (GI), renal, urinary, and integumentary systems function to eliminate metabolic byproducts and body wastes. This chapter discusses normal bowel and bladder function, normal developmental activities (such as, toilet training), and behaviors in children that are often self-limited but that may require intervention (e.g., encopresis and enuresis). Problems related more directly to GI and renal pathology are presented in Chapters 33 and 35. Dermatologic conditions are discussed in Chapter 37.

Healthy children demonstrate an extremely wide range of elimination patterns, and primary care providers have a responsibility to help parents understand what "normal" behavior is and what constitutes a problem. This can be a challenge because cultural and social expectations about elimination vary greatly, causing some parents to believe that their child has a problem when none exists and vice versa. This said, it is also important to realize that if a parent considers it a problem, providers must offer assistance because reassurance alone will not ease their concerns. Education is necessary. Also, developmental processes, such as toilet training, can lead to problems if not appropriately managed. Providers must conduct thorough and accurate assessments, provide anticipatory guidance for parents about what to expect as their child develops, and help parents know, understand, and facilitate healthy bowel and bladder function, because many parents have poor elimination habits themselves. Referral should be considered any time that an issue is complicated, out of normal developmental range, or causing significant distress to parents and/or child.

Standards

The American Academy of Pediatrics (AAP) and the U.S. Preventive Services Task Force (USPSTF) do not recommend routine urinalysis for asymptomatic children. Screening urinalysis should be conducted based on a specific clinical symptom or condition (Simon et al, 2014; USPSTF, 2014). The AAP recommends that toilet training begins when the child and the parent are ready, which is not before 18 to 24 months of age and may be closer to 3 years of age (Wolraich and Tippins, 2003).

Normal Patterns of Elimination: Bowel and Urinary

Infants

Bowel Patterns

Bowel patterns of infants are related to the frequency and amount of feeding and differ between formula-fed and breastfed babies. Breastfed infants commonly have many small stools per day in the first weeks of life; three to four loose stools per day in the neonate is an indicator of adequate breast milk. During the second month of life, infant stooling may decrease markedly, from a median of six stools to one stool per day. Nearly 40% of infants do not stool every day. Some older breastfed infants may stool as infrequently as once every 8 to 14 days (AAP, 2012). In exclusively breastfed infants, infrequent stooling is not a problem; if the infant is thriving, happy, and has no clinical signs (e.g., abdominal distention, irritability, vomiting), parents can be reassured that it is transient. The stools of breastfed infants are usually soft, sticky, or watery with a curd-like texture, light yellow, and have a "sour" but not unpleasant odor. Iron supplements can darken the stool and make it firmer.

Formula-fed babies have two to four stools each day in the first month. As patterns become established, the number of stools decreases, and older formula-fed infants may have one to three soft, semi-formed stools each day. Stools of formula-fed infants are firmer, darker, and smellier than those of breastfed infants. They may be brown, greenish, or dark yellow, depending on the type of formula and whether it is iron-fortified or if the child is given iron supplements. The stools of both breastfed and formula-fed babies become firmer, darker, and more predictable as solid foods are introduced but should remain soft enough that they are easy to pass for the infant. If there is a question of true constipation in an exclusively breastfed infant in the first months of life, referral to a specialist is indicated. It is important to explain to parents that it is the consistency of the stool that is passed that determines constipation, not the effort required, because grunting and straining can be normal.

Urinary Patterns

Urination is associated with fluid intake, increasing as infants take more fluids. Healthy, well-hydrated infants, whether breastfed or formula-fed, should urinate a minimum of six times a day but can void in small amounts as many as 15 to 20 times a day. The urine should be pale yellow or colorless. Fever in infants can quickly lead to dehydration, with less frequent urination.

Voluntary bowel and bladder control depends on myelination of the pyramidal tracts in the spinal cord, a process typically completed between 12 and 18 months of age. Infants 9 to 12 months old generally have regular patterns; they may have a bowel movement early in the morning or after feeding or stay dry for several hours and urinate immediately after waking from a nap. Parents may use these regular patterns to begin introducing the older infant to toilet training, and some parents will place the younger child on the "potty" when the child shows elimination cues. It is important to help the parent differentiate between helping the child associate cues with the potty and actually starting potty training, a process that should be determined individually according to the development of the child and the family.

Toddlers and Preschoolers

Bowel Patterns

Toddlers and preschoolers usually have regular elimination patterns. Although they typically have one to three stools a day, they should stool at least 5 to 7 days a week. Normal stools have an unpleasant odor and should be slender, light to medium brown, mushy, and easily passed by the child.

Urinary Patterns

By the time children are 2 years old, renal function is fully developed. The urinary pattern of toddlers and preschoolers is influenced by fluid intake, environmental conditions, perspiration, fever, and diarrhea with significant fluid loss. Toddlers typically urinate 8 to 14 times a day. Cold weather, excitement, and stress lead to increased frequency. A good guideline for water intake for children after 1 year of age is 30 mL/kg/day of water. Unless the parent has significant concern that the pediatric provider cannot alleviate or there are physical problems, there is no need to treat children who are wetting at night up to 5 years old.

School-Age Children

Bowel Patterns

Elimination patterns in school-age children approximate those of adults. Depending on intake, a child may have bowel movements from one to three times a day with typically five to seven bowel movements or more per week. Normal stools have an unpleasant odor and should be slender, light to medium brown, mushy, and easily passed by the child. School-age children should be completely toilet trained, although occasional soiling of underwear occurs as a result of poor hygiene or because children do not respond quickly to defecation cues. During the school-age years, it is important to be aware that children increasingly need independence and privacy; these needs extend into the arena of toilet management.

Urinary Patterns

The kidneys of school-age children are still small and accommodate a smaller urine volume at any one time than those of adults. Healthy bladder volume for school-age children is calculated as: age in years $\times$ 2 = bladder volume in ounces (multiplying the ounces calculated by 30 will give the volume in milliliters). Children should normally void six to eight times a day; three to four times a day is considered too infrequent. Dysfunctional voiding, daytime incontinence, or nocturnal enuresis warrant further evaluation, especially because these conditions can be associated with infection, dehydration, constipation, or sexual abuse. Although they are most often functional disorders due to bladder or bowel habits, referral to a pediatric urology specialist may be appropriate.

Adolescents

Bowel and Urinary Patterns

GI and renal functions are at adult levels in adolescents, and elimination patterns are similar to those of adults. It is important to determine not only frequency but character and effort to produce a bowel movement. Abnormal variation can occur in teenagers who have eating disorders. Adolescents are also susceptible to the demands of schedules, stress, school requirements, and irregular eating patterns. Sexual activity can contribute to changes in bowel or bladder function, including infections or constipation.

Assessment of Patterns

Assessment of elimination patterns begins with a thorough health history with questions being asked of the parent or the child, depending on the child's age and ability. It is very important to get information from the child, because parents may no longer be aware of habits, especially of older children. As variations of normal behavior become evident, relevant follow-up questions should be asked to clarify and complete the health picture.

Health History

Description of Current Status

The child's current elimination status can be assessed with the following questions:

- How often do you (asked of child) or does your child urinate? How many wet diapers does your baby have in a 24-hour period?

- How often do you (asked of child) or does your child have a bowel movement? Describe what the stools look, feel, and smell like. What is their size? How does your child act when having a bowel movement? Where do they have bowel movements? Do they use the toilet for both urine and stool? Do older children have aversions to school or public restrooms?
- Describe anything unusual about your child's elimination habits. Does your child resist going to the bathroom?
- Do you use any medications, including over-the-counter preparations or home remedies, to help your child with bowel movements?
- Describe your child's toileting habits. For example, at what time of day does your child have a bowel movement? Is this consistent?
- Ask of parents of a 9- to 12-month-old child: How do you think the process of toilet training will happen?
- Is your child toilet trained? When did training begin? Describe the process. How often do "accidents" happen? How do you (parent) feel toilet training is progressing? How stressed do you feel about the process and why?
- What names are used in your family for stool and urine, for body parts, and for the process of using the toilet? (Encourage accurate names when possible).

Birth and Early Infancy History

Determine whether any problems with the child's urine or stool were present at birth. For example, did the baby pass a meconium stool within 48 hours after birth? How soon after birth did the baby urinate? Was the baby breastfed? When were solids introduced and did that change stooling patterns or character?

Review of Systems

The review of systems should include the following questions:

- Has your child ever been constipated or had diarrhea? How do you define constipation and diarrhea? (See Table 12-1 for Bristol Scale of stool quality that reflects colonic transit time.) (Box 12-1 summarizes the Rome III criteria for functional constipation.) Is it chronic or only occasional? Did it start after a particular incident (e.g., illness, during toilet training, with a certain food or change in diet)? Providers need to remember that diarrhea can be a presenting symptom in constipation due to stool leaking around the more solid stool.
- Has your child ever had a urinary tract infection (UTI)? Describe the incident. Was there any fever, flank pain, or nausea and vomiting? Any workup (e.g., ultrasonography [US], urethrogram)? What were the findings, treatment, and follow-up?
- Has your child had any illness, injury, or operation related to the bowel or bladder? Describe.
- Does your child have a physical condition or chronic illness that affects voiding or bowel movements?

TABLE 12-1 Bristol Stool Form Scale

Type	Stool Description	Transit Description
Type 1	Separate hard lumps, like nuts	Slow colonic transit
Type 2	Sausage-shaped but lumpy	Slow colonic transit
Type 3	Sausage or snakelike but with cracks on surface	Normal colonic transit
Type 4	Sausage or snakelike, smooth and soft	Normal colonic transit
Type 5	Soft blobs with clear-cut edges	Normal colonic transit
Type 6	Fluffy pieces with ragged edges, mushy stool	Fast colonic transit
Type 7	Watery, no solid pieces	Fast colonic transit

Adapted from Choung RS, Locke GR 3rd, Zinsmeister AR, et al: Epidemiology of slow and fast colonic transit using a scale of stool form in a community, *Aliment Pharmacol Ther* 26:1043–1050, 2007.

• BOX 12-1 Rome III Criteria for Functional Constipation: Infants and Children

Child must have at least two of the following criteria for at least 1 month (infants to 4 years old) or for at least 2 months (children >4 years old), with no evidence of structural, metabolic, or endocrine disease:

- Two or fewer defecations per week
- At least one episode of fecal incontinence per week (after child is toilet trained)
- History of excessive stool retention, retentive posturing in children equal to or greater than 4 years old
- History of painful or hard bowel movements
- History of large diameter stools, could obstruct toilet
- Presence of large fecal mass in rectum

Rome Foundation: Rome III disorders and criteria (website): www.romecriteria.org/criteria/. Accessed September 1, 2014.

- Is there a history of bed-wetting? At what age did it resolve?
- What medications, including over-the-counter preparations, herbs, or complementary medications, does your child take?

Family History

Determine whether any family members, including parents, have had problems with urination or bowel movements, and describe them (e.g., chronic constipation or diarrhea, bed-wetting). Has the child or family traveled or lived outside the United States? Does the family residence use well water?

Environment and Psychosocial Issues

Environmental and psychosocial issues should be assessed, using questions such as:

- How do you, as a parent, feel about the issue of toileting?
- If appropriate, how often do you as a parent defecate/urinate?
- How do you interact with your child around toileting issues?
- How do you deal with toileting "accidents" (including bed-wetting)?
- What plans do you have for managing toilet training?
- Describe your child's typical diet.
- Tell me about the toileting facilities at your child's house, day care, and school. How do you think they affect your child's toileting habits?

Physical Examination

The physical examination includes external examination of the perineum, anus, and urinary meatus, including the base of the spine; and auscultation and palpation of the abdomen for bowel sounds, softness, masses, peristalsis, and tenderness. There should also be an age-appropriate gross motor neurologic examination performed.

Diagnostic Studies

Diagnostic studies may include:

- Urinalysis (with or without urine culture) as indicated based on symptoms
- Stool specimen, as indicated by history and symptoms
- Diagnostic imaging as indicated after initial laboratory workup and assessment/management considerations (see Chapters 33 and 35)

Management Strategies for Normal Patterns

Toilet Training

Toilet training occurs in the toddler and preschool years and is usually complete by the time the child is 4 years old, with the majority of children training between 2½ and 3½ years old. Successful toilet training requires sensitivity, understanding of development, good communication, hope, humor, and patience. In addition to becoming self-sufficient in their toileting, children should also learn that elimination is a natural and necessary process. As self-toileting is mastered, both parents and children should experience pride and satisfaction in having worked together to accomplish an important developmental task.

The health care provider plays an important role in providing anticipatory guidance to parents. Introduce the topic of toilet training at the 9-month visit and again at 12, 15, and 18 months; assess parents' expectations and plans, and provide ample opportunity for discussion and possible development of realistic toileting outcomes. It can also be useful to tell parents that age at toilet training is not related to or indicative of intelligence.

When to begin toilet training is a perennial question of parents. Providers can emphasize that every child is unique, and readiness cues should ultimately be used to decide when to begin training. Physiologic readiness develops by about 18 months. True voluntary sphincter control is a function of psychological and social development as well, so most children are not usually ready for independent toilet training until 24 months or even older. Guidelines for assessing toilet-training readiness include physical, cognitive, interpersonal or psychological, and parental skills (Table 12-2). It is also essential that parents understand and can express to children that the goal is to use the toilet, not to hold in urine or stool. This is an important distinction, and parents should not encourage holding of urine and/or stool, which can lead to bowel and bladder dysfunction (BBD).

As families from various cultural groups immigrate to the United States, health care providers need to understand family practices and be open to developing mutually agreed-upon approaches to toilet training. Early *assisted potty training*, for example, begins in the Vietnamese culture at about 3 months old, with most children trained by 24 months old (Duong et al, 2013).

If begun too early, toilet training can be very stressful for both parents and children and can contribute to family dysfunction. Starting independent toilet training before 24 or after 30 months has also been found to be related to

TABLE 12-2 Guidelines for Assessing Readiness to Toilet Train

Skill Type	Description
Child's physical skills	Has voluntary sphincter control Stays dry for 2 hours; may wake from naps still dry Is able to sit, walk, and squat Assists in dressing self
Child's cognitive skills	Recognizes urge to urinate or defecate Understands meaning of words used by family in toileting Understands what the toilet is for Understands connection between dry pants and toilet Is able to follow directions Is able to communicate needs
Child's interpersonal skills	Demonstrates desire to please parent Expresses curiosity about use of toilet Expresses desire to be dry and clean
Parental skills	Expresses desire to assist child with training Recognizes child's cues of readiness Has no compelling factor that will interfere with training (e.g., new job, move, newborn, and/or family loss or gain)

dysfunctional voiding and (in delayed training) constipation (Hodges et al, 2014).

Typically, children are trained first for nocturnal bowel control, and then daytime bowel control, daytime bladder control, and finally nocturnal bladder control. Average times for being fully trained are around 3 to 4 years old, with a normal age variation of up to a year for individual children.

There is little evidence regarding which, if any, toilet training strategy (e.g., early assisted; Brazelton's child-oriented approach [Brazelton and Sparrow, 2004]; operant conditioning, such as described in Azrin and Foxx's *Toilet Training in Less than a Day* [1974]) is most effective. When children and parents are ready to begin toilet training, several management techniques can be helpful (Box 12-2). If children resist training, the effort should be put on hold for a few weeks before trying again. It is important to stress to parents that none of these "holds" should be viewed as a failure for either parent or child. If toddlers seem to be toilet trained for a brief period and suddenly regress to wetting and soiling consistently, they should be placed back in diapers and the process begun again within a few weeks. It is extremely important that parents and children do not become engaged in a "battle for control" over toilet training. For example, providers should emphasize to parents that they should never ask the child, "Do you need to go potty, pee, and so on?" The answer will always be "No," and thus an immediate battle ensues that is not even about the actual toileting. Ultimately, it is the child's responsibility to control his or her bowel and urinary function, and toilet training is only one of the many tasks toddlers master on their way to independence. Parents have the responsibility to assist in the process by providing a positive environment and opportunities, teaching the techniques, and setting a positive example. It appears that a structured yet flexible approach that is responsive to the child's cues is likely to be most successful. Parents should be reassured that this needs to be individualized to each parent/child dyad and may be different for siblings.

Parents can become extremely frustrated if their expectations do not match the abilities and performance of their children, and child abuse related to toilet training may occur. Berkowitz (2011) asserts that issues around toileting are the second most prevalent factor precipitating fatal child abuse. Health care providers can play a crucial role in making the experience a positive one and preventing abuse by giving parents information about child development, techniques for managing the training process, and support and encouragement for their efforts. This includes proactively doing follow-up with families who express frustration or appear to be having difficulty with the toilet training process.

• BOX 12-2 Management of Toilet Training

- Keep child as clean and dry as possible:
  - Change diapers frequently.
  - Use training pants or underwear when child stays dry for several hours during the day; use diaper at night.
- Talk to child about toilet training:
  - Praise child for asking to have diaper changed.
  - Explain connection between being clean and dry and using toilet.
  - Emphasize that the goal is to produce in the toilet, not to hold to stay clean and dry.
  - Provide opportunity for child to use toilet, especially before going out to play, going on a trip, before naps, and at bedtime; set an example with adult behavior.
  - Do not ask child if they need to go, rather set up a time schedule of every 1½ hours for voiding and matter-of-factly state it is time to go.
- Teach child how to use toilet:
  - Allow child to observe while parents or older siblings use toilet.
  - Demonstrate how to sit on toilet with feet supported and knees spread with forward pelvic tilt, use toilet paper, flush, and wash hands.
- Provide practice time for child:
  - Provide a potty chair or portable toilet seat.
  - Allow child to sit on potty chair with clothes or diaper on.
  - Encourage child to use potty chair while parent uses regular toilet.
  - Have child sit on potty chair without diapers for 5-10 minutes at a time.
  - Practice at times the child usually urinates or defecates.
- Provide a comfortable, safe-feeling environment:
  - Seat child facing backward on a regular toilet or provide a footstool to rest the feet on with knees wide and forward pelvic tilt.
  - Never flush the toilet when child is sitting on it. Use sticky notes to stop automatic flush on public toilets.
  - Stay with child for safety reasons.
- Give consistent, positive feedback:
  - Praise child for trying and for success.
  - Be understanding of child's refusal to use toilet.
  - Never demand performance.
  - Never make child sit on toilet if child resists.
  - Ignore or minimize undesired behavior.
  - Never scold or punish if a child wets or soils.
  - Use star chart or other reward for success or effort; consider having the reward the child is working toward in the bathroom so that the job and reward are clearly connected for the child.
  - Do not praise excessively.

Altered Patterns of Elimination: Bowel and Bladder Dysfunction

Bowel and bladder dysfunction (BBD), formerly called *dysfunctional elimination syndrome* (Austin et al, 2014), is any abnormal pattern in bowel or bladder function at an age when an individual is developmentally capable of control. A number of factors contribute to BBD, and the close relationship between bowel and bladder function, due to the function of the pelvic floor, is key to understanding this complex and varied condition; it is, in reality, a set of conditions. The child may actively try to prevent bowel movements or urination (e.g., the school-aged child who has restricted access to bathroom facilities, the child who had a painful bowel movement and has decided that he or she does not want it to hurt, or the child who is "too busy" to stop and use the bathroom). The actual cause for each child is likely multifactorial; but in most cases, it is not necessary to know exactly why it happened. Parents can sometimes be very focused on the why and, although having that information may help to prevent the problem from recurring, it is not necessary in treating and resolving the issue.

Urgency, frequency, and urinary incontinence are common in BBD, and the child may have difficulty initiating urination or completely emptying the bladder. Persistent problems with incomplete emptying of the bladder can lead to UTI, vesicoureteral reflux (VUR), and (in severe or long-term situations) renal damage. Constipation can exacerbate bladder dysfunction by applying pressure to the bladder wall or restricting urinary flow. The child with BBD may experience stool incontinence (encopresis), either with or without constipation. Elimination problems also contribute to family difficulties, bullying, social isolation, emotional problems, and antisocial behaviors in families of children with fecal soiling (Kaugars et al, 2010; van Dijk et al, 2010).

The following sections discuss bowel dysfunction (fecal incontinence [encopresis] and stool toileting refusal [STR]) and urinary dysfunction (dysfunctional voiding and enuresis) in the healthy child who has no neurologic or structural defect that could cause the problem. These conditions are considered here as developmental problems of normal urinary and bowel habits. If assessment indicates a pathologic condition may be present, further investigation and different management, including referral, are necessary. It is also prudent to consider referral any time a parent or child suggests that it is an issue for them.

Encopresis/Constipation

A recent review of evidence-based data about encopresis and constipation in children, including definition, epidemiology, assessment, and management, has been presented by the North American and European Societies for Pediatric Gastroenterology, Hepatology and Nutrition (NASPGHAN and ESPGHAN). This discussion draws on that review (Tabbers et al, 2014).

Encopresis is defined as fecal incontinence after an age when the child should be able to control bowel movements, usually 4 years old. Fecal incontinence occurs at least once per month for at least 2 months prior to diagnosis. Primary, or continuous, encopresis is present in children who have never been toilet trained. Secondary, or discontinuous, encopresis is seen in those who were previously trained but who begin to soil. There are two subtypes of encopresis: (1) encopresis with constipation, associated with stool retention, constipation, and incontinence overflow (functional retentive fecal incontinence); and (2) encopresis without constipation, or functional nonretentive fecal incontinence, which is less common.

Encopresis may be more common than believed because many families hesitate to inform their health care provider about it due to social perceptions that the issue is related to either their parenting skills or abuse. The cause of encopresis is unclear, is usually multifactorial, and appears to differ among children. Both physiologic and psychosocial factors are involved.

Children with encopresis with constipation often have a history of an acute stool problem that was not adequately managed (e.g., the child had an illness that caused dehydration and constipation), leading to a cycle of constipation, painful defecation, stool retention, more severe constipation, more painful defecation, more stool retention, and so on. In encopresis with constipation, stool retention over time leads to distention of the colon and stretching of the rectum, ineffective peristalsis, decreased sensory threshold in the rectum, and weakened rectal and sphincter muscles. Stool becomes dry, hard, and difficult to evacuate (can be impacted), and bowel movements can be painful. Soft, semi-formed, or liquid stool from higher in the colon leaks around retained stool and passes uncontrollably through the rectum, causing soiling. The child is almost always unaware of the actual incontinence. Children with encopresis with constipation may either refuse or be willing to use the toilet.

Children with encopresis without constipation (functional nonretentive fecal incontinence) are not constipated, but have overflow incontinence or voluntary bowel movements in their clothing or other inappropriate places. Children with nonretentive encopresis appear to have more behavioral problems and externalizing behavior than children with retentive encopresis or those without stooling problems, although it is unclear which causes which. Some of these children may also have a developmentally delayed or faulty perception of the need to stool and will soil as a result (Pakarinen et al, 2006).

Physiologic

Possible physiologic factors related to encopresis with constipation may include the following:

- Inadequate fluid intake
- Dehydration caused by illness and fever or during active play in hot weather
- A change in diet, such as the introduction of solids or increased carbohydrates; there is conflicting information on the role of fiber intake pre- and post-constipation diagnosis (Tabbers et al, 2014)
- Secondary stool retention and constipation due to:
  - Painful bowel movements
  - Anal fissures
  - Paradoxic constriction of the external anal sphincter muscle during attempted defecation
  - Neurogenic conditions (e.g., aganglionic colon [Hirschsprung disease], cerebral palsy, myelomeningocele)
  - Endocrine and metabolic conditions (e.g., hypothyroidism)
  - Medications (e.g., opioids, iron supplements)

Psychosocial

Psychosocial treatment, which may include health education in the office setting or more formal counseling therapy, is indicated if these types of factors are present:

- Major family or life adjustments, such as loss of a parent, sibling, or other significant person
- Inappropriate toilet-training techniques leading to a power struggle; children who are pushed might rebel in the only way they can, by refusing to cooperate
- Irregular toileting patterns, often caused by travel, unfamiliar or unpleasant bathrooms, lack of regular routine, or child being absorbed in play or activities
- Physical abuse and sexual abuse
- Children who do not want to stop an activity to defecate

Clinical Findings

History

Early detection and treatment are important, so specific and directed questions need to be asked in well child visits. "Is pooping and peeing going okay?" is not a sufficient question to ask while obtaining history. The history can include the following:

- Reports of stained underwear, must differentiate between leakage and hygiene issue
- Report of fewer than three bowel movements per week
- Difficult or painful defecation
- Large-caliber or hard stool
- Child suddenly becoming still during play, attempting to hide when urge to defecate is felt
- Child attempting to retain stool (e.g., crossing legs, grimacing, or shifting from one foot to another)
- Reports of a bloated sensation, abdominal pain, or both (parents may notice that the waist bands of clothing fit differently based on stooling status)
- Odor of stool from leakage into underwear
- Streaks of bright blood on toilet paper or underwear
- Child attempting to retain urine
- Enuresis, nocturnal or diurnal
- UTIs
- Anorexia
- Avoiding using the toilet at school or other public places

Physical Examination

The NASPGHAN and ESPGHAN state that a digital examination is not supported by evidence (Tabbers et al, 2014). The physical examination should assess for the following:

- Overflow soiling
- Abdominal distention
- Abdominal tenderness on palpation
- Mass felt at the midline in the suprapubic area (descending colon)
- Anal fissures
- Sacral dimple or hair tuft
- Neurologic signs: absent or diminished abdominal, cremasteric, anal wink reflexes, and deep tendon reflexes (DTRs) in lower extremities may indicate a neurologic cause

Diagnostic Studies

X-rays and laboratory tests to identify structural or organic causes of constipation are not recommended by NASPGHAN and ESPGHAN (Tabbers et al, 2014). Results of an abdominal flat plate radiograph can indicate accumulation of stool in the sigmoid colon (see Chapter 33). Some parents may deny that their child is constipated, believing it may reflect negatively on their parenting skills. A flat plate radiograph can help parents better understand their child's problem.

Differential Diagnosis

The differential diagnoses for encopresis with constipation are as follows:

- Anorectal stenosis
- Spina bifida occulta, spinal cord dysplasia
- Hirschsprung disease
- Mental retardation
- Hypothyroidism
- Hypercalcemia
- Cerebral palsy
- Other organic causes of constipation (e.g., cystic fibrosis)
- The normal red-faced grunting and straining of infants on defecation

Management

In all cases, the goals of treatment are to establish a regular bowel routine, "demystify" the problem, alleviate blame, and gain cooperation for treatment plans. Treatment approaches for children with constipation have followed a pattern of:

- Bowel evacuation using oral polyethylene glycol (PEG) solutions, which are as effective as enemas but much less traumatizing to patients and families (Tabbers et al, 2014)
- Bowel retraining to establish a regular pattern of stooling
- Ongoing maintenance with medications as needed, normal physical activity as per AAP recommendations, and regular toileting hygiene to prevent recurring constipation

The emphasis in treating nonretentive fecal soiling is on behavioral therapy, educating the child and parent about normal stooling, and establishing a structured pattern of toileting. Box 12-3 outlines approaches to treating a child with encopresis without constipation (also see the Management subsection in the Stool Toileting Refusal section). Active pre-toilet training education can be used as a preventive option.

Children who have encopresis with constipation present a greater challenge. Education of parents and children is equally vital to successful treatment. A clear message to children and parents should be that the dynamics of encopresis (retention, colon stretching, decreased peristalsis, impaction, leaking) are not voluntary—no one is to blame; they can, however, be reversed through bowel rehabilitation.

Correcting them will take hard work, cooperation, and time, and the provider will work with the family to ensure success. Figure 12-1 can be used to educate parents and children about the bowel rehabilitation process involved in the treatment plan. Timed urination may also be helpful, because children who struggle to hold their urine activate the pelvic floor and, as a result, hold their stool as well.

In some cases, child mental health referral may be indicated but should not be the first referral and alone cannot cure the problem. This referral should be reserved for situations in which there are other indications that mental health interventions may be helpful to the child and/or family.

Figures 12-2 and 12-3 present algorithms primary care providers can use to manage constipation in children younger and older than 6 months. Table 12-3 provides guidelines to treating a child with encopresis with constipation, including appropriate medications. According to the ESPGHAN and NASPGHAN, although not U.S. Food and Drug Administration-approved for use in children, PEG is the first-line therapy for children presenting with functional constipation and/or fecal impaction. Further research is being conducted to determine the safety of long-term use in children (Tabbers et al, 2014; NASPGHAN Neurogastroenterology and Motility Committee, 2015). Enemas are recommended *only* if PEG is not available.

For maintenance, PEG is recommended as first-line therapy, although lactulose may be given if PEG is not available. Milk of magnesia, mineral oil, and stimulant laxatives may also be considered for maintenance or as second-line treatment. Enemas are not recommended. Maintenance medications need to be continued for a minimum of 2 months and should not be stopped until 1 month after resolution of the problem. At this time,

• BOX 12-3 Management of Children with Mild Encopresis without Constipation

- Monitor diet:
  - Ensure adequate fiber and water intake for age:
    - Recommended water intake is about 1 oz/kg/day.
    - Fiber recommendations: 4- to 8-year olds: about 25 g of fiber each day; 9- to 13-year-old girls: about 26 g of fiber each day; 9- to 13-year-old boys: about 31 g of fiber each day; 14- to 18-year-old girls: about 26 g of fiber each day; and 14- to 18-year-old boys: about 38 g of fiber each day. Legumes, vegetables, and some fruits are good sources of fiber.
  - Decrease milk to 16 oz/day.
  - Do not allow excessive dairy, rice, applesauce, bananas, white flour, or potatoes.
- Give child all responsibility for own toilet habits. Stop parental reminders to use toilet. Stop all encouragement and criticisms.
- Establish a regular toileting routine.
- Avoid use of stool softeners or laxatives.
- Encourage daily physical activity per American Academy of Pediatrics (AAP) recommendations.
- May use incentives or rewards to reinforce positive behavior. Have parent and child agree on reward beforehand so that it can be discussed as a positive, subtle reminder.

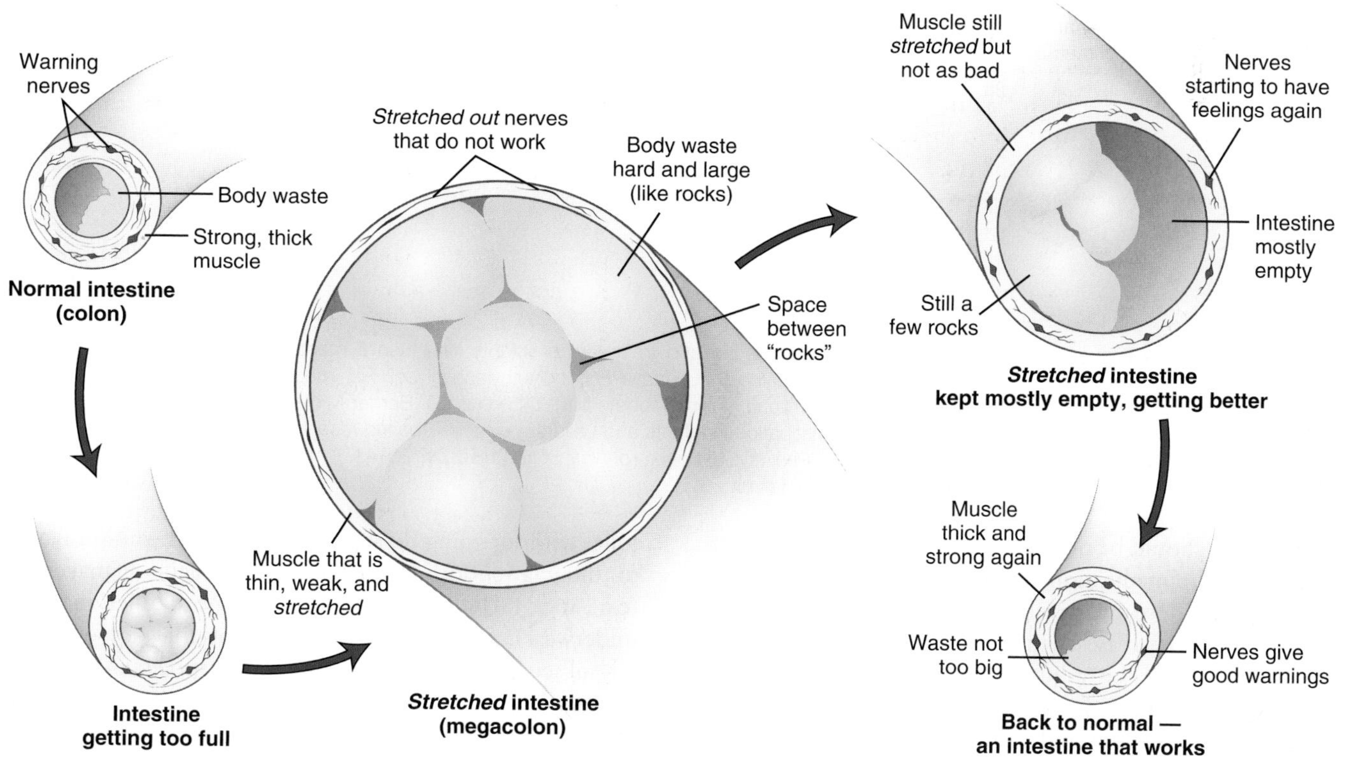

• Figure 12-1 Encopresis: Patient training diagram. (From Weissman L, Bridgemohan C: Bowel function, toileting, and encopresis. In Carey WB, Croker AC, Coleman WL, et al, editors: *Developmental-behavioral pediatrics*, ed 4, Philadelphia, 2009, Saunders.)

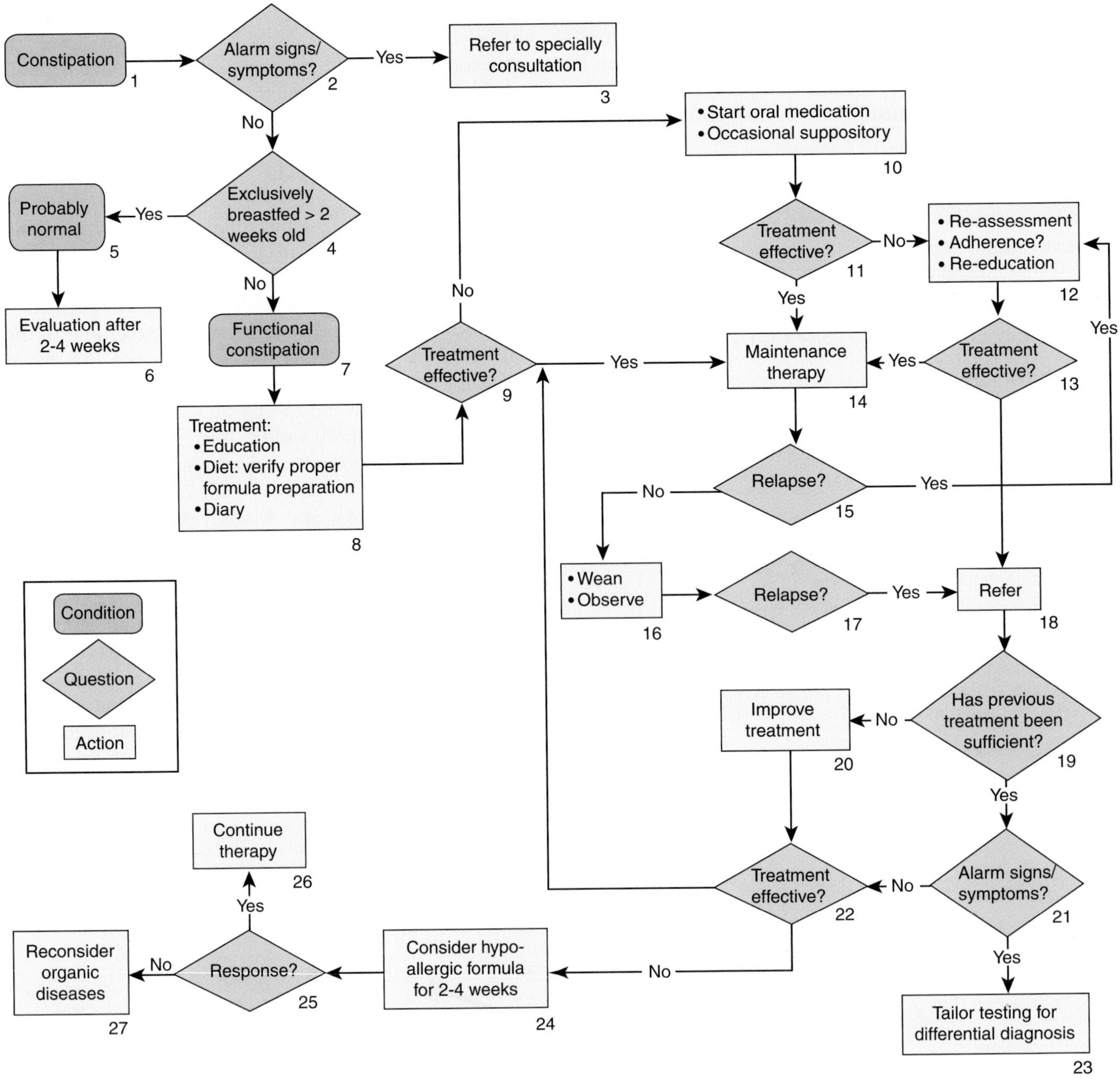

• **Figure 12-2** An algorithm for the evaluation and treatment of infants less than 6 months old. *Ca,* Calcium; *MRI,* magnetic resonance imaging; *Pb,* lead; *PEG,* polyethylene glycol; *Rx,* medication; T_4, thyroxine; *TSH,* thyroid-stimulating hormone. (From Tabbers MM, DiLorenzo C, Berger MY, et al: Evaluation and treatment of functional constipation in infants and children: evidence-based recommendations from ESPGHAN and NASPGHAN, *J Pediatr Gastroenterol Nutr* 58(2):258–274, 2014.)

medications should be decreased gradually and if any problems recur, the medication should be adjusted back to the last successful dose and given an additional 2 weeks before attempting to decrease again. Throughout the treatment, medications must be adjusted according to the clinical response, so the provider must be readily available for the family to ask questions and make modifications.

Because this problem often occurs in school-age children and the nature of the school setting can discourage children from using the restroom, providers should consult with the school nurse to ensure that children are allowed to use the toilet without going through extra steps and without having to draw attention to themselves. Hygiene management (e.g., may include access to a more private toilet and extra underwear) and psychological and emotional support in the school setting are important to a child's success in overcoming encopresis.

Complications

Persistent encopresis is an unpleasant condition, and children with encopresis often experience ridicule and shame. Age-group peers frequently treat children with scorn,

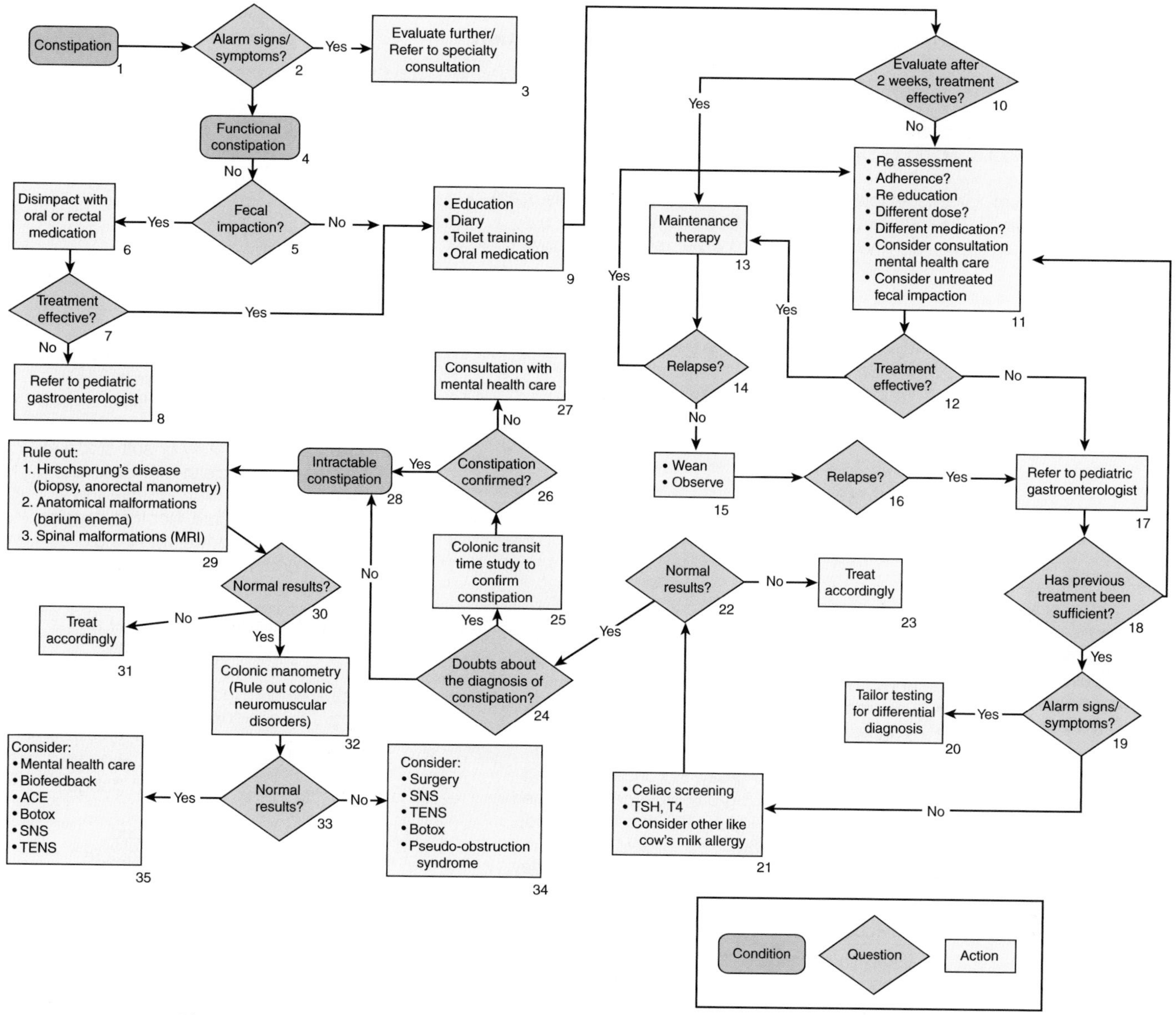

• Figure 12-3 An algorithm for the evaluation and treatment of infants 6 months old or older. *Ca,* Calcium; *MRI,* magnetic resonance imaging; *Pb,* lead; *T_4,* thyroxine; *TSH,* thyroid-stimulating hormone. (From Tabbers MM, DiLorenzo C, Berger MY, et al: Evaluation and treatment of functional constipation in infants and children: evidence-based recommendations from ESPGHAN and NASPGHAN, *J Pediatr Gastroenterol Nutr* 58(2):258–274, 2014.)

hostility, and rejection. Teachers and other adults might be disgusted by children with encopresis, and parents, dealing with anger, guilt, embarrassment, and helplessness, find their children and the condition extremely difficult to manage. Social, interpersonal, and family relations are at grave risk.

Intractable constipation, and even megacolon, can be seen in children with Down syndrome, cerebral palsy, or neurologic conditions. When medical management is unsuccessful, an antegrade continence enema procedure may be necessary.

Patient and Family Education

The best treatment of encopresis is prevention. If constipation or encopresis is caused by an underlying anatomic or organic cause (e.g., Hirschsprung disease, occult spina bifida, hypothyroidism), early diagnosis and referral is essential. The pediatric provider must understand the relationship between constipation and encopresis and/or diarrhea, recognize conditions that may contribute to each, and provide parents with anticipatory guidance related to toilet training and normal elimination habits in order to prevent problems. It is equally important to provide support during treatment. Although parents should be informed that treatment may be required for months or years, providers should emphasize that by following a clear, consistent, aggressive treatment protocol the condition can be managed. Finally, providers, parents, and the child must work together to prevent recurrence of symptoms after successful treatment.

TABLE 12-3 Management of Children with Encopresis with Constipation

Treatment Phase	Treatment Program	Comments
Phase I: Catharsis (bowel clean-out over 3 to 5 days; maximum of 6 consecutive days)	Oral clean-out administered at home (preferred): • PEG 3350: 1-1.5 g/kg/day in two to four divided doses *or* Enema (only if PEG is not available; infrequently used) • Sodium phosphate (Fleet) enema: 2-11 years: 6 mL/kg/day per rectum; may give up to 135 mL once a day in older children >11 years: An adult enema or 135 mL per rectum once a day	Home treatment is preferred, should take 3 to 5 days or until stool output is runny diarrhea. PEG can be premixed and stored in refrigerator for 48 hours. Catharsis may need to occur in the hospital if: • Retention is severe • Home compliance is poor • Parents prefer admission • Child needs enema for clean-out and parent should not administer Pediatric enema is 67.5 mL; adult enema is 135 mL. The child may have watery or soft stools for several days after clean-out. Child and parents should be informed that this does not indicate cure, but that ongoing maintenance and bowel retraining is essential for the bowel to return to normal functioning (see Fig. 12-1).

Phase II: Maintenance (regular bowel movements over 4 to 12 months)	**Oral Laxatives**
	• PEG 3350 starting at 0.4 and up to 0.8 g/kg/day PO in two divided doses
	• Lactulose 1-2 g/kg/day PO in two divided doses
	• Magnesium hydroxide
	  • 2-5 yr: 0.4-1.2 g/day, PO once or divided
	  • 6-11 yr: 1.2-2.4 g/day, PO once or divided
	  • 12-18 yr: 2.4-4.8 g/day, PO once or divided
	• Mineral oil 1-3 mL/kg/day PO once or divided, maximum 90 mL/day
	• Stimulant laxative Bisacodyl: 3-10 yr: 5 mg/day; >10 yr: 5-10 mg/day
	Behavioral Training
	• Establish daily toilet sitting 15-20 minutes after meals two to three times a day for 5-10 minutes
	• Provide positive reinforcement for toilet sitting and stooling
	• Keep a diary of bowel movements, recording time and amount
	• Ensure child has at least 1 hour of physical exercise per day; have child be active in the 15-20 minutes between mealtime and sitting on toilet
	Dietary Treatment
	• Ensure adequate dietary fiber intake
	• Ensure adequate fluid intake
		Adjust daily medications to achieve one to three soft, mushy stools per day.
		PEG has been shown to be safe and effective when used alone and more effective than lactulose (Gordon et al, 2013).
		Adding enemas to the chronic use of PEG is not supported by evidence (Tabbers et al, 2014).
		Use of senna is not recommended.
		Plan on 6 months of treatment before bowel regains normal function.
		Stimulant laxatives used as second- or third-line treatment.

Phase III: Weaning: Follow-up	• Continued treatment for at least 1 month after all symptoms are resolved. • Gradual tapering of laxative • Regular visits (about every 4-10 wk) depending on severity and need of family • Telephone availability to discuss progress and adjust doses • Counseling or referral as appropriate for psychosocial and developmental issues • Continued education regarding normal bowel function	Goals of follow-up visits: • Monitor compliance. • Provide encouragement and support. • Detect and treat relapse early if it occurs.

Adapted from Kehoe TD: The constipated 8-year-old. In Burns CE, Richardson B, Brady MA, editors: *Pediatric primary care case studies*, Sudbury, MA, 2010, Jones and Bartlett.
PEG, Polyethylene glycol; *PO, per os* (by mouth, orally).

Stool Toileting Refusal

STR is present when a child demonstrates a pattern of successfully using the toilet to urinate, but refuses to use the toilet for bowel movements. These children will usually defecate in a diaper, training pants, or "pull-ups." In some cases, children will retain stool or defecate outside the toilet. Encopresis without constipation also fits this description; the child defecates outside the toilet when beyond the age of expected training.

The incidence of STR has not been recently documented. Taubman (1997) found that 22% of healthy children between 18 and 30 months old experienced at least 1 month of STR. In a study of children who were trained at early ages (some as early as the first 6 months of life), there was a nearly 12% incidence of STR (Rugolotto et al, 2008). The cause of STR is unknown, but the presence of younger siblings in the household and the parents' inability to set limits for the child may be related. Constipation and painful bowel movements appear to precede rather than follow the problem.

Clinical Findings

History

Parents or caregivers report that the child demonstrates the following:

- Bladder control but refusal to defecate on the toilet
- A regular or irregular pattern of bowel movements
- Consistent signs from child that a bowel movement is imminent
- May have a history of hiding when defecating, either before or after toilet training begins

Physical Examination

The physical examination will be unremarkable.

- Examine the anus for fissures or irritation that may cause a child to refuse to defecate and the presence of an anal wink. A digital examination is not indicated.
- Check for signs of stool retention:
  - Abdominal distention
  - Abdominal tenderness on palpation
- Palpate for a mass in the sigmoid colon or at the midline in the suprapubic area (impaction).

Differential Diagnosis

The differential diagnosis includes stool withholding, constipation, and encopresis.

Management

Return the child to diapers and reintroduce toilet training in about a month or when the child indicates interest. Some children prefer not to wear diapers all the time, but will ask to have one put on when they feel the urge to defecate. If possible, have parents encourage the child to go into the bathroom for these diaper defecations. After having a bowel movement, the child asks to be changed and returns to wearing training pants. This pattern may continue for several weeks or months. When parents refrain from expressing negative messages about stooling or fecal matter and matter-of-factly clean up the child after defecating in the diaper, the duration of STR appears to shorten (Taubman et al, 2003). For older children, schedule a daily time for the child to sit on the toilet for 5 to 10 minutes when the child typically has a bowel movement; have these times be positive, never punitive or forced. Never flush the toilet while the child is sitting on it. If in a public restroom, have parents keep sticky notes with them to cover automatic flush sensors. Incentives and positive feedback when the child successfully uses the toilet for bowel movements may be effective (e.g., the parent can use star charts or cards on the wall and the child can remove them and turn them in for a prize), but excessive praise is not recommended, because the child is simply doing what is to be expected (Howard, 2013). If the child has constipation, fecal impaction, or both, initial bowel clean-out is necessary using PEG. Then a daily dose adjusted to clinical response is recommended until toilet training is complete.

Complications

Refusal to use the toilet for bowel movements may lead to stool withholding, constipation, and impaction, which are conditions that result in primary encopresis. Psychological complications include embarrassment, shame, conflict, and stress between children and parents, especially as the child becomes older. Child maltreatment can be a significant complication.

Patient and Family Education

Prevention through appropriate toilet training is key (see Box 12-2). If a child refuses to defecate on the toilet, use of punishment or force can complicate the problem. Parents should be alert for signs of constipation (see Box 12-1; Table 12-1) and should be encouraged to contact the pediatric provider sooner rather than later if there is any concern.

Dysfunctional Voiding

Dysfunctional voiding is defined by the International Children's Continence Society (ICCS) as a problem of bladder emptying. During voiding, the child contracts the external urethra in a "staccato pattern," resulting in intermittent flow, prolonged micturition time, and, often, incomplete emptying of the bladder, or there is a "plateau pattern" related to continuous, tonic sphincter contraction that results in a dynamic bladder outlet obstruction. Either detrusor overactivity or underactivity may be present. A long-standing pattern of incomplete emptying can lead to overextension of the bladder and subsequent underactive detrusor function. As a result, UTI, symptoms of urgency, frequency, and overflow incontinence can occur (Chase et al, 2010).

The cause of dysfunctional voiding is unknown, but it is believed to be multifactorial and is often accompanied by constipation. UTI, structural abnormalities, stress, and abuse must also be considered.

Clinical Findings

History

Because of the varied problems associated with dysfunctional voiding, children have a history of differing symptoms, including the following:

- Infrequent voiding
- Cluster voiding where they void a lot after a period of not voiding during each day (e.g., not voiding at school)
- Holding maneuvers
- Sudden daytime incontinence after having been dry
- Urgency
- Frequency
- Inability to stop the voiding stream
- Occasional nocturnal enuresis, but usually daytime wetting
- Incontinence after voiding (e.g., vaginal voiding)
- Constipation
- UTI

The history should also include information about the child's general development, achievement of developmental milestones, pattern of toilet training and elimination (i.e., frequency and volume of voiding and stooling as well as timing of episodes of any incontinence), any stressors experienced following toilet training, family history of problems with voiding, and the child's behavioral patterns, including the child's and family's emotional response to the condition. It is important to get direct information from the child because parents are often unaware of their older, toilet-trained child's elimination patterns.

Physical Examination

A complete physical examination should be done, including checking females for labial adhesions, which can be caused by and lead to vaginal voiding. Males should be checked for meatal stenosis, which can lead to a deflected stream that sprays upward. Consider, particularly, the possibility of constipation and check for abdominal masses indicating retained stool.

Diagnostic Studies

Urodynamic diagnostic procedures are not routinely done. The following tests are indicated:

- Urinalysis
- Urine culture and sensitivity
- Bladder US done by a urologic provider to measure post-void residual urine volume
- Renal and bladder US if structural abnormalities are suspected; an abnormal US can show a normal upper renal system and a thick-walled bladder
- Voiding cystourethrogram (VCUG) ordered by pediatric urology provider
- Uroflowmetry may be done by a urologic (preferably pediatric) provider
- The qualities of the uroflow include flow rate, pattern, and duration

Differential Diagnosis

The differential diagnoses for dysfunctional voiding are as follows:

- UTI
- Structural abnormality, such as abnormal sphincters, ectopic ureter, duplicated urethra, or urethral valves
- Neurogenic bladder
- Non-neurogenic neurogenic bladder (Hinman syndrome), which starts as behavioral and psychological disorders in which the child holds urine, leading to obstruction of the urinary tract and subsequent problems that mimic neurogenic bladder
- Asymptomatic VUR that does not cause voiding symptoms
- Trauma or abuse
- Urethritis (which may be caused by chemicals in soaps, bubble baths)

Management

The goal of management is to prevent or break the cycle of urinary dysfunction and its complications. Intervention includes the following:

- Treat any UTI if present (see Chapter 35).
- Treat constipation if present. This may eliminate the entire problem but can take months to adequately correct (see Encopresis/Constipation). Parents must be aware of the possible need for long-term treatment.
- First-line treatment should involve urotherapy (Box 12-4). At the start of the program, the family should focus on children doing the "jobs" given to them and not on successful resolution of the issue (Chase et al, 2010). There is conflicting evidence on the addition of biofeedback to urotherapy. Implementing biofeedback also has the drawback of needing multiple visits, which families may find difficult to attend and can be very costly.
- Second-line treatment combines urotherapy with pharmacotherapeutics. The ICCS has noted that use of medications is "an off-label method" (Chase et al, 2010), and a pediatric urology referral is indicated before using medications. Anticholinergics may be used, but in many children their side effects can be significant (e.g., constipation). Some pediatric urology providers have done trials using alpha blockers, but these are also off label. Pediatric urologists have also tried investigational use of botulinum toxin A (BtA) to inhibit acetylcholine release.
- Treat skin breakdown if present. Vinegar sitz baths can be very effective.

Patient and Family Education

Effective toilet training can prevent BBD, especially if children learn to be sensitive and responsive to cues to urinate and defecate. Parents should be instructed that holding urine is not the goal; because, paradoxically, if a person activates the pelvic floor to hold urine, often a feedback loop

• BOX 12-4 Urotherapy for Dysfunctional Voiding and Enuresis

- Educate parents and child on how the bladder works: Describe filling and emptying process, especially as it is related to problem of external sphincter contraction during voiding.
  - Explain the relationship between abdominal, pelvic floor, and external sphincter muscles; how to be aware of and to relax muscles to allow complete voiding.
  - Explain the relationship of bladder and bowel function as they are connected by the pelvic floor.
- Implement bladder retraining:
  - Establish a consistent, structured regimen of toileting: Set a timed-voiding schedule, usually every 2 hours, 1½ if actively treating, because the goal is to void before bladder contractions activate the pelvic floor; void before going to bed and immediately upon rising in morning.
  - Use correct toilet posture: Sit comfortably with hips abducted, knees wide, and feet and buttocks well supported with a pelvic tilt.
  - Void with relaxation: Have child take a deep breath and relax the sphincter when exhaling; use a straw to breathe through.
  - Void to completion: If not accomplished on the first voiding, double void by having child void and count to five and void again and repeat until no further urine is produced.
  - Avoid Credé maneuver.
- Give lifestyle advice related to diet and fluid intake.
  - Encourage 1 oz/kg/day of water to be consumed at regular intervals between breakfast and dinner. (This most often eliminates evening thirst.)
- Monitor progress:
  - Keep frequency and volume charts or a voiding diary.
- Actively manage bowel dysfunction.
- Implement behavioral interventions as indicated, based on child and family history.
- Neuromodulation and catheterization may be appropriate in resistant cases.

to the brain is activated and one feels the need to go less and less. Parents should be instructed to be alert to signs of dysuria. If urination is painful, children often struggle to retain urine or void incompletely. Early treatment for UTIs is essential to prevent renal dysfunction. Teaching elimination norms should be done at every well child check.

Enuresis

Enuresis is defined as voluntary or involuntary urination into bed or clothes at an age when toilet training should be complete. Children who have never established control have primary enuresis. Secondary enuresis is present when children have been dry for more than 6 to 12 months and begin wetting. Nocturnal enuresis is incontinence during sleep. If a child has normal daytime elimination with no concerns, then nighttime wetting is called *monosymptomatic nocturnal enuresis (MNE)*. More commonly, children with nocturnal enuresis have BBD symptoms during the day as well; this type of nocturnal enuresis is *non-monosymptomatic nocturnal enuresis (NMNE)*. Diurnal enuresis, daytime wetting, occurs during waking hours.

Diagnosing enuresis can be a challenge. According to the ICCS, using ICD-10 and DSM-V, a diagnosis of enuresis requires a minimum age of 5 years old, and one episode a month for a duration of 3 months. The ICCS goes on to state that enuresis is frequent if it occurs four or more times a week and infrequent if it occurs four or less times a month (Austin et al, 2014). It is important to remember that the age at which urinary continence is normally achieved varies greatly and thus children should be evaluated on a case-by-case basis, taking into account the child and family dynamics and developmental stages and the amount of duress the issue is causing. Regardless of the numbers, if the parent or child asks for help, they should receive it.

The cause of enuresis varies among children and can be difficult to determine. A number of factors have been found to be associated with enuresis, including the following:

- Constipation: It cannot be overemphasized how important it is to determine if constipation or impaction exists before treating nocturnal enuresis.
- Familial disposition: Even if there is a presumed genetic predisposition based on parental history, many of these children have constipation; and if that is treated, they have improvement.
- Neurologic developmental delay
- Behavioral comorbidities (e.g., externalizing behaviors): There appears to be a strong association between enuresis (especially daytime enuresis) and attention-deficit/hyperactivity disorder (ADHD) (von Gontard et al, 2011).
- Functional small bladder capacity: In some children, bladder capacity appears normal during the day but is functionally reduced at night (Godbole et al, 2011).
- Sleep disorders: Obstructive sleep apnea and disordered sleep patterns are associated with increased incidence of nocturnal enuresis (Godbole et al, 2011).
- Stress and family disruptions: Some examples are a divorce, move, or a new family member.
- Polyuria: This can be caused by nocturnal drinking as well as caffeine intake (Godbole et al, 2011).
- Inappropriate toilet training: This is especially common when parents are overly demanding or punitive of the child.

Clinical Findings

The goals of assessment are to (1) determine if there are comorbid or underlying conditions that require pediatric urology referral and (2) establish the best approach to treating this particular child's condition.

History

It is essential to gather the most honest nighttime *and* daytime history of elimination habits possible, both urine and bowel. Parents should be asked about the following:

- Voiding characteristics:
  - Urgency, dysuria, or dribbling
  - Are there voiding or stooling postponement behaviors?
  - Number of voids per day: Is nocturia present?

- Cluster voiding: For example, is the child waiting until after school?
- Frequency of wetting—day and night
- Type of urinary stream
- These findings warrant referral to a pediatric urologist (Nevéus et al, 2010):
  - Weak or interrupted urinary stream
  - Need to use abdominal pressure to urinate
  - Daytime incontinence and nocturnal enuresis combined
- Fluid intake, how much and when
- UTI
- History of enuresis, treatment, and age of resolution for other family members, including parents
- History of toilet training: What age was toilet training begun? How was it handled? Was the child ever dry? For how long?
- Effect of enuresis on child and parents
- Manner in which family deals with the enuresis: For example, is the child punished? Who changes the bed? Any previous medical treatment?
- Bowel patterns: What is the frequency? Is there constipation? Is there fecal incontinence? What is the quality of stool (see Box 12-1)?
- Sleep patterns: Look for indications of obstructive sleep-disordered breathing or apnea. Reassure parents that deep sleep is not a cause for nocturnal enuresis.
- General health:
  - Prenatal and perinatal history
  - Is child tired? Has child lost weight? Does child have excessive thirst or hunger (e.g., diabetes)?
  - Has the child been diagnosed with a neuropsychological condition (e.g., ADHD)?
- Presence of other behavior problems
- Changes in the home, family, or school environment: Be sure to determine if the enuresis was present before any disruptive changes occurred.

Physical Examination

The physical examination includes the following:

- Assess the external genitalia for signs of irritation, infection, labial fusion, and/or meatal stenosis.
- Check for fecal impaction.
  - Examine the abdomen for masses, especially at the suprapubic midline and in the left lower quadrant.
- Examine the lower back for dimples and hair tufts.
- Assess for neurologic function and DTR.

Diagnostic Studies

A urinalysis is recommended in all children with enuresis. A culture should be done if there are clinical symptoms to warrant it. More sophisticated testing is usually not necessary.

Differential Diagnosis

The differential diagnosis includes daytime extraordinary urinary frequency (pollakiuria), which is a benign condition of excessive urination (more than 8 to 12 times per day, often as frequent as every 15 to 30 minutes) seen in previously toilet-trained children who do not need to void at night. Pollakiuria has no known cause, but it may be associated with viral cystitis or urethritis, stress, and hypercalciuria. Although considered self-limited because it does not typically respond to medication, pollakiuria can persist for months or even years; however, it typically lasts about 6 months (Farber, 2013).

Organic causes of enuresis must be identified. The most common organic cause is UTI that may be related to BBD. Following is a list of other organic causes to consider, and worsening incontinence, development of neurologic signs (e.g., weakness in legs), and increased urine volumes or dilution warrant referral to specialists for further evaluation.

- Diabetes mellitus
- Diabetes insipidus
- Sickle cell disease, in which treatment by means of forced fluids may lead to increased urine output
- Chronic renal failure, in which the kidneys are unable to concentrate urine
- Structural anomalies, such as ectopic ureter (constant leakage is noted) or a vesicovaginal fistula
- Neurologic abnormalities, including neurogenic bladder
- Hypercalciuria
- Obstructive uropathy other than that due to BBD
- Vaginitis
- Sleep apnea

Management

The goals of treatment are to establish normal bladder function and prevent both physical and emotional or psychological complications. A thorough examination to distinguish between organic and nonorganic causes is the first crucial step. Intervention is then based on the underlying cause and involves behavioral modification, medication, treatment of comorbid or organic conditions, or a combination of these modalities. Treatment of daytime urinary dysfunction and constipation should be done before treating nocturnal enuresis (Van de Walle et al, 2012). Referral to a pediatric urology specialist may be necessary. Outcomes of treatment are categorized as:

- No response: Less than 50% decrease in enuresis
- Partial response: 50% to 99% reduction
- Complete response: 100% reduction

Over the long term, outcomes include:

- Relapse: More than one symptom relapse per month
- Continued success: No return of symptoms in 6 months
- Complete success: No return of symptoms after 2 years

Because functional enuresis is largely self-limited, there is consensus to delay aggressive treatment until the child is 6 to 8 years old. Treatment strategies for children 6 years old or older include the following:

- *Urotherapy:* A non-pharmacologic, nonsurgical intervention, urotherapy is basic to treatment of enuresis (see Box 12-4). Urotherapy increases daytime urination by establishing a regular voiding schedule—not waiting until the micturition urge is felt. It also limits nighttime urine production by regulating fluid intake. The goal is for the bladder to be able to hold urine produced overnight. Children should void before going to bed and again immediately upon waking in the morning. Proper posture while urinating is important to help the child be more sensitive to cues of a full bladder and to control urination. This approach has been used effectively for children with hyperactive bladders and may make medication unnecessary for many children. Urotherapy also involves aggressive treatment of constipation.

- *Enuresis alarms:* According to the ICCS, use of enuresis alarms and desmopressin medication are equivalent first-line therapies that can be used to treat enuresis (Nevéus et al, 2010); the decision to use an alarm should be made after discussion with the child and family and be based on their preference. Alarm therapy seems to be more effective in children with "decreased maximal voided volumes" (Maternik et al, 2015). A review of the research literature indicates that long-term alarm therapy is more effective than desmopressin for treatment of primary MNE (Perrin et al, 2013), and an enuresis alarm is considered first-line treatment when conditions such as diabetes, kidney disease, or urogenital malformations have been ruled out (Nevéus, 2011). Use of an alarm requires commitment and effort on the part of parents and extensive support from the primary care provider.
- *Drug therapy:* Drug therapy (see Table 12-4 for dosing and comments) can be combined with urotherapy and/or alarm therapy, but it is not curative. It usually has high initial success rates. Unfortunately, drug therapy can be expensive, and high relapse rates can occur when the drug is discontinued. When the wetting recurs, it can be very upsetting to the child, which is a factor that needs to be considered when prescribing. However, it can be very useful for overnight stays (e.g., camp) when staying dry is important to the child.

Desmopressin has an antidiuretic effect and appears to be most effective in children with large nocturnal urine production and normal nocturnal bladder capacity. Its effect is immediate and it can be taken only on nights that the child wants to be sure to stay dry (Nevéus et al, 2010). Desmopressin is available in three forms: nasal spray, oral tablets, or oral lyophilisate preparation (MELT) (sublingual administration). Nasal spray has led to hyponatremia, has a black box warning from the FDA, and is not recommended for routine use (Robson, 2009). Patients should be cautioned to avoid high fluid intake with the oral medication, to be sure that the correct dosage is given, and to discontinue the medication if headache, nausea, or vomiting occurs (Robson et al, 2007; Van de Walle et al, 2010). Use of the MELT preparation reduces fluid intake and has been shown in one study to reduce bed-wetting by a factor of two over use of the tablet form (Juul et al, 2013). Desmopressin may be more effective when combined with urotherapy.

Other drugs are not recommended as first-line treatment. These include anticholinergics (antimuscarinic drugs [also used for treatment of overactive bladder]: oxybutynin, tolterodine, and solifenacin), which can cause constipation and could complicate the problem; botulinum toxin type A (BtA); and imipramine, which should only be used as third-line therapy at tertiary care facilities, if at all, due to its cardiotoxic side effects.

Sacral nerve stimulation for children with severe voiding dysfunction that has not responded to aggressive urotherapy and medical interventions is currently being studied.

Complications

Enuresis contributes to poor self-esteem and disrupted family interactions and threatens the child's ability to

TABLE 12-4 Drug Therapy for Children 6 Years or Older with Monosymptomatic Nocturnal Enuresis

Medication	Dosing	Comments
Desmopressin acetate (DDAVP)	Oral: 0.2 mg tablet once daily at bedtime; can be adjusted up to maximum of 0.4 mg/day Oral: 120 mcg MELT once daily at bedtime; this is the bioequivalent of 0.2 mg tablet; can be adjusted up to 240 mcg/day	Effective in children with nocturnal polyuria and normal bladder volume. Short-term treatment only (4-8 weeks). Not recommended in children younger than 6 years. Not recommended to use nasal spray. Caution must be used with patients who are hypertensive or have a potential for fluid-electrolyte imbalance (e.g., children with cystic fibrosis susceptible to hyponatremia). Use least amount effective. Take on empty stomach; avoid caffeine, chocolate, NutraSweet, and carbonated beverages. Children must be wakened to urinate within 10 hours of taking the medication.
Oxybutynin chloride, Immediate release Oxybutynin chloride, Extended release	5 mg once daily at bedtime; increase as tolerated in 5 mg increments to maximum of 20 mg daily	Effective in children with daytime enuresis. Not recommended in children 5 years old or younger.

establish strong peer relationships. Parents of children with nocturnal and diurnal enuresis rate those children as having more problem behaviors than do parents of children without enuresis; these parents also rate their own stress level as higher (De Bruyne et al, 2009); children with enuresis are at risk for child abuse. Effective treatment improves behavior and self-concept, suggesting that enuresis precedes behavior problems.

Patient and Family Education

Supportive, proactive education of parents and positive reinforcement of children's efforts can help prevent enuresis. For 3- to 5-year-old children, a nonjudgmental attitude of "benign neglect" in the face of accidents is the best approach. For older children with enuresis, aggressive, long-term interventions are appropriate; wetting is a common phenomenon, and parents should be reassured that it rarely indicates disease. Dealing with a child who wets frequently can be frustrating, however, and parents need to know that the provider is committed to working closely with them until the child is dry.

For a complete list of references, please visit http://evolve.elsevier.com/Burns/pediatric/.

13

Physical Activity and Sports for Children and Adolescents

MICHELE L. POLFUSS, KAREN G. DUDERSTADT, MAXINE FOOKSON, AND CATHERINE G. BLOSSER

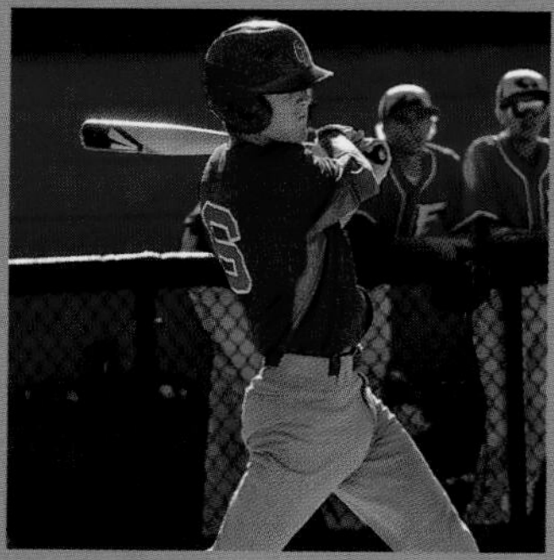

The importance of physical activity for all children during infancy, childhood, and adolescence, including those with chronic health conditions and special health care needs, cannot be overstated. Strong evidence suggests that engaging in physical activity improves cardiorespiratory and muscular fitness, cardiovascular and metabolic biomarkers, bone health, and body composition. Maintaining a healthy level of activity in combination with eating a healthy diet are the two most important factors in preventing disabling and chronic disease (U.S. Department of Health and Human Services [USDHHS], 2012). In the United States, children and adolescents fail to meet the recommended national physical activity goals. Globally, the rest of the world's population is not fairing any better. The levels of physical inactivity are increasing across the globe, adding to the burden of noncommunicable diseases and impacting general worldwide health (World Health Organization [WHO], 2015).

This chapter focuses on the importance and impact of physical activity on the health and well-being of children and youth. Physical activity guidelines and recommendations from early childhood through young adulthood, the impact of physical activity on the chronic conditions of childhood, the importance of nutrition and strengthening in young athletes, the preparticipation sports physical examination guidelines, and recommendations for safe play, whether engaging in competitive sports or recreational activities, are included.

Physical Activity: Overview

Physical activity is defined as "any bodily movement produced by skeletal muscles that requires energy expenditure—including activities undertaken while working, playing, carrying out household chores, travelling, and engaging in recreational pursuits" (WHO, 2015). Physical activity is not to be confused with *exercise,* which is a subcategory and denotes planned, structured, and repetitive activities.

In the United States, one-half of all boys and approximately one-third of all girls demonstrate adequate levels of cardiorespiratory fitness. The overall percentage of youth from 12 to 15 years old with *inadequate* levels of cardiorespiratory fitness has increased 10% in the past decade. Furthermore, there is a known relationship between cardiorespiratory fitness and body weight—as weight increases, cardiorespiratory fitness decreases (Gahche et al, 2014). The Centers for Disease Control and Prevention's (CDC's) biannual Youth Risk Behavior Surveillance System (YRBSS) monitors health risk behaviors of high school youth, grades 9 through 12, and compares the results against the Healthy People 2020 goals. The 2013 Youth Risk Behavior Survey (YRBS) showed that physical activity goals for children and youth were not being met and sedentary behaviors in youth were increasing (CDC, 2014). Data showed that females remain less physically active than males across all age groups. In addition, the percentage of youth who:

- Attended physical education (PE) classes on 1 or more days in an average school week decreased from 51.8% (in 2011) to 48% (in 2013).
- Attended PE classes on all 5 days in an average school week decreased from 31.5% (in 2011) to 29.4% (in 2013).
- Played on at least one sports team (run by their school or community groups during the 12 months before the survey) decreased from 58.4% (in 2011) to 54% (in 2013).

Additional United States surveys (National Health and Nutrition Examination Survey [NHANES] in conjunction with the National Youth Fitness Survey) found approximately 25% of youth 12 to 15 years old were engaged in the recommended 60 minutes of moderate-to-vigorous physical activity daily (Fakhouri et al, 2014). When physical activity and screen time were studied concurrently, fewer than 4 in 10 children met the recommendations for both physical activity and screen time daily (Fakhouri et al, 2013). This inactivity in childhood translates into increasing medical costs in the billions of dollars spent in the United States to manage and treat chronic diseases that later emerge in adulthood, such as heart disease and diabetes (American Diabetes Association, 2013; Go et al, 2014).

Globally, 3.2 million people die annually from risk factors related to physical inactivity. In developing urban societies, poverty, high crime rates, structural barriers in the environment (e.g., lack of safe recreational areas, high traffic density, and overcrowding), and poor air quality contribute to inactivity in children and youth (WHO, 2015).

Promoting Physical Activity: Guidelines and Standards

Health-enhancing physical activities are those activities that produce health benefits when added to baseline daily activity, such as brisk walking, jumping rope, dancing, playing soccer, and climbing on playground equipment. Aerobic activity, also called *endurance activity*, improves cardiorespiratory fitness and includes walking, running, swimming, and bicycling. The following guidelines and recommendations are complementary to one another.

The 2008 Physical Activity Guidelines for Americans provide specific clinical recommendations that address and promote physical activity for children from 6 years old through early adulthood. The guidelines stress the importance of engaging children and adolescents in a variety of physical activities that are age appropriate, enjoyable, and encourage sustained interest and participation. Recommendations include the following (USDHHS, 2015):

- Children and adolescents should strive for 60 minutes of physical activity daily; the minutes do not necessarily need to be contiguous.
- Physical activity should be of moderate to vigorous levels and include vigorous-intensity physical activity at least 3 days per week.
- Physical activity should include each of the following on 3 or more days per week:
  - Aerobic activity for cardiovascular and respiratory fitness
  - Resistance activities for muscle strengthening
  - Weight loading for bone strengthening

The Healthy People 2020 goals are broad-based collaborative efforts to address 10 high-priority public health issues in the United States; physical activity is one of these indicators. The following objectives relate to physical activity and fitness in children/adolescents (USDHHS, 2010). They focus on:

- Increasing the proportion of:
  - Adolescents who meet current physical activity guidelines for aerobic and for muscle-strengthening activity
  - Public and private schools that require daily PE
  - Adolescents who participate in daily school PE
  - School districts that require or recommend elementary school recess for an appropriate period of time
  - Children and adolescents who do not exceed recommended limits for screen time
  - The nation's public and private schools that provide access to their physical activity spaces and facilities for all persons outside of normal school hours (i.e., before and after the school day, on weekends, and during summer and other vacations)
  - Physician office visits that include counseling or education that address physical activity
  - Trips made by walking or by bicycle (developmental objectives)
- Increasing the number of states with licensing regulations for physical activity provided in child care
- Increasing legislative policies for the built environment that enhance access to and availability of physical activity opportunities (developmental objective)

The Joint Commission Ambulatory Care National Patient Safety Goals has a standard (NPSG 07.01.01) that addresses skin hygiene and frequent hand washing to prevent communicable skin infections, such as those spread during contact sports like wrestling. The guidelines written by the CDC or WHO are utilized as standards for meeting this goal.

The American Academy of Pediatrics (AAP) policy statement on promoting physical activity includes the following recommendations (AAP Council on Sports Medicine and Fitness and AAP Council on School Health, 2010). Physicians and health care professionals should:

- Participate with schools to set and implement goals to develop wellness policies for healthy nutrition, physical activity, and other strategies that promote wellness of students.
- Advocate for school curricula that emphasize the health benefits of regular physical activity and for recreational programs that promote the use of community and school facilities after hours by children and youth and at reasonable costs.
- Advocate for the reinstatement of compulsory, quality, and daily PE classes for kindergarten through 12th grade that are enjoyable and help students develop attitudes and skills for lifelong active lifestyles; maintain school recess, and promote extracurricular physical activity programs before and after school hours.
- Promote recreational facilities, parks, playgrounds, bicycle and walking paths, sidewalks, and marked crosswalks.
- Inquire about nutritional intake, plot body mass index (BMI), promote healthy eating and physical activity, and note and discuss the limitation of sedentary activities with children and youth.

- Encourage a culture of family physical activity by advocating that parents act as role models, incorporate physical activity into their own lives, and support their children in age-appropriate sports and recreational activities.
- Suggest that overweight children initially participate in activities that place less stress on weight-bearing joints, such as swimming, water polo, strength training, and cycling.

Health Benefits of Physical Activity

In addition to the aforementioned benefits gained from physical activity, there are specific benefits relevant to some chronic health conditions seen in children. Health care providers can use these known benefits as powerful promotional tools when counseling children with the following health conditions:

- Asthma: Moderate to vigorous exercise by children with mild and well-controlled asthma improves aerobic and anaerobic fitness that in turn benefits lung function and improves health outcomes (Conley et al, 2014). Exclusion from sports for all children with asthma is not indicated as long as the child's asthma is well controlled; those with moderate to severe asthma may require exclusion from participation in regular physical activity until asthma control is achieved. There is no evidence that physical activity substantially improves overall pulmonary function status (Crosbie, 2012).
- Cognition, depression, and well-being: Cognitive development and a sense of psychological well-being may also be positively influenced by physical activity (USDHHS, 2012). Children who engage in the recommended moderate to vigorous physical activity score significantly higher on measures of self-esteem than less active children and are more likely to report better well-being (Breslin et al, 2012). Regular participation in physical activity programs in schools may be protective against the onset of depression and beneficial for reducing depressive symptoms in youth (Brown et al, 2013).
- Academics: Research has demonstrated an association between improved academic performance (better grades, higher scores on standardized test scores, improved memory and concentration) and participation in regular physical activity. Any form of physical activity reduces sedentary time and is linked to increased academic and social maturation in children (Chin and Ludwig, 2014; Murray et al, 2013).
- Hypertension: For hypertensive youth, regular to vigorous physical activity (30 minutes, 3 days per week) reduces blood pressure and improves physical fitness. Resistance training coupled with aerobic exercise is beneficial for maintaining blood pressure within the normal range once the hypertension is resolved (McCambridge et al, 2010).
- Metabolic syndrome, insulin resistance, type 2 diabetes: For individuals with metabolic syndrome, engaging in moderate to vigorous regular physical activity has the positive effects of increasing high-density lipoproteins (HDLs) and reducing triglycerides and insulin levels. Exercise has not been shown to reduce total cholesterol or low-density lipoproteins (LDLs); however, regular moderate to vigorous physical exercise helps control weight, and even modest weight loss has been shown to reduce insulin resistance (Gebel, 2011). Additionally, a strong body of evidence suggests that regular physical activity and exercise alone reduce insulin resistance in overweight and obese youth and that both aerobic and resistance exercise (without weight loss or calorie restriction) achieve this result (Kim and Park, 2013).
- Obesity: Children who engage in physical activity have a lower adiposity, or accumulation of body fat, and improved health care outcomes. One study demonstrated that obese youth who engaged in moderate to vigorous physical activity for a minimum of 20 minutes per day 5 days per week over 12 weeks reduced adiposity, metabolic risks, and type 2 diabetes (Davis et al, 2012). Low-cost interventions in some school districts that involved simply increasing physical activity during the school day resulted in an increase in the level of physical fitness by 52% and helped combat obesity (Chin and Ludwig, 2014; Dobbins et al, 2013).

Physical Activity and Children with Special Health Care Needs

Many children and adolescents with intellectual and developmental disabilities (including those with Down syndrome, fragile X syndrome, Turner or Klinefelter syndromes, and autism) are capable of performing exercise or strenuous activities. Children with special health care needs and youth with disabilities require special focus in order to ensure that they have access to participate in sports and can be physically active at levels that offer health benefits. Benefits of physical activity for children and adolescents with disabilities are physiologic and psychological—improved self-esteem and sense of well-being, greater independence, improved social skills, and improved physical functioning.

Participation in sports for children with special needs has increased; however, research about participation of children with specific disabilities remains limited. By classifying a child as having a disability, parents, schools, and coaches are better able to allow children with similar abilities to participate; such classification also encourages activity and equipment adaptations that allow for greater participation. These children are at particular risk for obesity, which in turn leaves them susceptible to developing chronic diseases, including heart disease, stroke, hypertension, and diabetes. With regular exercise, many of these issues can be addressed.

Although the Special Olympics organization highlights global competitive games, the organization's enduring focus is to educate those with disabilities to make healthy lifestyle choices to improve their overall long-term health. The

Special Olympics organization provides guidelines for healthy nutrition, lifestyle choices and ways to increase one's level of physical fitness, and holds sports health screening clinics. It also serves as a resource for community and health care professionals to learn about athletic participation and how to address health care disparities of children with special needs (see Additional Resources).

Special Consideration: Atlantoaxial or Atlanto-Occipital Instability (AAI)

Youth with Down syndrome require special consideration because up to 40% can have a hypermobility or instability between C1 to C2 (atlantoaxial joints), and up to 61% can have occipitoatlantal hypermobility (Spiegel and Dormans, 2011). Under certain circumstances—with sudden or extreme flexion or hyperextension of the head and neck—subluxation and spinal cord compression can occur as a result of the vertebral anatomy and lax ligaments. Box 13-1 lists activities that should be avoided by those individuals with these vertebral instabilities. They may, however, engage in most of the listed noncontact sports. If the pre-participation physical examination reveals that there are symptoms suggestive of spinal cord compression and/or AAI, clearance for Special Olympics requires an additional thorough neurologic examination by a qualified physician. If that qualified physician certifies that the athlete may participate in the activity and the athlete (or parent/guardian of a minor) signs a waiver provided by Special Olympics, the athlete may choose to participate in the sport of the athlete's choice (Special Olympics, 2015).

• BOX 13-1 Sports Contraindicated for Youth with Down Syndrome Who Have Symptoms* or Confirmation of Atlantoaxial Instability

- Contact/collision sports (e.g., football, soccer)
- Artistic gymnastics
- Diving
- Butterfly stroke, individual medley events, diving starts
- High jump
- Pentathlon
- Powerlifting (back squat)
- Equestrian events
- Snowboarding
- Judo
- Alpine skiing
- Certain warm-up exercises that involve head or neck flexion-extension

*Symptoms of possible spinal cord compression or atlantoaxial instability can include neck pain, localized neurologic pain, weakness, numbness, spasticity (unusual "tightness" of certain muscles) or change in muscle tone, gait difficulties, hyperreflexia, change in bowel or bladder function, or other signs or symptoms of injury to the spinal cord (Special Olympics, 2015).

Data from Patel DR, Greydanus DE: Sport participation by physically and cognitively challenged young athletes, *Pediatr Clin North Am* 57(3):795–817, 2010; Special Olympics: Article 1: addendum F: participation by individuals with Down syndrome who have atlanto-axial instability, 2009, www.specialolympics.org/uploadedFiles/09_article_1.pdf. Accessed September 16, 2015.

Strategies to Support Physical Activity for Children and Adolescents

Motivation and Barriers to Maintaining Physical Activity

A number of factors affect an individual's motivation to become physically active and/or maintain a physically active lifestyle. Physical activity, like any behavior, operates on a socioecologic model. Table 13-1 describes the different levels at which a clinician can promote physical activity. The effect of socioeconomics, race/ethnicity, gender, and the individual's community must be considered in order to effectively and equitably address the barriers and resources for physical activity (Crespo et al, 2013; Millstein et al, 2011).

Can Health Care Providers Influence Lifestyle Behaviors?

Health care providers have the opportunity to impact the individual's lifestyle by focusing on components of healthy lifestyles, such as exercise, nutrition, and stress reduction. Familiarity with the theories of change, motivation, and motivational interviewing will provide practitioners with clinical skills to support behavioral change. (See Chapter 9 for a discussion regarding techniques for motivational interviewing.) If these techniques are used appropriately, the practitioner can support patient-centered care, educate the child and family, and increase motivation for the individual to competently manage their own health.

In randomized controlled trials and meta-analyses, active lifestyle interventions (e.g., establishing behavioral goals that are tracked weekly, learning to find solutions to barriers, and evaluating progress over time) have been shown to be more beneficial than no-treatment controls or education-only strategies (Wilfley et al, 2011). In addition to discussing lifestyle interventions with children and their families, clinicians can promote a fitness-oriented clinical environment and encourage clinic staff to model and promote healthy lifestyles. Examples of this include adding signs that encourage the use of stairs; providing water fountains; advertising and participating in healthy community events (e.g., farmer's markets, bike clubs, and fun runs); making educational materials accessible; and using and promoting the use of pedometers or other wireless activity tracking devices (Wilfley et al, 2011).

Counseling Families about Organized Sports for Their Children

Being physically active is best achieved as a lifelong habit when it is encouraged from infancy. Unstructured play, which builds creativity and dexterity, should be encouraged; however, this play has decreased in children's lives as parents

TABLE 13-1 Socioecologic Model for Effective Promotion of Physical Activity by Health Care Providers

Level of Intervention	Examples
Individual Level	
Carried out one on one during clinic visit to influence behaviors, knowledge, attributions, and beliefs.	Work with children and families to educate and promote a positive outlook toward physical activity: • Assess child's baseline physical activity level as a "vital sign" at all patient visits. • Discuss physical activity recommendations as part of healthy lifestyle counseling when providing obesity prevention, education, or obesity treatment. • Use motivational interviewing techniques to address and promote behavioral change for increasing physical activity. Base intervention on "stages of change" theory as a collaborative patient/provider model. See Chapter 9 for a discussion of these techniques. • Role model a healthy lifestyle.
Interpersonal Level	
Includes individuals' interactions with one another and relationships shared within social networks, such as families, peer groups, and friendship-based social networks.	• Recommend peer groups or walking groups to encourage accountability of its members. • Initiate family goals to participate in physical activity regularly and together. • Role model a healthy lifestyle and promote engagement in physical activities among clinic staff.
Organizational Level	
Promote activities on an institutional level that encourage physical activity through policies and rules specific to assemblies of individuals. Common examples of assemblies include schools, religious or faith-based institutions, and the workplace.	Support activities that encourage organizational physical activity promotion, for example: • School programs, such as walk or bike to school days (e.g., International Walk to School Day that occurs yearly in October; see www.walkbiketoschool.org/) • Screen time awareness week • Intramural programs • Advise child care centers about ways to increase physical activity for children and staff • Advise schools and parents about importance of recess and physical education (PE) • Encourage schools *not* to withhold recess as a punishment for misbehavior
Community Level	
Communities include individuals who participate in interpersonal relationships within various local groups of institutions and organizations. Communities may be defined geographically, politically, culturally, or by other common characteristics.	Promote activities that help communities structure public space and promote physical activity: • Ensure safe and easily accessible park and playground space. • Advocate for affordable organized activities (e.g., scholarships to pay for team sports, after-school activities for low-income youth and local recreation department or YMCA offerings). • Advocate for bike lanes and walking trails in the community. • Advocate for vehicular speed control along major routes to schools to encourage walking/cycling safety. • Promote programs that teach bike safety and distribute low-cost helmets. • Advocate for keeping school buildings open after school for supervised physical activities. • Volunteer to sit on school boards or be a part of school parent teaching associations to advocate for physical activity within the realm of school.
Structure, Policy, and Systems Level	
Represents the local, state, and federal structures and systems that affect the built environment, surrounding communities, and individuals.	Advocate for changes in public policy: • Testify at hearings on importance of maintaining PE in schools. • Address zoning issues to maintain or increase green spaces, such as parks, bike trails, and walking trails. • Work with planners to ensure that communities are designed to promote family friendly physical activity (e.g., adequate sidewalks/crosswalks, residential areas within walking distance to neighborhood schools, and adequate lighting at playfields and parks).

Some data from Centers for Disease Control and Prevention (CDC): Addressing obesity disparities: social ecological model, CDC (website), 2013, www.cdc.gov/obesity/health_equity/addressingtheissue.html. Accessed July 28, 2014.

endeavor to fill up their child's time with goal-oriented activities. Parents may believe that children benefit by building athlete skills at an early age through participating in athletic opportunities or risk falling behind athletically. This can lead to children often participating in a structured and specialized single sport athletic activity at an inappropriate young age, which may be detrimental physically and mentally (Malina, 2010). Structured sport play that is promoted in an age or developmentally appropriate manner supports a child's physical, cognitive, and emotional health. Table 13-2 and Figure 13-1 provide guidance for a developmentally appropriate approach to sports activities.

Strength Training

Strength training refers to the progressive use of a variety of resistive loads, movement speeds, and modalities to increase muscular strength and endurance. Modalities may include free weights, weight machines, elastic bands, and one's own body weight (e.g., plyometrics involve exercises that use a combination of body weight and rapid movements [e.g., hops and jumps] to enhance power and "explosiveness"). Strength training can be used for several reasons: to enhance performance in a particular sport, as a component of rehabilitation after some injuries, and, for some, to enhance muscle mass for appearance. A strength training program should be designed to fit the needs, goals, and abilities of the child or adolescent. The design criteria should take into consideration training age, existing motor skills and muscle strength, and technical proficiency in combination with biologic age and psychosocial maturity.

In the past, medical providers expressed concern that the lack of sufficient circulating androgens (needed for muscular strength and mass) could lead to damage of open growth plates, causing premature closure of epiphyses. However, current consensus is that strength training is advantageous, even for young athletes, provided that it is done in a safe and supervised manner (Milone et al, 2013). Strength training must be differentiated from weight training, weight lifting, or Olympic powerlifting (which employs maximal or supramaximal lifts). With strength training or resistance training, submaximal weights can be lifted by children and adolescents to improve performance safely under proper instruction and supervision. However, powerlifting and

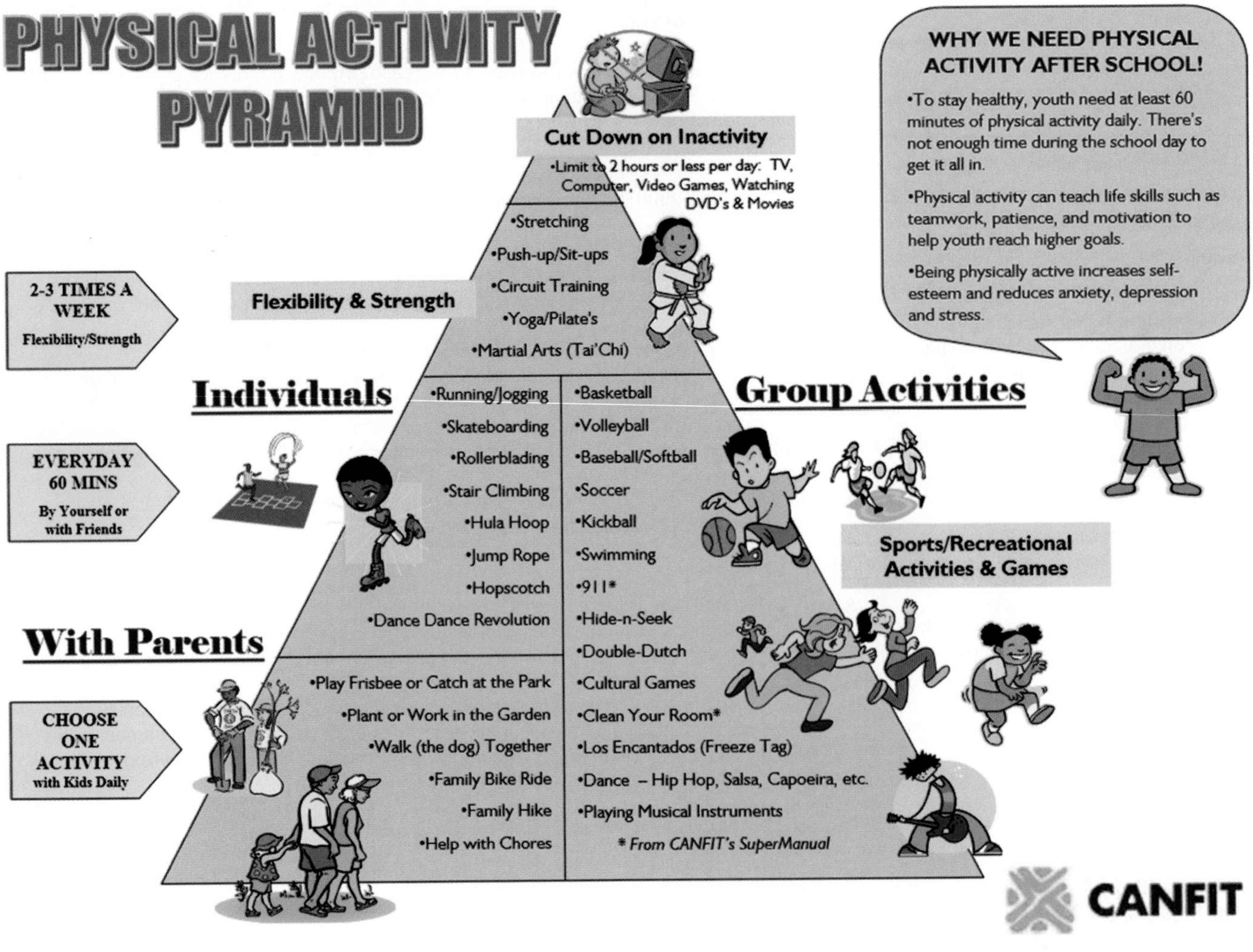

• **Figure 13-1** Children's physical activity pyramid. (By Barbara Willenberg, Associate State Food and Nutrition Specialist. © 1999 University of Missouri. Published by University Extension, University of Missouri-Columbia.)

TABLE 13-2 Appropriate Fitness Activities by Age Group

Age Group	Fitness Activities	Family Fitness Fun
Infant	• Encourage "tummy time." • Provide safe and clean spaces for infant to start rolling, playing, crawling, and doing other large muscle activities. • Place safe objects slightly out of reach (lightweight, cannot be swallowed, no sharp edges, brightly colored, nontoxic, textured).	• Bring the infant to new environments. • Play "patty-cake" and "peek-a-boo." • Place objects of interest (toys, rattles, and so on) out of the infant's reach; continue to move the object to encourage mobility and range of motion. • Continue close supervision. • Interact with infant when he or she is alert and attentive through use of brightly colored objects, facial expressions, and verbalization to encourage infant's participation. • Avoid overuse of strollers and walkers.
Toddlers	• Unstructured play that focuses on participation, not competition: hopping, jumping, tumbling, swinging, climbing, sandbox play, supervised water play, riding toys, walking, running, and so on.	• Stimulate toddler with music and interactive play. • Provide safe environments for the toddler to explore. • Continue close supervision, especially in public places (playgrounds) and environments with water. • Role model physical activity participation from all family members. • Begin to engage in household chores (e.g., setting table, putting toys away, gardening, and helping with laundry).
4 to 6 years	• Ride bike with training wheels (away from traffic); play catch and games, such as kickball, jumping rope, hopscotch, swimming, skating, and tag.	• Offer family time with walking, playing, running, tennis, skiing, dancing, scavenger hunts, supervised water play, ice skating, hiking, and bike riding. • Emphasize variety over one particular activity. • Continue close supervision, especially with activities in public places (playgrounds) or by water. • Enroll child in swimming lessons. • Encourage physical activity in short bursts throughout the day. • Monitor/limit sedentary time (videos, video games, television, and computer use). • Role model physical activity participation from all family members.
6 to 12 years	• Does well with organized games and sports. • Enjoys both noncompetitive and competitive games, such as swimming, bike riding, gymnastics, tumbling, martial arts, baseball, soccer, tennis, and basketball. • Avoid sports specialization until >10 years. • Is able to start strength training (7 years and older) with proper supervision (see Strength Training).	• Offer ample opportunities with families and friends to participate in walking, bike riding, camping, hiking, tennis, skiing, dancing, ice skating, and swimming. • Monitor playground equipment and water sports. • Follow safety guidelines for all activities (e.g., wearing helmet, athletic supporter, baseball pitching and throwing limitations). Review pitching limitation guidelines. • Monitor/limit sedentary time (videos, video games, television, and computer use). • Encourage healthy eating from all four food groups with good portion control. • Monitor for disordered eating patterns and increased interest on weight or dieting. • Role model physical activity participation from all family members.
13 to 18 years	• Any activity, including competitive and noncompetitive sports. • Encourage strength training (with proper form and supervision) to increase flexibility, strength, and reduce injuries (see Strength Training).	Continue all of the aforementioned plus: • Support participation in individual and team sports, such as track and field, tennis, swimming, basketball, baseball, and soccer. • Monitor for use of supplements or performance enhancing drugs.

Data from Centers for Disease Control and Prevention (CDC): Healthy schools: youth physical activity guidelines toolkit, CDC (website), 2015, www.cdc.gov/healthyyouth/physicalactivity/guidelines.htm. Accessed September 15, 2015; Hagan JF, Shaw JS, Duncan PM, editors: *Bright futures: guidelines for health supervision of infants, children, and adolescents*, ed 3, Elk Grove Village, IL, 2008, American Academy of Pediatrics, pp 147–154; West Virginia Department of Education, Office of Child Nutrition: Developmentally appropriate physical activity ideas, www.wvde.state.wv.us/child-nutrition/leap-of-taste/physical-activity/physical-activity-ideas/. Accessed September 15, 2015.

maximal weight training are not recommended for prepubescent children (Barbieri and Zaccagni, 2013).

Benefits of strength training include improved cardiovascular fitness, strength, flexibility, body composition, bone mineral density, blood lipid profile, and mental health (Lloyd et al, 2014). Additionally, strength training is an important component to weight management programs, because it has been shown to improve body composition and reduce skinfold thickness (Barbieri and Zaccagni, 2013). Strength training that is part of a well-rounded conditioning program has been shown to reduce blood pressure in hypertensive youth; when included in the preseason conditioning and training program for many sports, it correlates with a decrease in sports injuries (Lloyd et al, 2014; Young and Metzl, 2010).

Young athletes engaged in strength training should be supervised; however, there are fewer injuries from strength training than from the sports themselves. Box 13-2 lists general guidelines for strength training by the preadolescent. Restrictions on who can safely do strength training include youth with severe hypertension (Anyaegbu and Dharnidharka, 2014), those receiving chemotherapy with anthracyclines or any other potentially cardiotoxic medication, youth with some forms of cardiomyopathy (particularly hypertrophic cardiomyopathy), individuals with moderate to severe pulmonary hypertension (at risk for acute decompensation with a sudden change in hemodynamics), and those with Marfan syndrome and a dilated aortic root. Youth with seizure disorders should be withheld from strength training programs until clearance is obtained from a neurologist (AAP et al, 2011a).

Preseason Conditioning and Injury Prevention

A variety of strategies can be used to reduce the incidence and severity of injuries and heat-related illnesses and dehydration (see also Chapter 40). Some of the more typical injury conditions that can be avoided with simple prevention strategies are included in Table 13-3. Readiness can be addressed from two perspectives—developmental readiness and preseason conditioning readiness. Developmental readiness has been previously discussed.

• BOX 13-2 Safe Practices for Strength Training for Youth Athletes

General Guidelines

- Train under the supervision of a coach or trainer familiar with appropriate training regimens for different age groups and with the equipment and its use.
- Youth ready to play in organized sports (e.g., Little League baseball, soccer) should participate in some form of strength-related activity (e.g., push-ups and sit-ups for younger children). Females (especially prior to menarche) benefit from strength training to build bone mass.
- Strength training is only one component of a well-rounded fitness program.
- Prior to starting a formal strength training program, the youth should ideally have a physical examination, especially if he or she has any known or suspected health condition.
- Balance exercise among all muscle groups, including core muscles.
- Ensure adequate fluid intake during training.
- Begin and end training sessions with a period of warm-up/cool-down exercises (10 to 15 minutes) that include stretching and dynamic movement (slow jog, jumping, skipping).
- Advise athletes and families of the dangers of using performance-enhancing drugs.

Exercise and Equipment Selection

- Child-sized equipment (e.g., light barbells, small dumbbells, and elastic resistance bands) should be used.
- Youth should be able to properly and safely execute exercises using correct techniques.
- Resistance can be in the form of the child's own bodyweight, weight machines, resistance bands, free weights, and medicine balls.

Training Volume and Intensity

- *Volume* refers to the total number of times of an exercise multiplied by resistance used (kg) within any given training session.
- *Intensity* is the resistance (load or weight) needed to overcome gravity during a single repetition.
- The greater the intensity (weight), the lower the number of repetitions (volume) that should be completed.
- Choice of the appropriate training intensity is often a percentage of an individual's one repetition-maximum (1 RM).
- Initially, when the individual does not have prior experience with strength or resistance training, start with low volume (one to two sets) and low to moderate training intensities (≤60% 1 RM). Gradually increase as the youth gains competence.
- Number of sets and repetitions chosen can be flexible from session to session.
- Proper lifting technique, form, and safety take precedence over heaviness of weight.

Rest Intervals

- Build rest periods between sets into the training session(s). Allow about 1 minute minimum, increasing the period (e.g., 2 to 3 minutes) as the intensity of training increases.

Training Frequency

- Strength or resistance training is recommended two to three times per week on nonconsecutive days to allow for recovery and optimal strength building.
- Training frequency may increase as the child ages but needs close monitoring.

Data from American Academy of Pediatrics (AAP) Council on Sports Medicine and Fitness, McCambridge TM, Stricker PR: Policy statement: strength training by children and adolescents, *Pediatrics* 121(4):835–840, 2008; reaffirmed 2011; Faigenbaum AD, Lloyd RS, Myer GD: Youth resistance training: past practices, new perspectives, and future directions, *Pediatr Execr Sci* 25(4):591–604, 2013; Hatfield D: Strength training for children, a review of research literature, www.issaonline.edu/blog/index.cfm/2011/6/1/Strength-Training-for-Children-a-review-of-research-literature. Accessed September 15, 2015; Lloyd RS, Faigenbaum AD, Stone MH, et al: Position statement on youth resistance training: the 2014 International Consensus, *Br J Sports Med* 48(7):498–505, 2014.

TABLE 13-3 Common Injuries and Prevention Strategies

Medical Condition	Prevention Strategies	Comments
Muscle soreness	• Warm up body temperature before gentle stretching to maintain flexibility. • Start with lighter weights and fewer repetitions when starting a new regimen.	• Soreness should be minor, resulting from microscopic muscle or connective tissue damage; it is a normal result of muscles that are adapting to a new exercise program. • Clinicians should explain this soreness ahead of time so that new exercisers do not use this condition as an excuse to stop their fitness regimen.
Strains and sprains	• Participate in a preseason conditioning program. • Tape site of previous injury. • Warm up body temperature before stretching. • Maintain playing surfaces. • Use proper footwear. • Limit practice time.	• These injuries are mostly related to pivoting sports, such as basketball, football, and volleyball. • Knee braces should not replace adequate conditioning specific to the sport. They should only be used after a formal diagnosis and management plan is in place following consultation with a provider or athletic trainer; braces should be only one aspect of acute or overuse injury treatment. Categories of knee braces include sleeves (help with swelling and support but infer no real stability; may have extra knee padding that helps with prevention in sports at high risk for blows to the knee); PTO brace or patellar strap/bands for added patellar stability; and hinged-knee braces (include prophylactic braces [protection of knee ligaments during contact sports]; and functional or rehabilitative [intended to prevent reinjury after torn knee ligaments or postoperatively]). Braces should not replace rehabilitation and surgery, if required (AAP, 2015a).
Fractures	• Do strength-conditioning exercises. • Use proper techniques. • Take safety precautions. • Use protective gear that fits well, such as wrist guards.	• These injuries most commonly involve the upper extremities, such as when falling on an outstretched hand. Lower-extremity fractures can occur with sports such as soccer.
Stress fractures	• Use soft running and playing surfaces. • Use proper footgear. • Do strengthening exercises. • Stop activity when pain occurs.	
Lacerations/contusions/ abrasions (also see Chapter 40)	• Protective equipment is essential.	• These injuries are mostly related to baseball (contusion/abrasion), soccer, cycling, and ice hockey (lacerations).
Anterior leg pain syndrome (shin splints)	• Stretch before and after activity. • Pronate and supinate feet while standing. • Use soft playing surface. • Use proper footwear (proper fit, impact-absorbing sole, support for hindfoot). • Avoid sudden increase in activity. • Limit forceful, extensive use of foot flexors.	
Plantar fasciitis	• Use proper footwear (cushioned with fitted heel counters or lifts). • Stretch calf and Achilles tendon. • Do ice massage after event. • Correct biomechanical errors. • Limit hills and speed work; increase soft-surface running.	

Continued

TABLE 13-3 Common Injuries and Prevention Strategies—cont'd

Medical Condition	Prevention Strategies	Comments
Blisters (also see Chapter 40)	• Wear socks. • Wear properly fitted shoes. • Use powder, petroleum jelly, an anti-friction product (highly recommended), or Second Skin on at-risk or reddened area(s).	
Head and neck injuries	• Have appropriate supervision and coaching that teaches proper skills, such as tackling. • Adhere to safety rules of the game. • Strengthen neck muscles. • Use appropriate equipment: helmets and face and mouth gear. • Follow concussion guidelines for RTP after injury (see Table 13-10).	• Greatest risks for these injuries are from cycling, diving, equestrian sports, football, gymnastics, ice hockey, wrestling, trampolines, football, rugby, and cheerleading. • Risks increase with age.
Eye trauma	• Wear headgear and protective glasses.	• Eye injuries are most commonly related to baseball and ice hockey.

PTO, Patellar tracking orthosis; *RTP,* return-to-play.

Preseason conditioning (e.g., preparatory muscle conditioning and plyometrics) trains the central nervous system to react quickly to muscular stretching and shortening. Such conditioning has been demonstrated to be an effective method for decreasing overall injuries (Lloyd et al, 2014). Proper preseason conditioning should focus on enhancing strength, flexibility, endurance, and improving natural sport specific movements and agility (Nationwide Children's Hospital, n.d.a.). Conditioning also lessens overuse injuries (e.g., stress fractures, bursitis, and tendinopathies) and the amount of time needed for rehabilitation, helps strengthen bone, facilitates weight control, improves balance and coordination, adds muscle mass, and improves performance. Players as young as 10 to 12 years old benefit by being able to establish overall motion patterns when they participate in warm-up programs. Such conditioning is not sport specific and should not to be confused with weight lifting or body-building training. Coaches and fitness instructors should be certified and knowledgeable about age-specific training techniques and safety; adult training techniques should never be applied to children.

Use of Helmets for Cycling and Winter Sports

In the United States, approximately 900 people die annually in bicycle accidents; 75% are due to head injuries. Those individuals who wear an approved bicycle helmet have an 88% lower risk of brain injury compared with those without such a helmet. States that have helmet laws have significantly lower mean unadjusted fatality rates in children younger than 16 years old involved in bicycle accidents (Meehan et al, 2013). The AAP recommends that all cyclists wear properly fitted bicycle helmets whenever they ride. Health care providers should educate parents and children about wearing helmets and support state legislation when possible. Likewise, helmets should be worn when a child or youth is involved in skateboarding or inline skating, when riding all-terrain vehicles, motorcycles, or scooters, and when engaging in winter sports such as sking, ice hockey, or riding snowmobiles (AAP, 2015b; Lovejoy et al, 2012). Valuable information about bike safety for children is available from the National Highway Traffic Safety Administration. Proper use starts with proper helmet fitting. Some guidelines are listed here:

- Try on several sizes and models to find the best fit that:
  - Places the helmet low on the forehead.
  - Positions the brim so that it is parallel to the ground when the head is upright: The child should be able to see the brim when looking up. This may require removing or installing inside pads to enable a snug fit, or it may require adjusting the sizing ring.
  - Securely fastens the chin strap to the point where the helmet will not shift over the eyes, rock side to side, or come off when the child shakes his or her head.
- Helmets should carry a U.S. Consumer Product Safety Commission (USCPSC) sticker.
- Throw away any helmet involved in any substantial blow that resulted in marks on the outer surface; do not purchase secondhand helmets.
- Replace helmets every 5 years or sooner, depending on the manufacturer's recommendations.
- Children are more likely to wear helmets if a parental rule exists about its unconditional use, if parents wear helmets during cycling activities, and if there is a mandatory state helmet law. Unfortunately, state laws related to bicycles usually only apply to children 16 years old or younger.

Adult skiers who wear helmets serve as role models for children. During skiing and snowboarding, wearing a helmet reduces the individual's risk of serious injury and death by 60% (Fenerty et al, 2013). Skiers say they do not wear helmets because they want to take risks or the helmets impair their vision and hearing, although no association between helmet use and impaired vision or hearing has been found (Ruedl et al, 2012).

Basic Metabolic and Nutritional Needs and Abuses in Athletes

Youth athletes are less energy efficient when physically active than adult athletes which results in higher energy requirements per kilogram of body weight in youth (Jeukendrup and Cronin, 2011). Sufficient caloric intake ensures that body weight is maintained and/or modified and provides the energy and nutrients necessary for the individual to benefit from the effects of training. Without adequate energy intake, there is the risk of muscle loss, fatigue, injury, illness, and prolonged recovery process. Likewise, excess energy intake can result in increased body weight and body fat that can lead to increased risks of fatigue, injury, and poor performance.

Youth athletes should be able to meet 100% of their dietary needs from a balanced nutrition plan that includes a focus on the athlete's performance, hydration, and recovery. Supplements should only be used in selected medical conditions with known nutritional deficiencies, such as iron, calcium, or vitamin D (American College of Sports Medicine [ACSM], 2013). Nutrition recommendations are summarized in Table 13-4. Additional information follows about certain metabolic requirements during exercise.

Carbohydrates

Energy is gained through the consumption of a combination of carbohydrates, proteins, and fats. Short-term, high-intensity activities (i.e., anaerobic activity, such as high jumping or diving) exclusively use carbohydrates (glucose) as a fuel source, whereas longer-term activities (i.e., aerobic activity, such as running or cross-country skiing) use all three sources, carbohydrates, fats, and proteins. Complex carbohydrates (e.g., fruits, nuts, cereals, grains, pasta, and dried beans) are preferable to simple carbohydrates (such as, cookies, sugary foods, ice cream, and some crackers) because, although providing readily available energy, they do not cause the rapid rise in blood glucose levels with resultant insulin rebound that simple carbohydrates do. Hypoglycemia can result from insulin excess, which is counterproductive to the energy needed for sport participation. Sufficient carbohydrate intake to maintain body weight is required to adequately utilize proteins.

In general, carbohydrates are most effectively converted into needed energy if they are consumed several hours before the athletic event or practice. Approximately 3 to 4 grams per kilogram body weight of carbohydrate-rich solid food, 3 to 4 hours prior to exercise are recommended. Ingesting fluid carbohydrates (1 gram per kilogram of body weight) just before activities may improve performance (ACSM, 2013). Carbohydrate loading has not been studied in children and is generally not recommended (Jeukendrup and Cronin, 2011). After competition, carbohydrate intake is again important to improve the muscle glycogen resynthesis that occurs most rapidly in the first 30 minutes to 6 hours after exercise. Consuming complex carbohydrates in the form of snacks or fluids postexercise typically achieves this resynthesis.

Protein

Protein provides energy when stored glycogen and fat are depleted during endurance exercise and aids muscle synthesis and repair. Amino acid/protein supplements do not increase muscle mass or decrease body fat. Hypercalciuria with calcium loss and dehydration can occur if protein intake is too high, because excess nitrogen, and hence water, is excreted. Additionally, eating too much protein may lead to an underconsumption of adequate carbohydrates and fats, causing the excess protein to be stored as fat.

Fats

Dietary fats serve as high-calorie sources of energy. Athletes who are restricting nutritional intake of fats may underconsume them, thus becoming deficient in fat-soluble vitamins (A, D, E, and K).

Intentional Weight Loss

Weight loss by adolescent athletes can be a dangerous practice. Youth athletes may believe the need to control weight through dieting and intense exercising is part of a normal and acceptable routine for competitive athletes (Bratland-Sanda and Sundgot-Borgen, 2013). Wrestlers may try to lose weight to be eligible to compete in a lower weight class; runners sometimes vomit to run lighter; and female gymnasts may practice significant nutritional control to maintain weight and size. Dancers, divers, figure skaters, and cheerleaders also control weight for appearance advantages. Bodybuilders, rowers, distance runners, and swimmers often try to control their weight. Starvation can lead to suppressed growth hormones, can interfere with pubertal gonadal hormone changes, and may result in eating disorders. Nutritional counseling is essential, including a reminder that muscle weighs more than fat, and that during adolescent growth, weight gain is normal.

Wrestlers often engage in repeated bouts of excessive weight loss or weight cycling. Such transient weight cycling can reduce immune function, cause a reduction in glycogen stores, mood alteration, structural alterations in muscles, cognitive dysfunction, and decreased cardiac function, as well as alter the body's ability to maintain body temperature (ACSM, 2013). This practice is to be discouraged because of the risk of these short-term effects and long-term dysfunctional eating. Measurements of body composition before and during the wrestling season can help coaches and parents stay alert to risky behavior. Furthermore, any planned weight loss should involve

TABLE 13-4 Nutrition Recommendations for Athletes

Nutrient	Recommendations
Calories (from carbohydrates/fat/protein): For energy	• Maintain same for all people: 50% to 70% carbohydrate; 20% to 35% fat; 10% to 35% protein (see Chapter 10). • Do not decrease caloric intake during sports season. • May need 1500 to 3000 kcal more than recommended dietary allowance to meet activity requirements. To avoid weight loss, female athletes should not consume less than 1200 to 1400 calories per day; male athletes should not consume less than 1500 to 1700 calories per day. • Allow appropriate vegetarian diets, ensuring adequate micronutrients.
Vitamins and minerals: For energy production, hemoglobin synthesis, maintenance of bone health, immune function, and antioxidant protection	• Athletes diets are often low in calcium, vitamin D, B vitamins, iron, zinc, magnesium, and antioxidants, such as vitamins C and E, beta carotene, and selenium. • Follow RDA guidelines; do not take megadoses. • Adolescent girls may need to bring calcium (1200 to 1500 mg/d), vitamin D (400 to 800 IU), and iron intake up to recommended range. • Do not take salt tablets, because hypernatremia and delayed gastric emptying can result.
CHOs: Help maintain blood glucose levels and replenish muscle glycogen stores	• 6 to 10 g/kg body weight per day. • Use nutritious foods, such as fruits, vegetables, grains, and milk sugars. • Postexercise, ingest 1.0 to 1.5 g/kg of body weight in the first 30 minutes and again after 2 hours.
Protein and/or amino acid supplements: Facilitate muscle synthesis and repair	• No protein supplements needed; hypercalciuria with calcium loss and dehydration can occur if protein intake is too high. • Postexercise, ingest 10 to 20 g of protein 2 hours after exercise, along with the carbohydrates noted earlier.
Fats: For energy and to aid vitamin absorption	• Fat sources should be ⅓ polyunsaturated, ⅓ saturated, and ⅓ monounsaturated with zero trans fats. • Ensure adequate consumption of fat soluble vitamins (A, D, E, and K). • Pre-exercise intake high in fat and fiber can result in gastrointestinal distress.
Fluids with/without CHOs: For hydration, thermoregulation, may provide calories	• Plain water before, during, and after activity if physical exertion lasts no more than an hour. • If exertion lasts more than an hour, fluids should contain CHOs; if exertion lasts more than several hours, fluids should also contain added sodium to maintain hydration and performance. • Avoid carbonated drinks; they can delay gastric emptying and intestinal absorption. • Postexercise, replace 16 to 24 oz of fluid for every pound lost during exercise (determined by pre- and post-practice weights). Thirst is not a good indicator of fluid status. • Avoid caffeine drinks, because they can increase diuresis. • Key ingredients of a sports drink for athletic performance: 6% to 8% CHO (14 to 19 g per 8 oz, not to exceed 6% to 8%) and 110 to 165 mg sodium per 8 oz.

Data from American Academy of Pediatrics (AAP) Committee on Sports Medicine and Fitness: Policy statement: medical concerns of the female athlete, *Pediatrics* 106(3):610–613, 2000; reaffirmed 2008; American College of Sports Medicine (ACSM): Selected issues for nutrition and the athlete: a team physician consensus statement, *Med Sci Sports Exerc* 45(12):2378–2386, 2013; Greydanus DE, Omar H, Pratt HD: The adolescent female athlete: current concepts and conundrums, *Pediatr Clin North Am* 57(3):697–718, 2010.
CHO, Carbohydrate; *RDA,* recommended daily allowance.

appropriate dietary changes and exercise training. Wrestlers, coaches, and parents may elect to sign a contract requiring that the child eat three meals a day, that fluid be available at all times, and that no artificial means be used to remove fluids from the body (e.g., sauna or sweatsuit, laxatives, diuretics, diet pills, licit or illicit drugs, nicotine, prolonged fasting, over-exercising, or vomiting).

Is There a Role for Sports Drinks?

Sports drinks and energy drinks should not be confused with each other. They are heavily promoted by beverage companies with claims that they will improve performance and replace fluid (sports drinks) and boost energy, decrease fatigue, and enhance concentration and alertness (energy drinks). Sports drinks are flavored beverages that often contain carbohydrates, minerals, electrolytes, and sometimes vitamins or other nutrients. Energy drinks usually contain stimulants, such as caffeine and guarana, with varying amounts of the other ingredients found in sports drinks. There is no sufficient evidence to show that carbohydrates or electrolytes in these beverages are needed in place of water in the typically active child who maintains a balanced diet and who is engaged in routine physical activity on the school grounds (AAP Committee on Nutrition and Council on Sports Medicine and Fitness, 2011b; Cohen, 2012; Seifert et al, 2011). In addition, for nonathletic youth, sports drinks add a considerable number of unnecessary calories and can lead to tooth decay. The ingredients in these widely available drinks often contain greater than 8% carbohydrates (glucose, sucrose, and fructose). Some formulations also contain complex carbohydrates (e.g., maltodextrin) and amino acids. Energy drinks should be discouraged. See Table 13-4 regarding the appropriate use of sports drinks during vigorous sports participation and the discussion later in this chapter about performance-enhancing drugs and "energy drinks." An estimated 62% of youth report drinking a sports drink on a daily basis (O'Malley, 2012).

The Preparticipation Sports Physical Examination for Sports

More than 7.5 million youth participate in competitive high school athletics annually in the United States (Galas, 2014), and many more participate in recreational sports in school and community programs. Most youth involved in competitive sports are required to have medical clearance. This requirement provides an important opportunity for pediatric health care providers to assess the health and health behaviors of youth by conducting the preparticipation sports physical examination.

For many youth, the preparticipation physical examination (PPE) is their only health assessment during the adolescent years. It serves as an entry into the health care system and enables the primary care provider (PCP) to schedule a follow-up visit to address other health risks and concerns noted during the visit. However, PPEs are not required for many recreational activities in which youth engage. To encounter these children, it has been recommended that *all* children (not just those in structured sports programs) be encouraged to have a PPE. In this way, health and fitness will be promoted and assessed in all children (American Academy of Family Physicians [AAFP] et al, 2010).

Benefits of the Preparticipation Sports Physical Examination

The PPE historically served as a vehicle to provide liability protection, satisfy insurance regulations, and detect cardiovascular risks for sudden death. Over the years, other objectives have been identified that include:

- Evaluating health status (primary care prevention), including fitness level
- Detecting injuries, conditions, and illnesses that might limit competition and lead to significant morbidity or mortality and require further evaluation and treatment (including anticipatory guidance about safety equipment for athletic participation)
- Recommending alternative sports activities, as appropriate, or recommending exclusion of the child or youth from certain sports
- Identifying lifestyle risk factors and promoting healthy choices
- Documenting an athlete's age, grade-level eligibility, and emotional maturity level
- Collecting medical data for emergencies
- Recommending ways to improve athletic performance
- Interacting with youth on a variety of health-related issues, including mental health

By covering all of these facets, the PCP adopts a more comprehensive approach to the PPE and broadens the focus of the examination. Children with special health care needs and disabilities require a distinct focus in order to provide clearance for appropriate sports participation and fitness (see earlier discussion on children with special health care needs; a downloadable history form for athletes with special needs is available at the AAFP website [see Additional Resources]).

The PPE includes a prescreening health questionnaire targeting previous sports injuries, respiratory and cardiac health history, and the completion of standard PPE forms. The PPE monograph (AAFP et al, 2010) contains the recommended questionnaire, PPE, and clearance forms; many of the forms are available for download at the AAFP website. The complete monograph also contains guidelines for clinicians evaluating children with special needs and the female athlete (see Box 13-1 regarding youth with Down syndrome and atlantoaxial or atlanto-occipital instability).

Less than 1% of athletes are disqualified from participation based on the findings of the PPE; between 1% and 8% require further evaluation in order to be cleared (Landry, 2011). The majority of findings that disqualify a potential athlete or require further evaluation are musculoskeletal injuries, followed by cardiovascular symptoms or a cardiac murmur and neurologic symptoms or complaints. Positive cardiac findings on the health history, family history, or on the physical examination warrant a referral for pediatric cardiac evaluation prior to sports clearance.

Frequency of Preparticipation Examinations

State requirements vary regarding the frequency of the PPE; at the very least, a focused, annual interim PPE should be done on healthy young athletes in middle and high schools and college (Landry, 2011). The National Collegiate Athletic Association (NCAA) guidelines require confirmation of sickle cell status (either by test results or a written waiver declining the test) as well as a PPE prior to participating in an intercollegiate athlete program (NCAA, 2013).

Medical Clearance and Liability Issues

The PPE, including all health history and physical examination findings, must be fully documented in the medical record. The Health Information Portability and Accountability Act (HIPAA), Family Educational Rights and Privacy Act (FERPA), and professional liability need to be taken into consideration. Detailed cardiovascular findings should be clearly and comprehensively documented in the medical record and when providing clearance for participation in high or low impact sports. It is best to use phrasing, such as "I can find no medical reason why ____ should not participate in _____," rather than "It is safe for ____ to participate in ____" (McKeag and Moeller, 2007). Consultation with specialists related to the child's or adolescent's health condition should be obtained before giving athletic clearance or recommending any specific modification or adaptation to athletic participation.

Should the athlete, athlete's family, or guardian disagree with the provider's advice against participation in a certain chosen sport, the provider needs to obtain the athlete's, parent's, or guardian's signed informed consent statement acknowledging understanding of the advice and potential dangers of participation and releasing the provider and organization from liability. The final decision rests with the athlete, parents/guardians rather than with the health care provider (Sanders et al, 2013). Counseling about more appropriate alternative sports should occur and be documented. In addition, the athlete and parents should be counseled that:

- Even though the examination appears "normal," data on the exact risks of a known sport are often limited.
- Sudden cardiac death (SCD) is rare. See the discussion later in this chapter.
- Safety and conditioning are paramount for prevention; injury is a more common cause of morbidity and mortality in sports than medical causes.
- Use of performance-enhancing drugs and sports nutritionals and energy drinks are potentially dangerous or ineffective.

The AAP has classified the most common sports activities into three types: contact and collision, limited contact, and noncontact (Table 13-5). Table 13-6 provides recommendations and guidance on safe sports for various medical conditions and can be a useful reference for complex

Text continued on p. 250

TABLE 13-5 Classification of Sports According to Contact

Contact	Limited Contact	Noncontact
Basketball*†	Adventure racing[a]	Badminton
Boxing†[b]	Baseball	Bodybuilding[c]
Cheerleading	Bicycling	Bowling
Diving	Canoeing or kayaking (whitewater)	Canoeing or kayaking (flat water)
Extreme sports[d]	Fencing	Crew or rowing
Field hockey†	Field events	Curling
Football, tackle*†	Floor hockey	Dance
Gymnastics	Football, flag or touch	Field events: Discus, javelin, shot-put
Ice hockey[e]	Handball	Golf
Lacrosse†	High jump	Orienteering[g]
Martial arts[f]	Horseback riding	Powerlifting[c]
Rodeo	Martial arts[f]	Race walking
Rugby†	Pole vault	Riflery
Skiing, downhill	Racquetball	Rope jumping
Ski-jumping	Skateboarding	Running
Snowboarding	Skating: Ice, inline, roller	Sailing
Soccer†	Skiing: Cross-country, water	Scuba diving
Team handball	Softball	Swimming
Ultimate frisbee	Squash	Table tennis
Water polo	Volleyball	Tennis
Wrestling*†	Weight lifting	Track
	Windsurfing or surfing	

From Rice SF, American Academy of Pediatrics (AAP) Council on Sports Medicine and Fitness: Medical conditions affecting sports participation, *Pediatrics* 121(4):841–848, 2008; reaffirmed 2012. Used with permission.

*Most hazardous for causing injuries (Kocher MS: Pediatric sports medicine: the young athlete. In Miller MD, Thompson SR, editors: *DeLee & Drez's orthopaedic sports medicine: principles and practice*, vol II, ed 4, Philadelphia, 2015, Elsevier/Saunders, pp 1545–1554).

†Most frequent cause of concussions (Petteys RJ, Nair NM: Head and spine diagnosis and decision making. In Miller MD, Thompson SR, editors: *DeLee & Drez's orthopaedic sports medicine: principles and practice*, vol II, ed 4, Philadelphia, 2015, Elsevier/Saunders, pp 1478–1483).

[a]Adventure racing has been added since the previous statement was published and is defined as a combination of two or more disciplines, including orienteering and navigation, cross-country running, mountain biking, paddling, and climbing and rope skills.

[b]The American Academy of Pediatrics (AAP) opposes participation in boxing for children, adolescents, and young adults.

[c]The AAP recommends limiting bodybuilding and power lifting until the adolescent achieves sexual maturity rating 5 (Tanner stage V).

[d]Extreme sports has been added since the previous statement was published.

[e]The AAP recommends limiting the amount of body checking allowed for hockey players 15 years old and younger to reduce injuries.

[f]Martial arts can be subclassified as judo, jujitsu, karate, kung fu, and tae kwon do; some forms are contact sports and others are limited-contact sports.

[g]Orienteering is a race (contest) in which competitors use a map and a compass to find their way through unfamiliar territory.

TABLE 13-6 Medical Conditions and Sports Participation*

Condition	May Participate
Atlantoaxial instability (instability of the joint between C1 and C2)	
Explanation: Athlete (particularly if Down syndrome or juvenile rheumatoid arthritis with cervical involvement) needs evaluation; assess risk of spinal cord injury during sports especially with trampoline use.	Qualified yes
Bleeding disorder	
Explanation: Athlete needs evaluation.	Qualified yes
Cardiovascular disease	
• Carditis (inflammation of the heart) *Explanation*: Carditis may result in sudden death with exertion.	No
• Hypertension (high blood pressure) *Explanation*: Those with hypertension >5 mm Hg above the 99th percentile for age, gender, and height should avoid heavy weightlifting, power lifting, bodybuilding, and high-static component sports. Those with sustained hypertension (>95th percentile for age, gender, and height) need evaluation. See Chapter 31.	Qualified yes
• Congenital heart disease *Explanation*: Consultation with cardiologist. Children with mild forms may participate fully in most cases; those with moderate or severe forms or who have undergone surgery need evaluation.	Qualified yes
• Dysrhythmia (irregular heart rhythm) • Long QT syndrome • Malignant ventricular arrhythmias • Symptomatic Wolff-Parkinson-White syndrome • Advanced heart block • Family history of sudden death or previous sudden cardiac event • Implantation of a cardioverter-defibrillator *Explanation*: Consult with cardiologist. If symptoms (chest pain, syncope, near-syncope, dizziness, shortness of breath, or other symptoms of possible dysrhythmia) or evidence of mitral regurgitation on physical examination, refer for evaluation. All others may participate fully.	Qualified yes
• Heart murmur *Explanation*: If murmur is innocent, full participation is permitted. Otherwise, refer for evaluation (see structural/acquired heart disease, especially hypertrophic cardiomyopathy and mitral valve prolapse).	Qualified yes
• Structural/acquired heart disease	Qualified no
• Hypertrophic cardiomyopathy	Qualified no
• Coronary artery anomalies	Qualified no
• Arrhythmogenic right ventricular cardiomyopathy	Qualified no
• Acute rheumatic fever with carditis	Qualified no
• Ehlers-Danlos syndrome, vascular form	Qualified yes
• Marfan syndrome	Qualified yes
• Mitral valve prolapse	Qualified yes
• Anthracycline use *Explanation*: Consult with cardiologist because most of these conditions carry a significant risk of sudden cardiac death (SCD) associated with intense physical exercise.	Qualified yes
• Vasculitis/vascular disease • Kawasaki disease (coronary artery vasculitis) • Pulmonary hypertension *Explanation*: Consult with a cardiologist. Risk on the basis of disease activity, pathologic changes, and medical regimen.	Qualified yes
Cerebral palsy	
Explanation: Evaluate to assess functional capacity to perform sports-specific activity.	Qualified yes

Continued

TABLE 13-6 Medical Conditions and Sports Participation—cont'd

Condition	May Participate
Diabetes mellitus	
Explanation: All sports can be played with proper attention and appropriate adjustments to diet (particularly carbohydrate intake), blood glucose concentrations, hydration, and insulin therapy. Monitor before exercise, every 30 minutes during continuous exercise, 15 minutes after completion of exercise, and at bedtime.	Yes
Diarrhea, infectious	
Explanation: Unless symptoms are mild and athlete is fully hydrated, no participation is permitted (risk of dehydration and heat illness) (see fever).	Qualified no
Eating disorders	
Explanation: If eating disorder present, athlete needs medical and psychiatric assessment before participation.	Qualified yes
Eyes	
• Functionally one-eyed athlete • Loss of an eye • Detached retina or family history of retinal detachment at young age • High myopia • Connective tissue disorder, such as Marfan or Stickler syndrome • Previous intraocular eye surgery or serious eye injury *Explanation*: Boxing and full-contact martial arts are not recommended for functionally one-eyed athletes, because eye protection is impractical and/or not permitted. Some athletes who previously underwent intraocular surgery or had a serious eye injury may have increased risk of injury because of weakened eye tissue. Availability of eye guards approved by the American Society for Testing and Materials (ASTM) must be judged on an individual basis.	Qualified yes
• Conjunctivitis, infectious *Explanation*: If active infection, exclude from swimming.	Qualified no
Fever	
Explanation: Elevated core temperature may indicate pathologic medical condition (infection or disease).	No
Gastrointestinal	
• Malabsorption syndromes (celiac disease or cystic fibrosis) *Explanation*: Individual assessment for malnutrition or specific deficits; if treated adequately, may permit full activity.	Qualified yes
• Short-bowel syndrome or disorders requiring specialized nutritional support *Explanation*: Individual assessment for collision, contact, or limited-contact sports. Presence of central or peripheral, indwelling, venous catheter may require special considerations for activities and emergency preparedness for unexpected trauma to the device(s).	Qualified yes
Heat illness, history of	
Explanation: With likelihood of recurrence, needs assessment for presence of predisposing conditions; develop a prevention strategy for sufficient acclimatization, conditioning, hydration, and salt intake, as well as protective equipment and uniform configurations.	Qualified yes
Hepatitis, infectious (primarily hepatitis C)	
Explanation: Ensure protection with hepatitis B vaccination before participation; cover skin lesions; use universal precautions.	Yes
Human immunodeficiency virus (HIV) infection	
Explanation: As athlete's state of health allows (especially if viral load is undetectable or very low); cover skin lesions, use universal precautions; avoid sports likely to cause skin breaks/bleeding (e.g., wrestling and boxing). If viral load is detectable, avoid high-contact sports.	Yes
Kidney, absence of one	
Explanation: Assess for contact, collision, and limited-contact sports; protective equipment may allow participation in most sports.	Qualified yes

TABLE 13-6 Medical Conditions and Sports Participation—cont'd

Condition	May Participate
Liver, enlarged	
Explanation: Acutely enlarged liver: no participation because of risk of rupture; chronically enlarged or liver function compromised: individual assessment and sport dependent.	Qualified yes
Malignant neoplasm	
Explanation: Individual assessment.	Qualified yes
Musculoskeletal disorders	
Explanation: Individual assessment.	Qualified yes
Neurologic disorders	
• History of serious head or spine trauma or abnormality *Explanation*: Individual assessment for collision, contact, or limited-contact sports.	Qualified yes
• History of simple concussion (mild traumatic brain injury), multiple simple concussions, and/or complex concussion *Explanation*: Individual assessment; no athletic participation while symptomatic and/or exhibiting deficits in judgment or cognition; graduated return to full activity.	Qualified yes
• Myopathies *Explanation*: Individual assessment.	Qualified yes
• Recurrent headaches *Explanation*: Individual assessment.	Yes
• Recurrent plexopathy (burner or stinger) and cervical cord neurapraxia with persistent defects *Explanation*: Individual assessment for collision, contact, or limited-contact sports; regaining normal strength is benchmark for return to play.	Qualified yes
• Seizure disorder, well controlled *Explanation*: Risk of seizure during participation is minimal.	Yes
• Seizure disorder, poorly controlled *Explanation*: Individual assessment for collision, contact, or limited-contact sports. Avoid archery, riflery, swimming, weightlifting, power lifting, strength training, and sports involving heights.	Qualified yes
Obesity	
Explanation: Increased risk of heat illness and cardiovascular strain; needs acclimatization, hydration, and potential activity and recovery modifications during competition and training.	Yes
Organ transplant recipient (and those taking immunosuppressive medications)	
Explanation: Individual assessment	Qualified yes
Ovary, absence of one	
Explanation: Risk is minimal.	Yes
Pregnancy/postpartum	
Explanation: Individual assessment with modifications to usual exercise routines in later stages. Avoid fall risk activities and scuba diving. After birth, physiologic changes of pregnancy take 4 to 6 weeks to return to baseline.	Qualified yes
Respiratory conditions	
• Pulmonary compromise, including cystic fibrosis *Explanation*: Individual assessment; sports may be played if oxygenation remains satisfactory during graded exercise test; need acclimatization and hydration with cystic fibrosis.	Qualified yes
• Asthma *Explanation*: If controlled and with education, only those with severe asthma need to modify their participation. If using inhalers, have written action plan and use peak flowmeter daily. Scuba diving is a high-risk activity.	Yes
• Acute upper respiratory infection *Explanation*: Individual assessment for all except mild disease (see fever).	Qualified yes

Continued

TABLE 13-6 Medical Conditions and Sports Participation—cont'd

Condition	May Participate
Rheumatologic diseases	
• Juvenile rheumatoid arthritis *Explanation*: Individual assessment depends on involvement: cervical spine C1 and C2, risk of spinal cord injury; HLA-B27-associated arthritis; cardiovascular assessment for possible complications during exercise; if micrognathia, mouth guards; if uveitis, risk of eye damage from trauma.	Qualified yes
• Juvenile dermatomyositis, idiopathic myositis • Systemic lupus erythematosus • Raynaud phenomenon *Explanation*: If cardiac involvement, cardiology assessment required; if on systemic corticosteroid therapy, at higher risk of fractures and avascular necrosis; if on immunosuppressive medications, risk of serious infection; if myositis, active risk of rhabdomyolysis during intensive exercise with renal injury; photosensitivity with need for sun protection; if Raynaud phenomenon, risk to hands and feet with exposure to cold.	Qualified yes
Sickle cell disease	
Explanation: Individual assessment; as illness status permits, all sports may be played; avoid sport or activity that entails overexertion, overheating, dehydration, chilling; or takes place at high altitude, especially when not acclimatized.	Qualified yes
Sickle cell trait	
Explanation: If sickle cell trait (SCT), generally no increased risk of sudden death or other medical problems; if high exertional activity, performed under extreme conditions of heat and humidity or increased altitude, complications can occur; need to progressively acclimatize.	Yes
Skin infections, including herpes simplex, molluscum contagiosum, verrucae (warts), staphylococcal and streptococcal infections (furuncles [boils], carbuncles, impetigo, methicillin-resistant *Staphylococcus aureus* [cellulitis and/or abscesses]), scabies, and tinea	
Explanation: During contagious periods, gymnastics or cheerleading with mats, martial arts, wrestling, or other collision, contact, or limited-contact sports not allowed.	Qualified yes
Spleen, enlarged	
Explanation: If acutely enlarged spleen, participation avoided due to risk of rupture; if chronically enlarged, individual assessment needed.	Qualified yes
Testicle, undescended or absent	
Explanation: May require a protective cup depending upon sport.	Yes

From Rice SG, American Academy of Pediatrics (AAP) Council on Sports Medicine and Fitness: Medical conditions affecting sports participation, *Pediatrics* 121(4):841–848, 2008. © American Academy of Pediatrics, 2008. Used with permission.

*This table is designed for use by medical and nonmedical personnel. "Needs evaluation" means that a physician with appropriate knowledge and experience should assess the safety of a given sport for an athlete with the listed medical condition. Unless otherwise noted, this need for special consideration is because of variability in the severity of the disease, the risk of injury for the specific sports, or both.

decision-making and making specific recommendations as to which sports are appropriate for youth with identified health problems.

Where the Preparticipation Physical Examination Should Take Place

The PPE ideally should be provided by the child's or adolescent's PCP in the health care clinic. This allows the best opportunity for anticipatory guidance related to sports participation and injuries, as well as follow up of health concerns noted during the visit. Scheduling the examination a few weeks prior to the beginning of the sports season allows time for any subsequently medical follow-up, consultation, or referral. However, mass screenings are common in many school districts as an efficiency measure or because some youth may not have access to regular health care or may have difficulty making an appointment. Although mass screenings allow youth to participate in sports who may not otherwise have the opportunity, the chance for providers to follow up on health care needs identified during the examination can be compromised. Communication with parents, coaches, and trainers following the PPE is essential so that they are aware of the athlete's health status and any issues that may arise during participation.

Components of the Preparticipation Physical Examination

Health History

The AAFP PPE history form is recommended and seeks information about the following:

- General medical history
- Prior surgeries and any sequelae
- Previous trauma, especially musculoskeletal or central nervous system injuries (notably head injuries)
- Family history of cardiac risk factors, including unexplained drowning or unwitnessed car accidents (These can indicate an undiagnosed heart problem.)
- Specific cardiovascular disease questions (Box 13-3)
- Prior heat-intolerance episodes
- Asthma or other allergic reactions
- Loss of function or absence of any paired organs (eyes, testes, kidneys)
- Seizure disorder or any other unexplained loss of consciousness
- Infectious mononucleosis (IM)
- Skin infection
- Anatomic abnormalities, Down or Marfan syndrome, or history of Marfan syndrome in the family (See Box 13-4 for specific history questions for youth with Down syndrome.)
- Obesity
- Medications, including supplement use, herbal remedies
- Immunization status
- Nutritional history—rapid weight changes, dieting, body perception
- In females—menstrual history (see Box 13-8 regarding screening questions for the female athlete triad)

When performing the history portion of the PPE, health care providers should also obtain the following history in order to better understand the scope of sports participation prior to clearance:

- The particular sports activity planned, the extent of participation, level of competition, and training schedule
- Coaching and supervision: Is there a team health care provider? What is the level of certification of the trainers, coaches, and team health care provider?
- Hazardous playing and field conditions
- Plans for the sports activity in the future
- Injury prevention strategies, including level of preparticipation conditioning

• BOX 13-3 The 14-Element Cardiovascular Screening Checklist for Congenital and Genetic Heart Disease

Personal History

1. Chest pain/discomfort/tightness/pressure related to exertion
2. Unexplained syncope/near-syncope*
3. Excessive exertional and unexplained dyspnea/fatigue or palpitations, associated with exercise
4. Prior recognition of a heart murmur
5. Elevated systemic blood pressure
6. Prior restriction from participation in sports
7. Prior testing for the heart, ordered by a physician

Family History

8. Premature death (sudden and unexpected, or otherwise) before age 50 attributable to heart disease in one or more relatives
9. Disability from heart disease in a close relative <50 years of age
10. Hypertrophic or dilated cardiomyopathy, long QT syndrome, or other ion channelopathies, Marfan syndrome, or clinically significant arrhythmias; specific knowledge of certain cardiac conditions in family members

Physical Examination

11. Heart murmur†
12. Femoral pulses to exclude aortic coarctation
13. Physical stigmata of Marfan syndrome
14. Brachial artery blood pressure (sitting position)‡

Modified with permission from Maron BJ, Thompson PD, Ackerman MJ, et al: Recommendations and considerations related to preparticipation screening for cardiovascular abnormalities in competitive athletes: 2007 update: a scientific statement from the American Heart Association Council on Nutrition, Physical Activity, and Metabolism. Endorsed by the American College of Cardiology Foundation, *Circulation* 115(12):1643–1655, 2007. Used with permission of the American Heart Association.

*Judged not to be of neurocardiogenic (vasovagal) origin; of particular concern when occurring during or after physical exertion.

†Refers to heart murmurs judged likely to be organic and unlikely to be innocent; auscultation should be performed with the patient in both the supine and standing positions (or with Valsalva maneuver), specifically to identify murmurs of dynamic left ventricular outflow tract obstruction.

‡Preferably taken in both arms.

• BOX 13-4 History and Physical Components of Preparticipation Physical Examination for Youth with Down Syndrome

History

- Congenital heart disease
- Visual and/or hearing impairment
- Intellectual disability
- Diabetes mellitus
- Hypothyroidism
- Epilepsy
- Arthropathy of Down syndrome

Physical

- Atlantoaxial or atlanto-occipital instability or subluxation*
- Anomalies and disorders of the odontoid
- Occipitoatlantal instability
- Cervical spondylolysis
- Developmental dysplasia of the hip
- Hip dislocation
- Patellar instability
- Neuromuscular scoliosis
- Slipped capital femoral epiphysis
- Obesity

Data from Patel DR, Greydanus ED: Sport participation by physically and cognitively challenged young athletes, *Pediatr Clin North Am* 57(3):797–817, 2010.

*Lateral radiographic views of the cervical spine in flexion, extension, and neutral position; an atlantoaxial separation >4.5 mm or a neural canal width <14 mm may result in exclusion from competitive sports. (Prior to exclusion a magnetic resonance imaging [MRI] and consultation/referral to an orthopedist may be indicated to minimize the risk of spinal cord injury.)

- Nutritional changes needed for participation
- Risk behaviors present in child's life, not just related to sports, such as increased alcohol consumption, driving while intoxicated, lack of seatbelt use, lack of helmet use during extreme recreational sports activities (e.g., inline skating, skateboarding, snowboarding), use of drugs or performance-enhancing substances (including energy drinks, steroids [dehydroepiandrosterone (DHEA), androstenedione], creatine, gamma-hydroxybutyrate [GHB], gamma-butyrolactone [GBL], 1,4-butanediol [BD]), smoking, and sexual history
- Family involvement
- Psychological issues, such as recent life changes, stress management during the competitive season, and how success will be measured
- Strategies to maintain schoolwork

Physical Examination

The PPE should be a comprehensive head-to-toe physical examination with particular focus on cardiovascular, musculoskeletal, and neurologic systems (see also Chapters 7 and 8). The 90-second musculoskeletal screening examination is recommended for all youth participating in sports (Fig. 13-2). It is standardized to detect 90% of significant injuries and has 51% sensitivity and 97% specificity (AAFP et al, 2010). The examination focuses on musculoskeletal alignment, flexibility, and proprioception, which are effective measures of abnormalities and injury sequelae. Table 13-7 describes the components that should be included for different organ systems, including elements of the cardiovascular examination (also review red flags of the cardiovascular examination listed in Box 13-3). The provider needs to include a genital examination. This examination provides information with regard to sexual maturity (Tanner stage or sexual maturity rating [SMR]; see Chapter 8) and provides an opportunity for counseling about general development. The SMR level is important in sports in which weight and strength are of consideration, as well as required weight training for high contact sports. SMR reflects muscle and spine maturity. As the adolescent achieves greater sexual maturity, the risk of participation of high contact sports decreases although athletic injury remains a concern. Adolescents also may have greater muscle mass in comparison with a less mature, but equal weight teen at a lower SMR. The PPE also provides an opportunity to discuss with youth the important issues of reproductive health, risks of sexually transmitted infections, how to do a self-testicular examination and the risk of testicular cancer for males.

Diagnostic Studies

The use of echocardiographic screening has been proposed by cardiologists and others concerned about SCD, the risk for youths who have a predisposition to this condition, and liability in sports participation. Despite the merits of augmenting the health history and physical examination with a screening electrocardiogram (ECG) and echocardiogram, their use as universal screening tools for youth participating in competitive sports remains controversial (Galas, 2014). ECG, echocardiogram, or exercise stress tests are not recommended as a requirement for all PPEs (AAFP et al, 2010). However, many European countries outside the United States routinely screen with an ECG (Chandra et al, 2013).

Other diagnostic tests that may be indicated or mandated as part of the PPE health screening include:

- Urinalysis: Not routinely recommended. Certain amateur or professional organizations may require one as part of a drug screening policy.
- Hematocrit or hemoglobin: Not recommended for adolescent males but may be indicated for adolescent females with heavy menstrual cycles or history of iron deficiency anemia.
- Human immunodeficiency virus (HIV) testing: Encouraged if the athlete has any risk factors. Certain amateur or professional organizations may require screening.
- Sickle cell: Test for sickle cell trait (SCT) in high-risk groups (see later discussion).

Evaluation and Management of Sports Participation for Athletes with Specific Health Conditions

Table 13-6 summarizes the AAP's recommendations regarding sports participation for youth with specific health conditions. The provider's recommendations should be communicated to the youth and their parents and recorded in the student's medical record; the form should be returned to the school or sports facility. Several high-risk conditions (chronic and acute) and worrisome symptoms are discussed in the following sections in terms of their influence on decision-making and for the purposes of counseling and health management.

Chronic Medical Conditions

Asthma

Comprehensive management of intermittent and persistent asthma and exercise-induced bronchospasm (EIB) is discussed in Chapter 25. The goal is to achieve adequate asthma control so that the youth can fully participate in recreational or organized competitive sports. Exercise can act as an additional trigger for bronchospasm in those with underlying reactive airway disease, or exercise may serve as the only trigger for bronchospasm. Teachers and coaches should be aware of the youth's asthma or EIB. A written school sport management plan should be in place.

Cardiac Conditions

The goal for the health care provider is to recognize athletes who are at risk of significant morbidity or mortality from preexisting cardiac conditions. The need for increased cardiac output and oxygen demands varies by sport. The clinician needs to consider the effect of the athlete's stress level and emotional temperament during competition, as

Text continued on p. 257

- Appropriate for interscholastic, intramural, and extramural sports activities.
- A screening evaluation created to direct attention to problems but not evaluate the problems.
- Identifies the following conditions that might be adversely affected by athletic participation:

  a. Congenital problems

  b. Acquired problems

Questions such as the following are to be answered by the athlete and signed by BOTH the athlete and parent:

- Have you ever had an illness, condition, or injury that required you to go to the hospital, either as a patient overnight or in the emergency room or for x-rays; required an operation; caused you to see a doctor; caused you to miss a game or practice?
- Are you now or have you been under the care of a physician for any reason?
- Do you currently have any medical problems or injuries?
- Have you ever had a broken bone, joint sprain or ligament tear, muscle pull, head injury, neck injury or nerve pinch, dislocated joint, back trouble or problems?

ACTIVITY 1

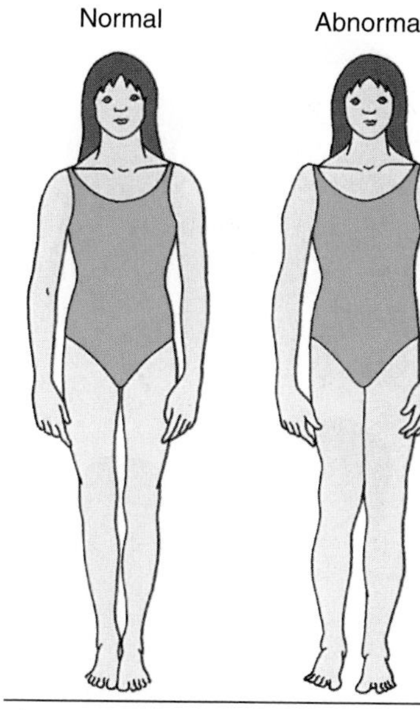

Instructions to patient:
"Stand up straight and face me."

What is screened:
Acromioclavicular joints, symmetry of extremities

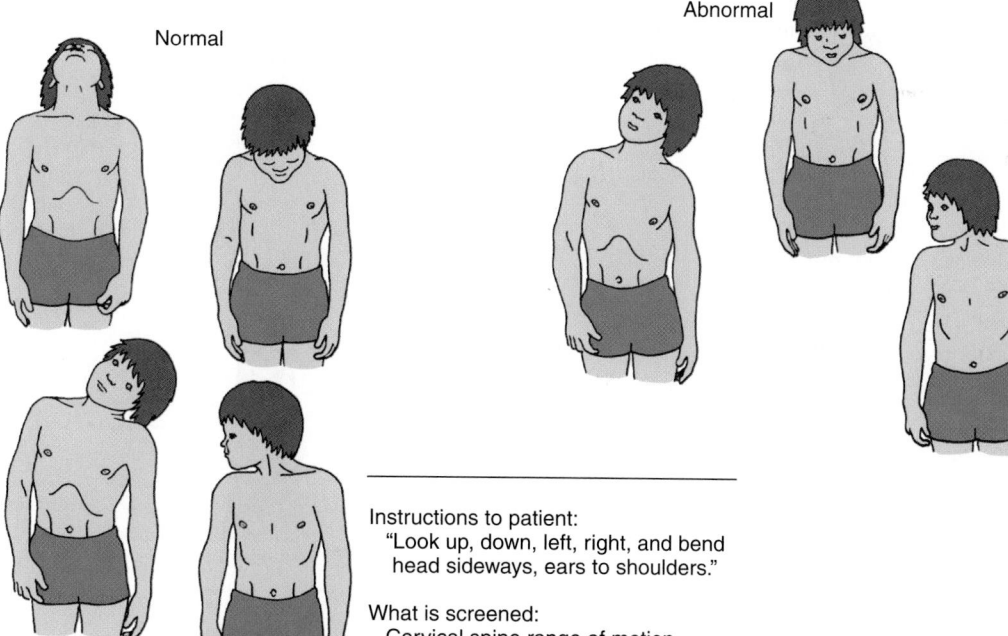

ACTIVITY 2

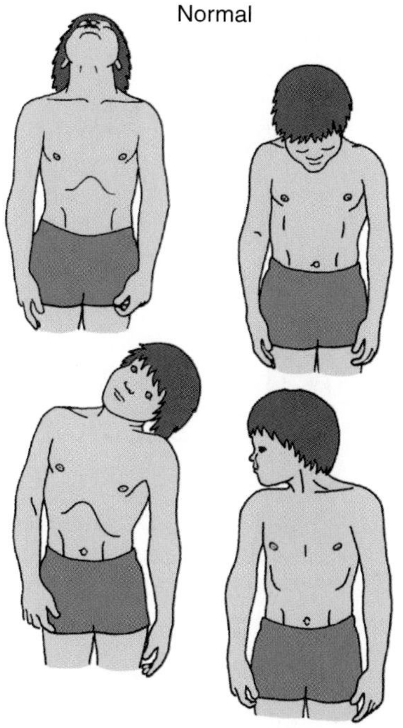

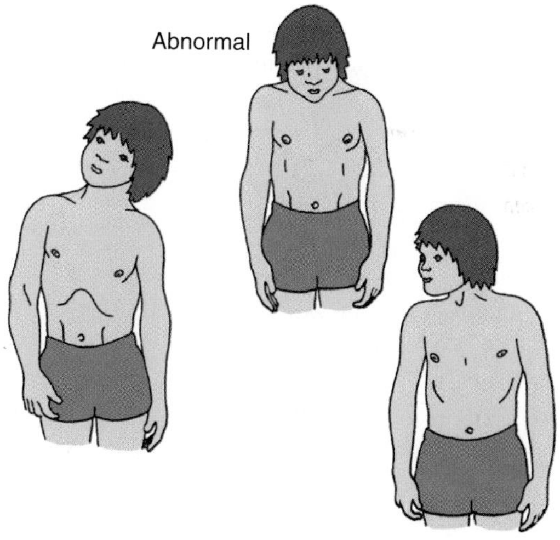

Instructions to patient:
"Look up, down, left, right, and bend head sideways, ears to shoulders."

What is screened:
Cervical spine range of motion

• **Figure 13-2** Illustration of the 90-second sports musculoskeletal examination. (Adapted from Ross Products Division, Abbott Laboratories, Columbus, OH, 43216. From For the practitioner: orthopaedic screening examination for participation sports. © 1981 Ross Products Division, Abbott Laboratories. Text adapted from Garrich JG: Sports medicine, *Pediatr Clin North Am* 24:737–747, 1977.)

Continued

ACTIVITY 3

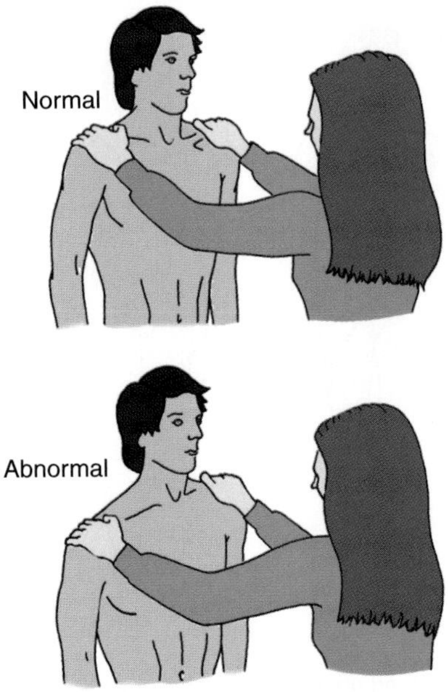

Instructions to patient:
"Shrug your shoulders." (Against resistance by examiner)

What is screened:
Trapezius strength

ACTIVITY 4

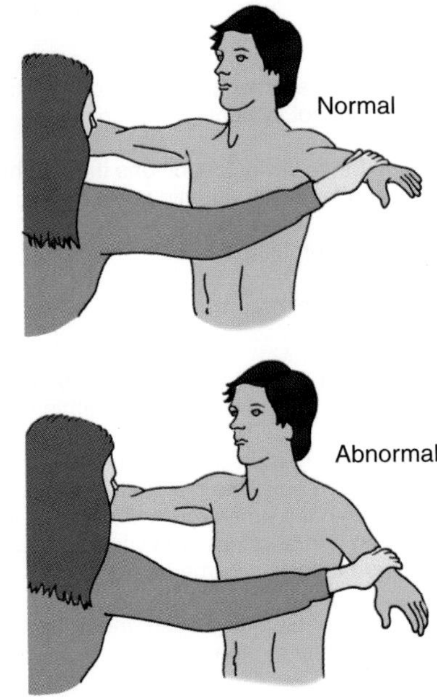

Instructions to patient:
"Hold arms outstretched from your sides and lift them." (Against resistance as examiner pushes down)

What is screened:
Shoulder range of motion

ACTIVITY 5

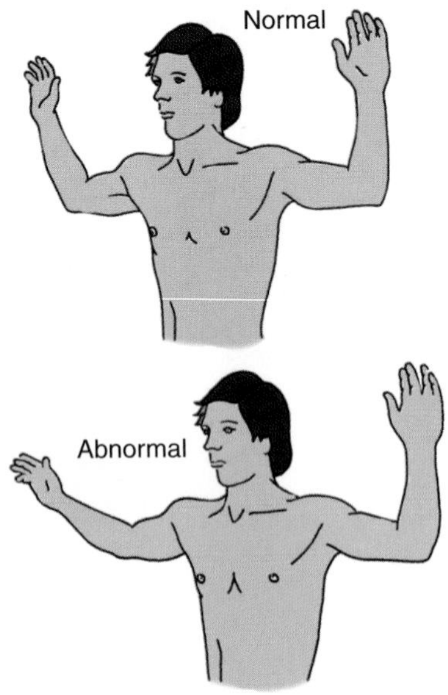

Instructions to patient:
"Raise your elbows at your sides 90 degrees. Rotate your hands backwards."

What is screened:
Deltoid strength
Shoulder rotation

ACTIVITY 6

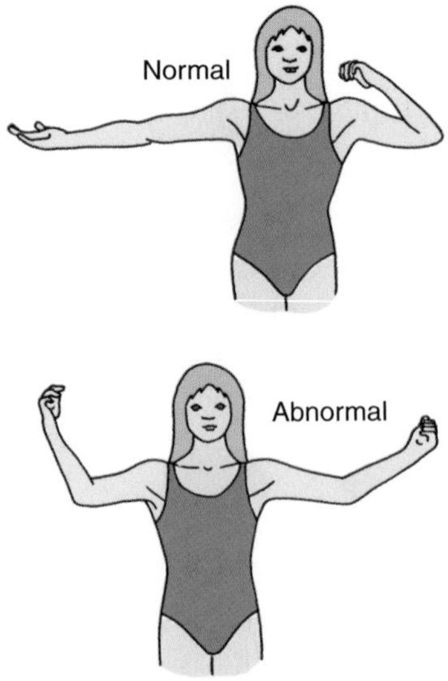

Instructions to patient:
"Hold arms straight out from sides, palms up. Flex and extend your elbows."

What is screened:
Elbow range of motion

• Figure 13-2, cont'd

ACTIVITY 7

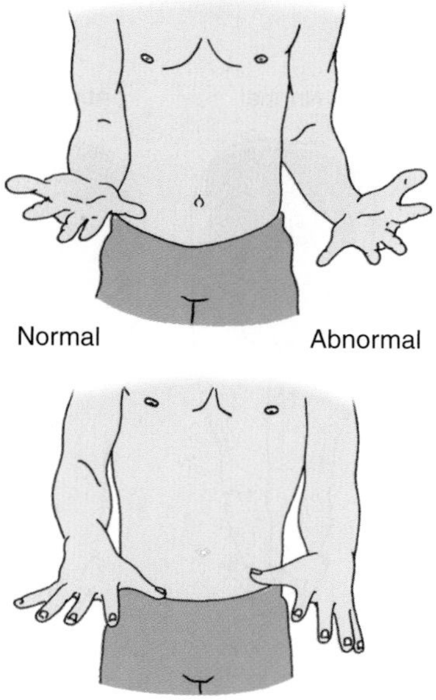

Instructions to patient:
"Let your arms down again. Flex your elbows so that your hands reach straight out. Rotate your wrists, palms facing up, then down."

What is screened:
Wrist range of motion (pronation/supination)

ACTIVITY 8

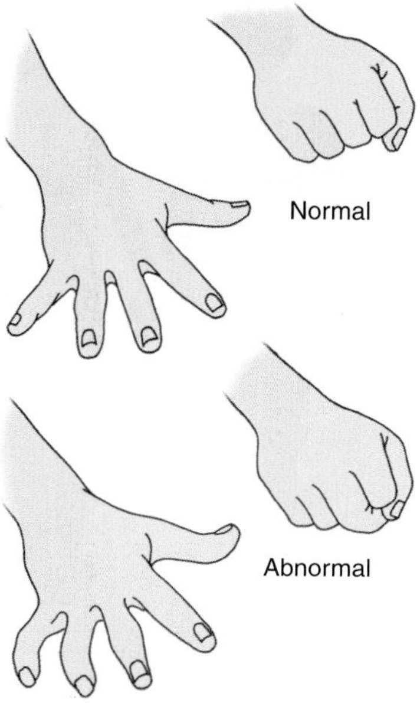

Instructions to patient:
"Show me your hands. Spread your fingers out (examiner resists spreading). Make a fist and squeeze."

What is screened:
Hand/finger range of motion and strength

ACTIVITY 9

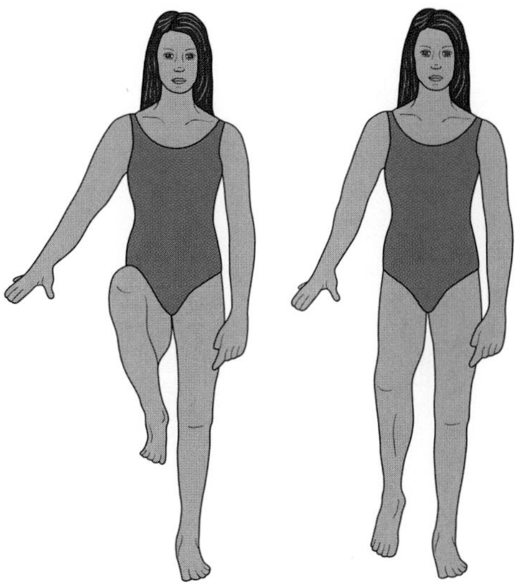

Instructions to patient:
"Lift your right leg up, bent at the knee. Repeat using the other leg."

What is screened:
Leg symmetry, knee or ankle effusion

ACTIVITY 10

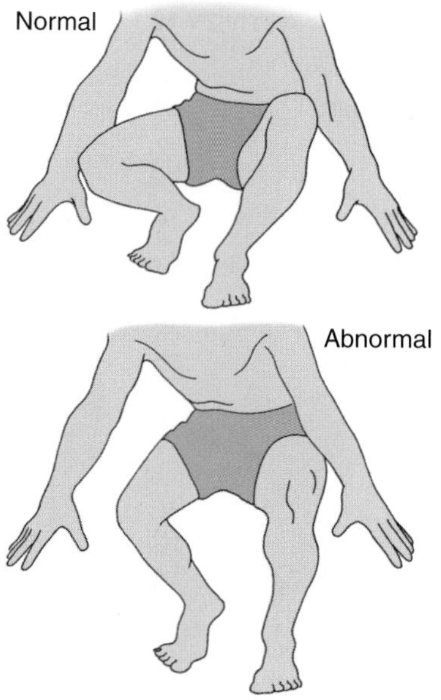

Instructions to patient:
"Squat like a duck, and walk four steps away from me."

What is screened:
Hip, knee, and ankle range of motion

• **Figure 13-2, cont'd**

Continued

ACTIVITY 11

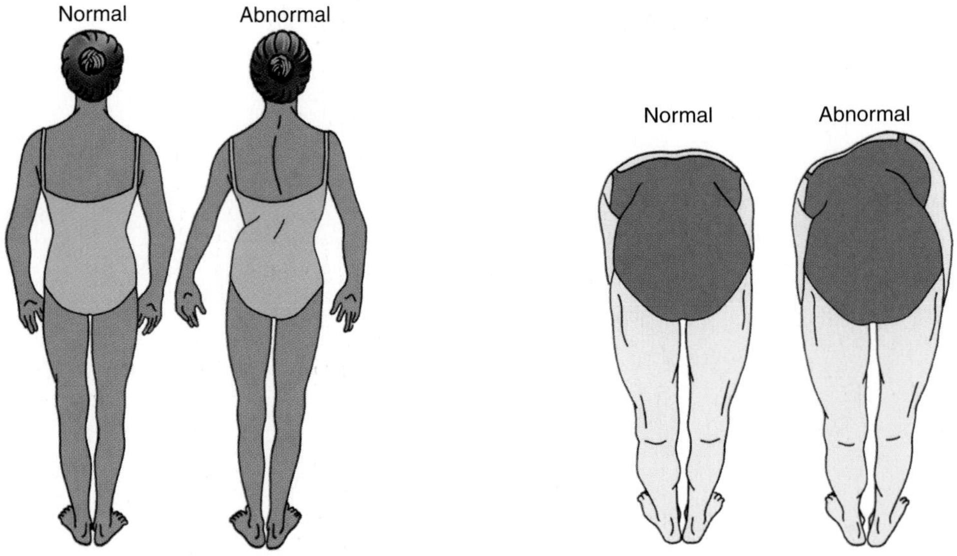

Instructions to patient:
"Stand up straight. Keep your knees as straight as you can, and try to touch your toes. Straighten slowly."

What is screened:
Shoulder symmetry, scoliosis, hip range of motion, hamstring tightness

ACTIVITY 12

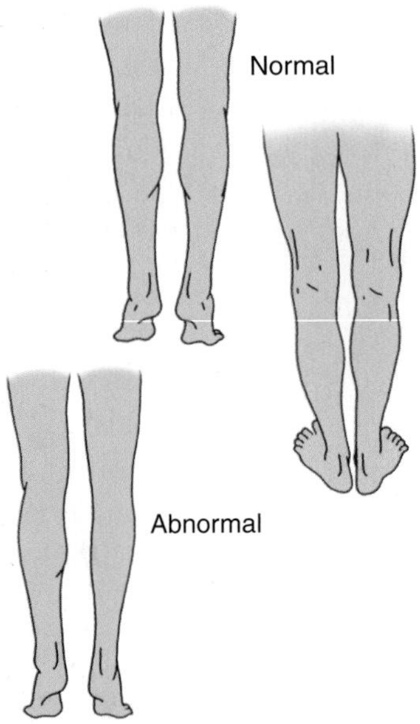

Instructions to patient:
"Stand up on your tiptoes."

What is screened:
Calf symmetry, leg strength

• **Figure 13-2, cont'd**

TABLE 13-7 Example of an Appropriate Preparticipation Physical Examination

Examination Feature	Comments
Height and weight; BMI	Establish baseline and monitor for eating disorders, steroid abuse.
Blood pressure, pulse	Assess in the context of participant's age, height, and sex.
General appearance	Excessive height and excessive long-bone growth (arachnodactyly, arm span greater than height, pectus excavatum) suggestive of Marfan syndrome.
Eyes	Important to detect vision defects; one of the eyes should have greater than 20/40 corrected vision. Lens subluxations, severe myopia, retinal detachments, and strabismus are associated with Marfan syndrome. Document anisometropia; absence of one eye can limit sport choices.
Cardiovascular (see Box 13-3)	Increased intensity and displacement at PMI suggests hypertrophy and CHF, respectively; murmur that intensifies with standing or Valsalva maneuver suggests hypertrophic cardiomyopathy; simultaneous delay between femoral and radial pulses or femoral pulse diminishment suggests aortic coarctation.
Respiratory	Observe for accessory muscle use or prolonged expiration, and auscultate for wheezing. EIB requires exercise testing for diagnosis.
Abdominal	Assess for masses, tenderness, or organomegaly (especially liver, spleen, and kidneys). In females, assess for any pain, enlargement over hypogastric area or pelvis that might suggest pregnancy or gynecologic problem; proceed with further workup as indicated.
Genitourinary	Hernias and varicoceles do not usually preclude sports participation. Check for single, undescended testicle, and/or masses.
Musculoskeletal	Use the 90-second orthopedic examination (see Fig. 13-2). Consider supplemental shoulder, knee, and ankle examinations as indicated specific to the chosen sport's injury prone areas.
Skin	Evidence of molluscum contagiosum, herpes simplex, impetigo, or lesions suggestive of MRSA, tinea corporis, or scabies would temporarily prohibit participation in sports where direct skin-to-skin competitor contact occurs (e.g., wrestling, martial arts).
Neurologic	Gross motor assessment with attention to equality of strength, especially with a history of recurrent stingers/burners, head injury. Usually sufficiently assessed during the 90-second musculoskeletal examination.

Data from American Academy of Family Physicians (AAFP), American Academy of Pediatrics (AAP), American College of Sports Medicine (ACSM), et al: Pre-participation physical evaluation form, 2010, www.aafp.org/dam/AAFP/documents/patient_care/fitness/ppephysicalexamform2010.pdf. Accessed September 10, 2014; Hess CJ, Mistry DJ, Herman D: Team medical coverage. In Miller MD, Thompson SR, editors: *DeLee & Drez's orthopaedic sports medicine: principles and practice*, vol I, ed 4, Philadelphia, 2015, Elsevier/Saunders, pp 173–184.

BMI, Body mass index; *CHF,* congestive heart failure; *EIB,* exercise-induced bronchospasm; *MRSA,* Methicillin-resistant *Staphylococcus aureus; PMI,* point of maximal impulse.

well as oxygen demands placed upon the cardiovascular system during high elevation competition, with underwater sports, or from extremes in temperatures during athletic training or participation. A valuable aid for making a clinical decision on the eligibility or disqualification of an athlete based on the demands placed upon the cardiovascular system and available oxygen by a particular sport can be found online at http://content.onlinejacc.org/article.aspx?articleid=1136519 (Figure 2; Mitchell et al, 2005).

Cardiac Murmurs

Because cardiac murmurs are a common finding in children, it is important to distinguish between benign and pathologic murmurs. For the PPE, evaluate heart sounds and listen for murmurs in each of four areas of the heart (see Chapter 31). Auscultate the chest with the youth supine and standing; have them perform a Valsalva maneuver and then squat and stand during auscultation. Squatting increases venous return to the heart, thus increasing left ventricular size and stroke volume; increased stroke volume usually causes murmurs to be louder. Standing or doing a Valsalva maneuver, on the other hand, decreases venous return and stroke volume, and usually causes the murmur to be quieter. If the reverse is heard, that is, softer with squatting and louder with standing or doing a Valsalva, then hypertrophic cardiomyopathy or mitral valve prolapse must be ruled out (Patel and Luckstead, 2013). Features of murmurs that require further evaluation include diastolic murmurs or systolic murmurs (grade 3 or greater); radiation of the murmur; or wide or fixed splitting of S_2.

Diabetes Mellitus

The goal for children and adolescents with both type 1 and type 2 diabetes mellitus (DM) is to support athletic participation consistent with the individual's goals and desires. Type 1 and type 2 DM are discussed in Chapter 26,

BOX 13-5 Recommendations for the Care of the Athlete with Type 1 Diabetes Mellitus

1. Schedule physical examination with health care provider.
   - May need to adjust blood testing schedule, insulin dosing, and general recommendations for safe participation in sport.
2. Meticulously test and record blood sugars as recommended and as needed (often before, during, and after training or competition). Note conditions present during different training or competition sessions.
3. Follow insulin dosing schedule, but be prepared for adjustments depending on level of physical activity.
   - Avoid injecting insulin into the limb that is most active in the exercise performed (i.e., inject at a distant site) to avoid overly rapid insulin absorption.
4. Plan snacks appropriately.
   - May need to increase snacks before, during, or after activity.
5. Pack supplies accordingly.
   - Pack extra testing supplies, pump supplies (if using pump), snacks, and water.
   - Wear medic alert bracelet.
   - Have emergency contact information readily available.
   - Have copy of diabetes management plan available.
6. Take control.
   - Tell coaches about diabetes diagnosis.
   - Educate coaches and teammate of signs and symptoms of hypo- and hyperglycemia.
     Hypoglycemia: Sweating, light-headedness, shaking, weakness, anxiety, hunger, headaches, problems concentrating, and/or confusion. If severe, watch for fainting or seizures.
     Hyperglycemia: Increased urination, dehydration, increased thirst, fatigue, weakness, and/or blurry vision.
   - Empower the youth to put diabetes first; it is okay for them to interrupt coaches, take breaks, or ask for help if needed.
   - Do not exercise alone (use the "buddy system").

Data from Kirk SE: The diabetic athlete. In Miller MD, Thompson SR, editors: *DeLee & Drez's orthopaedic sports medicine: principles and practice*, vol I, ed 4, Philadelphia, 2015, Elsevier/Saunders, pp 242–250; Nemours Foundation: Sports, exercise, and diabetes, Kidshealth (website), 2012, http://kidshealth.org/parent/diabetes_center/living_diabetes/sports_diabetes.html#. Accessed August 29, 2014.

including the management and monitoring issues for the two types in terms of an individual's level of participation in sports. Youth with DM should follow the same physical activity guidelines as all children—striving for 60 minutes of physical activity daily. It is essential that coaches, trainers, or other athletic staff be aware of the young athlete's diabetes care plan and be trained in aspects of care as outlined in the recommendations found in Box 13-5. This is particularly important in children with type 1 DM, because athletic activity can increase short-term complications of hypoglycemia or significant hyperglycemia.

Hypertension

Hypertension is the most common cardiovascular condition seen in competitive athletes (McCambridge et al, 2010). Table 13-8 summarizes the recommendations for sports participation of individuals with hypertension. Additionally, the athlete must:

- Be counseled to avoid anabolic steroids, growth hormone, illicit drugs (especially cocaine), nonprescribed stimulants, over-the-counter medications (e.g., pseudoephedrine and ephedra [ma huang]), alcohol, tobacco, caffeine, energy and sports drinks (see Recognition and Prevention of Performance-Enhancing Drug Use), and high-sodium foods.
- Be aware that with strenuous exercise and excessive sweating a total-body sodium deficit can occur. Therefore, care must be taken to rehydrate with salt-containing fluids and foods to ensure greater body water retention and distribution to all fluid compartments. A sports nutritionist or trainer can assist with proper rehydration.
- Be aware that for some athletic governing bodies, use of diuretics and beta-blockers is prohibited. These drugs have been shown to possibly decrease athletic performance in some individuals. Medication adaptations and registration of medications with the sport governing body may be required.

Seizures

Generally, all children and adolescents with seizure disorders should be encouraged to participate in the majority of sports. Exclusion would be based on the rationale that having a seizure would put the individual or others at significant risk. There are many benefits for the individual with a seizure disorder that occur due to regular participation in physical activity or sports. These include psychosocial and physiologic benefits as well as a possible reduction in seizure activity (Knowles and Pleacher, 2012). To date, studies do not demonstrate that exercise triggers seizures or that altered antiepileptic medication metabolism occurs during sports (Otallah et al, 2015).

If the seizures are well controlled, few restrictions are placed on the sports. If the seizures are poorly controlled, there needs to be an individualized decision, but generally the person should be excluded from contact, limited-contact, or collision activities or hazardous sports until control has been achieved. Although contact sports have not been shown to provoke seizures, head injury is always a risk. Guidelines provide that individuals whose seizures are well controlled may be involved in supervised contact sports, such as football, hockey, and wrestling (Gordon et al, 2010; Knowles and Pleacher, 2012). Skydiving and scuba diving are prohibited. Youths participating in some other activities (such as, cycling and those involving heights) should use common sense and follow recommendations given to them after considerable discussion about safety risks. Water sports and swimming should be allowed under direct supervision of trained individuals; the individual should avoid swimming in open or murky water and should use personal flotation devices (Knowles and Pleacher, 2012).

A decision about participation in a specific sport should be made with information about the type and frequency of

TABLE 13-8 Recommendations for Sports Participation by Athletes with Hypertension

Hypertensive Status	Sports Activity Limitations	Management
Normotensive	No limitations to competitive sports	Counsel to adopt healthy lifestyle behaviors: regular physical activity, healthy diet, and avoid drugs, tobacco, and alcohol.
Prehypertensive	No limitations	Blood pressure checks every 6 months; counsel as above.
Stage 1 hypertension—no end-organ damage, including left ventricular hypertrophy (LVH) or concomitant heart disease	No limitations or restrictions	Recheck blood pressure in 1 to 2 weeks, or sooner, if symptomatic. Refer to a specialist if patient is symptomatic, has any signs of cardiovascular disease, or has persistently elevated blood pressure on two additional occasions. Counsel on healthy lifestyle as above.
Stage 2 hypertension—no end-organ damage, including LVH or concomitant heart disease	Restrict from sports with high static and dynamic components until blood pressure is in the normal range.	These athletes must be evaluated by a specialist immediately if symptomatic, or within 1 week, even if asymptomatic.
Hypertensive with concomitant cardiovascular disease	Eligibility is usually based on the type and severity of the underlying cardiovascular disease.	Management dependent upon recommendations of cardiac specialist.

Data from McCambridge TM, Benjamin HJ, Brenner JS, et al: Policy statement: athletic participation by children and adolescents who have systemic hypertension, *Pediatrics* 125(6):1287–1294, 2010.

seizure, antiepileptic medication compliance, and presence of any comorbid conditions. Discussions ought to include the youth, parents, coaches or trainers, and a neurologist. In addition, consideration must be given to possible side effects (e.g., cognitive or behavioral changes, diplopia, dizziness, general fatigue, sedation, ataxia, tremors, hypohidrosis, dyskinesis, weight changes, decreased bone density) from anticonvulsant medication that could impair performance or put the individual at risk (Otallah et al, 2015).

Sickle Cell Trait

Sickle cell trait (SCT) is discussed in Chapter 41. Though typically asymptomatic under most circumstances, it can have implications for competitive athletes. Under conditions of intense exertion during sports (coupled with heat stress and dehydration), severe hypoxemia, acidosis, hyperthermia, and red cell dehydration are induced that can lead to sickling of the red blood cells. Small vessels supplying vital organs become blocked, resulting in ischemia and muscle breakdown (rhabdomyolysis); the athlete collapses, and death can occur unless treatment is begun immediately. Illness and altitude can further induce sickling (Harris et al, 2012). Persons with SCT appear to be at greatest risk when they are in a deconditioned state and perform short bursts of repetitive, high-intensity activity (e.g., sprints) (Grove and Gómez, 2015).

Athletes with SCT can participate in all sports, but it is important to know who they are in order to ensure safety in training and in all aspects of participation. The NCAA Legislative Council stipulates that all athletes participating in NCAA Division I and II sports must have sickle cell testing performed; show proof of sickle cell testing; or sign a waiver demonstrating that they understand the importance of testing for sickle cell, decline testing, and thereby release their institution from any liability related to declining testing. Those who do not agree with screening for sickle cell cite that the testing is potentially discriminatory; hematologists have rejected mandatory SCT screening and have chosen to recommend universal training interventions (Harris et al, 2012). Educating families about the risks of SCT and providing the option of SCT screening so that youths are aware of their SCT status are considered optimal practices.

Athletic trainers need to be cognizant of the following preventive measures to reduce the risk of sickling crisis (Casa et al, 2012a):

- Ensure preseason strength and conditioning training.
- Build up slowly in training, allowing for periods of rest and recovery between repetitions. Allow the athlete with SCT to self-pace in training.
- Follow preseason heat acclimatization guidelines for training and for any changes in climate or altitude during competitions.
  - Adjust athletes' work and rest cycles on an individual basis accounting for climate and altitude.
- Athletes with SCT should avoid performance tests in activities such as mile runs and serial sprints.
  - Activities such as repetitive high-speed sprints or interval training that produce lactic acid buildup should be accompanied by extended recovery periods.
- Ensure adequate hydration.

- Athletes with SCT should not train or compete when ill.
- Stop the workout *immediately* at onset of symptoms of muscle cramping, pain, swelling, weakness, tenderness, fatigue, or inability to catch one's breath.
- Educate the athlete, trainers, and coaches about how to handle a sickle cell emergency.
- Have an emergency medical plan written and on site.
- A sickling collapse is a medical emergency; emergency care/transport (911) must be called promptly. Field-side first aid includes monitoring vital signs, emergency respiratory and cardiac support as needed, cooling the athlete if overheating has occurred, and administering oxygen.

Acute Infectious Conditions

Infectious Mononucleosis

The peak age groups affected by infectious mononucleosis (IM) are adolescents and young adults. IM is covered in more depth in Chapter 24. With regard to athletes, splenomegaly (which occurs in about 50% of cases of IM) is the most concerning clinical issue (Krafczyk and Vikram, 2012). There is less than 0.5% risk of splenic rupture in those playing sports with this condition (Becker and Smith, 2014). Splenic rupture can occur spontaneously (rare), but the risk of rupture increases when participating in a contact or collision sport or a sport in which there is an increase in intraabdominal pressure (e.g., rowing and weightlifting that require Valsalva maneuvers). Diagnosing splenomegaly can be a challenge. Athletes often have well-defined and firm abdominal musculature. This makes palpation of the spleen difficult and unreliable as a diagnostic tool. However, imaging is not recommended as a routine diagnostic measure or in return-to-play (RTP) decisions because there is great variance in normal spleen size; the only way to accurately diagnose splenomegaly on ultrasound is to get baseline and serial images over time (Becker and Smith, 2014). If uncertain as to when the onset of IM was, Epstein-Barr virus (EBV) titers can be obtained. If Epstein-Barr virus nuclear antigen (EBNA) is found, then the individual has had IM for at least 6 to 8 weeks. If the titers are equivocal, then the provider can time the onset of IM to the presentation of symptoms. Recommendations for RTP for the athlete with IM are as follows:

- Advise the athlete to avoid any form of exertion, including all sports during the first 3 weeks (minimum) after onset of symptoms when the spleen is more likely to enlarge.
- At 3 weeks after symptom onset, assuming the athlete is afebrile and symptom-free, he or she may return to light, noncontact activities. No sport should be played if there is risk of chest or abdominal contact or if it involves increased intraabdominal pressure or Valsalva maneuvers.
- Fully returning to play should be made on a case-by-case basis and is generally considered safe at 4 weeks after symptom onset, assuming the patient's physical stamina has returned and all symptoms have resolved. If the sports involved increases intraabdominal pressure, a longer recovery time is suggested (Krafczyk and Vikram, 2012).

Skin Infections

Communicable dermatologic conditions are a common concern in sports. Many sports involve close body-to-body (skin-to-skin) contact, involve sharing training equipment, or have the potential of compromising skin integrity from abrasions and injuries. Prevention of infection is key. Box 13-6 lists the most effective measures to prevent transmission of common skin infections among athletes. Table 13-9 outlines RTP recommendations for athletes with several of the more common communicable skin infections.

Human Immunodeficiency Virus and Other Blood-Borne Viral Pathogens

The health care provider must consider the effect of playing a sport on the well-being of not only the individual athlete with an infectious blood-borne pathogen but also of other athletes with whom that person may come in contact. The emphasis for the student athlete and the athletic program team (including the health care consultant) should be placed predominately on educating youth about the traditional routes of transmission of infections from lifestyle behaviors off the athletic field, where they are more likely to be encountered. HIV, hepatitis B virus (HBV), and hepatitis C virus (HCV) are discussed here.

There is no epidemiologic evidence of transmission of HIV infection through sports contact; the highest risk for an athlete becoming positive for HIV occurs off the field (Abalos and Petri, 2015). There is no evidence that moderate intensity physical activity or the stresses of athletics are detrimental to the athlete with HIV. If the athlete is asymptomatic and without evidence of deficiencies in immunologic function, then the presence of HIV infection alone does not preclude participation.

HBV is more stable due to its ability to survive outside the body for longer periods of time and its resistance to alcohol, drying, temperature fluctuations, and many detergents. It has a higher risk of transmission than HIV. Nonetheless, the chance of transmission is considered extremely low, and no exclusion for asymptomatic carriers is recommended. Sustained, close physical contact sports (e.g., wrestling) carry some risk, although minimal, of transmitting HBV. There have been two documented cases of HBV spread in sports (i.e., in a Japanese sumo wrestling club and in an American football team) (Harris, 2011). Some sports organizations (e.g., NCAA, International Olympic Committee) differ on their policies concerning athletes' HBV status or titers. It may be prudent to exclude athletes with an acute HBV infection until there is an absence of HBV e antigen (HBeAg). Those with chronic HBV infections who are HBeAg positive should be excluded indefinitely (Harris, 2011; Jaworski et al, 2011).

• BOX 13-6 Prevention of Transmission of Communicable Skin Infections among Athletes: Prevention at an Individual Level

- Perform frequent hand washing using good technique (with soap or non-water alcohol hand sanitizer with an ethanol content of at least 60%) by all athletes and trainers.
- Shower immediately after practice and game (preferably with antimicrobial soap, especially if doing a body contact sport, such as wrestling, rugby, football); do not share soap or towels.
- Wash clothing, uniforms after each use (completely dry in a dryer).
- Regularly clean all personal equipment (e.g., helmets, body pads, knee/ankle sleeves, and braces).
- Wear protective clothing or gear designed to prevent skin abrasions or cuts.
- Keep cuts and abrasions covered with clean dry bandages or other dressings until healed.
- Do not share personal care items (e.g., bar soap, ointments from open containers, razors, towels, and/or cosmetics).
- Place a barrier (such as, clothing or a towel) between skin and shared equipment during weight-training, sauna, and steam-room benches.

Institutional or Sports Organizational Preventive Measures

- Institutions and sports clubs must follow guidelines for cleaning and disinfecting all commonly used equipment. See "Cleaning & Disinfecting Athletic Facilities for MRSA" at the CDC website (www.cdc.gov/mrsa/community/enviroment/athletic-facilities.html) for information about cleaning common equipment.
- Coaches and training staff must be knowledgeable about communicable disease issues for their sport.
- Coaches should educate athletes about infectious disease guidelines including exclusion-from-play; RTP; hand washing, and showering expectations; bagging up and uniform laundering expectations.
- Refer students to appropriate resources (e.g., team physician, athletic trainer, school nurse, or PCP) when infection is suspected.

Data from Centers for Disease Control and Prevention (CDC): Methicillin-resistant *Staphylococcus aureus* (MRSA) infections: cleaning and disinfecting athletic facilities for MRSA, CDC (website), 2013, www.cdc.gov/mrsa/community/enviroment/athletic-facilities.html. Accessed August 29, 2014; CDC: Methicillin-resistant *Staphylococcus aureus* (MRSA) infections: prevention information and advice for athletes; what to do if you think you have MRSA, CDC (website), 2013, www.cdc.gov/mrsa/community/team-hc-providers/advice-for-athletes.html. Accessed August 29, 2014.
CDC, Centers for Disease Control and Prevention; *MRSA,* methicillin-resistant *Staphylococcus aureus; PCP,* primary care provider; *RTP,* return-to-play.

HCV has the highest likelihood of being transmitted through blood or blood products, injecting drugs, or needle stick exposures. There have been no documented cases of sports-transmitted HCV infection (Abalos and Petri, 2015). Athletes with either acute hepatitis B or C may participate in sports once they are symptom-free and physically well.

Refer to Box 13-7 for a summary of standard blood-borne pathogen infection control measures for trainers and coaches. See Chapter 24 for a more in-depth discussion about these infectious diseases.

• BOX 13-7 Recommendations for Trainers and Coaches to Prevent the Transmission of Blood-Borne Pathogens in the Sports Environment

- The health status of all athletes with regard to HIV and hepatitis status should be held in confidence (as is all other health-related information).
- Individuals who care for injured or bleeding athletes should be trained in first aid and standard precautions.
- Standard precautions (blood, body fluids, secretions, and excretions regardless of whether visible blood is present) with the exception of sweat, has replaced universal precautions (blood and body fluid).
- Have appropriate supplies and equipment that comply with standard precautions available (e.g., gloves, googles, masks, bandages, appropriate waste containers, disinfectants).
  - Any "sharps" or contaminated bandages, dressings, equipment, or clothing should be properly handled and disposed of consistent with facility guidelines.
- Athletes need to be instructed to report any bleeding wound obtained during an athletic event. If bleeding, the athlete should cease playing until the bleeding has stopped, and only return to play when the wound is covered with an activity resistant covering. A contaminated uniform needs to be replaced before returning to play.
  - If blood or body fluids were transferred to another individual with intact skin, the skin should be wiped first with an antimicrobial (*not* a chemical germicide for use on surfaces), then soap and water as soon as possible. Postexposure evaluation by a licensed health care professional should occur after any incident involving the athlete having non-intact skin, eye, mouth, mucous membrane, or parenteral (under the skin) contact with blood or other potentially infectious material.
- All athletes should be fully immunized against HBV.
- Educate about all the routes of transmission, particularly risky behaviors practiced when off the field of competition.

Data from National Collegiate Athletic Association (NCAA): *2013-2014 NCAA sports medicine handbook*, Indianapolis, 2013, National Collegiate Athletic Association Publishing.
HBV, Hepatitis B virus; *HIV,* human immunodeficiency virus.

Exercise-Induced Dyspnea

Youth athletes may complain of breathlessness (including "can't catch my breath"), wheezing, coughing, or feeling like they cannot take a deep breath. Although these symptoms are commonly found in those with asthma or exercise-induced bronchospasm (EIB), there are other differential diagnoses that the health care provider must take into consideration. During exercise, there is an increase in ventilation and cardiac output, so both systems need to be evaluated in order to reach a diagnosis. Cardiac conditions causing exercise-induced dyspnea (EID) include pulmonary hypertension, hypertrophic cardiomyopathy, and cardiac dysrhythmias. Non-cardiac conditions (besides asthma and

TABLE 13-9 Recommendations for Return to Play for Athletes with Communicable Skin Conditions

Condition	Return-to-Play Guidelines
Tinea corporis	• Minimum 72 hours on a topical fungicide • Lesions must be covered with a gas-permeable dressing followed by underwrap and stretch tape
Tinea capitis	• Minimum 2 weeks systemic antifungal therapy
Herpes simplex (primary)	• Free of systemic symptoms of viral infection, fever, malaise, and so on • No new lesions for at least 72 hours • No moist lesions; all lesions must be covered with a firm, adherent crust • Minimum 120 hours on a systemic antiviral therapy, if prescribed (fully formed, ruptured, crusted-over lesions will not be affected by antiviral therapy) • Active lesions cannot be covered to allow participation
Herpes simplex (recurrent)	• No moist lesions; all lesions must be covered with a firm, adherent crust • Minimum 120 hours on a systemic antiviral therapy, if prescribed (fully formed, ruptured, crusted-over lesions will not be affected by antiviral therapy) • Active lesions cannot be covered to allow participation
Herpes simplex (questionable)	• Tzanck stain and/or HSV antigen assay • No play until results of tests known
Molluscum contagiosum	• Lesions must be curetted or removed • Localized or solitary lesions may be covered with a gas-permeable dressing followed by underwrap and stretch tape
Furuncles, carbuncles, folliculitis, impetigo, cellulitis, or MRSA	• No new lesions for at least 48 hours • Minimum 72 hours of antibiotic therapy (see also Chapter 37) • No moist, exudative, or draining lesions • Active lesions cannot be covered to allow participation

Adapted from National Collegiate Athletic Association (NCAA): *2013-14 and 2014-25 NCAA wrestling: rules and interpretations: Appendix A: skin infections in wrestling*. Indianapolis, 2014, NCAA; Wilson EK, deWeber K, Berry JW, et al: Cutaneous infections in wrestlers, *Sports Health* 5(5):423–437, 2014.
HSV, Herpes simplex virus; *MRSA,* methicillin-resistant *Staphylococcus aureus.*

EIB) include gastric reflux, vocal cord dysfunction, poor physical fitness, physiologic limitations, anemia, subclinical pulmonary embolism, and hyperventilation syndrome. Acute illnesses that can present with EID include rhinitis, sinusitis, bronchitis, and pneumonia (Newsham, 2013). The reader is encouraged to consult the appropriate sections of this textbook for assessing and managing these conditions and referral guidance.

High-Risk Conditions for Sports Participation

Sudden Cardiac Death in Young Athletes

In young athletes (i.e., younger than 35 years old), SCD is most commonly caused by underlying, often congenital, cardiac disease. The incidence is estimated to vary between 2.3 to 4.4 per 100,000 youth athletes per year; males are at greater risk than females and there is greater incidence in basketball and football athletes (Chandra et al, 2013). When the athlete is under exertion, an underlying cardiac condition can produce malignant ventricular dysrhythmias (ventricular tachycardia or ventricular fibrillation). Many athletes are totally asymptomatic until the traumatic event of SCD occurs. Screening for family history of risk factors, history of syncope, and history of cardiac disease or cardiac murmur in a child or adolescent are essential components of the PPE, yet these screening measures do not provide 100% assurance of determining risk of SCD (Chandra et al, 2013). The latest American Heart Association (AHA)/American College of Cardiology scientific statement continues to advise against the use of the 12-lead ECG as a universal screening tool (Maron et al, 2014). The ECG or other tests, such as echocardiograms, are indicated if the youth is at higher risk based on the 14-element questionnaire (see Box 13-3). See Chapter 31 for a discussion about the major underlying cardiac conditions that increase the risk for SCD. Other causes of SCD include:

- Anabolic steroids: Cardiac anomalies and possible myocardial damage remain under study (Statuta and Vaughan, 2015)
- Commotio cordis: A rare situation in which an athlete suffers a direct blow to the precordium by a projectile object, such as a baseball or softball, hockey puck, or lacrosse ball. If this happens at a vulnerable period of the cardiac cycle, it can trigger ventricular fibrillation. It is more common in children (mean age of 12 years old,

perhaps due to an underdeveloped thorax) (Battle et al, 2015).
- Exercise-induced bronchospasm (EIB): Although EIB may produce symptoms described as chest pain or chest discomfort, this can also be a sign of left ventricular outflow tract obstruction or coronary artery anomalies and should be further evaluated if the history and physical examination suggest a history of EIB.
- Premature coronary artery disease

Although SCD often occurs without warning, secondary preventive measures are advocated in school districts and community settings. These measures include increasing awareness of the incidence of SCD in youth in competitive sports, recognition of early symptoms of SCD, athletic personnel trained to provide effective cardiopulmonary resuscitation (CPR), and access to an automated external defibrillator (AED) in school, sports fields, and community settings. When secondary prevention programs are implemented, the ability to successfully resuscitate youth increases for those previously diagnosed and undiagnosed with cardiac disorders (Galas, 2014).

Musculoskeletal

Overuse or Traumatic Injuries

Overuse injuries are becoming more common in young athletes because of early sport specialization, year-round sports participation in multiple sports in the same season, and the increased demands put on young athletes by parents, coaches, and school settings (Wilson and Rodenberg, 2011). A common overuse injury unique to the skeletally immature athlete is apophysitis, resulting from repetitive irritation, inflammation, and microtrauma at the growth plate. The apophysis is a secondary ossification center that serves as the attachment site for a muscle-tendon unit, and it is the biomechanically weak point of the muscle-tendon-bone attachment. It is subject to injury in the growing athlete from repetitive stress and comprises a significant proportion of musculoskeletal complaints in youth involved in competitive sports (Wilson and Rodenberg, 2011). An avulsion fracture can occur in youth with apophysitis as a result of a forceful muscle contraction displacing a small piece of bone from its origin. Apophysitis may present as a persistent or worsening pain symptom after a specific history of injury or with gradual onset of pain without specific injury. Radiographs are generally not indicated. Persistent pain indicates the need for further diagnostics and referral.

Understanding the demands of a specific sport enables the PCP to more completely consider the various differential diagnoses, management, and a RTP plan. Many protocols are available that address RTP for specific sports. In general, for RTP, the health care provider should assess the injury for:
- Minimal swelling or joint effusions; some mild discomfort, swelling, and/or stiffness can be expected during initial reentry into activity
- Pain-free full range of motion
- At least 90% to 95% of normal strength
- Ability to perform all motions and actions of the required sport

Successful RTP includes regaining strength and conditioning of the injured area. A program of gradual return to play with a trial of sports activities may be necessary before full RTP is accomplished.

Other common musculoskeletal injuries from overuse or trauma in youth involved in competitive and recreational sports include sprains, subluxations, dislocations, and muscle contusions. Level of pain with physical activity and compromised range of motion, strength, endurance, and joint and ligament stability dictate the need for further evaluation with radiograph studies. See Chapter 38 for a more thorough discussion concerning the diagnosis and management of these conditions.

Baseball/Softball

Young baseball/softball throwers and pitchers are at particular risk of overuse injury or apophysitis. There are specific guidelines that address this issue for pitchers (American Sports Medicine Institute [ASMI], 2013; Rice et al, 2012; Zaremski and Krabak, 2012):
- Do not pitch more than 100 innings in any calendar year
- Refrain from throwing overhead for 2 to 3 months (4 months is preferred) per year; no competitive pitching for a least 4 months per year
- Watch and respond to signs of fatigue
- Do not play in both pitcher and catcher positions
- Follow daily and weekly pitch limits based on age: These limits are available on the American Sports Medicine Institute (ASMI) and Little League websites (see Additional Resources).
- Do not use radar guns
- Pitchers should not pitch for more than one team at a time
- Do not pitch on 3 consecutive days

Burners and Stingers

Burners and stingers are nerve root or brachial plexus compression or traction injuries and generally cause unilateral symptoms. This is a common injury in contact or collision sports, notably football and wrestling. The names derive from the sensation of a burn, stinging, electric, or "lightning bolt" sensation down an arm to the hand. The sensation can last seconds to minutes, but up to 10% can last hours, days, or longer. They may require a more extensive evaluation if weakness lasts more than a few days, there is a symptom of neck pain, the burners or stingers occur in both arms, or there is a prior history of recurrent burners or stingers.

Youth with mild to moderate burners or stingers must be free of all symptoms before given sports clearance; they should not be allowed to play if any neck pain or arm weakness remains.

Neck Injury

After neck injuries, the athlete should be free of neck and arm pain, have full range of neck motion, and have full neck strength before RTP. Neck radiographs and magnetic resonance imaging (MRI), if done, should not reveal abnormal position, disk disease, or spinal stenosis; refer for positive findings.

Head Injury/Concussions

See Chapter 28 for a full discussion regarding the evaluation and management of traumatic brain injury and concussion. An estimated 3.8 million concussions occur each year in the United States as a result of sports and physical activity that involve head trauma (Broglio et al, 2014). The sports posing the highest risk for head injuries include football, boxing, bicycling, basketball, and soccer. American football and Australian rugby have the highest incidence of concussion in competitive sports for males; for females, the rate of concussion is highest in soccer. Helmets for rugby provide some protection, but to date no football helmet has been found to be more protective than another (Giza et al, 2013). All 50 states in the United States have enacted concussion laws that cover education, assessment and emergency plans, athlete removal from play, and expert medical evaluation with RTP guidelines (Broglio et al, 2014).

Less emphasis is now placed on loss of consciousness, posttraumatic amnesia, and retrograde amnesia as ways to diagnosis and classify the severity of concussion. These only appear in a minority of injured athletes. Key points for sideline personnel and health care providers to remember include the following (Rossetti et al, 2015):

- Recognize that a concussion may have occurred.
- Most athletes show no obvious indications of concussion.
- Baseline (preseason) neurocognitive testing should be done on all athletes and used to compare any sideline assessments after an injury to avoid erroneous conclusions.
- Sideline assessment is imperative for any athlete who receives a significant head blow or is not "acting themselves" no matter the degree of impact.
- Concussion assessment needs to be carried out by a certified trainer or health care provider who has been trained to evaluate and manage concussions. The Sport Concussion Assessment Tool 3 (SCAT3) is recommended by the 4th International Conference on Concussion in Sport as a sideline concussion assessment tool (see Additional Resources).

Both physical and cognitive rest is indicated after the diagnosis of a concussion in youth. Cognitive recovery may lag behind physical symptom resolution, and cognitive recovery is a key factor in RTP decisions. Once symptoms resolve, the athlete can progress through steps to gradually RTP. Table 28-10 (see Chapter 28) lists the signs and symptoms of concussion; Table 13-10 describes the recommended step-wise RTP protocol.

Transient Quadriplegia

This condition can pose a significant problem and generally appears with bilateral symptoms. If a youth has symptoms,

TABLE 13-10 Graduated Return-to-Play Protocol after a Concussion

Rehabilitation Stage*	Functional Exercise at Each Stage of Rehabilitation	Objective of Each Stage
1. No activity	• Complete physical and cognitive rest (includes schoolwork, video gaming, and texting). • High school aged and younger youth should not return to sports until they have successfully returned to academics.	Recovery
2. Light aerobic exercise	• Walking, swimming, or stationary cycling keeping intensity <70% MPHR. • No resistance training.	Increase HR
3. Sport-specific exercise	• Skating drills in ice hockey, running drills in soccer. • No head impact activities.	Add movement
4. Noncontact training drills	• Progression to more complex training drills (e.g., passing drills in football and ice hockey). • May start progressive resistance training.	Exercise, coordination, and cognitive load
5. Full-contact practice	• Following medical clearance, participate in normal training activities.	Restore confidence and assess functional skills by coaching staff
6. Return to play	• Normal game play.	

From McCrory P, Meeuwisse WH, Aubry M, et al: Consensus statement on concussion in sports: the 4th International Conference on Concussion in Sport held in Zurich, November 2012, *Br J Sports Med* 47(5):250–258, 2013.
HR, Heart rate; *MPHR*, maximum predicted heart rate.
*Stay at each stage for 24 hours before progressing to next stage, as long as asymptomatic. If symptoms evolve at any stage, drop back to prior stage.

there should be no further participation in contact and collision sports until he or she is fully evaluated and/or if any objective structural problems are found. All transient quadriplegia muscle function and strength must have returned prior to clearance to resume play. Rehabilitation may be needed to achieve this.

Hernia

Hernias should be repaired. However, the teen with a hernia need not be restricted from sports participation but should be aware of the symptoms of incarceration.

Absence of Paired Organs

When a youth has an impairment or absence of one of a paired organ and wishes to participate in a sport, the PCP should take several factors into consideration. These include the quality and function of the organ; the probability of injury to that organ by participation in the sport; what, if any, protective equipment is available; and the effectiveness of that equipment (NCAA, 2013). A signed letter of understanding and waiver release by the student, parent, or guardian for the athlete's record are indicated.

Sports that involve objects, sticks, racquets, or aggressive play (such as, football or basketball) have greater risks for eye injuries. Baseball is the most dangerous eye sport; serious eye injuries from hockey have dramatically decreased with the mandatory use of face masks. Approved eyewear is available for all sports except boxing, wrestling, and full-contact martial arts. All youth participating in organized sports should wear the appropriate protective eyewear that is specified by the American Society for Testing and Materials (ASTM) or other organization with standards specific to football and lacrosse. Street-wear glasses and industrial education safety protective lenses are not appropriate substitutes. Contact lenses afford no protection. The child who has one eye or best-corrected vision in one eye worse than 20/40 *and* a small face to fit should be required to wear molded polycarbonate sport frames (American National Standards Institute [ANSI] Z87.1 frames) with 3-mm-thick polycarbonate lenses, However, even these are not ideal. It is better for the parent and child to choose a sport less likely to endanger the child's eye(s). For other functional one-eyed individuals, only participation in sports in which the use of eye protection is possible should be approved. For collision sports involving headgear (such as, football, hockey, or lacrosse) the same safety ASTM-approved eyewear should be worn under the cage shield or mask. A history of detached retina is significant, and participation should be limited to non-strenuous sports until consultation with an ophthalmologist is complete (see also Table 13-6).

Young men with a single testicle can be adequately protected with the use of a hard-cup athletic supporter for contact and collision sports and those sports in which objects are projected at high speed. Young women with one ovary should not be restricted (NCAA, 2013).

Special Considerations for the Female Athlete

Injuries and the Female Athlete

During a sport season, it is estimated that greater than one-third of high school female athletes will have an injury (Elliot et al, 2010). Anterior cruciate ligament (ACL) injuries will occur two to eight times more in the female athlete than the male athlete (Michaelidis and Koumantakis, 2014). This ACL injury typically occurs during deceleration, landing, pivoting, or contact with another athlete. Sports that increase this risk are basketball, tennis, field hockey, lacrosse, skiing, and soccer. It is theorized that the increased risk is due to several factors, including biomechanical, greater joint laxity in females, and hormonal effects on connective tissue (Groeger, 2010). Many girls' sports teams are incorporating some version of an ACL injury prevention training as part of their warm-ups, but these programs have shown mixed results in the reduction of injuries, partially related to the widely varied programs and attendance rates of the participants (Noyes and Barber-Westin, 2014). Components of a well-rounded prevention program should include "plyometrics, dynamic stabilization, strength training (trunk, upper and lower body), sport-specific agility training, education, and feedback on correct technique" (Michaelidis and Koumantakis, 2014, p 206).

Other injuries common in the female athlete include those of the patellofemoral joint and shoulder (sustained during diving, gymnastics, swimming, throwing, and volleyball) (Stracciolini et al, 2014). Stress fractures must be suspected in female athletes with low body weight and/or amenorrhea. The female athlete who is amenorrheic has a four times greater risk of stress fracture than does the athlete with normal menses (Groeger, 2010).

Intensive sport training does not appear to delay the growth and sexual maturation of young female athletes. This concern has been repeatedly raised at every world Olympics in regard to female gymnasts. However, studies conclude that the differences in growth and maturation are more likely due to genetics and physique preselection rather than to extended, intensive training (AAP Committee on Sports Medicine and Fitness, 2014).

The Female Athlete Triad

The female athlete triad consists of three entities: (1) low energy availability with or without a disordered eating pattern, (2) menstrual dysfunction (amenorrhea or oligomenorrhea), and (3) low bone mineral density (osteopenia or osteoporosis) (De Souza et al, 2014). At the root of this triad is the emphasis (either real or perceived by the athlete) on a lean body, maintaining a low weight, and/or retaining one's prepubertal physique. Girls who participate in sports that emphasize leanness are at the greatest risk of the triad of disorders, including distance running, gymnastics, dance/dance team, figure skating, and cheerleading (Barrack et al, 2013; House et al, 2013). It is estimated that the incidence of the female athlete triad in female high school athletes is 1.0% to 1.3% with a combined range of up to 15.9% for

• BOX 13-8 Screening Questions for Female Athlete Triad

Menstrual History

- Have you had a menstrual period?
- What was your age when you had your first period?
- When was your last period?
- How often do you have your periods? How many in the past year?

Medications

- Are you taking hormones (estrogen, progesterone, birth control pills)?

Weight

- Are you concerned about your weight?
- Are you trying to lose or gain weight?
- Are you on a diet or do you avoid certain foods?
- What have you done to try and control your weight (purging, binging, fasting, diet pills or other botanicals)?

Musculoskeletal

- Have you had a stress fracture?
- Have you been told that you have low bone density?

Data from DeSouza MJ, Nattiv A, Joy E, et al: 2014 Female Athlete Triad Coalition consensus statement on treatment and return to play of the female athlete triad, *Clin J Sport Med* 24(2):96–119, 2014.

• BOX 13-9 The Female Athlete Triad: Recommendations for the Clinician

- Screen for all elements of the triad at the PPE and at annual physicals (see Box 13-8).
- If one component of the triad exists, screen for others.
- Treatment should be multidisciplinary; may include mental health professional, nutritionist, and coach or trainer.
- If an eating disorder is suspected, refer the athlete to a nutrition professional and a mental health professional for screening/treatment (if necessary).
- Diagnosis of amenorrhea—screen for other causes (see Chapter 36). Functional hypothalamic amenorrhea (from the events of the triad) is a diagnosis of exclusion.
- Screen bone mineral density:
  - After a stress or low-impact fracture
  - After a total of 6 months of amenorrhea or oligomenorrhea
  - As part of the assessment of a disordered eating pattern
- Initial goal of treatment is to increase energy intake and decrease energy expenditure.
- Preventive counseling for all athletes should include nutritional (energy) needs for sports; importance of bone mineralization during child and adolescent years; bone health throughout life; and importance of physical activity, calcium, and vitamin D.

Data from De Souza MJ, Nattiv A, Joy E, et al: 2014 Female Athlete Triad Coalition consensus statement on treatment and return to play of the female athlete triad, *Clin J Sport Med* 24(2):96–119, 2014.
PPE, Preparticipation physical examination.

high school students and premenopausal women (Gibbs et al, 2013). Symptoms of the triad occur along a continuum rather than in unison; therefore, the identification of the early existence of an eating disorder, weight loss, or menstrual irregularities from a PPE history or examination should alert the provider to take a more thorough history and initiate early treatment in order to prevent development of the full triad (Deimel and Dunlap, 2012; De Souza et al, 2014) (see Box 13-8 for the PPE screening questions). Inadequate bone mineralization during the critical adolescent years puts the teen at lifelong risk of osteoporosis, which increases the risk of stress fractures during adolescence and throughout life and skeletal problems at menopause.

Disordered eating patterns can be due to either intentional caloric restriction (an eating disorder that may or may not encompass all the criteria for an anorexia or bulimia diagnosis) or an inadvertent insufficient intake in calories to meet the athlete's metabolic demands of her sport. Disordered eating, whatever the cause, leads to low energy availability. It is thought that when one's energy deficit reaches a critical low threshold, a cascade of hormonal and biochemical events occur that negatively affect the menstrual cycle and skeletal integrity (House et al, 2013). Box 13-9 lists recommendations for evaluating and managing an individual identified as having the female triad.

Heat and Humidity

Core body temperature is a balance of heat generation and heat dissipation (see also Chapter 40). A major contributor to core body temperature is the heat generated by muscle contractions. Exercising muscle generates 10 to 20 times the amount of heat of resting muscle, and sweating is the main mechanism that is used to rid the body of excess heat (AAP, 2015c). If the body is unable to rid itself of the excessive heat, body temperature will rise. Under ideal conditions, this can result in an increase of core body temperature of 1.8° F (1° C) in 5 minutes. When environmental heat or humidity excesses are added to the equation, the body must dissipate the heat at increased rates. Unless the usual heat dissipation mechanisms are properly working, heat stroke can result within 15 to 20 minutes. Heat is dissipated through evaporation (20% to 25%), convection (15%), and radiation (60%). It is dissipated only through evaporation when the environmental temperature exceeds body temperature and the humidity is 75% or less. There is no evaporation at 90% to 95% humidity. Thus, the combination of high heat and high humidity greatly taxes the body's ability to effectively lower core temperature.

Previously, it had been thought that children were less effective at regulating their body temperature during episodes of exercising in the heat when compared to adults. More recent research indicates that children (9 to 12 years old) have sufficient cardiovascular capacity, effective thermoregulation, and exercise tolerance as long as they are sufficiently hydrated (Bergeron, 2013). With these new findings, there is now a higher focus placed on modifying factors (such as, intensity and duration of activity) as long as ample hydration is provided. At the same time, it is imperative that the exercising youth be monitored appropriately because their metabolic heat production, heat storage, and body core temperature can rise quickly (Bergeron, 2013).

Inadequate heat acclimatization, heavy uniforms and gear, inadequate exercise recovery, too closely scheduled exercise sessions, and specific sports put the young athlete at further risk of heat-related injury. Athletes who are dealing with current or recent illnesses, especially gastrointestinal distress (e.g., vomiting and diarrhea) and/or fever may experience an increased risk of exercising in the heat due to hydration status and dysregulation of body temperature. Chronic illnesses such as diabetes insipidus, SCT, type 2 DM, obesity, juvenile hyperthyroidism, cystic fibrosis, and anticholinergic drugs or other medications (such as, dopamine reuptake inhibitors or diuretics) can all contribute to having a decreased heat tolerance and increased heat illness risk (Bergeron et al, 2011). Additionally, decreased sweat production may occur with spina bifida, quadriplegia, scleroderma, severe eczema, and sunburn among other conditions. These individuals need particular supervision because they might not recognize early warning signs of heat effects and may not hydrate adequately.

Heat illness is recognized as a leading cause of death and disability in the United States for high school and college athletes. Football is the most common activity leading to heat-related emergency room visits for individuals 19 years old or younger (CDC, 2011).

Sports Training Acclimatization for Prevention of Heat-Related Illnesses

Heat-related illnesses are totally preventable. *Heat acclimatization* is the training process by which athletes are exposed gradually to exercising in high-temperature environmental conditions. This training requires a minimum of 10 to 14 days (Lopez et al, 2011). By adhering to a carefully prescribed schedule, athletic performance improves, and the risk of later exertional, heat-related illness is reduced. For that reason, many sports associations at both the high school and collegiate levels require heat-acclimatization periods in their initial training schedules (Bergeron, 2013). Specific heat-acclimatization guidelines for athletic training are available from the National Athletic Trainers' Association (see Additional Resources).

Dehydration

Dehydration increases body temperature primarily due to the reduced blood volume along with increased demand for perfusion to the exercising muscle and skin. The decreased perfusion of the skin leads to decreased evaporation, which increases the body temperature (Casa et al, 2012b). The young athlete can prevent dehydration by drinking cool water before, during, and after activities. Performance and normal thermoregulation can decrease with as little as 1% dehydration, and most athletes enter their activity in a hypohydrated state. Thirst should not be the only guide to hydration needs (Arnaoutis et al, 2014). Coaching staff should play a role in educating, monitoring, and supporting the athlete's ability to maintain hydration and should be proactive in providing drink breaks, having water bottles accessible, and reminding players to drink. Even with proper education, athletes often will not drink enough and will be in a voluntary dehydrated state (Cleary et al, 2012; Williams and Blackwell, 2012). After competition, rehydration is important. Small amounts of sodium and carbohydrates found in sports drinks (see prior discussion regarding sports drinks) enhance rehydration; additional sodium supplements are not recommended. Drinking fluids with caffeine should be avoided because these beverages increase urine output, causing further dehydration.

Use of Ergogenic Drugs and Supplements

Ergogenic drugs refer to any legal and illicit substance used to enhance athletic performance (performance-enhancing drugs or nutritional muscle-building or sports supplements). Athletes use these substances because they are purported to have a variety of effects, such as increasing energy; prolonging sports endurance; increasing lean body mass and decreasing adipose tissue; increasing or decreasing weight; improving cardiovascular status; and enhancing overall performance in a given sport. Such claims and beliefs about these substances serve as powerful enticements to young athletes. The steroid precursors, growth hormone, and ephedra substances have not been proven to enhance performance, and they can have serious side effects of which youth are often unaware. Street names include gym candy, pumpers, weight trainers, stackers, roids, juice, and Arnolds.

There are a number of issues regarding the safety and moral questions that arise from use of ergogenic substances. Due to the Dietary Supplement Health and Education Act of 1994, many steroid precursors can be sold over the counter without stringent regulation. Although competitive sports can be positive when they promote teamwork, cooperation, and an increase in the athlete's confidence level, they can turn negative when they promote a win-at-all-cost association (Mulcahey et al, 2010). The use of such muscle-building or performance-enhancing substances takes away the element of fair competition and puts the individual's health at risk (Dandoy and Gereige, 2012).

The preponderance of ergogenic drug use can be attributed to many modern influences. These include the message conveyed by top athletes and sports icons who are using ergogenic drugs that these substances are acceptable, the emphasis and status placed on sports by society, canvassing ever younger players by sports scouts, and pressure to fund college education via sports scholarships. Adolescents at higher risk of using performance-enhancing drugs include males who are involved in sports that demand strength, power, and speed, such as football, wrestling, gymnastics, baseball, basketball and weight training. Additional risk factors include peer pressure, exposure to sports media, parents using these substances, history of depression, negative body image, and comparing one's body to others' (Dandoy and Gereige, 2012; Mulcahey et al, 2010).

Recognition and Prevention of Ergogenic Substance Use

All high school and collegiate sports associations have strongly worded policies prohibiting the use of performance-enhancing substances. They issue and actively enforce no-tolerance policies and endorse the U.S. Anti-Doping Agency regulations and world anti-doping code. It is important for clinicians to be aware of and communicate these positions to young athletes and their parents. Anticipatory guidance and education are essential in this area. Education needs to include both benefits and risks, and the educator needs to be well informed to be credible. "Clean" team members can provide leadership by disavowing performance-enhancing drugs and emphasizing the integrity (fair play) of sports competition. Parents and coaches should intervene whenever necessary. Nutrition and strength-training techniques, as previously discussed, are important aspects of "natural" athletic performance enhancement programs.

Given the prevalence of these drugs, clinicians must be alert to youth who use them. Although the use of these drugs is not always easy to detect, providers should be alert for rapid changes in lean body mass, muscle bulk, and concerns with behavioral or mood changes (Dandoy and Gereige, 2012; Mulcahey et al, 2010). Box 13-10 suggests several interviewing questions to assess the use of performance-enhancing substances.

Anabolic-Androgenic Steroids

The term *anabolic* refers to the drug's ability to stimulate protein synthesis; *androgenic* refers to the stimulation of male secondary sexual characteristics. Anabolic-androgenic steroids (AASs) react with a variety of receptors in the body, including glucocorticoids, progestin, estrogen, and androgen. Endogenous anabolic steroid production starts adolescent development in the prepubertal male. The exogenous drug used by both sexes for performance enhancement or appearance is derived from testosterone. It produces changes in the endocrine/reproductive, cardiovascular, hepatic, musculoskeletal, and neurologic systems. The AAS drugs are Class III controlled substances. AASs are often taken in amounts from 10 to 100 times the normal therapeutic dose (O'Malley, 2013).

According to 2013 National YRBSS data, 3.2% of students in 9th through 12th grade took steroid pills or shots without a doctor's prescription one or more times during their life; more males (4%) than females (2.2%) reported using steroids (CDC, 2014). Not all anabolic steroids users are involved in sports; an estimated 30% to 40% of teenagers who use steroids are non-athletes who are focused on their body's appearance (Mulcahey et al, 2010). Athletes participating in the following sports have been shown to be at most risk of using/abusing these substances: football, wrestling, weight training, baseball, and basketball (Dandoy and Gereige, 2012).

Clinical effects can be irreversible and extremely serious in males and females. Mild effects can include acne, weight gain, deepening voice, accelerated puberty, gynecomastia in males, or premature balding. With sustained use, some of the more serious side effects include cardiac failure, impotence, edema, testicular atrophy, liver dysfunction and possible malignancy, and tendon or muscle injuries (due to disorganized collagen fibril alignment). Premature epiphyseal closure can leave the immature athlete shorter than expected. In females, AAS use can cause irreversible menstrual irregularities and breast atrophy, virilization (enlargement of the clitoris, hirsutism, male pattern baldness, deepening of the voice with larynx changes), and amenorrhea. Mood swings, violent behavior, heightened aggression, and depression severe enough to be linked with suicide have been described. Mortality or life-threatening event statistics attributed to steroid use may be inaccurate as they can be masked by the diagnoses of cardiac arrest, liver, or kidney failure (Dandoy and Gereige, 2012; Mulcahey et al, 2010; O'Malley, 2013).

Steroid users may use the substance in three preparations: oral, injected, or transdermal. The oral forms are shorter acting and excreted over days; the injectables are more potent and last longer. Withdrawal effects can occur up to a year or more after use has stopped. Generally used in the off-season (to gain strength and prevent detection), these drugs are taken in cycles of use lasting 4 to 12 weeks each. Sometimes more than one type of steroid is used at a time ("stacking"), or the steroids are dosed incrementally and used in both the oral and injectable forms and then tapered at the end of a cycle ("pyramiding") (Dandoy and Gereige, 2012). Newer, "designer" synthetic steroids (e.g., tetrahydrogestrinone [THG], gestrinone, and trenbolone) were produced in an attempt to prevent detection by doping

BOX 13-10 Screening Youth for the Use of Body-Building and Other Performance-Enhancing Substances*

1. Are you using any substances or supplements to improve your performance in your sports(s)?
2. Do you use any substance to improve your body's appearance, weight, or strength?
3. How do you feel you are doing at your sport? Is your performance where you would like it to be? Are you satisfied with how you are doing? If not, how are you planning to improve?
4. What are your goals with regard to your sport?
5. Are there people in your life (coaches, parents, self) who are pressuring you to improve your performance?
6. Do you know of any athletes or other peers who are using performance-enhancing substances?
7. What questions do you have about drugs or supplements or other things athletes might use to enhance performance?

Adapted from Holland-Hall C: Performance-enhancing substances: is your adolescent patient using? *Pediatr Clin North Am* 54(4):651–662, 2007.
*Be sure to include questions about all drugs,body-building and other nutritional supplements, alcohol use, and needle use as per general adolescent health guidelines.

tests; however, newer doping tests can identify these synthetic steroids. Drugs used to mask the detection of steroids may include uricosuric agents (probenecid), diuretics (spironolactone, furosemide), and epitestosterone.

Androstenedione and Dehydroepiandrosterone

Androstenedione ("andro") and related dehydroepiandrosterone (DHEA) are prohormones that are converted to either testosterone or estrone. Androstenedione is a Class III controlled drug and DHEA may be purchased over the counter. These steroid precursors are used because of the mistaken belief that they will increase testosterone and produce the same effects on muscles and performance as seen with anabolic steroids. Studies, however, have not demonstrated any convincing measurable changes in athletic performance. Rather than show increases in testosterone levels, steroid precursors can significantly increase androstenedione and estradiol levels, causing the adverse changes seen with anabolic steroids. Changes include androgenizing effects in females, such as virilization; in males the changes include male pattern baldness, gynecomastia, acne, and testicular atrophy. In both genders over time, there can be adverse alterations in lipid levels and stunted growth (Dandoy and Gereige, 2012).

Growth Hormone

Human growth hormone (HGH) (available in a biosynthetic, injectable form) is often used one or more times a month and is banned by sporting leagues. Youths take it in the mistaken belief that it will enhance athletic performance through anabolic mechanisms of increasing lean body mass and decreasing fat mass. However, it appears to worsen exercise capacity by increasing exercise-induced lactate levels. Potential negative effects related to high-dose HGH use include diabetes, cardiomyopathy, hepatitis, and renal failure. Athletes who take it report a "feel-good" sensation (probably caused by fluid shifts within tissues) and decreases in subcutaneous fat for a fit appearance.

Creatine and Other Supplements

Creatine is involved in the production of energy for muscular contraction and is found in fish, meat, milk, and other foods in small amounts. Synthetic creatine is an over-the-counter supplement used in the belief that it enhances athletic endurance by improving muscular contraction strength and performance. It increases (by approximately 20%) stores of muscle phosphocreatine that in turn release initial energy for muscle contraction in short, high-intensity activities (e.g., wrestling), quickening phosphocreatine replenishment during recovery, and delaying fatigue onset. The exercise must be maximal and anaerobic and last long enough to deplete the stores nonusers would have. If the duration of the activity is too long (more than 60 seconds), other sources of energy supplant the creatine effects and benefit is not seen.

An adolescent's total daily requirement is 2 g per day; athletes typically take two to three times this amount in an attempt to improve their athletic performance (Dandoy and Gereige, 2012). Athletes generally take a cycle of 5 g, four times daily for 4 to 6 days and then a maintenance dose of 2 g per day for the following 3 months. A month of abstinence then is practiced. It is important for those taking creatine to drink 6 to 8 ounces of water to prevent dehydration. Carbohydrate-rich fluids increase the absorption, and caffeine impairs uptake.

Side effects of creatine supplementation can include weight gain due to water retention, poorer performance, anxiety, fatigue, headaches, rashes, dyspnea, muscle cramps, mild gastrointestinal distress, and elevated serum creatinine and renal disease (rare). Recent study results suggested a possible causal relationship between the use of muscle-building supplements (creatine, protein, and androstenedione or its booster) and a 65% increase risk of testicular cancer in men ages 18 to 55 years. The risk more than doubled in those who had taken the supplements for more than 3 years, who took multiple types of supplements, or who started before they were 25 years old. Further study is indicated to discern exactly what ingredients or possible contaminants may lead to the increase incidence. Thirty different types of MBS powders or pills were included in the study (Li et al, 2015). There are no other studies showing the effects of long-term use, the effect of supplementation on the other creatine storage organs (brain or heart), or effects in those younger than 18 years old. Studies in adults, however, validate that the benefits to taking creatine are limited to short, high-intensity activities, as discussed earlier (Dandoy and Gereige, 2012). Creatine is the most popular nutritional supplement sold (Dandoy and Gereige, 2012). Thirty-four percent of participants in a national survey who were younger than 18 years old reported using creatine in the prior 30 days to improve their sports performance (Evans et al, 2012).

Ephedra

Ephedra is a naturally occurring herb; ephedrine is the main active ingredient. Ephedrine has a chemical structure similar to amphetamine. It enhances the release of norepinephrine and stimulates the central nervous system. The herbal form is ma huang. Ephedra was banned as an energy enhancer and diet aid in 2004 by the U.S. Food and Drug Administration (FDA). A nationwide effort in 2006 focused on curbing the retail sale of pseudoephedrine, but some products that contain ephedra were not banned. Also, since the ban, ephedra has been replaced by other sympathomimetics that act similarly. Traditional Chinese herbal medicines, herbal teas, and medications that contain chemically synthesized ephedra are among the products not banned. Dietary supplements for bodybuilding and weight loss are readily available over the Internet and can include ephedra as a listed or unlisted ingredient. The ephedra may be combined with a botanical source of caffeine, notably guarana (Paullinia cupana), Kola nut (Cola nitida), or yerba mate.

Adverse reactions include tachycardia (most often), hypertension, dysrhythmias, anxiety, tremors, insomnia, paranoid psychoses, stroke, and sudden death. The active ingredients in ephedra are known to have serious interactions with amphetamines (e.g., dextroamphetamine used for attention-deficit/hyperactivity disorder [ADHD]), antidepressants (tricyclics and monoamine oxidase inhibitors [MAOIs]), blood thinning medications, blood pressure medication, caffeine, narcotics, and theophylline (used for asthma).

Energy Drinks

As previously discussed, energy drinks and sports drinks are different and can be classified by their ingredients. Under certain circumstances, sports drinks have a role to play to maintain hydration and aid in muscle glycogen resynthesis during and after periods of strenuous physical activity lasting more than an hour. However, *there is no role for energy drinks under any circumstances* for children or adolescents (AAP Committee on Nutrition and Council on Sports Medicine and Fitness, 2011b; Seifert et al, 2011).

Energy drinks contain substances that are nonnutritive stimulants, such as caffeine, guarana, taurine, ginseng, L-carnitine, creatine, yohimbine hydrochloride, and/or glucuronolactone, as well as sugar, carbohydrates, minerals, and electrolytes. They are marketed to improve energy, weight loss, stamina, athletic performance, and concentration. Energy drinks can have from 50 to 505 mg of caffeine per serving compared with a 12-oz soda that provides 34 to 54 mg of caffeine. It is estimated that 30% to 50% of adolescents drink an energy drink daily (O'Malley, 2012).

The medical concerns regarding energy drinks are numerable, including the fact that the excess sugar found in these drinks can result in an increase in calories, obesity, and dental caries. Increased bone demineralization may occur based on either caffeine interfering with intestinal calcium absorption or less calcium being ingested if milk is being replaced by energy drinks. When consumed in combination with alcohol, the depressant effects of the alcohol can be masked by the stimulating effect of the energy drink; users may feel wide awake and possibly underestimate their level of intoxication or impairment. When consumed in large amounts, the high caffeine content of energy drinks causes tachycardia, anxiety, and insomnia. If prolonged consumption occurs, additional symptoms can include agitation, tremors, and gastrointestinal distress. Energy drinks will exaggerate the adverse risks in individuals who have a history of seizures, mood disorders, diabetes, hyperthyroidism, cardiac disease, eating disorders, or ADHD (O'Malley, 2012; Seifert et al, 2011). Many European countries have imposed restrictions on where the energy drinks may be sold, banned them, or required that they carry a health warning statement.

Nutritional Supplements

Nutritional supplements are readily available to aspiring athletes who believe that they will perform better if using them. They generally are composed of one or more of the following: a vitamin, a mineral, an herb or other botanical, an amino acid, a dietary supplement that raises the total daily intake or a concentrate, metabolite, constituent, extract, or a combination of the last four ingredients. Approximately 70% of children younger than 18 years old have taken dietary supplements (Evans et al, 2012). Nutritional supplements are not well regulated. The Dietary Supplements and Health Education Act of 1994 allows supplement companies to make claims regarding the effect of the product on the body's function (e.g., improves performance), but they cannot claim that the product will be able to diagnose, treat, prevent, or cure a specific medical condition. Studies have shown a broad inconsistency in the accuracy of labeling ingredients and amounts, contamination, and the inclusion of dangerous substances (e.g., steroids), which is concerning. Nutritional supplements in children and adolescents should be discouraged unless taken under the direction of a health care provider or registered dietician; vitamins and minerals are best gained through a healthy, well-balanced diet.

Recreational Activities: Safety Issues

Recreational activities play a key role in maintaining and promoting physical activity and health. Health care providers should ask children and youth about all of their physical health activities and update this information regularly. Some activities may be a form of independent transportation (e.g., skateboarding, cycling), may serve as a cross-training method for another sport, and may be relatively inexpensive versus organized sports. Many of these activities may be associated with significant risks related to mortality (e.g., from spinal cord or head trauma) and morbidity (e.g., general body trauma, fractures, torn ligaments, concussions) unless undertaken safely. Table 13-11 identifies hazards linked to various recreational activities and related safety measures that providers can discuss with parents and children.

Many recreational activities take place outdoors, encouraging children to engage actively with the environment. As a result, environmental health and safety concerns must be considered. The health care provider should discuss environmental safety during the PPE, including exposure to toxic compounds, use of protective equipment, traffic and pedestrian safety, and lightning safety. Box 13-11 provides guidelines addressing lightning hazards during outdoor athletic events (see the National Lightning Safety Institute website for guidelines when participating in other outdoor activities, such as hiking and camping, golfing, boating, or swimming).

For a complete list of references, please visit http://evolve.elsevier.com/Burns/pediatric/.

TABLE 13-11 Recreational Activities: Their Hazards and Safety Recommendations

Activity and Hazards	Safety Measures
All-terrain vehicles (ATVs) • Loss of control	• No one <16 years old should drive or ride on ATVs. • Those ≥16 years old should take a hands-on training course offered by certified instructors. • Wear protective clothing (boots, goggles helmet, long pants, and reflective outerwear). • Have flags, reflectors, and lights on ATVs. • Never carry passengers. • Never ride on public or paved roads or at night (AAP, 2013; AAP, 2015b; Nationwide Children's Hospital, 2014).
Motorcycles, motor scooters, mopeds, minibikes, minicycles, trail bikes • Collisions; inability to accelerate when mixing with other traffic; inadequate brakes	• Wear a helmet at all times. • Teenage motorcyclists should receive *at least* 30 hours of professional instruction, including 10 hours of driving in moderate to heavy traffic (AAP, 2015b). • Discourage motorcycles for youth transportation. • Off-road vehicles (minibikes, minicycles, trail bikes) should not be used on the street.
Riding lawnmowers • Collisions or falling off when a passenger or operating; playing in vicinity of operating mower	• Be at least 16 years old and take an ATV course prior to operating riding mowers (AAP, 2015b).
Snowmobiles • Collisions, rollovers (teenage boys and young males account for 75% of all collisions)	• *No one* <16 years old should operate snowmobiles. • Adequate instruction/supervision by an adult is paramount. • Wear protective clothing (boots, goggles, helmet, insulated outwear, and reflective clothing). • Travel only on designated trails, and avoid roads, railroads, waterways, and pedestrians.
Personal watercraft (jet skis/water scooters) • Collisions; turn-overs; ejections (some models can carry up to three passengers and reach speeds up to 60 mph)	• No one <16 years old should operate a personal watercraft (PWC). • Wear a U.S. Coast Guard–approved flotation device. • Do not jump waves. • Do not operate a PWC if under the influence of alcohol. • Never operate in swimming areas or after sunset (AAP, 2015b; Personal Watercraft Industry Association [PWIA], 2011).
Golf carts • Collisions; loss of control; turn-overs	• Restrict drivers to those ≥16 years old. • Limit the number of riders. • Drive only at safe speeds; wear seat belts; use helmets. • Limit use to designated areas.
Community/school playgrounds • Falls, collisions	• Equipment and surfaces should be regularly inspected (includes sharp protrusions, detached matting, exposed concrete footings, tripping hazards) and maintained by schools and cities; all equipment should meet U.S. Consumer Product Safety Commission (USCPSC) guidelines. • Maintain good sight lines for supervision of child, based upon child's height. • Maintain barriers between playground and street. • Instruct children in proper use of equipment; monitor and enforce playground rules. • Surfaces should be constructed out of shock-absorbing, single-unit materials (double-shredded bark mulch, shredded tires, or sand). Asphalt and concrete are unsuitable. • Separate areas for active and quieter play (e.g., swings from sandboxes) and by age. Have adequate entry and exit space around equipment so that children do not collide with each other or equipment. • Avoid metal or wood seats (best plastic or rubber); ensure equipment has no openings that could entrap a child's head (American Academy of Orthopaedic Surgeons [AAOS], 2009).
Roller sports (skateboards, scooters) • Falls, collisions (boys injured more than girls)	• Wear a helmet and other protective gear (e.g., wrist guards, elbow and knee pads). • Do not ride in or near traffic; utilize and promote skateboarding parks. • Check skating area for holes, bumps, and rocks; do not ride on uneven surfaces. • Limit skateboarding to daylight hours. • Children <5 years old should not use skateboards; 5- to 10-year-olds should be under an adult's supervision. • If riding on ripsticks, follow the same safety tips as children on skateboards (Nationwide Children's Hospital, n.d.b.).

Continued

TABLE 13-11 Recreational Activities: Their Hazards and Safety Recommendations—cont'd

Activity and Hazards	Safety Measures
Swimming • Drowning (due to drain entrapment/entanglement; lack of swimming skills; inadequate supervision; lack of cardiopulmonary resuscitation [CPR] training by bystanders)	• Swimming pools should have drain covers, safety vacuum-release systems (SVRS), filter pumps with multiple drains, or other pressure-venting filters. Home pools should have pool alarms, fences, and covers. • All children should get swimming lessons and demonstrate proficiency. Non-swimmers require constant "arms-length" and "touch supervision." • If possible, swim where there are stationed lifeguards. • Parents, caregivers, and swim instructors should have CPR training (Weiss, 2010).

Trampoline
• Falls; doing acrobatic maneuvers (somersaults, flips); colliding with others using trampoline
	• Trampolines cannot be recommended for home use.
	• General recommendations:
	  • Extend padding to the frame, hooks, and springs.
	  • Prohibit ladders; install netting.
	  • Prohibit somersaulting, multiple jumpers, and jumping onto trampoline from a higher surface.
	  • Restrict use to children ≥6 years old.
	  • If trampoline is >20 inches off the ground, no one <6 years old should use it; clear any surrounding hazards (e.g., low-branching tree limbs).
	  • Frequently inspect and replace protective elements; discard trampoline if parts are worn or damaged and replacement parts are unavailable.
	  • Children should be actively supervised and guidelines enforced; adults should be ready to respond to medical emergencies (AAP Council on Sports Medicine and Fitness et al, 2012).

Winter sports (skiing, snowboarding) • Falls; collisions; suffocation; drowning	• Dress warmly (insulated outerwear, hat, gloves, and slip-resistant snow boots); wear safety goggles when skiing, snowboarding or snowmobiling. Wear sunscreen. • Wear special helmets made for skiers, snowboarders, and snowmobilers. When ice skating or sledding, wear a multi-sport or bicycle helmet if a ski helmet is unavailable. • Receive instruction from certified ski and snowboarding schools. • Use proper equipment; knee and elbow pads should be worn when ice skating; wrist guards should be worn by snowboarders. • Children <5 years old should only sled with an adult. • Children <7 years old should not snowboard; children <6 years old should not ride on snowmobiles without an adult. • Do not sled in or near streets or in areas with trees, fences, ponds, or light poles. Do not skate on river ice or ice that has thawed and refrozen. • Only one person should ride on a sled, unless child is riding with an adult. • Sit up and face forward; avoid sledding head first. • Steerable sleds are safer than snow disks or inner tubes. • Never ride a sled being pulled by a car, ATV, snowmobile, or other motorized vehicle. • Ice skate in designated skating areas (Nationwide Children's Hospital, n.d.c.).

BOX 13-11 Lightning Safety for Outdoor Athletic Events

- Designate a person to monitor weather conditions, starting 24 hours prior to the event. (Use The Weather Channel, NOAA Weather Radio, or local television stations.)
- Develop a policy about suspending and resuming the event if lightning danger is present.
- Identify safe shelters and evacuation sites (e.g., fully enclosed metal vehicles with windows up, substantial buildings, low ground, clumps of bushes or trees of the same height, ditches, and/or trenches).
- Avoid these shelter areas:
  - Outdoor metal objects, such as flag poles, fences, gates, high light poles, metal bleachers, golf carts, and machinery
  - Trees, water (including swimming pools/lakes/ocean), open fields, and high ground
- Practice the 30 second/30 minute rule:
  - If lightning occurs first, count until the thunder occurs (if ≤30 seconds, storm is within 6 miles and area is positively charged for a lightning strike). Suspend play and seek safety immediately.
  - Allow 30 minutes to pass since last flash or thunder before resuming event.
  - A good motto is: "If you see it (lightning), flee it. If you can hear it (thunder), clear it."
- If your hair feels like "it is standing on end" and/or you hear "crackling noises" *immediately* remove metal objects (including headgear and caps), put feet together, tuck head low, and maintain low, crouching position with hands on knees or over ears; position yourself 15 to 20 feet apart from others.
- People struck by lightning can be touched; administer CPR, and call 911.

Prepared by the National Lightning Safety Institute: Personal lightning safety, Louisville, CO, 2014 for reprinting and distributing. Available at www.lightningsafety.com/nlsi_pls.html. Accessed September 16, 2014.
CPR, Cardiopulmonary resuscitation; *NOAA,* National Oceanic and Atmospheric Administration.

14 Sleep and Rest

SUSAN HINES

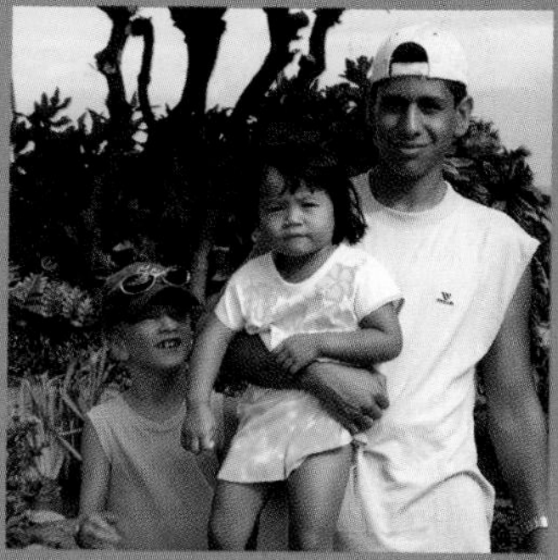

Adequate sleep is a necessary process for normal emotional, physiologic, and mental functioning in child development. Sleep affects every aspect of a child's development; insufficient sleep has been shown to have a negative impact on memory, learning, attention span, and executive functioning, as well as daytime behavior and temperament regulation (Johnson et al, 2013). Infants and young children spend a majority of time asleep, suggesting that sleep is a fundamental part of physical and mental development.

Sleep difficulties can pervade many areas of a child's health. Children with sleep disordered breathing (SDB) can manifest a continuum from simple snoring and upper airway resistance to obstructive sleep apnea (OSA) (Marcus et al, 2012a). Children who experience behavioral sleep problems (BSP) and/or SDB in the first 5 years of life are more likely to have special education needs by 8 years of age (Bonuck et al, 2012). Children with SDB are also found to have more frequent oxygen desaturations, pulmonary hypertension, systemic hypertension, and growth problems (Faruqui et al, 2011). Recent literature has also revealed a relationship between fragmented sleep, headaches, motor vehicle accidents, and, specifically, obesity, which is a mounting problem in our country (Faruqui et al, 2011). Pediatric sleep problems can also impact family members by causing interrupted sleep, which may lead to increased stress, decreased coping ability, and impaired daily functioning.

Sleep difficulties, which are a common concern of parents, are experienced by approximately 25% to 30% of all children and adolescents, regardless of age (Maintehran et al, 2012). Common sleep problems include behavioral insomnia, insufficient sleep, SDB, parasomnias, nightmares, periodic limb movements (PLMs), excessive sleepiness, and narcolepsy. Children with neurodevelopmental disorders (NDDs), such as autism spectrum disorders (ASDs) or attention-deficit/hyperactivity disorder (ADHD), experience more sleep disorders than typically developing children, with an estimated 50% to 95% meeting criteria for a sleep disorder (Cordum et al, 2014). The most prevalent concerns reported by parents of both NDD and typically developing children are difficulty falling asleep and frequent night awakenings.

Despite the clinical importance and high prevalence, sleep disorders are underrecognized by primary care physicians. Among 600 community pediatricians surveyed, about 20% do not routinely screen for sleep issues in school-age children during well-child visits (Amintehran et al, 2013). Another study found that only 20% of pediatricians have received formal sleep disorder training, a barrier to counseling youth and their guardians regarding sleep problems (Faruqui et al, 2011).

Sleep is traditionally considered a time of renewal for the mind and body, but it is not simply a state of rest. The brain is more active during certain periods of sleep than it is in wakefulness, and researchers believe sleep is essential for brain development, which may be one reason that infants and young children spend the majority of their time asleep. Growth, healing, learning, processing of information, and many other functions are facilitated by the sleep state. Sleep restriction results in an increase in daytime sleepiness and poorer performance on vigilance and memory tasks (Gruber et al, 2012). In normally developing children, 7 to 11 years old with no reported sleep problems, a cumulative sleep extension of 27 minutes has been associated with detectable improvement in emotional lability, impulsive behaviors, and daytime sleepiness, whereas a cumulative sleep restriction of 54 minutes was associated with a detectable deterioration in the same measures (Gruber et al, 2012). These findings are significant because they demonstrate how seemingly minor sleep changes can impact a child's academic performance.

Sleep issues and obesity have been linked in a variety of studies. Short sleep duration in adolescents has been demonstrated to increase the risk of obesity. One study prospectively followed nearly 800 children from preadolescence to early adolescence, third grade to sixth grade, and showed that shorter sleep in preadolescence increased the risk of being overweight by the sixth grade (Shochat et al, 2014). Furthermore, insufficient sleep was recently found to increase the risk of obesity in adolescents, regardless of physical activity (Iglay-Reger et al, 2014). Interestingly, the same study found that naps did not counteract the obesity effect, even when added into the total sleep duration.

OSA has been suggested to be a contributing factor to the pathogenesis of obesity by inducing leptin resistance and increasing ghrelin levels. Leptin is a key hormonal regulator of appetite and metabolism; it promotes a sense of fullness leading to reduced food intake. Ghrelin is a hormone secreted in the gut that increases appetite. Leptin resistance and increased ghrelin levels can potentiate cravings of high-calorie comfort foods (Tan et al, 2013). OSA generally causes insufficient sleep, compounding this metabolic insult.

Normal Sleep Stages and Cycles

Circadian Rhythm and Establishment of Normal Sleep Patterns

The circadian rhythm is an internal, endogenous clock that exists in all living organisms. This natural rhythm is synchronized to the 24-hour light-dark cycle, is genetically determined, and typically lasts slightly longer than 24 hours (American Academy of Sleep Medicine, 2014). Circadian rhythms emerge at about 2 to 3 months of age and are affected by melatonin secretion from the hypothalamus. A special center in the hypothalamus, called the *suprachiasmatic nucleus (SCN),* releases melatonin in response to darkness, as perceived by a nerve pathway from the retina in the eye. This melatonin cycle is established between 4 to 6 months of age. The SCN initiates signals to other parts of the brain that control hormones, body temperature, and other functions that play a role in making us feel sleepy or wide awake (National Sleep Foundation, 2015a).

Sleep Cycle

Normal sleep can be divided into two distinct phases: rapid eye movement (REM) sleep and non-rapid eye movement (NREM) sleep. NREM sleep can be further divided into three distinct stages as defined by changes in EEG patterns. NREM sleep constitutes of about 75% to 80% of total time spent in sleep, with the remaining 20% to 25% spent in REM sleep. These sleep stages make up sleep cycles, each lasting approximately 90 minutes, with about six of these cycles occurring per night.

Non-Rapid Eye Movement Sleep

Stage 1 (NREM1 or N1)

N1 sleep is a state of drowsiness and occurs at the transition to sleep. Aside from newborns and children diagnosed with narcolepsy, the average child's sleep stage begins in N1 sleep. There may be eye-rolling movements, decreased body movements, and possibly opening and closing of the eyelids. Individuals may believe they are awake, but they cannot accurately report events that occurred during this time. N1 sleep typically accounts for 3% to 8% of the total sleep time.

Stage 2 (NREM2 or N2)

N2 sleep is somewhat deeper than N1, although a person can still be easily aroused. There is a slowing of eye movements, breathing, and heart rate during N2. Muscles weaken also, but a child can still reposition himself. N2 sleep accounts for approximately 45% to 55% of total sleep time.

Stage 3 (NREM3 or N3)

N3 sleep is also known as *deep, delta,* or *slow-wave sleep (SWS).* During this stage of sleep, a child is even less responsive to the outside environment, and it can be very difficult to awaken a child during this stage. N3 sleep occurs in longer periods during the first half of the night, particularly during the first two sleep cycles, and represents around 15% to 20% of the total sleep time. Historically, NREM stage 4 (NREM4 or N4) was recognized, but, following the guidelines of the American Academy of Sleep Medicine (AASM), it is now included in the N3 sleep stage (American Academy of Sleep Medicine, 2014).

Rapid Eye Movement Sleep

REM sleep is characterized by increased electroencephalographic (EEG) activity and bursts of REMs similar to a wake state. Individuals experience vivid dreams, with simultaneous muscle paralysis that is thought to protect the person from physically acting out the dream. REM sleep is considered a time for the brain to learn from the experiences of the day. The amount of REM sleep is highest at infancy, around 55%, and decreases to about 20% to 25% by 5 years old. The majority of REM sleep occurs during the latter portion of the night.

If children are deprived of REM or SWS, pressure to restore that particular phase of sleep mounts. A rebound pattern develops as the body shortens other stages of sleep to obtain the stage that it has been lacking. Furthermore, patients deprived of REM sleep become excitable and anxious, and those deprived of SWS often present with intense fatigue. It may be that REM is related to psychological recovery and NREM is related to musculoskeletal recovery.

Sleep Cycle Processes

The sleep cycle order is normally N1, N2, N3, and REM. There is a greater amount of deep sleep (stage N3) earlier in the night, while the proportion of REM sleep increases in the last two cycles just before natural awakening. Individuals often have brief arousals between sleep cycles; most are so brief that they cannot be recalled.

Sleep Patterns by Age Group

Sleep changes with age, in duration, cycling, and habits. The average duration is seen in Table 14-1. Differences in sleep

TABLE 14-1 **Average Sleep by Age**

Age	Nighttime Sleep (hours)	Daytime Sleep (hours)
1 week old	8.25	8.25
1 month old	8.5	7
3 months old	10	5
6 months old	11	3.4
9 months old	11.2	2.8
12 months old	11.7	2.4
18 months old	11.6	1.8
2 years old	11.4	
3-5 years old	12.5	
5-11 years old	11	
12-17 years old	8-9	

Adapted from Dewar G: Baby sleep requirements: a guide for the science-minded, Parenting Science (website), 2008. www.parentingscience.com/baby-sleep-requirements.html. Accessed January 10, 2010; Dewar G: Newborn sleep patterns: a survival guide for the science-minded parent, Parenting Science (website), 2008. www.parentingscience.com/newborn-sleep.html. Accessed January 10, 2010; Jenni O, Molinari L, Caflisch J, et al: Sleep duration from ages 1 to 10 years: variability and stability in comparison with growth, *Pediatrics* 120(4):e769–e776, 2007; Rodriguez AJ: Pediatric sleep and epilepsy, *Curr Neurol Neurosci Rep* 7(4):342–347, 2007.

are described in this section, although the trends vary from child to child. There are no clear differences in sleep patterns as children move from one age group to the next; changes occur gradually.

Newborns

Newborn sleep is different from the sleep of older infants and children. Infants younger than 6 months old spend 50% of their sleep time in active REM sleep, compared with 20% to 25% in older children. REM sleep can be active in newborns with audible suckling. Newborns often enter REM sleep initially, unlike older children and adults who don't typically experience REM sleep until at least 90 minutes into the sleep cycle, and the sleep cycles are closer to 60 minutes. Active REM emerges more often during a sleep cycle in infants, resulting in shorter sleep cycles. By 6 months old, the infant's sleep architecture closely resembles that of an adult's.

Newborns sleep a total of 10.5 to 18 hours per day on an irregular schedule with periods of 1 to 3 hours spent awake (National Sleep Foundation, n.d.b). Sleep in newborns can last a few minutes to several hours, and they are often active during sleep with sucking, smiling, and twitching of arms and legs. Newborns need to feed frequently, and breastfeeding has been proposed to be one of the most prominent reasons for bed sharing. Nighttime feedings are usually not necessary by 6 months old, and many children will begin sleeping through the night; 70% to 80% will do so by 9 months old (National Sleep Foundation, n.d.b).

Sudden Infant Death Syndrome and Sleep Positioning

Deaths from sudden infant death syndrome (SIDS) have drastically decreased since the American Academy of Pediatrics (AAP) recommended that all infants sleep on their backs. However, sleep-related deaths from other causes, including suffocation, entrapment, and asphyxia, have increased. Therefore a new policy statement and technical report providing recommendations was released (AAP, 2011). Three important additions to the recommendations include:

- Breastfeeding is recommended and is associated with a reduced risk of SIDS.
- Infants should be immunized. Evidence suggests that immunization reduces the risk of SIDS by 50%.
- Bumper pads should not be used in cribs. There is no evidence that bumper pads prevent injuries, and there is a potential risk of suffocation, strangulation, or entrapment.

The largest ever meta-analysis of individual cases of SIDS evaluated and compared home sleeping arrangements of infants in 19 studies across the United Kingdom, Europe, and Australia. Breastfed infants younger than 3 months old who were bed sharing had a fivefold increase in the risk of SIDS even with nonsmoking and non-drug taking parents. Smoking, alcohol, and drugs greatly increased the SIDS risk when bed sharing in infants younger than 3 months old (Carpenter et al, 2013).

Toddlers

Toddlers need about 12 to 14 hours of sleep in a 24-hour period, and most toddlers transition to one nap around 18 to 22 months of age (National Sleep Foundation, n.d.b; Weintraub et al, 2012). Sleep difficulties are common in this age group and include resisting going to bed and nighttime awakenings because of toddlers' innate need for independence, as well as their increases in motor, social, and cognitive abilities. They are able to physically get out of bed, and this can become problematic. Separation anxiety, which is a normal developmental stage for children, ages 6 months to 2 years, can also contribute to resistance at bedtime (AAP, 2015). Nighttime fears and nightmares are also common in this age.

Some families co-sleep with their toddlers for cultural reasons, and other families co-sleep when they are unsuccessful at getting children to sleep in their own beds. Bed sharing is more common in Hispanic and black families (Barajas et al, 2011).

Preschoolers (3 to 5 Years Old)

Preschoolers typically sleep 11 to 13 hours each night, and most do not nap after they are 5 years old. As with toddlers, difficulty falling asleep and waking up during the night are common. With further development of imagination, preschoolers commonly experience nighttime fears and nightmares. In addition, sleepwalking and night terrors (or sleep terrors) peak during preschool years. Regular daytime routines promote regular sleep patterns too (Kouroglioti et al, 2014).

School-Age Children (5 to 12 Years Old)

Children from 5 to 12 years old need 10 to 11 hours of sleep. Some 5-year-olds still require a nap, but this need typically declines by first grade. If children still need naps in grade school, further evaluation is needed. Demands from school (homework), sports, and other extracurricular activities increase during this time. In addition, school-age children typically become more interested in TV, computers, and the Internet and also consume more caffeine products. All of these factors can lead to difficulty sleeping (Cespedes et al, 2014).

Older Children and Adolescents

Adolescents are notorious for not getting enough sleep. Most get less than the 8 to 9 hours recommended by the Centers for Disease Control and Prevention (CDC) (Matthews et al, 2014). Black males got the least amount of sleep. Adolescents have multiple reasons for not getting enough sleep including:

- A natural shift in their sleep schedule: After puberty, a biologic shift occurs in an adolescent's internal clock of about 2 hours, making it difficult to fall asleep early.
- Early high school start times: In most school districts, the move to high school is accompanied by an earlier school start time, which can be as early as 7:00 AM. Teens often have to wake up by 5:00 AM to get ready.
- Social and school obligations: Teens spend 30 to 35 hours per week on average in class and an additional 4 to 5 hours per week doing homework (Shochat et al, 2014). After-school activities, sports, and socializing often lead to late nights, adding to the problem. As a result, most adolescents can be sleep deprived.

Sleep Across Cultures

Mindell and colleagues (2013) conducted a large study of 10,085 children from 14 countries. Parents of Asian children reported significantly more sleep problems than parents in predominantly Caucasian nations. Chinese parents reported the highest rates of perceived sleep problems in both younger children (0 to 3 years old, 52%) and older children (3 to 6 years old, 44%).

Assessment of Sleep

History

Chief Complaint

Evaluation of potential sleep problems involves a comprehensive history of the child's 24-hour routine, focusing on bedtime habits, sleep environment, and daytime behavior. The family medical history along with the caregiver's attitudes and beliefs about what constitutes normal sleep are vital and can guide the investigation and treatment. The following topics should be addressed with the family:

- Routines used for getting the child to sleep, sleep resistance, and parental response to objections.
- Sleep aids (such as, pacifiers, blankets, and stuffed animals) and patting or rocking.
- Room environment, including co-sleeping, room temperature, and electronics used in the room.
- Nighttime behavior, such as prolonged awakening, night terrors, sleep walking, sleep eating, seizures, and head banging.
- Nighttime complaints of leg pain, restless sleep, and kicking, which can be associated with PLMs.
- SDB, such as snoring, gasping, apneas, cyanosis, headaches upon awakening, loud breathing, mouth breathing, neck hyperextension, and frequent position changes.
- Excessive secretions/drooling.
- Wake up times and daytime symptoms, such as difficulty waking up, falling asleep in class, hyperactivity, and overall emotional and cognitive functioning.
- Medications, caffeine intake (effects of caffeine can last up to 8 hours), exercise, and diet.

When sleep difficulties are noted, it is important to ask about the age when the problem began; precipitating events; presence of the symptoms on the weekends, holidays, and vacation; and if aggravating and alleviating factors are present. It is also necessary to ask about the effects on the child's daily living, as well as the impact on family members.

General Health History

Past Medical History and Review of Systems

Medical problems of the child are often associated with sleep difficulties. Pain and discomfort are important factors to consider. Assess the following:

- Obesity with sleep disordered breathing (SDB).
- Neurologic disorders (such as, ADHD, autism, cerebral palsy, and neuromuscular disorders) are associated with both BSP and SDB.
- Respiratory conditions, such as hypoxemia, asthma, laryngomalacia, and allergic rhinitis. OSA and asthma are highly prevalent respiratory disorders and are frequently comorbid (Prasad et al, 2013).
- Gastroesophageal reflux, which contributes to OSA especially in newborns and infants.
- Nocturnal enuresis, which can be associated with SDB.
- Dermatologic problems causing discomfort, such as itching (Chang et al, 2014).
- Pulmonary hypertension can be caused by untreated SDB and is important to assess.
- Failure to thrive secondary to increased caloric expenditure from increased work of breathing.
- Developmental delays, which can affect the child's ability to learn appropriate sleep behaviors.
- Epilepsy: Children with a seizure disorder are at increased risk for sleep disorders.
- Depression, anxiety, or other psychiatric problems can be significant in insomnia.

Family Assessment

Assess the following:

- Parental knowledge and expectations about infant and child sleep patterns.
- Parental ability and willingness to modify sleep hygiene.
- Family history of sleep disorders: SDB is often familial, which is important information for clinicians (Lundkvist et al, 2012).
- Recent divorces, separation, family, or close friend death or other family stressors.
- Recent changes in the living arrangements.

Physical Examination

A thorough physical examination should always be conducted, especially evaluating for signs of illness or pain in an individual presenting with a sleep issue. Vital signs should be obtained, including pulse oximetry, weight, body mass index (BMI), and blood pressure. Neurologic evaluation, including the child's muscle tone, needs to be completed because abnormal muscle tone can contribute to SDB. Special attention to obvious hyperactivity, anxiety, and/or depression is needed to fully evaluate the child.

Physical findings that may indicate sleep apnea include swollen turbinates, deviated septum, nasal polyps, open mouth posture, adenoid facies, large tonsils, narrow oropharynx, low hanging palate, high arched hard palate, micrognathia, or retrognathia.

Diagnostic Studies

Some sleep studies are practical for primary care providers. Others are ordered by sleep clinics where more technical measures are necessary.

A sleep-feeding-activity record for infants (Fig. 14-1) or a 2-week sleep diary (Fig. 14-2) can be useful for primary care providers and caregivers to identify patterns of awakenings and routines and is helpful when evaluating children with insomnia.

Sleep clinics may do studies, such as actigraphy. *Actigraphy* measures light exposure and activity over a period of time (typically 1 week) in the home environment. A device is worn on the wrist that resembles a watch band. In general, there is a good correlation between the polysomnogram (PSG) and actigraph-defined total sleep time, sleep latency, and sleep efficiency (percentage of time in bed spent sleeping) (El Shakankiry, 2011). Actigraphy is also helpful for evaluating the effectiveness of insomnia treatments, because total sleep time is measured. Actigraphy is often utilized along with a personal sleep diary recorded by the child (if age appropriate) or the parent. Furthermore, actigraphy offers objectivity and can dispel sleep misperceptions, which

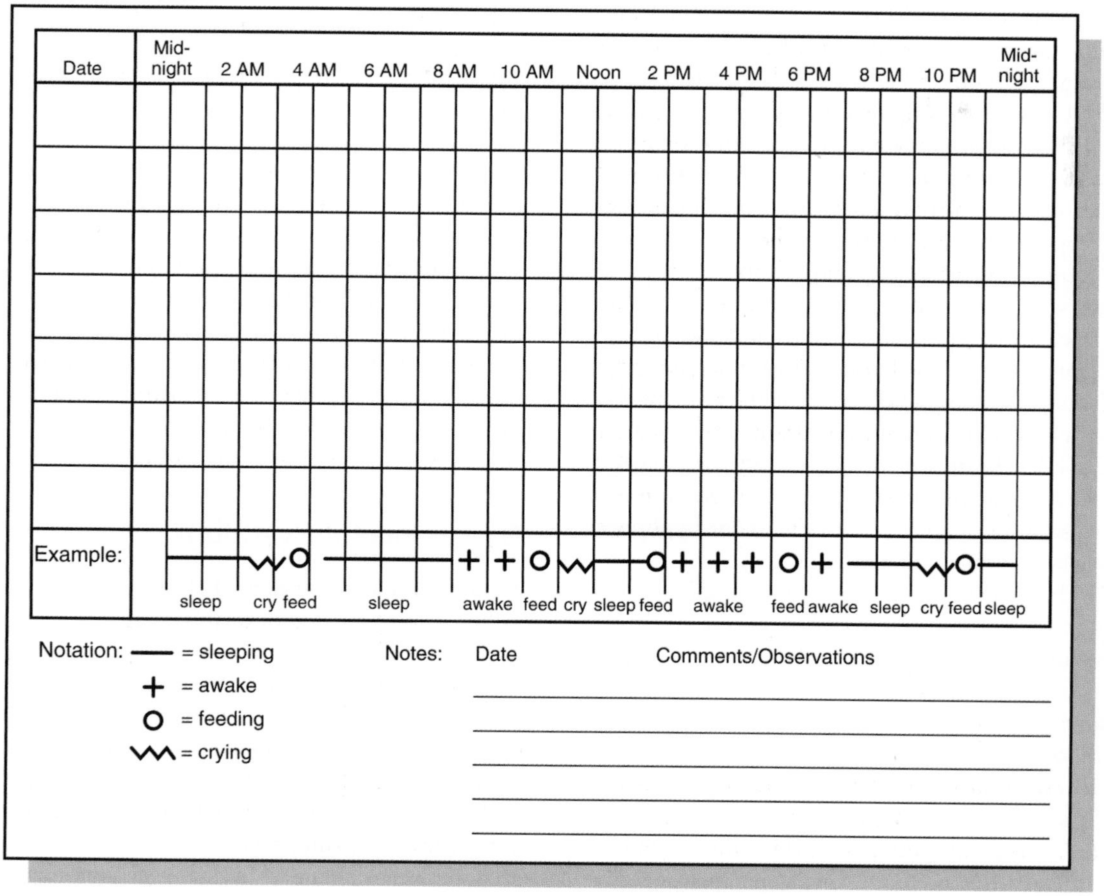

• **Figure 14-1** Example of a sleep-activity-feeding record.

Two-Week Sleep Diary	
Week 1:	Week 2:
Mon	Mon
Tue	Tue
Wed	Wed
Thu	Thu
Fri	Fri
Sat	Sat
Sun	Sun
Instructions: Describe your child's sleep each day. How long does your child sleep? What is the time it took to go to sleep? What are the hours of sleep? Describe issues during the night.	

• **Figure 14-2** Two-week sleep diary.

are common in some pediatric populations. For example, some adolescents will report being awake most of the night when they are actually sleeping a fair amount of time. Parents are not always able to quantify the amount of sleep of their children, because they are sleeping as well.

Diagnosing SDB in children can be a challenge, because the history and physical have a poor predictive value and have been shown to be equivalent to that of tossing a coin (Tan et al, 2013). Therefore, the AAP recommends that children with symptoms of OSA should be referred for further investigation with either a PSG or a referral to an ear, nose, and throat (ENT) surgeon or sleep provider. Either the PCP can order the PSG prior to referral or start with a referral, depending on their own comfort level with the decision and the process. A PSG is an overnight sleep study in a sleep lab that evaluates the child's breathing by identifying central, obstructive, and periodic breathing abnormalities with continuous pulse oximetry, heart rate, respiratory rate, end-tidal carbon dioxide, and video monitoring. It is considered the gold standard for the diagnosis of OSA (Marcus et al, 2012a). PLMs, which can be associated with both SDB and arousals, can also be identified. An expanded EEG can be added to the sleep study if seizures are suspected. A PSG will provide specific information on how many obstructive and/or central apneas or hypopneas are noted per hour during the night.

In 2011, the AASM recommended that all children undergoing an adenotonsillectomy (TA) have a nocturnal in-lab sleep study to evaluate for the presence and severity of SDB, because the history and physical are not completely reliable (Owens et al, 2012). The AASM also recommends follow-up sleep studies for children at risk for residual SDB, such as obesity, craniofacial abnormalities, and severe baseline SDB (Cielo and Brooks, 2013). Performing a PSG before surgery allows the surgery team to understand the severity of the OSA so that perioperative and postoperative complications can be anticipated. Additionally, a preoperative PSG helps determine which patients need a repeat PSG after surgery (Cielo and Brooks, 2013). Overnight pulse oximetry studies in the home are convenient and less expensive than PSGs. However, home pulse oximetry studies can be inaccurate secondary to detachment from the patient, especially in young children, and can yield erroneous data.

Strategies for Prevention and Management of Sleep Problems

Sleep Hygiene Promotion

Prevention of sleep problems involves promoting good sleep hygiene and can be established early by providing a dark, quiet, and slightly cool room for sleeping and a consistent sleep routine. Parents can use a variety of cues to set the sleep cycle, including daylight, darkness, meals, and activities. Making these cues clear to infants and children to help them establish healthy bedtime and sleep patterns is important. Exposure to light, even for brief periods of time, can prevent the secretion of melatonin, which is needed for sleep. Sleep promotion is discussed further in Chapter 5.

Dyssomnia Interventions

Dyssomnias are disorders of sleep related to the process of falling asleep, putting oneself back to sleep from an arousal, and sleeping on a regular basis at a reasonable time. Causes can be organic, such as SDB, narcolepsy, pain, illness, seizures, or adjustments to a new environment. However, many children learn poor sleep hygiene habits early and prevention is the best key. Although there are no data showing the best age at which to start behavioral strategies for sleep implementation, clinical experience suggests that between 3 and 4 months of age may be an ideal time (Thomas et al, 2014). Behavioral interventions before

3 months old are not recommended because infants may still need to feed frequently. Placing infants into their crib drowsy but still awake allows them to initiate sleep independently in their own environment and enables them to return to sleep independently throughout the night. This strategy has been found to be the most important recommendation for parents in multiple studies (Kuhn, 2014). Developing regular daytime and bedtime routines is also important to start at this stage of development. Have a relaxing bedtime routine that ends in the room where the child sleeps. The child should also sleep in the same sleeping environment every night, in a room that is cool, quiet, and dark—and without a TV.

Some schools in the country have delayed school start times with a resulting improvement in overall academic performance, less fighting between students, and improved attendance. A study from the University of Minnesota (2014) found that there was a 70% drop in the number of car crashes involving teen drivers at Jackson Hole High School in Wyoming, which shifted to the latest start time of the eight schools (8:55 AM). Recently, the AAP has recommended that schools make efforts to optimize sleep in students, aiming to make start times later. Effects anticipated include physical and mental health, safety, academic performance, and quality of life (AAP Adolescent Sleep Working Group, 2014).

Primary Care Interventions for Dyssomnias

When parents need further intervention strategies for sleep, several techniques have been shown to be helpful. They center on behavioral therapy.

Unmodified Extinction

Unmodified extinction is also known as *sleep training* or *systematic ignoring,* and it allows the child to cry it out. Parents implement a scheduled, pre-sleep bedtime routine, placing children in bed and ignoring all subsequent sleep interfering behaviors until the morning. This method does not appeal to all families and relies on strict structure. Most families see results in approximately 3 nights.

Graduated Extinction

Graduated extinction incorporates the same philosophy of establishing a bedtime routine but allows the parents to implement brief, planned checks on their child, assuring safety but with minimized parental attention (verbal and physical). The visits are systematically reduced until the child initiates and maintains sleep independently. This approach may take a few days to a few months.

An alternate form of graduated extinction allows the parent to sit with the drowsy child and then leave before the child falls asleep, promising to return. The parent may start by leaving for only several seconds but always returns, gradually extending the absences. The goal is for the child to fall asleep independently when the parent is out of the room. This approach can also take time but is beneficial for some families.

The Bedtime Pass

The bedtime pass is a novel variant of graduated extinction that targets bedtime resistance in children who are preschool to school age. The pass is a ticket and can be anything appreciated by the child; it is often helpful to have the child help make the pass. For example, asking the child to pick out pictures of his or her favorite movie character and laminating the pictures can act as bedtime passes. Parents inform their child that the pass may be exchanged for one visit in the child's room after bedtime by a parent or one opportunity to come out of the child's room. The child is told that once the pass is used, he or she cannot come out or call out from the room again that night. If the child uses the pass but then stays in his room until morning, the child can have a treat, such as a favorite breakfast. After some time, parents can supplement the rules and if the child does not use the pass at all, they get a "free reward" (e.g., 10 minutes of screen time or a sticker chart). Providing an immediate reward instead of later in the day is more effective.

Sleep in Children with Developmental and Neurologic Conditions

Children with ADHD and autism have the highest rates of sleep problems of all children with mental challenges, and like normally developing children, behavioral insomnia is the most common complaint. Resistance to bedtime and insufficient sleep in this population have been attributed partially to intrinsic dysregulation of neurotransmitters affecting sleep and wake patterns. In addition, this population of children can have difficulty understanding and implementing sleep routines, which are necessary for proper sleep hygiene (Cordum et al, 2014). Comorbid psychiatric disorders are common in these groups and contribute to the sleep difficulties.

Children with ADHD and sleep problems have been found to have poorer outcomes than children without sleep problems, including negative impacts on behavior, cognitive functioning, and family functioning. This is understandable considering that normally developing children with sleep deprivation have ADHD-like behaviors, such as inattention and short-term memory problems. Autistic children are especially prone to communication deficits, and sleep-onset delay has been found to be the strongest predictor of this, as well as stereotypical behavior (Cordum et al, 2014). Because of the high prevalence of sleep problems in this population, all children with NDDs should be screened for sleep problems.

Behavioral therapy is also the most effective intervention for managing insomnia in children with NDDs. However, a modified, staged approach is recommended to help these children secondary to their various abilities to comprehend. Furthermore, children with NDDs may benefit from a visual schedule or a "to do" list with pictures, words, or both to help remind them of each step.

Medications

Medications are not generally recommended as a first-line therapy for children with sleep problems. Behavioral therapy and establishing good sleep hygiene are the mainstays for any child with difficulties sleeping and need to be incorporated even if medication is used (Cordum et al, 2014).

Melatonin has been shown to be beneficial for sleep disorders of different etiologies—not only primary but also associated with mental, neurologic, or other medical disorders (Sanchez-Barceló et al, 2011). Although melatonin is the most commonly prescribed medication for insomnia, wide variation exists in the dosing used, and this suggests an urgent need to develop clear guidance for providers (Heussler et al, 2013). Hypnotic drugs, such as benzodiazepines, are discouraged because of the problems with dependence and because they are used for their sedative adverse effects rather than for primary effects on sleep-wake cycles or hyperarousal.

Antihistamines have not been studied for sleep effectiveness when used for long periods, and diphenhydramine, which is commonly used for its sedation properties, can encourage parasomnias in those children prone to them. A review of pharmacologic treatment of insomnia in children found that zolpidem (Ambien) produced high levels of side effects and was not effective in increasing total sleep time or decreasing sleep latency (Barrett et al, 2013).

Common Sleep Problems

Parasomnias: Night Terrors, Sleepwalking, and Nightmares

Parasomnias describe a group of sleep disorders that occur during NREM and REM sleep. NREM parasomnias include confusional arousals, somnambulism or sleep walking, night terrors, rhythmic movement disorders, benign neonatal sleep myoclonus, bruxism, and nocturnal enuresis. REM parasomnias include nightmares.

Precipitating factors for all NREM parasomnias include SDB, PLM, sleep deprivation, stress, fever, being overheated at night, full bladder, and use of central nervous system depressant medications. These factors can interrupt sleep; and when this interruption occurs during deep sleep, it can cause a partial awakening resulting in a parasomnia (scary dream). Benadryl, in particular, is a common medication used in children, which is known to precipitate parasomnias, because it increases N3 sleep. Identification and treatment of primary sleep disorders, such as PLMs and OSA, often results in the resolution of parasomnia symptoms (Haupt et al, 2013).

Non-Rapid Eye Movement Parasomnias

NREM parasomnias occur during N3 sleep and typically occur in the first third of the sleep cycle because that is when the majority of NREM sleep occurs. Furthermore, most NREM parasomnias occur at the end of the first sleep cycle or about 90 minutes into sleep. Most children have no memory of the events. Most episodes are brief, but they may last as long as 30 to 40 minutes. Waking up the child during any parasomnia is not recommended, because it can prolong the episodes. NREM parasomnias are often inherited. The movements exhibited during NREM parasomnias can be very complex. Confusional arousals, night terrors, and sleep walking can all be normal for children; but if they occur frequently, become prolonged, or pose a threat to safety (sleep walking), further evaluation is warranted.

Confusional Arousals

Confusional arousals occur when a child is awakened from a deep sleep during the first part of the night and is also known as excessive sleep inertia or sleep drunkenness (El Shakankiry, 2011). Children will sit up in bed, appear dazed, and often react slowly to questions. Confusional arousals occur around 2 years old and are typically benign but frightening for the parents. They generally diminish by 5 years old.

Sleep Walking

Sleep walking or stalking typically begin as confusional arousals but can also begin with the child getting out of bed and running with complex movements. The child typically appears dazed with open eyes, and the speech is mumbled and slurred. Sleep walking is common, occurring in approximately 1% to 15% of children, and is usually benign. These parasomnias are common around 4 years old and resolve around 8 years old (El Shakankiry, 2011). Of the parasomnias, sleep walking has the potential to be the most dangerous to the child (American Academy of Sleep Medicine, 2014).

Night Terrors

Night terrors are characterized by an extreme state of agitation when the child awakens from N3 sleep screaming. Dilated pupils, increased heart rate, and sweating are common. Like other arousals, they are typically short lived but can be prolonged with parental interference. Night terrors are reported in 1% to 6% of children, typically occurring after 18 months of age and resolved by 6 years old (El Shakankiry, 2011).

Rapid Eye Movement Parasomnias

Nightmares are frequently confused with night terrors, but they are distinctly different. Nightmares occur during REM sleep and are characterized by a sudden arousal from sleep to a fully awake state, whereas night terrors occur during N3 sleep and the child is, in reality, asleep during the event without recollection. Nightmares are typically recalled in detail even the next day. The average onset of nightmares is 36 to 72 months old, affecting between 25% and 50% of all children 3 to 6 years old (El Shakankiry, 2011).

Nightmares typically occur during the last portion of the night, whereas night terrors occur mostly in the first third of the night. Occasional nightmares are common during childhood and reassurance is generally effective. However, recurrent nightmares can be associated with daytime stressors, and further psychological evaluation may be needed (Haupt et al, 2013).

Assessment of Parasomnias

History

The health history for parasomnias should include the following topics:

- Characteristics of the event, including timing in relation to sleep onset, frequency, and length
- Symptoms of SDB or PLM
- Temperature of sleeping environment and sweating status of child despite the temperature
- Family history
- Medications
- Sleep patterns (how much sleep is obtained)
- Memory of the event

Treatment of Parasomnias

Parasomnias can be normal in all children, but if they are frequent, prolonged, or causing potential harm (such as, a sleep walking episode where the child leaves the house), further evaluation is warranted. If SDB is present, evaluation with a sleep study or referral to a sleep provider or ENT surgeon is needed.

Normalizing sleep patterns and calmly guiding the child back to bed (if sleep walking) without attempting to awaken the child seem to be the most effective actions for parasomnias (Haupt et al, 2013). Placing a bell on the child's bedroom door to alert parents that the child is leaving the room and making sure the house is secure are needed for somnambulism.

Sleep Cycle Problems (Circadian Rhythm Disorders)

Delayed Sleep Phase

The sleep cycle begins at a late hour and is followed by a late awakening. The child's internal clock for sleep and rest is not consistent with appropriate hours for sleep. Excessive naps or late morning waking may be related factors, especially for school-age children and adolescents.

Differential Diagnoses

The differential diagnoses are prolonged bedtime routine and oppositional disorder, which both involve active resistance to going to bed rather than inability to fall asleep.

Management

Three approaches are suggested:

1. Keep the nighttime routine in place, but awaken the child earlier each morning in 15-minute increments.
2. For the adolescent or older child who is off schedule by many hours (e.g., at the end of summer when beginning the school year will require getting up earlier), it could take weeks to back up the cycle appropriately using 15-minute increments. In this case, it is better to go forward in time. In other words, have the child remain awake until the next evening and then go to bed at the desired hour, beginning the desired routine from that point.
3. Have the child or family keep a sleep log to document gradual change.

Advanced Sleep Phase

The sleep cycle begins too early with correlated early rising.

Management

Meals, naps, and bedtime should be delayed until the desired times. The early waking resolves itself.

Inappropriate or Unpredictable Schedules

Some people have a poorly organized sleep-wake cycle. This is described by some as a temperament problem of rhythmicity.

Management

The routines of eating, activities, and sleeping should be kept as regular as possible. The older child may need to learn to play quietly in bed until others awaken or until a clock radio begins to play. At night, the child may need to learn to read or listen to music in bed when bedtime comes.

Nocturnal Enuresis

Nocturnal enuresis is a common complaint in children and widely regarded as a parasomnia by most sleep researchers, because it occurs only during NREM sleep. Primary enuresis occurs in children who have never attained dryness at night, whereas secondary enuresis occurs in children who have previously been potty trained. Similar to other disorders, there is a strong family predisposition for enuresis. SDB has been associated with enuresis, which is possibly due to the frequent arousals associated with SDB that often cause a lack of arousal for the child who needs to void. In 2010, the International Children's Continence Society (ICCS) published evidence- and consensus-based recommendations for evaluating and treating monosymptomatic enuresis. The ICCS recommends screening for symptoms of OSA during the initial evaluation of children with enuresis who snore loudly, because their enuresis may remit once their OSA is successively treated (Kotagal et al, 2012). See Chapter 12 for a further discussion of enuresis.

Restless Legs Syndrome and Periodic Limb Movements

Restless leg syndrome (RLS) has long been identified as a parasomnia in adults. RLS is a sensory and motor disorder characterized by irritating sensations in the legs accompanied by an irresistible urge to move the legs, which typically helps. PLMs are repetitive jerks, typically in the legs, that are found by PSG to occur every 5 to 90 seconds. RLS and PLMs usually occur together, but PLMs may occur without RLS.

The prevalence of PLMs in school-age children has been estimated to be 1.9% to 3.6%; however, the presence is often unrecognized in younger children or those with delays secondary to communication deficits. The exact etiology still remains partly unclear, but genetic factors, dopaminergic dysfunction, and low iron storage status have shown to play important roles (Tilma et al, 2013). Altered brain acquisition of iron has been identified as a major factor in RLS (Connor et al, 2011), although blood iron levels may be normal. Peripheral neuropathy and uremia are also causes of secondary RLS. Medications such as antidepressants, selective serotonin reuptake inhibitors (SSRIs), sedating antihistamines, and dopamine receptor antagonists may worsen or precipitate cases. PLMs and nighttime arousals are increased with sertraline (Zoloft) treatment, so clinicians should pay more attention to PLMs during SSRI treatment (Zang et al, 2013).

Clinical Findings and Diagnosis

Children will often complain of leg pain or itchy, crawly sensations. Affected children may complain to their parents that spiders or bugs are in their bed, and parents will find some improvement with massage. Sleep onset may be normal followed by arousal with the symptoms shortly thereafter. A recent study found the most striking single symptom of RLS or PLMs was awakening after 1 to 3 hours of sleep followed by screaming, crying, kicking, and slapping the legs or by verbally expressing that the legs hurt (Tilma et al, 2013). RLS and PLMs are associated with fragmented sleep, unrefreshed sleep, insomnia, daytime sleepiness, and hyperactivity. Generally, the child has a normal physical and neurologic examination. Diagnosis of PLMs/RLS is often based on the history and physical examination. If there are suspicions for SDB, a PSG is warranted; and if five or more PLMs per hour are experienced, PLMs are diagnosed. Growing pains, leg cramps, and Osgood-Schlatter disease are differential diagnoses.

Laboratory Studies

Ferritin level is a measure of one's iron supplies and can be a helpful laboratory test for PLMs. Ferritin levels less than 50 have been associated with RLS and PLMs in children, and supplementation with ferrous sulfate 3 mg/kg per day has been shown to drastically improve symptoms (Tilma et al, 2013).

Treatment

Clonazepam and gabapentin are sometimes used if ferritin levels are normal and other organic causes have been ruled out, but this should be initiated by a sleep specialist.

Head Banging and Bruxism

Rhythmic movement disorders involve head banging and body rocking and occur as the child is attempting to fall asleep. (It can repeat throughout the night when the child is trying to return to sleep.) Head banging and body rocking are the most commonly seen and can present before 2 years of age. The disorder is typically transient and self-limited and rarely requires intervention (El Shakankiry, 2011).

Sleep bruxism is stereotypic grinding or clenching of the teeth during sleep. Some believe there may be some relationship to stress. It frequently appears between 10 and 20 years old, although there is a short-lived infant version. Bruxism is seen in 8.2% of the population. Seizure disorder is a differential diagnosis. A dental referral may be useful (Carra et al, 2012). (Also see Chapter 34.)

Fear and Anxiety Dyssomnias

Evidence suggests that life stress and a predisposition to arousability are among the strongest predictors of insomnia (Harvey et al, 2014). Arousability has been indexed via cortisol output, increased brain activation, and increased heart rate, which further implicates the role of stress in the development of insomnia syndrome (Harvey et al, 2014). Evidence also points to a heredity component for insomnias.

A large study examining sleep in children and adolescents with anxiety disorders found that 88% had at least one sleep-related issue with insomnia, nightmares, and refusal to sleep alone (Kuhn, 2014). Exposure-based cognitive therapy is the method of choice for children with anxiety disorders and uses the gradual separation techniques to teach children how to master their own fears. This approach takes time, and many parents are reluctant because they are sleep deprived themselves. However, it can teach lasting coping strategies.

Depression and Sleep

Depression, oppositional defiant disorder, and generalized anxiety disorder are linked to sleep problems (Shanahan et al, 2014). A study investigating the link between sleep and depression found that gradual sleep extension combined with sleep hygiene advice had a beneficial effect on depressive symptoms of adolescents with chronic sleep reduction (Dewald-Kaufmann et al, 2014).

Epilepsy and Sleep

Children with epilepsy are two to three times more likely to have sleep problems than the general pediatric population. Children with a seizure disorder need careful evaluation of SDB, because their seizures may be increased by untreated SDB. Sleep deprivation is a trigger for seizures, and the drugs used for epilepsy may also disturb sleep. Furthermore, sleep activates the electrical charges in the brain that result in seizures, and seizures are timed according to the sleep-wake cycle (National Sleep Foundation, n.d.c). Rolandic epilepsy is benign epilepsy of childhood that occurs only during sleep and can cause awakenings that are sometimes confused with insomnia (National Sleep Foundation, n.d.a). Finally, children with seizures may have comorbidities (such as, NDDs), which make behavioral therapy the first-line treatment for this group also.

Sleep Disordered Breathing

Sleep disordered breathing (SDB) describes a group of disorders characterized by abnormal respiratory patterns (Walter et al, 2013). SDB ranges from primary snoring, where gas exchange is normal and there is no interruption in sleep, to OSA. OSA in children is defined as a disorder of breathing during sleep characterized by prolonged partial upper airway obstruction and/or intermittent complete obstruction, which disrupts the normal ventilation during sleep and normal sleep patterns (Marcus et al, 2012b). Primary snoring is common in approximately 3% to 15% of children, and OSA is prevalent in about 1% to 4% of children (Walter et al, 2013). SDB is also associated with lower socioeconomic status, such as parental education and employment, as well as maternal cigarette smoking, birth weight, and gestational age (Bonuck et al, 2012).

Clinical Findings

Signs of SDB can include snoring, gasping, apneas, increased work of breathing with paradoxical respirations, neck hyperextension, night sweating, tachycardia, tachypnea, restless sleep, and disrupted sleep. Following arousals caused by SDB, the child will typically drift back to sleep with the cycle repeating itself throughout the night, resulting in sleep fragmentation and non-restorative sleep. Some children experience insomnia because of SDB either at sleep onset or awakenings after sleep onset. Symptoms may include behavioral problems, hypertension, failure to thrive, ADHD, and/or daytime sleepiness. Risk factors include enlarged tonsils and/or adenoid, obesity, craniofacial anomalies, gastroesophageal reflux, and neuromuscular disorders. Children with neuromuscular disorders might not snore and should be evaluated with other criteria, specifically increased work of breathing, tachycardia, nocturnal sweating, and daytime symptoms.

Diagnostic Studies

The American Academy of Otolaryngology—Head and Neck Surgery suggests that a PSG should be obtained before adenotonsillectomy (TA) in children with obesity, Down syndrome, craniofacial abnormalities, neuromuscular disorders, sickle cell disease, or mucopolysaccharidosis. This same group of children is at increased risk for OSA after surgical procedures (Cielo and Brooks, 2013). OSA has been shown to cause excessive daytime sleepiness and fatigue, both of which are likely to reduce physical activity. Furthermore, OSA has been shown to promote inflammatory responses, leading to cellular death and end organ morbidities (Tan et al, 2013).

Surgical and Medical Treatment of Sleep Disordered Breathing

Tonsillectomy, adenoidectomy, or both are recommended as the first-line treatments of OSA and are performed by an otolaryngologist (Tan et al, 2013). TA has been shown to be cost effective and improve the Apnea Hypopnea Index (AHI) and quality of sleep and life in children (Marcus et al, 2012a). Additionally, TA is a relatively safe procedure, and as many as 93% of patients have no intraoperative or postoperative problems. The most common risk factors are pain and poor oral intake with more severe complications including hemorrhage, dehydrations, infection, and respiratory complications (Cielo and Brooks, 2013). For children younger than 1 year old, OSA is typically treated with an adenoidectomy (if enlarged) without the tonsillectomy secondary to increased risk of bleeding and anesthesia (Ramos et al, 2013). Additional risk factors for experiencing TA postoperative complications include obesity, young age, and severe preoperative OSA (Ramos et al, 2013).

Other surgical options include partial tonsillectomy, craniofacial surgery (mandibular distraction) for micrognathia, and tracheostomy in severe cases. These therapies may not be curative, and a repeat sleep study to evaluate the efficacy is typically needed.

At times, surgery is not an option—possibly because of a lack of tonsillar or adenoid hypertrophy, young age, morbid obesity, family or surgeon preference, or other risk factors. Nonsurgical options include positive airway pressure (PAP), nasal steroids and leukotriene receptor antagonists (montelukast [Singulair]), rapid maxillary expansion, oral appliances, weight loss, and supplemental oxygen (Cielo and Brooks, 2013).

Nasal steroids and montelukast can be effective in mild or moderate OSA. They work by reducing the size of lymphoid tissue, especially the adenoids. PAP therapy includes continuous positive airway pressure (CPAP), BIPAP (bi-level support), and AVASP (volume support). CPAP is typically used to treat SDB, except in children with neuromuscular disorders or in those needing extra support with tidal volume. CPAP delivers air pressure through a nasal mask and ranges from 4 cm of water pressure to 24 cm of water pressure.

A PSG with a PAP titration is necessary to determine the amount of pressure to administer. Pediatric sleep centers manage this therapy instead of the PCP. Although PAP therapy is highly effective, it is not always tolerated, and parental involvement is necessary. However, despite suboptimal adherence use, one recent study found a significant improvement in the neurobehavioral function of children after 3 months of PAP, even in developmentally delayed children (Marcus et al, 2012b). Additional sleep studies with repeat titrations are needed for the growing child depending on their age.

Central Sleep Apnea

Central sleep apnea (CSA) refers to absences of airflow that are related to failure of the ventilatory control system to stimulate a breath (American Academy of Sleep Medicine, 2014). Unlike OSA, CSA is not associated with a snore or gasp and is common in children intermittently, especially following a sigh. When CSA occurs frequently or results in oxygen desaturations, it is considered pathologic. CSA is more common in premature children or those with neurologic conditions, such as cerebral palsy, brainstem lesions, or Chiari malformations. CSA can also be induced by narcotic use.

A life-threatening condition called *congenital central hypoventilation syndrome* can present in newborns and should prompt immediate investigation and treatment. Premature infants typically outgrow CSA, and oxygen is often used to stimulate the ventilatory system. If hypoventilation is involved with CSA, bi-level ventilatory support with a backup rate is often used to restore normal gas exchange during sleep.

Narcolepsy

Narcolepsy is a disorder characterized by excessive daytime sleepiness, fragmented nocturnal sleep, and signs of REM-sleep dissociation—the most specific of which is cataplexy. Narcolepsy is an imbalance among wakefulness, REM, and slow wave sleep states that can range from mild to severe. Cataplexy is a brief sudden loss of skeletal muscle tone, which is typically brought on by laughter but can also be stimulated by other strong emotions. Neck and knee weakness and sagging of the jaw are common complaints. Respiratory muscles are not affected; however individuals sometimes describe feeling short of breath (American Academy of Sleep Medicine, 2014). Individuals retain consciousness during cataplexy events, which can help differentiate it from some types of seizures. Not all people with narcolepsy have cataplexy. Furthermore, excessive sleepiness, which is typically the first symptom to manifest, may present years before the cataplexy (American Academy of Sleep Medicine, 2014).

Other manifestations of narcolepsy include sleep onset paralysis and hypnogogic hallucinations. Sleep paralysis is the total inability to move any muscles when falling asleep or waking up. Normal individuals may experience occasional sleep paralysis upon awakening, which is often due to sleep deprivation or even SDB; however, sleep onset paralysis suggests narcolepsy. Hypnogogic hallucinations are vivid dreamlike visual or auditory experiences that occur just as the patient is falling asleep. Children often complain of feeling someone whispering nonsense into their ear or breathing on their neck. Rarely can the child determine what the person is saying. Weight gain, PLMs, and REM behavioral disorder are also common in people with narcolepsy.

Narcolepsy with cataplexy is caused by a deficiency of hypothalamic hypocretin (orexin) signaling, which is measured in the cerebral spinal fluid. The exact cause is unknown but recent studies have shown an increase in antibodies against beta-hemolytic streptococcus, which were strongest around onset of narcolepsy and decreased with disease duration, suggesting that strep infections may trigger the event (American Academy of Sleep Medicine, 2014). Reports of narcolepsy occurring after receiving the H1N1 vaccine have also been noted, but a definite causal relationship has not yet been established.

Narcolepsy with cataplexy occurs in 0.02% to 0.18% of the United States and western European populations. There is a low prevalence of familial cases. Narcolepsy typically occurs between 10 and 25 years old; however, it is seen in children as young as 5 years old.

Diagnosing narcolepsy is complex, and a referral to a sleep specialist is warranted. Untreated narcolepsy can result in academic and social failure in children. The fragmented sleep can make school and work attendance difficult as well. Treatment of narcolepsy is focused on treatment of the symptoms because there is no cure.

For a complete list of references, please visit http://evolve.elsevier.com/Burns/pediatric/.

15 Sexuality

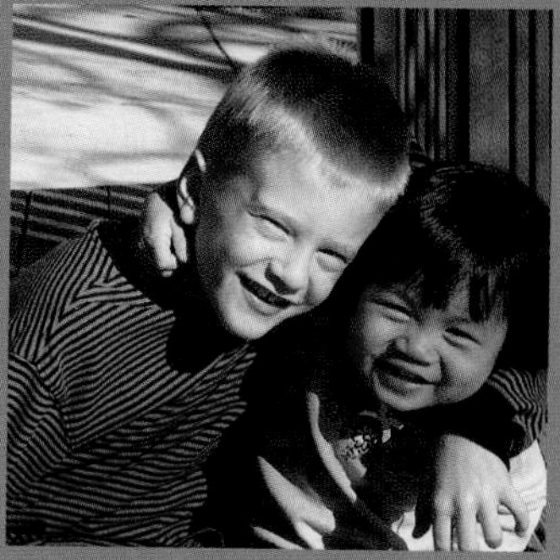

TERAL GERLT AND CATHERINE G. BLOSSER

Sexuality is the sexual knowledge, beliefs, attitudes, values, and behaviors of individuals. Its various dimensions involve the anatomy, physiology, and biochemistry of the sexual response system; identity, orientation, roles, and personality; and thoughts, feelings, and relationships. Sexuality is influenced by ethical, spiritual, cultural, and moral concerns. All persons are sexual, in the broadest sense of the word (SIECUS, 2014). Sexuality extends beyond genital sex to include gender-role and socialization, physical maturation and body image, social relationships, and future social aspirations (Murphy and Elias, 2006). The process of achieving a sense of one's sexuality in its broadest sense begins with conception and continues throughout life. Despite what parents may want to think, their children will become sexual people. The primary care provider (PCP) can play a crucial part in educating parents to anticipate, recognize, and guide their children through the stages of sexual development. The primary care visit gives parents a chance to ask questions and solicit advice from the child's provider. Also, at age-appropriate times, the primary care visit provides children and adolescents with opportunities to explore questions they have about their sexuality. Much of the literature on sexuality deals with problems. This chapter focuses on health promotion, emphasizing that sexual development is a normal and healthy part of human growth.

Standards

Performing Preventive Services: A Bright Futures Handbook, developed by the American Academy of Pediatrics (AAP; Tanski et al, 2010); the U.S. Preventive Services Task Force (USPSTF) children and adolescent recommendations (USPSTF, 2014); and the still-used *Guidelines for Adolescent Preventive Services (GAPS),* developed by the American Medical Association (AMA, 1997), offer the most comprehensive evidence- and consensus-based strategies concerning clinical preventive counseling and screening for adolescents. Together, these guidelines include many interventions that promote healthy sexual development and can prevent negative consequences of sexual behaviors. Additionally, the updated Centers for Disease Control and Prevention (CDC), *Sexually Transmitted Diseases Treatment Guidelines,* 2015, recommend behavioral counseling for all sexually active teens at risk for sexually transmitted infections (STIs) and human immunodeficiency virus (HIV) (Frieden et al, 2015). Strategies include:

- Ensuring a confidential environment in which the adolescent and health provider can freely exchange information
- Assessing and providing guidance toward the healthy accomplishment of physical, sexual, social, moral, cognitive, and emotional developmental tasks
- Supporting parental behaviors that promote healthy adolescent adjustment
- Providing health guidance that promotes wellness and healthy lifestyles, such as responsible sexual behaviors (e.g., abstinence, limiting the number of sex partners, and the modification of sexual practices)
- Educating about the use of latex condoms to prevent STIs, including infection with HIV
- Educating about appropriate methods of birth control with instructions on how to use them effectively
- Interviewing annually about involvement in sexual and other lifestyle behaviors (e.g., alcohol and drug use) that may result in unintended pregnancy and STIs, including HIV infection
- Asking questions that explore the adolescent's sexual orientation, number of sex partners in the previous 6 months, if the individual has exchanged sex for money or drugs, pregnancy, and STI history
- Assessing sexual maturity stages for normal progression
- Screening sexually active adolescents for STIs (chlamydia and gonorrhea) and providing pregnancy and partner notification and referral for treatment; those initiating sex early in adolescence, those residing in detention facilities, those who attend STI clinics, young men who have sex with men, and those using injection drugs are particularly at risk (Frieden et al, 2015)
- Providing confidential HIV and syphilis screening of adolescents at risk for infection
- Initiating routine cervical cytology screening at age 21 (American Congress of Obstetricians and Gynecologists [ACOG], 2012; American Cancer Society, 2014; USPSTF, 2014) and annual interviews about any history

of emotional, physical, and/or sexual abuse by caregivers, friends, or intimate partners
- Initiating the series of hepatitis B vaccinations for those 11 years and older if series not already completed
- Recommending routine human papillomavirus (HPV) vaccination for females and males age 11 or 12 years old—vaccination is also recommended for females between 13 and 26 years and males between 13 and 21 years if not yet vaccinated. There are three types of HPV vaccine: (1) HPV2, bivalent vaccine (Cervarix) includes HPV types 16 and 18 (2) HPV4, quadrivalent vaccine (Gardasil) includes HPV types 6, 11, 16, and 18, and (3) HPV9, including HPV types 6, 11, 16, 18, plus 31, 33, 45, 52, and 58. Both HPV4 and HPV9 are recommended for males and protect against the HPV types that cause 90% of genital warts in males and females (Markowitz et al, 2014).

Normal Patterns of Sexuality

Historical and Cultural Context of Sexuality

The term *psychosexual development* is often used to describe the continuum of sexual development from infancy to adulthood. Historically, however, Freud first used this term as an integral concept in his theories of personality development—and eventually psychoanalysis. His concern was focused on the "sexual desires" that he believed were intrinsic formative drives, instincts, and appetites that led to one's behaviors and beliefs. The interplay between expressing these sexual desires and the perceived need to repress them led to his five psychosexual stages of normal sexual development: *oral*: 0 to 18 months old; *oral*: 0 to 18 months old; *anal*: 18 to 36 month old; *anal*: 18 to 36 months old; *phallic*: 3 to 6 years old; *latency*: 6 years old to puberty; and *genital*: puberty and beyond. The developmental characteristics and the ages at which he assigned the stages varied as Freud advanced his theory throughout his career.

Among others, Erik Erikson furthered the discussion of sexual development by maintaining that children develop in predetermined stages. The stages were based on socialization and the effect this had on a child's personality, interactions with others, and self-esteem. Unsuccessfully fulfilling one stage prevented one from progressing to the next, until resolved. Successful completion of Erikson's stages related to the eventual healthy development of sexuality in terms of one's gender-role socialization, body image, social relationships, attitudes, values, and self-esteem.

Societal socialization norms and values provide males and females with rules about how they should behave. In Western cultures (although this is becoming less absolute), a person's sexual orientation has often been used to define the entire personality and identity. Other cultures and societies differ markedly on this last point. They may allow for greater gender diversity, viewing sexual roles, sexual assignment, and sexual behaviors on more of a continuum, or they may have strict laws (cultural or religious) against the practice of anything other than heterosexuality. Global Internet technology is also changing the way world views are disseminated, and individuals now have increasing opportunities to communicate their current social realities with others regarding sexual values, norms, relationships, and behaviors.

Contemporary Definitions

Sexuality has been defined by the Sexuality Information and Education Council of the United States (SIECUS, 2010) as encompassing "the sexual knowledge, beliefs, attitudes, values, and behaviors of individuals. Its various dimensions involve the anatomy, physiology, and biochemistry of the sexual response system; identity, orientation, roles, and personality; and thoughts, feelings, and relationships. Sexuality is influenced by ethical, spiritual, cultural, and moral concerns."

Murphy and Elias (2006, p 398) extend the definition to include gender-role and socialization, physical maturation and body image, social relationships, and future social aspirations.

Both definitions illustrate the multidimensional process of sexual development. The complexity of sexuality hinges on the key notion of gender. The following contemporary definitions explore this notion more fully:

- *Gender identity:* The knowledge of oneself as being male or female. It is believed to evolve from a combination of genetic, prenatal and postnatal endocrine influences, and postnatal psychosocial and environmental experiences (Cohen-Kettenis, 2010; Meininger and Remafedi, 2008; Murphy and Elias, 2006). It usually relates to anatomic sex, but not always (e.g., transgendered persons). One's gender identity develops in stages according to age, stage, and cognitive development, which are discussed later. Many theorists argue that gender identity is not fully established until a child has mastered the concept of gender permanency (5 to 7 years old). Others believe gender identity is achieved in the toddler and preschool years. Research of children with complex genital anomalies suggests that genital appearance alone may not be a crucial determinant in the formation of gender identity (Cohen-Kettenis, 2010).
- *Gender role:* The outward expression of maleness or femaleness; it usually relates to anatomic sex, but not always, such as with transvestites. This process begins at preschool age and continues into adulthood. It is characterized by the emergence of behaviors, attitudes, and feelings that are labeled as male, female, or neutral. Previous research suggests that gender role behavior is dependent on testosterone and estradiol exposure. Testosterone levels, measured in amniotic fluid, appear to predict male-typical behavior in childhood. Other behaviors that have been linked to the amount of testosterone exposure prenatally include core gender identity, physical aggression, and empathy. However, in a large prospective

cohort study, Robinson and colleagues (2013) did not find a consistent relationship between cord blood testosterone levels and internalizing or externalizing behavior difficulties. In fact, boys with increased levels of testosterone had lower scores for attention problems.

- *Gender assignment:* Gender assignment generally occurs at birth based on genital appearance and is the keystone in many societies for future gender socialization (i.e., gender identity). In most cases, genital appearance is determined from conception and is based on the 46XX and 46XY chromosome karyotypes and the appropriate masculinization effect of prenatal steroid exposure (testosterone and dihydrotestosterone). In approximately 1 in 4500 births, gender assignment may be difficult to assign at birth as a result of complex genital anomalies. In these cases, chromosomal analysis may be only one step in the process of assigning gender, because gonadal dysgenesis can lead to karyotype variations. Also in these cases, gender assignment is done after careful consideration of the pathologic conditions of the clinical syndrome (fetal exposure to prenatal steroids and degree of masculinization), long-term psychosexual and psychosocial functional outcome of surgical correction, and androgen support (see Chapter 26).
- *Gender attribution:* This is a subjective perception of person based on a number of cues (e.g., manner of dress, hairstyle, gait, mannerisms, and choice of occupation).
- *Gender or sexual orientation:* ("Whom do I love?") This refers to an individual's feelings of sexual attraction and erotic potential. Meininger and Remafedi (2008) define sexual orientation as an individual's attraction to the same or opposite sex. Sexual orientation is not dichotomous, and individuals tend to fall along a continuum of sexual expression and desires rather than into exclusive categories. The phrase *sexual preference* implies choice and should not be used in reference to sexual orientation.

Heterosexuality, homosexuality, and bisexuality are part of the normal spectrum of human sexuality and are equally valid and healthy developmental outcomes for youth (American Psychological Association [APA], 2008; Bidwell, 2009). Sexual orientation is not known to be caused by any particular factor or factors. Possible genetic (neuroanatomic), hormonal (neurophysiologic), developmental, social, and cultural influences have been postulated but have not been definitively identified. Most people have little or no sense of choice about their sexual orientation (APA, 2008; Remafedi, 2011). Adolescents may express different sexual behaviors, including short-term homosexual experiences. Teens may actually not be sexually active but label themselves as gay, lesbian, or bisexual because of whom they are physically or emotionally attracted to.

Sexual Health

The current working definition of *sexual health* as put forth by a group of international experts and reported by the World Health Organization (WHO), Department of Reproductive Health and Research (2006, p 5) states that: Sexual health is a state of physical, emotional, mental, and social well-being in relation to sexuality; it is not merely the absence of disease, dysfunction, or infirmity. Sexual health requires a positive and respectful approach to sexuality and sexual relationships, as well as the possibility of having pleasurable and safe sexual experiences, free of coercion, discrimination, and violence. For sexual health to be attained and maintained, the sexual rights of all persons must be respected, protected, and fulfilled.

Sexual function incorporates the biologic component of the human sexual response cycle and refers to the ability to give and receive sexual pleasure. *Sexual self-concept* is the psychological component of sexuality, the image one has of oneself as a man or a woman, and the evaluation of one's adequacy in masculine and feminine roles. *Sexual relationships* refer to the social domain of sexuality and include the interpersonal relationships in which one's sexuality is shared with others.

Stages of Developmental Patterns of Sexuality

The PCP is in a unique position to incrementally educate parents about their child's sexual maturation starting in infancy, as well as to help parents distinguish between normal and problematic sexual behaviors. Anticipatory guidance not only enables parents to accurately understand their child's normal sexual development but also provides a structure for healthy parent-child sexual discussions in an ongoing open manner throughout the child's life. Table 15-1 discusses the components of development and behavior related to sexuality.

Infancy to 2 Years Old

Newborn infants are reflexive beings, responding to their physical environment without hesitation or cognition. Sexual reflexes are present prenatally and are easily stimulated in the infant. It is not uncommon to observe a penile erection in prenatal ultrasounds or in the nursing child. Just as infants are fascinated by and explore their hands and feet, they explore their genitalia. Touching the genitalia—even masturbating—is pleasurable and soothing, is a natural part of exploring their environment, and begins as early as 3 to 5 months old. The provider should point out the spontaneity of this reflexive behavior so that a parent does not assign an adult sexuality interpretation to it.

Healthy parent-infant bonding requires physical contact and social interaction. Parents must hold, cuddle, stroke, talk to, look at, and respond to children if children are to develop a sense of trust on which intimacy and a positive self-image will be based in later years.

By the end of the first year, the child can differentiate between the sexes; some may even discriminate between sex-assigned toys. As society furthers its influence, children form their identities early and learn about their gender roles

TABLE 15-1 Sexual Behaviors, Self-Concept, and Relationships from Infancy Through Young Adulthood

	Normal Sexual Behaviors	Sexual Self-Concept	Sexual Role and Relationship
Infancy (birth through 1 year)	• Orgasmic potential present • Erectile function present • May explore genital area during diaper changes	• Gender identity reinforced	
Toddler	• Genital pleasuring and exploration • Sensual activity (e.g., hugging, stroking mother's breasts or other body parts)	• Association of sexuality and good and bad • Distinction between self and others	• Sex role differences learned • Discrimination between male and female role models • Sexual vocabulary learned
Preschool	• Sex play—exploration of own body and those of playmates; taking clothes off; showing genitals to other children or adults • Self pleasuring (masturbation) especially when tired	• Gender identity understood as a permanent condition	• Sex roles learned • Parental attachment and identification
School age (5 to 11 years)	• Masturbation (may occur more in public) • Sex play between peers (playing "house" or "doctor"); exploration through looking at and touching genitals • Asking questions and talking about sex • Dressing up as the opposite sex as part of dramatic play	• Curiosity about sex • Sexual fears and fantasies • Interest in aspects of sexual development • Self-awareness as sexual being	• Same-sex friends • Off-color humor related to sexuality
Adolescence, prepubertal	• Menarche (female) • Seminal emissions (male)	• Concerns about body image	• Same-sex friends • Sexual experiences as part of friendship
Adolescence, early	• Awkwardness in first sexual encounter • Masturbation, petting • May or may not be sexually active • May be aware of or question sexual orientation	• Anxiety over inadequacy, lack of partner, virginity	• Appropriate sex friendships • Dating
Adolescence, late	• May or may not be sexually active • May be aware of or question sexual orientation	• Responsibility for sexual activity	• Intimacy in relationships learned
Young adult	• Experimentation with sexual positions, expressions • Exploration of techniques	• Responsibility for sexual health (e.g., contraception, STI prevention) • Development of adult sexual value system, tolerance for others	• Giving and receiving pleasure learned • Long-term commitment to relationship developed

Data from Hillman JB, Spigarelli MG: Sexuality: its development and direction. In Carey WB, Crocker AC, Coleman WL, et al, editors: *Developmental-behavioral pediatrics*, Philadelphia, 2009, Saunders.
STI, Sexually transmitted infection.

from the reinforcement of behaviors expected of males and females.

Two to 5 Years Old

Toddlers are able to recognize and pronounce themselves "I'm a girl" or "I'm a boy," but they can easily confuse gender in others and sometimes in themselves. Changing one's style of clothes, for example, can be perceived as a change in gender. Children cannot integrate gender identity into their self-concept until they understand that gender is a permanent condition. The age at which this notion occurs is around 4 or 5 years old. Theorists argue that gender identity is fully attained between 5 and 7 years old, at which time this identity truly motivates sex-appropriate gender behavior. Children in this age group are extremely curious about their environment; they love to explore and experiment. Up to the age of 5 years, the variety and frequency of sexual behaviors increase and then start decreasing (Kellogg and Committee on Child Abuse and Neglect AAP, 2009). Children have a cognitive awareness of the pleasure that self-stimulation gives them and frequently masturbate, but, as with infants, they attribute no erotic or sexual meaning to their actions. They lack the concept of personal space and how their behavior may be misinterpreted as being sexual or improper. This is a good time for parents to discuss the notion of "private parts" and begin to teach the child that self-stimulation is acceptable but should be done in private. Parental redirection is usually all that is required.

The combination of curiosity and lack of self-consciousness characteristic of toddlers can contribute to embarrassing social incidents for their parents. They may be curious about what others look like under their clothes, touch other children's bodies, "play doctor," pretend to be Mommy and Daddy, and enjoy running around naked. By 4 years old, children may attach themselves more to the parent of the opposite sex.

Parents should be encouraged to use the appropriate names for body parts and bodily functions, even though they may also be using slang words. This enables children to better comprehend discussions with health providers, teachers, or health educators when the anatomical and physiologic terms are used.

Because children at this age interpret statements literally and have "magical" thinking, their understandings of the physical self can be distorted, and lengthy explanations about body functions can be misunderstood. Parents should help children understand that their bodies come in different shapes, sizes, and colors; that all of these are equally important; that boys and girls also share the same parts, but different genital parts; and that sharing and respect are important aspects for developing friendships. It is appropriate for parents to introduce the notion of germs and hygiene, such as washing hands. This helps establish a framework for parents to advance the discussion to include STIs later in life.

Situational factors can induce an increase in observed sexual behaviors in this age group, such as the birth of a new sibling, watching their mother breastfeed, and viewing another child's or adult's nudity. It has also been noted that children who spend more time in child care environments have demonstrated a larger number and frequency of observed sexual behaviors (Kellogg and Committee on Child Abuse and Neglect AAP, 2009).

Five to 9 Years Old

School-age children continue to have a high level of curiosity about sexuality, their bodies, and their environment. They are aware of the pleasure stimulation gives and continue to actively seek autoerotic arousal for enjoyment. Again, reassure parents that this behavior is not associated with sexual fantasies. Contact with other children may give them new ideas about sex, and sex games are typical (e.g., playing house or doctor) between same-age children, either of the same or opposite sex. This is normal behavior as long as a child is not emotionally distraught by the encounter or if it involves one child who is older than the other. Parents should avoid being overly alarmed if they witness this play. It is appropriate for parents to redirect the play to other activities. They should then discuss the situation later with their child to explore the experience, ascertain if the child was uncomfortable, and again emphasize the notion of privacy and respect for one's body. Box 15-1 discusses sexual actions beyond self-stimulation and sex play that can indicate possible sexual abuse.

By 5 to 7 years old, the use of sexual or "potty" language becomes evident—often to test parental reaction. Children at this age identify more with the same-sex parent; they tend to cluster into same-sex groups if given the opportunity. They are curious about where babies come from.

By the time children are about 8 years old, they begin to understand the significance of sexuality. They learn more about their body and body functions and "giggle" with children of their same sex when talking about sexuality, perhaps because they conceive that sex is a secretive topic. Unless parents actively communicate with their children, sexual lessons will be learned from peers, the media, jokes, and movies.

Some children may begin pubertal changes during this time and may be embarrassed by them. Acne, oily skin, and sweating may occur. As their bodies change, they become curious and want to see others' bodies. Masturbation is still

• BOX 15-1 Signs That Sexual Play May Go Beyond Normal

- The behavior is not age-appropriate.
- The behavior is prolonged.
- The child looks anxious or guilty or becomes extremely aroused.
- Child is being forced into sexual play through bribes, name-calling, and/or physical force.
- Child knows more about sexual matters than is appropriate for his or her age.

a normal way for them to explore their bodies. Sexual language is often used more to insult others or appear smart in front of their friends.

Parents and teachers are in key positions to teach children that their sexual curiosity and feelings are normal, to help boys and girls better understand how sexual development is an integral part of growing up, to use respectful language, and to reinforce that they are always available for questions (De Melker, 2015). Simple discussions about the body can introduce further discussions about hormones and reproductive systems. Establishing a good history of communication about sexuality and other subjects lays the groundwork for being accessible to update information as the child matures. This is also a good time for parents and others to reinforce the notion that there is diversity in families within which parents and adults love and care for children.

Preadolescence

Preadolescence is marked by the onset of pubertal changes. About this time, children understand sexuality as a normal part of life. Both males and females understand the changes that are occurring in each other's bodies and by 10 to 12 years old are ready to discuss sexual behavior and reproduction. Self-stimulation as a result of sexual reflexes may now become connected to sexual fantasies, sexual behavior, and sexual relationships. It is still common for preadolescents to socialize and develop close relationships mostly with members of the same sex. Both sexes often become uncomfortable or embarrassed about the changes in their bodies, particularly girls because breast development is more obvious to others. Privacy becomes more important.

Parents should discuss menstruation before it occurs so as not to cause undue alarm and have the child be caught "off guard." Being mindful of their values and beliefs, parents should discuss abstinence, STIs (including HIV), birth control, the HPV immunization for both sexes, consequences of early sexual activity (including teen pregnancy), and the influence of peer pressure. This is also a good time to discuss sexual orientation.

Adolescence

Adolescence is a period of rapid physical, emotional, and social change that presents a developmental challenge to both children and parents. In terms of sexuality, adolescents fit their sense of sexual being into their evolving self-image and personal identity; they learn about their bodies' (sometimes unexpected and embarrassing) sensual and sexual responses to stimulation, and they develop a sense of the moral significance of sexuality. The Guttmacher Institute (2014) reports that on average most adolescents will experience their first sexual intercourse at age 17 years and that 71% of both sexes will have had sexual intercourse by the time they reach their 19th birthday. Privacy is essential for the adolescent to explore this emerging self. Activities such as group social functions, dating, participation in sports, and interactions at work and school provide opportunities to learn social and interpersonal skills of intimacy.

Learning how to communicate about sex, how to set limits, how to prevent misunderstandings, and how to say yes or no are important skills for adolescents. Equally important is the process of developing a set of sexual values. Whether the adolescent practices abstinence, has a double standard for men's and women's sexual behavior, or is exploitative or nurturing in close personal relationships is a reflection of the adolescent's sexual values.

Sexuality in Individuals With Intellectual and Physical Developmental Disabilities

The sexual development of youth with intellectual and physical developmental disabilities (I/P/DD) is the same as those without such physical or cognitive limitations. The clinician needs to focus on the developmental level rather than chronological age when determining appropriateness of sexual behavior. For example, an individual with a cognitive level of a preschooler will normally exhibit sexual behaviors consistent with that developmental level.

The provider must also recognize that I/P/DD individuals have the same desires to make decisions and foster fulfilling relationships with others. Their abilities to develop healthy sexual identities and engage in sexual behaviors often largely hinge on society's comfort and proactive support concerning their right for healthy sexual expression, rather than on their disability itself. Individuals with I/P/DD may be viewed by society (including health providers, teachers, and parents) as being childlike, asexual, sexually inappropriate, having uncontrollable sexual urges, or being sexual deviants. Institutional isolation, overprotection, lack of awareness by others of their sexual needs, and pessimism about their potential often end up inhibiting the healthy sexual and psychosocial development of these individuals. As a consequence, many people with disabilities are vulnerable to sexual abuse and exploitation by those who house, employ, and take care of them. A person with a disability is three times more likely to be a victim of physical and sexual abuse; those with intellectual and mental disabilities are more vulnerable (WHO Department of Reproductive Health and Research and UNFPA, 2009). This victimization can lead to low self-esteem, anxiety, depression, and adjustment disorders (Murphy and Elias, 2006).

People with I/P/DD largely acquire their sex education from formal educational programs and the media rather than from family or friends. Females may obtain such education in the form of abuse. These individuals are less likely to share their thoughts, feelings, and experiences with family and friends. Unless healthy sexuality is taught and supported, unhealthy and abusive sexuality can occur. Sex education can be effective for those with I/P/DD, and topics should include those listed in Box 15-2. The depth and length of discussion should vary depending on the type of disability (e.g., sex education taught to a child with autism would have a different focus than that taught to a

• BOX 15-2 Sexual Education Topics for the Individual with Intellectual and Physical Developmental Disabilities

- Body parts
- Concepts of privacy and choice
- Masturbation
- Sexual abuse prevention
- Menstruation
- Homosexuality
- Marriage
- Sexual interaction
- Dating and intimacy
- Appropriate social behaviors
- Birth control, pregnancy
- Sexually transmitted infections
- Self-esteem
- Attitudes and values
- Sexual responsibility and privileges and consent

child with Down syndrome). Excellent resources and books for parents, teachers, and clinicians can be accessed from Planned Parenthood, SIECUS, and the Center for Parent Information and Resources (CPIR).

Factors That Can Alter Sexual Behaviors

Other factors can influence the frequency and number of different sexual behaviors exhibited by children. These include exposure to family nudity, co-bathing, limited privacy, exposure to readily accessible pornographic materials, exposure to sexual acts, extent of adult supervision, stressors (e.g., violence, parental absence due to incarceration, criminal activity, death, illness), sexual and physical abuse, neglect (can result in indiscriminate affection-seeking or interpersonal boundary problems), and psychiatric diagnoses (e.g., conduct disorder, attention-deficit/hyperactivity disorder [ADHD], oppositional defiant disorder) (Kellogg and Committee on Child Abuse and Neglect AAP, 2009).

Assessment of Normal Patterns of Sexual Development

Sexual development, questions, and concerns are present throughout childhood. Although for many children, the onset of their first sexual intercourse is the cornerstone of their "sexuality." Assessment of sexuality and sexual maturation should be integrated into the health history, interview and discussion, and physical examination at all health maintenance visits. A useful tool for the clinician is the Child Sexual Behavior Inventory (CSBI; available at www4.parinc.com/products/ProductIC.aspx?ProductID=IC-CSBI). This tool is completed by parents and can help evaluate normal and age-appropriate sexual behaviors for those 1 to 12 years of age. It was developed to aid in evaluating whether a child has been or may have been sexually abused. However, it can provide assistance to the provider dealing with a parent who is concerned about their child's sexual behavior.

Confidentiality

Research has shown clear evidence that sexuality education leads to a reduction in early onset of sexual intercourse and risky sexual behaviors. The AMA, AAP, Society for Adolescent Health and Medicine (SAHM), ACOG, Association of Women's Health, Obstetric and Neonatal Nurses (AWHONN), National Medical Association, and the American Academy of Family Physicians (AAFP) have endorsed policies advocating confidential medical visits for adolescents (AWHONN, 2010; AAFP, 2013). The National Association of Pediatric Nurse Practitioners (NAPNAP) supports confidentiality regarding sexual orientation and gender identity in accordance with state regulations regarding confidentiality of minors (NAPNAP, 2011). Despite these outstanding policies, many adolescents are not seeking health care due to concerns for confidentiality. Lehrer and colleagues (2007) found a strong correlation between youth concerns about confidentiality and certain risk characteristics. The odds of avoiding medical care due to confidentiality concerns increased in the presence of poor parental communication, high depressive symptoms, and suicidal ideation and/or attempt in the past year for both sexes. Females also had a significant correlation between forgoing medical care due to confidentiality concerns when their histories included sexual intercourse, no birth control used with last sexual encounter, prior STI, or any alcohol use in the past year.

Health providers need to be clear about their policy of confidentiality with both the youth and parent before the need arises. This discussion needs to include confidentiality boundaries (i.e., severe mental health issues and safety) and billing statements that may be sent to parents.

History

Functions of the Sexual History

The sexual history achieves several purposes. In addition to being a tool to collect information, the process itself gives permission to the child, adolescent, or parent to ask questions and receive reliable information regarding issues of sexual concern. It sets the stage to incorporate accurate, sexuality-specific education as a normal component of anticipatory guidance.

Types of Sexual Histories

The sexual history can be either comprehensive or problem-oriented. The comprehensive sexual history (Box 15-3) is detailed, encompassing all aspects of sexual information about individuals, their family of origin, siblings, and peer relationships. A comprehensive history is lengthy and may not be accomplished at the first visit or in a single interview; it can be anxiety-producing to have the client disclose such

• BOX 15-3 Comprehensive Adolescent Sexual and Reproductive History

Background Data

Adolescent name, age (birth date), and sex
History of risky behaviors (e.g., drug history: onset, duration, and frequency of use of cigarettes, alcohol, and/or other illicit drugs)
Parents ages
Religions
Educational levels
Occupations
Marital status
Affectional relationship (parent to parent)
Child's feelings toward parent(s)

Childhood Sexuality

What were your parents' attitudes about sexuality when you were a child?
How did your parents handle nudity?
When do you first recall seeing a nude person of the same sex? Opposite sex?
Who taught you about sex, sex play, pregnancy, intercourse, masturbation, homosexuality, sexually transmitted infections (STIs), birth?
How often did you play doctor or nurse or have other sex play with another child?
Tell me about any other sexual activity or experience that had a strong effect on you.

Adolescent Sexuality

Girls

Onset of breast development?
When did pubic hair appear?
Onset of menstruation (age, regularity of periods [initially, now])?
When was your last normal menstrual period (LNMP)?
What hygienic methods are used (pads, tampons)?
How were you prepared for menstruation? By whom?
What were your feelings about early periods? Later periods?
Have you had unusual bleeding or pains?

Boys

How were you prepared for adolescence? By whom?
Age of first orgasm (ejaculation)?
What were "wet dreams" like? How did they make you feel?
When did pubic hair appear?

Body Image

How do you feel about your body? Breasts? Genitals?
How much time do you spend nude in front of a mirror?

Masturbation

How old were you when you began?
What are others' reactions to your masturbation?
What methods do you use?
What are your feelings about it?

Necking and Petting

How old were you when you began? How often?
How many partners do you currently have?

Intercourse

How often have you had intercourse?
How many partners?
How often do you initiate sex?
How often do you currently have sex?
How often have you had oral sex?
Are your partners male, female, or both?
Type of intercourse: Penile-vaginal, orogenital, penile-anal, oral-anal

Contraceptive Use

What kinds of contraceptives have you used?
What are you using now?
Do you have any problems with contraceptives?
Do you use condoms?
How do you communicate about contraception with your partner?

Gender Identity and Expression

What does it mean to be lesbian, gay, bisexual, or transgender?
Do you think you might be lesbian, gay, bisexual, or transgender?
Do you think you need to have sex to find out?
Have you known any homosexual or transgender individuals?
How long have you had homosexual or transgender feelings?
How often have you been approached?
How often have you had homosexual experiences? What kinds of experiences? What were the circumstances?

Seduction and Rape

When have you seduced someone sexually?
When has someone seduced you?
Have you been raped?
Have you raped someone? How often have you forced someone to have sex?

Incest and Abuse

What kinds of touching did you receive in your home?
From your mother? Father? Brother(s)? Sister(s)? Other relatives? Others?

Prostitution

What feelings do you have about prostitution?
Have you ever accepted money for sex?
Have you ever had sex with a prostitute?

Sexually Transmitted Infections

How old were you when you learned about STIs?
Have you ever had an STI? Gonorrhea? Syphilis? Chlamydia?
Do you have any signs or symptoms of STIs now?

Pregnancy

Have you ever been pregnant? At what age?
How was it resolved—miscarriage, abortion, adoption, marriage, single parenthood?
Do you think there is a chance you are pregnant now?
Have you caused a pregnancy?

Abortion

What are your feelings about abortion?
Have you (or a partner) had an abortion? If yes, at what age? What were your feelings?
What about your feelings now? What about your feelings immediately afterward? What about your feelings after 1 year?

• BOX 15-4 Problem-Oriented Adolescent Sexual History

Describe the sexual concern, problem, issue, or difficulty that you have. Include the following history:

- Type of sex—oral, anal, and/or vaginal
- Condoms—consistency of use, for which sexual practices
- Previous sexually transmitted infections (STIs); medication allergies
- Most recent sexual encounter; number of partners in past 2 months
- Use of illegal drugs and alcohol by self and partner (include which drugs, frequency, route)
- Does patient and/or partner have sex with men, women, or both?
- Recent travel and location
- Any symptoms of dysuria, frequency, hematuria; adenopathy; fatigue; weight loss; night sweats; unexplained diarrhea; fever; rectal discharge, bleeding, constipation, pain?
- *Women only:* Additional symptoms of:
  - Vaginal discharge, bleeding, color of discharge; skin rashes, lesions, sores and location; pruritus (vulvar, anal, oral, other); pain (abdominal, vaginal, vulvar, anal, headache, joints)
  - Last normal menstrual period (LNMP), description, changes
- Birth control method(s), consistency of use
- *Men only:* Symptoms of:
  - Penile discharge; lesions and/or pruritus (penis, scrotum, urethra, oral cavity); pain in testes
- How do you feel about discussing this problem?
- How long have you had it? When did this problem begin?
- What do you think caused you to have this problem?
- What might be contributing to this problem?
- What kinds of things have you done to treat or solve this problem?
- What health professionals have you seen?
- What, if any, medication have you taken or are you taking?
- Have you talked to a friend or relative?
- Have you read any books to solve this problem? What books?

a level of detail during early visits, and clients can become fatigued by one lengthy interview.

In contrast, the problem-oriented sexual history (Box 15-4) usually focuses on the current complaint or assessment of specific behaviors, such as the risk of exposure to pregnancy or the acquisition of STIs. Problem-oriented sexual histories are shorter, more direct, and specific to the issue at hand.

Approach to Taking a Sexual History

The interviewer should do the following when taking a sexual history:

- Reassure the client that asking sexual questions is a normal part of clinical practice: "I'm going to ask you a few personal questions about your life and well-being that I ask all my teen patients."
- Give appropriate, factual information; use medical-sexual terminology rather than slang, unless the client cannot relate to medical terms.
- Use language that validates the client's understanding of terms and concepts. For example, when talking with adolescents, the question "Are you sexually active?" seeks information regarding current activity on a planned and regular basis. The adolescent who has concrete cognitive abilities may respond negatively. However, the question "Have you ever had a romantic relationship with a boy or a girl?" allows for a more inclusive description of sexual activity. Define "sex" as oral, vaginal, or anal.
- Use open-ended questions. Questions that contain "why" can require a level of analysis beyond the capabilities of teens operating at a concrete level of cognition.
- The question "When you think of people to whom you are sexually attracted, are they males, females, both, neither, or are you not sure yet?" opens up a conversation for youth struggling with their sexual orientation (Murphy and Elias, 2006).
- Phrase questions that may be emotionally laden in a way that lets clients know that their experience may not be exceptional (e.g., "Many people have been sexually abused or molested as children; has this happened to you?").

When asking sensitive questions, phrasing the question in a way that normalizes it makes answering the question easier: "How often do you masturbate?" is better than "Do you masturbate?"

Physical Examination

The physical examination serves to identify normal variations of sexual anatomy, the stage of sexual development (Tanner stages), and any pathologic condition. The physical examination should include examination of the breasts, pattern of body hair growth, and external genitalia. In sexually active adolescents or when an abnormality is suspected, a pelvic and/or rectal examination may be indicated. Laboratory studies are performed only as indicated and can include cervical, urethral, rectal, and/or pharyngeal cultures; urine-based nucleic acid amplification test (NAAT); blood work for STIs (see Chapter 36); or genetic studies.

The physical examination should be performed with care and sensitivity to the child's or adolescent's feelings. Very young children and toddlers make no distinction between examination of external genitalia and other body parts; young school-age children can be extremely modest, act embarrassed, and resist taking off their clothes for the examination. Older school-age children and adolescents can misinterpret the examination procedures and may feel violated or abused. The child needs to feel an element of control during the examination. By taking the time to provide clear explanations of procedures, using straightforward techniques, and involving the child in the examination (e.g., asking if the child wishes to have the parent or another adult present), the clinician can better achieve the fine balance necessary to perform a thorough, respectful examination.

TABLE 15-2 Red Flags for Abnormal Sexual Behavior of Children and Adolescents

Age	Can Occur in All Children but Assess Child's Environment for Violence, Abuse, Neglect	Red Flags
12 years or younger	• Asking peer/adult to engage in sexual act(s)* • Simulating foreplay with dolls/ peers (e.g., petting, French kissing) • Inserting objects into genitals* • Imitating intercourse* • Touching animal genitalia*	• Preoccupied with sexual play • Engaging in sexual play with children who are 4 or more years apart • Attempting to expose others' genitals (e.g., pulling another's pants down) • Precocious sexual knowledge • Sexually explicit proposals or behaviors that induce fear/threats of force or that are physically aggressive (including written notes, graffiti) • Compulsive masturbation; interrupts tasks to masturbate • Chronic peeping, exposing self, using obscenities, exhibiting pornographic interests • Simulating intercourse with dolls/peers/animals with clothing on or off • Oral, vaginal, anal penetration of dolls, peers, animals • Sexual behaviors that are persistent and cause anger in child if they are distracted
Older than 12 years	• Pornographic interest • Sexually aggressive themes/ obscenities; may embarrass others with these • Sexual preoccupation/anxiety interferes with daily activities • Single occurrences of peeping, exposing self, simulating intercourse with clothes on	• Chronic, public masturbation • Degrading or humiliating self or others with sexual themes • Grabbing or trying to expose others' genitals • Chronic occupation with sexually aggressive pornography • Sexually explicit talk or sexual behaviors with children 4 or more years younger (sexual abuse) • Making sexually explicit threats (including written) • Obscene phone calls, voyeurism, exhibitionism, sexual harassment • Performing rape or bestiality • Genital injury to others

Data from Hillman JB, Spigarelli MG: Sexuality: its development and direction. In Carey WB, Crocker AC, Coleman WL, et al, editors: *Developmental-behavioral pediatrics*, Philadelphia, 2009, Saunders/Elsevier; Kellogg ND, Committee on Child Abuse and Neglect, American Academy of Pediatrics: Clinical report—the evaluation of sexual behaviors in children, *Pediatrics* 124(3):994–998, 2009.
*Uncommon but can occur in children 2 to 6 years.

Management Strategies

The health provider has two primary goals related to management of sexual development in children: first, to help children achieve a healthy sexual identity and function, and second, to provide support for parents to enable them to guide their children through the process. Both goals can be achieved by counseling parents about children's sexual development. Anticipatory guidance about sexual development and maturation that is age-appropriate should be provided to parents and their children as a matter of course. In particular, the provider must:

- Assess the parent's level of understanding regarding normal physical and psychosocial sexual development in children
- Provide or clarify information as needed
- Provide strategies and support for teaching children about sexuality
- Assist the parent to connect to community-based resources

"Normal sexual behavior" is not always clear, and the range is especially wide in the 2- to 6-year-old child. Tables 15-1 and 15-2 provide information to help distinguish between the common, uncommon, and abnormal displays of sexual behavior.

Setting the Stage

When working with children, the provider focuses on establishing and maintaining a positive relationship based on mutual trust and respect. The child needs to feel validated and comfortable revealing concerns and asking questions. In addition to using a constructive approach to taking a sexual history, a positive relationship can be achieved by:

- Asking questions to give the message that the child is expected to be changing and is aware of and curious about those changes (e.g., "How are you feeling?" "How's your body?" "Do you notice that you're getting taller?" "Have you noticed your breasts getting any bigger?" "Boys' penises begin to get longer and wider as they become teenagers. Have you noticed any changes in yours?")

- Listening thoughtfully and carefully to the child's input
- Responding positively by answering the child's questions as fully as possible; being nonjudgmental, calm, friendly, and open; and having a sense of humor, yet taking the child seriously
- Using appropriate teachable moments during the health visit (e.g., when examining a 3-year-old for inguinal hernia, the clinician can discuss appropriate and inappropriate touching with the child and his or her parent)
- Providing accurate information and referral resources as appropriate
- Respecting the child's need for privacy (e.g., knocking before entering the examination room, providing appropriate gowns, examining the child semi-clothed)
- Maintaining confidentiality as appropriate, especially with an adolescent; however, children of any age may give information that need not be shared with the parent

Sex Education

For a child, developing healthy sexuality means gaining knowledge about physical changes; shaping a positive gender identity; clarifying one's sexual identity as a boy or a girl; establishing close, intimate relationships with others; and demonstrating the ability to make healthy judgments about sexuality and sexual activity. The questions a child asks and the behaviors displayed can embarrass some parents—who may respond in a manner that frightens, shames, or confuses the child. Children are born as sexual beings, and parents, whether or not they are aware of it, are constantly providing lessons in sex education. The way parents respond to a child's innate sexuality (innocent curiosity about sex, gender, and body parts and functions) and allow it to unfold is the core of a child's sex education. This response does more to mold that child's mature sexual behavior than all the information or misinformation parents may provide.

Parents should be encouraged to take advantage of teaching opportunities in normal childhood sexual play and to answer questions simply and directly at the child's level of understanding (Box 15-5). Box 15-6 outlines what children should know about sexuality at different ages.

Research has shown clear evidence that comprehensive sexuality education leads to a reduction in the early onset of sexual intercourse and risky sexual behaviors (Suellentrop, 2011). Yet, sex education in the schools remains controversial and subject to federal, state, and local mandate as to content. With the passage of the Patient Protection and Affordable Care Act, signed into law in March 2010, there are now funds available for comprehensive sex education. States may apply for grants from the State Personal Responsibility Education Program (PREP) but must use evidence-based elements in the curriculum (Administration of Children and Families, U.S. Department of Health and Human Services [HHS], 2014). See Box 15-7 for criteria of effective curriculum-based comprehensive programs.

• BOX 15-5 Approaches to Teaching Your Child About Sex

- Find out what your child already knows. Understand the question before answering. Check to be sure your answer is understood. Make sure you answer the question that is asked, and give your child a chance to ask more questions.
- If your child asks a question about sexuality at an inconvenient time, set a time and place as soon as possible to answer the question.
- Discuss sex in a matter-of-fact way.
- Use correct terminology when talking about body parts; use dolls and books as guides.
- Keep the topics short and to the point. Keep the child's attention span in mind.
- Do not worry about telling children too much about sex. They tune out what they do not understand.
- Encourage questions. Never embarrass children or tell them they are too young to understand or that they will learn that when they grow up.
- Include values, emotions, feelings, and decision-making in your discussion. Do not focus only on biologic facts.
- Let your child know that people have different beliefs about sexuality.
- Bring up topics of STIs, including HIV/AIDS.
- Discuss anticipated changes of puberty before they occur. Do not wait until your child is a teenager. Discuss menstruation with both girls and boys.
- If you do not know the answer to your child's question, say so, and then look it up. Ask your pediatric PCP.
- If your child is masturbating in public or engaging in sex play, redirect him or her to other activities. At a later time, discuss where a more appropriate private place is for the child to masturbate.
- When your child uses obscene or derogatory words, calmly explain what they mean, why it is not appropriate to use them, and that use of certain words can be insulting (e.g., "gay"). Do not laugh or joke about your child's use of such words, because this can serve as encouragement.

AIDS, Acquired immune deficiency syndrome; *HIV,* human immunodeficiency virus; *PCP,* primary care provider; *STI,* sexually transmitted infection.

In 2004, SIECUS published the third edition of *Guidelines for Comprehensive Sexuality Education: Kindergarten-12th Grade.* These guidelines are organized around six key concepts (human development, relationships, personal skills, sexual behavior, sexual health, and society and culture), and these concepts are discussed at four developmental levels. The basics of these guidelines are still in use, and SIECUS holds a repository of lesson plans and resources on its website (see Additional Resources; SIECUS, 2004).

Many professional nursing and medical organizations have policy statements or position papers that support comprehensive sex education in the schools and at home (AAFP, 2012; AAP, 2014; ACOG, 2014; SAHM et al, 2014). They encourage abstinence as the adolescents' best choice to prevent pregnancy and STIs; they also encourage parental involvement. However, all state that counseling and education on contraception, STIs, and HIV/acquired immune deficiency syndrome (AIDS) are essential.

BOX 15-6 Sexual Development: What Should Children Know?

By 5 Years Old, Children Should

- Use correct words for all sexual body parts.
- Be able to understand what it means to be male or female.
- Understand that their bodies belong to themselves, and they should say "no" to unwanted touch, but that having their private parts touched (for hygiene purposes by a parent) and during physical examinations by their health care provider when accompanied by a parent is normal.
- Know where babies come from; how they "get in" and "get out."
- Be able to talk about body parts without feeling "naughty."
- Be able to ask trusted adults questions about sexuality.
- Know that "sex talk" is for private times at home.

Elementary School Children (6 to 9 Years Old) Should

- Be aware that all creatures grow and reproduce.
- Be aware that sexuality is important at all ages, including at their parents' and grandparents' ages, and that it changes over time.
- Know and use proper words for body parts—their own and those of the opposite sex.
- Understand that there are many kinds of caring family types so that they do not see a single model of family as the only possible one.
- Be aware that sexual identity includes sexual orientation: lesbian, gay, heterosexual, bisexual, transgender.
- Understand the basic facts about how an individual acquires HIV/AIDS.
- Take an active role in managing their body's health and safety.

Nine- to 13-Year-Old Children/Young Teens Should

- Be informed about human reproduction.
- Be aware of changes they can expect in their bodies before puberty (by 9 to 11 years old).
- Know how normal developmental changes begin, including normal differences and when those events occur for males and females.
- Know how male and female bodies grow and differ.
- Understand the general stages of the body's growth.
- Understand the facts about menstruation and wet dreams.
- Know that emotional changes are very common during this time.
- Understand that human sexuality is a natural part of life (by 12 to 13 years old).
- Be aware of how behavior can be seen as sexual and how to deal with sexual behavior (by 12 to 13 years old)
- Be aware that sexual feelings are normal and okay.
- Know how to recognize and protect themselves against potential sexual abuse and how to react to such dangers.
- Be able to recognize male and female prostitution and its dangers.
- Know how babies are made and what behaviors are likely to lead to pregnancy.
- Know that it is possible to plan parenthood.
- Understand that having a child is a long-term responsibility and that every child deserves mature, responsible, loving parents.
- Be aware that contraceptives (birth control methods) exist (and should be able to name some).
- Know what abortion is.
- Know what STIs are.
  - Understand how a person can get STIs.
  - Be aware of how a person can protect himself or herself from STIs.
  - Know how STIs are treated.

Look for more detailed information and information about what older teens should know and understand about sexuality at www.plannedparenthood.org/parents/talking-to-kids-about-sex-and-sexuality.

AIDS, Acquired immune deficiency syndrome; *HIV,* human immunodeficiency virus; *STI,* sexually transmitted infection.

BOX 15-7 Criteria of Effective Curriculum-Based Comprehensive Sexuality Education Program

- Focus on clear health goals.
- Focus narrowly on specific types of behavior leading to the health goals.
- Address sexual psychosocial risk and protective factors that affect sexual behavior.
- Create a safe social environment.
- Include multiple activities to change each of the targeted risk and protective factors.
- Use instructionally sound teaching methods that actively involve participants, help them personalize information, and are designed to change the targeted risk and protective factors.
- Use activities, methods, and messages that are appropriate to the teens' culture, developmental age, and sexual experience.
- Cover topics in a logical sequence.
- Select educators with the ability to relate to young people and then train and support them.

Counseling of the Adolescent

Today's adolescents face multiple influences, including societal expectations that are at odds with the media's portrayal of sexuality; cultural norms, beliefs, and attitudes of the family of origin; peer group pressure to conform; and the individual's own values and belief system. All these influences need to be considered and addressed when counseling the adolescent.

The health care provider should use the answers given by the adolescent in the sexual history to further guide the counseling and educational needs of that individual. It may take several visits for the trust relationship to grow before the adolescent is willing to divulge certain aspects of his or her sexual self. The provider's job is to assure the adolescent of the confidential nature of the relationship and provide opportunities for trust to develop.

Adolescents should be counseled that abstinence is the most effective strategy for the prevention of pregnancy, STIs, and HIV/AIDS. Further, they need to know that it is a choice to remain abstinent and a choice to become sexually active, not just something that happens; with that choice comes responsibilities. Open communication and respect for self and their partner will lead to choices that include protection from STIs and pregnancy.

When counseling adolescents, the provider's approach needs to be appropriate for the psychosocial developmental stage of the teen. Using Piaget's stages of development as the basis, counseling may be tailored accordingly. Early adolescents (12 to 14 years old) are concrete thinkers and cannot get to the abstract thought of "what if." Counseling language needs to be in simple concrete terms. Using pictures and direct questions and statements helps facilitate this. Middle adolescents (15 to 17 years old) are starting to understand abstract concepts but will often regress to concrete thinking in stressful situations. An adolescent at this age may demonstrate mature thought processes at one point in time yet revert to concrete thinking at another. The provider needs to adjust the approach to middle adolescents accordingly, help them to identify the inconsistencies in their thought processes, and guide them through to the logical consequences. Late adolescents (18 to 21 years old) generally have abstract thought more firmly established and are future oriented. However, this ability varies, as with the general adult population.

Contraceptive and Safer Sex Counseling

It is important to use gender-neutral phrasing when discussing safer sex and contraception and not assume heterosexuality. Providers who provide contraceptive and safer sex counseling to adolescents should understand that the successful use of any method requires a complex process of knowledge, decision-making skills, and public behaviors. To use contraceptives and/or protective barriers successfully, an individual must master the following:

- *Knowledge.* For most adolescents, this means mastery of a barrier method (e.g., male or female condoms) to prevent an STI, in addition to a variety of hormonal methods for contraceptive purposes.
- *Ability to plan for the future.* Planning for the future requires self-admission that the adolescent will have sex in the future and the ability to take the steps necessary to use a method consistently and correctly.
- *Willingness to acquire needed contraceptive and/or barrier methods publicly.* The adolescent must be willing and able to be public with requests for contraceptive and/or protective devices (e.g., to purchase condoms at a local pharmacy or to seek services at the local clinic, school-based health facility, or private practice) (see Chapter 36 for more in-depth information on contraceptive methods).
- *Communication skills.* Adolescents must have the ability to communicate with another person, such as their partner, health care provider, pharmacist or salesperson, about their individual contraceptive and/or protective barrier needs.

Special Counseling Needs

Children's sense of self; personality; relationship to others and to the physical world; cognitive, emotional, and spiritual abilities; perceptions; and expressions are all influenced by and, in turn, influence their sexual development. If children experience challenges with sexuality, all other aspects of development are affected. Issues of major concern include child sexual abuse (see Chapter 17) and adolescent pregnancy (see Chapter 36).

Lesbian, Gay, Bisexual, Transgendered, and Questioning Youth

The concept of sexual orientation includes at least three distinctive components: (1) sexual imagery (fantasies or attraction), (2) actual sexual behavior responsiveness, and (3) the person's self-identification as heterosexual, bisexual, or homosexual. Transgender individuals identify themselves as the gender opposite of their biologic sex. Their sexual orientation may be heterosexual, homosexual, or bisexual.

Adolescent-specific data on sexual orientation are sparse. Remafedi and colleagues (1992) surveyed a representative sample of 34,706 Minnesota junior and senior high school youths and reported that 10.7% were unsure of their sexual orientation, 88.2% described themselves as exclusively heterosexual, and 1.1% described themselves as bisexual or primarily homosexual. In 2011, Kann and colleagues, analyzing data from the 2001-2009 Youth Risk Behavior Survey (YRBS), found a median of 1.3% identified as gay or lesbian, 3.7% as bisexual, and 2.5% were unsure. In the almost two decades since Remafedi and colleagues' early work (1992), the percentage of adolescents that are questioning is down by almost 8%, and those that identify as homosexual or bisexual in CDC data is at approximately 5% of the population. These data suggest that today's adolescents are able to self-identify earlier than in the past and spend less time feeling unsure as to their sexuality. Indeed, anecdotal data do seem to indicate that lesbian, gay, bisexual, and transgendered (LGBT) youth are coming out at younger ages (SAHM et al, 2014). The etiology of sexual orientation is unknown, and the sequential developmental phases from childhood to adulthood are debated (Bidwell, 2009). Sexual orientation tends to unfold with an awareness of same-sex attraction by the child's prepubertal years (Remafedi, 2011). As mentioned earlier, the development of sexual orientation is probably multifaceted and the result of a combination of genetic, biologic, and environmental factors that may affect males and females differently (Remafedi, 2011). Some postulate that it is a purely biologic phenomenon, largely determined in utero, as evidenced by the high concordance of homosexuality among monozygotic twins (especially in males). Researchers have studied prenatal androgen exposure, loci on the X chromosome, and neuroanatomical differences in the brain (especially in females) (Remafedi, 2011). The work of Bell and colleagues (1981) served to rule out many psychosocial components when the researchers concluded that homosexuality does not result from a cold, distant father; poor peer relationships; sexual abuse; or sexual experimentation in childhood.

Clinical Findings

The development of a minority sexual orientation involves a process of acknowledging and integrating one's sexual identity. The gold standard model of homosexual identity formation includes the following (Troiden, 1988):

- *Sensitization* occurs during childhood when individuals identify themselves as feeling different from others of the same gender. Girls describe themselves as "unfeminine," whereas boys often report feelings of disinterest in sports and a proclivity for artistic endeavors. Boys state that they are often called "sissies."
- *Identity confusion* usually occurs during adolescence when individuals begin to question whether they may be homosexual. On average, this occurs for males at 17 years old and for females at 18 years old. Feelings of inadequacy, insecurity, self-deprecation, poor self-esteem, and depression can result from unresolved identity confusion.
- *Identity assumption* is the stage at which the child assumes a homosexual identity that is shared with others. The age at which this occurs varies by gender (males at an average age of 19 to 21 years and females 21 to 23 years). Exploration of the homosexual role can lead to multiple sexual experiences with accompanying risks of acquiring STIs and HIV. In contrast, the individual can develop close long-term relationships with the same relationship problems as his or her heterosexual counterparts.
- *Commitment* is an internalized pledge to live as a homosexual and enter into a same-sex relationship. This process can be referred to as "coming out." External disclosure to others who are not homosexual may vary, depending on what is perceived to be safe to the individual. A stigma management strategy of blending, or acting in a "gender-appropriate" manner, may be adopted in an attempt to be safe in environments that are not tolerant or accepting of homosexuality.

Management

The goal of the provider working with adolescents who are LGBTQ is the same as with any adolescent: promote healthy sexual development, assess social and emotional well-being, and encourage physical health through healthy lifestyle choices. It is important to support and validate the adolescent throughout the process of developing his or her awareness of and commitment to a sexual orientation and provide a safe environment in which to access health care (SAHM et al, 2014).

The counseling needs of LGBTQ youth are much the same as with any adolescent. Specific interventions include the following: ensuring confidentiality, using gender-neutral nonjudgmental language, displaying information that is important to LGBTQ youth, and providing information about available resources for support. Encourage abstinence, promote safer sex for those who are sexually active, and counsel about the association between substance abuse and unsafe sexual practices.

For many LGBTQ youth, the process unfolds without event, especially those with family support (Ryan et al, 2010), whereas others have a rockier transition and engage in risky behaviors and experience complications (Remafedi, 2011; Russell and Toomey, 2012). Family support and acceptance have been associated with increased levels of self-esteem, social support, and overall health. They have also been found to be protective against depression, suicidal ideation and attempts, as well as substance abuse (Ryan et al, 2010). Maturity, access to accurate information, positive role models, and social support influence the LGBTQ youth's self-acceptance and success with intimate relationships (Remafedi, 2011).

Complications

Many sources report that LGBTQ youth engage in high-risk behaviors and face stress and victimization at a higher rate than their heterosexual peers (Kann et al, 2011; National Research Council, 2011; Russell et al, 2014; SAHM et al, 2014), which may lead to poor health outcomes for these adolescents. Providers need to be aware of the increased risks surrounding LGBTQ youth and address these needs through education and counseling at every health visit. There are many great resources available.

For a complete list of references, please visit http://evolve.elsevier.com/Burns/pediatric/.

16

Values, Beliefs, and Spirituality

ARDYS M. DUNN

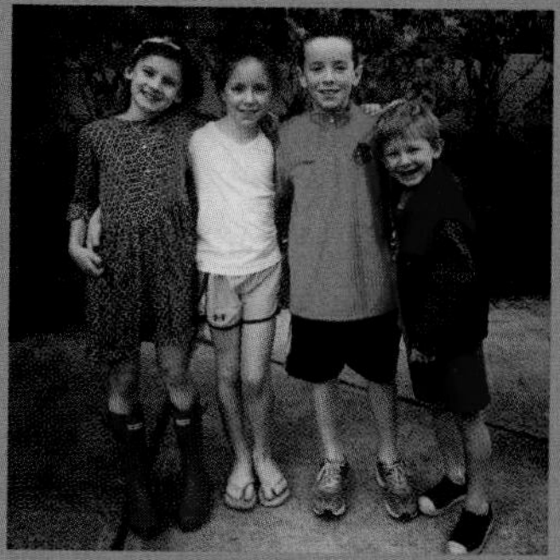

The health and well-being of children and adolescents are not limited to physical measures alone. There is growing recognition of the importance of attending to matters of the mind and spirit in the health care of all individuals. In addition, new discoveries in how the brain relates to physical, cognitive, perceptual, and affective functioning lend insight into the complexity of human responses to health and illness. The use of meditation, prayer, relaxation, and other mind-body therapies is known to facilitate healing. Holistic pediatric care includes assessment of social, cultural, and spiritual dimensions of the child, family, and community. It considers the effect of values and beliefs on health care decisions and explores ways to support those values, beliefs, and subsequent actions that promote health. Pediatric primary health care providers must be aware that beliefs, spirituality, faith, and religion can affect children's health. It is essential that primary pediatric care providers incorporate spiritual care into their practice. Doing so offers children, adolescents, and their families an invaluable resource to find meaning, comfort, and healing.

Standards of Practice

Health care in the United States has tended to focus on physical health and illness rather than the integration of mental, emotional, and spiritual health. When individuals have received care in the spiritual realm, they have traditionally been referred to chaplains, pastors, or other religious leaders in their faith community. However, the importance of health care providers being able to address the spiritual element of care has become widely acknowledged, and guidelines related to spiritual issues in health care are being developed.

The Society of Teachers of Family Medicine has published spiritual care competencies for the family resident education program that focus on knowledge, skills, and attitude. The spiritual and child health initiative of the Department of Pediatrics, Boston Medical Center and Medical Anthropology articulated guidelines for general pediatric practice. Together, these groups suggest that health care providers should (Anandarajah et al, 2010; Barnes et al, 2000):

- Have a conceptual framework of spirituality in their clinical care
- Understand the differences between spirituality and religion, the influence of beliefs on patient care, and ethical issues between patient and provider
- Anticipate patients will have spiritual or religious concerns
- Become broadly familiar with the religious worldview of the patient groups for whom they care
- Be skilled at assessing spiritual components of client systems, listening with attention to spiritual needs, and providing a therapeutic, compassionate presence to support healing; develop strategic interviewing skills
- Know where and how to access resources for spiritual care (e.g., chaplains); develop a resource list and network of local consultants, and make appropriate referrals
- Demonstrate respect for patients and colleagues
- Develop mindfulness to personal spiritual beliefs and perspectives, caring for the self and using practices that strengthen their healing intention as providers of patient care

Courses such as The Healer's Art, taught in nearly half of all medical schools across the country, can provide the framework for developing such competencies (see Additional Resources).

The Joint Commission requires spiritual assessments of patients admitted to tertiary care hospitals (The Joint Commission, 2010), and clinical guidelines for palliative care have been developed by the National Consensus Project for Quality Palliative Care (NCPQPC, 2013). Depression may have a spiritual connection, and the U.S. Preventive Services Task Force has recommended screening adolescents (12 to 18 years old) for major depressive disorders (USPSTF, 2009); this recommendation is currently being researched and may be revised (see Additional Resources).

Much of the focus on spiritual needs of children and families has been related to critical or palliative care or end-of-life decisions; and addressing spiritual beliefs may be particularly important for families facing life-threatening illnesses that seem unfair or that have no reasonable explanation. However, these discussions should be a standard part of well-child visits, as well as care of children who are acutely or chronically ill. Spirituality is essential to all human life and is a critical part of every child's healthy development.

Normal Patterns of Behavior

Definitions of Values, Beliefs, Faith, Spirituality, and Morality

Values have been defined as perceptions held about the worth or importance of a certain thing, person, or idea. *Beliefs* are attitudes that one holds that something is true. Values and beliefs influence actions, both consciously and unconsciously. They are guides that individuals use as they make decisions. Values and beliefs are learned phenomena, and recognition and acceptance of shared values and beliefs are fundamental to the integrity of the individual, the family, and the social group (see Chapter 3). Although perceptions, attitudes, values, and beliefs are transmitted from one generation to another, they remain open to change and are responsive to social contexts and situations. Values clarification is the process by which one examines behavior in light of values and changing circumstances and asks why a certain action is taken or whether that action is consistent with the values one claims to have. Change in values, beliefs, and behavior can result from the process of values clarification.

According to Fowler and Dell (2004), *faith* is the basis for developing beliefs, values, and meaning. Faith "(1) gives coherence and direction to persons' lives; (2) links them in shared trusts and loyalties with others; (3) grounds their personal stances and communal loyalties in a sense of relatedness to a larger frame of reference; and (4) enables them to face and deal with the challenges of human life and death, relying on that which has the quality of ultimacy in their lives" (Fowler and Dell, 2004, p 17). In this broad conceptualization, faith encompasses a wide range of religious and spiritual expression.

Closely related to faith, *spirituality* has been defined as an awareness of and commitment to a sacred, unifying force that gives meaning to life; the recognition of a nonmaterial higher power that encompasses all of life's affairs and is mediated through the individual's relationships to others, to the community, and to the environment (McLeod and Wright, 2008). Characteristics of spirituality are listed in Box 16-1. Spirituality and religion should not be confused. Religion is the organized expression of values, beliefs, and spirituality through religious activities, rituals, and behaviors. Children's expression of their spirituality depends on their experiences with faith language, ritual, and organization. For example, those children raised in families where prayer, discussion of religious beliefs, and participation in religious rituals and events are the norm will express their faith and spirituality differently from children raised in a more secular family system.

• BOX 16-1 Characteristics of Spirituality

Inner Resources and Identity

Those who possess inner resources have a sense of wholeness, competence, and direction. They are capable of responding to crises or turmoil and draw on inner strengths to maintain a sense of stability and control. They have values that give them courage and hope.

Interconnectedness

Interconnectedness is the sense of being an integral part of the world and attached to others, to one's environment, and to a universal or supreme being.

Purpose or Meaning of Life

A sense of direction and meaning and a reason for existence are developed in the relationships individuals have with others and their world.

Transcendence

The ability to go beyond, or transcend, the experiences of daily life is evident in the expression of hope, meaning, and direction when an individual is faced with fear, inability to effect change, uncertainty, and ambiguity.

Morality is the quality of being that encompasses that which is right (justice or fairness) and that which is good (empathy or kindness). Moral integrity involves demonstrating an *understanding* of right and wrong (moral cognition); engaging in *reflection* on ethical issues of justice and fairness (moral judgment); expressing a *sense of responsibility* to oneself, others, and the environment (moral sensitivity and emotions); and taking *action* based on one's moral values (moral character). Empathy, a fundamental moral emotion, is an expression of the ability to understand the condition of another and to experience a visceral or emotional reaction to that condition; to quite literally take the perspective of another.

This ability to take the perspective of another and both understand (cognitive) and feel (emotional) what the other is experiencing is fundamental to developing moral maturity. Mature morality is constructed through social interactions in which individuals mutually "reverse" their thinking: each strives to understand and feel how the other is thinking and feeling, and, as a result, each deepens his or her own understanding and emotions. Individuals capable of "putting themselves in another's shoes" are able to move beyond egoistical thinking (e.g., "What's in it for me?") to a basic concern for the greater good—of others, of societies, and of the environment (Bloom, 2013). This process of mutual *reciprocity* is "fundamentally distinct from culturally relativistic socialization, learning, or internalization processes" (Gibbs, 2014, p 96). Morality is not something that can be taught as a "cultural norm" or "expected behavior." Mature morality is a socially constructed phenomenon that goes beyond the rules, rituals, expectations, and norms of any one culture or society. Behavior that is unjust or evil (e.g., female genital mutilation) cannot be excused or tolerated simply because it is based in a cultural history.

Children's values and beliefs are reflected in different behaviors at different ages as they gain greater cognitive and social skills. In general, "adaptive, competent functioning" reflects positive values and development (Kochanska et al, 2010a). In particular, the development of moral integrity (or conscience) and spirituality (or faith) is expected of the healthy child. As they develop moral integrity and spiritual values, healthy children achieve a positive sense of self, learn to value themselves and their contribution to the family and larger social system, and feel a sense of understanding and belonging.

Development of Moral Integrity or Conscience

The development of moral integrity is an evolutionary process, likely derived from a "biologically-based predisposition" to altruism (Hoffman, 2000); it is influenced by prenatal, genetic, physical, neurologic, emotional, and social factors; and it continues through adulthood. Even infants and very young children demonstrate concern when confronted with a stressful situation (e.g., another child crying) and they may try to provide comfort (i.e., act "altruistically") or seek comfort themselves. As children grow—if given opportunities, guidance, and positive role models—these intrinsic expressions of concern and altruistic behaviors become more sophisticated. Moral reasoning is evident as children develop friendships, learn to care about others, and begin to understand that rights and responsibilities are essential to societal functioning. The ability to reflect on their own behavior and that of others is seen in the preschool years, and by middle childhood, children begin to assess the moral value of behaviors and make moral decisions.

Ongoing research continues to identify specific characteristics, dynamics, and determinants of the process of developing moral integrity. Recent discoveries in neurobiology and epigenetics, in particular, provide an exciting window into the ways children develop, often making connections between psychological and developmental processes and physical phenomena. Some of the theories include:

- *Developmental theories:* Research on the ways children gain moral integrity has primarily been based in developmental theory. Kohlberg's notion that moral development proceeds sequentially through phases related to intellectual development and social interactions is probably the most well known of these theories (Kohlberg, 1969), although other developmental perspectives have been offered and Kohlberg's work has been expanded upon (Gibbs, 2014; see Chapter 4). Freud, for example, asserted that children develop a conscience through identification with a significant caregiver mediated by the processes of guilt and shame. Piaget claimed that children's moral development parallels their intellectual development and ability to reason. And social learning theory (e.g., Vygotsky) states that positive role modeling and active social engagement with others teaches moral behavior.
- *Attachment, temperament, and reciprocity:* Kochanska and colleagues have conducted extensive research on how toddlers and preschool children develop a moral identity, a sense of their "moral self" that guides their future conduct. Secure attachment to the primary caregiver early in life is a critical determinant; this attachment supports an "eager, willing stance" toward the parent, and facilitates internalization of parental rules and standards as well as a sense of empathy with others (Kochanska et al, 2010b). In fact, secure attachment may override genetic effects as children develop the ability to self-regulate (Kochanska et al, 2009). Temperament can affect the child-parent interaction and the development of conscience in two ways. First, the natural temperament of the child may lend itself to internalization of parental values. Children with a naturally fearful temperament tend to more quickly internalize their parents' message and, as a result, require gentle parenting with "subtle discipline" for healthy development. Second, temperament may be difficult or conflictive between parent and child and require more directive socialization strategies. Children who demonstrate a "fearless" temperament appear to function best when there is a "mutually positive, responsive, binding, and cooperative orientation between parent and child" (i.e., reciprocity) (Kochanska and Aksan, 2006). When the parent is responsive to the child, the child tends to be more cooperative; children who are actively engaged in a supportive, reciprocal relationship with their parent are more likely to want to do what the parent suggests and healthy development is strengthened (Kochanska et al, 2010a; Leclère et al, 2014).
- *Gender:* Some theorists contend that gender plays a significant role in the way children interpret situations and make choices based on moral judgment (Gilligan, 1990), and there is evidence that girls are likely to be more empathic and more highly skilled in emotional judgments than boys (Fumagalli et al, 2010) or more likely to demonstrate giving behavior (Ongley et al, 2014). The relationship among genetics, neurobiology, and environment (including socialization) as determinants of this gender difference remains to be explained.
- *Neurobiology:* Recent research explored the role of neural development on moral behavior, particularly empathy (Gonzalez-Liencres et al, 2013; Herpers et al, 2014). Empathy, it appears, may be grounded in the brain. Three primary areas of brain circuitry process emotions, memory, and the cognitive functions that integrate behavioral responses:
    - The limbic system (amygdala, thalamus, and hypothalamus in particular) stores emotional memory,

transmits messages of stress (fight or flight), and appears to enable emotions of bonding, affiliation, and (their negative counterpart) separation. Activity in the amygdala (emotional memory) in particular stimulates activity in the orbital frontal cortex and ventromedial prefrontal cortex, centers of emotional learning, judgment, and decision-making.

- The mirror neuron system functions to encourage imitation and is activated when pain is experienced. Imagining, anticipating pain, or observing others' experience of pain also activates this system. Research on how mirror neurons shape infants' physical actions and how those actions, in turn, influence the infants' ability to perceive and analyze the actions of others may help explain how judgment evolves (Woodward and Gerson, 2014).
- The paralimbic system (insula and anterior cingulate cortex [ACC]) connects the limbic and mirror neuron systems with peripheral physiologic stimuli—both physical and emotional. The insula is activated by negative arousal, for example, pain, bad smells or taste, or fear. Conflict activates the ACC, which works with the insula, connecting physical arousal to emotions and engaging the memory of the limbic system to evaluate, judge, and (ultimately) act, all in an effort to relieve distress. Real and imagined arousal activates the paralimbic system, as does the perception of arousal in others.
- Functional deficits in these areas of the brain limit the individual's ability to feel emotion—in self or others, to make good judgments or decisions, and to demonstrate empathic, morally integrated behavior (Blair, 2013). Responsive parenting and positive physical experience (e.g., gentle touch, nurturing, and comfort) early in childhood appear to strengthen these areas of the brain, stimulating positive vagal nerve function, and contributing to feelings of calmness and compassion (Narvaez, 2010).
- *Epigenetics:* Findings of early research in the area of epigenetics suggest that epigenetic changes may mediate the effect of prenatal and infant environment on mental health and disease in older children and adults (McGowan and Szyf, 2010). In animal studies, behavior of a high-nurturing parent stimulates the gene that encodes glucocorticoid receptor proteins and relieves stress. A study of suicide victims who were abused as children revealed that they had decreased levels of this marker, suggesting that child abuse may have an epigenetic effect that leads to prolonged stress and mental disorders (McGowan et al, 2009).

Development of Spirituality

Although it has been argued that children are intrinsically spiritual, the development of spiritual expression in children is largely seen as paralleling cognitive and moral development (Fowler, 1981). Table 16-1 presents a developmental perspective of faith and outlines age-specific interventions to enhance healthy growth. Infants and toddlers are engaged in the processes of gaining trust and establishing autonomy or separateness of self from the parent. They are becoming

TABLE 16-1 Developmental Outcomes and Appropriate Interventions Related to Values and Beliefs by Age

	Infant (0-12 months old)	Toddler and Preschooler (1-5 years old)	School-Age Child (6-12 years old)	Adolescent
Moral integrity and conscience (right and wrong; sense of responsibility to oneself, others, and the environment)	Develops sense of trust in caregivers (Erikson, 1963); learns to adjust to family routine (e.g., sleeping, eating)	Believes rules are absolute; behaves well for fear of punishment or to receive rewards (Kohlberg, 1969); develops sense of autonomy, initiative, and purpose; differentiates self from others (Erikson, 1963)	Believes rules exist to keep order and protect people and that everyone benefits from them; behaves well to please others, to avoid guilt, and to maintain status of "good" child (Kohlberg, 1969); develops sense of industry, faith in self-competence; explores, creates, collects; understands cause and effect (Erikson, 1963); begins to understand and manage strong feelings, and develop and express moral decision-making	Rules are based on ethical judgment; believes individual answers to personal conscience, has moral obligation to a social contract; behaves to maintain respect of self, peers, and larger community (Kohlberg, 1969); integrates personality and develops sense of identity, loyalty to group and significant others (Erikson, 1963)

TABLE 16-1 Developmental Outcomes and Appropriate Interventions Related to Values and Beliefs by Age—cont'd

	Infant (0-12 months old)	Toddler and Preschooler (1-5 years old)	School-Age Child (6-12 years old)	Adolescent
Faith development (Fowler, 1981 as cited in Mueller, 2010)	Undifferentiated faith based on trust in relationships with parents and caregivers; infant develops object permanence, sense of trust, attachment, and sense of being nurtured	Intuitive-projective faith based on images, feelings, and symbols; children use imagination to make meaning of their world; egocentric thinking may contribute to misconceptions; child begins to participate in family's religious practices and rituals	Mythic-literal faith, with more concrete beliefs, a more rigid system of order and activities; faith as assent, as child learns to master the environment and become competent; child begins to explore ultimate issues, develop understanding of the meaning of life	Synthetic conventional faith—ideas about spirituality are synthesized through interpersonal relations with peers, parents, other significant adults, and life experiences; adolescent explores identity and personal meaning of faith; faith becomes source of identity as child seeks understanding of self in the world (Quinn, 2008); adolescent demonstrates self-reflection, insight, sense of inner spiritual process and presence in the world, and continues to more fully develop understanding of ultimate questions, life's meaning
Experienced faith (infancy through early adolescence) Affiliative faith (late adolescence)	Children experience faith through relationships with others and others' faith traditions			Adolescent actively participates in a faith community, feels a sense of belonging, awe, and wonder; acknowledges authority of faith community
Parental Interventions to Foster Healthy Development				
	Respond to infant's physiologic and emotional needs promptly and adequately; demonstrate loving, gentle approach in communication and interaction	Treat child with respect and acceptance; provide security, love, and companionship; set realistic limits on behavior, using positive discipline rather than punishment; remove temptation from environment; provide positive role model; provide guided opportunities to interact with adults and other children and active play alone; be patient; involve child in family religious practices; begin to establish regular tasks for child in family activities	Treat child with respect and acceptance; set realistic limits on behavior; provide opportunities for active play alone and with other children; encourage peer group activity; allow children to make decisions as appropriate, helping them to explore meanings of feelings, events, and interactions; choose narrative stories related to children's experience of moral dilemmas to explore right and wrong and to help child develop values; establish regular tasks for child as member of family; help child be successful in the family; teach family values and standards; encourage continued participation in family religious practices	Treat adolescent with respect and acceptance; set realistic limits on behavior; model and encourage family's moral standards; encourage involvement in family activities; allow children to make more of own choices regarding values and beliefs; allow appropriate experimentation in dress, hair, makeup as child develops sense of self; do not overreact to adolescent "crises"; provide opportunities to discuss values, ethics, and moral behavior; provide support and encouragement for successes and failures in school, social, athletic, and work activities; encourage continued participation in family religious practices

a part of a larger culture (i.e., the family). Preschool and early school-age children gain an understanding of the meaning of life through fantasy play, active engagement with their environment, strong attachments to their parents, and growing relationships with their peers. Although they have achieved the task of defining themselves as separate individuals, the thinking and behavior of preschool and early school-age children in relation to faith issues are expressions of the family's faith and practice. School-age children and adolescents define life's meaning within the context of their self-sufficiency, competence, and role differentiation and in their relationship to both peers and adults. Adolescents are moving from the secure, dependent stage of childhood toward the independence expected of adults. This period of transition can be disorienting, turbulent, even painful—one in which the adolescent actively searches for meaning and purpose (Haley, 2014a). Exploring their understanding of the ultimate questions in life, adolescents are interested in issues such as life, death, war, evil, good, and creation and develop increasing wisdom as they discuss and reflect on these important matters.

Assessment of Normal Patterns

The goals of assessing values and beliefs include the following:

- Identify the nature of the child's and family's belief system.
- Identify ways that the family interacts (internally, with a faith community, and with the larger community) to support these beliefs.
- Clarify how beliefs affect decisions and behaviors related to health and illness.
- Develop an understanding of how this particular illness or health issue challenges the child's and family's belief system.
- Determine how the provider can best address values, including spiritual or religious issues when giving care.

For younger children, assessment questions are often directed to the parent or caregiver. This can yield a wealth of information, but it may not accurately or completely assess the child's needs or understandings. Children may not be able to understand what is happening to them and they cannot always express themselves clearly or use the words or symbols related to values, beliefs, faith, or spirituality that are more familiar to adults. As a result, it may be difficult or even impossible to accurately interpret and understand the emotional and spiritual meaning a given experience has for a child. Adolescents, engaged in the process of developing a self-identity, including identifying, clarifying, and articulating their values and beliefs, are more capable of exploring assessment questions with the provider (Haley, 2014a).

History

Moral Integrity or Conscience

The focus of an assessment of moral integrity will vary depending on the age of the child, and it requires looking at the ways family members interact; the messages parents give to their children about what is just, fair, right, and good; as well as the child's behavior and responses to questions. The following points can guide the assessment:

- How does the child define right and wrong? How does the child's behavior reflect his or her moral understanding? How does the child demonstrate moral reasoning?
- What are family attitudes or beliefs about what is right and wrong?
- How are parents teaching their child about right and wrong?
- What other influences affect the child's concept of right and wrong (e.g., day care, teachers and counselors, peer group)?
- How do parents set limits on the child's behavior?
- How does the child respond to discipline and limits?
- What messages do parents give about the value and importance of the child's contribution to the family and the community?
- What messages do parents give about the value of respecting other people, ideas, property, and the environment?
- What opportunities do parents give the child to make independent, age-appropriate decisions?
- What traditions and family-centered activities does the family have? How is the child included in these activities?

Spirituality

Most spiritual assessment tools have been developed for use with adults, typically in critical or palliative care. Some, however, have been used with children and families (Table 16-2). An initial screening can determine if more in-depth assessment or pastoral intervention is appropriate. Grossoehme (2008) developed such a tool to be used by chaplains when initially interviewing hospitalized children or adolescents. Use of the screening tool appears to generate productive "deeper conversation with the patients" (Fig. 16-1). Assessment of spirituality can address general issues as well as the particular characteristics of spirituality (see Box 16-1), with questions being primarily addressed to parents and adapted to adolescents.

General. How are the following issues influenced, if at all, by your religious or spiritual beliefs:

- Family relations, gender roles, and children's and parents' responsibilities
- Sexuality issues (e.g., responsible sexuality, male and female roles, homosexuality, transgender issues, premarital sex)
- Dietary restrictions
- Rituals (e.g., prayer at mealtime, bedtime, or during times of crisis)
- Use of drugs, alcohol, or tobacco
- Medical treatment

Inner Resources and Identity. The following questions focus on internal strengths and qualities:

- What are your child's goals in life? Your family's goals?
- What are your child's strong points? Your family's strong points?

TABLE 16-2 Spiritual Assessment Tools

Tool Name (Acronym)	Questions Related to Tool	Citation
HOPE	Where does client find **H**ope, peace, and comfort? Does client participate in **O**rganized religion? What are **P**ersonal spiritual practices? What **E**ffect do these behaviors have on the client's health decisions?	(Anandarajah and Hight, 2001)
BELIEF	What is client's **B**elief system? **E**thics or values? **L**ifestyle behaviors (e.g., diet, rituals)? **I**nvolvement in a spiritual community? Religious **E**ducation and knowledge? **F**uture events and decisions about health that will be affected by religious beliefs?	(McEvoy, 2000)
SPIRIT	**S**piritual belief system (religious affiliation)? **P**ersonal spirituality (beliefs that child/family accept)? **I**ntegration and involvement with a religious community? **R**ituals and restrictions? **I**mplications for medical care (beliefs provider should take into consideration when discussing medical care)? **T**erminal events planning (e.g., advance directives, contacting clergy)?	(Highfield, 2000)
FICA	**F**aith and belief: Do you consider yourself religious? What gives your life meaning? Helps you cope with stress? **I**mportance: How important is your faith or beliefs? How do they influence your health or how you have managed this illness? **C**ommunity: Are you a part of a spiritual or religious community? Does this support you? Is there a group of people you love and who are important to you? **A**ddress: How would you like me, as your health provider, to address these issues in giving you care?	(Puchalski and Romer, 2000)

- What do you like about yourself? Your child? Your family?
- How important is faith or spirituality in your child's life? In your life?
- What brings you, your child, and your family joy and peace? Where do you find hope and comfort?

Interconnectedness. The following questions relate to connections the child and family have with each other and the larger community:

- What do you do as a family to show love for each other?
- Who are significant people in your child's and your family's life?
- Whom do you ask for support when your family needs help?
- How do members of your family share feelings with others?
- Do you feel that you and your family are part of a community? Of a larger world or universe?
- Does the family belong to a religious or spiritual group?
- With whom does your child/adolescent talk about values, beliefs, and spirituality?

Purpose or Meaning of Life. The following questions examine the child and family's sense of purpose:

- What are your family's religious, spiritual, and cultural beliefs? What ethics or values are important in your family's life? How do you express these beliefs (e.g., religious rituals or spiritual practices)?
- What gives life meaning? What is the most important thing in life to you?
- How do you teach your child about values and beliefs? How else does your child learn about values and beliefs?

Transcendence. The following question looks at ways the family overcomes challenges and fears:

- How do members of your family deal with spiritual distress during a crisis?

Physical Examination

Objective assessment of values and beliefs is largely based on observation of behavior, and, although subject to interpretation, these observations can indicate the child's sense of valuing others, self, and the environment. Observe the child's behavior, especially noting interaction with parents, other adults, and peers. The healthy child exhibits the following behaviors:

- Appears at ease, although behavior may vary (e.g., shy, quiet, active, talkative, engaging) depending on developmental level and temperament
- Engages actively, spontaneously, and affectionately with parent or caregiver

Child/Adolescent Spiritual Screening Tool

Name: ______________________________ Age:________

Please draw a circle around the answer below each statement.

How often do you think that...

1.	A good God watches over me.					
		Never	Rarely	Sometimes	Often	Always
2.	I have to live with God's punishment.					
		Never	Rarely	Sometimes	Often	Always
3.	I feel God's love in my life.					
		Never	Rarely	Sometimes	Often	Always
4.	Embarrassment plays a big role in my life.					
		Never	Rarely	Sometimes	Often	Always
5.	My hope tells me life's got to get better.					
		Never	Rarely	Sometimes	Often	Always
6.	I wish my family were with me more right now.					
		Never	Rarely	Sometimes	Often	Always
7.	I have friendships with kids in church.					
		Never	Rarely	Sometimes	Often	Always
8.	My loneliness makes life hard.					
		Never	Rarely	Sometimes	Often	Always
9.	Prayer helps me.					
		Never	Rarely	Sometimes	Often	Always
10.	God feels very far away from me.					
		Never	Rarely	Sometimes	Often	Always
11.	Having my parents nearby helps me when life is hard.					
		Never	Rarely	Sometimes	Often	Always
12.	My religion tells me my sickness (or my problem) is my fault.					
		Never	Rarely	Sometimes	Often	Always
13.	People show their love for me.					
		Never	Rarely	Sometimes	Often	Always
14.	My God is an angry God.					
		Never	Rarely	Sometimes	Often	Always
15.	I love who I am.					
		Never	Rarely	Sometimes	Often	Always
16.	Betrayal is part of my life story.					
		Never	Rarely	Sometimes	Often	Always
17.	I have lost a lot in life.					
		Never	Rarely	Sometimes	Often	Always

• **Figure 16-1** Spiritual Screening Tool for Children and Adolescents. Odd numbered items 1 through 15 indicate spiritual strengths; even numbered items 2 through 16 and item 17 indicate spiritual needs. Extent to which needs outweigh strengths may be one indication of how much an individual needs spiritual counseling. (From Grossoehme DH: Development of a spiritual screening tool for children and adolescents, *J Pastoral Care Counsel* 62(1):71–85, 2008.)

- Responds to parent or caregiver cues; follows directions and conforms to limits set without demonstrating guilt or fear of punishment
- Shares toys, depending on age
- Respects people and property
- Is not physically aggressive, depending on age
- Is able to articulate moral reasoning (older child)
- Is able to articulate a faith statement, depending on spiritual, religious, and cultural background (older child)

Management of Normal Patterns

The goals of management are to facilitate the development of moral integrity (including moral identity, judgment, and conduct) and a sense of spiritual self within the major areas of spirituality: self-awareness as a spiritual being and relationships with others, the environment, and with a sacred or transcendent entity.

Parents can encourage their child's development of moral integrity in the following ways:

- Be a loving, responsive, and accepting presence in their children's lives. This responsibility cannot be overemphasized; children's understandings and expressions of self-concept, spirituality, and moral integrity derive in large part from the quality of their interactions with significant adults.
- Set realistic standards or limits for right and wrong behavior.
- State what is acceptable and what is unacceptable behavior.
- Provide a rationale for limits set; the explanation varies depending on the cognitive and developmental level of the child.
- Articulate personal values, beliefs, and faith statements for the child. Give clear, age-appropriate explanations and spiritual lessons.
- Be a role model for constructive and positive behavior; be the model of what you want your child to be.
- Reinforce positive behavior and attempts at positive behavior.
- Hold children accountable for negative behavior; use "consequences" that are age-appropriate and that fairly suit the behavior being sanctioned.
- Teach children strategies to avoid misbehavior; teach constructive coping skills.
- Use creative parenting strategies (e.g., distraction, diversional activities) to help children avoid misbehavior.
- Provide a developmentally appropriate environment to minimize children's misbehavior. It is easier, for example, to remove a breakable object from a table than to repeatedly say "no" or to punish a child for breaking it.
- Provide opportunities for children to make age-appropriate decisions independently.
- Praise children in front of others.
- Do not give false praise.
- Articulate and reinforce messages that children belong and are valued for themselves, not just for their behaviors.
- Establish family traditions and projects that actively involve children (e.g., family outings or family value sessions, during which family members share a meal with directed conversation). Do not expect perfection.
- Involve children in the family's religious and cultural practices.
- Provide and encourage opportunities for children to engage with the larger community in activities that support the child's interests and reinforce family values.
- Engage the child in nature-based activities (e.g., walks, visits to parks, outdoor camps) that strengthen a sense of ecologic connection and responsibility.
- Provide opportunities for the child to explore moral and ethical dilemmas and to develop possible solutions.
- Discuss moral and spiritual implications of events in the child's life (e.g., death of a grandparent, birth of a sibling, sharing, stealing, and violence portrayed in media).
- Listen to and answer the child's questions.

Primary health care providers should do the following:

- Be aware of their own values and beliefs.
- Distinguish between moral, spiritual, and medical advice. Be willing to offer all advice, while recognizing that personal proselytizing is inappropriate in the provider-patient relationship.
- Recognize and respect differences between their values and client's values.
- Provide an opportunity for parents to express values and beliefs and to discuss questions and/or concerns they may have about their child's moral and spiritual development.
- Provide an opportunity for adolescents to think about and express their spiritual values and beliefs.
- Create an environment that allows and supports the child, adolescent, and/or parents to express doubts, questions, fears, and uncertainties.
- Provide information about parenting strategies, discipline, and effective communication between child and parents.
- Assist parents and child in values clarification as appropriate.
- Provide a role model of positive behavior.
- Offer an understanding, compassionate, and accepting presence. Be "mindfully present" with children, adolescents, and families (Haley, 2014b).
- Listen and respond to the unique condition of each individual.
- Modify the treatment plan as appropriate to meet spiritual and religious needs.
- Refer the family for religious or spiritual counseling and support as indicated or requested.

Altered Patterns

Lack of Moral Integrity or Conscience

Although lack of moral integrity is not a clinically defined condition, some children demonstrate lack of an age-appropriate capacity to respect others or the environment, to judge behavior as right or wrong, and to express empathy or remorse. They frequently engage in antisocial behaviors (see Chapter 19 for a fuller discussion of social aggression, conduct disorder, and oppositional defiant disorder). A multitude of factors contribute to poor moral reasoning and antisocial behaviors, including temperament, negative experiences in infancy and childhood (e.g., maternal depression, unresponsive parenting, and abuse), and environmental damage to neurologic systems.

Assessment

See Assessment of Normal Patterns.

Clinical Findings

Many behaviors seen are typical of normal children, depending on age, developmental, and cognitive levels (e.g., lying, hitting, and refusing to share), but the child who lacks conscience expresses little or no remorse for negative behavior, demonstrating a callous demeanor (Viding et al, 2014); lacks internalization of a sense of justice, fairness, or right and wrong; fails to develop an ability to self-regulate behavior; and continues antisocial behaviors beyond the expected developmental age.

Differential Diagnosis

Attention-deficit/hyperactivity disorder (ADHD), social aggression, conduct disorder, oppositional defiant disorder, autism, developmental delay, and depression are differential diagnoses.

Management

Early and assertive intervention can help many children develop a more healthy sense of their moral self and decrease antisocial behaviors, especially if treatment emphasizes developing moral judgment and correcting "self-serving cognitive distortion" (Barriga et al, 2009; Gibbs, 2014). In addition to strategies listed here, see the discussion of management strategies for normal moral development in this chapter and for social aggression, conduct disorder, and oppositional defiant disorder (see Chapter 19). In some cases, referral for psychiatric management may be necessary.

- Use storytelling, especially the personal narrative (the child's own story), to explore moral and ethical issues.
- Encourage interaction with older children who demonstrate higher levels of moral reasoning.
- Watch films, television, videos, and DVDs together with children, discussing moral dilemmas and behaviors; discuss books with adolescents.
- Monitor, discuss, and limit child's access to Internet and computer games.
- Assist child or adolescent to clarify values (e.g., ask child or adolescent to talk about what is most important to them; or to describe what characteristics of other people [and themselves] they see as being the "best" or most desirable).

Complications

Antisocial behavior and delinquency are behavioral disorders in which lack of moral integrity is a key component.

Moral and Spiritual Distress

Moral distress is defined as the "response to the inability to carry out one's chosen moral or ethical decision or action"; it is characterized by feelings of anxiety, powerlessness, frustration, and/or guilt (North American Nursing Diagnosis Association International [NANDA-I], 2014, p 368). Spiritual distress is an "impaired ability to experience and integrate meaning and purpose in life through connectedness with self, others, art, music, literature, nature, and/or a power greater than oneself" (NANDA-I, 2014, p 372).

Spiritual or moral distress can result from a number of factors. For children, issues of death and dying and serious illness are major causes, but any crisis can threaten the sense of meaning that is fundamental to the individual's moral and spiritual integrity. For infants and very young children, the simple fact of being hospitalized and removed from the routine and comfort of family life can lead to distress. Other factors that can contribute to this distress may include but are not limited to:

- Trauma or violence, to self or to significant others
- Witnessed violence (to others or in the media)
- Loss of significant other, especially parent or sibling
- Debilitating disease
- Chronic disease
- Separation of child from his or her family
- Isolation
- Homelessness
- Recommended medical therapies in conflict with child's or family's religious or spiritual beliefs (e.g., Christian Scientist)
- Barriers in the health care setting to practicing spiritual rituals (e.g., hospital routines that ignore patient's need to worship)
- Beliefs of health care providers, family members, or peers that conflict with those of child or parent

Assessment

See Assessment of Normal Patterns.

Clinical Findings

The following may be seen in spiritual or moral distress:

- Depressive behavior
- Suicidal ideation
- Withdrawal
- Lack of participation in usual religious practices
- Disparaging family's spiritual beliefs and values
- Questioning one's own value, meaning, and purpose of life

- Expressions of anger, resentment, or fear of God
- Expressions of fear of suffering or death
- Expressions of inner conflict and doubts about beliefs
- Expressions of sense of emptiness
- Sleep disturbance
- Somatic complaints
- Behavior changes with mood swings
- Request for spiritual assistance

Differential Diagnosis

Depression, poor coping mechanisms, conduct disorders, antisocial behavior, and posttraumatic stress disorder are differential diagnoses for spiritual distress.

Management

Spiritual integrity is fundamentally a sense of meaning and purpose: One has a direction, control, and promise in a future. Moral integrity reflects a sense of value in one's life choices: There is fairness and goodness in how one lives. Health crises can easily undermine this integrity. Management goals focus on helping children and families make sense of the events they are experiencing, to better understand what is happening to and with them, to regain control if possible, and to find ways to live that maximize what is right and "good." McLeod and Wright (2008) present a model of spiritual care practice using conversations to generate new understandings that ultimately relieve suffering and help families live with "unanswered" and "unanswerable" questions. This model assumes an open-ended, evolving interaction, with questions, dialogue, and reflection to explore difficult issues about the meaning of life. It assumes that each family system is unique and must be met with honor and respect. The process includes:

- "Calling forth and gathering" the family's and child's story of the illness; what has happened to them, how it has affected their faith or belief system
- "Opening space" in which feelings, ideas, and thoughts can be examined and interpreted, and where reflection is invited
- Using imagination and metaphor to hear and express meaning; this is often accomplished by telling stories, especially the patient's or similar stories, and offering hypothetical beliefs
- Listening with "open silence" so that the patient and family can express themselves freely
- Providing rituals that lead to conversation about the suffering being experienced (e.g., doing a genogram; asking the "one-question question" ["If you could have just one question answered in our work together, what would that question be?"]) (McLeod and Wright, 2008, p 126)

Meaning is generated in the conversations; in the interaction of questions, reflection, and answers; and clients express comfort even if the health outcome is ultimately beyond their control (McLeod and Wright, 2008).

In the process of developing a spirituality screening tool, Grossoehme (2008) found that adolescents identified several critical spiritual strengths and needs when they were confronted by a health problem:

- Strengths: Talking with parents, the presence of parents, and believing in a loving God
- Unfilled needs: Feeling isolated from one's family, feeling betrayed, and lacking a sense of purpose in life

Other management strategies can draw on these strengths, address these needs (and others), and ease distress:

- Identify and change situational factors that exacerbate distress. Assist parents to help their child process experiences contributing to distress. Engage the child or adolescent in conversation. Referral may be necessary in cases in which the child is experiencing significant psychological trauma. An integrated team composed of primary care provider, psychologist, clergy, and parish nurse can be appropriate. If children are hospitalized, hospital chaplains can be especially helpful to some families, and crisis therapy (e.g., response play therapy) can be effectively used when children are not able to verbally express their distress (McPherson, 2004).
- Provide comfort and security to allay fears and reassure child. Providers who work with children and adolescents who are hospitalized or who undergo long-term outpatient treatment for chronic illness should ensure that they have the same staff caregiver and have parents stay with them as much as possible.
- Encourage child and adolescent to participate in spiritual practices as desired. Adolescents who demonstrate positive spiritual coping tend to have fewer psychological problems (e.g., depression and conduct disorders) (Reynolds et al, 2014).
- Encourage child and adolescent to express feelings about what is happening to him or her.
- Encourage child and adolescent to talk about beliefs and understandings of stressors, such as death and illness.
- Answer questions honestly, according to the child's age and developmental level.
- Work with parents to help them process the experience from their perspective (see previous model of conversations: What is the parent's answer to the "one-question question"?)
- Advocate for the child and parent when they express beliefs in conflict with those of other health care providers or other family members.

Occasionally parents will refuse treatment for their child based on religious beliefs. Adolescents also may be emancipated or deemed by a court to be a "mature minor" (i.e., capable of making independent decisions) and may refuse care. If treatment is refused, the provider should:

- Ensure that the parents (or adolescent) are fully informed and fully understand the medical concern, course of the illness or condition, prognosis, and treatment.

- Provide or facilitate a discussion of the reasons behind the decision, the implications of the decision, and the parents' and child's or adolescent's feelings.
- Provide opportunity for parents and family to express negative feelings.
- Discuss possible use of complementary and alternative therapies (see Chapter 43).
- In some cases, providers may feel compelled to obtain a court order for care or temporary guardianship if necessary to treat the child.

Complications

Depression, suicide, and conduct disorders can be complications of spiritual or moral distress.

For a complete list of references, please visit http://evolve.elsevier.com/Burns/pediatric/.

17 Role Relationships

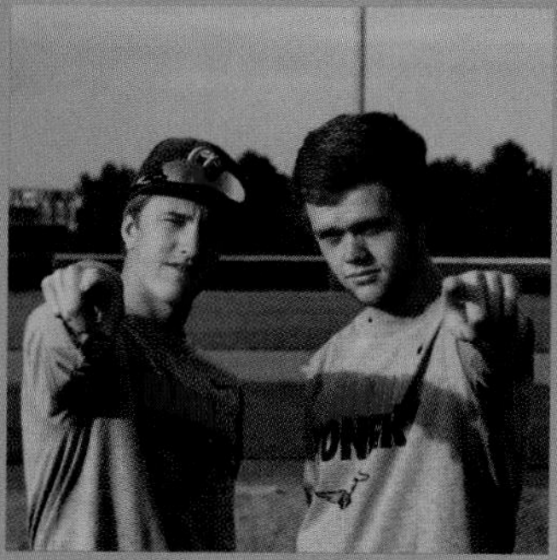

GABRIELLE M. PETERSEN, NOELLE NURRE, AND ARDYS M. DUNN

Children come with families, whether a nuclear unit of mother, father, and children or a more typical extended family in a social network of relatives and other significant individuals. In some cases, families are "blended" when two families join together as one. Currently, first-time parents are older, age of marriage is at an all-time high, and cohabitation (not marriage) is the typical first type of union. Births to unmarried women have risen from 5% in 1960 to about 40% in 2014. Divorce and remarriage remain common. These family arrangements can have major consequences for children's health and well-being (Olson, 2011).

Whatever the makeup of the family system, the pediatric primary care provider serves a crucial role in helping children and their families achieve optimal growth. Although parents and other family members are responsible for their children's daily health and welfare, pediatric providers offer necessary assessment and/or treatment when a child is physically ill or has emotional problems, and they advise and counsel children's caregivers on how to effectively handle issues that may arise as the child grows and develops. It is important that children develop the ability to interact well with others as well as understand, adopt, and carry out various social roles and responsibilities. Providers can help parents learn key communication and interaction skills in order to handle relationship issues with children at home, in school, and in the community. The pediatric provider must be sensitive to the roles that parents or caregivers, siblings, extended family members, peers, and the larger community have in shaping the developing child.

Chapter 2 outlines important considerations and appropriate tools to be used when assessing family systems. This chapter provides a foundation for the clinician to use as a reference when evaluating the complex encounters of families. In addition, it covers the assessment and management of situations or events that the provider is likely to see in a primary care setting related to family relationship problems, sibling rivalry, violence, and child maltreatment or neglect. Preventive interventions for role-relationship problems are identified.

Standards of Care

The Center for the Study of Social Policy (n.d.) introduced the Strengthening Families Approach and Protective Factors Framework in 2003 as a research-informed, strength-based initiative for preventing child abuse and neglect. Five protective factors have been identified that help keep all families strong and on the pathway of healthy development and well-being. The five factors include:

- Parental resilience
- Social connections
- Knowledge of parenting and child development
- Concrete support in times of need
- Social and emotional competence of children

Many children are abused, neglected, and exposed to violence in the United States and worldwide, with subsequent long-term effects of disease, injury, family and societal dysfunction, crime, and suicide. Every pediatric provider should have the goal of eliminating all violence, abuse, and neglect. In an effort to reach that goal, *Healthy People 2020* addresses issues of violence and abusive behavior and their negative effect on children, families, and society (U.S. Department of Health and Human Services [HHS] Office of Disease Prevention and Health Promotion, n.d.) with the following recommendations:

- Reduce children's exposure to violence.
- Reduce bullying and sexual violence with dating.
- Decrease the percentage of public middle and high schools with a violent incident.
- Reduce physical assaults and physical fighting among adolescents.
- Reduce weapon carrying by adolescents (grades 9 to 12) on school property.
- Reduce morbidity and mortality related to child maltreatment.
- Increase the reporting to child fatality review teams deaths among children 17 years old or younger that are due to external causes and all sudden and/or unexplained deaths of infants.

Child maltreatment is recognized as a significant public health problem. Current research indicates that one in eight children in the United States will experience maltreatment before their 18th birthday (Wildeman et al, 2014). Although the ideal goal for pediatric providers is zero, the target goal of *Healthy People 2020* is no more than 2.1 child maltreatment *deaths* per 100,000 children 17 years old or younger. The goal for nonfatal child maltreatment is 8.5 per 1000 children 17 years old or younger (HHS Office of Disease Prevention and Health Promotion, 2014). National, state, and local efforts must be dedicated to reducing preventable death and disability and to enhancing the quality of life for all children. Health professionals in their individual practice settings and as a collective group must commit to improving the quality of life by incorporating health promotion and disease prevention as integral components of health care for children and their families. Identification of at-risk families and referral for intervention must be priorities.

Family Functioning

Dimensions of Family Functioning

Common themes exist within all families, and six key dimensions, which are described in Box 17-1, have a significant effect on family functioning, contributing to cohesiveness, adaptability, and positive communication. To assist parents and children across the family life cycle and especially during times of stress, the provider must carefully assess these elements.

BOX 17-1 Six Key Dimensions Affecting Family Functioning

Resources that are available to the family include a social support network of extended family members, friends, and community, in addition to financial and other material assets. Families with limited resources or social support networks are more vulnerable to stressful life events than are families with resources and support systems in place.

Stresses and changes the family faces are numerous and can include financial strains, illness, marital strain, family transitions, losses, and lack of effective coping strategies. Life brings transitions that necessitate change. Many transitions are normal, some are anticipated, and others are unexpected; all can have a significant effect.

Childrearing styles are composed of parenting behaviors and beliefs that influence the environmental milieu in which the child learns about the world. Certain childrearing styles (e.g., an uninvolved, permissive, or strict authoritarian parenting style) are ineffective and have dire consequences for the emotional health of a child.

Values shared by family members provide a framework to guide, explain, and understand events being experienced and within which to find comfort, joy, and solace. Spiritual beliefs are one example of values that can support a family in its everyday life and in times of challenge.

Roles and structures vary greatly from one family to another, within an individual family, and as family members grow and develop. Role responsibilities and structures often change in response to external demands experienced by the family; shifts in the role of one family member can affect the role functions of other family members.

Coping style of the family speaks to the ways that demands are met, transitions handled, and concerns resolved. Positive or effective coping is characterized as a creative response to a change or stressor that results in a new behavior or attitude. Coping styles reflect habitual patterns of action. Over time, coping effort develops into a coping style.

Family Life Dynamics

The family is a dynamic social system that is usually the most powerful and constant influence shaping a child's development and socialization. The family provides emotional connections, behavioral constraints, and modeling that affect the child's development of self-regulation, emotional expression, and expectations regarding behaviors and relationships. Changes in one family member's behavior affect everyone else in the family unit.

Healthy families are cohesive and adaptable, with positive communication patterns. *Family cohesion* is an indication of the strength of the emotional bonding between family members. *Family adaptability* is the ability of a family system to appropriately change its power structure, role relationships, and relationship rules in response to the situational and/or developmental stress experienced. *Communication patterns* range from positive communication skills that convey messages (such as, empathy, reflective listening, and supportive comments) to negative communication that reflects double messages, double binds, criticism, and minimizes opportunities to share feelings. Communication is one of the most crucial elements within an interpersonal relationship. Family cohesion and adaptability are threatened and thwarted with negative communication patterns. The result of negative communication can be a chaotic household marked by high levels of family distress.

Each family has its own unique pattern of growth and development, and family systems evolve and change, demonstrating different dynamics depending on the stage of the family's life cycle. Just as a child goes through stages of development, so too do family units. Family life with young infants and preschool children is vastly different from family life with school-age children, with early versus late adolescents, or with young adults. Also different types of family units—nuclear, single parent, divorced, or blended—express different styles or patterns of family life.

The Interactive Family

A family is interactive, both within the family circle and between the family and its community. Within the family each member influences all other family members and is likewise affected by them. Although there are many different styles of parenting, adaptive behaviors are promoted by parenting styles that nurture the child (provide love, emotional support, and safety); maintain age-appropriate limits; grant age-appropriate autonomy; encourage the expression of feelings, thoughts, and desires; and facilitate the child's strengths and interests. Maladaptive patterns of interaction among family members (e.g., the family unit that fails to help the child learn self-discipline and the ability to socialize with others) can place a child and family at risk for negative outcomes.

There are many factors that are protective and foster resiliency in children. Certain temperaments, a caring relationship and/or social support outside the immediate family, community resources and opportunities, and effective parenting can counter the negative effects of adverse risk factors and contribute to a child's positive mental health. The degree of satisfaction as a couple and as parents is an important outcome measure of how well the family is functioning as a family unit. Single-parent households may face many challenges that can have a negative effect on the family unit but can be enhanced by developing nurturing relationships in both the parent's and the child's life. Children are at risk for developing mental health problems as a result of environmental factors, such as living in poverty, living in a community with a high crime rate, living in a home marked by marital conflict or domestic violence, living in a home in which they or their siblings are the victims of child maltreatment or neglect, or having a parent who abuses alcohol or other substances, or has a mental illness.

Assessment of Family Relationships and Dynamics

In addition to stressful issues that may arise with "typical" family relationships, providers are likely to encounter a variety of concerns that may include relationship problems, violence, child maltreatment, and/or neglect. Families and children who are experiencing or who are at risk for stressful situations must be identified. Assessment of families is also discussed in Chapter 2.

Family strengths and attributes that sustain and help families effectively deal with any level of stress are important factors to evaluate. In an assessment of family dynamics, the health care provider must investigate the relationships between the child, parent, or caretaker, as well as the social and environmental factors. Each factor must be analyzed separately, with its various components identified. The interactive effect of these factors must then be explored. The goal of assessment is to determine factors that have a positive or negative effect on the child's growth and development. Though the list is not exhaustive, Table 17-1 includes significant child, parent or caregiver, and social and environmental factors that can be used to alert the provider to areas that need further investigation.

Management for Health Promotion and Disease Prevention

Parents often approach primary care providers with concerns about developmental or role-relationship issues that can be managed with healthy parenting and effective communication (see Chapters 4 through 8). A supportive health care professional is in a strategic position to prevent problems and empower parents and children by providing anticipatory guidance, education, motivational support, resources, and opportunities for counseling.

Providers typically engage in *universal preventive interventions* related to both physical and mental health issues. Universal preventive interventions address the population as a whole with a goal of strengthening the parent-child

TABLE 17-1 Significant Factors for Assessment of High-Risk Family Relationships and Dynamics

Child Factors	Parent/Caregiver Factors	Social and Environmental Factors
Chronologic age and developmental level Present or past history of physical, emotional, or cognitive problems Personality traits, characteristics, and temperament Prior maltreatment or adverse life events, early toxic life stress Special care needs School performance	Physical, intellectual, or emotional functioning, illnesses, or limitations Current or previous history of substance abuse Financial resources, especially if poverty or limited finances is an issue Level of involvement in child care and life events of child Level of parenting skills, childrearing style, and communication skills Beliefs about discipline and corporal punishment Parental role and supports Parental history of experienced dysfunctional childrearing practices or any maltreatment or neglect A victim or perpetrator of domestic violence	Sibling assessment Type and strength of family social support network or social isolation Peer group relationships Stresses, crises, or conflicts in the home environment Cultural belief system Environmental condition of home and surrounding community Violence and poverty in the neighborhood environment Availability and accessibility of community support systems and partnerships

relationship by promoting wellness and improving communication. In contrast, *selective interventions* are directed at individuals or groups at risk for the development of mental health and/or relationship problems. Lastly, *indicated interventions* are for high-risk individuals who are experiencing symptoms or who have biologic markers for mental illness. Selective and indicated preventions often use a multidisciplinary approach, with community resources and other professionals from various social fields working together. The provider must develop a plan of action with goals and outcome measures and specific criteria that indicate when there is need for referral to a mental health or other professional.

Family Units

Two-Parent Families

Two-parent families include married couples with children, unmarried couples with children, and remarried couples with blended or stepfamilies. Approximately 66% of children in the United States live in two-parent families. Two-parent families experience the same stressors as single-parent families, but children in two-parent families tend to have social, economic, and health advantages. Parent educational levels, economic status, and health status are generally higher in two-parent families than in single-parent families (Annie E. Casey Foundation, 2014). However, several studies show that children's well-being depends more on the composition of the household (how invested and involved in the child's life the others are) and not just the number of adults present.

Single-Parent Families

A single parent and children living alone constitute a single-parent family; they are distinguished from multigenerational families, in which the single parent or two parents live with their children, their parents, their in-laws, or their grandchildren. Currently, about one third of children in the United States live in a single-parent household. Although the vast majority of single parents are women, increasingly fathers are raising their children in single-parent homes. In 2013, 26% of children in the United States lived in families with their mother as a single parent, whereas 8% lived in single father–parent families. African American children are more likely than children from all other racial groups (67%) to live in a single-parent household (Annie E. Casey Foundation, 2014). Single mothers are overrepresented among the very poor and those needing social assistance. The incidence of single-parent families varies by geographic, racial, and ethnic demographics. Numerous circumstances lead to single-parent households, including unemployment, divorce, births to unmarried mothers, abandonment of the family by a parent, incarceration of a parent, or death of a parent.

Single parents across all socioeconomic strata may have as many child-related demands on their time as married parents do; however their households have half as many adults to meet those demands (Bianchi, 2011). Even with help, the weight of responsibility is felt and exacerbated by lack of time and role strain. Single mothers who are employed experience more distress than partnered employed women, but factors such as income adequacy, psychological work quality, and work-family conflict also affect the outcomes (Dziak et al, 2010). A parent's work-related stress has a particularly strong effect on children in single-parent families (Heinrich, 2014). The Affordable Care Act of 2010 (ACA) helped remove barriers for families previously unable to purchase health insurance, and many children have been enrolled in health care plans or are covered under expanded Medicaid programs and the Child Health Insurance Program (Hamel et al, 2014).

Although single parenthood and cohabitation have increased in prevalence and have become more of an accepted societal norm, research shows that children in single-parent homes continue to fare worse than children born into married-couple households. The Fragile Families and Child Wellbeing study demonstrated that children in single-parent families are at an elevated risk for poor health outcomes, poor school achievement, and social and emotional behavior problems (Waldfogel et al, 2010). Research also suggests that children living in single-parent or cohabitating households are at greater risk for child maltreatment and neglect (Turner et al, 2013).

Clinical Findings

The provider must understand the household composition, family structure, and caregiving or living arrangements. This information gives insight into the protective supports, as well as stressors facing the families being served (Fiese et al, 2013). Several key areas are important to assess when working with single parents and their children. These areas can be divided into parent- and child-related factors.

Parent-related factors include the following:

- Screening for depression and other mental health concerns provides key assessment data related to emotional and physical well-being of the parent
- Availability of emotional support from their social network
- Living situation, presence of financial difficulties, and insurance coverage
- Availability of financial and emotional support from a noncustodial parent
- Availability and quality of child care for parents who must work
- Opportunities for the single parent to have a social life and relationships or personal time
- Ability of the parent to maintain consistency in discipline, in addition to a positive outlook and commitment to parenting

Child-related factors include the following:

- Role of the child in the family; responsibilities for taking care of siblings
- Relationship with custodial parent

- Relationship with the noncustodial parent
- Availability of opportunities to accomplish age-appropriate developmental tasks (e.g., Is child doing well in school? Does he or she have friends? Is child participating in sports or club activities?)
- Signs of problem behavior at school, at home, or with social activities
- Presence of children in the home with special needs (e.g., developmental disability, cognitive delay, or chronic illness)

Management

Many single-parent families cope well with the demands they face, benefiting from advice, anticipatory guidance, encouragement, and support of the provider. The availability of a social support network and positive communication patterns are important (Box 17-2). Social organizations, such as Big Brothers Big Sisters, offer a supportive role model for children in single-parent families. Parents Without Partners is a national organization that offers social activities and support for single parents. If parents request specific help or demonstrate signs of being exhausted, depressed, overwhelmed, burdened, or socially isolated, a referral for more specialized services (such as, counseling) may be appropriate. Similar signs in children plus deviant behaviors, emotional adjustment problems, or school disciplinary, academic, or behavioral problems can be indicators for mental health referral.

Patient and Family Education and Prevention

Although individual families may be helped to gain better coping skills, significant positive change in the quality of life of single-parent families depends on restructuring and increasing economic, educational, and family support resources in the community. Primary care providers should be informed about the effect that social service legislation has on the families that they serve and be willing to advocate for policy changes.

BOX 17-2 Significant Determinants for Successful Childrearing in a Single-Parent Home

- Support persons in the child's life who:
  - Collaborate with the single parent
  - Develop quality relationships with the child
  - Are available for the child
- Adults in child's community who provide support, including teachers, school officials, health care providers, and support person(s) for the parent
- Capacity of parent to communicate with child in open, direct, and understanding manner
- Ability of parent to recognize child's need for opportunities for enjoyment and accomplishment outside the home and to provide for the child
- Economic stability and well-being that is adequate to meet family's needs

Children Living with Grandparents or Extended Family Members

In 2011, 1 in 10 children in the United States was living in the same household with a grandparent. Of these 7.7 million children, about 3 million were primarily cared for by a grandparent. Among racial and ethnic groups, 8% of black, 4% of Hispanic; 3% of white; and 2% of Asian children are cared for primarily by a grandparent (Livingston, 2013). The reasons why grandparents assume responsibility for parenting their grandchildren vary but may include death, illness, or disability of a parent, teen pregnancy, parental abuse, parental substance abuse, and incarceration.

Grandparents face significant legal issues around custody, adoption, guardianship, and foster care. In addition, not every state provides financial assistance to grandparents. Grandparents may have difficulty accessing and paying for health care. For example, some insurance carriers do not allow grandchildren as dependents. A high percentage of grandparents do not receive social security or public assistance. The Pew Research Center noted that children who are primarily cared for by a grandparent are more likely to live below the poverty line (28% vs. 17%) and have lower median household incomes ($36,000 vs. $48,000) than children who are cared for primarily by a parent (Livingston, 2013). An estimated 2.5 million grandparents are raising their grandchildren in the United States (American Association of Retired Persons [AARP], 2014). Because there were only about 400,000 children in the United States in foster care in 2013 (HHS Administration for Children and Families, Administration on Children, Youth and Families, Children's Bureau, 2014), most of these 2.5 million grandparents do not have the benefits given foster parents—for example, child care, remuneration, developmental assessments, and tutoring.

Grandparents may still be active in the workforce either in part- or full-time employment, or they may have been enjoying their retirement and new challenges. Some may be thrilled to be parenting again, whereas others may be highly stressed—even clinically depressed. Health status is poorer among caregiving grandparents than non-caregiving grandparents. Compounding the practical, legal, economic, and health issues are the psychological and emotional responses of all involved. Grief, anger, confusion, resentment, and depression are reactions of grandparents and their grandchildren. At the same time, relief that the grandchildren are safe, loved, and nurtured can be present. Sensitivity and openness to grandparents can allow them to express their ambivalence and concerns. Expressed respect and appreciation can help form a working partnership (Hadfield, 2014).

Knowledge of resources can be especially helpful. The American Association of Retired Persons (AARP) has a website for grandparents, which lists excellent resources and information for grandparents parenting grandchildren, including information about financial assistance (e.g., the Temporary Assistance for Needy Families [TANF] program), online and community-based support groups, books and other literature, and a wide range of other resources. Support groups have been shown to be helpful in reducing the stress of raising grandchildren.

Providers should be alert to the following as they work with grandparents who are caregivers:

- Often children have lived with one or two biologic parents before either voluntary or court-ordered placement with the grandparent.
- Children can be involved in continuing conflict with their biologic parent or parents and may experience emotional reaction to separation from or abandonment by the parent(s).
- Children can experience the loss of friends, schoolmates, and familiar surroundings.
- Children need a supportive environment and consistency in routines including discipline.
- These families may need significant support from social service agencies, the educational system, and health care providers.

Children Living with Two Unmarried Parental Figures—Cohabitation

Children can be the biologic children of two adults who decide not to marry but live together, the biologic children of one of the adults but not the other, or children who live with their guardian and the guardian's unmarried partner. In each of these family situations, the development of a high-quality parent-child relationship, consistency in routines, and a continued commitment to the child are hallmarks of successful parenting and childrearing. Children born to cohabiting parents, however, are more likely to have health issues than other children. A study by Fiese and colleagues (2013) indicates that these children are at increased risk for receiving a diagnosis of asthma and, to a lesser extent, for developing obesity. Households with one biologic parent and one social parent often have fewer shared resources of time and money, and they have a higher risk of child abuse and neglect. Adolescents living in cohabitating households are more likely to smoke and drink alcohol in comparison with adolescents living in married or single-parent households. The reasons for these health disparities are unclear, but children face significant developmental risks if they sense a lack of permanence or certainty in their lives; if family life is characterized by conflict or poverty; or if there is inconsistency in who lives in the home, frequent breakups, new adult relationships, or frequent changes in living arrangements. Children also can be affected emotionally if other significant adults in the children's lives (other biologic parents, grandparents, or other extended family members) express distress about the relationship between the unmarried adults.

Children Living with Homosexual Parents

The American Academy of Pediatrics (AAP) affirms after extensive review of the literature that children's well-being is affected more by their relationships with their parents, their parents' sense of competence and security, and the presence of social and economic support than by the gender or the sexual orientation of their parents (AAP Committee on Psychosocial Aspects of Child and Family Health, 2013). Increasing numbers of same-gender couples are raising children today, a trend that will likely increase in the future. According to the 2010 U.S. Census, same-gender couples are parents to approximately 115,000 children under 18 years old (AAP Committee on Psychosocial Aspects of Child and Family Health, 2013). In fact, gay and lesbian parents are a part of the earlier discussions regarding single-parent, two-parent, grandparent, and cohabiting-parent households. As in any family, children living with homosexual parents may come from former heterosexual relationships; they may have been adopted; or they may have been conceived by assisted reproduction (i.e., egg or sperm donation, artificial insemination). These families reflect every ethnic, racial, and socioeconomic group in the United States. Children do well if the family relationships are healthy and parents support each other and the child. Children find it easier to deal with questions posed about their parents if they learn about their parents' sexual orientation during childhood rather than during adolescence. Finally, children are not at risk of developing a homosexual orientation because of their living situation.

Adolescent Parents

Teen (ages 15 to 19) birth rates in the United States have declined from 61.8 per 1000 births in 1991 to an historic low of 26.6 per 1000 births in 2013 (Hamilton et al, 2014). However the United States continues to have a higher number of teen births compared to other developed countries (Pinzon et al, 2012), and adolescent parents and their children represent populations at high risk for medical, psychological, developmental, and social problems. Predictors of teen motherhood are listed in Box 17-3 and adolescent pregnancy is discussed in Chapter 36.

Adolescents who become parents generally face the problems inherent when a major role is assumed before the individual is developmentally ready. Adolescent parents have developmental needs of their own and, not infrequently,

BOX 17-3 Predictors of Teen Motherhood

- Victim of sexual abuse as a child
- Adverse events in childhood
- Being a child of an addicted parent
- Family history of mental illness
- Lack of family involvement; an intolerable home situation as defined by the teen
- Poor academic achievement or school dropout
- Loss of a parent by death, separation, divorce, or foster placement
- Living in an impoverished social environment where adolescent pregnancy is commonplace and accepted
- Confusion about own sexual orientation

their needs are in conflict with those of their children. Often adolescent mothers feel isolated, exhausted, and depressed. Children of adolescent mothers are more likely than children of older mothers to have a low birth weight, to have ongoing health problems during childhood, to grow up in homes without fathers, and to be raised in poverty or near poverty. There are teens who can successfully parent their infant if given support; however, preexisting family and individual factors that lead a teenager to become a mother before completing the educational and developmental tasks necessary for adult life are more relevant predictors of successful parenting.

Clinical Findings

In order to better understand the environment in which a child will be raised, providers should ask about the adolescent parent's support system, their attitudes toward parenting, and sources of parenting advice they use. In addition, providers should determine the adolescent's school status, child care arrangements, financial situation, and plans for the future. Assessment of at-risk status varies, depending on the stage of the teen. Addressing these issues on an ongoing basis can contribute to more successful parenting and prevention of problems later in the child's or teen parent's life.

Infancy

Factors to assess when the teen is the mother of an infant include:

- Adolescent mother-infant attachment: Is there evidence of healthy attachment or emotional or physical neglect?
- Confidence and ability of teen mother to care for her infant
- Conflicts between the teen's needs and those of her infant: Is the mother more interested in reestablishing her adolescent lifestyle or caring for her infant?
- Living arrangements: With whom and where are the teen mother and baby living?
- Degree of involvement of the social support network in the mother's and infant's life: Is the baby's father invested in the child? Support from extended family?
- Return to school or the workforce: What are the child care arrangements?
- Adequacy of financial resources

Later Years

Toddler years are challenging, particularly for teens who themselves are survivors of abuse or neglectful parenting. Typically the teen mother and young child, if living with family, move out on their own or move in with the teen mother's partner. Factors to assess include:

- Mother's knowledge level of child development and ability to cope with the variety of toddler behaviors
- How well the family unit is functioning
- Progress made by the mother toward reaching her life goals

As the child gets older, the teen mother is thought of as a young mother. Children of these mothers, especially those who are poor and living in urban settings, are more likely than their peers to have behavioral problems. When their own children are adolescents, they find this a particularly difficult period, and often they become young grandmothers because the teen pregnancy circle is perpetuated.

Management

Key points in management include the following:

- Maintain regular and frequent contact with the teen mother during the child's infancy and early childhood. Remember that the teen mother and the infant or child have their own separate needs for health supervision and guidance.
- Provide a supportive environment for the teen mother. Have a plan for follow-up so that teen mothers do not get lost in the system. Emphasize the strengths of the teen mother and praise her positive efforts. Involve other family members (e.g., grandparents, the father) in discussions about child-rearing issues depending on the teen's wishes.
- Facilitate further education to minimize effects of poverty on child rearing.
- Refer to a community health nurse for home visits early in pregnancy and postpartum. This intervention has proven most successful in delaying subsequent pregnancy and improving healthy parenting and family life.
- Provide referrals for resources and community agencies that can assist teen mothers (e.g., parenting classes or literature; support groups; special clinic programs that see both infants and teen mothers; Woman, Infants, and Children [WIC] program; early child intervention programs provided by school districts and Head Start).
- Intervene early when warning signs of potential neglect or abuse are evident, and refer as necessary.

Families with Special Circumstances

Adoptive Parent Families

Adoption is the legal process that gives individuals who are not birth parents legal and permanent parental responsibility for children. Birth parents terminate their rights, and the adoptive parent(s) are awarded legal custody. Thus a new nuclear family is created.

Adoptions occur in a variety of different family makeups—married couples, single parents, intra-family adoption, subsidized adoption of children with special needs, gay and lesbian parents, grandparents, or other extended family members. Independent, identified, and international adoptions; surrogacy arrangements; and open adoptions are other examples of forms of adoption. Public and private agencies, independent adoption through attorneys, and foreign adoption services are potential avenues to assist in the placement of children.

Since 1975, with the dissolution of the National Center for Social Statistics, there have been no federal agencies or nonprofit organizations collecting data on the annual number of total adoptions in the United States. The Adoption and Safe Families Act of 1997 requires states to collect information about the adoptions of children in public foster care. During the 2013 fiscal year, over 50,000 children in the child welfare system were adopted with public child welfare agency involvement (HHS Administration for Children and Families, Administration on Children, Youth and Families, Children's Bureau, 2014a). According to the National Survey of Adoptive Parents 2007 data (the most recent data available), of the 1.8 million adopted children living in the United States in 2007, 38% were private domestic adoptions, 37% were foster care adoptions, and 25% were international adoptions (Vandivere et al, 2009).

Assessment

Assessment of adopting families includes the following:

- Legal status, arrangements, and circumstances surrounding adoption process
- What, if any, contact will the birth parent or parents have with the child? Will other family members (e.g., grandparents, aunts and uncles) have contact?
- Timing of finalization of the adoption and length of waiting period; how old was the child?
- Decisions about how and when to tell the child about being adopted
- Support services available for the adoptive family
- Any known or suspected medical (including growth and development) problems of child
- Any known medical, genetic, or psychosocial concerns related to birth parent or family
- Information about the pregnancy, delivery, and neonatal period or subsequent medical problems

Children adopted from foreign countries can be at risk for medical problems. Routine recommended screening tests are outlined in Box 17-4 (see Chapter 3 for discussion of medical examination of immigrants). If the reliability of prior vaccination history is questionable, it is acceptable practice to repeat the vaccinations (Centers for Disease Control and Prevention [CDC], n.d.).

Management

Schedule a preadoption consultation if possible to review any issues or concerns. Providers may need to do outreach to inform potential adoptive parents of the pediatric services that they provide (e.g., anticipatory guidance, information about child development and the adoption process). Support and guidance through the process before adoption is finalized is crucial, because there may be many hurdles facing parents. Once adoption is finalized, close monitoring and support by the primary care provider during the initial adoption period are important. According to the AAP, all adopted children should have a comprehensive medical evaluation immediately after their adoptive placement. The medical evaluation should include age-appropriate vision, hearing, dental, and behavioral/developmental screenings (Jones and Committee on Early Childhood, Adoption, and Dependent Care, 2012). Scheduling additional or more frequent health supervision visits is appropriate even when all appears well, but especially if high-risk situations or conditions are identified. If problems arise, prompt referral to specialty medical services, mental health, or social service agencies is imperative. Children with known special needs who are adopted are often eligible for federal and state financial support and services.

The presence of a social support network is important for adoptive families. Adoptive parents face the same parenting challenges as biologic parents do when their child passes through the various developmental stages of childhood. In addition, adoption is a lifelong commitment that can present special challenges for parents. Families adopting children with special needs may require extra assistance with family bonding and behavioral, mental health, and physical needs. Such families may first seek social support informally and, when other interventions have been found inadequate and a crisis looms, look for professional help. These families need preventive resources, reassurance of competence, and encouragement to strengthen social support networks.

Patient and Family Education and Prevention

When considering adoption, parents often have many questions about the initial adoption period and the

BOX 17-4 Recommended Screening Tests for Children Adopted from Foreign Countries

- Complete physical examination with developmental, dental, hearing, and vision screening
- Newborn metabolic screening panel (all infants)
- Complete blood count with differential, platelet count, and indices
- Iron studies (ferritin, serum iron, iron saturation)
- 25-Hydroxy vitamin D, calcium, phosphorus
- Thyroid stimulating hormone, free thyroxine
- Urinalysis
- Lead level
- Tuberculin skin test, despite any previous BCG vaccination; if positive result, obtain chest x-ray (see Chapter 24)
- Stool for ova and parasites, *Giardia* antigen, and *Cryptosporidium*
- Hepatitis B panel, including surface antibody and antigen and core antibody
- Hepatitis C antibody
- Syphilis serology
- HIV ELISA
- Hemoglobin electrophoresis (Asian, Latin American, and African children)
- G-6-phosphate dehydrogenase assay (Asian, Mediterranean, and African children)
- Malaria (PCR) (children from tropical or subtropical regions and those with fever of unknown origin)
- Rickets (radiograph) (Chinese children)
- Lactose intolerance (black, Latino, American Indian, and Asian children)

BCG, Bacille Calmette-Guérin; *ELISA,* enzyme-linked immunosorbent assay; *HIV,* human immunodeficiency virus; *PCR,* polymerase chain reaction.

establishment of a family relationship. Issues that the provider should address with parents include the following:

- There should be a gradual disclosure of the adoption to the child. Such disclosure should be done earlier rather than later, and children should always be told the truth about where they came from and why they were adopted.
- Discussions of the adoption should be open, keeping in mind the child's developmental stage, cognitive abilities, and emotional needs. It is important for adoptive parents to reassure the child in words and actions that he or she is loved, and the adoptive parents will always be there for the child.
- Discussions with the parents should address any myths, concerns, or fears that the parents might have about adoption and their adopted child.
- Parents need to understand that their child's wish to know about or seek out the biologic parents is not a rejection of them.
- Adolescence can be difficult for adoptive children as they seek their own identity and deal with the fact that they are adopted.
- Adoption of an older child may present an extra challenge, especially if the child has been shuffled between homes or emotionally scarred by abuse or neglect. Telling parents about such challenges can help them to be better prepared to handle some of the difficulties that may lie ahead for their family and seek counseling early if needed.

Children Living in Foster or Group Homes

Children are generally placed in family foster care or a group home because of concerns of child maltreatment in their birth family or because their biologic parents are unable to care for them. Some children are placed in foster care because they need specialized medical, psychiatric, or mental health care and developmental assistance beyond the ability of their biologic parents to provide. Other children may need to be removed from a chaotic and unsafe family environment, or they may have been abandoned or orphaned. These children are at high risk for deep-seated feelings of insecurity, loss, and anger. In 2012, about 400,000 children were engaged in the United States foster care system. Nearly half of all foster children live in foster homes with nonrelatives; about 28% live with relatives (Child Welfare Information Gateway, 2013a).

Assessment of foster families includes exploring the child's history that resulted in foster family placement, identifying physical or mental health issues that precipitated or resulted from separation from the birth parents, and evaluating the foster parent.

- Children frequently have a history of chronic stress, hardship, and emotional trauma in their family life.
- Children can experience multiple placements and separation from siblings.
- Foster children are often involved in family reunification programs and are placed back with their parents under the supervision of the child protective services.
- Foster children are placed under legal mandates in foster homes that mirror the children's ethnic, racial, and cultural identities as much as possible.
- Foster children often receive disjointed health care. In 2008, the Fostering Connections to Success and Increasing Adoptions Act (HR 6893) mandated that each state develop a plan for the ongoing oversight and coordination of health care for foster children. The Medical Home model, a concept introduced by the AAP in 1967, has been proposed as a way to ensure that foster children's medical needs are addressed (Jaudes et al, 2012).
- Research indicates that a disproportionate number of foster children have weight problems, medical issues, or developmental delays (Schneiderman et al, 2011). Therefore, careful assessment of weight, medical, and developmental problems of children in the foster care system is recommended.
- Children are emancipated from the foster care system at 18 years old and need to be prepared for this major life change. A limited number of states extend foster care until age 21 years.

Foster parents have a difficult role in society. They want to be treated with respect and to have their care and knowledge of their foster child acknowledged. They want to have the assistance needed to provide the best care possible to the children in their care. The Child Welfare League of America has excellent information and resources about and for family foster care providers. In addition, the National Foster Parent Association provides support and caregiving information for foster families (see Additional Resources).

Families with a Premature Infant

Low-birth-weight and premature infants present special issues for new parents. There may be an extended time between the birth of the child and when parents are able to bring their infant home. Concerns about the child's physiologic vulnerability may arise. Almost certainly, costs and time commitments around the care of the infant will be increased. Parents may have the same concerns as parents of a full-term newborn, but their fears and anxieties about being responsible for a seemingly fragile newborn may be magnified. Similar to the situation of a multiple birth, exploring who is caring for the child and who is helping the parents is a priority.

Families with Multiple Births

A family faced with caring for newborn twins, triplets, or more, even while delighted, can be quickly overwhelmed by the responsibility and amount of work involved. Assessing parents' level of fatigue, ability to seek and accept support, and plans for ongoing care is important for both the provider and the parents. Behavioral issues and the children's own unique relationships can be a challenge (Box 17-5).

• BOX 17-5 Characteristics Unique to Multiple Birth Children

- Develop a special sibling relationship marked by loyalty and cooperative play
- Have periods in which they get along well or quarrel with each other just as other siblings do
- Work out relationships among themselves
- Function more independently, needing less parental attention
- Develop their own language among themselves as young children
- Display sibling rivalry, especially if they are fraternal rather than identical twins

Advise parents who have multiple births to do the following:

- Breastfeed if possible. Twins can be breastfed at the same time or one right after the other. Develop a plan to rotate breastfeeding if the mother has more than two infants.
- Organize the home for daily activities, and plan ahead to have sufficient supplies and toys.
- Attempt to get twins or triplets on the same schedule (awake, sleep, feeding) as much as possible.
- Schedule daily activities to accomplish all that needs to be done.
- Take time out for themselves and as a couple.
- Keep a sense of humor.
- Promote individuality of each child. Spend individual time with each child.
- Seek out support people to help (e.g., enlist the aid of extended family members or neighbors) during early infancy when the tasks of physically caring for multiple infants can be overwhelming.
- Contact support groups.

When the children are school age, there is no exact recommendation for classroom placement for multiples. Children of multiple births may find it easier to develop a sense of self and make their own friendships if in separate classrooms. If there are older siblings, encourage parents to be aware of and attentive to their needs and feelings.

Children with Chronic Illness or Special Needs

Children with special health care needs (CSHCN) have been defined as "those who have or are at increased risk for a chronic physical, developmental, behavioral, or emotional condition and who also require health and related services of a type or amount beyond that required by children generally" (McPherson et al, 1998, p 138). Approximately 11.2 million (15.1%) children in the United States have disabilities or special needs (HHS Administration for Children and Families, Administration on Children, Youth and Families, Children's Bureau, 2013b). National surveys suggest that approximately 30% of all children have some form of chronic medical condition. Asthma, attention-deficit/hyperactivity disorder (ADHD), and obesity are common chronic health issues for children. Type 2 diabetes is also increasing in children, as are mental health diagnoses, including depression and anxiety. Increasing survival rates for children who were born prematurely, have congenital anomalies, or have genetic disorders contribute to the increased numbers of CSHCN as well. Lack of medical insurance or concerns about health care costs can also negatively affect children's overall health status.

Parents caring for a child with a significant medical or developmental challenge, whether it is a chronic illness, a disabling condition, or a developmental disability, are responsible for their child's daily medical care, monitoring, and management. The care can be minimal or consume hours of every day and night. The monitoring can be casual or meticulous; the management can be routine or complex. Survival may be a realistic concern. Parents may play multiple roles, including advocate, care coordinator, and care provider.

The effect of a chronic illness or disabling condition on a family, including the child, parents, siblings, and extended family, is influenced not only by the diagnosis and its sequelae, but also by the meaning it has for the family and individual members. Families experience grief (both at the time of diagnosis and as a chronic state), deal with a wide range of changing emotions, question their abilities to handle the situation, and are eager for information and support. Specific, ongoing issues for families of children with disabilities can be grouped into four areas: access to information and services, financial barriers, school and community inclusion, and family support (Resch et al, 2010).

Providers can address these areas with parents by:

- Giving expert information on the condition and what parents and child can expect over time. Referral to and/or consultation with specialists may be necessary.
- Providing the opportunity for child and family to explore the meaning of the condition in their lives and to acknowledge and accept the child with special needs.
- Helping families define what is "normal" for them; exploring ways to have the child and family participate in everyday normal activities.
- Connecting families to support groups and resources, including parenting interventions (Morawska et al, 2014).
- Advocating for the child and family with school placements and interventions.
- Assisting the family to meet financial needs; referral to community health resources or medical social work may be appropriate.

Providers working with families of children with chronic illness should also assess family systems for stress and its consequences, most notably maltreatment of the child. Chapter 21 discusses issues for care providers to consider when working with children who have chronic illness and their families.

Parents often become medical experts in their child's diagnosis and management, as well as in their child's idiosyncratic responses. They expect to be treated seriously and with respect, and they set high standards for their child's health care providers. In a classic paper, Thorne and Robinson (1988) described three phases of the relationship between health care providers and health care recipients or family caregivers. *Naive trusting* is the first stage, a time when the family assumes that its perspective is shared by the professionals who care for their family members, the family members' involvement as caregivers is respected and acknowledged, all professionals would be highly knowledgeable and skilled, and that communication would be honest and direct. As ongoing interactions with health care professionals teach families that these assumptions are not always valid, a second phase, characterized by *disenchantment,* occurs. Anger reflects the loss of trust in health care providers, and family members move toward trying to protect their family member. Finally, but not inevitably, family members move to a phase called *guarded alliance.* The no longer naive family members are able to reconstruct trust on a more sophisticated level, sharing it only with individual professionals who earn it.

Dynamics Affecting Family Life

Working Parents

In 2013, more than 63% of mothers with preschool-age children (younger than 6 years) were employed and about 72% of those worked full time. During the same year, nearly 75% of women with children between 6 and 17 years old were employed (U.S. Department of Labor Bureau of Labor Statistics, n.d.).

When both parents in a two-parent family work outside the home, their roles need to be coordinated to promote positive family outcomes. Making arrangements is an important task for the family, and parents may express concern about placing their child in a day care center. However, research indicates that children who spend time in non-maternal care (day care or child care facilities) do not develop differently than those who are cared for exclusively by their parents. This research also finds that parent or family characteristics have a stronger effect on children's cognitive and language development than the characteristics of the child care providers (Eunice Kennedy Shriver National Institute of Child Health and Human Development, 2006) (see Chapter 5 for a discussion of how to select child care).

Separation and Divorce

Divorce or the separation of parents can be emotionally stressful and extremely complex for families and can lead to significant emotional disruption and disequilibrium for all family members. It is important to understand that divorce is an ongoing process rather than a concrete event. Children may perceive it as a dramatic and painful time in their lives, and they will experience grief, because divorce is a loss of family as the child knows it. Behavioral changes are an expected reaction as the child attempts to adjust to the changing family situation.

Custodial and visitation arrangements for children vary and may change as the child grows. Joint custody is an option that allows both parents the opportunity to participate in mutual decision-making about their child's life and welfare. Various living arrangements and visitation rights are possible with joint custody. In some instances, however, single custody is in the best interest of the child, and the noncustodial parent may have limited or no contact and involvement in the child's life. Custody disputes and exposure to parental conflict place additional stress on children and can increase their feelings of insecurity (American Academy of Child and Adolescent Psychiatry [AACAP], 2013).

Children (and parents) tend to make a more successful adjustment if there has been a stable parenting foundation in the child's early years, if parents provide warmth and praise for the child through the divorce, and if the child knows that both parents will remain involved in their lives. Divorce is typically less stressful for a child when parents are able to develop a civil relationship with each other that focuses on what is best for the child.

Clinical Findings

The goal of assessment of the family experiencing separation or divorce is to determine both the needs and strengths of the family in order to assist the family with healthy coping. Child-related factors to consider include the developmental stage of the children and common psychosocial reactions to divorce likely at that stage. Additionally, the psychosocial effect of the divorce on the parents and the economic consequences of divorce on the family unit must be determined (Box 17-6).

Management

Anticipatory guidance given to parents who are in the process of separating and divorcing is outlined in Table 17-2.

Patient Education and Prevention

The goal of health education for children and parents experiencing divorce is to help restore a sense of wholeness and integrity in children's lives. Providers must stress those factors that have been shown to significantly affect whether the child will experience a healthful adjustment to the divorce (Box 17-7). Successful efforts implemented during initial periods of disequilibrium and reorganization will strengthen normal development and prevent future psychological trauma. In an early research study, Wallerstein (1983) identified six psychological tasks that children of divorce must master beginning from the time of parental separation and culminating in young adulthood, which are described in Box 17-8. These tasks continue to be relevant for children whose parents are divorced. If these psychological tasks are not achieved, the child's mastery of normal developmental tasks is negatively affected. Long-range and preventive interventions need to focus on helping the child achieve these tasks or goals.

• BOX 17-6 Assessment Factors in Divorce

Developmental Stage of Children

Age and developmental stage of children greatly affect their response to separation and divorce of parents.

Common reactions of children to divorce by age group:

- 2-5 years: Regression, irritability, sleep disturbances, aggression
- 6-8 years: Open grieving and feelings of rejection or being replaced; whiny, immature behavior; sadness; fearfulness
- 9-12 years: Fear and intense anger at one or both parents
- >13 years: Worried about own future, depressed, or acting-out behaviors (e.g., truancy, sexual activity, alcohol or drug use, suicide attempts)

Economic Consequence of Divorce

- Often devastating economic hardships and decline in living standards (especially for women)
- Nonpayment or delinquency in payment of child support

Common Issues for Children of Divorcing Parents

- Continued tension, conflict, and fighting between parents
- Litigation disputes over custody and visitation arrangements
- Abandonment by one parent or sporadic visitation (decreased availability) vs. denial of visitation
- Diminished parenting resulting from factors, such as availability issues or emotional inaccessibility, distress, or instability
- Limited social support system outside nuclear family
- Feelings of loneliness or emotional abandonment, or both

TABLE 17-2 Key Anticipatory Guidance Issues for Families Experiencing Divorce or Separation

Anticipatory Guidance Issue	Discussion Points with Parents
Advise parents to prepare the child for the impending breakup.	If possible, tell the child in advance of the breakup. Children who are appropriately prepared may cope better with the separation and change in family structure. Discussions should focus on supporting the child's needs for reassurance and stability, not on blame, recriminations, or the parent's needs.
Explain to parents the need to discuss these key issues with their children.	Discuss what arrangements have been made for the children to see departing parent unless visitation is not possible or problematic. Consider whether the children will be best served by continuing to see the departing parent when possible. Explain what divorce means in language appropriate to the child's cognitive and developmental level; offer an explanation of reasons for the divorce in the same terms. Reassure children that they did not cause the divorce or separation, that they cannot correct their parents' unhappiness in the marriage, and that the divorce is the parents' decision. Explain what the family structure will look like afterward and what changes will be necessary in the way the family functions. Explain the visitation arrangements as soon as they are established. Reassure children that they will be cared for, and they are not being abandoned by either parent, unless a parent has disappeared or refuses involvement. Tell children that feelings of sadness, anger, and disappointment are normal; encourage them not to "take sides," but love both parents. Discuss how to handle special circumstances, such as when the "other parent" abandons the child or does not visit.
Discuss the need for consistency.	Parents should strive to maintain consistent daily routines between the two households; encourage the use of security items that the child may depend on or carry familiar items between the homes during the transitional period. Be consistent in disciplinary practices.
Suggest self-help measures.	Children and parents may benefit from attending divorce recovery workshops, classes about families in transition, or peer support groups. School counselors, religious groups, or community and social service agencies may be helpful resources.
Acknowledge grief.	Providers should acknowledge the grief that both the parent and child are experiencing, and provide support.
Discuss when referral for mental health counseling might be indicated.	Children often demonstrate internalized or externalized psychosocial problems in response to divorce. Counseling may be indicated for the family members.

• BOX 17-7 Factors Affecting a Child's Ability to Achieve Healthy Adjustment to Divorce in His or Her Family

- The opportunity for continued participation of the noncustodial or visiting parent in the child's life on a regular basis
- Custodial parent attempts to make visits with the other parent a routine event so that there is consistent contact (phone, visiting, email)
- The ability of the custodial parent to handle and successfully parent the child
- The ability of parents to separate their own feelings of anger and conflict and resolve their own hostility toward each other so that the child's need for a relationship with both parents is met; divorced parents should not put the child in the middle
- The child does not become involved in parental conflict and does not feel rejected
- The availability of a social support network
- The ability of parents to meet the child's developmental needs and to help the child master the developmental tasks before him or her
- The child's overall personality and personal assets and deficits

• BOX 17-8 Six Psychological Tasks Children of Divorce Must Master

1. Acknowledge the reality of the marital breakup.
2. Disengage from parental conflict and distress and resume customary pursuits.
3. Resolve loss of familiar daily routine, traditions, and symbols and the physical presence of two parents.
4. Resolve anger and self-blame.
5. Accept the permanence of the divorce.
6. Achieve realistic hope regarding relationships—the capacity to love and be loved.

It may be a good idea to schedule additional visits or telephone contacts with the family to monitor their adjustment. Support can be provided by focusing on the family's positive strengths and resilience.

Remarriage: The Blended Family

A blended family is one in which two adults create a reorganized family by joining with their children from previous relationships. This term describes families created by remarriage after divorce or after the death of spouses. The introduction of a stepparent and possibly stepsiblings can be beneficial for a child or can be a time of difficult adjustment. The majority of children within blended families gradually adjust well to their new family situations.

Clinical Findings

Assess how the children are coping with significant life changes and realignment of family roles, and carefully consider any behavioral concerns (Box 17-9). This information

• BOX 17-9 Assessment of and Counseling Tips for Children in Blended Families

Assessment

Developmental Stage of Child

- Age and developmental stage of child greatly affect child's response to the remarriage and ability of child to cope with change and new family relationships.
- Early adolescence is often a time of greatest difficulty in adjustment to remarriage.
- A mother's subsequent pregnancy is often a time of increased frequency and intensity of problems with young children.

Common Issues for Children in Blended Families

- Complex relationship with new family members
- Altered relationships with own family members and possible feelings of betraying other biologic parent or being torn between parents
- Possible relocation and separation from family members and friends
- Continued or new tensions between parents and tensions between stepparents; rivalries between parents and stepparents
- Jealousy among stepsiblings
- Establishing new family traditions and values
- Continuing to respect earlier family history, traditions, and loyalties that may be in conflict with new family ties
- Unrealistic expectations by child of stepparent
- Unrealistic expectations by stepparent for instant love, respect, and obedience from child
- Tensions within blended family household, creating anxiety and fear of another family breakup

Characteristics of Problem Behaviors in Blended Families

- Problems can occur at home and at school.
- Children in divorced and blended families experience more behavioral, social, emotional, and educational problems than children from nondivorced families.
- Parental conflict, more than family structure, is the critical factor that influences both marital and family adjustment.

Counseling Tips

- Discuss upcoming changes with your child before remarriage and address possible fears, feelings, and expectations.
- Keep the marriage strong by a nurturing husband-and-wife relationship.
- Blended-family parents need to agree on discipline issues, how to set limits, and type of discipline; remembering to be consistent.
- Start new family traditions, such as weekly family meetings.
- Be patient and as flexible as possible; do not expect your child(ren) to have an immediate positive relationship with the new stepparent.
- Spend quiet, alone time with your child as much as possible and preferably every day.
- Do not force your child to align with the new parent and remember that a second parent does not replace the first; support and help maintain the relationship of your child with the other birthparent.

can help both the provider and the parents decide how to best focus their attention.

Management

The goal of primary care interventions is to foster positive parenting behaviors, protect the development of children, and enhance family functioning. Some counseling tips are listed in Box 17-9. Whether the family is given guidance and followed closely by the primary care provider or given a referral to mental health services depends on the presence of significant behavioral or mental health problems. Providers should investigate community services that assist blended families, such as a self-help group for stepparents or a parenting group. Written information including telephone numbers of community resources should be maintained in the practice setting.

Patient and Family Education and Prevention

Before remarriage, providers can counsel and guide parents regarding strategies for coping with transition in a blended family. Many children go on to develop strong and meaningful attachments to their stepparents if the relationship is cultivated over time with careful sensitivity to the needs of the child, parent, and family.

Military Deployment

In 2012, about 1.9 million children lived in military families and approximately 225,000 had a parent who was deployed at that time (Tozer, 2012). As United States military involvement changes, these numbers increase or decrease, but the needs of children in these families remain as compelling as ever and must be addressed. Having a parent sent to an active combat zone with an undetermined return date may rank as one of the most stressful events of childhood. Children in such situations may be vulnerable, especially as the coping resources of the remaining parent (or guardian) may be compromised by his or her own distress and uncertainty. Chandra and colleagues (2010) found that children with a deployed parent had more emotional difficulties compared with their peers; older youth and girls of all ages reported significantly more school, family, and peer-related difficulties if a parent was deployed. The longer the parental deployment and the poorer the non-deployed caregiver's mental health, the more likely it is that children will experience role-shifting and behavior problems during deployment and reintegration. Additional risk factors include history of rigid coping styles, family dysfunction, young families (especially first military separation), families recently moved to a new duty station, foreign-born spouse, families with young children, families without unit affiliation, pregnancy, and dual-career or single parents (Safran n.d.). Protective factors include resilience, family preparedness, active coping style, and positive psychological and mental health status of the at-home parent (DoD, 2010). Primary care providers are in a unique position to recognize the psychological strain on these children and their families, initiate referrals to mental health providers when indicated, and provide support and resources.

Children Living in Poverty

Families in the United States are facing poverty in increasing numbers, and children are the most at risk. In 2012, over 16 million (or more than 20%) of children in the United States lived in poverty. Children of color are disproportionally poor, with nearly one third of children of color living below the poverty line in 2012 (Children's Defense Fund, 2014). In some states, welfare reform has created a class of the working poor—those who make too much to qualify for subsidized health care, having to choose between keeping a job that helps feed their family or meeting their children's health care needs (Annie E. Casey Foundation, 2014). Impoverished women enrolled in the TANF program, which was intended to bring welfare mothers back into employment, have faced significant problems in many places. The low-wage jobs that most TANF recipients are prepared for do not pull them out of poverty. Further, they face the conflict of working to pay for food and shelter versus overseeing the health, safety, and education of their children. Few have employer health insurance, few can pay for quality day care, and many work two jobs to make ends meet—further separating them in time, place, and energy from their children. If women terminate from the TANF program, they have neither work nor welfare support.

Displaced or Homeless Children and Their Families

The number of homeless children in the United States is growing, with substance abuse and poverty as prime reasons for this increase. According to the National Alliance to End Homelessness (2014), on a single night in 2013, there were about 610,000 homeless individuals. Thirty-six percent of the homeless population is comprised of families. Although the national homeless rate fell in 2013 to 19 homeless persons per 10,000, some state's homeless rates increased significantly (National Alliance to End Homelessness, 2014).

Characteristics of homeless children include:

- Living in poverty because of limited employment opportunities, low wages, lack of affordable housing, no medical insurance (available, but often not signed up for), and inadequate social support services
- Living in families with a history of substance abuse, domestic violence, mental illness, or unexpected family or economic crisis
- The majority of these children are younger than 5 years old
- Runaway adolescents who are often victims of child abuse or neglect or teens alienated from their parents for multiple reasons
- Living in a variety of environments, such as a car, motel, makeshift shelters, or homeless shelters; often children and parents in families are separated

• BOX 17-10 Health Care Problems for Which Homeless Children Are at Risk

- Tuberculosis
- Multiple caries
- Impetigo
- Social isolation at school because of an unkempt appearance
- Poor hygiene
- Substandard living conditions leading to possible unsanitary conditions
- Mental health problems, including social isolation at school (e.g., due to unkempt appearance)
- Early initiation of and sustained substance abuse
- Sexually transmitted infections (STIs) for runaway teens and for those who prostitute themselves; pregnancy
- Abuse due to increased vulnerability in multifamily/people habitation and family stress

• BOX 17-11 Key Features Characteristic of Violence

Continuity: Once it is used as a coping mechanism, violence becomes a habit that is hard to break.
Reciprocity: Violence generates violent behavior in others, increasing tension and eliciting negative responses.
Sameness: One form of violence becomes as acceptable as another. As its use becomes more common, violence permeates all of one's life.
Addiction: Violence gives a sense of power and control that, although temporary, is addictive.
Limitations of options or alternative actions: Reasoning is difficult in violent situations, and problem-solving abilities are not used.
Escalation: Violence begets more frequent and more intense violence, with potential for serious sequelae.

- Poor school attendance: only 77% of homeless children attend school regularly
- Health care problems (Box 17-10)

Homeless children and their families have difficulty with the most basic needs of food, shelter, and clothing. Accessing education (requires registration) and health care (via the ACA) is possible but may not be taken advantage of by the parents due to many complex factors—many of which are related to their homelessness. The health care visit may be in response to a crisis that could not be denied, but assessment should include well-child care, including immunizations, on the operating principle that every child should receive the maximum health care possible.

Disaster Affecting the Family

There are many disasters or traumatic events that can affect children and their families. These can include natural disasters, such as hurricanes, tornados, floods and fires, or unintentional injuries, school or community shootings, or other disastrous incidents. Children and adolescents will need assistance in coping with feelings of fear, anxiety, and confusion that they may have. Children may feel sorry for those affected or afraid that something similar could happen to them (Schonfeld, 2013). Disastrous events usually come without warning; therefore, families are often not prepared to deal with the fallout that results.

Providers should educate parents and community members on the best ways to help children cope when disasters occur. Flexibility is essential, as children react to and cope with these situations in a variety of ways depending on their age, developmental status, and individual traits. It is important to ask children if they have any specific questions or concerns about the event, and provide answers in simple, direct, and age-appropriate terms. Avoid providing too much graphic or detailed information that may cause more distress to the child. Parents should also be aware that children may exhibit behavior or mood changes. They may display regressive behaviors (e.g., new separation anxiety), have sleep problems, or begin to complain of physical symptoms, including headaches or stomachaches (Schonfeld, 2013). Children may also develop posttraumatic symptoms, depression, or anxiety. Providers should be aware of community mental health resources for families when these symptoms are present.

Death in the Family

Death in families is discussed in Chapter 19 as a grief and bereavement issue.

Role-Relationship Problems

Violence

Violence is the outcome of aggressive behavior that becomes destructive and results in physical injury to people or damage to property. Characteristic features of violence are listed in Box 17-11.

Four main categories of violence can have an effect on children and their families:

- Interpersonal violence, including child abuse, corporal punishment, sibling violence, and intimate partner abuse
- Predatory violence (e.g., a crime or assault)
- Peer violence, such as dating violence, fighting, gang violence, and bullying (that can become violent)
- Sexual assault and rape, including date rape

Violence has been acknowledged as a major social and public health problem in the United States. A national survey on children's exposure to violence revealed that, in 2011, 60% of children and adolescents in the United States were exposed to violence in their daily lives and 41.2% experienced an assault-related injury (Finkelhor et al, 2013). Although there are major differences in rates of violence-related injuries and death by ethnic groups, the majority of homicides involve people who know each other and are of the same race. The typical scenario is played out as follows: an argument occurs, alcohol or drugs have been consumed, a weapon is available and used, and a serious injury or homicide is the end result. Boys are more likely to perpetrate and be victims of physical violence, whereas girls are more frequently victims of sexual assault and dating violence (Hickman, 2013). Of note is that recent trends indicate that crime and violence have been declining in the child and youth population (Finkelhor et al, 2014a).

There is no one cause of violent behavior. Violence can be preceded by situational crisis (e.g., unemployment) and risk factors have been identified that increase the likelihood of violent behavior (e.g., substance abuse). Developmental and environmental factors contribute to violence (e.g., impulsivity in young children; poverty, substandard living situations, and limited resources); however, not all individuals exposed to such factors resort to violence. Violence is a behavior that is learned by example and can become part of a child's methods of social interaction. Effective management of violence in families and communities depends on understanding major influences and key risk factors that contribute to or sustain violence.

Exposure to violence can lead to behavior problems and developmental issues, and it can significantly affect the physical and mental health of an individual. Homicide or serious injury can be the end result of violence. Although murders of children have decreased significantly in the past few years, they continue to be the third leading cause of death for all individuals 15 to 24 years old and the leading cause of death for African Americans 10 to 24 years old (David-Ferdon et al, 2013). The direct and indirect costs of violence in medical expenses, loss of productivity, and decreased quality of life are immense.

Clinical Findings

The assessment of youths who are victims of, witness to, or perpetrators of violent crime should focus on certain key pieces of historical information and the presence of risk factors to help determine the child's current safety and potential for future violence (Box 17-12). If possible, the youth and parent(s) should be interviewed separately, which may need to be done in conjunction with law enforcement personnel.

History of the episode:

- What seemed to cause the incident?
- Did the child or family know who was involved, or was this a random event?
- Were alcohol and/or drugs involved?
- Did either the victim or the perpetrator have or threaten to use a weapon? If yes, what type of weapon?

Past history:

- Have there been previous incidents of violence or assault?
- What is the usual pattern of drug or alcohol use?
- Does the child have a history of mental health problems?
- Was the youth a victim of child abuse?
- Does the youth have a criminal or police history?
- Is he or she a loner with weak social ties? Do the youth's friends engage in antisocial or delinquent behavior?
- Is there gang involvement or affiliation?
- Does the youth or peers have access to or carry a weapon or weapons?

Family and social history:

- Does the youth feel safe at home and in his or her neighborhood? How is the youth supervised by his or her parent(s)?
- Is there a family history of child abuse, substance or alcohol abuse, domestic violence, mental illness, or fighting at home?
- Are there firearms or other weapons in the home?

• BOX 17-12 Risk Factors for Serious Youth Violence

Individual Risk Factors

- Attention deficits, hyperactivity, or learning disorders
- Deficits in social cognitive or information-processing abilities
- Poor behavioral control
- History of early aggressive behavior
- Low IQ
- High emotional distress
- History of treatment for emotional problems
- Antisocial beliefs and attitudes
- Involvement with drugs, alcohol, or tobacco
- Exposure to violence and conflict in the family
- History of violent victimization

Family Risk Factors

- Authoritarian childrearing attitudes
- Harsh, lax, or inconsistent disciplinary practices
- Low parental involvement
- Poor monitoring and supervision of children
- Low emotional attachment to parents or caregivers
- Poor family functioning
- Low parental education and income
- Parental substance abuse or criminality

Peer and Social Risk Factors

- Association with delinquent peers
- Involvement in gangs
- Social rejection by peers
- Lack of involvement in conventional activities
- Poor academic performance
- Low commitment to school and school failure

Community Risk Factors

- Diminished economic opportunities
- High concentrations of poor residents
- High level of transiency
- High level of family disruption
- Low levels of community participation
- Socially disorganized neighborhoods

IQ, Intelligence quotient.

Adapted from Centers for Disease Control and Prevention (CDC): *Youth violence: risk and protective factors, CDC* (website): www.cdc.gov/violenceprevention/youthviolence/riskprotectivefactors.html. Accessed August 18, 2014.

- Are there school issues: attendance, academic difficulties, and/or behavioral problems?
- How does the youth spend free time? Employment? Socialization? Delinquency?
- Are siblings or other family members involved in gangs?
- Do siblings or other family members have criminal histories?
- Have any family members ever been victims, witnesses, or perpetrators of crime?

Management

The primary care provider is likely to become involved with the health care management of minor trauma resulting from assault, counseling after an incident of violence or threat of violence, and the prevention of youth violence.

In brief, the following are the key points in the management of minor assaults:

- Treat minor trauma or refer for necessary treatment
- Screen for alcohol and drugs
- Report the incident to law enforcement
- Refer to a social worker or mental health professional and to community programs as appropriate
- Work with parents and child to identify ways to prevent violence (e.g., discuss how the family can incorporate protective factors into their family life [Box 17-13])

Prevention of Youth Violence

Prevention of youth violence requires use of a public health model that addresses the complexity of causes and risk factors behind the problem. Some issues can be addressed in the primary care setting, whereas others require more active involvement in the community as a child and family advocate.

Primary Prevention

Strengthen families:

- Provide parents with skills for effective parenting (see Chapters 4 through 8 and 18).
- Support parents to be actively involved with their children, to supervise youths and their activities, and to monitor the child's peer group (having friends who engage in conventional, nonviolent behaviors is a protective factor).
- Connect families to needed community service resources.
- Educate parents about the effect of violence on their children (media and technology); discuss ways to minimize exposure.
- Teach about gun safety.

Strengthen developmental competencies of youth:

- Educate youths about violence and its prevention at an early age.
- Teach anger management and strategies for preventing a fight (role-playing).
- Promote self-defense strategies, such as learning a martial art.
- Discuss ways to manage a difficult or potentially violent situation (Boxes 17-14 and 17-15).

• BOX 17-13 Protective Factors Against Youth Violence

- Frequent shared activities with parents
- Ability to discuss problems with parents
- Connectedness to family or adults outside of the family
- Perceived parental expectations for school performance that are high
- Religious affiliation
- Positive social orientation
- Commitment to school and involvement in social activities with peers
- Consistent presence of parents during key portions of the youth's day

Centers for Disease Control and Prevention, Injury Prevention & Control Division of Violence Prevention: *Understanding and preventing violence: Summary of research activities Summer 2013, CDC* (website): www.cdc.gov/violenceprevention. Accessed August 11, 2014.

• BOX 17-14 Practical Hints for Talking with Teens about How to Keep Out of Trouble

Do not carry a weapon; instead, "fight clean" (i.e., discuss the issue in conflict). Carrying weapons only makes one less safe; pulling out a weapon begins a cycle of retaliation.

Do not go into harm's way. Avoid being around fights because the cycle of escalation and retaliation often involves innocent people.

Avoid being caught alone; stay with friends.

Do not be provoked into fighting. Words are said and names are called, not because the names are true, but rather to provoke anger and a fight.

If one becomes involved in a fight, try to end the incident on equal ground; that way anger is more likely to be diffused. The person who wins often takes on the aggressor role; the loser then becomes the scapegoat. Thus violence continues and becomes cyclic.

Suggest discussions with friends about ways to handle potential situations in which a gun or knife might be brandished.

Do not join gangs or associate with individuals who turn to violence as a way of settling differences.

Report threats of school violence to adults.

• BOX 17-15 Talking with Teens about Sexual Abuse/Assault

Males as well as females can be victimized.

Alcohol intoxication or the use of drugs is a major factor in sexual assault. Prevention includes not placing oneself in harm's way by using such substances.

Manipulative verbal threats and physically trapping the victim are common tactics used by perpetrators.

Reluctance to report gang or date rape is common. However, keeping the rape a secret only leads to self-doubt and delays healing. The teen should report the rape immediately and seek professional counseling.

Improve the environment:
- Support diversity training and bullying prevention programs in schools.
- Support after-school programs for youth and work for community commitment to youth programs.
- Make neighborhoods and schools safe places for youth.
- Involve the community in a commitment to prevent violence.
- Address the issues of media violence and of condoning violence as a way of life.
- Enforce current sale regulations and encourage additional sale regulations of consciousness-altering substances (e.g., alcohol, marijuana) to youth.
- Support legislation to regulate and control guns.
- Limit access to and carrying of weapons.

Secondary Prevention

Screen for potential problems:
- Assess for violence risk factors at all health supervision and illness visits.
- Screen for alcohol abuse problems.
- Ask about weapons in the home—their presence, use, storage, and access.

Care for children exposed to or threatened by violence:
- Address any physical or emotional problems resulting from violence in the primary care setting. Early intervention can prevent more serious problems later; referral may be necessary.
- Refer to community programs that make home visits to mothers of new babies, especially those in low-income and teen-mother families.
- Advocate for support groups for children who have suffered trauma or loss or witnessed violence (e.g., school counseling for traumatic experiences).
- Refer families to community support programs, such as Big Brothers Big Sisters of America.

Tertiary Prevention

Treatment and rehabilitation programs for offenders and treatment for victims and their families can be difficult and costly and yield only mixed results. The National Center for Victims of Crime has a Youth Initiative that offers help for this population (see Additional Resources).

Intimate Partner Violence (Domestic Violence)

Intimate partner violence (IPV) is violence that occurs between individuals in a close relationship. Although IPV generally occurs between adults, some teens do as well, and children who witness this violence are often significantly victimized as well. IPV can include physical violence, sexual violence, and/or emotional abuse and threats. According to the National Center for Injury Prevention and Control, over 12 million people are victims of IPV annually in the United States (CDC National Center for Injury Prevention and Control Division of Violence Prevention, 2014b). IPV can leave physical and emotional injuries to the victim. Children can also be physically injured during intimate partner disputes either by getting "caught in the crossfire," or in attempts to intervene. Children who witness violence between those who should be in a protective role are almost always emotionally traumatized. Studies have documented that exposure to IPV can lead to poor academic and social outcomes. There appears to be a dose-response relationship between IPV and poor outcomes; the more severe or chronic the exposure, the poorer the outcomes (Garner et al, 2012).

Clinical Findings

Although most professional organizations recommend screening for IPV, the effectiveness of screening is unclear, and it is difficult to identify families where IPV occurs. Intimate partner abuse occurs in all strata of society and, when presented with screening questions, many victims are reluctant to disclose their victimization due to fear of the consequences.

Management

For the pediatric primary health care provider, managing a child's exposure to IPV can be problematic. In most states, health care providers are mandated to report a child's exposure to IPV to child protective services (CPS) because it is considered a form of emotional child abuse (Campbell and Hibbard, 2014). State agencies can then further assess the family functioning and can offer resources to help the perpetrator, the adult victim, and the children who are also being victimized.

In all cases, care of families experiencing IPV requires a multidisciplinary, well-coordinated approach; referral and consultation with specialty treatment centers, social workers, and community health agencies are essential.

Patient Education and Prevention

The goal is to prevent IPV before it starts. Educating children about healthy behaviors and relationships can assist them in avoiding dating relationships that include violence. Primary care providers should also review the negative effects of children witnessing conflict between adults, specifically parents (Franchek-Roa, n.d.). Much less is known about preventing IPV in adults and further research is needed in this area.

Bullying

Bullying is a form of youth violence; it is defined by the CDC as any unwanted aggressive behavior(s) by another youth or group of youths. Bullying involves an observed or perceived power imbalance and the behaviors are repeated or likely to be repeated multiple times (CDC, 2014c). Bullying can include physical, verbal, or relational/social (e.g., spreading rumors or isolating one from the group) aggression. Due to the advent of social media and electronics, cyber-bullying is now considered another facet of bullying. Although the CDC definition of bullying excludes siblings and dating partners, abuse that occurs in a dating relationship may take the form of bullying, and there is growing evidence that siblings can be perpetrators of bullying that leads to long-term health problems (e.g., depression, self-harm) (Bowes et al, 2014).

In the United States bullying is, unfortunately, a common problem in the school setting. According to a 2011 nationwide survey on youth violence, during the 2009 to 2010 school year, 23% of public schools reported that bullying occurred among students on a daily or weekly basis. A higher percentage of middle school students reported being bullied than high school students. The same survey found that, in 2011, about 9% of all youth 12 to 18 years old reported being cyber-bullied either at school or away from school; girls reported being bullied electronically more often (6%) than boys (2%) (Robers et al, 2012).

Bullying behaviors can cause harm or distress to a targeted youth that includes physical and psychological manifestations. These behaviors can cause the targeted youth to feel socially isolated from his or her peer group and can potentially derail academic performance. Although most youth who are bullied do not consider suicide, the stress of bullying presents an increased risk of suicide for some young people (CDC National Center for Injury Prevention and Control Division of Violence Prevention, 2014a).

Youth engaging in bullying behaviors can be viewed as a perpetrator, victim, or both—a category known as the "bully/victim." There are a number of factors that can increase the risk of a youth engaging in or experiencing bullying, including (CDC, 2013):

- An attitude that is tolerant of violence
- Harsh parenting by caregivers
- Externalizing behaviors, such as disruption and defiance
- Low self-esteem
- Poor peer relationships
- Perception of being different

Clinical Findings

Youth rarely report bullying to an adult or care provider. Often it is not reported because the incidents typically occur when an adult is not present or has not witnessed any aggression. When an incident of bullying comes to the attention of the primary care provider, determine if the youth is considered the perpetrator, victim, or a combination of both. Evaluation of the youth's risk factors, family system, school performance, and the general presentation of the youth will determine in which category the youth may be.

It is ideal to interview the youth separately from the parent; however, it is necessary to gather the history from both. When talking with the youth, it is recommended to use the Home, Education and employment, Eating, Activities, Drugs, Sexuality, Suicide/Depression, and Safety (HEEADSSS) assessment (see Chapter 8). This psychosocial evaluation tool can help identify any concerns for bullying as well as relevant sequelae (Klein et al, 2014).

A history of the episode includes:

- Gathering details of what occurred to the youth: The use of open-ended questions, such as, "Tell me what happened," will aid in getting details as well as hearing the story in the youth's own narrative.
- Asking about past incidences and what occurred
- Assessing for any drug or alcohol use
- Assessing for weapon use: If a positive response is given, ask for specific type of weapon either used or threatened.

Management

The primary care provider is likely to become involved when an injury has occurred, when there are mental health concerns, or during the well-child examination when red flags arise during the psychosocial assessment. In general, the primary care provider should treat and manage any injuries, refer to mental health or social work for continued follow-up, and report to both CPS and/or law enforcement when necessary.

Patient and Family Education and Prevention

The ultimate goal is to stop bullying before it starts. There are many school-based bullying prevention programs, as well as community intervention programs, that are being implemented around the nation (see Additional Resources). It is important for the primary care provider to become familiar with the resources available in the community in which they practice and advocate in both the school and community settings for anti-bullying policies and bystander intervention trainings.

Child Maltreatment

Child abuse is an all too common pediatric problem. Until the late twentieth century, the issue of child abuse and neglect was often unrecognized or even ignored due to antiquated notions of children as "property" and ineffective social services. Since the seminal publication in 1962 of *The Battered-Child Syndrome* by Kempe and colleagues, great strides have been made in our medical, legal, and social approaches to child maltreatment. Children are a vulnerable, easily traumatized, powerless group, and it is the responsibility of all those who work with them to provide protection and care.

Child maltreatment is defined by the federal Child Abuse Prevention and Treatment Act (CAPTA) as "any recent act or failure to act on the part of a parent or caretaker which results in death, serious physical or emotional harm, sexual abuse or exploitation; or an act or failure to act which presents an imminent risk of serious harm" (Child Welfare Information Gateway, 2012). These are considered minimal standards and serve as guidelines for states to define and manage child maltreatment. Child maltreatment can be broken into four subcategories: neglect, psychological maltreatment, physical abuse, and sexual abuse.

According to information published by the Children's Bureau, there were an estimated 3.8 million total referrals to CPS in the United States in 2012; some children are reported more than once. Over 2 million of these referrals were responded to by CPS, and an estimated

686,000 children (9.2 per 1,000) were found to be victims of abuse or neglect. Children less than 1 year old had the highest rate of victimization, with a rate of 21.9 per 1000. Slightly more than one half (50.9%) of child victims were girls, whereas 48.7% were boys. Nearly one half of all maltreatment victims were Caucasian (44%), 21.8% were Hispanic, and 21% were African American. When stratifying the data, as in prior years, the most common form of abuse was neglect (78.3%), followed by physical abuse (18.3%) and sexual abuse (9.3%). A child may suffer from multiple forms of abuse. Based on reports from 49 states, a total of 1640 children in the United States were estimated to be the victims of fatal abuse (2.2 per 100,000) in 2012. Of these children, 70.3% were less than 3 years old. The fatality rate for girls (1.94 per 100,000) was lower than for boys (2.54 per 100,000). Most children who died suffered neglect (69.9%), but nearly 45% suffered physical abuse exclusively or suffered a combination of maltreatment. The perpetrator of fatal abuse is most commonly a biologic parent of the child (80%) (HHS Administration for Children and Families, Administration on Children, Youth and Families, Children's Bureau, 2013).

Child maltreatment in all its forms has been identified as a significant contributor to poor health outcomes across the lifespan. Earlier research found that Adverse Childhood Experiences (ACE), which include all forms of child abuse, have been found to significantly affect the physical and mental health of these adults (Felitti, 1998). More recent research has confirmed and expanded our understanding of the significant negative effects of early life trauma or toxic stress (Johnson et al, 2013).

General Assessment Guidelines

The importance of early identification and intervention cannot be overemphasized in order to minimize each child's exposure to ACE. Pediatric providers need to be alert to the possibility of child maltreatment. Thus, when an infant or child presents with certain injuries or behaviors, a careful and detailed history and physical examination must be conducted to identify all abusive injuries as well as to exclude all other possible etiologies. Box 17-16 lists behavioral signs that should alert the provider to the possibility of abuse that should be investigated further.

General Management Strategies

Pediatric primary care providers are in a unique position to identify children who are maltreated and to institute strategies for primary prevention aimed at high-risk families. The provider should know when and how to refer families and victims for further assessment, treatment and therapy when needed, as well as to perform anticipatory guidance and prevention in the general office setting.

All states have mandatory reporting laws that require health care professionals to report *suspected or known* child maltreatment to the appropriate agencies. If the history or physical examination is suspicious for child abuse, the provider should report to either CPS (also known as social services, department of human services, or department of family and youth services) or law enforcement. If the child is in imminent danger, a report should be made to both CPS and law enforcement. The burden to report minor injury or emotional maltreatment is just as great as the burden to report significant trauma resulting in grave bodily injury. Although the severity of injury is always an important consideration in treatment and disposition of the child, it does not determine, per se, whether intervention by protective services or law enforcement will occur. Nonetheless, providers should be educated to know that only reasonable suspicion of abuse, not certainty, is required to make a report. All clinic personnel (including unlicensed staff) need to be aware of their role in reporting possible abuse. (Abuse may be observed in the waiting or examination rooms.) Both civil and criminal immunity is ensured to mandated reporters who are acting within their professional role in making a required report. Because each state has its own reporting laws and procedures, providers should contact their state agency charged with protecting children for written guidelines about reporting laws and procedural policies related to child abuse. The telephone number for reporting suspicion of abuse should be readily available in each practice setting. If in doubt about the need to file a formal report regarding a particular situation, consult with staff at the local abuse reporting agency or with a child abuse specialist. The practice should have a list of child abuse resources in the community that can be accessed for guidance when needed.

Primary health care providers play a significant role in identifying injuries that are suspicious for abuse. Research has found that 21% of primary health care providers do not report injuries that child abuse experts would have reported (Sege et al, 2011). A common error of those who provide medical care for children is to assume that two-parent families or families that present well could not be abusive. Therefore, it is important that providers be willing to assess their own biases when determining if a report to CPS is warranted.

• BOX 17-16 Behavioral Signs Associated with Child Maltreatment

- Repeated injuries that are unexplainable or unusual
- Overly compliant or exhibits exaggerated fearfulness
- Clingy or indiscriminate attachment
- Extremes in behavior (aggressive or passive)
- Wary of physical contact with adults
- Frightened of a parent or another caretaker
- Exhibits drastic behavioral changes in and out of parental or caregiver presence
- Withdrawal from family or friends, poor school performance, depression or sadness, anxiety, aggressive or destructive behavior, or mistreating an animal or pet
- Suicidal (suicide attempts or plans) or engages in self-mutilation
- Displays sleep or eating disorders

Neglect

Neglect refers to the negligent treatment or maltreatment of a child that can harm or threaten to harm a child's health or welfare. Neglect by the parent or caregiver can be severe or subtle in its forms and effects, but occurs when children are not protected from danger, are placed in situations that threaten their health, or fail to receive adequate nurturance, supervision, clothing, shelter, food, education, and/or medical or dental care (Hornor, 2104). Examples would be when the parent or caregiver exposes the child to drugs in their environment; fails to respond to cries and physical needs of the child (e.g., diaper changes); fails to supervise young children playing in public areas; or consistently misses medical appointments. A key factor in neglect is the extreme or persistent presence of these conditions in the child's environment.

Neglect is the most common form of child maltreatment (HHS Administration for Children and Families, Administration on Children, Youth and Families, Children's Bureau, 2012) and the consequences of neglect are lifelong, extending well into adulthood. Recent literature has shown causal relationships between children experiencing adverse events in childhood and adult morbidities and chronic illness, such as heart disease and depression and other mental disorders (Gilbert et al, 2015).

Clinical Findings

The goal of assessment is to determine if neglect is occurring and whether the child's safety and welfare are threatened. General indicators of neglect are divided into child, home, and supervision factors (Box 17-17). In the primary care setting, providers can assess child factors. Home and supervision factors are more difficult for the provider to assess from the clinical setting. Questions and discussion about the home situation, however, should be included in the history (e.g., How are roles in the family divided? Who takes care of younger children? Who prepares the meals? Does the family get food stamps or WIC? Does the child have unusual behaviors [e.g., hoarding food, stealing]?). If the child is attending Head Start, the provider can consult with Head Start staff who, in turn, can conduct a home assessment. However, if providers even suspect neglect, they should call the local child protective service agency for guidance. A report to CPS may warrant an investigation in which child protective workers look at home factors with a focus on a safe and sanitary environment. To determine the degree of adult supervision, factors such as the child's age and level of functioning, the length of time the parent is away, where the parent goes, whether the parent leaves a plan of supervision (e.g., relative or adult living next door or nearby who was readily available to the child), and how often the child is left alone, are investigated. Most CPS hold parents to the standard of a "reasonable or prudent" parent. Economic factors are also considered when making judgments about parents' efforts to provide adequately for their children.

• BOX 17-17 General Indicators of Neglect: Child, Home, and Supervision Factors

Child

- Dirty, malnourished, poor hygiene, inadequately dressed for weather
- Inadequate medical and dental care (has multiple caries/decay)
- Always sleepy (chronic fatigue) or hungry
- Exhibits food insecurity behaviors (hiding, bingeing, stealing)

Home

- Fire hazards or other unsafe conditions
- Exposure to illegal substances
- No heating or plumbing
- Nutritional quality of the food inadequate
- Meals not prepared; food spoiled in refrigerator or cupboards

Supervision

- Child has history of repeated physical injuries or ingestion of harmful substances with evidence of poor supervision by adult caregiver
- Child cared for by another child
- Child left alone in the home, car, or anywhere without supervision (typically defined as a child younger than 12 years old who is left unsupervised during the daytime or a child less than 16 to 18 years old left unsupervised by an adult at night)

Differential Diagnosis

Differentiating willful neglect from neglect resulting from poverty, mental retardation, or mental illness is necessary. An example of willful neglect is a situation in which a parent was educated on how to seek resources for their family (such as, food stamps or rooming at a homeless shelter in severe weather conditions) but refuses to do so. Educational neglect (parent makes no provisions for the child to attend school) differs from truancy or elopement (i.e., when the child is sent to school but never arrives).

Management

If neglect is suspected, a report to CPS should be made and may lead to an investigation. Consultation with Head Start (if the child is enrolled) or referral to Head Start, a community health nurse for home assessment, or other social service agencies may be appropriate.

Psychological Maltreatment

Psychological maltreatment is defined as harm to a child's emotional stability or psychological capacity. It can take the form of acts of omission or commission, involve verbal or nonverbal communication, and can be done with or without intent to harm (Hibbard et al, 2012). Failure to adequately nurture children with support and affection is an example of emotional deprivation or an act of omission. Parents or caregivers who do not provide the normal experiences necessary for a child to feel loved, wanted, secure, or worthy are depriving their child of the emotional security that is critical for positive self-esteem. Parents or caregivers actively *commit* emotional abuse when they subject children to cruel statements and acts or reject, terrorize, ridicule, isolate, and corrupt the child. Torture, confinement, exposure to violence (witnessing IPV), and deprivation of food and water are extreme examples. Psychological maltreatment accounts for slightly over 8% of abuse reports (HHS Administration for Children and Families, Administration on Children, Youth and Families, Children's Bureau, 2012).

Parents or caregivers can ignore or reject their child for many reasons, including substance use, mental health disorders, personal problems, poor coping skills, poor parent role modeling, high stress levels or other preoccupying situations, or a personal history of emotional maltreatment. Children with chronic illness or those who are "different" from their siblings may become targets in the family system. Psychological maltreatment may contribute to failure to thrive (FTT), speech or sleep disorders, or a wide range of behavioral and emotional problems in children (e.g., withdrawal, aggressiveness, conduct and/or attachment disorders, depression).

Clinical Findings

A range of behavioral and physical indicators can lead to a suspicion of psychological maltreatment. Consistent or recurrent negative parental behaviors, willful cruelty, or unjustifiable emotional punishment are key indicators of psychological maltreatment, but the signs and symptoms can be more subtle and may not indicate abuse. Therefore, a careful history is important. It is essential to interview parents, caregivers, and any child older than 3 years old.

History

The history can include the following:

- Past health history: Might be suggestive of neglect (e.g., little or no health care supervision, immunizations not up-to-date, earlier removal of a sibling for neglect)
- Interview with caregiver: Might reveal caregiver's negative feelings toward child, a state of feeling overwhelmed or depressed, plus feelings of being deprived or unloved; caregiver may be cognitively delayed
- Behavior problems with child in school, among peers (e.g., bullying, being picked on, withdrawal)
- Feeding and dietary history should be obtained, but may not be truthful: Can be helpful in distinguishing formula-preparation error from neglect
- Financial hardships: May be related to inability to provide for basic needs, especially food

Physical Findings

Physical assessment of psychological maltreatment can be difficult. Nonorganic FTT can be related to physical and psychosocial factors, and both should be considered because they may be concurrent. Assessment of FTT is discussed in Chapter 33. Assessment for possible psychological maltreatment should include:

- *Child's behavior:* Child may avoid eye contact, resist physical contact, or have an expressionless face.
- *Parent-child interaction:* Parent may indicate a lack of attachment or presence of anger or dislike of child; may ignore, belittle, tease, or verbally abuse child.
- *Associated developmental delays:* Results from deficient psychosocial stimulation.

Differential Diagnosis

Intentional mental injury should be distinguished from that caused by parental deficits, such as cognitive, psychological, and economic limitations. Psychopathology in the child resulting from other causes is also in the differential diagnosis.

Management

Because psychological maltreatment is generally difficult to prove, the provider must carefully document what was said in the interview and what behavioral indicators were found. Reporting concerns to the appropriate CPS agency is essential, as is close supervision of these families. Referral to a community health nurse for in-home assessment may be appropriate. Referral to a mental health professional for evaluation should be considered to determine whether the behaviors or psychopathology, or both, in the child are due to parental emotional abuse or deprivation. Family therapy may be necessary, and parents can benefit from parenting support and education, in addition to social service support to cope with demands on the family system (e.g., child care, nutritional education, access to economic resources, Early Head Start). The child may need to be placed out of the home.

If a child has FTT, the condition must be treated clinically (see Chapter 33). Close and long-term health care supervision and follow-up plus psychosocial intervention and local case management by CPS are needed.

Patient and Family Education and Prevention

Prevention of emotional abuse generally involves the same prevention strategies as identified in the Physical Abuse section. Early recognition and intervention are the keys to preventing subsequent mental health problems. Frequent health visits to monitor the height and weight of infants who are falling behind are essential to prevent significant growth and development problems.

Physical Abuse

Physical child abuse is defined as maltreatment involving "physical acts that cause or could have caused physical injury to the child" (HHS Administration for Children and Families, Administration on Children, Youth and Families, Children's Bureau, 2012, p 118). All acts of physical abuse may not be done with the intent to injure the child. In some instances, the injury is a result of the parent or caregiver shaking, striking, or throwing the child in a moment of frustration or anger. Physical abuse can also be due to unreasonably severe corporal or unjustifiable punishment; or caused by intentional, deliberate assault, such as burning, biting, cutting, poking, twisting limbs, or torturing.

Child physical abuse also occurs place when a parent or caregiver falsifies the history or fabricates an illness in a child in order to receive attention from the medical community. This more rare form of abuse is known as *medical child abuse,* or previously *Munchausen syndrome by proxy,* and has been defined as "a child receives unnecessary and harmful or potentially harmful medical care at the instigation of a caretaker" (Roesler and Jenny, 2009). Medical child abuse can lead to significant injury or harm to a child and is associated with high morbidity and mortality (Flaherty et al, 2013). Identifying medical child abuse can be difficult, and providers should be alert to some possible indicator, including a caregiver who frequently seeks another medical opinion when the child is not diagnosed with an illness, who doesn't accept reassurance that the child is healthy, or who doesn't accept normal results. Evaluation for medical child abuse often requires an extensive medical records review; therefore, concerns of medical child abuse should be referred to a child abuse specialist who can assist in the process.

Clinical Findings

Determining the presence of physical abuse can be difficult. A child or parent may disclose a history of an inflicted injury, or there may be suspicious behavior or specific physical findings. Behaviors are not definitive signs of physical abuse but are important areas to investigate for additional information. Specific physical findings are often the key to a diagnosis of physical abuse. The provider should have a high level of suspicion if there are discrepancies in the reported history of the injury and the child's age and developmental capabilities do not match or are unusual for either the type and or severity of injury. For example, infants who are not yet independently mobile (e.g., cruising or crawling) should not have bruises.

History

The history should assess for the following:

- Child's statements about the cause of injury.
- Injury that is unusual for a specific age group.
- Injuries are unexplained or implausible (e.g., parent or caregiver cannot explain injury, is vague about how the injury occurred, gives discrepant accounts of what happened, or blames someone else); explanation does not match the type or mechanism of injury; or child is not developmentally capable of reported injurious behavior.
- Parent or caregiver delays seeking care for the child, seeks inappropriate care (e.g., for something other than the true issue), or age of injury is inconsistent with the history (e.g., bruises are in late stages of resolution yet parent states injury occurred a few hours earlier).
- Child, parent or caregiver, or both, hide injury (e.g., child wears excessive layers of clothing), or child is kept out of school (isolated).
- There is presence of triggering behaviors, such as an inconsolable colicky infant, toilet-training accidents, or sleeping or discipline problems that may have led to a violent response by a caregiver.
- There is a report of a crisis or stressful time for the family (e.g., financial difficulties) or IPV.
- There is a problem with substance abuse in the family.
- Family has a history of von Willebrand disease, hemophilia or clotting disorder, or osteogenesis imperfecta.

Physical Findings

Tables 17-3 and 17-4 describe common sites of injury and common characteristics of physical abuse by type of injury. Key considerations of abuse that should guide the physical examination include the following:

- Location of the injury
- Type of injury: Bruising, burns, fractures, or head trauma
- Pattern of bruises, abrasions, lacerations (i.e., does it resemble a known object?)
- Presence of multiple injuries, particularly in different stages of healing
- Signs of other forms of abuse or neglect
- Multiple mechanisms of injury (burns, fractures, and/or bruises)
- Severity of injury, especially as related to history given: Most infant falls do not result in significant injury. Falls of less than 5 feet (1.5 m) in vertical height have

TABLE 17-3 Common Sites of Injury in Physical Abuse of Children

Location of Injury*	Common Physical Finding
Head area	Eyes—bilateral black eyes Earlobe—pinch and pull marks Cheek—slap marks, squeeze marks Upper lip and frenulum—lacerations or bruises Scalp—bare and broken hair, bruises
Neck	Choke marks
Trunk	Trunk—bite marks, fingertip encirclement marks, hand slap, pinch mark, belt mark Buttocks and lower back—paddling and strap marks
Anogenital	Pinch marks, penile wrapping with constrictive materials
Extremities	Upper arms—grab marks Ankles or wrists—tethering, friction burn marks Feet—pin or razor tattoo marks

*The shins, elbows, and knees are the most typical sites of accidental, non–child abuse injuries where bruises, cuts, and abrasions are most commonly seen.

TABLE 17-4 Common Characteristics of Physical Abuse by Type of Injury

Type of Injury	Key Considerations
Bruises, abrasions and lacerations—surface and soft tissue	Pattern, shape, outline, or image of an object (e.g., handprint, cord, or buckle shapes) Location—sites other than over bony prominence (knees, shins, elbows, forehead) Number—more than one body surface or plane Multiple bruises
Burns—superficial or deep	Location: Burns on palms, soles, flexor surface of thighs or perineum; positive image of the shape of the object used to burn the child (e.g., curling irons, cigarette lighters, cigarettes, irons) Patterns, such as sharply demarcated or circumferential (e.g., sock, glove, zebra, branding, doughnut or cigarette shape) Cigarette burns—7.5- to 10 mm round lesion, raised edges and deep eschar
Human bite marks	Oval-shaped pattern, such as doughnut or double-horseshoe shape; can be on any part of the body; can have discrete tooth marks within the arcs or central ecchymosis between the arcs
Ligature marks	Typically, around neck or extremities; linear image at site where tool placed
Central nervous system/abusive head trauma	Radiographic findings (e.g., subdural hematomas, subarachnoid hemorrhages, skull fractures, suture spread), retinal hemorrhages; head trauma can have symptoms of irritability, lethargy, seizures, apnea, or coma Additional injuries may include posterior rib fractures and metaphyseal fractures
Internal organ trauma	Liver, bowel, spleen, pancreas, kidney damage consistent with blunt-force trauma May be no visible marks or bruises on abdomen May have symptoms of shock/sepsis Internal injury is second leading cause of death in child abuse
Skeletal fracture	Spiral fractures of long bones, avulsion of metaphyseal tips, multiple rib fractures in different stages of healing, subperiosteal proliferation reaction, unexplained fracture, especially in a young, nonambulatory child; fractures from birth injuries typically heal by 4 months
Poisoning or ingestion of medication	Deliberate poisoning or exposure to substance abuse via breast milk, passive inhalation of marijuana or other drugs
Medical child abuse (Munchausen syndrome by proxy)	Caregiver creates a fictitious illness or induces illness in child; signs and symptoms stop when perpetrator no longer has unsupervised contact with child

a less than one in a million chance of death (Chadwick et al, 2008).

Diagnostic Studies

These should include:

- Blood coagulation studies: Platelet count, bleeding time, prothrombin time, partial thromboplastin time, von Willebrand panel on any child who is severely bruised, has a history of "easy bruising" and suspicious bruises, or has intracranial bleeding
- Serum calcium, phosphorus, and alkaline phosphatase levels are useful measurements if bone disease is suspected
- Urinalysis, liver enzymes (aspartate aminotransferase [AST], alanine amino transferase [ALT]), amylase and lipase to rule out abdominal trauma
- Radiographic studies:
  - If physical abuse is suspected, any child under 12 months old should undergo radiologic skeletal survey. Skeletal survey should be strongly considered in children 12 months to 3 years old. An older child with limited range of motion or bony tenderness on examination should have a local radiologic evaluation. Table 17-5 gives details of which images are requested in a complete skeletal survey.
  - Computed tomography (CT) scan and/or a magnetic resonance imaging (MRI) study should be ordered

TABLE 17-5 Skeletal Survey

Area of Body	X-Ray View Requested
Skull	AP and lateral views
Spine	AP and lateral views
Chest/ribs	AP, lateral, and oblique views
Pelvis	AP views
Long bones	AP and lateral views
Hands	Oblique views
Feet	AP views

AP, Anterior-posterior.

whenever trauma to the face or head is suspected or on the basis of physical findings or symptoms.
- Abdominal CT if visceral injury is suspected.

Other studies are ordered depending on physical findings.

Differential Diagnosis

Differential diagnoses are identified by type of injury:
- Normal bruising from accidental injuries that typically involve the knees, anterior tibia, and forehead
- Mongolian spots
- Cultural practices, such as coining *(cao gio)* or spoon rubbing *(quat sha),* sometimes practiced by Southeast Asian groups
- Burns, impetigo, bullous impetigo, or toxic epidermal necrolysis (scalded skin syndrome)
- Fractures: Osteogenesis imperfecta and rare bone diseases, such as rickets, scurvy, congenital syphilis, and neoplasms
- Head injuries: Metabolic disorders and accidental causes
- Bruising or bleeding (hematologic disorders, such as vitamin K deficiency, von Willebrand disease, hemophilia)

Management

Medical treatment of specific types of injuries is discussed in this text under the appropriate illness-related heading. If physical abuse is suspected, certain general management strategies should be followed. The provider must:
- Report suspicions of physical abuse to CPS or law enforcement agencies, or both.
- Carefully document findings and any statements made by parent or caregiver or child, or both.
- Secure photographic documentation of soft tissue injury or burn injury; this may be done by law enforcement personnel, CPS, or health care providers, as appropriate.
- Refer for appropriate medical treatment of injuries depending on type and severity of injury.
- Refer to local Child Advocacy Center for specialized assessment and diagnosis if appropriate.
- Refer for mental health therapy. The need for long-term or intermittent therapy often depends on the individual child, the severity of the physical and emotional injuries, and other life events.

Patient and Family Education and Prevention

At-risk families have certain characteristics. A key to education and prevention is to identify families that have:
- A parental history of abuse during childhood or a history of exposure to interpersonal violence: Pursue affirmative responses with further questions as to what, if any, intervention(s) were taken.
- A family history of child maltreatment, including child death (categorized as extremely high risk), drug abuse, violent behavior, or serious mental illness.
- A mother or primary caregiver who does not show attachment to her infant, makes negative remarks about the child, or lacks basic parenting knowledge, skill, and motivation.
- Evidence of physical discipline of young infants.
- Family history of substance abuse and/or criminal activity.
- A lack of social support networks: Is the parent isolated?

The following interventions are recommended for at-risk children and families:
- Report immediately to CPS if abuse is suspected.
- Make early referrals for supportive services, including social service referrals, parenting classes, self-help groups (e.g., Parenting Support Programs or Alcoholics Anonymous plus battered women's services), respite care, public health nurse visits, or a combination of these.
- Provide close primary care supervision and ill-child follow-up visits.
- Use a multidisciplinary team approach to manage at-risk or high-risk families. A team approach gives objectivity to a situation.
- Use the services offered by community Child Advocacy Centers or child abuse prevention programs.

Sexual Abuse, Assault, and Date Rape

Sexual abuse is a complex form of child maltreatment. Child sex abuse definitions vary across disciplines, social systems, research efforts, and laws. Sex abuse can be defined to include acts of sexual assault or sexual exploitation of minors, or both. These acts can occur over an extended period of time or be a one-time incident; they may or may not involve force; they can involve threats of physical harm to a child or others in the family or emotional entrapment of the child; and the perpetrator often frames the incident as a secret between the victim and the perpetrator. In cases of child sexual abuse, multigenerational abuse is common. The perpetrator is usually known to the child and is often a "trusted" adult. For most policy makers and members of the public, child sexual abuse connotes sexual offenses at the hands of an adult. However, it has been reported that juveniles represent a growing group of perpetrators who commit sexually aggressive acts; recent research indicated that over half of the total estimate of sexual offenses were at the hands of juvenile perpetrators, many of them peer acquaintances (Finkelhor et al, 2014b). Children normally explore their developing sexuality, but some children engage in sexual behaviors that go beyond harmless curiosity. Some, but not all, of these children have a history of being sexually abused themselves. Intervention is necessary when children demonstrate problem sexual behaviors that are inappropriate or harmful to themselves or others (Box 17-18).

Sexual abuse of children and adolescents involves a range of acts, including rape, rape by multiple perpetrators, incest, sodomy, lewd or lascivious acts on a child younger than 14 years old (e.g., fondling or touching of genital areas and breasts or inappropriate kissing), oral copulation, and penetration of genital or anal openings by a foreign object. Sexual exploitation includes activities such as pornography depicting minors and promoting prostitution by minors. A group of children who are victims of sexual abuse are

• BOX 17-18 Sexual Problem Behaviors in Children

- Are clearly beyond the child's developmental stage (for example, a 3-year-old attempting to kiss an adult's genitals)
- Involve threats, force, or aggression
- Involve inappropriate or harmful use of sexual body parts (for example, inserting objects into the rectum or vagina)
- Involve children of widely different ages or abilities, such as a 12-year-old "playing doctor" with a 4-year-old
- Are associated with strong emotional reactions in a child, such as anger or anxiety
- Interfere with typical childhood interests and activities

National Child Traumatic Stress Network (NCTSN): *Understanding and coping with sexual behavior problems in children—information for parents and caregivers* PDF online: http://nctsn.org/nctsn_assets/pdfs/caring/sexualbehaviorproblems.pdf. Accessed November 22, 2014.

those children who are sexually exploited for commercial purposes, primarily through sex trafficking. Many of these victims are children who have run away. National estimates show that one in seven endangered runaways who were reported to the National Center for Missing and Exploited Children in 2013 was likely to be a sex trafficking victim. Sixty-seven percent of these children were in the care of social services or foster care when they ran (National Center for Missing & Exploited Children, 2014). Nationally, it is known that about 1 in 10 children (1 in 7 girls and 1 in 25 boys) will be sexually abused before they turn 18 years old (Townsend and Rheingold, 2013).

Clinical Findings

The pediatric primary care provider is likely to become involved in a child sexual abuse case in any of the following circumstances: there is a spontaneous disclosure by the child; a parent voices concerns about the possibility of abuse or reports a disclosure by the child; there are suspicious physical or historical findings, or both; or laboratory tests indicating sexually transmitted infections (STIs) are positive.

The child or adolescent who has been sexually assaulted by a stranger usually discloses the abuse and comes to a provider for an immediate evaluation. This type of assessment is straightforward and involves the usual taking of a history and performing the medical examination (see Chapter 36) with collection of possible evidence if the incident occurred within 72 hours. These children are often seen in the emergency department of a local hospital or, ideally, at a special center that treats victims of child sexual abuse, such as a local designated child abuse center.

Some children have been molested in the past but have only recently disclosed the abuse; in many instances, sexual abuse occurs over several years before the child discloses it. In other cases, the provider may only suspect that a child is being or has been sexually abused. Assessment of these children should focus on three areas: behavioral indicators, physical indicators, and the interview of the child (Table 17-6).

Ideally, an expert in the medical examination of children who have been or are suspected of being sexually abused should evaluate the child, so referral is essential. However, disclosure of sexual abuse may occur in the primary care setting, and the health provider must respond. The provider should attempt to gather information from the child and parent separately. When interviewing the child, the provider needs to be nonjudgmental, use language that the child understands, identify the words the child uses for the genital and rectal areas, have the child report what happened in his or her own words, and ask open-ended questions. Leading questions should never be used. The provider must document what was said accurately and in words used by the child and/or parent.

After reporting the case to the local child abuse hotline, the provider should work with CPS to ensure that a thorough assessment is conducted. This assessment includes a medical evaluation at a designated child abuse center with a complete physical examination and a forensic interview by a social worker, psychologist, or other trained professionals. The primary care provider must also assure the child and family that he or she will continue to be a support, advocate, and resource for them. Recanting a disclosure of sexual abuse is not uncommon because of fear of what disclosure can bring to the family or child; so reporting the case, referring to appropriate child abuse support services, and following up with the family are essential.

Diagnostic Studies

Any sexual abuse of children that involves oral, genital, rectal, or penile contact or penetration within the previous 72 hours requires that appropriate forensic specimens be collected (e.g., saliva, semen, nail scraping, and head and pubic hair), and testing for STIs should be done. It is best to discuss what types of diagnostic testing should be done with a child abuse expert prior to obtaining samples. Testing for *Neisseria gonorrhoeae, Chlamydia trachomatis,* and syphilis should be considered in all children with a history of sexual abuse. Cultures are still the gold standard in testing for STIs; however, research suggests that, in some cases, nucleic acid amplification tests (NAATs) on urine might be adequate to use for diagnosing *N. gonorrhoeae* and *C. trachomatis.* NAATs can be used as an alternative to culture with vaginal specimens or urine from girls, but culture remains the preferred method for urethral specimens or urine from boys and for extragenital specimens (i.e., pharynx and rectum) from all children. All positive specimens should be retained for additional testing (Workowski et al, 2010).

When evaluating a child or teen who has experienced an acute sexual assault within the 72-hour time frame, it is important to assess the risk of possible human immunodeficiency virus (HIV) exposure. The current recommendations by the CDC state that each case should be discussed with a local HIV/infectious disease specialist to determine if postexposure HIV prophylaxis is needed. Each case is

TABLE 17-6 **Behavioral and Physical Indicators of Sexual Abuse**

Behavioral Indicators	Physical Indicators—Nonspecific	Physical Indicators—Specific	Lack of Significant Physical Findings
Loss of bowel and bladder control Regressive behaviors, such as newly manifested clinging and irritability in young children, thumb sucking, renewed need for a security object Sleep disturbances, inability to sleep alone, bed-wetting after having been dry at night Overeating or lack of appetite; compulsive behaviors or unusual fears and phobias Change in school performance; loss of concentration or easy distractibility Sexualized behavior or play inappropriate for developmental level (see Chapter 15, Table 15-2) Depression or inactivity, poor peer relationships, poor self-esteem, acting-out, excessive anger Runaway, suicide attempts, prostitution or promiscuity, substance abuse, teen pregnancy, psychosomatic, gynecologic, and gastrointestinal complaints	Pain on urination; vaginal or penile discharge; vaginal, rectal, or penile bleeding Enuresis and encopresis Urethral or lymph gland inflammation; genital or perianal rashes; labial adhesions Pain in anal, gastrointestinal, pelvic, and urinary areas Genital injuries or signs, such as bruising, scratches, bites, grasp marks, swelling of the genitalia that are unexplained or inconsistent with history	Blunt-force trauma (lacerations, bruising, abrasions, tears) to the genital or rectal areas, or both, that is inconsistent with the history or these same findings with a history of sexual contact or penetration Commonly encountered STIs: • Diagnostic of sexual abuse—gonorrhea (by culture) and syphilis if not perinatally acquired, nondelivery-related or nonpregnancy-related chlamydia (culture is the only reliable diagnostic method), HIV, and herpes type 2 • Highly suspicious: *Trichomonas vaginalis* • Suspicious: Condyloma acuminatum (appearing after 3 years old and not perinatally acquired) • Possible: Herpes type 1 and nonvenereal warts (may be due to autoinoculation in the genital or anogenital area) • Uncertain: Bacterial vaginosis and *Mycoplasma* Pregnancy, sperm, and semen are certain indicators of sexual abuse in young children	Lack of findings is often the result of delayed disclosure and the nature of the abuse. Most sexual abuse of young children does not involve penetrating trauma. "It's normal to have a normal examination". Even in cases in which a perpetrator was convicted for sexual abuse and perpetrators report penile-genital contact, a majority of victims had normal or nonspecific examinations.

HIV, Human immunodeficiency virus; *STI,* sexually transmitted infection.
Note: Most child victims of sexual abuse do not have any significant physical findings.

considered based on multiple factors, such as risk of exposure, single versus multiple perpetrators, and potential of complying with the recommended treatment protocol and follow up with an HIV specialist. For further detailed information on medication regimes and follow-up, please refer to the current CDC treatment guidelines for a child with acute sexual assault.

Testing for STIs in children who were molested in the past (more than 72 hours previously) is based on the history provided and physical findings (e.g., genital discharge). Recent exposure and the possibility of penile contact are key indicators for whether specimens need to be collected. A colposcopic examination of the genital and rectal areas by an expert in the field is often recommended to help determine whether there is evidence of acute traumatic or past healed injury to the genital or rectal area.

Differential Diagnosis

Differential diagnoses include straddle injury to the genitalia or rectal area, which produces labial ecchymosis, abrasions, or tears; penetrating vaginal trauma from accidental injury, such as jumping from dresser onto bedpost (needs careful investigation and should have an easily identifiable history); perinatally acquired STIs or STIs acquired through close contact but not sexual abuse; lichen sclerosus, poor hygiene, and pinworm infestation that leads to vulvar skin irritation; and foreign body (frequently toilet paper) and other nonsexually transmitted bacteria causing vaginal discharge.

Management

An immediate forensic examination for a chain of evidence is required if trauma is present or the child gives a history that sexual abuse, including ejaculation, occurred within 72 hours. Colposcopy examination and specimen collection for semen, STI, pregnancy, and other evidence is done according to the local law-enforcement protocol for the evaluation of child sexual abuse or adolescent rape.

If the primary care provider is the first health care provider to see the child, he or she is likely to become involved in the following management issues:

- Careful documentation of the history and physical examination findings for medical-legal purposes
- Reporting of the case to law enforcement and social service agencies as required by law
- Referral for medical and psychosocial evaluation by experts in the field of child sexual abuse
- Referrals for crisis counseling of the child and other family members as needed
- Referrals for therapy, in addition to support and encouragement, for the child and family
- Treatment of STI: consider postexposure prophylaxis; follow-up STI cultures or blood work as indicated (e.g., HIV screening at the appropriate timelines)

The child who demonstrates inappropriate sexualized behavior (i.e., beyond child behavior seen as a part of normal developmental curiosity—see Box 17-18) should be referred to a mental health specialist trained in child development, child mental health, sexuality, and cultural variations regarding sexuality. Family therapy and education may also be necessary, because parents will benefit from specific strategies (guided by the therapist), support, and counseling to cope with the situation and best help their child.

Patient and Family Education and Prevention

Prevention of later psychological problems related to child sexual abuse and revictimization is important. Prevention of sexual abuse involves the following steps:

- Instruct parents and caregivers about the need for early and consistent education of their children regarding:
  - Good, bad, and secret touching of private parts
  - How to say no or the use of self-defense techniques (e.g., yelling, kicking, or fighting back) if someone inappropriately touches them
  - Telling a responsible adult
  - Not to keep secrets
- Parents should bring up this subject again as their child progresses through the various developmental stages. Young children who have been molested by a trusted adult often do not disclose for many years, because they were threatened not to tell anyone or they interpreted the sexual activity (if it is not painful) as a sign of affection from the trusted adult and not as molestation. Later feelings of guilt, fear, and betrayal can emerge when children realize they were molested.
- Emphasize to parents that they must not place their child in high-risk situations (e.g., a parent who was abused by her father may have kept this a secret, blaming herself for what happened; she may erroneously believe that the perpetrator will not sexually abuse her child and leaves her daughter with him). Counsel that children are never safe around a pedophile.
- Provide families with information and educational reading materials about the topic of sexual abuse of children. Teaching should be tailored to the child's cognitive and learning abilities.
- Report promptly any suspicion of sexual abuse.
- Support efforts to target high-risk groups for intervention to prevent the continued spread of child abuse (e.g., children who have exhibited sexual curiosity beyond the bounds of normal or have experimented with but not yet victimized other children; hence they become a juvenile perpetrator acting out the sexual activity or violence done to them) (see Chapter 15 regarding normal sexual exploration and activities).
- Support public education efforts and community child sexual abuse prevention programs.
- Educate parents about the need to talk to their children about their daily activities, especially what their children did during the time they were not with the parents.

For a complete list of references, please visit http://evolve.elsevier.com/Burns/pediatric/.

18

Self-Perception Issues

NANCY BARBER STARR

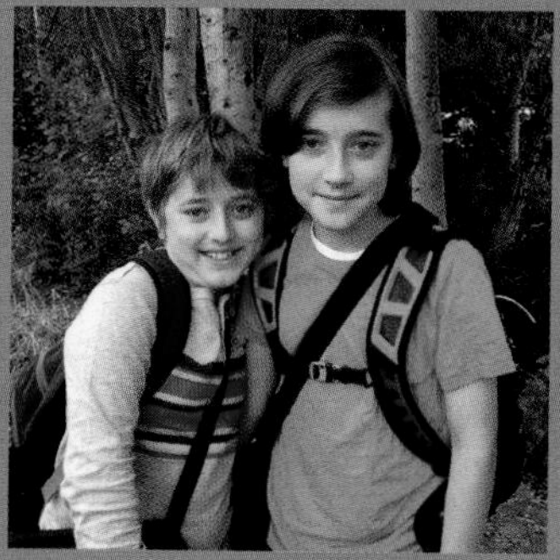

All people—children and adults—have mental pictures of themselves that steer the course of their lives. This mental picture, self-perception, begins to develop at birth, emerges in childhood, is refined and crystallized in adolescence, and continues to evolve throughout life. Self-perception is often used as an indicator and even a predictor of mental health or illness. It has to do with how individuals think and feel about themselves, their abilities, and their bodies. It is influenced by their interactions with others and the response of others to them. This perception, in turn, influences their attitude and the actions or choices each person makes throughout life.

Self-perception is a critical indicator of quality of life. It affects happiness, academic performance, relationships, creativity, healthy risk-taking, perseverance, resilience, and problem-solving. A positive self-perception is a precious gift that provides the confidence and energy to take on the world and achieve one's goals, withstand crises, and focus outside oneself. It enhances the building of relationships and giving to others. People with a positive self-perception tend to be responsible, committed to goals, genuine, forgiving, and positive. A positive self-perception is protective because it enhances children's abilities to deal with risk and learn to cope effectively. Adolescents, in particular, with a positive self-perception have a significant protective factor to minimize the risk of suicide (Sharaf et al, 2009).

In contrast, people with a negative self-perception tend to focus on their own needs, be self-critical, hypersensitive, and indecisive. A negative self-perception interferes with building relationships, drains energy, and often causes the person to feel like a victim. People with a negative self-perception tend to be unhappy, anxious, impatient, irritable, and negative or pessimistic. Children and adolescents with low self-perception have limited ability to respond to daily and developmental challenges and are more likely to participate in negative behaviors, such as school absence, smoking, drinking, drug use, and delinquency.

Multiple factors affect a child's self-perception, so assessment and management are not straightforward tasks but rather an intricately woven piece of both data collection and management planning. It may be helpful to think of self-esteem as including cognitive, affective, and behavioral aspects. The *cognitive* element emerges as an individual thinks about the ideal self and the perceived self. The *affective* component refers to the feelings that emerge when considering the discrepancy between the two selves. The *behavioral* aspect is seen in traits, such as assertiveness, resilience, and being decisive and respectful of others. Routine anticipatory guidance, education, and counseling, individualized to the child and family, give the provider the opportunity to facilitate the development of positive self-perception and to assist in preventing potential problems. Problems with self-perception are often hidden within somatic complaints, and the provider must maintain an awareness and sensitivity to the child or adolescent in order to identify and intervene appropriately. If done successfully, the child's life can be positively affected.

Standards of Care

Bright Futures: Guidelines for Health Supervision (Hagan et al, 2008) integrates self-perception with overall health supervision. The comprehensive practice guide and toolkit have a section in each developmental chapter that focuses on self-esteem. *Bright Futures in Practice: Mental Health* (Jellinek et al, 2002) and the *NAPNAP Mental Health Guide* (Melnyk, 2013) focus on prevention of psychosocial problems and early recognition of mental disorders. Although the U.S. Preventive Services Task Force (USPSTF) concludes that current evidence is insufficient to determine the benefit and harm of assessing for depression in adolescents in primary care, depression and suicide are potential complications of negative self-esteem and a significant risk in the adolescent population (USPSTF, 2015). *Healthy People 2020* objectives address the need to decrease both major depression and potential suicide in adolescents, and these issues should be considered by every primary care provider (HHS, 2015). Chapter 19 provides a comprehensive look at these issues.

Normal Patterns of Self-Perception

Components of Self-Perception

The term *self-perception* may be used interchangeably with terms such as *self-concept*, *self-esteem*, *self-efficacy*, and *self* or

• BOX 18-1 Definitions

Self-Concept (Think)

- The collection of beliefs, attitudes, knowledge, and ideas about oneself
- Based on academic, gender, racial, sexual, social, behavioral, and athletic attributes
- Competence/adequacy: "Who am I?" "I can do it!"
- Cognitive, descriptive: "I am a good runner."

Self-Esteem (Feel)

- The personal evaluation or judgment of self, including the emotional feeling (respect, regard, and self-confidence)
- Judgment of ability to face challenge, right to happiness and respect; self-confidence
- Worth, success: "I am okay." "I like and respect myself."
- Evaluative, opinionated: "I feel good about being a fast runner."

Self-Efficacy (Believe)

- Self-confidence or belief in one's ability to successfully perform a specific activity or task
- Influenced by multiple factors: Previous performance, behaviors of others, verbal encouragement from others, and physiologic reactions
- Low: Fear of risk and uncertainly, feelings of failure, impression management
- High: Willingness to take risks, sense of accomplishment, self-confidence

Self/Body Image

- One's picture of and feelings regarding one's body
- Affects emotions, thoughts, relationships, and behavior
- Physical appearance strongest correlate of global self-worth

• BOX 18-2 Enhancing Self-Perception: The Cycle of Learning

- Curiosity results in exploration.
- Exploration results in discovery.
- Discovery results in pleasure.
- Pleasure leads to repetition.
- Repetition results in mastery.
- Mastery results in new skills.
- New skills lead to confidence.
- Confidence contributes to self-esteem.
- Self-esteem increases sense of security.
- Security results in more exploration.

From Perry BD: Creating novelty, *Scholas Parent Child* 9:67–68, 2001. Copyright 2001 by Scholastic Inc.

body image. See Box 18-1 for a differentiation. Most important, it is essential to be aware that self-perception, being personal and subjective, includes both a description of the self and an evaluation of that description. The description a person draws and the evaluation a person makes come from thoughts and feelings, beliefs and convictions, observations, understanding, insight, and awareness received both from the self and from others. Three key components of self-perception are:

- Significance: "I am loved." (Parent: "I love you, no matter what.")
- Worthiness: "I like and respect myself." (Parent: "I accept and respect you.")
- Competence: "I can do it." (Parent: "I believe in you. You can do it.")

Significance comes from having a sense of belonging; feeling loved and lovable; feeling secure, cared for, and supported; and being accepted and understood unconditionally for whom one is, not what one does. This is the most important component in developing and maintaining a healthy self-esteem. Females are more likely to channel their self-perception into feeling desirable especially through relationships (Slattery, 2005).

Worthiness comes from understanding that as an individual you have a purpose in life. It is feeling valuable, acceptable, meeting personal moral standards, and respecting and feeling good about oneself. It also has to do with being respected and accepted by others. Feeling unconditional love, "no strings attached," is the cornerstone of self-worth.

Competence comes from feeling capable, confident, adequate, in control, and able to approach new tasks and deal with life optimistically, hopefully, and with courage. Active learning begins with a child's natural curiosity that leads to mastery and accomplishment, resulting in a growth in self-esteem and resilience (Box 18-2). Competence is often measured in terms of cognitive, physical, or social skills. Males are more likely to channel their self-perception into feeling capable especially through significance and achievement (Slattery, 2005).

Children who experience significance, worth, and competence confidently initiate activities, explore the environment, take risks, and rebound from disappointments. Appreciating themselves, they are able to reach out to and interact with others, accepting and offering love, respect, and encouragement.

External measures, such as those listed in Box 18-3, are often used by children who do not feel significant, worthy, or competent in order to try to create a positive self-perception. Physical attractiveness, socioeconomic status, and intelligence (academic achievement) are the three measures most frequently used by society. Excessive emphasis on external measures causes children to unduly compare themselves with others and often leads them to feel and describe themselves as insecure (unloved), inferior (unworthy), and inadequate (incompetent). Attempting to prove themselves, they often become both bossy and aggressive, or people pleasers and approval seekers.

The concept of *mindset* is an important part of a child's self-perception, not only in developing and stabilizing self-perception, but also in repairing any perceived damage. Children with a *growth mindset* have been taught to believe that hard work is at the crux of success and that effort and practice are contributing factors that lead to continued (or expanded) growth. Children exposed to this type of mindset typically receive praise for their process (i.e., effort, concentration, approach, or patience) that allows them to focus on learning rather than performing. An expandable mindset provides stable self-esteem and resiliency in dealing with failure; challenges can become opportunities for growth, not fearful experiences of failure.

In contrast, a child with a *fixed mindset* believes that success is due to a certain fixed trait or talent, and when failure or challenge occurs, it must be due to lack of that trait or talent. Children with a fixed mindset have often received praise in the form of appreciation for a certain talent or trait (e.g., intelligence, musical or athletic ability), and their performance has become their measure of worth. When they experience a perceived failure, they have nowhere to turn, because the talent is all they believe they have. They expend their energy trying to bolster their own self-perception by looking for an excuse, blaming someone, or comparing themselves to someone who has not done as well as they have. Table 18-1 shows clinical indicators of mindset.

• BOX 18-3 External Measures Used to Build Self-Perception

Physical appearance or attractiveness: How do I look?
Intelligence: What do I know?
Performance: How do I do?
Importance: Whom do I know? Who knows me?
Financial status: What and how much do I have?
Control: What and who do I control?

Developmental Stages

The development of a child's self-perception is closely tied to normal growth and development. Each stage of growth and development provides different opportunities to learn about the self and interact with and observe others and the environment. Transient periods of low self-perception are a normal part of development and can occur when a child sets new goals or is working on mastering new skills. One theoretic perspective that can be useful clinically is to view the development of self-perception as occurring in two stages (Box 18-4). The first stage, *emergence of the self,* occurs in infants, toddlers, and preschool-age children with parents and caretakers playing a key role laying the foundation for self-development. This is best accomplished in a supportive environment where infants come to view the world (their parents and caretakers) as responsive to their needs, both physical and emotional. Toddlers, with their new motor, cognitive, and language skills, thrive with positive acceptance, praise, and guidelines that set limits while allowing them to make choices. As preschoolers gain skills, feelings of competence emerge and, with better self-recognition, they internalize parents' demands; siblings and peers play an increasingly important role. Parents and teachers can begin to coach early problem-solving skills.

Refining the self, the second stage of self-development, occurs in school-age children and adolescents as they become more self-aware. Friendships, peers, and time spent in various activities play increasingly larger roles in shaping the child's character and personality and thus self-perception. Cultural stereotypes, such as those found in magazines, television, billboards, social media, and the Internet, influence the child's perception of society's "ideal" self. School-age children are preoccupied with evaluating themselves on the basis of external evidence: cognitive and physical skills,

TABLE 18-1 Clinical Indicators of Mindset

Indicator	Growth Mindset	Fixed Mindset
What does the individual think it takes to succeed?	Effort, practice	Intelligence, talent
What does the individual think makes a genius?	Hard work	Innate ability
What is the individual's typical response to new challenges?	Yes, please	No, thank you
How does the individual respond to setbacks?	The individual looks for new approaches and strategies	The individual blames others, becomes defensive, or gives up
What might you see if the individual experiences failure?	The individual tries again with a new approach	The individual lies about performance, makes excuses
What might you expect if you know the test is very difficult?	Sustained effort at studying	Cheating, procrastination

From Dweck CA, Master A: Self-concept. In Carey WB, Crocker AC, Coleman WL, et al, editors: *Developmental-behavioral pediatrics*, ed 4, Philadelphia, 2009, Elsevier.

• BOX 18-4 Developmental Stages of Self-Perception

Emergence of Self (First Stage)

Infants: View the world as responsive or unresponsive to their needs and learn that they are separate individuals who affect others by their behavior.

Toddlers: Explore their capabilities and limits and make others aware of their needs, desires, and concerns.

Preschoolers: Begin to use personal pronouns and pretend play, become aware of discrepancies in abilities, discover their bodies, move from seeing themselves as the center of the world.

Refining the Self (Second Stage)

School-age children: Become more confident of their own self-evaluation, evaluate self on the basis of external evidence, compare themselves with others, increasingly depend on peers for self-evaluation, and criticize and ridicule deviations from normal.

Early adolescents: "Try-on" images, finalize body image, focus on physical and emotional changes with peer acceptance determining self-evaluation, and use interpersonal self-description.

Late adolescents: Refine and crystallize self-perception (physical, social, spiritual) with values, goals, and competencies in place to guide their future.

achievements, physical appearance, social abilities and acceptance, and a sense of control. They are particularly prone to comparing themselves with others, making them vulnerable to social pressure. Any deviation from what society considers "normal" is subject to criticism and ridicule. Early school-age children, kindergarten through second grade, use observable characteristics to describe themselves and often overestimate their capabilities. Jellinek (2008) identifies points in a child's development where self-esteem is especially vulnerable. The first of these is in kindergarten or first grade where the child first encounters the "real world"—gold stars given to some students, not being invited to a birthday party, or clusters of friends that may not be inclusive. This begins the process of comparing themselves to peers testing their feelings of worth. By grades 3 through 5, children are becoming more aware of their strengths and weaknesses and are able to show feelings of pride and shame.

A second period of vulnerability occurs during preadolescence (at about age 9) with leveled reading and math groups, competition for positions on the athletic field and in the band room, and as cliques form, especially with girls. These events challenge the child's feelings of competence and significance. By middle school, grades 6 through 8 or 9, children are acutely attuned to the approval of their peers and beginning to form their own identity. This third period of vulnerability, according to Jellinek, is perhaps the greatest challenge, not only because of the great variation in physical and emotional maturity, but also with the increasing competition and comparison in the classroom, on the athletic field, and in social circles. The child who finds an identity in being a good student, or in the popular group, or as part of the athletic team is supported in the transition to young adulthood.

Overall, self-concept may decline across late childhood and early adolescence but then becomes increasingly differentiated as the child matures. Adolescents are defining who they are, where they are going, and how they are getting there. Early adolescents provide descriptions of themselves with interpersonal implications that lack flexibility and detail their sense of self based on relationships, with personal characteristics as the basis and reason for relationships. Early adolescents are still highly dependent on cultural stereotypes and peer acceptance, with physical and emotional changes being the main focus of self-evaluation. It is worth noting that puberty has different effects on males and females. The changes that a male experiences in puberty bring him closer to society's ideal body shape and can lead to a more positive satisfaction with body shape. Conversely, females widen at the hips and increase body fat, a change that is just the opposite of the Western culture ideal, often decreasing their satisfaction with body shape (Benowitz-Fredericks et al, 2012).

Middle adolescents, not yet comfortable with their bodies, spend much time focused on their appearance, trying on various looks. Part of the development of body image includes developing a sense of sexual self or becoming comfortable with one's sexuality, assuming culturally defined sexual roles, behaviors, and activities. Body image formation, a crucial element in shaping identity, is often finalized at this stage and is derived more from peers than parents. Any defect, disability, or discrepancy between what is seen and what is visualized as ideal is magnified and significant in the adolescent's eyes. Middle to late adolescents face another period of vulnerability because they may experience rejection from potential romantic partners, elite sports teams, musical ensembles, or college admission offices (Jellinek, 2008).

In the late adolescent years, as teens mature behaviorally, emotionally, and cognitively, they are increasingly able to integrate family, peer, education, social, cultural, and community aspects into their own self-perception. Establishing vocation, relationships, and values lead to a unique, independent, more stable self-identity in which they may begin to develop their own life story with important memories that help to make sense of their past, present, and future.

Developmental Assets, Family Assets, Sparks, and Developmental Relationships

Developmental Assets

In 1990, based on extensive research studies, the Search Institute identified 40 assets related to child and adolescent development, risk prevention, and resiliency (Search Institute, 2014a). These assets are listed in Table 18-2. Developmental assets are skills, experiences, relationships, and behaviors evidenced as support, strengths, and noncognitive skills in self, family, school, and the community. These

TABLE 18-2 **Forty Developmental Assets**

External Assets	Internal Assets
Support	**Commitment to Learning**
1. Family support	21. Achievement motivation
2. Positive family caring	22. School engagement
3. Other adult relationships	23. Homework
4. Caring neighborhood	24. Bonding to school
5. Caring school climate	25. Reading for pleasure
6. Parent involvement in school	
Empowerment	**Positive Values**
7. Community values youth	26. Caring
8. Youth as resources	27. Equality and social justice
9. Service to others	28. Integrity
10. Safety	29. Honesty
	30. Responsibility
	31. Restraint
Boundaries and Expectations	**Social Competencies**
11. Family boundaries	32. Planning and decision making
12. School boundaries	33. Interpersonal competence
13. Neighborhood boundaries	34. Cultural competence
14. Adult role models	35. Resistance skills
15. Positive peer influence	36. Peaceful conflict resolution
16. High expectations	
Constructive Use of Time	**Positive Identity**
17. Creative activities	37. Personal power
18. Youth programs	38. Self-esteem
19. Religious community	39. Sense of purpose
20. Time at home	40. Positive view of personal future

From Search Institute, www.search-institute.org.

become building blocks that help children and adolescents grow into healthy, happy, and contributing members of society. Assets are applicable to all young people regardless of gender, culture, socioeconomic situation, or geographic location. Research shows that the more assets a young person has, the more likely he or she is to make wise decisions and choose positive lifestyles while avoiding harmful or unhealthy choices. The latest initiative of the Search Institute is focused on identifying the "gateway assets," or those that help young people more readily acquire the full complement of assets, providing all who work with them more concrete ways to help them thrive.

A 2010 survey of 89,000 United States youth grades 6 through 12 showed that the average child had 19 of the 40 assets. Less than 11% had more than 31 of the 40 (Search Institute, 2014a). This study showed that those youth with the greatest number of developmental assets exhibited school success, persistence in the face of adversity, healthy behaviors, financial responsibility, a value of diversity, and leadership. The assets have been shown to be protective against the following high-risk behaviors: problem alcohol use, violence, illicit drug use, and sexual activity, with some positive protective effects on tobacco use, antisocial behavior, depression, and attempted suicide (Search Institute, 2014a).

There are developmental asset lists for adolescents (ages 12 to 18), middle childhood (ages 8 to 12), grades K to 3 (ages 5 to 9), and early childhood (ages 3 to 5). Common threads and unique features for each developmental age group are reflected in the asset lists. The middle childhood assets include the transition toward emerging self-hood and self-regulation. The early childhood assets respond to early childhood issues with essential ingredients that relate to school readiness, school success, and a happy productive life. The asset lists have been translated into 14 different languages and are accessible without charge on the Search Institute website (www.search-institute.org).

Family Assets

Family assets are the relationships, interactions, opportunities, and values that help families thrive. Developed using research in family systems theory, resiliency, and adolescent development, five dimensions and 21 specific qualities that strengthen families were identified by the Search Institute (Table 18-3) (Search Institute, 2014b). These assets were studied with a group of 1511 racially, ethnically, economically, geographically, and structurally diverse American families with a 10- to 15-year-old, including both the child and parenting adults. The results show that families are more alike than different, with an average score of 47 out of 100. Thus, although the average American family does demonstrate about half the desired assets, there is room for growth. Reassuring was the fact that these strengths were more commonly associated with young people's well-being than was family structure, income, education, immigrant status, community type, or other demographic factors. The more assets a family has, the more likely they are to take better care of their health, contribute more to their community, and have higher satisfaction with their families and lives. The best news is that development of these assets can be intentionally nurtured within a family. The Search Institute website has great online tools to assist families and providers in this endeavor.

Sparks

Another concept identifying why some kids flourish instead of just "getting by" is the concept of thriving, which "focuses on how an individual is 'doing' at any given point in time as well as the path he or she is taking into the future" (Benson, 2008). *Sparks* are the key dimension of thriving and are defined as those interests, talents, and passions that motivate young people to grow, learn, and contribute (Search Institute, 2014c). Sparks help a young person make positive choices about their activities and use of time, while leading them to express their unique personalities

TABLE 18-3 Family Assets

Types of Family Assets	Description
Nurturing Relationships	
Healthy relationships begin and grow as we show each other we care about what each of us has to say, how we feel, and our unique and shared interests.	• Positive communication • Affection • Emotional openness • Support for sparks
Establishing Routines	
Shared routine, traditions, and activities give a dependable rhythm to family life.	• Family meals • Shared activities • Meaningful traditions • Dependability
Maintaining Expectations	
Expectations make it clear how each person participates in and contributes to family life.	• Openness about tough topics • Fair rules • Defined boundaries • Clear expectations • Contributions to family
Adapting to Challenges	
Every family faces challenges, large and small. The ways families face and adapt to those changes together help them through the ups and downs of life.	• Management of daily commitments • Adaptability • Problem solving • Democratic decision-making
Connecting to the Community	
Community connections, relationships, and participation sustain, shape, and enrich how families live their lives together.	• Neighborhood cohesion • Relationship with others • Enriching activities • Supportive resources

From Search Institute, www.search-institute.org/familyassets.

and contribute to the world. Kids who thrive have both knowledge of their sparks and adults who support the development of those sparks. These kids evidence higher grades, better school attendance and physical health, empathy and social competence, a concern for the environment, a desire to help others, and a sense of purpose. The 10 most common sparks identified by American teenagers are listed in Box 18-5.

Developmental Relationships

The first gateway asset, and the latest focus of Search Institute research (Search Institute, 2014d), is the presence of developmental relationships. Though caring adult relationships have always been a part of the assets, a developmental relationship is a broader and deeper concept. Each person contributes to and benefits from the interaction. A developmental relationship is often with an adult but can also be with a close friend, sibling, or other peer. It enriches, transforms, and "propels young people on a path towards success and thriving" (Roehlkepartain, 2014). Five elements critical to these relationships are:

1. Express CARE: Show that you like me and want the best for me.
2. CHALLENGE growth: Insist that I try to continuously improve.
3. Provide SUPPORT: Help me complete tasks and achieve goals.
4. Share POWER: Hear my voice and let me share in making decisions.
5. Expand POSSIBILITIES: Expand my horizons and connect me to opportunities.

Within these five groups, 20 actions have been identified that make a relationship developmental. The framework is being examined nationally and results from these studies can also be found on the Search Institute website.

• BOX 18-5 The 10 Most Common Sparks Identified by American Teenagers

1. Creative arts
2. Athletics
3. Learning (e.g., languages, science, history)
4. Reading
5. Volunteering (e.g., helping, serving)
6. Spirituality, religion
7. Nature, ecology, environment
8. Living a quality life (e.g., joy, tolerance, caring)
9. Animal welfare
10. Leading

Factors Influencing Self-Perception

A variety of factors influence the development of self-perception (Fig. 18-1). Some of the more noteworthy ones include significant relationships and parenting style; attachment, temperament, and stress and trauma; health, cultural and spiritual identity, race, and ethnicity; social experiences; and media and technology.

Significant Relationships

Significant relationships are a key component in a child's development of self-perception. Parents or parent figures, siblings and other family members, ongoing caretakers and/or caring, involved adults (e.g., teachers, coaches, mentors) all play a role. A sturdy foundation is built with positive relationships where children feel, see, and hear repeated positive reinforcement that allows them to internalize or know that they are significant, worthy, and competent. Time spent with and encouragement given to the child, both in being together and in doing things, in addition to sharing life's happenings (listening, talking, and problem-solving), are essential ingredients. However, acceptance and

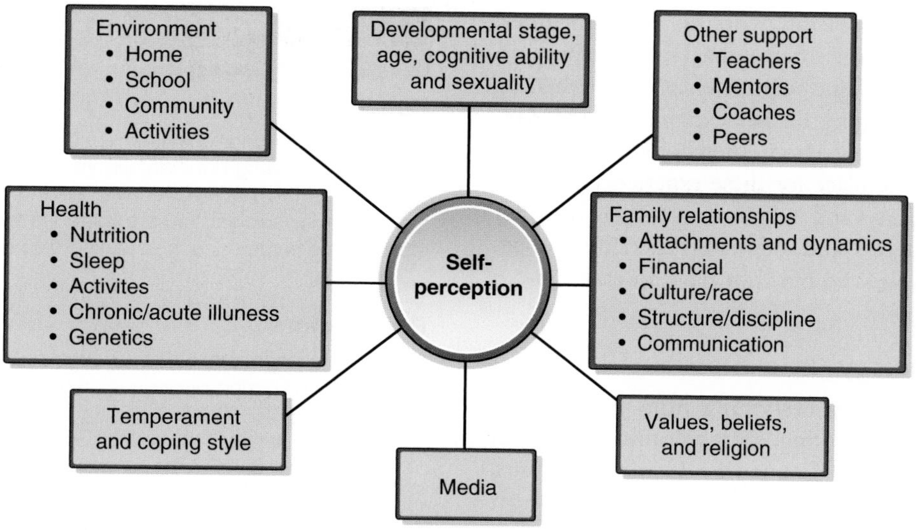

• **Figure 18-1** Factors that influence self-perception.

love, empathy, and an attitude of understanding need to be coupled with appropriate limits, boundaries, challenges, and the development of a growth mindset (discussed in the earlier section). This is especially true during the transition to adolescence; teens who perceive their parents as being accepting (parent-involved), with some degree of strictness (supervision), along with the granting of psychological autonomy have the strongest self-perception. Of note, studies have shown that first-born children tend to have higher levels of self-worth and that there are differences between boys and girls. Boys tend to focus more on achievement, whereas girls look to relationships. Girls look to their mothers as role models, and boys look to their fathers. At the same time, a father's positive interaction with his daughter helps her to feel cared for, protected, and respected. A mother's positive interaction with her son helps him to build confidence, believe in himself, and set his own goals (Slattery, 2008).

Parent-Child Attachment, Temperament, and Stress and Trauma

Parent-child attachment, the child's temperament, and the stress and trauma that the child and/or family endure all play a role in the development of the child's brain, with resultant effects on the development of the child's self-perception. Chapter 19 discusses these concepts in greater detail.

Health and Chronic Conditions

Health and chronic conditions of the child or a family member can also affect self-perception. Family appearance, intelligence, and other characteristics, including alcoholism, mental illness, and disfiguring disease, are to be considered, as are living conditions, such as poverty and homelessness (see Chapter 17). Children with disabilities may have emotions or beliefs about their appearance and capabilities that can negatively affect their self-perception. Other health factors such as physical activity, diet quality, weight, and lifestyle choices also play a role in a child's or adolescent's self-perception. It has been long thought (but not much studied in children) that obesity has a negative effect on self-perception. A longitudinal study done in Canada showed that low self-esteem did not predict excess weight, but that over a 4-year period, excess body weight did predict low self-esteem (Wang et al, 2009). A meta-analysis looking at self-perception in children with chronic health conditions who attended a camp for their condition found small improvements in self-perception (Odar et al, 2013).

Cultural Identity, Race, and Ethnicity

Cultural identity, race, and ethnicity are factors that have been studied over the past 50 years. Racial socialization is an important goal in raising children to develop cultural pride and well-being and learn to cope with racial discrimination. Adolescence is a critical time for racial-ethnic identity (REI) formation, and success in establishing an identity is positively associated with self-esteem. If successfully done, this becomes a protective factor and translates into doing well in school. A United Kingdom program with multi-heritage children who were considered at risk for multiple problems including low self-esteem had a positive effect on the children overall (as measured by self-esteem, well-being, and behavior), but interestingly not a significant effect on self-esteem alone as measured either by self-report or by parental perception (Phillips et al, 2008). In spite of social exclusion, high levels of family breakdown, underachievement in school, and distinct patterns of racism, the children did not suffer from low levels of self-esteem as measured either before or after participation.

Social Experiences

Children's social experiences provide opportunities to observe the world, test skills and abilities, interact with others, and try various roles. Positive experiences, such as success in solving problems, working out difficulties, and learning to carry on after setbacks, contribute to significance, self-worth, and competence, strengthening confidence and encouraging further exploration and risk-taking. The school setting (from preschool through late adolescence) is a prime place for these experiences. Clubs, sports, and community and religious avenues also offer opportunities for success and alternate experiences, especially for young people who may not have an easy time in school.

Media and Technology

Media, which encompasses everything from television to cell phones to social networking, exert a dominant force in the lives of children (AAP Council on Communications, 2013). Time engaged in media use is greater than time spent in school, and media have become the main leisure time activity for many young people. By providing opportunities for interaction and affiliation, as well as positive messages that teach pro-social attitudes and behaviors, media have the power to influence identity formation as well as a child's health and development. But media can also provide unhealthy feedback through the violence, sex, drugs, and body images portrayed in television shows and movies (Strasburger, 2010). Young people are especially vulnerable to these often indirect messages about body size and shape and sexuality. The bombardment of images of models and movie stars, as well as the promotion of beauty products, has the greatest effect on girls. Boys tend to be influenced to use products that claim to be able to improve their muscular appearance. Texting and various social media can have a positive effect on self-perception if adolescents receive positive feedback on their profile, but a negative effect if feedback is negative (Finn, 2010). Video game playing, which typically occurs more commonly in males, tends to show a lowered self-esteem and self-concept (Jackson et al, 2009). (See Chapter 8 for more information on social media.) It takes commitment and effort on the part of parents to monitor and help interpret these influences on children.

Red Flags and Risk Factors for Self-Perception

Identifying low self-perception as early as possible in a child's life is essential, because the younger the child is, the easier it is to take steps to make changes. Some of the red flags and risk factors for poor self-perception are listed in Box 18-6. Additionally, there are certain parent behaviors that can erode a child's self-perception. Although no parent deliberately undermines his or her child's self-esteem, many unintentionally chip away at a youngster's self-worth by committing the common errors listed in Box 18-7.

Assessment of Self-Perception

The goal of assessing self-perception is to know how children describe and evaluate themselves and to identify the sources that provide the input that they use to develop their sense of self. These assessments then lay the groundwork for planning interventions for the child and family. Corresponding assessments of the parent's, caretaker's, and peer's perception of the child are important.

• BOX 18-6 Red Flags and Risk Factors for Self-Perception Problems

Red Flags

Constantly asking for reassurance: Do I look okay? Am I fat?
Constantly showing bravado: Do you know I know so and so? Do you know I'm involved with such and such?
Depression or suicide: You are better off without me.
Obsessive disorders, such as eating disorders, alcohol or drug use

Risk Factors

Physical alterations, including body image: Chronic illness (visible or not), disfiguring disabilities, sensory disabilities, obesity, anorexia
Mental and emotional alterations: School problems, such as slow learner, semiliterate, underachiever, culturally deprived, late bloomer, difficult temperament, emotional or mental illness or abuse
Environmental and relational alterations: Disrupted families and family relationships or inability to meet basic needs, unrealistic expectations or faulty thinking, temperament or personality misfits, attachment disorders, social disorders, stress, past experiences of failure, rejection, criticism

• BOX 18-7 Common Errors That Erode Self-Esteem

Negating a child's feelings: Children's feelings are an important part of their identity. When parents reject their children's emotions, it feels like the parent is rejecting them.
Frequent criticism and dwelling on negatives: Disappointment in children makes them disappointed in themselves. Whereas parents may forget their critical remarks, children often take such comments literally and internalize them.
Using put-downs and derogatory labels: Negative labels damage a child's self-image and often become self-fulfilling prophecies. Parents should choose positive nicknames that convey affection and their high opinion of their child, such as Ace, Champ, Precious, or Pal.
Typecasting or stereotyping: Although children enjoy having a unique identity, typecasting can restrict their sense of possibility and narrow their expectations.
Expecting too much: Unrealistic expectations create excessive pressure and feelings of inadequacy. "Just a little bit better" gets translated as "not good enough." Praise a child for what he does well instead of focusing on what could be better.
Tying children's character or personal worth to their performance or behavior: Verbal blasts, such as "I'm so disappointed in you," make the parent's love feel conditional and subject to cancellation when the child's behavior does not measure up. Focus on the problem behavior rather than criticizing your child. Unconditional love means that nothing your child could ever say or do would cause you to withdraw your love.

TABLE 18-4 General and Component-Specific Questions to Assess Self-Perception

General Questions	Questions Specific to Components
For the Child • What do you like about yourself? How do you describe yourself in two or three words? (*Home, sports, school,* and *activities* may be clue words.) • What are your best qualities? How do you describe yourself (body image)? • What do you do well? What are you better at than most people? What are you proud of? • How do you respond to failure? How do you respond to new challenges? • Do you have a close friend(s)? • Do you feel in control of your life? What are your plans for next year? For after high school? • What motivates you? Gives you confidence? Are you willing to continue even after a setback? **For the Parent** • How does your parenting style (e.g., personality, patience, energy level, talents) compare with your child's? • Are you setting reasonable or attainable expectations for your child?	**Significance** • Does the child feel loved, lovable, cared for, secure, supported, accepted, and understood? • Is this love conditional or unconditional? Is this based on who the child is or what the child does? **Worthiness** • Does the child feel valuable, acceptable? • Are self-respect and self-liking evident? • What beliefs or convictions does the child have about himself or herself? Are these beliefs or convictions realistic? Do they match the child's lifestyle? **Competence** • Does the child feel capable, adequate, optimistic overall? • Does the child approach new tasks with confidence? • What are the child's cognitive, physical, and social strengths?

Assessment of self-perception is not a simple task. It cannot be observed directly or obtained from questioning alone but must be inferred from observed behavior, self-statements, and other relevant information. Self-rating, observational scales, draw-a-person tests, and puppet interviews are other means of assessment. The draw-a-person test, used with younger children, asks the child to draw a picture of himself or herself and a picture of another child. A comparison of the two drawings often gives an idea of the child's self-perception. Somewhere between fourth and sixth grades, self-esteem inventories can be considered. The Rosenberg Scale (1965), perhaps one of the better-known measures, was initially developed to assess adolescents. This 10-item questionnaire using a four-point Likert scale reflects current feelings, has proven reliability and validity, and is translated into more than 50 languages. A comprehensive meta-analysis of other measures of self-esteem for young children is available (Davis-Kean and Sandler, 2001) as are a variety of measures for adolescents (Schott and Bellin, 2001).

It is important, especially in adolescence, to evaluate self-concept over multiple domains, which may include academic achievements (scholastic competence), athletic achievements, peer (social) acceptance, physical appearance and attributes, relationships and interpersonal acceptance (close friendships, romantic appeal), participation in activities, moral behaviors as compared with internal standards, and a sense of control over personal accomplishments. When children and adolescents are asked to give a self-description, they use physical, social, and psychological dimensions referring to home, school, friends, sports, or activities in which they are involved. A study evaluating social leadership in elementary students showed positive self-perception as an important quality evidenced by any of six domains: scholastic, peer acceptance, athletic, physical, conduct, or self-worth (Scharf and Mayseless, 2009). For adolescents, parental perception of competence is often based on scholastic and behavioral parameters, whereas peer perceptions rely on physical appearance and social and athletic competence.

History

It is very helpful to routinely ask children to describe themselves during health supervision visits. At younger ages, questions may be focused, gradually becoming more open-ended as children mature. Asking parents similar questions is also beneficial. The questions in Table 18-4 can be used to assess a child's self-perception in the clinical setting.

The developmental and family assets, sparks, and developmental relationships frameworks are helpful tools for parents and children to compare their perceptions, identify strong and weak areas, and plan for areas of growth. The Search Institute has multiple resources, including questionnaires for various ages in many languages to assist the clinician (see Additional Resources).

To some extent the clinician must synthesize information collected over the entire visit in order to get a more complete picture of the child's self perception. This includes considering the details listed in Box 18-8.

Observations During the History and Examination

Direct questioning about all of the areas previously listed gives the provider information about the child. However,

• BOX 18-8 Questions for Other Pertinent Areas of Self-Perception

Parental/Family Influences

- Who is primarily responsible for parenting the child? How do parents describe themselves? Perceive their role?
- How do other family members (e.g., siblings, grandparents) relate to the child?
- How does the parent describe the child? How valued is the child? How is that shown?
- What are parental expectations for the child? Is the child given age-appropriate guidance, responsibilities, and freedoms?

Significant Others Outside Family

- Who are they? Peers? Teachers? Neighbors? Authority figures? Social supports? Networks? Mentors?
- What are the relationships like?

Environment and Social Experiences

- What is the child's environment like? What experiences or opportunities are there? Within the family? In the neighborhood? More formal activities (e.g., play groups, extracurricular activities)?
- What experiences or opportunities are there within the family and in the community to test skills and abilities? Interact with others? Try new roles? Is this encouraged?
- How protected is the child?

Discipline

- How is the child disciplined? What methods are used? Is guidance given?
- Are limits and consequences clear?
- Is the child allowed to try without having unrequested assistance provided too soon or being rescued?

Communication

- What messages is the child receiving? For example, "You are a helper," or "You are a bad boy."
- Is he or she listened to? Are feelings acknowledged?
- What does the child say about himself or herself? For example, describes self as "good" or "bad," "smart" or "dumb."
- What and how much media is the child viewing?

observation of the child and interactions between the child and the accompanying person(s) throughout the office visit are equally important.

- What is the relationship between the two?
- What actual words are said? With what tone of voice?
- What kind of nonverbal interaction occurs? What kind of physical interaction?
- Is the child encouraged to answer questions and perform tasks? Is rescuing occurring? Is guidance given?
- What expectations are voiced?
- How is discipline conducted within the examination setting? What limits are set?

Management Strategies for Developing Positive Self-Perception

Anticipatory guidance, education, and counseling are strategies that the provider uses to guide and direct the family, child, and adolescent in developing a healthy self-perception. If problems are significant and the child or family is in distress, mental health intervention may be necessary (see Chapter 19).

When working with the child and family, choose specific strategies to improve self-perception, keeping in mind that familial, generational, ethnic and cultural practices, stress, history of trauma, and chronic illness all influence the strategies that will be acceptable to the child and family. The strategies detailed here are often already a part of anticipatory guidance but are included because they have a specific effect on self-perception. General categories include facilitating good parenting; maintaining appropriate expectations of the child; using discipline techniques that enhance self-perception; communicating positively and with respect; providing helpful strategies for the child, adolescent, and parent; and encouraging asset building, spark development, and developmental relationships.

Facilitate Good Parenting

Facilitating good parenting includes the following:

- Know yourself: Parental self-perception, either positive or negative, has a significant effect on the child's self-perception. "If Mama ain't happy, ain't nobody happy." Parents should be encouraged to understand and accept themselves, acknowledge their strengths and accept their uniqueness, take care of themselves, treat themselves with respect, and be aware of their own feelings.
- Know your child/children: See what they see; feel what they feel; hope what they hope. This provides needed empathy. Children have their own personality, temperament, dreams, and opinions and need to be known, loved, accepted, and respected for who they are.
- Value your child/children: Appreciate and praise who they *are* rather than what they *do*. Show belief in their ability to learn, improve, and grow. Look in their eyes when you talk to them. Recognize their unique means of self-expression. Delight in their discoveries. Contribute to their collections. Identify their strengths, focus on their efforts, structure situations for success, and offer thanks for what they do. Avoid shame, criticism, and humiliation.
- Avoid comparing children: Children are individuals who grow and develop in their own way and at their own rate. Celebrate their accomplishments. Tell them how terrific they are. Their individuality needs to be respected, and comparisons with siblings or peers should be avoided.
- Be available to the child both physically and emotionally, teaching the child, modeling behavior, and helping the

child learn to relate to others: A sense of security and belonging occurs as you meet basic needs and spend time together, enjoying the child, having fun, touching, talking, and watching.
- Make them believe you are always on their team: Do things with them, not just for them. Show up at their concerts, games, and events. Visit their schools. Presence endorses the child's involvement and reinforces the importance of their efforts.
- Take time; avoid being hurried, especially during times of transition: Schedule times to be together. Play with your children, and let them choose the activity and set the pace. Spend at least 20 minutes each day giving them undivided attention. Consider whether dawdling, acting out, or feeling bad may be related to being hurried and feeling lack of emotional support.
- Insist on family meals: Time together sharing about everyone's day has been shown to enhance significance, worth, belonging, and safeguard both children and teens.
- Know their friends: Encourage positive involvement with friends and activities. Help find the right niche (e.g., length of time, type of activity) that fits the child. Show an interest in friends (e.g., host a sleepover, take a group to the zoo). Steer them away from less constructive friends and activities.
- Accept mistakes: Mistakes are a normal part of being human, especially growing up. Being involved means making mistakes, but it also allows for success.
- Let go: Empower them to make decisions. Trust them. Give them responsibility. Develop a gradual, planned granting of freedom and responsibility, beginning in infancy and ending in late adolescence. Letting go offers trust, provides opportunities, gives choices, instills confidence, and refrains from rushing to aid a struggling child. As part of this process, each year the child should make more decisions and assume more routine responsibilities than during the prior 12 months.

Maintain Appropriate Expectations of the Child

Maintaining appropriate expectations of the child includes the following:
- Keep expectations involving tasks, toys, and roles appropriate to the child's age. Expectations that are too high lead to pressure on children and a constant feeling of failure even when children are doing their best. Expectations that are too low diminish children's value and make them feel as if the parent has no faith in them. Expecting their best can be overly demanding because no one can consistently "do their best" all the time.
- Set expectations that are appropriate to the child's unique qualities. Each child's individual personality, temperament, strengths, and weaknesses must be considered. Parent-driven versus child-driven expectations need to be identified. Although this is a sensitive issue, knowing where expectations begin (with parent or child) and how they fit the child and family is important. Recognize differences between the parent's style and abilities and the child's.
- Identify limits and consequences clearly and follow through. Encourage flexible limit setting. For example, "You have to wear a coat, but you may choose the blue or red one."
- Clearly state expectations so that both the child and parent understand. This provides security for the child and prevents frustration, distrust, and further problems.
- Develop resilience in children by helping them learn to view failure or mistakes as chances to learn. Mistakes are accepted and expected. A realistic assessment of the child's performance, emphasizing strengths and discussing strategies that could lead to success, prepares children to approach future obstacles and disappointments constructively.

Use Discipline Techniques That Enhance Self-Perception

Using discipline techniques that enhance self-perception includes the following:
- The goal of discipline is to teach children, not punish them. The manner and intent of providing discipline are as important as the techniques used.
- Help the child learn to choose acceptable behaviors and learn self-control. Establish house rules. Catch the child being good and offer praise. Be sincere.
- Foster problem-solving to build confidence. Begin by providing opportunities to make choices and decisions. Teach the steps to problem-solving (stating the problem, expressing needs, considering alternatives, agreeing on a solution, and implementing and following through with the agreed-on solution). Take time and let the child work through the process.
- Consider utilizing a collaborative problem-solving approach (more recently known as Collaborative & Proactive Solutions, Greene, 2015; Lewis, 2015) especially with difficult or challenging behaviors. (See Lives in the Balance website in the Additional Resources list.)
- Provide guidance, but avoid rescuing children. Respect their choices, allowing them to persevere, learn, and work through frustration. This helps them learn independence and empowers them for further success. Rescuing (providing unrequested assistance too soon) must be differentiated from guiding, encouraging, and being an ally to the child. Guidance helps children understand themselves and the surrounding world, develop a conscience, and steer clear of potential problems.
- Think about where you are in the four phases of parenthood (Hostetler, 2008):
  - Commander: In the first years, encouraging a child's growth from discipline to self-discipline by explaining the reason for limits.

- Coach: In the early and middle school years, teaching growth from parent-direction to self-direction.
- Counselor: In the teen years, encouraging growth from dependence to independence.
- Consultant: In the early adult years, means letting go, yet being available to help as requested.

Communicate Positively and with Respect

Communicating positively and with respect includes the following:

- Listen to children. Good listening means taking them seriously, being interested, and letting them finish what they are saying. Show love in the way the child most appreciates. This may be through touch (giving hugs and back rubs), verbally (encouraging words and tone of voice), or nonverbally (positive facial expressions or high-fives). Say "I love you" often and in a variety of ways.
- Be aware of the words you use, in addition to the tone of voice, the intent of the words, and body language. Avoid negative messages that are sent in comparisons, put-downs (e.g., "You are such a baby."), humiliation (e.g., "You can't do anything right."), labeling (e.g., "You're such a slob."), and fault-finding.
- Use communication techniques that convey respect. Ask open-ended questions to encourage dialogue. Listen with empathy. Apologize and ask forgiveness when appropriate. Use "I" messages to express anger or frustration.
- Show respect by providing choices, asking their opinion, and allowing them to do what they want with their possessions.
- Praise and encourage children often, especially as they undertake new challenges or roles. Say "thanks" for their cooperation. Catch them doing well (e.g., "I like the way you…"). Acknowledge their help (e.g., "I appreciate…"). Love their person (e.g., "I love being with you…").
- Maintain a strength-based approach. Look for what the child does well and help them cultivate those strengths. Summer camps and special opportunities should be structured around these areas.
- Talk to kids about the reality of disappointment in everyone's life. Not everyone will always like you, nor will every effort always result in success. Frame "failure" in context of the child's effort and what could be done differently next time. Share parent's disappointments. Were they as serious as imagined? Were there long-term effects?
- When correcting, focus on specifics regarding lifelong learning and improvement academically, socially, culturally, and occupationally. Use believable, positive statements. For example, "Can I show you a way that might get better results?"
- Help children identify, handle, and express their feelings by accepting and acknowledging them. Avoid statements that deny children's feelings (e.g., "You don't really hate your sister.") or that give false reassurance (e.g., "You'll get over it in a few minutes. Stop complaining."). Instead, use reflective statements. For example, "Your sister really upsets you when she gets into your things," or "It's hard having to wait your turn, isn't it?" Listen. Share your own feelings and failures. Intervention may take place at the thought and behavior level after feelings are brought forward.
- Use "I" statements, not "you" judgments. This separates performance from worth and validates children's behavior while still allowing the behavior to be modified. Use "and," which tends to connect words, instead of "but," which tends to negate what was said before. For example, "I like your drawings, *and* I need you to color on the paper, not on the wall."
- Be aware of children's "self-talk." What children say to themselves not only reflects what they believe but also gives further definition to who they are. Positive statements enhance self-perception and minimize stress children feel. Negative statements reflect low self-perception and require intervention.
- Nurture curiosity and exploration to encourage mastery of new skills and help children reach their potential.

Provide Helpful Strategies for the Child, Adolescent, and Parent

Some helpful strategies for the child, adolescent, and parent are:

- Support early and ongoing self-assertions as means of children expressing themselves. For example, allow a preschooler to wear the outlandish outfit chosen unless it is totally inappropriate (e.g., a bathing suit in November) or a school-age child to create the menu one night a week.
- Offer genuine encounter moments (GEMs) (Hall, 1998). A GEM is a mutually agreed-on time that is set apart for 100% attention and love, focused attention, or direct involvement. The child takes the lead in how the time is spent.
- Use the 10-20-10 strategy (spending 10 uninterrupted minutes in the morning, 20 uninterrupted minutes after school or in the afternoon, and 10 uninterrupted minutes in the evening) to give one-on-one undivided attention (Forbes and Post, 2010).
- Remember the 20-second rule. When your child wants attention, even if you are really busy, you can almost always pause for 20 seconds to appreciate what they want to show you or share, and the child is often content with that.
- Assume the best in your child and focus on the positives. Make a list of positive attributes and strengths, and let your child hear you speak positively about him or her.
- Encourage a healthy connectedness. Children need to belong to and feel that they are a part of their family and groups outside their family through social activities and links within their community, ethnic group, or geographic area.
- Every child has interests and abilities that can be developed and displayed to provide the child with a sense of

success and a defense from failure. Identify what the child is interested in and good at and encourage and praise those skills, talents, efforts, and achievements. Seven kinds of intelligence have been identified: linguistic, mathematic, spatial, musical, bodily, interpersonal, and intrapersonal (see Chapter 20), and any or all can be used to build and affirm the child's island of competence.
- Help your child compete (Dobson, 1999). A child needs encouragement to develop skills, opportunities to use the skills, and second chances when failure occurs. A child is empowered by having an ally in these endeavors.
- Help your child develop a sense of purpose, knowing that he or she can affect the outcome of events in life. Children feel more effective and less bored and resentful if they feel they are contributing. Provide opportunities to make choices, solve problems, and develop responsibilities. Help them set goals and make plans. Follow their progress and talk about what happened.
- Promote a sense of ownership. Children who are given responsibility for themselves and their actions are also given a sense of control over their life.
- Teach a growth mindset. Praise effort, challenge seeking, and commitment. Emphasize hard work, perseverance, and courage.
- Counter sibling rivalry by focusing on each individual's strengths and differences. This helps diffuse the complaint that "it's not fair" and focus on each individual's need.
- Strengthen the home-school connection. Help with (but don't do) homework. Attend parent-teacher meetings. Support extra-curricular activities, and introduce local resources.
- Keep a close eye on the classroom. Problems in the classroom are often symptoms of other problems in a child's life. Temporary rough spots are normal and must be distinguished from more pervasive problems that require intervention.
- Defuse feelings of inferiority. Throughout the school years and adolescence, comparisons are the norm, and feelings of inferiority often result. Children aware of this fact who have learned to compete and compensate are more likely to believe in themselves despite feelings of inferiority.
- Remember the seven Cs of resilience in children: Competence, confidence, connection, character, contribution, coping, and control are tools that allow children to respond to challenges and adversity with a positive mindset (Ginsburg, 2015).
- Prepare for adolescence. A special time set aside to talk with preadolescents about the coming physical, social, and hormonal changes helps prepare them to handle the transitions with greater ease.
- Affirm that good lifestyle choices (physical activity, healthful diet) are boosters to self-perception.
- Act as "coach" for your children rather than being authoritarian. Encourage building life skills and increasing parent-child connection—communication, support, problem-solving, help-seeking—especially in the adolescent years or with children or adolescents struggling with low self-perception.

Encourage Asset Building, Sparks, and Developmental Relationships

Encourage asset building, sparks, and developmental relationships by doing the following:
- Foster identification and building of developmental and family assets.
- Adopt a thriving perspective, and help preteens and teens recognize their own spark(s).
- Involve everyone in the child's life (i.e., child, parents, teachers, health care providers, and community members), and encourage the growth of any developmental relationship that blossoms. Relationships are critical, and the process is ongoing.
- Use intentional redundancy, because hearing the same positive messages over and over again from many different people is important.
- Refer to the wealth of information available from the Search Institute.

Complications of Self-Perception

If a child's self-perception is chronically low, mental health issues often develop. Internalized problems (e.g., anxiety and depression) or externalized problems (e.g., anger and aggression) are seen. See Chapter 19 for discussion of these issues. Physical issues (e.g., somatic complaints and obesity) that overlap with the mental illness can also be seen.

Specific Self-Perception Problems in Children

Self-Esteem Problems

Description

When a child's sense of *significance* is disturbed and when the child is unsure of belonging and being loved, cared for, and accepted, self-esteem problems arise. The child has a loss of confidence and feelings of insecurity are evidenced. The child may question "Am I loved?" Self-esteem problems may be situational, transient, or chronic. Low self-esteem often results when love is conditional or when a child is accepted primarily for what he or she does rather than who he or she is. Attachment problems may be found in the family system. Child maltreatment, especially emotional and physical abuse, also interferes with the development of a healthy self-esteem (see Chapter 17) as does peer rejection.

Assessment

The child with self-esteem problems seeks attention, importance, and security. There may be a history of rejection or a dysfunctional family. Parental insensitivity, fatigue and time pressure, guilt, and rivals (e.g., siblings) may all

TABLE 18-5 Counterproductive Coping Strategies: Signs of Low Self-Esteem

Behavior	Example
Quitting	Ending a game before it is over to avoid losing
Avoiding	Not even trying something for fear of failure
Cheating	Copying answers from someone else on a test
Clowning around	Acting silly to minimize feeling like a failure
Controlling	Telling others what to do
Bullying	Putting others down to hide feelings of inadequacy
Denying	Minimizing the importance of a task
Rationalizing or making excuses	Blaming the teacher for failing a test

contribute. Self-destructive behaviors (e.g., suicide, eating disorders, teen pregnancy) may be present. Self-absorption or obsession with external markers of self-worth may be evident (see Box 18-3). Because of the desire for acceptance and love, these children are often people pleasers, seeking constant positive feedback. Position and status are attempts to prove importance. Counterproductive coping strategies may be used (Table 18-5). Being insecure, these children are fragile and defensive, especially vulnerable to criticism, and reacting negatively to any correction.

Differential Diagnosis

Differential diagnoses include personal identity problems, role performance problems, and body image problems.

Management

Unconditional love, acceptance, belonging, and security are needs that are not being met. Making time for one-on-one activities with a parent, finding a group that the child fits into, or fostering a nurturing or a developmental relationship can be helpful. See the Management Strategies for Developing Positive Self-Perception section for specific ideas to achieve these, especially "parental roles," "know your children," "limits and consequences," and the "10-20-10 strategy." Children with chronic illness may be helped by participating in groups with others dealing with similar issues. Providing education and treatment for adolescents with acne may be a relatively simple way to boost self-esteem.

Complications

Attention-seeking may be extreme, causing aggression and leading to behavior problems. Girls with low self-esteem are significantly more likely to initiate sexual intercourse than girls with high self-esteem. A relationship between acne and poor self-esteem (probably because of the effect on body image) has been demonstrated. Anxiety, attachment disorders, behavior problems, nonsuicidal self-destructive behavior (e.g., cutting), depression, disruptive behavior, social withdrawal, suicide, eating disorders, teen pregnancy, and violence are complications of self-esteem problems.

Personal Identity Problems

Description

When children are uncertain of their *worth,* do not receive respect as individuals, and are not valued for who they are, personal identity is shaky. Children may feel confused about who they are and may question, "Am I okay?" The child relies almost exclusively on how others define them, never knowing for sure who he or she is. This leads to internalizing others' negative perceptions and feelings of inferiority are manifested. Potential parental factors that contribute to these feelings of inferiority include insensitivity to the child in words or attitude, unrealistic expectations, fatigue and time pressure, guilt, and rivals for love.

Clinical Findings

Children with personal identity problems do not feel good about themselves and often lack self-respect, feeling as if they have not lived up to adult expectations. They may talk about themselves in degrading terms. There is a struggle to prove "I am okay." If overly burdened with unrealistic expectations, they may no longer have any initiative to keep going. Coping may take the form of withdrawal, fighting, clowning, denying there is a problem, or striving for conformity (see Table 18-5). Attachment problems may be found in the family system. There may be a history of the child being criticized, embarrassed, shamed, or humiliated, or of familial mental illness or abuse.

Differential Diagnosis

Self-esteem problems, role performance problems, and body image problems are differential diagnoses for personal identity problems.

Management

Self-respect, self-value, and feeling good about oneself are aspects of self-perception that are not developed in these children. See the Management Strategies for Developing Positive Self-Perception section for specific ideas to work on these aspects of self-perception, especially "value children," "maintain appropriate expectations of the child," and "defuse feelings of inferiority." Helping the child learn to compensate can conquer low self-esteem (see the Provide Helpful Strategies for the Child, Adolescent, and Parent section about finding the "island of competence"). The "10-20-10 strategy" to ensure one-on-one interaction is also helpful.

Complications

Anxiety, depression, suicide, guilt, anger, and hostility are complications of personal identity problems.

Role Performance Problems

Description

When children feel *incompetent* or are unable to perform expected activities or behaviors because of physical, mental, or cognitive disability, role performance problems emerge. These children do not feel adequate, confident, or in control and may think, "I can't do it." Role performance problems can occur in cognitive, social, and physical arenas. A typical scenario involves a child with school problems.

Clinical Findings

Children with role performance problems may retreat and be hesitant to approach new opportunities and experiences, or they may be perfectionists, always striving to prove competence. A history of failure, or being a slow learner, semiliterate, an underachiever, a late bloomer, or culturally deprived may be found.

Differential Diagnosis

Self-esteem problems, personal identity problems, body image problems, and actual physical, mental, learning, or cognitive problems are differential diagnoses for role performance problems.

Management

Because the child has feelings of incompetence, inadequacy, and lacks confidence and a sense of control, strategies to develop these skills are needed. See the Management Strategies for Developing Positive Self-Perception section for specific ideas to work on these aspects of self-perception, especially "find and build on the 'island of competence'" (a key) and "help your child compete." Working with the school and the parents to achieve these goals is helpful. Teacher support of the individual child, not just as one of many in the classroom, has been shown to have a positive effect on self-perception (Spilt et al, 2014).

Complications

Complications of role performance problems include anger and aggression, anxiety, behavior problems, depression, withdrawal, somatic complaints, and school failure.

Body Image Problems

Description

When there is a discrepancy between how children perceive their bodies, how they actually are, and how they want them to be, the result is body image problems. The discrepancy may be temporary or permanent, seen or unseen, and occurring in terms of size, function, appearance, or potential. Attitudes, feelings, and fantasies play a role in body image.

Disturbance in body image arises from varied sources, including physical illness or disability, chronic illness, emotional disturbances, abuse, attitudes conveyed by others, or perception of what is "normal" from the media. Body image problems are most common in adolescence, which is when teenagers are most concerned about physical appearance in comparison with that of their peers. Sexuality, especially in female adolescents, is a part of a teenager's developing body image. Body image problems also occur in younger children; an example can be seen when a young child suffers a fractured bone, is immobilized, and is unable to cope with not being able to master his or her environment.

Clinical Findings

Children with disturbed body image may have concerns related to appearance, body size, function, or potential. These may be noted by questioning or techniques, such as the puppet interview or draw-a-person. An adolescent body esteem questionnaire is available (Mendelson et al, 2001).

Possible behaviors include the following:

- Eating disorders (see Chapter 19)
- Actual or perceived change in structure and function of body or body part
- Refusing to look at or touch an altered or missing body part
- Preoccupation with the loss or change
- Overexposure or hiding of body part
- Feeling shame and embarrassment
- Distorted perception of a normal body
- Fear of rejection or unwanted attention from others

Differential Diagnosis

Self-esteem, personal identity, or role performance problems are differential diagnoses for body image problems.

Management

The discrepancy between the real and the desired body, in addition to the cause of the discrepancy, must be identified. Severity and cause of the discrepancy guide the intervention. If the discrepancy is developmental and not severe, education and counseling should help. If the problem is significant, referral for mental health care is often necessary.

Practices to develop appropriate ideas about appearance and value include the following:

- Explore parental feelings about their child's appearance. Look for ways to broadcast healthy attitudes.
- Prompt children to determine where attitudes originate. Appreciate concern about physical appearance, but discuss extremes. Favorite television shows or movies are good starting points.
- Teach that happiness and beauty do not go hand in hand. Discuss feeling beautiful (outward changes) and being beautiful (inward growth).
- Stress the need to celebrate each family member's uniqueness. Focus on personality traits and attitudes about life, school, and people—not on externals.

Other helpful interventions include the following:

- Encourage regular physical activity, especially with other family members. Developmentally focused youth sports programs (Girls on the Run and Girls on Track) showed positive self-esteem and body image findings (DeBate et al, 2009).

- Point out ways the child or adolescent is on target developmentally, and identify what can be expected over the next year. Emphasize the fact that there is a high degree of variability in development.
- Make family connections: Look for features similar to other family members; include talents and internal characteristics as well.
- Play the appreciation game: Name body parts and say something nice about that part. For example, "Thanks, ears, for letting me listen to my iPod."
- Go to the Don't Buy It: Get Media Smart website (see Additional Resources).
- Stay positive: Don't make or allow disparaging comments, and give compliments often.
- Identify areas where assistance is needed; refer to counselors, dietary therapy, occupational therapy, or physical therapy as appropriate.
- Collaborate with the school nurse or teacher to plan for the child at school.
- Involve the child in a peer group with similar problems.
- Verbalize acceptance; use play therapy to encourage verbalization.
- Teach new ways of handling situations to accommodate for loss or change.
- Discuss ways to camouflage areas of concern (e.g., wig or scarf for hair loss).
- Compliment behaviors that indicate acceptance.
- Provide ongoing support and encouragement as a primary care provider with focus on positive aspects of body and functioning.

For a complete list of references, please visit http://evolve.elsevier.com/Burns/pediatric/.

19

Coping and Stress Tolerance: Mental Health and Illness

DAWN LEE GARZON

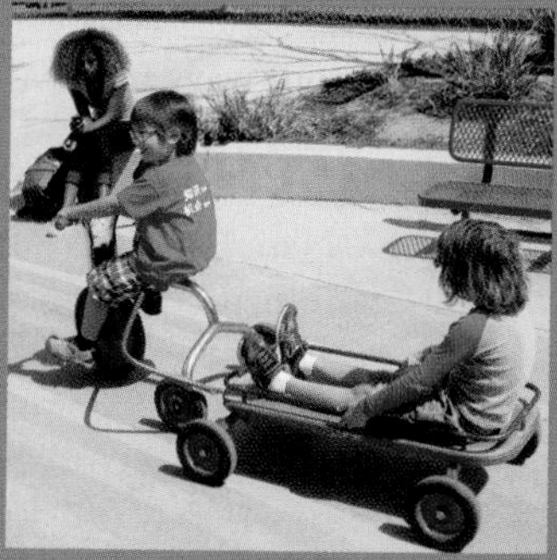

Mental health promotion begins at birth with nurturing, responsive caregiving; continues into the preschool years as young children learn to manage a range of emotions; is fostered through healthy family and peer relationships; and is maximized through child's and caregiver's emotional and social skills. Infancy and toddlerhood are particularly critical times in mental health development. Trust development and a sense of security begin with effective, timely parental response to the infant's needs. Contrary to popular belief, responsive parenting results in children who are able to self-regulate their behavior and who are confident and competent rather than clingy. As children become more mobile and autonomous late in the first year, parents should begin to use limit-setting strategies that include reasoning, explanations, and distractions. Effective use of discipline and a teaching-based style enhance the self-regulation development and foster strong self-concept and social competence (see Chapters 4 and 16).

The term *mental health disorders* describes conditions that affect behavioral, emotional, and neurologic development; a psychiatric illness; and stress and altered coping resulting from difficult life circumstances (Committee on Psychosocial Aspects of Child and Family Health and Task Force on Mental Health, 2009). The term *behavioral health issues* includes emotional health issues, substance use and abuse, and mental health disorders. There are many reasons for behavioral health issues in childhood and adolescence, including exposure to environmental toxins, such as lead and mercury; genetic inheritance; caregiver neglect or abuse; and exposure to violence. Anxiety and depression stem from genetic predispositions, neurohormonal influences, and the stresses and strains of modern family life. An increasing body of evidence indicates that epigenetics, or the role of nongenetic influences of gene expression, may be a significant contributor to mental illness. Known epigenetic influences include trauma, toxic stress, parenting style, nutrition, hormones, social support, drugs, and family interactions (Mahgoub and Monteggia, 2013; Shonkoff et al, 2012). Common childhood stressors that can negatively impact child mental health include parental divorce or separation, domestic violence, child abuse or neglect, death of a parent or sibling, natural disasters, familial mental illness, exposure to media reports of traumatic events, school problems, interpersonal conflict, and military deployment of a loved one.

The 2015 America's Children: Key National Indicators of Well-Being showed that 5% of responding parents identified their 4- to 17-year-old children as having definite or severe difficulties with emotion, concentration, behavior, or the ability to get along well with others (Wallman, 2015). Significant problems were identified for 6% of males and 4% of females and were more likely to occur for children living in families with incomes at 100% of the federal poverty level (8%) than those with incomes at or above 200% of the federal poverty level (4%). Children living with only their mother (8%) were more likely to have significant problems compared with children living in two-parent families (4%). Lastly, 43% of parents reported seeking help from a general physician, whereas 55% consulted a mental health specialist for their child's treatment.

Children and adolescents in the United States are not getting the mental health care that they need. National estimates indicate that 13% to 20% of American children require mental health services and that those with a psychiatric diagnosis represent those with severe impairment; those with mild symptoms often go unrecognized. Yet only half of the children and adolescents who meet diagnostic criteria for a mental health disorder have visited a health care provider for treatment of their condition in the past year, and fewer than 20% receive the treatment that they need (Wallman, 2015). As of 2012, there were only 8300 child psychiatrists, although it was estimated that 30,000 would be needed by 2000 (American Academy of Child and

Adolescent Psychiatry [AACAP], 2013b). The need for these professionals is especially acute for those who live in rural areas and who have low socioeconomic status (AACAP, 2013b). National estimates show that only 45% of adolescents with mental health issues received help in the previous year, with schools (23.6%) and specialty mental health (22.8%) as the most common settings for care. Only about 10% receive care in primary care settings (Costello et al, 2014). Primary care providers (PCPs) must take more active roles in the identification and early intervention of children and adolescents with mental health disorders (Foy et al, 2010a; National Association of Pediatric Nurse Practitioners [NAPNAP], 2013). Bright Futures and the American Academy of Pediatrics (AAP) call for assessment of family psychosocial functioning at all routine health supervision visits and routine screening for mental health issues using validated instruments for older school-age children and adolescents (Foy et al, 2010a; Hagan et al, 2008). Barriers to the creation of a mental health care home include insufficient provider education, time constraints, limited reimbursement for services provided, provider lack of familiarity with screening methods, and social stigmas that affect the child, family, and providers (Foy et al, 2010b).

Mental Health Influences

Neurobiologic Context

Early mental health influences include the child's genetic composition and the intrauterine effects on the developing fetus. Maternal nutrition, especially vitamin B_{12}, folate and folic acid intake, and stress hormone levels are among the most documented influences on the structure and function of the evolving central nervous system (Marques et al, 2013). Severe prenatal nutritional deficiency is associated with the development of schizophrenia, schizoaffective disorders, and congenital central nervous system abnormalities (Tottenham et al, 2010).

Risk and protective factors for psychopathologic conditions emerge from the interaction of genes and environmental experiences. The protective effect of nurturing parenting is evident in animal research and in an emerging body of human studies that demonstrates nurturing caregiving is associated with decreased hypothalamic-pituitary-adrenal (HPA) stress response (Kundakovic and Champagne, 2015; Marques et al, 2013). Children exposed to physical abuse, sexual abuse, verbal abuse, and/or neglect are more likely to have altered white matter development than their nonabused peers (Choi et al, 2009). The number and combinations of risk and protective factors for any individual are likely to determine behavior patterns, comorbidities, severity, and course of psychopathologic conditions during childhood, adolescence, and adulthood.

Functional magnetic resonance imaging (fMRI) and positron emission tomography (PET) scans allow for the identification and description of patterns in brain structure and function in normal children and adolescents. These imaging techniques also document altered patterns of structure and function in children and adolescents diagnosed with psychopathologic conditions. From infancy through early adulthood, changes in the limbic system, specifically the amygdala and hippocampus, influence emotional development and the emergence of affective disorders, substance abuse, and high-risk behaviors. However, none of these brain differences alone appear to be necessary or sufficient for psychopathologic conditions to occur. Rather, environmental strengths and vulnerabilities and cumulative life experiences more strongly influence the number and severity of symptoms and the adaptive competencies that the child displays at any age (Mahgoub and Monteggia, 2013).

Research demonstrates the profound effects of stress and environmental deprivation on the young child's brain development. Activation of the HPA axis triggers release of cortisol, feeding the fight-or-flight response. Elevated serum cortisol levels act as a toxin on neurons in the central nervous system, inhibiting the growth of dendrites and neurons and causing the death of neurons. Research also demonstrates the profound effects of the use-it-or-lose-it phenomenon on the number of neurons and dendritic growth and interconnections. In the final phase of brain growth, known as *differentiation,* the brain prunes away unused neurons and dendritic connections. Brain imaging of children exposed to the chronic stress of emotionally and materially deprived environments shows reduced brain volumes compared with the brain size of age- and sex-matched children from nondeprived environments (Tottenham et al, 2010). In short, all forms of material and interactive experiences actively shape children's brain architecture.

Chronic triggering of the HPA stress response hones the speed and intensity of a neurologic response. Chronic stress leads to swift, strong expressions of distress to even minor stressful stimuli. For example, preterm infants respond with a strong cry to even minor chilling or discomfort. Infant and child crying has profoundly negative effects on normal adults, triggering the adult's own stress response. Thus excessive and prolonged crying is a significant risk factor for child abuse and the development of problems in the parent-child relationship. Normal developmental changes add an important layer of influence and complexity to the interaction between the genetically driven biology of the child and his or her interaction with the environment.

Not all mental health problems are the result of parenting and environmental effects. Genetic links have been found for conduct disorder (CD), bipolar disorder, depression, schizophrenia, attention-deficit disorder (ADD), substance abuse, antisocial behavior, generalized anxiety disorder (GAD), and obsessive-compulsive disorder (OCD) among others (Mahgoub and Monteggia, 2013).

Mental Health in Primary Care

The mental health status of children and adolescents has profound effects on child development, family functioning, and society as a whole. PCPs, as health care home providers, are ideal mental health advocates because of their (Committee on Psychosocial Aspects of Child and Family Health and Task Force on Mental Health, 2009; Kolko and Perrin, 2014; NAPNAP, 2013):

- Established therapeutic relationships with children and families
- Capacity to engage in mental health promotion and anticipatory guidance
- Familiarity with normal child development and healthy parenting
- Experience coordinating care with other health care specialists
- Familiarity with chronic care principles and practice improvement

Prevention

Primary Prevention

Primary prevention of mental health problems occurs through positive, nurturing parent-child relationships. Children need to experience a secure attachment relationship and a sense of self-worth and being worthy of love. This serves as a foundation for developing social, emotional, and cognitive competence. Additional protective factors (Foy et al, 2010a) that promote resilience and mental wellness include:

- Responsive, thoughtful caregivers
- Supportive families
- Clear behavioral standards
- Parental recognition of individual achievements, efforts, and improvements
- Healthy peer relationships
- High-quality preschool, elementary, and secondary schools
- Faith
- Sense of control over one's life
- Sense of one's purpose and clear self-identity
- Opportunities to interact with positive peers and adults
- Freedom from racism, sexism, discrimination, and poverty

Pediatric providers must consistently screen for parent depression at health visits beginning with the prenatal visit, because parental depression threatens healthy parenting. A large body of research supports the significant negative effects of maternal depression, including prenatal depression, on the behavior and development of infants and young children (Phelan et al, 2014). See Chapter 5 for a discussion on postpartum depression.

Healthy parenting strategies result in parents who are positive in tone and regard for the child, responsive to the child's autonomy and individuality, neutral in response to unwanted behavior, and attentive to the child's needs (Boxes 19-1 and 19-2 and see Chapters 4 and 17). Parents who have not experienced this type of nurturing often need education and coaching in positive parenting behaviors.

Timely anticipatory guidance allows families to handle predictable life events that impact children, such as day care or school changes and moves. Increasing the caregiver's

• BOX 19-1 Caregiver Education to Maximize Child Mental Health

Teach caregivers that their responsiveness to their child's social and emotional needs fosters healthier behavior, improved school performance, and better interpersonal relationships.

Responsive and stable caregiving positively influences brain development. This is believed to be due to a unique interaction between stress hormones, genes, and the developing brain.

Educate caregivers about normal child development. It is especially important to foster realistic expectations for behavior and coping, and there should be special emphasis on developmental stress points and transitions.

Emphasize that predictable home, child care, and school routines are essential to a child's mental health.

Provide anticipatory guidance related to healthy prenatal care, diet, and exposures during routine preventative care.

Help caregivers to develop healthy caregiving skills and support them as those skills emerge.

Educate parents that early mental, verbal, and emotional abuse is especially toxic to the young child; it changes the child's brain and may result in lifelong issues and/or problems.

Adapted from *Report of healthy development: a summit on young children's mental health: partnering with communication scientists, collaborating across disciplines and leveraging impact to promote children's mental health*, Washington, DC, 2009, Society for Research in Child Development.

• BOX 19-2 Positive Parenting Strategies

Attend to the Child Individually

Allow the child to make reasonable choices.

Respond to child's bids for attention with eye contact, smiles, and physical contact.

Comment on child's appropriate and desirable behavior frequently and positively throughout the day.

Provide guaranteed special time daily: No interruptions, no directions, and no interrogations.

Prevent secondary gains for the child's minor transgressions by having no discussion, physical contact, perhaps even eye contact; be neutral and simply state the preferred behavior.

Listen Actively

Paraphrase or describe what the child is saying.

Reflect the child's feelings.

Share the child's affect by matching the child's body posture and tone of voice.

Avoid giving commands, judging, or editorializing.

Follow the child's lead in the interaction.

Convey Positive Regard

Communicate positive feelings (e.g., love) directly.

Give directions positively, firmly, and specifically.

Provide notice before requiring the child to change activities.

Label the behavior, not the child.

Praise competency and compliance; say thank you.

Apologize when appropriate.

Avoid shaming or belittling the child.

Strive for consistency.

awareness of the child's developmental and temperamental needs can facilitate the identification of strategies to effectively facilitate transitions. Providers should assist them to find ways to help their children use developmentally appropriate coping strategies. For example, caregivers can encourage symbolic play in preschoolers or use discussion about developmentally appropriate books or movies with older children to help them express feelings and worries and gain control of their situation.

Secondary Prevention

Secondary prevention, or early detection and intervention, addresses unanticipated life events. Social, emotional, or behavioral problems may emerge even in the context of positive childrearing approaches. Early recognition of pediatric stress and mental illness is easier when caregivers have a realistic understanding of their child's development and PCPs actively screen for developmental red flags. Secondary prevention involves working collaboratively to identify and implement appropriate management strategies or to explain and reinforce the value of mental health recommendations.

Medication may be necessary to manage some pediatric mental health problems but such problems require a combined approach of psychotherapy and medication, and studies show combination therapy is superior to medication alone. Use of medication to treat pediatric mental health problems is increasing, but there are concerns about which pharmacologic interventions should be used by PCPs. There are few randomized control trials involving children that demonstrate pharmacotherapeutic safety and efficacy. Existing research shows that medications that are effective in the management of adult mental health conditions are less effective or may be completely ineffective in children with similar diagnoses, likely due to differences in the organization and function of the developing brain of children at different ages. Many drugs used to treat mental health conditions have serious adverse side effects and require ongoing physiologic monitoring (Table 19-1). PCPs assess for interactions between medications used in treating mental health conditions and commonly prescribed medications also used in primary care, such as antibiotics and contraceptives, which may result in impaired drug effectiveness or toxic side effects.

Tertiary Prevention

Tertiary prevention and intervention address major losses and trauma (e.g., victimization through sexual or physical abuse, parental marital problems, divorce, substance abuse, and parental psychopathologic conditions). It is also necessary for all children with significant behavioral symptoms that impair daily functioning. Major losses and trauma are not the only causes of mental health problems in children. Even in the absence of behavioral manifestations of distress, a referral to a mental health specialist for further assessment and intervention is suggested because of the short- and long-term problems that result from traumatic experiences. In these cases, parents may not understand the need for referral. It is helpful for the pediatric provider to frame the behavior problem as a "normal response" to stress and/or trauma with the goal of referral being to maximize the child's growth and development. A release of information allows direct contact with the consultant to ensure follow-through. Ongoing follow-up is essential with children, families, and other professional providers.

Approaches to Children by Developmental Level

Special Approaches from Infancy Through Early Childhood

The early childhood years are the most critical for mental wellness. It is important for infants, toddlers, and preschoolers to have nurturing, supportive environments with ample opportunities for physical, emotional, and social growth. Healthy attachment is critical to the development of healthy, happy, and self-confident children. Infants and young children with good attachments develop the confidence to explore their world and learn cognitive and social skills. Caregiver strategies that foster good attachment include using loving verbal and nonverbal communication, providing consistent routines, having frequent "fun" and play time, accurately reading child signals, and providing timely response to the child's needs.

By early infancy, attentive parents describe their baby's likes and dislikes, sensitivities, and signals. Many babies comfort themselves for brief periods. Babies who receive prompt responses to their needs typically provide less intense distress signals and develop the ability to wait for care. Caregivers face the challenge of becoming effective, adaptive teachers for their changing baby.

Caregivers should provide older infants, toddlers, and preschoolers the opportunity to develop an "emotional IQ." This can be achieved by allowing the child to express and recognize the full spectrum of human emotion, from good to bad, and to develop skills to cope with negative emotions. Children learn empathy when the child receives sensitive empathic care. Signs of caregiving that impede mental wellness include difficulty with limit setting, frustration and negativity with toddler behavior, limited or absent verbal communication with the child, hurtful teasing, and multiple bruises and injuries, suggesting inadequate supervision, abuse, or neglect of the child (Hagan et al, 2008).

Physical, emotional, and verbal abuse are especially toxic to the young child who is developing self-identity and learning how to relate to others. Therefore, it is important for PCPs to educate parents about strategies that can be used when they are overwhelmed, and how to communicate with their child in a developmentally appropriate manner. Nurse home visitation programs are effective for improving parenting skills, enhancing parental social support, decreasing emotional/behavioral problems, and improving parent-infant attachment in at-risk families (Olds et al, 2014). Suspicions of child abuse or neglect need to be reported because PCPs are mandatory reporters.

TABLE 19-1 Evidence-Supported Drug Therapy for Common Mental Health Conditions in Childhood

Drug Class and Examples	Conditions Treated	Primary Care Drug Interactions	Common Side Effects
Selective Serotonin Reuptake Inhibitor			
Fluoxetine (FDA approved)	Anxiety; MDD, OCD, selective mutism	Multiple drug interactions Contraindicated drugs: MAOIs, tryptophan, St. John's wort, thioridazine, and TCAs	Headache, nervousness, insomnia or sedation, fatigue, nausea, diarrhea, dyspepsia, appetite loss Diet: Avoid tryptophan supplements, grapefruit juice, and alcohol
Escitalopram (FDA approved)	Depression, anxiety	Same as above but better drug interaction profile	
Fluvoxamine (not approved for children younger than 18 years old)	OCD	Increased risk of bleeding: NSAIDs, aspirin, warfarin	
Sertraline (only approved for OCD)	OCD		
Mood Stabilizer			
Lithium	Bipolar disorder, CD	Multiple drug interactions Risk for toxic drug levels: NSAIDs, metronidazole, and a wide range of antihypertensives	Weight gain, acne, sedation, tremors, GI upset, hair loss Diet: Limit caffeine, alcohol; ensure good fluid intake; maintain salt intake
Anticonvulsants Used as Mood Stabilizers			
Carbamazepine	Bipolar disorder	Multiple drug interactions Decreased effectiveness: corticosteroids, oral and subdermal contraceptives, and doxycycline Risk for toxic drug levels: Clarithromycin, cimetidine, erythromycin, ketoconazole, itraconazole, and loratadine	Drowsiness, restlessness, nausea, vomiting, diarrhea, dyspepsia, tremor Diet: Avoid alcohol and grapefruit juice
Valproic acid	Bipolar disorder	Multiple drug interactions Risk for toxic drug levels: Aspirin-containing products	Drowsiness, irritability, restlessness, headache, ataxia, dizziness, nausea, vomiting, diarrhea, dyspepsia, weight gain, pancreatitis, thrombocytopenia, carnitine deficiency, tremor, liver failure, diplopia, blurred vision Diet: Increase foods high in carnitine (red meats and dairy products)
Second-Generation Antipsychotics			
Risperidone (FDA approved)	Aggression CD ODD Schizophrenia Tourette syndrome	Multiple drug interactions Avoid: St. John's wort Potentiates: Antihypertensives	Hypotension, syncope, tachycardia, insomnia, agitation, headache, dizziness, seizures, rash, weight gain, nausea, vomiting, diarrhea, polyuria, weight gain, elevated lipids, hyperglycemia, rhinitis, sedation Diet: Oral solution not compatible with cola or tea
Olanzapine	Bipolar disorder		
Quetiapine (FDA approved)	Bipolar disorder Schizophrenia		

Takemoto CK: *Pediatric and neonatal dosage handbook*, ed 21, Hudson, OH, 2014, Lexicomp.

CD, Conduct disorder; *FDA,* U.S. Food and Drug Administration; *GI,* gastrointestinal; *MAOI,* monoamine oxidase inhibitor; *MDD,* major depressive disorder; *NSAID,* nonsteroidal anti-inflammatory drug; *OCD,* obsessive-compulsive disorder; *TCA,* tricyclic antidepressant.

Special Approaches During the School-Age Years Through Adolescence (Level 3)

Children at this age normally have significant abilities to control their emotions, behavior, and attention. The child's social roles and behavior expectations change dramatically at home, at school, and among peers. The child's self-concept and self-esteem face daily challenges in comparisons with peers' performance in academics, sports, and social interactions. Caregivers should support their child's self-esteem and exploration of a wide range of interests, and protect the child from early engagement in competition for which he or she is not emotionally ready.

Stress is a known risk factor for mental illness. It is important to allow older children and adolescents opportunities for "downtime" and relaxation. Healthy parenting during these ages involves modeling and teaching healthy ways to deal with stress. PCPs can improve coping by using strategies to improve resilience and communication skills. Special care should be paid to avoid child "overscheduling." All children and adolescents need time to relax and to mentally recharge from the stresses of school, work, and extracurricular activities. Family interventions that improve communication and foster healthy coping include family game nights and shared, sit-down meals.

It is important for caregivers to recognize that although adolescents' cognitive skills are nearly at adult levels, their ability to make good decisions under the influence of strong emotions is not as developed. Girls are especially vulnerable to affective disorders. Social roles and behavior expectations change dramatically with sexual maturation. On the positive side, altruism and idealism emerge, leading many adolescents to significant achievements. Providing accurate and timely information, sensitive support, and appropriate limits to the adolescent is important.

High-risk adolescent behaviors include sexual activity, alcohol and drug use, driving while intoxicated, tobacco use, aggressive or hostile behavior, depressed mood, and school absenteeism or academic failure (see Chapter 8 for a discussion of risk behaviors). Failure to set appropriate limits and expectations, lack of pride in the adolescent's achievements, negative affect toward the adolescent, frustration or anger with the normal adolescent mood lability, and failure to support the adolescent's positive engagement in the community and school signal problems in the caregiver-adolescent relationship.

Temperament Influences on Mental Health

Temperament is an inborn characteristic that involves an individual's characteristic style of emotional and behavioral response across situations. Although biologic in origin, temperament characteristics evolve and develop over time and are influenced by and patterned by the social environment. Short- and long-term psychosocial adjustments are shaped by the goodness-of-fit between the individual's temperament and the social environment. Goodness-of-fit refers to the congruence of a child's temperament with the expectations, demands, and opportunities of the social environment, including those of parents, family, and day care or school setting (see Table 19-2 for information about temperament types).

Temperament as a Risk Factor

Difficult temperaments are often associated with behavior disorders, although temperament alone is not a risk factor for maladjustment. Rather, temperament exerts an influence on children's psychosocial adjustment by affecting caretaker-child interactions. Difficult temperamental features tend to engender parental criticism and irritability, power struggles, and restrictive parenting. Critical mediators of the role of temperament in the development of behavioral disorders include parental psychological functioning, marital adjustment, childrearing attitudes and practices, and social support factors. Although temperament is unrelated to intelligence quotient (IQ), it affects academic outcomes, and some children are clearly disadvantaged by their more difficult temperaments in the majority of school environments.

Temperament Management

The goal for the PCP is to help caregivers achieve goodness-of-fit for their children. Specific strategies for intervening with temperament issues have been developed for parents (see Table 19-2). It is important for those who care for children (e.g., parents, teachers, and other caregivers) to:

- Recognize the child's innate behavioral qualities as temperament expressions. This can be facilitated by interviewing about child responses (e.g., changes in activities, new situations, changes in routines, new people) or by completing a standard temperament questionnaire.
- Understand how temperament relates to behavior and is not amenable to change. Allow parents to express their feelings about their child or their child's behavior and assist them to reframe their assessment more positively. Members of the extended family who advise parents may need to be included to help alleviate parental feelings of failure.
- Develop temperament-based management strategies, especially ways to deal with the more challenging temperaments. Such strategies can be applied to new situations as the child develops and becomes more autonomous, including those that occur in toddlerhood and preschool, such as mealtime and bedtime, or during school-related activities, such as doing homework.

Assessment and Management of Mental Health Disorders

A mental health disorder is a sustained behavior change that results in functional impairment. Because mental health

TABLE 19-2 Strategies to Help Parenting of Children with Different Temperaments

Temperament Characteristic	Strategy
Activity	Recognize the child's activity level and plan high-energy activities (such as long walks, family outings) with naps and the child's energy levels in mind. Plan for activities to keep high-energy children busy in situations when quiet is required (such as during religious services).
Rhythmicity	Keep the child's normal sleep, wake, and feeding schedule in mind when planning activities and outings. Avoid activities during "normal" naptimes. Use normal elimination patterns as a guide during toilet training.
Approach or withdrawal	Teach young children skills to deal with discomfort felt while meeting new people or having new experiences. Provide opportunities for children with approach/withdrawal problems to experience new situations and to meet new people in a supporting and loving environment. Recognize that new situations may be stressful.
Adaptability	Teach young children how to deal with disappointment. Provide reassurance when things don't go as planned.
Threshold of response	Recognize that not all children require the same amount of stimulation for calming. Adapt redirection strategies to the child's personal response threshold. Modify approaches to the situation (i.e., serious situations require a more firm approach when the child is in danger) and use care to not overrespond to more mild situations (e.g., when juice spills or things break).
Intensity of reaction	Help children to recognize their responses to positive and negative emotions. When an overresponse occurs, teach children how to modify their behavioral response to their feelings. Do not avoid situations in which frustrations may occur; part of developing emotional maturity is experiential.
Quality of mood	Use positive reinforcement for good mood responses to situations. Ignore negative mood responses.
Distractibility and attention span/persistence	Take a child's development and distractibility into consideration when doing tasks that require concentration (i.e., homework, quiet time). Teach the child strategies to help stay on track. Help parents set realistic expectations of the child's attention span.

problems cover a broad range of behavioral, emotional, and psychological disorders, many of which include genetic influences, the accurate identification of emotional, social, behavioral, and mental health status requires a thorough history and a physical examination. The physical examination detects underlying physical conditions that can result in behavioral or emotional changes. PCPs must recognize that common illness symptoms, such as fever, can change a child's behavior because of malaise, arthralgias, pain, or other physical symptoms. A series of laboratory, developmental, and psychological tests may also be required. Suggested areas to explore with relation to a child's stress and coping or mental health problems are reviewed in the following sections.

Assessment

Approaches to Children of Different Ages

During all health visits, the PCP should assess the quality of the verbal and nonverbal exchanges between infants, children, and adolescents and their parents and the health care provider. Specific attention should be paid to the child's emotions and energy, and the presence or absence of interaction among those present in the examination room.

The manner in which the provider conducts the history and physical examination is as important as the information obtained. Many caregivers and adolescents share their concerns only after a long period of trying to solve the problem themselves. They may be upset, worried, or frustrated. Many people are reluctant to discuss symptoms because of social stigmas against mental illness.

Providers are more likely to get a clear picture of what is happening and gain the family's trust if they take the time to sit down and actively listen at length to both the caregiver's and child's concerns and perceptions. It is critical to avoid rapidly firing questions, restricting the history to only using a preprinted schedule of questions (even though validated screening tools provide critical information), or taking notes that detract from giving full attention to the child and family. Sufficient time should be scheduled for the history and physical. If a potentially significant but nonemergent problem is uncovered in the course of an episodic visit, a lengthier appointment should be scheduled to avoid hurrying the assessment and potentially missing important data. It is essential to obtain information from the child's perspective and to use age-appropriate strategies.

Infants

Observations of babies and toddlers with their caregivers in structured and unstructured situations offer valuable clues to the strengths and limitations of each partner in the interaction. Even unstructured observations allow the observer to appreciate the emotional exchanges and the presence or absence of sensitive and contingent interactions between the infant and caregiver.

Toddlers and Young Preschoolers

Playing with figures, dolls, and toys gives older toddlers and young preschoolers a way to spontaneously express their feelings and emotions. It provides the opportunity for the professional to ask questions within the nonthreatening context of play. Play also helps evaluate the history provided by caregivers. If the caregiver identifies situations or people who provoke troubled behavior, the provider may select toys that are likely to elicit the child's story in play. For example, if the concerning behaviors began shortly after the birth of a new sibling, a baby doll, mother and father dolls, and a doll the child's age and gender could be selected.

School-Age Children

Older preschoolers and young school-age children can be assessed by offering them the opportunity to draw a picture of themselves and their family and asking them to tell a story about their picture. This allows the professional the opportunity to evaluate the child's feelings and emotions and, if problems and concerns become apparent, clarify details from the child's perspective in a nonthreatening and familiar way.

Adolescents

The PCP should interview the school-age child and adolescent separately from their caregivers. It often takes school agers 20 to 30 minutes and adolescents 30 minutes or more to share their perspectives and feelings. If mental health issues are uncovered during a brief (15 or 20 minute) visit, follow-up visits can be scheduled to allow sufficient time to explore their thoughts and concerns. Most children are comfortable talking about their feelings and experiences if they have a supportive listener. It is important to clarify issues related to confidentiality with both the adolescent and caregiver prior to initiating a mental health assessment. Tailor questions to the child's or adolescent's level of understanding, keeping questions simple and providing examples to younger children. Sample questions include:

- "Tell me about some of the things you do very well. What types of things do you have a hard time doing?"
- "You look very sad to me. Is there something that is making you sad?"
- "Many children have things they worry about. What worries you most?"
- "How are things going in your family?"
- "How is school going?"
- "How are your relationships with other people? Do you feel like other people understand you and see you for who you really are?"
- "Everyone feels angry at times. What makes you angry? What do you do when you are angry?"
- "If you could change one thing in your life, what would it be?"
- "Tell me what you think the problem is from your point of view."

History

Correctly pinpointing stress/coping issues and mental health disorders requires a more thorough history than does the diagnosis of many physical health problems. Following the comprehensive health history model found in Box 2-2 will be helpful because daily living (functional health), disease, developmental, and family domains must all be addressed.

The Symptom Analysis: Behavioral Manifestations

Caregivers are keen observers of their children, so it is wise to listen carefully to their observations and concerns. Behaviors that concern a caregiver may include those that are developmentally normal for the child, they may be abnormal, or they may represent extremes of the range of normal behavior. By obtaining a clear idea of the caregiver's concerns, the PCPs assess the parent's knowledge level about child development and behavior, clarify which behaviors are developmentally normal (but distressing to the caregiver), and confirm which behaviors fall outside the range of normal. Eliciting information from teachers and other caregivers reinforces caregiver reports and provides a contextual understanding of child behavior.

Family Domain: Common Family-Related Stressors

Common stressors that should be identified through the history are discussed in this section. Questions and specific examples of stressors are found in Table 19-3.

Recent Changes. It is helpful to specifically ask about recent changes in the family, work, school, and other settings because caregivers may not perceive some changes as sources of stress for their child. For example, a caregiver may welcome a job promotion that includes the need for travel and a significant pay increase. However, this same change may stress the child who is old enough to worry about how life will change with a traveling parent. Most recognize that the addition of a new family member is life changing for children already in the home, but other family changes like having a grandparent move in or an older sibling move out can be equally stressful. It is important to consider the developmental context of events and whether most children of a similar age would find the incident threatening or upsetting.

TABLE 19-3 History Taking: Areas for Assessment of Mental Health

Topic	Sample Questions	Potential Stressors
Behavioral manifestations: Symptom analysis	Describe your child's behavior. What seems to make it better or worse? How have you tried to help your child? How does the behavior make you feel? How do think your child feels?	Unrealistic parental expectations for child behavior Increasing frequency or severity of behavior Unpredictable situational context that elicits or maintains problem behavior (setting, timing, who is present, triggers) Behavior negatively affects relationships or child functioning Negative peer and/or teacher responses to and consequences of problem behavior Parents' feelings hurt by the behavior Parents unable to empathize with how the child feels Parents unsure about what the parent needs and what the child needs to improve the situation
Recent changes	What events or changes have occurred in your family in the past year?	
Contextual changes within the family	Who lives in your home? Have there been any recent changes at home or changes in family relationships?	Changes in household composition (e.g., births, expansion of household to include elders) Risk of loss or loss of attachment figure(s) Changes in family relationships (e.g., death, separation, divorce, older sibling moving away) Separation from the parent for foster care or care by others Return to the biologic family from kinship care or foster care Family violence Witness to trauma or violence New role or responsibilities presenting a psychological challenge (e.g., birth of a sibling) Sibling with special health care needs Mental health problems of parents, especially maternal depression Child's chronic illness or handicap
Recurring experiences	Tell me about the things you find difficult or stressful as a parent, especially in caring for this child.	Parental overprotection or neglect Restrictive or over permissive parenting Control struggles Ineffective conflict resolution Lack of effective parental supervision Parental failure to protect child in risky situations Ineffective limit-setting strategies Use of harsh discipline practices Parental mental or physical illness Reliance on the child by the parents for emotional comfort and support
Parents' personal history of being parented	Tell me about your most favorite and least favorite memories of growing up. How is your parenting similar to and different from the parenting you received as a child? What are your expectations for your child?	Parent abused or neglected as a child or exposed to violence or trauma as a child Parent adopted or in foster care as a child Unhappy parent childhood, poor role models Poor family communication patterns in family of origin Any indicators of parental psychopathologic condition, particularly maternal depression The parents' perception of the child, especially temperament, poor fit with parent The parents' knowledge and beliefs about harsh discipline or coercive parent-child interactions The parents' knowledge and beliefs about the development of autonomy and self-esteem, especially in relation to parenting strategies (e.g., praise and affection) and conflict resolution Parental strategies to facilitate the child's coping, given developmental level and temperament Unrealistic academic, athletic, or social expectations of the child

Contextual Changes in the Family. Contextual changes are more enduring changes in life circumstances, either for better or worse, which provoke changes in the child's perception of self, family, or feelings of relationship security. Examples include caregiver separation or remarriage, moving, and the birth of a sibling. These changes may result in self-blame or may create a sense of betrayal, because they stem from the actions of other family members, especially parents.

Parent Stress and Mental Illness. All caregivers face stress and feelings of being overwhelmed. It is important to assist caregivers to identify situations in which they know the risk of stress is greatest. For example, certain developmental stages are commonly more taxing than others, and many young children have increasing behavioral problems in the late afternoon hours as fatigue increases and energy levels lag. Anticipatory guidance provides interventions to help caregivers predict and minimize these "at-risk" times. Those with mental illness are at risk for increased role strain and parenting difficulties because of how their condition affects their perceptions and coping skills.

Impaired Parenting. Impaired parenting occurs when there is a mismatch between caregiving behaviors and a child's developmental or situational needs. This may result in inappropriate stimulation, inconsistent care, inappropriate supervision, developmentally inappropriate behavioral expectations, harsh words, child abuse or neglect, or child rejection. Parenting assessment includes exploring the influences that impact why caregivers parent the way they do. Caregivers face a tremendous challenge to adapt their parenting skills to the individual development and behavior of each child in their family. This may be evidenced by verbalization of dissatisfaction with their role, exacerbation of tensions between the parent and child, or inappropriate communication with the child. Child behaviors that may indicate impaired parenting include acting-out, developmental regression, and other aberrant behaviors.

Parents' Personal History of Being Parented. A significant body of research confirms the effect of the caregivers' personal history of being parented on the quality of parenting provided to children and indicates that those who had poor parenting as a child are more likely to have children who develop mental illness (Mahedy et al, 2014). Caregivers' recollections of how they were parented are powerful influences on their perceptions of child behavior, beliefs about children and childrearing, and ultimately the parenting behaviors used in the home. It is important to have the caregivers share memories, good and bad, of their childhood and what they liked and disliked about the parenting they experienced (see Table 19-3).

Family Health History. A thorough history of mental and developmental disorders in family members should be conducted and include school failure, delinquency, substance abuse, learning disorders, reading problems, mood disorders, personality disorders, schizophrenia, attention-deficit/hyperactivity disorder (ADD), autism, genetic syndromes, and birth defects.

Disease Domain

Prenatal and Birth History. History should include whether the pregnancy was planned and/or desired; maternal illness, exposures to toxins, substance use or stress during pregnancy; complications during labor or delivery; infant's postnatal course (including prematurity, illness, difficulty feeding, excessive irritability or lethargy); parent and family history of mental health problems; results of newborn screening; signs of genetic disorders; childhood illnesses and traumatic injuries, especially neurologic injuries and soft neurologic signs; and evidence of developmental delay.

Developmental Domain: Developmental Progress and Daily Living Domain

Achievement of milestones, level of social skills, relationships with peers, emotional maturity (e.g., ability to deal with the full spectrum of emotions), and school progression and issues should all be explored. All areas of the daily living domain need to be explored because behavior may affect all areas of daily life—nutrition, elimination, sleep, activities, relationships with others, communication patterns, sense of self, cognitive perceptual behaviors, and so on.

Physical Examination

The practitioner should complete a thorough physical examination with particular attention to recognition of physical anomalies, neurologic system evaluation, and evaluation of affect, cognition, and mental status.

Diagnostic Studies

Pertinent laboratory tests (hemoglobin, anti-streptolysin O [ASO] titer, blood lead level, serum electrolytes, drug tests for alcohol or illicit substances, or urinalysis) can rule out physical health problems with behavioral manifestations. The family history and findings on the physical examination may warrant genetic studies. Imaging of the central nervous system may be recommended, depending on family history, developmental, and neurologic findings.

Behavioral/Developmental Screening and Assessment Tools

A structured developmental screening or assessment is critical to the diagnosis of behavioral and/or mental health issues. If warranted by suspicious or ambiguous findings, a referral for a thorough developmental evaluation by a skilled psychologist or multidisciplinary developmental assessment team is appropriate. Behavioral rating scales or checklists are valuable screening tools, especially those with established reliability and validity that provide norms as a basis for comparison. See Chapters 5 through 8 for a listing of age-appropriate developmental screens with sound reliability and validity. The Achenbach Child Behavior Checklist is an excellent behavioral screen with established reliability and validity and has been used successfully with a wide variety of clinical populations. Available in English and

Spanish, it provides separate checklists for assessment of children 18 months to 5 years old and 6 to 18 years old, with norms provided by age and gender, and separate report forms for parents and teachers. Other checklists with clinical utility include the Pediatric Symptom Checklist (PSC) for children at least 11 years old. Even if children's scores do not reach a clinical level by normative standards, attention must be paid to notably high scores, stable problem behavior, and attending circumstances.

Maternal PPD can negatively affect infant development, so routine screening for symptoms of PPD is merited during episodic health visits in early infancy (Hagan et al, 2008). Further discussion of PPD screening is found in Chapter 5.

Temperament assessment can be useful for infants, toddlers, preschoolers, and school-age children. Caregiver reports of temperament reflect the caregivers' perception and may not accurately reflect objective reality. However, accurate or not, the caregivers' perceptions influence their behavior and feelings toward the child and must be taken seriously.

A behavioral diary or log kept by caregivers, by the school-age child or adolescent, and by the teacher informs the practitioner and family about the situational context for and severity of the behavior. Often this monitoring process itself serves as an effective intervention.

Making Mental Health and Behavioral Diagnoses

Making mental health diagnoses is often difficult. One must decide whether behaviors are within normal limits for age, temperament, family, health, and other factors. Comorbidities are common. In practice, several things may need to be addressed: the behavior, the family effects, nutrition, sleep, and other interrelated issues. In many cases, a mental health specialist such as a clinical psychologist or psychiatrist may be required to assist in diagnostic decision-making.

Management Strategies

After the diagnostic list is made, the PCP needs to decide how to manage and/or co-manage problems with other pediatric specialists. Pediatric PCPs manage more mental health problems than ever before, largely because of the scarcity of mental health services or inadequate insurance coverage that makes mental health care out of reach for many families. However, many PCPs lack adequate education to manage complex problems. In addition, it is financially difficult for many busy primary care practices to offer the extended appointments needed for high-quality mental health care, and mental health service reimbursement is different than that provided for medical care.

As a rule, if the cause of the problem is a life event with acute, short-term consequences (such as, the death of a pet or a friend moving away) or a common developmentally normal but troublesome behavior (e.g., temper tantrums or sibling rivalry), it can be managed in the primary care setting. More enduring problems, such as loss of a parent or major depression, require collaboration or consultation with or referral to a pediatric mental health specialist.

Appropriate care of pediatric mental illness always requires an interdisciplinary approach. Pharmacotherapy alone is never appropriate, nor should it be used without a thorough mental health evaluation. Clinical practice guidelines further emphasize the need for treatments to be evidence-based and inclusive of short- and long-term follow-up plans. All ethical issues regarding consent and assent are especially important in mental health care. Caregivers and patients should be aware of treatment risks, benefits, and alternative options.

Common Mental Health Problems

Special Problems of Infancy and Early Childhood

For many years, it was believed that infants and young children could not have mental health problems. It was as though pediatric health care providers believed that young children were protected from even the most adverse experiences. Research clearly demonstrates that this is not the case. Regulation disorders of sensory processing are discussed in Chapter 20.

The Shy Child

Shyness is a pattern of social inhibition with unfamiliar people, with novel objects, or in unfamiliar situations. Shy children are slower to approach peers or initiate play with an unfamiliar child and often spend more time observing the situation and other children in play before engaging. Infants show inborn bias to respond to unfamiliar events with anxiety, distress, or disorganization and retreat and withdrawal from social stimulation. In toddlerhood, inhibition persists, evidenced by irritability, withdrawal, and clinging to the caregiver in new situations. Many toddlers are shy, but this diminishes normally by school age. School-age shy children continue to make fewer social approaches. Shyness is caused by a temperamental disposition toward withdrawal that is linked to family factors and is common. Behavioral inhibition in social situations may be adaptive if handled effectively by the caregiver and can indicate optimal self-regulation and conscience development. Viewed by their peers as likable but shy, these children may be neglected by their peers. Although most shy children do not develop later internalizing disorders, extremely shy toddlers may be at risk for social withdrawal in later childhood and for developing an anxiety disorder in adolescence.

Differential Diagnosis

Children with social withdrawal rather than shyness have a lower rate of social interaction overall and do not warm up to social situations.

Management

Parenting strategies that provide warmth, sensitivity, and responsiveness to the child's inhibition and shyness foster security in attachment relationships and facilitate social competence. In preschool and school-age children, insensitivity and a lack of responsiveness foster a sense of insecurity and predict social withdrawal and associated internalizing disorders, including depression and adolescent anxiety. It is helpful to have caregivers prepare shy children for new situations by visiting new settings, identifying a sensitive adult to whom they may turn with requests or concerns, and negotiating for them to be allowed to watch and observe before engaging in play or other activities.

Bereavement

Grief is a feeling of distress, sorrow, and loss, whereas *bereavement* is the process of dealing with loss. Many people use grief and bereavement terms interchangeably. *Mourning* is the psychological process set in motion by loss of a loved one. The death of someone important to a child is considered one of the most stressful events to be experienced. For children and adolescents, death of a parent or sibling is the most disturbing loss.

The clinical picture of bereavement and grief depends, to some extent, on the concept of death. In infancy and toddlerhood, death is perceived as separation or abandonment, with no real cognitive understanding of death or the emotional resources to deal with loss. The central issue is the sense of loss or abandonment that can be due to temporary causes (e.g., caregiver travel, sibling hospitalization, natural disaster), long-term causes (e.g., caregiver separation, foster care placement), or permanent (e.g., death). Loss of a family member is particularly difficult because it results in the loss of the love and support from that person, significant effect on family functioning and resources, and changes in routines. Preschoolers and those younger than 6 years old tend to perceive death as a continuation of life under different circumstances. Death is personified and perceived as a punishment. From 6 to 11 years old, children grasp the irreversibility and finality of death although they struggle with understanding the specific loss of the loved one. Preadolescents and adolescents are able to be more abstract and philosophical about death. At any given developmental stage, a child can resolve the effect of the death only at that developmental level. Thus bereavement resurfaces, and the significance of the loss needs to be reworked at each subsequent developmental stage. It is expected that most children and adolescents experience at least one significant loss before they reach adulthood. It is estimated that 5% of children lose one or both parents to death before 15 years old.

Clinical Findings

Infants and toddlers cry out or search for the absent caregiver, refuse the attempts of others to soothe them, withdraw emotionally, appear sad, and no longer engage in age-appropriate activities. Sleep and feeding are disturbed; they display developmental regression and demonstrate extreme reactions to reminders of the missing caregiver through apathy, anger, or crying.

For the preschool and older child, grief is a process that unfolds over time. Initially children may seem emotionally unmoved, but the initial shock and denial give way to depressive symptoms that can last for weeks or months. A normal reaction to loss, depressive symptoms include sadness, feeling depressed, vomiting, bed-wetting, poor appetite, weight loss, insomnia, crying, internalizing symptoms (e.g., headache and stomachache), anxiety, guilt, and idealization of the person who died. Rage is a common reaction to the death of a parent, typically directed at the surviving parent and others in the immediate family. Angry behavior may also be directed at peers, compounding a sense of inferiority and alienation. Fears of dying, disease, and growing old are often stimulated. Identification with the deceased is common and needs to be assessed to determine whether this furthers or inhibits development. Similarly, a fantasy connection to a dead parent can develop and may be helpful. Guilt and responsibility are typical issues for children but are less problematic for adolescents. Adolescents often manifest a sudden "maturity" along with numbness, regrets, disorganization, and despair before closure and reorganization are achieved. It is not unusual for adolescents to develop stronger ties with friends and to distance from family while grieving.

Differential Diagnosis

Children at high risk for pathologic bereavement or depression generally have a previous history of individual and family problems. Symptoms of bereavement that should concern the provider and merit immediate referral to a mental health specialist include the following:

- Long-term denial and avoidance of feelings
- Suicidal wishes and preoccupation with death
- Distressing guilt about actions taken or not taken
- Preoccupation with worthlessness
- Persistent anger
- Decline in school performance
- Social withdrawal
- Persistent sleep problems
- Hallucinations beyond transitory experience of hearing the voice of, or seeing the image of, the deceased

Management

Caregiver education facilitates effective bereavement management in children and adolescents. Many question whether children and adolescents should attend the funeral or memorial service. Children need to participate in the rituals around death as much as they choose. Such services and rituals provide even young children with an important way to grieve, especially if such involvement is supportive, appropriately explained, and congruent with the family's values.

Children need caregiver help to understand the facts of death and to correct misunderstandings as they develop;

however, children cannot understand beyond their cognitive level. Caregivers often need to be reassured that showing their own feelings (e.g., disbelief, guilt, sadness, and anger) is normal and helpful to children; sharing feelings about and memories of the family member who died is helpful as well. Sensitivity to the child's reactions of grief and restlessness is important, as is support for the child's assimilation and mastery of the loss and emotional experience. Children need to express and work through feelings and fantasies related to the loss; communication is a must.

There are many books about death, loss, and grieving for children and adolescents that are geared to the various developmental levels. It is critical for children to have an attachment to an adult who can be an effective source of support and involvement, as well as a focus for reactions to loss. The child must be sensitively prepared for any changes occurring at the same time as the death, with the family advised to minimize these as much as possible. Any parental loss before 5 years old probably warrants treatment. Because bereavement resurfaces at subsequent developmental phases, early parental loss should be determined and current symptoms assessed as a possible manifestation of recurring bereavement issues.

Fears, Phobias, and Anxieties

Fears and Phobias

Fear is the occurrence of various avoidance responses to particular stimuli; it is a state of apprehension in response to a threatening situation. In contrast, a phobia is a persistent, extreme, and irrational fear triggered by the presence or anticipation of the presence of a specific person, object, or situation. The onset of fears occurs normally during late infancy and early toddlerhood and manifests as separation anxiety and stranger anxiety.

Childhood fears are a normal part of development. Fears have a developmental function, and predominant fears vary with age. Specific phobias occur in about 5% of the population and in 15% of children referred for anxiety-related problems. Phobias are determined by multiple factors including genetic influences, temperament, parental mental health problems, and individual conditioning histories.

Clinical Findings

Infants typically react fearfully to loss of physical support, heights, and unexpected stimuli. Toddlers experience separation anxiety and fear physical injury and strangers. Preschoolers fear imaginary creatures, animals, darkness, and being alone; they also demonstrate some persistent separation anxiety. Fear of animals and darkness extends into school age, but safety, natural events, and school- and health-related fears dominate. In preadolescence and adolescence, fears of bodily injury, economic and political catastrophes, and social fears are central. Fear and phobic reactions typically involve symptoms of autonomic arousal. The symptoms of autonomic arousal in those with phobias may evolve into panic attacks or phobic-avoidant reactions.

Differential Diagnosis

Distinction must be made between abnormal fears and normal developmental fears. Clinical phobias are defined on the basis of persistence, magnitude, and maladaptiveness.

Management

Most fears are short-lived, are not serious, and do not predict adult mental health problems. Parents must be cautioned against using fears as a form of behavioral control (e.g., threats of abandonment with toddlers or threatening a school-age child with an immunization) or as a discipline strategy (e.g., leaving a preschooler alone in a dark room). When the fear negatively affects the child's functioning, developmental progress, learning experiences, and level of comfort, referral is necessary. Treatment for fearful and phobic infants, toddlers, and preschoolers focuses on improving caregiver mental health, caregiver–child behavior management skills, and caregiver role satisfaction and self-efficacy. Various management strategies are available for treatment of phobias in children older than 5 years, including contingency management, cognitive-behavioral therapy (CBT), and family interventions. Contingency management is a therapeutic approach based on the idea that behavior is predictable in certain situations and that, in these situations, caregiving approaches can be planned using a combination of positive reinforcement of desired behaviors, noncontingent reinforcement where rewards (e.g., hugs, attention, and praise) are given regardless of child behavior, extinction where behavior results in no response, and discipline.

Anxiety

Anxiety is a diffuse apprehension in response to less specific stimuli; fear stimuli are more specific. It is a normal developmental phenomenon that is experienced by every person at some point. Anxious responses include somatic symptoms mediated by the autonomic system. These responses include physiologic changes, such as increased heart rate and blood pressure, tremor, sweating, and enhanced vigilance and reactivity. Anxiety that persists at high levels and causes maladaptive behavior warrants diagnosis and treatment. Anxiety disorders include conditions associated with childhood, like separation anxiety, and those also associated with adulthood like GAD, OCD, and posttraumatic stress disorder (PTSD). Children diagnosed with anxiety disorders tend to have multiple problems, are impaired in important areas of social functioning, and live with parents who experience symptoms of anxiety or mood disorders. Anxiety disorders typically first appear in the preschool years. The earlier the onset of these disorders, the greater the impairment in social and personal development, thus leading to a much greater likelihood of poor subjective views of their personal mental and physical health, social relationships, career satisfaction, and home and family relationships (Kessler et al, 2010).

Risk factors include: (1) genetics, (2) temperamental disposition for behavioral inhibition and/or shyness, and

(3) social environment or life circumstances (e.g., parental distress or dysfunction or trauma), especially during vulnerable developmental periods (e.g., attachment or separation-individuation) (Rapee et al, 2010). Youngsters with anxiety disorders are at high risk for subsequent anxiety disorders, comorbid mood disorders, and adolescent substance abuse. Anxiety disorders distinctly cluster in families.

Separation Anxiety Disorder

The essential feature of separation anxiety disorder is an abnormal reaction to real, impending, or imagined separation from major attachment figures, home, or familiar surroundings. Separation anxiety is a normal developmental phenomenon from about 7 months old through the preschool years. Some infants and toddlers experience excessive levels of distress with separation from their major caregiver, and they cry persistently and cannot be comforted or refuse to be cared for and comforted by a competent, substitute caregiver. Alternatively, older infants, toddlers, and preschoolers may act aggressively toward the substitute caregiver or intentionally injure themselves.

Separation anxiety disorder, in which reactivity to separation interferes with daily activities and developmental tasks, manifests from 5 to 16 years old; the mean age for clinical presentation is 9 years old. Separation anxiety disorder is a risk factor for the future development of panic disorder and depression in adolescence or adulthood (Sarvet and Brewer, 2011).

Separation anxiety disorder evolves from a poor attachment relationship or the interaction among physiologic, cognitive, and overt behavioral factors in response to life events that threaten safety or primary relationships, or both. It is probably the most common anxiety disorder from older infancy through the school-age years and the most common mental health reason for referral affecting 4% to 5% of children (Sarvet and Brewer, 2011). Among infants and young children, only about 10% of those affected by separation anxiety are referred for care despite the concerns of the majority of parents. Older children are usually brought to the health care provider when the disorder results in school refusal or somatic symptoms. A significant number of children with school refusal have separation anxiety disorder, and many of these have comorbid depression. Sleep problems and impaired social interactions are also common for children with separation anxiety disorder (Brewer and Sarvet, 2011).

Clinical Findings

The following are found in separation anxiety disorder:

- Developmentally inappropriate or excessive anxiety about separations
- Unrealistic worry about harm to self or attachment figures or about abandonment during periods of separation
- Reluctance to sleep alone or sleep away from home
- Persistent avoidance of being alone
- Nightmares about separation
- Physical complaints and signs of distress in anticipation of separation
- Social withdrawal during separations
- Environmental stress, parental dysfunction, and maternal depression are risk factors for separation anxiety disorder, especially with panic disorder or agoraphobia

The Spielberger State-Trait Anxiety Inventory for Children (STAIC) is a 20-item, self-report scale useful with children 9 to 12 years old; it can also be used with high reading–skill younger children and low reading–skill adolescents. The Screen for Child Anxiety Related Disorders (SCARED) is a 41-item self-report scale in the public domain for use in 8- to 18-year-olds.

Differential Diagnosis

Anxiety disorder not associated with separation is a differential diagnosis. Anxiety may occur as a response to trauma or as a manifestation of PTSD. It is essential to identify cues that a traumatic experience or situation (e.g., sexual or physical abuse) is the source of the anxiety symptoms. Depression and ADD are also common comorbidities. Common comorbidities with separation anxiety include social phobia and overanxious disorder. Problems at home can cause or exacerbate school refusal. For instance, a child may want to stay at home if the child worries about the caregiver's safety when she is alone.

Management

Anxiety disorder is best treated as a family system or relationship-based problem. Symptom relief is the first priority in school-age children. Identifying and treating the sources of the problem is the first line of treatment for infants through preschoolers and a secondary focus of treatment for school-age children. Note the role of attachment figures, and refer the child to a child therapist for early intervention with psychoeducational, behavioral, and cognitive-behavioral interventions as the best management approaches. Eighty percent to 90% of children respond to a combination of psychoeducation and parental education/training. PCPs can help children identify their anxious feelings and physical responses to their anxiety. Caregivers benefit from learning how to help their children identify feelings of anxiety and by supporting them during exacerbations. Pharmacotherapy is not particularly helpful in reducing symptoms and should only be used if the child fails to respond to nonpharmacologic intervention and has considerable impairment in function, thus meriting referral to a psychiatrist (Brewer and Sarvet, 2011).

Generalized Anxiety Disorder

GAD is cognitive and obsessive in nature. The child experiences excessive anxiety, worry, and apprehensive expectations generalized to a number of events or activities. These anxieties do not focus on a specific person, object, or situation, nor are they the result of a recent stressor. Children with GAD are characterized as "worriers." The exact onset is not known, but the diagnosis occurs most often among older children and adolescents 9 to 18 years old.

GAD is one of the most prevalent psychiatric disorders, affecting as many as 15% of older children and adolescents and is the second most common pediatric anxiety disorder. However, only 22% of adolescents who meet diagnostic criteria for GAD are diagnosed by PCPs (McBride, 2015). There are clear genetic influences of GAD, especially in females (Vendlinksi et al, 2014).

Clinical Findings

Major symptoms of GAD are:

- Worry about future events
- Poor-quality sleep
- Irritability and tantrums in young children
- Preoccupation with past behavior
- Overconcern about competence and marked preoccupation with performance
- Significant self-consciousness
- Restlessness, difficulty concentrating
- Somatic complaints without a physical basis
- Unexplained fatigue
- Unusual need for reassurance
- Comorbidity with other anxiety disorders, ADD, or mood disorder

Differential Diagnosis

Differential diagnoses are separation anxiety, adjustment disorder associated with a specific stressor, and ADD. It is important to attend to cues that might point to traumatic experiences or conditions as the source of anxiety symptoms and the presence of pediatric autoimmune neuropsychiatric disorders associated with streptococcal infections (PANDAS) (see Obsessive-Compulsive Disorder).

Management

The treatment of preschool children and toddlers generally focuses on behavioral and family interventions with the best response coming from interventions that incorporate cognitive behavior therapy with a caregiver component (Fig. 19-1). Preschoolers may benefit from play therapy. Refer the older child or adolescent to a pediatric mental health therapist for treatment of symptoms using relaxation techniques or cognitive-behavioral therapy (CBT) (Brewer

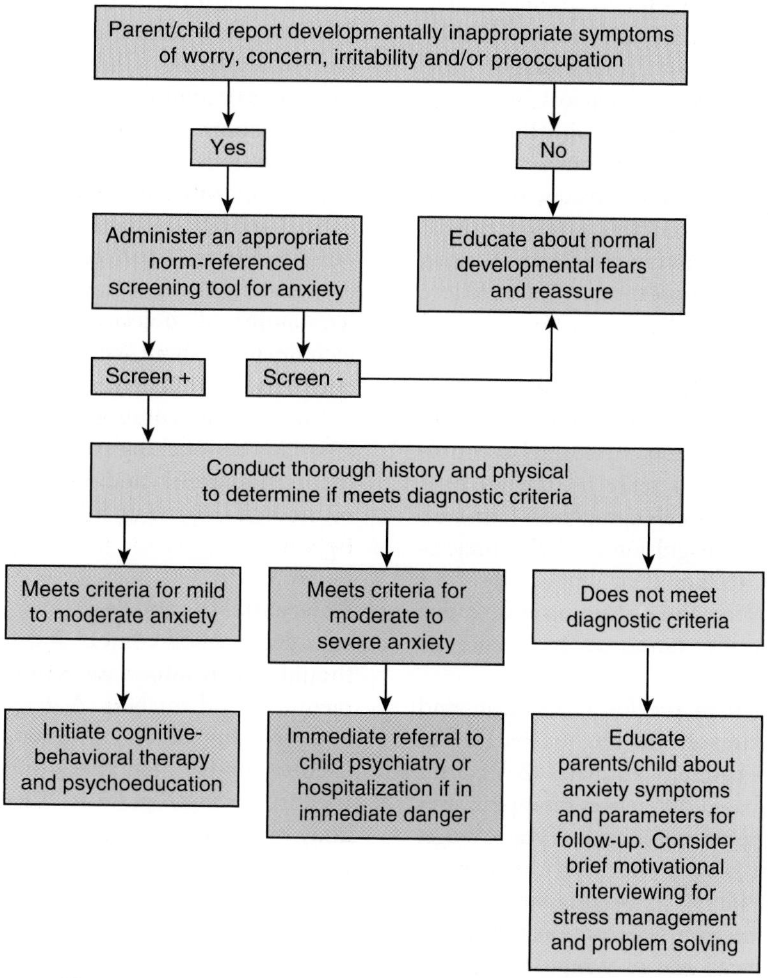

• **Figure 19-1** Primary care management of pediatric anxiety disorders.

and Sarvet, 2011). Individual and/or family counseling can be used to identify the source of anxiety. Treatment outcomes are more positive when parents are involved in interventions that target familial contextual processes. Younger school-age children seem to benefit from a combination of cognitive-behavioral strategies and family intervention (Brewer and Sarvet, 2011). Individual and group treatments or child- and family-focused treatments are equally effective, and follow-up data demonstrate that treatment gains are maintained up to several years after treatment.

Although clinicians administer selective serotonin reuptake inhibitors (SSRIs) and other psychotropic medications to children as young as 2 years old, there are no efficacy data, and long-term developmental sequelae of these treatments are unknown. Pharmacologic intervention in combination with CBT is advisable for older children and adolescents (McBride, 2015). Evidence points to the safety and efficacy of the SSRIs, especially fluvoxamine and fluoxetine, and other medications like buspirone (McBride, 2015). Benzodiazepines are not recommended because of cognitive impairment and concerns about tolerance and dependency.

Obsessive-Compulsive Disorder

Obsessions are recurrent thoughts, images, or impulses that are disturbing to the child and difficult to dislodge. They often involve a sense of risk or fear of harm to the child or family members; concerns about contamination are common. Compulsions are repetitive behaviors or mental acts that the child feels driven to perform with the aim of reducing the anxiety associated with obsessions and include behaviors such as washing (e.g., hands, objects, or body), counting, or arranging objects. Recurrent worries, rituals, and superstitious games are common in children at various stages of development; these behaviors result in mild anxiety but do not cause distress. OCD differs from normal child behavior in that it results in marked distress, is time consuming (individuals often spend a minimum of 1 hour a day engaged in the behavior), and interferes with the child's social, familial, or academic function. Abnormal compulsive behavior is distinguished by a sense of urgency or a profound discomfort until the ritual is completed. Children often deny the fear and lack recognition of the "senselessness" of the ritual and seem to hide their illness. Obsessive thoughts are intrusive, recurrent, and disturbing and, unlike anxious worries, are generally unrelated to events or situations.

OCD is more common than previously thought, and international prevalence estimates are 1% to 2% (Geller et al, 2012). OCD is more common in males (3:2) prior to adolescence, but gender-based differences disappear after puberty. OCD can be diagnosed as young as 2 years of age, especially in children with play or interests that have a compulsive or ritualistic quality (e.g., playing with objects in only one certain sequence with interruption producing intense distress), but the mean age of symptom onset is 10 years old (Brewer and Sarvet, 2011). Most adults with OCD report experiencing initial symptoms in late childhood or adolescence. Like most psychiatric conditions, OCD is a chronic disease, and if untreated can result in lifelong disease and significant loss of quality of life.

There are strong familial patterns of transmission, and the link between genetics and OCD is strong (Geller et al, 2012). A subgroup of pediatric patients with OCD and Tourette syndrome is diagnosed with pediatric autoimmune neuropsychiatric disorders associated with streptococcal infection (PANDAS), a condition believed to be the result of autoimmune responses following group A beta-hemolytic streptococci (GABHS) infection (Esposito et al, 2014; Geller et al, 2012). PANDAS diagnostic criteria include dramatic onset of OCD or tic disorder in children between 3 years old and puberty shortly following GABHS infection and symptom exacerbation. However, it is important to note that this diagnosis has been controversial since it was first established in the mid-1990s (Sarvet and Brewer, 2011). OCD is a chronic condition, and about half of all affected individuals have comorbid psychiatric conditions, typically other anxiety disorders, major depression, ADD, or substance abuse disorder (Geller et al, 2012). Disruptive behavior disorders and learning disorders are also common comorbidities.

Clinical Findings

OCD is characterized by obsessions and compulsions, as previously defined. Children may not recognize that their obsessions or compulsions are excessive or unreasonable, so determination of insight into the behaviors is important. The obsessions and compulsions are time consuming and may significantly interfere with the child's or adolescent's normal routine, academic performance, and social functioning. The most common obsession is fear of contamination that results in compulsive washing and avoidance of "contaminated" objects. Other common obsessive worries include fears about safety (their own or their parents'), exactness or symmetry, and religious sinfulness (scrupulosity). Common compulsions include repetitive counting, arranging or touching patterns, and compulsive rechecking (doors, homework, and exam items). High anxiety levels are common if they are unable to perform their obsession "until I get it right."

Differential Diagnosis

In order to assess context and severity of symptoms, PCPs should obtain information from the child, parents, family members, and teachers. A diagnosis of OCD is warranted if the content of the obsessions and compulsions is unrelated to another mental health disorder (e.g., social phobia, trichotillomania, pervasive developmental disorder, and body dysmorphic disorder). Medical conditions that mimic OCD include carbon monoxide poisoning, tumors, encephalitis, traumatic brain injury, Prader-Willi (compulsive eating), drug side effects (stimulants), and rheumatic fever. Providers should assess developmental history to determine delays and/or difficulties. School performance may be impaired, and OCD may mimic learning disorders when children have compulsions to reread or rewrite or have pathologic perfectionism. Caregivers of children with secretive rituals may bring their child to primary care with complaints of skin rashes (dermatitis, chapped hands), temper tantrums, declining school performance, or sudden food or activity aversions. Individuals with self-injurious behavior (see Chapter 8) physically harm themselves in order to decrease mental anguish; however, this disorder is distinct from the rituals of OCD.

Assessment should include symptom description and context, frequency, and effect on daily functioning. The National Institute for Health and Clinical Excellence (2005) guidelines indicate that six screening questions can be used to determine OCD pathology (Box 19-3). Children with suspected PANDAS and unclear history of recent upper respiratory tract infection should have confirmation of streptococcal infection either by throat culture or ASO titer. Clinical findings that differentiate PANDAS from classic OCD are urinary frequency, hyperactivity, impulsivity, and worsening handwriting (Bernstein et al, 2010).

Management

Decisions regarding treatment of OCD should center on the degree of child impairment. If the child's symptoms do not interfere with the child's life and do not cause undue distress, treatment can be deferred. Optimal treatment involves an individualized and developmentally appropriate approach that centers on child and family therapy to help the child learn to manage his or her anxiety and distress (Mancuso et al, 2010). CBT provides the best long-term effectiveness for OCD and is considered first-line therapy for all children and adolescents with mild to moderate OCD (Geller et al, 2012). Individuals with moderate to severe disease (e.g., causes excessive distress, leads to significant social isolation or inability to perform developmentally normal tasks, or that occurs with significant comorbid psychopathology) should receive pharmacologic management (Geller et al, 2012). SSRIs are first-line pharmacologic agents and have demonstrated effectiveness and improvement in quality of life in randomized controlled trials (Geller et al, 2012). Drug therapy results in an average of 25% decrease in symptoms severity. Evidence suggests that SSRIs (sertraline, fluoxetine, and fluvoxamine) provide the best pharmacologic effects with the greatest drug safety margin (Mancuso et al, 2010). Individuals who fail to respond to CBT, who experience increasing symptom severity during treatment, who show signs of psychosis and/or suicidality, and who fail to respond to SSRI should be referred to child psychiatry.

Research indicates that antibiotic treatment can help rapidly diminish tics in a subgroup of children with PANDAS; however, routine penicillin prophylaxis is not recommended. Individuals with severe symptoms may benefit from plasma exchange and immunoglobulin administration, but this treatment combination remains controversial (Mancuso et al, 2010).

• BOX 19-3 Quick Screening Questions for Obsessive-Compulsive Disorder

Do you wash yourself or clean more than most people?
Do you feel the need to check or double-check things often?
Do you have thoughts that bother you that you would like to get rid of but can't?
Do you find yourself spending a lot of time doing things (brushing teeth, getting dressed)?
Does it bother you when things are not lined up or are not in order?
Do these problems bother you?

Tic Disorders

Tic disorders are characterized by repetitive, fast, unconscious movements or vocalizations. Motor and verbal tics that persist for more than 1 year are called *Tourette syndrome.* All children have some repetitive habits (such as, finger sucking or hair twirling), and many of these are adaptive behaviors that help decrease stress or provide a sense of calm. Habits are considered pathologic when they have no clear purpose and result in physical or social impairment. Tic disorders cause significant anxiety for affected children and often result in impaired self-esteem, bullying, and emotional or academic problems.

Provisional (previously called *transient*) tics are fairly common and occur in up to 7% of school-age children, whereas chronic tics—those that last for more than 1 year—occur in 0.5% to 3% of the population. Half of all motor tics begin by age 7, and half of all vocal tics begin by age 9 (Murphy et al, 2013). There is some evidence that children with developmental disorders have greater risk of developing tics than their nonaffected peers. Tourette syndrome has clear genetic influences and affects approximately 0.7% of the population (Knight et al, 2012).

Clinical Findings

Motor tics can be simple (involving a single muscle group) or complex (complicated movements like jumping or a series of simple tics). Common simple tics include blinking, twitching of hands or limbs, shoulder shrugging, tongue thrusting, or squinting. Verbal tics include vocalizations or pushing air through the nose. Grunting sounds or clearing the throat are common. Obscene gestures and swearing are rare. Symptoms generally worsen during periods of stress, fatigue, or anxiety. Most children with tic disorders can suppress vocal tics when they intensely concentrate on other things like homework, games, and so on or when social pressure against verbalizations is high (Murphy et al, 2013). Other common tic disorders include trichotillomania (pulling out hair), bruxism (tooth grinding), skin pulling, and nail biting.

Differential Diagnosis

There is considerable diagnostic overlap between tic disorders, learning disorders, ADD, autism spectrum disorders, and OCD. Differential diagnoses include OCD, PANDAS, ADD, seizure disorders, central nervous system space occupying lesions, and dyskinesias.

Diagnostic Studies

There are a number of potential organic causes of new onset tic disorders, especially with disorientation and/or loss of fine motor skills (e.g., loses ability to draw figures or penmanship becomes impaired) (Murphy et al, 2013). Laboratory testing for hemoglobin, ferritin, renal function, hepatic function, thyroid function, and substance use are appropriate at the time of diagnosis (Murphy et al, 2013).

Management

Mild tics do not require treatment. Children with moderate to severe tics that disrupt their self-esteem or impair their socialization best respond to psychotherapy, specifically CBT. The focus of treatment is to extinguish the tic, to increase children's awareness of the behaviors, and to teach another behavior to engage in when they feel they are about to have a tic behavior. Best responses are often obtained with older children and adolescents. Common reminder strategies include using an elastic bandage over a digit to discourage thumb sucking, using an elastic hair band to make it difficult to grasp hair, or placing a rubber band that can be gently pulled when a child is aware of engaging in a tic behavior. Positive reinforcement is another effective extinguishing strategy. It is important to note that tics cannot be extinguished when the child is not interested in stopping the habit. For moderate to severe symptoms, common psychopharmaceuticals include SSRIs, atypical antipsychotics (e.g., risperidone), antihypertensives (e.g., clonidine), and anticonvulsants (Murphy et al, 2013). Immunoregulatory therapy (intravenous immunoglobulin, plasma exchange) and long-term antistreptococcal prophylaxis for prevention or to treat exacerbations are not recommended until more standardized diagnostic criteria and research are developed (Esposito et al, 2014).

Posttraumatic Stress Disorder

PTSD describes a characteristic set of symptoms that develops following actual or threatened exposure to a severe stressor or trauma. The trauma may result from a single event ("one sudden blow" trauma) or variable, multiple long-standing events, such as ongoing maltreatment. According to the *Diagnostic and Statistical Manual of Mental Disorders,* fifth edition (DSM-5), the criteria for PTSD include (American Psychiatric Association [APA], 2013):

- Witnessing or experiencing a traumatic event(s) that resulted in risk of death or serious injury to oneself or a loved one
- Event(s) that resulted in fear, helplessness, recurrent distress, agitation, or irritable behavior (the latter two are part of the diagnostic criteria for children younger than 6 years old)
- Symptoms that cause increased arousal, excessive startle, altered mood and emotional response, or intrusive thoughts or recurrent dreams and continued avoidance of reminders of the trauma
- Symptoms that last at least 1 month and cause significant impairment in social, cognitive, or school functioning
- Acute symptoms that last less than 3 months and chronic symptoms that last more than 3 months

Exposure to trauma is a key feature of the diagnosis of PTSD. Unfortunately, there are those who are skeptical about whether children suffer from PTSD. Parents and teachers frequently minimize traumatic effect, perhaps to relieve themselves of vicarious distress or to reassure themselves that their children have not suffered harm. Others, including mental health professionals, rationalize that children are too young to remember the trauma or too immature to be affected. However, the clinical descriptive and empirical evidence documents PTSD symptoms and other psychological difficulties experienced by children in various catastrophic situations and in situations of maltreatment.

Substantial PTSD rates are documented for children in foster care who were sexually or physically abused. This evidence leads to a better understanding of the clinical manifestations of PTSD in children. Three factors consistently influence the severity of the response: (1) severity of the trauma exposure, (2) parental distress related to the trauma, and (3) temporal proximity to the event.

Retrospective reports of adults with mental health problems indicate that PTSD is more common than previously believed. Estimates of prevalence in the United States are 4% for males and 6% for females (Cohen et al, 2010). The rate of PTSD is high among those who have been physically and sexually abused. The closer the perpetrator is in relation to the victim, the greater the trauma (e.g., PTSD is more likely when the perpetrator is a member of the immediate family as opposed to an extended family member, family friend, or stranger).

Clinical Findings

A diagnosis of PTSD requires that the child demonstrate specific behaviors following trauma, as follows (APA, 2013):

1. The child repeatedly re-experiences a set of symptoms from each of three following categories:
   - Recurrent and intrusive memories of the trauma
   - Nightmares of monsters or threats to self or others or distressing dreams about a specific event
   - Distress caused by cues that symbolize or resemble an aspect of the trauma, including physiologic reactivity
2. The child demonstrates three of the following symptoms, reflecting avoidance of stimuli associated with the traumatic event(s) and numbing of general responsiveness. These symptoms must not have been present before the trauma:
   - Avoidance of reminders of the trauma
   - Efforts to avoid thoughts, feelings, or conversations linked to the trauma
   - Amnesia for an important aspect of the trauma
   - Detachment or estrangement from others

- Emotional constriction (restricted range of affect)
- Diminished interest in or participation in usual activities
- A sense of a foreshortened future

3. Two persistent symptoms of increased arousal must be new to the child, present for at least 1 month, and cause clinically important distress or negatively affect functioning. These symptoms include the following:
   - Sleep disturbances
   - Hypervigilance
   - Difficulty concentrating
   - Exaggerated startle response
   - Agitated or disorganized behavior
   - Irritability or angry outbursts, extreme fussiness or tantrums

Among infants, toddlers, and preschoolers, symptoms must be understood within the context of the trauma itself, the child's temperament and personality, and the caregiver's ability to support the child and provide a sense of safety and protection. Table 19-4 includes a listing of PTSD symptoms by age group.

PTSD assessment in children requires careful and direct clinical interviews with the child and caregivers. If the identified traumatic event involves a caregiver as the perpetrator of child maltreatment or domestic violence, the non-offending caregiver or other caretaker should be interviewed. During assessment, do not use prompting or leading questions. Instead ask questions about whether someone has invaded the child's privacy, how it may have happened, and how the injuries came to be. Assessment should ascertain that a trauma has occurred, the nature of the trauma, and the consequent symptom pattern. Standardized assessment can include use of the Abbreviated University of California at Los Angeles PTSD Reaction Index (Cohen et al, 2010).

TABLE 19-4 Posttraumatic Stress Disorder Symptoms by Age Group

Age Group	Common Symptoms
Infancy	Feeding problems, failure to thrive, sleep problems, irritability
Preschool age	Sleep problems, nightmares, developmental regression, aggression, extreme temper tantrums, anxiety symptoms, sudden worsening of fears, irritability, avoidance symptoms
School age	Sleep problems, nightmares, developmental regression, repetitive themes in play, social withdrawal, may have partial amnesia of events, new onset anxiety or fears, panic attacks, impaired concentration, impaired school performance, avoidance symptoms or hypervigilance, somatic complaints
Adolescence	"Acting-out," nightmares, insomnia, extreme startling, social withdrawal, fears, anxiety, panic attacks, depression, anger or rage, internalizing, suicidal ideation, impaired concentration, impaired school performance, hypervigilance

Differential Diagnosis

The stressor must be of an extreme nature to warrant a diagnosis of PTSD. However, the stressor can be of any severity in an adjustment disorder (e.g., moving, starting a new school, birth of a sibling, divorce). Anxiety disorders, the most common differential diagnosis, are distinguished by not being precipitated by a traumatic event. Acute stress disorder is distinguished by the symptom pattern occurring and resolving within a 4-week period after the traumatic event. Recurrent intrusive thoughts occur in OCD but are experienced as inappropriate and are not related to an experienced trauma as they are in PTSD. Flashbacks also connect to the event and involve a feeling of reliving the event in PTSD, whereas hallucinations and other perceptual disturbances are unrelated to exposure to trauma. Comorbid conditions in preschoolers differ from those of adults and older children. Oppositional defiant disorder (ODD) is most common, followed by separation anxiety disorder and ADD. Major depressive disorder (MDD) is very unlikely.

Management

Referral to a pediatric mental health specialist is crucial and a report to social service agencies is essential for children younger than 18 years who have witnessed or experienced violence. Many child abuse intervention centers are prepared to accept referrals, assess, and direct management of children who have witnessed violence.

Beta-blockers like propranolol may be effective at decreasing somatic symptoms (e.g., racing heart rate and hyperpnea) associated with posttraumatic stress responses. Anxiety and depressive symptoms respond well to SSRIs (Cohen et al, 2010).

Crisis intervention is often necessary for the child as well as the parents. The PCP should educate parents about trauma and PTSD. Most pediatric psychiatrists use medications to treat PTSD, preferring SSRIs and alpha-adrenergic agonists. Child psychiatrists tend to prefer psychodynamic or cognitive-behavioral approaches, and nonmedical therapists tend to prefer the modalities of cognitive-behavioral, family, and nondirective play therapy. Symptom patterns persist, so consistent follow-up assessment is important. Early intervention and management are associated with the best long-term outcomes.

Mood Disorders

Depression

There are three categories of depression that occur during childhood and adolescence: (1) major depressive disorder (MDD), (2) dysthymic disorder, and (3) adjustment disorder with depressed mood. MDD is defined as either a depressed or irritable mood or a markedly diminished interest and pleasure in almost all of the usual activities, or both, for a period of at least 2 weeks. A dysthymic disorder is characterized by depressed or irritable mood for the majority of days in the past 2 years that is less intense but more chronic than major depressive episodes. Adjustment disorder with depressed mood typically occurs within 3 months after a major life stressor, involves less-severe symptoms, and is relatively mild and brief.

MDD has three subclassifications: (1) psychotic depression, (2) seasonal affective disorder, and (3) atypical depression. Children and adolescents with psychotic depression (e.g., affected individuals have hallucinations or delusions) have a greater incidence of adverse long-term outcomes, resistance to psychopharmacotherapy, and a much higher risk of developing bipolar depression. Atypical depression affects approximately 15% of children with depression and is characterized by hypersomnia, increased appetite, psychomotor retardation, and weight gain (Garzon et al, 2009). Seasonal affective disorder is most common during the fall and winter months when there is less daylight.

Depression rates increase with age. Although depression occurs in children younger than 5 years old, the true incidence is unknown given the limits of cognitive and language skills to communicate feelings. The prevalence of prepubertal depression is low (under 1%) but rises to approximately 5% for adolescents (AACAP, 2013a). Interestingly, the cumulate possibility of experiencing depression is 5% in early adolescence but rises to as high as 20% by late adolescence (Thapar et al, 2012). This rate increase for adolescents is thought to be linked to biology (e.g., sexual maturation and the influence of the sex hormones), social environment (e.g., greater social and academic expectations, greater exposure to negative events), and developmental factors (e.g., increased autonomy and abstract thinking). Vulnerability to depression involves interplay of genetic, biologic, biochemical, and psychosocial forces. Genetic factors underlie the risk for major depression, especially for earlier onset. The offspring of depressed parents are three to four times as likely to be diagnosed with depression, with a peak incidence at 15 to 20 years old (Thapar et al, 2012).

Three biologic theories of depression are used to understand the psychopharmacology of depression: (1) impaired neurotransmission, (2) endocrine dysfunction, and (3) biologic rhythm dysfunction. Given a biologic predisposition, certain life events may trigger the onset of depression. These include loss of a parent or significant other, losses that accompany a disability or injury, family dysfunction, chronic adversity, exposure to traumatic events, and physical or sexual abuse. There is a high risk of recurrent depression persisting into young adulthood. Cognitive vulnerabilities are implicated as factors related to depression. These include negative inferential styles about causes, consequences, and the self; the tendency to ruminate in response to depressed mood; low resiliency; and self-criticism (Thapar et al, 2012).

An important feature of early-onset depressive illness is the potential for the condition to switch from unipolar depression to bipolar depression. As many as one-third of preadolescent children who meet criteria for major depression develop bipolar depression (Garzon et al, 2009). Psychiatric comorbidity with depression is to be expected. The most common comorbidity with depression is an anxiety disorder (up to 70%) that occurs two or three times more often than CD. Other comorbid conditions include dysthymia, disruptive behavior disorders, eating disorders, substance abuse and/or dependence, learning disorders, stress disorders, and ADD (Thapar et al, 2012). Comorbid conditions may also occur with a variety of medical conditions, especially those with a neurologic component, such as brain injury, learning disorder, migraine headaches, and epilepsy.

Clinical Findings

Older children and adolescents with depression usually present with symptoms similar to those of adults. However, many children with depressed mood actually do not admit to feeling sad, but rather present with irritability, fluctuating mood, temper tantrums, social withdrawal, somatic complaints, agitation, separation anxiety, or behavioral problems. Males are more likely to have externalizing symptoms (e.g., aggression, acting-out, anger), and females are more likely to have internalizing symptoms (e.g., somatic complaints, feelings of sadness). Major depression symptoms represent a persistent change that occurs across settings, activities, and relationships and causes the child distress, impaired functioning, or developmental alteration. Infants and young children may present with failure to thrive, speech and motor delays, repetitive self-soothing behaviors, withdrawal from social interaction, poor attachment, and loss of developmental skills. Infants may not respond to extra efforts to soothe or engage them.

Toddlers and preschoolers may lack energy, be too eager to please others, be excessively or unusually clingy or whiney, and have developmentally inappropriate problems with separation. Preschoolers with MDD may present with sad or grouchy mood, lack of pleasure in play or activity, poor appetite and weight loss, sleep problems, low energy and activity levels, low self-esteem, or increased death or suicide play or talk.

School-age children may be irritable, angry, or hostile or have externalizing behavior, such as hyperactivity, difficulty handling aggression, or reckless behavior. Frequent absences from school, perhaps because of school phobia, or poor performance and other school problems are common. On the other hand, school-age children may have internalizing symptoms, such as boredom, lack of interest in playing with friends, social withdrawal, somatic complaints (e.g., stomachaches, headaches, muscle aches, or tiredness), eating or sleeping disturbances, enuresis, or encopresis. Some children with depression describe themselves in negative terms, whereas others, in an effort to compensate for feelings of poor self-worth, become preoccupied with attempting to please others.

Depression symptoms in adolescents include impulsivity, fatigue, hopelessness, antisocial behavior, substance use, restlessness, grouchiness, aggression, hypersexuality, and problems with family members or at school. Social withdrawal, manifested as shyness, boredom, or a lack of motivation, is common. Substance abuse is a problem for about 20% of these adolescents (Thapar et al, 2012).

Talking directly with the child or adolescent is essential because it is thought that half of depression cases are missed when only parents are interviewed. The following symptoms are common:

- Depressed mood: Sad, "blue," down, angry, bored
- Loss of interest and pleasure in usual activities
- Change in appetite or weight (loss or increase)
- Insomnia or hypersomnia
- Low energy and fatigue
- Difficulty concentrating; indecision
- Feelings of worthlessness or inappropriate or excessive guilt
- Recurrent thoughts of death or suicidal ideation

A diagnosis of MDD is made if there have been at least 2 weeks of depressed mood or loss of interest and at least four additional symptoms of depression. The symptoms cause considerable distress and impairment in social and academic functioning and cannot be caused by bereavement. Therefore, it is important to assess the following:

- Recent life events and losses
- Family history of depression or other psychiatric disorders
- Family dysfunction
- Changes in school performance
- Risk-taking behavior, including sexual activity and substance use
- Deteriorating relationships with family
- Changes in peer relations, especially social withdrawal

Mild depression causes impact in daily life, but affected individuals are still able to function and complete normal tasks although doing so requires a lot of energy because of lack of motivation. In moderate depression, what began as a decreased interest in engaging in activities becomes a complete lack of interest, and affected individuals often express concern about their inability to function and complete tasks. Severe depression is demonstrated by increased agitation, psychosis, and suicidality and will often demonstrate all the aforementioned depression symptoms. Undiagnosed and untreated/undertreated depression can be fatal. Suicide is the second leading cause of death for 14- to 24-year-olds (Centers for Disease Control and Prevention [CDC], 2013). Possible warning signs for suicide are listed in Table 19-5.

TABLE 19-5 Warning Signs for Suicide

Area of Functioning	Signs*
Changes in behavior	Accident prone or risk taking Drug and alcohol abuse Physical violence toward self, others, or animals Loss of appetite Sudden alienation from family, friends, coworkers Worsening performance at work or school Putting personal affairs in order Loss of interest in personal appearance Disposal of possessions Writing letters, notes, or poems with suicidal content; talking about suicide Buying a gun or other weapon
Changes in mood	Expressions of hopelessness or impending doom Explosive rage Dramatic swings in affect Crying spells Sleep disorders Talking about suicide
Changes in thinking	Preoccupation with death Difficulty concentrating Irrational speech Hearing voices, seeing visions Sudden interest (or loss of interest) in religion
Major life changes	Death of a family member or friend (especially by suicide) Separation or divorce Public humiliation or failure Serious illness or trauma Loss of financial security Recent relationship loss (e.g., first love)

*These signs must be interpreted in context. Many of them are common outside the realm of pre-suicidal behavior.

Depression Scales

Both patient self-report and clinician-completed rating scales are available. Table 19-6 contains a listing of these scales.

Differential Diagnosis

Some medications and certain chronic illnesses (hypothyroidism, adrenal insufficiency, epilepsy, metabolic disease, sleep disorders, hepatitis, multiple sclerosis, inflammatory bowel disease, and type 1 diabetes) predispose children and adolescents to depression. If a substance (e.g., medication, toxin, or drug of abuse) is related to the mood disturbance, a substance-induced mood disorder is diagnosed. Medications that commonly cause depressive symptoms include beta-blockers, benzodiazepines, nonsteroidal anti-inflammatory drugs (NSAIDs), stimulants, clonidine, corticosteroids, oral contraceptives, and isotretinoin. Infections, lead intoxication, anemia, eating disorders, mitral valve prolapse, premenstrual syndrome, and neurologic disorders can mimic depression in children and adolescents. In general, a physical examination and screening laboratory tests are necessary to rule out organic causes. Suggested diagnostic testing for an individual with new symptoms of

TABLE 19-6 Diagnostic Rating Scales for Depression Diagnosis

Scale	Appropriate Ages
Child Behavior Checklist (CBCL)	1.5 to 5 and 6 to 18 years old
Children's Depression Rating Scale-Revised (CDRS-R)	6 to 12 years old
Reynolds Child Depression Scale (RCDS)	6 to 12 years old
Children's Depression Inventory (CDI)	6 to 18 years old
Beck Depression Inventory (BDI)	Adolescents
Reynolds Adolescent Depression Scale (RADS)	Adolescents
Center for Epidemiologic Studies-Depression Scale (CES-D)	Adolescents
Depression Self-Rating Scale	Adolescents
Pediatric Symptom Checklist (PSC)	4 years old to adolescent
Patient Health Questionnaire-9 (PHQ-9) and PHQ-9 Modified for Teens	6 to 10 years old and 11 years old to adolescent

depression include complete blood count (CBC), pregnancy testing, Epstein-Barr titers, thyroid panel, liver function testing, urinalysis, and drug screening.

Depressive symptoms in response to a psychosocial stressor are diagnosed as adjustment disorder, which has a good short-term prognosis and does not predict later dysfunction. With separation anxiety disorder, depressive symptoms usually arise only in the context of separation and resolve quickly with reunion; however, concomitant depressive disorder is not uncommon. A depressive episode with irritable mood can be difficult to distinguish from a manic episode with irritable mood; careful evaluation of the presence of manic symptoms (e.g., excessive activity, inflated self-esteem, little need for sleep, talkativeness) is required. Many adolescents and adults who develop mania had preponderantly depressive symptoms in childhood. Family history of bipolarity is an important risk factor. Depression can be differentiated from the irritability and inattention of ADD in that children with MDD are not usually impulsive. In addition, they typically have a normal attention span before the onset of symptoms.

Management

The first goals of management are to determine suicidal risk and intervene to prevent suicide. Suicidal risk is greatest during the first 4 weeks of a depressive episode. Patients with acute suicidal intent that includes a plan, psychosis, risk of abuse, and unstable behavior require immediate psychiatric evaluation. Cumulative suicidal risks—prior suicidal behavior or attempts, depression, and alcohol, tobacco or drug abuse/dependence—require psychiatric intervention as well, and immediate referral must be made. Attention must also be paid to establish a safe environment (e.g., removal of firearms, knives, and lethal medications, including tricyclic antidepressants [TCAs]). Families of adolescents with depression may be noncompliant with recommendations to remove guns from the home in spite of compliance with other aspects of treatment. Vigilant follow-up in this regard is crucial. Other management strategies by the PCP include referral to community resources, such as hotlines, and commitment to a no-suicide agreement by which the adolescent agrees to refrain from harming himself or herself and promises to notify the caretaker or health care professional if suicidal ideation returns. It is important to note that suicidal ideation often increases during the treatment phase known as *emergence.* Emergence occurs in the first week to month of treatment when the patient's energy levels increase, but feelings of hopelessness and helplessness have not yet receded.

A major depressive episode requires intervention by a mental health specialist. Unfortunately only about half of all individuals with depression achieve full remission of their symptoms. Therapies typically include CBT in a group or individual psychotherapy format. Group CBT may help adolescents. Often, family therapy or psychoeducation is indicated. See Figure 19-2 for primary care management of pediatric depression.

A central issue in psychopharmacologic approaches is that children and adolescents are not usually included in clinical drug trial research, and safety and efficacy data from the literature about adults are often extrapolated to children. Available studies do not support the efficacy of TCAs for depression in young children, and they may actually be harmful. Although the 2004 "black box" warning for SSRIs occurred because of concerns of increased suicidality with use of these medications, randomized controlled trials of pediatric depression consistently demonstrate that best treatment responses come from combinations of CBT and SSRIs (Garzon et al, 2009). CBT appears to have a protective effect against suicide. Currently, fluoxetine and escitalopram are the only SSRIs with U.S. Food and Drug Administration (FDA) approval for use in children 12 years old and older. The FDA specifically recommends against the use of paroxetine in children and adolescents because of the 3.5-fold increased risk for suicide. Activation (e.g., elevated energy without mood change) and mania can occur in patients secondary to treatment with antidepressants. Therefore, it is critical that parents be taught about symptoms that merit immediate evaluation, including decreased impulse control, marked elevated mood, acting-out, fearlessness, and risk taking (Garzon et al, 2009). For children with psychosis, child psychiatrists often add antipsychotics like risperidone or olanzapine to the therapeutic drug plan (Cheung and Jensen, 2009).

Close follow-up is recommended for all children and adolescents with depression, especially when symptoms are significant enough to merit pharmacotherapy. Providers

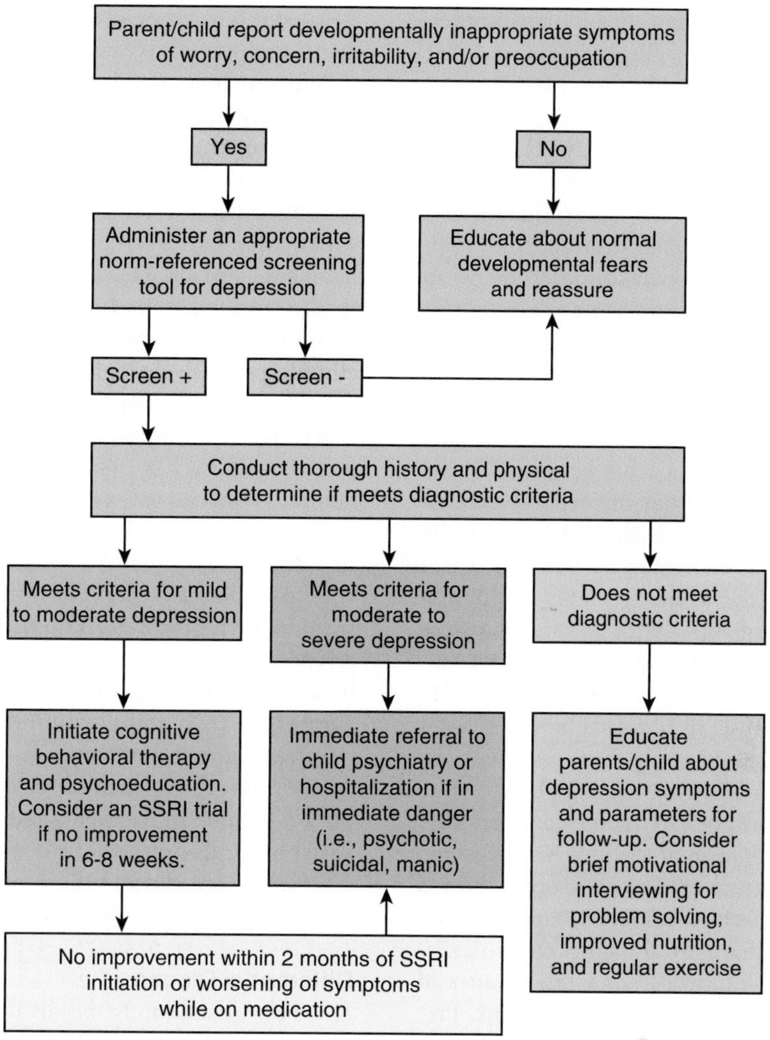

• **Figure 19-2** Primary care management of pediatric depression. *SSRI,* Selective serotonin reuptake inhibitor.

should make phone contact with the patient and/or family within 3 days and see the patient weekly until stable with the first 4 weeks of treatment being critical. Once stable, maintenance visits can occur at 3-month intervals.

Prognosis

MDD is a chronic condition with a high rate of recurrence. Although most children and adolescents will recover from an MDD episode, the probability of recurrence is 60% within 2 years and 75% by 5 years. Poor long-term outcomes are associated with severe or frequent disease, and in patients with significant family dysfunction, low socioeconomic status, and history of abuse or family strife (Birmaher et al, 2007).

Bipolar Disorder

Bipolar disorder, formerly known as *manic depression,* is characterized by unusual shifts in mood, energy, and functioning and may begin with manic, depressive, or a mixed set of manic and depressive symptoms. The majority of adults with bipolar disorder report their initial symptom was depression, and those who develop symptoms in childhood are significantly more likely to develop severe disease, to be hospitalized frequently, and to have a less favorable life course (Coryell et al, 2013). It is a recurrent disorder, and nearly all of those (90%) who have a single manic episode will have future episodes. Approximately 4% of children younger than age 18 meet the diagnostic criteria for bipolar disorder (Shain and Committee on Adolescence, 2012). The risk of suicide in bipolar depression is the highest of all the psychiatric disorders.

A characteristic pattern usually evolves for a particular person, with manic episodes preceding or following major depressive episodes. Most individuals with bipolar disorder return to a full level of functioning between episodes; 20% to 30% experience persistent mood lability and interpersonal difficulties (APA, 2013). Sometimes psychotic symptoms develop after several days or weeks of manic symptoms. Such features tend to predict that the individual with subsequent manic episodes will again experience psychotic symptoms.

Multiple theories explain the cause of bipolar disorder, but no definitive cause is known. Imaging studies reveal that there are structural changes commonly found in the third ventricle, the white matter, the prefrontal cortex, the amygdala, and the basal ganglia (Vederine et al, 2011). Genetic factors (specifically, defects on chromosomes 1, 6, 8, and 22) account for almost 60% of bipolar cases. There is evidence of a genetic influence for bipolar disorder from twin studies and adoption studies; bipolar disorder tends to cluster in families. Parents who are bipolar are at greater risk for having bipolar children. Fifty-nine percent of adults with bipolar depression report onset of symptoms during childhood or adolescence, but the onset of symptoms before 10 years old is rare (0.5%) (McClellan et al, 2007). The most common onset of symptoms occurs between 15 and 19 years old. There is no differential incidence based on race, ethnicity, or gender. Children with ADD seem to be vulnerable to bipolar illness, or it may be that ADD is a misdiagnosed early sign of the mania to come. If children are also bipolar, treatment of ADD with psychostimulants or antidepressants may precipitate a manic episode. Antidepressants in depressed children (6 to 12 years old) may also precipitate mania and the onset of bipolar illness.

Clinical Findings

Bipolar disorder in childhood or early adolescence appears to be a different, more severe form of the illness than occurs with late adolescent or adult onset. The early-onset form is characterized by irritability and continuous, rapid-cycling, and mixed-symptom state that may also co-occur with disruptive behavior disorders (e.g., ADD or CD); features of ADD or behavior disorder are often early symptoms. Prepubertal and early adolescent bipolar disorder is a fairly homogeneous phenotype, with no differences according to gender, puberty, or comorbid ADD. In the late adolescent or adult form, the hallmark features include classic manic episodes, episodic patterns of mania and depression, and relative stability between episodes. Symptoms include the following (Chang, 2009):

- Severe mood changes—extreme irritability or overly elated and silly
- Inflated self-esteem or grandiosity
- Increased energy and physical agitation
- Decreased need for sleep (sleeps few hours or no sleep for days without tiring)
- Talkativeness or compulsion to talk; frequent topic changes or cannot be interrupted
- Distractibility, with attention moving constantly from one thing to another
- Increase in goal-directed activity (socially or at school)
- Risk-taking behaviors or activities; taking "more dares"
- Hypersexuality in talk, thoughts, feelings, or behaviors
- Suicidal thoughts and behaviors in 76% of cases and suicidal attempts in 31% of cases

More than half of adolescents experience depression as their initial symptom (Chang, 2009). The most common symptoms of mania include irritable mood and grandiosity, elevated mood, decreased sleep, racing thoughts, poor judgment, flight of ideas, and hypersexuality.

With mania, children appear to be the happiest of people, but the happiness and laughter do not match the situation or context. Grandiosity may manifest in efforts to correct teachers or critique their efforts, seeing themselves as above rules and laws, or devoting time to an activity for which they have no talent. Children's sleep difficulties (a hallmark sign) are reflected in high activity levels before bed (e.g., rearranging the furniture), whereas adolescents need little sleep at all. Risk-taking behavior ranges from children climbing excessively high trees or hopping between rooftops to adolescents driving recklessly and speeding. In adolescents, manic episodes are more likely to include psychotic features and may be associated with school truancy, school failure, substance use, or antisocial behavior. No laboratory findings diagnostic of a manic episode have been identified, so a careful history and a thorough assessment are crucial.

The child or adolescent who has depression but also manifests symptoms of ADD that seem severe (e.g., extreme temper outbursts and mood changes) should be evaluated by a child psychiatrist with experience in bipolar disorder. Symptoms are manifested in relatively age-specific ways.

Assessment for comorbid conditions is important. Anxiety disorders, including panic disorder, affect about 30% of prepubertal patients and 10% of adolescent patients with bipolar disorder. Other common comorbidities include CD, substance abuse, ODD, disruptive behavior disorder, and personality disorders (Birmaher et al, 2007).

Differential Diagnosis

A manic episode must be distinguished from a mood disorder caused by a medical condition (e.g., brain tumor) and a substance-induced mood disorder (e.g., laughing fits with marijuana, amphetamine highs followed by withdrawal "crashes," perceptual distortions or hallucinations of hallucinogens). Distinguishing bipolar disorder from ADD can be a challenge. ADD, like mania, is characterized by excessive activity, poor impulse control and judgment, and denial of problems. However, ADD lacks a clear onset or episodes, mood disturbances, and psychotic features. Recent evidence suggests that children with ADD are vulnerable to bipolar disorder and that pharmacological treatments may precipitate manic episodes, so providers should carefully evaluate and refer any child treated for ADD who does not respond to therapy or who experiences a sudden worsening of agitation while using ADD medications.

Management

Referral to a child psychiatrist or child mental health care provider is critical. Current recommendations for pharmacologic treatment include the use of mood stabilizers, such as lithium, alone or in combination with antiseizure medications (e.g., valproate, divalproex) and atypical antipsychotics (e.g., risperidone). Neither antidepressants nor stimulants have proven effective. Antidepressant use may potentiate manic responses. The use of lithium must be carefully monitored. Data strongly support long-term maintenance on lithium to prevent relapse of bipolar symptoms (Birmaher et al, 2007).

The best clinical responses occur when pharmacotherapy is combined with individual and family psychotherapy (Shain and Committee on Adolescence, 2012). Therapy should focus on minimizing comorbidities, enhancing problem-solving and communication skills, and reducing negative self-thoughts. Other nonpharmacologic interventions with proven effectiveness include stress reduction, healthy diet, routine exercise, and developing good sleep hygiene.

Attention-Deficit/Hyperactivity Disorder

ADD, the most common of all child and adolescent behavioral disorders, commonly managed in primary care settings, is discussed in Chapter 20.

The Aggressive Child

Social Aggression

Social aggression is a pattern of social behavior with the intent to harm others (Leff et al, 2009). Onset may occur as early as toddlerhood. It can be overt (e.g., hitting or pushing) or covert (e.g., gossiping or socially ostracizing).

Approximately 5% to 6% of American children have behavioral problems with aggression and 1% to 10% of children meet criteria for ODD (Barbaresi, 2009). Males are more likely to be aggressive than females, and aggression peaks during adolescence. Females are more likely to be socially or covertly aggressive, whereas males are more likely to be overtly aggressive. Acute, stressful life events or transitions can precipitate a brief period of social aggression. Significant risk factors include a history of maltreatment; inconsistent or harsh discipline, or both; lack of maternal responsiveness; separations from parents; and shifts in parental figures or parental rejection. Social aggression can be a precursor to CD or ODD. Research indicates that there is an inherited pattern of susceptibility aggressiveness (Leff et al, 2009).

Clinical Findings

During preschool, social aggression manifests as oppositional or defiant behavior and is considered clinically significant if it interferes with normal developmental functioning. The pervasiveness, intensity, and persistence of irritable, argumentative, defiant, and easily annoyed behaviors identify a pathologic condition and may be precursors to ODD. In the preschool period, children have a beginning understanding of the effect of their behavior on others and can control their behavior on the basis of internalized norms and developing self-regulation. When social aggression becomes a pattern, peer rejection is common. Aggressive behavior involves the following:

- Destruction of property
- Name-calling
- Physical pestering and deliberately annoying others
- Hitting, biting, kicking, fighting
- Frequent conflict with peers
- Temper tantrums
- Misinterpreting social cues and responding aggressively
- Lack of problem-solving in social situations
- Use of bad language, swearing, obscene language and gestures
- Arguing for long periods
- Inappropriately suggestive or aggressive sexual behaviors

Differential Diagnosis

ODD is a pattern of open defiance and noncompliance toward authority figures. ODD symptoms emerge during the preschool years and persist for a minimum of 6 months. CD is a clear pattern of behavior established over a 6-month period, typically diagnosed at school age. CD differs from ODD in that it involves serious aggression toward people or animals, willful destruction of property, or theft. However, there is growing evidence that preschool children manifest clinically significant disruptive behavior problems, and valid diagnoses of ODD and CD can be made even in young children. Typical and atypical problems can be differentiated, and children with these problems can be identified with a developmentally based DSM-5 framework (APA, 2013).

Management

It is important to ascertain whether a difficult temperament underlies the behavioral difficulty, especially in conjunction with a lack of fit with parental temperament. A difficult temperament may account for a child's being difficult to discipline, having social behavior problems in school (e.g., poor fit with the teacher), or having poor academic achievement. In these situations, the use of positive parenting strategies does not have to change, but supportive counseling for the parents should be provided regarding temperament, its manifestations, and strategies for managing transitions and other difficult times or behaviors. A teacher conference may provide similar information and explore strategies to facilitate the child's learning and positive behavior.

When social aggression is a response to acute stress, the problem usually resolves if parents use positive parenting strategies and facilitate developmentally appropriate coping efforts. If peer relationship development is hampered, close monitoring of and intervention with peer interactions by day care, preschool, and school personnel, especially with the parents present for observation, enhances appropriate social behavior and competence. Changing schools in an effort to ameliorate problems is not advised because children carry their social difficulties with them and assume the same roles in new groups. It is helpful to work with teachers to ensure that they are supportive and facilitative.

When social aggression becomes a pattern of social behavior, referral for intervention is critical. Negative behavior in preschool playgroups is predictive of externalizing behavior problems in kindergarten. Substantial research literature supports the stability and persistence of disruptive behavior and aggression from toddlerhood to school age (Barbaresi, 2009). Early intervention is essential. Parental education should focus on reestablishing positive parent-child interactions, use of consistent limit setting, and teaching parents to use effective discipline.

Conduct Disorder

CD is a repetitive and persistent pattern of behavior in which the basic rights of others or major age-appropriate societal norms and rules are violated (APA, 2013). The onset of aggressive behavior is observed in toddlerhood. Early-onset conduct problems are diagnosed from 4 to 6 years old, and a formal diagnosis is typically made when the child is 7 years old or older. The cause of the disorder rests in chronic negative circumstances, as described for social aggression. CD is frequently associated with a history of harsh discipline, abuse, or neglect. Prevalence rates range from 1% to 10% (Leff et al, 2009). CD is more common in males than females (3 : 1). However, it is thought that the prevalence data do not accurately reflect the occurrence of CD for females, because the diagnostic criteria emphasize physical aggression.

Behavioral dysregulation tends to become notable during the transition from early to middle childhood and is mediated by changes in the structure and demands of the social environment—peers and school settings. There is a high rate of comorbidity with major depression, and the joint presence of CD and depression increases the risk for substance abuse and suicide. ADD negatively influences the development, course, and severity of CD.

Clinical Findings

Clinical features fall into four main subgroups: (1) aggressive behavior that threatens or results in physical harm to other people or animals, (2) nonaggressive behavior that causes property damage, (3) lying or stealing, and (4) serious violation of rules or laws. Several factors are relevant to practitioners for their prognostic importance:

- How atypical the behaviors are for age or gender
- How overt versus covert the behaviors are
- The nature of any aggression
- The presence of early antisocial or psychopathic-related symptoms

Most commonly, referrals for clinical treatment are for aggressive behavior patterns. Physical aggression toward others includes the following:

- Hitting, kicking, fighting
- Physical cruelty to animals or people
- Physical destruction (including fire setting)
- Frequent temper tantrums
- A high rate of annoying behavior, such as yelling, whining, or threatening
- Disobedience to adult authorities
- Lying, cheating, covert stealing
- Truancy and running away from home
- Blaming others for mistakes
- Use of or selling illegal drugs
- Engaging in deviant sexual behaviors (e.g., sexual assault)
- Academic problems

There is growing evidence that preadolescent and adolescent girls manifest CD more indirectly through verbal and relational aggression, including alienation, ostracism, and character defamation directed at the relationships between friends. With CD, social role functioning tends to be impaired with poor academic performance, poor family and peer relationships, and poor self-management. Childhood CD may predict antisocial personality disorder in adulthood. Poorer prognoses are associated with increased symptom severity.

Differential Diagnosis

ODD is characterized by more disobedience than aggressiveness and is evidenced in preschool or early school age. ADD is characterized by inattention, impulsiveness, and hyperactivity, but willful destruction is uncommon. CD is distinguished from isolated acts of aggressive behavior by degree of aggression exhibited, the presence of willful defiance, and by the persistence of symptoms for a minimum of 6 months (APA, 2013). A thorough physical examination is essential to rule out organic causes of behavior and to identify evidence of abuse, neglect, and substance abuse disorders.

Management

If aggressive behavior is identified before a CD develops, preventive efforts can be implemented. Successful programs are multifaceted, including a parent-directed component (e.g., parent education and support for positive parenting strategies and healthy, consistent approaches to discipline), social-cognitive skills training, proactive classroom management and teacher training, and group therapy (Leff et al, 2009). Effective education includes conflict resolution strategies and development of coping and resiliency skills. Once a CD is evident, referral for child and family intervention is crucial.

Safety is a priority in caring for children with aggressive and oppositional disorders. Because of the strong association of child abuse and neglect with CD, it is critical to determine if the child is in safe living conditions. If there is evidence of abuse or neglect, prompt referral to child protective agencies is mandatory. The practitioner must also determine whether other family members are safe from the child's or adolescent's aggressive behavior. Potential interventions when family safety is at risk include referral for inpatient psychiatric evaluation, police notification of criminal activity, supporting the family to petition the juvenile court for services, and referral to community health services.

Family therapy can be helpful for adolescents with CD. Collaboration between the family and the school is of critical importance, and the PCP can assist with strategies. Isolated individual treatment is not superior to parent intervention programs. Education about problem-solving skills may also be effective.

Psychopharmacologic intervention is reserved for explosive aggression and includes mood stabilizers, typical and atypical antipsychotics, clonidine, and stimulants. However, PCPs should refer patients to a mental health specialist for drug therapy given the high risk for substance abuse in those with CD.

Oppositional Defiant Disorder

ODD is a pattern of negative, hostile, and defiant behavior that is excessive compared with other children of the same age (APA, 2013). Symptoms often occur in early childhood, from 3 to 7 years old with the disorder typically beginning by 8 years old.

Etiologic factors include many of the parenting and family dysfunctions identified for social aggression. Precursors to the disorder are common in early childhood, especially defiance and negativism. More common in boys before puberty, the gender distribution is approximately equal thereafter. Community prevalence rates range from 2.6% to 15.6%, but clinical sample prevalence rates are much higher (28% to 65%) (Fraire and Ollendick, 2013).

Clinical Findings

The essential feature of ODD is a recurrent pattern of behavior that is negative, defiant, disobedient, and hostile toward authority figures. Behavior is typically directed at family members, teachers, or peers that the child knows well. The child manifests the following behaviors to an extent that leads to impairment (APA, 2013):

- Actively defies or refuses adult requests or rules
- Is argumentative, angry, resentful, touchy, or easily annoyed
- Easily loses temper; is vindictive
- Blames others for own mistakes or difficulties
- Deliberately does things to annoy others
- Children often see their own behavior as justifiable, not oppositional or defiant

Differential Diagnosis

CD involves more serious violations of the rights of others and a more willful disregard of authority.

Management

Attend to the early signs of defiant and oppositional behavior or aggression, or both, and educate parents about positive parenting strategies and exercising consistent, healthy discipline, which is similar to the management of CDs. Because these children typically do not perceive themselves as having a problem and rest the cause with the family system, referral for intervention is indicated. As described for CD, parent training programs are more successful if they include information about child behavior in multiple environments (e.g., school and home) and target dysfunctional family processes. Child training groups provide added benefit if combined with parent training groups. Again, collaboration with the school is important. These multiple approaches, conducted simultaneously, are most effective.

Autism Spectrum Disorder

This complex disorder, diagnosed using DSM-5 criteria, is discussed in Chapter 20.

Eating Disorders

Eating disorders cause abnormal eating behaviors that are secondary to altered body image (dysmorphism). Anorexia nervosa (commonly called *anorexia*) and bulimia nervosa (commonly called *bulimia*) are the primary eating disorders of concern; however, there are other conditions in this diagnostic cluster, including eating disorder not otherwise specified, rumination disorders, pica, and feeding disorders of infancy. Some believe obesity should be classified as an eating disorder because of the correlation between self-soothing and eating, and because many obese individuals have feelings of loss of control over their eating and symptoms of body dysmorphism. Eating disorders are complex conditions that are very difficult to treat and are associated with significant medical and mental health comorbidities. Anorexia has the highest mortality rate of all the mental health conditions. The 5-year mortality rate for anorexia is 15% to 20%, and the majority of these deaths are caused by electrolyte imbalance, malnutrition, and suicide (Miller and Golden, 2010). Due to the complexity of these disorders, specialty care is needed; however, PCPs play a critical role through detection and early intervention, case coordination, and monitoring for complications.

Lifetime prevalence rates for anorexia and bulimia are approximately 1% each (Miller and Golden, 2010). Both disorders affect females at much greater rates than males (9:1). Symptom onset usually occurs during mid to late adolescence, but preadolescent cases do occur and are associated with significantly higher morbidity and mortality. Athletes are more likely to develop eating disorders, especially those who compete in sports that are based on weight divisions (e.g., wrestling), long distance running, and those with emphases on aesthetic lines and flexibility (e.g., dancers, gymnasts, and ice skaters). Other individual risk factors include middle to high socioeconomic status, divorced families, chronic disease (e.g., diabetes mellitus, cystic fibrosis, depression, obesity, and substance abuse), recent weight loss in a previously obese person, personality disorders (e.g., borderline, narcissistic, and antisocial), strong will, and history of child abuse. Children and adolescents with eating disorders are more likely to have parents who have a weight or fitness focus, are substance abusers, have high achievement expectations, who comment on their child's physical appearance, have difficulty expressing emotions, or who are overprotective or enmeshed with their children. Like most mental illness, there is an increasing body of evidence suggesting a strong genetic component to anorexia and bulimia that results in altered serotonin and dopamine receptors.

Clinical Findings

Diagnosing anorexia or bulimia can be difficult. Some clinical findings characteristic of these disorders occur in the healthy adolescent. For example, it is not uncommon for a 14-year-old girl who is neither anorexic nor bulimic to express concern about her body appearance, stating that she is too fat or ugly. Additionally, anorexic or bulimic adolescents and their families commonly hide their condition and actions, deny problems, or present a mature, self-sufficient, and successful facade. Early in the disease process, the family system may appear to be coherent, making it difficult to collect accurate data about family relations and behavior patterns that contribute to eating disorders.

Many consider anorexia and bulimia to be part of a disease continuum with categories that are more arbitrary than actual. Clinical presentations vary depending on the disease severity. Both anorexia and bulimia are associated with disordered eating and body dysmorphism with or without purging (e.g., laxative abuse, enemas, diuretics, and induced vomiting). Generally there is no loss of appetite or sense of hunger. Affected individuals often link feelings of self-worth with weight or the ability to restrict food intake despite being hungry. Diagnostic criteria for anorexia are (APA, 2013):

- Refusal to maintain body weight at least 85% expected for age and height or failure to gain weight during growth periods so that weight drops below 85% expected
- Intense fear of weight gain and "being fat"
- Body dysmorphism
- Binge eating/purging subtype, which is associated with frequent purging although bingeing episodes are rare

Diagnostic criteria for bulimia are (APA, 2013):

- Consuming large quantities of food in a short period of time (within 2 hours)
- Loss of control during binge episodes (e.g., can't control the amount of food they eat or are shocked at amount consumed)
- Engaging in repeated behaviors to lose weight, including purging, excessive exercise, or fasting
- Bingeing or purging behaviors that occur at least once a week for at least 3 months

Individuals with anorexia are underweight, but children and adolescents with bulimia are often average weight or overweight. In addition to the regular primary care monitoring of weight and growth, it is important to include routine screening to detect the red flags (Table 19-7). Also helpful is the SCOFF questionnaire (Kirkby and Brown, 2007). This five-item screen asks the following questions:

1. Do you make yourself **S**ick because you feel uncomfortably full?
2. Do you worry that you have lost **C**ontrol over what you eat?
3. Have you lost **O**ver 10 pounds in the last 3 months?
4. Do you believe you are **F**at when others say you are thin?
5. Would you say **F**ood dominates your life?

TABLE 19-7 Red Flags and Signs That Indicate Need for Eating Disorder Treatment

Red Flags	Needs Treatment Signs
Reads diet books or clips dieting articles	Regularly fasts or skips meals
Visits pro-anorexia or bulimia websites (pro Anna or pro Mia)	Stops eating with family or friends
Intense focus on diet or regular dieting	Misses two or more periods during weight loss
Sudden desire to be a vegetarian	Reports binge eating
Sudden picky eating	Reports purging
Visits bathroom regularly during or after meals	Parents find laxatives or diet pills
Showers multiple times a day	Excessive exercise
Skips meals because "I ate at school" or other place away from home	Refuses to eat non-diet foods
Large amounts of missing food	Refuses to eat meals prepared by others Extreme calorie counting or portion controls

Patients with suspected eating disorders need a thorough history and physical examination and evaluation for comorbid depression, anxiety, suicidality, and risk of physical harm. Common history findings include:

- Menstrual irregularity
- Altered body perception, may manifest as feelings of being fat even though not overweight
- Preoccupation with food; often fixes elaborate meals but does not eat; rituals associated with food
- Desire to lose weight, and history of dieting or food rituals
- Weight fluctuation or loss
- Guilt about eating
- Hides eating or lies about having eaten or amount eaten
- Displays social isolation and mood changes: Irritable, sullen, hostile, introverted, unhappy, intolerant of others, can have suicidal ideation
- Fixed, highly structured schedule; inflexible to change
- Cold intolerance, fatigue, myalgias
- Constipation, diarrhea, abdominal bloating, gastrointestinal (GI) distress
- Sleep deprivation
- Sore throat
- Dizziness, syncope

- Other destructive behaviors: Shoplifting, substance abuse, self-harm
- Family history of chaos, abuse, sexual abuse

Common physical findings that may indicate an eating disorder are:

- Altered growth
- Round face with parotid gland enlargement
- Fluid retention, facial edema
- Thin body type, low body temperature
- Hypotension, bradycardia, orthostatic hypotension, shallow respirations
- Dental enamel erosion, dental caries
- Russell sign (e.g., knuckle cuts/calluses/abrasions from inducing vomiting)
- Thinning hair, alopecia, decreased deep tendon reflexes
- Abdominal distention, altered bowel sounds
- Lanugo, dry skin
- Muscle atrophy
- Mental torpor

Differential Diagnosis

Inflammatory bowel disease and peptic ulcer disease result in chronic pain and microscopic or gross bleeding. Central nervous system lesions cause focal neurologic signs. Hormonal and metabolic diseases cause symptoms like polyphagia, polydipsia, polyuria, abnormal hair growth, and goiter. Immune disorders are associated with frequent, rare, and opportunistic infections. Other mental health differential diagnoses include OCD, substance use disorder (SUD), and major depression.

Diagnostic Studies

Laboratory testing is done to ascertain the degree of electrolyte imbalance and malnutrition and to rule out other causes of weight loss and amenorrhea. Suggested diagnostic testing for an individual with a newly diagnosed eating disorder includes CBC (anemia), serum electrolytes (potassium, sodium, and acid-base imbalance), fasting glucose (diabetes), thyroid studies (hyperthyroidism), liver function testing, follicle-stimulating hormone (FSH), luteinizing hormone (LH), urinalysis electrocardiogram (ECG) (premature ventricular contractions and QT elongation), and bone density (if amenorrheic to look for osteopenia).

Management

Management of children and adolescents with anorexia or bulimia is difficult, in part because the child, family, and even the health care provider often deny the significance of the problem. Therefore, referral to mental health specialists is needed. Even though early detection and treatment are helpful in reducing physical complications, diagnosis can be delayed and treatment may be inadequate. Because the issue is not food, but rather sociopsychological dynamics of control in the child's life, effective treatment is complex and long term. Eating disorders are managed with a multifaceted approach with emphasis on nutritional rehabilitation, pharmacotherapeutics (e.g., antidepressants, atypical antipsychotics), and individual, family, and group therapy. Intensive, inpatient management is warranted for medical instability, psychosis or self-destructive behavior, and failure to improve with outpatient therapy. The evidence for CBT is strong, and family therapy clinically improves weight gain and parental control of re-nutrition (Campbell and Peebles, 2014).

Many children and adolescents with eating disorders require inpatient management, especially if there are fluid and electrolyte imbalances, cardiovascular instability, or significant mental illness. Individual and family therapy is critical. Pharmacologic approaches include antidepressants and atypical antipsychotics, but their use is controversial in many cases. The role of the PCP in the management of eating disorders is primarily that of screening and early identification. Weight gain during refeeding is expected to occur at 1.1 pounds (0.5 kg) per week (Campbell and Peebles, 2014). Close monitoring for refeeding syndrome is warranted. This is a rare, potentially life-threatening condition that occurs in the first days of enteral or parenteral feeding and results in severe fluid and electrolyte imbalance. Symptoms include confusion, severe irritability, organ dysfunction, and seizures.

Complications

Anorexia has the highest mortality rate of all mental health disorders. The complications of anorexia or bulimia include death, usually secondary to cardiac arrhythmia, hypokalemia, congestive heart failure, or suicide; altered metabolism (chronic); alcohol and drug addictions; osteoporosis; GI disturbance: ulcers, motility disorders; fertility problems; gynecologic problems related to prolonged amenorrhea; growth retardation; and dehydration.

Substance Abuse

Substance use is a precursor to abuse or dependence, and regular use clearly increases the risk for developing a SUD. However, the use of substances per se is not sufficient for a diagnosis of SUD. Substance abuse is a maladaptive pattern of the use of alcohol or drugs manifested in significant impairment or distress. The criteria for substance dependence in the DSM-5 is divided into specific categories (alcohol, cannabis, inhalants, and so on), and in adults it includes tolerance, withdrawal, and compulsive substance use (APA, 2013). For children and adolescents, tolerance and loss of control are not good indicators for a diagnosis. Instead, substance-related blackouts, craving, and impulsive sexual or risk-taking behavior tend to be more important criteria. Tobacco use is discussed in Chapter 42.

The cause of SUD is multifaceted. Many contributing factors exist, including the following:

- Genetic vulnerability (family history)
- Parental substance use
- Dysfunctional family relationships, such as rigidity, distant relationships, neglect, or lack of supervision
- Negative life events

- Psychiatric conditions (e.g., CD, ADD, depression)
- Low self-esteem, poor body image, ineffective coping (poor emotional regulation, poor problem-solving skills) or poor sleep hygiene
- School failure
- Low religiosity
- Latchkey child
- Sexual activity, homosexuality, bisexuality
- Competitive athleticism

Precipitating life events tend to center around loss of relationships (e.g., parental separation, divorce, or death; death of a close friend) and chronic negative circumstances (e.g., parental substance abuse, maltreatment).

Data from the Youth Risk Behavior Survey indicate that 35% of teens reported drinking alcohol and 23% reported using marijuana within the previous month (Kann et al, 2014). Approximately 21% of high school students binge drink, almost 19% of students drank alcohol for the first time before they were 13 years old, and about 21% reported having five or more drinks in a row during the past year. Nearly half of problem drinkers are thought to have tried alcohol by 10 years old and two-thirds by 13 years old. The majority of adolescents who use drugs do not progress to abuse or dependence. Peer influence seems to be less significant to the cause of substance abuse than previously thought. Boys tend to be more involved in use of both alcohol and drugs of all kinds than girls are at the same age. It is estimated that for both boys and girls, abuse of alcohol and other drugs is negligible from 10 to 13 years old, but doubles between adolescence (12 to 16 years old) and late adolescence (17 to 20 years old), peaks between 18 and 25 years old, and declines thereafter. The percentage of students reporting lifetime use of alcohol, marijuana, steroids, methamphetamines, and hallucinogenic drugs has decreased in the past decade, although the percentage of those reporting current use of cocaine and amphetamines has not changed significantly (Kann et al, 2014).

Clinical Findings

Identifying an adolescent's problem with substance abuse requires a careful assessment, conducted with an accepting, nonjudgmental, nonthreatening, matter-of-fact attitude. The covert nature of substance abuse and the dynamic of denial make it crucial to avoid a critical tone (see Chapter 8 for discussion of adolescent risk behavior).

Interviewing the adolescent with the parents is a key strategy for obtaining information about etiologic factors and behavioral, cognitive, emotional, and physical changes that they have observed in the adolescent. However, it is essential that the adolescent also be interviewed alone at every visit to assess mental health and family issues.

When talking about substance use with an adolescent, it is important to begin with general questions that are not overly personal. Begin by asking the adolescent about acquaintances or friends who smoke, drink, or use drugs; whether anyone in the family has had problems with these; and what the adolescent does with friends when they get together. It is helpful to ask about experimentation, under what circumstances it occurs, and the adolescent's feelings about it. To obtain a chronologic history of tobacco, alcohol, or drug use, it may be helpful to approach the subject by inquiring about prescription drugs and moving to illicit substances. The key is to remain nonjudgmental to elicit information that will indicate whether the adolescent is experimenting, a regular user, or dependent on substances. Ask about the adolescent's source of drugs or alcohol; the adolescent who uses substances provided by a friend or acquaintance is less advanced than one who purchases them directly. The practitioner should ask, "What? How much? How often? When? How? Where? With whom? Does the patient use substances at parties, home, school, alone, or with friends?"

The CRAFFT questionnaire is an appropriate screening instrument for substance abuse in the primary care setting (See Chapter 2). Positive responses to two or more items indicate a high likelihood for substance abuse and merits further evaluation and treatment.

Significant behavioral changes that may reflect drug use include the following (Foy et al, 2010b):

- Infants and young children: Excessive crying; poor feeding or failure to thrive; irritability, jitteriness, or excessive lethargy; poor eye contact; sleep disorders
- Older children and adolescents: Decreased school performance; lethargy, hyperactivity or agitation, hypervigilance, decreased attention; disinhibition; deviant or risk-taking behavior; repeated absences or suspensions from school; loss of interest in previously enjoyed activities; withdrawal from family and usual friends, or change in friends to those involved in drugs and alcohol; irritability, fighting or acting-out; hypersexuality; exaggerated mood swings; sleep pattern changes or nightmares; altered menstruation; and change in appetite (from anorexia to unusual hunger)

Mood changes include swings from depression to euphoria, nervousness, unreasonable anger, and frequent expressions of hopelessness or failure. Low self-esteem typically characterizes those who abuse substances.

Physical signs that indicate a substance use problem include the following:

- Weight loss
- Red eyes, associated with marijuana use
- Hoarseness, chronic cough, wheezing with use of inhalants and cocaine
- Frequent "colds" or "allergy" symptoms, epistaxis, and perforations of nasal septum with cocaine and inhalant use
- Accidents, trauma, injuries
- Intoxication
- Complete or partial amnesia for events during intoxication with alcohol and date rape drug use
- Dilated or constricted pupils
- Gynecomastia, irregular periods, small testes with marijuana
- Needle tracks occur with intramuscular (IM) steroids or intravenous (IV) heroin use

- Generalized pruritus with opiate use
- Reflux, diarrhea, gastritis, and constipation with opiate and alcohol use
- Perioral sores or pyodermas from huffing and bagging

Differential Diagnosis

Substance abuse is distinguished from social drinking or nonpathologic substance use by the presence of compulsive use, craving, or substance-related problems. SUDs are comorbid most often with CD, depression, and anxiety.

Diagnostic Studies

Urine toxicology can be helpful to verify adolescent truthfulness, although a positive drug screen result does not indicate substance abuse or dependence; it only indicates substance use. A negative drug screen result does not rule out an SUD. The approximate duration that drugs can be detected in the urine is as follows (Bukstein et al, 2005):

- Stimulants—1 to 2 days
- Cocaine and its major metabolite—1 to 3 days
- Sedative-hypnotics—1 day to 1 week
- Barbiturates—2 to 4 weeks
- Quaaludes—2 to 3 weeks
- Opiates—1 to 2 days
- Marijuana—up to 30 days

Duration of detection from last substance use varies according to the laboratory and type of test used. The AACAP recommends that to obtain a valid result, a positive result on immunoassay should be followed by confirmation with a more sensitive method, such as gas chromatography or mass spectrometry.

Management

Exposure to tobacco and alcohol and illicit substances begins in early childhood. The pediatric PCP should discuss parental modeling for the use of alcohol, tobacco, and other substances in early childhood during routine well-child visits. It is important to educate school-age children and their parents about substance use and its consequences. For adolescents, a direct assessment and an interview about substance use are essential. Parents should be advised not to involve their child in their own substance use. Something as seemingly innocuous as "getting dad a beer from the refrigerator" gives the child practice in alcohol use.

Substance abuse must be treated, and referral to a substance abuse program is crucial. The initial goal is to help adolescents take positive steps toward changing their substance use and abuse behavior. If the adolescent denies any problem, efforts should focus on helping the adolescent acknowledge problems. Clarifying reported negative consequences, creating doubts about substance use, and raising awareness of the risks related to current use are motivational interviewing strategies that may be helpful. It is important to remain empathic and yet emphasize the adolescent's responsibility to make healthy choices. If the adolescent has not reached a level of chronic use, prevention of harm is the goal of the intervention. Guide the adolescent to examine his or her substance use responsibly and identify ways to prevent harmful consequences.

If the adolescent progresses to chronic substance use, a number of options exist. Outpatient or day treatment programs are effective for those who can live and be managed at home. For adolescents with more serious addiction, comorbid psychiatric conditions, or suicidal ideation, residential treatment or hospitalization may be necessary. Given the prominence of family dysfunction and family life events in the cause of the problem, family-based treatment programs are essential. Family treatment, rather than family psychoeducation or family support groups, has been shown to be superior to other modalities. Follow-up assessments should include substance use issues and other predictors of use: stress or negative life events, depression or negative affect regulation, and the presence of positive support within or outside of the family. Self-help or 12-step groups are thought to be an essential element in the recovery process.

For a complete list of references, please visit http://evolve.elsevier.com/Burns/pediatric/.

20 Cognitive-Perceptual Disorders

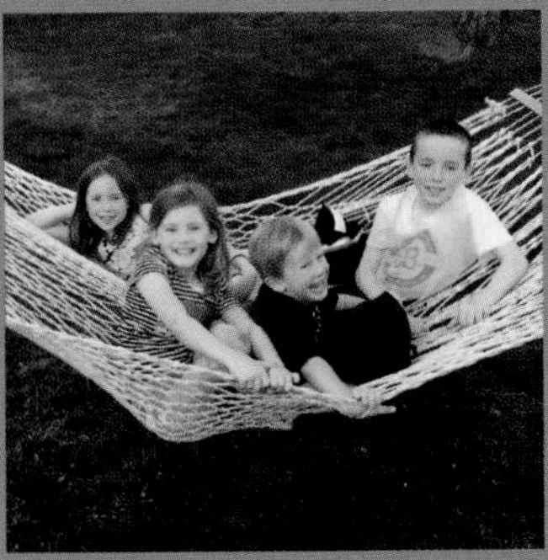

NANCY BARBER STARR AND CRISANN BOWMAN-HARVEY

Cognition is the acquisition, processing, and use of information. Successful development in this domain requires memory (encoding, storing, and retrieving information), representational competence (the ability to create and manipulate a mental image of an object or idea that is not seen), attention (learning how to focus and shift focus), as well as processing speed, which may be considered the key factor because it links the other three together (Wilks et al, 2010). Cognition and general knowledge represent the accumulation and reorganization of experiences that result from participating in a rich learning setting with skilled and appropriate adult interventions. From these experiences, children construct knowledge of patterns and relations, cause and effect, and methods of solving problems of everyday life. Perception is the organization, identification, and interpretation of sensory information in order to represent and understand the environment. Traditionally the focus on learning has been on visual or auditory input; however, the sensory processing theory, also known as *sensory integration,* holds that vestibular and proprioception are sensory components that are critical to learning. The multiple intelligence theory expands our focus to include a broader range of potential than the traditional ones.

Facilitating and monitoring cognitive-perceptual developmental progress as well as ensuring the maximum function of all the senses are integral parts of primary care. Screening hearing and vision is a recognized standard of care. Following cognitive development in infancy and early childhood is primarily done by monitoring language and problem-solving domains integral to the other developmental parameters and should be performed with standardized screening tools. Monitoring the adaptation to and performance in school is key. Soliciting information about school performance from preschool through high school assesses the child's mastery of educational tasks and academic challenges. Primary care providers (PCPs) may be consulted for guidance about appropriate timing and school placement for a child, performance that is better than or worse than expected, school problems, and the need for further assessment. As developmental experts, PCPs need to be able to work with the family and school to assess problems; advise, counsel, and educate parents; participate on interdisciplinary teams for diagnosis and management; and mediate and advocate for children and their learning needs.

Standards for Care

Healthy People 2020: Health Promotion and Disease Prevention Objectives for the Year 2020 supports the need for visual and hearing screening in children (U.S. Department of Health and Human Services [USDHHS], n.d.). Objectives include "increase the proportion of children who are ready for school in all five domains of healthy development," "increase educational achievement of adolescents and young adults," "increase the proportion of adolescents who consider school work to be meaningful and important," and "increase the percentage of young children with autism spectrum disorder (ASD) and other developmental delays who are screened, evaluated, and enrolled in early intervention services in a timely manner" (USHHS, 2014).

The U.S. Preventive Services Task Force's (USPSTF) (n.d.) Recommendations for Primary Care state that "the current evidence is insufficient to assess the balance of benefits and harms of screening for speech and language delay and disorders in children age 5 years or younger." *Bright Futures: Guidelines for Health Supervision of Infants, Children, and Adolescents* (Hagan et al, 2008) endorses surveillance and screening for the early identification and intervention of any problems with physical, cognitive, or social-emotional health. Specific cognitive skills in infancy, early childhood, middle childhood, and adolescence are identified in the child development sections. Screening for vision and hearing is recommended and considered effective.

Cognitive-Perceptual Development

Cognitive development at each stage of childhood is discussed in the earlier developmental chapters and is the basis for intelligence. There are many theories of cognitive development, but Piaget's theory of cognitive development (discussed in Chapter 4) is one of the classics. *Information processing (IP)* looks at human learning with a computer as a model. *Social cognition* looks at the spectrum of social behaviors and affiliation with others. *Neurodevelopmental functioning* of the brain uses a model of a toolkit full of basic instruments (functions) that work in clusters (like tools) in different areas of learning. The concept of *multiple intelligences* describes different ways children may be hardwired to process information. Societal, family, and individual elements can all affect a child's ability to learn and are combined in a matrix described by Wegner (2009).

Piaget: Cognitive Development

Piaget's key concepts include *assimilation* (taking in information through any and all the senses), *accommodation* (taking one's current abilities and understanding and modifying them to adjust to the new circumstance or challenge), *schema* (organizing this into a new mental structure or physical action), and *equilibrium* (a new level of cognition). See Chapter 4 for a more detailed examination of this theory.

Information Processing Theories

IP is another way to describe thinking or problem solving. It looks specifically at intellectual capabilities—how information is presented, processes used to transform information, and memory limits that constrain the amount of information that can be represented and processed. A child's ability to encode—identify and use critical information to create internal representations—is critical. If children fail to identify or comprehend critical elements or do not know how to encode them efficiently, they do not learn from potentially useful experiences. The structural components of IP include a sensory component with visual and auditory registers (like input devices for a computer), short-term storage/memory (like the central processing unit of a computer), and long-term storage/memory (like hard drive storage). Process components of IP include rehearsal activity (which is used to keep information in the short-term store [the working memory; automatic processing] and transforms information outside the direct control of the individual to retain information not consciously remembered) and the task environment or the context of the child—for example, a particular solution to a problem may create moral conflicts and thus alter the child's options. Fig. 20-1 illustrates an information-processing model.

Social Cognition

Social cognition, also called *intuition* or *common sense,* is the ability to interpret behavior and emotions of the self and others. It is not well documented and it is difficult to measure or assess, so it exists on a spectrum. There is a neural overlap with intellectual cognition, but social cognition also has distinct processes. Components of social cognition include the ability to understand thoughts, intentions, and emotions of self and others; to follow the rules of social play; to regulate one's own responses to unstructured or ambiguous social environments; to understand/anticipate how peers feel (empathy); to communicate and comprehend social meaning; and to understand body language and perceive faces.

There is a spectrum of social cognition developmental skills for each age cluster (Hansen and Ulrey, 2009). These include the following:

- Infancy—eye contact, social smile, reaching, emerging joint attention, and use of others' emotions to regulate self
- Toddler/preschool—emerging empathy, understanding social rules, constructing narratives, and reciprocity in play
- School age—functioning successfully and flexibly in both structured and unstructured situations and being "street smart"
- Adolescence—forming social group affiliations, emerging sexual identity, and social testing and teasing

Neurodevelopmental Framework

A neurodevelopmental framework is a model of learning based on a synthesis of research from neuroscience, cognitive psychology, and child and adolescent development, explaining how the brain functions and how these functions affect student learning and performance. Every person has strengths and weaknesses that influence learning, as well as particular affinities—subjects, ideas, and pursuits that they're drawn to. "Collectively, these strengths, weaknesses, and affinities shape both how we learn and what engages us—which, in turn, influence how much we actually learn and thrive in a given situation" (All Kinds of Minds, n.d.). There are eight constructs to the neurodevelopmental framework, which are listed in Table 20-1. Identifying a child's strengths and weaknesses by using these constructs provides a method to describe, organize, and address the individual child's learning needs.

Multiple Intelligences

In 1983, Dr. Howard Gardner identified eight different intelligences to account for the broad range of human potential in children and adults (Table 20-2). Gardner believed the traditional measure of intelligence based on intelligence quotient (IQ) testing was inadequate and left many talented and intelligent children and adults foundering (Smith, 2008).

Executive Functions and the Prefrontal Cortex

Executive functions are the cognitive, metacognitive, and behavioral skills required to organize purposeful goals and learn and function in school and in life. This complex

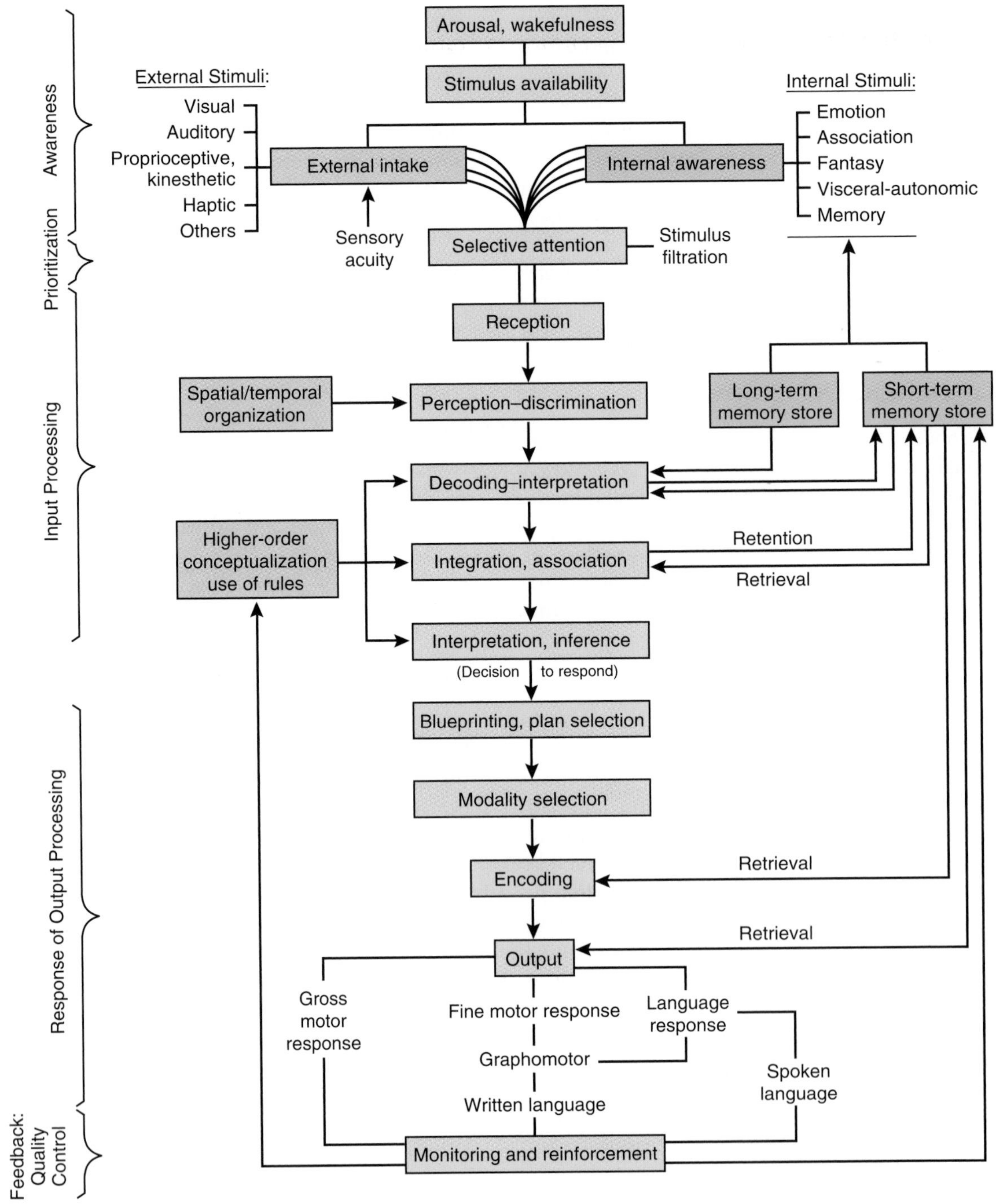

• **Figure 20-1** Information-processing model. (From Levine M, Brooks R, Shonkoff J: *A pediatric approach to learning disorders*, New York, 1980, Wiley, p 480.)

neurobiologic activity takes place in the prefrontal cortex (PFC), a highly specialized region where organization and regulation of information and stimuli occur. Specific activities include organizing and making sense of input received, sustaining focus on relevant stimuli, suppressing irrelevant stimuli (distractions), drawing on memory to understand stimuli, planning and organizing for future goals and consequences of actions, and regulating emotional and behavioral responses. These mental processes and behaviors enable self-regulation and metacognition (Barkley, 2012; Hasselhorn and Labuhn, 2011). Components of self-regulation include inhibition (the ability to stop or delay a first response, interrupt an inappropriate behavior, and resist interference by distracting thoughts or stimuli), flexibility (the ability to shift or transition between activities or thoughts), and emotional control (the ability to modify emotional expression to the most adaptive). Metacognition, the ability to think about thinking or use knowledge from the past and merge it with new tasks or challenges, is used to reflect, plan, and execute, as well as organize, be insightful, make logical

TABLE 20-1 Constructs of the Neurodevelopmental Learning Framework

Construct	Description
Attention	Maintaining mental energy for learning and work, absorbing and filtering incoming information, and overseeing the quality of academic output and behavior
Higher-order cognition (complex thinking)	Comprehending concepts, generating original ideas, and using logical approaches to address complex problems
Language	Understanding incoming oral and written information and communicating ideas orally and in writing
Memory	Briefly recording new information, mentally juggling information while using it to complete a task, and storing and then recalling information at a later time
Neuromotor functions (controlling movement)	Using large muscles in a coordinated manner, controlling finger and hand movements, and coordinating muscles needed for handwriting
Social cognition (making and keeping friends)	Knowing what to talk about, when, with whom, and for how long; working and playing with others in a cooperative manner; and nurturing positive relationships with influential people
Spatial ordering (visual thinking)	Understanding information that is presented visually, generating products that are visual, and organizing materials and spaces
Temporal-sequential ordering (keeping track of time/order)	Understanding the order of steps, events, or other sequences; generating products arranged in a meaningful order; and organizing time and schedules

From All Kinds of Minds: Learning framework, All Kinds of Minds (website), available at http://allkindsofminds.org/learning-framework. Accessed November 28, 2014.

TABLE 20-2 Multiple Intelligences

Intelligence	Description
Linguistic	Sensitivity to language; language-based function (word smart)
Logical/mathematical	Abstract reasoning, manipulation of symbols, detection of patterns, logical reasoning (number/reasoning smart)
Musical	Detection and production of musical structures and patterns; appreciation of pitch, rhythm, musical expressiveness (music smart)
Spatial	Visual memory, visual-spatial skills, visualization (picture smart)
Body/kinesthetic	Representation of ideas, feeling in movement; use of body, coordination, goal-directed activities (body smart)
Naturalistic	Classification and recognition of animals, plants (nature smart)
Social/interpersonal	Sensitivity and responsiveness to moods, motives, intentions, and feelings of others (people smart)
Personal/intrapersonal	Sensitivity to self, feelings, strengths, desires, weaknesses, and understanding of intention and motivation of others (self smart)

decisions, and complete complex activities. Components of metacognition include working memory—verbal (self-talk, blending, and organization) and nonverbal (mental representation and manipulation of visual-spatial information), problem-solving, and monitoring—task or self. Executive function disorder can occur independently but often occurs along with learning disorders, attention-deficit/hyperactivity disorder (ADHD), and ASD, as well as in children with a history of medical conditions, such as prematurity, prenatal drug and alcohol exposure, and traumatic brain injury.

Sensory Processing

Information is received from the environment through the senses: vision, hearing, touch, taste, smell, position (proprioception), and movement (vestibular). Sensory processing has to do with how individuals respond to, process, and/or organize sensory information for use in functional daily life routines and activities. Three processes of sensory integration have been used to describe sensory modulation (Miller et al, 2009):

- The regulation of responses to sensory stimulation
- Sensory discrimination—interpreting the specific characteristics of sensory stimuli (intensity, duration, spatial, and temporal elements)
- Sensory-based motor, which includes balance and core stability, as well as motor planning and sequencing movements

Social and Emotional Skills that Lead to Academic Success

Five key social and emotional skills or competencies have been identified that play a key role in shaping student achievement and future adult success: (1) self-control, (2) persistence, (3) mastery orientation, (4) academic self-efficacy, and (5) social competence (Child Trends, 2014). Self-control is the ability to manage and regulate emotion and behavior, inhibit negative responses, and delay gratification. Persistence is the ability to continue toward a goal in spite of obstacles, difficulties, or discouragement. Mastery orientation happens when a child wants to learn to increase competence or abilities rather than just to perform. Academic self-efficacy happens when children believe that they can not only perform a variety of academic tasks successfully but also understand that their actions influence outcome. Social competence is the set of skills necessary to interact successfully with others (teachers, peers, and other school officials). Although each of the skills has its own specific characteristics, they also reinforce each other.

Elements of Learning

Intelligence is the ability to learn or understand and deal with new situations. Learning occurs when there is observation (taking in information) and accommodation (revising existing mental structures). Intelligence is often measured by tests that evaluate problem-solving, language, attention, memory and IP. Language, memory, and attention are critical to achievement in school. Listening comprehension, oral expression, reading comprehension, and written expression are components of language that are important to learning. Likewise, each of the four levels of memory—(1) short-term, (2) active working, (3) consolidation in long-term, and (4) retrieval from long-term—plays a critical role in learning especially as the child progresses through school. Attention involves the ability to concentrate over time in the face of distraction, as well as the ability to shift focus when required. It is impacted by the specific task, the perceived need, and motivation. In adolescence, there is a wide variation in the ability to think and process information that is believed to be due to a complex interaction between overall cognitive ability and environmental experience.

Metacognition helps adolescents navigate the vast array of new thoughts, experiences, and emotions that they experience. However cognitive development and school achievement are dependent on a complex interweaving of society, family, and child elements. Wegner (2009) used these factors to develop a matrix that offers a way to examine the interplay of a child's individual profile, family factors, and community characteristics. Individual characteristics affecting academic performance include the following:

- Cognition—considered the predictor of academic success
- Developmental skills—play a role in contributing to intelligence
- Resilience—contributes to a child's motivation to succeed or ability to persevere through failure
- Desire for education—a personal belief that education is important and contributes to the future

Family factors that influence student educational achievement include the following:

- Community acceptance of varied types of family structures
- Family values at odds with the larger community, causing missed opportunities for the child
- Performance expectations out of line with a child's capabilities, either too high or too low
- Parental academic abilities that not only genetically influence a child's capability but also affect the home support a child may receive

Societal factors that influence educational systems include the following:

- Economic—the affluence of the community affects resources and experiences, as well as, potentially, the quality of teachers attracted
- Political—politicians may be hesitant to promote tax increases to provide needed resources for schools
- Religious—a preponderance of a specific religious group may exert influence on a school's curricula, policy, and procedures
- Cultural—as with religion, ethnic and cultural groups may exert pressure on a school

Assessment of Cognitive-Perceptual Development

Assessment of cognitive-perceptual development should be incorporated at every well-child visit from birth through young adulthood. This includes consideration of risk factors and current performance as elicited by history, screening tools, direct observation of the child and caregiver, and review of school data.

History

Risk factors that may be related include the following:

- Genetic elements—any disorder, condition, or malformation with identifiable cognitive effect (e.g., trisomy 21, velocardiofacial syndromes)
- Prenatal factors—maternal/paternal age at conception; use of tobacco, alcohol, or other substances; maternal hypertension and other complications; fetal hypoxemia or suboptimal growth

- Birth and perinatal events—adverse events during delivery; prematurity; prolonged neonatal complications, such as hyperbilirubinemia or infection
- Infancy to 3 years old—maternal depression; family wellness indicators; parental literacy; child illness or injury (e.g., traumatic brain injury, meningitis); deprivation, neglect, or abuse
- Three years old through kindergarten entry—aforementioned factors plus child interaction difficulties in larger group settings; lack of independent play or sustained interest in preferred activity, lack of expanding conversation and interactions with adults
- School age and adolescence—the aforementioned factors plus difficulties in academic settings, problems with interactions with peers or in large group settings

Screening

Monitoring hearing and vision is a crucial piece in assessment of perception. Additionally a developmental screening tool should be used consistently throughout the first 6 years of life to monitor for any lagging performance or delay. It is of note that children with cognitive-perceptual variations may achieve motor milestones on time, but experience delays in speech, social, and emotional areas of development. Developmental screening is discussed in greater detail in Chapters 4 through 8. Screening for autism using a tool such as the Modified Checklist for Autism in Toddlers (M-CHAT) is recommended at 18 and 24 months old (see the Autistic Spectrum Disorder section). If there are concerns about a child's ability to deal with sensory input, there is also a screen for that (see the Sensory Processing Disorder section).

As the child enters school, evaluation of the acquisition of academic skills, school achievement, and the child's social skill interactions becomes important. Early elementary grades (1 through 3) lay the foundation for the remainder of a child's schooling. Differentiating early struggles due to temperament, environment, or cognitive-perceptual weaknesses may be difficult but is essential. Later elementary education (grades 4 through 6) is characterized by increasing demands and need for independence. Complaints of being bored (gifted versus an overwhelmed child) and difficulty with emerging complex social hierarchy and peer influences are important to detect. During middle school, demands for independent functioning increase, whereas parental and teacher direction decreases. At the same time, significant physical and cognitive changes occur. As expectations ramp up, some children struggle academically and may have poor outcomes due to peer influence. This in turn may negatively impact any underlying chronic health condition. High school demands result in greater academic pressure as students compete for university and vocational school placements and scholarships. The need for autonomy and individuation as well as identification of personal strengths and goals are significant. Screening provides the opportunity to identify problems or concerns early in order to obtain further evaluation. School performance screeners are discussed in the Learning Disorders and Neurodevelopmental Dysfunctions section.

Management Strategies for Cognitive-Perceptual Development

Primary Care Strategies and Interprofessional Collaboration

A comprehensive, family-centered health care home needs to be the basis of care for any child with a cognitive-perceptual problem. This comprehensive approach ensures that the family/patient can access, coordinate, and understand services that are important for the child. This is discussed further in Chapter 21. The PCP has several important roles in this context. The first is to help the child/family demystify the condition or understand and clarify the issues with an upbeat positive approach. In addition to demystifying, the PCP can lead the identification and mobilization of the child's strengths. Although the caregiver can and should be the child's primary advocate, the PCP also serves to anticipate issues that may arise, providing management suggestions, fostering optimism along the way, defending the child's basic rights, and protecting the child from humiliation. All of this is done in the context of monitoring the child on an ongoing basis over time. Medication will at times be part of the management plan, and it may be handled by the PCP or in collaboration with other team members. The PCP helps families identify appropriate expert professional teams, serves as a case manager, and ensures that primary health care needs and special services are integrated. Additionally PCPs help parents explore options, develop plans of action, or act as a conduit to help parents find others who have solved similar problems. The use of a variety of professionals, including medical specialists, physical and occupational therapists, social workers, teachers with special education, psychologists, and mental health professionals provides the best resources for children with cognitive-perceptual needs.

Educational Strategies

If delays are suspected, it is extremely important to get the child quickly into early-intervention services. PCPs are in an ideal place to be able to identify and refer infants, toddlers, and preschoolers who show any concerning signs. When children reach school age, decisions should be made collaboratively between parents and school personnel about the best school placement of the child (mainstream classroom, special classroom, or combination of settings). The PCP may be involved in this decision by providing information related to the child's development in a relatively informal basis, or quite directly by advocating for the child and contributing in detail to specific plans. Children with cognitive-perceptual problems are often entitled to special education opportunities to maximize their learning potential. A wealth of information about these legal rights and provisions can be found on the Internet. The two most important federal laws, the Americans with Disabilities Act of 1990 and the Individuals with Disabilities Education Act (IDEA), reauthorized in 1997, provide mandates for reasonable accommodations that schools must provide to help children with disabilities achieve meaningful, equal opportunity to benefit from educational services. Free and Appropriate Public Education (FAPE) and Least Restrictive Environment (LRE) are parts of the special education system. A response to intervention (RTI) approach is a three-tiered response to determining if a child has a disability and qualifies for special education. It is more effective in identifying students with learning disabilities than the traditional IQ discrepancy model.

Once a child has been identified with special needs, an individualized education plan (IEP) or a Section 504 plan are two means of delineating help and accommodations for the child. Table 20-3 provides a differentiation of these two plans.

- The IEP originates from the IDEA and is designed for children who demonstrate a gap between learning potential and actual academic performance. It is a written plan defining the child's disabilities, current level of educational performance, educational needs, and specific annual goals as developed by a multidisciplinary team with parent involvement. An IEP includes specific academic, communication, motor, learning, functional, and socialization goals.
- The Section 504 plan specifies "reasonable accommodations" to help children with disabilities benefit from their education. Eligibility is based on the existence of an identified physical or mental condition that "substantially limits a major life activity" (in this case, learning). Each school district handles 504 plans differently, but there should be a 504 coordinator who oversees the process. Many children with ADHD and learning disabilities who do not have cognitive deficits but do have learning weaknesses or behavioral or emotional problems that interfere with learning are eligible for a 504 plan.

Regardless of whether or not a child with cognitive-perceptual challenges needs a formalized plan, it is essential to maintain a strengths-based approach. Helping children to identify and build upon their strengths contributes to their motivation and self-esteem. Helping the child (and family and teachers) understand and demystify whatever dysfunction or disability the child struggles with requires thoughtful analysis and input from various sources. It may be necessary at times to advocate for curriculum modifications, such as timing of a foreign language or

TABLE 20-3 Section 504 Plan and Individualized Educational Plan

Americans with Disabilities Act of 1990/Section 504 Plan	Individuals with Disabilities Education Act/Individualized Education Plan
Which Plan Fits the Child?	
For simple accommodations or minor changes Easier, faster, more flexible	Needs a wide range of services or protections More involved with mandated parental participation
Eligibility	
Based on identification of psychological or physical disorder that "substantially limits" a "major life activity" (learning and/or behavior)	Must meet criteria of qualified disability (ADHD not included); often OHI; developmental delays, emotional disturbances, or SLD that seriously affect learning or behavior and "by reason thereof" needs special education and/or related services
Evaluation	
An evaluation (not formalized testing) compiled by the school from a variety of sources to confirm assumption No money to cover evaluation or support/sustain accommodation Can occur without parental knowledge or participation	A complete evaluation compiled by a team of professionals including testing and information from a variety of sources Federally funded Must have written consent to perform
Provisions	
A plan with individualized accommodations such as extra time to complete assignments, a copy of notes, providing a quiet place to take tests, or assistive technologies No legal requirements for what is included in a 504, for parent involvement, or for mandated reevaluation	An individualized IEP describes the child's learning problems, details services to be provided, sets annual goals, and defines how progress will be measured Changes made only in meeting and in collaboration with team Special provisions if suspended or expelled Reevaluation mandated every 3 years

ADHD, Attention-deficit/hyperactivity disorder; *IEP*, individualized education plan; *OHI*, other health impairments; *SLD*, specific learning disability.

selection of math and science courses, to avoid memory overload. Remediation of skill sets is another helpful strategy that can be achieved with specialists or tutors in school resource rooms or learning centers. Although work on academic skills may be necessary, it is often just as essential to help with study skills, organizational habits, and cognitive strategies.

Family Support Strategies

Living with a child with a cognitive-perceptual problem requires an environment that offers consistency for the child. The family may be called upon to provide additional physical, emotional, and psychological support while ensuring appropriate education (advocacy, conferencing, and monitoring). Social and recreational opportunities can at times be a challenge. This can be overwhelming for not only the caregivers but also the siblings. The family must develop a structure with organization to support the child without becoming overprotective or intrusive and with consideration for the needs of all the family members. It can be helpful to parents for the PCP to provide education related to their rights and entitlements and to help them advocate for their child. Social support from community resources, parent training groups, and local support groups and national organizations that provide information and expert advice offer significant benefits to families. Support and relief may also be obtained by engaging the family with a counselor that can help them through more difficult times. Many of these resources are listed in Resources on the Evolve website.

Social and Adaptive Strategies

Social and adaptive strategies are intended to help children achieve maximal independence in living and learning in order to get along with family members and others in a variety of social environments. The family may need help to know what social and adaptive developmental steps children should master at various ages. Strategies to engage the child in learning new skills are often learned by trial and error but can also be gleaned from parents of children with similar challenges.

Children with cognitive-perceptual disorders often struggle to exhibit appropriate behaviors with other children and their peers. Social skills groups, sometimes available in schools, provide an avenue for children to learn how to better get along. Exercise and physical activity bring about biologic changes that make the brain ready to learn, be more focused and attentive, and be less moody and stressed (Brooks, 2014). Although exercise is useful for any child, it is critical for children with cognitive-perceptual issues, enabling them to relax, focus, and learn. Musical training is a useful tool to improve academic performance by increasing executive brain function, which provides inhibition, problem solving, goal direction, and cognitive flexibility (Barclay, 2014).

Cognitive-Perceptual Problems of Children

Attention-Deficit/Hyperactivity Disorder

ADHD is one of the most commonly diagnosed disorders in childhood. It is considered a neurodevelopmental disorder because it has a clear neurologic base with symptoms that can profoundly affect the behavior of individuals across many settings in their lives. Additionally, it is a chronic condition with persistence in many individuals into adolescence and adulthood. The symptoms of ADHD affect cognitive, educational, behavioral, emotional, and social functioning. Core symptoms of ADHD are inattention, hyperactivity, and impulsivity occurring at a developmentally inappropriate level observed in at least two settings (home, school, or work) with clear evidence of clinical impairment in social, academic, or occupational functioning. There is a range of severity of symptoms from one individual to the next (mild, moderate, and severe), and the scope and severity of behaviors may change within an individual as maturation occurs. Criteria defining ADHD established by the American Psychiatric Association (2014) in the *Diagnostic and Statistical Manual of Mental Disorders,* fifth edition (DSM-5) are listed in Table 20-4. These criteria are used to differentiate between three different ADHD presentations or specifiers, formerly called *subtypes* (Box 20-1).

ADHD affects self-regulation and executive functions. Self-regulation is action an individual takes that results in a change in behavior in order to modify the likelihood of a future consequence or attainment of a goal (Barkley, 2012). It requires intact executive functions of which six have been identified as being present in children with ADHD. They include the following (Brown, 2013b):

- *Activation*—organizing, prioritizing, and getting started
- *Focus*—sustaining and shifting attention to task
- *Effort*—regulating awareness, sustaining effort, and processing speed
- *Emotion*—managing frustration and modulating emotions
- *Memory*—utilizing working memory and accessing recall
- *Action*—monitoring and self-regulating action

Additionally, ADHD can have a significant impact on social relationships. Children may present with struggles in the classroom, difficulties with peers, or trouble regulating their behavior or emotions.

Prevalence in the United States

ADHD prevalence rates vary depending on the source, criteria used to make the diagnosis, and the ages sampled. A historical view provides the necessary context to understand changes in what is known about ADHD. Estimates of the incidence of ADHD in the United States range from 5% (American Psychiatric Association, 2014), to 8% (AAP et al, 2011), to 7.2% (Thomas et al, 2015 from their meta-analysis), and to 11% (13.2% male and 5.6% female;

TABLE 20-4 DSM-5 Criteria for Attention-Deficit/Hyperactivity Disorder

Domain	Criteria
Essential features	Several inattentive or hyperactive-impulsive symptoms were present before age 12 years. Several inattentive or hyperactive-impulsive symptoms are present in two or more settings (e.g., at home, school, or work; with friends or relatives; in other activities). There is clear evidence that the symptoms interfere with or reduce the quality of social, school, or work functioning. The symptoms do not happen only during the course of schizophrenia or another psychotic disorder. The symptoms are not better explained by another mental disorder (e.g., mood disorder, anxiety disorder, oppositional defiant disorder, dissociative disorder, or a personality disorder).
Inattention traits	Six or more symptoms of inattention for children up to age 16, or five or more for adolescents 17 years old and older and adults; symptoms of inattention have been present for at least 6 months, and they are inappropriate for developmental level: • Often fails to give close attention to details; makes careless mistakes in schoolwork, at work, or during other activities (e.g., overlooks or misses details, work is inaccurate) • Often has difficulty sustaining attention in tasks or play activities (e.g., has difficulty remaining focused during lectures, conversations, or lengthy reading) • Often does not seem to listen when spoken to directly (e.g., mind seems elsewhere even in the absence of any obvious distraction) • Often does not follow through on instructions and fails to finish schoolwork, chores, or duties in the workplace (e.g., starts tasks but quickly loses focus and is easily sidetracked) • Often has difficulty organizing tasks and activities (e.g., difficulty managing sequential tasks; difficulty keeping materials and belongings in order; messy, disorganized work; has poor time management; fails to meet deadlines) • Often avoids, dislikes, or is reluctant to engage in tasks that require sustained mental effort (e.g., schoolwork or homework; for older adolescents and adults, preparing reports, completing forms, reviewing lengthy papers) • Often loses things necessary for tasks or activities (e.g., school materials, pencils, books, tools, wallets, keys, paperwork, eyeglasses, mobile telephones) • Is often easily distracted by extraneous stimuli (for older adolescents and adults, may include unrelated thoughts) • Is often forgetful in daily activities (e.g., doing chores, running errands; for older adolescents and adults, returning calls, paying bills, keeping appointments)
Hyperactivity/impulsivity traits	Six or more symptoms of hyperactivity/impulsivity for children up to age 16, or five or more for adolescents 17 years old and older and adults; symptoms of hyperactivity/impulsivity have been present for at least 6 months to an extent that is disruptive and inappropriate for the person's developmental level: • Often fidgets with or taps hands or feet or squirms in seat • Often leaves seat in situations when remaining in seat is expected (e.g., leaves his or her place in the classroom, in the office or other workplace, or in other situations that require remaining in place) • Often runs about or climbs in situations in which it is inappropriate (Note: In adolescents or adults, may be limited to feeling restless) • Often unable to play or engage in leisure activities quietly • Is often "on the go," acting as if "driven by a motor" (e.g., is unable to be or uncomfortable being still for an extended time, such as in restaurants, meetings; may be experienced by others as being restless or difficult to keep up with) • Often talks excessively • Often blurts out an answer before a question has been completed (e.g., completes people's sentences; cannot wait for turn in conversation) • Often has difficulty waiting his or her turn (e.g., while waiting in line) • Often interrupts or intrudes on others (e.g., butts into conversations, games, or activities; may start using other people's things without asking or receiving permission; for adolescents and adults, may intrude into or take over what others are doing)

From American Psychiatric Association: *Diagnostic and statistical manual of mental disorders*, ed 5, Arlington, VA, 2013, American Psychiatric Association.

CDC, 2015). The percentage of children 4 to 17 years of age with a diagnosis of ADHD increased by 42% between 2003 and 2011 (CDC, 2014). However another review and meta-regression analysis done across three decades of data found that there was no evidence to suggest an increase in the number of children meeting the criteria of ADHD if standardized diagnostic procedures were followed. Instead the variability in prevalence estimates was a reflection of increasing awareness, access to treatment, or changes in clinical practice (Polanczyk et al, 2014). The average age of

• BOX 20-1 Attention-Deficit/Hyperactivity Disorder Diagnostic Presentations

ADHD, Combined Type

Significant number of symptoms from both inattention and hyperactivity/impulsivity are present

Accounts for the majority of ADHD cases

ADHD, Predominantly Inattentive

Significant number of inattentive symptoms identified, but not significant number in hyperactivity/impulsivity

Accounts for about one-third of ADHD cases

ADHD, Predominantly Hyperactive/Impulsive

Significant number of hyperactivity/impulsivity symptoms identified, but not significant number in inattention category

Accounts for less the fewest ADHD cases

ADHD, Attention-deficit/hyperactivity disorder.

diagnosis is 7 years old, with children who have severe ADHD diagnosed earlier. ADHD diagnosis prevalence varies substantially by state—from a low of 5.6% in Nevada to a high of 18.7% in Kentucky. Boys are identified with a higher prevalence than girls (2 : 1 in childhood, 1.6 : 1 across the lifespan), and girls are more likely to have the inattentive features (Brown, 2013a).

Cross-Cultural Considerations

There are racial/ethnic disparities in diagnosing ADHD. Children who are African American, Hispanic, or of other races/ethnicities are 69% less likely to be diagnosed with ADHD than white children. Morgan and colloeagues (2013) found that by eighth grade, 7% of white children had a diagnosis of ADHD compared to 3% in African American, 4.4% in Hispanic, and 3.5% in other races/ethnicities. Internationally, there is growing agreement across cultures about the presence of ADHD. Prior to the 1990s, diagnosis and treatment occurred in very few countries outside of the United States. Conrad and Bergey (2014) studied the diagnosis of ADHD in the United Kingdom, Germany, France, Italy, and Brazil and identified several vehicles that they felt facilitated what they called the "migration of the ADHD diagnosis." These elements included the transnational pharmaceutical industry, the influence of Western psychiatry, moving from the International Classification of Diseases (ICD) to DSM diagnostic criteria, the role of the Internet with easily accessible online screening checklists, and advocacy groups. A European Expert Roundtable on ADHD held in Brussels in 2012 developed a white paper identifying ADHD as one of the most neglected and misunderstood psychiatric conditions in Europe. The paper stated that although ADHD was estimated to affect approximately 1 in 20 children and adolescents across Europe, very few people received appropriate diagnosis due to the lack of public awareness and the widespread social stigma, as well as the lack of appropriate community frameworks (Young et al, 2013).

Effect of Attention-Deficit/Hyperactivity Disorder on Individuals, Families, and Communities

Because ADHD symptoms cross over so many settings and often persist into adulthood, this condition has a major effect on the individual, as well as on the family and community. Families report significantly higher levels of stress. Individuals have difficulties with peer relationships (21% vs. 3% of controls), increased nonfatal injuries (4.5% vs. 2.5% of controls), and issues with driving (traffic violations and accidents) (CDC, 2015). There are significant direct and indirect costs, including days of missed work due to the child's school and medical appointments, evaluation and treatment that are often not covered by health insurance (e.g., psychological or educational testing beyond that done at the school), and cost of medication and mental health care. Table 20-5 summarizes impairments across the lifespan.

Genetics and Neurobiologic Pathophysiology

Attention is a complex and multilayered neurologic activity requiring the function and interconnection of a number of different areas of the brain. No single cause for ADHD has been identified, although neurobiologic research is focused on understanding this condition. It is generally agreed that ADHD is primarily a genetic disorder with environmental factors modulating the predisposition to underlying biochemical vulnerability. A meta-analysis of over 1800 genetic studies determined inheritability to be between 75% to 91% (Zhang et al, 2012). It is likely that a group of genes impact the physiology of ADHD, not just a single gene, combined with in utero and early-life stressors. Genetic variations include deletions and duplications of DNA segments (copy number variants) associated with the manufacturing and regulation of the catecholamine (noradrenergic) neurotransmitters, noradrenaline and dopamine. The net result is that these neurotransmitters are less available in certain brain regions in individuals with ADHD. Both dopamine and noradrenaline (dopamine more strongly in ADHD) are essential for healthy brain function, especially for alerting to and maintaining attention, maintaining an appropriate level of internal arousal, and inhibiting external distraction.

Brain imaging studies have identified structural and functional differences in the frontal lobes and subcortical structures of the brain, indicating that ADHD brain development is significantly different from normal. However findings of a recent 15-year National Institute of Mental Health study of 446 children, half with ADHD and half without, found that the basic brain biology of children with ADHD was intact, following a normal, not disrupted, but rather delayed pattern of maturation until 3 years old (Sripada et al, 2014). This finding offers an explanation for those children whose symptoms improve or resolve as they get older.

TABLE 20-5 Summary of Attention-Deficit/Hyperactivity Disorder Impairments Across the Lifespan

Life Stage	Impairment
Childhood	Academic difficulties including: • Needs for special education (high comorbidity with learning disabilities) • Grade retention • Classroom behavior management issues • Difficulties with friendships and peer relationships • Behavioral difficulties at home and other settings (child care, sports, after-school programs) • High comorbidity with other childhood psychiatric problems • Associated difficulties (at higher rates than non-ADHD children) with sleep disorders, enuresis, encopresis
Adolescence	Academic difficulties including: • Needs for special education (high comorbidity with learning and emotional disabilities) • School failure and dropout • Social difficulties with peer relationships • Substance abuse (in untreated ADHD) • High comorbidity with other psychiatric disorders (depression, anxiety, conduct disorder) • High-risk behaviors leading to greater accident rates • Involvement in juvenile criminal activities
Adulthood	Difficulties include: • Fewer employment possibilities and higher rates of unemployment • Higher risk of tobacco, drug, and alcohol abuse • Higher risk of motor vehicle accidents • Marital discord and higher divorce rates • Increased incidence of criminal involvement

ADHD, Attention-deficit/hyperactivity disorder.

Environmental Factors

Although ADHD is primarily a genetic disorder, genes are usually expressed in interaction with the environment. As such, environmental factors may contribute to ADHD, and some genetic components may provide increased susceptibility to environmental stressors. Certain gestational and neonatal exposures seem to be significant contributors to ADHD. Although the interplay has not been well defined, potential links have been found with cigarette smoking and alcohol use during pregnancy, difficulties during birth, premature birth and low birth weight, and maternal psychosocial stress. In childhood, lead exposure, maternal malaise and depression, caregiver emotional distance, and criticism are correlated with ADHD (NIMN, 2012). Analysis of data from the 2011 National Survey of Children's Health Researchers found that many children with ADHD experience significantly higher rates of trauma than those without ADHD. This was evaluated by assessing nine adverse childhood experiences (ACEs): poverty, divorce, death of a parent/guardian, domestic violence, neighborhood violence, substance abuse, incarceration, familial mental illness, and discrimination. Children dealing with four or more ACEs were almost three times more likely to use ADHD medications compared to children with three or fewer adverse experiences. They also were more likely to have a parent rate their ADHD as moderate to severe compared to children with three or fewer ACE (AAP, 2014). Additionally, due to the genetic component, parents often have ADHD themselves, which makes it more difficult for them to provide structure and consistency. The biologic link in most of these risk factors is the stress response causing overstimulation in the developing brain as it is overexposed to catecholamines (DeSimone and Busby, 2014).

The faster pace and demands of society also impact the child with ADHD. Schools have longer school days, increasingly complex tasks, a higher pupil to teacher ratio, more lecture versus active learning, increased homework, emphasis on timed tasks and tests, and reduction of art, music, and physical education classes. The ubiquitous nature of video games on computers, game systems, and smartphones has both positive and negative effects but mostly negative. Although video games increase visual attention and the processing of information, the stimulation exceeds anything that normal life can offer, leading to impaired attention and greater impulsivity (Gentile et al, 2012). Problematic (addictive) video game use in boys with ADHD also puts them at greater risk for inattentive symptoms (Mazurek and Engelhardt, 2013).

Clinical Findings

Often, the child presents to the provider after having been referred by a child care provider, the school, or the parent/guardian. Concerns may be related to the ability to sustain attention, curb activity level, or inhibit impulsivity (core symptoms). However, concerns can also be related to memory, emotional control, organization, planning or inhibiting thoughts or actions (executive functions or cognitive control), and/or difficulty with friends and peers, following classroom rules, or regulating behavior (social relationships). ADHD symptoms affect the very life domains where children and adolescents are working on developmental mastery—school, peers, family life, sports, and recreational activities. It is important for the provider to inquire about all of these areas of the child's or teen's life.

The components of the ADHD assessment include the following:

- Interview of parent and child or adolescent for history
- Physical examination
- Information from standardized ADHD behavioral assessment scales from several different sources (parents,

caregivers, teachers, child care programs, and/or sports coaches)

- Other pertinent evaluations, such as school testing and psychological or other mental health evaluations

There is no one assessment tool to diagnose ADHD, although a number of tools and evidence-based practice guidelines are available to help clinicians develop an organized, efficient, and safe practice in assessing, diagnosing, and caring for children and adolescents with ADHD. Links to the main guidelines can be found in the Additional Resources list.

History and Physical Examination

A comprehensive history for ADHD assessment is outlined in Table 20-6. A physical examination consists of the following:

- Vital signs—weight, height, body mass index (BMI), blood pressure, pulse, and head circumference in young children
- Vision and hearing screen (if not up to date with school testing)
- General observation of child's behavior (may or may not present with ADHD symptoms in a structured clinical setting); observations of parent-child interaction
- General—dysmorphic stigmata suggestive of genetic syndrome or prenatal exposure to drugs or alcohol
- Skin—café au lait spots; signs of abuse
- Ear, nose, and throat (ENT)—signs of past recurring otitis media (scarring of tympanic membranes), signs of respiratory allergies, enlarged tonsils, sleep apnea
- Cardiovascular—heart sounds and rhythm, murmur, pulses
- Neurologic—general screening examination—mental status, speech and language, motor skills, and general cognition and mental process as appropriate for age
- Screening for anemia, lead, and thyroid dysfunction, if indicated

TABLE 20-6 Attention-Deficit/Hyperactivity Disorder History

Assessment Area	Suggested Topics to Explore
Chief complaint and history of present problem	Major areas of concern and beliefs about causation of problem First awareness of problem and previous evaluations and results Medication history for behavioral, emotional, or learning problems
Birth history*	Prenatal history; maternal health; use of medications, recreational drugs, alcohol, and tobacco during pregnancy Birth and postpartum complications, prematurity, low birth weight or intrauterine growth retardation, anoxia, difficult delivery, birth defects Neonatal behavior: Feeding, sleep, temperament problems
Medical history	Chronic diseases, ongoing medications, environmental allergies Hospitalizations, prolonged illness Trauma history (head injury, frequent injuries) Poisoning or lead or environmental exposures Neurologic status, seizures, tics, habit spasms, uncontrolled twitches, outbursts of uncontrollable sounds or words Cardiovascular history
General health*	Vision, hearing
ADHD history	Attention: Paying attention, sustaining attention, listening, following through, organization, reluctant to engage in activities that need sustained attention, loses things, distracted, forgetful Activity: Fidgets, leaves seat, runs or climbs when inappropriate, has difficulty with quiet games, talks excessively, has problems waiting turn, interrupts, "on the go"
Developmental history*	Milestones: Motor, personal/social, language, cognitive Strengths (e.g., personality, activities, friendliness) and weaknesses
Behavioral history*	Frequency with which child complies when told to do something Methods used at home to improve behavior and effectiveness Parenting skills and style, cultural beliefs, and agreement about child management Counseling history for child or family (or both)
Academic history	Child's progress at each grade level (strengths seen) Adjustment problems at school, child's history with peers, friendships Difficulties with specific skills: Reading, writing, spelling, math, concepts Performance problems: Attention, grades, participation, excessive talking, disturbing others, fighting, bullying, teasing, abusive language, not completing work School assistance: Tutoring, counseling, special help

Continued

TABLE 20-6 Attention-Deficit/Hyperactivity Disorder History—cont'd

Assessment Area	Suggested Topics to Explore
Functional Health Patterns	
Feeding	Not able to sit through a complete meal, messy and clumsy with utensils, dishes, and glasses Inadequate caloric intake can be result of symptoms and further exacerbated by medications used to treat ADHD Gastric distress may be a side effect of stimulant medication
Elimination	Enuresis, encopresis
Sleeping	Difficulty falling asleep, night waking, needs less sleep than other family members Complains about fatigue interfering with completion of tasks
Activity	Difficulty maintaining routines for activities of daily living
Cognitive	Level of performance is below potential for achievement Tends to miss the point of conversations and activities Often does things the hard way in absence of established routines
Self-concept	Struggles with low self-esteem, moodiness
Role relationships	General family relationships (child and parents/siblings) Home, day care, and school environments Births, deaths, marriage, and family transitions, recent moves; parental deployment, separation, divorce, remarriage Violence: Domestic, current or past abuse of parent or child; problems with the law; weapons in the home Inadequate social and relational skills Lies, steals, plays with fire, hurts animals, is aggressive with other children, talks back to adults
Coping and stress tolerance	Family stress (e.g., parent job loss or change, financial problems) and coping patterns Outbursts of temper, low tolerance for frustration Moody, worried, sad, quiet, destructive, fearful or fearless, self-deprecating Somatic complaints
Family and environmental history*	ADHD, neurologic problems, learning difficulties Mental health history of close family members, health or behavior problems in other family members Genetic disorders: Cognitive disabilities, growth disorders, neurofibromatosis Drug or alcohol abuse (current and/or past), involvement with law enforcement, weapons in the home
Teacher history	Obtain information from school about child's problems, strengths, weaknesses, academic management of issues

ADHD, Attention-deficit/hyperactivity disorder.
*These must be included in the assessment.

Attention-Deficit/Hyperactivity Disorder Standardized Assessment (Behavior) Scales and Other Diagnostic Tools

Evidence-based practice guidelines recommend the use of ADHD-specific behavior rating scales. These scales should be completed independently by individuals who know the child or adolescent from at least two different domains of life (e.g., home, school, and day care). They provide the most objective data to assess the scope and severity of the symptoms. It is essential to include school data in the evaluation process. As children get older and attend middle or high school, it is appropriate to obtain information from teachers who work with the student throughout the school day. This information provides valuable insight into symptom variation at different hours of the day, as well as clues to possible learning difficulties in specific subjects.

Behavioral rating scales are also extremely useful to monitor change once treatment has begun. A number of different behavioral scales have been developed to evaluate ADHD, some that also screen for executive function and comorbidities. Commonly used ones include the Vanderbilt ADHD Scales, the ADHD Rating Scale IV, Conners Parent and Teacher Rating Scales, and the Child Attention Profile. All can be found online, some at no charge. It is generally recommended that a provider consistently use one scale to become familiar with its scoring and interpretation.

Objective measures of ADHD are mostly used in research rather than clinical practice. Computerized tests, such as the Test of Variables of Attention (TOVA), Gordon Diagnostic, Conners CPT, the Quotient ADHD test, and the Neuropsychiatric EEG-Based Assessment Aid (NEBA) System are examples.

Differential Diagnosis and Comorbidities

There is a high incidence of other disorders that coexist with, or look similar to, ADHD. It is important to assertain if the symptoms being reported are caused by ADHD with comorbidity or the comorbid disorder is masquerading as ADHD. The approach to treatment may be very different. Additionally, some of these coexisting conditions may manifest over time, so monitoring for these conditions after assessment is critical. Sleep disorders occur in up to half of children with ADHD, and the co-occurrence must be differentiated from solely sleep pathology. Having disrupted sleep can worsen ADHD symptoms. Learning disorders, especially language and reading, occur in almost half of children with ADHD. Emotional or behavioral disorders are common and include reaction to trauma, anxiety (25%), mood disorders like depression or bipolar depression (20%), and oppositional defiant or conduct disorder (35%) (AAP, 2015).

Management

Diagnostic Formulation and Initial Meeting with Family and Child

Once the provider obtains data from the complete history and physical examination, behavioral rating scales from the various domains, and any other evaluations (school reports, psychoeducational testing, mental health assessment), it is important to assess the onset, duration, and settings where impairment is present, as well as the nature and degree of symptoms and functional impairment. A clinical judgment is required about the effect of core and associated symptoms on academic achievement and classroom performance; family, peer, and authority relationships; sports and recreation participation; and behavioral and emotional regulation with thoughtful consideration of the possibility of coexisting conditions. This review leads to a preliminary diagnosis: (1) findings that are all within a normal range of development; (2) findings that are consistent with a different diagnosis; (3) findings that are mildly or inconsistently elevated compared to peers but not associated with any functional impairment; or (4) findings that fit with the diagnosis of ADHD in one of the sub-presentations—predominantly inattentive, predominately hyperactive/impulsive, or combined.

After evaluating all of the information it is imperative to set aside sufficient time to discuss the findings with the family in detail. This discussion should be comprehensive and use a biopsychosocial framework so that the parents clearly understand their child's attentional difficulties as part of an inclusive picture of his or her functioning at school, home, and in the community. Families need education about associated coexisting mental health diagnoses and issues, academic performance issues, learning disabilities, developmental concerns, medical diagnoses, social concerns, family issues, and stressors (Dobie et al, 2012). For those children not meeting the criteria for ADHD and who do not have another condition identified, it is equally important to meet with their families to review findings and establish a plan that includes close monitoring and further evaluation of their learning or behavior problems.

Although the discussion of ADHD is often one of identifying difficulties and vulnerabilities in many dimensions of a young person's life, it is imperative for clinicians to identify the child's and family's strengths and to build on those during the entire diagnostic and treatment process. It is also worthwhile to share the perspective that, although some of these traits are a problem in childhood, the high energy, creativity, humor, and flexibility in ideation can actually lead to a successful career. Note some of the very famous and successful people with ADHD (e.g., Albert Einstein, Michael Jordan, and Walt Disney).

ADHD occurs within a sociocultural framework, and keeping this perspective while working with families is helpful. As a culture we value attention and control of impulsivity and are continually raising educational standards. Perceptions about parenting and childrearing, beliefs about medication and the health care system in general, family and social networking roles in managing child behavior problems, and parents' own experiences with school are all factors that shape the approach to seeking care, diagnosis, and treatment. Families may have differing understandings of what constitutes behavior problems. Providers who are most successful in working with families are open and honest in the discussion of diagnoses and all treatment options and include key family members in collaborative decision-making, striving to become more aware of the community and cultural values of the populations with which they work.

Educating Child, Family, and School Personnel

The parents should receive information on common features of ADHD and how they relate to the child's previous and current problems, as well as future expectations of the clinical course and intervention strategies. The importance of teacher selection each year should be emphasized. For the child, a developmentally appropriate explanation and demystification of ADHD are essential—knowing how attention works and identifying their own strengths and attributes, as well as the areas of weakness that need support. Communication with the school personnel is imperative in order to provide specific teacher-focused information about diagnosis and difficulties in all identified areas and to address appropriate intervention strategies and modifications.

Families need to be well educated about the disorder as a large part of the treatment for ADHD involves parent-child management techniques. The chronic nature of ADHD has a tremendous effect on family functioning and treatment compliance. Conversely, family factors play a part in the outcomes for children with ADHD. Parents often have to educate others about the special needs of their child. Because children with ADHD manifest a great variety of behaviors, parents are the experts who ultimately manage the problems and impact the outcome for their child. There are many excellent resources for reliable patient education about ADHD. Likewise, education of the child or adolescent, the parents, teachers, and other caregivers is critical. Providers should have several resources available that they are familiar with and comfortable recommending to families.

Plan of Care, Special Health Needs Status, and Medical Home

After review of data with the family, it is important to recognize that the child has special health care needs and is best served within a health care home. Ideally the PCP serves as care coordinator with strong family-school partnerships. Establishing a long-term, comprehensive plan of care with a focus on the areas of functional impairment (academic achievement; relationships—parent, peer, sibling, and adult authority; social skills—sports and recreational participation; and behavior and emotional regulation) is the next step. A key element of the plan is short-term target goals—approximately three key, specific, measureable items at a time from the areas that are most impaired, incorporating the child's strengths and resiliency (Box 20-2). The plan of care focuses on three major areas: pharmacologic (or medication) management, behavior management, and supportive services for functional areas. The health care home ensures that appropriate, regular follow-up care occurs.

Pharmacologic Management

Medications effectively reduce core symptoms and are recommended for, and limited to, children who meet the diagnostic criteria of ADHD. Stimulants are considered the most effective medications, but three non-stimulants (one selective norepinephrine-reuptake inhibitor and two α_2-adrenergic agonists) are also efficacious. Medication selection depends on the age of the child, the desired timing and length of coverage, other coexisting conditions, and insurance coverage. Current available and approved medications are listed in Table 20-7. The PCP's initial focus needs to be on finding the medication and dosage that best fits the child's needs.

Stimulants. The first-line medications for uncomplicated ADHD treatment are the stimulants, methylphenidate and amphetamine compounds, which are each equally effective and available in a variety of forms. The stimulants work by increasing the availability of neurotransmitters at the neuron synapses by blocking the transporters that remove dopamine and norepinephrine in the pathways in key areas of the brain where ample bioavailability of these compounds is essential but decreased. This action is theorized to allow the child to exhibit more purposeful, goal-oriented behavior by focusing attention, lessening impulsiveness, and decreasing motor activity. Between 70% and 90% of children respond positively to one of the stimulant medications (see Table 20-7), although there is no predictor for which one will be better for any individual. If treatment at the highest tolerated dose of one stimulant group does not help (the child is a non-responder), the recommendation is to try a medication from the other group, or a different medication from the same group.

Special Considerations in Choosing a Stimulant. Because both compounds of stimulants are equally efficacious and the side effect profiles are the same, consider the severity of impairment, coexisting conditions or vulnerabilities, and whether an extended-release or short-acting form is the best fit. Children with predominantly inattentive presentation often respond well to lower doses, whereas children with predominantly hyperactive presentation have a more positive response at moderate to high doses. In general, the long-acting forms are preferred because no midday school dosing is required, thus providing smoother coverage, greater convenience, improved compliance, and less stigma. The second-generation, extended-release preparations have one of two delivery mechanisms: bimodal—beaded formulation with short- and long-acting beads, and ascending—capsule with multiple layers and an osmotic pressure delivery system that increases the blood level as the day goes on (Cook, 2014). A short-acting medication might be chosen if dosage titration or side effects are of concern.

When working with the adolescent, it is important to assess for substance abuse and, if identified, refer for treatment prior to prescribing stimulants for ADHD. If no risk is detected but there are concerns about stimulant diversion (e.g., selling the drug to other students), lisdexamfetamine or dermal methylphenidate are stimulants that make this less likely due to their pharmacokinetics. Alternatively, one of the non-stimulant drugs can be chosen. Additionally, the provider must be thoughtful about the risks that an adolescent ADHD driver faces and the long and late hours when studying often occurs, and consider which medications best provide coverage for these situations.

Preschoolers, 4 to 5 years old, are also a special consideration, and the diagnosis must be approached with care. Symptoms in preschoolers are often related to other conditions, such as language disorders, hearing loss, low intellectual functioning, or other psychopathology. Behavioral therapy, most often in the form of group parent training, is the first line of treatment and has been shown more effective than methylphenidate in a comprehensive review (Charach et al, 2013). However, medication can be considered for a child who has moderate to severe dysfunction, whose symptoms have persisted for at least 9 months, and whose dysfunction has manifested not only at home but also in preschool or child care and/or who has an inadequate response to behavioral therapy medication (AAP et al, 2011). However, there are medication issues that need consideration. Dextroamphetamine is approved by the U.S. Food and Drug Administration (FDA, 2011) for children younger than 6 years old with ADHD, but there is a paucity of research about its safety in this age group. Early, classic studies show safety and efficacy using methylphenidate in this age group (Pliszka and AACAP Work Group on Quality Issues, 2007), but the FDA has not approved it for children younger than 6 years old, making its use off-label. Because of the low dose (0.15 to 0.3 mg/kg/day of methylphenidate given two or three times a day [maximum at 1 mg/kg/day in studies]), only short acting forms are available (Horst,

• BOX 20-2 Ideas for Family Support, Home Management, Friends, and Activities for Children with Attention-Deficit/Hyperactivity Disorder

Family Support

- *Routines, rules, and family relationships* are key areas. Home should be a respite, and feeling valued is critical. Life with ADHD is stressful for the child and the family, and remembering to keep these areas in good shape helps ease the stress.
- *Family meetings* provide opportunity to discuss structure, rewards, and consequences, as well as plan and problem solve.
- *Support and advocacy groups* can offer understanding and specific expertise in managing daily problems that come from living with a diagnosis of ADHD (see Resources on the Evolve website).
- *Family therapy or counseling* is frequently used short term with goals specific to the family's situation. It is especially helpful if there is aggressive behavior or problems related to anxiety, self-esteem, and depression or if other family members (especially siblings) are in need of psychological assessment or support.
- *"Coaching"* assists a child or adolescent develop skills that are difficult. Problem solving, time management, and organizational skills, as well as learning strategies (how to be an active learner, learning how to learn, and learning how to organize learning) are areas in which coaching is successful.
- *Consistent inconsistency* is the rule—it is not poor attitude or lack of motivation, it is part of the biology of ADHD.

Home Management

- *Environmental management:* A calm, predictable home with clear, consistent morning and evening routines is extremely helpful for the child with ADHD. An organized place for everyday things to go is another way to provide structure.
- *Homework support* is essential (Box 20-3). Mental fatigue should be monitored.
- *Exercise:* Aerobic exercise has been shown to improve clinical, cognitive, and scholastic performance, because it increases dopamine and norepinephrine levels, as well as serotonin. Scheduling daily time to be active and expend energy especially in the morning before school is extremely important in helping children with ADHD stay regulated. Tai chi and karate, which demand discipline and self-control, are especially useful.
- *Downtime or senseless fun:* Children with ADHD need more time than most children for normal activities of childhood, including time to do nothing and daydream. Time in less-structured activities improves self-directed executive function (Barker et al, 2014).
- *Computers:* Many children with ADHD have a very positive view of computers; they are "unconditionally accepting, produce neat results, never criticize, offer second and third chances, can help with spelling and organization, and provide much needed fun and relaxation" (Jellinek, 2008, p 41). Keep an open mind to their use with the parameter that they should not be used to the point of social isolation.
- *Nutrition:* Regular mealtimes with normal portion sizes provide structure in eating healthy, appropriate meals that provide necessary energy. Saltine crackers with the morning dose of stimulant medication can decrease complaints of stomachaches. Instant breakfast drinks and other high-calorie foods supplement calories when the child has low caloric intake because of difficulty sitting through meals or side effects of medications. Cyproheptadine (Periactin) is sometimes used as an appetite stimulant.
- *Sleep:* Many children and adults with ADHD do not require as much sleep as other people or have trouble initiating sleep or staying asleep. It is important to ask if the child is sleeping well and staying in bed the entire night. Ritualized bedtime routines are important; massage, deep breathing, and relaxation techniques are sometimes helpful. Melatonin (2 to 6 mg/day), low dose clonidine, or an antihistamine may be helpful; however, long-term use of these agents is not supported by clinical evidence or efficacy.
- *Patience, unconditional love, and support* are especially important for children with ADHD, because they face so many challenges in getting through their day. Plan a daily "time in" for 15 to 20 minutes with undivided parent attention focused on a child-selected activity.
- Complementary treatments may also have some benefit (see Chapter 43).

Friends and Activities

- *Social skills training:* This training is intended to increase knowledge about appropriate and inappropriate social behaviors. Maintaining eye contact, initiating and maintaining conversation, sharing, and cooperating are often target skills. Social skills groups may be through school or other community resources. Research on the efficacy of teaching social skills to children with ADHD has been disappointing; the difficulty seems to be not a lack of knowledge of what behavior is appropriate but rather a lack of ability to act on what is known.
- *Areas of strength* should be developed (music, sports, computer) rather than always focusing on areas of weakness. Camps, clubs, and appropriate work can provide avenues for development of skills and new friendships.
- *Activities* of the child's choosing in areas of strength or developmentally appropriate work can help build peer relationships and self-esteem.
- *Friendships* may come more easily if structure is provided (going to a movie or a sporting event) and the time frame is consistent with what the child can handle.
- *Musical training* has been shown to facilitate development and maintenance of certain executive functioning skills that may be helpful to children with ADHD (Barclay, 2014).

ADHD, Attention-deficit/hyperactivity disorder.

2013). Consider that the rate of metabolism for stimulant medications in this age group is slower, so the starting dose should be lower and the dose increase smaller. Careful monitoring for side effects and an off-medication trial after 6 months are recommended (Ghuman and Ghuman, 2014).

When dosing stimulants, it is important to remember that:

- Dose response is unique to each child/teen and should be adjusted for age, body weight, degree of impairment, and specific symptoms targeted for improvement

TABLE 20-7 Stimulant Medications Used to Treat Attention-Deficit/Hyperactivity Disorder Symptoms

Medication	Dosing Form/Units	Duration and Pattern of Release	Starting Dosage (Maximum Dosage)	Approved Age	Comments
Amphetamines (0.3 to 0.8 mg/kg/day; maximum 1.5 mg/kg/day; rare to exceed 0.8 mg/kg/day)					
Amphetamine and dextroamphetamine (Adderall XR) (mixed amphetamine salts)	Daily 5-, 10-, 15-, 20-, 25-, 30-mg capsule	8 to 12 hours; 50% immediately released; 50% released 4 hours later	10 mg; increase 10 mg weekly (40 mg)	6+	May sprinkle on applesauce and swallow without chewing
Amphetamine and dextroamphetamine (Adderall) (mixed amphetamine salts)	bid or tid 5-, 7.5-, 10-, 12.5-, 15-, 20-, 30-mg scored tablet	4 to 6 hours; 100% released immediately	5 mg daily or bid; increase 2.5 mg/wk (40 mg)	3+	FDA approved for 3- to 5-year-olds
Dextroamphetamine (Dexedrine)	bid or tid 5-, 10-mg tablet	4 to 5 hours; 100% released immediately	5 mg daily or bid; increase 5 mg/wk (40 mg)		FDA approved for 3- to 5-year-olds, 2.5 mg daily with increase of 2.5 mg/wk
Dextroamphetamine (Dexedrine Spansule)	bid 5-, 10-, 15-mg spansule	4 to 8 hours; 40% released immediately; 60% released continuously	5 mg daily; increase 5 mg/wk (40 mg)	3-16	May sprinkle on applesauce and swallow without chewing
Lisdexamfetamine (Vyvanse)	Daily 10-, 20-, 30-, 40-, 50-, 60-, 70-mg capsule	10 to 12 hours; released continuously	20 mg daily (70 mg)	6-12	May sprinkle contents in glass of water; needs to be drunk immediately
Methylphenidates (0.5 to 1.0 mg/kg/day; maximum 2.0 mg/kg/day; rare to exceed 1.0 mg/kg/day)					
Methylphenidate (Concerta)	Daily 18-, 27-, 36-, 54-mg tablet	9 to 12 hours; 22% released immediately; 78% released continuously ascending pattern	18 mg daily; increase 18 mg/wk (72 mg)	6+	Non-crushable; must be swallowed whole
Methylphenidate (Daytrana); skin patch	Daily 10-, 15-, 20-, 30-mg transdermal patch	10 to 12 hours; released continuously ascending pattern; higher plasma levels than oral	Apply 2 hours before desired effect (30 mg)	6+	Remove after 9 hours (may remove earlier); drug effect continues for 3 hours after removal Skin hypersensitivity especially if patch not removed after 9 hours
Dexmethylphenidate (Focalin)	bid or tid 2.5-, 5-, 10-mg tablet	4 to 6 hours; 100% released immediately	2.5 mg bid; increase 2.5-5 mg increments (20 mg)	6-17	

Dexmethylphenidate (Focalin XR)	Daily or bid 5-, 10-, 15-, 20-, 30-mg capsule	6 to 10 hours; 50% released immediately; 50% released in 4 hours; bimodal pattern	5 mg; increase 5 mg/wk (20 mg)	6+	May sprinkle on applesauce and swallow without chewing
Methylphenidate (Ritalin)	bid or tid 5-, 10-, 20-mg tablet	2 to 4 hours; 100% released immediately	5 mg (60 mg)	6+	Rapid onset, rapid termination of action
Methylphenidate (Ritalin LA)	Daily 10-, 20-, 30-, 40-mg capsule	6 to 10 hours; 50% released immediately; 50% modified release; bimodal pattern	10 mg daily; increase 10 mg/wk (60 mg)	6+	May sprinkle on applesauce and swallow without chewing
Methylphenidate (Quillivant XR)	Daily 25 mg/5 mL liquid	8 to 10 hours; 20% immediate-release and 80% extended-release	20 mg daily; increase 10-20 mg/wk (60 mg)	6+	Only time-released liquid Shake bottle well before use Refrigerate
Non-Stimulant and Alpha-Agonists					
Atomoxetine (Strattera)	Daily or twice daily 10-,18-, 25-, 40-, 60-, 80-, 100-mg capsule	18 to 24 hours; immediate-release	<70 kg: 0.5 mg/kg/day; increase every 3 days to 1.2 mg/kg/day (1.4 mg/kg/day or 100 mg) >70 kg: 40 mg; increase every 3 days to 80 mg (100 mg)	6+	May take 2 to 4 weeks for peak effect; must be taken 7 days a week Give with food to minimize adverse effects
Guanfacine (Intuniv)	Daily 1-, 2-, 3-, 4-mg tablet	Extended-release	1 mg for the first week; then increase by 1 mg/week (4 mg)	6+	Monotherapy or adjunct to stimulant; may need to take for 2 weeks for effect Do not give with high-fat meal; do not discontinue abruptly
Clonidine (Kapvay)	Initiate therapy HS: as increase dose, split dose to equal dose twice daily or higher dosage HS 0.1-, 0.2-mg tablet; week-long patch 0.1 mg/day, 0.2 mg/day, 0.3 mg/day	Extended-release	Begin with 0.1 mg HS; increase 0.1 mg/wk	6+	Monotherapy or adjunct to stimulant; may take 1 to 2 weeks to appreciate effect; typically requires bid dosing; do not discontinue abruptly

bid, twice a day; *FDA,* U.S. Food and Drug Administration; *HS,* at bedtime; *tid,* three times a day.

- Dosing begins at the low end and can be titrated up every 1 to 3 weeks with monitoring for symptom improvement and side effects at each dose change
- Approximately one third of children/teens respond at the low dose, one third at mid-dose range, and one third require the higher doses for maximum benefit
- The dosing goal is maximum reduction of ADHD core symptoms with minimal side effects
- If the child or teen arrives at the maximum dose without benefit or experiences side effects, change to a different medication, the other stimulant group, or a non-stimulant medication
- Families should be instructed to monitor for benefit and adverse effects so that the lowest effective dose can be recognized

When a change in medication is needed, consider the following (Cook, 2014):

- An amphetamine is roughly 1.5 times as potent as methylphenidate
- Focalin products are roughly two times more potent than regular methylphenidate products, and Daytrana is roughly 1.5 times immediate release methylphenidate
- Vyvanse potency is less than other amphetamine products with estimated 30 mg = Adderall 10 mg; Vyvanse 50 mg = Adderall 20 mg; Vyvanse 70 mg = Adderall 30 mg
- Consider augmenting a stimulant medication with an extended release α-agonist (see later) if there is benefit from the stimulant but still some residual symptoms at maximum dosage

Side Effects, Contraindications, Cardiac Warning, and Tics. Common adverse effects for any of the stimulants include decreased appetite, weight loss, insomnia, stomachache, and headache. With time, these symptoms often resolve but must be monitored. If they persist, they may be dealt with by decreasing the dose, switching the medication, or adding a medication. Concerns about the effect of stimulants on growth exist, but a recent longitudinal study showed that stimulant medication is not associated with any differences in adult height or changes in growth (Harstad et al, 2014b). Emotional lability and irritability, especially if persistent and not just the result of the medication wearing off, can indicate the need to adjust the dose, change the medication, or revisit at the diagnosis. Contraindications to stimulants include psychosis or any previous untoward reactions to stimulant medication. If using transdermal methylphenidate, the skin may be irritated where the patch is applied; alternating sites, good skin care, and moisturization will usually take care of the irritation. The use of a topical steroid may be useful for irritation or itching.

Cardiac Warning. The FDA published a study in 2011 showing that there was no association between the use of certain ADHD medications, including stimulants and atomoxetine, and adverse cardiovascular effects—stroke, myocardial infarction, or sudden cardiac death. The recommendations from this study state that the medications should be used according to the professional prescribing label, and generally the stimulant medications and atomoxetine should not be given to anyone with serious heart problems or for whom an increase in blood pressure or heart rate would be problematic. Screening for cardiovascular risk prior to initiating treatment with any of the ADHD medications includes: (1) a cardiac history for any shortness of breath with exercise, exercise intolerance, fainting or seizures with exercise, palpitations, elevated blood pressure, previously detected cardiac abnormalities, rheumatic fever, cardiomyopathy, and/or dysrhythmia; (2) a family cardiac history for sudden unexplained or cardiac death before age 35, or any rate, rhythm, or structural cardiac problems in the family, and (3) complete physical examination with special attention to the cardiovascular system. A screening tool for sudden death risk factors among children starting stimulant medication is available online (https://www.icsi.org/_asset/60nzr5/ADHD-Interactive0312.pdf) (Dobie et al, 2012). If the cardiac history and examination are negative, no further tests are recommended prior to starting ADHD medication. If there are any positives in the history or examination, a consultation with a pediatric cardiologist is necessary before initiating medication.

Tics and Tic Disorders. Approximately 20% of all children develop tics, although often these are mild and simple in complexity and typically resolve within a year. Children with ADHD are more likely to have tics, with up to 20% developing a chronic tic disorder. Likewise, over half of children with Tourette syndrome or chronic tic disorder have coexisting ADHD, and typically ADHD emerges before onset of tics. Although the FDA issued a contraindication to the use of methylphenidates and a warning for amphetamine use in patients with preexisting tic disorders or those with a family history of Tourette syndrome, stimulant medication is unlikely to evoke or exacerbate tics and may even improve tic symptoms and reduce oppositional behaviors. However, stimulants may exacerbate anxiety disorders and thus worsen the tics. No one drug is less likely to cause or exacerbate tics, but methylphenidate has been studied more. The recommendation is to start with a low dose of short-acting stimulant and then switch to a long-acting stimulant if tolerated. If ineffective or intolerable, try the alternate stimulant or the addition or substitution of an α-agonist. Atomoxetine (Strattera), although not as well studied in this population, is considered a satisfactory drug (Myers and Zinner, 2013). If tics emerge after medication is started, are not severe or disturbing to the child or adolescent, and the medication is having a net benefit, it is acceptable to continue treatment with the stimulant. If the tics worsen, are disturbing, or become chronic, switching to an alternate medication or adding an α-agonist is an option.

Atomoxetine. Atomoxetine is a noncontrolled, nonstimulant medication approved as a first-line medication for ADHD for children older than age 6 years. Atomoxetine is a norepinephrine reuptake inhibitor that works to increase norepinephrine availability in key areas of the brain. Unlike the stimulants, the effects of atomoxetine are not immediate, and patients need to be advised that it may take up to 6 weeks of regular use before effects are noted. It is usually dosed once a day, but it can be given twice daily. Although it is not as effective as either methylphenidate or amphetamine, atomoxetine may be a preferable first choice if the family prefers a non-stimulant medication, a substance abuse concern exists in the family, a child has had side effects with the stimulants, or tics, anxiety, or sleep initiation difficulties. Additionally, it provides the benefit of 24-hour coverage, but it must not be discontinued abruptly.

Side Effects and Warnings. Common adverse effects of atomoxetine include decreased appetite, gastrointestinal complaints (nausea, anorexia), somnolence and dizziness, and mild increase in blood pressure or heart rate. Most of these resolve with time—headaches are the most likely to persist—and can be managed with dose reduction or change of medication.

Warning: Liver Toxicity. There have been a few reports of an idiosyncratic reaction causing liver toxicity in patients taking atomoxetine. Currently, there is no recommendation to do liver studies prior to initiating treatment. However if evidence of jaundice or elevated liver function is found, the medication should be stopped. Patients may be cautioned to report dark urine, flulike illness, fatigue, abdominal pain, or nausea.

Warning: Suicidal Thinking or Attempts. There have also been a few reports of an increased risk of suicidal ideation or attempts in children and adolescents being treated with atomoxetine. Although the risk is small, parents and patients should be advised that if there is any change in mood—depression, mood lability, agitation, suicidal thoughts or gestures—they must get care immediately. Preexisting and development of suicidal thoughts, hallucinations, psychosis, or mania are absolute contraindications. These children need referral to a qualified mental health clinician.

Warning: Severe Cardiovascular Disorders. Because of the possibility of increased blood pressure or heart rate that could be clinically important (for example, a 15 to 20 mm Hg rise in blood pressure or 20 beats per minute increase in heart rate), the FDA has recommended that atomoxetine should not be used in those individuals with tachyarrhythmias or hypertension (FDA, 2014).

Second-Line or Adjunct Medications. Extended-release guanfacine (Intuniv) and extended-release clonidine (Kapvay) are approved for treatment of ADHD in children 6 years old and older, although evidence of efficacy is not as strong as for the stimulants or atomoxetine. Intuniv is the first ADHD medication to improve oppositional symptoms in addition to ADHD core symptoms, especially impulsivity. Kapvay is especially helpful in children with sleep issues. Like atomoxetine, these medications do not worsen tics, are not typically abused, and may be especially effective with children who have trouble sleeping or conduct disorder symptoms. It takes approximately 2 weeks to appreciate any effect; once a day dosing and more stable plasma concentration are benefits. Additionally, both of these have FDA approval as adjunctive therapy to stimulant medications and can provide additional symptom reduction.

A cardiovascular history and full physical examination are recommended (see section on Stimulants) prior to initiating these medications. The most common adverse effects of these α-agonists include sedation, bradycardia, and abdominal pain. With guanfacine, these effects tend to resolve over time. Monitoring blood pressure and heart rate is important, but decreases in either do not require discontinuation of medication unless the child becomes symptomatic (e.g., hypotensive or bradycardic). Instruct the family not to abruptly discontinue the medication because of the possibility of rebound hypertension.

Behavior Management

Behavior management is a set of specific interventions with the goal of modifying the physical and social environment to alter behavior. There are a variety of parenting programs that help caregivers give differential attention to and set up rewards and reinforcers for positive behavior, give clear and effective commands and structure, and establish safe and consistent discipline strategies. Although behavioral management modalities are not as powerful as medication in reducing core ADHD symptoms, these treatments are clearly effective. Behavior management exclusive of medication should be used if the child is younger than 6 years old, symptoms are mild, and/or DSM criteria are not met. Medication paired with behavior management is used when there is a poor response to medication alone, there are psychosocial stressors or coexisting conditions, or when the parents desire it. Children receiving both medication and behavior management have more reports of parent and teacher satisfaction, as well as lower dosages of medication, than children receiving only medication or behavior management (AAP, n.d.).

Parent Skills Training and Cognitive-Behavioral Therapy. The goal of parent skills training is for parents to learn ways to set children up for success by giving the child direction, setting goals and limits to improve compliance, increasing self-esteem, enhancing the parent-child relationship, and reducing struggles in the home. Three essential components include: (1) increasing positive parent-child interactions, (2) practicing different scenarios with one's own child, and (3) learning time-out/disciplinary consistency. If parents disagree about management or do not get along, this approach is not likely to work.

Thoughts and beliefs exert an influence on and are influenced by emotions, experiences, and actions. Cognitive-behavioral therapy (CBT) utilizes psychoeducation, direction, and new skills to modify behavior. CBT specific to ADHD includes organization and planning, managing distractibility, using adaptive thinking, and application of skills to improve procrastination.

Classroom Management, Adaptive Technology, Peer Interventions, and Neurofeedback. Behavior management can also be used in the classroom with the goal of improved attention to instruction and work productivity, as well as decreased disruptive behavior. Common techniques include increased structure with the use of behavior contracts with goals and reinforcement. Using token economy (earning or losing points that can be exchanged for privileges or items) or creating a periodic behavior report card are common examples.

There are multiple different ways that adaptive technology can be used to assist the child with ADHD. Voice-activated software that helps with writing papers, note-taking pens that allow note taking that then downloads into a computer, visual thinking tools, word prediction software, electronic organizers, and cell phones with timers and reminders are a few of the options.

Using peer intervention strategy, a peer is paired with the child with ADHD to help reduce inappropriate or disruptive behavior. The intervention may also occur in a group with the focus on improving peer interactions and relationships.

Neurofeedback retrains the brain to a more self-regulated state using electroencephalographic (EEG) feedback. Used in conjunction with computer attention training, it can result in prompt and greater improvement in ADHD symptoms that are sustained at 6-month follow-up (Steiner et al, 2014).

Supports and Services: Family, Home, Friends, Activities, and Self-Esteem

It is necessary to initially help parents understand the complexity of the diagnosis, to deal with feelings of shock or confusion, and to cope with guilt. The diagnosis of a child is often the first clue to the eventual diagnosis of an older sibling or a parent who is experiencing similar difficulties. ADHD symptoms can impact the already complex relationships within a family, so ongoing support is important. Children with ADHD have a constant struggle with self-esteem as they strive to meet expectations placed on them. It is crucial to identify their areas of strength and pleasure and provide opportunities to develop those areas rather than constantly focusing on remediating areas of weakness. Box 20-3 has some specific management ideas, and Chapter 18 has information on self-perception.

School Management. As discussed earlier in this section and chapter, it is essential that the PCP work with the family and the school to set reasonable expectations and develop a plan for the child to be successful in school. Many teachers are familiar with ADHD, and many schools have strategies in place to work with these children, including behavior management programs or interventions to enhance academic and social functioning (e.g., daily or weekly progress notes, behavior cards, and/or study or organizational skills training). The child will likely benefit from either an IEP or 504 plan for academic learning or behavior (see earlier section and Box 20-4 for ideas about classroom adaptations). Schools have several specialists that may be utilized—school psychologists, counselors, and special educators—to help modify the classroom, plan accommodations, and identify triggers and reinforcers. School should also be a place to focus on developing strengths outside of the academic arena—theater, music, sports, art, and clubs are great options. Sometimes the family will seek support outside of the school system for assessment or treatment. The PCP can help facilitate such referrals and incorporate recommendations into the overall plan.

BOX 20-3 Tips for Home-Based Homework Support

1. Provide a quiet location where work will be done with minimal distractions. Set up a work station equipped with necessary materials.
2. Establish a homework time as early as possible to prevent the child from being too tired.
3. Establish a homework plan: Review assignments and make a schedule for completion, breaking into small, manageable pieces.
4. Help the child to get started. Monitor without taking over. Praise effort; do not insist on perfection.
5. Use a timer to help with time management. Structure time for breaks as often as every 15 minutes if needed. Encourage movement during breaks.
6. Permit time for editing so the child does not to lose points due to editing errors. Help to study for tests.
7. Provide incentives to help motivation.
8. Identify another student to contact for clarification.

Follow-Up Care

The health care home model provides for the essential and regular follow-up of the child and family with ADHD, including medical, psychosocial, and educational factors. Follow-up management includes reassessment of core symptoms, functioning, and target goals; review of medication regimen; provision of anticipatory guidance and further education; care coordination and advocacy; and assessment of family functioning, and need for family support or other resources. Box 20-5 provides questions to help the PCP develop and revise the plan of care.

Reassessment of the Child, Family, and Care Coordination. Regular reassessment of the child's core symptoms and functioning should occur at least twice a year with communication from the family, the school, and anyone else involved. In addition to assessment of medication effectiveness, it is important to include a more comprehensive look at the child's functioning in school, at home, with peers, and activities. Assessment of family functioning, including the reasonableness of parental expectations, should also be completed with a focus on areas where additional resources or support is needed. Reassessment involves collecting and evaluating information and then sitting down with the family to review and make adjustments to the target goals and plan. The Vanderbilt Scale has a follow-up version for parents and teachers that collects information about the core ADHD symptoms, level of impairment, potential side effects, and comorbid

BOX 20-4 Suggestions for Classroom Accommodations for Children with Attention-Deficit/Hyperactivity Disorder

Memory and Attention

Seat the child close to the teacher away from heavy traffic areas (e.g., doorways).
Keep oral instructions brief with repetitions; avoid multiple commands.
Provide written directions—broken down or simplified if needed.
"Walk" the child through assignments to be sure they are understood.
Break tasks and homework into small tasks.
Use visual aids, hands-on, and experiential teaching methods rather than strict lecture style.
Teach active reading with underlining and active listening with note taking.
Provide remedial help in small sessions.
Teach subvocalization (saying words in your head while reading) to aid memorizing.
Establish a signal that reminds the child to focus and return to task.
Allow non-distracting motor activity during tasks requiring concentration (e.g., squeezing a ball or fingering Velcro to replace pencil tapping).
Allow earplugs for auditory processing issues.

Impulse Control

Allow for freedom of movement as much as possible (e.g., classroom helper).
Never punish the child by taking away physical education, recess, or other physical outlets.
Teach the child to monitor quality of work before turning it in.

Classroom Atmosphere

Provide a structured classroom with clear expectations.
Use moderate, consistent discipline.
Rely on positive reinforcement for good behavior.
Provide a quiet place to work in the classroom (headsets with select music may block out distractions).

Organizational Skills

Establish a daily checklist of tasks.
Use a daily planner. List homework assignments with due date and needed resources.
Divide notebook into three sections: work to be completed, work completed, and work to be saved.
Color code class material to help organize.
Follow up on homework not turned in.
Allow extra time for gathering necessary items, packing backpack, and so on.
Provide an extra set of textbooks for use at home.
Teach strategies for time management and basic study skills.
Develop preview and planning skills.

Productivity Problems

Divide worksheets into sections.
Reduce the amount of homework and written classwork.
Modify the number of math problems to be completed.
Provide test modification—quiet location and extra time.
Use assistive technology—word processor, calculator, audio books, and note taker pen.

Written Expression

Give extra time to complete written tests and assignments.
Provide help with handwriting.
Allow child to dictate reports and take tests orally.
Reduce the quantity of written work required.
Grade papers on content rather than untidy work, spelling errors, or poor handwriting.

Self-Esteem

Reward progress.
Encourage performance in areas of child's strength.
Avoid humiliation.
Give hand signals only the child can see as private reminders of appropriate behavior.

Social Relationships

Provide feedback about behavior involving other children.
Make sure other children do not believe that the child is doing less or is allowed unacceptable behavior; change the rules for all children if necessary.

symptoms. Often families think things are going fairly well when indeed they may benefit from treatment modifications. It is also important to monitor growth, sleep, appetite, and the development of any significant symptoms, such as aggression or tics, at these visits.

Medication Monitoring. When initiating medication treatment and any time there is a dose or medication change, the provider should meet with the family to assess the effectiveness. Sometimes this can be as often as every 1 to 3 weeks. These visits focus on symptom reduction, monitoring the duration of relief, and managing side effects. Once the individual is stable on an effective dose, medication monitoring should occur at a minimum of every 3 to 6 months. The visit should include vital signs with height, weight, blood pressure, and pulse, and an abbreviated physical examination with a focus on the cardiac system.

Medication modification may include dose adjustment, a change in the timing of the dose, or adding an adjunct medication. Many of the minor side effects can be minimized by having children and teens eat a healthy meal before taking their medication, taking the medication with food, or eating soon after the dose. Advising about sleep hygiene, considering a safe medication (e.g., melatonin at bedtime), or reminding about use of a mild analgesic (such as acetaminophen for headache complaints) are simple strategies that can make a difference.

Some children taking stimulants experience "rebound" moodiness as the medication wears off. This often happens

• BOX 20-5 Questions to Consider When Developing the Plan of Care for a Child/Adolescent With Attention-Deficit Hyperactivity Disorder

- Does the family need further assistance in understanding the core symptoms of ADHD and their child's/adolescent's target symptoms and coexisting conditions?
- Does the family need support in learning how to establish, measure, and monitor target goals?
- Have the family's goals been identified and addressed in the care plan?
- Does the family have an understanding of effective behavior management techniques for responding to tantrums, oppositional behavior, or poor compliance to requests and commands?
- Is help needed for normalizing peer and family relationships?
- Does the child/adolescent need help in academic areas? If so, has a formal evaluation been performed and reviewed to distinguish work production problems secondary to ADHD from coexisting learning or language disabilities?
- Does the child/adolescent need help in achieving independence in self-help or schoolwork production?
- Does the child/adolescent or family require help with optimizing, organizing, planning, or managing schoolwork flow?
- Does the family need help in recognition, understanding, or management of coexisting conditions?
- Is there a plan in place to systematically educate the child/adolescent about ADHD and its treatment as well as the child's/adolescent's own strengths and weaknesses?
- Is there a plan in place to empower the child/adolescent with the knowledge and understanding that will increase his or her adherence to treatments and has that begun as early as possible and been addressed at the child's/adolescent's developmental level?
- Does the family have a copy of a care plan that summarizes findings and treatment recommendations that can be updated and used in school settings and other professional settings so that the history and treatment plan does not need to be constantly reinvented?
- Is the follow-up plan sufficient to provide comprehensive, coordinated, family-centered, culturally competent, and ongoing care?

Taken from American Academy of Pediatrics (AAP): Implementing the key action statements: an algorithm and explanation for process of care for the evaluation, diagnosis, treatment, and monitoring of ADHD in children and adolescents. Available at http://pediatrics.aappublications.org/content/suppl/2011/10/11/peds.2011-2654.DC1/zpe611117822p.pdf. Accessed December 23, 2014.
ADHD, Attention-deficit/hyperactivity disorder.

in the afternoon after school. It is felt to be due to waning medication effects, tiredness, and the post–school day stresses. These symptoms can be treated by giving a low dose of the same short-acting stimulant that the child is taking in the afternoon.

A trial without medications may be considered if the child is stable and doing well. It is best done at a time when there will be few transitions, and definitely not at the beginning of the school year, especially the junior/senior year of high school. There should be close follow-up during the first 4 weeks off medications.

Complementary Therapies

A 2012 comprehensive review of dietary methods of treatment of ADHD concluded that additive-free and oligoantigenic/elimination diets are difficult, time consuming, disruptive to the household, and only indicated in selected patients. However, adopting the "healthy diet pattern" rich in fish, vegetables, legumes, and whole grain foods instead of the "Western diet pattern" high in total fat, saturated fat, refined sugars and sodium with decreased omega-3 fatty acids, fiber, and folate may be useful. Zinc and iron should only be used in patients who have a proven deficiency, but omega-3 supplements (300-600 mg/day) or omega-6 fatty acids (30-60 mg/day) for 2 to 3 months may be helpful, although benefits are not clearly demonstrated (Millichap and Yee, 2012). Vayarin is a prescription-strength form of omega-3 fatty acids classified as a medical food for use in dietary management of ADHD. It is not regulated, approved, or registered with the FDA, but it may be a treatment strategy for families resisting traditional pharmacotherapy or as a supplement (Iannelli, 2014).

Patient and Family Education and Prevention

An important part of the health care home is providing both the child/adolescent and the parent with ongoing psychoeducation and anticipatory guidance about ADHD and the changes that occur. As the child matures, so does the brain, and symptomatology and coexisting conditions may change. PCPs must be attuned to these changes and provide anticipatory guidance and modify treatment plans as needed. Empowering children/adolescents as they are ready to understand their condition and impairments is essential. Essential components include management strategies, continuing to clarify that ADHD is not a lack of intelligence, and helping them to build on strengths. Parents should be equipped with proactive strategies for the home and dealing with transitions to middle school, high school, and college or vocational studies. Anticipatory guidance includes immediate and long-term expectations, study and organizational skills, and guidance on behavior management. Families are often under stress because of the ongoing challenges, and helping them learn how to cope with the stress or access mental health services is important.

Referral, Complications, and Prognosis

It is important for the PCP to know when to refer a child or adolescent to a mental health specialist or psychiatrist. Reconsider the accuracy of the diagnosis, and refer if a child or adolescent is a nonresponder to medication trials at therapeutic dose levels with at least two of the first-line medications, has side effects or preexisting conditions that would be contraindications to ADHD treatment with any of the first-line medications, and/or has high levels of comorbidities that may be more challenging to treat and require mental health and/or educational specialists.

Untreated, children with ADHD can struggle with education and learning, social relationships, self-management and self-esteem, employment (lower socioeconomic status, higher unemployment rates), higher rates of traffic violations and motor vehicle accidents, difficult family interactions including marital discord and divorce, as well as an increased risk of substance abuse, depression, and anxiety. Medication interactions and side effects are also potential complications, especially in children with concurrent diagnoses of emotional disorders and chronic illness. With different providers prescribing medications, side effects can be missed because they mimic symptoms already present in a confusing and complicated disorder. A cumulative effect can be seen when relationships at home, school, and in the community deteriorate, putting the child or adolescent with ADHD at risk for engaging in delinquent or socially unacceptable behaviors. However, adolescents who are adequately treated for their ADHD are less likely to abuse drugs or alcohol than untreated peers with ADHD and have a lower dropout rate and are more likely to report success in setting and completing goals (Harstad et al, 2014a). A study of the diagnostic stability (no change in diagnosis) of ADHD revealed several factors that appeared to be related to an ongoing diagnosis of ADHD in children initially diagnosed before 6 years old (Law et al, 2014). These factors included the severity of externalizing (acting out, misbehaving) and internalizing (being withdrawn, not participating), the mental health history of the parents, and the socioeconomic status. Additionally over half of the children who lost their diagnosis were diagnosed with other disorders, such as anxiety, autism, and learning disorders.

Learning Disorders and Neurodevelopmental Dysfunctions

As discussed in the beginning of this chapter, cognition and learning are complex processes that require the child to deal with the input, integration, memory, and output of information. Input, getting the information in, can have associated visual auditory components and often has to do with receptive language. Integration is making sense of the information usually by sequencing, abstraction, or organization. Memory, the storing and retrieving of information, involves the working memory, long-term memory, or short-term memory. Output, how the information gets back out, usually involves expressive language or motor issues. Problems typically interfere with a child's reading, writing, and/or math skills, but can also cause problems with higher level skills, such as organization, time planning, and abstract reasoning.

Assessing the eight constructs in the neurodevelopmental model (see Table 20-1) is one way to look at a child's areas of difficulty. This approach creates a profile of neurodevelopmental strengths and weaknesses with problems classified according to degree as a variation, dysfunction, disability, or handicap (Box 20-6). Most children with academic struggles have more than one dysfunction that results in delayed or difficult acquisition and reduced productivity. Identified strengths are used to balance out the difficulties.

• BOX 20-6 Hierarchy of Neurodevelopmental Status

Variation: An unusual pattern of neurodevelopmental function (e.g., a higher divergent mind)
Dysfunction: A distinct weakness within a neurodevelopmental function (e.g., a weak retrieval area)
Disability: A performance deficiency caused (at least in part) by a neurodevelopmental dysfunction (e.g., trouble throwing a ball)
Handicap: A disability occurring in a much-needed or critical performance area (e.g., a significant reading problem)

The theory of multiple intelligences (see Table 20-2) begs us to remember that although school focuses primarily on linguistic and logical-mathematical intelligence, and many cultures esteem highly articulate or logical people, there are other types of intelligence. Unfortunately many children with other types of intelligence do not receive much reinforcement in school, and in fact, may end up being labeled "learning disabled" or "underachievers," when in actuality their unique ways of thinking and learning are not addressed by the typical classroom.

Learning disabilities are manifested by consistent, significant difficulties in acquiring and using reading, writing, listening, speaking, reasoning, math, and social skills. Some of the most common learning disorders as defined by the National Institute of Child Health and Human Development (NICHHD) are listed in Box 20-7. Learning disorders are traditionally defined as discrepancies between aptitude (intelligence) and achievement (learning output) on standardized tests, with the diagnoses of reading disorder, mathematics disorder, disorder of written expression, and learning disorder not otherwise specified (NOS) given. However the American Psychiatric Association (2014) DSM-5 simplified learning disabilities into one diagnostic spectrum with subtypes (specifiers) that take into account individual deficits. Additionally the requirement for discrepancy between IQ and achievement was eliminated and replaced with four criteria (key characteristics, impairment, onset, and disorders that must be ruled out) that must be met. Language-based learning disorders are most typically due to problems with decoding (the ability to turn printed symbols into sounds and words) or comprehension (the ability to extract meaning from those words). Decoding requires word analysis skills and an adequate sight vocabulary. Comprehension is impossible without decoding, but it also requires verbal comprehension, memory, and higher cognitive skills (e.g., abstraction, reasoning). Inaccurate spelling can also be an issue, and it is often accompanied by other developmental dysfunctions. Dysfunctions in children who have trouble with writing may be due to fine motor issues, memory weaknesses, language disabilities, or organization. Poor math performance can be linked with weak nonverbal reasoning, language disability, memory dysfunction, and

BOX 20-7 Common Learning Disorders

- Dyslexia: This condition causes problems with language skills, particularly reading. Children with dyslexia may have difficulty spelling, understanding sentences, and recognizing words they already know.
- Dysgraphia: Children with dysgraphia have problems with their handwriting. They may have problems forming letters, writing within a defined space, and writing down their thoughts.
- Dyscalculia: Children with this math learning disability may have difficulty understanding arithmetic concepts and doing tasks, such as addition, multiplication, and measuring.
- Dyspraxia: This condition, also termed *sensory integration disorder,* involves problems with motor coordination that lead to poor balance and clumsiness. Poor hand-eye coordination also causes difficulty with fine motor tasks, such as putting puzzles together and coloring within the lines.
- Apraxia of speech: Sometimes called *verbal apraxia,* this disorder involves problems with speaking. Children with this disorder have trouble saying what they want to say correctly and consistently.
- Central auditory processing disorder: Children with this condition have trouble understanding and remembering language-related tasks. They have difficulty explaining things, understanding jokes, and following directions. They confuse words and are easily distracted.
- Nonverbal learning disorders: Children with these conditions have strong verbal skills but great difficulty understanding facial expression and body language. In addition, they are physically clumsy and have trouble generalizing and following multistep directions.
- Visual perceptual/visual motor deficit: Children with this condition mix up letters; they might confuse "m" and "w" or "d" and "b," for example. They may also lose their place while reading, copy inaccurately, write messily, and cut paper clumsily.
- Aphasia: Aphasia, also called *dysphasia* is a language disorder. Children with this disorder have difficulty understanding spoken language, poor reading comprehension, trouble with writing, and great difficulty finding words to express thoughts and feelings. Aphasia occurs when the language areas of the brain are damaged. In adults, it often is caused by stroke, but children may get aphasia from a brain tumor, head injury, or brain infection.

Data from Eunice Kennedy Shriver National Institute of Child Health and Development (NICHHD): Learning disabilities: condition information, National Institutes of Health (NIH) (website), 2014, available at www.nichd.nih.gov/health/topics/learning/conditioninfo/Pages/default.aspx. Accessed January 31, 2015.

attention deficits. Disorders of the executive functions result in a disruption of the mental processes and behaviors that enable self-regulation and metacognition. They are seen most commonly with prematurity, prenatal drug and alcohol exposure, and traumatic brain injury.

Learning disorders result from a variety of genetic, constitutional, or neurodevelopmental factors—anything that disrupts the central nervous system. Problems are often present from birth and often inherited. Although specific causes of learning disorders unknown, there are differences in the part of the brain that deals with language (Eunice Kennedy Shriver NICHHD, 2014). Genetic linkage analysis suggests abnormalities on chromosomes 2, 3, 6, 5, and 16 (Rimrodt and Lipkin, 2011). Environmental factors (such as, alcohol and drug use, exposure to toxins, poor nutrition, family involvement, emotional disturbances, and cultural differences) play a role. The National Center of Educational Statistics reported 4.8% of students in 2010 to 2011 had a specific learning disability (U.S. Department of Education [USDE], 2013), with 80% representing reading disability, which makes it almost as common as pediatric disorders like asthma (Rimrodt and Lipkin, 2011).

Clinical Findings

Language processing, visual and auditory processing, memory, motor coordination, and spatial and temporal orientation difficulties are hallmarks of the condition, although a child will probably not have difficulties in all areas. Common struggles with reading include difficulty decoding unfamiliar words, poor comprehension and retention, and slow reading rate. With mathematics, there can be difficulty remembering number facts and solving practical problems. Poor and labored handwriting, faulty spelling, and grammar and syntax errors are indicative of writing problems. Signs of academic distress can be identified in three stages (Rimrodt and Lipkin, 2011). The first signs are increased learning effort as a child's coping abilities are overcome by increasing school demands. Specific findings may include spending increased time on homework compared to classmates, school anxiety, class clown behavior, and complaints that school is boring. If intervention does not happen at this point, signs of school distress (failing grades; absences; social disengagement; detention, suspension, aggression, and bullying behavior) begin to appear. School failure, the third stage, results in retention, expulsion, and dropping out.

Assessment

Assessment includes identification of risk factors, observation for characteristics of learning disorders, and consideration of other causes for the learning problems. Family history may include dyslexia or other learning disability (frequently familial), decreased academic achievement, attention deficits, and grade retention or school dropout. Medical history may include prematurity or low birthweight, early developmental concerns or delays, especially speech/language issues, head injury, seizure disorder, or a chronic health condition. Significant child assessment issues to consider include connectedness to school (feels accepted, valued, respected, and included); description of school and effort; perception of the cause of the problems; experiences at school with teachers, peers, homework, and temperament; coping skills; and social competence. Components of the parent interview deal with the child's functioning at home versus school; school coping; psychological, behavioral, and stress responses to the problems; ability to attend to and complete tasks; and strengths and weaknesses

• BOX 20-8 Level I School Performance Prescreening Questionnaire

1. Do you have any concerns about your child's learning or school performance?
2. Do you have any concerns about your child's attention, concentration, impulsivity, and/or overactivity?
3. Do you have any concerns about how your child is doing in certain subjects at school? If yes, is it reading? Writing? Math? Other?
4. Do you have any concern about how much your child is enjoying school compared with friends or classmates?
5. Does your child have any problems completing homework?

of the child. School and teacher history should include teacher's report of academic performance, absences, engagement, behavioral information, and results of any educational testing. The physical examination should include behavioral observations, hearing and vision evaluation, sensory processing screening, and a focus on any signs of neurologic problems, dysmorphic features, or minor congenital anomalies.

Screening

Developmental surveillance is an ongoing part of routine health care in the preschool years. It is equally important as children move through their school years to continue surveillance of a child's school performance in order to identify difficulties that may not arise until the child faces the school challenges. The school performance prescreening questionnaire (Box 20-8) is a five-item instrument that can be administered at every well-child check. If the prescreening questionnaire shows no evidence of school problems, screening should occur at the next routine visit. If school problems are suspected, a school performance screener should be administered. The school performance screener (Box 20-9) is a more comprehensive assessment tool for follow up of a positive prescreening questionnaire; it is used in conjunction with samples of school work, report cards, and previously administered tests. Additionally the National Center for Learning Disabilities has a Learning Disabilities Checklist (available online), which is organized by skill set and age group and free to download.

Differential Diagnosis

Behavioral and mental health problems (especially ADHD and anxiety) and problems with social interactions may be associated but are separate conditions. Cognitive limitations, visual or hearing problems, school absence, environmental deprivation in preschool, fetal alcohol syndrome, lead or other toxic exposure, and fragile X syndrome are included in the differential diagnosis. ACEs, bereavement, developmental problems, and sleep deprivation also need to be differentiated.

• BOX 20-9 Level II School Performance Screener

1. In what area(s) does your child have problems in school performance? Learning/achievement? Attention/concentration/memory? Behavior?
2. Subjects/activities of difficulty: Reading? Math? Spelling? Writing? Speaking? Listening? Remembering? Science? Social studies? Language/grammar? Following directions? Inconsistency? Transferring knowledge from one situation to another? Organizing?
3. Current grade? What grade did problems become evident? Did child repeat a grade? Was the child ever in danger of repeating a grade?
4. Grades on report card? Performance on standardized testing? Is excessive amount of help needed to do homework? Is excessive amount of homework due to child not completing in school? Would grades be lower without a great amount of extra work being done at home with parents? Is homework a battle each night?
5. Stressors? None? Current? At time of onset of school problems? With family? Peers? At school?
6. Medical concerns? Frequent ear infections? Hearing problem? Vision problem? Prenatal/perinatal problems? Allergies? Loss of consciousness? Sleep problem? Describe.
7. Strengths? Reading? Math? Spelling? Writing? Speaking? Listening? Remembering? Science? Social studies? Language/grammar? Other? Learns better by seeing versus hearing or vice versa?
8. How does the child get along with peers? Involved in extracurricular activities? Type? If so, how does he or she do?
9. Emotional issues: Lack of motivation? School avoidance? Homework avoidance? Seems lazy? Irritable? Anxious? Volatile? Down on self? Aggressive? Gives up easily? Refuses to work in class? Doesn't turn work in? Oppositional? Angry?
10. Tested by school system? If yes, eligible for services? Receives services (types)? Found ineligible? Has received services, but they have been discontinued?

Management

The PCPs role is to monitor children's development from birth through adulthood, with a focus on early identification of any school issues that may need further workup. If concerns arise, the family may need support and direction through the assessment process, which is often lengthy and emotional (see the Educational and Adaptive Support section). This process involves interprofessional collaboration with colleagues in both medical and educational fields as the child undergoes evaluation. Once a child receives a diagnosis, the PCP should serve as case manager. In this role, it is important to build trust and optimism and to reinforce strengths of the child and family. Tasks may include helping parents and children understand the implications of a particular learning disability and how it affects interactions with peers and everyday life; exploring ideas and acting as a conduit to help parents find reliable resources and others who have solved similar problems; and identifying the child's strengths, affinities, and interests in order to develop passions and areas of expertise.

Educational and Adaptive Support

The psychoeducational evaluation should include identification of strengths and weaknesses, determination of cognitive ability, assessment of perceptual strengths and weaknesses, examination of communicative ability, and assessment of social and emotional adaptation. Out of that evaluation, an IEP or a 504 plan (see the Educational Strategies section) can be developed with appropriate plans and accommodations, such as a resource room and bypass interventions. Assistive technologies (e.g., read-aloud devices from text and computer programs) to help remediate deficiencies may be helpful. Calculators and word processors may help circumvent handwriting problems. Providing acknowledgment of a child's aptitude, initiative, spirit, industry, and self-efficacy is a way of providing tangible support.

Family and Social Support

Parents may need help devising an organized approach to respond to their child's struggles (Box 20-10). It is especially important to provide a child with a learning disability support with homework at home (see Box 20-2). Helping parents maintain a positive perspective is sometimes necessary, as is referral for counseling to deal with the demands and stresses. Encouraging the parents to do research and become experts on their child's needs proves helpful, especially in planning for school. Finally, provide gentle reminders to the parents that their influence on the child outweighs anything else.

Complications

School distress (avoidance, acting-out, disengagement, or alienation) and school failure (retention, expulsion, and dropping out) are possible complications of learning disability. Lowered self-esteem and coexisting mental health problems, such as anxiety and depression, can also be experienced.

• BOX 20-10 A Parent's Response to a Learning Disability

- Know your child's strengths.
- Collect information about your child's performance.
- Have your child evaluated.
- Work as a team to help your child.
- Talk to your child about learning disabilities.
- Find reasonable accommodations that can help.
- Monitor your child's progress.
- Know your legal rights.
- Organize information about your child's learning disability—a folder with letters and material, copies of school files, samples of work that demonstrate difficulty as well as strengths; keep a contact log; keep a log of own observations.

Patient and Family Education and Prevention

Starting early in life, children need to be exposed to language—reading and talking. The Reach Out and Read program, in which health care providers give books and encourage reading, has proven to be a successful strategy. Dolly Parton's Imagination Library provides guidance for establishing a community program to provide free books to children from birth to age 5 (see Resources on the Evolve website). Student engagement in school is defined as participation, performance, and identification with the school. Research supports the fact that attendance, completion of school work, and participation in extracurricular activities leads to positive school performance.

Sensory Processing Disorder

The brain and nervous system function to perceive, integrate, interpret, and then facilitate appropriate coordinated motor and behavioral responses. This includes visual, tactile, auditory, olfactory, gustatory, vestibular (movement), and proprioceptive (muscle and joint position) information. Attention, learning, regulation of energy levels and emotions, motor skill development, and social function in children are dependent on this input. Sensory processing disorder (SPD), the inaccurate or imprecise detection, modulation, and/or integration of sensory input, occurs in a wide spectrum of neurodevelopmental disorders and can disrupt everyday life (Sensory Processing Disorder Foundation, n.d.). Children with SPD do not have cognitive delays and may even be intellectually gifted; their brains are just wired in a different manner. Sensory processing problems fall into three main diagnostic patterns (Box 20-11).

• BOX 20-11 Patterns of Sensory Processing Disorders

- Sensory modulation disorder: Difficulty regulating and organizing the intensity and nature of responses to sensory input so that they can be appropriately graded to changing experiences (sensations considered pleasurable or positive in most individuals are perceived as painful, irritating, and unpleasant)
  - Sensory over-responsive: Responds too much, for too long, or to stimuli of weak intensity
  - Sensory under-responsive: Responds too little, or needs extremely strong stimulation to become aware of the stimulus
  - Sensory seeking/craving: Responds with intense searching for more or stronger stimulation
- Sensory discrimination disorder: Difficulty interpreting the specific characteristics of sensory stimuli (e.g., the intensity, the duration, the spatial, and the temporal elements of sensations); present in any of the seven sensory systems
- Sensory-based motor disorders
  - Postural disorder: Problems in balance and core stability
  - Dyspraxia: Difficulties in motor planning and sequencing movements

Sensory integration disorder was first identified in the 1960s by A. Jean Ayres. Now called *sensory processing disorder,* SPD is frequently found in premature children, gifted children, and those with ASD, ADHD, developmental coordination disorder, and fragile X syndrome. Additionally SPD is found with environmental factors, such as institutionalization (overseas adoptees), severe physical or sexual abuse, poverty, lead poisoning, alcohol and drug exposure, and newborn hospitalization for medical conditions. There is controversy about whether SPD is an actual disorder of the sensory pathways, or only a deficit associated with other developmental and behavioral disorders (AAP, 2012). Both the Zero to Three Diagnostic Classification of Mental Health and Developmental Disorders of Infancy and Childhood Revised (Zero to Three, 2014) and the *Diagnostic Manual for Infancy and Early Childhood of the Interdisciplinary Council on Developmental and Learning Disorders* (Interdisciplinary Council on Developmental and Learning Disorders, 2005) include a classification for SPD. Like many neurodevelopmental disorders, specific causes have not been identified. Two recent studies using an advanced magnetic resonance imaging (MRI) technique to study the white matter microstructure of the brain showed decreased connectivity in areas of sensory perception as well as the auditory, visual, and tactile systems involved in sensory processing (Chang et al, 2014; Owen et al, 2013).

Clinical Findings

Children with SPD face many challenges in everyday life. Motor clumsiness, behavioral problems, and difficulties with abilities needed for school success are not uncommon. Children who are over-responders have difficulties with clothing, physical contact, light, sound, and food. Children who are under-responders have little or no reaction to stimulation, pain, and extreme hot or cold and can risk injuring themselves. Children who are sensory seekers are on perpetual overdrive and often in trouble with friends and family. When there is muscle and joint impairment (postural disorder), posture and motor skills are affected (can be described as floppy babies, a klutz, a spaz). These children have difficulty with changes in ground surfaces, may appear to be uncoordinated, or may have delayed oculomotor control. Children with dyspraxia do not do well when asked to recognize and distinguish shapes and textures, may have poor handwriting, or may present with an altered ability to do things like tying shoes, using buttons, or dressing themselves.

Sensory problems in infants often become behavioral problems in preschoolers caused by others' negative reactions to their behaviors. Adolescents and adults may have difficulty with close relationships, recreation, and performing routines and activities involved in school or work.

Assessment

History and Physical Examination

The history and physical examination may reveal relationships between behaviors and specific sensory experiences. Infants may be colicky or fussy babies, fearful of movement, resist being held or comforted, and may have eating and sleeping difficulties. Preschoolers may not engage in purposeful interactive play; have delayed skill development; be defiant, irritable, and stubborn; resist transitions and certain activities; and have issues with feeding, dressing, and sleep. The school-age child has trouble with handwriting, figuring out steps in a game, organizing school work, and spontaneous play interaction; trouble with handling change and transition; and is easily frustrated. Adolescents report trouble with social interactions, learning in the classroom, and physical skill development.

Screening and Evaluation

Red flags for SPD are found in Box 20-12. Any suspicious differences in development or parental concerns warrant screening. A more complete SPD Checklist and Sensory

• BOX 20-12 Red Flags for a Sensory Processing Disorder

If more than a few of the symptoms listed here fit the child, refer to the complete Sensory Processing Disorder (SPD) Checklist. A Spanish-language copy of the red flags is available at www.spdfoundation.net/about-sensory-processing-disorder/symptoms/.

Infants and Toddlers

____ Problems eating or sleeping
____ Refuses to go to anyone but a specific person
____ Irritable when being dressed; uncomfortable in clothes
____ Rarely plays with toys
____ Resists cuddling, arches away when held
____ Cannot calm self
____ Floppy or stiff body, motor delays

Preschoolers

____ Overly sensitive to touch, noises, smells, other people
____ Difficulty making friends
____ Difficulty dressing, eating, sleeping, and/or toilet training
____ Clumsy; poor motor skills; weakness
____ In constant motion; in everyone else's face and space
____ Frequent or long temper tantrums

Grade Schoolers

___ Overly sensitive to touch, noise, smells, other people
___ Easily distracted, fidgety, craves movement; aggressive
___ Easily overwhelmed
___ Difficulty with handwriting or motor activities
___ Difficulty making friends
___ Unaware of pain and/or other people

Adolescents and Adults

___ Overly sensitive to touch, noise, smells, and other people
___ Poor self-esteem; afraid of failing at new tasks
___ Lethargic and slow
___ Always on the go; impulsive; distractible
___ Leaves tasks uncompleted
___ Clumsy, slow, poor motor skills or handwriting
___ Difficulty staying focused at work and in meetings

Integration Observation Guide 0-12 Months can be found at www.spdfounation.net. The Short Sensory Profile is available for purchase through Pearson Assessments. Screening should result in one of three findings: (1) no further evaluation needed, (2) watch and re-screen, or (3) complete evaluation recommended. Evaluation is usually conducted by a specially trained occupational therapist using questionnaires, observational tools, and standardized tests (Schaaf et al, 2014).

Differential Diagnosis and Comorbidities

Differential diagnoses include other developmental or cognitive delays, including Down syndrome, anxiety, aggression, and other mental illness. There is a much higher prevalence of SPD in children who have ADHD, ASD, and fragile X syndrome, although ADHD and ASD are considered unique disorders with distinct symptoms.

Management

The AAP Policy Statement on Sensory Integration Therapies recommends that, when sensory symptoms are present, providers consider and evaluate for other developmental disorders, usually by referral to a developmental and behavioral specialist (AAP, 2012). Early diagnosis and treatment for SPD not only increase the chance of successful intervention especially as related to acquiring skills for school, they also help minimize the secondary issues that develop when children receive inappropriate labels and begin to feel like they are "failing." If an occupational therapy referral is made, it is best to select a therapist with sensory integration training. Treatment is expensive and not always covered by insurance, so monitoring the effectiveness is a role of the PCP. The goal of therapy is to develop appropriate and automatic responses to sensations so that the child can function competently in play, at school, in daily living, and in self-care routines. Therapy includes the use of sensory stimuli in one domain to affect performance in another, usually taking place in a sensory-rich environment, providing what is called *sensory nourishment* or a *sensory diet.* Over time, new neurologic connections are established, allowing regulation of arousal and attention, formation of attachment and social relationships, and organization of actions in the physical world.

It is helpful for families with children with SPD to know that these children may be able to perform in school but may come home and fall apart; often try to control in an attempt to manage what is happening inside their brains; can sometimes accomplish something if they put 100% effort into it but can't always perform at 100%; often have trouble with transitions, family gatherings, parties, and vacation (things considered fun); do best with an environment that is predictable and routine and the same from day to day; and may be sensitive to touch and pull away from hugs and cuddling.

Complications

Complications include the inability to make friends, poor self-concept, academic failure, being labeled clumsy, uncooperative, disruptive, and out of control. Anxiety, depression, aggression, or other behavior problems are not uncommon. Caregivers may be blamed or criticized for the child's behavior.

Autistic Spectrum Disorder

ASD is a complex neurobiologic and neurodevelopmental disorder characterized by patterns of delay and deviance in the development of social, communicative, and cognitive skills that arise in the first years of life (Volkmar et al, 2014). According to the DSM-5, ASD is characterized by two diagnostic domains:

- Deficits in social communication and interaction across multiple contexts
- Restrictive, repetitive patterns of behaviors, interests, and activities

These symptoms must be present in the early developmental period, cause significant impairment, and not be better explained by intellectual disability. Box 20-13 lists the complete DSM-5 criteria. The disorder varies considerably in severity, and part of the DSM-5 criteria includes specifying severity level. Table 20-8 identifies criteria for severity levels.

The DSM-5 criteria state that a patient must show symptoms from early childhood even if the symptoms are not recognized until later in life. This encourages early diagnosis of ASD but also allows for later diagnosis if symptoms are not fully recognized at an early age. The DSM-5 reclassifies Rett disorder as a genetic disease, includes unusual sensory behaviors as criteria, and no longer recognizes pervasive developmental disorder NOS, Asperger syndrome, and childhood disintegrative disorder as separate conditions.

ASD causes lifelong disability that usually becomes apparent in the first 3 years of life. Development is uneven, with occasional talent in a limited area, such as music or mathematics, coupled with severe deficits in other areas. Many autistic children have other impairments, such as sleep problems, gastrointestinal problems (diarrhea, constipation, and abdominal pain), and irritability. Additionally, it is not uncommon to have co-occurring diagnosis of intellectual disability (50% severe, 35% mild to moderate), anxiety/phobias (up to 50%), obsessive compulsive behaviors, ADHD, depression, disruptive disorders (aggression, tantrums, and self-injury), and seizures (20% to 25%) (Harrington and Allen, 2014; Volkmar et al, 2014). Identification of comorbidities is essential.

Although the cause of ASD is still unknown, both genetic and environmental causes are being investigated. Certain genetic disorders (fragile X syndrome, neurofibromatosis, tuberous sclerosis, Angelman syndrome, and Rett syndrome) are often associated with ASD and should be considered in the evaluation. Genetic research has unveiled multiple possibilities about the role of genetics in the cause of ASD. "Hot spots" have been found on almost every chromosome, as well as disruption in intervening sequences and extra synapses (the lack of pruning). Immune system dysfunction has also been implicated and may be related to

• BOX 20-13 Diagnostic Criteria for Autistic Disorders

A. A total of more than six items from the following criteria with at least two from criterion 1 and one each from criteria 2 and 3:
   1. Qualitative impairment in social interaction as manifested by at least two of the following:
      a. Marked impairment in the use of multiple nonverbal behaviors, such as eye-to-eye gaze, facial expression, body posture, and gestures to regulate social interaction
      b. Failure to develop peer relationships appropriate to developmental level
      c. Lack of spontaneous seeking to share enjoyment, interests, or achievements with other people (lack of showing, bringing, or pointing out objects of interest)
   2. Qualitative impairments in communication as manifested by at least one of the following:
      a. Delay in or total lack of development of spoken language (not accompanied by an attempt to compensate through alternative modes of communication, such as gesture or mime)
      b. In individuals with adequate speech, marked impairment in the ability to initiate or sustain a conversation
      c. Stereotyped and repetitive use of language or idiosyncratic language
      d. Lack of varied, spontaneous make-believe play or social imitative play appropriate to developmental level
   3. Restricted, repetitive, and stereotyped patterns of behavior, interests, and activities as manifested by at least one of the following:
      a. Encompassing preoccupation with one or more stereotyped and restricted patterns of interest that is abnormal either in intensity or focus
      b. Apparently inflexible adherence to specific, nonfunctional routines or rituals
      c. Stereotyped and repetitive motor mannerisms (e.g., hand or finger flapping or twisting, or complex whole-body movements)
      d. Persistent preoccupation with parts of objects
B. Delay or abnormal functioning in at last one of the following areas with onset before 3 years old:
   1. Social interaction
   2. Language as used in social communication
   3. Symbolic or imaginative play
C. Disturbance not better accounted for by Rett disorder or childhood disintegrative disorder

From American Psychiatric Association: *Diagnostic and Statistical Manual of Mental Disorders*, ed 5, Arlington, VA, 2014, American Psychiatric Association.

the excess number of synapses. However, even with rigorous testing, up to 75% of children show no measurable genetic abnormality (Dixon-Salazar et al, 2014; Harrington and Allen, 2014; Tang et al, 2014). The Childhood Autism Risk from Genetics and Environment (CHARGE) study looks for interaction between genes and the environment, hoping to identify both prenatal and postnatal influences. One study identified increased risk for ASD from maternal metabolic conditions (diabetes, obesity, and hypertension) (Krakowiak et al, 2012). Rzhetsky and colleagues (2014), using congenital malformations as a surrogate measure of environmental effect, found a strong link between ASD and rates of congenital malformations. In the United States, for every 1% increase in the incidence of congenital malformations of the reproductive system in males above the mean, the incidence of ASD increased by 283%. The same study also looked at nonreproductive congenital malformations in males and found a 31.8% increase in ASD for every 1% increase in incidence above the mean in the United States. The CDC is conducting a multi-year, multi-site Study to Explore Early Development (SEED), with the aim of helping to identify factors that put a child at risk for ASD and has identified the following risk factors:

- A critical period before, during, and immediately after birth
- Maternal ingestion of valproic acid and thalidomide during pregnancy
- Children born to older parents
- Children with certain genetic or chromosomal conditions, such as fragile X syndrome or tuberous sclerosis

Other factors associated with increased risk for ASD include prenatal infections, such as congenital rubella or cytomegalovirus, neonatal infections; untreated phenylketonuria; prematurity; and twin or multiple pregnancy. The CDC (2014) reports that if one identical twin has autism, the other is affected 60% to 96% of the time. The risk decreases from 0% to 24% for nonidentical twins. In addition, parents who have a child with an ASD have a 2% to 8% chance of having a second child who is affected. There continues to be a great deal of negative and high-profile media attention (not supported by evidence) concerning a risk of autism associated with mercury exposure or bacterial or fungal contamination in vaccines—in spite of overwhelming evidence that no such association exists.

The CDC's Autism and Developmental Disabilities Monitoring Network (ADDM) reports autism in all racial, ethnic, and socioeconomic groups with an incidence of 1:68 children, and an almost 5:1 ratio of male-to-female children, or 1 in 42 males and 1 in 289 females. Although evidence indicates there is no difference in prevalence according to race, the most recent ADDM report shows Latinos and African Americans are more likely to be misdiagnosed, diagnosed at a later age (if at all), and diagnosed with more severe symptoms (CDC, 2014). Regional centers that are part of the Centers for Autism and Developmental Disabilities Research and Epidemiology (CADDRE) Network are involved in ongoing research related to autism.

Clinical Findings

In general, children with ASD demonstrate problems with social interactions, communication, and language skills shown by their unusual ways of relating to people, objects, and events; abnormal responses to sensory stimuli, usually sound; and restricted, repetitive, or stereotyped behaviors and echolalic speech.

Infants

An autistic infant may be a passive, non-engaging, quiet, floppy infant or a difficult, colicky, stiff baby with poor eye

TABLE 20-8 Severity Levels for Autism Spectrum Disorder

Severity Level	Social Communication	Restricted, Repetitive Behaviors
Level 3 "Requiring very substantial support"	Severe deficits in verbal and nonverbal social communication skills; very limited initiation of social interactions; minimal response to social overtures. e.g., few words of intelligible speech; rarely initiates interaction and, when child does, makes unusual approaches to meet needs only; responds to only very direct social approaches.	Inflexibility of behavior, extreme difficulty coping with change, or other restricted/repetitive behaviors markedly interfere with functioning in all spheres. Great distress/difficulty changing focus or action.
Level 2 "Requiring substantial support"	Marked deficits in verbal and nonverbal social communication skills; social impairments apparent even with supports in place; limited initiation of social interactions; reduced or abnormal responses to social overtures from others. e.g., speaks simple sentences; interaction limited to narrow special interests markedly odd nonverbal communication.	Inflexibility of behavior, difficulty coping with change, or other restricted/repetitive behaviors appear frequently enough to be obvious to the casual observer and interfere with functioning in a variety of contexts. Distress and/or difficulty changing focus or action.
Level 1 "Requiring support"	Without supports in place, deficits in social communication cause noticeable impairments. Difficulty initiating social interactions atypical or unsuccessful response to social overtures. e.g., able to speak in full sentences and engages in communication but to-and-fro conversation with others fails; attempts to make friends are odd and typically unsuccessful.	Inflexibility of behavior causes significant interference with functioning in one or more contexts. Difficulty switching between activities. Problems of organization and planning hamper independence.

From American Psychiatric Association (APA): *Diagnostic and statistical manual of mental disorders*, ed 5, Arlington, VA, 2014, American Psychiatric Association.

contact. Attachment problems are often present, and there is failure to respond to name or gestures. Autism is usually not identified in infancy, although some studies looking at early findings (such as, vocalization and eye tracking) are currently in process (Hack, 2014; Jones and Klin, 2013).

Toddlers

During the toddler stage, parents often become convinced that something is wrong with their child. Language delays, lack of social relatedness, and severe behavior problems are common. Expressive language is delayed. If speaking, echolalia, the repetition of words or phrases spoken by another, is present, or the child will only talk about specific interests and have trouble modulating tone of voice. Socially the child exhibits detachment, decreased eye contact, a lack of reciprocity or initiating conversation, lack of fear, and poor creative play skills. Persistent and excessive temper tantrums; repetitive movements; a preference to line, stack, or spin toys; and insistence on routines are commonly observed behaviors. Children affected by ASD have relative strengths in visual-motor problem-solving.

Preschoolers

Language delays include lack of meaningful speech, decreased gestures, and gaze disturbances. Social interaction disturbances such as lack of fear of strangers, invasion of others' space, preference to be alone, and lack of social awareness are often seen. Persistent and insistent behaviors are common. Symbolic play is limited. The child may have precocious or average development of rote memory skills but often without comprehension of concepts.

School-Age Children

School-age children with autism often lack reciprocal friendships and continue with language, social, and behavioral problems. Transitions from place to place and activity to activity can be difficult. Behaviors are ritualistic.

Adolescents

Adolescents usually continue with similar behaviors. Rote learning is possible, but comprehension lags. It should be noted that some high-functioning autistic children are mainstreamed and do very well in regular classrooms. Mildly affected persons may be academically successful but have social relationship problems.

Assessment

Every child should have developmental surveillance routinely done in early childhood to assess for red flags of ASD (Box 20-14), and providers should be sensitive to parental concerns. Developmental history is essential and family history may reveal other members with ASD, speech delay or language deficits, mood disorders, or mental retardation. The review of systems should investigate seizures, hearing loss, head injury, and meningitis. The child should have a complete physical examination with a focus on any findings

• BOX 20-14 Red Flags for Autism

Does not respond to his or her name by 12 months old
Does not point at objects to show interest (pointing at an airplane flying over) by 14 months old
Does not play "pretend" games (pretending to "feed" a doll) by 18 months old
Avoids eye contact and wants to be alone
Has trouble understanding other people's feelings or talking about their own feelings
Has delayed speech and language skills (no babbling or gesturing by 12 months old; no single words by 16 months old; no two-word [not echolalic] phrases by 24 months old)
Repeats words or phrases over and over (echolalia)
Gives unrelated answers to questions
Gets upset by minor changes
Has obsessive interests
Flaps their hands, rocks their body, or spins in circles
Has unusual reactions to the way things sound, smell, taste, look, or feel
Fails to meet childhood developmental milestones
Has a sibling with autism
Has loss of any language or social abilities at any age

suggestive of genetic syndromes (e.g., skin findings) or neurologic abnormalities (e.g., macrocephaly, hypotonia).

Screening and Specialty Referral for Diagnosis

The AAP recommends doing screening for autism at 18 and 24 months of age. The Checklist for Autism in Toddlers (CHAT) is the best known, most commonly recommended, validated tool for screening children between 16 to 30 months old for ASD. *The Modified Checklist for Autism in Toddlers, revised with follow-up (M-CHAT-R/F)* (Robins et al, 2014), is the latest version and and can be found at www2.gsu.edu/~psydlr/M-CHAT/Official_M-CHAT_Website_files/M-CHAT-R_F.pdf. The Infant and Toddler Checklist was designed to screen for communication delays but is now used for autism screening (9 to 24 months old). The Childhood Autism Screening Test (CAST) can be used for children over 3 years old. The Autism Mental Status Exam (AMSE) is an observational assessment tool that structures the way the provider observes and documents signs and symptoms of ASD. Children who fail routine developmental screening should begin an early identification process using DSM-5 diagnostic criteria. This process includes analyzing family and provider concerns, descriptions of behavior, medical history, and questionnaires like the M-CHAT.

If there is a concern that a child has an ASD, referral for a comprehensive diagnostic assessment should be done by a multidisciplinary team, ideally at a specialty center, addressing core symptoms, cognition, language, and adaptive, sensory, and motor skills. Specialty assessment includes developmental, behavioral, and IQ testing; audiologic evaluation and testing for lead exposure; and fragile X syndrome and comparative genomic hybridization array. Neuroimaging, EEG, and metabolic testing are done as indicated by examination and history. Once diagnosis and severity of ASD have been determined, assessment of any comorbidity or other diagnosis is determined.

Differential Diagnosis

Pragmatic social disorder, language disorder with ADHD, intellectual disability with visual impairment, and harsh psychosocial conditions (posttraumatic stress disorder [PTSD], reactive attachment disorder, and abuse in childhood) are all conditions in the differential diagnosis.

Management

After a diagnosis of autism is made, it is important to provide education about the diagnosis, obtain resources and support, and identify the child as one with special health care needs who is best served in a health care home with family-centered, continuous, and comprehensive care. The PCP is an ideal care coordinator, ensuring that an appropriate, long-term, comprehensive plan of care is in place. The AACAP recommends a plan with the following four components: (1) appropriate, evidenced-based, and structured educational and behavioral interventions; (2) pharmacotherapy only for a specific target symptom or comorbid condition; (3) active role in long-term therapy; and (4) inquiring about the use of complementary or alternative therapies (Volkmar et al, 2014). Management of children with ASD is complex and requires a multidisciplinary approach. Intensive psychological and educational interventions are primary treatments. Team members may include a behavioral-developmental pediatrician or nurse, a gastroenterologist or allergist, a dietician, and/or speech and occupational therapists. Levels of severity change over time, and an ongoing relationship with someone who knows the child is helpful in assessing those changes and modifying the plan to ensure the child is receiving the correct services. A review by the Autism Evidenced-Based Practice Review Group investigated thousands of studies to determine which ones were worthy of being called evidence-based. Twenty-seven interventions were identified with substantial research to confirm their findings, and another 24 had some support. The full report is available online (Wong et al, 2015).

Behavior/Mental Health

The most important aspect of autism management is behavioral training. The target behaviors vary according to age, developmental level, and disruptiveness of behaviors. The applied behavior analysis (ABA) approach is considered an optimal strategy and is the most well researched. It focuses on the development of socially appropriate behaviors while decreasing challenging behaviors. However, ABA requires extensive parental education, is very time intensive and expensive, and is often not covered by insurance, thereby limiting its use by many families. Social skills training, one on one or in small groups, early and intense developmental work, and, most recently, parenting strategies are part of management. The parenting role has come to the forefront with a focus on parents being important collaborators at all stages—from assessment through goal development and treatment delivery.

Educational System

Extensive assessment and early intense intervention are necessary to maximize educational abilities and enhance learning for children with autism. Early intervention programs for preschoolers, school-based special education, and information and assistance for school personnel are essential. Children need educational classrooms that range from full- to part-time special education, as well as the availability of resource rooms. Planning for care requires cognitive testing to identify the child's strengths and weaknesses, in addition to social, behavioral, and language assessment. Every child with ASD needs an IEP or 504 plan in place with a focus on strengths as well as weaknesses. When special abilities are discovered in children with autism, attempts should be made to encourage opportunities for success in those areas. Accommodations are necessary, and parents and school personnel need to become skilled advocates for the child. Protection from unrealistic expectations of social competence is often necessary to help the child with autism to succeed. The long-term goal should be to permit the child to function as effectively and comfortably as possible in the least restrictive environment.

Medication

Although there is no medication available for the treatment of the core symptoms of autism, medications used to treat behaviors associated with autism have shown moderate success. The AACAP position statement on ASD states that there is limited benefit and significant limitations to the use of medication, although it may be an important tool offered for specific target symptoms of co-occurring mental health conditions (Volkmer et al, 2014). The most common symptoms addressed by pharmacotherapy are attentional difficulties, hyperactivity, affective difficulties (e.g., anxiety or depression), compulsive behaviors or interfering repetitive activity, irritability, aggression, self-injurious behavior, and sleep disruption. Usually, autistic children do not benefit from stimulant medications unless they also suffer from an attention deficit. Selective serotonin reuptake inhibitors (fluoxetine) may be helpful because some children have abnormal serotonin function if they are depressed or anxious. About one-quarter of autistic children also have seizures and may be given anticonvulsants. Atypical antipsychotics, such as risperidone or aripiprazole, are sometimes used for irritability, physical aggression, or severe tantrums. Citalopram is not recommended for repetitive behaviors in autism (Volkmar et al, 2014). Improvement in social impairment has been shown with investigational drugs like oxytocin that work on glutamate receptors, but further studies are warranted (Cassels, 2013).

Diet, Nutrition, and Complementary and Alternative Therapies

There are many ongoing studies looking at various aspects of nutrition and its effects on ASD, although to date none have strong enough data to become evidenced-based treatment. Nonetheless, it is useful for the PCP to be familiar with some of the information that families may hear or ask about. Nutritional strategies are either additive (supplementing with vitamins [A, C, B_6, and B_{12}], magnesium, folic acid, fatty acids, or probiotics), or they are subtractive (eliminating based on food intolerance, allergy, yeast-free, gluten-free, casein-free, ketogenic, or specific carbohydrate). Not only is there lack of evidence-based research to support the effectiveness of these diets, they are costly, take time to prepare, have an effect on other family members, and a few studies have shown resulting amino acid depletion and bone loss. Special diets also complicate school participation. Further information on nutrition and autism can be found in the articles by Stewart and colleagues (2015), Nievengarten (2014), and Nigg and colleagues (2012). The bottom line is to ensure that the child is getting well-balanced nutrition even though that is often difficult due to atypical food preferences, food selectivity, and disruptive mealtime behaviors.

It is important to be at least somewhat familiar with complementary or alternative therapies that are available and to ask families what they are using or considering, because patients of families often do not volunteer this information (Kramer, 2014). While maintaining a nonjudgmental approach, encourage the family to thoroughly research the approach they are considering, know what specific behavior they are hoping to affect, and attempt only one treatment at a time. Teaching and supporting families in their decisions about care while assessing the effectiveness, risks, and monitoring for possible side effects of such treatments are elements of care. Chapter 43 discusses complementary alternatives that have been scientifically evaluated.

Family Counseling and Support

Families need a great deal of support and training to manage children with autism, and siblings may need help dealing with the time and attention focused on the child with ASD. Referral for supportive counseling may be helpful. Groups and mentors can also be of assistance for both support and concrete management ideas. Although the prognosis for children with autism is highly variable, long-term care needs to be addressed, because few autistic children become fully independent, employed adults.

Hearing Impairment

Hearing impairment is a cognitive-perceptual problem. Information related to the etiology of hearing loss, prevalence, risk factors, assessment of hearing loss, differential diagnosis, as well as other ear problems is found in Chapter 30. Hearing loss is typically classified as mild, moderate, severe, or profound, and it is described as unilateral or bilateral, pre-lingual (before learning to talk) or post-lingual (after learning to talk), symmetrical (same in both ears) or asymmetrical (different in each ear), progressive or sudden, fluctuating (better or worse with time) or stable, and congenital or acquired/delayed onset. Additionally,

TABLE 20-9 Developmental Milestones for Hearing Impaired Children

	Developmental Milestones
Infants (0-1 yr)	Sensorimotor stage normal Language development: Deaf children exposed early to sign language develop language similarly to hearing children exposed to spoken language Deaf children exposed to both spoken and sign language learn both and progress as hearing children Deaf children exposed only to spoken language have language delays Language output decreased around 6 to 9 months old
Toddlers (12 mo-2 yr)	Sensorimotor stage normal Language output decreased
Preschoolers (3-5 yr)	May have preoperational delays Symbolic play may be delayed if language skills are decreased
School-age (6-12 yr)	May have concrete operations delays Decreased self-concept
Adolescents (13-19 yr)	Increased adjustment problems and decreased social maturity Decreased self-concept May have formal operations delays

hearing-impaired children often suffer from genetic conditions with multisystem problems and comorbidities, such as cerebral palsy, visual deficits, and intellectual disabilities.

Clinical Findings and Developmental and Behavioral Effects

Developmental milestones for hearing impaired children can be found in Table 20-9. Most hearing-impaired children have some usable hearing. Factors affecting the behavioral and developmental outcomes include the type and degree of hearing loss, the etiology of the loss (with comorbidities), the age at onset of deafness and age of identification of hearing loss, the timing and appropriateness of educational interventions, and the family environment. The four main areas affected by hearing loss are: (1) delay in the development of receptive and expressive communication skills, (2) reduced academic achievement due to language deficit causing learning problems, (3) communication difficulties causing social isolation and poor self-concept, and (4) impact on vocational choices. Box 20-15 lists the red flags for hearing impairment. Children who do not hear have difficulties with language development, which in turn affect their ability to communicate their needs and thoughts. Inner language development and the ability to translate experiences into verbally mediated thoughts and memories are also affected. They generally do well on nonverbal and performance measures of intelligence but fall short wherever abstract concepts and language abilities are required. Because early schooling focuses on development of communication, these children may have less time focused on instruction in other areas, and they often score lower on reading comprehension and mathematical tests. Box 20-16 lists the effects of hearing loss on the development of the child.

• BOX 20-15 Red Flags for Hearing Loss

Infancy

- Does not startle at loud noises
- Does not turn to the source of a sound after 6 months of age
- Does not say single words, such as "dada" or "mama" by 1 year of age
- Turns head when he or she sees you but not just to voice
- Seems to hear some sounds but not others

Childhood

- Delayed or unclear speech
- Difficulty following instructions
- Teacher concerns about paying attention
- Often saying "Huh?" or "What?"
- Turning the volume on television or radio up very high

Hearing-impaired children may manifest more behavioral and emotional problems than normal-hearing children, with impulsivity and aggression most commonly seen. Unless their families focus on methods for joint communication, children with hearing loss may not receive the same nurturing and social support as their hearing cohorts receive from their parents. For example, if a child learns American Sign Language (ASL) but his or her parents do not, that communication opportunity is lost. Teens with hearing loss often face identity confusion because they compare themselves to their hearing peers, have academic challenges because they miss information and have a difficult time in class discussion, and experience depression or low self-esteem from the feelings of being different.

Assessment

National standards recommend universal hearing screening of all neonates before 1 month of age, with follow-up of abnormal results by 3 months of age. Early identification and intervention by 6 months of age are recommended because hearing impairments significantly affect the child's development, language acquisition, and academic achievement. Additional screening is recommended with any risk factor, and it is recommended routinely at ages 3, 4, 6, 8, 10, 12, 15, and 18 years. Appropriate methods for hearing assessment can be found in Chapter 30. It is imperative to pay close attention to parental concerns about their child's hearing.

Additionally, it is vital that thorough vision screening is done, because deaf individuals are extremely dependent on good sight. It is also essential that development is routinely monitored, especially in linguistic and cognitive areas.

• BOX 20-16 Effects of Hearing Loss on Development

Vocabulary

- Vocabulary develops more slowly
- Learn concrete words more easily (e.g., "cat," "jump," "five," and "red") than abstract words (e.g., "before," "after," "equal to," and "jealous").
- Difficulty with function words (e.g., "the," "an," "are," and "a").
- The gap in vocabulary between children with normal hearing and those with hearing loss widens with age; there is no catch up without intervention.
- Has difficulty understanding words with multiple meanings (e.g., "bank" can mean the edge of a stream or a place where we put money).

Sentence Structure

- Comprehends and produces shorter and simpler sentences.
- Has difficulty understanding and writing complex sentences—for example, relative clauses ("The teacher whom I have for math was sick today.") or passive voice ("The ball was thrown by Mary.").
- Often cannot hear word endings, such as "-s" or "-ed," leading to misunderstandings and misuse of verb tense, pluralization, non-agreement of subject and verb, and possessives.

Speaking

- Often cannot hear quiet speech sounds, such as "s," "sh," "f," "t," and "k," and may not include them in their speech, making the child difficult to understand.
- May not hear their own voices when they speak, thus speaking too loudly or not loud enough, speak in too high a pitch, or sound like they are mumbling because of poor stress, poor inflection, or poor rate of speaking.

Academic Achievement

- Difficulty with all areas, especially reading and mathematical concepts.
- Children with mild to moderate hearing losses, on average, achieve one to four grade levels lower than their peers with normal hearing, unless appropriate management occurs.
- Those with severe to profound hearing loss usually achieve skills no higher than the third- or fourth-grade level, unless appropriate educational intervention occurs early.
- The gap in academic achievement between children with normal hearing and those with hearing loss widens as they progress in school.
- Level of achievement is related to parental involvement and the quantity, quality, and timing of the support services children receive.

Social Functioning

- Severe to profound hearing loss children often report feeling isolated, without friends, and unhappy in school, particularly when their socialization is limited with other children whose hearing loss is limited.
- Social problems appear more frequently in children with a mild or moderate hearing loss than severe to profound loss.

From the American Speech-Language-Hearing Association: effects of hearing loss on development, American Speech-Language-Hearing Association (website), available at http://www.asha.org/public/hearing/disorders/effects.htm. Accessed October 27, 2014.

Management

The child with hearing impairment should be in a health care home and the PCP is ideal as case manager, ensuring that all team members and needed pieces are in place for the best care of the child. The multidisciplinary team should include a PCP, an audiologist and a speech and language pathologist, a sign language specialist, developmental linguist (provides training in listening and proper use of assistive devices), and/or possibly a teacher of the deaf. Genetics counselors, social workers, and other specialists can also be useful. The PCP plays a vital role in providing emotional support and help to parents, encouraging discussion of development, assessing the effect on siblings, providing information about relevant parent support groups and national/local organizations, sharing knowledge related to school-based and community resources and eligibility requirements for special services, communicating regularly with the specialists, and helping the family with developmental transitions, such as beginning school, adolescence, and independent living.

From an information-processing perspective, much of the management of the deaf child is directed at providing stimuli that the infant and child can use to understand and interact with the environment. Visual stimuli are the primary substitute for auditory deficits. Key components of care include subsequent early intervention by 6 months old for identified infants with hearing loss, ongoing hearing, developmental, and language assessments, and continued communication with the multidisciplinary team or pediatric otolaryngologist. It is imperative that children are exposed to good language models in both visual and auditory modalities as soon as the hearing loss is detected and throughout the child's life to ensure adequate cognitive, emotional, social, and educational development. Families must be encouraged to ensure that the child participates with other children in a multitude of experiences and not lead a sheltered life. Parents may be confronted with many choices and, due to a variety of factors including depression, may defer decisions regarding treatment for a period of time. PCPs need to encourage families to proceed with language and communication strategies from the time of identification.

Habilitation and Assistive Devices and Amplification Devices

Many technologic advances are available to help those who have hearing impairments. Alerting and warning devices, such as strobe lights, vibrating wake-up alarms, text messaging, email, closed-captioned television and movies, phones with captioning capabilities, hearing guide dogs, and social networking sites on the Internet are helpful. If children sign, they should be provided with an interpreter during health care visits. Children with hearing loss may have inadequate health care information and knowledge because of poor communication between provider and child.

Amplification from a very early age is crucial to improvement in speech and language and thus cognitive abilities of hearing-impaired children. Different types of hearing amplification have different purposes, and wireless and Bluetooth technologies have vastly improved the flexibility and use of amplification devices. Hearing assistive technology systems (HATS), including FM systems, infrared systems, induction loop systems, and one-to-one communicators, may be used with or without hearing aids or cochlear implants. Sound field systems amplify sound throughout a room, not just to an individual. The body box may be used for children younger than 3 years old and for those in need of more powerful or durable amplification. Postauricular (as early as 4 weeks of age) or external canal (as children get older) devices are frequently used. If external ear devices are used, the ear molds must fit well and need revision every 3 to 6 months initially, and annually by the time the child reaches 4 to 6 years of age. Ear molds should be washed with soap and water each night and cleaned carefully to avoid clogging. External otitis media can be avoided with adjustment of molds to reduce irritation and use of petroleum jelly to decrease friction. If an infection occurs, it can usually be managed by using an antibiotic ointment and leaving the molds out for 1 to 2 days. For fungal infections, antifungal drops should be used and the molds left out for 3 to 5 days.

Cochlear implants provide direct electrical stimulation to the auditory nerve. They are used most often for children with bilateral, sensorineural, and severe to profound hearing loss; they require a dedicated family and educational support system. A cochlear implant center provides care for the patient from identifying appropriate children to implanting the device to providing appropriate training and follow-up care. Bone-anchored hearing implants may be used when auricular or postauricular aids cannot be used. They increase audibility in noisy situations, improve speech understanding, and help with sound localization—all by conducting sound directly through the temporal bone to the cochlea.

Educational System and Family Support

Early intervention for children with hearing loss should be in place by 6 months of age with an individualized family service plan (IFSP) or educational plan (IEP or 504) in place to ensure proper services. Language development is important because language serves not only as a communication device but also as a system for storing and using information. Identification of each child's strongest modalities helps to plan the best strategies. Educational services need to be family-centered and culturally sensitive. There are several schools of thought related to education of the hearing impaired. Cued speech or language, ASL, use of captions, or total communication (spoken and ASL) are different strategies. Oralists focus on amplification, speech reading, and speech training and do not support exposure to sign language. Those who believe in the total communication approach counter that ASL links the deaf to one another and the deaf community, and it increases their acquisition of language and functioning in adulthood. Total communication methods include amplification, sign language, finger spelling, speech reading, and speech training. However, the use of cochlear implants is rapidly changing the perceptual environment of hearing-impaired children so that these arguments may be less relevant.

Families experience stress and grieving when the diagnosis is made. Parents benefit from advice, information, contact with other parents in the same situation, a deaf mentor, and a listener or counselor who supports them in the acceptance and parenting of their child with hearing loss. Facilitating bonding in the early years is especially critical. Parents of deaf children experience stress with different stages of their child's life, because there are always special issues (e.g., child care and transportation). Siblings, grandparents, and extended family must be considered, as they need to cope with a child who has a disabling condition as well. Many families find that learning to celebrate every small step and milestone and recognizing that small steps eventually become larger ones helps them make healthy adjustments to the child's multiple needs.

Visual Impairment

Vision relates to cognitive functioning in that it triggers curiosity, helps integrate information, and invites exploration more than any other sense. Visual impairment impacts an individual's ability to successfully complete the activities of everyday life. Visual impairment as it relates to cognitive functioning is discussed in this chapter. Information related to the etiology of visual loss, prevalence, risk factors, assessment of vision, differential diagnosis, as well as other visual problems is found in Chapter 29. Visual loss may be congenital or acquired (visual memory is retained). *Vision impairment* is defined as having vision that is 20/40 or worse in the better eye even with eyeglasses. *Partial vision* is defined as best corrected visual acuity between 20/70 and 20/200. *Legal blindness* is distant visual acuity of 20/200 in the better eye or a visual field that includes an angle not greater than 20 degrees. *Amaurosis* is the medical term for partial or total loss of vision. The National Federation of the Blind (2014) defines a blind individual as anyone whose sight is bad enough even with corrective lenses that they must use alternative methods to engage in any activity that persons with normal vision would do using their eyes. The impact of the visual impairment is tied to the onset, the severity, and the type of visual loss, as well as to any coexisting conditions. In addition to decreased visual acuity and visual field, a number of other vision problems may also impact visual functioning. There may be issues with sensitivity to light or glare, blind spots in visual fields, or problems with contrast or certain colors. Factors such as lighting, the environment, fatigue, and emotional status also impact visual functioning.

More than half of the children with significant loss of vision have comorbid chronic or neurologic conditions, including mental retardation, autism, cerebral palsy, seizure disorders, hearing loss, chronic lung disease, cardiac conditions, and metabolic disorders. Congenital cataracts, congenital glaucoma, high refractive errors, retinopathy of prematurity (ROP), detached retina, neurologic conditions involving cranial nerve II, cortical blindness, and optic atrophy are causative factors as are retinoblastoma, trauma, infection, hydrocephaly, and genetic conditions. There is increased risk for low-birth-weight, small-for-gestational age, and large-for-gestational age babies. The major causes of blindness in children around the world are determined by socioeconomic development and the availability of primary health care and eye care services. Approximately half of these children have underlying causes that could have been prevented or eye conditions that could have been treated to preserve vision. All countries deal with cataracts, glaucoma, congenital abnormalities, and hereditary retinal dystrophies. In high-income countries lesions of the optic nerve and higher visual pathways are most common; in middle-income countries, ROP is the most common; and in low-income countries, corneal scarring from measles, vitamin A deficiency, the use of harmful traditional eye remedies, and ophthalmia neonatorum are most common (World Health Organization, 2014).

The American Printing House for the Blind (n.d.) polls each state annually for the data on the number of legally blind children through age 21 in the United States eligible to receive free reading material in Braille, large print, or audio format. In 2014, the total number of students was reported at 60,393.

Clinical Findings and Developmental and Behavioral Effects

The age at which vision is lost is important, because children with even a short time of visual experience perceive the environment as a place with different dimensions. Loss of vision interferes with social interactions and may delay bonding. Gross and fine motor functions, balance and spatial concepts, language and learning, and sleep are impaired. Developmental milestones for children with visual impairment are found in Table 20-10. Children with visual impairment plus other handicapping conditions have even greater developmental delays.

Assessment

Assessment of vision is discussed in Chapter 29. Important components include the prenatal and birth history, especially prematurity with diagnosis of ROP; family history are genetic visual impairments; developmental history (attachment, midline play, reaching, gross motor skills, language skills); and sleep patterns. It is wise to pay close attention to parental concerns about their child's vision, because they may note concerns that might otherwise be missed. Box 20-17 provides examples of red flags for visual impairment. Hearing screening and routine developmental assessment are important in order to maximize other aspects of the visually impaired child's life.

• BOX 20-17 Red Flags for Visual Impairment

- Failure to fix and follow a moving object
- Lack of smiling in response to visual stimuli
- Poking the eyes or waving the hands in front of the face
- Failure to blink at a camera flash in front of the face
- Fixed or intermittent strabismus persisting longer than 6 months old
- Timidity, clumsiness, or behavioral change may be initial signs in young children
- Deterioration in school performance and indifference to school activities in the older child

Providing special cues for these children helps them to understand their environment and what is going on around them. Talking softly, warning before gently touching, and paying attention to body cues rather than visual or facial signals are helpful. For older children, the following tactics are helpful:

- Address the child by name
- Describe what you plan to do and how
- Warn the child before touching and of any discomfort
- Let the child touch or examine instruments

Management

The child with visual impairment should be in a health care home and the PCP is ideal to serve as case manager, ensuring that all team members and needed pieces are in place for the best care of the child. The multidisciplinary team should include the PCP, ophthalmologist, special certification teacher, and orientation and mobility specialist. Once a vision problem is diagnosed, the next step should be a low vision examination focused on function in order to determine appropriate interventions. The PCP can play a vital role in providing emotional support and help to parents, encouraging discussion of development, assessing the effect on siblings, and helping the family with developmental transitions, such as beginning school, adolescence, and independent living. Additionally, providing information about relevant parent support groups and national/local organizations, sharing knowledge related to school-based and community resources and eligibility requirements for special services, and communicating regularly with the specialists can be key roles.

From an information-processing perspective, much of the management of the visually impaired child is directed at providing stimuli that the infant and child can use to understand and interact with the environment. Communication is less affected than adaptive motor skills, and language serves as a main bridge toward helping children understand the world they live in. Sensory compensation is not automatic but must be developed and taught. For example, parents may find that smiles in infants are muted or fleeting, so they must identify other cues that their baby wants and needs them, such as reaching out to touch. Table 20-11 details developmental interventions for children with vision impairment.

TABLE 20-10 Developmental Milestones for Visually Impaired Children

Age Group	Communication	Gross Motor Skills	Fine Motor Skills	Social and Emotional	Cognitive
Birth to 3 months old	• Differentiated cries (has different cries for different wants) • Responds to familiar voices • Reacts to sudden sounds • Ignores certain sounds and attends to others	• Holds head steady while being moved • Lifts head up when on belly • Elevates self by arms when on belly (totally blind or light perception only babies may not do this until after they roll from back to belly)	• Plays with hands • Uses hands for purposeful action • Retains object placed in hand • Plays with toys that produce sound	• Recognizes caregiver's voice • Can be soothed by voice or touch • Smiles when played with	• Recognizes primary caregiver • Plays with rattle • Cries when hungry or uncomfortable
4 to 6 months old	• Turns toward sound • Makes three different vowel sounds • Imitates vocalization	• Sits with some support • Rolls from belly to back, from back to belly • Sits alone steadily • Pulls to standing (while holding your hands) • Moves forward through crawling, creeping, or any other method	• Reaches for object in contact with body with one hand (rather than two) • Places objects in mouth • Uses pads of fingertips to grasp small objects • Transfers object from hand to hand • Brings object to midline • Pulls objects out of container	• Initiates request for attention	• Turns toward sound • Places objects in mouth • Shows preference in play materials • Reaches for object in contact with body
7 to 9 months old	• Produces vowel-consonant combinations (e.g., ga-ga or ba-ba) • Recognizes familiar sounds or phrases	• Pulls self to sitting position • Pulls to standing position (using furniture) • Sits down • Attempts to walk (while holding your hand) • Creeps forward on hands and knees for a distance of 3 feet or more • Takes coordinated steps (while holding your hand)	• Explores different textures • Places object in container • Pulls string to activate toy • Plays pat-a-cake	• Differentiates between familiar and unfamiliar people • Shows "stranger anxiety" • Shows fear of separation	• Explores different textures • Uncovers toy • Pulls string to activate toy • Searches briefly for object lost from grasp but not in contact with body • Reaches for object based only on sound cue • Places object in container upon request

Continued

TABLE 20-10 Developmental Milestones for Visually Impaired Children—cont'd

Age Group	Communication	Gross Motor Skills	Fine Motor Skills	Social and Emotional	Cognitive
10 to 12 months old	• Uses gestures • Responds appropriately to familiar requests • Jabbers expressively • Begins to name things	• Stands alone • Bends down to pick up object • Walks sideways holding on to furniture • Walks alone (three steps) • Walks alone with good coordination (five steps) • Pushes small obstacles out of the way • Walks about house or yard independently	• Places one peg repeatedly into hole	• Uses gestures • Cries when caregiver leaves • Begins to enjoy social games like peek-a-boo	• Moves or gestures toward you when called • Locates fixed (constant) object (e.g., highchair, table, and so on) • Puts many objects in container • Learns that an object exists even if it is out of sight • Works to solve simple problems • Begins to understand cause and effect
13 to 15 months old	• Anticipates routines in response to a familiar request • Uses two words appropriately	• Moves around large obstacle • Walks up stairs with help; walks down stairs with help			• Uses two related objects (e.g., strikes drum with stick) • Uses object to perform social action (e.g., brushes hair, puts on necklace, and so on)
16 to 18 months old	• Uses words to make wants known				
19 to 21 months old	• Uses eight words appropriately • Strings two words together (e.g., "ma-ma bye-bye")				
22 to 24 months old	• Uses two- and three-word sentences	• Squats	• Stacks large objects	• Imitates caregiver • Plays alongside other children • Asks others when needs help	• Matches objects • Pays attention to activities longer
3 years old	• Understands most simple language • Communicates clearly	• Runs, jumps, climbs	• Uses hands for complex tasks • Throws a ball	• Enjoys helping around the house • Likes to be praised after doing simple tasks • Is aware of people's feelings	• Fits shapes into matching holes • Sorts objects • Takes things apart and puts them together
5 years old	• Talks about what he or she has done • Asks many questions	• Easily walks backward • Hops on one foot	• Copies simple shapes	• Plays with other children • Understands rules • Expresses many feelings	• Follows simple directions and does simple puzzles • Understands counting

TABLE 20-11 Developmental Interventions for Visually Impaired Infants and Children

Age	Psychosocial	Cognitive	Motor
Infancy	Hold and talk to the infant to promote recognition through tactile and auditory modalities. Respond to other social cues from the infant besides smiling.	Stimulate the hands and mouth. Provide a cradle gym so that reaching and touching give feedback. Provide toys with feedback, such as sound, interesting textures, or tastes.	Encourage the prone position at times while awake, a position that blind children do not generally like because they have no reinforcement visually for lifting the head. Encourage head turning. Bring the hands into midline. Exercise the legs and massage during baths and diaper changes. Put bells on booties.
5-8 mo	Stranger anxiety occurs early. Parents need to be available. Provide predictable routines.	Provide finger foods. Provide new temperatures, textures, toys with various sounds and sensations. Talk to the child. Call attention to music and other sounds in the environment. From infancy, provide labels for objects.	Encourage outdoor play and on the floor. Dance and move the child actively. Sleepy behavior may be an indicator of insufficient sensory stimulation.
9-12 mo	Provide predictable routines. Touch and voice are important. Cuddle.	Encourage reaching to find a sound source. Provide toys that respond to the actions of the child to develop cause-effect concepts. Name and describe the activities and items in the environment.	Encourage creeping about, which will occur after the child can reach for a sound. Help to stand and cruise. Touch and name body parts.
Toddler	Stranger anxiety continues. Reassure toddler of return. Regression and tantrums are frustration responses. Guide behavior into more appropriate responses. Reduce frustrations when possible.	Continue to work on object permanence concept, which is delayed. Noncontingent sounds, such as television or radio, are not helpful. Articulation may be normal but the child may not easily progress to meaningful sentences. Pair lessons with hands-on activities.	Walking should begin. Crab walking is a common problem that needs to be eliminated. Walking with the child's feet on the adult's feet can help develop the reciprocal pattern. "Blindisms" may appear and can be altered with teaching. Walk together both indoors and outdoors.
Preschool	Interactions with peers and sighted children. Establish behavioral limits as with sighted children. Teach self-help skills, such as hygiene, feeding, and dressing.	Teach games with directional concepts. Provide experiences in a variety of settings: park, grocery, and so on. Give verbal descriptions of play areas and activities of other kids in the space.	Develop motor skills, such as walking, climbing, and swimming.
School age and adolescent	Continue to develop social skills and develop self-esteem through opportunities to be successful in activities. Provide opportunities to be with other children. Continue to develop self-help skills.	School with additional supports for the visually impaired in the following areas: • Orientation and mobility • Social interaction skills • Independent living skills • Recreation/leisure skills • Career education • Use of assistive technologies • Self-determination	Specific mobility training with balance, coordination, strength, visual-motor control, and finger dexterity content.

Data from Lewis V: Development and disability, Philadelphia, 2003, Blackwell; Teplin S: Visual handicaps. In Green M, Haggerty R, editors: *Ambulatory pediatrics*, Philadelphia, 1999, Saunders; Teplin SW, Greeley S, Anthony TL: Blindness and visual impairment. In Carey WB, Crocker AC, Coleman WL, et al, editors: *Developmental-behavioral pediatrics*, ed 4, Philadelphia, 2009, Elsevier, pp 698–716.

Habilitation and Assistive Devices

Sleep patterns are likely to be disturbed because visually impaired children take longer to get to sleep and have longer and more frequent night awakening than their normally sighted peers. Many visually impaired children benefit from taking melatonin at bedtime. Difficulty with daily living skills may include dressing, eating, hygiene, use of the telephone, and handling money. An orientation and mobility specialist teaches the visually handicapped child to travel with a sighted guide, use a cane, and use public transportation. Physical education and fitness are as important to visually impaired children as to other children. Generally, individual sports, such as gymnastics and swimming, are more successful endeavors for a blind child than team sports, even if the child is partially sighted. The Special Olympics and Junior Blind Olympic organizations hold competitions for the visually impaired in an array of sports activities.

A variety of technologic devices are available for children with visual impairment with the goal of improving function through the use of devices and/or adaptive skills. Glasses, high-powered spectacles or hand-held magnifiers, a telescope, or spectacle-mounted telescope may be used to assist with low vision. Special optical devices, Braille devices, low vision devices, phone accessibility, screen readers and magnifiers, voice synthesizers, reading systems, digital books, and mobility devices are some options. The Internet provides easy access to many different options. For children who have visual and hearing loss, the National Deaf-Blind Equipment Distribution Program provides great alternatives (see on the Evolve website).

Educational System

Early intervention for children with visual impairment should be implemented with an appropriate IFSP or educational plan (IEP or 504) in place as appropriate to ensure proper educational services as soon as possible after a child is identified. Infant early education and developmental preschool programs are essential, and an IFSP with parent involvement provides the structure for this. When children are ready to enter elementary school, there are specific psychological assessments using tests designed for visually impaired children to ensure correct educational placement and appropriate educational support systems. From this, the IEP or 504 plan is developed and reviewed annually, with input from parents and school officials.

Educational programs for visually handicapped children may include some of the following components. Children with peripheral losses may have to be taught to scan with their head and eyes to gain more awareness of their environment. Accommodations may include a preferred seat in class or supplying larger print materials. Both parents and teachers may have to be educated to expect and encourage the child to hold reading materials close enough to see them. Learning to read Braille begins when sighted children learn to read, and learning to write Braille involves learning to use a special keyboard in the early elementary grades. By fourth grade, visually impaired children should also learn to use a regular keyboard. Developing additional listening skills and gaining proficiency in the use of computers with aids are also essential skills. Full-time classes for visually impaired children may be available and taught by teachers with special certification—teachers of visually impaired (TVI). Some schools have resource room programs in which the child spends part of the day with a specially trained teacher and the remainder of the day in a regular classroom. Some school districts provide itinerant programs in which a specially trained teacher works with several teachers in regular classrooms, consulting with them about the learning needs of the visually impaired children in their classrooms. An orientation and mobility specialist can be used to help the child learn to navigate independently. Schools for the blind are generally reserved for children with multiple handicaps.

Family Support

As with other disabling conditions, parents want to be told as soon as possible about their child's visual impairment, and they want not only the diagnosis but also resources and direction about where to get more information. Because visual cues are so important in language and social interactions, there may be difficulties with attachment resulting from failure of eye contact and facial expressiveness. Families of children with visual impairment benefit from education and specialized anticipatory guidance designed to facilitate development throughout childhood. Families learn to adapt in a variety of ways. Parent support groups are valuable, and national organizations provide helpful resources. Some families benefit from counseling.

For a complete list of references, please visit http://evolve.elsevier.com/Burns/pediatric/

UNIT 4

Approaches to Disease Management

21 Introduction to Disease Management

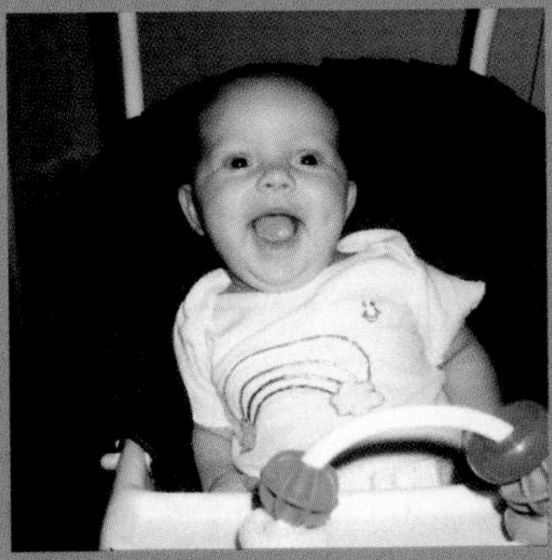

RITA MARIE JOHN AND MARGARET A. BRADY

Respiratory and gastrointestinal infections are the most common illnesses seen in pediatric practice settings and may present as minor or life-threatening acute illnesses (Smith, 2011). Noninfectious diseases can also present as acute or chronic conditions, such as those seen with inflammatory or allergic responses, trauma, malignancies, or autoimmune diseases. This chapter provides an overview of the care of the child with acute or chronic diseases and moves into a general discussion on assessment, management, and educational approaches applicable to all diseases. One of the major roles for the primary care provider is to arrive at a diagnosis and management plan that is consistent with pediatric standards of practice; this may involve telephone triaging in addition to providing care in ambulatory practice or urgent care settings. Two areas also deserve special consideration in pediatrics—fever and pain—because these problems can be a part of the clinical presentation. Pain is addressed in Chapter 23; fever and its management are addressed later in this chapter.

Key Concepts in Illness Management in Children

The health care provider begins management of an acute illness by obtaining a clear understanding of the presenting complaint and taking a complete history. The provider must always remember that these two elements, plus an accurate assessment, diagnosis, and successful management plan are contingent on the following eight factors:

1. Development of a trusting relationship.
2. Careful observation of the child and the family with the aim of getting to know the family and the child.
3. Attention to pertinent positive and negative historical and physical findings, avoiding skewing questions toward a particular diagnosis (van den Berge and Mamede, 2013).
4. Knowledge of physiologic functions and developmental considerations that vary by age.
5. Careful consideration of the differential diagnoses with deliberate reflection during the diagnostic process (Thammasitboon and Cutrer, 2013; Weiss, 2011) (see diagnostic process discussed in Chapter 2 and Determining an Accurate Diagnosis later in this chapter).
6. Tailoring information and promoting thoughtful discussion to involve the parent and/or patient in shared decision-making. This concept depends on input and feedback from the parents or caregivers and, if appropriate, the child. The resulting partnership takes into consideration culture, patient choices, social milieu, and specific needs, and, as a result, improves adherence to a management plan (Epstein, 2013; Fiks et al, 2010) (see Shared Decision-Making as Part of Child- and Family-Centered Care).
7. Use of health literacy concepts. It should not be assumed that medical terms used by the parent and provider are shared. For example, a parent's definition of fever may be any temperature greater than 99° F (37.2° C), or wheezing to a parent may in fact be rhonchi. Health literacy is discussed later in this chapter and in Chapter 9.
8. Feedback from the family and child needs to be obtained in order to ensure that there is understanding and agreement about the diagnosis and etiology of the problem, if known, and the acute illness management plan.

When satisfied that these eight parameters have been given adequate attention, an action or management plan is formed that is acceptable to the parent or guardian, child, and provider.

Shared Decision-Making as Part of Child- and Family-Centered Care

Shared decision-making (SDM) involves a provider and the patient's family working together to find a health care decision that is acceptable to both parties (Légaré and Thompson-Leduc, 2014). Charles and colleagues (1999) point to four key characteristics that need to be present in a shared decision: (1) Both patient and providers participate in the phases of shared decision; (2) information is shared between parties; (3) the expressed treatment preference is shared between the parties; and (4) agreement is reached. Patients who feel that they have been an active participant in the SDM process have improved health outcomes (Hirsch et al, 2010; Shay and Lafata, 2014).

A review of studies investigating preference-match strategies in physician patient communication conducted through 2004 revealed that 71% of subjects preferred an active role in decisions about their health (Kiesler and Auerbach, 2006). A recent study found that a provider's positive attitude toward SDM positively influences a patient's ability to engage in SDM (Légaré et al, 2011). A Cochrane review found that using decision aids (i.e., interventions to support decisions) to assist patients in making decisions about their health did not necessarily involve a significant amount of time being added to the health encounter visit, with a median of 2.5 additional minutes. The additional provider intervention included identifying the needed decision, providing information about treatment or screening choices and their associated outcomes, and comparing these choices to usual care and/or alternative interventions (Stacey et al, 2014). The SDM partnership varies with different situations and requires different levels of involvement from the provider; however, the goal is to jointly make decisions consistent with the patient's wishes as appropriate (Kon, 2010).

SDM requires a collaborative approach in which the provider neither assumes a paternalistic approach, in which provider decisions are explained without choices left to parent or child, nor a "hands-off" approach, in which the provider offers options but gives no guidance regarding best choices. Further, in some cases, a SDM approach is not appropriate (e.g., decisions to be made about emergency care after a life-threatening accident). The SDM approach is somewhere in the middle; the provider, family, and child jointly decide the course of action. A good example of SDM might involve the decision to order diagnostic testing. The decision needs to consider family, child, and provider preferences, because there are many courses of action that can lead to the same end. Parents of a 6-year-old may pressure the provider to order blood work and imaging studies when the diagnosis is clearly primary enuresis and not related to a kidney abnormality. In this situation, ordering extensive laboratory and other diagnostic studies would not be the best course of action for the child. Similarly, if the diagnosis appears to be nephrotic syndrome, the child would be better served by being referred to a pediatric nephrologist for confirmation of the initial diagnosis, ordering of laboratory tests, and treatment.

A Cochrane review failed to come to any firm conclusion on how best to encourage professionals to adapt SDM into their practice (Légaré et al, 2010). Nevertheless, SDM is a key point in the management of both acute and chronic illness. (See the Additional Resources at the end of the chapter for a list of programs on SDM.)

Overview of Parent and Child Education: Illness Management and Prevention

Health Literacy

Health literacy has been shown to have a significant impact on health outcomes (Berkman et al, 2011) and is an important issue to consider in all areas of pediatric health care (see Chapter 9 for a full discussion). The development of treatment plans in disease management requires special attention to the health literacy of clients. Written instructions and easy-to-read handouts with simple illustrations are useful for parents, caregivers, and children. Simply giving oral or written instructions is not enough; the provider needs to make sure that the receiver understands them. In designing handouts, using plain, conversational language, simple words, and short sentences without medical jargon increases comprehension. Whether a practice setting develops its own instruction sheets or uses information sheets from other resource texts, it is important that the instructions be written in the family's native language and at a reading level appropriate for the individual family. Several different tools assess reading level and ease of readability of material, such as a patient handout (e.g., the Gunning Fog Index, the SMOG Readability Formula, and Flesch-Kincaid test). The best tool to estimate reading level appears to be the SMOG Readability Formula (Fitzsimmons et al, 2010), and a level no higher than fifth grade is best for patient materials. In addition, the U.S. Department of Health and Human Services (HHS) Office of Disease Prevention and Health Promotion (2010), recognizing the importance of health literacy, has a National Action Plan to Improve Health Literacy. The goal of the plan is to deliver person-centered health services together with accurate and actionable information in order to promote lifelong learning and health. Links to websites for these tools and the National Action Plan can be found in the Additional Resources section in Chapter 9.

A number of books written for the lay public are excellent resources to suggest to parents (Schmitt, 2005). The care provider should develop a list of appropriate books and websites to give to parents based on the literacy level and unique characteristics. Select books that offer guidance about common infections of childhood, preventive pediatrics, common behavioral problems, and other frequently encountered pediatric concerns. Each practice setting should have its own list of books and supply of handouts, brochures, pamphlets, and other printed resources to share with families in their practice. The Centers for Disease Control and Prevention (CDC) offers health education information through their "An Ounce of Prevention" Campaign that addresses common pediatric infectious diseases and their prevention (www.cdc.gov/ounceofprevention/).

Health Care Education

Primary care providers' effectiveness is enhanced by their ability to educate children and their families about the prevention of disease and the management of common acute illnesses or exacerbations of chronic conditions, such as asthma or eczema. The child-parent educational component of the management plan must be individualized using all the characteristics of the child and family that make them unique—age, education, health literacy, cultural background, family structure and function, economic status, stress, community support and resources, and others. Education planning can be short term, as in discharge education, or long range to help families understand, manage, and cope with long-term chronic conditions.

Discharge Education

When children are going home from a health care visit for an illness, they need information to make decisions related to the condition, where it came from, how it can be expected to resolve, how to manage it, complications to look for, and strategies for preventing its recurrence or transmission to others. Because most patients and families will remember only about three main points from a discussion, written instructions are essential. The key points to cover related to management of all disease conditions should include the following essential points with strong consideration of health literacy concepts. Of course, it is important to consider where the patient and family are in the trajectory of disease diagnosis and management. They may not need all of the information during one visit.

1. Diagnosis information:
   - Information about the cause, if known, and epidemiology of infectious or noninfectious illnesses or medical conditions, communicability issues, and prevention guidelines, if applicable
   - The rationale for and procedures involved with diagnostic testing, including laboratory, radiographic, or imaging tests and the meaning of results
   - Estimations of the length of time or time frame before laboratory or imaging results are available, especially when there will be long waiting periods (these are particularly frustrating for parents)
   - Information about the length of time that it can take before the child improves and symptoms wane; description of what the course of the disease or illness is likely to be and signs of improvement
   - Recognition and discussion of cultural practices and beliefs about the illness or condition
2. Management information:
   - Specific, written instructions about when to return for any necessary follow-up or when to be available for a scheduled telephone conference
   - Written instructions to make sure that families truly understand special treatment or therapy, how to use adaptive devices, and how to perform home monitoring tests
   - Careful instructions about the proper dosing of medication, the potential need to switch medications during treatment, and the side effects of both prescription and over-the-counter (OTC) drugs (see Chapter 22 and Medication and Illness later in this chapter)
   - Plan for administration of medications at school; all appropriate forms must be completed, and school personnel must be instructed on key issues related to pharmacologic therapy
   - Specific information about any dietary needs or changes, special hydration needs (i.e., electrolyte solutions or an increase in fluid intake), plus any changes in eating patterns that can be expected
   - Information about any potential benefit or harm from specific folk medicine or complementary and alternative medicine (CAM) practices (including herbal, dietary supplements, or botanical preparations) if used either alone or concurrently with prescribed or OTC medications
   - Information for the working parent about resources for sick care in the community that are convenient (accessible) and affordable
   - Information about the safety and appropriateness of day care during the illness
3. Complications information:
   - Written information about specific signs and symptoms that indicate worsening of the illness, the need for immediate medical attention, or for a return visit sooner than planned (e.g., a newborn with a fever of 100.4° F [38° C]; a child with severe lethargy, tender abdomen, labored breathing, stiff neck, bluish lips, purple "dots" on the skin, severe pain, inability to walk, or fever greater than 104° F [40° C])
4. Prevention information:
   - Information about prevention and recurrence risk
5. Barriers to care issues:
   - Determination of impediments that prevent the parent or child from complying with the management plan (e.g., limited financial resources, inability to read, dysfunctional family, and/or transportation problems) and discussion about steps to correct these difficulties

When discussing the management plan with parent(s) and/or child, sit down and make eye contact with them if this is culturally appropriate. The parents' or caregivers' understanding of instructions should always be assessed by asking them to repeat what they have been told. By doing this, any misunderstandings can be addressed. One of the ways to obtain this feedback is by using the three questions in the "Ask me three" plan (National Patient Safety Foundation, 2014):

- What is my main problem?
- What do I need to do?
- Why is it important for me to do this?

Parents and caregivers would adapt these questions to their child's unique situation and say:

- What is my child's main problem?
- What do we need to do for our child?
- Why is it important for us to do this?

Education for Chronic Illnesses of Children

Education should be directed to the parent and/or caregivers as well as to the child. The family's ability to understand the health plan needs to be considered in designing educational strategies. A clinician has a wide range of options in providing education during encounters. They include using strength-based counseling, audio and visual media aids, electronic communication, touch points, child-centered communications, and family-centered concepts (Schor, 2009). The severity of the illness or disease and the child's age, maturity, and cognitive level are key factors that determine the child's degree of involvement in self-care activities related to acute illness and chronic disease management. Children should be taught basic health promotion and disease prevention behaviors (e.g., hand washing) from early childhood. Likewise they should be involved in the management of their illness to the fullest extent possible, considering their developmental capabilities and the complexity and severity of their illness. The pediatric provider also might be called on to be a liaison with school district personnel about the child's illness or medical condition in order to optimize the child's educational and social experience at school. Providers must be involved in helping to educate and prepare parents and children and youth with special health care needs (CYSHCN) related to transitions to adult care, including selection of health care providers and living arrangements if necessary.

Provider Considerations for Care of Children with Illnesses

Parents as Observers of Illness

Most parents are alert to subtle changes in their children, so it is important to listen attentively when parents voice their concerns. A sick child who is considered high risk due to physical, mental health, or social problems merits closer observation and follow-up than does the average thriving child who becomes ill. If the child returns and is not significantly improved or is more symptomatic, the initial evaluation and diagnosis should be revisited by carefully analyzing the symptoms, investigating problems related to compliance or adherence, repeating the physical examination, reviewing likely differential diagnoses, and confirming the diagnosis before deciding on another management plan. Be sure to have the family's current or contact telephone number in case a telephone contact needs to be made regarding the results of diagnostic studies that come back or to monitor the course of the child's condition.

Medications and Illness

Parents often need help to understand certain principles related to medication use and illness management if they may advocate for a medication to quickly cure their child's illness. Based on the child's diagnosis, the provider may need to discuss the importance of allowing time for the body's natural defense system to fight disease; such is often the case with viral illnesses in young children. Premature and excessive pharmacologic therapy can result in needless iatrogenic disease or resistance to antimicrobial agents and often confuses the clinical picture. The drug of first choice—the one that is least harmful—should be given time to work. Busy parents may not be receptive to this fact. Prematurely changing to a new drug, adding additional drugs, and using more toxic drugs are dangerous practices for the provider to engage in and can decrease confidence in the provider (Ledford et al, 2010).

Day Care and Illnesses

Another issue to consider is attendance in day care. The number of infants and young children in day care is expanding as the number of women in the workforce increases. This phenomenon creates several issues:

- The disease pattern in this cohort of children is often related to group exposure to illnesses.
- The issue of multiple caregivers can complicate history taking. It is critical to collect as much information as possible from as many sources. When the person bringing the child is not the caregiver, the provider should use the phone to communicate with the actual caregiver.
- Sometimes parents express feelings of guilt because they must work and their child is exposed to various communicable illnesses at day care. Simply explaining that children do get sick during childhood may help relieve stress for parents and should be part of the educational information given to parents.

Working with Non–English-Speaking Families

With the diversity of dialects spoken in the United States, language issues can be a barrier to providing optimal health care. If a practice setting does not have access to an interpreter or native speaker, interpreter services can sometimes be obtained from local telephone services. It is important that both the health care provider and the parent or caregiver can communicate with and understand each other (see Chapter 3).

Emergency Department Utilization

Educating families about how and when to use an emergency department (ED) is also important—not only for continuity of care but also for better management of health care dollars. A 2012 study in the United States revealed that 24.8% of children from birth to 17 years old with Medicaid visited an ED at least once over the previous 12 months. This was in comparison with 15.7% who were uninsured and 12.9% with private insurance. The EDs were more often utilized for the treatment of nonserious illnesses by families with Medicaid than those with private insurance. Seventy-five percent of the ED visits occurred at night or on weekends regardless of the insurance status; most nonserious illness visits were attributed to the medical office not being open (Gindi and Jones, 2014). Children with medically complex conditions are more likely to have ED visits and utilize more resources in hospitals (Hudson et al, 2014). Health care providers working in EDs must adhere to illness assessment and management protocols and provide critical documentation outlining their physical examination and diagnostic findings, assessment, and management strategies, including parental education and indications for needed follow-up in primary care settings or for when to return to the ED if the child's condition worsens or does not improve.

Chronic Disease Management Issues

The types and characteristics of chronic diseases in children are varied and include a spectrum of rare conditions and genetic or prenatal conditions. Some chronic conditions are not permanent, serious, or obvious, whereas others are irreversible, involve acute exacerbations and remissions, and are readily apparent.

In 2010, the United States spent $2.6 trillion on health care, an increase of 3.9% from 2009, and 17.9% of its gross domestic product, with 83% of medical costs related to chronic illness. The number of children and adolescents diagnosed with a chronic medical condition has been steadily increasing over the past 20 years due to an increase in the prevalence of obesity, asthma, and advances in medical care that increased survival rates in certain diseases (i.e., cystic fibrosis, kidney transplant) (McGrady and Hommel, 2013). The number of children with chronic conditions also varies depending on the definition and methods used to classify a chronic condition (Allen, 2010).

Children and Youth with Special Health Care Needs

CYSHCN are defined by the HHS Health Resources and Services Administration, Maternal and Child Health Bureau (2013) as those children with one or more chronic physical, developmental, behavioral, or emotional conditions that require health and related services of a type or amount greater than the average child. This definition remains the guiding principle to identify children eligible for federal and state assistance because of their chronic health condition. The need for services, rather than medical diagnosis, is the key factor or criterion that labels a child as having special needs.

According to the HHS statistics, 15.1% of all children have special health care needs. The prevalence of CYSHCN increases markedly with age, with 9.3% of infants to 5 year olds classified as CYSHCN and 18.3% of all children designated as having special health care needs (HHS, 2013). The health care services provided to this unique group of children represent nearly 25% of all outpatient pediatric visits (Hing et al, 2010).

There can be great variability in the presentation and the course of illness among children with special needs. They and their families often face a range of problems that are as diverse as the conditions that cause these difficulties. A variety of genetic, congenital, and acquired conditions can lead to permanent or persistent problems that have a significant effect on the child's and family's lifestyle. Health care providers must remember that family members are the ones who bear the major daily burden of care. There are several key points to keep in mind when working with these children and their families:

- Early intervention from the time of birth and afterward to prevent secondary psychosocial difficulties is crucial; the developmental aspects of long-term illness must be addressed.
- Counseling may be needed for the child and family to handle psychosocial and behavioral problems or to discuss their emotions and feelings.
- The child, the family, and school personnel must be consulted to ensure that the child is able to attain realistic developmental milestones. Involvement with schools and community agencies is part of the role of the provider working to coordinate care for CYSHCN.
- Integrate clinical practice guidelines as part of the care for patients with special health care needs. These are available at www.guidelines.gov and include guidelines published by the National Association of Pediatric Nurse Practitioners (NAPNAP) and the American Academy of Pediatrics (AAP).
- Early identification of the condition or disease is of paramount importance.
- Prevention of special health problems is a primary goal of care and includes the following:
  - Early prenatal care for all pregnant women
  - Genetic counseling as indicated
  - Elimination of environmental triggers or toxins
- Provision of primary care services—regular health maintenance supervision and anticipatory guidance—must not be overlooked.

Legislative and Governmental Support for Children and Youth with Special Health Care Needs

There are a number of laws and governmental agencies that support CYSHCN:

- The Patient Protection and Affordable Care Act of 2010 (ACA) contains provisions that impact CYSHCN. The ACA does not allow private insurance companies to deny claims based on preexisting conditions, and patients previously denied private coverage due to preexisting conditions can now access health insurance. The coverage for the latter does vary from state to state, meaning cost of coverage, copays, deductibles, and out-of-pocket limits will vary. In addition, the individual must be uninsured for at least 6 months before he or she is eligible. The cap for annual and lifetime benefits have been removed, and young adults can stay on their parents' plan until they are 26 years old. Patients with life-threatening conditions who have a life expectancy of less than 6 months are eligible for hospice care without having to forgo potentially curative care (Rosenthal et al, 2010).
- Laws related to appropriate educational support in school as a right:

- Public Law 94-142, the Education of All Handicapped Children Act of 1975, mandates an appropriate education for all school-age children with developmental disabilities in the least restrictive environment. This law was amended by the Individuals with Disabilities Education Act (IDEA) in 2004 and in 2008. The final version was published in the Federal Register in 2011 (U.S. Department of Justice, 2010). This law covers children with special needs from 3 years old to 18 or 21 years old. It also provides for early intervention services from birth to 3 years old (Billimoria and Kamat, 2014). A component of IDEA, Free and Appropriate Public Education (FAPE), is required under IDEA and mandates that schools allow any child who needs specialized education services to receive them free of charge. Children with disabilities must also receive educational services in the least restrictive environment.
- Public Law 99-457 (1986) provides states with the opportunity to extend benefits of Public Law 94-142 to children from birth to 2 years old.
- Prevention of discrimination is a right and is mandated under legislation related to individuals with disabilities. The Americans with Disabilities Act (1990) is a law that provides federal protection in the areas of employment, transportation, public accommodations, and communication for individuals with disabilities (U.S. Department of Justice, 2014). The scope of protection covers both private and public sectors.
- Section 504 of the Rehabilitation Act of 1973 for children with disabilities in regular education/inclusive settings prevents discrimination and provides safeguards and support for reasonable accommodations in the school settings, such as ramps, use of assistive technology, special seating arrangement, and permission to hand in assignments late due to illness. The Americans with Disabilities Act and Section 504 of the Rehabilitation Act of 1973 provide for modifications in the school environment that students need in order to learn; such modifications are based on the individual student's disability requirements. If the modifications are not included in the individualized education plan (IEP), then the modifications are covered under IDEA.

- Agency and support services:
  - Each state has programs (Title V) to assist CYSHCN with medical care and to provide links to social services, state vocational rehabilitation programs, and state school-to-work projects.
  - Social service support is essential to help determine financial eligibility for Supplemental Security Income (SSI) or state program benefits (e.g., Medicaid) for individuals with physical, mental, and developmental disabilities, or specific chronic diseases.
  - Advocacy for children with chronic conditions and their families includes assisting them to secure coordinated and comprehensive health care and community-based services as needed. The Office of Developmental Disabilities can provide services to families who care for children with developmental disabilities. The services vary from state to state and are not guaranteed. The provider should refer families to this office for case management. Each state manages its own program, and providers must check with their individual states for a list of provided services and whether particular services are funded, including the level of funding.

Emotional Support for Children and Youth with Special Health Care Needs and Their Families

Helping parents and children more effectively handle the emotional stress associated with a chronic illness and condition is a major focus of care. Key points to be cognizant of include:

- The time of diagnosis and periods of exacerbations of illness are viewed as times of crisis and added stress. *Chronic sorrow* is a phenomenon that involves feelings of sadness, anger, guilt, or failure. Parents of a child with a chronic condition may experience these feelings at various times during their child's life. The term was coined by Olshansky (1962) to describe cyclical, recurring feelings of sadness during one's lifetime that are of differing degrees of intensity. It involves grieving without finality. It is not pathologic and does not occur uniformly within families (Vitale and Falco, 2014). There are four main components of chronic sorrow: (1) recurrent or intermittent, (2) having no end, (3) an increase in intensity over time, and (4) can be triggered by predictable internal or external effects.
- Developing a trusting relationship with these children and their families involves being respectful and accepting of their varied emotional needs.
- Engaging parents and their children in the treatment plan is a major and essential task (see Shared Decision-Making as Part of Child- and Family-Centered Care earlier in this chapter). Professional empathy by the provider is associated with a higher level of agreement with the treatment plan (Parkin et al, 2014). Self-management of the disease whenever possible empowers the child, parents, or both depending on the child's age and cognitive ability.
- Research has demonstrated that more paternal involvement in illness-related support is associated with better family and maternal outcomes in families of children with chronic illness; hence in a two-parent household, participation by both parents in their child's care and health care visits should be encouraged (Gavin and Wysocki, 2006).
- Partial or poor adherence to complex treatment regimens should be addressed. Motivational interviewing techniques can be a useful tool. Nonadherence issues should be dealt with in a collaborative, "blame-free" problem-solving approach.

- Parents of children with chronic diseases are more likely to think about using, or are using, CAM practices (Adams et al, 2013). Respecting their reaching out for additional treatments is important. However, it is not common practice for parents to reveal this to their conventional pediatric providers, so it is important that the health care provider ask about such practices. Some of these treatments may be ineffective or harmful (see Chapter 43).

Family-Centered Care for Children with Chronic Conditions

Family-centered care is a key concept that should be used to empower the family. Parents who have infants and young children with chronic conditions should be viewed as therapeutic partners in the management plan. Communication with parents should be open and honest. They should be treated with respect and dignity and allowed to vent their emotions and to use coping mechanisms that work for them. Likewise, as the older child and adolescent mature, their partnership role emerges.

Relapses in adherence behavior are problematic but not unusual in situations involving complex treatment plans. Problems of adherence to the management plan can lead to serious medical complications, increased rates of hospitalization, greater length of hospital stay, and increased health care costs. The use of educational approaches combined with behavioral approaches is more likely to be effective in increasing adherence rates than use of educational interventions alone (Dean et al, 2010). Therefore, the provider should explore with parents and children what can help them become more adherent using motivational interviewing, linking medication taking with established routines, offering rewards for adherent behavior, or using smartphone applications (Schwartz, 2010; Vervloet et al, 2012). Box 21-1 outlines categories and key factors to consider when addressing concerns about adherence (see Chapter 22).

Training in motivational interviewing, in which the interviewer seeks to ascertain the individual's level of readiness to change, is a promising technique to use in situations of less than optimal adherence. The key tenets of motivational interviewing are to establish and express empathy, to provide the choice to change or not, to work with patients and families to identify their own personal treatment goals, to work with resistance, to assist in the removal of barriers to change, to provide feedback, and to advocate for the development of patient self-efficacy (Coleman and Pasternak, 2012; Shay and Lafata, 2014). There is a brief self-management support tool that providers may find useful in working with parents and adolescents in developing an action plan for change that is available at www.chcf.org/publications/2009/09/selfmanagement-support-training-materials (see Chapter 9 for more information).

Family support groups are often beneficial; they offer an opportunity to interact with others who have experienced many of the same challenges, difficulties, sorrows, and triumphs. The provider must address sibling issues and feelings, such as anger or embarrassment; a sense of being overwhelmed with added responsibilities; or believing they need to be the protector for their brother or sister. These groups can be face-to-face or Internet-based depending on patient preferences.

• BOX 21-1 Key Factors that Affect Treatment Adherence in Children and Adolescents with Acute Illnesses or Chronic Diseases or Conditions

Illness

- Severity of the illness and its predictability
- Length of illness and prognosis
- Effect of illness on functional and social activities of daily living

Management

- Complexity of treatment plan
- Length of time for each treatment, how often, and for what length of time treatments must continue
- Visibility of assistive equipment

Family

- Support network and size of family
- Financial resources; knowledge base and the understanding of illness or condition; overall cognitive skills; communication style
- Coping ability and skills; problem-solving skills
- Family's belief system and spiritual base

Child or Teen

- Age
- Cognitive, social, and emotional level of development; temperament
- Peer group; coping ability

Health Care Provider and Environment

- Communication style of health care providers with child, family, and other health care providers; belief in empowerment of parent and child/teen, as appropriate
- Organization of clinic or office setting to be child, teen, and family friendly; need for adaptive modifications in their environment
- Number of health care providers involved in the child's care; team member collaboration and partnership among themselves and with the family
- Open and "blame-free" approach when adherence issues arise

Challenges in the Patient-Centered Health Care Model

Primary Care for Chronically Ill Children

Children with chronic conditions have unique health and psychosocial needs. The health care provider may give care to a child with a rare disease or disorder or be involved with the management of a child with a much more common chronic condition, such as asthma or cerebral palsy. Of note, an increasing number of primary care providers are involved in the specialty care of these children. Children with chronic illnesses deserve a pediatric health care home where they, as unique children and families, can receive comprehensive, patient-centered, culturally effective, community-based, family-centered coordinated health care with accessible services in an organization committed to quality and safety (Peikes et al, 2011). Although the present language still points to the medical home with a physician as leader, more recent literature uses the term *clinician,* thus allowing for other members of the team to lead the team (Scholl et al, 2014). Nurse practitioner organizations have asked for a change in the language within the medical home model.

The critical issue in health promotion and disease management for children with special health needs is to ensure an organized and coordinated approach to provide appropriate treatment for the child's specific chronic disease or condition and to ensure that the child's primary health care needs are met. The goals of patient-centered medical or health care home should be to (1) provide family-centered care; (2) provide clear, unbiased information about medical care, management, and community resources; (3) provide all-encompassing primary care that is available on an in-patient and outpatient basis 24 hours a day throughout the year; (4) provide care over an extended period of time that allows for transitions to adult care; (5) provide appropriate referrals to subspecialists and care coordination with the team; (6) maintain a record of pertinent information; (7) interact with educational systems including early intervention programs; and (8) provide developmentally appropriate and culturally competent counseling to ensure optimal outcomes (Medical Home Initiatives for Children with Special Needs Project Advisory Committee and AAP, 2002).

Pediatric health care settings should work to establish a medical home with a multidisciplinary team model and care coordination. These teams offer the expertise of many individuals in a united approach. In ideal situations, the involvement of a clinical social worker, a community health nurse, or a nurse case manager is important to secure essential community resources for the child and family. Parents or guardians are a crucial part of the team. All team members must remember to respect the knowledge that parents or caregivers have about their child, their child's condition, and how the child is likely to respond physically and emotionally to new therapeutic interventions or treatments, situational changes, or exacerbations of illnesses. Other principles coming out of the health care home model are to:

- Develop a database for CYSHCN who require additional contact time outside of the typical scheduled time frame for either sick or well visits, and be sure to flag their charts. An electronic medical record (EMR) system may provide a function for this. This will help in scheduling additional visit time and alert the office staff when scheduling visits.
- Designate a care coordinator for each special care needs patient and train the staff about the medical home concept.

Health care management for children with special health needs includes: (1) assessing their needs; (2) planning comprehensive health care to provide for physical and psychosocial needs; (3) facilitating and coordinating services; (4) following up and monitoring services given and the child's progress; and (5) empowering the child and family through education, counseling, and support.

Child and Family Issues about Quality of Life

Addressing issues up front about quality of life should always be part of the assessment process in chronic pediatric illness management. Child and/or parent perceptions about quality of life issues, such as physical and emotional pain and discomfort, may not be the same as those held by the health care provider. It is vitally important to determine how the child and the parent feel—physically, emotionally, and socially—by listening to them and asking for their input, rather than assuming that all is going well based on outward appearances. Health care management of children with chronic disease is about empowering them to live their lives to the fullest potential.

Chronic Care of Children and the Health Care System

The Chronic Care Model identifies essential elements of a health care system that encourages high-quality chronic disease care utilizing the community, the health system, self-management support, delivery system design, decision support, and clinical information systems (Coleman et al, 2009). The care within these health care homes is proactive and centered around the patient with a prepared team that adheres to the latest clinical guidelines and promotes patient safety.

Providing quality pediatric care for CYSHCN requires that providers follow clinical practice guidelines that are available and congruent with the family's and child's values and beliefs. For example, recently released guidelines about care of the child with sickle cell disease should include annual transcranial Doppler ultrasound evaluations from 2 to 16 years old and long-term transfusion therapy to prevent stroke in patients with abnormal results (Yawn et al, 2014). Therefore, a key component of the medical home is prevention of further disability by ensuring that screening and clinical practice guidelines for chronic disease management are meticulously adhered to and faithfully followed.

The level or type of involvement in the treatment and management of a child with a specific chronic disease may vary depending on the unique situation of the child and family and the health care provider's subspecialty training and education. Strategies related to fostering the child's psychosocial development should be addressed at each health care encounter. A holistic approach to care is a major tenet of the medical home model. Certain situations may require additional advocacy when CYSHCN and their families are in a particularly vulnerable position (e.g., if the parent of a child with special needs loses his or her job or suffers significant illness or injury and cannot adequately provide for the child). Children with chronic conditions do well when family functioning is high and there is positive family adaptation. Thus, the goal for the pediatric health care home is to provide for open communication between parent, child, and provider and to advocate for effective and efficient coordinated health care services.

Common Concerns of Children and Families Related to Chronic Illness Care

Although chronic illnesses are diverse in their severity and effect on the child, certain issues are often common concerns for children with chronic conditions and their families and their health care management. By using a medical home model, members of the health care team can communicate about a variety of issues. They include the following:

- The high cost of treatment—the potential need for financial assistance
- Lack of, or difficulties and barriers in, acquiring health care insurance
- Family lifestyle alterations that may be required of parents, siblings, or both, in caring for the child
- The need to overcome system barriers that families may face navigating through the maze of agency paperwork
- The need for supervised care by multiple health care providers and the frequent lack of coordination of services in providing continuity of care
- Unpredictability of the condition and the potential for complications, frequent medical visits, hospitalizations, and death
- The desire to be kept informed of their child's condition and progress
- Treatments or procedures that may be embarrassing, painful, or time consuming
- The developmental effect that chronic disease can have on a child, especially during adolescence and early adulthood (periods of increased vulnerability)
- Longevity concerns—ability to live and function independently as an adult, including the need for career and vocational counseling
- The level of knowledge parents need about the pharmacologic management of pain and the disease process or other therapeutic treatments, including nutritional support for the at-home care of the child
- The effect of stress on emotional and psychological well-being of the child and family members—parents or caregivers, siblings, and possibly the extended family support network
- Acceptance by peers
- Parental striving to successfully normalize their child's life by acknowledging the child's condition and its effect on family lifestyle while actively engaging in accommodations to focus on the child and not the condition
- Dealing with feelings (e.g., anger, sorrow) while attempting to cope with chronic illness
  - Children with chronic conditions have a greater risk for developing psychological comorbidities of maladjustment, depression, and anxiety compared with their well peers (Perrin et al, 2012). The National Center for Telehealth and Technology has developed a tool (T2 Mood Tracker) for patients to track symptoms of mental health disorders, such as depression, anxiety, posttraumatic stress, as well as a general well-being. It is available at http://t2health.dcoe.mil/apps/t2-mood-tracker.
- Developing advocacy skills for these children to access services through schools, state and community agencies, or special federally sponsored programs
- Securing special illness-related equipment (e.g., movement and mobility aids—such as, walkers, wheelchairs, or braces) or acquiring communication aids, such as hearing aids or special computers with voices
- Finding respite care or transitional care for the dependent adult child
- Legal conservatory issues and the concern about who will care for the child as an adult when parents are no longer capable of providing physical care or are deceased
- Problems of nonadherence

Assessment and Management of Children with Acute or Chronic Illnesses

History and Physical Examination

Chapter 2 discusses the complete history and physical examination of children from infancy through adolescence. In addition, each of the pediatric disease management chapters in this unit focuses on key questions to ask in history taking and highlights significant findings to be alert to if found on the physical examination. Careful attention must be given when analyzing the signs and symptoms of a child's illness, including the presentation of clinical findings, the course of the disease process, and its associated manifestations. A clear history of the illness is essential and requires a comprehensive description of any symptom or sign of illness.

The physical examination is often a challenge when a young child is ill and uncooperative. Patience is important when examining children who are sick. The sick child should be carefully assessed so that significant physical findings are not missed during a hurried or cursory examination. The parts of the physical examination that are especially bothersome or frightening to a child, based on either historical information, observation, or age factors, should be performed last. Often examining the child on the parent's lap can be helpful in these situations. Repeating parts of the examination or observational reassessment is often useful (e.g., after an infant is breastfed). Distraction is critical in accomplishing the physical examination. Using a variety of distractions from bubbles to smartphone applications that distract children can make the process smooth.

• BOX 21-2 Indicators for Assessing Severity of Illness in Pediatric Patients and a Scoring Guide

1. Level of consciousness or quality of cry
   - Strong cry with normal tone or content and not crying (NL)
   - Whimpering or sobbing (MI)
   - Weak or moaning or high-pitched cry (SI)
2. Hydration
   - Skin normal; eyes and mouth moist (NL)
   - Skin and eyes normal and mouth slightly dry (MI)
   - Skin doughy or tented and eyes may be sunken; dry eyes and mouth (SI)
3. Color
   - Pink (NL)
   - Pale hands, feet, or acrocyanosis (MI)
   - Pale or blue or ashen gray or mottled (SI)
4. Respiratory status
   - Normal (NL)
   - Nasal flaring, tachypnea, oxygen saturation of ≤95%, crackles (MI)
   - Grunting, tachypnea with more than 60 breaths/min, moderate or severe chest in-drawing (SI)
5. Reaction to stimulation by parent or health care provider—how a crying child reacts when held, patted on back, jiggled on lap, or carried
   - Strong cry and normal tone or content and not crying (NL)
   - Crying on and off (MI)
   - Cries continuously or minimal response (SI)
6. Sleep-to-awake or awake-to-sleep state
   - If awake then stays awake or, if asleep and stimulated, wakens quickly (NL)
   - Eyes close briefly then awakens or awakens but needs prolonged stimulation (MI)
   - Not able to arouse or falls to sleep (SI)
7. Response to social cues (being held, kissed, hugged, touched, quietly talked to, or comforted)—for infants 2 months old or younger use alert ratings
   - Smiles or alerts (NL)
   - Either briefly smiles or alerts to cue (MI)
   - No smile, face anxious, dull look, expressionless, or no alerting (SI)

Data from McCarthy, PL: Evaluation of the sick child in the office and clinic. In Kliegman RM, Behrman RE, Jenson HB et al, editors. *Nelson textbook of pediatrics*, ed 18, Philadelphia, 2007, Saunders; National Institute for Health and Clinical Excellence (NICE): Feverish illness in children under 5 years, 2013. Available at www.nice.org.uk/guidance/CG160/chapter/1-Recommendations#/. Accessed August 12, 2015.
MI, Moderately impaired; *NL,* normal; *SI,* severely impaired.

To help assess the severity of illness in infants and young children, careful attention must be given to judging key indicators during the history and the physical examination (Box 21-2). These indicators are an important part of the assessment and the evaluation process when determining the management plan. They include level of consciousness, hydration, color, respiratory status reaction to stimulation, sleep-to-awake or awake-to-sleep state, and response to social cues. The ability of the child to be comforted is part of the assessment process. The child's overall appearance is very important but if the child has a fever and looks ill, giving an antipyretic and reevaluating are key (Saunders and Gorelick, 2011).

Considerations about Diagnostic Studies

Laboratory Studies

Chapter 27 contains a detailed discussion of the complete blood count (CBC) and provides insight as to the information that can be gained from a CBC, in addition to indications for ordering this basic laboratory study. Coagulation studies are also discussed. Chapter 24 discusses the laboratory workup for young children with a fever of undetermined origin. All disease entities or conditions addressed in this text include information about diagnostic studies and laboratory tests. Diagnostic studies and tests can be valuable, but it should be remembered that no diagnostic test or study is 100% sensitive and specific. False positives and false negatives occur; therefore, these tests are only one part of the entire database. Tests should be ordered only when the results are necessary to guide clinical decision-making.

Imaging Studies

When deciding whether to order diagnostic imaging studies, the provider should keep the following goals in mind: order only those tests that give the most information for the least money, are the least invasive, are crucial in the establishment of a concrete diagnosis, and are critical elements in the development of the treatment plan. There is a campaign to "image gently" in order to avoid unnecessary radiation exposure during childhood. The American College of Radiologists has information about appropriateness criteria for providers to use as an aid in ordering the proper diagnostic studies based on the patient's symptoms. This website (https://acsearch.acr.org/list) provides a pediatric section with links to narrative and evidence-based information.

There are several useful points to remember about common imaging tests:

- Conventional radiographs
  - Useful diagnostic tools if correctly ordered (e.g., the type of view[s] needed)
  - Least expensive of the imaging tests
  - Readily available
  - Involves radiation
- Computed tomography (CT) imaging
  - Best for detecting calcifications and fresh blood; shows greater bone detail than magnetic resonance imaging (MRI) (Smith, 2011)
  - Can be used with contrast material (taken by mouth, rectum, or injected via vein) for special evaluations, such as abnormalities affecting blood vessels; check for allergies to iodine or seafood, kidney disease, or prior reaction to contrast materials
  - Shows relationships well; images can be presented in the frontal, transverse, or sagittal planes or obtained in three-dimensional (3D) imaging
  - May require sedation or anesthetic for infants and young children

- Requires radiation exposure, which increases cancer risk (Goske et al, 2014; Johnson et al, 2014); it is therefore important that CT examinations be performed only when absolutely necessary
  - Costly
- MRI
  - Detects neuronal migrations, soft tissue lesions, and abnormalities of brain structure, ventricular size, as well as chronic subdural effusions
  - Provides excellent images of soft tissue without exposure to ionizing radiation; MRI shows greater tissue detail than CT (Smith, 2011)
  - Often requires sedation or anesthetic in infants and young children because immobilization is necessary
  - Advanced MRIs include diffusion MRI, magnetization transfer MRI, fluid-attenuated inversion recovery (FLAIR), magnetic resonance angiography, magnetic resonance gated intracranial cerebrospinal fluid (liquor) dynamics (MR-GILD), magnetic resonance spectroscopy, functional MRI (fMRI), real-time MRI, and interventional MRI; usually ordered by specialists
  - Expensive
- Ultrasonography
  - Gives two-dimensional (2D) images and measurements of internal organ systems; however, air-filled lungs and gas-filled bowel loops are impenetrable to ultrasound
  - With Doppler ultrasound blood flow direction and velocity can be measured; a still picture of the image can be recorded as a permanent record, or sonography can be viewed as the image is being projected onto a video screen
  - Highly dependent on operator skill and experience
  - No sedation required
  - No radiation exposure; noninvasive

Determining an Accurate Diagnosis

Following the history and physical examination, possible diagnoses need to be generated. The management plan will be the direct result of the working diagnosis and the differential.

Diagnostic errors are more common than realized. Elstein (2009) estimated diagnostic error at 15%; Berner and Graber's (2008) review of diagnostic error rate for specific conditions was 10% to 69%. They concluded that the rate of diagnostic error is unacceptably high. Diagnostic errors come from faulty data gathering or verification, as well as inadequate knowledge (Thammasitboon and Cutrer, 2013). Graber and colleagues (2005) identified three common types of errors:

1. Context error (limiting diagnostic possibilities)
2. Availability errors (choosing a familiar diagnosis over a rare one)
3. Premature closure (failure to fully consider other diagnoses)

Diagnostic errors remain a leading cause of malpractice claims (Nurses Service Organization, 2014). With increasing time constraints in clinical practice, difficulty in keeping track of patients in large group practices, and the development of the full clinical picture that may only become evident over time, it is important to use every available resource to elucidate difficult diagnoses.

A more reflective thought process by the clinician can help to avoid errors (Cutrer et al, 2013; Thammasitboon and Cutrer, 2013; Thammasitboon et al, 2013a; Weiss, 2011). Strategies to improve differential diagnostic skills fall into three major categories: (1) expanding clinical expertise, (2) avoiding cognitive processing errors, and (3) using cognitive aids in diagnostic decision-making. In terms of expanding clinical expertise, providers must be lifelong learners, increasing their expertise in both the science of diagnostic decision-making and closing the gaps in their knowledge about a variety of diseases. In terms of avoiding cognitive errors, the clinician must develop skills to avoid questions that are biased toward a particular diagnosis, as well as understanding the importance of reflective practice. By using evidence-based medicine and understanding the common errors of clinical practice, clinicians will improve their ability to make accurate diagnostic decisions. There are several types of diagnostic aids, including using group decision-making and seeking a second opinion on error-prone diseases, such as appendicitis. The use of algorithms, diagnostic decision support, checklists, as well as point-of-care knowledge bases within EMRs or smartphones can improve the likelihood of a correct differential diagnosis. In addition, the system that the clinician works in must provide a way for laboratory testing to be promptly noted by providers (Thammasitboon and Cutrer, 2013). A tracking and follow-up system for diagnostic studies is critical. Empowering patients by making sure that they engaged in the diagnostic process is also very important (Thammasitboon et al, 2013b). Whereas a complete review of the numerous and various methods to reduce error is outside the scope of this chapter, an essential point to remember is that *reflective practice leads to improvement in diagnostic accuracy over time.* Consulting with or referring difficult patients to a more experienced health care provider and using a computerized diagnostic decision support may be helpful when dealing with a challenging pediatric situation and/or illness presentation.

Data suggest that computerized diagnostic systems may give useful suggestions, provided that all symptoms are entered correctly into the database. Internet-based decision support systems allow providers to consider a wider variety of differential diagnoses and formulate an appropriate plan. They are noted in the Additional Resources section of this chapter. Diagnostic decision support systems do not make a diagnosis but expand the list of differentials based on age, gender, geographic area, symptoms, and signs.

Management Considerations

Acute Illness

The plan of care following a sick visit is organized according to diagnostic studies, medications prescribed, education, follow-up, and referrals. Each visit plan needs to consider the patient's or parent's desires; the most appropriate, if any, diagnostic study needed to evaluate the presenting problem; the follow-up needed; and whether referral is needed.

Chapter 24 identifies specific infectious diseases and assessment criteria for illnesses or problems commonly seen in childhood. It also discusses an overall assessment and management plan for sick, febrile children. In general, with infectious diseases, the age of a child is a significant factor to consider when doing an assessment and creating a management plan. For example, the immune response in infants from birth to 90 days old is particularly ineffective because of their immature immune system. Therefore, infants and young children are at increased risk for overwhelming bacteremia with any infection. Therefore, blood, urine, and cerebrospinal fluid cultures, including hospital admission, are the recommended management of febrile neonates (28 days old or less), although there is significant variation in treatment from these evidence-based recommendations that occurs in EDs across the United States (Jain et al, 2014).

Management of an ill child can include a short stay in an outpatient clinic, private office, or emergency or urgent care department for intravenous hydration, pulmonary therapy, medication, and/or close observation. For infants between 1 and 2 months old, admission depends on the results of diagnostic studies, the appearance of the infant, and whether the infant can be adequately followed up within 24 hours (Ishimine, 2007; Nield and Kamat, 2011). Administration of ceftriaxone can be considered in these patients on a case-by-case basis. After 2 to 3 months of age and before 3 years of age, admission again depends on history, symptomatology, and laboratory results (e.g., an abnormal chest x-ray). Typically children in this age group have more frequent outpatient management and close follow-up visits than younger children. Before sending an ill infant or child home from the office (rather than admitting the child to the hospital), the provider must carefully assess the parent's ability to cope with a significantly ill child and recognize signs and symptoms of worsening illness.

Medication Management

Prescribing Pharmacologic Agents

When prescribing pharmacologic agents or recommending OTC drugs, it is important to be knowledgeable of the pharmacodynamics and pharmacokinetics of the drug, the usual dosage, adverse reactions, drug interactions, and the indications and contraindications for its use in children. The provider must have a clear purpose in mind for using a particular drug and should not prescribe or recommend agents because of pressure from a parent or any other individual. Chapter 22 discusses pediatric medication management and medication adherence, and Chapter 23 discusses pain medication.

Pediatric patients are at increased risk for adverse drug reactions for numerous reasons, which highlights the need for individualized doses based on the patient's age, weight, and clinical condition and changing pharmacokinetic parameters at various ages and stages of maturational development. Selecting the appropriate pharmacologic agent to adequately treat an illness or condition and minimizing the risk of medication errors are important. Lists of current medications and dosages for prescription and OTC drugs, herbals, dietary supplements, and botanical preparations should be in a standard place in the patient's chart or EMR. Allergies to medications, with the identified adverse response, should be highlighted in a place that is easily visible. Advise the parents to have their child wear an Allergy Alert bracelet or necklace if they are subject to a life-threatening allergy (e.g., a severe peanut allergy).

In addition, some prescription plans or health care settings may require that a diagnosis and allergies to medication be listed on the prescription form. Do a SCRIPT analysis after writing a prescription for any medication. This helps the provider review the pharmacologic management plan and evaluate whether all five points have been considered and adequately covered. SCRIPT is a useful mnemonic to remember and stands for the following:

- **S**ide effects
- **C**ontraindications
- **R**ight medication, dosage, frequency, route, and duration
- **I**ndications
- **P**ediatric considerations
- **T**ransmittal of all necessary information on the prescription

Parental Education Related to Medication Use

Before patients and their parents or caregivers leave the health care setting, they should have a basic understanding about the pharmacologic effect of any medication, OTC drug, or medicinal product that is prescribed or recommended. Points of information that should be emphasized include the following:

- The purpose of the drug, how much should be given, and the frequency of administration and whether it is given on an empty stomach
- Compatibility issues: Possible drug-drug or drug-nutrient interactions, precautions, or adverse reactions that can occur
- Instructions about the indications for using a drug that is given on an "as necessary" basis or under specific circumstances (e.g., a rescue plan for the child with asthma whose symptoms are worsening)
- Signs or symptoms that indicate that a drug is either effective or not producing the desired effect or effects
- The need for refrigeration or storage (e.g., exposed to light)
- If applicable, any monitoring parameters that are required for safe administration of the drug or to maintain effective therapeutic blood levels
- Pregnancy risk factor of a drug (refers to the U.S. Food and Drug Administration's [FDA's] A, B, C, D, or X categories that indicate the potential of a systemically absorbed drug causing birth defects) and the need to screen for pregnancy when giving specific drugs to female teenagers

- For children who take multiple medications, the importance of always carrying with them an up-to-date list of medications (prescription, OTC, herbal products, vitamins, and minerals), their strengths and dosages, in addition to a list of medications the child cannot take in case of an emergency or if the child is seen by another health care provider
- Tips to help parents administer medications that may be difficult to get the child to take (e.g., how to hold an infant or small child when administering a medication)
- How to mask the flavor of unpleasant medications, if appropriate, based on the medication

Return demonstration can be a useful adjunct to evaluate the ability of the parent or child to administer a drug or drugs in the desired fashion. Return demonstration is a desired teaching tool in many situations. Examples of such circumstances include the following:

- Administering oral suspensions to infants and young children
- Measuring small or exact dosages (e.g., when a syringe is needed to measure amounts)
- Giving injectable, intravenous, gastrostomy, or nasogastric tube medications
- Instilling ophthalmic drops or ointments or nasal sprays or drops
- Using a metered dose inhaler (MDI), spacers, or inhalation equipment
- Ensuring that parents with limited cognitive abilities can safely administer medication to their children
- Administering multiple medications to ensure that the correct dose of the correct medication is given (e.g., 3 mL of amoxicillin suspension and 1 mL of metoclopramide syrup and not the reverse)

Referral and Consults

On many occasions, pediatric care providers identify clinical or behavioral problems that they are uncomfortable with or unprepared to manage. Clear communication is important to a successful referral or consult. Although the two terms tend to be used interchangeably, there is a difference between a consult and a referral. *Referral* implies that patients will be assessed and managed by the provider that you referred them to, whereas a *consult* implies that the primary care provider wishes to continue to manage the patient's care but seeks consultation about particular aspects of the case. The goals of both processes are to enhance patient outcomes and improve patient care. Whether the primary care provider refers the child and family to, or consults with, another health care expert, certain information must be shared with the referral or consultant provider in an organized, logical fashion. Guidelines for presenting this information are as follows:

- Give the child's name, age, tentative or actual diagnosis, and what you want the consultant to do (e.g., "newly diagnosed type 2 diabetes mellitus; needs initial insulin control and diet and physical activity recommendations").
- In a sentence or two briefly discuss why the child or family is being referred or the reason that a consultation is being requested.
- Give a synopsis of the history, clinical findings, prior management plan, and outcome of treatment if applicable. Clearly identify whether this is a referral or a consult.
- Identify any pertinent past medical history, such as chronic illnesses or conditions.
- Provide pertinent family, educational, or social information, including insurance coverage if this is problematic.

In addition, the primary care provider and the referral specialist must coordinate their services, being clear on who is responsible for which services (e.g., follow-up testing, monitoring, and treatments); clear communication and shared information between the two providers are essential. The provider should maintain a listing of specialty providers in the local area who take referrals from their work setting. If the provider is employed in a large health maintenance organization, there should be a list of pediatric specialty providers within the organization. The child's insurance coverage is often a major factor in referral, and often prior authorization from an insurance carrier is needed for a referral. Important information to gather about specialty providers includes their specialty or subspecialty practice area, evaluation of their effectiveness (can be an informal notation, such as "great resource person"), and, if applicable, their fees for service (e.g., full fee or sliding scale) and which insurance plans will reimburse for their services.

The primary care provider may ask a specialist to provide guidance through informal, "curbside" consults, but, due to malpractice concerns, many specialists are not open to do this. In addition, providers getting an informal consult may not be given all the needed information. If an informal consultation is provided, the primary care provider should present information about the patient, as listed previously, and discuss potential management options. At the end of the informal consultation, the primary care provider should summarize in the patient's chart, the key areas that were discussed, and the agreed on recommendations.

Often overlooked sources of free consultation are state and local public health departments or agencies, health-related professional organizations, and some major medical centers that provide telephone consultation for providers in their service area. Again a notation should be placed in the child's chart or EMR if the case is discussed with a consultant in such an agency. Connecting with colleagues on the Internet must be done securely; new laws carry heavy fines for transmitted information that is not done with encryption over a secure server (Neatherlin, 2014).

When a patient is referred to another provider, the primary care provider must explain the reason for the referral to the child and parent, how the transfer of care will be managed, and when the patient is to return to see the primary care provider. The information should be presented in such a manner as to dispel fears of abandonment or giving up. The bond between the child, the parent, and the primary care provider is typically a strong relationship that individuals rely on. If the primary care provider plans to seek a consultation, the child and parent should be informed by explaining the need for a second opinion or the desire to collaborate with others to ensure that nothing has been missed. After the consultation parents should be informed about what the consultant and primary care provider decided was the best course of action. Finally, the parent may seek consultation with another health care provider. If so, treat this as the parent's need to collaborate in the child's care and listen to the recommendation by this consultant. Be sure that the consultant's reports are duly filed in the child's chart.

Referral to National and Local Organizations and Resources for Chronic Medical Issues

Parents and their children with specific disease entities or health conditions can benefit from the educational materials, resources, and support that national health organizations provide. Learning to live with a chronic disease or handicapping condition presents a special challenge to families. Most national organizations provide written materials that parents and children can easily understand about the cause, management, and treatment of the particular disease in question. These materials also help parents explain their child's condition to teachers and others. Many of these national organizations can guide parents and children to support groups with other families and children who are similarly challenged and to health professionals and other related groups who specialize in the treatment of a particular disease entity. Likewise these organizations can assist parents in accessing unique services to benefit their children (e.g., enrolling in special camps and sports activities, learning about the various legal rights of children with disabilities or handicapping conditions, and acquiring special adaptive equipment).

Many national and local health organizations and foundations provide educational materials and valuable information designed for health professionals about a variety of subjects related to their target population of children. For children with rare disorders, the National Organization for Rare Disorders (NORD) may be able to assist parents and offer information about the child's condition or disease (www.raredisease.org). Often these national organizations can provide up-to-date information about new treatment modalities or management strategies. A list of some excellent websites that provide education about a variety of pediatric problems is located in the Additional Resources section of this chapter. Health care providers should take advantage of the services that these organizations offer. In addition, every clinical or practice setting should have a listing of local community resources. One can compile a personal local resource guide and keep this information along with a listing of national organizations.

Tips Regarding Documentation: Patient Visit and Follow-Up

There are several important rules for the primary care provider to remember regarding documentation when charting. Many malpractice claims against care providers are due to a lack of documentation. The old adage, "If it isn't in writing, then it wasn't done" has been used more than once to find care providers liable and render a judgment in favor of the plaintiff. Good documentation practices include:

- Being alert to a complaint or combination of complaints that are red flags for more serious illness (e.g., abdominal or chest pains, headache, syncope). Be sure to note pertinent positive and negative history and physical findings relative to these complaints when charting.
- Identifying differential diagnoses and ruling out the worst possible illness first. Be sure to gather enough data to either rule in or out the diagnosis based on history, physical findings, or diagnostic studies. If you put "rule-out" on your assessment, you have to include a management plan to do so (i.e., it cannot be listed as a diagnosis or a differential diagnosis if you don't plan to do anything about "ruling it out").
- Conveying the seriousness of the issue to the family or caretaker if there is the probability of a serious illness and the child needs to return for additional visits or have diagnostic studies done. Be sure to document that conversation.
- Revisiting an unresolved problem until it is resolved. This can be accomplished by:
  - Rescheduling a follow-up examination.
  - Telephone or email contact as appropriate with the family to determine if the complaint or illness has been resolved.
- Knowing patient or family risk factors and screening for them through diagnostic studies or history.
- Ensuring that there is a system in place in the practice setting to follow-up and secure the results of diagnostic studies that were ordered. There should be a mechanism to ensure that the test or procedure was done and that the provider was given the results and documented reviewing them.
- Following up all abnormal test results. There should be a note placed in the chart that the abnormal results were discussed (and with whom) and the plan of action.
- Following up on referrals to other health care professionals or agencies and documenting the recommendations or treatments implemented from these referral sources.
- Making sure that results of newborn screenings are in the chart.

Chart audits should be a regular part of practice quality improvement. Look for such things as omissions of information, whether problems identified in earlier visits were addressed at subsequent visits until resolved, compliance with routine health maintenance screenings, and adherence to evidence-based practice guidelines.

Telehealth Management of Illnesses

Multiple communication technologies are available to interact with patients and family. The use of brief electronic communication via text messaging, Facebook, email, Twitter, or Instagram have become increasing popular. Patients have expressed considerable interest in communicating with their providers over these new media. This section reviews telephone triage, text messages, and social media websites and discusses possible problems associated with the new media and what can be done to overcome them.

Telephone Triage Systems

All primary care providers should ensure that their practice settings have a standardized approach to telephone triage. Triage protocols classify problems into one of several categories. These include life-threatening, emergent, urgent, nonurgent, recurrent, or mildly ill. Protocols may vary slightly, but the major aim is to provide safe advice while avoiding unnecessary visits to an urgent care center or ED. Protocols may use a standardized algorithm in order to obtain history, leading to a patient disposition to manage specific health concerns (Schmitt, 2012). Several excellent resources address telephone triage management of illnesses in children (Briggs, 2011; Hertz, 2011; Schmitt, 2012). Telephone triage can also be called *telehealth, telephone advice services, telephone consultations,* or *telenursing.* Many insurance companies offer telephone triage services as part of the benefits to their insured to avoid unnecessary ED visits. Nurse-run telephone triage services have been shown to be a safe and cost-effective way to triage children to provide effective screening and appropriate dispositions about the type of care needed regarding an illness-related concern (Blank et al, 2012; Bunn et al, 2008; Huibers et al, 2011).

A major benefit of telephone triage is to provide convenient access to health care professionals and health care advice. The major difficulty in providing telephone advice is the difficulty of accurately assessing a situation without visual input. Families are asking for FaceTime communications, sending pictures of the problems via email, and asking to Skype instead of, or as a supplement to, telephone interaction. However, the risk of a Health Insurance Portability and Accountability Act (HIPAA) security breach must be considered prior to initiating such interactions.

Steps of an Effective Triage System

Management-by-telephone protocol in an individual practice setting should accomplish the following objectives:

- Allow the telephone triage person to manage ill-child calls safely; prevent harmful triage or recommendations.
- Provide a standard of care and improve the quality of care.
- Prevent omissions resulting from provider forgetfulness or fatigue.

The method of interaction, screening questions to ask, expressing concern, and reflective listening are important considerations. The individual doing the telephone triage must be receptive to the parent's call, stressing that the call is as important to the provider as it is to the parent. Parents can be anxious and find it difficult to calmly state the problem. The triage person needs to be a perceptive, conscientious, and calm individual who carefully listens to the caller; ask questions as dictated by protocol and by judgment; process the information; determine the correct management protocol to use for a particular situation; give the necessary instructions to parents; offer comfort and understanding to help the parent manage the illness; and document the encounter within a relatively short period of time.

The sequence of steps that one must go through in using telephone protocols includes the ability to do all of the following:

- Collect data about the symptoms through open-ended and direct questioning.
- Identify the problem or main symptom.
- Develop a working assessment.
- Decide on a triage category for the patient.
- Select the correct protocol.
- Correctly advise the patient about the course of action.

Questions should be asked in an effort to narrow the problem clinically and to assist the parent to be clear and focused. In addition, questions should be clustered by area of concern, should move from most to least serious, and should follow a logical sequence based on initial data obtained. When using protocols, the nurse needs to make sure that each question is asked but can add additional questions if needed. Screening questions that should be asked of parents include the following:

- Duration: How long has the problem been present?
- Description: Tell me about the problem. What signs and symptoms are present?
- Clinical changes: How has the child's behavior or activity level changed (e.g., eating, sleeping, playing, interaction with peers and family members)?
- Appetite: Has there been a change in the child's drinking or eating habits?
- Elimination: Have there been associated changes in bowel or bladder habits?
- Sleep pattern: Has there been a change in the child's normal sleeping habits?
- Environmental problems: Has there been any recent exposure, change, or stress in the child's environment?
- Cause: What does the parent believe is contributing to or causing this condition?
- Management: What has the parent done for the condition, and with what effect?
- Feelings: Does the parent feel anxious about how the child is behaving?

Keep in mind that protocols are a tool and should not override one's own professional judgment. If the provider feels that the patient needs to be seen despite what the telephone triage advice protocol states, then the patient should be seen. The provider's preference needs to be made clear to those triaging (Rutenberg and Greenberg, 2012).

If the office or clinic is not using a standardized telephone triage reference source (such as that by Schmitt, 2012), office protocols should be developed to ensure an effective telephone management system. Office protocols may be prewritten and should be regularly reviewed and modified by the clinician. There are also a wide variety of Internet-based telephone triage programs that will record the answers as the questions are asked.

Nonemergent calls to a practice about a sick child during the day are usually routed through a telephone receptionist—who can make an appointment, if appropriate, or transfer the call to a triage nurse or primary care provider. They in turn can determine the urgency of the need to see the child, give home care advice, or refer to the primary care provider for care. If home care advice is given, the triage person should use standards of care or telephone advice protocols discussed previously. An office telephone triage system needs to have a protocol in place to route triage notes to the appropriate primary care provider so that the provider can be alert to any significant issues with the child (e.g., increasing calls indicating exacerbation and poor control of asthma).

After-hours or call centers are another avenue that pediatric practices use for handling sick calls after office hours. These centers may employ nurses and/or nurse practitioners who use telephone protocols to guide parents in the management of their child's illness until their regular health provider is available. Call centers alleviate the burden of night call and are set up to use telephone protocols and a software program for documentation. It is incumbent on pediatric health care providers within their practice setting to evaluate whether such a center would effectively meet their standards of care for after-hours management of children.

Documentation of Triage Telephone Calls

Documentation of telephone triage calls and their disposition is an important element in a successful system for managing telephone calls for sick children. All documentation systems should be part of the EMR. Written paper or electronic documentation must be scanned into the EMR so that other providers know about a child's problem. Documentation ensures a medicolegal defense; a method to review medical records for quality improvement and assurance purposes; an avenue to assist in complaint resolution if parents are upset about the advice given to them; and a tool to use when making follow-up calls to the family. Important items to include in any documentation of a telephone communication are:

- Date and time
- Patient data—name, age, sex, and telephone number—and history of chronic disease or condition
- List of medications and their dosage if prescribed by the health care providers
- The chief complaint and a brief list of symptoms and signs, including their duration and frequency
- Documentation of sleeping pattern; activity level, appetite; and bowel and bladder elimination
- Diagnosis or working assessment
- Triage category (life-threatening, emergent, and so on)
- Instructions given about follow-up
- An "other" section for any additional comments that are deemed important information

When using telephone protocols in a practice setting, training is essential and ensures consistency in the use of the system. Staff sessions, designed to review the written or electronic documentation, are also useful teaching tools and should be encouraged. Perhaps the most important point to emphasize about the use of any telephone management system is the need to assess the comfort of the parent with the advice given. Parents should be asked at the end of the telephone contact whether they are comfortable with the advice and plan. If the parent is not satisfied or is uneasy about the plan, primary care provider consultation should be an option. Finally, parents should be told to call back if their child's condition worsens or the problem persists too long.

Texting

Short message system (SMS) text messages have been increasing steadily since the emergence in smartphone technology. Although the figures vary from website to website, the number is clearly over 2 trillion in the United States alone. There are no HIPAA compliant texting devices (per se) available on the market; however, texting back and forth can be used, providing there are adequate controls in place and used. Although texting can be an efficient means of communication, there are potentially considerable privacy and security risks associated with this means of communication. HIPAA was originally enacted in 1996—before text messaging or Facebook was available. As a result, the recently enacted Omnibus rule has regulated these communications; and effective September 23, 2013, all providers need to have the ability to have secure health care communications with an encryption protection platform as part of their mobile device. If there is a loss of a mobile device, the user can be disconnected from the system to avoid a data breach (Hardiman and Edwards, 2013). In addition, protected health information is not allowed to be stored on personal mobile devices if a personal mobile device is used on an open Wi-Fi network (where a data breach can easily occur). Secure health care communications can be stored on an encrypted messaging platform and, if loss of the device occurs, the user can be disconnected from the system. However, such platforms have not yet been approved by a government agency as HIPAA compliant. Traditional SMS messaging is not HIPAA compliant, can be forwarded to anyone, and can stay forever on the sender's and receiver's server. The Joint Commission has banned the use of SMS for transmitting confidential health information.

The average cost of a HIPAA data breach was reported to be $2.0 million per organization and, although the number of data breaches has decreased, the number of organizations with at least one data breach was 90% (Ponemon Institute, 2010). The penalty for each violation can range from $100 to $1,500,000 for each calendar year (HHS, 2013). Thus, practices need to decide whether the risk of a data breach is worth the convenience.

If text messaging is used by a provider who is evaluating a child's problems, it would be important to ensure that the same information that would normally be asked in a telephone conversation is ascertained in the text message before giving any recommendations. Most SMS communications are used to send appointment reminders, give educational messages, provide support to patients between visits, and track lab results; however, text messages can also be sent that provide emotional support for patients between visits.

Not all patients want to receive SMS; therefore patients also must agree to the use of SMS messaging prior to a practice sending out reminders or tests. These agreements need to be reviewed by a lawyer prior to initiating their use and updated at each visit or at a regularly scheduled period of time. Renewal of such agreements is critical; for example, parents or a teen may give old phones to family members that could result in a risk of breach of confidentiality. Some organizations have banned texting as a form of communication with patients, whereas others have asked for encryption, passcode protection, registration of devices, secure disposal of devices, and third-party secure messaging programs. Each organization needs to have a patient communication policy that parents or teens need to sign.

Social Media Websites

Many parents and youths spend more time on email, Twitter, Facebook, Google Plus, Instagram, YouTube, and LinkedIn than talking on the phone. A provider may be asked to connect as a friend on Facebook; however, there is a risk of disclosing personal patient information on these websites, leading to breaches in the patient-provider relationship. As a result, it is suggested that clinicians avoid social media relationships and do not accept invitations from patients or their parents. Providers should also avoid looking up their patients on social media websites in order to respect their privacy (Guseh et al, 2009; Roett and Coleman, 2013).

It is critical that health care providers not post any pictures of patients or post information about patients on a social media website, because this is a clear HIPAA violation. Photographs of patients should not be placed in open view in an office setting. Omitting a patient's name does not guarantee that the person cannot be identified due to the uniqueness of a disease or a time or date of visit.

Email

As with SMS, emailing patients can be very convenient, but it has the same problems associated with SMS text messaging. Therefore, it is important to limit this type of communication to encrypted networks in which the mobile device can be turned off if it is lost. Again, there is a significant risk of data breach in emails, and there are no HIPAA secure devices for this purpose at this time.

Educating Parents about Office Telephone and Electronic Messaging Policy

Practice settings should have an electronic messaging or telephone call policy about sick calls and should acquaint parents with this policy. The policy should cover basic information about the office protocol for handling calls, requests for advice sent electronically about sick children, or other child-related concerns during office hours, such as well-child questions, prescription refills, nighttime (after-hours) calls, and weekend and holiday calls. Who screens calls, when calls are returned (e.g., during the noon hour or from 4 to 5 PM), and after-hours coverage are points to cover in the policy. Likewise, a policy about staff's role in answering electronic messages should be in place.

Parents should be encouraged to handle minor illnesses at home without unnecessary calling in for advice. Home instruction sheets for managing fevers (including medication dosage charts) and common childhood illnesses or books on common pediatric illnesses designed for parents are excellent resources to provide to parents. Pamphlets can be given to parents at anticipatory guidance visits. In addition, NAPNAP has several handouts that can be accessed from its website, and there is also a parent section on the AAP website, which is an excellent resource. During illness visits, parents should be told what to expect when their child is ill, preparing them for the increasing temperature, vomiting, or diarrhea, in addition to what to do if they occur.

Parents need to know what type of situations require a call for emergency medical services or the poison control center. If sick care is necessary after scheduled office hours, parents will need to give the following information about their child:

- The main symptoms
- Any chronic disease or health problem
- Temperature (and route it was taken)
- Approximate weight
- Names and dosages of current medications
- Type of insurance coverage
- Preferred name of pharmacy and phone number

Box 21-3 provides general rules for parents when calling a health care provider. Box 21-4 gives parental guidelines for deciding when to call.

Illness Prevention

Prevention of illness and communicable diseases is a significant goal when providing primary health care services for children or managing the care of children with chronic diseases or conditions. Health care providers must be vigilant in their practice settings to prevent or reduce the possibility of exposure to communicable diseases and to control the spread of infectious diseases that are a threat to infants, children, and youth. Using the following guidelines can further the goal of prevention:

- All children should be appropriately immunized against vaccine-preventable diseases according to the

• BOX 21-3 General Guidelines for Parents When Contacting the Primary Care Provider

- When calling for *nonurgent* matters, such as well-baby advice, prescription refills, or appointments, call during office hours whenever possible.
- When calling for an *urgent issue,* tell the receptionist or answering service that your call is an urgent call.
- Give the following *information on every call:* your child's name, age, sex, major problem, and telephone number where you can be reached.
- Be ready to give *information related to your child's problem* as briefly and clearly as possible:
  - What are the signs and symptoms?
  - How long has the problem existed?
  - What have you done for the problem?
  - How did your child respond to what was done?
  - How do you feel about your child's condition? What is your intuition? Is your child getting better or worse?
- Be ready to give information about your child's general health.
  - Does your child have any chronic illnesses that need to be considered?
  - Is your child receiving medications for this problem or another problem? Has your child recently received immunizations?
  - Does your child have any allergies?
- If you do not talk to your provider directly, before hanging up, ask when your call will most likely be returned.
- If you do not receive a return call within a reasonable amount of time, call back to make sure your message was taken correctly.
- If your provider decides not to examine your child, before hanging up make sure you determine the following:
  - The most likely cause of your child's condition
  - Which medicines or treatments should be given
  - What signs or symptoms to watch for
  - When you should call back for more advice or to report changes in your child's condition
- If you do not understand the instructions, ask to have them repeated or call back for clarification.
- If you are instructed to come to the office or go to an emergency department (ED), make sure you have clear directions on how to get there. If you are too anxious to drive, ask a friend or neighbor to drive or call a taxi. If an ambulance is necessary, the provider may be able to call it for you.

• BOX 21-4 Guidelines for Parents for When to Contact the Primary Care Provider

When to call immediately for an infant younger than 3 months old*:

Baby has the following symptoms:
- Is unusually sleepy
- Has a rectal temperature of 100.4° F (38° C) or higher
- Refuses to eat three or four times in a row
- Has repeated bouts of diarrhea or vomiting
- Has a labored, wheezing, or grunting breathing pattern that lasts longer than half an hour
- Has an illness associated with a rash that looks like bleeding under the skin
- Baby's eyes, hands, or feet have a yellow, jaundiced color or the baby develops pumpkin-colored skin
- You feel very nervous about your baby's illness or general condition

When to call immediately for an older child (child has the following symptoms):
- Seems unresponsive, does not make eye contact with you, or has cold and clammy skin that is not associated with vomiting
- Looks much sicker than usual with a routine illness
- Has an illness with a rash that looks like bleeding under the skin (purple blotches or spots)
- Has any symptom that you believe to be unusual or frightening; this includes trouble breathing, stiff neck, severe headache, or very high fever

When to call immediately after trauma or injury:
- Child has struck his or her head and has either lost consciousness momentarily, has nausea or vomiting, or complains of severe headache; also call if there is mental confusion, unbalanced walking, poor coordination, loss of memory, or a discharge coming from one or both ears
- There is continued swelling, tenderness, or a strange look to the injured part
- Child refuses to use an injured extremity for more than half an hour
- There is a deep puncture wound, a cut longer than 0.5 inch, or your child has not received a tetanus shot within the past 5 to 10 years
- There is injury to an eye that causes redness, pain, or tearing for more than 15 minutes
- Child has been bitten by an animal, and the bite has gone through the skin
- You need first aid instructions to control bleeding or other problems
- You believe that your child may have swallowed a toxic or poisonous substance

When to call about symptoms:
- You are concerned about how your child looks
- Symptoms seem to be getting worse or last longer than expected
- Fever of more than 101° F (38.3° C) has lasted longer than 24 hours
- Cough, cold, sore throat, or runny nose has lasted longer than 48 to 72 hours
- Vomiting has lasted longer than 8 hours or diarrhea longer than 24 hours or when there is blood in the stool or vomit
- Child has severe stomach pains lasting longer than 4 hours
- Symptom seems more severe than it has in the past
- Child has a rash or other problem, and you are not sure what is causing it
- You are not certain whether the child needs to be seen by the health care provider

When to call Emergency Medical Service (911) immediately and not your primary care provider:
- An infant younger than 3 months* who:
  - Is difficult to arouse
  - Has poor color, looks blue, difficulty breathing
  - Is limp and unresponsive

*Infants younger than 3 months, especially newborns, can quickly become acutely and gravely ill needing careful assessment by health providers.

recommendations of the Advisory Committee on Immunization Practices (ACIP), the AAP, and the American Academy of Family Physicians (AAFP). See Chapter 24 for the recommended immunizations and schedules.
- Communicable diseases need to be identified and treated appropriately and reported in a timely fashion to public health departments as required by law.
- Develop practice setting policies about the following: Segregate infected children from well children as quickly as possible; avoid crowded waiting rooms, shorten waiting times, and minimize sharing of toys; wash hands before and after each patient contact; wipe the body of otoscopes or ophthalmoscopes regularly with alcohol; clean ear curettes after each use or use disposable ones, use alcohol wipes to clean stethoscope heads after each patient use, and disinfect with bleach solution or alcohol or sterilize any non-disposable tool if used between patients or contaminated with blood or other body secretions. Use gloves as appropriate when exposure to body fluids is a consideration.

Child Care Settings and Infectious Diseases

In the United States, over 23.7 million preschoolers routinely spend "care time" in settings outside of their homes (Waggoner-Fountain, 2011). This population is more immunologically susceptible to illness because of their ages, hygiene habits, dietary factors (including nutritional deficits that may be a result of hunger), frequent viral illnesses, and close proximity to one another. Transmission depends on the prevalence in the population, infectivity, and survival characteristics of the organism. The environment enhances easy exposure to many infectious agents, whether spread from diapers, airborne, or from play surfaces. Although any illness can present and spread in a child care setting, the diseases are primarily due to respiratory and gastrointestinal etiologies. Day care in a small day care home is associated with less spread of infectious disease than is day care provided in a larger center. Some general guidelines for recommending whether a child should or should not be excluded from child care are included in Table 21-1.

In addition to educating parents about ways to decrease the incidence and transmission of infectious diseases, including the vaccination of children, health care providers can be a valuable resource for helping establish written policies for child care settings in their communities. These policies should address prevention and control of infectious agents and include:
- Record keeping of current immunization documents of children and staff
- Written hand hygiene policies and procedures for monitoring adherence to these policies
  - Hand washing procedure should take 40 to 60 seconds (World Health Organization, 2009). Teach parents and children the importance of washing their hands, especially after toileting, blowing their nose, and

TABLE 21-1 Deciding When to Exclude a Child from a Child Care Setting

Exclude	Do Not Exclude
Illness prevents the child from participating in program activities	Yellow or green nasal discharge
Illness results in greater care need than the care staff can provide without compromising the health and safety of the other children	Nonpurulent conjunctivitis without fever or behavioral change
Child has fever, unusual lethargy, irritability, behavioral changes, persistent crying, difficulty breathing, intermittent abdominal pain, or other signs of possible severe disease	Exanthem without fever or behavioral changes; erythema infectiosum (fifth disease) in an otherwise healthy individual
Diarrhea (defined as an increased number of stools in comparison with the child's normal pattern, with increased stool water or decreased form) that is not contained by diapers or toilet use; blood or mucus in stool	Fever lower than 101° F (38.5° C) without other illness symptoms
Persistent abdominal pain lasting more than 2 hours	HB carrier status
Vomiting more than two times in the previous 24 hours	Most viral infections (e.g., CMV, mononucleosis)
Mouth sores associated with an inability to control drooling of saliva	Nits, if being treated
Rash or known MRSA infection with fever or behavioral changes	HIV infection
Purulent conjunctivitis with fever and/or behavioral changes	Scabies, after treatment started
Scabies prior to starting treatment	

Data from Pickering LK, Baker CJ, Kimberlin DW, et al: Children in out-of-home child care. In *Red book: 2009 Report of the Committee on Infectious Disease*, ed 28, Elk Grove Village, IL, 2009, American Academy of Pediatrics.
CMV, Cytomegalovirus; *HB*, hepatitis B, *HIV*, human immunodeficiency virus; *MRSA*, methicillin-resistant *Staphylococcus aureus*.

before eating. The CDC has excellent materials that can be used with families (see Additional Resources).

- Guidelines for appropriate environmental sanitation practices
  - Disposing of waste (e.g., blood, urine, feces, vomit, saliva) should be practiced appropriately along with proper cleaning and disinfection of equipment, toys, toilets, eating areas, and diaper-changing surfaces. There should be a regular schedule of cleaning—in addition to cleaning when items are contaminated.
- A timeline to ensure regular updating of blood-borne pathogen training of staff
- Formalize protocols to reduce respiratory spread of disease
  - Cough into one's sleeve and minimize use of handkerchiefs; cover mouth when sneezing or coughing, dispose of tissue after wiping nose, and wash hands immediately; discourage habits of touching the mouth, nose, and eyes; eliminate passive smoke and provide adequate ventilation.
- Mandates prohibiting raw or undercooked eggs or meats from being served
- Promotion of appropriate handling, preparation, sanitation, and storage of food
  - Those primarily handling food should not change diapers.
- Development of a plan of action that promotes prompt identification and reporting of infectious diseases
- Reducing exposure to communicable disease by separating sick children from well children
- Educating youth about the prevention of sexually transmitted infections (STIs)
- Educating young children and teenagers to not share food, liquids, personal hygiene products, cosmetics, hair coverings, grooming products, or towels with others
- Discouraging children from kissing pets and playing in areas of animal fecal contamination (e.g., sandboxes)
- Providing preventive health guidance about avoiding secondhand smoke

Caring for Our Children: National Health and Safety Standards: Guidelines for Early Care and Education Programs by the AAP, American Public Health Association, and National Resource Center for Health and Safety in Child Care and Early Education (2011) offers guidelines for preventive health practices that promote a safe environment for infants and children. This resource addresses the issues of disease prevention and management in family and group day care homes and child care centers (see Additional Resources) and is available online at http://nrckids.org/default/assets/File/Products/Infant%20and%20Toddler/Caring%20for%20Infants%20and%20Toddlers%20Final.pdf. In addition, several out-of-home day care resources are listed in Box 21-5. Preventing and controlling the spread of illness in these group settings are important issues in maintaining health.

• BOX 21-5 Organizational Resources for Illness Prevention and Out-of-Home Day Care

Early Education and Child Care Initiatives (www.healthychildcare.org/index.html)

- Programs for teaching care providers how to administer medications
- Quality child care
- Quarterly newsletter for health care providers, teachers, and providers

KidsHealth (http://kidshealth.org/)

- Parent-, child-, teen-, and teacher-friendly information about general pediatric health topics
- Provides information about staying helathy and safe

National Resource Center for Health and Safety in Childcare and Early Education (http://nrckids.org)

- Goal is to help foster health and safety in out-of-home educational settings

Child Care Aware (www.childcareaware.org)

- Helps parent identify child care resources

Fever in Children

Fever Assessment

Fever is one of the most common reasons that parents seek health care advice (Cunha, 2012). It is a complex systematic inflammatory response that involves modification of the body's thermoregulatory center (hypothalamus) set point. The pathophysiology of fever is a result of an alteration in the thermoregulatory center of the preoptic nuclei of the anterior hypothalamus. Within the center is a group of neurons that maintain the body temperature. These neurons are sensitive to cytokine-mediated responses, as well as acute phase reactants, such as toxins and products of viral or bacterial metabolism. Antigen-antibody complexes and complement components also act as pyrogens, causing monocytes to activate to become macrophages and other inflammatory cells to release cytokines. Cytokines are a critical factor in the fever and the inflammatory response, releasing prostaglandin E that raises the thermoregulatory set point (McIntyre, 2011). Heat production is caused by increased cellular metabolism, involuntary shivering, autonomic responses (such as, vasoconstriction), and behavioral responses (such as, covering oneself).

Most pediatric sources define *fever* as a rectal temperature higher than 100.4° F (38° C) (Nield and Kamat, 2011). The measurement of fever can be done in several ways, as discussed in the next section. The differential diagnosis in a febrile child includes infectious and noninfectious causes. Although viral infections are responsible for most children's fever, the differential for fever includes bacterial infection, malignancy, reaction to immunizations, and connective tissue disease. Thus, a careful history and physical examination are important to develop a differential diagnoses.

Types of Thermometers and Measurement Sites

In an attempt to measure the core temperature of the body reflected by the temperature around the hypothalamus, several noninvasive methods have been developed. Although there are invasive devices that measure core body temperature by measuring the pulmonary artery temperature (Barnason et al, 2012), these methods are too invasive to be used in routine pediatric practice. The types of thermometers used at the present time include glass thermometer with mercury (in developing countries), chemical thermometer (phase change), electronic digital thermometer, infrared-sensing ear thermometer, and infrared forehead thermometer. Body temperature can be measured at the tympanic membrane; temporal area; and axillary, oral, and rectal sites. Table 21-2 lists the thermometers available and temperature measurement sites.

Both tympanic and temporal thermometers are well tolerated and easy to use; however, rectal temperature remains the gold standard unless it is contraindicated for a medical reason. A rectal temperature more closely approximates body core temperature readings than do axillary, oral, temporal, or tympanic measurements. Stein and colleagues (2012) studied the relationship between axillary and rectal temperatures in children younger than 1 year old and reported marked inconsistencies between the axillary and rectal route. They concluded that the rectal route was more accurate in children younger than 1 year of age. Although axillary temperatures are recommended in the neonatal period, after this period, the method is not effective and is influenced by sweating. An oral temperature is a more comfortable method for children over 5 years of age and is more accurate than axillary measurement. The results of oral readings are slower and influenced by tachypnea, hot and cold drinks, exercise, mouth breathing, and thermometer position.

The tympanic membrane and hypothalamus share the same blood supply from the internal and external carotid arteries, but there are additional sources of blood supply to the tympanic membrane and the reading can be affected by poor positioning, cerumen, and otitis media. When the thermometer tip is not securely fitted in the canal, the reading measures the temperature of the ear canal, skin, or cerumen. However, with proper use the reading is rapid, clean, convenient, and risk-free (Avner, 2009).

TABLE 21-2 Types of Thermometers and Measurement Sites

Type of Thermometer	Measurement Site
Mercury in glass (in developing countries)	• Axilla • Oral • Rectal
Chemical thermometer (phase change)	• Axilla • Oral
Contact electronic	• Axilla • Oral • Rectal
Non-contact infrared forehead	• Forehead • Naval, if forehead is not available
Infrared tympanic membrane	• Ear

The new infrared thermometer measures the temperature at the surface of the skin on the forehead. An infrared non-contact thermometer (Thermofocus) allows caregivers to measure temperature without touching the child by pointing the thermometer to the center of the forehead. The light-emitting diode (LED) system emits two beams of light that meet to form one image when the thermometer is at the correct distance. The naval can be used if the forehead is not assessable. Teran and colleagues (2011) reported 97% sensitivity and specificity; however, an earlier study found the device overestimated fever in afebrile children and underestimated fever in children with high fever (Fortuna et al, 2010). Another study compared rectal temperatures to infrared non-contact thermometer (Thermofocus) and tympanic thermometers and found significant differences between rectal temperature measurements and those of both the tympanic thermometer and the Thermofocus. These findings lead researchers to advise continuation of rectal temperatures in febrile children (Paes et al, 2010). Clearly more research is needed before adopting any one method exclusively.

Physiologically the child's heart rate increases 10 to 15 beats per minute and respiratory rate increases three to five breaths per minute for each elevation of degree centigrade (C) (Avner, 2009). There is a normal diurnal variation in body temperature with a low point between 4 and 8 AM and a peak later in the day at 4 to 6 PM. Body temperature also varies by age (younger infants have a higher temperature), gender, physical activity, and surrounding air temperature. Environmental conditions (e.g., swaddling an infant) may produce transient elevated temperatures, and it may be necessary to take several readings to verify whether an elevated temperature is due to an environmental or a pathologic cause.

Parental concern can be a factor in a decision to use an antipyretic. Parents with "fever phobia" need reassurance, because they may believe that high temperatures cause brain damage or, if not treated, will go higher. Cellular damage does not occur until temperatures reach more than 105.8° to 107.6° F (41° to 42° C). Fevers less than 105.8° F (41° C), per se, are not associated with brain damage. Parents need to know that, except for temperatures higher than 104° F (40° C), fevers are a body defense mechanism. Fevers are thought to impart a beneficial effect by enhancing immunologic responses, such as increasing phagocytosis and leukocyte migration, and interfering with viral replication and virulence of some microbes.

However, there are potential adverse effects from fevers, including increased metabolic rate with associated fluid loss, oxygen consumption, and increased caloric needs. In addition, febrile seizures are the most common convulsive event in children younger than 5 years old and occur in children at a rate of 2% to 5% (AAP, Subcommittee on Febrile Seizures, 2011). Seizure events are very worrisome for parents and fever concern heightens in parents whose child has had a prior febrile seizure event. Although the fever-associated symptoms of headache, malaise, anorexia, and irritability are uncomfortable for the child, the overall state of the child needs to be determined by complete history and physical and prompt follow-up.

Many health care providers treat fever to provide comfort to a child and use pharmacologic agents when a temperature exceeds 101°F (38.3°C). Some clinicians use temperatures greater than 101.5°F (38.6°C) as their guide to treatment. Suppressing a fever in a young child who is ill can also assist in clinical decision-making if the irritability, tachypnea, and tachycardia associated with a fever resolve after administration of an antipyretic; however, a febrile child's reduction in fever after antipyretic administration should not be the sole criterion to judge whether a child has a significant illness. Rather, the overall clinical appearance of the child after fever reduction is the more accurate way of evaluating a child with a fever and determining management (Avner, 2009; Ishimine, 2007). A toxic appearing child is considered at risk until proven otherwise and needs a thoughtful workup. The appearance of a child who has a benign illness and a high fever usually is better (i.e., does not appear as ill), whereas a child with a serious infection will still appear ill after fever reduction (Avner, 2009).

The presence of fever without a known source is always worrisome particularly during infancy. The management of infants and children less than 36 months of age with fever without localizing signs is based on age (i.e., younger than 1 month old, 1 to 3 months old, and 3 to 36 months old), temperature 101°F (38.3°C) or higher, appearance (toxic or well appearing), and diagnostic study results that may include any or all of the following: CBC, body fluid cultures (urine, stool, and cerebrospinal fluid), chest radiograph, and other tests (Nield and Kamat, 2011). Chapter 24 discusses the evaluation and management of children with fevers without focus and fevers of unknown origin and includes algorithms. These children merit careful evaluation that may include consultation with pediatrician colleagues based on the child's at-risk status.

Fever Management

Management strategies for fever control include the following:

- Nonpharmacologic measures:
  - Provide adequate hydration.
  - Provide reassurance to parents and advice that not all fevers need to be treated.
  - Provide appropriate clothing; do not bundle in additional clothing or coverings.
  - Provide ambient environment temperatures of around 72°F (22°C).
  - Sponge with tepid water for temperatures greater than 104°F (40°C). Sponging should be stopped if the child starts to shiver. Ice-water baths and alcohol sponging should not be done.
- Pharmacologic measures:
  - Antipyretic agents: Refer to Table 21-3. Acetaminophen and ibuprofen work in the same manner by inhibiting prostaglandin synthesis without affecting the baseline body temperature (Taketomo et al, 2014). Alternating these antipyretics carries with it an increased risk of medication errors and possible toxicity. Therefore, before using this regime, careful consideration of the risk versus the benefits must be weighed taking into consideration parental abilities (Section on Clinical Pharmacology and Therapeutics et al, 2011).
  - Acetaminophen, 10 to 15 mg/kg/dose every 4 to 6 hours by mouth, not to exceed five doses in 24 hours; temperature generally is reduced by 1° to 2°C within 2 hours. At an oral dose of 15 mg/kg/dose, it is as effective as ibuprofen at 10 mg/kg/dose. Acetaminophen is the drug of first choice.

TABLE 21-3 Antipyretics: Infants and Children (12 Years Old and Younger)

Drug	Dosage	Comments*
Acetaminophen	10 to 15 mg/kg every 4 to 6 hours PO (not to exceed five doses/24 hr) *or* 10 to 20 mg/kg every 4 to 6 hours per rectal suppository as needed (not to exceed five doses in 24 hr)	Temperature reduced by 1.8° to 3.6°F (1° to 2°C) within 2 hours; 15 mg/kg/dose as effective as ibuprofen at 10 mg/kg/dose; drug of choice
Ibuprofen	For temperatures <102.5°F (39°C): 5 mg/kg/dose every 6 to 8 hours as needed For temperatures ≥102.5°F (39°C): 10 mg/kg/dose every 6 to 8 hours as needed	Use in children 6 months old to 12 years old; maximum daily dose of 40 mg/kg; temperature stays lower for a longer period of time with ibuprofen vs. acetaminophen. Use with caution if decreased liver function, asthma, or coagulation disorder.

PO, Per os (by mouth, orally).
*Educate parents that the goal of antipyretics is to make the child more comfortable.

- Ibuprofen in children 6 months to 12 years old: For temperature lower than 102.5° F (39.2° C), 5 mg/kg/dose every 6 to 8 hours; for temperature 102.5° F (39.2° C) or higher, 10 mg/kg/dose every 6 to 8 hours with a maximum daily dose of 40 mg/kg/day. The duration of fever response with ibuprofen may be longer than with acetaminophen. Thus the temperature remains lower for a longer time with ibuprofen.
- Naproxen sodium is marketed as a "fever reducer." However, it has not been well studied as an antipyretic in children and should not be used for this purpose.

For a complete list of references, please visit http://evolve.elsevier.com/Burns/pediatric/.

22
Prescribing Medications in Pediatrics

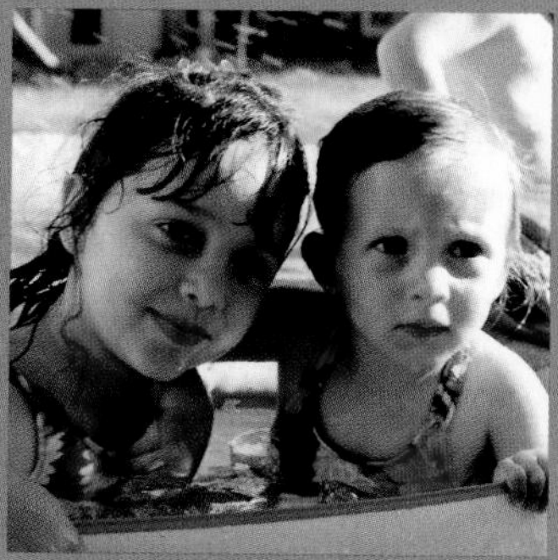

CATHERINE G. BLOSSER

This chapter is designed to enable the health care provider to have a better understanding about prescribing pharmaceuticals for the pediatric population, including ways to enhance adherence. It is assumed that the reader has taken a pharmacology course and has a strong grasp of biochemical principles. The reader is directed to consult a comprehensive pediatric drug reference, the U.S. Food and Drug Administration (FDA), or pharmaceutical manufacturers regarding specific drugs, their classification, preparation, indications, dosing, side effects, interactions, and other considerations.

National Safety Goals Regarding Prescribing Medications

The Joint Commission has published the National Patient Safety Goals (NPSG) that address several concerns regarding medication practices in ambulatory health care clinics. In 2008, the NPSG focused on the dispensing of sample medications. In 2014, the goals stressed the importance of reconciling medication information. The Joint Commission directs health care providers to review what medications are prescribed, ask about what is actually being taken, be aware of possible drug interactions between medications, inquire if the medication is producing the desired effect, and inquire about side effects. Likewise, providers should be in a practice setting that has a system in place to communicate medication-related information among providers working with the same individual (The Joint Commission, 2015). (See Additional Resources—The Joint Commission website regarding further information about the NPSG for ambulatory care.)

Regulation and Safety of Pharmaceuticals

Less than 50% of drugs approved by the FDA in the United States have been specifically tested for use in some subset of the pediatric population (American Academy of Pediatrics [AAP], Committee on Drugs, 2014). This historical lack of drug testing in the pediatric population stems from several factors, which include unprofitability of the pediatric pharmaceutical market (it is relatively small, except for vaccines and some cough/cold medications); difficulty setting up child-friendly environments within which to carry out testing; difficulty taking biologic samples; inability to obtain informed consent from children and adolescents; questionable use of placebo controls in children; possible discomfort, risks, and liability; and difficulty in formulating acceptable medication delivery systems (e.g., tablets, liquids) for specific pediatric age groups (Edmunds and Mayhew, 2013; Thaul, 2012).

In 1997, landmark legislation in the United States (the Food and Drug Administration Modernization Act [FDAMA]) required pharmaceutical companies to survey existing data and determine whether there was sufficient support to use various drugs in the pediatric population with pediatric indications and dosages included in the labeling. If such support was demonstrated, controlled clinical studies that supported pediatric use did not need to be done. If there was insufficient information to support a pediatric indication, the labeling statement "safety and effectiveness in pediatric patients have not been established" was allowed. Since 1997, the FDA has issued significant amendments to the FDAMA.

Drug safety and efficacy for pediatric use is currently addressed in the United States by two legislative acts, both of which were introduced in 2003 and permanently renewed in 2012: the Best Pharmaceuticals for Children Act (BPCA) and the Pediatric Research Equity Act (PREA). The BPCA grants a patent extension when drug companies voluntarily study a known or new drug in children. The PREA gives the FDA more leverage over the types of new drugs developed for children, and the pharmaceutical companies can be required to conduct pediatric studies if the FDA declares a drug as possibly beneficial to ill children or one that might be used by a substantial number of children. Additionally, the FDA can require pediatric studies if a new drug application is for a new indication, contains a new active ingredient in an already marketed drug, proposes a change in dosage, or a new route of delivery. Under the BPCA, if companies refuse to conduct studies for children on off-patent drugs (i.e., generics), the Foundation for the National Institutes of Health (FNIH) can be requested to conduct the appropriate research or contract out the research. Following this mandate the FNIH, in collaboration with the FDA and pediatric researchers, identifies drugs and therapeutic areas of highest priority for study in pediatric populations every 3 years and issues a Priority List of Needs in Pediatric Therapeutics. There are 17 therapeutic areas (e.g., infectious disease, dermatology, neurology, and cancer) within which there is a list of drugs that require further research. The list can be found on the BPCA website: http://bpca.nichd.nih.gov/prioritization/status/Documents/Priority_List_07082014.pdf.

An internal review committee (Pediatric Advisory Committee [PAC]) at the FDA evaluates the post-market safety of all pediatric drugs, biologic products, and medical devices granted patent exclusivity by the FDA. The PAC can request labeling modifications, areas where further investigation is efficacious, areas where further clinical trial data are necessary, and clinical trial design.

Under BPCA and PREA auspices, there have been over 500 pediatric labeling changes (e.g., ibuprofen now lists doses for those 6 months to 2 years and ranitidine includes accurate dosing information for use in infants). Loratadine, gabapentin, and famotidine required similar labeling changes based upon age group. For updates on pediatric drug labeling changes, consult the FDA website (see Additional Resources).

Pharmaceutical labeling is required to make drug information easily accessible and comprehensive for providers. The most important prescribing information about the benefits and risk of a drug, the date of initial product approval, and the phone number and website address to report adverse effects are now placed at the beginning of prescribing information and package inserts in a section called *Highlights*. Similar formatting must be included in electronic prescribing tools and other information resources. The American Academy of Pediatrics offers an online, subscription-based continuing education program (PediaLink) for providers that includes information about labeling changes.

The PAC recommends that pharmaceutical labels carry warnings about suicide, neonatal withdrawal/toxicity, and risks of off-label use for some drugs in pediatrics. However, many clinical adverse effects of drugs in this age group may go unreported, and the true nature of a drug's safety may not be fully understood. Providers are responsible for reporting adverse effects and for monitoring the use of off-label drugs. All providers are encouraged to report adverse effects to the FDA MedWatch website (see Additional Resources).

In the European Union, any company that applies to the European Medicines Agency (EMA) is compelled to include a pediatric investigation plan or obtain a waiver if a drug is not applicable for use in children. This provision, the Pediatric Regulation, also provides funding to study off-patent drugs in children, with the results made available to the public.

Safety Issues with Pharmaceutical Manufacturers

An estimated 40% of over-the-counter (OTC) and generic drugs sold in the United States are manufactured by pharmaceutical firms in India (Harris, 2014); China is also a major exporter of drugs. Concerns with counterfeiting, manufacturing safety lapses, substandard products, and falsified drug test results have led to an increase in FDA investigations, penalties, and enforcement measures within those countries. (Chapter 43 also discusses safety and regulatory issues of imported herbs, botanicals, and dietary supplement products.)

Ethical Issues with Pharmaceutical Testing

More than one third of the published drug trials in pediatrics have been carried out, at least partly, in developing countries. This practice raises an ethical issue, because many of the drugs may involve vulnerable populations, may not be made available or affordable to the participating countries despite their efficacy, or the results may be pertinent only within the population studied (Pasquali et al, 2010).

Guidelines for Writing a Prescription

Prescriptions must be written in a manner that conveys accurate information to the pharmacist, the child and/or parent/caregiver, and other clinicians accessing the child's chart. Illegible or poor handwriting and distractions when writing prescriptions are major causes of medication dispensing errors. Electronic prescribing or e-prescribing (i.e., a computer-generated system) can greatly reduce many errors (e.g., can cross-check the prescription against known allergies; calculate appropriate drug dosing based upon weight and/or body surface area; and note dosage limits, drug-drug interactions, and duplications) (Johnson et al, 2013). If a handwritten prescription is necessary, the clinician must dedicate time to ensure that the prescription is written clearly and succinctly so that the correct drug and directions are conveyed to the pharmacist, child, and/or caregiver. Accuracy can be enhanced by following the guidelines listed in Box 22-1.

General Prescribing Guidelines

When prescribing pharmacologic agents or recommending OTC drugs, it is important to be knowledgeable of the pharmacodynamics and pharmacokinetics of the drug, the usual dosage, adverse reactions, drug interactions, and the indications and contraindications for its use in children. There must be a clear purpose in mind for using a particular drug, and pressure from parents or other individuals should not be a determining factor. Some general points to keep in mind when prescribing drugs or OTC medications include:

- Assess renal and hepatic systems for degree of maturation and function.

• BOX 22-1 Guidelines for Accurately Writing a Prescription*

- Limit each prescription to one medication.
- Prescriptions should be preprinted with names of prescribers in your practice setting; circle your name. (Pharmacist will know who to contact for questions/clarifications should the signature be illegible.)
- Eliminate drug abbreviations (e.g., TCN could mean triamcinolone or tetracycline).
- Use computer-generated prescriptions whenever possible. If a handwritten prescription is needed, print out name of medication in block letters rather than write out the name in cursive.
- Provide concise dosage information:
  - Use metric measures, such as milligrams rather than designating tablet, vial, teaspoon, tablespoon, or dropper. Most parents, including those who are non-English speakers or who have low literacy, can follow instructions on the use of metric measures (Yin et al, 2014).
  - Write "unit" rather than a "U," which can be mistaken for a zero or a number.
  - Write "international unit" rather than IU, which can be mistaken for IV or the number 10.
  - Write "daily" rather than qd, which can be mistaken for qid.
  - Write "every other day" rather than qod, which can be mistaken for qid and qd.
  - Avoid a trailing or terminal zero (e.g., 9.0 mg), because the decimal point may be missed. Write 9 mg instead.
  - Lead with a zero before a decimal point (e.g., 0.15 mg) so that the decimal point is not missed.
  - Avoid using decimal points whenever possible (e.g., write 300 mg instead of 0.3 g).
- Do not use abbreviations for body parts (e.g., o.d. for right eye).
- Avoid vague instructions that might cause confusion when patient is taking several drugs (e.g., avoid "take as directed" or "prn" without stipulating how often drug should be taken).
- Use generic, official, or trademarked name; avoid chemical names or coined names.
- Add the patient's age and weight to orient pharmacist and help ensure age-appropriate prescription and dosage (e.g., tetracycline should not be prescribed to a 5-year-old).
- Specify number of pills to be dispensed rather than stating a time duration. Adding refills for an acute treatment confuses duration of therapy and may preclude patient returning for a necessary recheck appointment.
- State indication or purpose of drug (alerts pharmacist and other physicians to appropriateness of medication and aids in counseling). This can be as simple as stating it is for a respiratory or skin condition (preprint the body system directly on the prescription for easy check-off).
- Add supplemental information (e.g., avoid sun exposure; do not take with grapefruit juice; take with food).
- Remain alert to lethal doses and compromising pathologic conditions (e.g., compromised renal or hepatic functions) that might affect drug levels.

Data from Edmunds MW, Mayhew MS: *Pharmacology for the primary care provider*, ed 4, St. Louis, 2013, Elsevier/Mosby; Jenkins RH, Vaida AJ: Simple strategies to avoid medication errors, *Fam Pract Manag* 14(2):41–47, 2007; Teichman PG, Caffee AE: Prescription writing to maximize patient safety, *Fam Pract Manag* 9(7):27–30, 2002.

IV, Intravenous; *q.d., quaque die* (every day); *q.i.d., quater in die* (four times a day); *q.o.d., quaque altera die* (every other day).

*A complete list of abbreviations to avoid when writing prescriptions is available from www.ismp.org/tools/errorproneabbreviations.pdf

- Use clinical practice guidelines, if available.
- Be aware of the influence of advertising in prescribing practice. The newest agent may be more expensive, and there may be no evidence that its use will lead to a better outcome.
- Use a decision-support system to investigate the possibility of drug interactions and side effects (e.g., an electronic medical record support system; smartphone application like CheckRx; or an online program, such as Epocrates).
- Check for interactions between pharmacologic agents and any herbs, botanicals, or dietary supplements being taken concurrently.

Prescribing Medications for Children

The dosage for pediatric patients has typically been determined by extrapolating from the adult dose and proportionately reducing the dose based on the child's weight and drug side effect profiles. However, this does not take into account developmental changes in pediatric metabolism, the drug's pharmacokinetics, adverse effects (e.g., the connection between selective serotonin reuptake inhibitors [SSRIs] and potential suicide risk in adolescents), and medication delivery form. The fields of ethnopharmacology and pharmacogenetics/genomics provide health professionals with a better understanding of how variations of certain phase I enzymes, for the oxidation or reduction of drugs (e.g., CYP450), are influenced by genetics (e.g., CYP2D6 gene is located on chromosome 22), age, and developmental level of organs, the immune system, and metabolic rates. CYP2D6 is responsible for the metabolism and elimination of approximately 30% of clinically used drugs (Edmunds and Mayhew, 2013).

The maturing child is physiologically dynamic. Such factors as size, age, renal function, cardiac output, hepatic flood flow, concomitant drugs, diseases, individual characteristics (including race), and maturation/development/genetics of body systems can lead to specific pharmacokinetic differences that affect any given drug effect and dosing decisions. Again, it is beyond the scope of this chapter to cover the broad topic of the pharmacokinetics and pharmacodynamics of medications used in children. However, a few fundamental principles are worth summarizing:

- Absorption of drugs: For injectables, absorption rates will vary depending upon the blood flow to muscular or subcutaneous tissues, muscle mass, the quantity of adipose tissue, and muscle activity at the injection site. The immature, mature, or compromised gastrointestinal (GI) tract varies in permeability, gastric acid production, rates of peristalsis and gastric emptying, intestinal flora, enzyme function, and transport mechanisms. All of these can affect drug absorption. The younger the child, the more the absorption may vary.
- Drug distribution: The inherent physicochemical properties of a drug and the complex processes involved with growth and development in children affect drug distribution. Body weight (amount attributed to fat, protein,

and intracellular water), bone and teeth maturation (e.g., tetracycline is deposited in growing teeth and can cause permanent staining), and pathologic factors that alter physiologic function also must be taken into consideration. This is particularly important when prescribing for infants and young children (e.g., some drugs more easily cross the blood-brain barrier; a premature infant's blood-brain barrier is more permeable; and some conditions [e.g., meningitis, brain tumors, cranial trauma] can affect central nervous system permeability). Alterations in protein binding increases some drug distribution. The provider also needs to be aware of drugs contraindicated during breastfeeding (see Chapter 11 for suggested references).

- Drug metabolism: Biotransformation processes change drugs into inactive, less active, or active compounds in the body. Such reactions produce metabolites that vary in their rates and degree of elimination from the body (e.g., penicillins are not metabolized, are poorly absorbed, and are eliminated unchanged) (Brunton et al, 2010). Most drug metabolism occurs in the liver. Therefore, the provider needs to be aware of the maturation level of the liver when prescribing drugs metabolized by that organ. Infants generally metabolize drugs more slowly than older children due to decreased levels of oxidases and conjugating enzymes. However, the rate of drug metabolism by the liver in children exceeds that of adults between 2 and 6 years of age, reaching adult rates when the child is 10 to 12 years of age. This means that certain drugs may need to be administered more often or at higher doses to younger children. The GI tract, kidney, and plasma may also play a role in biotransformation but to a lesser extent (Edmunds and Mayhew, 2013).
- Elimination: The maturity of a child's renal excretion system has a significant effect on drug elimination. The glomerular filtration, tubular secretion, and tubular reabsorption rates are reduced in neonates and preemies; adult rates may be reached as early as 6 months of age in healthy infants. Common drugs cleared by the renal system (e.g., penicillin, digoxin) require dosage and dosing schedule changes and close monitoring in ill or immature infants. Changes in urinary acidity can either increase or decrease the excretion rate of drugs as well. As an example, sodium bicarbonate alkalinizes the urine and increases the excretion rate of certain drugs, such as phenobarbital and nitrofurantoin.

Pharmaceuticals Used In Pediatrics: Off-Label Prescribing

Despite the lack of studies in the pediatric population and lack of pediatric labeling, an overwhelming number of drugs are prescribed for children. Such "off-label" use does not mean that the drug is being prescribed improperly or unethically for the condition or age. Evidence for the pharmaceutical use and safety in the pediatric age group may not have been submitted to the FDA, or the drug does not meet the "level of substantial evidence" needed for FDA approval.

For example, many antibiotics, asthmatic medications, dermatologics, ophthalmologic drops, and anti-psychotropic drugs are commonly prescribed off-label.

Perils of Prescribing Off-Label

The practice of prescribing off-label is not without risk. Providers must balance patient safety against their judgment that the patient will derive the intended benefit. Some general guidelines include the following (AAP, Committee on Drugs, 2014; Buppert, 2012):

- Consult the *Physician's Desk Reference,* Epocrates or other reputable pharmacology application (app), or the package insert when prescribing.
- Do not base the decision to use a particular drug solely on what "somebody" or "everyone else" may be doing.
- Check the FDA website for any warnings about the drug.
- Discuss recommendations with the patient or family to treat with off-label medications; document the decision-making process and the patient's/family's consent in the medical record.
- Be mindful about the precautions that come with each drug, heeding warnings and contraindications.

Other Factors to Consider in Medication Management

Prescribing medications for pediatric patients presents a special challenge. Decisions about which drugs to use are not based simply on which one will be most effective in treating the child's clinical condition or which drugs are most typically prescribed. Ethical considerations must also be taken into account when prescribing, particularly where evidence of efficacy is weak or anecdotal and safety is a concern. Family social and functional issues must also be considered, as well as factors that influence adherence, such as taste, dosing regimen, and collaborative decision making (Table 22-1). (Parental education related to medication use is discussed in Chapter 21, and the reader is encouraged to review this discussion.)

A child's developmental level and age affect the amount of influence parents have over the administration of and adherence to a medication regimen. For *infants* it is important to take the following into consideration:

- The parent should be taught how to properly administer medications.
- Determine whether other caregivers will be administering the medication.
- Determine whether a simplified dosing schedule is necessary for a family (e.g., with children in day care).

Toddlers and *preschoolers* are beginning to exert their independence, and administering medication to this age group can be challenging. The keys to success with this age group are to:

- Choose a medication regimen with the fewest problems associated with administration.
- Take into account palatability and doses per day

TABLE 22-1 Factors That Influence Adherence to Taking Prescribed Pediatric Medications

Factors That Influence Adherence	Interventions That Improve Adherence
Length of treatment: Longer treatment contributes to poorer adherence.	*Shorten length of treatment if possible* (e.g., use 5 days of therapy for otitis media rather than 10; this can be accomplished with a number of antibiotics [azithromycin and cefpodoxime at all ages; amoxicillin in children over 5 years of age]).
Medical condition: Adherence rates vary with chronic illnesses, frequency of medication changes, lack of physical symptoms, need of mastering techniques of medication administration, lack of immediate benefits of medication.	*Develop creative solutions to encourage adherence* (e.g., sticker charts, pill boxes, calendars, link dose to a personal daily habit, such as teeth brushing). Determine how drug regimen will fit into child's lifestyle and try to modify it to fit the child in order to increase adherence; repeat short educational instructions at every visit (include verbal and written instructions); assess for depression. Discuss barriers (e.g., does child have other priorities; does treatment create a negative identity; does child want to avoid unpleasantness) and their underlying assumptions. Provide continuity of care.
Doses per day: The more doses of a medication that need to be administered per day, the poorer the adherence rate. This is particularly true with working parents and children in school who often miss midday doses.	*Simplify dosing regimen*. Prescribing medications that require once or twice daily dosing increases adherence (Bell, 2008). When the child needs to take the medication at day care or school, dispense two bottles: one for school and one for home. This will ensure fewer missed doses due to forgetting to transport the medication back and forth.
Palatability and ease of ingestion: Unpalatable medications are resisted by children, especially young children. Some children have difficulty swallowing some formulations (e.g., pills).	*Choose the best-tasting medication, prescribe chewables, or mask the taste*. If a medication has the same efficacy profile, the best-tasting (though that may not mean it tastes good) medication will be easier to administer to young children. Most pharmacies in the United States offer FLAVORx (for a small fee), which allows children or parents to custom choose how their liquid medicine will taste by masking or overriding the existing flavor (see Additional Resources). There is also the option of using flavoring syrups or crushing tablets, such as prednisone, and mixing with palatable semi-solid foods, such as chocolate syrup, jam, applesauce, or pudding. Before crushing any tablet or mixing a medication with syrup, the provider should check with a pharmacist to determine if the food is compatible with the medication. *Facilitate swallowing of pills and capsules*. Place pill in mouth and take a mouthful of water; turn head as far to the right as possible and swallow. Repeat on the left side and rotate sides, depending upon the number of pills in the treatment regimen.
Expense: Out-of-pocket costs may be difficult for some families to meet.	*Choose the medication that has the lowest out-of-pocket expense for the family*. Prescribe generics when appropriate and offer information on insurance coverage and resources (e.g., discount cards, mail-order pharmacies, and medication assistance programs).
Beliefs systems: The following can affect adherence: religious and spiritual beliefs concerning medication ingredients of animal origin; concern with the safety profile and long-term effects of medications; medication viewed as a "crutch," or child/teen views self as an "addict."	*Counsel medication use issues with ethical and cultural sensitivity, especially in multi-faith communities*. Specifically address safety and side effects of drug regimen and elicit concerns. Use motivational interviewing techniques (see Chapter 9). Assess literacy/health level.
Family/social factors: Issues such as working parents, poor transportation, homelessness, lack of social support, fatigue, family disruption, dysfunction, risky behavior (alcohol consumption and drug abuse), and level of literacy/health literacy can affect the ability to understand and adhere to a treatment regimen.	*Assess the family for issues that affect successful outcome*. If there is poor or less than expected outcome with a treatment regimen, the provider should determine if family issues are a barrier to adherence and address interventions to assist the family in identifying strategies that improve success. Assess literacy/health levels.

School-age children developmentally are industrious, and they are often the most willing to take medications. Education should focus on:

- Both the parent who will administer the medication *and* the child who will be taking the medication.
- Letting the child choose the formulation if possible (liquid, chewable, or pills to swallow).
- Avoiding dosing during school hours if possible.

Adolescent patients often administer their own medication. The provider needs to closely collaborate with adolescent patients regarding their medication regimen by:

- Allowing them to have input about the dosing schedule and what will work best for them.
- Assisting the family with the transition from parent to teen administration.

Medication Adherence

The 2010 survey data regarding ambulatory health care sponsored by the Centers for Disease Control and Prevention (CDC) found that approximately 72% of pediatric visits resulted in a drug being provided or prescribed (CDC, 2014)). Only 72% to 78% of prescriptions may have actually been filled with the highest rate (84%) for those 18 years and younger (Fischer et al, 2010). Yet, 50% to 55% of pediatric patients do not consistently take their medication for chronic medical problems, with adherence rates declining more after the first 6 months of diagnosis (American Psychological Association [APA], Society of Pediatric Psychology, 2014). Medication nonadherence increases the utilization of health care services by children/adolescents with chronic medical conditions, such as asthma, epilepsy, human immunodeficiency virus (HIV), and inflammatory bowel disease (McGrady and Hommel, 2013). In addition, the lack of health insurance also contributes to poor adherence rates in those with chronic diseases.

Historically, whether or not a patient was taking the recommended pharmaceutical or following a recommended treatment regimen was referred to as *compliance* or *noncompliance*. The term *adherence* is currently used more often in the medical literature. Providers need to assess the child's/parent's barriers to medication adherence. Nonadherence needs to be proactively managed in order to improve clinical outcomes and cost effectiveness. Table 22-1 discusses general factors that predispose to lower adherence rates and suggests strategies to increase those rates. Some objective measurements can be used to access adherence (e.g., laboratory measurements, dosage count, medication diaries, and refill rates). A myriad of research studies about adherence have led to the following conclusions:

- Providers obtain a better idea of the actual adherence rate if the question they ask is nonjudgmental, open-ended, and framed in terms of nonadherence, such as "How many doses did you miss?" or "What difficulties are you having with your medication?" rather than "Did you take all of your medicine?" (Bell, 2008).
- Adolescents are less likely to be adherent. Adherence rates in this age group can be increased by directly observing therapy for depressed youth (Gaur et al, 2010), involving the mother more in the treatment regimen (Reed-Knight et al, 2011), acknowledging the need for a future life on medication for those with a chronic illness (Longhofer and Floersch, 2010), experiencing the rewards of treatment (improvement in symptoms, school performance, and family relationships) (Hamrin et al, 2010), and improving the teen's or parent's understanding of the medication and how to manage it if it conflicts with other activities (Edgecombe et al, 2010). Additionally, Duncan and colleagues (2013) demonstrated that youth have greater adherence rates if they and their parents share the responsibility for disease management and learn methods that address parent-child/teen conflict and promote family problem sharing while promoting youth independence.
- Adherence is not a steady state; therefore, adherence needs to be assessed as part of each office visit.
- Individuals take into consideration the perceived risks and benefits for each medication separately (McHorney and Gadkari, 2010).
- A provider's credibility (trustworthiness and expertise) influences a patient's perceptions about the need for prescribed therapy. Providers need to be clear about the treatment plan, efficacy of treatment, and expectations for finding the appropriate drug (Ledford et al, 2010).
- Incorporate all modes of teaching styles: videos, written materials, demonstrations, and oral instructions.
- Ascertain who the child and family believe is the best support person (family member, outside friends, and so on) to work with to promote adherence to the medication regimen.
- A provider is more effective when practicing active listening, providing emotional support, using plain language, giving brief but complete instructions and having the child/parent repeat instructions or "teach back," allowing adequate time for visits, using pictograms, and involving office staff in teaching activities.
- Providers and staff also need to self-critique any biases they have toward ethnically and socially diverse populations and overcome any cultural barriers (American College of Preventive Medicine [ACPM], 2014).
- Providers and staff need to tailor education to the individual's level of understanding and health literacy level. Reading materials should be geared toward a sixth-grade or lower reading level (Kohler, 2009). Without administering a formal literacy test, providers/staff can assess literacy level by asking about the individual's confidence in completing medical forms, what assistance they need to read information, or how they would rate their own literacy level (Powers et al, 2010).
- Adherence rates can improve by scheduling more follow-up visits and spending more time discussing the child's/parent's perception about the disease process,

reasons for and benefits of the medication, and importance of adherence (Jones et al, 2014).

- Reinforcement techniques increase rates of adherence; have the child/adolescent and/or parents identify and use reinforcement strategies (e.g., stickers, special treats [a day at the zoo and so on]).
- Written instructions increase adherence rates. Consumer medication information (CMI) leaflets dispensed through retail pharmacies are written by drug information companies; they are not approved or regulated by the FDA. Patient package inserts (PPIs) are developed by the pharmaceutical manufacturer and discuss risk information in easier-to-read language.
- Establishing a provider/pharmacist collaborative management program for chronic treatment regimens increases adherence rates (Gums et al, 2014; Howard-Thompson et al, 2013).
- The use of tools and newer technologies are receiving more attention as a means to improve adherence rates. These include pictogram-based instruction sheets and logs that are language appropriate and include pill cards (photos of pills, why taken, and when to take); telephone counseling; video or mobile games to increase knowledge, disease management adherence, and clinical outcomes; mobile phone apps (see Additional Resources); short, weekly text messages (see Additional Resources); pill boxes and organizers; watch alarms; and smart pills that will report back exactly if and when the specific medicine was taken and record how one's body responded to the drug (under development by Proteus Digital Health]) (Arya et al, 2013; Deshazo et al, 2010; Madrigal, 2014; Puri, 2014).

Overprescribing Antibiotics; a Continuing Problem

Antibiotic misuse remains high, surging 36% worldwide from 2000 to 2010 (Van Boeckel et al, 2014). The growth in use has largely occurred in countries with a growing middle class that increasingly is able to afford these medications. At the same time, there is growing concern for public health because of a concurrent global increase in antibiotic resistance. Furthermore, antibiotics classified as "last resort" account for the most dramatic increase in use. Public awareness campaigns are believed to have effectively reduced the overall consumption of antibiotics in the United States and Europe, whereas their use has increased in Australia, New Zealand, high-income Asian countries, Brazil, Russia, India, and South Africa. It is concerning that less-affluent countries may be using antibiotics in lieu of implementing long-term preventive public health measures to deal with diseases (e.g., sanitation) (Van Boeckel et al, 2014).

A recent survey of patients and health care providers sheds light on the overprescribing of antibiotics and their misuse in the United States (Yox and Scudder, 2014). Survey results revealed that 17.6% to 18.6% of women's health care and pediatric providers prescribed antibiotics in the absence of diagnostic certainty. Reasons given included being "certain enough" of the need for the drugs, feeling more comfortable treating the infection in case its etiology was bacterial, and not having more information about the etiology because of slowness in getting lab results (Yox and Scudder, 2014).

The European Union is unique in its funding of a comprehensive plan to address the overuse issue (Bartlett et al, 2013). Efforts are being made in the United States to establish antibiotic stewardship programs to decrease the inappropriate prescribing of antibiotics. In-patient programs that utilize prescriber audits, feedback and some restrictive methods have shown success in decreasing inappropriate antibiotic use. Applying similar stewardship interventions (education, audits, and feedback over a year) to the outpatient setting, pediatricians decreased their use of antibiotics for some common respiratory illnesses (Gerber et al, 2013). Furthermore, physicians cited that they would be more likely to change their antibiotic prescription writing habits if there were improved and more rapid results for laboratory tests and if they knew community patterns of antibiotic resistance (Yox and Scudder, 2014).

Advances in Pharmacologic Research: Maximizing Therapeutic Efficacy

As previously mentioned, genetic variations of certain enzymes affect drug metabolism and an individual's response to a dosage. New research is also shedding light on "drug chronotherapy." This field of inquiry (chronobiology) is demonstrating that the metabolism and tolerability of certain drugs depend upon the body's own biologic timing (circadian rhythm) of certain organs, tissues, and cells. Advances have been made on discerning when certain pharmaceuticals should be taken to better align with these rhythms to produce better outcomes and allay side effects. Such chronopharmaceutics are behind the new regimens for treating certain cancers, rheumatoid arthritis, and congenital adrenal hyperplasia. Additional studies have investigated the best time to take certain drugs used to treat hypertension, asthma, hay fever, nighttime acid reflux, and osteoarthritis (Simon, 2013; Walsh, 2014). Further studies into chronotherapy coupled with genetics, age, and gender hold promise for improving the efficacy of many therapeutics (Kaur et al, 2013).

Disposal of Pharmaceuticals

Most OTC and prescription drugs should not be disposed of at home (e.g., flushed down the drain or toilet). Trace amounts have been found in rivers, streams, and treated water, creating health concerns related to hormone disruption, antibiotic resistance, and synergistic effects.

Community water treatment plants do not routinely filter out medicines. Providers should know which pharmacies in their area will take back unused or expired products or encourage patients to dispose of unused medications at hazardous recycling facilities or at a community-sponsored "take-back" program. Local cities, counties' Board of Health, or household trash/recycling service companies can provide information about drug take-back programs. If these actions are not possible, proper disposal of unused drugs is offered as an Environmental Health Tip on the inside back cover of this textbook.

For a complete list of references, please visit http://evolve.elsevier.com/Burns/pediatric/.

23 Pediatric Pain Management

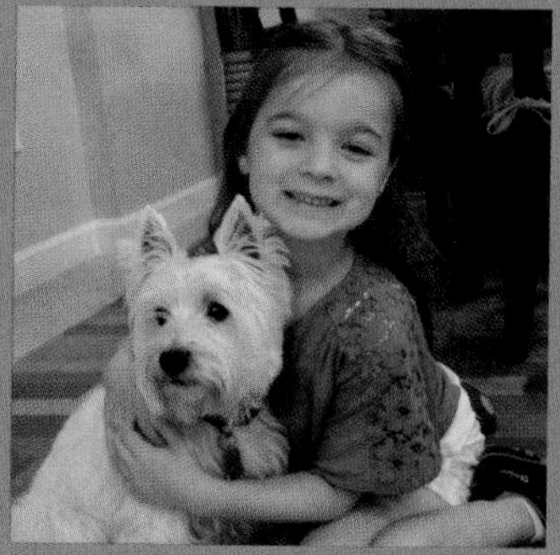

JENNIFER NEWCOMBE AND MARGARET A. BRADY

Health care providers must be familiar with the assessment and effective management of pain in the pediatric and adolescent populations. Many children undergo painful operative and diagnostic procedures. For example, 77% of pediatric patients presenting to an emergency department are in pain or require a painful procedure (Wente, 2013). Pain results from injury or disease or as a side effect from a diagnostic or therapeutic procedure or surgery. Preterm infants are a particularly vulnerable population who must undergo numerous painful procedures (Chidambaran and Sadhasivam, 2012). These early painful experiences are significant events, and pain studies document that unrelieved pain has negative physiologic and psychological consequences. Early pain stimuli and experiences can produce long-term consequences for the child. It is thought that early and prolonged pain may affect the child's pain systems, stress response and behavior, and learning, resulting in increased pain sensitivity (Chidambaran and Sadhasivam, 2012). Inadequate pain control during initial procedures can decrease the effectiveness of analgesia during subsequent procedures. Standards for pediatric care necessitate pain management be part of all treatment plans, from minor painful procedures to more serious illness or injury. Therefore, all health care management plans should include the elimination of preventable pain and reduction of unpreventable pain.

The importance of effective pain management in children cannot be overemphasized. To this end, a joint statement was issued by the American Academy of Pediatrics (AAP, 2001) and the American Pain Society (APS) reinforcing the need for health care providers to treat pain and suffering in all infants, children, and adolescents. This statement continues to be a relevant document today. Also, that same year, The Joint Commission recognized pain as "the fifth vital sign" and established standards requiring the assessment of pain in all patients (Phillips, 2000).

The focus of this chapter is minor pain assessment and management in primary and emergency care settings. The pediatric provider should seek other references for more in-depth discussions of chronic pain or cancer-related pain treatment in pediatric patients.

Pain in Children

Key factors influencing effective pain management in children include the following:

- Established pain is difficult to control; therefore, essential goals of pain management are prevention of and quick action in response to pain.
- Pediatric and adolescent patients and their families should be involved as much as possible in pain education—its assessment and management. Parents must be educated about their role in engaging and providing distraction and comfort to their child during and after painful procedures (e.g., needlesticks, ear examinations, incision and drainage procedures, and vaccinations).
- Culture and family learning patterns must be considered (e.g., beliefs about pain, folk remedies, how pain is expressed verbally, and language barriers).
- Genetic stressors may be responsible for differing levels of neurotransmitters or medication responses.
- Children's pain perceptions are influenced by individual, physiologic and psychological differences, memories, and prenatal and perinatal stressors.
- Chronic pain is rarely associated with sympathetic nervous system arousal. Therefore, children with chronic pain may not appear to be in pain. This may negatively affect their pain evaluation and treatment. To effectively treat chronic pain in children, physical and psychological manifestations of chronic pain should be considered.
- Developmental issues (e.g., cognitive, emotional, and physical), age, and temperament significantly affect how pain is interpreted, expressed, and controlled. Therefore, pain management must be tailored to the child's age and developmental level.
- Cognitive issues influencing pain perception include the child's memory and level of understanding, ability to control what will happen, attachment of meaning to a situation with regard to pain, and expectations of the intensity of pain.
- Emotional issues affecting a child's pain perception include anxiety, fear, frustration, anger, and depression.

- Social issues, including how others react to a child in pain, influence the treatment plan. Likewise, family harmony or conflict influences a child's pain.
- Pain perception involves complex neural interactions that send out impulses or noxious stimuli generated by tissue damage. Melzack and Wall's gate control theory of pain (1965) explains four processes necessary for pain to occur (Mendell, 2013):
  - Transduction: Painful or noxious stimuli are translated into electrical signals at sensory nerve endings and forwarded to the spinal cord via A-delta fibers and C fibers. The A-delta fibers are myelinated and when activated result in sharp, stinging sensations. In contrast, C fibers are unmyelinated, and their activation results in vaguely located dull or burning pain.
  - Transmission: Electrical impulses are forwarded through the sensory nervous system through both the peripheral and central nervous systems.
  - Modulation: Alteration of information by endogenous mechanisms results in lessening or amplification of the initial signal.
  - Perception: The emotional and physical experience of pain.
- A health care provider's fear of severe adverse events from pain medications, such as central nervous system and respiratory depression related to their use, often results in inadequate pain control (Chidambaran and Sadhasivam, 2012).
- For a variety of reasons (e.g., fear of getting a shot), some children do not report pain to health care providers.

The goal of acute pain management in pediatrics is to effectively control pain with minimal therapy and side effects. Positive outcomes of effective pain control are decreased suffering, increased satisfaction for the child and parents, an enhanced recovery process, and a positive script learned by the child related to pain and its management that can be used in the future. In some situations (e.g., after surgical procedures, severe burns, or with chronic pain issues), complete "freedom" from pain is not possible; however, much can be done to alleviate pain in these situations through the use of analgesic agents and other adjunctive therapies.

Barriers to Treatment of Pain in Children

The AAP Committee on Psychosocial Aspects of Child and Family Health (2001) and APS Task Force on Pain in Infants, Children, and Adolescents recognize the following barriers in the assessment and management of acute pain:

- Belief in the myth that children, especially infants, do not feel pain the way adults do, or if they do, there is no consequence
- Lack of assessment and reassessment for the presence of pain
- Misunderstanding of how to conceptualize and quantify a subjective experience
- Lack of pain treatment knowledge
- The notion that addressing pain in children takes too much time and effort
- Fears of adverse effects of analgesic medications, including respiratory depression and addiction
- Personal values and beliefs of health care professionals about the meaning and value of pain

Health care providers must be cognizant of these issues and the negative effect that these barriers exert on their pain management strategies. Effective management of pain is the responsibility of all health care providers, whether one is the sole manager of pain or one who refers the child to a specialized pediatric pain management team.

Overview of Pain

Pain perception develops early in fetal life. By the end of the second week of gestation, fetal skin and mouth sensory neurons develop, and these structures mark the foundations of neural pain transmission. At approximately 32 weeks of gestation, the beginning of the neuronal pain inhibiting mechanism appears and continues developing until the newborn period. It is postulated that newborns subjected to repetitive acute pain events experience central neural changes that program them to later pain vulnerability, cognitive effects, and opioid tolerance (Chidambaran and Sadhasivam, 2012).

Pain involves peripheral physiologic, cognitive, and emotional components of the central nervous system. It may be linked to actual tissue damage or associated with no demonstrable somatic pathology (Zeltzer and Krane, 2011). Pain can be an acute or chronic phenomenon. Acute pain often is associated with an identifiable injury that resolves in a predictable and expected time frame. Physiologic changes in the nervous system are responsible for chronic pain resulting from untreated or undertreated persistent acute pain. Factors not necessarily related to the initial cause of pain may perpetuate it. Pain is further classified as nociceptive or neuropathic. Nociception is the way the nervous system encodes and processes harmful stimuli in the body. *Nociceptive* pain occurs with special nerve endings, nociceptors, are irritated. It is subdivided into two subcategories that describe the physiologic structures associated with nociceptive pain—somatic and visceral. *Somatic* pain is well localized in skin and subcutaneous tissues but does not encompass bone, muscle, blood vessels, and connective tissue. Somatic pain is typically described as dull or aching. In contrast, *visceral* pain involves the internal organs of the body, is poorly localized, and is typically described as a continual aching sensation or a deep cramp or sharp, squeezing pain. Visceral pain results in referred pain that involves distant dermatomal or myotomal sites. The mechanisms associated with visceral pain include distention, stretching, compression, and/or infiltration of an organ. *Neuropathic* pain is associated with an injury to the peripheral nerves, spinal cord, or brain or an illness that results in a malfunction of the nervous system. This painful sensation is characterized as a shooting or stabbing pain superimposed on a backdrop of aching and burning. Key features are poor localization, paresthesias, and dysesthesia (Hauer and Jones, 2014).

Pain Assessment

Developmental factors must be considered in assessment of pain. Infant and toddler assessment must rely on pain-related behaviors, typically nonverbal responses (e.g., facial expression, limb movements, and crying). Most 2-year-olds can use their own words to indicate pain, can report its general location, but cannot describe pain severity. Three-year-olds can say they have "no pain, a little pain, or a lot," and around the age of 4, most children are able to rate the intensity of their pain using a four- to five-item pain discrimination scale. Around 8 years old, children can indicate the location, intensity, and quality of their pain (Srouji et al, 2010).

A systematic approach to the assessment of child and adolescent pain begins by obtaining a pain history from the child and or the parent. When talking with younger children, ask the parent what words the child uses for pain (e.g., "owie," "boo-boo," "ouchie," "hurting," "uncomfortable," "warm," or "stinging"), and use these words with the child. Behavioral observations and physiologic findings provide additional information necessary for a comprehensive pain assessment. Pain evaluation in children needs to be multidimensional. The provider must collect data about what children say related to their pain, assess for physiologic and emotional manifestations of pain, and investigate other pertinent factors contributing to the child's pain, as listed earlier.

Although self-report of pain intensity is an important parameter that the provider must consider when assessing pain, evidence suggests that self-report pain scores mean different things to different children. Using a standardized pain score threshold (or number) as the gold standard measure that a child must achieve via his or her self-report is not in the best interest of the child. Self-report should not be the sole determinant of the treatment plan or type of evaluation. Instead, an individualized approach to the interpretation and use of pain scores is required (Voepel-Lewis, 2013). For these reasons, the child's pain assessment is never complete until the provider considers self-report data as well as individual and contextual factors related to this child's clinical history, child and family preferences, and responses to previous treatments (Twycross et al, 2014).

Clinical Findings

History

A careful history is necessary and requires a systematic approach. An interval history and examination are needed when pain does not abate as expected or there is a change in quality, intensity, duration, or location. Pain has a sensory and emotional component. Because pain is a subjective phenomenon, it is best measured by self-report (Habich et al, 2012). The following information should be obtained during pain assessment:

- Pain history (symptom analysis)
  - Intensity (mild, moderate, severe, or overwhelming)
  - Location (including areas of radiation and referral)
  - Quality—how pain is described by child or parent (e.g., stinging, burning, throbbing or squeezing feeling, or "big ouchie") and any pain behaviors noted
  - Pain duration (present all the time or comes and goes)
  - Temporal features or chronology (when and how the pain started, precipitating factors, and any variations in intensity and quality)
  - Previous treatments or procedures
  - Aggravating or alleviating factors
  - Other associated symptoms, such as anxiety, tachycardia, or diaphoresis
  - Impact on daily activities
- Past pain experience, including the child's memory of a painful experience and the pain treatment
- Cultural beliefs about pain and its causes and treatment
- Self-reports of pain in the verbal child (if possible obtain pain history as noted). Self-reporting is dependent on a child's cognitive ability to understand pain severity on a continuum (Hauer and Jones, 2014). Children as young as 3 years old may be capable of quantifying their pain and translating it to a visual representation.
- Between 3 and 8 years old, children's ability to describe location, intensity, and quality of their pain increases. Introduction to the pain scale includes an explanation that this is one way for children to express how they hurt (Hauer and Jones, 2014). Providers should select reliable, valid, sensitive, and easily understood instruments that can be used consistently. The use of self-report tools, patient pain journals, and other objective pain measures helps to quantify pain before treatment and serves to evaluate the outcome of treatment. Web-based tools (e.g., Pain QuILT) and smartphone apps (e.g., the painometer) to assess pain intensity are new tools under investigation. Selected common pain scales are shown in Table 23-1.
- Factors that influence self-report of pain include:
  - Situational influences may modify children's pain scores (i.e., setting, person asking, or what they expect to happen as a result of their answer).
  - Children may underreport pain if they lack knowledge that pain can be treated or if they fear their complaint may upset their parents.
  - Some children may overstate their pain to receive increased attention.
  - Various factors and perceptions affecting a child's report of pain include nausea, anxiety, or fears, such as receiving an injection, talking to a health care provider, disappointing or bothering others, receiving a medication, or the need to be re-hospitalized. Younger children may confuse fear with pain. Adolescents may

TABLE 23-1 **Common Pain Rating Scales Used to Measure Pain in Pediatric and Adolescent Patients**

Pain Scale/Description	Instructions	Recommended Age/ Comments
Faces Pain Rating Scales		
Wong-Baker FACES Scale* (Wong, 1996; Wong and Baker, 1988): Consists of six cartoon faces ranging from smiling face for "no pain" to tearful face for "worst pain." Scale is 0 to 5. **The Faces Pain Scale–Revised (FPS-R)†** (International Association for the Study of Pain) is a self-report tool that children can use to rate their pain. It uses the 0 to 10 metric to rate pain and has no smiling or tearful faces.	*Brief word instructions:* Point to each face, using the words to describe the pain intensity. Ask the child to choose the face that best describes his or her own pain, and record the appropriate number. Tell the child that the faces show how much something can hurt or be painful. Start by pointing to the face that has "no pain." Continue pointing to each face, and say this face has more pain continuing to the last face and say this has "very much pain." Ask child to point to the face that shows how much pain or hurt he has.	Children as young as 3 years old. For coding purposes, numbers 0, 2, 4, 6, 8, 10 can be substituted for a 0 to 5 system. For age range 4 to 16 years old, do not use the words "happy" or "sad" to describe the faces.
Other Pain Rating Scales		
Oucher Scale (Beyer, 1989): Consists of six photographs of child's face representing "no hurt" to "biggest hurt you could ever have"; also includes a vertical scale with numbers from 1 to 100; scales for African American and Hispanic children have been developed (Villarruel and Denyes, 1991).	*Numeric scale:* Explains variations in pain intensity by pointing to each section of scale: "Zero means no hurt." "This means little hurts" (1 to 29 section). "This means middle hurts" (30 to 69 section). "This means big hurts" (upper part of scale, 70 to 99 section). "100 means the biggest hurt you could ever have." Score is actual number stated by child. *Photographic scale:* Point to each photograph on Oucher scale and explain variations in pain intensity saying: first picture from the bottom is "no hurt," second is "little hurt," third is "a little more hurt," fourth is "even more hurt than that," fifth is "pretty much or a lot of hurt," and the sixth is the "biggest hurt you could ever have." Score pictures from 0 to 5, with the bottom picture scored as 0. Obtain current pain score by asking, "How much hurt do you have right now?"	Children 3 to 13 years old. Use the numeric scale if child can count to 100 by ones and identify larger of any two numbers or by 10s (Jordan-Marsh et al, 1994). Determine child's cognitive ability to use photographic scale; should be able to seriate six geometric shapes from largest to smallest. Allow the child to select his ethnic version of Oucher scale or use the version that most closely matches the physical characteristics of the child.
Hester Poker Chip Tool‡ (Hester et al, 1989): Uses four red poker chips placed horizontally in front of the child.	Start by telling the child you want to talk about the hurt he or she may be having right now. Align the chips horizontally in front of the child on a firm surface. Tell the child, "These are pieces of hurt." Beginning at the chip nearest the child's left side and ending at the one nearest the right side, point to the chips and say, "This (first chip) is a little bit of hurt and this (fourth chip) is the most hurt you could ever have." For a young child or for any child who may not fully comprehend the instructions, clarify by saying, "That means this one (first chip) is just a little hurt, this (second chip) is a little more hurt, this (third chip) is more yet, and this one (fourth chip) is the most hurt you could ever have." Do not give children an option for zero hurt. Children without pain will indicate with responses, such as "I don't have any." Ask child, "How many pieces of hurt do you have right now?" After initial use of the poker chip tool, some children internalize the concept of "pieces of hurt." If a child gives a response, such as "I have one right now," *before* you ask or before you lay out the chips, record the number of chips on the pain flow sheet. Clarify the child's answer by words, such as, "Oh, you have a little hurt? Tell me about the hurt."	Children as young as 4 years old.

TABLE 23-1 Common Pain Rating Scales Used to Measure Pain in Pediatric and Adolescent Patients—cont'd

Pain Scale/Description	Instructions	Recommended Age/ Comments
Word-Graphic Rating Scale[§] (Tesler et al, 1991): Uses descriptive words (may vary in other scales) to denote varying intensities of pain.	Explain to the child, "This line has words to describe how much pain you may have. This side of the line means no pain, and over here the line means the worst possible pain." (Point where "no pain" is and run your finger along the line to "worst possible pain" as you say it.) "If you have no pain, you would mark like this." (Show example.) "If you have some pain, you would mark somewhere along the line, depending on how much pain you have." (Show example.) "The more pain you have, the closer to worst pain you would mark. The worst pain possible is marked like this." (Show example.) "Show me how much pain you have right now by marking with a straight, up-and-down line anywhere along the line." With a millimeter rule, measure from the "no pain" end to the mark and record this measurement as the pain score.	Children 4 to 17 years old.
Numeric Scale: Uses straight line with endpoints identified as "no pain" and "worst pain" and sometimes "medium pain" in the middle; divisions along line are marked in units from 0 to 10 (high number may vary).	Explain that at one end of the line is a 0—a person feels no pain (hurt). At the other end is usually a 5 or 10—the person feels the worst pain imaginable. Numbers from 1 to 5 or 10 are for a very little pain to a whole lot of pain. Ask child to choose a number that best describes his or her pain.	Children as young as 5 years old, if they can count and have some concept of numbers and their values in relation to other numbers. May use scale horizontally or vertically.
Visual Analogue Scale (Cline et al, 1992): Defined as a vertical or horizontal line that is drawn to a certain length (such as, 10 cm) and anchored by items that represent the extremes of the subjective phenomenon (such as, pain) that is measured.	Ask the child to place a mark on a line that best describes the amount of his or her pain. With a centimeter ruler, measure from "no pain" end to the mark, and record this measurement as the pain score.	Children as young as 4½ years old, preferably 7 years old. Vertical or horizontal scale may be used.
Color Tool (Eland, 1993): Uses colored markers for child to construct own scale that is used with body outline.	Present eight markers in random order. Ask the child, "Of these colors, which color is like (event identified as having hurt the most)?" Place the marker (represents severe pain) away from the other markers. Ask the child, "Which color is like a hurt, but not quite as much as (event identified as having hurt the most)?" Place the marker next to the marker chosen to represent severe pain. Ask the child, "Which color is like something that hurts just a little?" Place marker with the others. Then ask, "Which color is like no hurt at all?" Show the four marker color choices to the child in order from worst to the no-hurt color. Ask the child to show on body outlines where he or she hurts, using the markers. After the child colors the body part(s) where it hurts, ask if they are current hurts or hurts from the past. Ask if the child knows why the area hurts if it is not clear why the child says it does.	Children as young as 4 years old, if they know their colors, are not color blind, and are able to construct the scale if in pain.

Continued

TABLE 23-1 Common Pain Rating Scales Used to Measure Pain in Pediatric and Adolescent Patients—cont'd

Pain Scale/Description	Instructions	Recommended Age/ Comments
Non-Communicating Children's Pain Checklist–Revised (NCCPC-R) (Breau et al, 2002)	Observational tool with a suggested 2-hour period of assessment—present with the child for the majority of time. Six behavioral categories are rated using a scale of 0 = not at all; 1 = just a little; 2 = fairly often; 3 = very often, and NA = not applicable.	Children ages 3 to 18 years old who are cognitively impaired or disabled and cannot speak. Can be used in the home or a residential center by parent or others. Available at www.aboutkidshealth.ca/En/Documents/AKH_Breau_everyday.pdf

**Wong-Baker FACES Pain Rating Scale Reference Manual,* describing development and research of the scale, is available from the Mayday Pain Resource Center, City of Hope National Medical Center, 1500 East Duarte Road, Duarte, CA 91010; phone: (626) 301-8941.
†The Faces Pain Scale–Revised (FPS-R) Accessed at www.iasp-pain.org/Education/Content.aspx?ItemNumber=1519&navItemNumber=577.
‡Developed in 1975 by Nancy O. Hester, University of Colorado Health Sciences Center, School of Nursing, Denver, CO 80262. Also available in Spanish and French.
§Instructions for Word-Graphic Rating Scale from Acute Pain Management Guideline Panel: Acute pain management in infants, children, and adolescents: operative and medical procedures; quick reference guide for clinicians, AHCPR pub no 92-0020, Rockville, MD, 1992, Agency for Health Care Policy and Research (now the Agency for Healthcare Research and Quality [AHRQ]), Public Health Service, U.S. Department of Health and Human Services. Word-Graphic Rating Scale is part of the Adolescent Pediatric Pain Tool and is available from Pediatric Pain Study, University of California, School of Nursing, Department of Family Health Care Nursing, San Francisco, CA 94143-0606; phone: (415) 476-4040.

not want to miss an athletic event or disappoint their teammates, so they may underreport their pain or deny being in pain.

- Children with developmental delays may have difficulty reporting pain, may be less precise in their communications, or may be unable to verbally communicate their pain. Their pain expressions may be less precise, resulting in slower reporting of pain (Wolraich et al, 2008). However, if self-report is possible, it is always preferred over observational tools.
  - Children with developmental delays are no less sensitive to painful stimuli than children with normal development. Those with autism spectrum disorder may exhibit pain or discomfort as would a developmentally normal child, by crying, moaning, seeking comfort, and so on (Allely, 2013).
  - The revised FLACC scale is also valid for children from 4 to 19 years old with cognitive impairment (Hauer and Jones, 2014). This pain scale focuses on five behavioral components and is commonly used in children less than 3 years old. The acronym **FLACC** stands for assessment of the child's **F**acial expression, **L**eg movements, **A**ctivity level, **C**ry, and **C**onsolability.
  - The Non-Communicating Children's Pain Checklist–Revised (NCCPC-R) is designed for use with children, 3 to 18 years old, who have cognitive disabilities or impairments, whether or not physically impaired or disabled, and are unable to communicate through speech. This tool focuses on vocal, social, facial, activity, body and limbs, and physiologic behavioral clues to assess level of pain using a 0 to 4 point scale: 0 = not at all, 1 = just a little, 2 = fairly often, and 3 = very often. Scoring is typically based over a 2-hour observational period (Breau et al, 2002).
- Few scales are valid for intubated children. However, some intubated children are still able to self-report by using a faces pain tool or writing notes.
  - The comfort scale (Bear and Ward-Smith, 2006) has established validity and reliability for use in mechanically ventilated children. It combines six behavioral and two physiologic measures.
  - In intubated children, monitor physiologic parameters, such as increases in heart rate, blood pressure, respiration, and decreased oxygen saturation.

Pediatric pain assessment can be challenging given developmental and cultural considerations that influence pain expression. These include whether distressed behaviors manifested by either verbal or nonverbal children of various ages indicate pain or how other causative factors (such as, anxiety, fear, stress, or hunger) in the infant and young child affect pain and its expression. A detailed pain history is often essential and necessary.

Behavioral Indicators

Displayed nonverbal cues are important indicators of pain. Behavioral observations include vocalizations (e.g., crying, whimpering, and whining); social withdrawal; changes in sleep patterns (more or less); verbalizations; facial expressions of guarding, grimacing, tightly closed eyelids, grinding or clenching teeth, breath holding, vigilance, or anger; motor responses; body posture; and activity, such as rubbing or touching the painful site, avoiding the painful site, or guarding the affected area (e.g., not letting anyone touch the abdomen or withdrawal of an injured limb). These may be the only cues of pain in preverbal or nonverbal children. Infants in pain sleep less, are irritable and agitated, do not feed well or refuse to feed, and have increased muscle tone. It is important to remember behaviors in cognitively impaired children are very individualized and may not be those typically associated with pain.

Physiologic Indicators

Physiologic parameters (e.g., alterations in heart rate, oxygen saturation, respiratory rate and pattern, and blood pressure) are neither sensitive nor specific indicators of pain, particularly in children who experience chronic pain. Other physical indicators include findings such as diaphoresis, palmar sweating, and pallor. Pulse-oximetry readings may decrease due to increased oxygen consumption. Other physiologic responses to pain include changes in metabolic functioning (e.g., hypermetabolism, hyperglycemia, or lipolysis), decreased gut motility, sodium and water retention, and cytokine production.

Management

Because there are various types of pain—acute, chronic persistent, recurrent, nociceptive, neuropathic, and psychogenic (Table 23-2)—the choice of treatment depends on the type of pain, in addition to its intensity: fair, moderate, or severe. These factors guide pain management decisions. Table 23-3 provides management guidance using pharmacologic drugs. If pain is secondary to a known etiology or underlying disease, the pediatric provider must treat its underlying causes. Other measures may be needed to control pain symptoms. Principles of effective office-based pain management include the use of a combination of pharmacologic and nonpharmacologic measures. Due to a wide range of treatment options, Hauer and Jones (2014) suggest pediatric providers consider a child's prior experience with pain medications, including side effects; previous use of

TABLE 23-2 Origins and Classifications of Pain

Type	Description/Characteristics	Examples
Origin		
Acute	Brief; associated with tissue damage or inflammation; intensity steadily diminishes over days to weeks Often identifiable cause, predictable and expected time frame	Surgical pain, burns, fractures, infection (e.g., cellulitis, abscess), trauma (e.g., puncture wound, fracture), pharyngitis
Chronic persistent	Persistent or near-persistent pain lasting 3 months or longer with changes in the nervous system (central sensitization)	Arthritis, joint pain (e.g., juvenile arthritis, sickle cell crisis)
Recurrent	Repetitive painful episodes alternating with pain-free intervals	Headache; abdominal, chest, or limb pain
Categories		
Somatic	Pain due to stimulation of nociceptors in the peripheral nervous system from injury to or inflammation of tissues (e.g., skin, vasculature, fascia, joints) In skin and superficial tissues the pain is sharp, throbbing or pulsatile, well localized; in deep somatic tissues, pain is dull, throbbing or pulsatile, aching, and not well localized	Laceration, sunburn, burns, fractures, infections, inflammatory conditions
Visceral	Pain related to injury to or inflammation of visceral organs	Bowel distention, pancreatitis, appendicitis
Neuropathic	Persistent pain related to persistent or abnormal excitability in the peripheral or central nervous system from injury, inflammation, or dysfunction with no ongoing tissue injury; often described as "burning," "strange," or "pins and needles or electrical sensation" (dysesthesias) Shooting, stabbing over a background of aching and burning; not well localized	Amputation pain syndromes, plexus injuries, reflex sympathetic dystrophy; posthepatic neuralgia, sciatica Trigeminal neuralgia
Psychogenic	Persistent pain that is a manifestation of a psychiatric disease	Somatization disorder, somatoform pain disorder, conversion disorder

TABLE 23-3 Common Oral Pain Medications and Doses Used with Children (Less than 50 Kilograms)

Pain Medication	Dosage	Special Instructions	Comments
Acetaminophen	10-15 mg/kg every 4-6 hr	Do *not* exceed five doses/24 hr 24-hr maximum limit: Term neonates <10 days, 10-15 mg/kg/dose every 6 hr (60 mg/kg/day); term neonates >10 days, 10-15 mg/kg/dose (90 mg/kg/day)	Nonopioid No anti-inflammatory activity
Ibuprofen	4-10 mg/kg every 6-8 hr	Maximum daily dosage: 40 mg/kg/day	NSAID use in children ≥ 6 mo
Codeine	0.5-1 mg/kg every 4-6 hr	Maximum dosage for children: 60 mg/dose	Opioid (not recommended for routine use in young children) This is a high-alert medication with risk of harm if used in error; do not use for post T and/or A Decreased incremental analgesic effect with doses higher than 65 mg 10% of individuals cannot metabolize this drug, so does not always work well
Naproxen	5-7 mg/kg every 8-12 hr		In children >2 years old NSAID Oral liquid available
Acetaminophen with hydrocodone (moderate pain)	Dosage in children has not been well established Usual initial dosage based on hydrocodone: 0.1-0.2 mg/kg every 4-6 hr	Dosage is limited by appropriate dosage of acetaminophen and hydrocodone	Used for moderate pain Consider if acetaminophen or ibuprofen is not effective Hydrocodone is titrated for analgesic effect Use with caution in infants due to potential respiratory depression effect
Oxycodone	Initial dosage: 0.1-0.2 mg/kg every 4-6 hr	Not used <6 months old	Opioid Used for moderate to severe pain relief This is a high-alert medication with risk of harm if used in error
Acetaminophen with oxycodone	10-15 mg/kg every 4-6 hr (of acetaminophen) or 0.1-0.2 mg/kg/dose of oxycodone	Maximum initial dosage of oxycodone: up to 5 mg/dose	This is a high-alert medication with risk of harm if used in error Manufacturer recommends every 6 hr
Methadone	Initial dosage: 0.1 mg/kg/dose every 4 hr for two to three doses, then 6-12 hr as needed or 0.7 mg/kg/24 hr divided every 4-6 hr	Maximum dosage: 10 mg/dose	Opioid Half-life is up to 96 hr; useful in chronic pain and with opioid-tolerant people Need to be weaned off, not abruptly stopped in order to avoid withdrawal symptoms
Aspirin	10-15 mg/kg every 4-6 hr	Maximum dosage: lesser amount of either 4 g/day or 120 mg/kg/24 hr in children	NSAID Used only in selective cases because of its association with Reye syndrome Inhibits platelet aggregation; may cause postoperative bleeding Do not administer to children with suspected or confirmed viral infection—used only in limited conditions

Data from Taketomo CK, Hodding JH, Kraus, DM: *Pediatric & neonatal dosage handbook*, ed 21, Hudson, OH, 2014, Lexicomp.
NSAID, Nonsteroidal anti-inflammatory drug; *T and/or A,* tonsillectomy and/or adenoidectomy.

nonpharmacologic interventions; coping skills; and social and spiritual influences.

Acute Pain Management

The goals of nonpharmacologic interventions are to reduce fear, decrease pain, and give children a sense of control (Wente, 2013). Common nonpharmacologic measures used with acute pain take into consideration the child's age and include the measures highlighted in the following sections.

Infants

Common nonpharmacologic measures used with acute pain in infants include:

- Sensorimotor techniques for infants, such as pacifiers (non-nutritive sucking), skin-to-skin contact, swaddling, holding, singing, calming music, and rocking (Srouji et al, 2010)
- Twelve percent sucrose solution (2 mL over a minute) via pacifier, gloved finger, or eye dropper. Administer 2 minutes before a procedure is started. Analgesic effect can last for 5 to 10 minutes (Hardcastle, 2010).

Children and Adolescents

Common nonpharmacologic measures used with acute pain in children and adolescents include:

- Cognitive-behavioral strategies, such as relaxation procedures (controlled breathing and progressive muscle relaxation), coping statements repeating a positive thought (e.g., "I am strong and can do this."), music, play therapy, modeling positive coping behaviors (e.g., practicing sessions prior to a procedure), parental coaching and positive reinforcement, and preparation/education/information before painful procedures or surgeries. To be effective, cognitive and behavioral strategies should appeal to the child's imagination, sense of play, and attention. It is important to consider the child's age as well as developmental abilities and preferences (Madhok et al, 2011).
- Physical strategies, such as application of heat (if muscle spasm) or cold (if swelling, bleeding, or pain), pressure, massage, breathing exercises, acupuncture, exercise, rest, or immobilization; physical therapy can be useful especially for children with musculoskeletal pain or children who are deconditioned from inactivity (Madhok et al, 2011).
- Distraction techniques have proven effectiveness. These include having the child watch a video, practice imagery, perform self-hypnosis, look out the window, or play with a toy, especially one that lights up; praising the child; giving the child a party blower, bubbles, or pinwheel and asking the child to blow the pain away; providing stickers or stamps; or gently stroking the child. Using squeeze balls with adolescents can provide distraction.

In addition to nonpharmacologic strategies, pain medications used in primary care settings typically include acetaminophen and ibuprofen. Ibuprofen is usually given first in order to allow for later usage of acetaminophen and narcotic-containing preparations (Madhok et al, 2011). This is helpful in preventing accidental acetaminophen overdose.

Prescribing appropriate pain medication at the appropriate dosage is critical. In addition, awareness of pharmacogenomics (i.e., the acquired or inherited genetic influences on drug response) for safe and effective analgesic therapy for children is another consideration that has gained attention. The clinician should consult a pediatric pharmacology reference for recommended dosing of analgesics because dosages and guidelines may change and for information about drug preparations, such as availability in liquid, tablet, or gel form and the corresponding concentration (milligrams per dose) of the various preparations:

Pharmacologic agents used in primary care settings for acute pain management include the following (see Table 23-3):

- Analgesic for mild to moderate pain (Taketomo et al, 2014): For infants and children, acetaminophen 10 to 15 mg/kg every 4 to 6 hours as needed not to exceed five doses in 24 hours with a maximum of 75 mg/kg/day and not to exceed 4000 mg/day. Adolescent and adult dosage is 325 to 650 mg every 4 to 6 hours or 1000 mg/dose three or four times a day (see manufacturer's recommendation as they may vary by product); maximum daily amount is 4 grams. In the United States, intravenous (IV) acetaminophen has been approved for children 2 years of age and older at the following dosages based on age and weight (Baley et al, 2014). Primary care providers may be involved in its administration in emergency departments. For children more than 2 years of age and less than 50 kg, the dosage is 15 mg/kg every 6 hours with a maximum daily dose of 75 mg/kg. For adolescents more than 13 years of age or more than 50 kg, the dosage is 1000 mg IV every 6 hours with a maximum total daily dose of 4000 mg. Anti-inflammatory agents are more effective if inflammation is a key factor that is causing pain, because acetaminophen has limited peripheral anti-inflammatory action. Acetaminophen is potentially hepatotoxic, so avoid its use in children with hepatic disease or dysfunction. Because acetaminophen is a component in many over-the-counter (OTC) preparations, be alert to the potential for overdose if several drugs with acetaminophen are being taken.
- Oral nonsteroidal anti-inflammatory drugs (NSAIDs): The usual pediatric dosages for children weighing less than 50 kg and dosages for children and adolescents 50 kg or more are listed in pediatric drug texts (Taketomo et al, 2014).
    - Aspirin 10 to 15 mg/kg/dose every 4 to 6 hours as needed up to a maximum of 4 g/day for children less than 50 kg. However, its use is contraindicated in children younger than 18 years of age. Because of its association with Reye syndrome, it should only be

TABLE 23-4 Management of Common Opioid Side Effects

Side Effect	Comments	Drug Dosage
Nausea	Exclude other processes, such as bowel obstruction. Consider switching to different opioid. Use antiemetics.	Metoclopramide and ondansetron: refer to a pediatric pharmacology text
Pruritus	Exclude other causes, such as drug allergy. Consider switching to different opioid. Use antipruritics.	Diphenhydramine: 0.5-1mg/kg every 6 hr (max 100 mg/day) Hydroxyzine: Children and adolescents, 0.5 mg/kg/dose PO every 6 hr (maximum single dose 50 mg)
Constipation	Encourage water, high-fiber diet if appropriate and vegetables. Regular use of stimulant and stool softener laxatives.	Docusate: Dosage by age (oral): • <3 yr: 10-40 mg/day • 3-6 yr: 20-60 mg/day • 6-12 yr: 40-150 mg/day Can give in one to four divided doses Teens and adults: 50-400 mg/day in one to four divided doses Bisacodyl rectal suppository: • <2 yr: 5 mg/day • >2-11 yr: 5-10 mg/day • >12 yr and adults: 10 mg/day Polyethylene glycol 3350 (MiraLax): Occasional constipation (0.5-1.5 g/kg/day with a maximum of 17 g/day) to severe impaction (>3 yr: 1-1.5 g/kg/day for 3 days; maximum dose 100 g per day)

Data from Zeltzer LK, Krane EJ: Pediatric pain management. In Kliegman RM, Stanton BF, St. Geme JW, et al, editors: *Nelson textbook of pediatrics*, ed 19, Philadelphia, 2011, Saunders/Elsevier, pp 360–375; Taketomo CK, Hodding JH, Kraus, DM: *Pediatric & neonatal dosage handbook*, ed 21, Hudson, OH, 2014, Lexicomp.
PO, Per os (by mouth, orally).

used in the management of selected pediatric conditions (e.g., juvenile arthritis and Kawasaki disease). Due to bleeding issues, aspirin should be discontinued 10 to 14 days before major invasive procedures or surgeries.

- Ibuprofen 4 to 10 mg/kg every 6 to 8 hours as needed for infants more than 6 months and children (less than 50 kg) with a maximum daily dose of 40 mg/kg/day and a maximum single dose of 400 mg; adolescent and adult: 200 to 400 mg/dose every 4 to 6 hours as needed with 1.2 g/day maximum. Avoid if there is an aspirin allergy, anticipated surgery, bleeding disorder, hemorrhage, gastritis, or renal disease. Use with caution in children not eating solids.
- Naproxen, older than 2 years: 5 to 7 mg/kg/dose every 8 to 12 hours; adolescents and adults for mild to moderate pain or dysmenorrhea: initial 500 mg dose and then 250 mg every 6 to 8 hours or 500 mg every 12 hours, maximum 1250 mg/day initially and then maximum daily dose 1000 mg/day. This medicine requires similar cautions as ibuprofen. Delayed-release preparations are not recommended for acute pain management.

- Opioid agonists are used for moderate to severe pain. All opioids produce a range of side effects including constipation, nausea and vomiting, pruritus, sedation, respiratory depression, and urinary retention. Side effects should be anticipated and treated aggressively. Consideration in dosing is needed for opioid-naive children. Although many of the common opioids are listed in this text, primary care providers may typically only use a select few of these medications in primary care settings. Common opioid side effects and management are listed in Table 23-4 and as follows (Taketomo et al, 2014):
  - Codeine: Of note, codeine toxicity is a concentration-dependent toxicity associated with pharmacogenomic factors linked to CYP2D6 variability in individuals who are ultrarapid-metabolizer. Because codeine use has been associated with deaths, though infrequent, in healthy children after procedures thought to be safe, its use in children is *not* recommended (Rieder and Carleton, 2014). Usual adolescent/adult dose is 30 mg; range per dose is 15 to 60 mg every 4 to 6 hours as needed. It is a highly constipating drug and associated with nausea, gastrointestinal distress, and vomiting. Usual adult dose is 30 mg; range per dose is 15 to 60 mg every 4 to 6 hours as needed.
  - Hydromorphone: The use of hydromorphone by primary care providers in the ambulatory management of pediatric pain should be limited to situations

of moderate to severe pain and in consultation with pain management specialists. It is a potent schedule II drug. Oral dosage, infants 6 months and less than 10 kg: Usual range is 0.03 to 0.06 mg/kg/dose every 4 hours as needed; children and teens less than 50 kg: 0.03 to 0.08 mg/kg/dose every 3 to 4 hours; children more than 50 kg and adolescents: 1 to 2 mg/dose every 3 to 4 hours as needed for opioid-naive children; those with prior opioid exposure may need a higher initial doses; usual adult dosage of 2 to 4 mg/dose with a maximum of 8 mg/dose.

- Methadone is a synthetic opioid that has a long duration of action (12 to 36 hours). Traditionally it is used with opioid-dependent patients (e.g., neonatal abstinence syndrome). Methadone is being increasingly used in cases of acute pain to provide stable levels of opioid analgesia. Methadone has a high bioavailability (85%) making it an attractive oral analgesic. Children: 0.1 mg/kg/dose orally every 4 hours initially for two or three doses and then every 6 to 12 hours as needed; it can also be dosed at 0.7 mg/kg per 24 hours divided every 4 to 6 hours. The maximum dose is 10 mg/dose. Methadone dosing must be individualized. Prior opioid exposure and withdrawal symptoms are key factors to consider. Patients must be carefully monitored to avoid overmedication with repeated doses. Abrupt discontinuation after prolonged use can result in withdrawal symptoms or seizures. Methadone has the potential to increase the corrected QT interval (QTc; the QT interval corrected for heart rate), so a baseline electrocardiogram is usually obtained (Taketomo et al, 2014).
- Hydrocodone (commonly combined with acetaminophen)—dose has not been well established in children and must be used with caution. Infants have increased sensitivity to hydrocodone with resulting respiratory depression. The dosing guidelines for opioid-naive children less than 50 kg who are in moderate or severe pain are as follows: Usual initial dose based on hydrocodone is 0.1 to 0.2 mg/kg/dose orally every 4 to 6 hours; for those more than 50 kg, the usual initial dose is 5 to 10 mg every 3 to 4 hours. Typically adolescents and adults dosage is 5 to 10 mg every 4 to 6 hours as needed. Hydrocodone is available in fixed combinations with acetaminophen. If given with acetaminophen, the maximum recommended dose of acetaminophen, for a child or adolescent, cannot be exceeded because of liver toxicity. Opioid-naive children typically require decreased dosage. Because of the misuse and abuse of opioid drugs, hydrocodone combination products are now schedule II drugs.
- Oxycodone—for infants 6 months or older and weight less than 50 kg: Oral initial dose, 0.1 to 0.2 mg/kg/dose every 4 to 6 hours for severe pain (available in liquid and in varied concentrations) for children as needed with a maximum of 5 to 10 mg/dose. For children 50 kg or more and adults experiencing moderate to severe pain, the usual initial dose is 5 to 10 mg every 4 to 6 hours as needed with a 20 mg/dose maximum. It comes in tablets, capsules, solution, and a controlled-release product that is available alone or in fixed combinations with acetaminophen. Oxycodone has restricted access with special U.S. Food and Drug Administration (FDA) training required to prescribe.
- Morphine—an oral dose of 0.3 mg/kg is recommended by some experts as an initial dose for the child (less than 50 kg) in severe pain (maximum is 15 to 20 mg/dose) with subsequent recommended dosing of 0.2 to 0.5 mg/kg/dose every 3 to 4 hours as needed. Adult dosage (greater than 50 kg) is 15 to 20 mg orally every 3 to 4 hours as needed. This drug is not used commonly in primary care settings for the management of acute pain.
- Topical analgesic creams, such as eutectic mixture of local anesthetics (EMLA) and iontophoresis delivery of drugs, are used with procedures involving skin punctures. Topical liposomal 4% lidocaine creams (LMX4) provides effective analgesia in 30 minutes, whereas EMLA takes 1 hour for full effectiveness. Subcutaneous injection of combinations of local anesthetics, such as lidocaine, epinephrine, and tetracaine (LET), are useful in suturing lacerations. It is recommended to use an occlusive dressing after applying LET to the wound. This prevents the LET from seeping out and allows the practitioner to visualize the wound for blanching on the margins. Blanching of the margins indicates adequate absorption of LET into the tissue (Madhok et al, 2011). Never use epinephrine-containing local anesthetics for digits or the penis because of end artery adverse effect.
- Benzodiazepines may play a role in the treatment of pain if spasms are a contributing factor to the pain experienced by a child (Hauer and Jones, 2014). Be mindful of drug and herbal interactions with benzodiazepines.

Pharmacologic Considerations

There can be interactions between herbal preparations and common pain relievers and anesthetics. Stop herbal supplements at least 1 week before any scheduled surgical procedure to prevent alterations in coagulation or interactions with anesthesia (see Table 43-3 for specific examples). Should the provider, family or patient wish to consider nonpharmacologic management of pain as an option, Chapter 43 provides some guidance.

An essential consideration in administering analgesics is whether there is a need to maintain certain serum concentration levels. In situations requiring a steady-state serum concentration for pain relief (e.g., following same-day surgery, fractures), around-the-clock dosing of pain medications for 48 to 72 hours is preferable to "as needed (pro re nata [PRN])" dosing, which is associated with drops in serum concentration levels. When the child is given a PRN dose of medication, a significant period may elapse before adequate analgesic effect occurs.

Factors that Produce Age-Related Differences in Analgesia Responses

Consider the following factors that produce age-related differences in analgesia responses:

- Neonates and young infants have delayed hepatic enzyme maturation resulting in altered drug metabolic inactivation. Analgesics metabolized in the liver, such as opioids, have a prolonged elimination half-life in newborns and young infants. Rates of maturation of individual enzyme functions vary, but most mature by approximately 6 months of age (Zeltzer and Krane, 2011).
- Glomerular filtration is reduced in the first few weeks of life, which results in slower elimination of opioids and their active metabolites (Quigley, 2012).
- Toddler's and preschool children's renal clearance of analgesics is greater than adults (Zeltzer and Krane, 2011).
- Neonates and young infants have decreased plasma protein binding for many drugs, resulting in greater concentrations of pharmacologically active unbound drug (Zeltzer and Krane, 2011).

Chronic Pain Management

Surveillance data for the pediatric population estimates that approximately 30% of children are living with chronic pain. Children and adolescents with chronic pain are at greater risk for anxiety and depression, especially girls, and experience more emotional and functional problems including more depressive symptoms than others of the same age. Chronic pain affects children's school attendance, participation in hobbies, appetite, and quality of life resulting in increased health services (Odell and Logan, 2013). Because it is not always feasible to totally eradicate the pain, return of function is often the goal.

The entire central nervous system is affected by chronic pain resulting in increased neuronal responsiveness to painful and nonpainful stimuli. This phenomenon is called *central sensitization* and is thought to be linked to the development and maintenance of many types of chronic pain (Woolf, 2011). Furthermore, if a child with chronic pain handles the pain by being very quiet or withdrawn, this coping mechanism may lead to inaccurate assumptions by providers that the child's pain is well controlled when just the opposite is true.

Chronic pain is differentiated from acute pain when the duration of pain lasts longer than the expected healing time for an injury or from 3 to 6 months or longer. A diagnosis of "pain disorder" is made when the primary complaint is severe pain that involves five key features: (1) pain in one or more anatomical sites that is the predominant focus; (2) significant distress involving social or other important functions; (3) psychological factors implicated in either the onset, severity, exacerbation, or maintenance of the pain; (4) the pain is not from a malingering or fictitious illness; and (5) a mood, anxiety, or psychotic disorder is not related to the etiology of the pain. Some of the most common causes of chronic pain in pediatrics include migraine, recurrent abdominal pain, and generalized musculoskeletal pain (Odell and Logan, 2013).

Health care providers may worry they will miss an organic cause when dealing with a child with recurrent or chronic pain in which the etiology may be in question. The first step in a chronic pain assessment should be a comprehensive evaluation that includes a thorough history of the pain with questions that can help uncover the possibility of comorbid conditions (e.g., depression, anxiety disorders, and contributing psychosocial factors). A focused physical examination is then performed. If warranted by historical and physical data, selected laboratory and/or radiographic studies can be conducted. There is no standard laboratory workup for the evaluation of chronic pain. Extensive laboratory investigations are not always needed or recommended and can be harmful. Having cautiously collected and evaluated the data, the primary care provider can better explain what is causing or adding to the child's pain and work in partnership with the child and parent to develop a comprehensive pain treatment strategy plan to effectively manage the child's pain (Box 23-1). Pharmacologic measures and nonpharmacologic techniques are used in the primary care setting for chronic pain management.

Pharmacologic Measures

Pharmacologic measures include (see Table 23-3):

- NSAIDs, acetaminophen, and tricyclic antidepressants (TCAs) are the primary treatments used to treat chronic pain unrelated to disease or trauma. Assess the efficacy of the pharmacologic therapy as follows:
  - Have the child or parent use a pain intensity rating scale and keep a diary of the child's activities and pain.
  - On follow-up visits, question whether symptoms have improved.
- Selective serotonin reuptake inhibitors (SSRIs), opioids, certain anticonvulsants, muscle relaxants (e.g., cerebral palsy), and other selected medications may be needed. Warnings about their use in primary care are discussed later in this section.
- Gabapentin is the anticonvulsant most frequently used to treat neuropathic pain associated with burning, stabbing, or aching. Due to few adverse side effects, it is often considered a first-line therapy. Children requiring these agents for the management of their chronic pain are best handled by referral to pain management specialists. The Lidoderm patch, a topical agent, is also useful in the treatment of focal neuropathic pain.

TCAs are used for phantom limb, peripheral neuropathy, migraine headaches, radiation-induced nerve injury, or tumor-associated nerve damage (Hauer and Jones, 2014) and are typically prescribed by pediatric specialists and not primary care providers. Use of tricyclics is contraindicated in patients with cardiac conduction disturbances. The pain dosage for TCAs (more commonly used in children with chronic pain) is lower than the dosage prescribed in the

• BOX 23-1 Key Strategies in the Evaluation and Treatment of Chronic Pain

Evaluation

History Key Points

Actively listen to the parent's and child's description of the pain experience; listen to their pain story.
Be sure to talk to the adolescent alone.
Ask questions related to the presence of psychosocial and developmental comorbidities or contributing psychosocial-developmental factors (e.g., school issues, family dysfunction, negative coping strategies, and/or depression).
Question about onset of pain; time of day; duration; frequency of pain episodes and if sudden or gradual onset; location and radiation; associated symptoms; description of the pain; what started the pain and/or keeps it going; what has been used to control the pain (medications, CAM, other modalities); how is pain affecting the child's and family's life (sleep, activities, appetite); what decreases the pain or makes it worse?

Physical Examination Focus Points

Note the child's appearance, posture, and gait.
Carefully examine areas of hypersensitivity and tender points in muscles or tendon insertion sites.

Laboratory and Imaging Studies (Limit Testing to Only What Is Needed)

Only tests needed based on history and physical examination and if not done recently.
Consider routine tests such as CBC with differential, sedimentation rate; obtain a urinalysis if child's physical examination suggests the need for such tests.

Treatment

Educate child and family about the nature of chronic pain and the reason for the child's pain.
Focus efforts on helping the child enhance his or her coping skills.
Identify a plan with the child and family on how to improve child's functional ability, emphasizing:

- Sleep: Improving sleep hygiene using psychological strategies and pharmacologic agents if needed
- Cognitive-behavioral therapy: Biofeedback, hypnotherapy, relaxation techniques
- School: Talk with the parents, child, and school personnel to develop a plan to help child reach potential in the school setting in academic, social, and physical activities
- Physical therapy and mental health referral if indicated
- Other treatments to reduce stress: Massage; art, aroma, music therapy; acupuncture, yoga
- Medication: As needed while remembering that nonpharmacologic strategies and interventions are also essential management tools

CAM, Complementary and alternative medicine; *CBC,* complete blood count.

treatment of depression. The FDA has not approved the use of these drugs for depression in pediatric patients (Taketomo et al, 2014); therefore, the primary care provider's role would be to refer to the appropriate pain management specialist for the initial assessment for such drugs and assist in the monitoring of children on TCAs. Tricyclics have significant adverse effects, such as sedation, orthostatic hypotension, dry mouth, constipation, and urinary hesitancy. These side effects typically subside as the child develops tolerance to the medication. The use of TCAs in children can result in serious, if not fatal, problems due to their heightened potential of toxicity in the pediatric population.

Patients treated with antidepressants require close monitoring and observation for worsening of depression, suicidality, and unusual behavior, especially during the first few months of therapy. Family members must be educated about closely observing the patient and communicating the patient's condition frequently to the health care provider.

Botulinum products are approved for certain chronic painful conditions in children such as seventh cranial nerve disorders, dynamic muscle contractures associated with cerebral palsy, and migraine headaches. FDA approval for the use of botulinum in children lists age requirements and condition restrictions. Its use is reserved for those who have failed conservative treatment. Pain specialists work with children and their families during the administration of this drug. The primary care provider should be familiar with adverse and life-threatening reactions associated with this drug to answer parents' questions if they care for children receiving this drug.

Nonpharmacologic Measures

Nonpharmacologic techniques and considerations include:

- Physical therapy, relaxation, massage, guided imagery, biofeedback, hypnosis, heat and cold, distraction, transcutaneous electrical nerve stimulation (TENS), music therapy, acupuncture, and psychological therapy, which are frequently used as adjuncts to pharmacologic therapy of chronic pain. Invasive techniques, such as neuroablative procedures and spinal cord stimulation, are occasionally used as a last resort. Hypnotherapy and biofeedback may be beneficial in the treatment of chronic pain.
- Critical factors in chronic pain assessment include level of child and family distress (including their level of anxiety, depression, and feelings of hopelessness), cultural beliefs, and pain perception.

Additional Measures

There are parental strategies that can encourage optimal coping with chronic pain issues. These include the following (Palermo and Zeltzer, 2009):

- Not giving excessive attention, special privileges, or treats when the child complains of pain.
- Encouraging normal activities, within reason, during pain episodes (e.g., going to school, doing chores).
- Spending time during the day doing quiet, low-key activities when the child cannot go to school or participate in other events. Activities, such as playing games all day and excessive time spent watching television or

videos, may reinforce the child in not wanting to participate in "well" activities.

- Lessening the focus on pain by not repeatedly asking the child about his or her pain. Children typically will let their parent know when they are in pain.
- Reinforcing the child's role in pain self-management through the use of nonpharmacologic strategies based on developmental appropriateness. When the child reports pain, ask, "What do you think you can do to help lessen your pain?" Then talk about the nonpharmacologic strategies. However, give breakthrough pain medication if the child requests it.

In providing chronic care management, the primary care provider must also be diligent in assessing for depression, situational anxiety, anxiety disorders, posttraumatic stress disorder, social anxiety, panic disorder, separation anxiety, and obsessive-compulsive disorder that are present or subsequently develop. These comorbidities, if present, affect the child's experience of pain and how he or she copes (Zeltzer and Krane, 2011).

Chronic pain is most successfully treated by a coordinated, planned, interdisciplinary approach. It is essential that all team members are communicating the same message in an integrated team approach format. Study results provide strong evidence-based support for using psychological interventions as key management components to reduce chronic pain in children. These strategies (e.g., relaxation techniques, parent interventions, and cognitive strategies) should be emphasized as essential components of the treatment plan because they reduce pain symptoms and disability posttreatment (Fisher et al, 2014; Palermo et al, 2010).

Table 23-5 outlines specific pain problems commonly seen in pediatrics, in addition to pain relief strategies. The health care provider should become familiar with clinical practice guidelines that address pain management related to common chronic pediatric conditions. Sickle cell anemia and juvenile arthritis are examples of chronic conditions marked by acute, chronic, and mixed (acute superimposed on chronic) pain. The National Heart, Lung, and Blood Institute published a key document titled *The Management of Sickle Cell Disease* (2002) that addressed a variety of disease-related issues, including pain management. This landmark document tackled the misconceptions about pain in children with sickle cell anemia and provided guidelines for the proper use of analgesia. Pain is a critical feature of this disease and can have significant negative effects on quality of life. The Evidence-Based Management of Sickle Cell Disease: Expert Panel Report, 2014 provides guidelines for the management of chronic pain in children and is available online (www.nhlbi.nih.gov/health-pro/guidelines/sickle-cell-disease-guidelines/index.htm). There is also information available from the Arthritis Foundation KIDS Get Arthritis, Too about the management of pain in children with juvenile arthritis. Knowledge of appropriate pain management resources and using pain control protocols are key elements in optimizing the care of children with chronic diseases and improving quality of life. Specific disease-related pain management is discussed in subsequent chapters of this text.

Partnership in Care

Several critical elements related to pain management and administration of pain medications must be emphasized to parents and children. They include:

- Pain medication should be taken exactly as prescribed.
- Myths related to addiction and the use of opioids for pain control should be discussed when these agents are needed for pain control.
- The use of other methods for relieving pain should be utilized, because they are essential components of the pain management plan. Medication alone is not sufficient to manage chronic pain; similarly, cognitive-behavioral therapies are helpful in acute pain situations.
- Teens should be warned about drinking alcohol with opioids.
- The health care provider needs to be kept apprised of all prescribed, OTC, and herbal medications taken.
- Pain medication taken over long periods of time may need to be tapered and not abruptly stopped.
- Pain medication works most effectively when taken before the onset of severe pain.
- Common side effects such as constipation, dizziness, nausea, drowsiness, sweating, and flushing occur with the administration of pain medications. The health care provider should be aware of these problems so that appropriate interventions can be applied.
- The provider and parent and/or child need to assess for overall improvement in control of pain and its related symptoms.
  - The provider and parent cannot be solely dependent on numbers attached to an assessment tool. Look at the broader picture, such as improvement in the amount of crying, facial grimacing, spasm, stiffening, and so on.
  - Consider whether the severity, duration, and frequency of the symptom(s) have decreased
- Have a follow-up plan in place that identifies a timeline as to when to expect improvement in pain control and or symptoms. This depends on a number of factors (e.g., the medication and its onset of action, symptoms, and the frequency of the pain or symptoms [i.e., daily or intermittent]).
- Establish a time frame for follow-up visits and discuss indications for earlier interventions if the situation is not improving or worsening.

Pain management requires comprehensive treatment strategies (Odell and Logan, 2013). A multidisciplinary approach should be used when partnering with patients and their families. Disciplines include medicine, psychology, physical therapy, occupational therapy, and nursing. Parents and their children report higher satisfaction when a multidisciplinary approach to pain management has been utilized. This is important because patient and parent

TABLE 23-5 Common Pediatric Pain Problems and Pain Relief Strategies

Pediatric Pain Problems	Pain Relief Strategies
Otalgia	Acetaminophen or ibuprofen Antipyrine and benzocaine otic drops Warmed compresses pressed against the ear
Pharyngitis	Acetaminophen or ibuprofen Antibiotics if GABHS Saltwater gargles Anesthetic lozenges for older child
Stomatitis	Ibuprofen Bland diet Saline mouth rinses for older children Benadryl-calcium carbonate (Maalox) (in a 1 : 1 preparation) to coat the mucous membranes Viscous lidocaine (remember the potential for aspiration and toxicity) Sucralfate
Musculoskeletal injury	**RICE**—**R**est, **I**ce, **C**ompression, and **E**levation Immobilization of affected area Cold for the initial 48 to 72 hours NSAIDs
Fractures and sprains	NSAIDs Narcotic analgesics if severe fracture or sprain Topical ibuprofen, ketoprofen, and felbinac give relief in soft tissue trauma, strains, and sprains; however, studies have involved only adults
Injection pain (e.g., immunizations)	Distraction and relaxation techniques EMLA cream (maximum recommended dose based on application area; it is also age and weight dependent)* Ice Spot pressure (press down into muscle where shot is to be given) Vapocoolants
Neonate and infant procedural pain	12% sucrose solution orally (can be placed on pacifier) Acetaminophen
In emergency department or urgent care settings: IV line placement or venipuncture, lumbar puncture, abscess drainage, joint aspiration	EMLA/LMX4 (prevent mucous membrane contact or ingestion)†
Laceration	Lidocaine, epinephrine, and tetracaine (LET) procedure: Use on open wounds that are simple lacerations of head, neck, extremities, or trunk that are <5 cm in length; use 3 mL max; place LET mixed with cellulose on open wound and cover with occlusive dressing, or place two cotton balls soaked with LET in the wound Contraindications: Allergy to amide anesthetics, gross contamination of wound; do not use on mucous membranes, digits, genitalia, ear, or nose

EMLA, Eutectic mixture of local anesthetics; *GABHUS,* Group A beta-hemolytic streptococcal infection; *IV,* intravenous; *NSAID,* nonsteroidal anti-inflammatory drug.

*EMLA is contraindicated in patients with congenital or idiopathic methemoglobinemia or in infants less than 12 months old who are being treated with sulfas, acetaminophen, benzocaine, chloroquine, dapsone, nitrofurantoin, phenobarbital, phenytoin, or quinine.

†EMLA/LMX4 (liposomal 4% lidocaine cream) contraindicated with nonintact skin, allergy to amide anesthetics, or in emergent situations.

satisfaction correlates with adherence to treatment recommendations (Odell and Logan, 2013).

Follow-up assessment determines whether optimal pain control is achieved, evaluates whether pharmacologic side effects are minimized or effectively managed, and ensures the causative factor of the pain was correctly identified. Follow-up assessment may be conducted via the phone or by appointment. The time frame for follow-up is individualized depending on the severity of pain, underlying health condition, and parent-child socioemotional factors (Odell and Logan, 2013).

For a complete list of references, please visit http://evolve.elsevier.com/Burns/pediatric/.

24

Infectious Diseases and Immunizations

CATHERINE G. BLOSSER, CATHERINE O'KEEFE, AND SUSAN K. SANDERSON

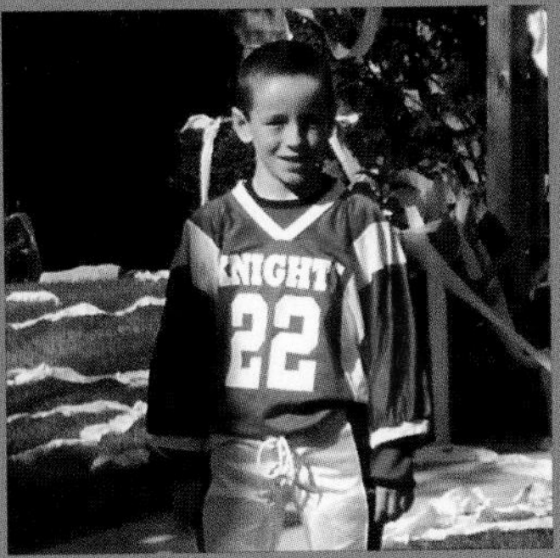

Infectious diseases are the leading causes of illness in infants and children despite advances in public and personal health, antimicrobials, and active and passive vaccination (Cherry and Adachi, 2014). The ability to distinguish serious infections from those that resolve with minimal or no intervention is an important skill for primary care providers (PCPs). Nearly as important as the medical care provided to the sick child is the ability to effectively communicate with, educate, and support the often frustrated and anxious parents. Additionally, the provider must include preventive education, including vaccinations, in the routine delivery of primary health care.

Pathogenesis of Infectious Diseases

Researchers from the National Institutes of Health (NIH) Common Fund Human Microbiome Project are mapping the normal microbial makeup of healthy individuals. This project has found that approximately 100 trillion microorganisms (mostly bacteria, but also viruses and fungi) abound in the body (the brain, spinal fluid, blood, urine, lungs, and tissues are inherently sterile) and for the most part live in harmony with their human hosts, contributing to human survival. Bacteria outnumber human cells by 10 to 1 and can weigh 2 to 7 pounds, depending upon an individual's size (NIH, 2013). In turn, viruses outnumber bacteria 10 to 1 and are common both in and on humans and in most ecosystems (Saey, 2014).

The normal human flora, or "normal microbiota" (Table 24-1), remain throughout life unless environmental changes affect them. Studies show that humans are losing some of their microbial diversity. It is believed that this loss is in part due to the overuse of antibiotics, cesarean sections, and modern sanitation. This loss may account for the increase in asthma, allergies, diabetes, obesity, and possibly some forms of cancer (Blaser, 2014).

It is estimated that only 10% of pathogens attributed to causing human diseases have been identified. Although viruses are the most frequent cause of childhood infectious illnesses, bacterial infections (particularly of the skin and mucosal surfaces) are also common. Bacteria are ubiquitous in the environment. They are intercellular microorganisms that carry all their requirements and mechanisms for growth and multiplication with them. Most can grow on nonliving surfaces. Some live at different temperature extremes. They have many shapes, including curved rods, spheres, rods, and spirals. Each bacterium has its own unique mode(s) of transmission and mechanisms of colonization and pathogenesis. Humans are inoculated with important bacteria on the skin (especially in moist areas) and mucosal surfaces (including the upper respiratory, urinary, and gastrointestinal [GI] tracts) during vaginal birth or shortly afterward.

Most bacteria are harmless and are the first line of defense against the colonization by potentially pathogenic organisms. Microbiotas are required for digestion, to degrade toxins, and help in the maturation of the immune system. Infectious disease results when the balance between harmless colonization and protective immunity is disrupted in favor of harmful proliferation of a microorganism. Bacteria are adept at adapting, as evidenced by increasing resistance to antibiotics.

In comparison, viruses (Latin noun meaning *toxin* or *poison*) are submicroscopic particles that invade a host cell, redirect the normal cell's functions, and effectively transfer genetic information (deoxyribonucleic acid [DNA] and ribonucleic acid [RNA]) to replicate viral particles. Viruses need to have a living host in order to multiply. Dangerous viruses are rare because of their inability to simultaneously meet three criteria necessary for virulence: (1) to inflict serious harm, (2) to go unrecognized by the immune system, and (3) to spread efficiently. Viruses can also control bacteria; these are referred to as *bacteriophages,* or "eaters of bacteria." These phages are numerous in the environment and practically harmless to humans. Vaccines can prevent the spread of viruses, and antiviral medications can help slow down their reproduction in some cases. Newer research

TABLE 24-1 Common Distribution Sites of Normal Microflora* Found in Humans

Bacterium	Very Commonly or Commonly Found in These Locations	Notes
Aerobic Bacteria		
Gram Positive		
Staphylococcus aureus	Skin, hair, naso-oropharynx, lower GI, cerumen, vagina	Rarely found in the anterior vagina and conjunctiva; trachea, bronchi, lungs, and sinuses are normally sterile; has potential for being a pathogen. A study shows that high levels of MRSA bacteria in the nose are indicative of MRSA colonization in the axilla, groin, perineum; if screening cultures are done, culturing the nose will produce reliable results of colonization in other areas (Mermel et al, 2011).
Staphylococcus epidermidis	Skin, hair, naso-oropharynx, adult vagina, urethra, conjunctiva, ear (including cerumen), lower GI	Occasionally found in the vagina of prepubertal females; found in low numbers in "normal" urine, probably as a result of contamination from urethra and skin areas.
Staphylococcus saprophyticus	Skin, mucous membranes, vagina, perineum	Most common cause of UTI in sexually active women. Has the potential of being a pathogen.
Streptococci		
• *S. mitis*	Skin, pharynx, mouth; less commonly in adult vagina and urethra; rare lower GI	
• *S. mutans*	Mouth, pharynx	Has the potential of being a pathogen.
• *S. pneumoniae* (*Pneumococcus, Diplococcus*)	Nasopharynx, mouth; rarely found in conjunctiva, nose, vagina	Common cause respiratory tract and ear infections; pathogen of sepsis, pneumonia, meningitis.
• *S. pyogenes* (group A)	Mouth, pharynx; rarely skin, conjunctiva, adult vagina, lower GI	Common cause of skin and pharyngeal infections.
Bifidobacterium bifidum	Lower GI	
Enterococcus faecalis	Lower GI, postpubertal vagina; mouth, anterior urethra; rarely pharynx	Has potential of being a pathogen.
Propionibacterium acnes	Skin (rarely seen in children prior to age of 10 years); external ear	Commonly involved in acne vulgaris during puberty.
Gram Negative		
Acinetobacter spp.	Skin; less commonly respiratory tract, mouth, GI	Successful at causing outbreaks and developing antibiotic resistance.
Corynebacterium	Skin, conjunctiva, naso-oropharynx, mouth, lower GI, anterior urethra, adult vagina	
Citrobacter diversus	Lower GI	Common cause of UTI.
Escherichia coli	Lower GI, vagina, mouth, anterior urethra; rarely found in conjunctiva, nose, pharynx	Has the potential of being a pathogen.
Haemophilus influenzae	Nasopharynx, mouth; rarely conjunctiva, ear	Cause of upper respiratory tract, ear, and eye infections.
Kingella kingae (formerly referred to as *Moraxella kingae*)	Pharynx	Has the potential of being a pathogen (cause of invasive infections in young children).
Klebsiella pneumoniae	Nose, colon, axillary area	Associated with neonatal sepsis; urinary tract infections.
Lactobacillus spp.	Pharynx, mouth, lower GI, adult vagina	
Moraxella catarrhalis	Nasopharynx	Implicated in otitis media.
Morganella morganii	Lower GI	

Continued

TABLE 24-1 Common Distribution Sites of Normal Microflora Found in Humans—cont'd

Bacterium	Very Commonly or Commonly Found in These Locations	Notes
Mycobacterium spp.	Skin, lower GI, anterior urethra; rarely nasopharynx	
Mycoplasma	Mouth, pharynx, lower GI, vagina; rarely anterior urethra	Implicated in upper and lower respiratory tract infections.
Neisseria spp. (e.g., *N. mucosa*)	Nose, pharynx (100% of population), conjunctiva, mouth, anterior urethra, vagina	Nonpathogenic species.
N. meningitidis	Nose, pharynx (100% of population), mouth, vagina	Significant cause of meningitis and sepsis in children.
Proteus spp.	Skin, nasopharynx, mouth, lower GI, vagina, anterior urethra; rarely in conjunctiva	
Pseudomonas aeruginosa	Lower GI; rarely in pharynx, mouth, anterior urethra; colonization in lungs of patients with cystic fibrosis (Murray et al, 2007); small numbers can be found on the skin	Has the potential of being a pathogen.
Anaerobic Bacteria		
Bacteroides spp.	Lower GI, anterior urethra; rarely adult vagina	Has the potential of being a pathogen.
Clostridium spp.	Lower GI; rarely mouth	Has the potential for being a pathogen.
Streptococcus spp.	Mouth, colon, adult vagina	
Spirochetes (a distinct form of bacteria)	Pharynx, mouth, lower GI	
Fungi		
Actinomycetes spp.	Pharynx, mouth	
Candida albicans	Skin, conjunctiva, mouth, lower GI, adult vagina	Can be found in voided urine, but is a contaminant.
Cryptococcus spp.	Skin	
Protozoa	Mouth, lower GI, adult vagina	

Data from Carroll KC: Normal human microbiota. In Brooks GF, Carroll KC, Butel JS, et al, editors: *Jawetz, Melnick, & Adelberg's medical microbiology*, ed 26, New York, 2013, McGraw-Hill, pp 165–174; Mermel LA, Cartony JM, Covington P, et al: Methicillin-resistant *Staphylococcus aureus* colonization at different body sites: a prospective, quantitative analysis, *J Clin Microbiol* 49(3):1119–1121, 2011; Murray TS, Egan M, Kazmierczak BI: *Pseudomonas aeruginosa* chronic colonization in cystic fibrosis patients, *Curr Opin Pediatr* 19(1):83–88, 2007; Todar K: The normal bacterial flora of humans, Todar's Online Textbook of Bacteriology (website), 2008–2012, available at www.textbookofbacteriology.net/normalflora.html. Accessed February 28, 2015.

GI, Gastrointestinal; *MRSA,* methicillin-resistant Staphylococcus aureus; *spp.,* species; *URI,* urinary tract infection.

*Normal microflora in humans consist of indigenous microorganisms that colonize human body tissues and live in a mutualistic state without producing disease. An individual's microflora depends on genetics, age, sex, stress, nutrition, and diet. A pathogen is a microorganism (or virus) than can produce disease. Normal flora can become pathogens when a host is compromised or weakened (endogenous pathogen); other microorganisms can invade a host during times of disease only (obligate pathogens) or lowered resistance (opportunistic pathogens). Skin microflora can also include yeast *(Malassezia furfur)*, molds *(Trichophyton mentagrophytes* var. *interdigitale*), and mites *(Demodex folliculorum)*. The type of normal flora found in the vagina depends on one's age, pH, and hormonal levels. Cerumen contains some antimicrobial elements to discourage growth of pathogenic *Pseudomonas aeruginosa* and *Staphylococcus aureus*. The cervix is normally sterile but can demonstrate flora similar to those in the upper area of the vagina. Greater than 500 species of bacteria have been identified in the colon. The flow of tears and inherent antibacterial lysozymes prevent the growth of flora in the conjunctiva.

is focusing on human resident viruses (human virome), and there is indication that viruses play a part in the human defense system (Saey, 2014).

The human immune system is complex and provides many layers of protection from disease. Skin and mucosal surfaces provide a barrier to invasion by microorganisms, and antibodies and immune cells allow the body to defend itself in general and specific ways against invasion by pathogens. Microorganisms may breach the immune barrier provided by skin and mucosa by binding to cell surface structures. For example, influenza virus uses its hemagglutinin protein to attach to cell membranes and invade respiratory mucosa. Disease caused by microbial pathogens can result from destruction of infected cells and tissues and from disruption of normal cell functions. Some disease symptoms are caused by the immune system's response to infection, which can result in local or systemic inflammatory responses. Biotechnology is being applied to developing bacterial-based treatments that harness the ability of some bacteria to enter into cells and trigger intense immune responses, much like vaccines. A variety of genetically engineered and modified strains of bacteria are being studied as possible treatments for certain bacterial infections (e.g., malaria, human immunodeficiency virus [HIV]) and cancers (Gaidos, 2014).

Clinical Findings

History

Most infectious illnesses in pediatrics are diagnosed solely based on history and physical examination. A comprehensive history generates and helps prioritize differential diagnoses for that particular individual based on symptomatology and history. Many symptoms are shared by different illnesses, and establishing a differential diagnoses can be challenging (e.g., fever is most commonly associated with infectious illnesses but also occurs with rheumatologic or oncologic diseases). Crucial aspects of the history that help distinguish infectious illnesses from other types of diseases or assist in determining the responsible pathogen include:

- The history of present illness with a careful analysis of the presenting symptoms: When did the symptoms start? What other symptoms were associated with the illness? Were there periods when the patient seemed improved or even back to normal?
- A comprehensive past medical history: Careful questioning makes certain diagnoses more or less likely. Determine place of birth and past acute or chronic illnesses. A history of asthma in a teenager with fever and cough, for example, is suspicious of atypical pneumonia.
- Current and recent medications: Recent antibiotic use may negate culture results or contribute to resistant infections (e.g., methicillin-resistant *Staphylococcus aureus* [MRSA] tissue infection). Include any nonprescription, herbal, or natural health products that may have recently been used.
- Immunizations: Adherence to recommended vaccine schedules (including age and spacing of vaccines) is an important consideration if the child's symptoms suggest a vaccine preventable disease.
- Family history, particularly regarding infectious illness: Important information includes a history of any relative (first or second degree) with a known immune deficiency, with numerous infections or difficulty recovering from infections, or with a history of recurrent miscarriages. Any of these may raise suspicion for an immune deficiency. A strong history of autoimmune disease in the family may suggest possible rheumatologic diagnoses as opposed to an infectious process.
- Social history: Attendance at day care or school or living in a crowded setting is associated with increased exposure to viral infections. A sexual history obtained under confidential conditions is very important for accurate assessment of the sexually active adolescent, including males who have sex with males and those who have high risk sexual practices.
- Exposure history, including any known contacts with individuals with similar symptoms: A comprehensive, in-depth exposure history can help in diagnosing infections consistent with epidemic illness (e.g., influenza) as well as those that might otherwise not be considered. Specific questions include any contact with individuals with known illnesses or at high risk for certain illnesses or contact with animals (e.g., at farms or animal markets) or animal by-products (e.g., hides, waste, blood), insects, or snakes (e.g., bites). A history of travel to tropical countries or areas with endemic illnesses is important (e.g., Lyme disease, malaria, dengue, or parasitic illnesses), as well as the lodging accommodations during travel (e.g., possible exposure to parasites). Other important exposures include environmental tobacco smoke or mold, swimming in rivers, flood waters, or other waterways.
- Complete review of symptoms: Some presenting features of the illness may be discounted or forgotten by children or parents and are recalled only when direct questions are asked.
- Diet history: Any ingestion of raw milk or raw or undercooked meats and/or fish; history of pica.

Physical Examination

A complete physical examination is necessary; however, the differential diagnoses generated during the process of taking the history can stimulate the examiner to focus on certain aspects of the examination. Physical findings that may be encountered with infectious diseases include:

- Abnormal vital signs (e.g., fever, tachypnea, low blood pressure [concerning for dehydration and/or septic shock]).
- Irritability is nonspecific in ill children, but may raise concern for meningitis or Kawasaki disease. Lethargy raises concern for meningitis and sepsis (particularly in infants and younger children).
- A stiff or painful neck (suggestive of meningitis).
- A new murmur (may herald the possibility of endocarditis or rheumatic fever).
- Refusal to walk (can be a manifestation of deep tissue infections [e.g., pyomyositis], osteomyelitis, septic arthritis, or meningitis).
- Skin or mucous membrane changes (exanthema or enanthema, respectively) are common with viral illness, and characteristic rashes are typically associated with specific illnesses (e.g., chickenpox).

Diagnostic Aids

Laboratory and Imaging Studies

The values obtained from laboratory studies are measurements of the "host-pathogen damage-response framework." Inflammation or tissue damage stimulates proinflammatory cytokines, which in turn activate proteins referred to as *acute-phase reactants.* There is no single marker with the necessary sensitivity, specificity, or predictive values to serve as a stand-alone test upon which to initiate therapy when serious infection is suspected. Likewise, testing cannot positively confirm when therapy can reliably be stopped in proven infection (Long, 2012). New types of biomarkers of bloodstream infections/sepsis are under investigation.

In selected circumstances, laboratory evaluation can help clarify a diagnosis or rule out a serious illness that may be under consideration. When in doubt as to which study to order, it may be helpful to consult with knowledgeable laboratory personnel or an infectious disease expert. The following should be taken in consideration when ordering diagnostic studies:

- The quality of the specimen sent to the lab strongly affects the reliability of the results. For example, pus aspirated from a skin infection is generally more likely to grow the pathogen of concern than is a surface swab; it has the added advantage of allowing the specimen to undergo a Gram stain. The collection site of the microbiologic specimen needs to be appropriately cleansed to minimize possible skin contamination (e.g., with sterile saline, 70% alcohol, and/or iodine).
- The timing of sample collection affects the accuracy of results. Bacterial cultures collected after the administration of antibiotics may remain negative even with active infection. Acute and convalescent titers or certain blood chemistries can help to make a diagnosis or monitor response to treatment.
- Laboratory tests require a certain volume or quantity to ensure valid and reliable results; be prepared to prioritize test requests when a limited quantity has been collected (e.g., if a catheterized urine specimen only yields 7 mL, it may be more important to get a urine culture than a urinalysis).
- Microbiologic samples may require special handling and should be transported to the laboratory promptly. The laboratory should be contacted if there is any question regarding the collection and transport of samples.

The CDC lists the notifiable infectious diseases and conditions that must be reported to local public health authorities or their agents at www.cdc.gov/mmwr/preview/mmwrhtml/mm6253a1.htm?s_cid=mm6253a1_e. In many cases this reporting is done by the laboratory, but there are some conditions for which the provider may treat and not send in a laboratory specimen (e.g., Lyme disease). Providers should be familiar with the list.

Complete Blood Count

From an infectious disease standpoint, the white blood cell (WBC) count is generally the most useful piece of information obtained from the complete blood count (CBC). It is often elevated (leukocytosis) in bacterial infections and may be decreased (leukopenia) in some viral infections. A differential WBC may further focus the diagnosis. Bacterial infections often (but not always) cause increases in the neutrophil (or polymorphonuclear cell) count and may elevate bands (immature neutrophils), whereas viral infections often cause elevated lymphocyte counts and/or atypical lymphocyte production (see Chapter 27 for a review of hematology). WBCs can be affected by long-term use of certain medications (some can decrease WBCs), age, steroid use (can increase WBCs), and clinical state (e.g., overwhelming sepsis can lead to decreased WBCs). Chronic inflammatory processes can cause a decrease in red blood cells (RBCs) (e.g., anemia).

Platelet Count/Mean Platelet Volume

The platelet count is elevated (thrombocytosis) during the active phase of acute infection and correlates with concurrent elevations in C-reactive protein (CRP) and erythrocyte sedimentation rate (ESR). However, mean platelet volume (MPV) is inversely related to elevations in CRP and ESR (Zareifar et al, 2014).

C-Reactive Protein

The CRP is among the serum acute phase reactants that increase in the presence of acute inflammation and specific pathogens. CRP is sometimes used as part of the workup for infants at risk of septicemia; however, its diagnostic value for influencing clinical judgment remains weak (Nabulsi et al, 2012). The value above which CRP is most highly predictive of bacterial infection has not been firmly established (Hofer et al, 2012), but sepsis is much less likely to occur with a CRP of less than 10 mg/L. Serial CRPs 24 to 48 hours after the onset of symptoms are recommended and can be beneficial for monitoring the body's response to treatment in certain infections (e.g., in neonatal sepsis and osteomyelitis). Inflammatory processes other than infection may lead to an elevated CRP, including maternal and perinatal factors, trauma, rheumatologic diseases, and oncologic diseases. Persistent elevations of CRP may be related to treatment failure and such conditions as adiposity, use of birth control pills, and pregnancy.

Procalcitonin

Serum procalcitonin (Pro-CT) is considered a biomarker for differentiating certain viral infections from serious bacterial infections. Procalcitonin is a protein that has activity similar to a hormone and a cytokine. It is produced by several cell types and many organs in response to systemic proinflammatory stimuli. Pro-CT levels tend to rise and fall more quickly than CRP during onset and control of bacterial infections. It may prove to be a valuable tool when the ability to draw and process blood cultures is limited (Galetto-Lacour and Gervaix, 2010). Levels are increased in children with bacteremia and can reflect the severity of the illness (Kaplan and Vallejo, 2014). Its usefulness has been studied for predicting pyelonephritis (higher sensitivity and specificity than CRP [Xu et al, 2014]), bacterial pneumonia, early-onset sepsis in premature infants, bacterial infection in febrile neutropenic children with cancer, diarrhea-associated hemolytic-uremic syndrome, bacterial causes of acute hepatic disease, bacterial versus aseptic meningitis, and various diseases or conditions that involve inflammatory processes (e.g., posttraumatic sepsis, Crohn disease) (Long, 2012; Steinberger et al, 2014). At this point, it should only be used in concert with other clinical and diagnostic data when making diagnostic and management decisions (Nabulsi et al, 2012). Rapid test kits are available.

Erythrocyte Sedimentation Rate

The ESR is another measure of inflammation and reflects the observation that RBCs settle more rapidly when acute phase proteins (such as, fibrinogen) are present in serum than when they are not. Although the ESR is not a specific test for infection, it is useful in helping evaluate fever of unknown origin (FUO) and, like CRP, can be used to monitor response to therapy. A low sedimentation rate (<10 mm/hr) is unlikely if the cause of prolonged unexplained fever is a bacterial infection. Viral infections result in mean ESR values around 20 mm/hr (90% <30 mm/hr), with the exception of adenovirus, which may be associated with values higher than 30 mm/hr. An ESR more than 50 mm/hr in children warrants further extensive evaluation (Long, 2012).

During the waxing and waning period of infection, the ESR tends to increase and resolve more slowly than CRP values. ESR is considered a useful marker to evaluate the effectiveness of therapy when long-term antibiotics are needed. It is used when managing diseases in which treatment effectiveness is judged, in part, by the normalization of the ESR (e.g., osteomyelitis). Like CRP, the ESR is often elevated in noninfectious conditions that cause inflammation (e.g., miliary tuberculosis [TB], bacterial arthritis, head/neck abscesses for which ESRs greater than 100 mm/hr can occur). Anemia also causes a nonspecific increase in the ESR.

Cultures, Stains, and Antimicrobial Susceptibility Testing

The usefulness of microbiologic testing is absolutely dependent on the quality of the sample and on the correct choice of test for the given clinical situation. Details of appropriate tests for given infections are discussed in the sections about specific infectious agents.

The presence of pus assists in the diagnosis of some infections. Staining methods can be useful in certain clinical situations, such as when fungal or other infections are suspected. Antigen detection immunofluorescence or antibody assays (e.g., complement fixation tests [CFTs], immunofluorescence techniques, and enzyme-linked immunosorbent assays [ELISAs]) are often used in the diagnosis of viral infections. There are many diagnostic staining methods available.

Specimens from fluids or tissue can be sent for bacterial, viral, or fungal cultures; however, the laboratory may need to be notified in cases of certain suspected pathogens to provide specific instruction for the most accurate evaluation of the sample (e.g., pertussis). Bacterial susceptibility testing to common antibiotics can be done on cultured samples, especially if organism resistance is suspected because of community resistance patterns.

Other Technologies

DNA and RNA testing have become increasingly common in the in-patient setting and are being used more frequently in clinical practice. These tests rely on using polymerase chain reaction (PCR). Multiple organisms can be screened using one sample. Pathogens that are commonly detected by PCR include *Neisseria gonorrhoeae, Chlamydia trachomatis,* HIV, *Bordetella pertussis,* herpesviruses, and enteroviruses. Newer technologies also include molecular finger printing for nosocomial infection and microarrays for differentiating between viral and bacterial pathogens.

Immunoserology

In specific situations, tests that rely on the generation of an antibody response may be useful. Various methods (e.g., hemagglutination, enzyme immunoassays, latex agglutination, complement fixation, immunofluorescence, and neutralization assays) can be used to detect the presence of antibodies to specific infectious organisms (e.g., HIV, West Nile virus [WNV], *Bartonella henselae,* and *Mycoplasma pneumoniae*).

Imaging Techniques

Radiographs, computed tomography (CT) scans, magnetic resonance imaging (MRI), echocardiography, and ultrasounds can be used to assist in the diagnosis of infections of the bone, sinus, lung, skin, viscera, brain, and heart (see Chapter 21). Several nuclear imaging techniques have been used to evaluate possible bone infections, as well as tumors, fractures, urinary backflow blockage, heart conditions, GI bleeding, and thyroid disorders.

General Management Strategies

Preventing the Spread of Infection

Thorough and frequent hand washing is the most effective means of preventing the spread of infection. In addition to educating parents and children on the importance of proper hand washing, it is crucial that health care providers practice proper hand washing. Alcohol-based hand rubs may be substituted for soap and water in most cases, as long as the ethanol content is at least 60% (Centers for Disease Control and Prevention [CDC], 2015a). Such alcohol products are ineffective against controlling the spread of *Clostridium difficile.* It is recommended that gloves and washing hands with soap and water be used after contact with children with *C. difficile*–associated disease and/or in outbreak settings (Dubberke and Gerding, 2011).

Specific guidance that should be given to children and parents includes:

- Wash hands after using the bathroom, before meals, and before preparing foods. The proper technique includes scrubbing with soap and water for at least 20 seconds (the time it takes to sing "Happy Birthday" twice), rinsing with warm water, and drying completely.
- Avoid finger-nose and finger-eye contact, particularly if exposed to someone with a cold.
- Use a tissue to cover the mouth and nose when coughing or sneezing to help prevent the spread of pathogens. If a tissue is unavailable, the upper sleeve should be used (not the hands).

Use of Antibiotics

In the United States, at least 2 million people each year become infected with antibiotic resistant bacteria, at least 23,000 people die as a direct result of this resistant, and others die from complications stemming from an antibiotic-resistant infection (CDC, 2013a). Antibiotics are often prescribed for conditions that do not require their use, and inappropriate prescribing patterns likely contribute to the emergence of resistant bacteria. This is particularly troublesome for children in group child care settings, given the increased incidence of resistant bacteria, including infections with *Streptococcus pneumoniae, Haemophilus influenzae, Escherichia coli,* and MRSA (Shane and Pickering, 2012). Providers are encouraged to educate children and parents about the role and efficacy of antibiotics and to assume a more "targeted therapy" approach when prescribing. The CDC provides brochures, posters, and information sheets that may be helpful in explaining the importance of judicious use of antibiotics. Knowledge about emerging resistance patterns, local epidemiology, and susceptibility patterns of bacterial agents within their practice communities will better arm the provider to appropriately prescribe antibiotics (see Chapter 22 for a further discussion about the overuse of antibiotics).

Prevention of Infection Through the Use of Vaccines

Childhood immunization is a mainstay of preventive disease control. It has reduced the burden of mortality and morbidity due to infectious diseases around the world and is extremely cost effective.

Immunization is the process by which the body is artificially induced to mount a defense against certain foreign antigens. In this way, the immune system is primed to provide future protection with the next exposure to these same antigens. This is achieved by either (1) *active immunization* that involves introducing either a live attenuated vaccine or a toxoid (inactivated toxin) or by (2) *passive immunization* that involves administering an exogenous antibody, such as an immunoglobulin.

Vaccines approved for use in the United States include *Haemophilus influenzae* type B (Hib), meningococcus, diphtheria, pertussis, tetanus, polio, measles, mumps, rubella, human papillomavirus (HPV), hepatitis A virus (HAV), hepatitis B virus (HBV), influenza, varicella, rabies, typhoid, zoster, Japanese encephalitis, rotavirus, yellow fever, and pneumococcus; all but five are on the routine recommended vaccine schedule for all or specific populations of children and adolescents.

Despite the availability of vaccines, continued efforts to promote vaccination and keep immunizations current must be maintained and strengthened. PCPs may still encounter children with these illnesses because not all routine vaccines have been given (see following discussion on parental refusal to vaccination). Many of these diseases rarely occur in the United States, but the high incidence of global travel leaves underimmunized populations vulnerable to reintroduction of preventable diseases from countries where the disease is endemic.

Barriers to Vaccination

PCPs are frequently faced with immunization issues: product recalls; new vaccines; shortages of vaccines; parental vaccine refusal, "hesitancy" or "shot limiters"; changing and complex immunization schedules; media misinformation; vaccine ineffectiveness for a specific circulating dominant strain of influenza; program funding issues; provider confusion; and unique immunization needs of special populations. Medical providers also report inadequate reimbursement, storage and stocking issues, documentation hassles, language barriers, counseling issues, and safety concerns as reasons for not offering vaccinations onsite. System barriers such as vaccine costs, a lack of centralized vaccine registry, and universal vaccination records can also affect immunization rates (Dombkowski et al, 2012; Gidengil et al, 2010; Keeton and Chen, 2010; Lieu et al, 2015).

Several demonstration and research projects have had success in raising immunization rates, including community partnerships that involve school-based immunization programs to reach a large population of underimmunized children. They also bypass difficulties, such as lack of adequate insurance or lack of priority on the part of families (Walker et al, 2014; Whitney et al, 2014).

Parents refuse vaccinations for their children for many reasons, most of which are not based in scientific fact. Specifically parents have expressed concerns that vaccines are not safe (including some of their ingredients), have not had adequate safety testing, may cause learning disabilities (e.g., autism), may overload or weaken the child's immune system, or are painful. Other parents feel that the child may be more vulnerable to adverse reactions given a family history, the child's prematurity, or an underlying medical condition. Some parents have had unsatisfactory past experiences with the health care system, distrust government agencies, have community support for underimmunization (live in a cluster community), have religious beliefs counter to immunization, lack information, lack insurance, or have state policies that make it easy to exempt their child (Frew et al, 2011; Institute of Medicine [IOM] Committee on Assessment of Studies of Health Outcomes Related to the Recommended Childhood Immunization Schedule, 2013; Maglione et al, 2014). In addition, parents may perceive that there are other effective measures to avoid infection (e.g., hand washing/face masks), that the potential risk of illness from preventable communicable diseases is overblown, or they may simply lack concern regarding the preventable illnesses (Frew et al, 2011).

Lieu and colleagues (2015) recently identified geographic clusters of underimmunized communities in northern California. Eighteen percent to 23% of children in these communities were underimmunized, compared to 11% in the general population. Whites, blacks, Hispanics, and other undesignated individuals had higher rates of underimmunization than Asians. Having higher incomes or higher percentages of Asians and Hispanics residing in certain blocks were associated with children being fully immunized. Having higher education levels (i.e., graduate degrees) and living in poverty were associated with lower immunization rates (Lieu et al, 2015).

A health care provider's verbal cues can affect whether or not a parent chooses to vaccinate. Opel and colleagues (2013) found that when a provider is more directive (e.g., "these shots are due today") rather than participatory (e.g., "what shots do you want your child to receive today"), there are fewer refusals by vaccine-hesitant parents. Some additional helpful points to cover when discussing immunizations with vaccine-hesitant parents include the following (Murray et al, 2013):

- Listen to and question parents' reasons for refusing or delaying vaccines.
- Be familiar with misconceptions and controversies regarding the dangers of vaccines and be prepared to address them. Inform concerned parents that all childhood vaccines are available in thimerosal-free forms.
- The infant's/child's immune system will not be overwhelmed by multiple vaccines being given at the same time. Mention that a healthy infant's/child's immune system capably fights off an estimated 2,000 to 6,000 germs (antigens) daily when playing, eating, and breathing. The number of antigens in any combination of vaccines on the current schedule is much lower (150 for the entire Advisory Committee on Immunization Practices [ACIP] schedule) (American Academy of Pediatrics [AAP], 2015a).
- Emphasize the balance between risk and benefits of vaccination and that the risk associated with diseases is greater than the risk of a serious adverse vaccine reaction. Clarify that vaccines have the same effect on the immune system that the active disease does—without the morbidity and/or mortality seen in active disease.
- Provide a vaccine information statement (VIS) or other printed educational materials from reliable sources; provide website resources (see Additional Resources on the Evolve site).
- If the parent refuses to vaccinate or delays vaccination, document discussion about risks, note that VIS was given, and have parent complete and sign a vaccine refusal form (see Additional Resources on the Evolve site). If the parent is unwilling to sign the form, make notation on form and have it witnessed by a clinic staff member; keep in the medical record. Some families may be willing to accept some vaccinations.
- Flag medical records of unimmunized or underimmunized children to alert provider(s) so that subsequent illness visits will include those communicable diseases in the differential diagnoses; the immunization discussion should be revisited each time.
- Providers are discouraged from dismissing families from their practice unless there is a substantial level of distrust, notable differences in the philosophy about care, or poor communication between provider and child/family. In such circumstances, advance notice in writing to parents must be given and medical care provided until a new provider is selected (AAP et al, 2015b).

Providers should also identify underimmunized sectors within their communities and be prepared to tailor their approach and interventions toward this sector, as well as work with public health officials to meet national vaccination benchmarks.

Adverse Reactions to Vaccines

The Institute of Medicine (IOM) has determined that there is no substantiated evidence of a causal relationship between thimerosal-containing vaccines or measles, mumps, rubella (MMR) vaccine and "pervasive developmental disorders," such as autism, attention-deficit/hyperactivity disorder (ADHD), speech/language delays, childhood disintegrative disorder, Asperger syndrome, or Rett syndrome (IOM et al, 2012; IOM Committee on Assessment of Studies of Health Outcomes Related to the Recommended Childhood Immunization Schedule, 2013). The IOM also reported finding no general connection, no biologic mechanism consistent with a relationship between immunization or an adverse event, or insufficient causal evidence between hepatitis B and demyelinating diseases of the central nervous system (CNS) and peripheral nervous system (e.g., multiple sclerosis, acute disseminated encephalomyelitis, optic neuritis, transverse myelitis, Guillain-Barré syndrome, and brachial neuritis). The IOM also investigated the role that multiple vaccines might play in causing type 1 diabetes or serious infections. After a review of dozens of scientific research studies, a causal relationship was dismissed.

However, vaccines are not without adverse effects, and the IOM recognizes that understanding such events is dependent upon learning more about the immune system, autoimmunity, and the effects of genetic variation on the immune response. The IOM and colleagues (2012) have found convincing evidence that:

- The MMR, varicella zoster, influenza, hepatitis B, meningococcal, and tetanus–containing vaccines can cause anaphylaxis.

- Vaccine injections can cause syncope, fainting, deltoid bursitis, shoulder pain, and loss of shoulder motion.
- After MMR, febrile seizures (benign and without sequelae) and measles inclusion body encephalitis (rare) in immunocompromised children can occur within a year of vaccination.
- Varicella zoster vaccine has a causal relationship to some adverse events (e.g., chickenpox rash; pneumonia, meningitis, hepatitis in children with immunodeficiencies; viral reactivation leading to meningitis or encephalitis).

Vaccines that are thimerosal-free or contain trace amounts are on the CDC's recommended list for childhood immunizations with two exceptions: (1) multidose vials of inactivated flu vaccine and (2) multidose vials of one meningococcal vaccine that contains thimerosal. There are thimerosal-free alternatives available for each of these products.

Vaccines for Children Program

The Vaccines for Children (VFC) program enables PCPs to obtain all or most ACIP-authorized vaccines without cost. These vaccines are provided free to children younger than 19 years old who are Medicaid-eligible, are uninsured, or who are Native American or Alaska Native. To date, the VFC program pays for 50% of all vaccines administered to children in the United States younger than 6 years old (Whitney et al, 2014). In addition, children whose insurance does not cover immunizations (underinsured) are eligible to receive vaccines at federally qualified health centers and rural health clinics. All states receive a set level of federal VFC funds. Some states augment that amount to cover more vaccines. Providers wishing to participate need only contact their local state Medicaid office to enroll; they need not be a Medicaid-participating provider. Free vaccines plus their shipping costs and an administrative fee, which varies from state to state, are included in this incentive package; there is a minimum of paperwork for the provider.

The Affordable Care Act stipulates that children younger than 19 years old who are enrolled in new group or individual private health plans with an in-network provider are immediately eligible to receive free vaccines that have been recommended by the ACIP prior to September 2009. Vaccines recommended by the ACIP after 2009 are covered in the plan 1 year after the recommendation.

Vaccine Shortages

The Vaccine Management Business Improvement Project (VMBIP) is in charge of addressing all problems related to vaccine shortages, including vaccine procurement, ordering, distribution, and management. In addition, federal legislative proposals are ongoing to ensure federal-private sector partnerships to provide necessary incentives and protections to quickly bring additional and better vaccines to market (Shrestha et al, 2010). Ongoing information regarding vaccine shortages and expected procurement data are available through the CDC (see Additional Resources on the Evolve site). Medical providers should develop a tracking system to recall patients whose vaccinations are delayed because of supply shortages. During such times, providers can check with the websites of AAP, ACIP, and National Immunization Program for recommendations regarding vaccine deferrals, prioritization of high-risk children, and suspensions of school and child care entry requirements.

Vaccine Safety and Resources for Providers

Informed consent is critical when discussing the benefits and risks of vaccination. The National Childhood Vaccine Injury Act of 1986 (Public Law 99–660, amended by Public Law 101–239) calls for standardized VIS consent forms. All practitioners are required to use these forms to fulfill their duty to warn the public about possible adverse events. VIS forms are available in 42 different languages on the CDC website. The law also requires that the vaccine lot number, site of inoculation, and name of the person administering the vaccine be included in the medical record. Some state laws require a parental signed consent form.

The National Childhood Vaccine Injury Act also requires health care providers to report adverse events that occur after immunization so that unexpected patterns and safety concerns can be addressed. The suspected events are to be reported to the Vaccine Adverse Event Reporting System (VAERS), using their standard confidential form. Information on which vaccine-associated injuries are reportable as well as official report forms can be downloaded from www.vaers.hhs.gov or from the U.S. Food and Drug Administration (FDA) website. Parents can also report adverse effects to VAERS.

In 2001, the CDC established the Clinical Immunization Safety Assessment (CISA) network in response to the fact that many adverse events became evident only after prelicensure studies of vaccines were completed and that many clinicians would not necessarily be aware of such events. CISA developed research protocols around adverse events in order to better understand the adverse event at an immunocompromised level or in certain targeted populations not covered in initial vaccine testing populations. Additionally, providers can submit specific cases to CISA for vaccine consultation and can receive vaccine safety information (e.g., managing postvaccine adverse events).

Vaccines on the Horizon

Modern vaccinology research (e.g., DNA vaccines and the nanoparticle approach) is addressing new vaccine development, including *Shigella* conjugate vaccine for children, vaccines for herpes simplex virus (HSV) types 1 and 2, cytomegalovirus (CMV) (to prevent congenital CMV); Marburg virus (a hemorrhagic fever disease), dengue fever, hantavirus, HIV, WNV, Lassa fever, drug-resistant pneumococci and staphylococci (MRSA), enterococci (for traveler's diarrhea prevention), severe acute respiratory syndrome (SARS), Ebola (outbreaks in West Africa accelerated efforts in Ebola vaccine development; two vaccines have entered into safety and efficacy trials), insulin-dependent diabetes, TB, malaria, *C. difficile,* universal influenza vaccine for year-round coverage, enterovirus 71 encephalitis, Lyme disease, norovirus, and urinary tract infections. Several different types of cancer vaccines are under investigation. Other studies are ongoing to develop a conjugate group B streptococcus vaccine for pregnant women to provide passive immunity to their fetuses, a vaccine to cover more serotypes of *H. influenzae,* and live and subunit parainfluenza type 3 vaccines. New vaccine delivery systems are being investigated that include skin-patch vaccines, edible vaccines, additional applications for nasal delivery, and needle-free injections. Additionally, vaccines are being developed for vulnerable individuals (infants, pregnant women, and the immunocompromised).

Acetaminophen Prophylaxis after Vaccination?

Although some studies have detected significantly lower antibody responses in infants and children who were given antipyretics prior to or after routine vaccinations, the lower antibody response did not influence persistent immunological memory (Prymula et al, 2013, 2014). Also, a systematic review concluded that the use of antipyretics prior to vaccinations reduced post-vaccine fever and discomfort and was not accompanied by a decrease in vaccine protection (Das et al, 2014). There is also insufficient evidence to support the recommendation of pretreatment with a combination of acetaminophen and ibuprofen; however, antipyretics can be used as needed to increase the comfort of the child (AAP et al, 2011).

Active Immunity

General Principles

Inoculating a child with all or part of a modified product from a microorganism evokes an immune response. Whole organisms (live, attenuated, or killed), modified proteins, and/or sugars are used to prepare certain vaccines. The response to a live attenuated vaccine can be as protective as the natural infection. Anti-invasive, anti-adherence, antitoxin, neutralizing antibodies, or other protective responses can be found soon after the vaccination is given. Live attenuated vaccines usually confer broader and longer-lived immunity than the inactivated types that require booster vaccines. Killed and inactivated vaccines can provide systemic protection (immune globulin G [IgG] antibodies) but may fail to provide local mucosal antibody (immune globulin A [IgA]). Thus, although protected from systemic illness, a recipient of a killed vaccine can have local colonization or infection that can be a problem during an epidemic. The active and inert vaccine ingredients differ among manufacturers; such ingredients are listed on the manufacturer's vaccine information sheets. One must be aware of these components (such as, antimicrobials) because of a patient's possible hypersensitivity.

Research is ongoing regarding the effect of environmental or inborne factors on the body's immune responses to vaccinations. Increased levels of prenatal and/or postnatal polychlorinated biphenyls (PCBs) have been correlated with lowered antibody response to tetanus and diphtheria vaccines in children at 18 months and 7 years old (Grandjean et al, 2012) but not at 6 months old (Jusko et al, 2010). Research to identify genetic factors that account for the variation in immune response to the flu vaccine can possibly help those with lower responses to vaccines boost their immunity (Franco et al, 2013).

The ACIP of the CDC, the AAP, and the American Academy of Family Physicians (AAFP) annually approve a new unified recommended childhood immunization schedule for the United States. Providers can download the most recent immunization schedules at the beginning of each calendar year from the CDC (see Vaccines under Additional Resources on the Evolve site). There are three schedules of recommended immunizations: (1) for children 0 to 6 years old; (2) children 7 to 18 years old; and (3) a catch-up schedule for children 4 months to 18 years old who start their vaccines late, who are delayed, or for whom an immunization history is unknown. Other countries may follow the same schedule or determine their own recommendations (see World Health Organization [WHO] in Additional Resources on the Evolve site).

Maternal antibodies neutralize certain vaccines, so some are delayed until the child is 1 year old (e.g., measles). Infants vaccinated in the first year of life require more inoculations than older children. Children who are not immunized in the first year of life should be vaccinated according to the most recent catch-up immunization schedule. Missed vaccinations should be given as soon as possible, and the entire series does not need to be repeated.

Vaccines given outside the United States are acceptable, as long as there is reliable written evidence of administration (including dates and number of doses), and the age and spacing are the same as CDC recommendations. It would be reasonable to check antibody titers or reimmunize the child if in doubt. Diphtheria and tetanus toxoids with pertussis (DTP), diphtheria-tetanus-acellular pertussis (DTaP), bacille Calmette-Guérin (BCG), poliovirus, measles, and hepatitis B vaccines are routinely given overseas, but Hib, *S. pneumoniae*, mumps, rubella, hepatitis A, and varicella are given less often.

The ACIP offers some general vaccination guidelines including:

- Routine vaccine doses may be given 4 days or fewer prior to the minimum intervals or ages to provide some schedule flexibility.
- If two live virus parenteral vaccines are given less than 28 days apart, the vaccine given second should be disregarded; repeat this second vaccine at least 4 weeks later.
- Do not aspirate the syringe before injection (unproven necessity); do not recap the needle after use.
- When multiple vaccines are given on the same extremity, the sites of injection should be at least 1 inch apart;

the anterolateral aspect of the thigh is the preferred site for this.

- Use only written, dated records. Parent or guardian recollection of a child's immunization status may not be reliable.
- Reimmunization of an immune individual is not harmful.
- Reduced or divided doses of vaccines should not be given.
- Techniques to decrease the pain of immunizations include applying pressure or rubbing near the injection site for about 10 seconds before vaccination; putting sucrose on the tongue or pacifier of an infant; having children blow a pinwheel or bubbles during the procedure; having child sit upright on caregiver's lap or hug caregiver chest-to-chest.
- Those administering vaccines should know how to recognize and respond to syncope and severe allergic reactions, including anaphylaxis. Individuals with severe allergy to latex should not be administered vaccines that come from vials or syringes that contain latex (vial stoppers and syringe plungers can contain latex; see package insert).
- Personnel should be designated to monitor and document storage requirements (temperature, safety precautions) daily. Failure to transport and store vaccines correctly can lead to vaccine failure. The manufacturer's package inserts provide this information.
- In some circumstances (e.g., imminent travel, delayed immunizations) an accelerated schedule is available from the ACIP.
- The major contraindication for any vaccine is anaphylaxis with a prior dose or to a vaccine component.

Considerations When Choosing Inactive Vaccines

Information about side effects, precautions, contraindications, and special case considerations of the various attenuated or killed vaccines is available from the CDC, from the manufacturers' package inserts, or from a current AAP Red Book. Some of the more general side effects from the vaccines include (AAP et al, 2015b):

- Mild to moderate fever and/or local reactions (swelling, pain, erythema), usually within the first 24 to 72 hours (e.g., to diphtheria-tetanus-acellular pertussis [DTaP], Td, or Tdap Hib conjugate, HBV, pneumococcal conjugate [PCV-13], and meningococcal [can include headache and irritability]). Fever and rash may occur 1 or 2 weeks after MMR or MMRV.
- Sterile abscesses due to a hypersensitivity response to the vaccine itself or to an adjuvant (notably alum) (DTaP).

A history of anaphylaxis after any vaccine is a contraindication, unless the child has undergone desensitization. Hypersensitivity reactions to components within vaccines may or may not preclude the administration of certain vaccines; allergy testing may be indicated. Vaccine package inserts should be consulted regarding hypersensitivities to ovalbumin, other egg white proteins, gelatin, yeast, and latex (nonsynthetic). Vaccine administration during pregnancy and following moderate to severe acute infections is also addressed in the vaccine package inserts.

Inactivated Vaccines

Diphtheria-Tetanus-Acellular Pertussis Vaccine

DTaP vaccines are used in the United States for children younger than 7 years old; tetanus-diphtheria-acellular pertussis (Tdap) is given to those 7 years old or older. Acellular pertussis preparations have fewer side effects than the whole-cell vaccine. The whole-cell product, diphtheria and tetanus toxoids with pertussis (DTP) vaccine, which is no longer available in the United States, may be available in other parts of the world. If given in another country, DTP is an acceptable alternative to DTaP; once the child is living in the United States, DTaP would be given to complete a primary series. Combination vaccines are available that include DTaP, Hib, and other vaccines; however, single DTaP products cannot be mixed with any other vaccine.

Universal immunization with DTaP (or DTP) is the only effective control measure for these illnesses. Diphtheria and tetanus toxoids are highly effective vaccines as proven by the rarity of these diseases in the United States. All of the available vaccines are equally effective but differ slightly in their components. The duration of immunity after pertussis infection has not been established, but it is not lifelong; vaccination is still warranted. Recent pertussis outbreaks among fully vaccinated individuals have raised concerns about the durability of protection conferred by the current acellular pertussis vaccines (Meade et al, 2014). Research findings suggest that to control pertussis in young infants, who are the most vulnerable to its life-threatening complications, older children and adults should receive a single booster with Tdap rather than with tetanus-diptheria (Td) (see the CDC website for current recommended immunization schedules). Waning immunity, as well as changing antigenic and genotypic characteristics of the circulating *B. pertussis* strains, have prompted vaccinologists to look into new pertussis vaccine formulations (Clark, 2014). Tetanus prophylaxis as part of wound management (Table 24-2) is based on age, nature of the wound, type of prior Td toxoid vaccine, and vaccine reaction history.

Polio Vaccine

Only inactivated polio vaccine (IPV) is available for use in the United States; seroconversion to each of the three serotypes of polio ranges from 99% to 100% after three doses. The need for booster dosages of enhanced IPV has not been determined; immunity is believed to possibly be lifelong. The CDC provides guidelines for when polio vaccinations should be considered for those who are immunocompromised or at risk of imminent exposure from travel or outbreak, including adults. Oral polio vaccine (OPV) is currently used for global eradication, but the goal is to switch over to exclusive use of IPV once all global wild poliovirus has been eradicated (Orenstein et al, 2015).

Haemophilus Influenzae Type B Vaccine

Of the six serotypes type B (Hib) is the most virulent, accounting for pneumonia, bacteremia, meningitis, epiglottitis,

TABLE 24-2 Tetanus Prophylaxis in Wound Management

Previous Tetanus Immunization	Clean, Minor Wounds	Other Wounds (Contaminated by Dirt, Feces, Soil, Saliva; Burns, Avulsions, Punctures; Due to Missiles, Crushing, Frostbite)
Uncertain or fewer than three doses	Td or Tdap only*	Td or Tdap* and TIG† within 3 days
Three or more doses	Td or Tdap* *only* if last dose >10 years ago	Td or Tdap* if last dose >5 years ago

Data from American Academy of Pediatrics (AAP) Committee on Infectious Disease: Policy statement: additional recommendations for use of tetanus toxoid, reduced-content diphtheria toxoid, and acellular pertussis vaccine (Tdap), *Pediatrics* 128(4):809–812, 2011; Pickering LK, Baker CJ, Kimberlin DW, et al: Tetanus. *Red book: 2012 report of the Committee on Infectious Diseases*, ed 29, Elk Grove Village, IL, 2012, American Academy of Pediatrics, p 709.

Td, Tetanus-diptheria; *Tdap,* tetanus-diphtheria-acellular pertussis; *TIG,* tetanus immune globulin.

*In those 7 years old or older (including anyone in contact with infants >12 months old and health care workers), Tdap is preferred for prophylaxis as a booster dose if not given prior (applies if Td has been previously given; there is no minimum interval necessary between Td and Tdap); any subsequently needed prophylaxis or catch-up doses would be given as Td per catch-up schedule or every 10 years if caught up. In children younger than 7 years old, use DTaP (DT if pertussis is contraindicated).

†If TIG is not available, intravenous immunoglobulin (IVIG) can be substituted.

septic arthritis, cellulitis, otitis media, purulent pericarditis, and other less common infections, notably in those younger than 4 years old. Until the advent of the first Hib polysaccharide vaccine in 1987, Hib was the most common cause of bacterial meningitis in children in the United States. Use of this vaccine resulted in a phenomenal 99% decrease in the incidence of overall Hib disease in children younger than 5 years old. Most new cases of infections due to this organism in the United States now occur in children who are underimmunized or in infants who have not completed their primary series (AAP et al, 2015b). Hib continues to be a problematic pathogen in countries that do not have this vaccine routinely available. Guidelines for chemoprophylaxis are available on the CDC website for exposed, unimmunized household contacts younger than 4 years old who are at risk of invasive Hib disease.

Hepatitis A Virus Vaccine

The primary HAV vaccine initiatives focus on children in order to prevent transmission to adults in whom the illness is likely to be serious. Current guidelines include universal vaccination for those 1 to 18 years old and for other subsets of the population.

HAV is currently given as a two-dose series. The two inactivated HAV vaccines licensed in the United States have seroconversion rates of greater than 99% after the first booster is given. It appears that the long-term protective levels of these vaccines last for 14 to 20 years in children and at least 25 years in adults (CDC, 2015g). Due to the long-term persistence of protective levels of hepatitis A antibodies, the need for a third dose has not been determined. In some cases (e.g., areas where hepatitis A is endemic), a single dose may be adequate to provide protection (Raczniak et al, 2013).

HAV vaccine can be administered simultaneously with other childhood vaccines, but it should be given at a separate injection site (e.g., intramuscular [IM] injection in the deltoid). The risk of vaccination to a pregnant woman is considered low to nonexistent. Seroconversion of immunocompromised patients (including those with HIV) may be suboptimal. Either immunoglobulin or a single dose of HAV vaccine shows equal efficacy for preventing symptomatic disease if given within 14 days of exposure.

Recommendations also target the following groups of individuals (CDC, 2013b; Immunization Action Committee, 2013; WHO, 2013):

- Those traveling to countries where HAV is endemic (see CDC under Additional Resources on the Evolve site)
- Children and adolescents residing in and in contact with others from communities with a high incidence or outbreak of HAV
- Children in diapers in day care centers with high rates of HAV
- Men who have sex with men
- Individuals with severe illness (e.g., chronic liver disease)
- Illicit-drug users (using injectable or noninjectable drugs)
- Those with blood-clotting disorders (e.g., hemophiliacs)
- Unvaccinated persons more than 1 years old who are household members and/or close contacts (including babysitters) of an international adoptee from a country of high or intermediate endemicity during the 60-day period after the adoptee's arrival

Hepatitis B Virus Vaccine

Two recombinant hepatitis B virus (HBV) vaccines, composed of hepatitis B surface antigen (HBsAg) protein, are licensed in the United States. They are equally immunogenic and interchangeable when used as directed according to the manufacturer's guidelines. The seroconversion rate is 90% to 95%, and immunogenicity appears to last 20 or more years. Routine booster doses are not recommended except for patients receiving hemodialysis or for other immunocompromised patients whose annual antibody to HBsAg level falls under 10 milli-international units/mL. Pregnancy and lactation are not contraindicated for vaccination. Test all pregnant women for HBsAg early in each pregnancy. The immunoprophylaxis management of newborns whose mothers are HBsAg positive is noted in Table 24-3.

Text continues on p. 489

TABLE 24-3 Immunoglobulins Used in Children in the United States

Immunoglobulin	Reference Name	Indications for Use	Comments
Botulism immune globulin intravenous	BIG-IV	Botulism toxin A or B in infants <1 year old	Available as BabyBig from California Department of Health Services (510-231-7600). A HBAT may be indicated for life-threatening food-borne botulism (other than infant botulism) but risk must be weighed against side effects (fever, serum sickness, anaphylaxis); only available from CDC (770-488-7100).
Cytomegalovirus immune globulin intravenous	CMV-IGIV	For stem cell or organ transplants. Studies ongoing to evaluate use for CMV transmission to newborns	Used in combination with IV ganciclovir to treat CMV pneumonia. In hematopoietic stem cell transplant recipients, CMV-IGIV and ganciclovir administered intravenously has been reported to be synergistic in treatment of CMV pneumonia.
Diphtheria antitoxin (from equine sera)		Life-threatening *Corynebacterium diphtheriae* disease	Only available from CDC to treat life-threatening diphtheria; preferred route of administration is IV. Anaphylaxis and delayed serum sickness are possible adverse reactions and need to be weighed against risks of disease. Tests for reaction to animal sera should be performed.
Hepatitis B immune globulin	HBIG	Prophylaxis for those unvaccinated or undervaccinated; who have discrete identifiable exposure to blood; exposed to body fluids that contain blood: • Newborns whose mothers are HBsAg positive • Household contacts <12 months old who have received only one prior HBV vaccine and the second dose is not due • Sexual contact or needle-sharing with known HBsAg-positive cases, including sexual assault or abuse victims • Individuals with percutaneous or permucosal exposure to body secretions of known cases	If mother's HBsAg status is unknown before delivery, infants should receive both HBV vaccine and HBIG within 12 hours of birth or 24 hours of blood exposure; vaccines administered after birth should be given at different injection sites. HBIG can be given within 7 days of delivery if mother tests positive for HBsAg postpartum but it is less effective. Sexual partners of known cases: give HBIG and HBV vaccine up to 14 days after last exposure; repeat vaccine at 1 and 6 months Household contacts <12 months old: HBIG and three doses of HBV vaccine. If >12 months old, follow index case's antibody profile (if a carrier, vaccinate all household members). If children and adolescents have documented Hep B series and unknown seroconversion status, a booster dose is indicated. Hepatitis B vaccine can also be used for postexposure prophylaxis if given within 12 to 24 hours after exposure.

TABLE 24-3 Immunoglobulins Used in Children in the United States—cont'd

Immunoglobulin	Reference Name	Indications for Use	Comments
Immune globulin	IG	Hepatitis A prophylaxis: • Household contacts and sexual partners of known cases • Persons accidentally inoculated with a contaminated needle • Newborn infants of infected, jaundiced mothers • People with open lesions directly exposed to body secretions of known cases • Children in schools where more than one case is reported • All children and employees of child care centers where a case is reported • Custodial care residents and staff in close contact with an active case • Persons traveling to developing countries for less than 3 months • HAV vaccine can be given concurrently with IG, if warranted, for those traveling internationally	Is given within 2 weeks of exposure; can be used in children <2 years old; is thimerosal-free; >85% effective; dosage for those with continuous exposure to HAV differs from that given for short-term exposure HAV vaccine can also be used for postexposure prophylaxis if given within 14 days of exposure
		Measles prophylaxis: • To prevent or modify infection in unvaccinated children <1 year old and others at higher risk of complications who have been exposed to measles • IGIV is recommended for pregnant women and the immunocompromised who are without immunity	Not indicated in those who have had one dose of vaccine at ≥12 months old, unless immunocompromised Given within 6 days after exposure; the dose for those immunocompromised differs according to the type and degree of immunodeficiency, whether IGIV has been given, and prior dosage amounts of immune globulin

		Rubella prophylaxis:
		• Modifies or suppresses the clinical manifestations of the disease, urine shedding, and decreases the rate of viremia.
		• For use in:
		  • Early pregnancy after confirmed exposure and only if termination of pregnancy is not an option
		  • Infants after maternal exposure
		  • Older children not vaccinated with known exposure or at serious risk (immunocompromised)
			If pregnant woman is exposed to wild rubella or as a result of being accidentally vaccinated within 28 days of conception, fetus has theoretic risk of 1.3% of congenital rubella; Refer to OB-GYN
			Administration of immune globulin and the absence of clinical manifestation of maternal rubella infection do not guarantee the infant will be born without congenital rubella syndrome. IgM antibody (not IgG) after immune globulin can be used to determine maternal infection after exposure

Continued

TABLE 24-3 Immunoglobulins Used in Children in the United States—cont'd

Immunoglobulin	Reference Name	Indications for Use	Comments
Immune globulin intravenous	IGIV	FDA-approved for treating primary immunodeficiencies, chronic lymphocytic leukemia, bone marrow transplantation, HIV in children, ITP, Kawasaki disease; IGIV contains measles antibodies sufficient for measles prophylaxis (see Immune globulin)	Off-label use, including treatment for toxic shock syndrome, has created shortages
Rabies immune globulin (human)	HRIG, RIG	For postexposure prophylaxis for rabies; used in conjunction with rabies vaccine	Prior to use, consult with local health authorities
Respiratory syncytial virus immune globulin	RSV-IGIV (RespiGam)	Reduces risk of RSV bronchiolitis or pneumonia in high-risk children Provides additional protection against other respiratory viral illnesses; may be preferred over palivizumab in children with immune deficiencies or for premature infants prior to discharge in the RSV season for the first month of prophylaxis	Palivizumab, a monoclonal antibody, is generally preferred over RSV-IGIV (see Chapter 32, Bronchiolitis)
Tetanus immune globulin	TIG	For individuals with tetanus-prone wounds who are under vaccinated (fewer than three tetanus toxoid vaccine doses) or whose vaccination status is unknown For individuals with tetanus infection in combination with antibiotics (metronidazole or penicillin G) For immunodeficient patients, including those with HIV; they should be considered under-vaccinated regardless of actual tetanus toxoid status	Tetanus-prone wounds include those contaminated with dirt (especially if around horses), feces, or saliva; puncture wounds; avulsions; wounds acquired as a consequence of missiles, burns, crushing, or frostbite In infants <6 months old without the initial three-dose series, decision to use TIG depends on mother's tetanus toxoid immunization history at the time of delivery and if the wound is tetanus prone (e.g., out-of-hospital delivery and umbilical cord cut with non-sterile implement). TIG is given IM plus a dose of tetanus toxoid vaccine If TIG not available, IGIV may be considered (not licensed for this use in the United States); equine TAT is another alternative to TIG (not available in the United States)—hypersensitivity testing required before use of TAT Smaller dose is administered for tetanus neonatorum
Vaccinia immune globulin intravenous	VIG-IGIV	Being held in reserve to prevent or manage complications of smallpox; can be used in individuals receiving an experimental vaccine that involves a vaccinia carrier virus	Only available from CDC

TABLE 24-3 Immunoglobulins Used in Children in the United States—cont'd

Immunoglobulin	Reference Name	Indications for Use	Comments
Varicella immune globulin	VariZIG (varicella-zoster immune globulin)	Given to those exposed to varicella infection who are most susceptible to varicella and most likely to develop the disease and in whom complications of the infection would result: • Household contacts • Playmates with face-to-face contact (5 minutes to 1 hour) • Infant whose mother had varicella onset 5 days or less before delivery or within 48 hours after delivery • Immunocompromised children and adolescents without history of varicella, varicella immunization, or known to be susceptible • Hospitalized preterm infants 28 weeks or more gestation whose mother lacks history of varicella or serologic evidence of protection • Hospitalized preterm infants less than 28 weeks' gestation or less than 1000 g birth weight exposed in neonatal period regardless of mother's history or VZV serologic evidence* • Other conditions: See CDC guidelines	Available from FFF Enterprises 24 hours/day (1-800-843-7477); strict adherence to forms and protocols required Administered within 96 hours after exposure; may be of benefit if given within 10 days (AAP, 2015b) Not indicated in infants whose mothers had zoster infection In the absence of VariZIG, IGIV or acyclovir may be considered*

Data from Meissner HC: Passive immunization. In Long SS, Pickering LK, Prober CG, editors: *Principles and practice of pediatric infectious diseases*, ed 4, New York, 2012, Elsevier, pp 37–43; Pickering LK, Baker CJ, Kimberlin DW, et al, editors: *Red Book: 2015 Report of the Committee on Infectious Diseases*, ed 30, Elk Grove Village, Il, 2015, American Academy of Pediatrics.

CDC, Centers for Disease Control and Prevention; *CMV*, cytomegalovirus; *FDA*, U.S. Food and Drug Administration; *HAV*, hepatitis A virus; *HBAT*, heptavalent equine antitoxin; *HBsAg*, hepatitis B surface antigen; *HBV*, hepatitis B virus; *HIV*, human immunodeficiency virus; *IG*, immune globulin; *IgG*, immunoglobulin G; *IgM*, immunoglobulin M; *IM*, intramuscular; *ITP*, idiopathic thrombocytopenia purpura; *IV*, intravenous; *IVIG*, intravenous immunoglobulin; *OB-GYN*, obstetrics and gynaecology; *RSV*, respiratory syncytial virus; *TAT*, tetanus antitoxin.

*Consult with an expert in infectious disease or the CDC.

Preterm infants weighing less than 2000 g should be immunized when they are 1 month old. All newborns weighing 2000 g or more should be vaccinated prior to hospital discharge. In addition to young children and adolescents not previously vaccinated, there are other specific individuals who should be screened and/or, depending upon screening status, receive the HBV series (AAP et al, 2015b):

- Hemophiliac patients and other recipients of certain blood products
- Intravenous (IV) drug users
- Individuals with HIV, chronic liver disease, or on hemodialysis
- Heterosexual persons with a history of multiple sex partners in the previous 6 months or with recent sexually transmitted infections
- Men who have sex with men
- Household and sexual contacts of those who are HBsAg positive
- Foreign-born individuals (including adoptees) where HBsAg prevalence is 2% or greater need screening for HBV despite their immunization history.
- Susceptible child who bit a person with chronic HBV infection.
- Staff and residents of residential institutions for the developmentally disabled
- Staff and attendees of nonresidential day care and school programs for the developmentally delayed if an identified HBV carrier is known to attend or poses risk of infecting others
- Health care workers and others with occupational risk
- International travelers who travel to areas where endemicity for HBV is 2% or greater and who otherwise may be at risk
- Inmates in juvenile detention and other correctional facilities if un- or underimmunized
- Individuals with diabetes mellitus between the ages of 19 and 59 years old

The HBV vaccine series plus hepatitis immune globulin (HBIG) or a HBV booster dose (if previously immunized) are recommended for postexposure immunoprophylaxis for those with percutaneous or sexual exposure to an HBsAg-positive individual if given within 12 to 24 hours of exposure.

Human Papillomavirus Vaccine

Two HPV vaccines are licensed for use in the United States. Gardasil (referred to as HPV4) is a quadrivalent vaccine that protects against the two primary oncogenic strains, types 16 and 18, as well as types 6 and 11. It is licensed for males (to prevent genital warts and male HPV-associated cancers) and females (to prevent cervical intraepithelial neoplasia) as early as 9 years old through 26 years old. The efficacy rate of Gardasil for prevention of the four strains of HPV-related disease in females is close to 100% after a series of three doses. In the United Kingdom, the recommended series is two doses, and this schedule is being evaluated for possible implementation in the United States. Duration studies have only been done through the first 5 years post-vaccination and no waning of protection has been seen (Markowitz et al, 2014). Immunogenicity trials show antibody responses greater for females and males 9 through 15 years old as compared with those 15 years old or older. Preadolescent females and all sexually active women benefit from the vaccine if they have not been exposed to any of the vaccine's HPV strains. It is unclear if there is cross-protection against cervical intraepithelial neoplasia types not included in the vaccine. There is no protection for HPV oncogenic types acquired prior to the vaccine (Markowitz et al, 2014). The vaccine is offered under the VFC program for females. The vaccine should not replace routine cervical cancer screening; prevaccine Papanicolaou (Pap) or pregnancy tests are not warranted.

Cervarix (referred to as HPV2) targets HPV types 16 and 18 and is only licensed for use in females 9 through 26 years old. It has shown some cross-protection against infection of other HPV vaccine types that cause cancer; its efficacy rate ranges from about 87% for HPV 18 to 98% for HPV 16 after a series of three doses (Markowitz et al, 2014).

Pre- and post-research studies show that both vaccines are safe with mild side effects (CDC, 2015b). Pregnant women should not receive the vaccine. Providers are encouraged to report any inadvertent exposure during pregnancy to HPV4 vaccine to Merck (1-877-888-4231) or to HPV2 to GlaxoSmithKline (1-888-452-9622); the CDC is tracking such exposure on VAERS. To date there is no evidence of spontaneous abortions or major birth defects from these vaccines (AAP et al, 2015b).

Influenza Vaccine

The influenza vaccine is formulated yearly based on epidemiologic forecasts. Usually one or two influenza A virus strains are changed based on the dominant influenza strain(s) projected to infect the population in the approaching flu season. Major changes in viral antigens generally occur at 10-year intervals. This process is called *antigenic shift*. Minor variations that occur are called *antigenic drift*. These changes within the virus can prevent the body's immune system from recognizing the altered strain and mounting an immunologic response thus requiring annual vaccination.

The ACIP recommends annual, universal vaccination for those 6 months old and older unless contraindicated. Influenza disease rates are highest among children younger than 2 years old, in those 65 years old and older, and in those with high-risk medical conditions. Children serve as a major vector for influenza transmission because of their own high rates for contracting the virus; they also shed the virus at higher rates and for longer periods than adults. After even one influenza illness, people remain susceptible to other influenza strains; severe epidemics have occurred historically. See Influenza Viral Infections later in this chapter.

The two influenza vaccines are available. They either contain three virus strains (influenza A [H3N2 and seasonal H1N1] and one lineage of influenza B virus)[trivalent]) or the two influenza A strains plus two lineages of influenza B viruses (quadrivalent). The inactivated influenza vaccine (IIV) is available intramuscularly as IIV3 or IIV4 for those 6 months old or older (those 18 to 64 years old may opt to have IIV3 administered intradermally), whereas the quadravalent live-attenuated inactivated vaccine (LAIV4) is restricted to healthy, nonpregnant individuals 2 through 49 years old. The LAIV is only available as an intranasal prefilled spray for these age groups (further information about restrictions is available from the CDC). The AAP has no preference for which formulation is used for the appropriate ages (AAP et al, 2015b). An alternative IIV3 (given intramuscularly) is manufactured without using eggs and is available to those 18 years or older. Follow package inserts to determine the number of doses and dosage amounts for the age of the child.

Because other common childhood viral agents can cause diseases that are similar to influenza, the effect of the vaccine is less likely to be evident in children. The efficacy rate ranges from 50% to 95% for IIV in healthy children older than 2 years (higher if the vaccine strain closely matches the circulating wild strain); the efficacy is lower in children younger than 24 months old. LAIV has shown an efficacy rate of between 86% and 96%, but may be lower in young children. Immunity wanes up to 50% within 6 to 12 months after vaccination (AAP et al, 2015b).

The vaccine should be given as soon as it becomes available before the onset of the yearly influenza season. It can be given any time until the anticipated end of the infective season to cover intermittent peaks (into May). It is acceptable to concurrently vaccinate with either IIV or LAIV and other inactivated or live vaccines.

Meningococcal Vaccine

Of the 13 serotypes of *Neisseria meningitidis,* serogroups B, C, Y, and W135 are most often associated with meningococcal disease. Serogroups B, C, and Y each cause one third of the diseases in the United States. Most infections in children younger than 5 years old are attributed to serogroup B, whereas C, Y, and W135 cause three fourths of infections in those 11 years old and older. Infections due to serogroup A are rare. Meningococcal disease is associated with high morbidity and mortality in those who are infected; less than 1,000 infections are reported annually in the United States (CDC, 2015c).

Until late 2014, when the FDA approved a vaccine for serogroup B, only serogroups A, C, Y, and W135 were covered by vaccines in the United States. The vaccines that provide immunity to serogroups A, C, Y, and W-135 include three conjugate meningococcal vaccines (MenACWY-D and MenACWY-CRM) (Menactra and Menveo) and a combination vaccine (HibMenCY/TT) (MenHibrix) that contains the routine vaccines for Hib and *N. meningitidis* serotypes A and C; and one meningococcal polysaccharide vaccine (MPSV4) (Menomune). Ages, dosages, and schedules vary between the vaccines, and the provider needs to be familiar with the recommended regimens. The two vaccines for serogroups B, Trumenba and Bexsero, are currently licensed for individuals 10 to 25 years old and have been used to help stem the spread of disease during outbreaks caused by serogroup B in communities (notably college campuses). Routine use of the serogroup B vaccines is not recommended until further consideration (AAP et al, 2015b). Consult the CDC/ACIP or manufacturers package instructions regarding the current indications, precautions, timing of doses, need for boosters, and age restrictions for each of the vaccines; with the addition of the newer vaccines that cover serogroup B, the ACIP recommended immunization schedule may change. MenACWY-CRM is currently recommended as part of the routine ACIP immunization schedule for those 11 through 21 years old. The other vaccines are given to those at high risk for contracting meningococcal infection, including all adolescents; unvaccinated or partially vaccinated college freshmen living in dormitories; military recruits; those with HIV, functional or anatomic asplenia, or persistent complement deficiencies (including infants as young as 2 months old [see ACIP indications for use of MenHibrix in this instance]); travelers to hyperendemic or epidemic countries; or those exposed during a community outbreak attributable to a vaccine serogroup.

Pneumococcal Vaccines

There are 91 known serotypes of pneumococcus, and there has been a shift in the pneumococcal strains responsible for illness. Pneumococcal conjugate vaccine 13 (PCV13) covers 13 of those serotypes. PCV13 was licensed in 2010, succeeding PCV7, and is recommended for all children 2 through 59 months old; children 24 through 71 months old with incompleted schedules and underlying medical conditions (sickle cell disease, asplenia, chronic heart of lung disease, diabetes mellitus, cerebrospinal fluid leak, cochlear implant, or other immunocompromising disorders); and those 6 to 18 years old who have immunocompromised disorders, asplenia, cerebrospinal fluid leak, or a cochlear implant.

Children 2 years old through 18 years at high risk of pneumococcal disease should also receive two 23-valent pneumococcal polysaccharide vaccine (PPSV23) immunizations as part of their pneumococcal vaccine schedule. PPSV23 confers broader coverage against 23 pneumococcal serotypes rather than the 13 in PCV13. The number of doses varies according to the number of prior PCV7 or PCV13 vaccines given and the age of the child. No more than 2 PPSV23 doses should be given prior to 65 years old.

Live Vaccines

Precautions Regarding Administration of Live Vaccines

It is important for providers to consult with infectious disease experts and authoritative reference resources when contemplating administering live vaccines to immunocompromised individuals. Recommendations may differ according to the child's type, degree of T-cell compromise, and anticipated length of illness (e.g., those with DiGeorge syndrome, HIV infection, cancer, immunosuppression, or other cellular immune problem). An individual with a low T-cell count or a cellular immunodeficiency can be seriously compromised if given an LAIV. After reduction or cessation of chemotherapy or administration of an immune globulin, the timing for the administration of inactivated or live-virus vaccine can vary; consult CDC/ACIP guidelines.

Bacille Calmette-Guérin Vaccine

Bacille Calmette-Guérin (BCG) live vaccine was developed in the early part of the twentieth century to prevent the spread of TB. The vaccines in use worldwide differ in composition and efficacy because of the differing attenuated substrains of *Mycobacterium bovis* from which they are derived. The vaccine is widely recommended at birth as a public health measure in more than 100 countries. The vaccine provides suboptimal protection against primary pulmonary TB or reactivation of latent infection. The efficacy of BCG in preventing disseminated and other potentially fatal effects from *Mycobacterium tuberculosis* disease (meningitis and miliary) in infants and children is approximately 80%. For all populations worldwide, the efficacy of BCG is close to 50%; the variation is believed to be due to genetic differences in substrains, populations, concurrent infection with other diseases, or handling of the vaccine (AAP et al, 2015b; WHO, 2009). Countries have their own immunization schedules and generally single dose of the vaccine is ideally given to non-HIV infected infants at birth. Until 2 months old, healthy non-HIV infected infants may be given BCG without having a tuberculin skin test (TST), unless suspected of having congenital infection; after 2 months, a TST is required prior to vaccination with BCG. In infants who are exposed to smear-positive pulmonary TB shortly after birth, 6 months of prophylactic isoniazid should be given prior to receiving the BCG vaccine (WHO, 2014a). New recombinant BCG and live attenuated TB vaccines are currently under development.

In the United States, BCG use is not recommended, but its use may be considered in infants and children with a negative tuberculin skin test (TST) who: (1) live with persons with infectious pulmonary TB who are untreated or ineffectually treated, cannot be removed from those persons, and are without a source of long-term primary treatment; or (2) live with persons who have drug-resistant forms of TB (to isoniazid and rifampin) and cannot be separated from those persons. Before administering BCG in the United States, pediatric TB experts should be consulted. Health care workers in high-risk settings also may be candidates for BCG (AAP et al, 2015b). A complete guideline for the use of BCG is available from the WHO (see Additional Resources on the Evolve site).

The TST and the newer interferon-gamma release assay (IGRA) test for detecting tuberculosis infection is discussed later in this chapter under Tuberculosis.

Measles-Mumps-Rubella Vaccine

MMR is a trivalent vaccine; this combination is also offered as a quadrivalent vaccine with varicella (MMRV). Due to vaccine manufacturing and availability, it may be difficult to obtain measles, mumps, and rubella vaccines individually.

The ACIP recommends that health care personnel demonstrate evidence of immunity to each of these diseases (Shefer et al, 2011).

Measles Vaccine. A live attenuated measles vaccine using a chick embryo cell culture is licensed for use in the United States. Efficacy of the first vaccine at 12 months old is about 95%; after the second vaccine, seroconversion is about 98% (AAP et al, 2015b). Children who do not receive the second dose at kindergarten should be revaccinated at the earliest possible time. Persons vaccinated with killed vaccine, live vaccine and IgG, and those vaccinated before 12 months old should be revaccinated twice more. In children receiving palivizumab (Synagis), the MMR vaccine can be given on schedule.

The measles component is responsible for almost all the adverse reactions to the MMR vaccine. Transient rashes and fever of 103° F (39.4° C) can occur approximately 5 to 12 days after vaccination. Those with fever usually have no other symptoms, and the fever generally resolves within 1 to 2 (up to 5) days. Newer studies have shown that when the combination MMRV vaccine is given for the primary dose, the risk for febrile seizures increases twofold. When a separate varicella vaccine is given at the same time as MMR but in a different site in children between 12 and 23 months old, one additional seizure in 2300 to 2600 children can occur (AAP et al, 2015b). The AAP recommends that health care providers discuss this increased risk with parents and offer either the MMR and varicella separately as the primary dose for this age group or the combination (MMRV) (the CDC-issued VIS reflects this information). The MMRV given as the second dose between 4 and 6 years is not associated with the same increased risk for a febrile seizure (Rowhani-Rahbar et al, 2013).

The contraindications to measles vaccine should be reviewed prior to administering the vaccine to those also needing a TST; who are pregnant or planning to become pregnant within the next 28 days; who have had an anaphylactic reaction to gelatin, egg, neomycin, or prior MMR vaccine; or who have a febrile illness. There are selected recommendations for giving MMR to those with compromised immune systems and for those who have received immunoglobulins and blood products. Guidelines are available from manufacturer package inserts or from the CDC. Encephalopathy and encephalitis are rare complications of the vaccine, and they occur at a much lower rate than after the natural disease.

Measles Exposure or Epidemics. Measles was deemed no longer endemic in the United States in 2000. However, measles outbreaks continue to occur largely due to unvaccinated individuals and importation of the disease from countries with endemic measles (CDC, 2015d). In cases of exposure to measles infection, the measles vaccine can provide some protection if given within 72 hours. Immunoglobulin can be used within 6 days of exposure to measles infection and prevents or modifies the infection in susceptible people (e.g., contacts younger than 1 year old, children and adolescents with HIV infection and children born to HIV-infected women whose own HIV infection status is unknown). During measles outbreaks or anticipated travel, immunization can begin as early as 6 months old. Two additional doses of the vaccine are then given at the routine recommended ages (AAP et al, 2015b).

Mumps Vaccine. The live-attenuated mumps vaccine is given in combination as MMR or MMRV. It is estimated to achieve an 80% seroconversion rate after one dose and 90% after two doses. However, a mumps outbreak in 2006 brought into question how long immunity lasts, which may be shorter than anticipated. Fever, parotitis, and orchitis have been rarely reported as side effects of the vaccine; causality has not been established for other effects, such as febrile seizures, rash, pruritus, nerve deafness, encephalopathy, encephalitis, purpura, or paralysis. These side effects occur at a much lower rate than they do after the natural disease. Contraindications are the same as for measles. Use of the MMR vaccine or immunoglobulin preparations are not effective as postexposure control measures; instead, infected individuals should be isolated for 5 days after the onset of parotitis (AAP et al, 2015b).

Rubella Vaccine. The live-attenuated rubella vaccine is given in combination with measles and mumps (MMR) or with added varicella (MMRV). The seroconversion rate is greater than 95% after one dose. Mild reactions to the vaccine include fever (5% to 15%), lymphadenopathy, rash (5%), joint pain (less than 1%) and arthralgia (usually seen more in unvaccinated postpubertal females; onset 7 to 21 days after vaccine), small peripheral joint pain, and paresthesias. Contraindications are the same as for the measles vaccine. If inadvertently given to a pregnant woman, it does not serve as an indication for termination of the pregnancy. However, the woman should be informed that the fetus is at a maximum theoretic risk of 1.3% of developing congenital rubella (AAP et al, 2015b). Refer to the AAP Red Book or the CDC for information regarding special vaccination precautions for children who are immunocompromised.

Females younger than 13 years old without documentation of rubella immunity (documented second dose of MMR or laboratory confirmation) should be the focus for vaccination. Routine prenatal screening for rubella susceptibility is warranted in postpubertal females, and they should be given the vaccine if indicated. Mothers found to be rubella-nonimmune during pregnancy should receive immediate postpartum vaccination.

Measles, Mumps, Rubella, and Varicella Vaccine

The combination MMR and varicella vaccine is as effective as when MMR and varicella vaccines are given separately, avoids potentially missing the administration of one of these vaccines, allows fewer vaccinations, and has excellent immunogenicity. See the earlier Measles Vaccine section regarding the increased risk of febrile seizures when the first immunization dose is given as the combined MMRV.

Varicella Vaccine

This LAIV from the Oka strain of varicella-zoster virus (VZV) is well tolerated and immunogenic. The seroconversion rates range from 85% after one dose to 98% after the second dose. Two vaccines are licensed for use in the United States: (1) a single-antigen vaccine and (2) a quadrivalent vaccine with measles, mumps, and rubella (MMRV).

A small percentage of vaccinees develop localized pain, erythema, and tenderness. Others may develop a mild, generalized maculopapular rash or a varicelliform eruption (generally non-vesicular) after vaccination. The varicelliform rash generally occurs within 2 weeks of vaccination, and wild-type VZV has been isolated from these lesions. A short period of fever may also occur 5 to 12 days after the vaccine. Given the low risk of secondary transmission, immunocompromised household contacts do not need to be isolated from recently vaccinated individuals. Those who contract varicella infection after being immunized usually have minimal fever, fewer than 50 lesions, and recover more rapidly than if they had not been vaccinated. These breakthrough varicella cases appear to be related to longer times since vaccination (Tafuri et al, 2014).

When to Consider Postexposure Prophylaxis for Varicella Disease. Postexposure varicella-zoster immune globulin (VariZIG) is available to those for whom exposure poses significant risk (see Table 24-3) and should be provided within 10 days of exposure (AAP et al, 2015b). As a substitute, IGIV, acyclovir within 7 days, or varicella vaccine (given within 3 to 5 days after exposure) can be considered. However, there are limited data on acyclovir as a postexposure prophylaxis measure for immunocompromised children (Gershon, 2014). Other individuals are also considered for prophylaxis if significant exposure to varicella or zoster occurs; guidelines are available from the CDC or current AAP Red Book.

The varicella vaccine should be given 5 months after VariZIG, unless varicella disease occurred despite VariZIG administration. Serologic testing to determine vaccine-induced antibody response may be unreliable and should not be used to determine susceptibility. The test is more reliable for diagnosing natural infection but not in those who are immunocompromised (AAP et al, 2015b).

Rotavirus Vaccine

An estimated four out of five children are likely to be infected with a rotavirus before they turn 5 years old. There are two rotavirus vaccines licensed in the United States, oral human-bovine reassortant pentavalent rotavirus (RV5) and oral human attenuated rotavirus (RV1), that have different dosing regimens; either a two- or three-dose oral series is recommended for infants between 6 to 32 weeks old. An increased risk for intussusception has been seen following both vaccines, usually occurring within 7 days following the first or second dose. In the United States, this means an estimated one in 20,000 to one in 100,000 might develop intussusception after either vaccine (CDC, 2015e). Both vaccines are effective and demonstrate similar safety and efficacy profiles. Ideally the same vaccine should be used for all doses, but this is not absolute if the prior vaccine name is not known or is unavailable. Infants in resource-poor countries do not appear to develop a robust response to either of the rotavirus vaccines. The reason for this is not well understood but may be related to maternal antibodies passed on to the infant either transplacentally or through breast milk (Shin et al, 2012). Contraindications include a history of intussusception or severe combined immunodeficiency disease. Refer to the CDC website or AAP Red Book for information on further contraindications, warnings and precautions, and immunization of children with specific health conditions prior to administration. Consultation with an immunologist may be helpful in particularly complex situations.

Smallpox Vaccine

The United States stockpiles smallpox vaccine in case of preexposure or postexposure situations, such as bioterrorism. The vaccine contains a live vaccinia virus and protects against variola major and variola minor. The vaccine is not routinely given. In the case of a smallpox outbreak, high-risk individuals will be vaccinated per CDC guidelines issued at the time. Measures to take to contain an outbreak can be found on the CDC website.

Passive Immunity: The Immunoglobulins

Passive immunization entails injecting an individual with a solution of preexisting antibodies to prevent or amend an infectious disease. These antibodies are derived from sera of pooled human immunoglobulin, illness-specific human immunoglobulin, antibodies formulated from animals, or monoclonal antibodies. Some of the more common passive immunizations and their uses given to pediatric patients are listed in Table 24-3.

Passive immunization is reserved for individuals who suffer from immunodeficiencies in whom a live or attenuated vaccine could be dangerous or for those who have a problem making antibodies. An immunoglobulin is also indicated for unimmunized or underimmunized patients who have been exposed to an infectious disease and whose incubation period is not long enough to allow complete active immunization. People at high risk for developing severe complications from an infectious disease should receive passive immunization when exposed. Some individuals who suffer from disease-produced toxins benefit from antitoxin passive immunization (e.g., a poisonous snakebite, tetanus, diphtheria, and botulism). All immunoglobulins manufactured in the United States are screened for HIV-1 and HIV-2, syphilis, human T-lymphotropic viruses (HTLV-1, HTLV-2), WNV, hepatitis B and C; most for *Trypanosoma cruzi* (Chagas disease); and selected ones for CMV. Additionally, the United States requires manufacturers of IGIV and other preparations administered IV or IM to undergo procedures to inactivate or remove viruses (AAP et al, 2015b).

Immunoglobulins are given either IM or IV (IGIV). Most adverse reactions involve localized pain at the injection site but can also include flushing, headache, chills, sweating, and shock; children should not be given a product to which they have had a prior adverse reaction. Systemic reactions may occur, so administering personnel should be prepared to handle acute reactions and, in specific individuals, vasomotor or cardiac complications (e.g., elevated blood pressure, cardiac failure, or both). Off-label use is discouraged.

Some hyperimmune globulin preparations from human donors provide "super immunity" because of their high antibody levels to certain infectious diseases. Such products include those for hepatitis B (HBIG), rabies (RIG), tetanus (TIG), varicella-zoster (VariZIG), botulinum antitoxin (BIG), and cytomegalovirus (CMV-IGIV). Equine-derived antisera are available for botulism, tetanus, diphtheria, and rabies. These can produce more severe adverse reactions (including fatal anaphylaxis). They should be used with caution and only after hypersensitivity testing to animal sera is completed by a specialist.

Respiratory Syncytial Virus Prophylaxis

Palivizumab (Synagis) is the only product on the American market for use in infants at high risk for adverse outcomes of a respiratory syncytial virus (RSV) infection. Palivizumab is a humanized mouse monoclonal antibody and has the benefit of being administered intramuscularly rather than intravenously. It is given in five (maximum) monthly IM injections during RSV season (usually November through March or April depending on the region) and is generally well tolerated. Palivizumab has been shown to be safe and effective in reducing RSV hospitalizations in high-risk infants by 39% to 82%. Recurrent RSV infection can occur in the same child—even if he or she has received palivizumab—due to more than one RSV circulating within any given community. It has a high cost-to-benefit ratio. Consider RSV prophylaxis for the following children (AAP et al, 2015b):

- Infants born before 29 weeks and 0 days of gestation during RSV season until they are 12 months old
- Children born prematurely at or before 32 weeks and 0 days of gestation who are younger than 2 years old with chronic lung disease (CLD) and who required treatment for their CLD within 6 months of the onset of RSV season (including oxygen therapy); prophylaxis can be given to 2-year-old children with CLD of prematurity who continue to require medical support during the 6 months prior to the onset of RSV season.
- Infants up to 12 months old with hemodynamically significant cyanotic or complicated congenital heart disease
- Infants up to 12 months old with neuromuscular disorder or congenital anomalies that compromise clearing of respiratory secretions

Consult the most current AAP Red Book or CDC for more specific recommendations, including the length of prophylaxis. Adverse reactions may include otitis media, rhinitis, upper respiratory tract infection, apnea, rash, and injection site reaction. Alanine amino transferase (ALT) and aspartate aminotransferase (AST) levels may increase and hemoglobin/hematocrit levels may fall. Once opened, a vial of palivizumab must be used within 6 hours (there is no preservative). It can be given concurrently with other vaccines.

Infections in Children in Child Care Settings

Children in child care settings are 2 to 18 times more likely to suffer from a myriad of infectious diseases, principally respiratory and GI in nature. Additionally, these children receive two to four times more antibiotic treatment and acquire antibiotic-resistant organisms more frequently than children not in child care (Waggoner-Fountain, 2011). Infections typically spread in these settings are listed in Table 24-4. Some general guidelines about which children to exclude or not to exclude in child care settings are listed in Table 21-1.

Specific Viral Diseases

Enteroviruses

Nonpolio Enteroviruses

Of the more than 100 serotypes of nonpolio RNA enteroviruses, 10 to 15 serotypes account for most diseases. They are grouped into four genomic classifications: human

TABLE 24-4 Pathogens and Modes of Transmission in Child Care Settings

Modes of Transmission	Bacteria	Viruses	Parasites, Fungi, Mites, and Lice
Respiratory	*Haemophilus influenzae* type B *Neisseria meningitides* Group A streptococcus (GAS) *Streptococcus pneumonia* *Bordetella pertussis* *Mycobacterium tuberculosis* *Kingella kingae* (also known as *Moraxella kingae*)	Adenovirus Coronavirus Influenza A and B Measles Mumps Varicella-zoster Metapneumovirus Parainfluenza Parvovirus B19 Respiratory syncytial virus Rhinovirus	
Fecal-oral	*Campylobacter jejuni* *Salmonella* spp. *Shigella* spp. *Clostridium difficile* Aeromonas Plesiomonas *Escherichia coli* O157:H7	Enteroviruses (including genus Klebsiella) Hepatitis A virus Rotavirus Calicivirus Astrovirus Norovirus (Norwalk) Enteric adenovirus	*Cryptosporidium* parvum Giardia lamblia Enterobius vermicularis
Person-to-person via skin contact	Group A *Streptococcus* (GAS) *Staphylococcus aureus*	Herpes simplex Varicella-zoster Molluscum contagiosum	*Pediculus capitis* *Sarcoptes scabiei* *Trichophyton* spp. *Microsporum* spp.
Contact with blood, urine, or saliva		Cytomegalovirus (CMV) Hepatitis B and C Herpes simplex Human immunodeficiency virus (HIV)	

Data from Shane AC, Pickering LK: Infections associated with group childcare. In Long SS, Pickering LK, Prober CG, editors: *Principles and practice of pediatric infectious diseases*, ed 4, New York, 2012, Elsevier, pp 24–31; American Academy of Pediatrics (AAP) Committee on Infectious Diseases, Kimberlin DW, Brady MT, et al, editors: *Children in out-of-home child care: Red Book: 2015 report of the Committee on Infectious Diseases*, ed 30, Elk Grove Village, IL, 2015, American Academy of Pediatrics, p 135.

enteroviruses (HEVs) A, B, C, and D. Coxsackieviruses and echoviruses are subgroups of HEVs. Hand-foot-mouth, herpangina, pleurodynia, acute hemorrhagic conjunctivitis, myocarditis, pericarditis, pancreatitis, orchitis, and dermatomyositis-like syndrome are manifestations of infection. These enteroviruses are the most common cause of aseptic meningitis and have also been associated with paralysis, neonatal sepsis, encephalitis, and other respiratory and GI symptoms. The specific serotype may not be unique to any given disease (Abzug, 2011).

As evidenced by the name, enteroviruses concentrate on the GI tract as their primary invasion, replication, and transmission site; they spread by fecal-oral contamination, especially in diapered infants. They are also transmitted via the respiratory route and vertically either prenatally, during parturition, or possibly by way of breastfeeding by an infected mother who lacks antibodies to that particular serotype. Transplacental infection can lead to serious disseminated disease in the neonate that involves multiorgan systems (liver, heart, meninges, and adrenal cortex).

Enteroviruses have worldwide distribution, occurring in temperate climates during the summer and fall and in tropical climates year round. In known cases, infants younger than 12 months old have the highest prevalence rate (>25%), and HEVs account for 55% to 65% of hospitalizations for suspected infant sepsis. Illness occurs more frequently in males; those living in crowded, unsanitary conditions; and in those of lower socioeconomic status (Abzug, 2011). Infection can range from asymptomatic to undifferentiated febrile illness to severe illness. Young children are more likely to be symptomatic. The incubation period is 3 to 6 days (less for hemorrhagic conjunctivitis). After infection, the virus is shed from the respiratory tract for up to 3 weeks and from the GI tract for up to 7 to 11 weeks; it is viable on environmental surfaces for long periods.

Nonpolio enteroviral infection is not a reportable disease, nor is it routinely tested for in the clinical setting, so the overall incidence rate is not known. The CDC administers the National Respiratory and Enteric Virus Surveillance System (NREVSS) and the National Enterovirus

Surveillance System (NESS) to monitor detection patterns of respiratory and enteric adenoviruses. The 2014 outbreak of an illness in children referred to as *acute flaccid myelitis* bears some similarity to infections caused by viruses, including enterovirus; epidemiologic studies are ongoing (CDC, 2015f).

Clinical Findings

History. General symptoms include:

- A mild upper respiratory infection (URI) is common and may include complaints of sore throat, fever, vomiting, diarrhea, anorexia, coryza, abdominal pain, rash, and headache.
- Nonspecific febrile illness of at least 3 days: In young children, there is an undifferentiated abrupt-onset febrile illness (101° to 104° F [38.5° to 40° C]) associated with myalgias, malaise, irritability; fever may wax and wane over several days.
- Onset of viral symptoms within 1 to 2 weeks after delivery for neonates infected transplacentally.

Physical Examination. General findings include mild conjunctivitis, pharyngeal infection, and/or cervical adenopathy. Other findings include:

- Skin: Rash may be macular, macular-papular, urticarial, vesicular, or petechial. May imitate the rash of meningitis, measles, or rubella.
- Herpangina: There is a sudden onset of high fever (up to 106° F [41° C]) lasting 1 to 4 days. Loss of appetite, sore throat, and dysphagia are common, with vomiting and abdominal pain in 25% of cases. Small vesicles (from one to more than 15 lesions of 1 to 2 mm each) appear and enlarge to ulcers (3 to 4 mm) on the anterior pillars of the fauces, tonsils, uvula, and pharynx and the edge of the soft palate. The vesicles commonly have red areolas up to 10 mm in diameter. This self-limiting infection usually lasts 3 to 7 days.
- Acute lymphonodular pharyngitis: This manifests as an acute sore throat lasting approximately 1 week.
- Hand-foot-mouth disease: This is a clinical entity evidenced by fever, vesicular eruptions in the oropharynx that may ulcerate, and a maculopapular rash involving the hands and feet. The rash evolves to vesicles, especially on the dorsa of the hands and the soles of the feet, and lasts 1 to 2 weeks (Fig. 24-1).
- Aseptic meningitis: There are the usual signs of fever, stiff neck, and headache. Altered sensorium and seizures are common. Most cases appear in epidemics or as unique cases; most patients recover completely.
- Paralytic disease: A Guillain-Barré–type syndrome has been described.
- Congenital or neonatal infection: The neonatal infection often manifests as a sudden onset of vomiting, coughing, anorexia, fever or hypothermia, rash, jaundice, irritability, cyanosis, tachycardia, and dyspnea. It is often mistaken for pneumonia. The latter three symptoms can progress to myocarditis and congestive heart failure (CHF). Infants can go into cardiac collapse, have hepatic and adrenal necrosis, suffer intracranial hemorrhage, and die. For those who survive severe disease, the recovery can be rapid.

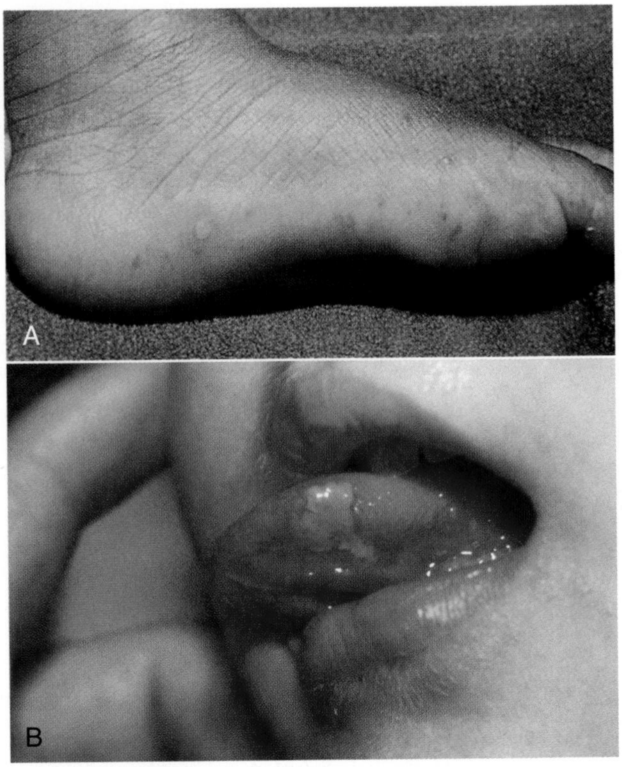

• **Figure 24-1 A** and **B,** Hand-foot-mouth rash.

- Acute hemorrhagic conjunctivitis: Characterized by sudden eye pain, photophobia, blurred vision, tearing, and conjunctival erythema and infection. Most patients recover in a few weeks.
- Pleurodynia (Bornholm disease or devil's grip): This condition usually occurs in epidemics, but some isolated cases can occur. It is most often caused by type B disease, but echoviruses have been implicated. There may be a prodrome before the onset of chest pain ushered in by headache, malaise, anorexia, and myalgia. The onset of chest or upper abdominal pain can be sudden, is pleuritic in nature, and is aggravated by deep breathing, coughing, or sudden movements. The pain occurs in waves of spasms that last several minutes to several hours and is described by individuals as feeling like being stabbed with a knife or being squeezed in a vise. It can be mistaken for coronary artery disease, pneumonia, or pleural inflammation. Low to high fever occurs, and a pleural friction rub often is heard. The disease generally lasts from 3 to 6 days (up to a few weeks).
- Orchitis: This type B infection is clinically similar to mumps.
- Myocarditis or pericarditis: HEVs are associated with 25% to 35% of cases of myocarditis and pericarditis of identified cause. Symptoms can range from mild to severe (sudden death), and male adolescents and young adults are particularly vulnerable (Abzug, 2011).

- Respiratory symptoms are frequently reported before the onset of fatigue, dyspnea, chest pain, CHF, and dysrhythmias. Wheezing, asthma exacerbation, apnea, respiratory distress, pneumonia, otitis media, bronchiolitis, croup, parotitis, and paroxysmal thoracic pain may be seen.

Diagnostic Studies. PCR assay is highly sensitive for all enteroviruses, results can be available in hours, and the test is more sensitive than cell culture. Cultures can be obtained from throat, stool, rectum, cerebrospinal fluid (CSF), urine and blood; sensitivities range from 0% to 80% (AAP et al, 2015b). CBC is usually normal. Serology for serotype-specific IgM antibody or other testing is less useful than culture or PCR.

Differential Diagnosis and Management

The differential diagnosis includes other causes of the aforementioned conditions (e.g., viral or bacterial infections [pneumonia, meningitis, sepsis], or connective tissue diseases).

There is no specific therapy available. IGIV has been used and proven helpful in some chronic and life-threatening infections. The use of antiviral therapy is under study or development, although none are commercially available at this time (e.g., pleconaril and pocapavir) (AAP et al, 2015b). Enteric precautions and good hand washing are the only efficient control measures.

Poliomyelitis Virus

The poliovirus is an enterovirus with three serotypes (types 1, 2, and 3). The disease ranges from an asymptomatic illness to severe CNS involvement. Humans are the only documented source of infection. Transmission is through fecal-oral and respiratory routes. Almost all cases in North America occur in individuals most likely exposed to children who had received oral poliovirus vaccine in another country (AAP, 2015b). There have been wild-type poliovirus importations into countries previously deemed polio-free (Europe, Africa, and Asia), and polio continues to be endemic in Pakistan, Nigeria, and Afghanistan. Through the efforts of the Global Polio Eradication Initiative the incidence of polio worldwide remains low; however, reemergence is a concern. Eighty percent of the world's people now live in polio-free areas, including India and WHO members in the Southeast Asia region (CDC, 2014a).

Poliomyelitis should be considered in any unimmunized or underimmunized child who has a nonspecific febrile illness, aseptic meningitis, or paralytic symptoms (paralysis occurs in under 1% of infections). Asymptomatic disease occurs in about 72% of those infected (AAP et al, 2015b); symptomatic but nonparalytic illness occurs in approximately 5% of cases (Simões, 2011).

The diagnostic test of choice is a viral culture from stool and throat (two samples taken 24 to 48 hours apart) as soon as polio is suspected and at least within 14 days of onset of symptoms. The wild-type virus needs to be differentiated from the vaccine-acquired type. The CSF may be normal or show changes based on the degree of CNS involvement. Antibody titers vary from the acute phase and those taken 3 to 6 weeks later.

Differential Diagnosis and Management

Polio is rare. Differential diagnoses include other conditions causing flaccid muscular weakness and/or paralysis: acute flaccid myelitis, Guillain-Barré syndrome, peripheral neuritis, transverse myelitis, encephalitis, vaccine-associated paralytic poliomyelitis (VAPP), rabies, tetanus, botulism, demyelinating encephalomyelitis, tick-bite paralysis, WNV, spinal cord tumors, familial periodic paralysis, myasthenia gravis, and hysterical paralysis. Conditions that cause decreased limb movement or pseudo-weakness are also differential diagnoses and include unrecognized trauma of the sciatic nerve, toxic synovitis, acute osteomyelitis, acute rheumatic fever, scurvy, and congenital syphilitic osteomyelitis.

Management is supportive and directed at minimizing skeletal deformity in the paralytic form of the disease. Both nonparalytic and mild paralytic cases can be managed on an outpatient basis but otherwise individuals should be hospitalized. During the early stages of the disease, individuals should be advised against increasing their physical activity, exercising, or becoming fatigued because these factors may increase the risk of paralytic disease (Simões, 2011).

Preventive measures include active and passive vaccination; the CDC provides guidelines for vaccination in individuals traveling to endemic countries.

Hepatoviruses

Hepatitis A Virus

HAV is an RNA-containing virus belonging to the Picornaviridae family, which comprises five genera (enteroviruses, rhinoviruses, hepatoviruses, cardioviruses, and aphthoviruses). HAV causes a primary infection in the liver. It is a highly contagious infection and commonly spreads through person-to-person contact and fecal-oral contamination of food and water; rarely is it transmitted by contaminated blood transfusion. It accounts for most of the acute and benign viral hepatitis in the United States and worldwide. There is no seasonal or geographic variance.

Transmission occurs readily in households and child care centers; risk factors also include personal contact with an infected individual, international travel, recognized food-borne outbreak, men who have sex with men, and illicit drug use. In children younger than 6 years old, about 30% are symptomatic; few of these have jaundice (CDC, 2015g). This high anicteric incidence allows considerable spread of disease to adult caretakers in child care settings. Infants are protected by maternal antibodies during the first few months of life. Older children and adults tend to have more symptomatic disease. The incidence rates are similar across all age groups and geographic regions.

The incubation period is 15 to 50 days (average 28 to 30 days). The period of contagion is as long as the virus is shed and usually lasts 1 to 3 weeks. The highest period of infectivity is from up to 2 weeks before the onset of illness until 1 week after the onset of jaundice, although neonates and young children may continue to harbor the virus in their stool for longer periods (Rios, 2014).

Clinical Findings

The following two phases may be seen:

1. Preicteric phase: This phase manifests as an acute febrile illness. Malaise, nausea, anorexia, vomiting, digestive complaints, fever (rarely higher than 102° F [38.9° C]), headache, and occasional abdominal complaints occur. This phase goes unnoticed in many children. There can be dull right upper quadrant pain; some children may have only mild URI and GI symptoms along with a transient fever.
2. Icteric phase: Jaundice appears shortly after the onset of symptoms (70% incidence in older children and adults) (AAP et al, 2015b) and can last from a few days to almost a month; it may be subtle in children. Urine darkens, and stools become clay colored. Often these are the only apparent signs of the illness. Diarrhea is common in infants, whereas constipation is more common in older children and adults. Patients feel sick. Infants have poor weight gain during the icteric phase. Mild hepatomegaly and tenderness, posterior cervical adenopathy, and a tender spleen (10% to 20% incidence) may occur (Rios, 2014).

Fulminant disease is rare. There is no chronic disease. Complete recovery can be expected within 1 to 2 months with occasional relapses lasting up to 6 months.

Diagnostic Studies. Serologic testing is widely available. IgM-specific antibodies indicate recent infection. These are replaced by IgG-specific antibodies 2 to 4 months later and serve as indicators of past infection. Elevations of AST and alanine aminotransferase (ALT) occur most consistently, may precede the symptoms by a week or more, and indicate the degree of inflammatory injury. Elevations are also seen in gamma-glutamyl transpeptidase (GGTP) and serum bilirubin (rarely above 10 mg/dL); mild lymphocytosis may be seen.

Differential Diagnosis

Any cause of jaundice is in the differential diagnosis of HAV.

- Infancy: Physiologic jaundice, hemolytic disease, galactosemia, hypothyroidism, biliary metabolic disorders, biliary atresia, alpha 1-antitrypsin deficiency, and choledochal cysts. Hypervitaminosis A causes a yellow pigmentation (carotenemia) of the skin often mistaken for jaundice in children. Infections, such as those referred to as TORCH (toxoplasmosis, other [syphilis, varicella-zoster, parvovirus B19], rubella, cytomegalovirus, and herpes infections), also cause hepatitis.
- Older infants, children, and adolescents: Hemolytic-uremic syndrome, Reye syndrome, malaria, leptospirosis, brucellosis, chronic hemolytic diseases with gallstone development, Wilson disease, cystic fibrosis, Banti syndrome, collagen-vascular disease (e.g., systemic lupus erythematosus [SLE]), infectious mononucleosis syndrome (IMS), CMV, coxsackievirus, toxoplasmosis, Weil disease, yellow fever, acute cholangitis, amebiasis, and hepatitis B, C, and D are in the differential diagnosis. Drugs and poisons such as pyrazinamide, isoniazid, valproic acid, acetaminophen overdose, zoxazolamine, gold, cinchophen, phenothiazines, and methyltestosterone also cause hepatitis.

Management, Complications, and Prevention

Therapy is supportive. Good hand hygiene after diaper changes is a crucial preventive measure, especially for child care personnel. The use of immunoglobulin or HAV vaccine within 2 weeks of exposure is discussed earlier in this chapter (see Table 24-3). Those with acute infections who work as food handlers or in schools/child care settings should be excluded for 1 week after onset of symptoms (AAP et al, 2015b). Although patients can become very ill, most cases of HAV resolve completely. Fulminant hepatitis with liver failure is rare. Prevention includes good personal hygiene and safe drinking water, in addition to routine HAV vaccine for those 12 months old and older.

Hepatitis B Virus

HBV is a DNA-containing hepadnavirus. It is highly contagious and causes severe liver disease. The most common method of transmission is percutaneous or permucosal exposure to contaminated blood/serum, semen, vaginal secretions, and other bodily fluids, including but not limited to amniotic, cerebrospinal, and pleural; it is not spread by the fecal-oral route. HBV can survive in a dried state for more than 1 week, but it is highly susceptible to common household disinfectants, such as 1:10 diluted bleach. Prolonged percutaneous contact with contaminated fomites, such as toothbrushes and razors, can be a source of infection.

The major reservoirs for HBV are healthy chronic carriers and patients with acute disease. Approximately 700,000 to 1.4 million people have chronic HBV in the United States, and approximately 240 million worldwide (CDC, 2015h; WHO, 2015a). Unimmunized children who have immigrated to the United States from sub-Saharan Africa and East Asia and other high endemic areas pose the highest infection risk. Transmission is rare within the United States because of the high HBV immunization coverage in children. Highest rates of infection in the United States across all age ranges are reported in men from 25 to 44 years old (CDC, 2015h). Perinatal transmission is highly efficient during the birthing process from female carriers (HBsAg-positive or hepatitis B e antigen [HBeAg]-positive, or both) to their newborn children. In utero transmission is rare because HBV is a large molecule and rarely crosses the placenta. The infection rate is 70% to 90% if both maternal antigen markers are positive, and 5% to 20% if the mother is HBsAg-positive but HBeAg-negative (AAP et al, 2015b).

Whether one eventually develops chronic infection depends on the age one is infected and the rate of loss of HBeAg. More than 90% of infected infants will develop chronic infection after exposure. Twenty-five percent to 50% of children who acquire the infection between 1 and 5 years old (as compared to about 5% exposed as adults) develop chronic HBV infection. Twenty-five percent of those chronically infected children die prematurely of cirrhosis or liver cancer (CDC, 2015h). Individuals who abuse IV drugs, engage in sexual activity with multiple partners, or have male-to-male sex have the greatest risk of acquiring HBV. Health care workers who are exposed to blood, blood products, or blood-contaminated body fluids and those working with the developmentally disabled are also at a high risk, as are chronic renal dialysis patients. Tattooing or body piercing with contaminated instruments is another route of infection. Breastfeeding is not contraindicated. All infants, children, and adolescents who missed the birth dose of HBV should be screened, especially if their parents were born in regions of high-HBV endemicity.

Clinical Findings

The incubation period is 45 to 160 days (average of 120 days). HBV has a range of illness from asymptomatic seroconversion to fulminating disease and death. HBV usually has a gradual onset. Most children who acquired HBV at an early age are asymptomatic. Some have minimal nonspecific constitutional complaints, such as fever, nausea, and minimal hepatomegaly. Arthralgia and skin problems, such as urticaria or other rashes, can be the first apparent signs. Papular acrodermatitis has been described in infants. Acute HBV infection is somewhat similar to the icteric phase of HAV, but it is usually more severe. Skin, mucous membranes, and sclerae are icteric. The liver is enlarged and tender.

Diagnostic Studies. Serologic tests include HBsAg, hepatitis B core antigen (HBcAg), HBeAg, and antibodies to these antigens; the results can be useful in determining the stage of infection (Table 24-5). Changes in liver enzymes indicate the degree of injury. There is elevation of serum transaminases (SGOT, AST, SGPT, and ALT). Prothrombin time can be elevated, especially in fulminating disease. Hybridization assays, nucleic acid amplification testing, and gene amplification techniques (e.g., PCR) are also available.

Differential Diagnosis and Management

Any cause of jaundice is included; refer to the Differential Diagnosis section of HAV.

Therapy for acute infection is supportive. The use of active and passive vaccination has been discussed. A specialist in hepatitis B in children should be consulted for management of suspected reactivation of HBV or for chronic hepatitis B due to the risk of developing hepatocellular carcinoma. The FDA has approved five medications for treatment of children with chronic hepatitis B: Interferon-alfa (>12 months old); lamivudine (>3 years old); adefovir and tenofovir (>12 years old); and entecavir (>16 years old). The choice of who should receive medication and the duration of therapy remain controversial and subject to more study (Sokal et al, 2013). The European Society of Pediatric Gastroenterology, Hepatology and Nutrition (ESPGHAN) has published a guideline with algorithms describing initial evaluation, monitoring, and criteria for treatment (see Additional Resources on the Evolve site). Those with chronic infection should receive yearly liver ultrasound,

TABLE 24-5 Interpretation of Serologic Markers for Hepatitis B Virus Infection

Serologic Marker				
HBsAg	Anti-HBs	IgM Anti-HBc	Total Anti-HBc	Interpretation
–	–	–	–	Susceptible; never infected
+	–	–	–	Acute infection, early incubation; transient, up to 3 weeks after vaccination
+	–	+	+	Acute infection
–	–	+	+	Acute infection, resolving
–	+	–	+	Past infection, recovered, and immune
+	–	–	+	Chronic infection
–	–	–	+	False positive (i.e., susceptible) past infection, or "low level" chronic infection
–	+	–	–	Immune from vaccination

From Byrd KK, Murphy TV, Hu DJ: Hepatitis B and hepatitis D viruses. In Long SS, Pickering LK, Prober CG, editors: *Principles and practice of pediatric infectious diseases*, ed 4, New York, 2012, Elsevier, Table 213-2.

Anti-HBs, Antibody to hepatitis B surface antigen; *HBsAg,* hepatitis B surface antigen; *IgM anti-HBc,* immunoglobulin M antibody to hepatitis B core antigen; *total anti-HBc,* total antibody to hepatitis B core antigen.

testing of liver function and alpha-fetoprotein concentration, and vaccination for HAV. Liver biopsies may be done to accurately monitor the effects of liver involvement. HBIG and corticosteroids are not useful (AAP et al, 2015b).

Complications and Prevention

Liver failure, cirrhosis, and hepatocellular carcinoma are complications of chronic infection. The initial infection can be prevented with hepatitis B vaccination. Transmission in utero or during labor to newborns and postexposure prophylaxis is covered in Table 24-3.

Hepatitis C Virus

Hepatitis C virus (HCV), a single-stranded RNA virus with seven genotypes and multiple subtypes in the Flaviviridae family, causes the chronic form of what used to be called *non-A, non-B hepatitis.* The virus is transmitted by contact with infected blood, blood supply products, or unsafe drug injection practices. The estimated prevalence in the United States is 1.3% (about 4 million people) and 170 million people worldwide (AAP et al, 2015b; Yazigi and Balistreri, 2011). The prevalence in children of all ages is difficult to establish with estimates ranging from approximately 0.1% to 0.4% (Hartwell et al, 2014). Those who do not go on to develop chronic hepatitis C (15% to 25%) will spontaneously clear the virus without treatment (CDC, 2015i). However, HCV infection has the highest rate of developing into chronic infection and liver disease (70% to 80% of adults) than all of the other hepatitis infections; the incidence of these complications in children is thought to be lower (AAP et al, 2015b).

Perinatal transmission is the major route for infecting children: approximately 6 out of every 100 infants born to HCV-infected mothers become infected (CDC, 2015i). Mothers who are HIV-positive have a twofold to threefold increased likelihood of transmitting the virus to their infants (Mack et al, 2012). Vaginal birth and breastfeeding do not contribute to higher rates of transmission, and women with HCV alone should not be discouraged from experiencing either (American College of Obstetricians and Gynecologists, 2013). Infants who acquire HCV per vertical transmission have a high rate of spontaneous resolution approaching 25% to 40%, usually by 24 months old but some as late as 7 years old. Older children experience a spontaneous resolution at a rate of 6% to 12% (Mack et al, 2012).

The most common means of HCV transmission in the United States is from injection drug use. An estimated one third of injection drug users between the ages of 18 and 30 years old are infected (CDC, 2015i). Men who have sex with men are also at increased risk of infection. Strict blood product screening and manufacturing practices in the United States have reduced the risk of transmission significantly.

Clinical Findings

HCV has an incubation period ranging from 2 weeks to 6 months (average 45 days). Onset of symptoms is often insidious; most children are asymptomatic. Flulike prodromal symptoms (jaundice, nausea, anorexia, upper right quadrant abdominal pain) may occur in 20% to 30% of older children and adults (Tohme et al, 2012). Chronic hepatitis with cirrhosis is a late occurrence, often 20 to 30 years later. Fulminant infection is uncommon. Teenagers may be discovered to be HCV-positive when being screened for other reasons (e.g., a school blood donation drive).

Diagnostic Studies. There is no serologic marker for acute infection. Confirmation of HCV using IgG antibody enzyme immunoassay for anti-HCV, enhanced chemiluminescence immunoassay (CIA), and HCV RNA PCR are used for screening and diagnosis. False negative results can occur, however, early in the infection. The majority of individuals seroconvert within 15 weeks postexposure or within 5 to 6 weeks after the onset of illness symptoms. A newborn can be anti-HCV-positive from maternal transfer for up to 18 months, so testing should ideally be done after that time. Liver function tests are indicated and liver enzymes may go up and down with some near normal levels for many years; liver biopsy is confirmatory (CDC, 2015i; Jhaveri, 2014). A table on the interpretation of results of tests for HCV infection is available from the CDC (see Additional Resources on the Evolve site).

Differential Diagnosis and Management

Differential diagnoses include HAV and HBV and other causes of chronic hepatitis. See the Differential Diagnosis section of HAV.

Treatment of acute HCV in children is supportive. Chronic HCV infections in children, 3 to 17 years old, respond to therapy with nonpegylated interferon alfa-2b and ribavirin. The newer anti-HCV agents are not applicable to the treatment for children at the present time (Jhaveri, 2014). HAV and HBV vaccines should be given to prevent further liver complications. Liver damage can be exacerbated by comorbid conditions, such as cancer, iron overload, thalassemia, or HIV. Drugs such as acetaminophen or antiretroviral medications need to be closely monitored; patients should have serum hepatic transaminases monitored closely. Children with HCV infection need not be excluded from child care facilities (AAP et al, 2015b). Individuals with HCV should be discouraged from using alcohol to prevent further liver injury and from sharing razors and toothbrushes; condom use should be encouraged.

Complications and Prevention

The course of HCV is generally mild even with cirrhosis. Liver transplantation is an option in severe cases although reinfection after transplant is common and progressive. The outcome of chronic HCV disease in children is less known. Immunoglobulin is not recommended for prophylaxis after exposure. Research into developing a vaccine is ongoing.

Hepatitis D Virus

Hepatitis D virus (HDV) is caused by an RNA virus that is structurally different from HAV, HBV, and HCV. HDV infection is uncommon in children but must be considered in cases of fulminant hepatitis or hepatic failure. It cannot cause infection unless the child also is infected with HBV, which it needs to replicate. Transmission is through parenteral, percutaneous, or mucosal contact (including sexual) with infected blood and can be acquired either as a coinfection with or superinfection in an individual with chronic HBV. Incubation is 2 to 8 weeks. In the United States, it is diagnosed most commonly in drug users, individuals with hemophilia, and immigrants from southern Italy and parts of Eastern Europe, South America, Africa, and the Middle East. Mother-to-newborn transmission is rare (AAP et al, 2015b). Infection is detected using IgM antibody to HDV. There is no vaccine against HDV. However, HBV vaccine is preventive of HDV because of its comorbidity with HBV. Those with chronic HBV should take precautions against being infected.

Hepatitis E Virus

Hepatitis E virus (HEV) is an RNA virus in the family Hepeviridae; certain strains can also have zoonotic hosts (e.g., swine, nonhuman primates). It is passed via the fecal-oral route. Contaminated water is the most common reservoir. It is an acute infection whose symptoms resemble those of other viral hepatitis. Symptomatic individuals are usually older adolescents and young adults; pregnant women (notably in the third trimester) are particularly vulnerable to more serious illness. Children are either asymptomatic or experience mild symptoms. If symptoms appear, they do so within 15 to 60 days (mean 40 days) after exposure. Endemic areas include India, the Middle East, parts of Africa, Southeast Asia, and Mexico. Most cases in the United States are found in immigrants or visitors from these locations. Clinical symptoms include jaundice, malaise, anorexia, fever, abdominal pain, and arthralgia; these are similar to symptoms of HAV but are often more severe. Laboratory studies include IgM and IgG anti-HEV, but these can be unreliable. Definitive diagnosis is determined by the detection of viral RNA in serum or stool using reverse transcriptase–polymerase chain reaction (RT-PCR) assay. Treatment is supportive; there is no approved vaccine in the United States. Good hand hygiene is crucial. Chronic infection is rare, and recovery is usually complete. The overall mortality rate is 4% or less; however, in pregnant women, the mortality rate can reach 25% (Teshale and Kamili, 2012).

Herpes Family of Viruses

The herpes family of viruses is large with several features in common: all infect humans, the viruses establish latency for the life of the host, and reactivation is controlled by immune function. Most active infections are self-limited. Infection becomes serious and life threatening when the cellular immune system is compromised or is naïve, such as in the newborn. This family of viruses includes HSV types 1 and 2, VZV, Epstein-Barr virus (EBV), CMV, and human herpesvirus 6, 7, and 8 (HHV-6, HHV-7, and HHV-8). HSV-1, HSV-2, and VZV are members of the α-herpesvirus subfamily with neurotropic characteristics and latency in the sensory ganglia.

HSV-1, HSV-2, VZV, EBV, HHV-6, and HHV-7 are discussed in the following sections. See Chapter 39 for a discussion of perinatally acquired CMV infection and other resources for a discussion about HHV-8.

Herpes Simplex Virus

HSV is among the most widely disseminated infectious agents in humans; it is a double-stranded DNA virus and there are two types. HSV-1 is associated with orolabial lesions or oral secretion and infects the mouth, lips, and eyes and can progress to the CNS. HSV-2 is shed from genital lesions and genital secretions and is most commonly associated with genital and neonatal infection. Both HSV types can be found in oral or genital sites depending upon the extent of oral-genital contact. Although HSV-2 accounts for 70% to 85% of neonatal cases, both types are equally devastating to a newborn (Straface et al, 2012). Type 1 virus typically is the causative agent in primary infections in children 6 months to 5 years old and most often presents as gingivostomatitis. Distribution is worldwide, but the infection is more frequent in crowded environments. It is spread by intimate, direct contact usually by an adult with or without symptoms. There is no seasonal variation.

HSV-2 infections usually occur as a result of sexual activity. Sexual molestation must always be ruled out when the infection is found in non-neonates; for this reason, determining the type of virus is always important. Neither type is transmitted by inanimate objects, such as toilet seats.

Neonatal HSV-2 infection is primarily transmitted from the mother as the infant passes through an infected birth canal with viral migration to the neonate's conjunctiva, nose and/or mouth mucosa, or broken skin due to forceps or a scalp electrode. Infection can also occur with cesarean births. Risk of infection for an infant born to a mother with a primary genital infection is 33% to 50%. The risk is reduced to 3% to 5% to an infant born vaginally to a woman with recurrent genital HSV infections and less than 3% if born to a woman with recurrent asymptomatic shedding at the time of delivery. However, about 60% to 80% of infants with congenital HSV infection are born to women without a history or clinical findings of active infection during pregnancy. The incidence is 1 in 3000 to 20,000 live births in the United States depending upon demographics and geographic area (Gutierrez et al, 2014). Although rare (5%), in utero transmission can occur. Postnatal transmission is described but is also less common (10%) than during the peripartum period (Pinninti and Kimberlin, 2014). Mothers can inoculate their babies from oral, breast, or skin lesions. Fathers also can inoculate infants with nongenital lesions from their mouths or on their hands. There can be lateral transmission from an infected baby in the nursery due to inadequate hand hygiene by hospital personnel.

Period of communicability for HSV-1 and HSV-2 (when not in the neonatal period) is 2 days to 2 weeks. Some cases of congenital infection occur more than 6 weeks after birth depending on when the fetus was exposed. Infection can be transmitted during either primary or recurrent infections, whether symptomatic or asymptomatic.

Clinical Findings

History and physical findings are determined by the port of entry of the host, age, state of health, and immune competence. Eczema alone or in combination with other manifestations is a complicating factor. Clinical findings, diagnosis, management, and treatment of some of the most commonly seen infections in children and adolescents due to HSV-1 and HSV-2 are discussed in other chapters (i.e., gingivostomatitis, neonatal herpetic infection, eczema herpeticum, herpes vulvovaginitis, herpes labialis, and herpes keratoconjunctivitis). A few general observations follow:

- Neonatal infection: The neonate is always symptomatic; infection is described by the extent and location of disease: disseminated (approximately 25% of cases); CNS (approximately 30% of cases); and skin, eye, and/or mouth (SEM) (approximately 45% of cases). Disseminated disease presents around day 10 to 12 of life with multiple organ failure; two-thirds develop concurrent encephalitis. Almost half of the infants with disseminated disease never develop the characteristic vesicular rash. CNS disease presents around 16 to 19 days of life with neurologic manifestations of focal/generalized seizures, lethargy and/or irritability, and poor feeding. The majority of these infants will develop herpetic lesions during the course of the illness. SEM manifests itself around day 10 to 12 of life (Pinninti and Kimberlin, 2014) (see Chapter 39).
- Traumatic herpetic infection: This is a localized infection that occurs in a susceptible child because of an abrasion, teething, finger sucking, laceration, or burn that is inoculated with herpesvirus by an orally infected parent who kisses the "booboo" or from auto-inoculation. Vesicles appear at the site of the lesion. There may be fever, constitutional symptoms, and regional lymph node involvement. Athletic activities such as wrestling and rugby have been implicated in mucocutaneous herpetic lesions.
- Acute herpetic meningoencephalitis: After the neonatal period, infection with HSV-1 is a leading cause of intermittent, nonepidemic encephalitis in children and adults in the United States. Encephalitis can be focal, mimicking a mass lesion. Diagnosis is made by brain biopsy. In contrast, HSV meningitis is usually a relatively benign disease most often caused by HSV-2.
- Recurrent infections: The body does not truly eradicate the virus; the virus lies dormant, and recurrent infections are common. Recurrent infections occur either as herpes labialis or genital herpes. Some incidence of recurrent aseptic meningitis can be attributed to HSV infection.

Diagnostic Studies

Intrapartum cultures from mother and child should be obtained no later than 12 and 24 hours after birth if neonatal infection is suspected. Tests may include viral culture, cytology-Pap smears, Tzanck stains, ELISA, fluorescent techniques, glycoprotein G assay, blood or CSF PCR in neonates, or histologic evaluation and viral culture from a brain biopsy in cases of encephalitis. Cultures in neonates need to be taken from skin vesicles, mouth, nasopharynx, eyes, blood, rectum, and CSF. Serologic tests are not helpful in neonates. If encephalitis is suspected, an electroencephalogram (EEG) and MRI of the brain are performed. In disseminated disease, elevated transaminase and/or radiographic evidence of HSV pneumonitis may be seen.

Differential Diagnosis and Management

The diagnosis is usually not a problem if vesicles are present. Coxsackievirus can cause a vesicular stomatitis. Neonatal HSV disease should always be suspected in cases of neonatal respiratory distress or sepsis.

The management of HSV infections is discussed in other chapters (i.e., gingivostomatitis, neonatal herpetic infection, eczema herpeticum, herpes vulvovaginitis, herpes labialis, and herpes keratoconjunctivitis). Parenteral acyclovir is the treatment of choice in life-threatening illness, neonatal infection, or disease in immunocompromised patients.

Oral acyclovir suppressive therapy for 6 months after parenteral treatment of any classification of acute neonatal disease has been shown to reduce the recurrences of mucocutaneous lesions and improve neurodevelopmental outcomes. The absolute neutrophil count (ANC) should be continuously monitored during the 6 months of suppressive treatment in these infants. If neutropenia should occur, acyclovir therapy should be stopped until the neutrophil count recovers; the acyclovir is then restarted. Any new lesion(s) suggestive of HSV should be cultured.

Infants born to women with active *recurrent* genital infection are generally not given empiric antiviral medication, but instead are closely monitored by parents/caregivers and providers over the following 6 weeks. Careful hand hygiene before and after handling newborns and refraining from kissing or nuzzling (masks can be worn until lesions have crusted) by those with active herpes labialis infection are basic preventive measures.

Complications

Most HSV infections are usually mild. However, bacterial superinfection is always a potential problem. Any child with evidence of HSV ocular involvement must be referred to an ophthalmologist immediately.

With aggressive antiviral therapy (acyclovir) the morbidity and mortality associated with neonatal herpetic infection has significantly improved. Treated appropriately, 1-year mortality has been reduced to 29% for disseminated disease and 4% for CNS disease. Poor neurologic outcomes have been reduced to 17% of neonates with disseminated disease and 69% with CNS disease. Aggressive acyclovir therapy has resulted in SEM infections remaining limited to the mucocutaneous lesions and not leading to disseminated or CNS disease (Pinninti and Kimberlin, 2013).

Patient and Family Education

- Toddlers and infants with primary gingivostomatitis who are drooling should be excluded from child care centers if they cannot control their saliva. Children with recurrent "fever blisters" may attend school. Covering recurrent HSV lesions with a bandage is appropriate for children with active nonmucosal involvement.
- Wrestlers should be excluded from competition until lesions have healed. (See also Chapter 13, Box 13-8 and Table 13-9).
- All pregnant women must be asked about HSV infection in themselves and all sexual partners. Signs and symptoms of HSV should be carefully monitored throughout pregnancy.
- During labor, all women must again be questioned about HSV and carefully examined for signs and symptoms of infection. Cesarean delivery is indicated in women with apparent infection unless membranes are ruptured for more than 4 to 6 hours. Scalp monitoring should be avoided.

Infectious Mononucleosis Syndrome

IMS is caused by EBV, a member of the γ-herpesviruses, in more than 90% of cases; the remaining cases are attributed to acute CMV, *Toxoplasma gondii,* adenovirus, viral hepatitis, HIV, and possibly rubella. Distribution of IMS is worldwide, with more than 95% of the population having been infected (Jenson, 2011). Almost all older children and adolescents in poor urban settings of developed countries or in developing countries are seropositive for EBV. In these children, primary exposure occurs in infancy or early childhood, tends to produce only mild symptoms, and is subclinical. Infection in children younger than 4 years old occurs less frequently in more affluent populations in developed countries; one third of cases occur during adolescence or young adulthood (Jenson, 2011). The mode of transmission is personal contact, usually from deep kissing; by penetrative sexual contact; or from the exchange of saliva among children. The virus can live outside the body in saliva for several hours. About 20% to 30% of healthy immune individuals shed EBV at any one time. From 60% to 90% of EBV-infected individuals on immunosuppressive therapy, including those on steroids, shed virus (Jenson, 2011).

Because IMS virus is found in the saliva and blood of both clinically ill and asymptomatic infected persons for many months, the period of communicability is difficult to assess. The period of incubation is thought to be from 30 to 50 days. It is only mildly contagious.

Clinical Findings

IMS is a disease of the primary lymphoid tissue and peripheral blood. Lymphoid tissue—regional lymph nodes, tonsils, spleen, and liver—is enlarged. Atypical lymphocytes are seen in the peripheral blood. Almost all body organs are involved, including but not limited to the lungs, heart, kidneys, adrenals, CNS, and skin. Symptoms are variable and can last up to 2 to 3 weeks. Clinical presentation typically occurs in three phases: *prodrome*, *acute*, and *resolution*. During the *prodrome* phase, symptoms are mild and may include malaise, fatigue, and possibly fever, and it is difficult to distinguish IMS from other viral infections. The acute phase follows with the classic symptoms of fever (100.4° F [38° C] to 104.9° F [40.5° C]), sore throat, malaise, and fatigue. Physical findings include discrete, nontender, nonerythematous lymphadenopathy, as well as tonsillopharyngitis (exudative in approximately half of the patients). Hepatomegaly and splenomegaly occur in about 50% to 60% of children and are more common in the younger child (Leach et al, 2014). Skin rash occurs in 3% to 15% of cases, usually on the trunk, arms, and palms. It can be maculopapular, urticarial, scarlatiniform, hemorrhagic (rarely), or nodular and usually occurs during the first few days of symptomatology onset and lasts 1 to 6 days. The rash occurs more frequently in those taking ampicillin or amoxicillin (up to 80%) and probably represents a form of arteritis or vasculitis rather than hypersensitivity to ampicillin. The rash typically starts 5 to 10 days after the drug has been started. Additionally, a symmetric rash of erythematous papules with or without coalescence on the cheeks, extremities, and buttocks (looks similar to atopic dermatitis) is associated with EBV infection and is referred to as the Gianotti-Crosti syndrome (Jensen, 2011). After several days (or up to 3 to 4 weeks), the *resolution* phase begins with gradual decrease of fatigue and fever; organomegaly may take 1 to 2 months to resolve (Leach et al, 2014).

Diagnostic Studies

The CBC provides a classic picture of lymphocytosis with more than 10% atypical lymphocytes; elevated liver enzymes are typical. Monospot and the serum heterophile test are positive in 85% of infected patients older than 4 years old (often negative in those younger than 4 years old). Children older than 4 years usually must be ill for approximately 2 weeks before seroconverting. Viral culture and Epstein-Barr–specific core and capsule antibody testing are usually used for diagnosis if the primary screening test results are negative and there is continued suspicion of IMS (e.g., in younger children). Depending on the specific EBV antigen system tested, levels can be detectable for years after infection.

Differential Diagnosis and Management

IMS is in the differential diagnosis of almost every infectious disease. Conditions and infections typically associated with a mononucleosis-like syndrome are gram-positive alpha-beta hemolytic streptococcal pharyngitis, leukemia, lymphoreticular malignancies, adenoviruses, toxoplasmosis, CMV, rubella, HIV, hepatitis, SLE, drug reactions, and diphtheria.

Treatment is supportive with adequate bed rest for debilitated cases, over-the-counter pain relievers, fluids, and increased calories. Corticosteroids and acyclovir are not recommended for routine uncomplicated disease; penicillin products should not be given. Contact sports and strenuous exercise should be avoided for 4 weeks and especially in those with hepatosplenomegaly (see Chapter 13 for return-to-play sports participation recommendations after hepatosplenomegaly). Symptoms generally resolve within 2 to 4 weeks; fatigue and weakness may persist for up to 6 to 12 months after severe infection. Complete recovery can be expected in more than 95% of cases without any specific treatment (Leach et al, 2014).

Complications and Patient and Family Education

Otherwise healthy children and youth experience few sequelae. Rare complications include splenic rupture, neurologic complications (from aseptic meningitis, encephalitis, myelitis, optic neuritis, cranial nerve palsies, Guillain-Barré syndrome), thrombocytopenia, agranulocytosis, hemolytic anemia, orchitis, myocarditis, or chronic IMS. The virus also seems to increase the risk for Hodgkin disease. Death is rare. There is no clear evidence that supports an association between EBV infection and chronic fatigue syndrome (Leach et al, 2014).

Persons with a recent history of IMS or an infectious mononucleosis-like disease should not donate blood or organs. Sharing food and drinks with infected individuals needs to be avoided in order to reduce the risk of acquiring EBV-associated IMS (Leach et al, 2014).

Roseola Infantum (Exanthem Subitum)

HHV-6 and HHV-7 are the members of the Roseolovirus genus in the Betaherpesvirinae subfamily of human herpesviruses. HHV-6 is responsible for the majority of cases of roseola infantum (exanthema subitum or sixth disease) and has been associated with other diseases, including encephalitis, especially in immunocompromised hosts. A small percentage of children with roseola have primary infection with HHV-7 (Caserta, 2011). Humans are the only natural reservoir. The method of transmission is not completely understood, but the virus is probably spread via the oral, nasal, and conjunctival routes of other family members, caregivers, or close contacts. Transmission is suspected to be either prenatal or during or after parturition. The disease is most commonly seen in children between 7 and 24 months old, after protective maternal antibodies have waned. It is rare in children younger than 3 months old or older than 4 years old (Cherry, 2014). Most children are HHV-6 seropositive by 4 years old, and about 85% are seropositive for HHV-7 by adulthood (AAP et al, 2015b). Reactivation of infection can occur in those who are immunocompromised. Visits to emergency departments are common as a result of the associated fevers, toxicity, and/or seizures associated with this disease in infants. The disease occurs worldwide, year round, and shows no gender preference (Cherry, 2014). The incubation period has a mean of 9 to 10 days. The period of communicability is probably greatest during the fever phase before the rash erupts.

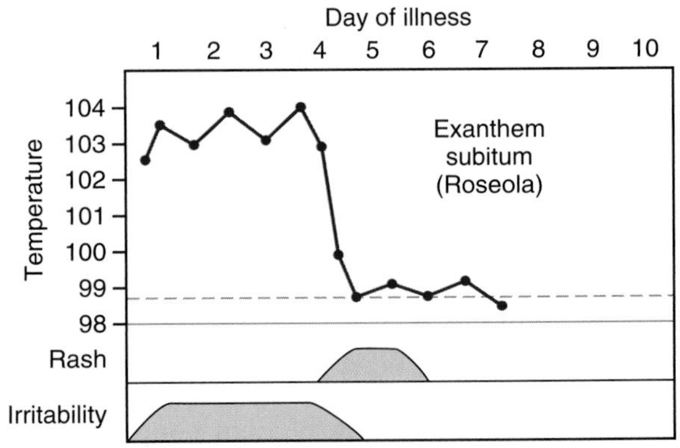

• **Figure 24-2** Schematic diagram illustrating the symptoms of roseola.

Clinical Findings

There is a sudden onset of fever from 101° F to more than 103° F (38.3° C to more than 39.5° C) for 3 to 7 days, but the child does not seem particularly ill. However, during high fevers irritability and malaise may be noted (Cherry, 2014). There may be signs of a URI; lymphadenopathy in the cervical and posterior occipital areas; lethargy; infected palpebral conjunctiva; eyelid edema; GI complaints; reddened TMs; and, occasionally, a febrile convulsion (10% to 15% of cases) (AAP et al, 2015b). As the fever breaks, a diffuse, nonpruritic, discrete, rose-colored maculopapular rash, 2 to 3 mm in diameter, appears (Fig. 24-2). It fades on pressure and rarely coalesces. The roseola exanthema is similar to the rash of rubella. The rash lasts from hours to 2 to 3 days, begins on the trunk, and spreads centrifugally. In the rare case of CNS involvement, the anterior fontanelle may bulge (Cherry, 2014).

Diagnostic Studies

The diagnosis of roseola exanthema can usually be made on clinical presentation alone, and diagnostic studies are not indicated. If serology is done (diagnosis is unclear or symptoms are severe or unusual), the WBC count is distinctive, showing a decrease for age initially, dropping further by the third or fourth day, and then returning into the normal range. It tends to follow the fever pattern. Other serologic testing may involve isolating HHV-6 for peripheral blood mononuclear cells and documenting a significant rise in antibody titer; however, test results can vary widely, so diagnosing unequivocal acute infection is problematic. Serial titers 2 to 3 weeks apart are more reliable. Fourfold increases in HHV-6 or HHV-7 IgG antibodies suggest active infection. Virus cultures can be helpful. A rapid HHV-6 culture is available. A RT-PCR assay can distinguish between the acute and latent infection.

Differential Diagnosis, Management, and Complications

The clinical course usually makes this illness easy to diagnose. Most viral rashes, scarlatina, and drug hypersensitivity are included in the differential diagnoses. A roseola-like illness is also associated with parvovirus B19, echovirus 16, other enteroviruses, measles, and adenoviruses. Until the rash develops, fever without focus and bacterial sepsis are in the differential diagnosis. If a febrile seizure occurs, meningitis is usually added to the differential diagnosis.

Management is supportive. Acetaminophen can be used if the child is uncomfortable with the fever. There is no practical means of prevention. Complications include febrile convulsions, meningoencephalitis, encephalitis, and hemiplegia.

Varicella

VZV is a common highly contagious virus belonging to the herpesvirus family. Chickenpox is the primary illness. It derives its name not from chickens but from the propensity of the lesions to resemble chickpeas. Shingles (herpes zoster) is the reactivation infection of latent VZV acquired during varicella infection (see Chapter 37).

Humans are the only reservoir of infection; illness is spread by direct contact, droplets, and airborne transmission. Victims of shingles are also infectious and can cause primary varicella illness. Immunity is usually lifelong. Symptomatic reinfection is rare, but asymptomatic reinfection occurs and symptoms are usually mild. Immunocompromised patients are at risk of developing generalized zoster. The disease tends to peak in those 10 to 14 years old, although the overall incidence has decreased in all age groups from prevaccine levels (after licensure in 1995, incidence declined 90% by 2005 with further reduction after the second dose was made routine in 2006) (AAP et al, 2015b). Distribution is worldwide and endemic in most large cities. Epidemics occur at irregular intervals; the greatest incidence is in late winter and spring in temperate climates. Mild varicella breakthrough infection occurs in approximately 10% to 20% of those previously vaccinated; however, the vaccine has been shown to be 97% protective against severe disease (Gershon, 2014).

The incubation period is 10 to 21 days (mean of 14 to 16 days). The period of communicability is 1 to 2 days before the rash erupts until all lesions have crusted over (about 3 to 7 days). Communicability can be prolonged in individuals who received varicella immune globulin or IGIV (AAP et al, 2015b).

Clinical Findings

The following two phases are seen in varicella:

1. Prodrome: Not always present. It is composed of low-grade fever, listlessness, headache, backache, anorexia, mild abdominal pain, and occasionally URI symptoms. These symptoms may occur 1 to 2 days before onset of the second phase.
2. Rash: Classic appearance. It is centripetal, beginning on the scalp, face, or trunk. Crops of generally highly pruritic lesions progress from spots to "teardrop vesicles" that cloud over and umbilicate in 24 to 48 hours. After a few days, all morphologic forms can be seen simultaneously. An average number of lesions is about 300 (LaRussa and Marin, 2011). Scabs last from 5 to 20 days, depending on the depth of the lesions. There can be high fever, to 105° F (40.6° C). The more severe the rash, the higher the fever. Lesions can develop on all mucosal tissues, mouth, pharynx, larynx, trachea, vagina, and anus. Breakthrough varicella disease can occur more than 42 days after vaccination and should be regarded as contagious irrespective of the number of vesicles that are present (LaRussa and Marin, 2011).

Diagnostic Studies

Since the incidence of varicella disease has decreased, many providers may be unfamiliar with the clinical presentation of the disease, especially in mild cases with few lesions. Diagnostic studies can play an important role in these instances. For both unvaccinated and vaccinated persons, the most reliable method for diagnosing VZV is the PCR (preferred) or direct fluorescent antibody (DFA) done from scrapings of a vesicle base during the first 3 to 4 days post-eruption. Tzanck smears of lesions demonstrate multinucleated giant cells containing intranuclear inclusion bodies but are not specific for VZV. A positive serologic test for varicella-zoster IgM antibody is also confirmatory. Serial IgG antibody titers from acute and convalescent samples can also be compared for diagnosis confirmation. The virus can be cultured from vesicular fluid, CSF, and biopsy of tissue but is less sensitive than the PCR. The WBC count is usually within normal limits.

Differential Diagnosis and Management

The rash is classic; therefore, the diagnosis is usually not a problem. Figure. 24-3 shows differences in distribution of the maculopapular eruptions and prodromal symptoms of scarlet fever, chickenpox, and smallpox. Occasionally, impetigo, cigarette burns, and insect bites can cause some confusion in children with a mild rash. Other infections that can be confused with varicella include eczema herpeticum, HSV, and Stevens-Johnson syndrome.

Chickenpox is usually a benign infection in normal children. Treatment is supportive and includes management of itching with antihistamines or oatmeal baths, acetaminophen for fever, and antistaphylococcal penicillin or cephalosporins for bacterial superinfections until the bacterial agent has been identified. Children with fever for more than several days, or increasing temperatures 4 or more days after the appearance of the rash, should be evaluated closely for invasive disease. Aspirin is contraindicated because of the possibility of Reye syndrome. The use of ibuprofen for fever has been questioned because of a possible causal relationship with bacterial superinfections (Gershon, 2014).

Intravenous acyclovir is efficacious for immunocompromised individuals and for those with severe disease. See Table 24-3 regarding use of varicella immune globulin; it is not effective after the disease has progressed. Oral acyclovir is expensive and is not routinely recommended for most children. When given to otherwise healthy children within

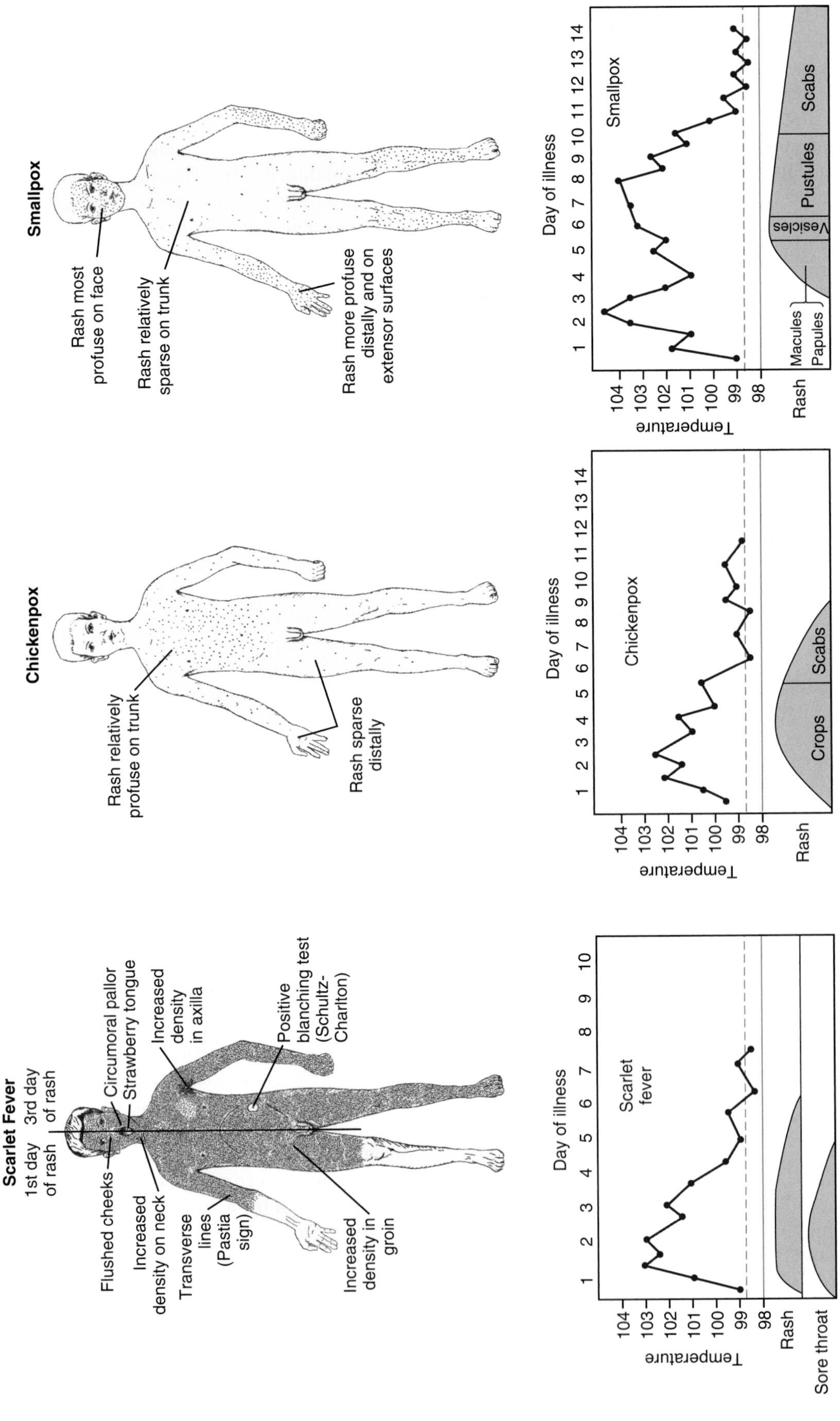

• **Figure 24-3** Differences in distribution of the maculopapular eruptions of scarlet fever, chickenpox, and smallpox.

24 hours after eruption of the rash, there is a modest decrease in the symptoms and duration of the illness. Indication for the use of oral acyclovir is available from the CDC and AAP Red Book (CDC, 2013b). It can also be considered for use in pregnant women with varicella, especially in their second or third trimester. The safety of acyclovir to the fetus in the first trimester is uncertain; however, one large study showed that exposure to acyclovir or valacyclovir in the first trimester of pregnancy was not associated with an increased risk of major birth defects (Pasternak and Hviid, 2010).

Complications

The following complications can occur: pyodermas (about a 5% incidence, causing serious invasive disease with *Streptococcus* and *Staphylococcus*); ITP (1% to 2%); pneumonia (with smoking as an increased risk factor); CNS complications (e.g., encephalitis and Reye syndrome); and, rarely, glomerulonephritis, orchitis, hepatitis, toxic shock, osteomyelitis, necrotizing fasciitis, myositis, myocarditis, arthritis, and appendicitis. Primary varicella is rarely associated with mortality since the licensure of the varicella vaccine; highest mortality is found in newborns and immunocompromised children (Gershon, 2014). Neonatal involvement is directly tied to the timing of the maternal infection with varicella. See Chapter 39 for a discussion about congenital varicella syndrome.

Patient and Family Education

- Children exposed to chickenpox can attend school for about 1 week. If they begin to show signs of illness, they must be kept home for 1 week. If they do not break out in a rash, they may return to school. Children with active disease are to be kept home until all lesions are dry.
- Exposed patients: Use of varicella immune globulin has been discussed and can cause asymptomatic infection. Individuals who received this immune globulin should obtain age-appropriate varicella immunization (unless contraindicated) in 5 months. See further recommendations regarding varicella immune globulin for the immunocompromised in the AAP Red Book or from the CDC. Varicella vaccine is previously discussed.

Influenza Viral Infections

Influenza virus is an orthomyxovirus of three antigenic types: A, B, and C. Types A and B are responsible for epidemic disease; type C is attributed to sporadic mild influenza-like illness in children. Type A is further classified into two surface proteins—hemagglutinin (H) and neuraminidase (N). Three hemagglutinin subtypes and two neuraminidase types are known to cause disease in humans (e.g., H1N1, HIN2, and H3N2). Variant influenza viruses can also infect humans and originate from swine and domestic or wild avian sources. Influenza is a highly contagious disease and is spread person to person by direct contact, droplet contamination, and fomites recently contaminated with infected nasopharyngeal secretions.

Typical Influenza

In temperate climates, typical influenza epidemics occur in the winter months, last approximately 4 to 8 weeks, and peak 2 weeks after the index case. Influenza illness circulates year round in countries closest to the equator. In recent years, some epidemics have lasted 3 months as a result of more than one strain of virus circulating within a community. Children, particularly those of school age, can shed the virus longer than adults (10 days versus 5 days) and, therefore, are particularly prolific transmitters within a community. After the emergence of a newly shifted subtype, the highest incidence of the illness occurs in healthy children 5 to 18 years old. Children younger than 2 years old (especially infants younger than 6 months old), individuals 65 years old and older, and those with chronic diseases have excessively high rates of hospitalization. Mortality rates in the United States from 1976 to 2006 ranged from 3,000 to 49,000 deaths per year (CDC, 2015j). Those 65 years and older account for the majority of deaths; children under 5 years old with high-risk conditions account for most deaths in children (AAP et al, 2015b).

The incubation period is 1 to 4 days. Patients become infectious 24 hours before the onset of symptoms. Viral shedding usually peaks by day 3 and ceases 7 days after the onset of illness.

Clinical Findings

Classic clinical symptoms include a sudden onset of high fever (102° F to 106° F [38.8°C to 41° C]), headache, chills, coryza, vertigo, sore throat, pain in the back and extremities, and a dry hacking cough that can resemble pertussis. Vomiting, diarrhea, and croup can occur in young children, as well as conjunctival infection and epistaxis. Infants can appear septic. In severe infection, there can be involvement of the lower respiratory tract with atelectasis or infiltrates. Severe influenza-associated myocarditis (evidenced by weak heart sounds and rapid, weak pulse) results in distention of the right side of the heart and CHF. Acute symptoms generally last 2 to 3 days, rarely over 5 days.

Diagnostic Studies. Rapid influenza diagnostic tests demonstrate limited sensitivities and predictive values. They are useful when determining the etiology behind a respiratory disease outbreak in certain settings (e.g., schools, camps, hospitals) or if the child has been in recent close exposure to pigs, poultry, or other animals and was possibly exposed to novel influenza A virus infection. A negative result should not be the determining factor when deciding on a clinical course of treatment (e.g., antiviral treatment), to stop an outbreak, or to protect others at risk for complications (CDC, 2015k). Special viral cultures taken from the nasopharyngeal or nasal cavity by swab, nasal wash, or aspirate (depends upon test used) within 72 hours of the onset of illness can isolate the virus in 2 to 6 days to confirm the diagnosis. Other tests for influenza virus include serology (uses acute and convalescent sera), PCR, immunofluorescent assay (IFA), and rapid molecular assays. A CBC may show leukopenia.

Differential Diagnosis, Management, and Complications

The differential diagnosis includes other viral respiratory infections (e.g., common cold, parainfluenza, respiratory syncytial virus, rhinovirus, avian flu based on risk factors), allergic croup, epiglottitis, and bacterial pulmonary infections (e.g., *M. pneumoniae*).

Treatment is supportive (bed rest, fluids, over-the-counter antipyretics, cough medications). Children and parents need to be advised of symptoms that would warrant further medical consultation (e.g., dehydration, difficulty breathing, muscle weakness). Hand hygiene, barrier protection (e.g., masks, gowns), and social distancing should be promoted. Five antiviral medications are approved for treatment or chemoprophylaxis of influenza A and B strains in the United States. However due to viral resistance to amantadine and rimantadine, the ACIP recommends that neither be used until susceptibility is reliable (CDC, 2015l). Treatment or prophylaxis with antiviral therapy (i.e., zanamivir, oseltamivir, or peramivir [restricted to those 18 years old or older] in the United States) should be reserved for the following children or adolescents (CDC, 2015l):

- Children with immunosuppression
- Children younger than 2 years old
- Children with chronic illnesses (pulmonary [including asthma], cardiovascular [excludes hypertension alone], renal, hepatic, hematological [including sickle cell disease], metabolic disorders [including diabetes mellitus], neurologic and neurodevelopment conditions [including seizure disorders], intellectual disability, moderate to severe developmental delay, muscular dystrophy, or spinal cord injury)
- Women who are pregnant or postpartum (within 2 weeks after delivery)
- Youth younger than 19 years old who are receiving long-term aspirin therapy
- American Indians/Alaska Natives
- Children who are morbidly obese (i.e., BMI is 40 or greater)
- Children in residential care facilities

When antivirals are indicated, treatment should be started within 48 hours of symptom onset and continued until the patient is asymptomatic for 24 to 48 hours. The FDA recommends oseltamivir to treat influenza in those 2 weeks old or older and for chemoprophylaxis in those 1 year old or older. The AAP and CDC endorse its use to treat influenza in those under 2 weeks old and as chemoprophylaxis in those 3 months to 1 year old (CDC, 2015m). The effectiveness of the antivirals can vary from year to year based on the virus and strains in play for that season. PCPs can consult the CDC website "FluView Interactive" (see Additional Resources on the Evolve site) for information regarding circulating strains and antiviral resistance patterns within their geographic regions during influenza season.

Complications include Reye syndrome, respiratory infections (acute otitis media [AOM], pneumonia), acute myositis, toxic shock, myocarditis, and cystic fibrosis and asthma exacerbations followed by bacterial superinfection, usually with *H. influenzae*. Do not give aspirin to influenza sufferers!

Patient and Family Education

Influenza vaccine should be widely promoted (see Influenza Vaccine section). Although not mandated by any professional organization, the Infectious Diseases Society of America (IDSA), the Society for Healthcare Epidemiology of America (SHEA), and the Pediatric Infectious Diseases Society (PIDS) recommend that all health care providers receive yearly influenza vaccine to protect themselves and prevent the spread of this disease to their patients and families. This action is viewed as an ethical obligation of all health care providers and personnel (IDSA, 2013).

Highly Pathogenic Avian Influenza

The highly pathogenic avian influenza A (HPAI H5N1 or, simply H5N1) virus has the potential to acquire genes from the influenza virus that affects other species. It is spread quickly and has morphed into a more pathogenic virus than when it first emerged in 1996. There is little natural immunity in humans; fortunately the disease in humans is still restricted and uncommon, and the virus has not yet mutated to be efficiently transmitted from person to person. To date, only humans who have had known direct contact with sick or dead poultry, wild birds, or who have visited live poultry markets are most at risk for acquiring the virus. The outbreak worldwide has not diminished significantly, and health care providers in the United States should remain on alert. Human cases have been reported in Asia, Africa, the Pacific, Canada, Europe, and Near East. The highest number of cases occur in Indonesia, Egypt, and Vietnam (CDC, 2015n).

Humans who acquire the disease may experience a range of mild to more severe symptoms. Symptoms include fever (often >100.4° F [38° C]), cough, sore throat, malaise, myalgias, abdominal pain, diarrhea, and respiratory symptoms progressing to pneumonia with shortness of breath, difficulty breathing, and hypoxia. Complications of severe infection include acute respiratory and multiorgan system failure leading to death. To date, the mortality rate in humans has been approximately 60% (WHO, 2015b). A vaccine for HPAI H5N1 has been recently developed. If avian influenza is suspected, CDC provides guidance in obtaining specimens, monitoring suspected cases, and advising precautions for those traveling to endemic locales. The United States has banned importation of birds (dead or alive) and bird products (including hatching eggs) from H5N1-affected countries (a list of countries is available from the CDC).

Other Viral Diseases

Human Immunodeficiency Virus

Human immunodeficiency viruses (serotypes HIV-1 and HIV-2) are retroviruses that cause disease in humans. Retroviruses are RNA viruses that must make a DNA copy of their RNA in order to replicate. HIV cells enter into a target CD4+ T cell and, using the reverse transcriptase enzyme, convert their RNA into DNA that integrates with the T-cell DNA within the cell nucleus, permanently infecting the host cell. Through processes of transcription, translation, and maturation the HIV genes convert into messenger RNA and leave the nucleus. Eventually new virions bud from the CD4+ T cells, infect other cells, and the cycle is repeated. HIV persists in infected individuals for life; latent virus protein remains in cells of the blood, brain, bone marrow, and genital tract even when the plasma viral load cannot be detected.

Both serotypes cause clinically indistinguishable disease; most of the infections worldwide are attributed to HIV-1 (HIV-2 is less common and generally limited to West African and India). In the United States, HIV-1 group M subtype B is the most prevalent, but non-subtype B and group O strains have been detected in infants whose mothers come from regions in Africa, India, Southeast Asia, or countries in proximity to these countries (U.S. Department of Health and Human Services [USDHHS], 2015).

The worldwide burden of HIV/acquired immune deficiency syndrome (AIDS) remains high with approximately 35 million individuals infected with HIV at the end of 2013. Sub-Saharan Africa remains the most affected region and accounts for approximately 90% of all children with newly diagnosed infection (Shetty and Maldonado, 2016). Antiviral treatment is increasingly available in low- and middle-income countries; however, pediatric coverage with these drugs is lagging as compared to coverage for adults (WHO, 2014b). Limited resources in some countries also make unscreened blood products a viable means of transmission.

In the United States (including the six dependent territories, and the District of Columbia) from 2008 through 2012, the annual estimated number of diagnoses of HIV infection remained stable while the overall estimated rate decreased using a confidential named-based reporting system. Rates were stable for children younger than 13 years old and 15 through 19 years old but increased for children 13 and 14 years old and individuals 20 through 29 years old. The rate of female infection decreased. Eighty percent of infections occurred in adolescent and adult males with over 50% of youth unaware they were infected. Because of the long incubation period (8 to 12 years), these adolescents may not experience symptoms until they are in their 20s or 30s.Transmission was greatest for males through male-to-male sexual contact and/or injection drug use (67%), or for females, through heterosexual contact (26%). Increased rates of infection were seen for American Indians/Alaska Natives and Asians, whereas there were decreased or stable rates for all other categories of ethnicity and race (CDC, 2015o, 2015p, 2015q). Vertical transmission from an infected mother to her infant occurs more often in non-Hispanic African Americans and Hispanics, although race and ethnicity are not risk factors alone (socioeconomic and injection drug use are suspected contributors).

Humans are the only known reservoir for HIV-1 and HIV-2. Although there are AIDS-like syndromes in other primates and felines, infection cannot be obtained from pets, animals, or insects. HIV has been isolated from blood (lymphocytes, macrophages, and plasma), CSF, pleural fluid, cervical secretions, human milk, feces, saliva, and urine. However, only blood, semen, cervical secretions, and human milk are implicated in transmission. Transmission is through intimate sexual contact, sharing of contaminated needles for injection (inconclusive mode for HIV-2), transfusion of contaminated blood or blood products, perinatal exposure, and breastfeeding. HIV-2 has lower transmissibility rates than HIV-1 (Luzuriaga, 2012). Accidental needlesticks in occupational settings rarely account for seroconversion with no confirmed cases of occupational transmission since 1999 in the United States. Transmission from accidental needlesticks from nonoccupational sources has not been documented. Transmission of HIV from a human bite (even when saliva is contaminated with blood) or from antibody-screened blood transfusions in the United States are extremely rare (CDC, 2015r). A small number of children have been reported to have acquired HIV from sexual abuse (Yogev and Chadwick, 2011).

The transmission of HIV to infants can occur in several ways. In utero transmission accounts for about 30% of infections (intrauterine transmission usually occurs by 10 weeks of gestation and is associated with early, severe disease in the newborn); via intrapartum transmission (at least 60%; from infected blood and cervicovaginal secretions in the birth canal or microtransfusions occurring between mother and fetus during labor); or postpartum transmission via breast milk (15%: transmission rates can range from 33% to 50% globally in resource-poor countries) (Shetty and Maldonado, 2016; UNICEF, 2015; Yogev and Chadwick, 2011). Risk of an untreated HIV-infected woman giving birth to an infected infant with HIV-1 is 25% to 35% (4% or less for HIV-2) (Luzuriaga, 2012). In vaginal twin deliveries, the firstborn twin has a greater risk of developing HIV than the second. Other risk factors for increased transmission include maternal drug use, premature rupture of membranes more than 4 hours before the onset of labor, low birthweight, and premature birth before 34 weeks (Shetty and Maldonaldo, 2016; Yogev and Chadwick, 2011). Transmission has been reported in infants who were fed premasticated food by HIV-1-infected caregivers (USDHHS, 2015).

Mother-to-child transmission has been virtually eliminated in the United States and other high-income countries due to rigorous universal antenatal HIV testing, use of combination antiretroviral treatment (cART), cesarean births (cesarean delivery reduces the risk of fetal infection by 87% if zidovudine is also given to both mother and infant), and abstaining from breastfeeding (Shetty and Maldonado, 2016).

Studies confirm that transmission rates increase with longevity of breastfeeding; infants exclusively breastfed until 6 months have one-third the risk of infection than those breastfed until 2 years old. Exclusive breastfeeding may offer some protective immune factors, and the concentration of HIV in breast milk has been found to increase when mixed feeding occurs and after weaning (Kuhn et al, 2013; UNICEF, 2015). In developing countries where pediatric AIDS is pandemic, treatment regimens—out of nutritional necessity—have traditionally included breastfeeding plus short-term antiretroviral drug treatment for women and infants.

The incubation period is variable. The onset of symptoms of HIV infection in infants untreated perinatally can occur as early as 5.2 months (Shetty and Maldonaldo, 2016). The infection can also have a latency period longer than 5 years. Disease progression and earlier mortality are more rapid in children born to mothers with advanced infection, low CD4+ T-lymphocyte count, and high viral loads. In sub-Saharan Africa, approximately 30% of children untreated with antiviral medication succumb to the disease by 1 year old, and more than 50% die before they turn 2 years old. Children untreated that live in the United States and Europe have a mortality rate between 10% and 20% (Shetty and Maldonado, 2016).

Clinical Findings

HIV infection is often experienced as an influenza-like illness (fever, rash, sore throat, lymphadenopathy, and myalgias) for 2 to 4 weeks. These symptoms can suggest a nonspecific viral process, and a provider may not consider HIV in the differential diagnosis. At this point, the asymptomatic infection may continue for a few months to up to 15 years, depending on the viral load. The CD4+ T cells start declining at an average rate of about 50 cells/μL/year.

There are four HIV clinical categories for children with HIV infection, ranging from "not symptomatic" to "severely symptomatic." These categories, paired with the degree of age-specific CD4+ T-lymphocyte count and total percentage of lymphocytes, are used to determine the stage of disease and management strategies. Newborn examinations are usually normal. Lymphadenopathy is often the first symptom, then hepatosplenomegaly. Some children have failure to thrive, chronic or recurrent diarrhea, pneumonia (*Pneumocystis jiroveci* peaks at 3 to 6 months of age), oral candidiasis, recurrent bacterial infections, chronic parotid swelling, and progressive neurologic deterioration. Those with high HIV loads develop symptoms earlier, including failure to thrive and encephalopathy. Other opportunistic diseases are *Mycobacterium avium* infection, severe CMV after 6 months old, EBV, VZV, disseminated histoplasmosis, RSV, *M. tuberculosis*, and measles (despite vaccination).

Children—other than infants—generally have more recurrent bacterial infections (20%), parotid gland swelling, lymphoid interstitial pneumonitis, or neurologic deficiencies that can progress to encephalopathy. *S. pneumoniae*, Hib, *S. aureus*, and *Salmonella* organisms are common infections in pediatric AIDS patients. Sinusitis, cellulitis, gingivostomatitis, herpetic zoster, glomerulopathy (especially in those of African descent), cardiac hypertrophy, anemia, CHF, and purulent middle ear infections are common. Malignancies are uncommon in pediatric AIDS (Yogev and Chadwick, 2011).

Diagnostic Studies

With newborn HIV screening, approximately 30% to 40% of those infected in utero will be identified within 48 hours of birth and nearly 93% by the time they are 2 weeks old. Those infected intrapartum might become positive 2 to 6 weeks after birth (Shetty and Maldonaldo, 2016). Most infants without other exposure risks (e.g., those breastfed) will lose maternal antibody between 6 and 12 months, but some can take as long as 18 or more months to serorevert (Yogev and Chadwick, 2011). Table 24-6 lists recommended tests and testing times.

Lymphopenia occurs as the disease progresses. There are decreased circulating CD4+ cells (T-suppressor, T-helper cells), and the helper-suppressor ratio is less than one. The CDC defines an individual as suffering from autoimmune deficiency disease (e.g., AIDS) when their CD4+ T cell count is less than 200/mm^3. Some AIDS patients become seronegative late in the disease because the weakened immune system cannot manufacture antibodies.

Partners and other children of the HIV-infected mother need to receive appropriate HIV screening. In cases where an infant is adopted or in foster care and when the HIV status of the mother is unknown, an appropriate HIV testing for age should be performed. HIV-infected pregnant women are advised to start antiretroviral treatment during pregnancy, irrespective of their CD4+ cell counts and HIV RNA levels, to help prevent vertical transmission (USDHHS, 2014a). Prior to starting a newborn on antiretroviral prophylaxis, a CBC and differential need to be taken, because anemia is often a side effect of some of the drugs.

If HIV infection is suspected because of history in a child over 18 months old, screening HIV antibody assays plus a confirmatory antibody test or virologic detection test are warranted. In cases of acute HIV infection or AIDs, antibody tests may be negative and different virologic testing is necessary. A pediatric HIV specialist should be consulted.

Differential Diagnosis

The differential diagnosis includes other causes of immunologic deficiency, such as recent therapy with an immunosuppressive agent, lymphoproliferative disease, congenital immunologic states, inflammatory bowel disease, DiGeorge syndrome, ITP, chronic allergies, cystic fibrosis, graft-versus-host reaction, congenital CMV, toxoplasmosis, ataxia, or telangiectasia.

Management and Complications

Treatment goals include suppressing viral replication to undetectable levels; restoring/preserving immune function; reducing HIV-associated sequelae; minimizing drug toxicity; promoting normal growth and development; promoting treatment regimen adherence; and improving quality of life. Any information about HIV and AIDS treatment in

TABLE 24-6 Testing Schedule for Human Immunodeficiency Virus in the Exposed, Non-Breastfeeding Infant¶ in the United States

Test*	Time After Birth
First HIV DNA PCR† or HIV qualitative RNA assay‡ from peripheral blood (not cord blood); confirm if positive using the same test on another blood sample	Within 48 hours
Optional, HIV DNA PCR† or HIV qualitative RNA assay‡; confirm if positive	14 to 21 days (some clinicians prefer this optional testing date)
Second HIV DNA PCR† or HIV qualitative RNA assay‡; confirm if positive	1 to 3 months
Third HIV DNA PCR† or HIV qualitative RNA assay‡; confirm if positive	4 to 6 months
Fourth§ HIV DNA PCR† or HIV qualitative RNA assay‡; confirm if positive	12 and 24 months

Data from U.S. Department of Health and Human Services (USDHHS): Guidelines for the use of antiretroviral agents in pediatric HIV infection: diagnosis of HIV infection in infants and children, AIDSinfo (website), 2015, available at http://aidsinfo.nih.gov/guidelines/html/2/pediatric-arv-guidelines/55/diagnosis-of-hiv-infection-in-infants-and-children. Accessed March 20, 2015.

DNA, Deoxyribonucleic acid; HIV, human immunodeficiency virus; PCR, polymerase chain reaction; RNA, ribonucleic acid.

*The following tests for HIV are not recommended for use in those younger than 1 month old: HIV culture; HIV p24 antigen assay; immune complex dissociated (ICD) p24 antigen assay. Those older than 18 months old can be tested using an HIV antibody assay. Most tests will detect both HIV-1 and HIV-2 infection but will not discern between the two. HIV-2 infection can be confirmed using other tests.

†HIV DNA PCR testing may be preferable for infants who are receiving combination antiretroviral treatment (cART) prophylaxis or preemptive treatment because HIV RNA assays may be less sensitive in the presence of such treatment.

‡The newer qualitative HIV RNA PCR assay detects HIV-1 non-type B or group O strain in infants and is recommended for infants born to mothers from Africa, India, or Southeast Asia or if infection is suspected and the initial HIV DNA PCR assay(s) are negative (HIV DNA PCR has limited sensitivity to this subtype/strain).

§This fourth test is an option to document loss of maternal antibodies in infants 12 to 18 months old with prior negative tests; or to definitely exclude or confirm HIV infection in infants 18 to 24 months with prior HIV-antibody positive tests.

¶Infant is considered infected if two separate samples test positive by HIV DNA PCR or qualitative HIV RNA PCR. Infant <18 months old and non-breastfeeding is considered *definitely negative* if two negative tests are obtained at ≥1 month and ≥4 months OR two separate negative tests are obtained at ≥6 months AND no other laboratory or clinical evidence that suggests HIV/acquired immune deficiency syndrome (AIDS).

children is subject to change, and the provider is advised to check with the CDC or AIDSinfo regarding updated guidelines for diagnosis, treatment, monitoring drug toxicity and adherence, and specific immunization precautions and regimens. Treatment decisions and laboratory studies should be made in consultation with a pediatric HIV specialist.

Current recommended drug regimens for cART include at least three oral antiretroviral drugs from at least two drug classes. Generally two nucleoside reverse transcriptase inhibitors (NRTIs) plus either a non-nucleoside reverse transcriptase inhibitor (NNRTI) or protease inhibitor (PI), often boosted with low-dose ritonavir, are used. Treatment regimens are individualized based on a number of factors (e.g., age, immune status, viral load, clinical categories, viral resistance, potential adherence issues, drug toxicity, and comorbid conditions); frequent laboratory studies and possible antiretroviral changes throughout the life of the individual are required. Such effective cART regimens have resulted in an 81% to 93% reduction in mortality from 1994 to 2006 in the United States and United Kingdom. Some children infected as infants are living into their third and fourth decades of life with the potential to live longer (USDHHS, 2015).

Established protocols for the HIV-infected mother and her newborn are available on the AIDSinfo website (see Additional Resources on the Evolve site). The prophylaxis protocol using zidovudine (or alternatives) for the HIV-exposed newborn from birth to 6 weeks old can be accessed at https://aidsinfo.nih.gov/contentfiles/lvguidelines/PerinatalGL.pdf, Table 8. Ensure blood work has been done before initiating the prophylaxis regimen. The infant should be discharged from the hospital with the full 6-week course of zidovudine in hand for the parent, not just a prescription, with complete instructions for administration. This helps ensure greater compliance and continuity of prophylaxis. Additionally, infants with known HIV exposure whose status remains unknown or who are HIV infected, should be prescribed trimethoprim-sulfamethoxazole as prophylaxis against *Pneumocystis jirovecii* at 4 to 6 weeks old until the child is 1 year old (administered either on 3 consecutive days a week or daily). If the newborn proves to be uninfected with HIV, the prophylaxis can be stopped. Alternative prophylaxis antibiotics are available on the AIDsinfo website (see Additional Resources on the Evolve site). Treatment of associated conditions with appropriate medical therapy is indicated using IGIV, antifungals, antivirals, antimycobacterials, and nutritional counseling. After delivery, mothers need to be encouraged to continue their cART, use a reliable method of birth control, and take precautions to prevent sexual transmission of the virus. At present, it is not clear from clinical and laboratory studies if in utero exposure to cART taken by the mother may have any long-term sequelae in the child/adolescent (USDHHS, 2014b).

Treatment of a child (versus newborn) infected with HIV also requires collaboration with pediatric HIV specialists because drug regimens are complex and are constantly being revised. Adolescents can present a particular noncompliance risk because of denial and fear of their infection, substance abuse and addiction, misinformation, distrust of and inexperience with the medical system, self-esteem issues, unstable living situations, and lack of familial and social support systems. It is important for the provider to be nonconfrontational yet discuss risk factors and advocate for family planning services and needle exchange programs, postexposure prophylaxis regimens, and prompt involvement in new treatments as they become available.

An important role of the PCP in HIV treatment is helping to boost adherence rates. In addition, side effects must be monitored closely because many of the antiretroviral drugs can interact with other commonly prescribed medications (including oral contraceptives). The treatment regimens are highly challenging for parents because of complex dosing schedules and unwillingness of children to take the required medications. Many preparations are not offered in liquid form or the taste is not attractive to children. See Chapter 22 for information about addressing and enhancing medication adherence rates in children and adolescents.

HIV becomes a multisystemic illness with multiorgan complications.

Prevention and Reduction of Perinatal Transmission of Human Immunodeficiency Virus

The CDC, WHO, and United Nations AIDS agencies are useful resources for current treatment regimens; recommendations may vary by country. WHO strategies for preventing the transmission of HIV to women and from mother to child include:

- Improve access to antiretroviral therapy for HIV-infected women and children. The use of cART to reduce perinatal transmission of HIV has become the accepted treatment standard in developed and underdeveloped countries. WHO recommends using a once-daily simplified triple antiretroviral drug regimen for all pregnant and breastfeeding women with HIV, with consideration of lifelong treatment (WHO, 2014c).
- Improve access to testing (less than 40% of people in United Nation Member States know their HIV status); encourage use of self-testing kits for early diagnosis and treatment (one has been approved by the FDA; others are under development).
- Increase blood/tissue/surgical/injection safety education.
- Expand maternal/newborn/child health care (to initiate earlier treatment and prevention education).
- Expand sexual and reproductive health education.
- Strengthen infant nutrition support.
- Use cesarean delivery if indicated.
- Promote exclusive breastfeeding by HIV-positive mothers.
- Increase availability of chemophylaxis for the neonate and infant until HIV status is known (WHO, 2011).

In the United States, guidelines for preventing transmission by HIV-infected women include discouraging breastfeeding, even if on cART. Delivery by cesarean is recommended, depending upon the mother's viral load (CDC, 2015p).

However, research in underdeveloped countries, notably from South Africa, demonstrates that a combination of exclusive breastfeeding and cART by the mother or infant can significantly reduce the risk of transmitting HIV through breast milk. Protection against HIV infection increases if the infant is breastfed exclusively prior to 6 months with continued breastfeeding to 12 months. HIV-positive women who are being treated with cART in developing countries are encouraged to breastfeed their infants (Langa, 2010).

Because cART is now standard treatment for HIV-infected pregnant women and their infants, adherence to the recommended postnatal HIV prophylaxis for both the mother and her infant can be problematic. One meta-analysis demonstrated that only 73.5% of pregnant women achieved an 80% or greater adherence rate; this rate decreased in the postpartum period. Reasons for lack of adequate adherence were attributed to the following factors (Nachega et al, 2012):

- Concern about the safety of antiretroviral therapy drugs on the fetus or woman
- Advanced AIDS stage and health-related symptoms of pregnancy (nausea, vomiting, fatigue)
- HIV disease
- Other physical or economic factors
- Depression (especially postpartum)
- Presence of alcohol or drug abuse
- The complexity and length of antiretroviral therapy drug regimens for woman or infant
- Lack of social support

More recent studies reinforced those of Nachega and colleagues and also found that other mental health issues, age, homelessness, poverty, inconsistent access to antiretroviral therapy, and HIV stigma were associated with lower adherence, whereas trust and/or satisfaction with the HIV care provider were correlated with higher adherence (Langebeek et al, 2014; USD-HHSHHS, 2014b) in the United States.

The following should be standard knowledge and practice for providers in terms of HIV:

- Health care providers need to be alert to the potential risk of transmission of HIV infection to infants in utero, in the postpartum period, and through human milk. Counsel caregivers against giving premasticated food to infants.
- Document routine HIV education and routine testing with consent of all adolescents seeking prenatal care; ensure that each adolescent knows her HIV status and the methods available to prevent the acquisition and transmission of HIV to her newborn.
- At the time of delivery, provide education about HIV and complete a rapid HIV testing with consent if HIV status is unknown.
- Women in the United States diagnosed with HIV infection just prior to labor or soon after delivery or those who have known infection risks (e.g., injection drug users) but whose status is unknown at delivery should be advised against breastfeeding. If a woman desires to breastfeed, she can be assisted to pump (and discard milk) until HIV testing is done and seronegativity is confirmed.

- There are no special precautions for handling expressed breast milk of HIV-infected women. No transmission to another infant has been reported after a single exposure to milk expressed by an HIV-infected mother (CDC, 2009). Pasteurization and donor screening ensures the safety of human milk banks. The nonprofit Human Milk Banking Association of North America (HMBANA) sets standards of testing for all their members' milk banks.
- Adolescents must be counseled about the risk of HIV transmission (e.g., sexual transmission, sharing of needles or syringes) and the use of condoms. Condom use during last intercourse was reported by 59.1% of adolescents, whereas only 12.9% report ever having had an HIV test (female rates are higher than for males) (Kann et al, 2014).
- School attendance for HIV-infected children: The benefit from attendance far outweighs the risks. Factors that must be taken into account include the risk to the immunosuppressed child from "normal germs" from healthy kids and school personnel. Because casual transmission is unknown, there is no real risk to other children as long as the infected child can control body secretions. Children who display biting behavior or have oozing wounds should be cared for in a setting that minimizes risk to others. The child's PCP is the only person with an absolute need to know the child's primary diagnosis. If the family decides to inform the school, those informed should maintain confidentiality. If the family chooses not to inform the school, parents should get assurance that the school will notify them of any communicable disease outbreaks (e.g., varicella, measles) or physical altercations with others.
- Routine screening of school-age children for HIV antibodies is not indicated.

Preexposure Prophylaxis for Certain High Risk Individuals

Preexposure prophylaxis (PrEP) is now recommended in the United States and by the WHO for those at ongoing, substantial risk of being infected with HIV. Individuals who would qualify for PrEP include those having male-to-male anal sex without a condom or with a diagnosed sexually transmitted disease in the past 6 months; those having sex with an HIV-positive partner; injection drug users who share equipment or who have been in a drug treatment program in the past 6 months; individuals not in a monogamous sexual relationship with partners who have not been recently tested and found to be HIV-negative; or heterosexual men or women who do not use condoms and have sex with high-risk partners (e.g., bisexual males, injection drug users). In studies, the rates of getting HIV ranged from 62% to 92% depending upon the risk factor noted earlier (CDC, 2015s). The prophylaxis regimen involves a fixed-dose combination of two antiretroviral drugs taken daily. The clinical practice guideline for PrEP is available on the CDC website (see Additional Resources on the Evolve site). The efficacy and safety for use in adolescents has not been established, so the risks and benefits are still being studied. A monthly-inserted vaginal ring with an antiviral and two long-acting injectable antiviral agents are under development as alternatives to daily PrEP.

Postexposure Prophylaxis After Nonoccupational Exposure

The PCP may be faced with having to assess and counsel parents after their child has had an accidental puncture wound from a discarded needle found in a public setting; from a wound obtained from a bite, a fight, or during a sports activity; or from sexual abuse. Though transmission is extremely rare, the PCP needs to be able to address the situation with a level of understanding of the risks and recommendations of the CDC.

The body fluids of an HIV-infected person do not all carry the same amount of viral load or risk. For example, exposure to blood of a known HIV-infected person carries the highest risk, whereas blood-free saliva, semen or vaginal secretions, and human milk carry a low risk; urine, feces, and vomitus are unlikely to transmit the virus. Syringes that might have been used and discarded by an HIV-infected, injection-drug user generate the most concern of parents. The following information is useful when counseling parents (Smith et al, 2005):

- HIV viability is vulnerable to drying.
- The smaller the needle bore, the more limited the amount of blood present.
- There has been no documented transmission of HIV from an accidentally found, discarded needle.
- One is more likely to face greater risk from biting an individual who is HIV-positive (saliva contaminated with HIV-infected blood) than from having been bitten by one infected with HIV (saliva not contaminated by infected blood).

The PCP and parent must weigh the unproven safety and benefits of participating in the postexposure prophylaxis (PEP) regimen against the significant toxicity of the drugs themselves. If instituted, PEP therapy ideally needs to start within 72 hours after exposure and continue for 28 days. Close follow up for support, medication monitoring (adherence and toxicity), and serial HIV antibody screening are needed (Box 24-1 provides some management strategies). The CDC provides an algorithm for evaluating and treating possible nonoccupational exposure and makes recommendations as to whether or not PEP is warranted. Consult the CDC website for current guidelines.

Measles (Rubeola)

Measles (rubeola) is a Morbillivirus in the Paramyxoviridae family and is similar to mumps and influenza and is a serious illness in children. There is only one antigenic type. Measles is characterized by a rash, indicating viremia. Worldwide, approximately 20 million people annually become infected with measles with 146,000 deaths. In the

• BOX 24-1 Management After Possible Exposure to Human Immunodeficiency Virus

1. Treat the exposure site.
   - Wash wounds with soap and water; flush mucous membranes with water. Give Td or Tdap booster if appropriate (see Table 24-2 and Table 24-3).
2. Evaluate the exposure source if possible to guide need for postexposure prophylaxis.
   - Determine the human immunodeficiency virus (HIV) infection status of the exposure source. If unknown, testing with appropriate consent should be offered if possible.
3. Evaluate the exposed person.
   - Perform HIV serologic testing to identify current HIV infection and hepatitis B and hepatitis C serologic testing as appropriate.
   - Provide or refer for counseling to address stress and anxiety.
   - Discuss prevention of potential secondary HIV transmission.
   - Discuss prevention of repeat exposure, if appropriate.
   - Report the incident to legal or administrative authorities as appropriate to the setting of the exposure and the severity of the incident.
4. Consider postexposure prophylaxis (not to be used for frequent exposures).
   - Explain potential benefits and risks.
   - Discuss issues of drug toxicity and medication compliance.
   - Measure complete blood cell count, creatinine, and alanine transaminase concentration as baseline for possible drug toxicity.
   - Begin postexposure prophylaxis as soon as possible after exposure, preferably within 1 to 4 hours; prophylaxis begun more than 72 hours after exposure is unlikely to be effective.
   - Arrange for follow up with HIV specialist and psychologist if appropriate.
   - Educate about prevention of secondary transmission (sexually active adolescent should avoid sex, or use condoms, until all follow-up test results are negative).
5. Choose therapy (should contain three [or more] antiretroviral drugs).
   - Consider drug potency and toxicity, regimen complexity and effects on compliance, and possibility of drug resistance in the exposure source.
   - Supply 3 to 5 days of medication immediately, instructing patients to obtain remainder of medication at follow-up visit (for total of 28 days).
6. Follow up.
   - Perform initial follow up within 2 to 3 days to review drug regimen and adherence, evaluate for symptoms of drug toxicity, assess psychosocial status, and arrange appropriate referrals, if needed.
   - Ensure has enough medication to complete 28-day regimen.
   - Monitor for drug adverse effects at 4 weeks with complete blood cell count and alanine transaminase concentration.
   - Evaluate for psychological stress and medication compliance with weekly office visits or telephone calls.
   - Consider referral for counseling if needed.
   - Repeat HIV serologic testing at 6 weeks, 12 weeks, and 6 months after exposure.

From Havens PL, Committee on Pediatric AIDS: Postexposure prophylaxis in children and adolescents for nonoccupational exposure to human immunodeficiency virus, *Pediatrics* 111(6):1475–1489, 2003, reaffirmed 2009; Kuhar DT, Henderson DK, Struble KA, et al: Updated US Public Health Service guidelines for the management of occupational exposures to human immunodeficiency virus and recommendations for postexposure prophylaxis, *Infect Control Hosp Epidemiol* 34(9):875–892, 2013.

United States, annual rates since 2000 have ranged from 37 (in 2004) to 668 (in 2014); a multi-state outbreak occurred in 2015 (CDC, 2015t). Most of the cases in the United States have originated in unvaccinated individuals who imported the measles after being in countries where large outbreaks have been reported (including, but not limited to, England, France, Germany, India, the Philippines, Asia, and Africa). The disease spreads within communities where there are larger numbers of unvaccinated or undervaccinated individuals and where herd immunity falls below a critical point.

Humans and primates are the only known reservoir of infection. The sources of the infection include respiratory secretions, blood, and urine of infected persons. Virus is transmitted through droplet contact, fomites, and, less likely, aerosol transmission. Peak incidence of infection in susceptible persons occurs during late winter and spring months. Once exposed, approximately 9 out of 10 susceptible individuals will develop the disease (CDC, 2015t).

The incubation period for measles is 8 to 12 days; for modified measles, as long as 21 days. A person is contagious 1 to 2 days before the onset of symptoms or 3 to 5 days before the rash, and 4 days after the appearance of the rash, or roughly 14 days (range 7 to 18 days). There is no carrier state; disease or two vaccinations usually confer lifelong immunity.

Clinical Findings

The clinical manifestations are divided into three stages:

1. Incubation period: There are no specific symptoms.
2. Prodromal period: This first sign of the illness lasts 4 to 5 days and consists of URI symptoms, low to moderate fever (greater than 101° F [38.3° C]), and cough, coryza, and conjunctivitis (the "three Cs" of measles). An enanthem (Koplik spots) can be found on the oral mucosa opposite the lower molars. They are small, irregular, bluish white granules on an erythematous background, last 12 to 15 hours, and are pathognomonic of measles infection.
3. Rash stage: The rash of unmodified measles usually appears on the third or fourth day of the illness. As the rash appears, temperature rises, often to 105° F (40.5° C).

The rash is maculopapular and first appears behind the ears and on the forehead. Papules enlarge, coalesce, and move progressively downward, engulfing the face, neck, and arms over the next 24 hours. By the end of the second 24 hours, the rash has spread to the back, abdomen, and thighs. As the legs become more involved, the face begins to clear. The entire process takes approximately 3 days. Respiratory symptoms are most severe on day 3 of the rash. The more severe the rash, the more severe the illness. It can become hemorrhagic. This type of measles can be fatal because of disseminated intravascular coagulation (DIC). The rash begins to fade after the fourth day. The disease peaks; defervescence occurs. After the rash clears, a residual desquamating light-colored pigmentation occurs, lasting approximately 1 week.

Modified measles illness can present in children who have been passively immunized with immunoglobulin after exposure to the disease, have residual maternal antibodies, or have received an improperly administered measles-containing vaccine. In these cases, the illness is an abbreviated version of the typical disease. The prodrome period can last 1 to 2 days with normal to low-grade fever. URI symptoms are minimal to absent. Koplik spots usually do not appear. The rash is so mild that it is often missed.

Diagnostic Studies

A single measles IgM antibody level is useful if drawn when symptoms appear; the reactivity is low after more than 30 days. Confirmation of disease can also be made by viral isolation from urine, blood, throat or nasopharyngeal secretions, or from serial IgG antibody titers that compare acute and convalescent serum specimens. Measles is a reportable disease in the United States within 24 hours of diagnosis.

Differential Diagnosis and Management

Any viral rash, toxoplasmosis, scarlet fever, Kawasaki syndrome, meningococcemia, Rocky Mountain spotted fever (RMSF), drug rashes, and serum sickness are included in the differential diagnosis.

Treatment is supportive (antipyretics, bed rest, adequate fluids, air humidification, warm room, darkened room if photophobia is present). No antiviral therapy is available, although ribavirin has been used off label to treat severe measles infections and in children who are immunocompromised (AAP et al, 2015b). Bacterial superinfections (e.g., ear infections, bronchopneumonia, and encephalitis) are treated with appropriate antibiotics. All children with encephalitis, severe pneumonia, or compromised immune systems should be managed in consultation with an infectious disease expert.

Children in the United States and in countries where malnutrition is an issue are at greater risk for death or morbidity with measles infection. These children, and those with severe measles, have lower vitamin A levels. The WHO recommends vitamin A for all children despite their country of residence. Dose once daily for 2 days: under 6 months old, 50,000 international units; 6 through 11 months old, 100,000 international units; 12 months old or older, 200,000 international units.

Care of Exposed Individuals

The measles vaccine should be given within 72 hours of exposure to those who are vaccine-eligible and who have been exposed. This is the first choice to prevent or modify the infection and may be given to infants 6 to 11 months old (AAP et al, 2015b). Immune globulin (IGIM or IGIV) given within 6 days of exposure can be administered to prevent or modify the disease in those susceptible (those without prior measles vaccine, infants younger than 12 months old, pregnant women, and immunocompromised individuals), regardless of their measles vaccination status.

Complications

Bacterial superinfection and viral complications can manifest as a URI, obstructive laryngitis, otitis, diarrhea, mastoiditis, cervical adenitis, bronchitis, transient hepatitis, and pneumonia (the largest cause of fatalities in infants). The causative organism can be the measles virus itself or group A beta-hemolytic streptococci (GABHS), pneumococci, *H. influenzae,* or *S. aureus*. Infection can exacerbate underlying TB. Other complications include myocarditis, purpura fulminans ("black measles," characterized by multiorgan bleeding), encephalitis and other neurologic sequelae, and subacute sclerosing panencephalitis (fatal complication of wild-type measles). There are usually no complications with modified measles.

Mumps

Mumps is an acute generalized viral disease with painful enlargement of one or more salivary glands (usually parotid glands). Mumps is in the Paramyxoviridae family. Only one serotype is known, and humans are the only natural reservoir. The source of infection is contact with the saliva and/or respiratory tract secretions of infected persons. Incidence of this illness has decreased by more than 99% in the United States since the advent of the mumps vaccine (CDC, 2015u). After two doses, the effectiveness of mumps vaccine ranges from 66% to 95%; higher rates of infection occur more often in individuals who are unvaccinated or undervaccinated. Infection occurs during all seasons but is most common during late winter and spring and in children younger than 10 years old; it affects both sexes equally. Mumps virus crosses the placenta; studies are inconsistent in determining whether or not infection during the first trimester increases the risk of spontaneous abortion or intrauterine fetal demise. Fetal malformations after prenatal mumps infection have not been demonstrated (AAP et al, 2015b).

The incubation period ranges from 12 to 25 days (usually 16 to 18 days). The period of communicability is about 1 to 2 days before glandular swelling and up to 5 days after the onset of swelling. About one third of patients are asymptomatic or only have URI symptoms. Lifelong immunity is usually conferred after one infection; rarely is a second infection seen.

Clinical Findings

There are two clinical stages:

1. Prodromal stage: Rare in children but can cause fever, headache, anorexia, neck or other muscular pain, and malaise.
2. Swelling stage: Approximately 24 hours after the prodromal stage, 31% to 65% of those affected will have painful swelling of one or both parotid glands. If both glands are affected, one generally swells before the other. The gland fills the space between the posterior border of the mandible and mastoid, pushing downward and forward to the zygoma. The ear is pushed forward and upward. Swelling can take a few hours to a few days. The enlarged glands usually return to normal size in 3 to 7 days. Rarely a maculopapular, pink discrete rash is seen on the trunk. Pain on the affected side can be elicited by having the patient eat something sour. This is known as the "pickle sign." The Stensen duct is red and swollen. The Wharton duct is frequently swollen. Fever is usually moderate; 20% are afebrile. Ten percent to 15% of cases involve only submandibular gland swelling. Little pain is associated with submandibular infection; however, the redness subsides more slowly. If sublingual salivary glands are involved, there is bilateral swelling in the submental region in the floor of the mouth. Edema caused by lymphatic obstruction of the manubrium and upper chest is reported. Orchitis may occur in individuals who contract mumps after puberty.

Diagnostic Studies

This virus can be detected from a buccal swab (Stenson duct exudate), throat washings, saliva, or spinal fluid using RT-PCR and serologic tests (mumps-specific IgM antibodies or serial acute/convalescent titers for IgG antibodies). Leukopenia with relative lymphocytosis and an elevated amylase are typical. Test results are more reliable for diagnosis when specimens are obtained within 1 to 3 days after onset of symptoms (AAP et al, 2015b).

Differential Diagnosis, Management, and Complications

Cervical or preauricular lymphadenitis, CMV, HIV, enteroviruses, tumor, suppurative parotitis by bacterial (e.g., nontuberculous mycobacterium) or viral (influenza A, coxsackievirus, parainfluenza 1 and 3, EBV) infection, idiopathic recurrent parotitis, parotid ductal obstruction, Mikulicz syndrome, uveoparotid fever, and cancer (especially lymphosarcoma) are included in the differential diagnosis.

Treatment is supportive (antipyretics, bed rest as needed, diet appropriate for chewing discomfort). Corticosteroids or nonsteroidal anti-inflammatory drugs (NSAIDs) are given to manage arthritic complications. Manage orchitis with bed rest and scrotal elevation. School and day care students should be kept home until 9 days after the onset of parotid swelling. Active and passive immunization have been discussed.

Complications include meningoencephalitis (mostly males older than 20 years old); orchitis and/or epididymitis (10% incidence in postpubertal males; sterility is rare); oophoritis (in postpubertal women; fertility is not affected); rarely pancreatitis, thyroiditis (uncommon in children), myocarditis, deafness (transient or permanent), arthritis (rare in children), thrombocytopenia, hemolytic anemia (usually self-limited), mastitis, and glomerulonephritis.

Erythema Infectiosum

Erythema infectiosum, or fifth disease, is caused by parvovirus B19. The virus is a member of the Parvoviridae family and is a single-stranded DNA virus that replicates in erythrocyte precursors. It is called *fifth disease* because it was the fifth childhood eruptive rash described historically. These rashes include measles, scarlet fever, rubella, Filatov-Dukes disease, erythema infectiosum, and erythema subitum (roseola infantum, sixth disease). Humans are the only reservoir. Erythema infectiosum is spread via vertical transmission from mother to fetus, by respiratory tract secretions, and percutaneous exposure to blood or blood products. Distribution is worldwide. It is a disease of childhood, highest in 5- to 15-year-olds, but infants and adults are not immune. Secondary spread to household contacts is up to 50% (AAP et al, 2015b). The disease occurs most commonly in late winter and early spring.

The incubation period is approximately 4 to 21 days; the rash and symptoms occur between 2 and 3 weeks after exposure. The highest period of communicability is before the appearance of the rash, joint pain or swelling (the latter two seen rarely in children). Chronic infection can occur in those immunocompromised or with most types of hemolytic anemias.

Clinical Findings

The following two phases are seen in erythema infectiosum:

1. Prodrome: Consists of mild fever (15% to 30% of cases), myalgia, headache, malaise, and/or URI symptoms.
2. Rash: Appears 7 to 10 days after the prodromal stage and occurs in three stages: It first appears on the face as an intense red eruption on the cheeks (slapped cheek) with circumoral pallor that lasts 1 to 4 days. Next a lacy maculopapular eruption appears on the trunk, and then moves peripherally to the arms, thighs, and buttocks. Palms and soles are generally spared. This phase can last a month. Finally, the rash subsides. Older children may have mild pruritus. There may be periodic recurrences precipitated by trauma, heat, exercise, stress, sunlight, or cold (Fig. 24-4). Children less commonly experience arthralgia (more often in the knees) than adults, who

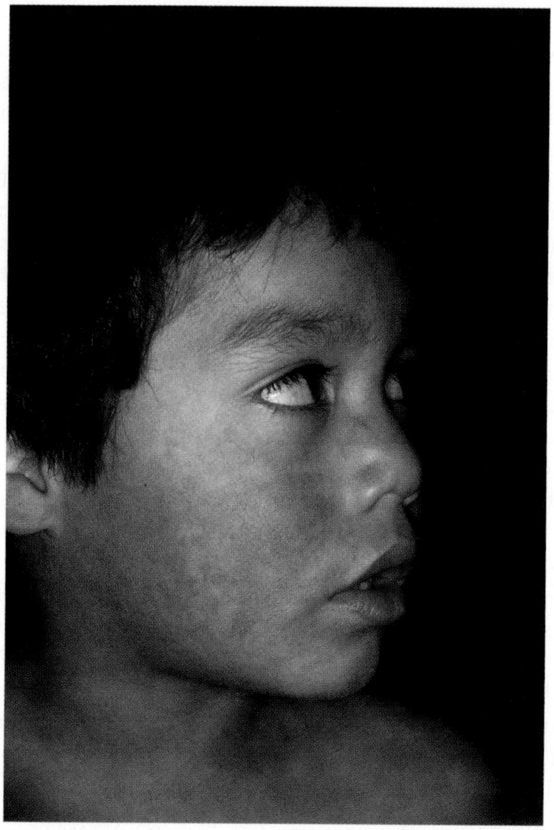

• **Figure 24-4** Erythema infectiosum, fifth disease.

may complain of symmetric polyarthropathy. Arthralgia most commonly resolves in 2 to 4 weeks. Those with hemolytic anemias or who are immunocompromised may have fever, pallor, tachycardia, and symptoms of heart failure.

Diagnostic Studies

Laboratory testing is not generally indicated because the diagnosis can be made clinically. Serum B19-specific IgM antibody confirms the presence of infection and persists for 6 to 8 weeks. Anti-B19 IgG confirms past infection. For immunocompromised individuals, PCR assay is the method of choice. Standard cultures are not useful.

Differential Diagnosis, Management, and Complications

This is not a difficult disease to diagnose. The differential diagnoses include rubella, enterovirus disease, lupus, atypical measles, and drug rashes.

There is no specific antiviral treatment. Those with hemolytic anemia or who are immunocompromised should be considered for transfusion. IGIV offers some help for those with immunocompromised conditions. Because there is widespread undetected infection in children and adults, avoidance of known exposure can reduce but not eliminate the risk of infection. Children in the rash stage may attend school.

Complications are few and typically not significant in all previously healthy patients; recovery is usually without sequelae. The most frequently reported complications include arthritis (hands, wrists, knees, and/or ankles occurring 2 to 3 weeks after onset of initial symptoms); chronic infection in those immunodeficient; aplastic crisis (more common in those with chronic hemolytic anemias, including sickle cell anemia, thalassemia, hereditary spherocytosis, or other types of chronic hemolysis); thrombocytopenic purpura or neutropenia; myocarditis (rare); papular-purpuric "gloves and socks" syndrome (fever, pruritus, purpura, painful edema, and redness in a glove-and-sock distribution pattern) followed by petechiae and oral lesions; or fetal hydrops and death or intrauterine growth retardation if exposed in utero (no reports of congenital anomalies) (AAP et al, 2015b). An exposed pregnant woman should consult with her health care provider.

Parainfluenza Virus

Human parainfluenza virus (hPIV), a paramyxovirus, is similar to the influenza and mumps viruses and is an important cause of laryngotracheobronchitis (croup), bronchitis, bronchiolitis, and pneumonia. This virus accounts for 7% of hospital admissions of children younger than 5 years old. In the United States, epidemiologic studies attribute hPIV to two thirds of croup cases, one quarter of tracheobronchitis, and 50% of URIs (colds, laryngitis, pharyngitis, otitis media) in children (Yogev and Breese Hall, 2014).

There are four antigenic types of hPIV. Types 1 and 2 usually strike children 1 to 5 years old and are most frequently associated with croup; outbreaks are seen more in summer and fall and in odd-numbered years; reinfections occur at any age. Type 3 is endemic, associated more with bronchitis, bronchiolitis, and pneumonia in those younger than 12 months old, results in shorter immunity (a particular problem for immunocompromised patients), and outbreaks tend to peak in the spring and summer (sometimes into fall months). Type 4 infections are less well pathologically and clinically understood, may be more pervasive than once thought, and can cause mild to severe respiratory illness. By the time most children are 5 years old, they have been exposed to all of the types. An individual can expect to have repeated infections due to hPIV during their lifetime as immunity is transient and limited.

This virus is spread by direct person-to-person contact through infected nasopharyngeal secretions or from fomite contamination. It replicates in the superficial ciliated epithelial cells lining the airways of the upper and lower respiratory tract and spreads readily. The incubation period is 2 to 6 days. Healthy children can shed virus for 4 to 7 days before symptom onset and up to 7 to 21 days after resolution of symptoms. The virus can live on nonporous surfaces for up to 10 hours (Yogev and Breese Hall, 2014).

Clinical Findings

Symptoms may include an acute onset of mild fever, sore throat, rhinitis, hoarseness, and cough (including a typical "croup" cough). Lower respiratory involvement symptoms include dyspnea, crackles, wheezing, and hyperaeration. In older children and adolescents, recurrent infection may manifest as a mild URI.

Diagnostic Studies

Routine testing is not needed. Specific RT-PCR assays are the standard diagnostic test when needed. The virus can be isolated from nasopharyngeal secretions; culture results are usually available within 4 to 7 days (or earlier) depending on the testing technique available. Sensitivities vary when rapid antigen identification is done by IFAs and enzyme immunoassays. WBC count may be normal or slightly elevated with a mild lymphocyte elevation.

Differential Diagnosis, Management, and Complications

The differential diagnosis includes other viral URIs, allergic croup, laryngotracheitis, bacterial tracheitis, retropharyngeal abscess, epiglottitis, laryngeal diphtheria, foreign body aspiration, or GI reflux.

The treatment is supportive; recovery is uncomplicated in most cases. Reliable studies using ribavirin are lacking; therefore, aerosolized ribavirin should only be considered for high-risk patients with severe lower respiratory involvement (Yogev and Breese Hall, 2014). With the newer outpatient guidelines for managing croup, few children progress to needing hospitalization (see Chapter 32). Antibiotics are reasonable in cases of severe infection when secondary bacterial invasion is suspected (e.g., otitis media, bronchitis, tracheitis, pneumonia). No vaccine is available; intravenous immune globulin is not helpful. Good hand hygiene is important.

Complications are infrequent. Those who are immunocompromised are more prone to developing secondary bacterial infections.

Rubella (German or 3-Day Measles)

Rubella is an acute disease of childhood that occurs either postnatally or congenitally. Rubella is an RNA virus of the genus Rubivirus, in the Togaviridae family. Humans are the only reservoir; disease is seen more in adolescents and young adults (Cherry and Adachi, 2014). Infection is spread through nasopharyngeal secretions or transplacentally during either apparent or silent infection. It is worldwide in distribution. The virus has been isolated in blood, breast milk, conjunctival sac, and urine of infected individuals.

One must have prolonged and repeated contact to become infected. The incubation period is 14 to 21 days (mean 18 days). The maximum period of viral shedding (and presumed transmissibility) is believed to be 5 days before to 6 days after the appearance of the rash. Males and females are equally affected. Genetic factors may play a role in the degree of transmissibility. Infants infected in utero can shed virus past their first birthday (Cherry and Adachi, 2014). In the United States, disease occurs during the winter and spring months, notably March, April, and May. There is lifelong immunity after naturally occurring disease; however, asymptomatic reinfection can occur. Because illness without rash exists, the actual number of reinfections is unknown. Reinfection is known to occur from wild-type virus and in those previously immunized.

Use of the rubella vaccine has eliminated endemic rubella infections in the United States and other countries with national immunization programs. Most cases in the United States now occur in those unvaccinated (including infants born to unvaccinated mothers), foreign-born, or immigrants from areas with poor vaccination coverage. Endemic rubella rates have increased and congenital rubella remains high in the Western Pacific, Southeast Asia, and some African regions where vaccination programs are not universal (Cherry and Adachi, 2014).

If primary maternal rubella infection occurs during the first 12 weeks of pregnancy, there is an estimated 61% risk of congenital defects (ophthalmologic, cardiac, auditory, or neurologic); the risk is 26% if maternal infection occurs in the second trimester (Cherry and Adachi, 2014). In pregnant women reinfection rarely results in congenital rubella syndrome. Accidental revaccination of a pregnant woman should not be considered a reason for pregnancy termination alone; surveillance demonstrates signs of infection in the infant but not congenital rubella syndrome (Cherry and Adachi, 2014).

Clinical Findings

Approximately 25% of infections are subclinical (Cherry and Adachi, 2014). Postnatal disease is marked by three stages:

1. Prodrome: The mild symptoms of fever (101.5° F [38.6° C], lower GI upset, sore throat, eye pain, arthralgia, malaise, and headache occur about 1 to 5 days prior to onset of stage 3 and are occasionally missed.
2. Lymphadenopathy: Usually begins within 24 hours, but can begin as early as 7 days before the rash appears, and can last for more than 1 week. The postauricular, posterior cervical, and posterior occipital are the primary lymph nodes involved. There is generalized lymph node involvement, and at times splenomegaly is noted.
3. Rash: An enanthem (known as Forchheimer spots) can appear before the general rash, consisting of small rose-colored to reddish spots on the soft palate. The enanthem is not considered pathognomonic. The rubella rash (discrete maculopapules that occasionally coalesce) is often the first obvious sign of illness, typically begins on the face, can fade before it spreads to the chest and caudally during the next 24 hours, and is usually gone by the third day. There can be itching without a rash or a fine, bran-like desquamation. A low-grade fever can occur during the eruptive phase and continue for up to 3 days. There is no photophobia; anorexia, headache, and malaise are rare. Exanthems occur less often in adolescents and young adults; there may be more pruritus. A facial rash acneiform in appearance is more likely found in adolescents (Cherry and Adachi, 2014).

Diagnostic Studies

Diagnosis is usually made by clinical symptoms. Real-time RT-PCR and RT-PCR of nasal or throat (preferred) specimens can be used to detect this virus. Serologic testing for confirmation of disease or immunity includes enzyme immunoassays and latex agglutination tests for rubella IgG and IgM antibodies. However, timing is everything; IgM may not be detectable before the fifth day after the rash appears. If the test is conducted earlier and yields negative results, it should be repeated after day 5. To detect IgG antibody, the specimen should be obtained as soon after symptom onset as possible, and then repeated in 7 to 21 days. Level of IgG antibody can also be used to determine immune status due to natural infection or vaccination. False-positive rubella IgM tests can occur due to the presence of rheumatoid factors or other viral infections. Leukopenia tends to occur.

Differential Diagnosis, Management, and Complications

The disease can be difficult to diagnose unless there is an epidemic. The rash can be confused with scarlet fever, mononucleosis, enterovirus, roseola, rubeola, erythema infectiosum, EBV, and drug eruptions.

Treatment is supportive (e.g., antipyretics for fever control) unless complications occur. Children with rubella should be kept home from school or child care for approximately 1 week after the rash erupts. Active and passive immunization have been discussed.

Complications in postnatal rubella in children are not common. These include arthralgia or arthritis and thrombocytopenia or encephalitis. The arthralgia/arthritis (fingers, knees, wrists) occur in those of postpubertal ages with females being afflicted more often than males. Onset is about a week after appearance of rash and symptoms last 3 to 28 days. Thrombocytopenia or encephalitis can occur within 4 days of onset of rash. Severe thrombocytopenic purpura can be managed with corticosteroid therapy and platelet transfusions. Myocarditis, pericarditis, follicular conjunctivitis, hemolytic anemia, and hepatitis are rare complications.

Mosquito-Borne Viruses

West Nile Virus

WNV is an arbovirus (family Flaviviridae) related to St. Louis and Japanese encephalitis viruses. Previously endemic to Africa, West Asia, and the Middle East, the virus has spread globally since 1999, including across the United States (with the exception of Alaska and Hawaii). It recurs yearly during warmer weather, when mosquitoes begin breeding. Temperate climates and drought conditions are believed to encourage mosquito-borne illnesses. WNV is mainly spread to people by bites from a variety of infected mosquitoes (most often the *Culex* genus in the United States). The mosquito feeds at dawn and dusk and breeds in standing water. Rarely, the virus spreads through organ transplantation, blood transfusions, placenta, breast milk, and possible aerosol transmission. The blood supply has been screened for WNV in the United States since 2003, but organ and tissue donation programs routinely do not screen (Denman and Hart, 2015).

Mosquitoes become infected by feeding on the blood of previously mosquito-infected birds. They then transfer the virus via saliva to other birds (including chickens and turkeys), horses, humans, and other animals (e.g., cats, dogs, squirrels). The level of viremia is amplified within the birds, and a hallmark of the presence of WNV in communities may be the die-off of specific bird species, notably ravens, crows, magpies, and jays; resistance may be developing in some avian species over time. Bird-to-human transmission is not believed to occur unless dead infected birds are handled without precautions to blood and tissues (Denman and Hart, 2015).

Symptoms in immunocompetent humans develop 2 to 14 days after being bitten by an infected mosquito. The disease more frequently affects children aged 10 and older. Morbidity and mortality rates are highest in individuals who have preexisting chronic diseases, are immunosuppressed, had organ transplants, or are older adults. Neuroinvasive disease affects less than 1% of cases, mostly older adults, but can be severe and deadly with a mortality rate of approximately 0.6% in children (Martin et al, 2014).

Clinical Findings

The provider needs to take seasonality, presentation, and virulence into consideration because symptoms can mimic those of influenza or GI infection and be misdiagnosed. Only about 20% of individuals exhibit signs and symptoms (Denman and Hart, 2015), which are nonspecific and typically include fever (100.4° F to 104° F [38° C to 40° C]); headache; muscle aches; eye pain; rash (typically on chest, back, arms; can occur in 50% of children); lymphadenopathy; weakness; anorexia; nausea; diarrhea, abdominal pain, and vomiting. Myocarditis and hepatitis can occur occasionally in children (Martin et al, 2014).

Those with mild disease experience symptomatic relief within a week, but fatigue may linger for a few weeks longer. Children with severe infection may experience typical symptoms plus neuroinvasive involvement. CNS symptoms, severe headache, change in mental status (disorientation), awkward gait or paralysis, optic neuritis, myelitis, polyradiculitis, stiff neck and nerve abnormalities, tremors or seizures, respiratory failure, stupor, or coma might be seen. Most pregnant women who contract WNV deliver infants who show no signs of congenital WNV involvement. However, the newborn should be closely examined for congenital anomalies, neurologic and hearing deficits, and signs of viral infection.

Diagnostic Studies. Consider testing children with a febrile or acute neurologic illness whose history includes exposure to mosquitoes, prenatal exposure with or without breastfeeding, recent blood transfusion, or organ transplant. The test of choice is IgM antibody capture–enzyme-linked immunosorbent assay (MAC-ELISA) from serum or CFS collected by day 7 or 8 (more likely detectable) of clinical symptom onset. Serial titers are then collected 2 to 3 weeks apart to compare acute and convalescent samples. Positive tests should be confirmed by other specific WNV tests. A blood count may be normal or show leukocytosis, leukopenia, lymphopenia, or anemia. In those with hepatitis or myositis, transaminases and creatine kinase may be elevated. MRI or CT scan (or both) are indicated if the individual has neurologic findings. A newborn exposed in utero to WNV should have either cord or infant serum tested for IgM after delivery.

Differential Diagnosis, Management, and Complications

Mild viral or influenza infection, GI viral infection, aseptic meningitis, poliomyelitis, Guillain-Barré syndrome, dengue fever, chikungunya, St. Louis encephalitis, and acute flaccid paralysis are included in the differential diagnosis.

For asymptomatic or mild cases, supportive treatment is indicated (rest, fever control, hydration, and perhaps control of nausea/vomiting). Hospitalization is indicated for those with symptoms of meningitis, encephalitis, or severe muscle weakness, paralysis, dysphagia, or dysarthria. Antiretrovirals are not indicated in routine cases. Closely follow cases occurring in the young, those with respiratory symptoms, or with comorbities.

With severe infection, complications include encephalitis, meningoencephalitis, meningitis, cardiac dysrhythmias, optic neuritis, uveitis, chorioretinitis, orchitis, myocarditis, pancreatitis, Guillain-Barré syndrome, respiratory muscle paralysis, and hepatitis.

Patient and Family Education

To prevent disease, one must avoid mosquito bites. Mosquito abatement programs have been instituted in communities to reduce mosquito breeding grounds. Counseling includes:

- Stay indoors during the mosquitoes' most active times—dawn and dusk; if one must be outdoors during these times, wear light-colored, long-sleeved shirts and long pants.
- Apply insect repellent with either N,N-diethyl-3-methylbenzamide (DEET; formerly N,N-diethyl-meta-toluamide), picaridine 5% to 10%, oil of lemon eucalyptus, or soybean oil to exposed skin (permethrin and DEET can be applied to clothing), Concentration of DEET depends on length of time of expected exposure to mosquitoes or ticks: 10% DEET confers approximately 2 hours of protection; 30% about 5 hours. Apply according to length of protection needed. Use sparingly and wash DEET off with soap and water when the child is inside (AAP, 2012).
- Do not use DEET on skin or clothing of children younger than 2 months old. Do not use greater than 30% strength DEET on children. Do not apply to face, hands, or open wounds/cuts.
- Do not use combination sunscreen and DEET products because sunscreen needs to be reapplied more frequently; the DEET component applied too frequently can be toxic.
- Inventory outdoor areas for standing water that serves as breeding areas for mosquitoes (e.g., old tires, pots or containers, birdbath [change once a week], neglected swimming pools, pool or spa covers). Keep pools and spas clean and chlorinated.
- Use tight-fitting screens on all doors and windows.
- Report any dead birds, especially crows, jays, hawks, magpies, and owls, to local health department or pest control agency.

A vaccine for humans is under development; equine vaccines are available and recommended for horses.

Dengue Virus

Dengue virus (DENV) is an RNA virus belonging to the Flaviviridae family with four serotypes (DENV1, -2, -3, and -4). There is no cross immunity between serotypes; in fact, cross-reactivity occurs between serotypes that can often intensify the disease on subsequent infections. Lifelong immunity is gained to specific serotypes once they have caused infection. Serotypes DENV1 and DENV4 cause primary infection more often; DENV2 and DENV3 are more likely to cause severe dengue hemorrhagic fever. The virus is transmitted to humans by a bite from an infected *Aedes aegypti* (less commonly *Aedes albopictus* or *Aedes polynesiensis*) mosquito. A human can pass along the virus through blood transfusions, organ transplants, percutaneous exposure to blood, or transplacentally. An infected person can transmit the virus 2 days before symptom onset and during the 7-day period of viremia (this can threaten the blood supply, which is not currently screened for WNV in the United States) (Rios, 2015). The incubation period is 3 to 14 days once transmitted to the human host.

Due to climate change, increased travel, returning military personnel, and emigration from tropical and subtropical regions, DENV and viral hemorrhagic fever are increasingly occurring in the United States, Europe, and other regions of the world. Multiple DENV serotypes make epidemics ubiquitous, occurring in more than 100 countries in the WHO regions of Africa, the Eastern Mediterranean, Southeast Asia, the Western Pacific, and the Americas. The latter three are the most seriously impacted regions. Endemic areas in the United States include Puerto Rico, the Virgin Islands, and American Samoa. Outbreaks have occurred in Texas, Hawaii, and Florida. Worldwide, approximately 284 million to 528 million people are infected each year (WHO, 2015c).

Clinical Findings

History and Physical Examination. If DENV infection is suspected, it is imperative that providers question children and families about travel or residence outside of the United States (including any military deployment), onset of fever, vaccination records, and any prior infections with DENV, WNV, St. Louis encephalitis virus, Japanese encephalitis virus, or yellow fever virus (these have cross-reacting antibodies). Inquire about past 24-hour fluid intake, changes in mentation or dizziness, urinary output, and diarrhea. Approximately 50% of infections are asymptomatic or may have undifferentiated fever (often these are seen in young children or in those experiencing their first infection) (CDC, 2014b). Three phases of infection occur:

- Febrile phase: Fever rises rapidly; can last 2 to 7 days; is greater than 102.2° F (39° C). This phase is typically classified as "dengue fever" and is comprised of the acute fever plus two or more of the following: headaches, retro-orbital pain, photophobia, general body ache, myalgia, arthralgia, facial flushing progressing to maculopapular or morbilliform rash, injected oral pharynx, leukopenia, anorexia, nausea/vomiting, diarrhea, mild epitaxis, bleeding gums, ecchymosis, bleeding at venipuncture sites, hepatomegaly, menorrhagia, or conjunctival injection. A positive tourniquet test points toward DENV (WHO, 2012). After this febrile phase, a person may start the recovery phase or continue into the critical phase.
- Critical phase (mild to severe plasma leak): Begins 4 to 7 days after viral transmission and lasts 3 to 10 days and begins after fever abates. The hallmark is increased capillary permeability as a result of plasma leakage. At this point, the infection may be classified as "dengue hemorrhagic fever." Dengue hemorrhagic fever has four requirements: prior fever of 2 to 7 days; spontaneous bleeding (a tourniquet test is sufficient); platelet count 100,000/mm^3 or less; and evidence of anemia or a progression to "dengue shock syndrome" (internal bleeding, shock, platelet count <50,000/mm^3, hematocrit values ≥20% of normal for age/gender) (Garcia et al, 2015). The increased hematocrit is an important early sign to indicate severe disease as plasma leaks into body tissues. Other warning signs of progressing disease include lethargy, restlessness, confusion, vomiting, severe abdominal pain (GI bleeding), respiratory distress (pleural effusion), ascites, hepatitis, encephalitis, myocarditis, and blood pressure and volume changes. The critical phase may last 24 to 48 hours. The mortality rate can reach over 20% without aggressive treatment at this stage (WHO, 2015c).
- Recovery phase: Reabsorption of extravascular compartment fluid occurs over the following 48 to 72 hours. Other symptoms start resolving; pruritus may occur; ascites, pulmonary and cardiac issues may arise if IV fluids have been given in excess; body systems and laboratory studies normalize.

Diagnostic Studies. A CBC, platelet count, and hematocrit are crucial monitoring studies. Progressive leukopenia is an early sign. A rapid and progressive decrease in platelet count and hematocrit rising above baseline are early signs of plasma leakage. Hematuria may occur. A serum urea more than 4.0 mmol/L (indicates dehydration) and total protein 67.0 g/L or less (indicates plasma leakage into tissues) signify a child is more at risk for hemorrhagic fever and shock syndrome (Garcia et al, 2015).

Isolation of the virus, serology, and molecular tests are available. However, it is a challenge to decide which test is most efficacious based upon the timing of symptoms, course of the disease, and if a specific serotype is needed. The CDC's Dengue Branch can be consulted to help with the decision.

Differential Diagnosis, Management, and Complications

Influenza, other hemorrhagic diseases, sepsis, meningococcemia, adenoviruses, HIV, chikungunya, infectious mononucleosis, measles, rubella, SARS, malaria, Henoch-Schönlein purpura, or other thrombocytopenic purpura syndromes may present with some similar symptoms. It is noteworthy that DENV does not involve upper respiratory symptoms. It is imperative that the provider elicit details about onset of fever, rash, and diagnostic studies to distinguish between the differential diagnoses.

Correct diagnosis and rapid treatment are crucial. In the United States, DENV is a nationally reportable disease to the CDC. Management is supportive, consisting of fluids to prevent dehydration (evaluate child's ability to take in adequate fluids and families ability to care for child), antipyretics, and stringent monitoring for urinary output and bleeding. Infants or children with coexisting conditions should be hospitalized. Children should be seen daily in the clinic during the febrile phase of this illness. Hospitalization is warranted for those showing signs of progressive disease (see Diagnostic Studies). WHO provides a downloadable guideline and useful algorithm for diagnosis and management (see Additional Resources on the Evolve site).

Dehydration and fever in children can result in neurological disturbances and febrile seizures. Severe dengue shock syndrome is a leading cause of serious illness and death among children younger than 5 years old in some Asian and Latin American countries. Myocarditis, pancreatitis, hepatitis, and neuroinvasive disease can occur. Aggressive treatment has brought the mortality rate down to less than 1% (WHO, 2015c).

Patient and Family Education

Prevention is similar to WNV. Community-wide efforts largely focus on controlling vectors with insecticides. Transgenesis and paratransgenesis to reduce insect vectorial capacity or eliminate DENV are being tested and show promise in trials (Mole, 2013a). There is an ongoing effort to develop a dengue vaccine.

Hantavirus Pulmonary Syndrome

Hantavirus pulmonary syndrome (HPS) was formerly referred to as *Hantavirus*. The causative agent is commonly Sin Nombre virus (SNV) in the United States, 1 of 23 Hantaviruses found worldwide that cause considerable morbidity and mortality (Chapman et al, 2014). The virus reservoirs include Old and New World rats, mice, voles, and lemmings, mostly in rural areas; the deer mouse is the most common reservoir in the United States and Canada. Disease is spread by aerosolization of the rodent's saliva, urine, and feces excretions. Because of the widespread distribution and the role of these rodents in biodiversity, eradication is neither feasible nor desirable. Most cases in the United States occur in the spring and summer months but this can vary depending on location and rodent population.

Incidence of HPS is rare in the United States; less than 7% of cases occur in children younger than 17 years old. Thirty-four states in the United States reported cases in 2013, with 95% of those states located west of the Mississippi River (CDC, 2014c). In 2011, HPS resulted in similar mortality rates of about 35% in both the United States and the Americas (Chapman et al, 2014).

Providers should suspect HPS infection in a child with an ill-defined febrile disease (or fever of unknown origin) with abdominal or back pain or myalgia, who lives in or has been in an appropriate rural, endemic geographic setting for HPS, who has thrombocytopenia or proteinuria, or has been exposed to rodents or engaged in an activity where rodent nests or excreta may have been disturbed (e.g., cleaning out barns or sheds). The incubation period is typically 4 to 42 days after exposure to infected rodent excreta. The illness typically involves a prodromal phase of abrupt fever, chills, headache, nausea, vomiting, diarrhea, and myalgia (notably of shoulders, lower back, upper legs) for 3 to 7 days followed by abrupt onset of pulmonary edema, cardiac decompensation, and hypotension. On physical examination, restlessness; flushed face, neck, and upper thorax; injected conjunctiva and pharynx; bradycardia; and petechiae may be seen. There is early thrombocytopenia and leukocytosis with a shift to the left; proteinuria and hematuria may also occur.

The diagnosis is confirmed by detecting hanta-specific IgG and IgM antibodies to SNV using ELISA; RT-PCR can also detect SNV RNA. A rapid diagnostic test is available. Those with suspected HPS need to be hospitalized for supportive management of pulmonary edema, hypoxemia, and hypotension. Generally, the acute illness is followed by a prolonged convalescence period of 3 to 6 weeks, then by complete recovery.

The differential diagnosis includes rickettsial diseases, leptospirosis, influenza, streptococcal pneumonia, legionellosis, *Yersinia pestis* infection (plague), meningococcemia, brucellosis, mycoplasmal and fungal pneumonias (including *Coccidioides immitis* and *Histoplasma* pneumonia), tularemia, psittacosis, and autoimmune disorders (including thrombotic thrombocytopenic purpura).

Human avoidance of rodent waste and nests is the goal in dealing with this disease. Before people work around mouse-infested basements or outbuildings they should read the guideline about cleaning up after rodents, which is available on the CDC website. Chemoprophylaxis or vaccines are not available.

Additional Noteworthy Viruses in Circulation

Human Pneumovirus (Metapneumovirus)

Metapneumovirus (human pneumovirus; hMPV) is a respiratory pathogen of the Paramyxoviridae family, discovered in 2001. Its antigenicity, symptomatology, and epidemiology are closely related to RSV, including a simultaneous (and expanded) seasonal pattern. This agent should be considered as a causative agent of acute respiratory infection among hospitalized children before their second birthday, especially in the late winter/early spring months in temperate climates. Incidence rates range from 5% to 25% in those with acute lower respiratory tract infections. Approximately 95% to 100% of all 5-year-olds are seropositive for this agent with the majority being seropositive by 2 years old (Schuster and Williams, 2014). Symptoms of hMPV may include fever, transient maculopapular rash, vomiting/diarrhea, rhinitis, wheezing/stridor, tachypnea, abnormal tympanic membranes, pharyngitis, hoarseness, rhonchi, rales, and hypoxia. Those with asthma may experience an exacerbation. Chest x-rays may demonstrate diffuse perihilar infiltrates, peribronchial cuffing, lobar infiltrates, or hyperaeration. Viral shedding is for approximately 7 to 14 days. The differential is RSV, parainfluenza, and influenza. Immunoassays, RT-PCR, and serology tests are diagnostic tests. Treatment is supportive; acute respiratory distress requires hospitalization. Ribavirin has had limited application in cases involving immunocompromised children (Schuster and Williams, 2014). A vaccine is under development. Complications can include AOM or later bacterial pneumonia.

Human Calicivirus Infections (Norovirus and Sapovirus)

Norovirus (also called *Hunter virus* and *Norwalk-like virus*) and Sapovirus belong to the Caliciviridae family. These viruses are highly contagious and occur in closed populations, such as in child care centers, schools, camps, cruise ships, hotels, or other closed facilities. Norovirus accounts for about 80% to 90% of the sporadic epidemics of gastroenteritis in children younger than 5 years old and 20% of hospitalizations due to diarrheal illnesses. Most children have antibodies by the time they are 5 years old (Lucero et al, 2014). Transmission is person to person by the fecal-oral route, through contaminated water, or by food contaminated by infected food handlers (notably salads, shellfish, ice, and a variety of ready-to-eat foods [e.g., prepared fruit, bakery products]). Children can also acquire norovirus from contaminated water in public swimming pools, wading pools, water parks, and from flooding where fresh water and sewage mingle. The incubation period is 12 to 60 hours (average 24 hours); the duration of illness is typically 24 to 48 hours (5 to 6 days in endemic settings); and the virus can be excreted for 15 days up to 2 months after onset of symptoms. Symptoms of infection include nausea, vomiting, nonbloody diarrhea, abdominal cramps, chills, headache, muscle aches, and fatigue; some individuals may experience a low-grade fever. Vomiting is more pronounced in children over 1 year old whereas diarrhea is more prominent in infants and adults (Lucero et al, 2014).

Stool specimens will be negative for bacterial, parasitic, or fungal pathogens. Diagnosis can be made with real-time quantitative RT-PCR assay. Enzyme immunoassays are readily available but useful only to screen during gastroenteritis outbreaks. In these circumstances, negative results do not exclude *Norovirus,* and the newer RT-PCR test should be performed.

Treatment is supportive, including rehydration, because dehydration can be a serious complication of norovirus infection. There is no antiviral treatment or vaccine. Preventive measures include child care and school personnel, food handlers, and children/caregivers being trained in good hand washing and other hygienic measures (surfaces should be cleaned with sodium hypochlorite solution or 70% ethanol). Precautions when in public recreational water facilities include not swimming with diarrhea; not swallowing the water; washing children's perianal area with soap and water before going into the water; and taking children for frequent bathroom breaks and diaper checks. This illness can recur.

Coronaviruses

Multiple strains of human coronaviruses (HCoVs) have been identified as causing a variety of respiratory tract infections in humans. Not all of the strains are understood epidemiologically or clinically. It has been postulated that a strain(s) of coronaviruses may also be an enteric pathogen and play a causative role in infants with gastroenteritis and necrotizing enterocolitis (Poutanen, 2012). HCoVs are likely transmitted by a combination of droplet and direct and indirect contact. After rhinoviruses, they are the most common cause of the common cold. Depending upon the strain, some may be associated with AOM, asthma exacerbations, croup, bronchiolitis, pneumonia, gastroenteritis, nausea/vomiting, and febrile seizures. The severe acute respiratory syndrome coronavirus (SARS-CoV) strain can lead to more severe disease.

SARS-CoV is one of the coronaviruses that is better understood, largely due to being the causative strain identified after a worldwide outbreak in late 2003 (no cases since 2004). After mucosal inoculation, this virus can replicate in the lung and GI tract and ultimately lead to clinical deterioration. Fortunately, children are infected less by this strain; when they are infected their illness is more mild than those of adolescents and adults. The U.S. National Select Agent Registry Program has declared SARS coronavirus as having the potential to pose a severe threat to public health and safety (CDC, 2013c).

The incubation period for HCoV strains is a few days (SARS-CoV ranges from 2 to 10 days); HCoV strains typically are transmitted in the first 2 to 5 days of illness (SARS-CoV transmission is more intense during the second week of illness). Outbreaks occur during the winter and spring in temperate climates (winter for SARS).

HCoVs are not typically diagnosed from respiratory tract specimens; however, some specialized laboratories offer comprehensive diagnostic testing based on RT-PCR and can identify HCoV. Antibody tests also are available for SARS-CoV.

Management is supportive for HCoV infections, although SARS-CoV infection involves strict isolation of the index case, respiratory precautions (hand hygiene, gloves, masks), and home isolation of index cases and their caregivers. Drug treatments are under development. Prevention of transmission is the same for other respiratory infections.

Potential Emerging and Reemerging Viruses on the Horizon

Based upon data and statistical modeling, there has been speculation about what "candidate diseases" might appear or reappear, taking into consideration such factors as: global climate changes, increasing international travel, known vectors, increasing drug resistance (notably to HIV, TB, malaria, and pathogens causing pneumonia, sepsis, skin and urinary tract infections), decreased vaccination levels (e.g., polio resurgence reported in 10 countries in 2014) (United Nations News Centre, 2014), importation of wild animals (that serve as vectors), and bioterrorism. Among others, the flaviviruses (dengue fever, Japanese encephalitis, and yellow fever [all with mosquito vectors]), chikungunya (an alphavirus, also with a mosquito as vector), and a new pandemic of influenza (H7N9) are likely to emerge in the United States (Kaye et al, 2010). Also of concern is the spread of the Asian tiger mosquito *(A. albopictus)* to the United States and Europe that carries the St. Louis and La Crosse encephalitis illnesses (Arnold, 2013). Other emerging and re-emerging viruses worldwide include Das-Congo hemorrhagic fever virus, HIV 1 and 2, monkeypox, and other hemorrhagic fever diseases.

Middle Eastern Respiratory Syndrome

Identified in 2012, to date all cases of Middle Eastern respiratory syndrome coronavirus (MERS-CoV) have been linked to countries in and near the Arabian Peninsula. Few cases have been diagnosed in the United States; those identified were found in health workers exposed to the virus in Saudi Arabia. The CDC is continuing to monitor and study this virus in efforts to better understand it because it has the potential to spread to the United States. In the Middle Eastern countries, the illness has occurred in all ages. Symptoms are predominately fever, cough, and shortness of breath progressing to acute respiratory illness. The mortality rate has ranged from 30% to 40% (CDC, 2015v).

Monitoring the Global Spread of Viruses

Global Viral (GV) (formerly the Global Viral Forecasting Initiative) is an international organization that monitors the emergence of deadly viruses spread from animals to humans in order to address the most important global infectious disease threats and detect pandemics as they begin. Among its current activities, the Global Viral Fellows Program supports international research, public health development and education, and scientific leadership. One GV goal is to increase the "bank of genetic information" from known viruses in order to develop vaccines to stop the spread of disease. Newer technologies are being developed to more quickly sequence and identify the genetic identity of viruses. The GV and global partners have numerous "viral listening posts" in sub-Saharan Africa and Southeast Asia where pandemics often start. Air travel and road development increase the transmission of these potentially dangerous viruses.

Parasitic-Caused Disease: Malaria

Malaria is spread worldwide by the bite of the nocturnal-feeding female *Anopheles* genus of mosquito. The mosquito is the vector for the typically five different species of the intraerythrocytic parasite, *Plasmodium,* that infects humans. Poorer tropical and sub-tropical areas of the world experience malaria in epidemic proportions. In the United States, infection is typically acquired from travel or residence from abroad, although anopheline mosquitoes are present in temperate regions of the country. Globally, an estimated 198 million cases of malaria were identified in 2013; 500,000 people died of malaria, mostly children in the African region (CDC, 2015w). Relapses of infection occur because of dormant liver stage parasites (hypnozoite) or chronic asymptomatic parasitemia.

Malaria presents as a febrile nonspecific illness without localizing signs from 7 to 30 days after exposure. Malaria should be suspected in a person with a fever who has recently traveled in an area where malaria is endemic. Antimalarial drugs taken as prophylaxis by travelers may serve to delay symptom onset for up to 12 months. Symptoms typically are high fever with chills, rigor, sweats, and headache, which may appear suddenly and in a cyclic pattern every 2 to 3 days. Nausea, vomiting, diarrhea, cough, pallor, jaundice, tachypnea, arthralgia, myalgia, abdominal and back pain, and hepatosplenomegaly may also occur. The disease can progress in severity and end in death as a result of neurologic compromise, renal and respiratory failure, metabolic acidosis, severe anemia, or vascular collapse and shock.

Diagnostic studies may show anemia, thrombocytopenia, elevated bilirubin, and aminotransferases. Diagnosis is confirmed by identifying the parasite microscopically. Negative smears should be retested every 12 to 24 hours during a 72-hour period. PCR, DNA probes, and RNA testing are also used. A rapid test for antigen detection is available.

Choice of treatment is dependent upon the identified species, possible drug resistance, and severity of disease. Assistance with diagnosis and management is available from the 24-hour CDC Malaria Hotline (770-488-7788). Research is focused on using imidazopyrazine chemicals to disable an enzyme necessary for replication within the parasite (Mole, 2013b). Vaccines and new drugs to combat malaria are under development and in clinical trials.

In malaria-epidemic regions, treatment and preventive efforts involve four measures: (1) case management (diagnosis and treatment), (2) insecticide-treated nets (ITNs), (3) intermittent preventive treatment of malaria in pregnant women (IPTp) and infants (IPTi), and (4) indoor residual spraying (IRS). Larval and other vector control and mass drug administration and mass fever treatment may also be used (see WHO in Additional Resources on the Evolve site for information regarding IPTp and IPTi). The CDC offers useful information regarding a traveler's risk assessment; availability and choice of antimalarial drug prophylaxis (vary) for children and adults; a malaria country map; and preventive measures (see Additional Resources on the Evolve site).

Tick-Borne Diseases

Lyme disease, ehrlichiosis, anaplasmosis, RMSF, tick-borne relapsing fever, babesiosis, tularemia, and African tick bite fever are common tick-borne diseases in the United States. It is important for providers to be aware of the specific tick vectors and epidemic geographic areas of the vectors. Only the first three diseases are discussed here (tularemia is a potential bioterrorism agent). A provider should be suspicious and include tick-borne diseases in the differential diagnosis when an individual complains of influenza-like symptoms (fever, headache, myalgia) during summer (an unusual time for such symptoms), especially if they live and recreate outdoors in endemic areas.

Lyme Disease

Borrelia burgdorferi (Bb), a spirochete, is the causative agent that is carried and transmitted to humans by infected species of *Ixodes* ticks. Lyme disease is the most commonly reported vector-borne infection in the United States and Europe and is a growing epidemic.

The ticks infected with *Bb* in the United States are predominantly found in the northeast, the mid-Atlantic states, Wisconsin, Minnesota, and Northern California (Moore, 2015). Scandinavian countries and central Europe (Germany, Austria, and Switzerland) also report incidences of LD. It is estimated that as many as 300,000 people are diagnosed in the United States each year (CDC, 2015x). When eastern black-legged deer tick *(Ixodes scapularis)* or western black-legged deer tick *(Ixodes pacificus)* larvae hatch in early summer, they are usually not infected. During their life cycle (nymphal and adult molt stages), the tick can feed on an infected host and become infected with *Bb.* In the east, the natural host for *Bb* is the white-footed mouse or deer; in the west, it is the western gray squirrel or western fence lizard, less so chipmunks and some bird species (these are relatively poor reservoirs which accounts for the lower rate of occurrence in the west). Tick vectors in Europe include ground-feeding birds and small and medium-sized mammals. The infected tick then transmits the organism to humans. The infection is more likely to be transmitted by immature ticks in the nymphal stage. The size of the tick in the nymphal stage is about 1 mm (poppyseed size); in the adult stages from 2.5 mm to 4 mm (sesame seed size).

There is varied risk of transmission, depending on the percentage of ticks actually infected with *Bb*. Annual confirmed incidence rates vary (in 2014 a high of 87 per 100,000 cases was reported in Maine) (CDC, 2015y). Boys 5 to 9 years old have higher incidence rates than all other ages (CDC, 2015z1). Coinfection with other tick-borne pathogens must be considered in endemic regions. The risk of human infection after an *Ixodes* tick bite is low, even in endemic areas (1.2% to 4.4% in United States studies) (Sood and Krause, 2014) and is related to how long the tick has fed. It takes hours for the tick to fully implant its mouth into the host's skin and days to become fully engorged. Nymphal ticks must feed for 36 to 48 hours or more and adult ticks for 48 to 72 hours before the risk of transmission of *Bb* is significant; many human victims have removed the tick before this time. However, because of the small size of the tick and possible location on the body where it is lodged (e.g., scalp), an engorged tick may not be noticed before it drops off. The disease is not regarded as being teratogenic to fetal development as long as the mother receives the appropriate antibiotic treatment (CDC, 2015z2). The majority of infections occur from June to August, less so from December through March.

Clinical Findings

Lyme disease can present with a variety of symptoms. Only 25% to 30% of people diagnosed recall having had a tick bite (Nichols and Windemuth, 2013). Classic Lyme disease can be divided into three stages:

1. Stage 1 (early localized disease): Generally within 1 to 2 weeks after the bite, a typical rash may appear at the inoculation site (range from 1 to 31 days; mean 10 days). Erythema migrans (EM) rash begins as a red, annular macule or papule at the site of the tick bite that progresses in 24 to 48 hours to being surrounded by a clearing and then a larger annular erythematous outer ring. It may appear as a "bull's-eye" and needs to be at least 5 cm in size to meet diagnostic criteria for EM (Fig. 24-5). Multiple lesions may occur in different sites; however, 10% of children in North America may not demonstrate EM (Sood and Krause, 2014). EM typically is warm and pruritic but not painful. The rash remains for a few weeks and fades even if untreated. In many cases, the rash does not follow this classic pattern but instead may resemble nummular eczema, tinea, granuloma annulare, an insect bite, or cellulitis; the rapid enlargement of erythema migrans helps distinguish it. Those without EM and 50% with EM may present with flu-like symptoms including fever, malaise, headache, arthralgia, myalgia, and stiff neck (Nichols and Windemuth, 2013). Without treatment, these symptoms, including the rash, may become intermittent, lasting for weeks to months.
2. Stage 2 (early disseminated disease): Through spirochetemia, the organism disseminates through hematologic or lymphatic channels. Secondary annular lesions (1 to

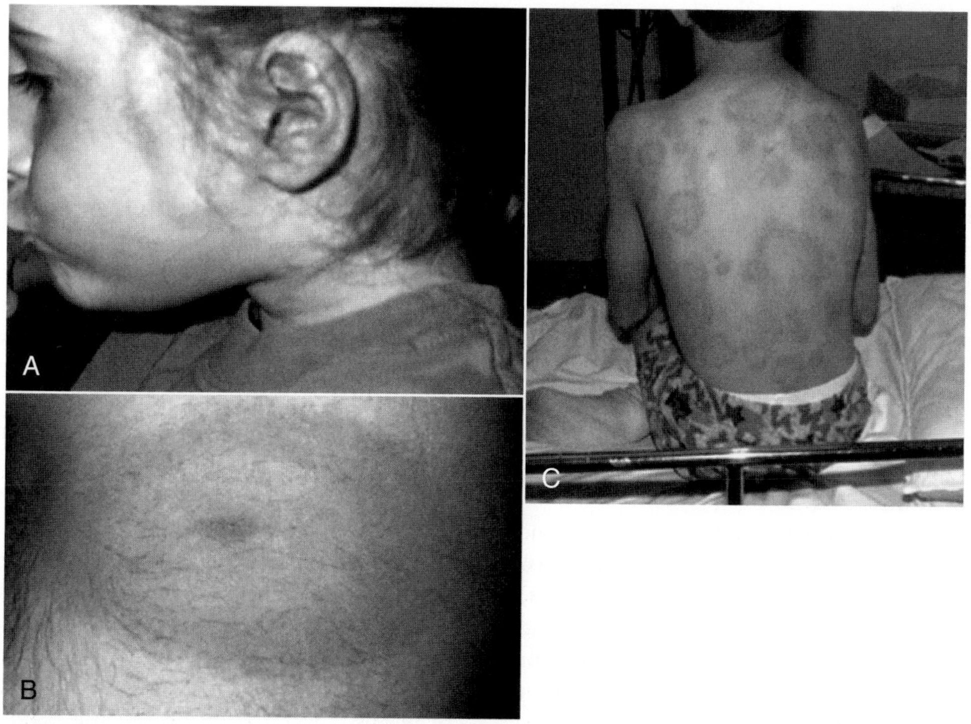

• **Figure 24-5** Erythema migrans (EM) of Lyme disease. **A,** EM scalp lesion only partially visible on the face. **B,** EM oval lesion. (See companion Expert Consult website for color version.) **C,** EM dark annular lesion. (From Cherry, JD, et al: *Feigin and Cherry's textbook of pediatric infectious diseases*, ed 7, Philadelphia, 2014, Saunders/Elsevier. **A** to **C,** Courtesy of Vijay Sikand, MD. All images reproduced from Sood SK, editor: *Lyme Borreliosis in Europe and North America*, Hoboken, NJ, 2011, John Wiley and Sons.)

3 cm) may also appear that are morphologically similar to, but smaller than, the EM lesion. Symptoms in children with disseminated disease may also present as neurologic (frequent headaches; lethargy; neck pain; mood swings; irritability; neuralgia; paresthesia, and motor or sensory impairment, mostly affecting cervical and thoracic dermatomes; cranial neuropathies [especially seventh nerve palsy in children]), cardiac (Lyme carditis, presenting as syncope and malaise), and generalized illness manifestations (stomachaches, urinary symptoms, migratory musculoskeletal pains). Stage 2 can last from weeks to 2 years without treatment. Most of the symptoms (including the rash) wax and wane during this time.

3. Stage 3 (late disease): Stage 3 usually begins with pauciarticular or monoarticular arthritis that occurs weeks to months after the initial tick bite; chronic neurologic symptoms also may occur in 5% of those untreated (cognitive and memory loss issues, numbness/tingling in hands and feet). The knees are most commonly affected. The joints are red, hot, and swollen, but not as painful as with other types of bacterial arthritis. Untreated, the arthritis initially resolves in a few weeks but becomes recurrent, migratory (but rarely to small joints), and chronic. Adolescents experience arthritis more severely and for a longer period of time (Sood and Krause, 2014). Untreated, late manifestation of the disease may appear months to years after the initial infection.

Diagnostic Studies

The IDSA and CDC provide guidelines for the diagnosis and treatment of LD. LD is best diagnosed by clinical and epidemiologic history and typical physical findings. The presence of EM is diagnostic; no serologic test is necessary. If the provider is suspicious for LD without EM, serologic testing is done keeping in mind several factors: First, serologic tests for IgM antibodies do not become positive for 2 to 4 weeks and IgG for 4 to 6 weeks after a bite. Second, serological tests should not be routinely used as screening tools because of the propensity for false-positive results. Finally, serologically positive results may indicate prior infection rather than present acute infection because IgM antibodies do not decline until 4 to 6 months after disease onset, and IgG antibodies can remain elevated for years (Nichols and Windemuth, 2013).

The CDC recommends a two-step approach to serologic testing. A single blood sample is drawn and tested. The first step tests the sample using enzyme immunoassay (ELISA) or (rarely) indirect IFA. If results are negative, the second step test is not needed. If the first test results are positive or equivocal, a second test using an IgM and IgG Western blot for *Bb* antibodies is done if the individual has had symptoms for less than 30 days. If symptoms have lasted longer than 30 days, just an IgG Western blot test is performed. A positive Western blot test is interpreted as reacting with 5 to 10 scored bands on the IgG assay and 2 to 3 on the IgM assay. The number of bands necessary for confirmation of LD is a controversial issue surrounding the diagnosis of this disease. The ELISA produces many false-positives because of cross-reactions with other spirochetes, lupus, and varicella organisms. After 4 weeks of symptoms, the IgG result should only be used to support the diagnosis (Sood and Krause, 2014).

Differential Diagnosis, Management, and Complications

The rash, if present, may suggest eczema, tinea, granuloma annulare, cellulitis, or an insect bite. Other differential diagnoses include osteomyelitis, WNV, parvovirus B19, relapsing fever, syphilis, leptospirosis, mycoplasma, septic arthritis, infectious hepatitis, nonresponsive lymphadenopathy, meningitis, multiple sclerosis, amyotrophic lateral sclerosis, juvenile arthritis, Bell palsy, other spirochete-caused diseases, thyroid disease, heavy metal toxicity, and vasculitis. Primary psychiatric disorders, in recalcitrant cases after appropriate treatment for Lyme disease, should also be considered.

Clinical judgment is crucial in determining whether to treat a patient. The earlier in the EM stage that treatment is started, the better the long-term outcome. In suspicious LD cases, delaying treatment until laboratory results are known decreases the chances of successfully treating this disease in its early stages. The provider is advised to study the literature from the CDC, IDSA, or consult with an infectious disease specialist if uncertain how to proceed.

A provider can feel confident about giving a prophylactic dose of doxycycline, amoxicillin, or cefuroxime in children when the history includes the following (Moore, 2015):

- Tick bite only: The tick is reliably identified as a nymph or adult *I. scapularis* species (providers in endemic areas should have this expertise of identification and most commercial and public health laboratories in endemic areas can make this determination), *and* the tick was attached for at least 36 to 72 hours (as indicated by size of engorgement or known time of exposure), *and* the tick was acquired in an endemic area. For treatment, see drugs and dosages under Early localized disease or EM.
  - If a tick has been removed but it cannot be identified as an *Ixodes* nor the timeline for attachment verified, prophylaxis should not be given. The child and caregivers should be given guidance about the signs and symptoms of EM and localized disease. Should these develop within 30 days, the child should be considered for diagnostic tests and treatment of the disease (Moore, 2015).
- Early localized disease (stage 1) or EM usually resolves within several days of starting treatment. Drugs and dosages (AAP et al, 2015b) include:
  - Younger than 8 years old: Amoxicillin 50 mg/kg per day, orally, divided into 3 doses for 14 days (maximum 1.5 g/day)

- 8 years or older: Doxycycline: single 200 mg dose daily or 4 mg/kg per day divided into two doses PO for 14 days (maximum 200 mg per day). Give a small snack with doxycycline to reduce nausea.
- For children unable to take amoxicillin or doxycycline: cefuroxime 30 mg/kg per day, orally, divided into two doses for 14 days (maximum 1000 mg per day) is preferable.

- Early or late disseminated disease: Consult with a Lyme disease specialist.

Post-Lyme disease syndrome is currently used to describe persistent subjective symptoms that some may experience after treatment. Some providers speculate that there may be a chronic form of the infection with its own diagnostic criteria and treatment approaches (Nichols and Windemuth, 2013). In children, lingering fatigue, musculoskeletal pain, or cognitive or short-term memory difficulties have occurred but may be due to persistent immune-mediated inflammation rather than continued infection with *Bb.* A child with chronic symptoms whose family attributes them to LD should be questioned about adherence to any prior treatments, reevaluated for reinfection, and referred to appropriate specialists as indicated by symptomatology. A positive serologic finding without other symptoms of clinical disease does not warrant the use of antibiotics (Sood and Krause, 2014).

Complications include Lyme meningitis, myocarditis, myopericarditis, left ventricular dysfunction, or cardiomegaly. Other tick-borne diseases can be co-transmitted with Lyme disease (human babesiosis and human granulocytic anaplasmosis).

Patient and Family Education

Avoid tick-infested areas whenever possible. If in such areas, follow tick skin repellent strategies using DEET as previously discussed. Shower after being outdoors, and inspect the entire body carefully every day during the tick season (special attention to armpit, groin, back, and scalp areas). Spray permethrin on clothing and wear light-colored long pants (tucked into socks or shoes), long sleeves, and a hat. Chronic absorption of insecticides can produce toxicity, especially in children; however, when used according to directions, children older than 2 months can safely use DEET. Picaridin (KBR 3023) and plant-based oil of eucalyptus are alternative repellents. Families should be taught how to remove ticks safely; any removed tick should be saved in a dry container and brought with the child for identification. Pets should be checked each day and ticks removed if found.

Ehrlichiosis and Anaplasmosis

Both ehrlichiosis and anaplasmosis are caused by distinct species of obligate intracellular bacteria carried by the lone star tick (*Amblyomma americanum,* of which there are two species, for ehrlichial infections) and the black-legged or deer tick (*I. scapularis,* for anaplasmosis). The southeast, south-central, and westward areas of Texas are common endemic areas for ehrlichiosis in the United States. Anaplasma infections are reported more commonly in the northeast and Midwest states and the same regions in which Lyme disease occurs; the provider must always consider a coinfection with Lyme disease or babesiosis when considering anaplasmosis. Any individual who has a history of tick exposure in an endemic area, a nonspecific rapid onset febrile illness from May through October, and some of the following symptoms should be evaluated for ehrlichiosis or anaplasmosis. Children are increasingly acquiring these diseases, which are most likely underreported (Lantos and McKinney, 2014). The incubation period for both diseases ranges from 7 to 14 days after a tick bite.

Both infections produce similar acute, systemic symptoms: fever, headache, myalgia, malaise, chills, nausea, and anorexia in about half of those infected. Less common symptoms include diarrhea and vomiting, weight loss, arthralgia, cough, and change in mental status. With ehrlichiosis, a rash is seen in about 60% of infected children; a rarely rarely occurs with *Anaplasma* (CDC, 2014d). The rash (petechial, macular, or maculopapular and distinguishable from that of RMSF) is variable in appearance, generally involves the trunk with sparing of the hands and feet, and appears about a week after the onset of other symptoms.

Diagnosis can be made using an IFA assay to determine IgG antibody specific titers on a blood sample tested during the acute and convalescent periods (2 to 4 weeks apart). Titers are then compared. The gold standard is a fourfold increase in the antibody titer between assays; titers may be negative in the first 7 to 10 days of the illness. DNA by PCR assay titer can also be used. Other laboratory tests show similar results: leukopenia (relative and absolute lymphopenia and a left shift), neutropenia, anemia, or thrombocytopenia with elevated hepatic transaminases in the first week of clinical illness. Pleocytosis with predominance of lymphocytes and increased total protein is commonly seen in CSF samples.

The differential diagnosis for ehrlichiosis and anaplasmosis includes RMSF, Lyme disease, other tick-borne illnesses (e.g., babesiosis, Colorado tick fever, relapsing fever, and tularemia), dengue, malaria, enteroviruses, adenoviruses, sepsis, and toxic shock syndrome.

The treatment of choice for both infections is doxycycline *for all* ages given the life-threatening nature of these illnesses: 100 lb (45.4 kg) or more: 100 mg twice daily PO or IV for 10 to 14 days in order to cover coinfection with Lyme disease; less than 100 lb, 2.2 mg/kg per dose twice daily PO/IV (maximum per dose is 100 mg). Data suggest that discoloration of permanent teeth is not significant if doxycycline is taken for 14 days or less (CDC, 2014d). A response to treatment should occur within 1 week. Treatment should be started before laboratory confirmation.

Systemic complications include pulmonary infiltrates, bone marrow hypoplasia, respiratory failure, encephalopathy, meningitis, DIC, spontaneous hemorrhage, and renal failure. The mortality rate for ehrlichiosis is about 3%, and it is about 0.5% for anaplasmosis (Lantos and McKinney, 2014). Recovery is usually complete after 1 to 2 weeks; some neurologic difficulties can remain in children who have had systemic disease. Prevention is the same for Lyme disease. Prophylaxis is not recommended due to the low risk of infection.

Rocky Mountain Spotted Fever

Rickettsia rickettsii, a nonmotile, pleomorphic, weakly gram-negative coccobacillus, is the etiologic agent of RMSF. In the United States, it is the most severe rickettsial disease and most common vector-borne disease after Lyme disease (Reller and Dumler, 2011). Vectors for *R. rickettsii* include the American dog tick *(Dermacentor variabilis)* found in the eastern and central United States, the Rocky Mountain wood tick (*Dermacentor andersoni;* also the vector for Colorado tick fever and tularemia) found in the Rocky Mountain states and west, and the brown dog tick *(Rhipicephalus sanguineus)* recently reported in eastern Arizona. Southwestern Canada, Mexico, and Central and South America also have reported cases.

In the United States RMSF was historically centered in northern Rocky Mountain states, but it is now found in all contiguous states except Maine and Vermont. Sixty percent of cases are located in North Carolina, Tennessee, Arkansas, Missouri, and Oklahoma (CDC, 2014d). The incidence continues to increase (6 cases per million in 2010 [CDC, 2013d]). RMSF is most common in spring and summer months when ticks are most active (peak is June and July). The incubation period is 2 to 14 days. The longer the tick is attached, the more likely *R. rickettsii* is to be transmitted. Prompt removal of a tick is important to lower the chance of infection.

Clinical Findings

Symptoms include the following: fever (104°F [40°C]; occurs in up to 98% of children), chills, severe headache, myalgias, malaise, GI upset/tenderness, diarrhea, cough, conjunctival injection, photophobia, and altered mental status. Focal neurologic deficits (e.g., paralysis, transient deafness) appear with disease progression. Most individuals (90%) develop a maculopapular rash, typically 2 to 5 days after fever onset (CDC, 2014d). The rash begins as small, flat, nonpruritic, faintly pink spots on the wrists, forearms, and ankles, then spreads to the trunk (sometimes to palms and soles). The rash may be easily missed in dark-skinned individuals. On day 6 or later, a petechial rash, a sign of progressive disease, may appear. Only 60% of individuals recall having removed an attached tick (Reller and Dumler, 2011).

Diagnostic Studies

The most rapidly available diagnostic aid is immunohistochemical staining or PCR testing performed on a skin biopsy of petechial or macular lesions to look for *R. rickettsii.* The conclusive diagnostic gold standard is IFA on paired serologic samples taken in the first week and 2 to 4 weeks later. A fourfold change in IgG-specific antibody titer is typical. However, antibody titers may be negative in the first 7 to 10 days of the illness.

Diagnostic studies also show diffuse vascular injury characterized by thrombocytopenia (<150,000 platelets/μL), mild to moderate hyponatremia (<130 mEq/mL), leukocytosis as the disease progresses with a left-shifted leukocyte differential, and anemia. Mildly elevated hepatic transaminase levels may be found.

Differential Diagnoses

The differential diagnoses include enteroviral infections, adenoviral infections, meningococcemia, influenza, gram-negative bacterial sepsis, toxic shock syndrome, measles, rubella, secondary syphilis, leptospirosis, typhoid fever, disseminated gonococcal infection, immune thrombocytopenic purpura, thrombotic thrombocytopenic purpura, immune complex vasculitis (e.g., SLE), infectious mononucleosis, hypersensitivity reaction to drugs, murine typhus, rickettsialpox, recrudescent typhus, and sylvatic *R. prowazekii* infection that is enzootic in flying squirrels (Lantos and McKinney, 2014).

Management

It is important to start antibiotic treatment prior to the onset of the rash and within the first 5 days if other clinical symptoms suggest RMSF, especially because of possible false-negative serology findings early in the disease. Without early treatment, the disease can rapidly progress to death. Lantos and McKinney (2014) provide the following guidance:

- If the child appears in the summer in an endemic area (with or without history of exposure to a tick or dog) with an acute fever of less than 2 days but without profound malaise/myalgia/headache, obtain a CBC and chemistry panel and monitor the child.
- If the fever goes into the third day and laboratory studies were suggestive of RMSF, or if the child appears more ill, empiric antibiotics should be started. Although conjunctival injection and peripheral edema may appear at the same time as the rash, their presence also points toward a diagnosis of RMSF.

Treatment consists of doxycycline *for all* ages for 7 to 10 days. Children under 100 lb [45.4 kg]: 2.2 mg/kg per dose given twice daily PO or IV; children over 100 lb: 100 mg twice daily PO or IV (maximum dose for all is 100 mg per dose). Doxycycline does not pose a significant risk considering the mortality associated with this disease (CDC, 2014d).

Complications and Patient and Family Education

Complications include neurologic deficits that can be long term (e.g., speech and swallowing dysfunction, global encephalopathy, gait disturbances, and cortical blindness). Loss of digits due to autoamputation can occur. Untreated, the fatality rate is about 20%; for those treated, the rate is about 5% (Lantos and McKinney, 2014). For prevention, see prior discussion under Lyme disease.

Bacterial Infections

Although less common than viral diseases, bacterial infections allow for interventions (including antibiotics) that can decrease the course of an illness and prevent subsequent complications. Many bacterial infections may be diagnosed clinically and treated empirically. A good understanding of the pathophysiology of common bacterial infections, and knowledge of the most likely organisms involved, allows for efficient and effective implementation of treatment. Bacterial infections of the skin and soft tissues, lymphadenitis, osteomyelitis, fasciitis, pneumonia, meningitis, infectious diarrhea, and UTI are discussed in other chapters relevant to the system affected; fungal infections and parasitic infections are also discussed in other chapters.

Community-Acquired Methicillin-Resistant *Staphylococcus Aureus*

Knowing the prevalence of community-acquired methicillin-resistant *S. aureus* (CA-MRSA) in a community is crucial for a provider to effectively treat severe pneumonia, cellulitis, osteomyelitis, myositis, bacteremia, endocarditis, empyema, meningitis, scalded skin syndrome, toxic shock syndrome, deep tissue abscesses (especially those that come on quickly), spider bites, skin and soft tissue infections, and necrotizing fasciitis. CA-MRSA is often the cause of purulent skin and soft tissue infections in the United States (CDC, 2013e). It is also increasingly being implicated as the causative agent in pneumonia in the younger age groups and in those without risk factors. CA-MRSA has novel elements. It has an altered penicillin-binding protein with decreased sensitivity to most beta-lactam antibiotics. With a combination of this protein and specific genetic encoding for cytotoxicity (affects the degree of virulence), the *S. aureus* strains are able to evade neutrophils and cause leukocyte, monocyte, and macrophage destruction and tissue necrosis (Daum, 2012; Liu et al, 2011).

The following history and physical findings place an otherwise healthy individual at risk of acquired CA-MRSA infection:

- Individual has a boil, furuncle, or abscess without draining pus that is erythematous, warm, painful; onset may have been rapid (key finding)
- Individual fails treatment with a beta-lactam agent. If individual has been in contact with a cat, consider cat-scratch disease as a differential diagnosis (it would have been unresponsive to beta-lactam treatment)
- Other family members have similar skin infections
- Individual has a recent history of skin infection, even if it was responsive to a beta-lactam agent
- Neonate with skin or soft tissue infection
- Skin lesion looks like a spider bite; larger lesions are more suspicious for MRSA
- Pus is present
- History of recurrent small, nontender, nonpruritic maculopapular lesions that become pruritic or painful; multiple lesions present
- Individual participates in contact sports (e.g., wrestling, football) where turf burns and abrasions are common, and athletes share lockers, bars of soap, towels, other equipment
- Individual may be of an ethnic minority, of lower socioeconomic status, in the military, homeless, recently incarcerated, living in a crowded environment, using illicit drugs, or participating in high-risk sexual behaviors
- Nonpregnant or pregnant woman has a breast abscess
- Individual has history in the past year of having been hospitalized, of having had surgery, or of having had a permanent indwelling medical device passing through the skin
- Child attends child care; is younger than 2 years old
- Individual has cystic fibrosis or progressive respiratory tract infection
- Individual has a head or neck infection (retropharyngeal abscess, mastoiditis, AOM, sinusitis, periorbital and orbital infections), osteomyelitis, myositis, pneumonias with empyema, sepsis, pustulosis in neonates

The provider can safely treat many superficial skin lesions (e.g., impetigo, localized pustulosis in an asymptomatic neonate) without a culture using topical bacitracin or mupirocin ointment applied to affected area three times daily for 7 to 10 days. Consider oral or IV antimicrobial therapy for widespread impetigo (Daum, 2012). In all cases, providers need to assess each case carefully and provide instructions to parents to return if the child is unresponsive to treatment. Anticipate complications and consider the clinical clues previously mentioned for skin and soft-tissue infection. The selection of a drug that covers MRSA should be made on the basis of the prevalence of MRSA within one's community, if infection was nosocomial, and the severity of the infection. See Chapters 37 and 40 for other discussions about MRSA.

Recommended management strategies (Fig. 24-6) include:

- Incision and drainage (I&D) with culture is the treatment of choice for any non-draining but fluctuant abscess; antibiotics alone are ineffective (performing I&D prior to localization of pus is not effective and may promote more serious infection). Antibiotics are not needed after draining the abscess in mild cases. Consider empiric treatment (PO or IV) for MRSA for those with severe local infection; for those with signs of systemic toxicity; or for those who failed to respond to prior oral treatment (Stevens et al, 2014). Those with a temperature higher than 100.4° F [38° C], heart rate higher than 90, tachypnea more than 24 breaths/minute, or WBC count more than12,000 or less than 400; who are immunocompromised or at risk of endocarditis may require IV antibiotics. Refer to an infectious disease consult.
- Send specimens to the laboratory for a Gram stain, culture and sensitivity, and "d-test" (indicates any

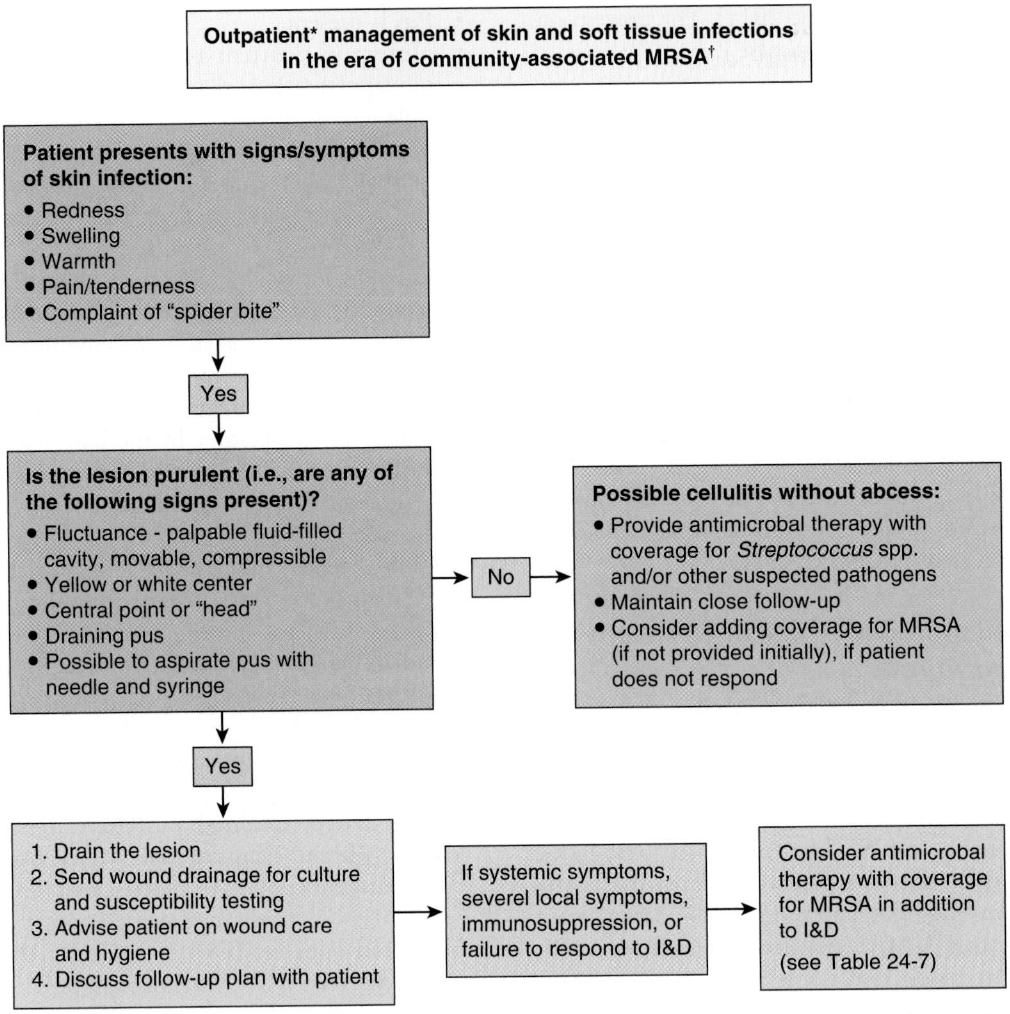

• **Figure 24-6** Algorithm for outpatient management of skin and soft tissue infections. *I&D,* Incision and drainage; *MRSA,* methicillin-resistant *Staphylococcus aureus; SSTI,* skin and soft tissue infection. *Severe infections (appears toxic, has unstable comorbidity or limb-threatening infection; sepsis or life-threatening infection [e.g., necrotizing fascitis]) require inpatient management; consult an infectious disease specialist. †Visit www.cdc.gov/mrsa for more information.

possible inducible resistance to clindamycin). Cultures should not be taken from superficial open surface wounds due to contaminating skin bacteria.

- For deep-seated infections without fluid fluctuation and without signs of bacteremia (e.g., fever, chills, malaise), warm compresses to localize pus are appropriate, and oral antibiotics can be considered. The individual should be instructed to return for further evaluation in 24 to 36 hours for I&D as indicated (providers need to have a way to contact patient regarding status).
- For uncomplicated soft tissue infection (e.g., bullous and non-bullous impetigo; secondarily infected eczema, ulcers, or lacerations) and without fluid fluctuation, empiric topical mupirocin 2% is usually sufficient. Using moist heat on small furuncles to promote draining may also be sufficient. Ecthyma and impetigo are treated with an oral antimicrobial for 7 days (Stevens et al, 2014).
- The use of oral antibiotic treatment for suspected methicillin-sensitive *S. aureus* infection is appropriate under the following circumstances, and providers should contact the child/family within 2 to 3 days to determine response to treatment (Table 24-7 lists recommended antibiotic choices):
  - Presence of abscesses (one or multiple sites) or rapidly progressing local infection with signs of cellulitis; systemic symptoms; comorbidities or immunosuppression; abscess is in an area difficult to incise/drain (e.g., face, hand, genitalia); or lack of response to incision/drainage (Stevens et al, 2014).
- Prevention measures for athletes and return to play guidelines are included in Box 13-6 and Table 13-9.
- For recurrent MRSA soft tissue infections:
  - Review hygiene and wound care.
  - Institute environmental hygiene measures (clean surfaces in contact with skin [e.g., doorknobs, bathtubs, counters, and toilet seats]).
  - Decolonization techniques (consider where ongoing transmission is occurring within a household despite

TABLE 24-7 Initial Outpatient Treatment Options for Mild to Moderate Suspected Community-Acquired Methicillin-Resistant *Staphylococcus aureus* Infections*

Antibiotic†	Comments	Precautions
Clindamycin	Treats serious infections (nonpurulent [mild] or purulent) due to *Staphylococcus aureus*. Additional d-test should be done on specimen by lab to ensure clindamycin susceptibility. Resistance seen in deep-seated infections (osteomyelitis, endocarditis, pneumonia). Do not use if local resistance rates exceed 10% to 15%.	Although uncommon, may cause *Clostridium difficile*-associated disease.
Doxycycline	For children 8 years old and older; treats *S. aureus*, but activity against GAS less well known.	Can cause photosensitivity; do not use in pregnancy.
Minocycline	For children 8 years old and older.	
Linezolid	For complicated skin/soft tissue infections, pneumonia.	Has been associated with myelosuppression, neuropathy, and lactic acidosis during prolonged therapy. Before using, consult with infectious disease specialist.
Trimethoprim-sulfamethoxazole (TMP-SMX)	Limited efficacy data for treating GAS so avoid using for initial treatment of cellulitis (AAP, 2015b).	Do not use in infants under 2 months old; do not use in third trimester of pregnancy.

Data from Stevens DL, Bisno AL, Chambers HF, et al: Practice guidelines for the diagnosis and management of skin and soft tissue infections: 2014 update by the Infectious Disease Society of America, *Clin Infect Dis* 59(2):e10–e52, 2014; Stewart EE, Fernald D, Staton EW: A toolkit to improve the treatment of CA-MRSA, *Fam Pract Manag* 19(5):21–24, 2012.

GAS, Group A streptococcus; *PO*, *per os* (by mouth, orally).

*Serious systemic symptoms (sepsis), severe local symptoms, immunosuppression or failure to respond to incision and drainage (I&D) require hospitalization. In typical cases, Gram stain and culture of pus or exudates from skin lesions of impetigo and ecthyma are recommended to identify *Staphylococcus aureus* and/or a β-hemolytic streptococcus; treatment without these studies is reasonable.

†Treatment recommendations do not apply to neonates. Antibiotic treatment is for 7 days, depending upon response. If response is low, treat for up to 10 to 14 days.

adherence to hygiene and wound care strategies). May include nasal decolonization with mupirocin 2% twice daily for 5 days (apply to groin and around rectal area of diapered infants/children); daily antiseptic body wash with a skin antiseptic solution (e.g., chlorhexidine) for 5 to 14 days or diluted bleach baths (¼ cup bleach for ¼ tub of water) for 15 minutes twice weekly for about 3 months. Oral antibiotics are not routinely recommended for decolonization. Consider an infectious disease consult for individuals with recurrent MRSA infections (Liu et al, 2011).

Other Emerging Drug-Resistant Bacterial Infections

At least 2 million people in the United States acquire a serious bacterial infection that is resistant to one or more antibiotics used to treat the infection, and approximately 23,000 deaths are attributed to those antibiotic-resistance organisms (CDC, 2013a). Multiple drug resistant gram-negative bacteria are a major concern. Enterobacteriaceae, *Pseudomonas aeruginosa,* and *Acinetobacter* have already gained resistance to virtually all antibiotics in hospital settings. Multi-drug resistance is emerging to gram-positive organisms as well (e.g., *Staphylococcus* and *Enterococcus*) but to a lesser degree. Resistance to anti-malarials, multiple drug-resistant tuberculosis (MDR-TB), and extensively drug-resistant tuberculosis (XDR-TB) are increasing (CDC, 2013a).

Antibiotics are among the most commonly prescribed drugs for people, with up to 50% of all prescribed antibiotics either dosed ineffectively or unnecessarily (CDC, 2013a). More than 70% of antibiotics are prescribed in ambulatory pediatrics for respiratory conditions; 23% of the prescribed antibiotics are for conditions without an indication for antibiotic treatment (e.g., asthma, viral conditions) (Hersh et al, 2011). Improving antibiotic prescribing/stewardship is an essential part of decreasing antibiotic resistance influenced by inappropriate and/or overuse of antibiotics (see Chapter 22 for a further discussion about the overuse of antibiotics).

Cat-Scratch Disease

B. henselae, a slow-growing, gram-negative bacillus, is the causative organism for cat-scratch disease. It is a common infection, and a common cause of chronic persistent (>3 weeks) lymphadenopathy in children. In 90% of cases, a cat (usually a kitten) is involved (occasionally a dog). The organism is transmitted to humans through a cat bite or scratch or from hands contaminated with flea feces that touch an open skin lesion or eye. The incidence is greater than 22,000 cases annually in the United States with the highest incidence occurring in the Southern states and in children younger than 5 years old (Howard et al, 2014). The disease is most prevalent in fall and winter except in tropical areas, where it shows no seasonal predilection. The incubation period between injury and primary skin lesion is 7 to 12 days. The lymphadenopathy may take 5 to 50 days to develop but averages 12 days.

Clinical Findings

Systemic illness is present in approximately one third of cases although the majority of patients are afebrile without constitutional symptoms (Schutze and Jacobs, 2012). The illness typically presents with cutaneous findings and other key characteristics that include:

- Erythematous papules (3 to 5 mm) arise approximately 1 week after inoculation, can persist for up to 4 weeks and are seen in about two thirds of individuals. They may follow a linear pattern that follows the cat scratch. The rash may be misdiagnosed as impetigo secondary to an insect bite. The cutaneous lesions heal spontaneously. One to 4 weeks after the inoculation, the axillary, cervical, submandibular, preauricular, epitrochlear, inguinal, and femoral nodes closest to the lesion begin to swell (in that general order). There can be single or multiple nodes involved. The node may swell to 1 to 5 cm. The area around the infected node is usually warm, tender, indurated, and erythematous during the first few weeks. Cellulitis is uncommon, but large nodes may suppurate up to 30% of the time (Schutze and Jacobs, 2012). The lymphadenopathy usually lasts 1 to 2 months and up to 1 year in some cases. Mucous membrane ulcers may occur. A fever of 100.4° F to 102.2° F (38° C to 39° C), malaise, anorexia, fatigue, and headache also accompany the lymphadenopathy in one third of patients.
- A small percentage of children may present with Parinaud oculoglandular syndrome (a painful nonsuppurative conjunctivitis) with preauricular lymphadenopathy. Inoculation is surmised to be from rubbing the eye(s) following handling a cat. Recovery is spontaneous in 2 to 4 months after onset without sequelae (Howard et al, 2014).
- Immunocompromised hosts can have persistent or relapsing fevers, bacteremia, weight loss and other systemic symptoms.

Diagnostic Studies

An IFA for serum antibodies is available from commercial labs, state health departments, or the CDC and shows good correlation with this disease. *B. henselae* is rarely recovered from cultures. A *Bartonella* DNA PCR can be performed on tissue and body fluids (pleural and CSF). CT or ultrasonography may identify hepatic or splenic abscesses and granulomas. The CBC may be normal or show mild leukocytosis. The ESR and CRP may be elevated early in the disease process; hepatic transaminases may increase with systemic disease. Lymph node biopsy may show nonspecific bacilli.

Differential Diagnosis, Management, and Complications

The differential diagnosis includes any cause of lymphadenopathy, but most commonly includes bacterial and viral infections (e.g., streptococci [especially group A beta-hemolytic], staphylococci, anaerobic bacteria, atypical mycobacteria, tularemia, brucellosis, CMV, HIV, EBV, systemic fungal infections, toxoplasmosis). Malignancy and neck masses from other sources (e.g., cystic hygromas, bronchogenic cysts, tumors) are in the differential.

Most cases of cat-scratch disease resolve spontaneously within 2 to 4 months, so symptomatic treatment is usually sufficient. Antipyretics can be used for a moderate fever. Painful nodes can be treated with moist wraps or needle aspiration. Needle aspiration can yield material for diagnostic testing. I&D of nonsuppurative lesions should be avoided because of the high risk of chronic draining sinuses. Antibiotics are not generally used unless there is concern for systemic cat-scratch disease or bacterial involvement of lesions. Azithromycin, clarithromycin, trimethoprim-sulfamethoxazole (TMP-SMX), rifampin, ciprofloxacin, and doxycycline are commonly used antibiotics. A 5-day course of oral azithromycin has shown to be of moderate benefit and can be given for localized disease to speed recovery (Howard et al, 2014). Treatment is recommended for the immunocompromised and may be beneficial for those with acute or severe systemic sequelae (e.g., hepatic or splenic involvement or painful adenitis). Treatment with one of the oral agents and parenteral gentamicin are effective. Optimal length of therapy is not known, but several weeks may be needed (AAP et al, 2015b).

Children should be discouraged from playing roughly with cats. Cat scratches should be washed thoroughly with soap and water. Immunocompromised individuals should stay away from cats that scratch or bite and avoid stray cats and cats younger than 1 year old. A small percentage of individuals manifest systemic illness. This can be associated with fever up to 106° F (41.2° C), malaise, fatigue, anorexia, weight loss, emesis, headache, hepatosplenomegaly, sore throat, exanthema, blindness secondary to stellate macular retinopathy, neurologic changes (bizarre behavior), seizures, and arthralgia. Enlarged mediastinal or pancreatic nodes can cause pleurisy, obstructive phenomena, and splenic and hepatic abscesses (may be associated with prolonged fevers). Other complications include encephalopathy (5% incidence after 1 to 3 weeks of lymphadenopathy), aseptic meningitis, severe chronic systemic disease, erythema nodosa, neuroretinitis, thrombocytopenic purpura, primary atypical pneumonia, relapsing bacteremia, breast mass, endocarditis, angiomatoid papules, and osteomyelitis. Almost all of these problems generally resolve completely over several months, rarely as long as a year (Schutze and Jacobs, 2012).

Kingella Kingae Infection

Kingella kingae is an important cause of invasive infections in children younger than 4 years old, but has not been reported in infants younger than 6 months old. The organism is part of the normal flora of the pharynx in children (over 6 months old) more than in adults; it can easily be transmitted among children in child care settings. The onset is usually insidious, which can result in delay of diagnosis (Murphy, 2015). The history often includes recent or concomitant gingivostomatitis or URI. Suspect *K. kingae* in culture-negative skeletal infections of young children; it is the most common cause of septic arthritis in children younger than 3 years old (Yagupsky, 2012). Septic arthritis usually involves the knee, hip, or ankle. Other invasive disease can include osteomyelitis (distal femur is the most common site), diskitis, endocarditis in children and adults with underlying cardiac disease (HACEK group of organisms [***H****aemophilus* spp., ***A****ctinobacillus actinomycetemcomitans,* ***C****ardiobacterium hominis,* ***E****ikenella corrodens,* ***K****ingella kingae*]), meningitis, occult bacteremia, and pneumonia. The organism is difficult to isolate in solid culture media. Recent studies show PCR dramatically enhances detection in bone and joint fluid samples (Porsch et al, 2014). The organism is susceptible to many antibiotics (penicillins, aminoglycosides, ciprofloxacin, and erythromycin) but is resistant to clindamycin and vancomycin. Most strains are susceptible to TMP-SMX despite resistance to trimethoprim alone. Standard hygienic preventive measures should be in place in child care settings to decrease risk of transmission (Porsch et al, 2014).

Meningococcal Disease

Many organisms can cause meningitis (group B streptococcus, *E. coli, Listeria monocytogenes,* enterococci, *S. pneumoniae, N. meningitidis,* and *H. influenzae*). The causative organism varies with age. Only *N. meningitidis* is discussed here (see Chapter 28 for a discussion of other CNS infections).

N. meningitidis is a gram-negative diplococcus. It is a common commensal organism in the human nasopharynx. Serotypes A, B, C, W-135, and Y (polysaccharide encapsulated organisms) are largely the causes of invasive disease worldwide. In the United States, serogroups B, C, and Y account for approximately 90% of invasive meningococcal disease and share equal incidence of disease. Infants and adolescents 16 to 21 years old have the highest incidence, although it can be found in all ages (CDC, 2014e). Serogroup B causes 60% of disease in infants and children under 5 years old. Serogroups C, Y, and W-135 affect the majority of cases in adolescents and young adults (AAP et al, 2015b). The organism is spread from person to person via respiratory tract secretions (large droplets) or contact with saliva (kissing). Asymptomatic carriers are the most common source of transmission with carriage of approximately 10% of the population at any given time (Granoff and Gilsdorf, 2011). Disease occurs most often during the winter season, but can occur sporadically; rates can increase in sub-Sahara Africa during the dry season. Epidemics occur in semi-closed communities (e.g., child care centers, schools, college dormitories [especially among college freshmen], and military barracks) and account for about 2 out of 100 cases of disease (CDC, 2014e). Children or youth with functional or anatomic asplenia, complement deficiencies (e.g., nephritic syndrome, SLE, hepatic failure), or properdin deficiency are at increased risk for invasive or recurring meningococcal disease (Pollard and Finn, 2012). The incubation period is 1 to 14 days. Individuals are contagious until 24 hours after initiation of treatment. Carriage can persist for weeks to months, although disease onset is usually days to a week after colonization (Granoff and Gilsdorf, 2011).

Clinical Findings

Meningococcal disease presentation varies widely from mild viral symptoms with fever to severe disease. Recognized patterns of disease include bacteremia without sepsis, meningococcemic sepsis without meningitis, meningitis with or without meningococcemia, meningoencephalitis, and specific organ infection. Presenting symptoms can include:

- Occult bacteremia: This appears in a febrile child with a URI or GI-like symptoms. There may be a maculopapular rash. Often these children are treated as having a viral illness. Bacteremia may resolve without antimicrobial intervention, but approximately 66% of cases with sustained bacteremia will progress to meningococcal meningitis (Pollard and Finn, 2012).
- Meningococcemia: Fulminant meningococcemia progresses rapidly over several hours starting with fever onset and may be accompanied by other signs of septic shock. Initial symptoms can include fever, headache, myalgia, chills, cold hands and feet, influenza symptoms, vomiting, and abdominal pain. Skin changes are characterized by prominent petechiae (Fig. 24-7) that may quickly progress to purpura fulminans. Other signs include hypotension, DIC, acidosis, adrenal hemorrhage, renal failure, myocardial failure, and coma. Death can occur within 12 hours of onset and most deaths are within 48 hours. Meningitis is present in 5% to 20% of meningococcemia cases (Atkinson et al, 2012).
- Meningococcal meningitis: The most common clinical findings are fever, headache, and stiff neck. Fever and irritability may be the only initial symptoms in young children, whereas fever and headache are more typical in older children and adolescents. Other symptoms may include nausea, vomiting, photophobia and altered mental status. Bacteremia is present in 75% of meningococcal meningitis (Atkinson et al, 2012).

Diagnostic Studies

The diagnosis is confirmed with a positive culture or Gram stain from normally sterile sites (blood, CSF, synovial fluid), sputum, or petechial or purpura lesion scraping. Blood and CSF cultures may be negative if the child has been

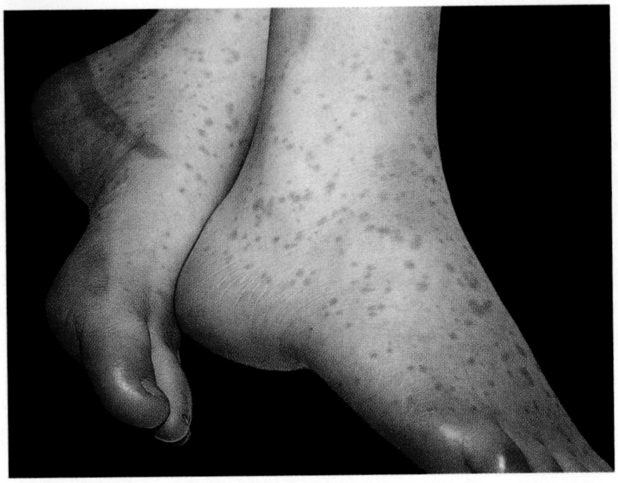

• **Figure 24-7** Petechiae of meningococcemia. (From Habif TP: *Clinical dermatology*, ed 5, Philadelphia, 2010, Mosby.)

pretreated with antibiotics. PCR assays can be used with CSF, serum, and plasma to detect meningococcal DNA; results are available in 4 to 8 hours. PCR is available in some public health and research laboratories, is widely used in the United Kingdom, and is useful when antibiotics are given before testing and organism growth has been suppressed. In a probable case, a positive latex agglutination test of CSF supports diagnosis if the clinical illness is consistent with meningitis. However, this test has poor sensitivity and specificity, especially for serogroup B, and is not recommended if the PCR (in addition to culture) is available. Other laboratory findings may include leukopenia or leukocytosis with increased presence of bands and neutrophils, hypoalbuminemia, hypocalcemia, metabolic acidosis with increased lactate levels, decreased platelets, and elevated ESR and CRP. Decreased prothrombin and fibrinogen and prolonged coagulation times are seen with DIC.

Differential Diagnosis

The list of differential diagnoses is long and includes septicemia caused by other invasive bacteria (e.g., pneumococcus or *H. influenza*), viral meningitis, TB brain abscess, chronic otitis media, and sinusitis. Collagen-vascular diseases, primary hematologic and oncologic disease, erythema nodosa, erythema multiforme, RMSF, mycoplasma, lead encephalopathy, coxsackievirus, echovirus, rubella and rubeola infections, Henoch-Schönlein purpura, ITP, viral exanthems, typhus, typhoid, toxic shock syndrome, rat bite fever, gonococcemia, *S. aureus* endocarditis, and Kawasaki syndrome are also in the differential diagnosis.

Management, Control Measures, and Complications

If the child is suspected of having meningococcemia, hospitalization is mandatory and IV antibiotics are started pending culture results. A 5- to 7-day treatment course is usually adequate in children.

Exposed contacts must be carefully monitored. Household, school, or child contacts who develop a febrile illness must be promptly evaluated for invasive disease. Household contacts have 500 to 800 times the risk factor of individuals in the general community (AAP et al, 2015b). Control measures include:

- Chemoprophylaxis is ideally given within 24 hours of identification of the index case regardless of immunization status (vaccines are not 100% effective). Individuals (including children in child care and preschool) who have had close contact with the index case 7 days before the onset of symptoms are at increased risk of invasive disease and should receive prophylaxis. Airline travel of more than 8 hours while sitting next to an infected individual qualifies one for prophylaxis (AAP et al, 2015b). Casual contact with the index case or with a high-risk contact is usually not considered high risk. Medical staff (unless they performed mouth-to-mouth resuscitation, intubation, or suctioning before antibiotics were started) are also not at high risk. Oral rifampin or ciprofloxacin are the antimicrobials of choice for infants and children. If the community has a pattern of ciprofloxacin-resistance to *N. meningitidi*, azithromycin as a single oral dose is effective (AAP et al, 2015b).
- Prophylaxis during outbreak: Vaccination, in conjunction with chemoprophylaxis, is advisable to prevent extended outbreaks only if the identified strain is contained in the vaccine (see the discussion under Meningococcal Vaccine for guidance). Vaccines are available for serogroups A, B, C, Y, and W-135.

Complications are caused by inflammation, intravascular hemorrhage, necrosis in multiple organ systems, and shock. Skeletal deformities and limb amputations are not infrequent. Meningitis can lead to ataxia, seizures, pneumonia, deafness (5% to 10%), arthritis and pericarditis, visual field defects, palsies and paralysis, developmental delays, and hydrocephalus. The fatality rate is about 10%. Even with aggressive treatment, meningococcemia has a fatality rate of approximately 5%. Survivors may experience such permanent sequelae as hearing loss (2% to 15%), neurologic damage (7%), or loss of a limb (3%) (Pollard and Finn, 2012).

Streptococcal Disease

Streptococci are gram-positive spherical cocci that are broadly classified based on their ability to hemolyze RBCs. Complete hemolysis is known as *beta-hemolytic.* Partial hemolysis is *alpha-hemolytic*; non-hemolysis is *gamma-hemolytic*. Cell wall carbohydrate differences further subdivide the streptococci. These differences are identified as Lancefield antigen subgroups A-H and K-V. Subgroups A-H and K-O are associated with human disease. Group A beta-hemolytic streptococcus is the most virulent, although group B beta-hemolytic streptococcus can cause bacteremia and meningitis in infants younger than 3 months old (rarely older). Group A streptococcus (GAS) are also subdivided into more than 100 subtypes based upon their M protein antigen located on the cell surface and fimbriae on the cell's outer edge. The virulence of GAS is greatly dependent upon their M protein. If the M protein is present, GAS strains are able to resist phagocytosis; if the M protein is weak or absent, the strains are basically avirulent (e.g., chronic GAS pharyngeal carriers). GAS also produces many varieties of enzymes and toxins that may stimulate specific antitoxin antibodies for immunity or serve as evidence of past infection but not confer immunity. There may also not be cross-immunity between antibodies for different GAS strains (e.g., scarlet fever is caused by three different pyrogenic exotoxins, so the illness can recur). Some general remarks about specific illnesses due to GAS and non-group A and B streptococcus infection are discussed in this chapter; cross-references to specific chapters are noted for other GAS caused infections.

Group A Streptococcus

Streptococcus microbes most commonly invade the respiratory tract, skin, soft tissues, and blood. Transmission is primarily through infected upper respiratory tract secretions or, secondarily, through skin invasion. Fomites and household pets are not vectors. Food-borne outbreaks from contamination by food handlers have been reported. Both streptococcus pharyngitis and impetigo are associated with crowding, whether at home, school, or other institution. Streptococcal pharyngitis is rare in infants and children younger than 3 years old, but the incidence rises with age and is most common in the winter and early spring in temperate climates when respiratory viruses circulate. Carrier rates in asymptomatic children are up to 20% (Arnold and Nizet, 2012). By contrast, streptococcus skin infection (impetigo, pyoderma) is more common in toddlers and preschool-age children. Those at increased risk for invasive GAS are individuals with varicella infection, IV drug use, HIV, diabetes, chronic heart or lung disease, infants, and older adults.

The incubation period is 2 to 5 days for pharyngitis and 7 to 10 days from skin acquisition to development of impetiginous lesions. In untreated individuals, the period of communicability is from the onset of symptoms up to a few months. Children are generally considered non-infectious 24 hours after the start of appropriate antibiotic therapy.

Clinical Findings and Diagnostic Studies

The following may be seen in GAS:

- Respiratory tract infection: Streptococcal tonsillopharyngitis (GABHS) and pneumonia are described in Chapter 32. Peritonsillar abscess, cervical lymphadenitis, retropharyngeal abscess, otitis media, mastoiditis, and sinusitis symptoms may be clinical features.
- Scarlet fever: This is caused by erythrogenic toxin. It is uncommon in children younger than 3 years old. The incubation period is approximately 3 days (the range is 1 to 7 days). There is abrupt illness with sore throat, vomiting, headache, chills, and malaise. Fever can reach 104° F (40° C). Tonsils are erythematous, swollen, and usually covered in exudate. The pharynx also is inflamed and can be covered with a gray-white exudate. The palate and uvula are erythematous and reddened, and petechiae are present. The tongue is usually coated and red. Desquamation of the coating leaves prominent papillae (strawberry tongue). The typical scarlatina rash appears 1 to 5 days following onset of symptoms but may be the presenting symptom. The exanthema is red, blanches to pressure, and is finely papular, making the skin feel coarse, with a sandpaper feel. The rash generally begins on the neck and spreads to the trunk and extremities becoming generalized within 24 hours. The face may be spared (cheeks may be reddened with circumoral pallor), but the rash becomes denser on the neck, axilla, and groin. Pastia lines, transverse linear hyperpigmented areas with tiny petechiae, are seen in the folds of the joints (see Fig. 24-3). In severe disease, small vesicles (miliary sudamina) can be found on the hands, feet, and abdomen. There is circumoral pallor and the cheeks are erythematous. The rash begins to fade and desquamate after 3 to 4 days starting on the face and slowly moving to the trunk and extremities and may include fingernail margins, palms, and soles; this process can take up to 6 weeks. Sore throat and constitutional symptoms resolve in approximately 5 to 7 days (average 3 to 4 days).
- Bacteremia: This can occur after respiratory (pharyngitis, tonsillitis, AOM) and localized skin infections. Some children have no obvious source of infection. Meningitis, osteomyelitis, septic arthritis, pyelonephritis, pneumonia, peritonitis, and bacterial endocarditis are rare but are associated with GAS bacteremia. (Neonatal sepsis due to group B streptococcus is discussed in Chapter 39.)
- Vaginitis and streptococcal toxic shock syndrome (see discussions in Chapter 36).
- Perianal streptococcal cellulitis: Symptoms include local itching, pain, blood-streaked stools, erythema, and proctitis. Fever and systemic infections are uncommon. Although infection is usually the result of autoinoculation, sexual molestation is in the differential.
- Skin infections (see Chapter 37); rheumatic heart disease (see Chapter 25); and necrotizing fasciitis (see Chapter 37).

Refer to disease-specific chapters for diagnostic studies of disease-specific conditions.

Differential Diagnosis, Management, and Complications

Many viral pathogens are on the differential for acute pharyngitis, including influenza, parainfluenza, rhinovirus, coronavirus, adenovirus, and respiratory syncytial virus. EBV is common and is usually accompanied by other clinical findings (e.g., splenomegaly, generalized lymphadenopathy). Other causes of bacterial upper respiratory disease include (though rare) diphtheria, tularemia, toxoplasmosis, mycoplasma, tonsillar TB, salmonellosis, and brucellosis (Gerber, 2011). Staphylococcal impetigo must be differentiated from GABHS pyoderma. Septicemia, meningitis, osteomyelitis, septic arthritis, pyelonephritis, and bacterial endocarditis can result from other bacteria causing similar infections.

Antimicrobial therapy is recommended for GABHS-caused pharyngitis to decrease the risk of acute rheumatic fever, decrease the length of the illness, prevent complications, and reduce transmission to others. See appropriate aforementioned site-specific chapters for recommendations for managing specific infections.

Complications are usually caused by the spread of the disease from the localized infection. Upper respiratory complications include cervical lymphadenitis, retropharyngeal abscess, otitis media, mastoiditis, and sinusitis if the primary infection is unrecognized or treatment is inadequate. Acute poststreptococcal glomerulonephritis can occur following skin or upper respiratory GAS infection, whereas acute rheumatic fever only occurs following GAS URIs. Poststreptococcal reactive arthritis can occur following GAS pharyngitis. Skin infection with GAS may progress to cellulitis, myositis, or necrotizing fasciitis. Other complications may be associated with invasive infections including pneumonia, pleural empyema, meningitis, osteomyelitis, and bacterial endocarditis.

Pediatric autoimmune neuropsychiatric disorders associated with streptococcal infections (PANDAS) is a group of neuropsychiatric disorders thought to result from the production of autoimmune antibodies; these include obsessive-compulsive disorders, tic disorders, and Tourette syndrome. See Chapter 19 for further discussion.

Non–Group A or B Streptococci

These streptococci or Lancefield groups (principally groups C and G) are associated with invasive disease in all age groups. They may cause septicemia, UTIs, endocarditis, respiratory disease (upper and lower), skin soft tissue infection, pharyngitis, brain abscesses, and meningitis in newborns, children, adolescents, and adults. The incubation period and communicability times are unknown. Positive culture from normally sterile body fluids is adequate for diagnosis. Penicillin G is the drug of choice with modification based on culture sensitivities. Pneumonia with empyema or abscess may respond slowly despite effective antimicrobial therapy with fevers lasting more than 7 days (Haslam and St. Geme, 2012).

Tuberculosis

TB is caused by *M. tuberculosis* and is a very slow-growing organism, taking up to 10 weeks to grow on solid media and 1 to 6 weeks in liquid media. The degree of infectivity depends on the intensity and length of exposure to and the burden of bacilli carried by the index case. For this reason, TB is regarded as moderately infectious under most situations (Fitzgerald et al, 2015). The bacilli are spread primarily by droplet contamination from coughing, sneezing, or talking. Droplets can stay suspended in the air for hours. Fomite transmission is uncommon; in more than 98% of cases, the portal of entry is the lung (Starke, 2012).

TB may be either latent (LTBI; the individual is infected but not contagious) or active (signs and symptoms of active disease are present and individual is contagious). Not all infected individuals will develop an active disease. Generally about 3% to 4% of those infected with the bacilli progress to active disease during the first year after infection; thereafter, an additional 5% progress to disease (Fitzgerald et al, 2015). These estimates are based on heavy exposures during disease-prone periods of life.

Globally, one third of the world's population is infected with the mycobacteria (Starke, 2012). Ninety-five percent of cases of active TB occur in countries where HIV/AIDS infection has been epidemic and health care is poor or inaccessible. Individuals in the United States with the highest incidence of active TB live in urban, low-income areas. Approximately 60% reported TB cases in the United States are foreign-born with 80% being Hispanic and non-Caucasian. High-risk groups include immigrants, international adoptees, those from or travelers to high-prevalence regions (Asia, Africa, Latin American, and former Soviet Union countries), the homeless, alcoholics, IV drug users, and individuals in correctional facilities or other close communal settings (AAP et al, 2015b).

Infection is typically detected by a positive Mantoux TST or a positive interferon gamma release assay (IGRA) in a child found to be at high risk. In certain circumstances a child may have findings suggestive of TB infection and not have a positive TST or IGRA.These tests are reactive within 2 to 10 weeks after initial exposure to an active TB case. Risk of progression to disease is highest in the first 6 months after infection. The risk continues to remain high for the subsequent 2 years after infection, but the infection may remain latent for years before progressing to disease. After treatment is started, infectivity in active cases may cease within days or take several weeks depending on the drugs prescribed and response of the organisms and other characteristics of the disease (e.g., for cavitary disease, response can take longer). In children younger than 10 years old, there is usually minimal cough and little expulsion of bacilli and, therefore, less contagion. Most infections in children are from adults.

The age at the time of infection is predictive of the likelihood an infection will evolve into disease. Progression to disease is highest in infants, individuals 15 to 25 years old, and older adults; those older than 14 years old have the highest risk of developing clinical disease. Children younger than 5 years old account for about 60% of American childhood cases; children 5 to 14 years old have the lowest rate of disease. Other factors that make an individual more prone to active disease include having had another TB infection within the prior 2 years; immune status (immunocompromised individuals [from a disease (e.g., HIV) or immunosuppressive drugs] are at higher risk); IV drug use; those with chronic diseases (e.g., Hodgkin disease, lymphoma, diabetes mellitus, chronic renal failure, malnutrition); and those receiving tumor necrosis factor-alpha antagonists to treat arthritis, inflammatory bowel disease, or other diseases.

Congenital TB is extremely rare. An infant would most likely become infected after delivery from contact with an infected mother or other person. Exposure in utero could occur from exposure to maternal bacteremia, seeding of the placenta by disseminated (miliary) TB from the mother that gained access to the fetal circulation, fetal aspiration of amniotic fluid at delivery if the mother had tuberculous endometritis, or in utero ingestion of infected amniotic fluid (Starke, 2012).

Clinical Findings Primary Pulmonary Tuberculosis

Table 24-8 describes a synopsis of clinical findings for the stages of TB in children and interventions. Most children ages 3 to 15 years with primary pulmonary TB are asymptomatic except for a positive TB skin test or interferon-gamma release assay (IGRA). An effective immune response eliminates most of the bacilli, although small numbers of bacilli can be spread throughout the body during the bacteremic phase.

Any symptoms in children are generally minor and slightly more evident in infants; up to 50% may exhibit radiographic changes but have no physical findings. Most children with disease first develop hilar lymphadenopathy then focal hyperinflation and atelectasis (Starke, 2011). Signs and symptoms typically occur 1 to 6 months after infection and may range from low-grade fever, and nonproductive cough and dyspnea (more common in infants) to malaise, decreased appetite, weight loss (failure to thrive in infants), night sweats, chills, erythema nodosum, and phlyctenular keratoconjunctivitis (a hypersensitivity reaction marked by elevated clear nodules with surrounding hyperemia near the limbus). Approximately 25% to 30% of children will present with extrapulmonary TB symptoms (e.g., meningitis and/or granulomatous inflammation of the lymph nodes, bones, joints, skin, and middle ear and mastoid) (Starke, 2011). Rarely, enlarging lymph nodes can compress and obstruct regional bronchus, causing respiratory distress; this is more commonly seen with infants. Compression of the esophagus (causing dysphagia or aspiration) and major arteries and veins (causing edema) can also occur. Recurrent cough, stridor, and wheezing are signs of increasing pulmonary infection.

Screening Tests for Infection

Low-risk groups do not need to be routinely screened for TB. Children are considered at high risk for TB if they meet any of the following risk criteria:

- Have close contact with others who have suspected or confirmed TB
- Was born in, or has traveled for more than 1 week to, TB-prevalent parts of the world (Asia, Middle East, Africa, Latin America, countries formerly part of the Soviet Union) (it is reasonable to wait 10 weeks after return from traveling to such areas for screening with the TST or IGRA if the child is well and has no history of exposure)
- Live in an area where there is a rise in TB infection
- Have clinical signs suggestive of TB on chest radiograph or other clinical evidence suggestive of TB infection
- Are HIV positive (beginning at 3 to 12 months of age; TST only), have an immunosuppressive disorder, or are being treated with immunosuppressive drugs
- Are homeless, reside in correctional or other residental institution, is a member of a migrant farm family
- Consider in children with Hodgkin disease, diabetes mellitus, chronic renal failure, malnutrition, and those receiving tumor necrosis factor antagonists.

TABLE 24-8 Characteristics of Tuberculosis in Children

	STAGE		
	Exposure	Infection (LTBI)	Disease
Mantoux skin test or IGRA (for children 3 years and older and in those who have received BCG). Use Mantoux if HIV infected	Negative (results not reliable in infants younger than 3 months)	Positive (TST: in 60% to 90% of cases)	Positive (TST: in 60% to 90% of cases)
Physical examination	Normal	Normal	Usually abnormal*
Chest radiograph	Normal	Usually normal†	Usually abnormal‡
Treatment	If <4 years old or with impaired immunity (e.g., HIV)	Always	Always
Number of drugs	One	One (additional regimens available)	Four

Data from American Academy of Pediatrics, Kimberlin DW, Brady MT, et al, editors: *Tuberculosis, Red Book: 2015 Report of the Committee on Infectious Diseases*, ed 30, Elk Grove Village, IL, 2015, American Academy of Pediatrics, pp 805–831; Starke JR: Tuberculosis *(Mycobacterium tuberculosis)*. In Kliegman RM, Stanton BF, St. Geme III JW, et al, editors: *Nelson textbook of pediatrics*, ed 19, Philadelphia, 2011, Saunders, pp 996–1011.

BCG, Bacille Calmette-Guérin vaccine; *HIV,* human immunodeficiency virus; *IGRA*, interferon-gamma release assay; *LTBI,* latent tuberculosis infection.

*More than 50% of infants and children with pulmonary tuberculosis have a normal physical examination.

†May reveal healed lesions (calcification in the lungs, hilar lymph nodes, or both).

‡Some children with extrapulmonary tuberculosis have a normal chest radiograph.

Mantoux Tuberculin Skin Test. Tuberculin skin testing is based on the delayed hypersensitivity to *M. tuberculosis* antigens. The Mantoux skin test is used, which is a purified protein derivative (PPD). If the child becomes infected with TB, the test usually becomes positive 4 to 8 weeks (between 3 weeks and 3 month) after inhalation of the bacilli (Starke, 2011). All children with positive TST need quick clinical and radiographic evaluation.

The Mantoux test uses 0.1 mL of 5 tuberculin units (TU) of PPD. It is injected intradermally into the volar surface of the forearm, producing a palpable wheal with 6 to 10 mm of induration (crucial for accurate testing). A multipuncture skin test should not be used. The Mantoux test is read 48 to 72 hours later by an experienced health care professional. The induration, not the erythema, is measured. Sensitivity to the TST generally persists for years even after effective antitubular drug treatment.

Children with prior BCG vaccination can receive the TST, and interpretation of the test is the same as for nonrecipients. Prior BCG vaccination can produce a mild to severe hypersensitivity reaction, however, depending on several factors: the age of the BCG vaccine itself, its quality, the strain of *M. bovis* used, the number of past doses of BCG vaccine received, nutritional status, immunologic factors, infection with environmental mycobacteria, and the frequency of skin testing (boosts the response). The degree of positivity decreases over time, depending on the age at vaccination.

All children with positive TST need quick clinical and radiographic evaluation. A Mantoux skin test is defined as positive for latent tuberculosis infection (LTBI) or TB disease if the following reactions occur (AAP et al, 2015b):

- Induration (5 mm or greater) in children who are in close contact with an individual with active or previously active TB cases, have a chest radiograph consistent with active or previously active TB, have clinical findings of TB, have an immunosuppressive disorder or HIV infection, or are receiving immunosuppressive drugs
- Induration (10 mm or greater) in children younger than 4 years old with any of the high-risk factors listed earlier
- Induration (15 mm or greater) in children 4 years old or older without any risk factors
- If the skin test shows onset of induration after 72 hours, it should be interpreted as positive

Skin testing is not always valid and can be negative in 10% to 40% of children with positive cultures. This decreased reactivity can occur in immunocompromised children (e.g., with HIV), infants younger than 3 months of age, those with poor nutrition, or those with other viral infections (notably measles, varicella, and influenza). Ten percent of those with progressive TB (up to 50% with disseminated disease or meningitis) will not react until several months after receiving drug treatment (AAP et al, 2015b; Starke, 2011). Additionally, a poor response to the skin test can occur due to inadequate handling of the Mantoux solution, improper injection technique, or interpretation error. Individuals sensitized to nontuberculous mycobacteria can cross-react and have a less than 10- to 12-mm reaction to TB skin testing.

Interferon Gamma Release Assays. IGRAs include QuantiFERON-TB Gold In-Tube and T-SPOT.TB. IGRAs are screening tests approved by the FDA for detecting T-cell response to specific *M. tuberculosis* antigens. They have the advantage over the Mantoux test of not being affected by prior BCG vaccination. Children with indeterminate IRGA may need to have the test repeated. IGRAs are recommended for the following circumstances (AAP et al, 2015b; CDC 2012a):

- Immunocompetent children 3 years old or older to confirm suspected LTBI or active disease. A positive result is indicative of TB infection; a negative IGRA is not to be interpreted as absence of infection or disease if clinical signs and symptoms suggest otherwise
- Children 3 years old or older who have received BCG vaccine
- Children 3 years old or older who are unlikely to return for TST reading
- If the initial TST is positive in children 3 years old or older who have received BCG vaccine, in whom additional evidence is needed to improve compliance, or if nontuberculous mycobacterial disease is suspected
- Might be used with other diagnostic tests in an infant suspected of having congenital tuberculosis

Diagnostic Studies

Chest radiography early in the disease may show only localized, nonspecific infiltrates. Inflammation of lung tissue and hilar lymph nodes continues as the disease progresses; this is quickly resolved in most children, but increased hilar adenopathy is usually seen in infants. The hallmark is disproportionately enlarged regional lymph nodes as compared with a relatively small pleural focus (Starke, 2012).

Radiography in older children shows inconspicuous pneumonitis in the lower and middle lung fields. In adolescents, apical or subapical infiltrates are seen, often with cavitations, and no hilar adenopathy (Fitzgerald et al, 2015). Extensive pulmonary infiltrates and cavitation can be seen if there has been erosion and necrosis from disseminated bacilli. Lesions may be the size of millet seeds; hence the name "miliary" TB.

Hilar adenopathy suggests TB, but culture of the organism is essential to establish the diagnosis. Specimens for culture may be obtained from gastric aspirates, sputum, bronchial washings, pleural fluid, CSF, urine or other body fluids, or biopsies. However, mycobacteria are isolated in less than 50% of children and 75% of infants with pulmonary TB (AAP et al, 2015b). Children older than 5 years old and adolescents can be induced to cough to produce sputum with aerosolized hypertonic saline. When age or ability to produce sputum is a factor, early morning gastric aspirates, collected on three separate mornings and analyzed by fluorescent staining, is an effective and sensitive testing method. Histologic examination for acid-fast bacilli (AFB) from biopsies can be helpful. Solid media cultures can take up to

10 weeks to grow with an additional 2 to 4 weeks for susceptibility testing, whereas liquid cultures take 1 to 6 weeks. Rapid DNA probes or high-pressure liquid chromatography of cultured organisms can be done to differentiate between *M. tuberculosis* and *M. bovis* based on pyrazinamide resistance that is characteristic of *M. bovis*.

If an isolate from an index case is positive for TB, culture material does not need to be obtained from an exposed child. However, a culture is necessary in the following circumstances: the index case is unavailable, the child has HIV infection or is immunocompromised, drug-resistant TB is suspected, or the child has extrapulmonary symptoms (AAP et al, 2015b). A nucleic acid amplification test (NAAT) on respiratory secretions has become standard practice when TB is suspected; it is not used as a definitive test to exclude TB. It is used to aid in the diagnosis of TB when symptoms suggest active TB infection, but it does not supplant an AFB smear and culture. Results are known 1 or more weeks earlier than a culture. Its use expedites the appropriate initiation of treatment (CDC, 2012b). Additional research needs to be done before NAATs can be approved for use in extrapulmonary or primary TB in children who cannot produce sputum (AAP et al, 2015b).

Differential Diagnosis

The provider should consider TB in children with symptoms of basilar meningitis, hydrocephalus, cranial nerve palsy, or stroke. Permanent neurologic dysfunction can result and has a worse prognosis in infants than in toddlers and older children. The differential diagnosis also includes mycotic infections, staphylococcal pneumonia, sarcoidosis, chronic pneumonia, and Hodgkin lymphoma. Differential diagnosis in lymph node diseases includes cat-scratch disease, tularemia, toxoplasmosis, tumor, brachial cysts, cystic hygroma, and pyogenic infection.

Management

A TB specialist should be consulted when a child has a positive TST or when TB is suspected or a child is a contact. TB is a reportable infectious disease. After index and contact cases are identified and diagnostic studies are done, the state and/or local health department often initiate treatment and follow-up. The treatment regimens are often in flux. It is advised that providers consult a pediatric TB specialist before initiating treatment for any type of TB infection to ensure that the most current treatment is prescribed; different regimens will be used if the child also has concurrent HIV infection.

Antitubercular drug treatment is focused on eradicating the bacilli and inhibiting their multiplication in LTBI and early pulmonary disease as quickly as possible. Rapid resolution of caseous or granulomatous lesions will not occur. It is imperative that strict adherence to drug combination regimens be followed to minimize drug resistance. This may need to be done under directly observed therapy (DOT). If the treatment regimen is prescribed by a TB specialist or health department, the primary care provider should be aware of the specific antitubercular drug regimen the child is on. The first-line drugs are administered orally and include isoniazid INH), rifampin (RIF), pyrazinamide (PZA), and ethambutol (EMB). The typical treatment regimens for children/families able to adhere to daily administration include:

- For prophylaxis after contact with person with active TB or for LTBI: INH, taken once daily for 9 months; if INH resistant, RIF is used once daily for 6 months.
- For pulmonary and extrapulmonary disease (miliary, lymph node, bone, joint infection): All four drugs are taken once daily for 2 months. INH and RIF are then continued for 4 months more and administered 2 or 3 times a week (duration of treatment may be extended if also has HIV).
- For hilar adenopathy only: INH and RIF are taken once daily for 6 months.
- For meningitis: All four drugs are taken once daily for 2 months. Ethionamide or an aminoglycoside is used instead of EMB in young children. INH and RIF are then continued for 7 to 10 months more, taken once or twice weekly (total of 9 to 12 months of treatment).
- Newborns suspected of having congenital TB: INH, RIF, PZA, and an aminoglycoside are used.

The treatment regimens are often in flux, and there are alternative regimens in use. Under some alternative regimens the drugs may be administered twice a week under DOT, provide for shortened durations of treatment, or use different combinations of drugs depending upon age, drug-resistance, extent of TB infection, and concurrent infections. The CDC, AAP Red Book, and WHO are excellent resources for drug regimens and recommended dosages.

Pregnant women who are diagnosed with TB disease or who have signs and symptoms or abnormal findings on chest x-ray consistent with TB during pregnancy should be promptly treated for TB and also tested for HIV. If the pregnant woman is found to have LTBI and a normal chest x-ray, she should be started on LTBI treatment for 9 months after the postpartum period, and the newborn would need no further evaluation or therapy (AAP et al, 2015b). If she is found to have active disease, some isolation may be recommended and the newborn evaluated for congenital TB disease. If congenital TB is excluded, the infant should be started on treatment for LTBI after birth for 3 or 4 months (at which time a Mantoux skin test should be given) even if breastfeeding and the mother is on concurrent therapy.

The exclusively breastfed infant receiving isoniazid should be given pyridoxine, although it is not routinely recommended for children and adolescents. It is also recommended for use in children whose diets are either deficient in meat or milk, if they also have HIV, and for pregnant adolescents; the tablets can be pulverized for easier administration. For children with meningeal, endobronchial, pleural and pericardial effusion, abdominal TB, and miliary TB, corticosteroids may be used to decrease the inflammation that is detrimental to organ function; its use also decreases mortality rates and neurologic disability.

Monitoring Response to Treatment

Tracking of index and contact cases is under the jurisdiction of state and local health departments. Initial evaluation, drug management, and follow-up may also take place in these centers. However, the PCP plays a crucial role in monitoring response to treatment. The following are general monitoring guidelines (AAP et al, 2015b):

- See all individuals monthly who are being treated for any stage of TB. Evaluate for antitubercular drug adherence and side effects, notably for symptoms of hepatitis if on isoniazid (a rare finding in healthy infants, children, and adolescents). Educate patients to call immediately if experiencing signs of hepatoxicity (e.g., vomiting, abdominal pain, and jaundice), peripheral neuritis, diarrhea, or GI irritation. Those on pyrazinamide may experience hepatoxicity, arthralgia, or GI disturbances. Rifampin may cause orange secretions in urine, vomiting, hepatitis, flulike symptoms, thrombocytopenia, and pruritus; those on oral contraceptives need to use a back-up birth control method.
- Routine lab monitoring is not recommended in children unless the child has severe TB disease, meningitis, or disseminated disease. In these cases, transaminases should be checked monthly for the first several months. Other indications for laboratory studies include current or recent liver or biliary disease, use of hepatotoxic drugs (e.g., HIV, seizure medications), clinical evidence of hepatotoxicity, and/or pregnant or within 12 weeks postpartum.
- A sputum specimen for AFB smear and culture is collected after 2 months of drug therapy to evaluate response; if sputum culture is positive after 3 months of therapy, the bacilli need to be rechecked for drug susceptibility.
- If cavitation is present on initial chest x-ray and a 2-month sputum culture is positive, treatment with INH and RIF should be extended an additional 3 months for a total treatment duration of 9 months.
- Repeat chest radiograph after 2 months; it is good practice to take one after therapy has been completed as a baseline for comparison against any subsequent films. Hilar adenopathy can persist for 2 to 3 years despite adequate therapy. Residual calcification of the primary focus or regional lymph nodes may be evident on x-ray.
- Extrapulmonary disease: Follow clinical symptoms.
- For those taking ethambutol, ask about presence of any visual disturbances (screen visual acuity and red-green color vision if dosages exceed 20 mg/kg/day or if on more than 2 months of treatment with this drug); if unable to test visual acuity, consider an alternate drug.
- Children can be given measles and other attenuated live-virus vaccines at age-appropriate times, unless they are on high-dose corticosteroids, are severely ill, or have another contraindication.
- If therapy is interrupted, treatment length should be extended. Consult with a TB specialist.

Complications

The following complications with their clinical findings can occur with TB:

- Progressive primary pulmonary disease: Rarely, primary TB can progress and disseminate. This occurs more frequently in infants and children younger than 5 years old, a result of their immune systems being immature or inadequate to the task of eliminating bacilli. The primary pleural focus enlarges and develops a large caseous center, and liquefaction forms a cavity that contains large numbers of bacilli. Symptoms in children with progressive disease are more acute and include high intermittent fevers, night sweats, severe cough, and weight loss. Pleural effusion, peritonitis, or meningitis can occur in as many as two thirds of individuals (Fitzgerald et al, 2015). In young adults, the infection is usually more chronic and onset is subtle. Nonspecific symptoms include fever, anorexia, weakness, and weight loss. The physical examination should include a careful skin examination, looking for cutaneous eruptions, sinus tracts, scrotal masses, and lymphadenopathy; hepatomegaly, splenomegaly, tachypnea, dyspnea, rales, wheezes, and stridor are often found. Inflamed nodes can erode through the endobronchial wall; fistulas can occur between the lymph node and the bronchial lumen and cause fibrosis, bronchiectasis, and pneumonia.
- Reactivation of pulmonary TB: There is potential for reactivation of pulmonary TB in those who acquired their initial infection when they were older than 7 years old. Reactivation is more likely to occur after the child reaches adolescence and can present with either few symptoms, or fever, anorexia, malaise, weight loss, night sweats, productive cough, hemoptysis, and chest pain. These individuals are highly contagious until effective treatment is started, but full recovery is excellent with appropriate treatment (Starke, 2012).
- Miliary disease: During the early stages of the primary disease, bacilli disseminate and reach the bloodstream directly from the initial focus or by way of the regional lymph nodes. Prior to effective drug therapy, this complication of primary pulmonary disease occurred more commonly in infants, children, and adolescents. It appears more often now in racial minorities, in those with underlying conditions that may compromise the immune system, and in older adults (Fitzgerald et al, 2015). Systemic signs such as anorexia, weight loss, and low-grade fever progress over weeks to lymphadenopathy, hepatosplenomegaly, higher fever, dyspnea, cough, rales, wheezing, frank respiratory distress, and pneumothorax or pneumomediastinum. Headache suggests meningitis; abdominal pain suggests tuberculous peritonitis (Starke, 2011).
- Lymph node disease: This is an extrapulmonary form of TB affecting the superficial lymph nodes; it is known as *scrofula*. It can be caused by drinking raw milk contaminated with *M. bovis* or after initial infection with

M. tuberculosis. The head, trunk, neck, and inguinal and lower extremity nodes are firm (but not hard), fixed to underlying tissue, and nontender. The lymphadenopathy is usually unilateral at first and can progress to multinode involvement. Tuberculin skin testing is usually positive; a chest x-ray is normal 70% of the time; cultures from lymph node biopsies reveal mycobacteria in about 50% of cases (Starke, 2011).

- Pleural effusions: Pleural effusion frequently occurs in primary disease, caused by an extension of the bacillus into the pleural space by subpleural foci or hematogenous spread, or both. It usually occurs 6 to 9 months after the primary infection. Symptoms include abrupt onset of low to high fever, shortness of breath, chest pain on deep inspiration, and decreased breath sounds. Response to treatment takes several weeks; radiographic changes can continue to be evident for months following treatment (Starke, 2012).
- Tuberculous meningitis: Meningitis is the most serious complication of TB. It generally follows primary pulmonary disease in 0.5% of untreated infants and young children 6 months to 4 years old (rare in infants younger than 4 months old). Meningeal infection is also common in miliary TB. Bacilli migrate to the subarachnoid space. Caseous lesions can enlarge, encapsulate, and form a tuberculoma that can act just like any other CNS mass lesion. Tuberculoma are rare and usually occur in children younger than 10 years old. Symptoms can evolve slowly or rapidly; infants and children generally experience rapid onset. Tuberculin skin testing is negative in 40% of cases with up to 50% also having negative chest x-rays (Starke, 2012). Diagnosis is via CSF AFB stain and culture. Symptoms include headache, fever, malaise, irritability, drowsiness, decreased developmental milestones, nuchal rigidity, positive Kernig or Brudzinski signs, hypertonia, vomiting, seizures, and other neurologic symptoms. The provider should consider TB in the differential diagnosis for any child who presents with basilar meningitis and hydrocephaly, cranial nerve palsy, or stroke without other apparent cause.
- Cutaneous TB: This variant occurs in 1% to 2% of all TB cases worldwide, but is rare in the United States (Starke, 2011). Individuals at high risk include those with HIV, those living in poor sanitary conditions, of low socioeconomic status, and the malnourished.
- Hematogenous spread of TB to other organs or body systems: Every body system can be affected by TB. Spread can be to endocrine and exocrine glands, urogenital tract, heart and pericardium, skeleton, eyes, abdomen, tonsils, adenoids, larynx, middle ear, and mastoids.
- MDR-TB is defined as resistance to isoniazid and rifampin. XDR-TB is defined as resistance to isoniazid and rifampin, one fluoroquinolone, and at least one aminoglycoside (capreomycin, amikacin, or kanamycin). Rates of drug resistance have risen from 3% to 9% in the past 30 years (Starke, 2012).

Helminthic Zoonoses

About 75% of emerging infectious diseases originate with animals, and approximately 60% of all human pathogens are zoonotic (transmitted from an animal to a human host) in origin (CDC, 2015z3). Transmission of zoonotic infections can occur by several routes:

- Direct infection by ingestion of eggs or the penetration of larvae into the body (infections such as tapeworms and roundworms are acquired from their eggs; hookworms penetrate the skin)
- Indirect infection by ingestion of larvae in food (e.g., fish, meat, snails, freshwater shrimp, land crabs)
- Exposure to an intermediary vector (e.g., mosquitoes, flies, fleas, ticks)

A large percentage of households in the United States have domestic pets (about 37% with dogs; 30% with cats); therefore, close contact is inevitable (American Veterinary Medical Association, 2012). Domesticated dogs, cats, and wild animals (e.g., raccoons) kept as pets can be infected with intestinal helminth parasites. Mild to severe illness can result when a helminth is transmitted to children, most often by fecal contamination. Only toxocariasis larva migrans, which may be encountered in primary care, is discussed here. (See Chapter 33 for a further discussion on intestinal parasites.)

Toxocariasis

Toxocariasis, or larva migrans, is caused by a parasitic helminth larvae (of the roundworm) found in dogs (*T. canis*) and cats (*T. catis*). The larvae can live for extended periods in human and animal organs and tissues causing an inflammatory condition. The most common clinical syndromes are visceral larva migrans (VLM), ocular toxocariasis (formerly called ocular larva migrans), and covert disease. *Toxocara* larvae rarely migrate to the CNS causing eosinophilic meningoencephalitis or granuloma formation (CDC, 2013f). They can be further classified as *asymptomatic* or *clinically unapparent*. *T. catis* causes less VLM than *T. canis*; *T. canis* can cause VLM, OLM, and, in severe cases, neural larva migrans.

Dogs or cats of any age can carry the *Toxocara* roundworm; worldwide, dogs (especially puppies) are a more common vector than kittens. Puppies are infected prior to birth (not true for kittens) or from their mother's milk. Ingestion of these hardy eggs (they can remain viable for months and in inclement weather conditions) occurs from contact with excreta in contaminated soil (e.g., in sandboxes, parks, playgrounds, schoolyards, public places where dogs and cats have visited), hands, toys, or in food. Once the eggs are ingested and hatched, the larvae can penetrate the intestines and migrate to the liver, lungs, heart, brain, and muscles. With initial or mild infestations, the larvae seem to be able to reach other locations, such as the brain and eye, more easily. In humans, the larvae cannot complete their maturation into adult worms (as they do in animals), so infected individuals do not pass eggs or larvae in their excreta.

The most recent study within the United States showed a prevalence rate of 14% for toxocariasis (Woodhall, 2012) with 4.6% to 7.3% of children infected (Dent and Kazura, 2011). Young children and those younger than 20 years old are most commonly infected (CDC, 2103f). VLM occurs in older children and adolescents but is most commonly seen in children 2 to 7 years old and in those with a history of pica. Ocular toxocariasis occurs more often in older children and adolescents (AAP et al, 2015b).

Clinical Findings

Symptoms result from the migrating larvae and from the induced eosinophilic granulomatous inflammation of organs and tissues. Symptom severity depends on the number of larvae ingested and degree of allergic response. Assess exposure history for pica or geophagia; exposure to dogs, cats, or environments where animals are known to frequent (parks, sandboxes); and recent travel. In the case of ocular toxocariasis, there may be no history of pica or previous VLM.

Toxocariasis should be considered in any child with a nonspecific history of recurrent abdominal pain, reactive airway disease, and allergies of unknown cause. The clinical history of VLM may include rash, abdominal and/or limb pain, anorexia, nausea/vomiting, lethargy, or respiratory symptoms (cough, wheezing). Ocular toxocariasis is usually associated with a history of a "wandering eye" or squinting, light sensitivity, a white pupil, swelling around an eye, or eye pain. Neural larva migrans often presents as soon as 2 to 4 weeks after ingestion of the larvae. The child's history can include weakness, incoordination, ataxia, irritability, seizures, altered mental status, stupor, and/or coma.

Physical Examination

- Ocular toxocariasis: Posterior or peripheral subretinal mass, decreased vision, pain, strabismus, or leukokoria
- VLM: Abdominal pain, hepatomegaly, irritability, respiratory symptoms (coughing, wheezing, pneumonia), cervical adenitis, urticaria, pruritic skin lesions or nodules, macular rash
- Neural larva migrans: Neurologic impairment
- Covert larva migrans: Chronic weakness, abdominal pain, allergic signs (asymptomatic eosinophilia or wheezing may be the only indicators of disease)

Diagnostic Studies

Eosinophilia is present in 50% to 75% of cases; a normal count does not rule out this infection (Dent and Kazura, 2011).

- VLM: CBC reveals leukocytosis, marked eosinophilia (>500/μL), hypergammaglobulinemia (IgG, IgM, IgE), and elevated A and B blood group isohemagglutinin titers. *Toxocara* ELISA antibody can be used for confirmatory testing; it does not, however, distinguish from past and active disease. Most symptomatic children will have titers of 1:32 or greater (Dent and Kazura, 2011).
- Ocular toxocariasis: Serologic testing done for VLM is not reliable because it is less sensitive. Diagnosis is usually based on typical clinical findings of a retinal scarring or granuloma formation with elevated antibody titers. *Toxocara* titers of a specimen of vitreous-aqueous fluid are usually higher than serum titers. CT and MRI may be used to detect granulomatous lesions.
- Overt larva migrans: May demonstrate eosinophilia and increased IgE.

Differential Diagnosis

Other helminths, hypereosinophilic syndromes, retinoblastoma, autoimmune disease, and allergic conditions are included in the differential diagnoses.

Management and Complications

Most individuals do not require treatment because symptoms are usually mild with spontaneous recovery occurring over a period of weeks to months (Dent and Kazura, 2011). Pediatric infectious disease referral for evaluation and treatment is indicated for patients with symptomatic VLM, ocular toxocariasis, or CNS disease. Management is based on controlling inflammatory reactions (corticosteroids) and use of appropriate anthelmintic therapy. Albendazole is the drug of choice with mebendazole as an alternative. Longer courses of 3 to 4 weeks are needed to treat disease with CNS and ocular involvement; systemic and intraocular corticosteroid therapy should be considered for ocular toxocariasis (managed by qualified ophthalmologist and infectious disease specialist). Family pets need evaluation by a veterinarian. Permanent ocular structural damage may result from ocular toxocariasis. Neural larva migrans may cause acute eosinophilic meningoencephalitis.

Patient and Family Education

Prevention of zoonotic infestations includes identifying possible sources of exposure, encouraging routine helminth testing for pets, decontamination of soiled environments, and prevention of further exposure. The last intervention includes education about safe pet fecal cleanup, the regular deworming of pets, good hand washing, behavioral modification in cases of pica and geophagia, and covering sandboxes when not in use. Communities should be encouraged to promote leash laws and responsible pet ownership (e.g., cleaning up pet fecal waste), to disallow dogs from playgrounds and parks where children play, and to restrict open access to sandboxes.

The Child Presenting with Fever

Fever is defined as an abnormally elevated rectal temperature of 100.4° F (38° C) or greater.

The normal physiologic hypothalamic set-point for body temperature is altered by many different agents (see Chapter 21 for a more complete description of the physiologic processes involved in fever mechanisms). Febrile illnesses in neonates are usually the result of congenital infections or infections acquired at delivery (e.g., late-onset group B streptococcal infection), in the nursery (especially in premature infants), at home (e.g., pneumococcal or meningococcal infection), and those acquired as a result of anatomic or physiologic dysfunction (e.g., renal). Causes of fever in children are related to bacterial and viral infections, vaccines, biologic agents, tissue damage, malignancy, drugs, collagen-vascular disorders, endocrine disorders, inflammatory disorders, and other disease states. Temperatures higher than 105.8° F (41° C) are rarely of infectious origin but are due to CNS dysfunction (e.g., malignant hyperthermia, drug fever, heat stroke).

There are two situations of invasive bacterial or viral infections that are a particular challenge for any provider dealing with neonates, infants, and children 36 months old or younger—*fever without focus*—and in all ages—*fever of unknown origin*. Each of these situations is discussed separately, and guidelines for their management are given. A fairly objective diagnosis can be reached by completing a careful history and physical examination and following diagnostic, assessment, and management guidelines based on age, symptoms, estimated risks, associated diseases, and immune status. A few general epidemiologic points are helpful for this discussion (Nield and Kamat, 2011):

- In infants younger than 3 months old with fever, 70% of causative agents can be identified—the majority being viral. A workup for bacterial disease is still necessary. The younger the infant, the greater the uncertainty about the possibility of a serious bacterial infection, and the greater the need to rule out this possibility.
- Viruses have a seasonal pattern: RSV and influenza A in winter; enterovirus in summer and fall.
- Bacteremia occurs in approximately 5% of previously well infants younger than 3 months old.
- Bacteremia can be an occult infection in young infants and children (i.e., nontoxic-appearing child whose blood culture is positive for a pathogenic organism).
- Occult bacteremia occurs in less than 0.5% in children between 3 and 36 months old who have been vaccinated with both conjugated Hib and *S. pneumoniae* vaccines. Otitis media, pneumonia, URIs, enteritis, UTIs, osteomyelitis, and meningitis more commonly account for infections in this age range.

TABLE 24-9 Age-Related Causes of Serious Bacterial and Viral Infections in Very Young Infants*

Age	Bacterial and Viral Infections
Meningitis	
<1 mo	Group B streptococcus *Escherichia coli* (and other enteric gram-negative bacilli) *Listeria monocytogenes* *Streptococcus pneumoniae* *Haemophilus influenzae* *Staphylococcus aureus* *Neisseria meningitidis* *Salmonella* spp. Herpes simplex Enteroviruses
1 to 3 mo	*S. pneumoniae* Group B streptococcus *N. meningitidis* *Salmonella* spp. *H. influenzae* *L. monocytogenes* *S. aureus*
Osteoarticular Infections	
<1 mo	Group B streptococcus *S. aureus*
1 to 3 mo	*S. aureus* Group B streptococcus *S. pneumoniae*
Urinary Tract Infection	
0 to 3 mo	*E. coli* Other enteric gram-negative bacilli Group D streptococcus (including *Enterococcus* spp.)

Data from Nield LS, Kamat D: Fever without a focus. In Kliegman RM, Stanton BF, St. Geme III JW, et al, editors: *Nelson textbook of pediatrics*, ed 19, Philadelphia, 2011, Saunders, pp 896–902; Shapiro ED: Fever without localizing signs. In Long SS, Pickering LK, Prober CG, editors: *Principles and practice of pediatric infectious diseases*, ed 4, New York, 2012, Elsevier, pp 114–116.
*In decreasing order of frequency.

Fever Without Focus in Infants and Young Children

Fever without focus is an acute febrile illness in which the etiology of the fever is not apparent after careful history and physical examination. Approximately 30% of febrile children 1 month to 36 months old do not have localizing signs of infection. In the vast majority of these children, the etiology is most often viral (Nield and Kamat, 2011). However, children between birth and 24 months old are at greatest risk for unsuspected occult bacteremia; it is less common in those older than 36 months.Table 24-9 provides a list of the most common pathogens causing bacteremia in infants younger than 3 months old. Since the advent of the Hib conjugate vaccine, this pathogen has become rare as a cause of bacteremia in children 3 to 36 months old; the incidence of *S. pneumoniae* bacteremia has decreased substantially since conjugate vaccine has been routinely in use (Nield and Kamat, 2011; Shapiro, 2012).

Clinical Findings

History and Physical Examination

The following should be included in the history of the illness:

- Duration and degree of fever (rectal temperature was 100.4° F [38° C] or greater?)

- Associated symptoms: Vomiting, diarrhea, respiratory symptoms, rash (especially petechiae or purpura), feeding pattern, irritability, inconsolability, change in play activities, lethargy (level of consciousness characterized by poor or absent eye contact or failure to recognize parents or interact with persons or objects in the environment)
- Review of known exposures (family illness, contacts with other ill children, day care contacts); recent travel history
- Recent vaccination
- Past medical history of malignancy, splenectomy, shunt, indwelling catheter, immunologic disorders, recurrent bacterial infections, serious bacterial infection
- Neonatal history of complications, prior antibiotics, prior surgeries, hyperbilirubinemia
- Chronic illness
- Current medications, including antipyretics, antibiotics, herbs, and dietary supplements
- Immunization history, particularly with Hib conjugate and pneumococcal conjugate vaccines

A complete physical examination should be done. Of special note are symptoms suggestive of serious bacterial illness (e.g., fever, bulging anterior fontanelle, respiratory system changes, lethargy and other CNS symptoms, evidence of skin infection or rashes, skin perfusion and turgor).

Diagnostic Studies

An algorithm for determining the diagnostic studies based upon specific age groups is found in Figure 24-8. Febrile infants younger than 1 month old or any febrile toxic appearing child 0 to 36 months old should be admitted to the hospital for a complete sepsis workup and given appropriate antibiotic treatment. The need for CSF from infants 1 month to 3 months old varies between different management guidelines if empiric antibiotics are being considered (Palazzi, 2014).

A negative, low-risk ambulatory workup is characterized by:

- CBC: WBC count less than 15,000/mm^3, absolute band count of fewer than 1,500 bands/mm^3; non-elevated ESR and/or CRP (may be included as part of workup in some standard guidelines)
- Catheterized urinalysis: Fewer than 10 WBCs/hpf spun sediment, negative leukocytes and nitrites
- When diarrhea is present: Fewer than 5 WBCs/hpf in stool
- If cough is present: Negative chest x-ray

Appropriate cultures should be obtained and monitored every 24 hours until final results are known. Viral testing should be done based on seasonality. Obtain HSV PCR from blood and CSF and PCR/culture from skin sites (mouth/throat, eyes, umbilicus, perirectal) if infant is 42 days old or less, has vesicular skin lesions, abnormal CSF, or seizures.

Differential Diagnosis

The differential diagnoses include upper respiratory tract disease (e.g., viral URI, otitis media, and sinusitis); lower respiratory tract disease (e.g., bronchiolitis, pneumonia); GI disease; musculoskeletal infections (e.g., cellulitis, septic arthritis, osteomyelitis); urinary tract infection (especially due to *E. coli*); and occult bacteremia due to other pathogens in children 3 to 36 months old (in those immunized with both Hib and pneumococcal conjugate vaccine, the rate of occult bacteremia is less than 0.5%) (Nield and Kamat, 2011). Serious bacterial agents are identified in approximately 10% to 15% of previously well neonates with fever and diagnoses of sepsis, meningitis, UTI, enteritis, osteomyelitis, or suppurative arthritis. Other possible illnesses to consider in this age group include pyelonephritis (more often occurring in uncircumcised boys, neonates, those with urinary tract anomalies, and females), otitis media, omphalitis, mastitis, and other skin or soft tissue infections (Nield and Kamat, 2011).

Management

Applying Risk Criteria

There are several criteria or protocols for identifying infants younger than 3 months old who have serious bacterial illness (e.g., bacteremia, UTI, meningitis, bacterial gastroenteritis, or pneumonia) that require empiric antibiotics and possibly hospitalization. The most widely cited guidelines include the Boston, Philadelphia, Milwaukee, and Rochester; all are based upon clinical assessment and laboratory studies (Moher et al, 2012). (See the algorithm for managing specific age groups based upon risk factors in Fig. 24-8).

High risk is regarded as any of the following:

- Any febrile infant younger than 1 month old; any toxic-appearing neonate, infant, or child regardless of age, risk factors, or degree of fever
- An infant 1 to 3 months old with a rectal temperature of 100.4° F (38° C) or greater
- An infant 1 to 3 months old with a chronic illness or underlying condition (including prematurity) with unreliable caretakers
- An infant younger than 3 months old even if diagnosed with otitis media (the workup is continued)
- Infants and children 3 to 36 months old with a rectal temperature of 102.2° F (39° C) and laboratory study results that place the child in a high-risk category
- Any aged child with fever and petechiae who appears ill

Immediate hospitalization and workup are indicated for high-risk cases. Any child younger than 36 months old who appears well with rectal temperature more than 102.2° F (39° C), WBC more than 15,000/mm^3, and who has not been vaccinated with Hib and *S. pneumoniae* conjugate vaccines should be started on empiric antibiotic therapy (Nield and Kamat, 2011).

Low risk is regarded as any of the following:

- An infant 1 to 3 months old who is nontoxic appearing with no clinical evidence of ear, skin, joint, or bones infections and who has low-risk diagnostic study results
- An infant 3 to 6 months old with a rectal temperature more than 100.4° F (38° C) but less than 102.2° F (39° C) who does not appear ill

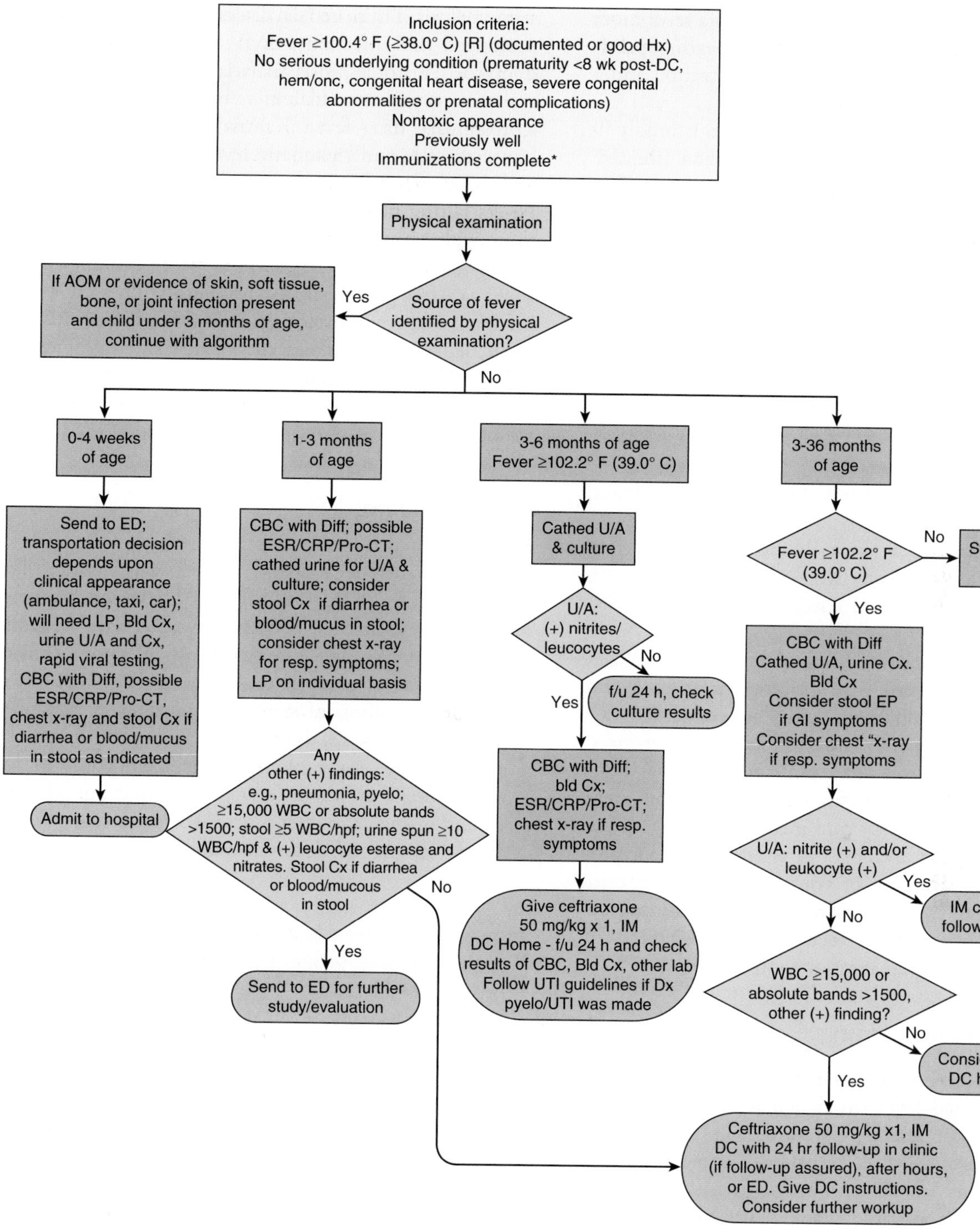

• **Figure 24-8** Fever without focus algorithm. *AOM*, Acute otitis media; *Bld Cx*, blood culture; *Cathed*, catherterized; *CBC*, complete blood count; *CRP,* C-reactive protein; *Cx*, culture, *DC*, discharge; *Diff,* differential; *Dx*, diagnosis; *ED*, emergency department; *EP*, enteric pathogens (culture); *ESR,* erythrocyte sedimentation rate; *f/u*, follow-up; *GI,* gastrointestinal; *h*, hours; *hem/onc*, hematologic/oncology issue; *hpf*, high power field; *Hx*, history; *IM*, intramuscular; *LP*, lumbar puncture; *Pro-CT*, procalcitonin; *pyelo*, pyelonephritis; *resp.*, respiratory; *U/A*, urinalysis; *UTI*, urinary tract infection; *WBC*, white blood cell count; *wk,* week. *Occult bacteremia can be as high as 5% if immunizations are incomplete (<1% if complete). (Updated and modified from Children's Hospital and Health Center: *R/O sepsis algorithm*, San Diego, 1998, Children's Hospital and Health Center. Additional data from Allen CH: Fever without a source in children 3 to 36 months of age, UpToDate (website), 2014, available at www.uptodate.com/contents/fever-without-a-source-in-children-3-to-36-months-of-age. Accessed March 10, 2015; Hui C, Neto G, Tsertsvadze A, et al: Diagnosis and management of febrile infants (0–3 months): Evidence Report/Technology Assessments, No. 205, Rockville, MD, 2012, Agency for Healthcare Research and Quality; Nield LS, Kamat D: Fever without a focus. In Kliegman RM, Stanton BF, St. Geme III JW, et al, editors: *Nelson textbook of pediatrics*, ed 19, Philadelphia, 2011, Saunders/Elsevier, pp 896–902; Smitherman HF, Macias CG: Evaluation and management of the febrile young infant (7 to 90 days of age), UpToDate topic 6072: Version 22.0, updated September 2015.)

- An infant or child 3 to 36 months old with a fever more than 102.2° F (39° C), who is nontoxic appearing, previously healthy with a non-focal bacterial infection and a positive rapid influenza A test
- An infant or child 3 to 36 months old who is mildly ill appearing with rectal temperature greater than 102.2° F (39° C) but less than 104° F (40° C) and low-risk diagnostic study results. There should be documented immunizations to at least two doses of both *H. influenzae* conjugate vaccine and pneumococcal conjugate vaccine (PCV7 or PCV13)

In light of the decrease in bacteremia caused by *H. influenzae* and *S. pneumonia,* a well-appearing nontoxic infant from 1 to 3 months old with no foci of infection, who meets low risk criteria, has good reliable caregivers and close follow-up does not need empirical antibiotics (nor a lumbar puncture) (Nield and Kamat, 2011).

Follow-up management criteria for any child not being hospitalized includes:

- Reevaluation in the clinic in 24 hours and access to emergency care if condition worsens.
- Daily follow-up on culture results (blood, urine, CSF) until results are final.
- If cultures become positive, infant/child needs to be seen for evaluation and appropriate antibiotic treatment based on organism and additional workup as needed.
- Parents of infants who are managed as outpatients need detailed instructions on signs and symptoms that indicate a worsening of their infant's illness. Symptoms that would prompt emergency care include: a change in or new rash; duskiness, cyanosis, or mottling; coolness of extremities; poor feeding or vomiting; irritability; cries with positional changes; difficulty in comforting or arousing; seizure activity (eye rolling or jerking of extremities); or bulging anterior fontanelle.

Fever of Unknown Origin

The definition of *fever of unknown origin (FUO)* in children is: (1) a documented fever (rectal temperature more than 101° F [38.3° C] or oral temperature more than 100° F [37.8° C]) present most days for 3 weeks or more without an etiology, despite 3 weeks of outpatient visits and extensive studies, and (2) no etiology after 1 week of evaluation in the hospital or as an outpatient (Long and Edwards, 2012; Nield and Kamat, 2011). The health care provider must frequently rethink and reevaluate historical, clinical, and laboratory data on a child with a FUO. An infectious disease consultation is recommended.

Many FUOs are atypical presentations of common disorders, notably infections (accounting for more than one third of cases) or rheumatologic and connective tissue diseases (e.g., juvenile rheumatoid arthritis, SLE). In the United States, infectious diseases associated with most diagnoses of FUO include EBV, cat-scratch disease *(B. henselae),* complicated UTIs, and vertebral and pelvic osteomyelitis (Long and Edwards, 2012). Other causative agents include salmonellosis, TB, rickettsial diseases, syphilis, Lyme disease, prolonged viral infections, CMV, viral hepatitis, coccidioidomycosis, histoplasmosis, malaria, and toxoplasmosis. Less common causes are tularemia, brucellosis, rat-bite fever, leptospirosis, drug fever, Kawasaki disease, inflammatory bowel disease, and rheumatic fever. Neoplastic conditions and AIDS generally have symptoms other than just fever. Fevers lasting more than 6 months have been reported in those with granulomatosis or autoimmune disease. In children younger than 6 years old, the most common causes of FUO are UTI/pyelonephritis, respiratory illnesses, localized infections (abscess, osteomyelitis), juvenile arthritis, and, rarely, leukemia. In adolescents, the most common causes include TB, inflammatory bowel disease, autoimmune disorders, lymphoma, as well as the causes listed for children younger than 6 years old (Nield and Kamat, 2011). Also see the differential diagnosis list that follows.

Clinical Findings

History

A careful history helps distinguish between recurrent fever episodes and those that need further evaluation. Recurrent fevers resolve with well periods between them, suggesting an etiology of multiple self-limiting infections. History should include:

- A careful analysis of symptoms or signs, a meticulous review of systems, history of the fever pattern, and patient's age. An adolescent with complaints of low-grade fevers, or whose fever has resolved but who feels ill and is unable to attend school or social activities may have "fatigue of deconditioning" (Box 24-2). These

• BOX 24-2 Typical Findings in Patients with Fatigue of Deconditioning

- Older than 12 years old
- Pre-illness achievement high (academic and social)
- Family expectations high (performance)
- Acute febrile illness with onset easily dated
- Family and outside attention high
- Multiple but vague complaints
- Odd complaints (e.g., 10-second "shooting" pains at multiple sites; 30-second "blindness"; stereotypic, sporadic, brief unilateral tremors, jerks, or "paralysis" lasting <1 minute)
- Tiredness, but no daytime sleep (or reversal of daytime and nighttime sleep)
- There is a model of chronic illness in family, recent loss of important person, and/or change in family dynamics
- Unusual cooperation and interest during interview and examination (or unusual fearfulness and dependency on parent)
- Preserved or increased weight
- Normal physical and neurologic examination
- Normal results of screening laboratory tests

From Long SS, Edwards KM: Prolonged, recurrent and periodic fever syndromes. In Long SS, Pickering LK, Prober CG, editors: *Principles and practice of pediatric infectious diseases*, ed 4, New York, 2012, Elsevier, pp 117–127.

children require the same careful medical evaluation, but rarely have a serious infection or medical condition (Long and Edwards, 2012).
- Note of past medical history of recurrent infections, surgery, transfusions, and contact with ill individuals
- Medication use, including over-the-counter and herbal/natural/dietary supplements
- Family medical history, including autoimmune disease or inflammatory bowel disorder; genetic background (inherited periodic fever syndromes [e.g., familial Mediterranean fever, hyperimmunoglobulinemia D with periodic fever syndrome], tumor receptor–associated periodic syndrome)
- Family pets including reptiles, pet immunization history, or exposure to wild or other domestic animals
- Unusual dietary habits (eating squirrel, rabbit, or other unusual animal meat)
- History of pica; history of travel (location; travel immunizations; water/food ingested; if returned home with travel souvenirs containing dirt, rocks, or earth-contaminated artifacts)

Physical Examination

Special attention needs to be paid to these areas:
- Skin: Presence of rashes, lesions, nailfold capillary abnormalities; presence or absence of sweating
- Mouth: Note a smooth tongue with absence of fungiform papillae; presence of candidiasis
- Throat: Exudate, erythema
- Local or generalized lymphadenopathy or hepatosplenomegaly
- Joint examination, and palpation of bones for tenderness, swelling
- Palpation/percussion of sinus and mastoid areas for tenderness; tap upper teeth
- Eye examination noting exudate, palpebral or bulbar conjunctivitis, conjunctival hemorrhages, papillary reaction; a complete ophthalmologic examination is indicated to fully evaluate for uveitis, chorioretinitis, proptosis
- Pelvic examination in adolescent females
- Rectal examination and guaiac test
- Deep tendon reflexes

Diagnostic Studies

Laboratory studies are dependent on a history and physical examination that point to a specific infection or area of suspicion. Studies might include:
- CBC with differential, ESR (>30 mm/hr needs further evaluation), CRP, or procalcitonin
- Serologic tests for specific diseases as suggested by history and examination
- Blood cultures obtained aerobically (may require serial specimens to rule out endocarditis, osteomyelitis, or deep abscesses)
- Urinalysis plus urine cultures
- Mantoux skin test or IGRA
- Chest, sinus, mastoid, and GI tract radiographs may be indicated
- Liver chemistries
- Heterophil antibody and antinuclear antibody titer in older children
- If bone marrow biopsy is obtained, send cultures for bacteria, AFB, and fungus
- Echocardiogram if subacute endocarditis is suspected
- Other tests may involve radionuclide scans, total body CT, MRI, ultrasounds, or biopsies

Differential Diagnosis and Management

Infectious diseases, collagen-vascular disease (e.g., juvenile arthritis, SLE), malignancies, drug fever (can be any drug), nosocomial, HIV-associated illnesses, diabetes insipidus, hyperthyroidism, inflammatory bowel disease, hematoma in a confined space, anhidrotic ectodermal dysplasia, and Munchausen syndrome by proxy are included in the differential diagnosis of an FUO.

An infectious disease consultation is advised with consideration of hospitalizing the child if there is evidence of systemic illness or failure to thrive, the child is very young, the parent(s) anxiety is extreme, or an extensive workup is planned. Otherwise, the child should be followed with frequent visits, documented fever pattern, and other specialized tests if screening tests indicate the need, or if other physical findings develop. Treatment is based on the underlying diagnosis. Empiric use of antibiotics should be avoided unless the child is critically ill and suspected to have disseminated TB (Nield and Kamat, 2011).

Infectious Agents Used in Bioterrorism

Agents of biologic warfare are categorized by the CDC according to their potential for aerosol transmission, susceptibility of the population, degree of person-to-person transmission, expected high morbidity and mortality rates, the likelihood for delayed diagnosis, and the lack of effective and efficacious treatments. Agents at highest risk to the populace are known as *category A weapons of bioterrorism.* These include specific bacteria (e.g., *Bacillus anthracis* [anthrax]; *Clostridium botulinum* [botulism]; *Francisella tularensis* [tularemia]; *Yersinia pestis* [plague]) and viruses (e.g., variola virus [smallpox]; viruses of hemorrhagic fever [Ebola, Marburg, Lassa fever]). Most of these diseases are rarely, if ever, seen in clinical practice settings. Refer to the CDC website for specific details about anticipated agents that might be used. The CDC has established a Laboratory Response Network to provide standardized diagnostic testing for selected agents and link state and local public health laboratories with other advanced-capacity laboratories (see Additional Resources on the Evolve site).

Children are at particular risk for exposure to and absorption of biologic warfare agents should they be employed (e.g., anthrax and botulinum toxin). Factors that predispose them to such risk include being within closer proximity to the ground, having faster ventilation rates and thinner skins, having an increased risk of dehydration, and having greater undeveloped cognition.

Providers can join other community health care providers in developing pediatric readiness plans to any large disaster (e.g., storms, earthquakes, acts of bioterrorism). These readiness plans should include triage, isolation and treatment/care facilities, transportation, communication, housing, and the establishment of vaccination clinics on a massive scale for children, especially in communities where health departments and/or emergency departments may not have the procedural skills to address a severely ill pediatric population. Health alerts can be requested by email from the CDC.

For a complete list of references, please visit http://evolve.elsevier.com/Burns/pediatric/.

25

Atopic, Rheumatic, and Immunodeficiency Disorders

RITA MARIE JOHN AND MARGARET A. BRADY

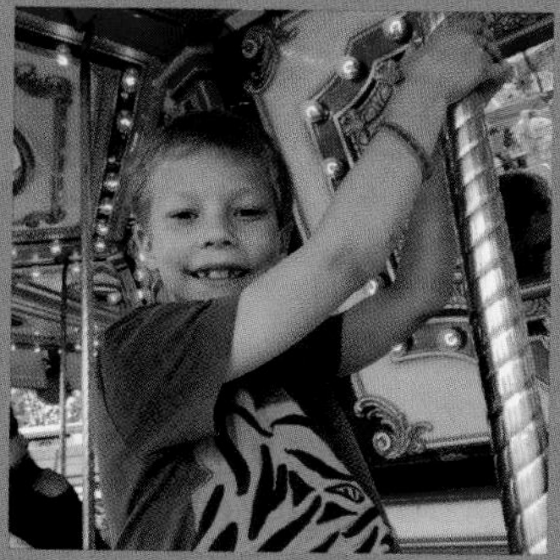

Atopic disorders, rheumatic diseases (collagen vascular or connective tissue diseases) of childhood, and immunodeficiencies share certain characteristics that lend to their combined discussion. Inflammation, chronicity, and genetic predisposition are common to these groups of disorders. The triad of atopic disorders that may or may not coexist consists of atopic dermatitis (AD), allergic rhinitis (AR) (or "hay fever"), and asthma. The two most common childhood rheumatic diseases that a primary care provider (PCP) is likely to encounter are juvenile idiopathic arthritis (JIA) and systemic lupus erythematosus (SLE). They are collagen-vascular disorders that have localized or generalized findings marked by inflammation and an autoimmune response. Vasculitis, an inflammation of the blood vessels, is characteristic of many of the rheumatic diseases.

Rheumatologic diseases can begin in childhood. Fibromyalgia is a rheumatic disease that causes chronic central pain characterized by widespread musculoskeletal pain with multiple painful tender points, fatigue, poor sleep, and cognitive impairment leading to academic problems (Kashikar-Zuck and Ting, 2014). Chronic fatigue syndrome (CFS), a somewhat controversial diagnosis, is also addressed. Although the incidence of rheumatic fever has diminished significantly in the United States, it is still a disease found across the globe. Henoch-Schönlein purpura (HSP), the most common systemic vasculitis syndrome of childhood, and Kawasaki disease (KD), the most common cause of acquired heart disease, are included in this chapter. The chapter ends with a synopsis of the more common primary immune deficiency disorders seen in childhood because early diagnosis and intervention are critical.

Pathophysiology and Defense Mechanisms

Atopic and Allergic Disorders

Allergies are acquired alterations in the body with an immunologic basis. An allergen acts as an antigen that triggers an immunoglobulin E (IgE) response in genetically predisposed individuals. The union of antigen and antibody creates a cascade of biochemical reactions. There are four types of allergic reactions:

- Type I: Manifested as typical allergic symptoms to the extreme of anaphylactic reactions
- Type II: Antibody cytotoxicity reactions
- Type III: Immune complex reactions with Arthus-reactions and serum sickness as examples
- Type IV: Cellular immune-mediated or delayed-T cell type hypersensitivity

All four types of allergic or hypersensitivity reactions are mediated by circulating or cellular antibodies and generally can occur in any individual (Leung and Akdis, 2011). Type I involves local and systemic manifestations, resulting from an interaction between antigen and tissue cells that have been sensitized with reaginic antibody, generally IgE (e.g., urticaria and angioedema). Type II involves reactions from antibody interacting with antigenic components on cell surfaces (e.g., hemolytic anemia and transfusion reactions). Type III is characterized by deposition of immune microprecipitates in or around blood vessels. Complement or toxic products are released. HSP is one example of type III–mediated reactions. A type IV allergic reaction is a delayed-type hypersensitivity interaction involving sensitized T-lymphocytic cells that results in the release of toxic lymphoid cell products. Cytokines are released, which stimulate bone marrow precursors to produce more leukocytes that become macrophages. Examples of type IV reactions are tuberculin skin test reactions and contact dermatitis (Leung and Akdis, 2011).

Atopy represents a complex interaction between multiple genes and environmental exposures. Atopic disorders are forms of allergic reactivity that occur only in certain susceptible individuals with an unknown and probably genetic predisposition. Environmental factors also play a role in atopy of these individuals who exhibit a hyperresponsiveness in target organs (lungs, skin, or nose). Certain antigens (e.g., cat dander, ragweed) are problematic for atopic individuals but not for others. These atopic individuals become sensitized to the offending allergen, resulting in an atopic disorder.

The development of an atopic disorder or allergic response involves a susceptible individual who is both exposed to an offending antigen and has a predisposition to selective synthesis of IgE when in contact with common environmental antigens. If these conditions are in place and contact with an offending antigen occurs, the following biochemical chain of cascading events unfolds:

1. There is a brisk proliferation of T-helper type 2 (Th2) cells that secrete cytokines: interleukin (IL)-3, IL-4, IL-5, IL-9, and IL-13.
2. Cytokines are involved in IgE synthesis and activation of eosinophils.
3. IgE binds to receptors on mast cells, basophils, and Langerhans cells.
4. Chemical mediators that cause biochemical reactions and allergic-related injury to target organs (skin and respiratory tract) are released. Examples of chemical mediators include but are not limited to histamine, tryptase, prostaglandins, leukotrienes, eosinophil chemotactic factor of anaphylaxis, and platelet-activating factor.
5. The end result of this biochemical process is target organ tissue injury. Examples of tissue injury include inflammation and hyperresponsiveness resulting in such symptoms as obstruction, increased mucus discharge, and pruritus.

Immediate allergic reactions can involve sneezing, hives, wheezing, vomiting, or anaphylaxis. Acute reactions (<30 minutes) can be followed by a late-phase response several hours (2 to 12) after the initial response. This late-phase response is due to the influx of other inflammatory cells (such as, basophils, eosinophils, monocytes, lymphocytes, and neutrophils) and their inflammatory mediators that are recruited to the site of the acute allergic reaction.

The pathogenesis of atopic diseases involves a complex interrelationship of genetic, environmental, and immunologic factors. The main defense mechanism to protect against atopic disorders is the elimination of the offending substance to prevent IgE development and antigen-antibody interaction. For example, if there is a family history of atopic disorders, breastfeeding offers the protection of limited exposure to cow's milk protein and the benefit of maternal immunoglobulin A (IgA) and immunoglobulin G (IgG) antibodies. Once chemical mediators are released, the body's protective responses reduce inflammation and repair tissue damage. Pharmacologic therapy cannot cure atopic disorders, but it reduces symptoms and checks the allergic process. For example, drugs may be used to control inflammation (corticosteroids), compete with histamine for receptor sites on target tissues (antihistamines), act as a selective leukotriene receptor antagonist (e.g., montelukast), and prevent mast cell degranulation and mediator release (cromolyn sodium).

Immune Deficiency

The pathogenesis of immune deficiency involves the primitive innate immune system in which phagocytic cells act against bacteria as a first-line defense amplified by the complement system. The innate system is composed of neutrophils, monocytes, macrophages, and natural killer (NK) cells. The complement system attracts the cells to the area of inflammation via chemoattractants and enhances phagocytosis by opsonins. The innate immune system is responsible for alerting the adaptive immune system to the presence of infection (Omenetti et al, 2012). The adaptive immune system provides a more specific response to the presence of antigens or foreign substances. Lymphocytes, a key player in adaptive immunity, are divided into T cells, B cells, and NK cells. The T-specific lymphocyte binds with the antigen and also triggers a response causing the release of humoral mediators, including cytokines and B-cell–produced immunoglobulins. The antibodies block the binding of antigens to cellular receptors and, therefore, neutralize microbes and microbial toxins (Omenetti et al, 2012). The T cells function as the cellular immune system, whereas the less numerous B cells serve as the humoral immune system. The role of killer cells in host defense is less clear.

Rheumatic Disorders

JIA and SLE are rheumatic disorders that can occur in childhood. They are connective tissue disorders marked by inflammatory changes in connective tissues throughout the body. The exact cause of these collagen diseases is not completely understood; however, an autoimmune basis is postulated as a key factor in rheumatic disease. Additional discussion related to etiology is presented under each disease entity. There are no natural defense mechanisms identified to prevent either of these diseases. Periods of remission do occur in some children with SLE for unknown reasons, and many children with JIA achieve complete remission with puberty (approximately 85% complete remission rate) (Wu et al, 2011). Inflammation is a significant factor in these two rheumatic diseases of childhood.

Overview of Laboratory Diagnostic Studies in Rheumatic Diseases

Although there is no laboratory test that has 100% sensitivity and specificity, the critical laboratory tests commonly ordered in child with or suspected of having SLE include the following: acute phase reactants, such as C-reactive protein (CRP), erythrocyte sedimentation rate (ESR), serum ferritin, platelets, and procalcitonin; tests for antinuclear antibodies (ANAs), anti–double-stranded deoxyribonucleic acid (DNA), and anti-Smith (Sm) antibody; and determination of serum complement levels. Urinalysis is frequently done in rheumatologic disorders known to have renal involvement. Other related blood, serologic, and urine laboratory studies are indicated depending on organ involvement (e.g., renal involvement is a frequent complication) (Mehta, 2012). The presence of anti-cyclic citrullinated peptide (anti-CCP) antibody is a surrogate marker and is helpful in diagnosing JIA in the early stages of disease (Mehta, 2012). Guidelines for the laboratory workup of SLE and JIA are discussed later in this chapter.

Imaging studies (magnetic resonance imaging [MRI] and radiographs) are done to assess and manage joint abnormalities keeping in mind the call by the American College of Radiology to "image gently." The future, increased risks of oncological disorders associated with some rheumatic diseases must be considered.

General Management Strategies

The atopic and rheumatic disorders and immune deficiencies tend to be chronic conditions with exacerbation and remission of symptoms. Individual management strategies are based on the specific disease process and are discussed in each of their respective sections. The following general measures should be part of the management of atopic, rheumatoid, and immune deficiency disorders:

- Encourage self-care and learning about one's disease.
- Address issues of burdens associated with living with a chronic disease, such as:
  - Financial burdens associated with the disease
  - School, peer, and family dynamics
  - Body image and pain management as needed
  - Child and adolescent adjustment and engagement leading to improved adherence
  - Child-parent role in management of a long-term illness or chronic condition
  - Nutrition and the avoidance of obesity, if activity is limited, or foods if they are known triggers
- Refer to parent and/or child support groups and professional organizations and resource groups

Rheumatologic Disorders

Juvenile Idiopathic Arthritis

JIA, formerly known as *juvenile rheumatoid arthritis (JRA),* now encompasses several disorders that have a common feature of arthritis (e.g., enthesitis-related arthritis and psoriatic arthritis) and had not been identified under the nomenclature of JRA (Wu et al, 2011). The diagnosis of JIA requires a persistent arthritis for more than 6 weeks in a pediatric patient younger than 16 years old. Table 25-1 shows the most current classification system.

TABLE 25-1 Juvenile Idiopathic Arthritis Subtypes and Clinical Joint Characteristics

Juvenile Idiopathic Arthritis Subtype	Clinical Joint Characteristics
Oligoarticular	Four or less joints with persistent disease never having more than four-joint involvement and extended disease progressing to more than four joints within the first 6 months
Polyarticular (RF negative)	Five or more joints with symmetrical involvement
Polyarticular (RF positive)	Symmetric involvement of both small and large joints with erosive joint disease
Systemic	Either polyarticular or oligoarticular disease
Enthesitis-related arthritis	Weight-bearing joints involved especially hip and intertarsal joints and a history of back pain, which is inflammatory in nature or sacroiliac joint involvement
Psoriatic arthritis	Asymmetric or symmetric small or large joints
Undifferentiated	

RF, Rheumatoid factor.

The underlying cause of most forms of JIA is unclear; however, it is a heterogenous disorder. It is likely environmentally induced in genetically predisposed individual. Human leukocytic antigen (HLA) class I and II alleles have been associated with JIA (Gowdie and Tse, 2012). This linkage points to the involvement of T cells and antigen presentation in the pathophysiology of the disease. An environmental trigger, such as infection or trauma, is also important in the pathogenetic process in JIA. The trigger results in an uncontrolled adaptive and innate response toward the self-antigen, the autoimmune reaction. The presence of autoantigens from cartilage and joint tissue leads to activation of the T cells and results in release of proinflammatory cytokines (Gowdie and Tse, 2012). In contrast, systemic juvenile idiopathic arthritis (SJIA), which does not have HLA gene association, may be the result of an autoinflammatory response from the innate immune system. SJIA is postulated to be the result of uncontrolled activity of the innate immune system, because this type of JIA disease is not associated with autoantibodies but rather uncontrolled activity of the phagocytes, including neutrophils, monocytes, and macrophages. The difference in the pathogenic processes may explain the differences in the clinical presentation of the disease.

In oligoarticular and rheumatoid factor (RF)-positive polyarticular JIA, there is autoimmunity with involvement of the adaptive immune system. The presence of positive ANAs and RF is associated with HLA genes. The humoral response is responsible for the release of autoantibodies (especially ANAs), an increase in serum immunoglobulins, and the formation of circulating immune complexes and complement activation. The cell-mediated reaction is associated with a T-lymphocyte response that plays a key role in cytokine production, resulting in the release of tumor necrosis factor alpha (TNF-α), IL-1, and IL-6. B lymphocytes are activated by T-helper cells and produce autoantibodies that link to self-antigens. The B lymphocytes infiltrate the synovium with the end result of nonsuppurative chronic inflammation of the synovium that can lead to articular cartilage and joint structure erosion.

The chronic arthritides of childhood present unique challenges to the child, family, and the pediatric provider. Approximately 1 in 1000 children are affected with oligoarticular JIA, the most common arthritic subtype. Certain histocompatibility complex antigens are more prevalent in the JIA population. Cytokine production, proliferation of macrophage-like synoviocytes, infiltration with neutrophils and T lymphocytes, and autoimmunity are thought to be the major pathologic processes causing chronic joint inflammation.

The rate of JIA is significantly higher in girls than in boys, typically in oligoarticular and pauciarticular JIA. The female to male ratio in systemic onset is equal. The approximate percentage of occurrence and age breakdown for each of the subtypes follows: systemic (10%) occurs at any age; polyarticular (40%) has a late (6 to 12 years old) or early childhood (1 to 4 years old) onset; and oligoarticular (50%) has a late or early onset. Adolescents tend to have more RF-positive disease (Wu et al, 2011).

Clinical Findings

History

The major complaints in all forms of JIA are from the arthritis characterized by:

- Pain—generally a mild to moderate aching
- Joint stiffness—worse in the morning and after rest; arthralgia may occur during the day
- Joint effusion and warmth

Systemic symptoms are found more commonly in systemic and polyarticular subtypes and include anemia, anorexia, fever, fatigue, lymphadenopathy, salmon-colored rash (SJIA), and weight loss. Growth abnormalities can result in localized growth disturbances, including premature fusion of the epiphyses, bony overgrowth (rheumatoid nodules), and limb-length discrepancies.

Physical Examination

Associated features are:

- Non-migratory monoarticular or polyarticular involvement of large or proximal interphalangeal joints for more than 3 months
- Systemic manifestations—fever, salmon-colored rashes, leukocytosis, serositis, lymphadenopathy, and rheumatoid nodules

Less commonly seen are ocular disease (e.g., iridocyclitis, iritis, or uveitis), pleuritis, pericarditis, anemia of chronic disease, fatigue, and growth failure, or leg-length discrepancy if the arthritis is unilateral.

Key physical findings are:

- Swelling of the joint with effusion or thickening of synovial membrane, or both, noted on palpation of the joint line
- Heat over inflamed joint and tenderness along joint line
- Loss of joint range of motion and function; child typically holds the affected joints in slight flexion and may walk with limp
- Uveitis may be present with ciliary injection and decreased vision. However, it is usually asymptomatic.

There are five major types of JIA (Gowdie and Tse, 2012):

1. Oligoarticular pattern: This type of JIA involves four or less joints, typically the weight-bearing joints within the first 6 months of diagnosis. The diagnosis is classified as persistent or extended disease, depending on the number of joints involved. About 50% progress to extended disease where there is involvement of four or more joints after the first 6 months of disease. This involvement primarily is in larger or medium joints, such as the knee, ankle, wrists, and elbow; however, systemic symptoms are rare. The synovitis may be mild and painless with asymmetric joint involvement and unremarkable laboratory values. Uveitis occurs in 30% especially if the child has a positive ANA (Gowdie and Tse, 2012).
2. Polyarticular pattern: This involves five or more joints and is divided into RF-negative and RF-positive disease. Involved joints can be large or small with an acute or insidious onset. RF-negative ANA positive polyarticular JIA is difficult to distinguish from extended oligoarticular pattern disease. Using the number of joints involved and the timing of onset of the arthritis can be helpful. In contrast, RF-positive disease can have chronic pain and symmetric joint swelling, low-grade fever, fatigue, nodules, and anemia of chronic disease. An acute form of uveitis occurs in this subtype. Polyarticular JIA typically involves small joints of the hands, feet, ankles, wrists, knees, and can also involve the cervical spine. Adolescents with this type differ from those with early onset in that they exhibit a positive RF. Adolescents who develop late-onset polyarticular JIA have a course similar to the adult entity. Both forms of the disease are more common in females.
3. SJIA: This is characterized by arthritis in one or more joints for 6 weeks' duration in a child younger than 16 years old with a fever of at least 2 weeks' duration with

at least 3 days of daily fever. In addition, there is also a fleeting erythematous rash, lymphadenopathy, hepatomegaly, splenomegaly, and serositis (Ringold et al, 2013). Myocarditis with pericardial effusion occurs in approximately 10%. RF is rarely positive and the ANA is only positive in 5% to 10%; however, there may be anemia, thrombocytosis, increased acute phase reactants, and elevated transaminase levels. About 10% of children with SJIA develop a life-threatening macrophage activation syndrome (MAS) with fever, organomegaly, cytopenia, hyperferritinemia (acute phase reactant), hypertriglyceridemia, coagulopathy, and hypofibrinogenemia.

4. Enthesitis-related JIA: This typically entails arthritis of the lower limbs especially the hip and intertarsal joints with the sacroiliac joints involved later in the disease. Enthesitis involves inflammation at the insertion of tendons, ligaments, or joint capsules and is characterized by swelling, tenderness, and warmth. Enthesitis may present with joint or foot pain. There is a risk of anklyosing spondylitis 10 to 15 years later. It tends to occur in late childhood and adolescence and acute symptomatic uveitis occurs in about 7%.
5. Psoriatic arthritis: This is more common between the ages of 2 and 4 and again between 9 to 11 years old. There is usually a family history of psoriasis, or the child has psoriasis; however, the arthritis can precede the psoriasis by years. There can be dactylitis or a sausage-like swelling of the digits; involvement in the small digits is not uncommon.

Diagnostic Studies

JIA is a diagnosis of exclusion. The diagnosis is based on physical findings and history of arthritis lasting for 6 weeks or longer. There is no diagnostic laboratory test for JIA. Most children with oligoarticular arthritis have negative laboratory markers. Those with polyarticular and systemic-onset typically have elevated acute-phase reactants and anemia of chronic disease. A positive result for RF by latex fixation may be present, but a positive RF occurs in less than 10% of children with JIA and rarely in those with SJIA. ANA may be present in up to 50% of children with oligoarticular disease. A positive ANA helps identify children at higher risk for uveitis. The anti-CCP antibody test can be added to the initial workup of JIA, because citrullinated residues are part of the essential antigenic components that are recognized by autoantibodies in rheumatoid arthritis (Mehta, 2012). The anti-CCP antibodies are associated with more aggressive disease and may be present before the onset of symptoms. The anti-CCP antibody is highly specific, but its precise role has not been established because it is found primarily in children with polyarticular JIA (Mehta, 2012). Useful laboratory tests include a complete blood count (CBC) (to exclude leukemia); ESR, CRP, Lyme titers, and liver function tests. The results may reveal lymphopenia, anemia, elevated transaminases, and hypoalbuminemia; however, laboratory studies may be normal in these children. Imaging studies (MRI) can help in managing joint pathologic conditions. Analysis of synovial fluid is not helpful in the diagnosis of JIA.

Differential Diagnosis

The various causes of monoarticular arthritis are part of the differential diagnosis. However, Lyme disease must be excluded and other differentials, including tumors, leukemia, cancer, bacterial infections, toxic synovitis, rheumatic fever, SLE, spondyloarthropathies, inflammatory bowel disease, septic arthritis, and chondromalacia patellae, need to be carefully considered.

Management

A specialist in pediatric rheumatology should follow children with severe involvement. Ophthalmology referral and evaluation is critical in a child with a positive ANA. Uveitis needs immediate ophthalmologic management. It is most common in oligoarticular JIA and is highly associated with a positive ANA. Other pediatric subspecialists, such as orthopedists, pain management specialists, and cardiologists, may be consulted as needed. Therapy depends on the degree of local or systemic involvement.

The main treatment goals are to suppress inflammation, preserve and maximize joint function, prevent joint deformities, and prevent blindness. Drug therapy is used to control the inflammation responsible for tissue injury with the goal of preventing permanent tissue changes, which is not always possible. Aggressive early treatment to induce a remission is a key consideration in JIA management in order to prevent deformity and improve outcomes and is now the goal of the practice guidelines for both polyarticular JIA and SJIA (Ringold et al, 2013, 2014). Aspirin therapy has largely been replaced with the use of nonsteroidal anti-inflammatory drugs (NSAIDs). Pharmacologic agents commonly used in the management of JIA include the following (Gowdie and Tse, 2012):

- NSAIDs: Children with oligoarthritis generally respond well to NSAIDs (Taketomo et al, 2014).
  - Ibuprofen: 30 to 40 mg/kg/day three to four divided doses (maximum single dose is 800 mg; maximum daily dose 2400 mg/day)
  - Tolmetin: 20 to 30 mg/kg/day divided in three to four doses (maximum dose is 1800 mg/day)
  - Naproxen: 10 mg/kg/day in two divided doses (maximum dose is 1000 mg/day)
  - Indomethacin: Older than 2 years old, 1 to 2 mg/kg/day divided in two to four doses (maximum dose is 4 mg/kg/day); adults, 25 to 50 mg/dose two or three times/day (maximum dose is 200 mg/day)
  - Celecoxib: Older than 2 years old and adolescents (≥10 kg to ≤25 kg), 50 mg twice daily; >25 kg, 100 mg twice daily
- Oral, parenteral, intraarticular corticosteroids:
  - Systemic arthritis: Can be used for 2 weeks as initial therapy for SJIA with involvement of more than four joints and a physician global assessment (using the Provider global assessment tool of disease activity) of

less than 5 or a Provider global score of more than 5 without care about active joint involvement. Corticosteroids can be used as bridging therapy until other medications take effect (Ringold et al, 2013)
  - All the other types of arthritis: Prednisone in the lowest possible dose with optional intraarticular steroid injection (Ringold et al, 2014)
- Disease-modifying antirheumatic drugs (DMARDs): Recent published guidelines vary related to the initiation of these agents depending on type of arthritis, joint involvement, and MD global assessment of functioning
  - Nonbiologic DMARD treatment: methotrexate, sulfasalazine, leflunomide (managed by pediatric rheumatologist)
  - Biologic DMARD treatment (managed by pediatric rheumatologist)
    - Short-acting agents: Anti-IL-1 anakinra is the first-line agent for SJIA with significant joint involvement and poor global functioning (Sterba and Sterba, 2013).
    - Long-acting agents: Rilonacept, canakinumab, and tocilizumab have long-acting activity (Sterba and Sterba, 2013). Rilonacept is a recombinant fusion protein with high affinity for IL-1β, IL-1α, and IL-1 receptors and a half-life of 8.6 days. Canakinumab is a humanized monoclonal antibody effective against IL-β with a half-life of 28 days. Tocilizumab is effective against IL-6 (Sterba and Sterba, 2013).
    - TNF-α agents: For example, etanercept (Enbrel, infliximab (Remicade), and adalimumab (Humira) soak up tumor necrosis factor, an immune-system protein, and block the inflammatory cascade. Methotrexate or anakinra is used in severe forms of JIA.
    - Intraarticular corticosteroid injections are used if there is severe joint involvement.
    - Pharmacologic therapy for uveitis is given as indicated by an ophthalmologist. Females with ANA-positive oligoarticular JIA are at high risk for uveitis and require slit-lamp examination every 3 to 4 months. The uveitis often does not correspond to the severity of the arthritis (i.e., uveitis may be present despite quiescent arthritis).
    - Physical therapy—range of motion muscle-strengthening exercises and heat treatments—is used for joint involvement; occupational therapy is beneficial. Rest and splinting are used if indicated.
    - Ophthalmologic follow-up every 3 months for 4 years (even if the arthritis has resolved) for all ANA-positive JIA children. They have a greater risk of uveitis that may not be clinically apparent but can lead to blindness if not detected and treated.

Complications and Prognosis

Systemic involvement can include iridocyclitis, uveitis, pleuritis, pericarditis, anemia, fatigue, and hepatitis. Residual joint damage caused by granulation of tissue in the joint space can occur. Children most likely to develop permanent crippling disability include those with hip involvement, unremitting synovitis, or positive-RF test.

The course of the disease is variable, and there is no curative treatment. Again, early aggressive treatment is critical; therefore, referral to a specialist is important. After an initial episode, the child may never have another episode, or the disease may go into remission and recur months or years later. The disease process of JIA wanes with age and completely subsides in 85% of children; however, systemic onset, a positive RF, poor response to therapy, and the radiologic evidence of erosion are associated with a poor prognosis. Onset of disease in the teenage years is related to progression to adult rheumatoid disease.

Patient and Parent Education and Prevention

The following education and preventive measures are taken:
- For children on aspirin therapy (not typically given), educate parents about the risk of Reye syndrome and its signs and symptoms.
- Recommend yearly influenza vaccine.
- Offer chronic disease counseling and encourage normal play and recreation.
- Educate about side effects of medications, in addition to splinting, orthotics, and bracing requirements.
- Instruct about need to follow up with an ophthalmologist. Frequency of follow-up for uveitis screening is based on subtype of JIA and is determined by protocol guidelines and ophthalmology.
- Ensure parent and child understand that physical therapy is a mainstay of treatment for chronic childhood arthritis and should be part of the child's daily routine. A daily plan should include passive, active, and resistive exercises.
- Water therapy and the use of heat or cold reduce pain and stiffness. Swimming is an excellent activity except for children with severe anemia and severe cardiac disease.
- Tricycle or bike riding and low-impact dance are other beneficial activities.
- Refer to the American Arthritis Foundation and the Juvenile Arthritis Association, which have excellent resources for family members and children.
- Instruct on the need to involve school personnel in the identification of required school-related services through an individualized education plan (IEP) or a 504.
- Discuss the challenge of pain management and its assessment in children with chronic arthritis and encourage parents to advocate for effective pain control on behalf of their child.

Systemic Lupus Erythematosus

SLE is a chronic, systemic rheumatic disease characterized by altered immune regulation that can involve inflammation in multi-organ systems, including the blood cells, kidneys, nervous system, and skin. Autoantibody formation is a key characteristic of SLE resulting in significantly increased numbers of circulating autoantibodies and impairment in the normal suppression of autoreactive B-cell clones. Cell-mediated autoimmune responses are part of the pathogenesis of SLE. Children with SLE exhibit a marked increase in the production of autoantibodies that attack the body's DNA. This leads to immune complex formation and tissue damage from either direct bonding in tissues, immune complex deposition, or a combination of both (Ardoin and Schanberg, 2011).

Various immune phenomena are associated with SLE, including altered immunologic reactions in the T- and B-lymphocyte function. There is a loss of T-lymphocyte control and hyperactivity of B-lymphocytes, resulting in nonspecific and specific antibody and autoantibody production. Because SLE is characterized by inflammatory damage to target organs brought on by autoantibodies attacking self-antigens, there is a strong link between a faulty immune mechanism and SLE. Its exact etiology is unknown, but many factors, including genetics in predisposed individuals, hormones, and environment, are linked to the immune dysregulation that occurs. Environmental factors thought to play a role in its pathogenesis are oral contraceptive use, pregnancy, microbials (viral agents mostly), temperate climates, exposure to ultraviolet light, and certain drugs (e.g., hydralazine and procainamide).

SLE is characterized by ANA production and deposition of immune complexes in various tissues of the body with impaired clearance. Deposits of immune complexes are abundant and can trigger a generalized inflammatory response and fibrinoid deposits in blood vessels walls that can lead to tissue damage, such as vasculitis and ischemia and numerous organ system abnormalities (commonly the heart and renal system) (Wu et al, 2011). There is variety in both the acuity and the course of the disease over time.

Childhood onset is rare with an incidence of 0.3 to 0.9 per 100.000. However, it is more acute and severe in children than in adults. There is a higher incidence in Asians, African Americans, Hispanics, and Native Americans. Most report a median age of onset between 11 and 12 years (Levy and Kamphuis, 2012). Females are preponderantly affected more than males with a 4:1 ratio before puberty and an 8:1 ratio after puberty (Ardoin and Schanberg, 2011).

Clinical Findings

The hallmark of SLE is a butterfly or malar erythematous facial rash, which increases in intensity in sunlight. Clinical findings depend on organ involvement. Its presentation may be abrupt or have a gradual, nonspecific onset. Fever, rash, fatigue, and joint pain are the most typical presentation in children.

History

The history may include the following:

- Joint involvement
  - Most common initial finding
  - Nonerosive arthritis with tenderness, effusion, and tenderness
- Arthralgia
- Systemic manifestations:
  - Constitutional symptoms: Low-grade fever (intermittent or sustained), weight loss, and lymphadenopathy
  - Painless, oral ulcers that tend to be in the mouth or nose
  - Skin disorder: Malar or discoid rash, photosensitivity, alopecia, Raynaud phenomenon, livedo reticularis, vasculitis with petechiae, palpable purpura, digital ulcers
  - Renal disorders with proteinuria and casts
  - Neurologic disorders with seizures, headache, or psychosis
  - Hematologic disorder with hemolytic anemia with reticulocytosis, leukopenia, lymphopenia, thrombocytopenia
  - Immunologic disorder with antibody to native DNA or Sm protein, antiphospholipid antibiotics
  - Pulmonary disorders with pleuritis leading to shortness of breath and chest pain
  - Cardiac disorders with pericarditis, myocarditis, noninfective (Libman-Sacks) endocarditis
  - ANA with a presence of ANA by immunofluorescence

Physical Examination

The following may be seen on physical examination (Ardoin and Schanberg, 2011):

- Skin manifestations
  - Pallor, livedo reticularis, petechia, palpable purpura, and digital ulcers
  - Malar or "butterfly" rash—scaly erythematous maculopapular rash covering malar areas extending over the bridge of the nose and cheeks; may spread down the face to the chest and extremities; "butterfly" rash and other lesions can be photosensitive; seen in approximately 95% of those with SLE
  - Mucous membrane manifestations (ulceration) of the mouth and nasal septum
  - Gingivitis, mucosal hemorrhage, erosions, ulcerations
  - Silvery whitening of the vermilion border of the lips or thickening, redness, ulceration, or crusting of the lips
- Joint tenderness
- Serositis
- Cardiac friction rub due to pericarditis
- Pleural friction rubs due to pleuritis
- Abdominal: Hepatosplenomegaly and lymphadenopathy

Diagnostic Studies

Initial laboratory testing includes CBC, ANA, ESR, CRP, serum chemical analysis (metabolic and protein screen), and urinalysis. The ANA test is positive in more than 97% of children who have active, untreated SLE; titers are usually high (Mehta, 2012). A negative ANA excludes SLE from the diagnosis except for the rare false-negative test. The sensitivity of the ANA is greater than 95%, but the specific is as low as 36%. An ANA may be followed up with testing for disease-specific types of ANA (e.g., antibodies to Sm, Ro, or La). The ANA autoantibody profile screens for anti-Sm, anti-Ro, anti-La, anti-double strand DNA, and anti-ribonucleoprotein (anti-RNP) antibodies (Mehta, 2012). Antibodies to double-stranded DNA are present in most patients with SLE and are generally exclusively seen in cases of SLE but not other disease states. Antibodies directed against Sm are diagnostic of SLE, but are only found in 30% of patients with SLE. Antiphospholipid antibodies may also accompany SLE and predispose to stroke (Levy and Kamphuis, 2012). Leukopenia or lymphopenia, hemolytic anemia, and thrombocytopenia are frequent laboratory findings. Other laboratory and radiographic studies depend on organ involvement and can include a chest x-ray, electrocardiogram (ECG), urine and serologic testing renal ultrasound, and histopathologic studies. Proteinuria and hematuria are hallmarks of lupus nephritis.

Differential Diagnosis

The differential diagnoses are infection, malignancy, or autoimmune/inflammatory disease. Infectious diseases that resemble SLE include bacterial infections, viral infections, and other infections, such as Q fever (Coxiella), tuberculosis, Lyme disease, or toxoplasmosis. Leukemia, lymphoma, neuroblastoma, and Langerhans cell histiocytosis are malignant differentials (Levy and Kamphuis, 2012). A host of other autoimmune diseases can mimic SLE, including acute rheumatic fever (ARF), autoimmune lymphoproliferative syndrome, and common variable immunodeficiency. A temporary, drug-induced SLE can be caused by several pharmacologic agents, including hydantoin compounds, hydralazine, isoniazid (INH), procainamide, and sulfonamides.

Management

Children with SLE need to be followed by a rheumatologist. Other pediatric subspecialists may be consulted. Therapy depends on the degree of local or systemic involvement. Sunlight is a known trigger of SLE. Therefore, ultraviolet A and B sunscreen is essential both indoors due to daylight fluorescent lighting and outdoors due to sun exposure. Prompt recognition and treatment of disease flares are essential to prevent systemic complications, so frequent clinical and laboratory monitoring is important. The following measures also may be helpful (Ardoin and Schanberg, 2011):

- NSAIDs are used for relief of musculoskeletal pain, arthritis, arthralgias, serositis, or pain. (If nephritis is present, use with caution.)
- Oral steroids are prescribed if renal, cardiac, pulmonary, or central nervous system (CNS) involvement is present. They were the mainstay of SLE for decades. The dose is adjusted depending on clinical and laboratory findings. Cautious tapering of steroids is often needed.
- Antimalarial drugs (e.g., hydroxychloroquine) may be used to treat cutaneous and musculoskeletal manifestations and are used as a maintenance therapy.
- Immunosuppressant agents, such as methotrexate and azathioprine (Imuran) may be used as steroid-sparing agents. Methotrexate is used for arthritis; azathioprine is used in treating cytopenias, vasculitic rash, or serositis. Mycophenolate mofetil (CellCept) is used to induce remission in lupus nephritis or maintenance of other organ involvement. Cyclophosphamide is only used for life-threatening symptoms.
- Use of other pharmacologic agents or therapies depends on the type and degree of organ system involvement. Rituximab (Rituxan) is a monoclonal antibody that binds and kills active B cells and has been used for cytopenias. Belimumab (Benlysta), a new monoclonal antibody approved in adults, is under study in children (Levy and Kamphuis, 2012).
- Vitamin D and calcium supplements are used to reduce the risk of osteoporosis related to chronic corticosteroid use.

Complications and Prognosis

SLE is generally considered a controllable disease in children; however, the severity of the illness varies. In disease flares, the child may experience poor sleep and daytime fatigue with decreased cardiovascular conditioning, resulting in increased pain. A diagnosis of SLE in childhood does not always mean a poor prognosis, especially if renal involvement or cerebritis is not present. Renal failure, CNS lupus, myocardial infarction, cardiac failure, and infection are the leading causes of death in children. Exposure to ultraviolet light may bring out or worsen skin lesions and result in exacerbation of systemic problems. Side effects resulting from chronic use of high-dose corticosteroids (e.g., osteoporosis, avascular necrosis) are a complication of treatment. SLE is a chronic disease with periods of waxing and waning of symptoms; however, complete remission can occur. Children with mild disease do well, but those with severe major organ involvement generally have a poor prognosis. Parents need education about the effect of sun exposure and the need for sunscreen protection and the need to rest between activities, because fatigue is a frequent problem.

Fibromyalgia Syndrome

Fibromyalgia is the term used to describe a chronic, idiopathic pain syndrome characterized by widespread, diffuse, nonarticular musculoskeletal pain and fatigue with multiple trigger points that are discrete painful sites. It is considered a subset of musculoskeletal pain syndromes. Age of presentation is typically during the adolescent years with a mean age of onset of 12 years old, with females affected more often than males (Giardino, 2013). Fibromyalgia is more common in adults but can occur in children, especially in those older than 12 years old. The prevalence of fibromyalgia in children has a variable incidence ranging from 1.2% to 6.2% (Buskila and Ablin, 2012; Durmaz et al, 2013).

The pathophysiology is not clear, but there is evidence that the CNS has increased pain or sensory feelings. Prolonged muscle stress may lead to amplification of pain. Changes in the central pathway may lead to heightened awareness of pain (Alfvén, 2012). There is a lack of clear criteria for diagnosing fibromyalgia in children, which may be confusing for the PCP (Buskila and Ablin, 2012; McLeod, 2014). The syndrome is also referred to as *myofascial pain syndrome, generalized pain syndrome, fibrositis,* and *pain amplification syndrome.* It is a complex syndrome that involves fatigue, poor sleep patterns with non-refreshing sleep, and generalized pain involving muscles, ligaments, and tendons. It is more common in Caucasians and adolescent females between 13 to 15 years of age (Giardino, 2013).

Symptoms are often vague and variable, with no major organ system abnormalities found. The presentation can range from a generalized increased sensitivity to pain to a more classic pattern of specific symptoms. It is a complex disease in which psychosocial stresses, environmental factors, and hypersensitivity to stimuli occur, leading to painful areas (Buskila and Ablin, 2012). The cause and pathogenesis of fibromyalgia are uncertain, but they are thought to involve CNS malfunction with amplification of pain transmission and interpretation. Genetic predisposition is also implicated because familial prevalence has been reported. Fibromyalgia can occur as a primary condition or in conjunction with other rheumatologic disorders (secondary fibromyalgia) (Kashikar-Zuck and Ting, 2014).

Clinical Findings

Pediatric diagnostic criteria were first defined by Yunus and Masi (1985). In 1990, the American College of Rheumatology defined fibromyalgia in adults citing the presence of widespread pain for 3 or more months, along with tender points in 11 out of 18 predetermined tender points (Wolfe et al, 1990). The Yunus and Masi criteria are seen in Box 25-1. The adult 2010 criteria for fibromyalgia evaluate widespread pain criteria and symptom severity using the Widespread Pain Index (WPI) and a symptom severity (SS) score (Wolfe et al, 2010). The disease waxes and wanes in severity and interferes with activities of daily living. The lack of clearly defined pediatric criteria leads to a delay in diagnosis. Some rheumatologists use the 1985 criteria and others use the 1990 criteria. Children with widespread musculoskeletal pain and painful point tenderness may have fibromyalgia and should be referred.

History

Pain history is the key finding because early on the associated symptoms of chronic fatigue, depression, or mood disorder may be lacking (Kashikar-Zuck and Ting, 2014). Stress may exacerbate the pain: therefore, a careful psychosocial history is a critical component to identify triggers. The history may include the following long-standing common symptoms:

- Pain at multiple sites, including muscles and in the soft tissues around joints
- Pain may awaken from sleep and interfere with routine activities
- Fatigue and malaise
- Paresthesias and complaints of headache
- Insomnia or prolonged night awakenings
- Depression (a significant number exhibit depressive symptoms) and anxiety
- School absence due to pain is not uncommon but keeps up with school work

• BOX 25-1 The Yanus and Masi Criteria for Juvenile Fibromyalgia

- Pain in at least three areas for more than 3 months without underlying cause and normal laboratory tests
- More than 5 of 18 tender points, which include occiput, low cervical spine, trapezius at the midpoint, supraspinous above the scapula near the medial border, second rib at the costochondral junctions, lateral epicondyle, upper outer quadrants of the gluteal muscle, posterior to greater trochanter prominence, and at the medial fat pad of the knee at the joint line
- Three of 10 minor criteria listed here:
  - Fatigue
  - Poor sleep
  - Irritable bowel syndrome
  - Chronic tension or anxiety
  - Soft tissue swelling
  - Pain affected by weather
  - Paresthesia
  - Pain affected by activity
  - Headache
  - Pain affected by anxiety and/or stress

Physical Examination

Local areas of painful (not just tender) trigger points in muscles (usually at areas of tendon insertion) with digital pressure are characteristic physical findings. Pressure causes pain at the site and in a circumferential or linear pattern surrounding the site. Common trigger points include the neck, back, lateral epicondyles, greater trochanter, and knees. Typically there is no evidence of arthritis or muscular weakness.

Diagnostic Studies

Laboratory studies are of little benefit. Blood count, liver functions, and muscle enzymes are normal. If secondary fibromyalgia is present, order appropriate tests to rule out a different rheumatoid disorder. Children with fibromyalgia can have a false-positive ANA, as do 20% of children without rheumatoid disorders.

Differential Diagnosis

Other underlying illness must be excluded, including inflammatory diseases (e.g., SLE, post-infectious fatigue that can follow Epstein-Barr virus [EBV] or influenza virus infections, or mood and conversion disorders). In CFS, tiredness lasting longer than 6 months rather than pain is the major complaint. Fibromyalgia initially may be mistaken for other rheumatoid diseases, but it does not have the associated rashes, weight loss, fever (more than 101° F [38.3° C]), or joint swelling. Lyme disease is also in the differential, but the course of the illness is not characterized by pain.

Management

Children and their parents need reassurance that fibromyalgia is not life-threatening, but it is a chronic condition that can be a lifelong problem. Treatment focuses on relieving symptoms and can include the following:

- Physical therapy for range-of-motion exercises, mild low-impact aerobic exercises (e.g., swimming, bicycling, and walking), and muscle strengthening
- Psychotherapy and relaxation techniques to help cope with this condition and stress
- NSAIDs can be prescribed for pain control
- Gabapentin can be prescribed to reduce pain sensitivity

Patient and Parent Education

Patients and parents should be educated about fibromyalgia and that it is not a psychosomatic disorder. In addition, guidance should be given about sleep hygiene and the possibility that this could be a chronic problem with periods of remissions followed by exacerbations.

Prognosis

The outcome of fibromyalgia in children varies, but studies demonstrate the persistence of fibromyalgia into adulthood (Buskila and Ablin, 2012; Kashikar-Zuck et al, 2010, 2014). However, fibromyalgia in children generally has a better prognosis than it does in adults (Kashikar-Zuck et al, 2014).

Chronic Fatigue Syndrome

Fatigue is a common complaint in adolescence; however, only a small number of children go on to have chronic issues of severe debilitating and overwhelming fatigue that presents the provider with the diagnostic challenge as to its etiology as does CFS. Children can develop idiopathic pain syndromes, which are characterized by the presence of severe disability despite the lack of physical or laboratory findings. The key complaint is fatigue of new onset that is unexplained, is not linked to ongoing exertion, and is persistent. Their fatigue is not substantially relieved by rest or sleep and results in substantial reduction in activity much lower than before the onset of their fatigue illness. About two thirds of pediatric cases have a reported onset of CFS after a preceding viral illness with pharyngitis and fever.

Clinical Findings

There are two criteria necessary for a diagnosis of CFS (Centers for Disease Control and Prevention [CDC], 2015a). The first is severe chronic and debilitating fatigue present for at least 6 months or longer that is not relieved by rest and another medical or psychiatric diagnosis does not explain this physical symptom. In addition to fatigue symptoms as just described, the child needs to have at least four of the following eight symptoms to meet CFS criteria:

- Self-reported impaired short-term memory or limitations in concentration (cognitive dysfunction) that results in impaired social, academic, occupational, or personal activities
- Recurrent sore throat
- Painful cervical or axillary lymph nodes
- Muscle pain (myalgia)
- Multiple joint arthralgia with no swelling or redness noted
- Headaches of a new pattern or severity
- Unrefreshing sleep
- Post-exertional malaise lasting for more than 24 hours

Other secondary complaints may include but are not limited to weight loss, night sweats, visual disturbances, dizziness, or fainting (CDC, 2015a). Complaints of low-grade fever may be reported but are generally not documented on examination. There may be a history of neuropsychiatric problems; however, in these cases, a psychiatric illness must first be excluded before a diagnosis of CFS can be made. Although EBV infection has been implicated in the cause of CFS, EBV does not explain all symptoms. No single immunologic abnormality has been consistently identified as the causative factor. The cause of CFS remains undetermined and may possibly represent the culminating effect of multiple factors, such as infectious disease, immunologic dysfunction, stress, and/or neurally mediated hypotension (CDC, 2015). Treatment is based on symptoms.

Differential Diagnosis

CFS is a diagnosis of exclusion, so other conditions need to be ruled out. Care must be taken in diagnosing this disorder in children, because other conditions (e.g., hypothyroidism, sleep apnea, hepatitis B or C, SLE, cancer, alcohol or drug abuse, Lyme disease, and major depressive and other psychiatric disorders) must first be ruled out. Kempke and colleagues (2013) found that self-reported childhood trauma (particularly emotional neglect and or abuse) by adults predicts increased levels of CFS core symptoms of daily pain and fatigue.

The child is best referred to a specialist in CFS for management.

Management

Pharmacologic intervention generally is not effective. Psychological support (stressing that this disease is not made up) and exercise are associated with reduced disability. Children and adolescents with chronic fatigue reporting illness may have symptoms that wax and wane over time. The majority of pediatric patients typically will have substantial improvement in their symptoms or complete recovery 1 to 4 years after diagnosis (Jones and Jenson, 2011).

Reactive Arthritis Related to Streptococcal Infection: Acute Rheumatic Fever and Post-Streptococcal Reactive Arthritis

ARF is an exaggerated autoimmune response in a susceptible host to group A streptococcus (GAS). Epitopes, the surface portion of certain subspecies of GAS, are similar to human myosin and the tissue of the mitral annulus and chordae. These sites act as antigens activating the immune response that results in antibody formation and initiation of the antibody/antigen response. Antistreptococcal immunoglobulins, stimulated by repeated streptococcal infections, attack the heart and joints, CNS, and cutaneous tissue. Greater organism virulence is associated with specific M protein types and a more "mucoid" capsule. There appears to be a strong genetic influence on susceptibility to GAS infection, with a family history of rheumatic fever and a lower socioeconomic status as known risk factors.

Today ARF occurs in developing countries as well as rural Australia (Kerdemelidis et al, 2010). The latency period from infection with GAS until symptom onset of ARF is usually 2 to 6 weeks. There is insufficient evidence to link streptococcal impetigo with ARF (Kerdemelidis et al, 2010). Recurrence of ARF following subsequent episodes of GAS pharyngitis (symptomatic or asymptomatic infection) is high. The most commonly affected age group in children is 5 to 15 years (Gerber, 2011).

Evidence of a prior GAS infection is needed for the diagnosis of ARF and post-streptococcal reactive arthritis (PSRA). Confirmation of a GAS infection by throat culture or rapid strep test cannot differentiate the carrier state from a true infection. Serologic testing for the presence of elevated or increasing antistreptococcal antibody titers (antistreptolysin O [ASO] test) or anti-DNase B testing will confirm a recent strep infection (Berard, 2012). One to 2 weeks following an acute GAS infection, the ASO titer and the anti-DNase B levels will rise. The ASO titer peaks in 3 to 6 weeks; the DNase B level peaks in 6 to 8 weeks (Berard, 2012). Both remain elevated for months after GAS infection, so increasing titers are the key to the diagnosis.

Post-Streptococcal Reactive Arthritis

PSRA can develop during or following an infection with GAS with a higher incidence in children who are HLA-B27 positive (Berard, 2012). It is associated with persistent joint arthritis of small or large joints or the axial spine. This form of arthritis is more persistent and less receptive to NSAID treatment. There are no specific criteria for PSRA, but a history of recent streptococcal infection documented using the titers discussed earlier is important.

In PSRA, the arthritis may occur sooner, is more persistent, and involves both large and small joints. There is no associated cardiac involvement. There is only moderate elevation in acute phase reactions, and the treatment of PSRA with NSAIDS may be more difficult (Berard, 2012). Eventually the arthritis resolves without joint damage.

Acute Rheumatic Fever

ARF is a nonsuppurative complication following a Lancefield GAS pharyngeal infection that results in an autoimmune inflammatory process involving the joints (polyarthritis), heart (rheumatic heart disease), CNS (Sydenham chorea), and subcutaneous tissue (subcutaneous nodules and erythema marginatum). Recurrent ARF with its multisystem responses can follow with subsequent GAS pharyngeal infections. Long-term effects on tissues are generally minimal except for the damage done to cardiac valves that leaves fibrosis and scarring and results in rheumatic heart disease. ARF is diagnosed based on a set of criteria called the *revised Jones criteria* (1992). These criteria are used for the initial attack of ARF. Further modifications of the Jones criteria are used for recurrent ARF.

Clinical Findings and History

The diagnosis of an initial attack of ARF is based on the following revised Jones criteria:

- Evidence of documented (culture, rapid streptococcal antigen test, or ASO titer) GAS pharyngeal infection
- Findings of two major manifestations or one major and two minor manifestations of ARF (Berard, 2012; Burke and Chang, 2014)

Major Manifestations

Children with fewer manifestations can also have ARF. Arthritis of large joints occurs in 65% of cases, carditis in 50%, chorea in 15% to 30%, cutaneous nodules in 5%, and subcutaneous nodules in less than 7%. There is some controversy regarding the use of the Jones criteria in developing countries where the ability for diagnostic testing may be limited; therefore, the World Health Organization (WHO) criteria (Box 25-2) may be used (Ferrieri, 2002; Seckel and Hoke, 2011).

- Carditis is common (pancarditis, valves, pericardium, myocardium) and can cause chronic, life-threatening disease (i.e., congestive heart failure [CHF]) with estimates of 30% to 80% of patients with ARF experiencing carditis; it is more common in younger children than adolescents. The symptoms of carditis may be vague and insidious with decreased appetite, fatigue, and pains. A high-pitched holosystolic murmur is heard at the apex with radiation to the infrascapular area, as well as tachycardia and often a gallop rhythm. Mitral and possibly aortic regurgitation occur in 95% of cases, usually within 2 weeks of RF illness. The mitral valve becomes leaky due to annular dilation and elongation of the chordate that attach leaflets to the left ventricle. With moderate to severe mitral regurgitation CHF develops; recurrent episodes of RF lead to worsening valve disease.
- Polyarthritis (migratory and painful) involving large joints and rarely small or unusual joints (e.g., vertebrae); it is the most common manifestation of ARF.
- Sydenham chorea is uncommon.

• BOX 25-2 2002-2003 World Health Organization Criteria for the Diagnosis of Rheumatic Fever and Rheumatic Heart Disease—Based on the Revised Jones Criteria

Diagnostic Categories

- Primary episode of RF*
- Recurrent attack of RF in a patient *without* established rheumatic heart disease†
- Recurrent attack of RF in a patient *with* established rheumatic heart disease
- Rheumatic chorea: Insidious onset rheumatic carditis†
- Chronic valve lesions of rheumatic heart disease (patients presenting for the first time with pure mitral stenosis or mixed mitral valve disease)‡

Criteria

- Two major or one major and two minor manifestations *plus* evidence of a preceding GAS infection
- Two minor manifestations *plus* evidence of a preceding GAS infection§
- Other major manifestations or evidence of GAS infection not required
- Do not require any other criteria to be diagnosed as having rheumatic heart disease and/or aortic valve disease

Major Manifestations

- Carditis
- Polyarthritis
- Chorea
- Erythema marginatum
- Subcutaneous nodules

Minor Manifestations

- Clinical fever, polyarthralgia
- Laboratory elevated acute phase reactants (ESR or leukocyte count)

Supporting Evidence of a Preceding Group A Streptococcal Infection within the Past 45 Days

- ECG: Prolonged PR interval
- Elevated or rising ASO or other streptococcal antibody *or*
- A positive throat culture *or*
- Rapid antigen test for GAS *or*
- Recent scarlet fever

From World Health Organization (WHO): *Rheumatic fever and rheumatic heart disease: report of a WHO expert consultation*, 2001. Available at www.who.int/cardiovascular_diseases/resources/en/cvd_trs923.pdf. Accessed January 11, 2015, Table 4.1, p 23.

ASO, Anti-streptolysin O; *ECG,* electrocardiogram; *ESR,* erythrocyte sedimentation rate; *GAS,* group A streptococcus; *RF,* rheumatic fever.

*Patients may present with polyarthritis (or with only polyarthralgia or monoarthritis) and with several (three or more) other minor manifestations, together with evidence of recent GAS infection. Some of these cases may later turn out to be RF. It is prudent to consider them as cases of "probable RF" (once other diagnoses are excluded) and advise regular secondary prophylaxis. Such patients require close follow-up and regular examination of the heart. This cautious approach is particularly suitable for patients in vulnerable age groups in high-incidence settings.

†Infective endocarditis should be excluded.

‡Congenital heart disease should be excluded.

§Some patients with recurrent attacks may not fulfill these criteria.

- Erythema marginatum manifested as pink macules on the trunk and extremities; nonpruritic; this sign is uncommon.
- Subcutaneous nodules associated with repeated episodes and severe carditis; this sign is uncommon.

Minor Manifestations

- Fever (101° F to 102° F [38.2° C to 38.9° C]), arthralgia, history of ARF

Diagnostic Studies

- Elevated acute-phase reactants (ESR, white blood cells [WBCs], CRP)
- Leukocytosis
- Prolonged PR interval on ECG

Children may be diagnosed with ARF without evidence of a preceding streptococcal infection in the following two situations: (1) a child with Sydenham chorea or (2) with acquired heart disease (commonly mitral valve regurgitation without a congenitally abnormal or prolapsed valve) that can only be linked to ARF. Approximately 80% of children with ARF have an elevated ASO titer. A combination of both DNase-B testing and ASO rising may confirm the recent infection.

Differential Diagnosis

ARF is a clinical diagnosis associated with rising antibody titers. Arthritis and arthralgia can accompany a variety of diseases including JIA; connective tissue diseases; viral infections, such as parvovirus; inflammatory bowel disease; bacterial infections, such as gonorrhea; hemophilia; infective endocarditis; and Lyme disease (Berard, 2012). A complete history and physical examination with appropriate diagnostic testing are critical to establish the diagnosis.

Management

The treatment of ARF includes the following:

- Antibiotic therapy to eradicate GAS infection: Primary prevention requires that a GAS infection be treated within 10 days of onset. Benzathine penicillin G is the drug of choice unless there is an allergic history; erythromycin is then the drug of choice. Azithromycin and cephalosporins are also sometimes used (Gerber, 2011). A patient with a history of ARF who has an upper respiratory infection should be treated for GAS whether or not GAS is recovered as asymptomatic infection can trigger a recurrence.
- Anti-inflammatory therapy: Aspirin can be used for arthritis after the diagnosis is established; it is usually

given only for 2 weeks and then tapered. It is also used to treat mild to moderate carditis. Aspirin and steroids provide symptomatic relief but do not prevent the incidence of chronic heart disease. Steroids have been beneficial in the management of severe carditis, reducing its morbidity and mortality. The association of Reye syndrome with aspirin use is always a concern and must be addressed with parents. Yearly influenza immunization is critical for children on aspirin therapy.

- Chest radiographs, ECG, and echocardiography are indicated; carditis usually develops within the first 3 weeks of symptoms.
- Referral for CHF treatment if needed: medical management and or valve replacement.
- Bed rest is generally indicated only for children with CHF. Children with Sydenham chorea may need to be protected from injury until their choreiform movements are controlled. Steroids in the absence of other symptoms are not useful in the treatment of chorea.
- Children with severe chorea may benefit from the use of antiepileptic agents, such as sodium valproate or carbamazepine.

Prevention of Acute Rheumatic Fever

- Treat GAS pharyngeal infections with appropriate antibiotics. Antibacterial prophylaxis for those with a prior history of ARF is required because of the greatly increased risk of recurrent ARF with subsequent inadequately treated GAS infections. Intramuscular penicillin G (1.2 million units) is more effective than daily penicillin V (Gerber, 2011) and must be given every 4 weeks (every 28 days) not monthly. It can be given every 3 weeks in high-risk children.
- Antibacterial secondary prophylaxis with penicillin is given every 4 weeks for 5 years after the last ARF episode in children without carditis or until 21 years old (whichever is longer). For those with carditis and persistent myocardial or valvular disease, treatment is 10 or more years and may be lifelong (Gerber, 2011). In the majority of patients, valvular disease will resolve if they are compliant in taking antibiotic prophylaxis after the first episode of rheumatic heart disease.

Complications

Chronic CHF can occur after an initial episode of ARF or follow recurrent episodes of ARF. Residual valvular damage is responsible for CHF. The risk of significant cardiac disease increases dramatically with each subsequent episode of ARF; thus prevention of subsequent GAS infections is critical. Engagement in the follow-up is essential to prevent the need for cardiac valvular repair.

Pediatric Vasculitis

Pediatric vasculitis is a complex group of disorders that are characterized by inflammation in the blood vessel (Weiss, 2012). Vasculitis can occur as a primary condition that can involve primarily large vessels (Takayasu arteritis), medium-size vessels (childhood polyarteritis nodosa, cutaneous polyarteritis, KD), and small vessel disease in a granulomatous form (Wegener granulomatosis, Churg-Strauss syndrome) or small vessel disease in a nongranulomatous form (microscopic polyangiitis, HSP, isolated cutaneous leukocytoclastic vasculitis, hypocomplementemic urticarial vasculitis). Secondary vasculitis can occur due to infection, malignancy, drugs, or connective tissue disease. The occurrence of primary vasculitis in pediatrics is approximately 23 per 100,000. Fever and diffuse pain associated with malaise may be early symptoms, along with elevated acute phase reactants (ESR, CRP, platelets, ferritin, procalcitonin). As the vasculitis progresses, there may be specific clinical findings, such as organ involvement, purpuric rash, or detection of antibodies known as *antineutrophil cytoplasmic antibodies (ANCAs)*. The presenting symptoms and signs depend on the organ involved (Weiss, 2012). The most common types of vasculitis are addressed in this textbook; readers should consult a rheumatology textbook for information regarding other less common types of vasculitis. All of these conditions require specialist care to prevent significant health problems.

Henoch-Schönlein Purpura

HSP is the most common vasculitis of children and is a leukoclastic vasculitis of the small vessels. Although 75% of affected children are younger than 10, most children are between 4 to 6 years of age with Caucasians having the highest incidence and African Americans the lowest incidence (Reid-Adam, 2014). An upper respiratory infection often precedes HSP. It can occur anytime from infancy (as early as 6 months old) to adulthood. The classic presentation includes abdominal pain, palpable petechial or purpuric rash on the lower extremity, arthritis, and renal disease (Weiss, 2012), but the cutaneous palpable purpura is the hallmark of the disease (Reid-Adam, 2014). HSP is seen slightly more frequently in males than females and occurs more frequently in winter months than other times of the year.

A skin biopsy shows leukocytic vasculitis with granulocytic infiltration of tissue along with IgA deposition within the vessel walls (Reid-Adam, 2014). Hemorrhage and ischemia are associated findings. With inflammation of the small blood vessels, extravasation of blood occurs into local tissue, resulting in a variety of skin manifestations, including a maculopapular rash or urticarial rash the first 24 hours, followed by purpura, bullae, or necrotic lesions.

The rash along with an oligoarticular, self-limiting, and non-destructive arthritis occurs in 75% of children. The lower extremities, typically the ankles and knees, are the most common arthritic sites. The gastrointestinal (GI) manifestations occur in 50% to 75% of children and include bleeding (33%), abdominal pain, and intussusception (1% to 5%) with the GI manifestations preceding skin signs by 2 weeks. The most common manifestation of renal disease is microscopic hematuria with or without proteinuria. Symptoms of renal involvement can occur in 20% to 60% of children. Renal manifestations include nephritic or nephrotic syndrome but rarely renal failure. Renal involvement usually occurs after the onset of a rash and can be an acute or chronic problem (Weiss, 2012).

Clinical Findings

The diagnosis of HSP based on the EULAR/PReS classification must include purpura or petechiae, predominantly in the lower extremities with one or more of the following: arthritis or arthralgias, abdominal pain, histopathology demonstrating IgA deposition, and/or renal involvement with either hematuria or proteinuria (Ozen et al, 2010).

History

The history of a preceding viral illness and the clinical presentation of the symptoms listed earlier support the diagnosis of HSP. It can also present with seizures, stroke, mental status change, hemoptysis due to pulmonary hemorrhage, or edema of the eyes, hands, or scrotum.

Physical Examination

- Skin rash: Starts as a pinkish maculopapular rash and progresses from red to purple to brown palpable purpura
- Arthritis
  - Warmth, swelling, and erythema over the joints
  - Periarthritis is common and involves the knees and ankles
- Diffuse abdominal pain on palpation
- Edema of the scrotum, eyes, or hands
- Hypertension: Repeated blood pressure measurement and follow-up due to subclinical disease (Reid-Adam, 2014)

Diagnostic Studies

The diagnosis of HSP is based on clinical findings. A urinalysis must be done to check for hematuria and proteinuria (a common sign of nephritis) and needs to be repeated on follow-up due to a high incidence of renal disease. Other studies include blood urea nitrogen (BUN) to evaluate renal function and stool guaiac for occult blood as the incidence of GI bleeding is high even in the absence of frank rectal bleeding. If GI obstruction is a consideration, abdominal radiographs should be ordered. Other tests (e.g., chest radiographs, computed tomography [CT] scans, or electroencephalographs) are ordered based on the signs and symptoms of complications, such as shortness of breath, seizures, mental status changes, or hypertension. Diagnostic studies are useful to identify specific organ system involvement and the severity of complications.

Acute phase reactants and WBC (nonspecific indicators of systemic inflammation) are elevated in HSP. This condition is associated with a nonthrombocytopenic purpura, the platelet count is normal or even high. Renal biopsy may be warranted if renal involvement is severe.

Differential Diagnosis

HSP must be differentiated from other diseases that cause purpura: immune thrombocytopenic purpura, poststreptococcal glomerular nephritis, hemolytic uremic syndrome, infections, SLE, serum sickness, or hypersensitivity vasculitis (Weiss, 2012). Other forms of vasculitides, such as Wegener granulomatosis and polyarteritis nodosa, although more common in adults, need to be considered (Rabinovich, 2011).

Management

Children with HSP need co-management with pediatric specialists, depending on organ system involvement. Hospitalization is necessary with moderate to severe GI and renal system involvement or if pulmonary, cardiac, or CNS manifestations are present. Treatment with corticosteroid has been shown to improve outcomes, especially in GI complications (Weiss, 2012; Weiss et al, 2007); however, prophylaxis with corticosteroids does not reduce the incidence of renal disease. In severe, life-threatening cases, treatment with immunophoresis may be instituted, followed by the use of other immunosuppressive agents including cyclophosphamide, azathioprine, or cyclosporine.

- Monitor for GI blood loss.
- Monitor for hematuria and proteinuria.
- Monitor and treat hypertension.
- Prescribe analgesics and NSAIDs for arthritis.
- Follow up and refer patients with HSP as complications arise.

Complications and Prognosis

Infrequent complications of HSP seen in children include myositis, orchitis, hemorrhagic cystitis, pancreatitis, cholecystitis, bowel infarction, perforation or stricture, intussusception, acute renal failure, seizures, ataxia, pulmonary hemorrhage, carditis, anterior uveitis, and episcleritis. Ileoileal intussusception is a complication marked by severe colicky abdominal pain.

The arthritis associated with HSP does not leave joint damage and typically does not recur (Weiss, 2012). HSP tends to last 3 to 4 weeks and then completely resolves in most cases without significant sequelae. However, the rash can wax and wane for 1 year; some children have recurrent disease. The presence of significant nephritis in the initial course of the disease (elevated BUN and persistent high-grade proteinuria) is a potentially serious complication with risk for long-term sequelae, such as hypertension or renal insufficiency. Less than 1% of children with HSP progress to end-stage renal disease (Weiss, 2012).

Patient and Parent Education

The provider should educate patients and parents about:

- The illness, its complications, and the risk of recurrence
- The need to closely monitor for nephritis for 1 year following the initial presentation and after resolution, including blood pressure and urinalysis testing (Weiss, 2012)

Kawasaki Disease

KD (also known as *mucocutaneous lymph node syndrome* or *infantile polyarteritis*) is the second most common childhood vasculitis with a varying incidence from country to country, with Japan having the highest incidence of 239.6 per 100,000. The incidence is increasing in Japan, the United Kingdom, and India (Saundankar et al, 2014). The disease is characterized by an acute generalized systemic medium vessel vasculitis occurring throughout the body. Although its cause is unknown, it is believed that an infectious agent activates the immune system in a genetically susceptible host. Genetics may explain the higher incidence in Asia as well as a higher incidence in children of parents or siblings with a history of the disease. Recent data suggest T-cell activation plays a role in disease severity and susceptibility (Scuccimarri, 2012).

KD exhibits geographic and seasonal outbreaks, in the late winter and early spring. Person-to-person spread is low. Referral of these children to a pediatrician is necessary. It is self-limited and the most common cause of acquired heart disease in children in Japan and the United States (Saundankar et al, 2014). The EULAR/PReS classification for KD includes a persistent fever for at least 5 days plus four of the following (Ozen et al, 2010):

- Bilateral conjunctival injection
- Changes of the lips and oral cavity
- Cervical lymphadenopathy
- Polymorphous exanthema
- Changes in the peripheral extremities (swelling of the hands or feet) or perineal area

Clinical Findings

Despite accepted KD guidelines, children can have atypical or incomplete KD with coronary anomalies shown by echocardiogram. Children younger than 6 to 12 months old may have more atypical findings. In atypical KD, the child may fulfill the criteria but has an additional feature that is not usually seen in KD. In incomplete KD, the fever may last for 5 days or more, but the child will only meet two or three of the other criteria. Incomplete KD is more common in children younger than 1 year old and older than 9 years old. Thus, incomplete KD without nodal involvement is possible. Coronary artery involvement is found more frequently in children with incomplete KD, so based on the frequency of the disease, an index of suspicion should be maintained in infancy and older school-age children (Scuccimarri, 2012). If KD is untreated, the normal course of fever is 10 to 14 days.

Other clinical features associated with KD include irritability, aseptic meningitis, mild acute iridocyclitis or anterior uveitis, otitis media due to inflammation rather than infection of the drum, urethritis, hydrops of the gallbladder, and facial nerve palsy. In children who have received BCG, there may be erythema and induration at the site of injection. Two rare complications are MAS and peripheral gangrene (Scuccimarri, 2012).

Stage 1: Acute Phase

The acute phase (days 0 to 14) begins with an abrupt onset of high fever (greater than 102.2° F [39° C]) that is unresponsive to antipyretics or antibiotics. Significant irritability, bilateral nonpurulent conjunctival injection, erythema of the oropharynx, dryness and fissuring of the lips, "strawberry tongue," cervical lymphadenopathy, a polymorphous rash, erythema of the urethral meatus, tachycardia, and edema of the extremities are typically noted. During the acute phase, there may be pericardial, myocardial, endocardial, and coronary artery inflammation. The child typically is tachycardic and has a hyperdynamic precordium with a gallop rhythm and a flow murmur. Rarely, children have low cardiac output syndrome from poor myocardial function.

Stage 2: Subacute Phase

The subacute phase (2 to 4 weeks after illness onset) begins with resolution of the fever and lasts until all other clinical signs have disappeared. Irritability may be prolonged throughout this phase. Desquamation of the fingers (at the junction of nail tip and digit) occurs first, followed by desquamation of the toes. Transient jaundice, abnormal liver function tests, arthralgia or arthritis, transient diarrhea, orchitis, facial palsy, and sensorineural hearing loss may occur. Coronary artery aneurysms appear during this period—more so in untreated children. Common sites for aneurysms, in order of frequency, are the proximal left anterior descending coronary, proximal right coronary, left main coronary, left circumflex, and distal right coronary artery.

Stage 3: Convalescent Phase

During the convalescent phase, all clinical signs of KD have resolved, but laboratory values may not have returned to normal. This phase is complete when all blood values are normal (6 to 8 weeks from onset). However, nail changes including Beau lines (deep transverse grooves across the nails) may be seen (Scuccimari, 2012).

Although some researchers note a chronic phase lasting from 40 days to years after illness onset, this phase is not present in all patients. Although coronary complications, if present, can persist into adulthood, a recent study of 564 patients with KD revealed a low incidence of side effects in children who were followed to 21 years of age (Holve et al, 2014).

Diagnostic Studies

KD is a diagnosis of exclusion. Results of lab investigations are not diagnostic but rather help rule in other diagnoses. Although the acute phase reactants (ESR and CRP) are usually increased, they may be normal early in the course of the illness. A CBC may show an increased WBC with a predominance of neutrophils with toxic granulation. Anemia may follow with prolonged inflammation. A marked thrombocytosis with values greater than 1 million follow in the second week of illness in the subacute phase. The comprehensive metabolic profile may show an increase in serum transaminases and hypoalbuminemia. Sterile pyuria may occur. Leukopenia and thrombocytopenia in

KD may occur in association with the life-threatening MAS.

- Stage 1 is typified by an elevated ESR and platelet count (as high as 700,000/mm^3), elevated CRP, leukocytosis with left shift, slight decreases in red blood cells and hemoglobin, hypoalbuminemia, increased α_2-globulin, and sterile pyuria. The platelet count may be initially normal with gradual increase after the seventh day of fever.
- Blood, urine, cerebrospinal fluid, and group A beta-hemolytic streptococci (GABHS) pharyngeal cultures may be indicated given the symptomatology (to rule out other sources of fever).
- Echocardiograms at acute illness, 2 weeks and 6 to 8 weeks after onset of fever, are performed to evaluate for coronary, myocardial, and pericardial inflammation. Angiography, MRI, and cardiac stress testing may be considered.

Differential Diagnosis

The differential diagnosis includes viral infections (e.g., measles, adenovirus, EBV, enterovirus, influenza, or roseola) and bacterial infections (e.g., cervical adenitis, scarlet fever, staphylococcal scalded skin syndrome, toxic shock syndrome, leptospirosis, or Rickettsia illness, such as Rocky Mountain spotted fever). Immune-mediated diseases may need to be considered and include Steven-Johnson syndrome, serum sickness, RF, SJIA or other JIA, or connective tissue diseases, such as SLE. Other differential diagnoses include mercury poisoning, or tumor necrosis factor receptor–associated periodic syndromes, such as hyper IgM syndrome (Scuccimarri, 2012).

Management

- Early diagnosis is essential to prevent aneurysms in the coronary and extraparenchymal muscular arteries. Treatment goals include: (1) evoking a rapid anti-inflammatory response, (2) preventing coronary thrombosis by inhibiting platelet aggregation, and (3) minimizing long-term coronary risk factors by exercise, a heart healthy diet, and smoking prevention. The child should be referred for initial treatment that includes the following medications and agents (Scuccimarri, 2012):
    - Intravenous immunoglobulin (IVIG) therapy (a single dose of 2 g/kg over 12 hours, ideally in the first 10 days of the illness) to reduce the incidence of coronary artery abnormalities. The use of immunoglobulin after the tenth day must be individualized. If a child is found to have an abnormal echocardiogram, fever, tachycardia, or other signs of inflammation beyond the tenth day, then immunoglobulin is still indicated. Retreatment with immunoglobulin may be useful for persistent or recurrent fevers.
    - High-dose aspirin is given for its anti-inflammatory properties (80 to 100 mg/kg/day in four divided doses—every 6 hours initially) until afebrile for at least 48 to 72 hours, then lowering the aspirin dose to 3 to 5 mg/kg/day until 6 to 8 weeks and then can discontinue if the echocardiogram is normal. If significant coronary artery abnormalities develop and do not resolve, aspirin or other antiplatelet therapy is used indefinitely.
    - For patients with IVIG-resistant disease as indicated by a persistent fever 48 hours after treatment with IVIG and aspirin, a second treatment of IVIG at 2 mg/kg over 12 hours is initiated. If this is not successful, then methylprednisone IV at 30 mg/kg over 3 hours once a day for 1 to 3 days may be initiated. Infliximab 5 mg/kg may also be used. If the patient is still febrile, then the opposite anti-inflammatory can be used. (Methylprednisone in the infliximab groups, or infliximab in the methylprednisone group.) Other options include cyclosporine A, methotrexate or cyclophosphamide (Saneeymehri et al, 2015).
- An echocardiogram should be obtained as soon as the diagnosis is established as a baseline study, with subsequent studies at 2 weeks and 6 to 8 weeks after onset of illness. If a child is found to have abnormalities, more frequent evaluations may be indicated.
- All children on chronic aspirin therapy should receive inactivated influenza vaccination. If varicella or influenza develops, aspirin treatment should be stopped for 6 weeks and another antiplatelet drug substituted to minimize the risk of Reye syndrome.
- Live virus vaccines should be delayed until 11 months after administration of IVIG (AAP Red Book, 2015).
- Children without coronary or cardiac changes should be followed by a cardiologist during the first year after the onset of KD. If there are no cardiac changes during that first year, then the PCP may follow the patient with no activity restrictions imposed at that point.
- Patients with any range of transient coronary artery dilation (including giant aneurysms) should be followed by a cardiologist for years; physical activity limitations may be imposed.
- Follow and counsel all KD patients about a heart-healthy diet.

Complications and Prognosis

The acute disease is self-limited; however, during the initial stage (acute phase), inflammation of the arterioles, venules, and capillaries of the heart occurs and can later progress to coronary artery aneurysm in 15% to 25% of untreated children (less than 5% when treated appropriately). The process of aneurysm formation and subsequent thrombosis or scarring of the coronary artery may occur as late as 6 months after the initial illness. Other possible complications include recurrence of KD (less than 2%); CHF or massive myocardial infarction; myocarditis or pericarditis, or both (30%); pericardial effusion; and mitral valve insufficiency. Mortality (1.25%) from KD occurs from cardiac sequelae 15 to 45 days after onset of fever. Children with coronary dilation or aneurysms (especially those greater than 4 mm) may have long-term coronary endothelial changes that place the child at risk for early ischemic disease;

they may also develop dyslipidemias (Wood and Tulloh, 2009). Studies from Japan raise concern about risk of early atherosclerosis (due to arterial damage, ongoing inflammatory process, and alteration in lipid profile and other atherosclerosis risk factors) even in children without coronary changes during acute febrile illness (Fukazawa and Ogawa, 2009).

The risk of coronary aneurysm is reduced in patients older than 1 year old if IVIG is given within 10 days of the illness. Aneurysm regression occurs in half of all patients who develop them, commonly by 1 year after the illness (80% resolve within 5 years), but vessels do not dilate normally in response to increased oxygen demand by the myocardium. Prompt treatment of chest pain, dyspnea, extreme lethargy, or syncope is always warranted. Surgical revascularization and transcatheter revascularization are used for some coronary sequelae of KD (Wood and Tulloh, 2009).

Atopic Disorders

Asthma

Asthma is a chronic respiratory disease characterized by periods of coughing, wheezing, respiratory distress, and bronchospasm. Asthma can occur with a persistent cough without significant wheezing. It is the most common chronic respiratory disease of children, with an incidence as high as 30% of children in the Western world, and it is the leading cause of emergency department visits (Jackson et al, 2011; Liu et al, 2011).

The pathophysiology is the result of immunohistopathologic responses that produce shedding of airway epithelium and collagen deposition beneath the basement membrane, edema, mast cell activation and inflammatory infiltration by eosinophils, lymphocytes (Th2-like cells), and neutrophils (especially in fatal asthma). The persistent inflammation can result in irreversible changes, such as airway wall remodeling. Inflammation causes acute bronchoconstriction, airway edema, and mucous plug formation. In addition, airway inflammation can trigger a hyperresponsiveness to a variety of stimuli, including allergens, exercise, cold air, and physical, chemical, or pharmacologic agents. This results in bronchospasm, which presents as wheezing, breathlessness, chest tightness, and cough that can be worse at night or with exercise. The airflow obstruction is often reversible, either spontaneously or with treatment. Remodeling of the airway can occur secondary to persistent fibrotic changes in the airway lining. The fibrosis alters the airway caliber, leading to decreased airflow with permanent changes starting in childhood, but become recognizable in adults. Recent advances have shown that there are different "phenotypes" of this disease with different clinical manifestations, and data suggest that children who have symptoms before 3 years old are more likely to have changes in lung functioning at 6 years old (Szefler et al, 2014).

Asthma in children is classified as intermittent, mild persistent, moderate persistent, or severe persistent depending on symptoms, recurrences, need for specific medications, and pulmonary function measurements (Table 25-2). Children classified at any level of asthma can have episodes involving mild, moderate, or severe exacerbations. Exacerbations involve progressive worsening of shortness of breath, cough, wheezing, chest tightness, or any combination of these symptoms. The degree of airway hyperresponsiveness is usually related to the severity of asthma that can change over time. A well-controlled child with asthma has only one exacerbation in 3 years on average (Jackson et al, 2011).

Many children experience early- and late-phase responses to their asthma episode. The early asthmatic response (EAR) phase is characterized by activation of mast cells and their mediators, with bronchoconstriction being the key feature. EAR starts within 15 to 30 minutes of mast cell activation and resolves within approximately 1 hour if the individual is removed from the offending allergen. The late-phase asthmatic response is a prolonged inflammatory state that usually follows the EAR within 4 to 12 hours after exposure to the allergen, is often associated with airway hyperresponsiveness more severe than the EAR presentation, and can last from hours to several weeks. Exercise-induced bronchospasm describes the phenomenon of airway narrowing during, or minutes after, the onset of vigorous activity. Most asthmatics exhibit airway hyperirritability after vigorous activity and display exercise-induced bronchospasm. For some children, exercise is the trigger for their asthma. Although asthma is not always associated with an allergic disorder in children, many pediatric patients with chronic asthma have an allergic component. Increased weight gain in pregnancy and the first 2 years of life may increase TNF-α, a proinflammatory cytokine implicated in asthma, which may be a predictive biomarker for asthma (Szefler et al, 2014).

It is not known for certain whether hyperresponsiveness of the airways is present at birth or acquired later in genetically predisposed children. However, the genetic predisposition for the development of an IgE-mediated response to common aeroallergens, known as *atopy,* remains the strongest identifiable predisposing risk factor for asthma. A combination of genetic predisposition and exposure to certain environmental factors are the necessary components responsible for the pathophysiologic response associated with asthma. Origins of asthma exacerbations include exposure to respiratory virus, seasonal patterns, exposure to mycoplasma pneumonia and *Chlamydophila pneumoniae,* pollution, smoking, pregnancy, and psychological stress (Jackson et al, 2011; Szefler, 2013). Asthma is rarely diagnosed before 12 months old due to the high rate of viral illness causing bronchiolitis (Nelson and Zorc, 2013). A diagnosis of asthma should be made with caution in a toddler who has only wheezing associated with viral infections (Mueller et al, 2013).

The morbidity and mortality statistics of asthma in childhood demonstrate an alarming increasing incidence of asthma and its complications with a lifetime prevalence of 13% (Nelson and Zorc, 2013). The prevalence rate for asthma is highest among children 5 to 17 years with the

TABLE 25-2 **Classification of Asthma Severity in Children: Clinical Features Before Treatment**

Classification and Step	Symptoms*	Nighttime Symptoms	Lung Function
Step 1: Intermittent	Symptoms two times or less per week Asymptomatic and normal PEF between exacerbations Requires SABA 2 days/week Exacerbations brief (few hours or days); varying intensity No interference with normal activity	Two times or less per month	FEV_1 >80% predicted Normal FEV_1 between exacerbations
Step 2: Mild persistent	Symptoms more than two times per week but less than one time per day Requires SABA more than two days/week but not more than one per day Exacerbations may affect activity (minor)	Three to four times per month	FEV_1 >80% predicted
Step 3: Moderate persistent	Daily symptoms Daily use of inhaled SABA Some limitations Exacerbations affect activity, two times or more per week; may last days	More than one time per week but not nightly	FEV_1 >60% but <80% predicted
Step 4: Severe persistent	Continual symptoms Requires SABA several times/day Extremely limited physical activity Frequent exacerbations	Often seven times per week	FEV_1 <60% predicted

Adapted from National Heart, Lung, and Blood Institute (NHLBI): *Full report of the expert panel: guidelines for the diagnosis and management of asthma, (EPR-3)*, Bethesda, MD, 2007, National Institutes of Health.
FEV_1, Forced expiratory volume in 1 second; *PEF*, peak expiratory flow; *SABA*, short-acting $beta_2$-agonist.
*Having at least one symptom in a particular step places the child in that particular classification.

highest rate among black children (Centers for Disease Control and Prevention, 2015). Minority children have fewer ambulatory care visits for asthma and are less likely to be on a controller medication. Occupational or environmental exposure can cause airway inflammation associated with asthma. Factors known to precipitate or aggravate asthma in children include the following:

- Atopic individual response to allergens—inhaled, topical, ingested
- Viral infections and bacterial infections with atypical mycobacterium
- Exposure to known irritants (paint fumes, smoke, air pollutants) and occupational chemicals
- Gastroesophageal reflux
- Exposure to tobacco smoke (for infants, especially smoking by mother)
- Environmental changes—rapid changes in barometric pressure, temperature, especially cold air
- Exercise and psychological factors or emotional stresses (e.g., crying, laughter, anxiety attack, or panic or panic disorder)
- AR and sinusitis
- Drugs (e.g., acetaminophen, aspirin, beta-blockers)
- Food additives (sulfites)
- Endocrine factors (e.g., obesity)

Allergen-induced asthma results in hyperresponsive airways. The majority of children with asthma show evidence of sensitization to any of the following inhalant allergens:

- House dust mites, cockroaches, indoor molds
- Saliva and dander of cats and dogs
- Outdoor seasonal molds
- Airborne pollens—trees, grasses, and weeds
- Food allergy, including egg and tree nut

Clinical Findings

History

In a primary care setting, asthma should be monitored using a standardized instrument, which may include the Asthma Control Test (ACT), Asthma Control Questionnaire, Asthma Therapy Assessment Questionnaire, Asthma Control Score, and other instruments as found in the guidelines summary (National Heart, Lung, and Blood Institute [NHLBI], 2007, p 17). The advantages of a standardized questionnaire are that it allows the health care provider to assess changes in the patient's asthma and alter the management plan as needed. However, data suggest the use of these tools is not effective in poorly controlled children in an acute setting (Szefler, 2014).

The assessment of asthma symptoms allows providers to determine if the asthma is well controlled, less well controlled, or poorly controlled (Mueller et al, 2013). Well-controlled children have symptoms less than 2 days a week and use short-acting $beta_2$-agonists (SABAs) less than twice a week, whereas less well-controlled patients have symptoms more than 2 days a week and likely need a step up in treatments. Poorly controlled children have symptoms during the day and may utilize SABAs several times a day.

In primary care settings and the emergency department, the initial presentation is assessed based on the ability to talk in sentences, breathlessness, and alertness (Nelson and Zorc, 2013). Critical points to cover in the history of a child being seen for asthma include the following:

- Family history of asthma or other related allergic disorders (e.g., eczema or AR)
- Conditions associated with asthma (e.g., chronic sinusitis, nasal polyposis, gastroesophageal reflux, and chronic otitis media)
- Complaints of chest tightness or dyspnea
- Cough and wheezing particularly at night and in the early morning or shortness of breath with exercise or exertion (characteristic of asthma)
- Seasonal, continuous, or episodic pattern of symptoms that may be associated with certain allergens or triggering agents
- Episodes of recurrent "bronchitis" or pneumonia
- Precipitation of symptoms by known aggravating factors (upper respiratory infections, acetaminophen, aspirin)
- Level of alertness

Physical Examination

Table 25-3 outlines the physical assessment findings correlated with asthma severity. Broadly speaking, the following may be seen on physical examination:

- Heterophonous wheezing (different pitches but may be absent if severe obstruction)
- Continuous and persistent coughing
- Prolonged expiratory phase, high-pitched rhonchi especially at the bases
- Diminished breath sounds
- Signs of respiratory distress, including tachypnea, retractions, nasal flaring, use of accessory muscles, increasing restlessness, apprehension, agitation, drowsiness to coma
- Tachycardia, hypertension or hypotension, pulsus paradoxus
- Cyanosis of lips and nail beds if hypoxic
- Possible associated findings include sinusitis, AD, and AR.

Diagnostic Studies

Laboratory and radiographic tests should be individualized and based on symptoms, severity or chronology of the disease, response to therapy, and age. Tests to consider include the following:

- Oxygen saturation by pulse oximetry to assess severity of acute exacerbation. This should be a routine part of every assessment of a child with asthma. Pulse oximetry measures the oxygen saturation (SaO_2) of hemoglobin—the percentage of total hemoglobin that is oxygenated.
- A CBC if secondary infection or anemia is suspected (also check for elevated numbers of eosinophils).

TABLE 25-3 Physical Assessment of Asthma and Asthma Severity

Severity of Asthma	Physical Assessment Findings
Mild	Wheezing at the end of expiration or no wheezing No or minimal intercostal retractions along posterior axillary line Slight prolongation of expiratory phase Normal aeration in all lung fields Can talk in sentences
Moderate	Wheezing throughout expiration Intercostal retractions Prolonged expiratory phase Decreased breath sounds at the base
Severe	Use of accessory muscles plus lower rib and suprasternal retractions; nasal flaring Inspiratory and expiratory wheezing or no wheezing heard with poor air exchange Suprasternal retractions with abdominal breathing Decreased breath sounds throughout base
Impending respiratory arrest	Diminished breath sounds over entire lung filed Tiring, inability to maintain respirations Severely prolonged expiration if breath sounds are heard Drowsy, confused

- Routine chest radiographs are not indicated in most children with asthma. Results are typically normal or only show hyperinflation. Again imaging should be ordered judiciously with consideration of the long-term risk. However, chest radiographs can be useful in the following situations: selected cases of asthma or suspected asthma or if the child has persistent wheezing without a clinical explanation. Children with hypoxia, fever, suspected pneumonia, and/or localized rales requiring admission are candidates for imaging. Infants with wheezing during the winter who have clinical bronchiolitis do not need imaging (Nelson and Zorc, 2013).
- If sinusitis is suspected as the trigger, no diagnostic radiographic testing is needed.
- Allergy evaluation should be considered, keeping in mind that history and physical examination are key in this consideration. (Refer child to pediatric allergist.)
- Sweat test should be considered based on history in every patient with asthma.
- Pulmonary function tests:
    - Spirometry testing is the gold standard for diagnosing asthma and should be used on a regular basis to monitor, evaluate, and manage asthma. Exercise challenges using spirometry can also be done to evaluate the child with exercised-induced asthma. Children older than 5 years can typically perform spirometry.

- To evaluate the accuracy of the spirometry, look for an initial sharp peak with an extension down to the baseline at the end of expiration that is reproducible at least two times. Compare the child's values with the predicted value for the child's age, height, sex, and race.
- Look at the forced expiratory volume in 1 second (FEV_1), which represents the amount of air exhaled in 1 second. The interpretation of percentage predicted is:
  - >75%: Normal
  - 60% to 75%: Mild obstruction
  - 50% to 59%: Moderate obstruction
  - <49%: Severe obstruction
- The forced vital capacity (FVC) represents the amount of air expelled:
  - 80% to 120%: Normal
  - 70% to 79%: Mild reduction
  - 50% to 69%: Moderate reduction
  - <50%: Severe reduction
- The FEV_1/FVC represents the amount of air expelled in the first second over the total amount of air expelled and should be greater than 90% of the predicted value. Spirometry testing is done prior to a breathing treatment and 10 minutes after the treatment. If the child's FEV_1 improves by 12%, the child likely has asthma because this illustrates hyperresponsiveness.
- The forced expiratory flow (FEF) (FEF_{25} to FEF_{75}) reflects the middle portion of the downward limb of the curve and is a good measure of smaller airway function. The interpretation of percentage predicted is:
  - >60%: Normal
  - 40% to 60%: Mild obstruction
  - 20% to 40%: Moderate obstruction
  - <10%: Severe obstruction
- Doing spirometry during well-child checks and for sick visits gives the practitioner an excellent indication of the amount of inflammation and bronchospasm present in the airway (Kamakshya, 2012). Table 25-4 represents abnormal spirometry patterns.
- Consider the use of more sophisticated pulmonary laboratory studies for the child with severe asthma.
- Peak flow measurements:
  - If spirometry is not an option, peak expiratory flow (PEF) can be used.
  - PEF can be used in some children as young as 4 to 5 years old. The values are instrument specific, so the child's personal best value is the best guide to help detect possible changes in airway obstruction. The predicted range for height and age can be substituted if personal best rate is not available (Table 25-5). Interpretation of PEF reading is as follows if PEF is in the:
    - Green zone: More than 80% to 100% of personal best signals good control.
    - Yellow zone: Between 50% and 79% of personal best signals a caution.

TABLE 25-4 Abnormal Spirometry Findings

	Obstructive	Restrictive
FVC	Normal or ↓	↓
FEV_1	↓	↓
FEV_1/FVC	↓	Normal or ↑

FEV_1, Forced expiratory volume in 1 second; *FVC*, forced vital capacity.

TABLE 25-5 Predicted Average Peak Expiratory Flow for Normal Children and Adolescents

Height (Inches)	Males and Females (L/min)	Height (Inches)	Males and Females (L/min)	Height (Inches)	Males and Females (L/min)
43	147	51	254	59	360
44	160	52	267	60	373
45	173	53	280	61	387
46	187	54	293	62	400
47	200	55	307	63	413
48	214	56	320	64	427
49	227	57	334	65	440
50	240	58	347	66	454
				67	467

From National Heart, Lung, and Blood Institute (NHLBI): *Executive summary: guidelines for the diagnosis and management of asthma, NIH Pub No 94-3042A*, Bethesda, MD, 1994, National Institutes of Health; adapted from Polger G, Promedhar V: *Pulmonary function testing in children: techniques and standards*, Philadelphia, 1971, Saunders.

• BOX 25-3 Use of the Peak Flowmeter and Its Interpretation

Steps to follow in using a peak flow meter:
1. Have child stand up.
2. Make sure that indicator is at the base of the numbered scale.
3. Ask child to take a deep breath.
4. Have the child place the peak flow meter in the mouth with the lips sealing the mouthpiece. Tell the child not to put his or her tongue in the hole of the mouthpiece.
5. Tell the child to blow out as hard and fast as possible.
6. Record the rate, but if the child coughs, do not write down that number.
7. Repeat steps 2 through 6, two more times.
8. Record the highest of the three values.

Peak Expiratory Flow Rate

Maximum flow rate that is produced during forced expiration with fully inflated lungs.

Personal Best Value

Highest value achieved in measuring peak expiratory flow (PEF) rate over a 2-week period when child's asthma is under good control is known as one's *personal best value* or *rate.* Good control is defined as when one feels well without asthma symptoms. To determine personal best, take readings twice daily, in the morning and late afternoon or evening, and 15 to 20 minutes after taking an inhaled short-acting beta$_2$-agonist (SABA). Using the personal best value is the most accurate gauge to use to interpret changes in peak flow measurements because the child's own scores are used as the standard for comparison.

    - Red zone: Between 0% and 50% of personal best signals major airflow obstruction.
    - Box 25-3 describes use of peak flowmeter and interpretation of results.
- Exhaled nitric oxide (Dweik et al, 2011):
  - A biomarker for the children with asthma is exhaled nitric oxide testing, which measures a fraction of exhaled nitric oxide (FE_{no}).
  - The test measures eosinophilic airway inflammation and helps to determine whether corticosteroids would be helpful in the management of the patient. It may support the diagnosis of asthma and can help determine compliance with corticosteroid therapy.
  - A FE_{no} value of more than 35 ppb in children indicates eosinophilic inflammation and likely responsiveness to corticosteroids, whereas 25 to 35 ppb should be interpreted with caution. There is still controversy about this test, although guidelines have been published.

Differential Diagnosis

Numerous conditions can cause airway obstruction and be incorrectly confused with asthma, especially in young children and infants. Differential diagnoses include:
- Acute bronchiolitis, laryngotracheobronchitis, bronchopneumonia, pneumothorax
- Bronchial foreign body aspiration
- Congenital malformations of the heart with CHF
- Congenital pulmonary abnormalities or bronchopulmonary dysplasia
- Genetic disorders, such as cystic fibrosis and alpha-1-antitrypin deficiency
- Tracheal or foreign body compression (e.g., vascular aortic ring, enlarged lymph nodes or tumors)
- Chronic lower respiratory tract infections caused by immunodeficiency disorders
- Congenital malformation of the GI system with resultant recurrent aspirations
- Vocal cord dysfunction
- Gastroesophageal reflux disease
- Exposure to toxic substance
- Anaphylaxis

Management

Management strategies are based on whether the child has intermittent, mild persistent, moderate persistent, or severe persistent asthma (see Table 25-3). A stepwise approach is recommended. If control of symptoms is not maintained at a particular step of classification and management, the health care provider first should reevaluate for adherence and administration factors. If these factors do not appear to be responsible for the lack of symptom control, go to the next treatment step. Likewise, gradual step-downs in pharmacologic therapy may be considered when the child is well controlled for 3 months. Inhaled corticosteroids may be reduced about 25% to 50% every 3 months to the lowest possible dose needed to control the child's asthma (NHLBI, 2007; Szefler et al, 2014).

Chronic Asthma

Treatment of chronic asthma in children is based on general control measures and pharmacotherapy. Control measures can include the following:
- Avoid exposure to known allergens or irritants.
- Avoid use of acetaminophen in children at risk for asthma (Jackson et al, 2011; McBride, 2011).
- Administer yearly influenza vaccine.
- Control environment to eliminate or reduce offending allergen.
- Consider allergen immunotherapy. Studies have pointed to reduction in health care cost and improved outcomes associated with allergy immunotherapy (Dretzke et al, 2013; Hankin et al, 2013).
- Treat rhinitis, sinusitis, or gastroesophageal reflux.
- Other pharmacologic agents that may need to be considered include:
  - Anticholinergics—to reduce vagal tone in the airways (may also decrease mucus gland secretion)
  - Cromolyn sodium—to inhibit mast cell release of histamine
  - Leukotriene modifiers—to disrupt the synthesis or function of leukotrienes
  - If needed, refer to pulmonology for omalizumab, a recombinant DNA-derived, humanized IgG monoclonal antibody that binds to human IgE on the

surface of mast cells and basophils. This anti-IgE monoclonal antibody is used as a second-line treatment for children older than 12 who have moderate to severe allergy-related asthma and react to perennial allergens. It is used when symptoms are not controlled by inhaled corticosteroids.

- Follow up with PCP after an exacerbation requiring emergency department care, and obtain a clear written asthma action plan.
- Education regarding asthma basics, including triggers and prevention with environmental modification, as well as the different treatment modalities includes the techniques of administration and dispelling any myths regarding asthma medication. In terms of coping, the child and family need to be able to understand their emotions, worries, and uncertainty, as well as when to contact their PCP. Developing and understanding the asthma action plan is very important during a well-child visit (Archibald and Scott, 2014).

The pharmacologic management of asthma in children is based on the severity of asthma and the child's age. The stepwise approach to treatment (Figs. 25-1 and 25-2) is based on severity of symptoms and the use of pharmacotherapy to control chronic symptoms, maintain normal activity, prevent recurrent exacerbations, and minimize adverse side effects and nearly "normal" pulmonary function. Within any classification, a child may experience mild, moderate, or severe exacerbations. NHLBI guidelines for assessing asthma control and initiating and adjusting asthma therapy for the various pediatric age groups are found in Figures 25-3 and 25-4.

Important considerations to note in the pharmacologic treatment of asthma include the following:

- Control of asthma should be gained as quickly as possible by starting at the classification step most appropriate to the initial severity of the child's symptoms or at a higher level (e.g., a course of systemic corticosteroids or higher dose of inhaled corticosteroid). After control of symptoms, decrease treatment to the least amount of medication needed to maintain control.
- Systemic corticosteroids may be needed at any time and stepped up if there is a major flare-up of symptoms.

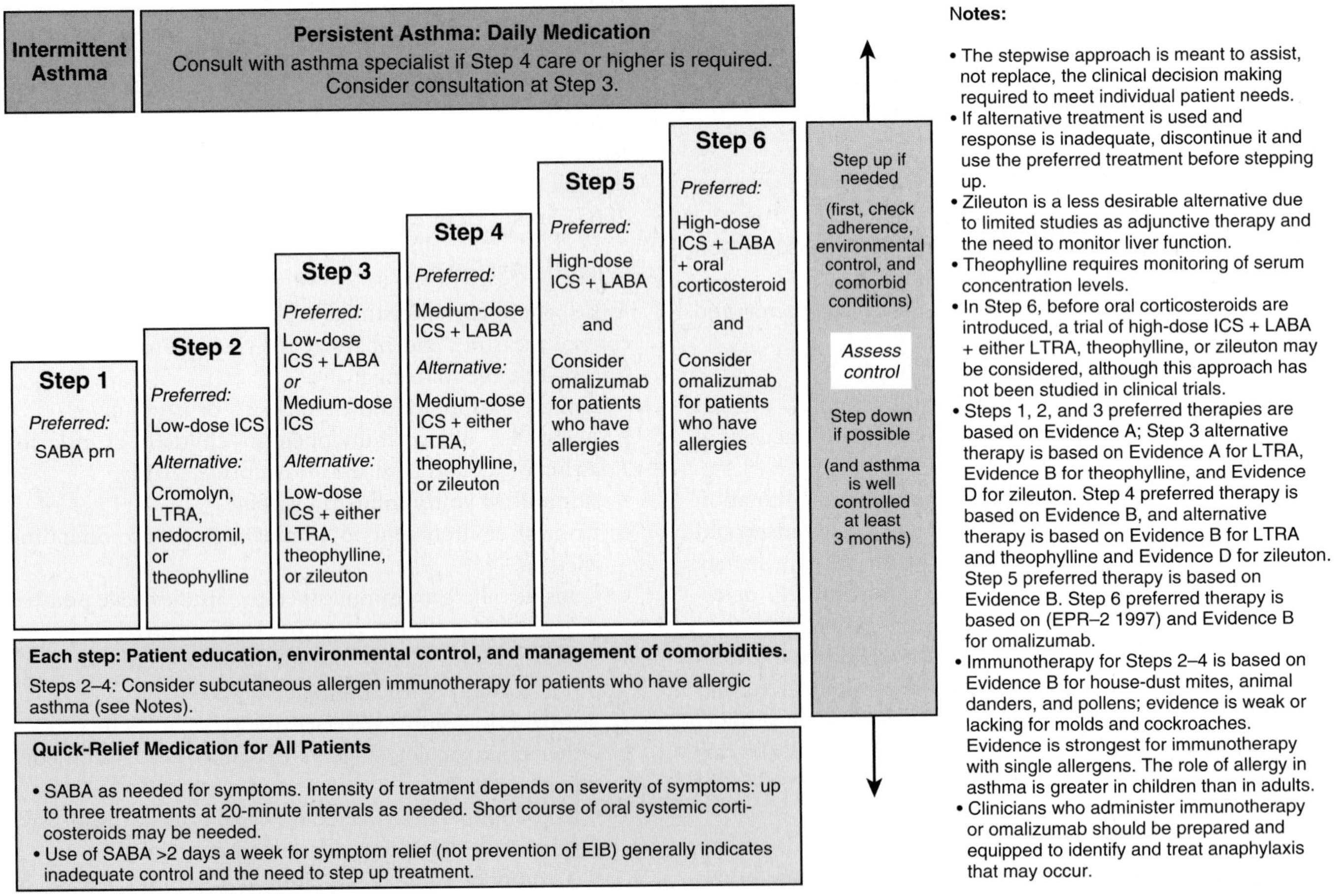

• **Figure 25-1** Stepwise approach for managing asthma in patients 12 years old and older and adults. *Alphabetical listing is used when more than one treatment option is listed within either preferred or alternative therapy. EIB,* Exercise-induced bronchospasm; *ICS,* inhaled corticosteroid; *LABA,* long-acting beta$_2$-agonist; *LTRA,* leukotriene receptor antagonist; *prn, pro re nata* (when necessary); *SABA,* short-acting beta$_2$-agonist. (From National Heart, Lung, and Blood Institute: *National Asthma and Prevention Program: expert panel report 3: guidelines for the diagnosis and management of asthma*, 2007. Available at www.nhlbi.nih.gov/guidelines/asthma/asthsumm.pdf. Accessed October 30, 2015, p 45.)

Step up if needed (first check inhaler technique, adherence, environmental control, and comorbid conditions)

Assess control

Step down if possible (and asthma is well controlled at least 3 months)

Children 0–4 years old

	Step 1	Step 2	Step 3	Step 4	Step 5	Step 6
	Intermittent Asthma	**Persistent Asthma: Daily Medication** Consult with asthma specialist if Step 3 care or higher is required. Consider consultation at Step 2.				
Preferred	SABA prn	Low-dose ICS	Medium-dose ICS	Medium-dose ICS + LABA *or* montelukast	High-dose ICS + LABA *or* montelukast	High-dose ICS + **LABA or montelukast** + **Oral corticosteroids ICS**
Alternative		Cromolyn *or* montelukast				
	Each Step: Patient Education and Environmental Control					
Quick-Relief Medication	• SABA as needed for symptoms. Intensity of treatment depends on severity of symptoms. • With viral respiratory symptoms: SABA q 4–6 hours up to 24 hours (longer with physician consult). Consider short course of oral systemic corticosteroids if exacerbation is severe or patient has history of previous severe exacerbations. Caution: Frequent use of SABA may indicate the need to step up treatment. See text for recommendations on initiating daily long-term-control therapy.					

Notes

- The stepwise approach is meant to assist, not replace, the clinical decision making required to meet individual patient needs.
- If an alternative treatment is used and response is inadequate, discontinue it and use the preferred treatment before stepping up.
- If clear benefit is not observed within 4–6 weeks, and patient's/family's medication technique and adherence are satisfactory, consider adjusting therapy or an alternative diagnosis.
- Studies on children 0 to 4 years old are limited. Step 2 preferred therapy is based on Evidence A. All other recommendations are based on expert opinion and extrapolation from studies in older children.
- Clinicians who administer immunotherapy should be prepared and equipped to identify and treat anaphylaxis that may occur.

Children 5–11 Years old

	Step 1	Step 2	Step 3	Step 4	Step 5	Step 6
	Intermittent Asthma	**Persistent Asthma: Daily Medication** Consult with asthma specialist if Step 4 care or higher is required. Consider consultation at Step 3.				
Preferred	SABA prn	Low-dose ICS	Low-dose ICS + LABA, LTRA, *or* theophylline *OR*	Medium-dose ICS + LABA	High-dose ICS + LABA	High-dose ICS + LABA + Oral corticosteroids
Alternative		Cromolyn LTRA nedocromil, *or* theophylline	Medium-dose ICS	Medium-dose ICS + LTRA *or* theophylline	High-dose ICS + LTRA *or* theophylline	High-dose ICS + LTRA *or* theophylline + Oral corticosteroids
	Each Step: Patient Education and Environmental Control, and Management of Comorbidities Steps 2–4: Consider subcutaneous allergen immunotherapy for patients who have persistent, allergic asthma.					
Quick-Relief Medication	• SABA as needed for symptoms. Intensity of treatment depends on severity of symptoms: up to three treatments at 20-minute intervals as needed. Short course of oral systemic corticosteroids may be needed. Caution: Increasing use of SABA or use >2 days a week for symptom relief (not prevention of EIB) generally indicates inadequate control and the need to step up treatment.					

- The stepwise approach is meant to assist, not replace, the clinical decision making required to meet individual patient needs.
- If an alternative treatment is used and response is inadequate, discontinue it and use the preferred treatment before stepping up.
- Theophylline is a less desirable alternative due to the need to monitor serum concentration levels.
- Steps 1 and 2 medications are based on Evidence A. Step 3 ICS and ICS plus adjunctive therapy are based on Evidence B for efficacy of each treatment and extrapolation from comparator trials in older children and adults—comparator trials are not available for this age group; Steps 4–6 are based on expert opinion and extrapolation from studies in older children and adults.
- Immunotherapy for Steps 2–4 is based on Evidence B for house-dust mites, animal danders, and pollens; evidence is weak or lacking for molds and cockroaches. Evidence is strongest for immunotherapy with single allergens. The role of allergy in asthma is greater in children than adults.
- Clinicians who administer immunotherapy should be prepared and equipped to identify and treat anaphylaxis that may occur.

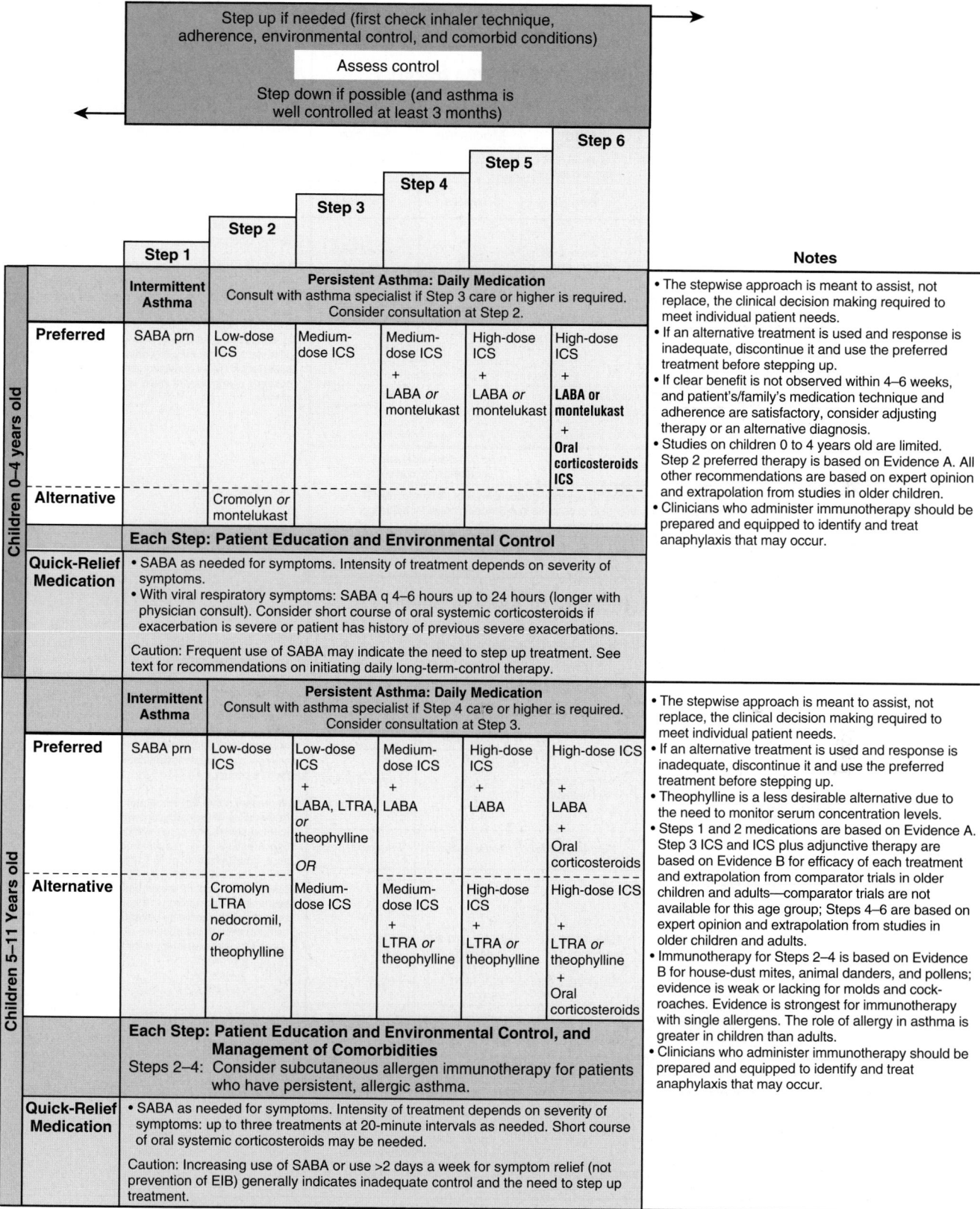

• **Figure 25-2** Stepwise approach for managing asthma in children 0 to 4 years old and 5 to 11 years old. *Alphabetical order is used when more than one treatment option is listed within either preferred or alternative therapy. EIB,* Exercise-induced bronchospasm; *ICS,* inhaled corticosteroid; *LABA,* long-acting beta$_2$-agonist; *LTRA,* leukotriene receptor antagonist; *prn, pro re nata* (when necessary); *SABA,* short-acting beta$_2$-agonist. (From National Heart, Lung, and Blood Institute: *National Asthma and Prevention Program: expert panel report 3: guidelines for the diagnosis and management of asthma*, 2007. Available at www.nhlbi.nih.gov/guidelines/asthma/asthsumm.pdf. Accessed October 30, 2015, p 42.)

Children 0–4 years old

Components of Severity		Classification of Asthma Severity: Intermittent	Persistent: Mild	Persistent: Moderate	Persistent: Severe
Impairment	Symptoms	≤2 days/week	>2 days/week but not daily	Daily	Throughout the day
	Nighttime awakenings	0	1-2x/month	3-4x/month	>1x/week
	SABA use for symptom control (not prevention of EIB)	≤2 days/week	>2 days/week but not daily	Daily	Several times per day
	Interference with normal activity	None	Minor limitation	Some limitation	Extremely limited
Risk	Exacerbations requiring oral systemic corticosteroids	0-1/year	≥2 exacerbations in 6 months requiring oral systemic corticosteroids, or ≥4 wheezing episodes/1 year lasting >1 day *and* risk factors for persistent asthma		
		← Consider severity and interval since last exacerbation. Frequency and severity may fluctuate over time. →			
		Exacerbations of any severity may occur in patients in any severity category			
Recommended Step for Initiating Therapy **(See Fig. 25-2 for treatment steps.)**		Step 1	Step 2	Step 3 and consider short course of oral systemic corticosteroids	
		In 2-6 weeks, depending on severity, evaluate level of asthma control that is achieved. If no clear benefit is oberved in 4-6 weeks, consider adjusting therapy or alternative diagnoses.			

Notes

- The stepwise approach is meant to assist, not replace, the clinical decision making required to meet individual patient needs.
- Level of severity is determined by both impairment and risk. Assess impairment domain by patient's/caregiver's recall of previous 2-4 weeks. Symptom assessment for longer periods should reflect a global assessment, such as inquiring whether the patient's asthma is better or worse since the last visit. Assign severity to the most severe category in which any feature occurs.
- At present, there are inadequate data to correspond frequencies of exacerbations with different levels of asthma severity. For treatment purposes, patients who had ≥2 exacerbations requiring oral systemic corticosteroids in the past 6 months, or ≥4 wheezing episodes in the past year, and who have risk factors for persistent asthma may be considered the same as patients who have persistent asthma, even in the absence of impairment levels consistent with persistent asthma.

Children 5–11 years old

Components of Severity		Classification of Asthma Severity: Intermittent	Persistent: Mild	Persistent: Moderate	Persistent: Severe
Impairment	Symptoms	≤2 days/week	>2 days/week but not daily	Daily	Throughout the day
	Nighttime awakenings	≤2x/month	3-4x/month	>1x/week but not nightly	Often 7x/week
	SABA use for symptom control (not prevention of EIB)	≤2 days/week	>2 days/week but not daily	Daily	Several times per day
	Interference with normal activity	None	Minor limitation	Some limitation	Extremely limited
	Lung function	• Normal FEV_1 between exacerbations • FEV_1 >80% predicted • FEV_1/FVC >85%	• FEV_1 >80% predicted • FEV_1/FVC >80%	• FEV_1 = 60-80% predicted • FEV_1/FVC = 75-80%	• FEV_1 < 60% predicted • FEV_1/FVC < 75%
Risk	Exacerbations requiring oral systemic corticosteroids	0-1/year (see Notes)	≥2/year (see Notes) →		
		← Consider severity and interval since last exacerbation. → Frequency and severity may fluctuate over time for patients in any severity category.			
		Relative annual risk of exacerbations may be related to FEV_1.			
Recommended Step for Initiating Therapy **(See Fig. 25-2 for treatment steps.)**		Step 1	Step 2	Step 3, medium-dose ICS option	Step 3, medium-dose ICS option, or step 4
				and consider short course of oral systemic corticosteroids	
		In 2-6 weeks, evaluate level of asthma control that is achieved, and adjust therapy accordingly.			

Notes

- The stepwise approach is meant to assist, not replace, the clinical decision making required to meet individual patient needs.
- Level of severity is determined by both impairment and risk. Assess impairment domain by patient's/caregiver's recall of previous 2-4 weeks and spirometry. Assign severity to the most severe category in which any feature occurs.
- At present, there are inadequate data to correspond frequencies of exacerbations with different levels of asthma severity. In general, more frequent and intense exacerbations (e.g., requiring urgent, unscheduled care, hospitalization, or ICU admission) indicate greater underlying disease severity. For treatment purposes, patients who had ≥2 exacerbations requiring oral systemic corticosteroids in the past year may be considered the same as patients who have persistent asthma, even in the absence of impairment levels consistent with persistent asthma.

• **Figure 25-3** Assessing asthma severity and initiating therapy in children 0 to 4 years old and 5 to 11 years old who are not currently taking long-term control medication. *EIB,* Exercise-induced bronchospasm; *FEV_1,* forced expiratory volume in 1 second; *FVC,* forced vital capacity; *ICS,* inhaled corticosteroid; *ICU,* intensive care unit; *SABA,* short-acting beta$_2$-agonist. (From National Heart, Lung, Blood Institute: *National Asthma Prevention Program: expert panel report 3: guidelines for the diagnosis and management of asthma*, 2007. Available at www.nhlbi.nih.gov/guidelines/asthma/asthsumm.pdf. Accessed October 30, 2015, pp 40–41.)

Children ≥12 years old

Components of Severity		Classification of Asthma Severity: Intermittent	Persistent: Mild	Persistent: Moderate	Persistent: Severe
Impairment	Symptoms	≤2 days/week	>2 days/week but not daily	Daily	Throughout the day
	Nighttime awakenings	≤2x/month	3-4x/month	>1x/week but not nightly	Often 7x/week
	SABA use for symptom control (not prevention of EIB)	≤2 days/week	>2 days/week but not daily, and not more than 1x on any day	Daily	Several times per day
Normal FEV_1/FVC: 08-19 years old 85% 20-39 years old 80% 40-59 years old 75% 60-80 years old 70%	Interference with normal activity	None	Minor limitation	Some limitation	Extremely limited
	Lung function	• Normal FEV_1 between exacerbations • FEV_1 >80% predicted • FEV_1/FVC normal	• FEV_1 >80% predicted • FEV_1/FVC normal	• FEV_1 >60 but <80% predicted • FEV_1/FVC reduced 5%	• FEV_1 < 60% predicted • FEV_1/FVC reduced >5%
Risk	Exacerbations requiring oral systemic corticosteroids	0-1/year (see Notes)	≥2/year (see Notes) →		
		← Consider severity and interval since last exacerbation. → Frequency and severity may fluctuate over time for patients in any severity category.			
		Relative annual risk of exacerbations may be related to FEV_1.			
Recommended Step for Initiating Therapy (See Fig. 25-1 for treatment steps.)		Step 1	Step 2	Step 3 and consider short course of oral systemic corticosteroids	Step 4 or 5 and consider short course of oral systemic corticosteroids
		In 2-6 weeks, evaluate level of asthma control that is achieved and adjust therpay accordingly.			

Notes

- The stepwise approach is meant to assist, not replace, the clinical decision making required to meet individual patient needs.
- Level of severity is determined by both impairment and risk. Assess impairment domain by patient's/caregiver's recall of previous 2-4 weeks and spirometry. Assign severity to the most severe category in which any feature occurs.
- At present, there are inadequate data to correspond frequencies of exacerbations with different levels of asthma severity. In general, more frequent and intense exacerbations (e.g., requiring urgent, unscheduled care, hospitalization, or ICU admission) indicate greater underlying disease severity. For treatment purposes, patients who had ≥2 exacerbations requiring oral systemic corticosteroids in the past year may be considered the same as patients who have persistent asthma, even in the absence of impairment levels consistent with persistent asthma.

• **Figure 25-4** Assessing asthma severity and initiating therapy in children 12 years old and older and adults who are not currently taking long-term control medication. *EIB,* Exercise-induced bronchospasm; *FEV_1,* forced expiratory volume in 1 second; *FVC,* forced vital capacity; *ICU,* intensive care unit; *SABA,* short-acting beta$_2$-agonist. (From National Heart, Lung, Blood Institute: *National Asthma Prevention Program: expert panel report 3: guidelines for the diagnosis and management of asthma*, 2007. Available at www.nhlbi.nih.gov/guidelines/asthma/asthsumm.pdf. Accessed October 30, 2015, p 43.)

Control of inflammation is a key principle in the management of asthma.

- The combination of inhaled corticosteroids with a long-acting beta$_2$-agonist (LABA) can further control asthma (Szefler, 2013).
- Children with intermittent asthma may have long periods in which they are symptom-free; they can also have life-threatening exacerbations, often provoked by respiratory infection. In these situations, a short course of systemic corticosteroids should be used.
- Variations in asthma necessitate individualized treatment plans.
- β_2 agonists can be administered with metered dose inhaler (MDI) therapy via spacer for children with mild and moderate exacerbations of asthma, but for children with severe airway obstruction who may have decreased deposition of drug in the base of the lung, a nebulizer may be better (Nelson and Zorc, 2013). There is need for more research on the use of MDI therapy and nebulizer therapy in the pediatric population (Szefler et al, 2014). A spacer or holding chamber with an attached mask enhances the delivery of MDI medications to the lower airways of a child. Spacers eliminate the need to synchronize inhalation with activation of MDI. Older children can use a spacer without the mask.
- Dry powder inhalers (DPIs) do not need spacers or shaking before use. Instruct children to rinse their mouth with water and spit after inhalation. DPIs should not be used in children younger than 4 years old.
- Different inhaled corticosteroids are not equal in potency to each other on a per puff or microgram basis. Tables 25-6 and 25-7 compare daily low, medium, and high doses of various inhaled corticosteroids used for children. Combination inhaled corticosteroid and LABA can be used in children from 4 years old (Taketomo et al, 2014).
- For treatment of exercise-induced bronchospasm:
  - Warm up before exercise for 5 to 10 minutes.
  - Use either an inhaled SABA or a mast cell stabilizer (cromolyn) or both prior to exercise. Combination of both types of drugs is the more effective therapy. A LABA can be used in older children.
  - Use two puffs of a β_2 agonist and/or cromolyn MDI 15 to 30 minutes before exercise. Tolerance may develop if a β_2 agonist is used more than a few times

TABLE 25-6 Estimated Comparative Daily Dosages for Inhaled Corticosteroids

Drug	Low Daily Dose		Medium Daily Dose		High Daily Dose	
	Child*	Adult†	Child*	Adult†	Child*	Adult†
Beclomethasone HFA (40 or 80 mcg/puff)	80-160 mcg	80-240 mcg	>160-320 mcg	>240-480 mcg	>320 mcg	>480 mcg
Budesonide (90 or 180, mcg/actuation) aerosol powder breath-activated inhalation	180-400 mcg	180-600 mcg	>400-800 mcg	>600-1200 mcg	>800 mcg	>1200 mcg
Budesonide inhaled suspension for nebulization (child dose) (0.25 mg/2 mL, 0.5 mg/2 mL)	0.5 mg		1 mg		2 mg	N/A
Flunisolide aerosol solution inhalation (80 mcg/spray)	160 mcg	320 mcg	320 mcg	>320-640 mcg	>640 mcg	>640 mcg
Fluticasone HFA: 44, 110, or 220 mcg/actuation	88-176 mcg	88-264 mcg	>176-352 mcg	>264-440 mcg	>352 mcg	>440 mcg
Fluticasone aerosol powder breath-activated inhalation: 50, 100, or 250 mcg/inhalation	100-200 mcg	100-300 mcg	>200-400 mcg	>300-500 mcg	>400 mcg	>500 mcg
Mometasone aerosol powder breath-activated inhalation (220 mcg/INH)‡	N/A	200 mcg	N/A	400 mcg	N/A	>400 mcg

Adapted from the National Heart, Lung, and Blood Institute (NHLBI): *Full report of the expert panel: guidelines for the diagnosis and management of asthma (EPR-3)*, Bethesda, MD, 2007, National Institutes of Health; Taketomo CK, Hodding JH, Kraus DM: *Pediatric dosage handbook*, ed 21, Hudson, OH, 2014, Lexi-Comp.
HFA, Hydrofluoroalkane; *INH,* inhalation; *N/A,* not approved and no data available for this age group.
*Child 5 to 11 years old.
†Adult 12 years old and older.
‡Note 220 mcg/inhalation provides 200 mcg of mometasone per actuation.

TABLE 25-7 Inhaled Corticosteroids in Children 0 to 4 Years Old

	Low Daily Dose	Medium Daily Dose	High Daily Dose
Budesonide inhaled suspension for nebulization (0.25 mg/2 mL, 0.5 mg/2 mL)	0.25-0.5 mg	>0.5-1 mg	>1 mg
Fluticasone HFA: 44, 110, or 220 mcg/actuation	176 mcg	>176-352 mcg	>352 mcg

Adapted from the National Heart, Lung, and Blood Institute (NHLBI): *Full report of the expert panel: guidelines for the diagnosis and management of asthma (EPR-3)*, Bethesda, MD, 2007, National Institutes of Health; Taketomo CK, Hodding JH, Kraus DM: *Pediatric dosage handbook*, ed 21, Hudson, OH, 2014, Lexi-Comp.
HFA, Hydrofluoroalkane.

a week; it should not be used as a controller monotherapy. Those who exercise regularly and develop symptoms of asthma should use controller medication, preferably an inhaled corticosteroid.
- Using a scarf or mask around the mouth may decrease exercise-induced asthma (EIA) induced by cold.

Table 25-8 identifies the usual dosages for long-term control medications (exclusive of inhaled corticosteroids) used to treat asthma in children. Quick-relief medications are listed in Table 25-9. Practice parameters are guides and should not replace individualized treatment based on clinical judgment and unique differences among children.

Acute Exacerbations of Asthma

The treatment of acute episodes of asthma is also based on classification of the severity of the episode. Acute episodes

Text continued on p. 579

TABLE 25-8 Long-Term Control Medications for the Treatment of Asthma

Medication	Dosage Form	Child Dosage*	Adult Dosage†	Comments
Inhaled Corticosteroids (see Tables 25-6 and 25-7)				
Systemic Corticosteroids—Applies to All Three Corticosteroids				
Methylprednisolone	2-, 4-, 8-, 16-, 32-mg tablets	0.25-2 mg/kg daily in a single dose in AM or every other day as needed for control; 60 mg maximum dose	7.5-60 mg daily in a single dose in AM or every other day as needed for control	For long-term treatment of severe persistent asthma, administer single dose in AM either daily or on alternate days (alternate-day therapy may produce less adrenal suppression). If daily doses are required, one study suggests improved efficacy and no increase in adrenal suppression when administered at 3 PM.
Prednisolone	5-mg tablets, 5 mg/5 mL, 1 mg/mL	Same as above	Same as above	
Prednisone	1-, 2-, 5-, 10-, 20-, 50-mg tablets; 5 mg/mL, 1 mg/mL	Short-course “burst”: 1-2 mg/kg/day in a single or two divided doses a day, maximum 60 mg/day for 3-10 days	Short-course “burst” to achieve control: 40-60 mg/day as single or two divided doses for 3-10 days	Short courses or “bursts” are effective for establishing control when initiating therapy or during a period of gradual deterioration. The bursts should be continued until patient achieves 80% PEF rate personal best or symptoms resolve. This usually requires 3 to 10 days but may require longer treatment. There is no evidence that tapering the dose following improvement prevents relapse.
Cromolyn				
Cromolyn	20 mg/ampule for nebulization solution, inhalation	Children ≥2 years old: 1 ampule four times a day initially; usual dose three times a day	1 ampule three or four times a day; usual dose three times a day	≥2 years old: Single dose of 20 mg 10 to 15 minutes before exercise or allergen exposure provides effective prophylaxis for 1 to 2 hours.

Continued

TABLE 25-8 Long-Term Control Medications for the Treatment of Asthma—cont'd

Medication	Dosage Form	Child Dosage*	Adult Dosage†	Comments
Inhaled Long-Acting Beta$_2$-Agonists—Should Not Be Used for Symptom Relief or for Exacerbations; Use with Inhaled Corticosteroids				
Salmeterol	DPI: 50 mcg/inhalation	≥4 years old: 1 activation/puff every 12 hours	1 activation/puff every 12 hours	Use with inhaled corticosteroid only. Do not use as a rescue inhaler for symptom relief or for exacerbations.
Formoterol	DPI: 12 mcg/single-use capsule	≥5 years old: 1 capsule every 12 hours apart	1 capsule every 12 hours	Do not take orally; must be used with aerolizer. Should be used with inhaled steroid.
Sustained-release albuterol	4-mg tablet‡ 8-mg tablet§	≥6 years old at 0.3-0.6 mg/kg/day in two divided doses; not to exceed 8 mg/day	4-8 mg/dose twice a day; can increase to 8 mg/dose twice a day	Not recommended treatment for asthma.
Methylxanthines				
Theophylline (numerous manufacturers)	Liquids Sustained-release tablets and capsules	Maintenance oral doses for chronic conditions. 1-9 years old: 20-24 mg/kg/day (maximum 600 mg/day); 9-12 years old: 16 mg/kg/day (maximum 600 mg/day); >12-16 years old: 13 mg/kg/day (maximum 600 mg/day) (dosing interval depends on product)	Maintenance dose for acute symptoms: 10 mg/kg/day divided every 8-12 hours; up to 900 mg maximum/day	Not recommended as long-term control medication. Routine serum theophylline level monitoring required (serum concentration 5-15 mcg/mL). Smoking alters dosage requirements.
Leukotriene Modifiers				
Montelukast	4- or 5-mg chewable tablet, 10-mg tablet; granules 4 mg/packet	12 months to 5 years old: 4 mg a day; 6-14 years old: 5 mg a day	≥15 years old: 10 mg a day Prevention of EIB: 6 to 14 years old: 5 mg; ≥15 years old: 10 mg at least 2 hours before exercise (no other doses should be given in 24 hours)	
Zafirlukast	10- or 20-mg tablet	5-11 years old: 10-mg tablet twice a day	>12 years old: 20-mg tablet twice a day	Take zafirlukast at least 1 hour before or 2 hours after meals.
Zileuton	600-mg tablet and 600 mg extended release		2400 mg daily (give tablets four times a day) or 1200 mg twice a day of the extended release	Less desirable because of the need to monitor hepatic enzymes (ALT); used in children older than 12 years old.

TABLE 25-8 Long-Term Control Medications for the Treatment of Asthma—cont'd

Medication	Dosage Form	Child Dosage*	Adult Dosage[†]	Comments
Combined Medication				
Fluticasone/ salmeterol	HFA: 45, 115, fluticasone 230 mcg/21 mcg salmeterol		HFA: ≥12 years old: Two inhalations twice a day of 45 mcg fluticasone/21 mcg salmeterol *or* 115 mcg fluticasone/21 mcg salmeterol	HFA adult dose not to exceed 2 inhalations of 230 mcg fluticasone/21 mcg salmeterol twice daily. Starting dose dependent on current steroid therapy.
	Diskus: 100, 250, or 500 mcg fluticasone/50 mcg salmeterol	Diskus: >4-11 years old: 1 inhalation twice a day of 100 mcg fluticasone/50 mcg salmeterol; dose depends on severity of asthma	Diskus: 1 inhalation twice a day of 100 mcg fluticasone/50 mcg salmeterol; dose depends on severity of asthma	Starting dose based on current steroid therapy.
Budesonide/ formoterol aerosol for oral inhalation	Aerosol: 80 mcg *or* 160 mcg budesonide/4.5 mcg formoterol	5-11 years old: 2 inhalations twice a day of aerosol 80 mcg/4.5 mcg, not to exceed 4 inhalations/day	≥12 years old: 2 inhalations twice a day of aerosol 80 mcg/4.5 mcg, not to exceed 4 inhalations/day; if not controlled may increase to 160 mcg budesonide/4.5 mcg formoterol inhalation twice daily not exceeding 4 inhalations day	

Adapted from the National Heart, Lung, and Blood Institute (NHLBI): *Full report of the expert panel: guidelines for the diagnosis and management of asthma (EPR-3)*, Bethesda, MD, 2007, National Institutes of Health; Taketomo CK, Hodding JH, Kraus DM: *Pediatric dosage handbook*, ed 21, Hudson, OH, 2014, Lexi-Comp.

ALT, Alanine amino transferase; *DPI,* dry powder inhaler; *EIB,* exercise-induced bronchospasm; *HFA,* hydrofluoroalkane; *PEF,* peak expiratory flow.

*Infants and children <12 years old.

[†]Adult, 12 years old and older.

[‡]Albuterol (Proventil Repetabs) come in 4 mg only.

[§]Albuterol (Volmax) comes in 4 mg and 8 mg.

TABLE 25-9 Quick-Relief Medications for the Treatment of Asthma

Medication	Dosage Form	Child Dosage*	Adult Dosage	Comments
Short-Acting Inhaled Beta$_2$-Agonists				
Metered Dose Inhalers				
Albuterol HFA	90 mcg/puff, 200 puffs	Acute exacerbation: 4-8 puffs every 20 minutes for three doses, then every 1-4 hours as needed Maintenance: 0-4 years old, 1-2 inhalations every 4-6 hours; >5 years old, 2 puffs every 4-6 hours prn	Acute exacerbation: 4-8 puffs every 20 minutes for 4 hours, then every 1-4 hours as needed Maintenance: 2 puffs every 4-6 hours prn	Not generally recommended for long-term treatment. Regular use on a daily basis indicates the need for additional long-term control therapy.

Continued

TABLE 25-9 **Quick-Relief Medications for the Treatment of Asthma—cont'd**

Medication	Dosage Form	Child Dosage*	Adult Dosage	Comments
Pirbuterol	200 mcg/INH, 400 INH	Acute exacerbation: 4-8 inhalations every 20 minutes for three doses, then every 1-4 hours as needed Maintenance: 2 inhalations three or four times/day	Acute exacerbation: 4-8 inhalations every 20 minutes for up to 4 hours, then every 1-4 hours as needed Maintenance: 2 inhalations three or four times/day	
Levalbuterol HFA	45 mcg/puff	Acute exacerbation: 4-8 puffs every 20 minutes for three doses, then every 1-4 hours Maintenance : ≥5 years old: 2 inhalations every 4-6 hours	Acute exacerbation: 4-8 puffs every 20 minutes for up to 4 hours, then every 1-4 hours as needed Maintenance: 2 inhalations every 4-6 hours	Not FDA approved for long-term, daily maintenance use. Use more than 2 days/week indicates need for long-term control therapy Non-selective agents (e.g., epinephrine, isoproterenol, metaproterenol) are not recommended because of their potential for excessive cardiac stimulation, especially at high doses.
Nebulizer Solution				
Albuterol	5 mg/mL (0.5%) 0.63 mg/3 mL 1.25 mg/3 mL 2.5 mg/3 mL	<5 years old: 0.63-2.5 mg in 3 mL NS every 4-6 hr prn >5 yr: 1.25-2.5 mg in 3 mL of NS every 4-8 hours prn	Adults: 1.25-5 mg in 3 mL of NS every 4-8 hours prn	May mix with cromolyn or ipratropium nebulizer solutions; may double dose for mild exacerbations.
Levalbuterol	0.31 mg/3 mL 0.63 mg/3 mL 1.25 mg/3 mL	Acute exacerbation: 0.075 mg/kg (minimum dose 1.25 mg) every 20 minutes for three doses, then 0.075-0.15 mg/kg (not to exceed 5 mg) every 1-4 hours as needed Maintenance: 0-4 years old: 0.31-1.25 mg every 4-6 hours prn; ≥5 years old and adults: 0.31-0.63 mg every 8 hours prn	Acute exacerbation: 1.25-2.5 mg every 20 minutes for three doses, then 1.25-5 mg every 1-4 hours as needed Maintenance: 0.31-0.63 mg every 8 hours as needed	Use more than 2 days/week indicates need for long-term control therapy

TABLE 25-9 Quick-Relief Medications for the Treatment of Asthma—cont'd

Medication	Dosage Form	Child Dosage*	Adult Dosage	Comments
Anticholinergics				
Ipratropium HFA (MDI) Ipratropium (Nebulizer solution)	17 mcg/puff, 200-puff canister 0.02% (2.5 mL)	Refer to a pharmacology textbook	Refer to a pharmacology textbook	Evidence is lacking that ipratropium HFA produces added benefit to β_2-agonists in long-term asthma therapy.
I				
Systemic Corticosteroids—Dosage Applies to All Three Corticosteroids				
Methylprednisolone	2-, 4-, 8-, 16-, 32-mg tablets	Short-course "burst": 1-2 mg/kg/day in divided doses once or twice daily, maximum 60 mg/day, for 3-10 days	Short-course "burst" to achieve control: 40-60 mg/day as single or two divided doses for 3-10 days	Short courses or "bursts" are effective for establishing control when initiating therapy or during a period of gradual deterioration.
Prednisolone	5-mg tablets, 5 mg/5 mL, 15 mg/5 mL			
Prednisone	1-, 2.5-, 5-, 10-, 20-, 50-mg tablets: 5 mg/mL, 5 mg/5 mL			The burst should be continued until patient achieves 80% PEF rate personal best or symptoms resolve; this usually requires 3-10 days but may require longer; there is no evidence that tapering the dose following improvement prevents relapse.

Adapted from the National Heart, Lung, and Blood Institute (NHLBI): *Full report of the expert panel: guidelines for the diagnosis and management of asthma (EPR-3)*, Bethesda, MD, 2007, National Institutes of Health; Taketomo CK, Hodding JH, Kraus DM: *Pediatric dosage handbook*, ed 21, Hudson, OH, 2014, Lexi-Comp.

FDA, U.S. Food and Drug Administration; *HFA*, hydrofluoroalkane; *INH*, inhalations; *MDI*, metered dose inhaler; *NS*, normal saline; *PEF*, peak expiratory flow; *prn*, *pro re nata* (when necessary).

*<12 years old.

are classified as mild, moderate, and severe. Signs and symptoms are summarized in Table 25-10. Early recognition of warning signs and treatment should be stressed in both patient or parent education, or both.

The initial pharmacologic treatment for acute asthma exacerbations is shown in Figure 25-5. It consists of inhaled SABAs (albuterol), two to six puffs every 20 minutes for three treatments by way of MDI with a spacer, or a single nebulizer treatment (0.15 mg/kg; minimum 1.25 to 2.5 mg of 0.5% solution of albuterol in 2 to 3 mL of normal saline).

If the initial treatment results in a good response (PEF/FEV_1 > 70% of the patient's best), the inhaled SABAs can be continued every 3 to 4 hours for 24 to 48 hours with a 3-day course of oral steroids at 1 to 2 mg/kg/day to a maximum of 60 mg per day. Reassessment is important to ensure an adequate response and to further assess asthma severity.

An incomplete response (PEF or FEV_1 between 40% and 69% of personal best or symptoms recur within 4 hours of therapy) is treated by continuing β_2 agonists and adding an oral corticosteroid. The β_2 agonist can be given by nebulizer or MDI with spacer. Parents should be taught to call their PCP for additional instructions. If there is marked distress (severe acute symptoms) or a poor response (PEF or FEV_1 <40%) to treatment, the child should have the β_2 agonist repeated immediately and should be taken to the emergency department. Emergency medical rescue (911) transportation should be used if the distress is severe and the child is agitated and unable to talk. If children experience acute asthma exacerbations more than once every 4 to 6 weeks, their treatment plan should be reevaluated.

TABLE 25-10 Classifying Severity of Asthma Exacerbations*

	Mild	Moderate	Severe	Respiratory Arrest Imminent
Symptoms				
Breathless	While walking Can lie down	While at rest (infant—softer, shorter cry; difficulty feeding) Prefers sitting	While at rest (infant—stops feeding) Sits upright	
Talks in	Sentences	Phrases	Words	
Alertness	May be agitated	Usually agitated	Usually agitated	Drowsy or confused
Signs				
Respiratory rate* (See guide below)	Increased	Increased	Often >30/min	
Use of accessory muscles; suprasternal retractions	Usually not	Commonly	Usually	Paradoxical thoracoabdominal movement
Wheeze	Moderate, often only end expiratory	Loud; throughout exhalation	Usually loud; throughout inhalation and exhalation	Absence of wheeze
Pulse/min* (See guide below)	<100	100-120	>120	Bradycardia
Pulsus paradoxus	Absent <10 mm Hg	May be present 10-25 mm Hg	Often present >25 mm Hg (adult), 20-40 mm Hg (child)	Absence suggests respiratory muscle fatigue
Functional Assessment				
PEF percentage predicted or percentage personal best	≥70%	Approximately 40%-69%	<40% predicted or personal best, or response lasts <2 hours	<25%
PaO_2 (on room air) *and/or*	Normal (test not usually necessary)	>60 mm Hg (test not usually necessary)	<60 mm Hg: possible cyanosis	
PCO_2	<42 mm Hg (test not usually necessary)	<42 mm Hg (test not usually necessary)	≥42 mm Hg: possible respiratory failure	
SaO_2% (on room air) at sea level	>95% (test not usually necessary)	90%-95%	<90%	

Guide to Normal Respiratory and Cardiac Rates

Normal Rates of Breathing in Awake Children

Age	Rate
<2 months old	<60/min
2-12 months old	<50/min
1-5 years old	<40/min
6-8 years old	<30/min

Normal Pulse Rates in Children

Age	Rate
2-12 months old	<160/min
1-2 years old	<120/min
2-8 years old	<110/min

From National Heart, Lung, and Blood Institute (NHLBI): *Full report of the expert panel: guidelines for the diagnosis and management of asthma (EPR-3)*, Bethesda, MD, 2007, National Institutes of Health.

$PaCO_2$, Partial pressure of carbon dioxide; *PaO_2*, partial pressure of oxygen in arterial blood; *PEF*, peak expiratory flow; *SaO_2*, oxygen saturation in arterial blood.

*The presence of several parameters, but not necessarily all, indicates the general classification of the exacerbation. Many of these parameters have not been systematically studied, so they serve only as general guides.

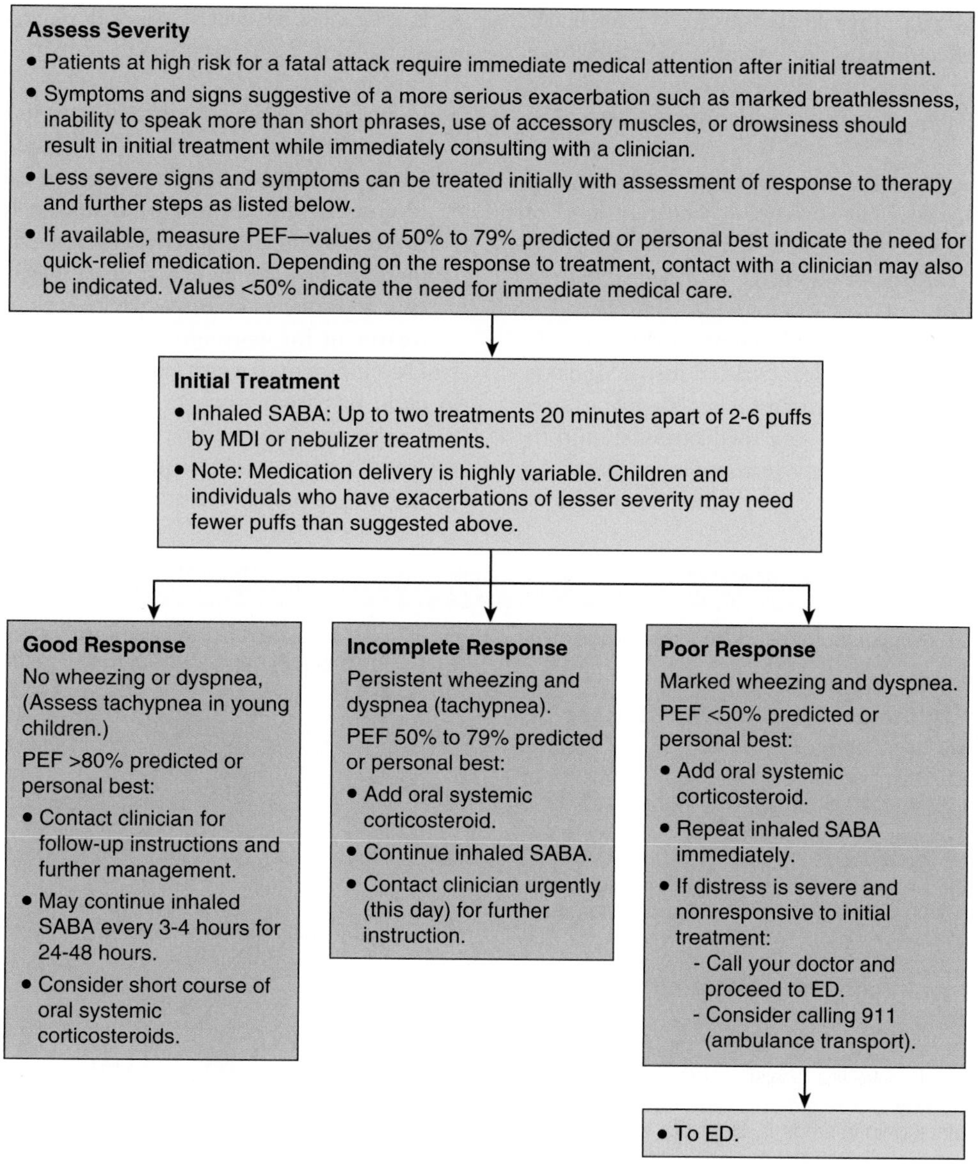
Assess Severity
• Patients at high risk for a fatal attack require immediate medical attention after initial treatment.
• Symptoms and signs suggestive of a more serious exacerbation such as marked breathlessness, inability to speak more than short phrases, use of accessory muscles, or drowsiness should result in initial treatment while immediately consulting with a clinician.
• Less severe signs and symptoms can be treated initially with assessment of response to therapy and further steps as listed below.
• If available, measure PEF—values of 50% to 79% predicted or personal best indicate the need for quick-relief medication. Depending on the response to treatment, contact with a clinician may also be indicated. Values <50% indicate the need for immediate medical care.
Initial Treatment
• Inhaled SABA: Up to two treatments 20 minutes apart of 2-6 puffs by MDI or nebulizer treatments.
• Note: Medication delivery is highly variable. Children and individuals who have exacerbations of lesser severity may need fewer puffs than suggested above.
Good Response
No wheezing or dyspnea, (Assess tachypnea in young children.)
PEF >80% predicted or personal best:
• Contact clinician for follow-up instructions and further management.
• May continue inhaled SABA every 3-4 hours for 24-48 hours.
• Consider short course of oral systemic corticosteroids.
Incomplete Response
Persistent wheezing and dyspnea (tachypnea).
PEF 50% to 79% predicted or personal best:
• Add oral systemic corticosteroid.
• Continue inhaled SABA.
• Contact clinician urgently (this day) for further instruction.
Poor Response
Marked wheezing and dyspnea.
PEF <50% predicted or personal best:
• Add oral systemic corticosteroid.
• Repeat inhaled SABA immediately.
• If distress is severe and nonresponsive to initial treatment:
- Call your doctor and proceed to ED.
- Consider calling 911 (ambulance transport).
• To ED.

• **Figure 25-5** Management of asthma exacerbations: Home treatment. *ED,* Emergency department; *MDI,* metered dose inhaler; *PEF,* peak expiratory flow; *SABA,* short-acting beta$_2$-agonist.

This chapter focuses on the outpatient management of patient with asthma. However, familiarity with other drug options used in more severe asthma is important. They include:

- Magnesium sulfate IV is used in emergency settings to decrease the intracellular calcium concentration. It causes bronchodilation due to respiratory smooth muscle relaxation.
- Ipratropium oral inhalation is an anticholinergic bronchodilator used to treat bronchospasms. Evidence of its long-term maintenance use to control bronchospasms is lacking (Taketomo et al, 2014)
- Epinephrine given subcutaneously or intramuscularly is still an option in severe asthma where the delivery of medication to smaller airways is limited due to bronchoconstriction.
- Heliox is a mixture of oxygen and helium, which can improve drug delivery in obstructed airways because helium has a lower density and less airway resistance (Nelson and Zorc, 2013).

Complications

Complications from asthma can range from mild secondary respiratory infections to respiratory arrest. Unresponsiveness to pharmacologic agents can lead to status asthmaticus and ultimately to death. Chronic high-dose steroid use leads to growth retardation and other related side effects.

Patient and Parent Education and Prevention

The PCP needs to support self-care management through in-depth education as appropriate. Easy to understand education needs to be tailored to meet the child's individual needs, family needs, and cultural beliefs using a "teach back" technique. Correct administration of inhaled medication should be demonstrated during initial training sessions and reevaluated in subsequent visits. Provide instruction on the following:

- Basic understanding of what asthma is, what is good asthma control, and what is the child's current level of symptomatology
- Environmental control of allergens or triggers, such as smoking and dust
- Basic understanding of what different medications do and how to use them: Give clear, written instructions on how to administer, how much and when to give, monitoring side effects, and how long medication should be taken. A written plan is highly recommended based on either symptoms or peak expiratory flow rate (PEFR).
- How to use inhalers, spacer devices, or aerosol equipment (Box 25-4) along with proper cleaning of aerosol equipment
- Identifying asthma symptoms that indicate a change in therapy is needed or necessitate immediate reevaluation; when and where to seek emergency care
- Home PEF monitoring or symptom monitoring: What to do if symptoms worsen (what medications to add or increase; how frequently to use inhaled medication; specific indications about when to seek additional medical treatment for worsening of symptoms)
- Development of a written action/treatment plan with the child or parent to cover these issues (Fig. 25-6 shows a sample form for home treatment plan.)
- Need to have an adequate supply of all medications (including oral corticosteroids) at home and medications

• BOX 25-4 How to Use a Metered Dose Inhaler

Using an inhaler seems simple, but most patients do not use it correctly.

Steps for Using an Inhaler for Children Younger than 5 Years Old

1. The use of a mask chamber with a MDI allows the delivery of inhaled medications even in an uncooperative child.
2. The child should be placed in the parent's lap, and the mask placed around the child's mouth.
3. Press down on the MDI while firmly holding the mask around the child's mouth. The child will eventually take a deep breath and inhale the medication.

Steps for Using an Inhaler for Children 5 Years Old or Older

Getting Ready

1. Take off the cap and shake the inhaler.
2. Breathe out all the way.
3. Hold the inhaler as shown in steps A, B, or C.

Breathe in Slowly

1. Start breathing in slowly through the mouth, and then press down on the inhaler one time. (If a holding chamber is used, first press down on the inhaler.) Within 5 seconds, begin to breathe in slowly.
2. Keep breathing in slowly, as deeply as possible.

Hold Your Breath

1. Hold breath for a slow count to 10 if possible.
2. For inhaled quick-relief medicine (β_2-agonists), wait about 1 minute between puffs. There is no need to wait between puffs for other medicines.
   A. Hold inhaler 1 to 2 inches in front of mouth (about the width of two fingers).

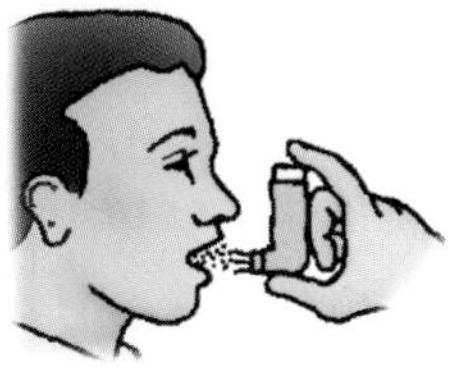

   B. Use a spacer/holding chamber. These come in many shapes and can be useful to any patient.

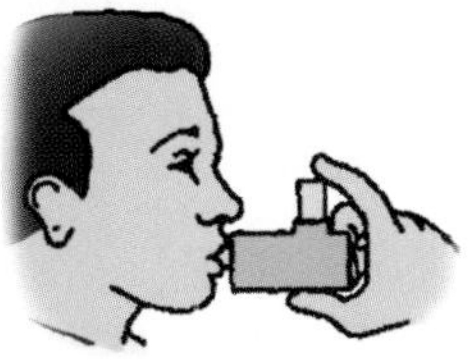

   C. Put inhaler in mouth. Do not use for steroids.

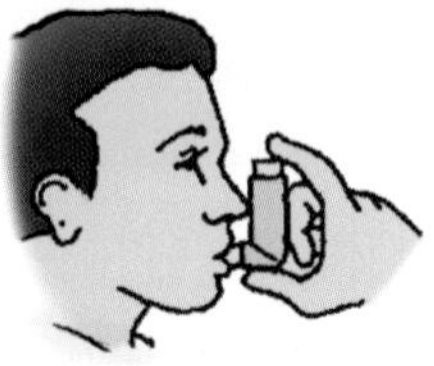

Step A or B is best, but step C can be used if patient has trouble with step A or B.

Clean Inhaler as Needed

Look at the hole where the medicine sprays out from inhaler. If "powder" can be seen in or around the hole, clean the inhaler. Remove the metal canister from the L-shaped plastic mouthpiece. Rinse only the mouthpiece and cap in warm water and let dry overnight. In the morning, put the canister back inside. Put the cap on.

Know When to Replace Inhaler

For medicines taken each day: As an example, a new canister has 200 puffs (number of puffs is listed on canister), and child is told to take 8 puffs per day: 8 puffs per day for 25 days equal 200 puffs in canister. So this canister will last 25 days. If child started using this inhaler on May 1, replace it on or before May 25. Write the date on the canister. For quick-relief medicine, take as needed and count each puff. Do not put canisters in water to see if empty.

MDI, Metered dose inhaler.

Asthma Treatment Plan

(This asthma action plan meets NJ Law N.J.S.A. 18A:40-12.8) (Physician's Orders)

The Pediatric/Adult Asthma Coalition of New Jersey
"Your Pathway to Asthma Control"
PACNJ approved Plan available at www.pacnj.org

Sponsored by AMERICAN LUNG ASSOCIATION. IN NEW JERSEY

NEW JERSEY DEPARTMENT OF HEALTH AND SENIOR SERVICES

THE GREAT SEAL OF THE STATE · NJDOE

(Please Print)

Name	Date of Birth	Effective Date
Doctor	Parent/Guardian (if applicable)	Emergency Contact
Phone	Phone	Phone

HEALTHY

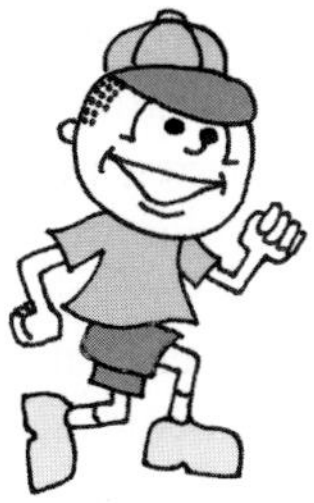

You have *all* of these:
- Breathing is good
- No cough or wheeze
- Sleep through the night
- Can work, exercise, and play

And/or Peak flow above ________

Take daily medicine(s). Some metered dose inhalers may be more effective with a "spacer" – use if directed.

MEDICINE	HOW MUCH to take and HOW OFTEN to take it
☐ Advair® ☐ 100, ☐ 250, ☐ 500	1 inhalation twice a day
☐ Advair® HFA ☐ 45, ☐ 115, ☐ 230	2 puffs MDI twice a day
☐ Alvesco® ☐ 80, ☐ 160	☐ 1, ☐ 2 puffs MDI twice a day
☐ Asmanex® Twisthaler® ☐ 110, ☐ 220	☐ 1, ☐ 2 inhalations ☐ once or ☐ twice a day
☐ Flovent® ☐ 44, ☐ 110, ☐ 220	2 puffs MDI twice a day
☐ Flovent® Diskus® ☐ 50 ☐ 100 ☐ 250	1 inhalation twice a day
☐ Pulmicort Flexhaler® ☐ 90, ☐ 180	☐ 1, ☐ 2 inhalations ☐ once or ☐ twice a day
☐ Pulmicort Respules® ☐ 0.25, ☐ 0.5, ☐ 1.0	1 unit nebulized ☐ once or ☐ twice a day
☐ Qvar® ☐ 40, ☐ 80	☐ 1, ☐ 2 puffs MDI twice a day
☐ Singulair ☐ 4, ☐ 5, ☐ 10 mg	1 tablet daily
☐ Symbicort® ☐ 80, ☐ 160	☐ 1, ☐ 2 puffs MDI twice a day
☐ Other	
☐ None	

Remember to rinse your mouth after taking inhaled medicine.

If exercise triggers your asthma, take this medicine________________ ____minutes before exercise.

CAUTION

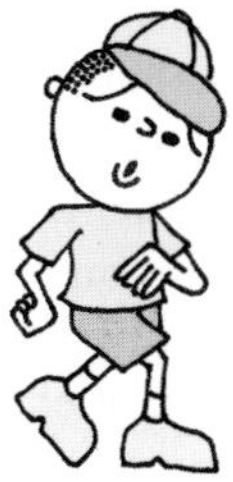

You have *any* of these:
- Exposure to known trigger
- Cough
- Mild wheeze
- Tight chest
- Coughing at night
- Other:__________

And/or Peak flow from______ to______

Continue daily medicine(s) and add fast-acting medicine(s).

MEDICINE	HOW MUCH to take and HOW OFTEN to take it
☐ Accuneb® ☐ 0.63, ☐ 1.25 mg	1 unit nebulized every 4 hours as needed
☐ Albuterol ☐ 1.25, ☐ 2.5 mg	1 unit nebulized every 4 hours as needed
☐ Albuterol ☐ Pro-Air ☐ Proventil®	2 puffs MDI every 4 hours as needed
☐ Ventolin® ☐ Maxair ☐ Xopenex®	2 puffs MDI every 4 hours as needed
☐ Xopenex® ☐ 0.31, ☐ 0.63, ☐ 1.25 mg	1 unit nebulized every 4 hours as needed
☐ Increase the dose of, or add:	
☐ Other	

➡ **If fast-acting medicine is needed more than 2 times a week, except before exercise, then call your doctor.**

EMERGENCY

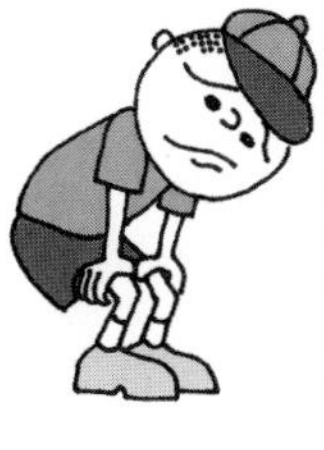

Your asthma is getting worse fast:
- Fast-acting medicine did not help within 15-20 minutes
- Breathing is hard and fast
- Nose opens wide
- Ribs show
- Trouble walking and talking
- Lips blue • Fingernails blue

And/or Peak flow below ________

Take these medicines NOW and call 911.
Asthma can be a life-threatening illness. Do not wait!

☐ Accuneb® ☐ 0.63, ☐ 1.25 mg	1 unit nebulized every 20 minutes
☐ Albuterol ☐ 1.25, ☐ 2.5 mg	1 unit nebulized every 20 minutes
☐ Albuterol ☐ Pro-Air ☐ Proventil®	2 puffs MDI every 20 minutes
☐ Ventolin® ☐ Maxair ☐ Xopenex®	2 puffs MDI every 20 minutes
☐ Xopenex® ☐ 0.31, ☐ 0.63, ☐ 1.25 mg	1 unit nebulized every 20 minutes
☐ Other	

Triggers

Check all items that trigger patient's asthma:
- ❑ Chalk dust
- ❑ Cigarette Smoke & second hand smoke
- ❑ Colds/Flu
- ❑ Dust mites, dust, stuffed animals, carpet
- ❑ Exercise
- ❑ Mold
- ❑ Ozone alert days
- ❑ Pests - rodents & cockroaches
- ❑ Pets - animal dander
- ❑ Plants, flowers, cut grass, pollen
- ❑ Strong odors, perfumes, cleaning products, scented products
- ❑ Sudden temperature change
- ❑ Wood Smoke
- ❑ Foods: ________
- ❑ Other: ________

This asthma treatment plan is meant to assist, not replace, the clinical decision-making required to meet individual patient needs.

The Pediatric/Adult Asthma Coalition of New Jersey, sponsored by the American Lung Association of New Jersey, and this publication are supported by a grant from the New Jersey Department of Health and Senior Services (NJDHSS), with funds provided by the U.S. Centers for Disease Control and Prevention (USCDCP) under Cooperative Agreement 5U59EH000206-3. Its contents are solely the responsibility of the authors and do not necessarily represent the official views of the NJDHSS or the USCDCP.

Although this document has been funded wholly or in part by the United States Environmental Protection Agency under Agreement XA97256707-2 to the American Lung Association of New Jersey, it has not gone through the Agency's publications review process and therefore, may not necessarily reflect the views of the Agency and no official endorsement should be inferred.

REVISED MAY 2009
Permission to reproduce blank form
www.pacnj.org

FOR MINORS ONLY:

☐ This student is capable and has been instructed in the proper method of self-administering of the non-nebulized inhaled medications named above in accordance with NJ Law.

☐ This student is not approved to self-medicate.

PHYSICIAN/APN/PA SIGNATURE________________ DATE________

PARENT/GUARDIAN SIGNATURE________________

PHYSICIAN STAMP

Make a copy for patient and for physician file. For children under 18, send original to school nurse or child care provider.

• **Figure 25-6** Sample asthma treatment plan form. (From the Pediatric/Adult Asthma Coalition of New Jersey: *Asthma treatment plan*, 2009. Available at www.pacnj.org/pdfs/asthmatreatmentenglish2010.pdf. Accessed October 30, 2015.)

readily accessible to the child at school or other settings where the child frequents
- Management of the child at school, camp, or other places away from home
- Need for regular follow-up every 1 to 6 months and as needed with exacerbations

The PCP should stress that asthma is a chronic disease that can be controlled—the goal of therapy is to maintain normal activity. The absence of symptoms does not mean the disease has disappeared, rather that it is well controlled. The child should wear a medical alert bracelet. Children and parents should be acquainted with local asthma education programs and activities, such as asthma camp. Written instructions and handouts should be provided for other significant individuals in the child's life, including caregivers and school personnel.

Prognosis

Asthma is a chronic disease that for most children can be successfully managed with proper pharmacologic therapy, allergen and environmental control, and patient education. Mild asthma is more likely to disappear with increasing age than is moderate or severe asthma.

Allergic Rhinitis

AR and asthma frequently are seen as comorbid conditions (Bousquet et al, 2012). The link between the upper and lower respiratory disease causes poorly controlled AR to lead to poorly controlled asthma. AR is a disorder that results in inflammation of the nasal epithelium and other related local manifestations caused by the release of chemical mediators from an antigen-antibody reaction. Most children with AR have moderate to severe AR; phenotypes of this disease can change over time (Bousquet et al, 2012). AR represents a type I IgE-mediated allergic response. It is a clinical diagnosis that is based on the presence of rhinorrhea, nasal pruritus and congestion, and sneezing. Manifestations can be seasonal or perennial depending on exposure to the offending agent and subsequent sensitization to the offending allergen (Leung and Akdis, 2011). There may be a related family or medical history of AD, AR, or asthma.

AR is second only to asthma as the most common atopic disorder. There is an increased incidence in families with an atopic history. Genetic (the presence of an abnormal sensitivity that is associated with IgE production) and environmental factors are linked to its cause. Repeated exposure to the offending allergen for a period of time is an important contributing factor necessary for sensitizing the immune system to produce an allergic IgE response. Many of the allergens that cause asthma produce AR in the same child; AR is postulated to be a distinct feature of the same inflammatory process that results in asthma. Thus to effectively treat asthma, AR must also be effectively managed with therapies aimed at symptom relief (Tsabouri et al, 2014).

AR is rare in children younger than 6 months old and, if present in infancy, is due to foods or household inhalants, not seasonal pollens. Food allergens can occasionally cause rhinitis. There is a reported lower incidence of AR in children who had early contact with children in the family or in day care, or early exposure to childhood pets, or growing up on a farm (Matheson et al, 2011).

In AR, the mucous membranes of the nose, eyes, eustachian tubes, middle ear, sinuses, and pharynx become inflamed. The nasal mucosa are particularly vulnerable to inhaled allergens with a resulting type I, IgE-mediated allergic response. The nasal mucosa of a susceptible individual comes into contact with an allergen that binds to a specific IgE antibody. Superficial mucosal mast cells and basophils then degranulate and release chemical mediators, such as histamine and tryptase, chymase, kinins, heparin, and newly generated mediators including leukotrienes, prostaglandins, and platelet-activating factors (Milgrom and Leung, 2011). This causes an early-phase reaction of edema, cellular recruitment, and increased vascular permeability with hyperemia and increased serous and mucoid secretions. A late-phase response can occur about 4 to 8 hours later resulting in additional release of chemical mediators from eosinophils, basophils, CD4 T cells, monocytes, and neutrophils that cause chronic nasal inflammation (Leung and Akdis, 2011).

AR tends to be seasonal, perennial, or episodic. Seasonal AR (hay fever or seasonal pollenosis) typically occurs after 3 years of age. Seasonal AR results from sensitization to airborne allergens, such as tree, grass, and weed pollen (ragweed and other weeds) and outdoor molds. There can be geographic variations in seasonal AR depending on climate and when allergens are released into the environment.

Perennial AR has year-round signs and symptoms that may be more severe in the winter. Onset of manifestations can occur before the second year of life, and offending substances tend to be indoor allergens, including the following:
- House-dust mites
- Cockroaches
- Feathers
- Allergens or dander of household pets
- Indoor mold spores and seasonal pollens

Episodic AR occurs with intermittent exposure to an allergen with a resultant rhinitis and is related to a distinct event, such as visiting a house where a cat dwells.

Clinical Findings

Common nasal symptoms and findings on physical examination include:
- Reduced patency from chronic or recurrent bilateral nasal obstruction as a result of congestion and inflammation
- Mouth breathing, snoring, nasal speech
- Pale to purplish and edema (bogginess) of nasal mucous membranes
- Clear, thin, watery to seromucoid rhinorrhea
- Nasal crease—horizontal crease across the lower third of the nose

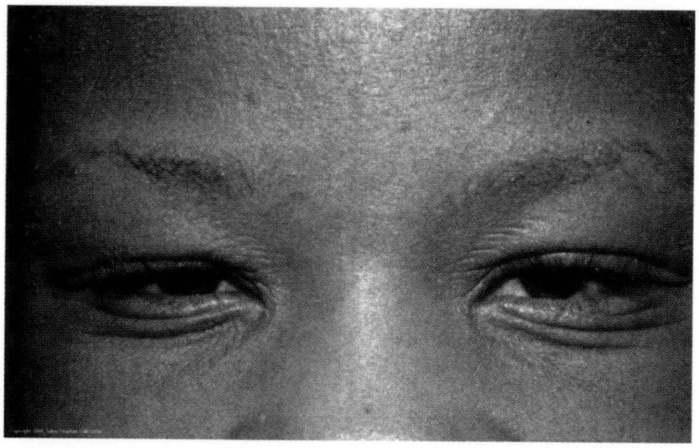

• **Figure 25-7** Dennie line, or Morgan line. (From Cohen B: *Pediatric dermatology*, ed 3, Philadelphia, 2005, Mosby.)

- Itching, rubbing of nose or "allergic salute"
- Nasal stuffiness, postnasal drip, paroxysms of sneezing, congested cough, or night cough
- Dennie lines, Morgan fold, or atopic pleats—extra groove in lower eyelid (Fig. 25-7)

Associated manifestations include the following:

- Itching of palate, pharynx, nose, or eyes
- High arched palate
- Hoarseness and frequent attempts to clear the throat
- Redness of the conjunctiva, tearing, lid and periorbital edema, infraorbital cyanosis or allergic shiners (dark periorbital swelling)
- Enlarged tonsillar and adenoidal tissue
- "Cobblestone" appearance of the pharynx or palpebral conjunctivae (or both) as a result of increased lymphoid tissue
- Malocclusion if problem is chronic
- Sleep disturbances are common in allergic disease (Koinis-Mitchell et al, 2012) with performance problems at school from in adequate sleep

Diagnostic Studies and Allergy Testing

Characteristic symptoms and clinical findings are the key to diagnosis. A history of atopy in the child or family member is helpful in making the diagnosis of AR. The presence of eosinophils on nasal smear can help substantiate the diagnosis, but is a nonspecific, non-universal finding. The presence of nasal eosinophilia often predicts a positive response to nasal corticosteroid sprays. Referrals for skin or serologic testing for IgE antibody to specific allergens should be reserved for the child with significant symptoms who does not respond to traditional management.

The American Academy of Pediatrics (AAP) established guidelines for allergy testing in childhood recommend against ordering large panels of allergen testing. This practice can lead to the diagnosis of an allergy that the child does not have and can result in unnecessary avoidance. It can also result in false reassurance in the face of a negative test when in fact the child's history is positive for an offending trigger. Neither positive skin testing nor positive allergen specific IgE blood tests should be the sole basis for telling a family that their child is allergic to a particular airborne antigen or food. History is critical to determine the test's accuracy (Sicherer et al, 2012).

Differential Diagnosis

Consideration in the differential diagnosis are the common cold, purulent rhinitis, sinusitis, adenoidal hypertrophy, foreign body obstruction, nasal polyposis of cystic fibrosis, nasopharyngeal tumors, choanal atresia or stenosis, and vasomotor rhinitis. Overuse of prescription or over-the-counter topical nasal decongestants can cause drug-induced rhinitis (rhinitis medicamentosa), as can the use of cocaine. Some individuals experience idiopathic rhinitis marked by nasal hyperresponsiveness to nonspecific triggers, such as strong smells (e.g., perfumes, bleach), tobacco smoke, or changes in environmental temperature and humidity. Hormonal rhinitis occurs during pregnancy, puberty, and in hypothyroidism; and food-induced rhinitis is associated with consumption of hot and spicy foods.

Management

The first line pharmacologic treatment for AR is the oral H_1 antihistamines and/or intranasal steroids. Pharmacologic therapy is one aspect of treatment, but other strategies need to include avoidance and education. Immunotherapy and other therapies should be used for children with more severe AR who fail to respond to traditional management.

Avoidance Strategies

Determining triggering factors if possible and avoiding exposure to the offending allergen or irritant as much as possible are essential. Allergens causing seasonal rhinitis are more difficult to avoid than are the indoor allergens, such as molds, because pollens are smaller and lighter and thus remain in the air longer. Determine triggering factors if possible. Key avoidance measures for indoor allergens and irritants include the following:

- Control house dust, paying special attention to the child's bedroom.
  - Use dust mite–proof mattress and pillow covers (allergen-impermeable encasement).
  - Wash bed linens in hot water (greater than 130° F [54.4° C]) weekly.
  - Minimize (if possible, eliminate) stuffed toys in child's bedroom.
  - Use vertical blinds instead of horizontal blinds or curtains.
  - Remove carpeting from bedroom.
  - Use plastic or wood furniture instead of cloth or upholstered furniture.
- Eliminate smoking from the child's environment; if household members still smoke despite education, emphasize smoking outside the house.
- Consider pets that are hairless because protein in pet saliva causes the reactivity of fur.

- Reduce mold; avoid damp basements and other sources of moisture from the home environment.
- Indoor humidity should be less than 50%; avoid vaporizers.
- Use dehumidifiers, air conditioners with efficient filters, and air-cleaning devices with an electronic precipitator or with a high-efficiency particulate air (HEPA) filter.
- Eliminate milk, egg, or wheat for infants with perennial AR if these prove to be offending substances.
- Vector control for cockroach elimination.

Pharmacologic Therapy

Treatment depends on the severity of the symptoms and the ability of the parent or child to comply with recommendations. Intranasal corticosteroids reduce inflammation, edema, and mucus production and are typically a key component in long-term therapy to manage symptoms associated with AR. Non-sedating antihistamines are frequently used to treat the symptoms of rhinorrhea, sneezing, and nasal and eye pruritus. Pharmacologic agents should be started 1 to 2 weeks before pollen season for children with seasonal AR. For perennial AR, start with the maximum recommended dose, and then taper to the minimum dose needed to control symptoms. Often children with AR benefit from a combination approach; some require only single-line therapy. Antibiotics should only be prescribed for secondary infections (sinusitis).

Oral Antihistamines.

- Oral antihistamines are divided into different classes; different classes of drugs may be more effective for different children (Table 25-11).
- Oral antihistamines are especially helpful in seasonal AR but do little to relieve nasal obstruction. The second-generation antihistamines are particularly effective in relieving symptoms of AR (nasal itching, sneezing, and rhinorrhea) by controlling the release of chemical mediators. They are often used to manage this problem.
- Drug dosage may need to be increased until relief of symptoms is obtained or side effects are experienced.
- Tolerance to a particular antihistamine can develop and may need to rotate drugs.
- If side effects with one antihistamine are experienced, another antihistamine in a different class or one in the same class but with different actions should be prescribed.
- Sedating antihistamines may interfere with daytime activities and negatively affect school performance; second-generation antihistamines (e.g., cetirizine, loratadine, and fexofenadine) are associated with less sedation effect.

Topical Nasal Antihistamine.

- Azelastine is a nasal antihistamine spray approved for use in seasonal AR in children 5 years old and older. Azelastine acts by competing with histamine for H_1-receptor sites; it has a bitter taste and is associated with sedation.

TABLE 25-11 Antihistamine Classes*

Class	Name	Comments
Ethanolamine	Diphenhydramine Clemastine Carbinoxamine	Sedation, dizziness, thickening of bronchial secretions Dry mouth, fatigue, headache, somnolence, bradycardia Drowsiness, CNS excitation and difficulty sleeping
Ethylenediamine	Pyrilamine	Not used in children
Alkylamines	Chlorpheniramine Brompheniramine	Drowsiness, sedation, dry mouth, GI symptoms Palpitations, weight gain, drowsiness, dizziness, headache
Piperazine	Hydroxyzine	Sedation, dizziness, dry mouth
Piperidine	Cyproheptadine	CNS depression or stimulation, weight gain, dry mouth
Nonsedating antihistamines	Loratadine	Dry mouth, fatigue, headache, somnolence Approved for children ≥2 years old
	Cetirizine	Dry mouth, fatigue, headache, somnolence Approved for children ≥2 years old
	Fexofenadine	Dry mouth, fatigue, headache, somnolence, dysmenorrhea, flulike signs Approved for children ≥6 years old

Data from Centers for Disease Control and Prevention (CDC): Infant deaths associated with cough and cold medications—two states, 2005, *MMWR Morb Mortal Wkly Rep* 56(01):1–4, 2007; U.S. Food and Drug Administration: *Using over-the-counter cough and cold products in children*, 2008. Available at www.fda.gov/ForConsumers/ConsumerUpdates/ucm048515.htm. Accessed October 30, 2015.

CNS, Central nervous system; *GI*, gastrointestinal.

*The CDC released a report warning about the use of cough and cold medications in children <6 years old. Products containing nasal decongestants (e.g., pseudoephedrine), antihistamines (e.g., carbinoxamine), cough suppressants (e.g., dextromethorphan), and expectorants are often used by parents of children in this age group; however, their use is associated with adverse side effects that may lead to death in children <2 years old. This warning now applies to children <4 years old.

- Olopatadine is a nasal spray approved for use in children older than 6 years old. Like nasal azelastine, it is effective in reducing itching, sneezing, rhinorrhea, and congestion (Sheikh, 2014).

Decongestants.

- Decongestants may help relieve nasal congestion; however, they have limited long-term benefit because of adverse effects associated with their use (Atkins and Leung, 2011).
- Decongestants may be used alone or in combination with an antihistamine.
- Topical decongestants can cause rebound rhinorrhea (rhinitis medicamentosa) if used for more than 3 to 5 days; errors in administration can cause systemic absorption and side effects of irritability, nervousness, and insomnia among others.
- Children younger than 4 years old should not be given decongestants.

Nasal Cromolyn.

- Cromolyn is an intranasal mast cell stabilizer used for seasonal or perennial AR. It is less effective than intranasal corticosteroids, and frequent dosing is needed. It is safe for children 2 years old and older.

Intranasal Corticosteroids.

- Corticosteroids are effective in reducing inflammation and subsequent nasal obstruction. Clear the child's nasal passages of mucus before use.
- Corticosteroids are considered one of the most effective treatments to manage AR and have been safely used in long-term management of this condition.
- Corticosteroids can be effective for relieving symptoms of nasal congestion, rhinorrhea, itching, and sneezing.
- Inhaled corticosteroids can take up to 4 weeks before clinical benefit is observed (Mueller et al, 2013).
- Side effects can include local burning, irritation, sneezing, or soreness (<10% experience these symptoms). Epistaxis is related to improper technique—spraying the nasal septum.
- Table 25-12 lists usual dosages per nostril for intranasal corticosteroid preparations (Taketomo et al, 2014).

Leukotriene Modifiers.

- Montelukast is approved for use in seasonal and perennial AR. It is approved from 6 months to 5 years at 4 mg packet (granules) once daily. It has a moderate effect when used alone. If patient has AR, administer dose in morning or evening; if patient also has asthma, give dose in evening.

Antibiotics.

- Treat secondary infections (e.g., sinusitis and otitis media) with appropriate antibiotics.

Allergy Immunotherapy and Other Treatments

Although allergy immunotherapy has been called *allergen-specific immunotherapy, specific immunotherapy, allergen immunotherapy,* and *allergy immunotherapy,* the latter is the term most recently recommended by the American and European Academies (Burks et al, 2013). Allergy immunotherapy is indicated when symptoms are not improved with avoidance measures and pharmacologic therapy or when complications of chronic or recurrent sinusitis or otitis media and hearing loss are problematic. A key feature of allergy immunotherapy is its potential to alter allergic disease, thereby, helping to prevent asthma (Burks et al, 2013). Therapy can be subcutaneous immunotherapy (SCIT) or sublingual immunotherapy (SLIT). The goal of both is to induce immune tolerance and cause a change in the immune response to specific antigens to produce longer lasting benefits without the need for daily medication (Burks et al, 2013). It causes a change in T-cell tolerance rather than B cells; therefore, IgE levels may not change and cannot account for decreased reactions to antigen.

SCIT adverse reactions can be local or systemic and include life-threatening reactions (Burks et al, 2013). The majority of the reactions occur within 30 minutes; therefore, the child should be monitored for 30 minutes afterward. It should be conducted in a facility that has both the necessary equipment and health care professionals who are prepared to treat anaphylaxis. SLIT has a better safety profile than SCIT; the most common adverse reactions are local, including mild oromucosal pruritus or edema (Burks et al, 2013). Oral immunotherapy (OIT) and SLIT have been used to induce desensitization to allergens, including milk, peanuts, eggs, and hazelnuts in small trials, but neither is approved for widespread use in food allergy.

The meta-analysis framework investigating the use of omalizumab in patients older than 12 years old with inadequately controlled and significant AR noted significant symptom relief and improved quality of life (Tsabouri et al, 2014). Occurrences of adverse reactions were not statistically significant.

Complications and Prognosis

Sinusitis may complicate AR due to associated swelling of the mucosal lining of the sinuses with secondary infection. Likewise eustachian tube dysfunction and its sequel, serous otitis media, are common complications. Malocclusion, the development of a high-arched palate, and the typical allergic facies can result from long-standing AR. Chronic AR may lead to chronic cough and postnasal drip. If a child has both AR and asthma, treatment of the child's AR is essential if the child's asthma is to be effectively managed.

Perennial AR can be a chronic problem unless offending allergens are identified and eliminated from the environment. If this is not possible, pharmacologic therapy is usually helpful in reducing symptoms. As the child grows and the nasal passages increase in size, symptoms may also lessen. Symptoms from seasonal AR often worsen from the adolescent years to mid-adulthood. Moving to a new environment often results in a short respite (1 to 3 years) from symptoms. However, the child frequently becomes sensitized to new airborne pollens and symptoms of seasonal AR return.

TABLE 25-12 Intranasal Corticosteroid Preparations Used for Allergic Rhinitis: Usual Dosages

Drug	Dosage	Age, Number of Inhalations or Sprays per Nostril and Daily Frequency
Beclomethasone, aerosol solution	80 mcg/actuation	≥12 years old: 320 mcg once daily (160 mcg/nostril or 2 sprays each nostril of 80 mcg)
Beclomethasone AQ, aqueous suspension	42 mcg/spray	≥6-12 years old: Initial, 1-spray/nostril (42 mcg/inhalation) twice a day (total single dose of 84 mcg); increase to 2 sprays/nostril (two 42 mcg inhalations) twice a day (total single dose of 168 mcg) if needed; decreases to 42 mcg (1 spray) each nostril twice a day with control. ≥12 years old: 84 mcg (1 spray/nostril) or 168 mcg (2 sprays/nostril) twice a day
Budesonide*	32 mcg/actuation	≥6 years old: Initial, 1 spray/nostril once daily (64 mcg total dose) Maximum dose: <12 years old, 2 sprays/nostril once a day (daily maximum dose of 128 mcg) ≥12 years old: 4 sprays/nostril once a day (daily maximum dose of 256 mcg)
Flunisolide	25 mcg/actuation	6-14 years old: Initial, 2 spray/nostril twice daily (100 mcg twice a day), or 1 spray/nostril three times a day (50 mcg three times a day) to a maximum of 4 sprays/ nostril daily (200 mcg/day); maintenance dose is 1 spray/nostril daily 15 years old: 2 sprays/nostril twice a day (total single dose of 100 mcg) to 2 sprays/nostril three times/day (total single dose of 100 mcg); max daily dose of 400 mcg); maintenance 1 spray/nostril daily
Fluticasone propionate (Flonase)	50 mcg/actuation	≥4 years old and adolescents: Initial 1 spray/nostril daily; 2 sprays daily if severe or poor response; reduce to 1 spray/nostril/day once symptoms controlled Adult: 2 sprays/nostril daily or 1 spray/nostril twice daily; may reduce to 1 spray/ nostril daily once symptoms controlled
Fluticasone furoate (Veramyst)	27.5 mcg/spray	2-11 years old: Initial, 1 spray/nostril once a day (total dose of 55 mcg/day), increase to 2 sprays/nostril once a day (total 110 mcg/day); reduce to 1 spray/ nostril a day with control ≥12 years old and adolescents: 2 sprays/nostril daily(110 mcg/day); reduce to 1 spray/nostril once daily (total 55 mcg/day)
Mometasone	50 mcg/actuation	2-11 years old: 1 spray (50 mcg)/nostril daily >12 years old: 2 sprays (100 mcg)/nostril daily
Triamcinolone (Nasacort AQ)	55 mcg/spray	2-5 years old: 1 spray (55 mcg)/nostril once daily 6-11 years old: Initial, 1 spray (55 mcg)/nostril once daily, can increase to 2 sprays (110 mcg)/nostril once daily; maintenance 1 spray (55 mcg)/nostril with control >12 years old: 2 sprays (110 mcg)/nostril daily; maintenance dose 1 (55 mcg) spray/nostril daily

Data from Taketomo CK, Hodding JH, Kraus DM: *Pediatric dosage handbook*, ed 21, Hudson, OH, 2014, Lexi-Comp.
*Reduce slowly every 2 to 4 weeks to smallest effective dose.

Patient and Parent Education and Prevention

Because AR is often a chronic problem, parents and children need to have specific information about controlling this disorder:

- Instruct on environmental control. Handouts and a review of ways to individualize this information are essential.
- Review pharmacologic therapy, including indications for and changes in medications, frequency of use, and common side effects and contraindications.
- Demonstrate, with return demonstration, how to use intranasal sprays or inhalers if prescribed.

Atopic Dermatitis

AD is a common chronic, pruritic, inflammatory skin disorder of childhood characterized by acute and chronic skin eruptions. The term *atopic eczema* is used interchangeably with *atopic dermatitis.* AD manifests a typical morphology and distribution of flexural lichenification or linearity in adults and facial and extensor involvement in infants and children. AD is frequently referred to as the "itch that rashes." With AD, the skin's ability to act as a protective barrier is impaired, resulting in xerosis (dry skin), cracking, increased skin markings, lichenification, and susceptibility to bacterial, viral, and fungal infections (Fig. 25-8).

The American Academy of Allergy and Immunology (Schneider et al, 2013), the American Academy of Dermatology (Eichenfield et al, 2014), and the AAP (Tollefson et al, 2014) have published AD guidelines. There are definite similarities between all the guidelines, but they do vary in frequency and length of certain treatment, such as bleach baths and skin therapy maintenance. Topical agents are the mainstay in all of the guidelines.

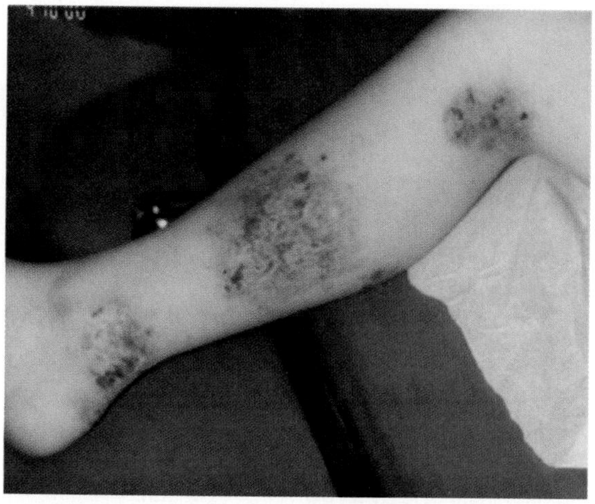

• **Figure 25-8** Acute atopic dermatitis (AD). (Photograph courtesy Peggy Vernon RN, MA, CPNP, Aurora/Parker Skin Care Center, CO.)

AD affects approximately 10% to 12% of the childhood population in the United States with higher incidence in other countries. AD develops in 85% of children within the first 12 months of life and in 95% of children before the age of 5 years. Approximately 0.9% of adults have AD; some of whom had an adult onset, but the majority had AD as a child. AD is often the first manifestation of the "atopic march" with asthma and AR following. Asthma also develops in approximately 30% and AR develops in 35% of those with AD. The incidence of AD is increasing in the United States (Schneider et al, 2013).

The exact etiology is unknown and may vary from individual to individual. Although many children have high IgE levels, an exact immune mechanism for this disorder is not evident. Newest information on pathophysiology of AD includes epidermal barrier defects and immune dysregulation of both aspects of the immune system—innate and adaptive. The exact role of IgE bearing Langerhans cells, atopic keratinocytes, eosinophils, mast cells and monocytes/macrophages, and the interaction with cytokines IL-4, IL-5, and IL-13 is complex and not fully elucidated (Schneider et al, 2013). Most children with AD have elevated IgE levels. The risk of secondary infection is higher due to inadequate response of the innate immune system to epicutaneous microbes, causing an increased susceptibility to *Staphylococcus aureus* and viruses, such as herpes simplex. The identification of the filaggrin (FLG) mutation has been identified as a risk factor for AD. The FLG is produced in the stratum granulosum and contributes to the natural moisture in the stratum corneum. The lack of stratum corneum hydration and an increase in the pH from a defect in the FLG cause an impaired barrier function (Wollenberg and Schnopp, 2010). A defect in the epithelial barrier integrity is a contributing factor to the onset of AD. If the barrier's integrity is impaired due to allergy and irritants, there is cytokine production, inflammation, and the development of lesions (Schneider et al, 2013). Abnormalities in histamine production (increased in the skin), chemotaxis, monocytes, and cytokines are associated with AD. This is a complex disorder caused by the interaction of genetic susceptibility and micro- and macro-environment, leading to tissue inflammation in the host (Schneider et al, 2013).

A positive family history of AD is common, as is a family history of atopic disease. Sweating increases itching in atopic skin, and transepidermal water loss is increased. A predisposition to the development of pruritus is believed to be a key factor with variability in the extent of the skin involvement and severity of presentation. Pruritus and relapsing eczematous lesions in the typical morphology are essential parts of making the diagnosis (Schneider et al, 2013).

Clinical Findings

The following are seen in AD (Schneider et al, 2013) (Table 25-13):

- Pruritus and eczematous changes reflecting typical age-specific morphologic patterns
- History of a chronic or relapsing skin condition
- More than one third of cases begin before 3 months old: Dry skin is the only initial sign. These infants are generally not brought in for health care until pruritus and the itch-scratch-itch cycle develops, generally around 2 to 3 months old.
- Acute manifestations (more common in infants) include:
  - Intense itching and redness
  - Papules, vesicles, edema, serous discharge, and crusts
  - Generalized dry skin (xerosis) with dry hair and scalp; diaper area usually spared
  - Lichenification is typically not seen
- Chronic manifestations (more common in children and adolescents) include:
  - Lichenification—thickened, leathery, hyperpigmented skin
  - Scratch marks
  - Generalized xerosis with flaky and rough skin: Table 25-13 is a description of the characteristics of AD at different ages.
- Other key features of AD:
  - Tendency toward dry skin and a lowered threshold for itching (itch-scratch-itch cycle)
  - Tendency to worsen during dry winter months or with heat in the summer
  - Chronic AD often secondarily infected with *S. aureus* (most commonly) or *Streptococcus pyogenes* (occasionally)
  - Hyperpigmentation may be noted especially in areas of lichenification
- Possible associated features:
  - Atopic pleats—extra groove in lower eyelid called *Dennie lines* or *Morgan fold* (see Fig. 25-7), crease across upper bulb of nose
  - Accentuated palmar and flexural creases
  - Allergic shiners, mild facial pallor, or dry hair
  - Keratosis pilaris—follicular papules occurring on the extensor aspect of the arms, anterior thighs, and lateral aspects of the cheeks

TABLE 25-13 Assessment of Atopic Dermatitis

Onset/Initial Presentation	Signs and Symptoms	Comment/Prognosis
<3 months old	Dry skin first sign	Often not noticed
2-3 months old	Itch-scratch-itch cycle starts	
Infantile phase	Acute presentation—common in infants: intense itching; redness, papules, vesicles, edema; serous discharge and crusts Cheeks, forehead, scalp, extending to trunk as symmetric patches or to the extremities; lateral extensor surface of arms and legs diaper area and groin are spared of lesion	Two thirds of cases resolve by 2-3 years Generalized xerosis
Childhood phase (starts 2 years old to puberty)	Pruritus is severe Lesions are dry and papular with circumscribed scaly patches Involves wrists, hands, popliteal and antecubital fossa; eyebrows thin and broken off with lack of the lateral third of the eyebrow (called *Hertoghe sign*); some only have feet involved; may have allergic-atopic facies and white dermatographism Flexural involvement	One third continue into teenage years—tendency to be chronic
Adolescent/adult phase	Begins at puberty and can commonly continue into adulthood Often involves the flexural folds (popliteal and antecubital fossae), face, neck, upper arms and back, dorsa of hands, fingers, feet, and toes Dry skin and lichenification are prominent findings Erythematous, dry-scaling papules and plaques with fewer exudates Postinflammatory hypopigmentation or hyperpigmentation that disappears	New or recurrence of a chronic condition

- Nummular eczema, dyshidrotic eczema, juvenile plantar dermatitis, nipple eczema, or ichthyosis vulgaris
- White dermatographism and some have an associated circumoral pallor (thought to be related to local edema and vasoconstriction)

Diagnostic Studies

The diagnosis of AD is based on characteristic clinical findings. A chronic or recurring rash that is pruritic and has a characteristic distribution and appearance, together with a family or personal history of atopy, are key to the diagnosis. Histologic examination of the skin is rarely needed and reserved only for cases that are difficult to diagnose and to exclude other diseases. There is a more severe subtype associated with IgE responses to allergens and a higher rate of secondary infection and a milder form lacking these features (Wollenberg and Schnopp, 2010). Immunologic testing (e.g., IgE, CAP-RAST, or prick test) is not needed to confirm the diagnosis or to monitor treatment. Skin testing and desensitization are not routinely recommended for children with AD only. If secondary fungal infection is suspected, collect scrapings and use potassium hydroxide (KOH) to look for fungal hyphae.

Differential Diagnosis

Other types of dermatitis, including seborrheic dermatitis, contact dermatitis, allergic contact dermatitis, nummular dermatitis, psoriasis, and scabies, are included in the differential diagnosis. A few genetic conditions are associated with similar skin eruptions (e.g., phenylketonuria, Wiskott-Aldrich syndrome, histiocytosis X, and acrodermatitis enteropathica). Pityriasis alba is also a differential diagnosis.

Management

Treatment strategy is based on the following key concepts:

- The itch-scratch-itch cycle must be interrupted.
- Dryness of the skin must be corrected by rehydrating the stratum corneum with lubrication as the first-line therapy to enhance skin moisturization (Eichenfield et al, 2014; Schneider et al, 2013). The choice of the moisturizer is dependent on the individual, but should be safe, free of additives, and inexpensive. Application of moisturizer should take place soon after bath to decrease transepidermal water loss (Eichenfield et al, 2014). Skin barrier protection starting at birth may be protective against the development of AD (Eichenfield et al, 2014).
- If moisturization does not control the disease, then topical corticosteroids (TCPs) are used with low potency corticosteroids for maintenance and higher potency for exacerbations (Eichenfield et al, 2014; Schneider et al, 2013).
- Use of non-soap surfactants and synthetic detergents, which are more acid, are often recommended but without good supporting evidence (Eichenfield et al, 2014).
- Eliminate any known offending agents (irritants and allergic triggers).
- Secondary bacterial or viral infections must be treated.

Acute versus chronic care management is also a consideration. The following therapies are key factors in the control of AD.

Pharmacotherapy

- Antihistamine agents have little direct effect on pruritus, but sedating doses at night help relieve pruritus, which is worse at night. They have limited effectiveness as monotherapy in AD. The following agents are often used:
  - Hydroxyzine has excellent antihistaminic qualities but can cause drowsiness and behavioral changes. If an antihistamine is needed throughout the day, the usual oral dose of hydroxyzine in children is 2 mg/kg/day divided every 6 to 8 hours (Taketomo et al, 2014). This dose may need to be increased.
  - Diphenhydramine hydrochloride is also a useful antihistamine, especially if sedation is also needed. The usual oral dose of diphenhydramine hydrochloride in children is as follows: 2 to 6 years old, 6.25 mg every 4 to 6 hours with 37.5 mg/day maximum; 6 to 12 years old, 12.5 to 25 mg every 4 to 6 hours with 150 mg/day maximum; children older than 12, 25 to 50 mg every 4 to 6 hours with 300 mg/day maximum (Taketomo et al, 2014).
  - Doxepin is a tricyclic antidepressant with strong antihistamine activity used by dermatologists for the treatment of itch. It is not approved for use in children, and the risk of suicidal ideation should be assessed if a child is on this drug. It is also available as doxepin 5% cream, but due to potential for sedation and overdose, this formulation is not used in children.
  - Nonsedating or low-sedating antihistamines may be considered (see Table 25-11).
  - Cutaneous antihistamines are not recommended.
- TCPs are a mainstay of therapy:
  - TCPs reduce inflammation and pruritus. The classification of the TCP should be known because potent and very potent TCPs are associated with more side effects, such as thinning of the skin or adrenal axis suppression, than milder preparations. Most children with AD do not need high potency topical steroids (Tollefson et al, 2014). A proactive approach to the treatment of AD includes twice weekly application of a low dose TCP for up to 4 months once the lesions are quiet (Eichenfield et al, 2014). The rationale for this approach is that the skin is actually not normal and has a defect in hydration, which can be treated using an intermittent approach (Eichenfield et al, 2014; Wollenberg and Schnopp, 2010).
  - Gels penetrate well, are somewhat more drying, and are effective in the management of acute weeping or vesicular lesions.
  - Ointments penetrate more effectively than creams or lotions and provide occlusion. They are beneficial in the management of dry, lichenified, or plaque-like areas; however, they may occlude eccrine ducts and lead to sweating.
  - Application
    - Fingertip method: The amount of steroid to be applied should be a strip of cream from the distal interphalangeal joint to the top of the adult finger for an area equaling two adult palms. Apply a thin layer of TCP to affected areas marked with acute exacerbations twice a day or once a day if using a newer formulation (Eichenfield et al, 2014).
    - When applied over large areas of dermatitis or if occlusion (covering with plastic wrap) is used, the possibility of significant systemic absorption is greatly increased, especially in infants and young children.
  - There are seven classes of steroid with Class 1 being very high potency to Class 7 being the lowest potency (Eichenfield et al, 2014). Greater caution is needed when applying the steroids to the face, neck, and skin folds because the skin is thinner and there is higher risk of systemic absorption (Eichenfield et al, 2014; Schneider et al, 2013). Tapering of the strength of the steroids should occur only once the outbreak is fully controlled. Then the child is switched to once or twice weekly application of a low dose TCS at areas of outbreak to reduce the relapse. Baseline moisturizing skin care should continue with a low strength TCS once to twice a week to reduce inflammation (Eichenfield et al, 2014). (See Table 37-1 for a listing of TCPs by potency rating.)
- Topical calcineurin inhibitors (TCIs)
  - TCIs are second-line therapy that is useful in both acute and chronic AD. Two agents are available—tacrolimus topical (Protopic) ointment 0.03% and 0.1% strengths and pimecrolimus topical (Elidel) 1% cream—have been shown to be as effective as mid-strength TCS. They can be combined with TCS in the treatment of children whose AD has not responded to TCS. They are considered steroid-sparing agents (Eichenfield et al, 2014; Schneider et al, 2013). Tacrolimus 0.03% and pimecrolimus 1% are approved for use at age 2 and older, whereas tacrolimus 0.1% is approved in children older than 15 (Eichenfield et al, 2014).
  - TCIs have black box warnings due to the higher rate of lymphoma in rats given high dosages of these drugs. These NSAIDs block calcineurin, a protein phosphatase that causes T-cell activation. The most common side effect is itching, stinging, or burning, which starts 5 minutes after the application and can last for an hour but usually decreases after 1 week (Schneider et al, 2013). It usually occurs during the first several days of administration and in severe cases of AD. TCIs are safe steroid-sparing agents and work well on thinner skin of the face, neck, groin, and axillae. Sun protection is needed with their use (Taketomo et al, 2014).

    - Parents need to be informed of the black box warning and the pros and cons of their use should be discussed. There is an increased theoretical risk of cutaneous viral infections with the use of TCIs (Eichenfield et al, 2014)
- Prescription emollient devices
    - Skin barrier repair and treatment: Drugs (i.e., EpiCeram and Eletone) that improve the skin's hydration barrier are available by prescription. They are used twice a day. The preparations have unique ratios of lipids that resemble endogenous compositions (Schneider et al, 2013). They are expensive and not covered by all insurance plans.
- Cool coal tar
    - Although these agents have been used in psoriasis, there are few studies in children with newer agents which are more cosmetically acceptable. However, the AD guidelines do not recommend their use.
- Wet wrap therapy (WWT)
    - WWT can be used in significant flares with recalcitrant disease. The usual topical agents are applied followed by a wet layer of tubular gauze or cotton pajama that is applied with a dry outside layer. The child sleeps overnight with the WWT (Eichenfield et al, 2014; Schneider et al, 2013).
- Topical antimicrobials and antiseptics
    - The immune dysregulation in AD results in a tendency for *S. aureus* to colonize the skin in AD, as well as viral infection, including herpes simplex. Reduction of colonization with staphylococcus, as well as treatment of infection, may be equally as important. The use of bleach baths in conjunction with intranasal topical mupirocin for 3 months may be helpful (Eichenfield et al, 2014). Schneider and colleagues (2013) recommend dilute bleach baths (⅛ to ¼ cup of chlorine bleach in a full tub of bath water) twice a week in children with recurrent infection.
    - Topical antibiotic preparations are contraindicated, although the use of mupirocin has been demonstrated to reduce colony counts of *S. aureus.*
    - Topical antibacterial scrubs are contraindicated because they dry out the skin and cause irritation.
- Oral antibiotics
    - Short courses of systemic antibiotic agents are essential if secondary skin infection with *S. aureus* or *S. pyogenes* is suspected. First-generation cephalosporins are most commonly used.
    - Be cognizant that community-based methicillin-resistant *Staphylococcus aureus* (MRSA) has been rapidly increasing.

Non-Pharmacological Therapy

- Skin lubrication
    - Emolliate with a moisturizer. Lubricants maintain the skin's hydration, and emollients are the treatment of choice for dry skin.
    - An ointment-based emollient (e.g., Vaseline, petrolatum jelly, Crisco, vegetable oil, whipped petrolatum, Aquaphor) can be applied just before getting out of the bath water or just after getting out of the bath while still damp. If the child does not like the greasy feel of an ointment, other topical creams (e.g., Vanicream, CeraVe, Cetaphil) can be used. This is also a good time to apply TCPs, because absorption of the agent is more effective if the skin is hydrated.
    - Emollients can be applied three or four times a day as needed, such as fragrance-free Eucerin cream, Crisco (plain, not butter flavored), Aveeno, Moisturel, Neutrogena, Dermasil, Curel, or petroleum jelly (an occlusive agent). If a child is sensitive to fragrances, scented creams, such as Nivea and Vaseline Intensive Care, should be avoided. TriCeram is a moisturizer that repairs the stratum corneum barrier function. Like CeraVe, it is a ceramide-dominant, lipid-based emollient. Urea-containing products, such as Aquacare cream or lotion and Ureacin Crème, soften and moisturize dry skin. Stinging is a side effect when using urea-containing products on fissured or flaring skin.
    - For some children with AD (xerotic individuals), frequent bathing may exacerbate their pruritus and thus aggravate their skin problems. Bathing must be limited in these patients and emollients used. If a child experiences stinging when bathing during acute exacerbations, adding 1 cup of table salt into the bath may reduce the stinging sensation.
- Avoidance of triggering factors
    - Avoid common irritating substances, including toiletries, wool, and harsh chemicals.
    - Keep fingernails short to decrease additional skin trauma from scratching.
    - Consider stopping the use of fabric softeners and using a sensitive-skin detergent (e.g., All Free Clear).
    - Evaluate for possible food triggers and if history is positive, testing is not needed (Schneider et al, 2013; Sicherer et al, 2012). The clinician should *not* do an extensive battery of allergy tests and then make recommendations for food elimination based on those tests, without history of food sensitivity.

Other Therapies

- Phototherapy
    - Ultraviolet narrow-band UVB light treatment may benefit and should only be done by dermatologists; however, it is rarely used because of the risk of skin cancer.
- Systemic immunomodulating agents
    - Immunomodulating agents (such as, cyclosporine, azathioprine, mycophenolate mofetil, and systemic corticosteroids) can provide help to patients with severe, refractory AD, but due to side effect profiles should only be used by a specialist after all other options have failed.

Environmental Management

- Decreased environmental humidity and an increase in antigen presentation are key causative factors. Therefore, increase environmental humidity and decrease exposure to antigens. Cool temperatures (e.g., through the use of air conditioning) help.
- Eliminate or avoid known or suspected offending agents. These include:
  - Non-breathable fabrics—nylon or wool; wool is irritating, whereas soft cotton clothing is not. Clothes should be loose fitting.
  - Overheating and overdressing (heat and perspiration are irritant triggers that increase pruritus).
  - Chlorine, turpentine, harsh soaps, fabric softeners, products with fragrances, and bleach.
  - Allergenic agents, such as feather pillows, fuzzy toys, stuffed animals, and pets.
  - House-dust mites—careful attention to the child's bedroom is important (e.g., encasing mattresses and pillows, washing bedding in hot water weekly, frequent vacuuming, removing carpets or at least frequent cleaning are recommended).

Dietary Management

- In infants, whey-protein partially hydrolyzed infant formula is not hypoallergenic and should not be given to infants who have milk allergy (Chung et al, 2012). Dietary restriction should only be done on the basis of a history of food allergy. Food allergens in older children and adults are not common triggers.
- The use of probiotics was not recommended by the guidelines (Eichenfield et al, 2014; Schneider et al, 2013) because of scant evidence of effectiveness (Grüber et al, 2010).

Refer to a dermatologist if a child is unresponsive to traditional therapy or has an unusual manifestation.

Complications and Prognosis

Secondary skin infections are a frequent complication of AD due to *S. aureus,* viruses (eczema herpeticum or disseminated herpes simplex), and fungi (culture or KOH to diagnose). Lichenification, a secondary skin change marked by thickening of the skin, is associated with chronic itching. Keratoconus is occasionally seen and is associated with chronic rubbing of the eyelids. In patients with AD, nocturnal melatonin levels are lower and may be responsible for sleep disturbances (Chang et al, 2014). With appropriate treatment, AD can generally be controlled. In two thirds of children, symptoms of AD become less severe, with complete remission in 20%; however, there is an adolescent and adult stage of AD. Risk factors for adult AD include widespread dermatitis as a child, family history of AD, early initial childhood age of onset, high serum IgE levels, and a history of asthma or AR (Leung and Akdis, 2011). Self-image problems may result if AD is severe.

Patient and Parent Education and Prevention

- Emphasize that AD is often a recurrent disease that can be controlled. The goal of therapy is to prevent the itch-scratch-itch cycle and hydrate the skin. Specific written instructions and handouts should include the following as the home management is complex. Parents need to understand:
  - The use of medications (when, how much, and how often to use; side effects; and proper application of topical preparations)
  - Care of the skin
  - Role of environmental controls of allergens or triggers
  - What to do if symptoms worsen or signs of secondary skin infection appear and when to seek additional medical treatment
- Precipitating factors
  - Extreme temperatures or humidity, excess sweat, and/or emotional stress
  - New clothes—wash with mild detergent (with no dyes or perfumes) before wearing them to remove formaldehyde and other chemicals
  - Harsh washing detergents—add second rinse cycle when washing clothes
  - Wearing coarse clothes
  - Excess soap and water
  - Cutaneous or systemic infection

Pediatric Immunodeficiency Disorders

Immunodeficiency is a failure of one part of the body's defense mechanism resulting in recurrent infection of variable degrees and associated with morbidity and mortality in a child. In order to understand immunodeficiency, one needs to understand the normal immune system and its defense system. There are three lines of defense against antigens: external barriers, innate immunity, and adaptive immunity.

Physiology of the Immune System

The external barriers that assist the immune defense system are physical and mechanical and include skin and the epithelial lining of the GI tract, genitourinary tract, and respiratory tract. The biochemical barriers include perspiration, tears, saliva, surfactant, hydrochloric acid in the stomach, and normal bacterial flora in our body. Innate immunity is more primitive and uses special cell pattern recognition to provide a line of defense. It responds without prior exposure and is activated when there is direct contact with specific microbial products, such as lipopolysaccharides, cell wall components, and microbial nucleotides. Innate immunity is mediated by neutrophils, macrophages, and complement and cytokines that provide a host defense to ward off infection.

The complement and cytokines signal specific cellular and humoral immunity to add in host defenses. Complement amplifies the innate immune response by providing critical factors to enhance phagocytosis via opsonin and attracts white cells to the site of inflammation, thereby acting as chemoattractives. Neutrophils form a first line of defense and ingest the infecting organisms, internalizing the organism into an intracellular compartment and releasing bactericidal products. The role of neutrophils in the early inflammation process is primarily phagocytic, resulting in the creation of pus at the site of infection. Monocytes appear at the site of inflammation 1 to 7 days after the initial neutrophil infiltration and turn to macrophages ingesting and disposing of foreign material, including bacteria. Eosinophils have mild phagocytic activity and help in the regulation of vascular mediators released by mast cells. They play an important role in hypersensitive allergic response seen in anaphylaxis (Buckley, 2011a, 2011b).

Adaptive immunity is a specific process of recognition in what the host responds specifically to a foreign substance, such as a bacterium antigen. The B and T cells play a major role in this system with T lymphocytes forming the cellular arm and B lymphocytes producing specific antibodies or immunoglobulins. In the initial primary exposure, the antigen exposure to B cells results in antibody formation. This reaction stimulates memory T cells to recognize the antigen for future exposures. Antibodies provide protection against bacterial infections and promote the ingestion of bacteria, as well as the neutralization of bacterial toxins and inactivation of virus. There are different classes of antibodies, with IgM and IgG providing protection against systemic infections and IgA providing protection at mucosa surfaces in the GI, genitourinary, and respiratory tract. Cytokines, although primarily acting locally, mediate innate and adaptive immunity and stimulate T-lymphocyte formation. The T-helper cells recognize antigen by binding to the antigenic fragment displayed by the HLA molecules. The T-helper type 1 (Th1) cells are the arm of cellular immunity and activate microphages, enhance cytotoxic T-cell function, produce cytokines, and recognize the infecting agent. Type 2 T-helper cells enhance antibody formation by B cells releasing cytokines and increases IgE production and mediating eosinophil recruitment and activation (Buckley, 2011b).

The soluble protein components of the immune system aside from antibodies IgA, IgG, and IgM include cytokines, complement, and surfaces moles known as *defensins* and *cathelicidins.* Cytokines, such as interleukin and interferon, are critical in the differentiation and maturation of immune cells. Interleukins are biochemical messengers produced by macrophages and lymphocytes and promote the production of leukocytes, induce leukocyte chemotaxis, and cause alteration of adhesion molecule expression on many cells. Interferons protect against viral infection but do not directly kill the antigen; rather they attempt to prevent further infection. They have no effect on cells already infected. Other cytokines, such as TNF-α, are secreted by mast cells and macrophages and initiate fever by the production of prostaglandins and other inflammatory serum proteins. Chemokines also promote leukocyte chemotaxis. The exact role of surface moles as host-defense molecules of innate immunity is not clear (Buckley, 2011a, 2011b).

Primary and Secondary Immunodeficiency Disorders

Given the complexity of the immune system, it is easy to understand why there are over 150 identified inherited immunodeficiency disorders. Immunodeficiency can be primary or secondary. A primary immunodeficiency disorder (PIDD) is generally genetic. In terms of distribution, 50% are B-cell deficiencies, 20% are T- and B-cell deficient, 10% are T-cell deficient, 18% are disorders of granulocytes, and 2% are complement deficiencies (Modell et al, 2011). They can also be divided by defects of the adaptive immune system either in the cellular and humoral arm or defects of the innate immune system, which primarily are cellular abnormalities but can also be soluble protein defects (interleukins, interferons, complement defects). Table 25-14 shows the immune deficiency and the common clinical presentation.

Common PIDDs include selective IgA, IgG subclass deficiencies, transient hypogammaglobulinemia of infancy, and DiGeorge deficiency. Uncommon immunodeficiencies include X-linked agammaglobulinemia, severe combined immunodeficiencies, complement deficiencies, as well as phagocytic disorders like combined granulomatous disease. Secondary immunodeficiencies can occur due to infections, drugs (e.g., corticosteroids), renal failure, human immunodeficiency virus (HIV), and leukemia and lymphoma (Buckley, 2011b).

The first immunodeficiency described was an X-linked agammaglobulinemia due to a deficiency of beta-ketothiolase (BKT) on the X chromosome. The condition causes deficiency of B cells that leads to a lack of immunoglobulins of all types. The infant presents with infection at 4 to 6 months old as the maternal antibodies start to wane, leading to pyogenic infections and to increased incidence of otitis media, pneumonia, sinusitis, and infections with encapsulated bacteria such as *Haemophilus influenzae and Streptococcus pneumonia* (Buckley, 2011b). Selected IgA deficiency is much more common (1:300-500) and is due to either a defect in the B-cell production of IgA or lowered production of specific cytokines (transforming growth factor beta [TGF-β], IL-5) or in B-cell ability to respond to these cytokines. Recurrent sinopulmonary infections, GI infections, and autoimmunity are signs of this deficiency.

Clinical Presentation

History

A history of unusual, frequent, or recurrent infections is crucial to identifying patients with primary immunodeficiencies. PCPs need to keep in mind that many children with PIDDs do not have any signs of dysmorphology. They may have a history of more severe, atypical, or persistent infections or autoimmune or rheumatologic manifestations, findings less commonly recognized in children with PIDDs

TABLE 25-14 Selected Pediatric Primary Immunodeficiencies and Their Clinical Presentation

Immunodeficiency	Clinical Presentation
Severe combined immunodeficiency (SCID)	In infancy, persistent thrush, failure to thrive, pneumonia, diarrhea, recurrent difficult to treat unusual infections
Wiskott Aldrich syndrome	Thrombocytopenia, bloody stools, draining ears, atopic eczema, recurrent infections with encapsulated organisms, EBV associated malignancy (Burkitt lymphoma)
Hyper-IgE syndrome	Staphylococcal abscess, pneumatoceles, osteopenia, unusual infection, recurrent otitis and sinusitis, recurrent pneumonias
DiGeorge syndrome	With partial thymic hypoplasia, may have normal course. If no thymus, resemble patients with SCID
Common variable immunodeficiency	Normal or enlarged tonsils, splenomegaly, alopecia areata, thrombocytopenia, Sprue-like disease, 438-fold increase in lymphoma
Selective IgA	Infections of respiratory, GI and genitourinary tracts

Adapted from text in Buckley RH: Evaluation of suspected immunodeficiency. In Kliegman RM, Stanton BF, St. Geme JW, et al, editors: *Nelson textbook of pediatrics*, ed 19, Philadelphia, 2011, Saunders/Elsevier, pp 715–722; Buckley RH: Primary defects of antibody production. In Kliegman RM, Stanton BF, St. Geme JW, et al, editors: *Nelson textbook of pediatrics*, ed 19, Philadelphia, 2011, Saunders/Elsevier, pp 722–728; Buckley RH: T lymphocytes, B lymphocytes, and natural killer cells. In Kliegman RM, Stanton BF, St. Geme JW, et al, editors: *Nelson textbook of pediatrics*, ed 19, Philadelphia, 2011, Saunders/Elsevier, p 722.
EBV, Epstein-Barr virus; *GI*, gastrointestinal; *IgA*, immunoglobulin A; *IgE*, immunoglobulin E.

(Torgerson, 2012). There may be a sibling who died from sepsis or meningitis, but no workup for immune deficiency was done. A complete family history should be obtained. The child may present with congenital infections but also may present later in infancy, childhood, or adulthood. Box 25-5 is a list of the 10 warning signs of immunodeficiency outlined by the Jeffrey Modell Foundation (Modell et al, 2011).

Physical Assessment

The child with an immunodeficiency may not have any distinguishing characteristic. Lack of palpable lymph nodes or lack of tonsils may be a sign of X-linked agammaglobulinemia. A child with defects of the great vessels combined with hypognathism (under developed chin) and low, cupped ears may have DiGeorge syndrome. Patients with cutaneous telangiectasias may develop ataxia in early childhood and have recurrent infections.

BOX 25-5 Warning Signs of Primary Immunodeficiency Disorders: Jeffrey Modell Foundation

- Four or more new ear infections within 1 year
- Two or more serious sinus infections within 1 year
- Two or more months on antibiotics with little effect
- Two or more pneumonias within 1 year
- Failure of an infant to gain weight or grow normally
- Recurrent, deep skin or organ abscesses
- Persistent thrush in mouth or fungal infection on skin
- Need for intravenous antibiotics to clear infections
- Two or more deep-seated infections including septicemia
- A family history of primary immunodeficiency

Diagnostic Testing

The child with an immunodeficiency disorder may present with a low lymphocyte count, low neutrophil count, or a low leukocytes count. It is important to calculate the total neutrophil count. A low IgA is likely to be the most common deficiency. The initial workup as outlined by the Jeffrey Modell Foundations includes a complete history and physical examination, a CBC with differential and platelet count, and quantitative immunoglobulins, including IgG, IgA, and IgM. If this is not helpful, referral to a specialist in immunology is needed for further testing, including IgG subclass; candida, pneumococcal, and tetanus skin tests; lymphocyte surface markers—CD3, CD4, CD8, CD19, CD15, and CD16—along with a neutrophil oxidation burst and mononuclear lymphocyte proliferation studies. Table 25-14 addresses the more common immunodeficiencies and their clinical presentation. By using the Jeffrey Modell Foundation warning signs, the PCP can refer to immunology with stage 1 workup already done (Modell et al, 2011).

Management

Children with immunodeficiency disorders have a higher risk of oncologic disorders as a result of their treatment, which in some cases requires granulocyte stimulation factor. The role of the PCP is to consider immunodeficiency disorders in children with recurrent, persistent, unusual infections and refer to specialists. These children and their families need coordinated health services in a pediatric health care home with providers who will support them and act as their advocate and educator for health supervision and health promotion services. It is also important to recognize that infections in children with immunodeficiencies may require consultation due to the unusual nature or more persistent course of the infection.

For a complete list of references, please visit http://evolve.elsevier.com/Burns/pediatric/.

26 Endocrine and Metabolic Disorders

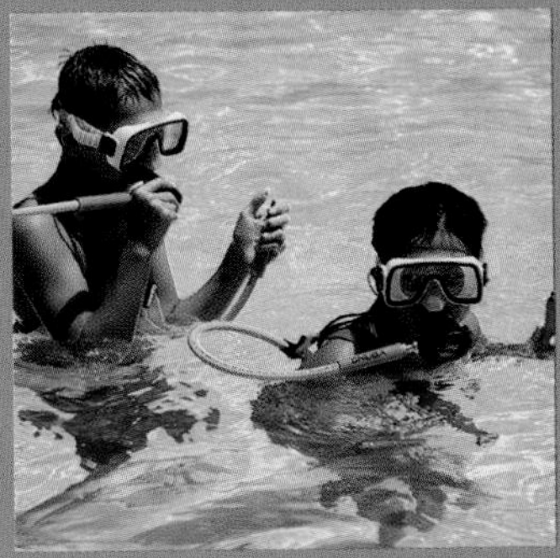

ARLENE SMALDONE, ROBERT D. STEINER, AND BECKY J. WHITTEMORE

Endocrine and metabolic disorders affect a large number of children and may be rare (e.g., nephropathic cystinosis) or relatively common (e.g., type 1 and type 2 diabetes mellitus). This chapter begins with an overview of anatomy, physiology, and pathophysiology of the endocrine and metabolic system and general issues related to assessment and management of the disorders. Following are two sections covering endocrine and metabolic disorders because many are managed by primary care providers in collaboration with specialists. Although a great degree of overlap happens in these disorders, distinctive processes occur in each, and as such, specific conditions may involve different approaches to assessment and management.

Anatomy and Physiology

The endocrine system regulates growth, pubertal development and reproduction, homeostasis of the individual, and the production, storage, and utilization of energy. Classically, the endocrine system was understood to function via hormones produced in glands with action at a distant site. Now, the understanding is that hormones may also act in a paracrine fashion affecting cells adjacent to the hormone-secreting cell or in an autocrine fashion in which the hormone affects the secreting cell by diffusion. Many endocrine glands are controlled by the hypothalamic-pituitary axis. Many of the hormones of the hypothalamic-pituitary axis (or molecules that are structurally similar to such hormones) are also made in the gut and other tissues.

Hormones are often activated by a feedback loop; for example, thyrotropin-releasing hormone (TRH) from the hypothalamus stimulates pituitary thyrotropin (thyroid-stimulating hormone [TSH]) secretion, which in turn stimulates thyroid hormone production (triiodothyronine [T_3] and thyroxine [T_4]). Thyroid hormone levels provide feedback to the hypothalamus and pituitary thereby suppressing TRH and TSH secretion so that a balance is reached. In similar fashion, the adrenal glands secrete corticosteroids and the gonads produce progesterone, androgens, and estradiol, all of which influence hypothalamic and pituitary hormone production. For some systems, the set-point changes as individuals develop. Hormone secretion can be regulated by nerve cells and by factors important in the immune system (e.g., cytokines interact with hormones that influence weight homeostasis).

Metabolic function in the body involves complex biochemical processes to transform essential amino acids, carbohydrates, and lipids to substances or energy that can be used at the cellular level; to produce molecules; and to perform cell functions. These biochemical processes or metabolic pathways are driven by enzyme activity.

Pathophysiology

Endocrine abnormalities occur when an alteration in regulation of the normal feedback system results in hyposecretion or hypersecretion of one or more hormones. Multiple factors cause alterations in hormone production. These factors include tumors, trauma, infection, systemic disease, genetic disorders, congenital malformation or agenesis of an endocrine gland, idiopathic causes, and iatrogenic causes (e.g., medications). The defect or problem can originate at the pituitary-hypothalamic level, in organ abnormalities, or for unknown reasons that lead to unresponsiveness to endogenous hormone. Hypothyroidism and hyperthyroidism are examples of disease entities in which the interrelationships of the hypothalamic-pituitary-thyroid axis may be altered at any one of these sites.

Metabolic diseases are generally considered inborn errors of metabolism (IEM). An alteration in genetic constitution results in disrupted biochemical functioning. For example, in children with phenylketonuria (PKU; a deficiency of the enzyme phenylalanine hydroxylase), the essential amino acid phenylalanine accumulates, resulting in intellectual disability if not treated within the first weeks of life.

Assessment

Endocrine and metabolic disorders disrupt organs throughout the body and can alter various body functions. Assessment requires a thorough family history, physical examination, and specific diagnostic testing for the suspected disorder.

History

- What is the child's growth pattern since birth?
- Has there been a recent alteration in growth pattern?
- Is the child taking any medications, including herbs and supplements, that could affect endocrine or metabolic function?
- Any signs or symptoms of endocrine or metabolic dysfunction?
- Any maternal exposure to radioiodine, goitrogens, or iodine medication during pregnancy?
- When did the child first show signs of sexual development?
- What is the child's diet and exercise history?
- Any family history of endocrine, autoimmune, or metabolic disorders (e.g., diabetes mellitus, thyroid disease)?
- Does the child have unusual odors, recurrent vomiting, or unexplained lethargy?

Physical Examination

A detailed examination should include the following:

- Measure stature: Supine length is preferred for children younger than 2 years old. Use a stadiometer for children older than 2 years. Plot height, weight, and head circumference on a standardized growth chart appropriate to the child's age and gender. It is currently recommended that the World Health Organization (WHO) growth chart be used to monitor growth in children younger than 2 years old and that the Centers for Disease Control and Prevention (CDC) growth charts be used for children from 2 to 20 years old (Graber and Rappoport, 2012). In addition, growth charts are available for children with certain genetic conditions, such as Down and Turner syndromes, and should be used to assess growth patterns of children with these conditions. Serial measurements are critical to assess growth patterns over time.
- Check for proportionate appearance: Measure sitting and standing heights for upper to lower segment ratio.
- Assess height age (the age corresponding to the child's height when plotted at the 50th percentile on a growth chart) and growth velocity (linear growth in centimeters or inches over the past year).
- Inspect the child's genitalia for signs of normal, abnormal, or ambiguous genitalia.
- Identify the stage of sexual development using Tanner sexual maturity rating (see Chapter 8).
- Note facial, axillary, and pubic hair for presence, distribution, and texture.
- Examine the skin for presence of striae and acanthosis nigricans of the neck, axilla, breast, knuckles, and skin folds.
- Palpate the neck for thyroid gland symmetry and size, noting enlargement or presence of nodules.
- Examine for presence of dysmorphic features.
- Examine the abdomen noting any organomegaly.
- Complete general neurologic examination.

Acquired endocrine disorders are often due to either hyposecretion or hypersecretion of a specific hormone or combination of hormones, and the child may or may not appear ill. Signs of dehydration, exophthalmos, and tachycardia are physical findings associated with endocrine pathology. Newborns with metabolic disorders may initially appear well, but physical signs develop with metabolic activity. Characteristic physical findings associated with specific disease entities are presented later in this chapter.

Diagnostic Studies

Measurement of hormone levels is a key tool in the diagnosis of endocrine disorders. Specific blood and urine studies that identify end products of abnormal metabolism or elevated or diminished levels of various substances such as ammonia, glucose, galactose, or amino acids are important in the diagnosis of metabolic disorders. Accurate interpretation of data requires strict adherence to laboratory protocol for collecting and managing specimens. Additionally, not all laboratories have the ability to conduct tests that are sensitive to the hormone or substance being measured (e.g., measurement of hormones in precocious puberty requires high sensitivity; measurement of ammonia levels requires strict procedures when obtaining the sample).

Radiographic and imaging studies (e.g., bone age, ultrasonography, computed tomography [CT], and magnetic resonance imaging [MRI]) are important diagnostic tools in evaluating certain endocrine and metabolic disorders.

Many of these studies are expensive and can put additional emotional stress on a family that is already uncertain about their child's condition.

Management Strategies

General Measures

Clinical consequences for the child affected by an endocrine or metabolic disorder vary from mild to severe. If undiagnosed and untreated, these disorders may lead to irreversible intellectual disability, physical disability, neurologic damage, and/or death. Early detection, accurate diagnosis, and timely intervention are necessary to achieve

favorable outcomes. Chronic disease issues and the effects of these diseases on lifestyle must also be addressed:
- Family, school, peer, and emotional adjustment
- Body image, self-esteem, and social competence
- Disease understanding, acceptance, and self-care
- Regimen adherence

A successful outcome depends on the patient and family receiving support and encouragement in self-care, learning about the disease, and understanding the patient-parent role in managing a long-term illness or chronic condition.

Genetic Counseling

Genetic counseling is often necessary. Implications are significant for the family of a child with endocrine or metabolic disorders that are genetically linked (see Chapter 41).

Medications

Pharmacologic therapy, including hormone replacement, whether temporary or lifelong, is often essential for management of these disorders. Often, medications must be administered via injection, creating distress in both the child and caregiver. Short, clear instructions about medications are important; how much to give, when and how to administer, possible side effects, and when to make adjustments in medication are key messages to convey. Long-term adherence to medications can become problematic with chronic illnesses and requires constant vigilance on the part of providers who interact with the child (see Chapter 22 for discussion about adherence and medications).

Dietary Considerations

Metabolic diseases often require strict adherence to dietary plans and restrictions. Parents, patients, caregivers, and school personnel must be aware of the dietary needs and restrictions and the effect of diet on the disease process. They must also be given support in order to adjust to the economic, social, and psychological demands created by such restrictions.

Patient and Family Education

Close supervision and frequent follow-up are necessary for children with metabolic and endocrine disorders. These children are best evaluated initially and periodically by a multidisciplinary team with expertise in pediatric endocrinology and metabolism or clinical genetics. Parent and patient education should include:
- Nature of the disorder
- Treatment plan
- Possible complications
- Plan for long-term follow-up, including the timing and process of transition to adult care services

The multidisciplinary team can provide the education and support needed. The primary care provider, as a part of this team, is in an ideal position to reinforce the plan of care. Additionally, essential primary health care needs and anticipatory guidance cannot be overlooked.

Disorders of Endocrine Function

Endocrine pathologies most commonly seen in children can be assessed by considering the following seven areas:
- Disturbance of growth
- Abnormalities of pubertal development
- Adrenal conditions
- Disorders of sexual maturation
- Thyroid conditions
- Diabetes mellitus, types 1 and 2
- Posterior pituitary gland dysfunction

Growth Disorders

Children grow in a predictable way, and deviation from a normal growth pattern can be the first sign of an endocrine disorder. Accurate serial growth data must be collected in order to assess a pattern of growth and current growth velocity. A child's predicted growth potential is based in large part on genetic potential and may change with altered nutritional status and illness patterns. An estimate of the expected stature (±2 standard deviations where 1 standard deviation equals 2 inches [4.5 cm]) for a particular child can be made by calculating a mid-parental target height:
- Target height for boys: (Mother's height + 5 inches [13 cm]) + (Father's height)/2
- Target height for girls: (Father's height − 5 inches [13 cm]) + (Mother's height)/2

Growth disorders may be classified as primary or secondary. Primary growth disorders include skeletal dysplasias, chromosomal abnormalities (e.g., Turner syndrome), and genetic short stature. Secondary growth disorders may result from undernutrition, chronic disease, endocrine disorder, and idiopathic (constitutional) growth delay (CGD) (Box 26-1). The following discussion focuses on growth hormone deficiency (GHD) and CGD (Table 26-1).

Growth Hormone Deficiency

Growth hormone (GH) is an anterior pituitary hormone released in response to sleep, exercise, and hypoglycemia. Secretion of GH occurs in a series of irregular and pulsatile bursts throughout the day and night with most GH activity occurring during sleep. GHD may be either congenital or acquired. Individuals may also be resistant to GH, and GHD increases with age and immunodeficiency.

Clinical Findings

History. A history obtained to evaluate the short or slowly growing child should include:
- Details of pregnancy, delivery, and newborn period
    - Mother's health during pregnancy
    - Birthing process, type, and presence of complications
    - Birth length and weight

TABLE 26-1 Short Stature: Characteristics of Growth Hormone Deficiency and Constitutional Growth Delay in Children

Condition	Etiology	Onset	Presentation	Endocrine/Metabolic Disturbance
Growth hormone deficiency (GHD)	Idiopathic (most common) Pituitary or hypothalamic disease Trauma Minor organic hypothalamic lesion Infection Radiation	Congenital or acquired	Slow growth rate with normal birth weight Signs and symptoms of increased intracranial pressure Microphallus Proportional short stature Delayed bone age	Deficiency or impairment in secretion of growth hormone-releasing hormone
Constitutional growth delay (CGD)	Variation of normal growth Not a disease	First years of life with impaired growth	Growth velocity is normal after 3 years of age Delayed puberty with pubertal growth spurt Delayed bone age Positive family history	None—final height is appropriate for parents' height

BOX 26-1 Classification of Growth Retardation

Primary Growth Abnormalities

Osteochondrodysplasia
Chromosome abnormalities
Intrauterine growth retardation
Dysmorphic syndromes

Genetic Short Stature

SHOX gene haploinsufficiency

Secondary Growth Failure

Malnutrition
Chronic illness
Endocrine disorders

- Hypothyroidism
- Cushing syndrome
- Pseudohypoparathyroidism
- Rickets
- IGF-1 deficiency
    - GHD
    - Growth hormone insensitivity
    - Defects in IGF-1 synthesis

Variants of Normal Growth

Constitutional delay of growth
Puberty

GHD, Growth hormone deficiency; *IGF-1,* insulin-like growth factor 1; *SHOX,* short stature homeobox.

    - Neonatal course, including history of prolonged jaundice, hypoglycemia, and/or microphallus (often diagnostic of congenital GHD)
    - Dysmorphia, especially midline facial defects or eye abnormalities
- Parents' and siblings' height, weight, and growth pattern
- Age at which growth decelerates
- Chronic illness(es)
- Symptoms of hypothyroidism or other known pituitary hormone deficiency
- Trauma or insult to the central nervous system (CNS)
- Treatment with cranial radiation
- Signs of an intracranial lesion

Physical Examination. Physical examination of the short child or child who is not growing well should include:

- Identification of clinical clues to chronic illness or dysmorphic syndrome (e.g., childlike face with large, prominent forehead)
- Presence of midline defect
- Evaluation of the fundi for signs of increased intracranial pressure
- Palpation of the thyroid gland for the presence of a goiter
- Evaluation of the stage of puberty
- Measurement of body proportions including arm span, height and upper-to-lower (U/L) body segment ratio to exclude a skeletal dysplasia (dwarfing condition): Interpretation of the U/L body segment ratio is dependent on the age of the child. Body proportion varies during childhood. At birth, the U/L ratio is approximately 1.7; 1.3 at 3 years old; and 0.89 to 0.95 in postpubertal age children.

Diagnostic Studies. If growth velocity is subnormal (including when prior heights are not available), initial evaluation should include:

- Hypoglycemia
- Complete blood count (CBC) and sedimentation rate (erythrocyte sedimentation rate [ESR])
- Urinalysis
- Screening for gastrointestinal illness when appropriate (e.g., celiac disease screening [serum IgA and transglutaminase], irritable bowel disease [ESR], stool for ova and parasites)
- Chemistry panel
- Growth factors (insulin-like growth factor 1 [IGF-1] and insulin-like growth factor–binding protein 3 [IGFBP-3])
- Thyroid function tests: Free T_4 and TSH should be obtained to exclude both pituitary TSH deficiency and primary hypothyroidism
- Bone age x-ray of left wrist and hand

- Karyotype to rule out Turner syndrome in girls: Girls with Turner mosaicism may not manifest the typical clinical findings of Turner syndrome (e.g., cubitus valgus, webbing of the neck), thus highlighting the importance of karyotyping all females presenting with short stature (Milbrandt and Thomas, 2013) (see Chapter 41).
- Measurement of GH production may be necessary: Because secretion of GH is pulsatile, random serum measurement of the hormone is inadequate; stimulation testing using agents (such as, arginine, levodopa, clonidine, and/or glucagon) is needed to accurately assess GH production.

Differential Diagnosis

Individual children with short stature may not fit nicely into a single category but may have multiple factors contributing to their stature. Many chronic illnesses can slow linear growth, likely through a variety of mechanisms including malnutrition, acidosis, anorexia, and deficiencies of minerals (e.g., zinc and iron) and vitamins necessary for growth (Box 26-2). Typically, children with poor growth as a result of chronic illness are underweight for their height; their weight gain slows prior to growth deceleration. Thyroid hormones are essential to growth during childhood; sex steroids are important for normal growth during the pubertal growth spurt. Deficiency of these hormones is characterized by subnormal growth velocity, normal to increased weight for height, and delay in bone age.

Management

Children should be referred to a pediatric endocrinologist if hypothyroidism, low IGF-1 and IGFBP-3 or other hormone deficiency is confirmed, or for unexplained persistent slow growth without evidence of chronic illness. The U.S. Food and Drug Administration (FDA) has approved eight indications for GH therapy (Box 26-3). GH dosing is based on a child's body weight with doses ranging from 0.15 to 0.30 mg/kg/week. When it was first introduced as a therapy, GH was administered intramuscularly three times a week; therapeutic response, however, is greater for children receiving daily subcutaneous injections, and daily dosing is currently the most frequently used regimen. During the first year of therapy, growth velocity may exceed normal growth rates as much as fourfold. Reported side effects of GH include glucose intolerance, pseudotumor cerebri, edema, growth of nevi, slipped capital femoral epiphyses, and scoliosis (Romero et al, 2013). The cost of GH therapy may present an economic burden to the family, and referral to a social worker to assist in finding financial support may be appropriate.

Constitutional Growth Delay

Constitutional delay of growth and puberty is a common growth pattern variation and should not be considered a disease entity. When the child has no evidence of chronic illness, has a delay in bone age, and is growing at a normal rate for bone age, the likely diagnosis is constitutional growth delay (CGD). These children generally reach normal adult height, although they may be slightly short compared to other family members.

Clinical Findings

History. The history may include the following:

- Normal length and weight at birth
- Slowed linear growth between 1 to 3 years old and then normal growth velocity; normal height velocity is the most critical factor in diagnosing CGD
- Height at or slightly below the third percentile on standardized growth charts
- Delayed pubertal development
- History of similar growth patterns in other family members: Often there is a family history of at least one family member who did not begin puberty until later than what would be expected.

• BOX 26-2 Chronic Illness Contributing to Growth Failure

Gastrointestinal disease
- Celiac disease
- Inflammatory bowel disease
- Cystic fibrosis

Cardiovascular disease
- Cyanotic heart disease
- Congestive heart failure

Renal disease
- Uremia
- Renal tubular acidosis

Hematologic disorders
- Chronic anemia

Inborn errors of metabolism
Pulmonary disease
Chronic infection
Anorexia nervosa

• BOX 26-3 FDA-Approved Indications for Growth Hormone Therapy

GHD
Growth failure caused by chronic renal failure
Turner syndrome
Prader-Willi syndrome
Intrauterine growth retardation with failure to catch up by 2 years old
Noonan's syndrome
SHOX-containing gene deficiency
Idiopathic short stature
- Height more than 2.25 standard deviations below the mean for age and gender
- Unexplained short stature with poor height prognosis

FDA, U.S. Food and Drug Administration; *GHD*, growth hormone deficiency; *SHOX*, short stature homeobox.

Physical Examination. Findings on physical examination include:

- Delayed bone age with growth velocity normal for bone age
- Final height prediction based on bone age within range of calculated target height
- Neurologic examination within normal limits

Diagnostic Studies. The same screening tests used to evaluate GHD are performed to rule out pathologic conditions. A bone age x-ray can often be helpful in distinguishing between CGD and idiopathic short stature. The child with CGD will have a bone age consistent with his or her height age, whereas the child with idiopathic short stature will have a bone age consistent with his or her chronologic age (Graber and Rappoport, 2012).

Management

Reassurance and support should be provided to the child and family regarding ultimate height and development. An endocrine referral may be necessary to differentiate CGD from GHD and for possible hormone replacement therapy.

Growth Excess

In contrast to those with CGD, some children are tall for their family as young children and enter puberty early, yet ultimately reach a height within the normal range for their family. Rarely will this accelerated growth require referral to a pediatric endocrinologist. Tall stature in comparison with parents' height or rapid growth velocity in childhood may represent an underlying abnormality. These include:

- Primary skeletal abnormalities, such as Marfan syndrome, Klinefelter syndrome, and other overgrowth syndromes
- Overnutrition that advances the bone age and the timing of puberty: In these children, weight gain occurs first, and weight percentile is further above the growth curve than height percentile.
- Excess adrenal androgens or gonadal steroids: These children will have physical examination findings of early puberty.

Pubertal Disorders

The physical changes of puberty occur in response to production of sex steroids by the ovaries or testes (see Chapter 8). Hypothalamic gonadotropin-releasing hormone (GnRH) regulates the release of luteinizing hormone (LH) and follicle-stimulating hormone (FSH) from the pituitary gland, which in turn stimulates gonadal hormone secretion.

By mid-gestation the fetal hypothalamic-pituitary-gonadal axis is intact; at term, the production of GnRH, LH, and FSH in this system are at low levels. When placental and maternal hormones are removed at delivery, unrestrained production of these hormones occurs in the newborn, and the infant experiences a "mini puberty" between 2 weeks and 3 months of postnatal life. After infancy, the hypothalamic GnRH pulse generator is more sensitive to feedback inhibition from the brain, and by 1 year of age, LH and FSH decrease to the prepubertal range, and the child enters a "latency" period, which will continue until the time of puberty. Puberty occurs when the feedback inhibition is released and GnRH is again produced. The timing of the release correlates better with bone age than chronologic age (Bordini and Rosenfield, 2011a).

The initiation of puberty in girls is earlier now compared to past decades (Loomba-Albrecht and Styne, 2012) and varies by race and ethnicity. Tanner 2 stage breast development is present in less than 5% of non-Hispanic white girls with normal body mass index (BMI) by the age of 8 years; however, thelarche (breast bud development) is a normal finding in non-Hispanic black and Mexican American girls before 8 years of age (Bordini and Rosenfield, 2011b). Although girls are starting puberty at a younger age than in past generations, the timing of menarche and reaching Tanner stage 5 has not changed dramatically. Menarche typically occurs within 3 years from the start of breast development. Ninety-five percent of girls will have signs of puberty by 12 years old and achieve menarche by 14 years old. Boys normally begin puberty anywhere from 9 years old to 14 years old. The first sign of puberty is increased testicular volume in 85% of boys. Clinicians should be concerned when puberty presents early or is delayed.

Early Puberty/Precocious Puberty

Early puberty is divided into four categories: premature thelarche, premature adrenarche, isolated menarche, and true precocious puberty.

Premature thelarche, isolated breast development without any other features of puberty, occurs in infant and toddler girls and is sometimes present at birth. This breast development, likely due to estrogens produced during the mini puberty of infancy or increased responsiveness of the breast primordia, resolves over time and rarely progresses to true precocious puberty.

Premature adrenarche is the early onset of pubic or axillary hair in either boys (prior to 10 years old) or girls (prior to 8 years old) not associated with other features of true puberty. Bone and height age may be slightly advanced in relation to chronologic age in children with premature adrenarche and plasma dehydroepiandrosterone (DHEA) values may be slightly elevated (Loomba-Albrecht and Styne, 2012). Premature adrenarche may be caused by a mild form of congenital adrenal hyperplasia (CAH), exposure to topical testosterone, or rarely, adrenal tumor. Most often, the condition is idiopathic. Children with idiopathic premature adrenarche are at increased risk for polycystic ovary syndrome and metabolic syndrome (Bordini and Rosenfield, 2011b).

Isolated menarche is an uncommon condition in which girls have one to a few episodes of vaginal bleeding without breast development. In this condition, sexual abuse, vaginal tumor, a functional estrogen-producing ovarian cyst, and primary hypothyroidism all need to be excluded.

• BOX 26-4 Disorders of Puberty

Central Precocious Puberty

Idiopathic
CNS disorder
- Hamartoma
- Tumor
- CNS radiation
- Infection
- Trauma

Hypothyroidism
HCG-secreting tumor

Peripheral Precocious Puberty

Girls

McCune-Albright syndrome
Ovarian cyst
Estrogen-secreting ovarian or adrenal tumor

Boys

Severe, non-salt wasting, CAH
Testotoxicosis (activating mutation of the LH receptor)
Testicular tumor

CAH, Congenital adrenal hyperplasia; *CNS,* central nervous system; *HCG,* human chorionic gonadotropin; *LH,* luteinizing hormone.

True precocious puberty refers to the onset of multiple features of puberty earlier than the normal range. It is defined as thelarche or pubarche (appearance of pubic hair) before 8 years old in girls and before 9 years old in boys, except in the case of non-Hispanic African American and Mexican American girls where thelarche is considered within the normal range after 7 years old (Bordini and Rosenfield, 2011b). Features of precocious puberty may include accelerated linear growth, breast development or penile enlargement, and pubic hair development. Depending on the duration of symptoms, the bone age may be advanced. Precocious puberty can be divided into two broad categories: (1) central, gonadotropin dependent; or (2) peripheral, gonadotropin independent (Box 26-4). Prolonged exposure to exogenous sex hormones (mother's birth control pills or father's topical testosterone) (Rodriquez and Dougan, 2013) and exposure to chemicals that disrupt endocrine function (see Chapter 42) can cause precocious puberty (Ozen and Darcan, 2011).

In the United States, the incidence of precocious puberty is 0.01% to 0.05% per year. Precocious puberty is more common in females compared to males and in African American children compared to Caucasian children (Rodriquez and Dougan, 2013). Any lesion that disrupts the normal connections between the brain and the hypothalamus can cause central precocious puberty. This condition is most often idiopathic in girls. Boys have a 30% incidence of CNS tumors in situations of central precocious puberty.

Clinical Findings

Many children who present with features of early puberty do not require treatment. All children who exhibit signs of puberty at a younger age than normal, however, should have an evaluation as to the etiology. Those children who start to develop signs of puberty at the early end of the normal range should be evaluated if they have rapid progression of pubertal signs resulting in a bone age more than 2 years ahead of chronologic age, or new CNS-related findings (e.g., headaches, seizures, and/or focal neurologic defects).

History. Evaluation includes the following:

- Age of onset
- Type, duration, and progression of pubertal symptoms (i.e., breast tissue, pubic hair, phallic enlargement, acne, body odor, oily scalp)
- Pattern of growth
- Any symptoms suggestive of a CNS lesion
- Family pattern of pubertal changes
- Exposure to topical estrogens or testosterone, oral estrogens, or environmental hormone disruptors

Physical Examination. Physical examination should include:

- Assessment of stature and growth velocity
- Description of the child's Tanner stage:
  - Breast development: Breast development should be evaluated by palpation rather than inspection to differentiate between the presence of true breast tissue versus fat deposition
  - Presence of pubic and axillary hair (girls)
  - Penile length, testicular volume, and pubic and axillary hair (boys) (see Chapter 8)

Diagnostic Studies. Diagnostic studies should include:

- Premature thelarche: No laboratory studies are necessary in the infant or toddler girl unless she has other features of true puberty or continued increase in breast size.
- Premature adrenarche: Serum 17-hydroxyprogesterone (17-OHP) to exclude CAH and a 24-hour urine collection for 17-ketosteroids or imaging of the adrenal glands to exclude an adrenal tumor.
- Isolated menarche: Thyroid function tests to exclude primary hypothyroidism, and pelvic ultrasound to rule out the presence of an ovarian cyst or pelvic tumor.
- True precocious puberty:
  - Bone age x-ray of left wrist
  - LH, FSH, and estradiol or testosterone: Use a laboratory with a sensitive assay that will detect early pubertal values at the lower end of the range.
    - If LH and FSH are high (in pubertal range: indication of central etiology), an MRI is indicated to exclude CNS tumor.
    - If LH and FSH are low (in prepubertal range: indication of peripheral puberty), complete a GnRH stimulation test to distinguish central from peripheral puberty.
  - If etiology is peripheral puberty:
    - Pelvic ultrasonography of girls
    - Testicular ultrasonography of boys
    - Serum 17-OHP to rule out a severe form of CAH

Management

Treatment of early puberty depends on the etiology and should always be done with the guidance of a pediatric endocrinologist. Management depends on the underlying disorder, age of the child, degree of advancement of the bone age, and the child's and family's emotional response to the condition. Radiation, surgery, or chemotherapy is indicated in the case of CNS tumors. A long-acting GnRH agonist may be used to bring serum sex steroids to prepubertal levels. Treatment of precocious puberty is important to increase final adult height.

Delayed Puberty

Puberty is considered delayed when a boy 14 years old or older or a girl 13 years old or older has no clinical features of puberty on physical examination or if puberty has not progressed within a timely basis. Girls should progress to menarche within 5 years of breast budding; boys should attain Tanner 5 pubertal development within 4.5 years of initiation of puberty. If puberty is either delayed or has failed to progress, the child should be referred to an endocrinologist for evaluation of hypogonadism (Loomba-Albrecht and Styne, 2012).

Any chronic condition that delays the bone age may cause delayed puberty, because the timing of puberty correlates better with bone age than chronologic age (Box 26-5). In addition, failure of any part of the hypothalamic-pituitary-gonadal axis may also delay puberty (Box 26-6). The most common cause of delayed puberty is CGD.

Clinical Findings

History and Physical Examination. History and physical examination should focus on clinical clues indicating a chronic illness, symptoms or signs of hypothyroidism (discussed later in this chapter), prior history of CNS insult, or new CNS symptoms suggesting hypopituitarism. Review of systems should include questions about pattern of growth, especially growth velocity, sense of smell, and galactorrhea.

• BOX 26-5 Etiology of Delayed Puberty

Chronic Illness

GI with poor weight gain
Chronic renal failure
Anorexia nervosa or bulimia
Chronic anemia
Respiratory or cardiac disease
Medication-induced poor weight gain

Constitutional Growth Delay

Endocrine diseases associated with delayed bone age
Hypothyroidism

Growth Hormone Deficiency

Failure of the hypothalamic-pituitary-gonadal axis

GI, Gastrointestinal.

Diagnostic Studies. Laboratory investigation should include:

- Focused screening for acute or chronic illness (CBC, sedimentation rate, C-reactive protein, urinalysis, liver enzymes, electrolytes [renal function])
- Bone age x-ray
- Free T_4 and TSH
- IGF-1 and IGFBP-3, if GHD is suspect
- Serum prolactin
- LH and FSH (when gonadal failure is present, LH and FSH are abnormally elevated)

Management

A referral to a pediatric endocrinologist is necessary to determine the etiology and necessary treatment. Hormonal replacement is the treatment of choice for hypogonadism, whereas youth with CGD require reassurance that puberty will occur spontaneously albeit later compared to some peers (Loomba-Albrecht and Styne, 2012).

Adrenal Disorders

Anatomy and Physiology

Adrenal gland steroid production is under the control of the hypothalamic-pituitary axis. The hypothalamus secretes corticotropin-releasing hormone (CRH) in a pulsatile fashion, which stimulates production and secretion of adrenocorticotropic hormone (ACTH) by the pituitary gland. ACTH regulates adrenal glucocorticoid (cortisol) and androgen production. Cortisol is produced in a series of enzymatic steps (Fig. 26-1) and is highest in the morning, low in the afternoon and evening, and lowest at midnight. Secreted in response to hypoglycemia, hypotension, pain, or other stressful events, cortisol has negative feedback on

• BOX 26-6 Failure of the Hypothalamic-Pituitary-Gonadal Axis

Hypothalamic Pituitary Dysfunction (LH/FSH Deficiency)

Multiple pituitary hormone deficiency

- Isolated gonadotropin deficiency
- Kallmann syndrome (anosmia and gonadotropin deficiency)
- Hyperprolactinemia
- Functional deficiency associated with lack of calories or extreme exercise

Gonadal Failure

Girls

Turner syndrome
Oophoritis
Galactosemia
Chemotherapy induced

Boys

Vanishing testes syndrome (in utero testicular torsion)
Chemotherapy or radiation

FSH, Follicle-stimulating hormone; *LH*, luteinizing hormone.

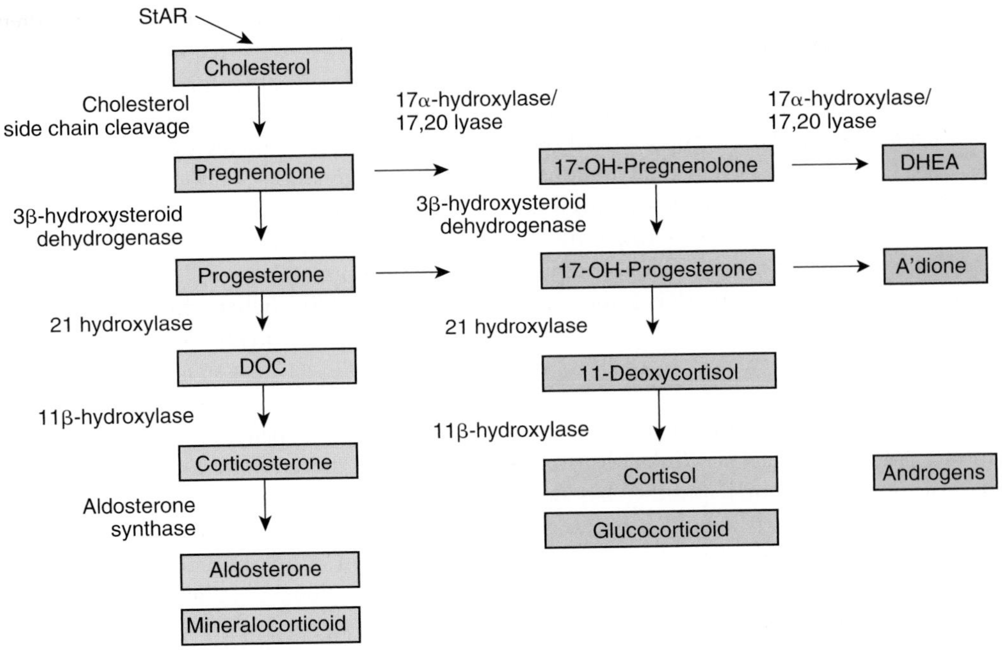

• **Figure 26-1** Adrenal steroidogenesis. After the steroidogenic acute regulatory *(StAR)* protein–mediated uptake of cholesterol into mitochondria within adrenocortical cells, aldosterone, cortisol, and adrenal androgens are synthesized through the coordinated action of a series of steroidogenic enzymes in a zone-specific fashion. *A'dione,* Androstenedione; *DHEA,* dehydroepiandrosterone; *DOC,* deoxycorticosterone. (From Stewart PM: The adrenal cortex. In Larsen PR, Kronenberg HM, Melmed S, et al, editors: *Williams textbook of endocrinology*, ed 10, Philadelphia, 2003, WB Saunders, p 495.)

the synthesis and secretion of CRH, vasopressin, and ACTH.

The adrenal gland also produces mineralocorticoid hormones (aldosterone), regulated by renal production of renin interacting with angiotensinogen, to create angiotensin. The renin-angiotensin system is involved in regulation of salts, especially sodium; blood pressure; and renal blood flow. Aldosterone production also occurs in enzymatic steps, many of which are common to the cortisol production pathway.

Adrenal Insufficiency

Adrenal insufficiency is characterized by a deficiency of hormones produced by the adrenal cortex; deficits of cortisol and aldosterone are perhaps the most detrimental to body function. In primary adrenal insufficiency (hypofunctioning adrenal gland), glucocorticoid (cortisol) *and* mineralocorticoid (aldosterone) hormones are deficient, whereas in secondary adrenal insufficiency (hypothalamic or pituitary defect), only a glucocorticoid deficit is found. Thus, children with both forms of adrenal insufficiency have hypoglycemia and hypotension caused by cortisol deficiency. Only those with a primary adrenal insufficiency are at risk for salt-wasting crisis (hyponatremia, hyperkalemia, acidosis, and dehydration) caused by aldosterone deficiency.

Primary adrenal insufficiency may be due to an inability to produce cortisol secondary to an enzyme defect in the adrenal steroid pathway (CAH), hypoplasia of the adrenal gland, or an acquired defect (Box 26-7). Lesions of the hypothalamus or pituitary lead to secondary adrenal insufficiency. Suppression of the hypothalamic-pituitary-adrenal axis secondary to steroid use can also lead to adrenal insufficiency. Infants born extremely prematurely (24 to 28 weeks' gestation) sometimes demonstrate symptoms of adrenal insufficiency because of immaturity of the hypothalamic-pituitary-adrenal axis.

• BOX 26-7 Adrenal Insufficiency

Deficiency of Corticotropin-Releasing Hormone or Adrenocorticotropin

- Isolated deficiency
  - Congenital
  - Acquired as a result of hypophysitis
- Multiple pituitary hormone deficiencies
  - Congenital (septo-optic dysplasia, midline defects, and so on)
  - Acquired (CNS trauma, infection, tumor, radiation)

Primary Adrenal

- Congenital
  - CAH (most common 21-OH deficiency)
  - Adrenal hypoplasia (X-linked, autosomal recessive, ACTH receptor defect)
- Acquired
  - X-linked, adrenoleukodystrophy
  - Autoimmune (Addison)
  - Infection

21-OH, 21-Hydroxylase; *ACTH*, adrenocorticotropin; *CAH,* congenital adrenal hyperplasia; *CNS*, central nervous system.

Secondary adrenal insufficiency can occur as a result of ACTH deficiency, as one of multiple hypothalamic-pituitary deficiencies, or rarely as an isolated problem. Most often the infant or child has a syndrome known to be associated with hypopituitarism (e.g., septo-optic dysplasia), has also been discovered to have GHD, or has a destructive lesion (e.g., tumor) or a history of prior radiation to the brain or CNS trauma.

CAH is caused by a deficiency of any of the enzymes in the cortisol pathway. In addition to interrupting normal cortisol production, the most common enzymatic abnormality, 21-hydroxylase (21-OH) deficiency, causes shunting of cortisol precursors to the androgen pathway, resulting in production of elevated levels of adrenal androgens in utero. Female infants born with classic CAH typically have ambiguous genitalia (e.g., enlarged clitoris and/or posterior fusion of the labia) from this excessive androgen exposure in utero. However, male infants have no signs of CAH at birth with the exception of subtle hyperpigmentation and possible mild enlargement of the penis (Trapp et al, 2013). About 75% of children with CAH caused by 21-OH deficiency will also have aldosterone deficiency. Newborn screening programs now routinely test for the presence of CAH caused by 21-OH deficiency to detect CAH early to avoid a potentially life-threatening salt-wasting crisis in affected infants.

Clinical Findings

History. Symptoms of cortisol deficiency include a history of:

- Poor appetite
- Failure to thrive or weight loss
- Weakness
- Vomiting

Symptoms of aldosterone deficiency include:

- Vomiting
- Poor feeding
- Lethargy
- Dehydration

Physical Examination. The following signs are often seen:

- Dehydration
- Hypotension
- Excessive pigmentation of the skin and mucous membranes (present only with primary adrenal insufficiency)

Diagnostic Studies. The following diagnostic studies are indicated:

- Serum glucose (hypoglycemia)
- Blood gases and bicarbonate (metabolic acidosis)
- Electrolytes (low sodium, elevated potassium with aldosterone deficiency)
- Serum cortisol: A cortisol value greater than 20 mcg/dL indicates adrenal sufficiency; a value lower than that must be interpreted in the clinical context in which the sample was drawn. Often an ACTH stimulation test, performed in collaboration with a pediatric endocrinologist, is needed to conclusively diagnose both primary and secondary adrenal insufficiency.
- Serum ACTH (elevated in primary adrenal insufficiency)
- Serum 17-OHP (diagnostic in children with suspected CAH caused by 21-OH deficiency)
- Serum renin level (elevated in aldosterone deficiency)
- Aldosterone level (low in aldosterone deficiency)

Plasma renin and aldosterone levels are interpreted best if they are drawn when serum sodium levels are low.

Management

Treatment of adrenal insufficiency includes hormone replacement and is best managed by a pediatric endocrinologist. An adrenal crisis is a medical emergency requiring immediate and vigorous administration of intravenous (IV) dextrose, normal saline, and stress doses of hydrocortisone succinate. IV stress doses of hydrocortisone succinate vary with age: 25 mg in children younger than 3 years old; 50 mg in children 3 to 12 years old; and 100 mg in children older than 12 years old, administered every 6 hours. Parents should be instructed regarding the need for stress doses of hydrocortisone succinate when their child has a febrile illness, surgery, or trauma; they should also be taught how to administer hydrocortisone succinate via intramuscular injection in case the child is vomiting or otherwise unable to swallow or retain oral medication. This injection allows parents extended time to seek further medical advice or intervention.

Long-term therapy of CAH includes oral hydrocortisone in replacement doses of 8 to 10 mg/M^2 (8 to 10 mg per square meter of body surface) in children with ACTH deficiency or primary adrenal insufficiency. Children with CAH tend to have higher hydrocortisone needs. If present, aldosterone deficiency must be treated with fludrocortisone acetate. Treatment of CAH requires a fine balancing act to replace steroids, thereby preventing androgen overproduction. Excess steroid intake can lead to delayed growth; not enough steroids contribute to rapid bone age growth and ultimate short stature. Individual treatment plans are essential to meet the specific needs of individual children. The primary care provider should be familiar with the medical endocrinology treatment plan and reinforce it at routine well- and sick-child visits.

Hyperadrenal States

Cortisol excess is most commonly caused by exogenous glucocorticoid treatment of an illness (e.g., serious asthma, to prevent rejection after a transplant, or as part of chemotherapy protocols). Endogenous cortisol excess may be due to a pituitary tumor producing ACTH, adrenal tumor, or to ectopic production of ACTH from a nonpituitary tumor (rare in children).

Clinical Findings

History and Physical Examination. Features of cortisol excess include:

- Weight gain
- Growth failure
- Osteopenia

- Hypertension
- Delayed puberty
- Plethora (hypervolemia)
- Skin: Acne, purple striae, hirsutism
- Compulsive behavior

Diagnostic Studies. In situations where growth is slow or growth data are missing and cortisol excess needs to be excluded by laboratory evaluation, a 24-hour urine collection for free cortisol or a late evening serum or salivary cortisol are the best screening tests.

Differential Diagnosis

Obesity is in the differential diagnosis, but almost all children with simple obesity are tall for their age and cortisol excess can be excluded on physical examination alone.

Management

When children receive glucocorticoids for underlying illness for longer than 7 to 10 days, the steroid dose should be weaned rather than abruptly discontinued to allow the hypothalamic-pituitary-adrenal axis to recover normal function and sometimes to prevent a flare up of the underlying disease. Procedures for tapering the dose are empiric, but in general, the longer the child has been on glucocorticoids, the longer the taper. Withdrawal plans are based on the goal of treating the child with the least amount of glucocorticoids in order to avoid long-term adverse effects while avoiding potential adrenal insufficiency during withdrawal. Decreasing the dose to a physiologic dose while monitoring the cortisol level is one method to wean. A morning cortisol value of 20 mcg/dL suggests it is safe to wean further or, if the child is already on half maintenance dose, discontinue the medication (Lansang and Hustak, 2011). Even after the steroid has been safely discontinued, the patient may not be able to respond adequately to severe stress for as long as 6 to 12 months.

Disorders of Sex Development

Abnormalities of sexual differentiation usually present in infancy with ambiguous genitalia. The spectrum of physical examination findings ranges from the appearance of a normal male penis and normal scrotum but without palpable gonads, to an infant who looks mostly female with mild enlargement of the clitoris. True hermaphroditism, in which the infant has both male and female gonadal structures, is rare.

Infants with 46 XY chromosomes who have complete androgen insensitivity (androgen receptor defect) have genitalia that appear female; these children are not detected in the newborn period unless a karyotype is performed for some other reason. Children with complete androgen insensitivity may not be identified until the time of an inguinal hernia repair when a testis is discovered or during the teen years when they fail to develop pubic hair or menstruate.

Disorders of sex development occur when the XX fetus is exposed to excess androgen in utero, the XY fetus is unable to produce or respond to androgens, or, rarely, true hermaphroditism. The most common cause of disordered sex development is CAH that exposes an XX fetus to excess androgens during fetal life (see Fig. 26-1). Less common virilizing conditions include aromatase deficiency or virilizing tumor in the mother. In an XY fetus, disordered sex development can result from inadequate androgen production or partial androgen insensitivity.

Clinical Findings

All infants should receive a complete genital examination before discharge from the nursery. The initial laboratory evaluation of an infant with ambiguous genitalia should be directed by a pediatric endocrinologist and includes:

- A karyotype test that can be done quickly (within 48 to 72 hours) if the cytogenetics laboratory is alerted to the urgency. Subsequent laboratory evaluation is based on karyotype results.
- In XY infants, measurement of the precursors of testosterone, testosterone, and dihydrotestosterone.
- In XX infants, serum 17-OHP to establish a diagnosis of 21-OH deficiency.
- Serum Müllerian inhibitory substance can also be measured or can be assessed indirectly by obtaining an ultrasound or genitogram.

Management

The family needs to be counseled immediately. The primary health care provider has a responsibility to document the abnormality and refer to a specialist team that includes a pediatric endocrinologist, medical geneticist, and pediatric urologist. The initial studies should be sent with the referral. The specialist team should meet with families and educate them about the normal process of genital development, the cause of their child's abnormality, the evaluation process, and the determination of gender for childrearing. Female is the appropriate sex of rearing for XX infants with CAH and for infants with complete androgen insensitivity. Sex of rearing in incompletely masculinized XY infants is complicated, and waiting to assign the sex of rearing until the evaluation is complete is imperative (Majumdar and Mazur, 2013). Treatment of the underlying cause, if known (e.g., CAH), is essential.

Thyroid Disorders

Anatomy and Physiology

The hypothalamic-pituitary-thyroid axis begins functioning in utero (Fig. 26-2). The hypothalamus produces TRH, which in turn stimulates pituitary production of TSH. TSH stimulates the thyroid gland to secrete primarily T_4. T_4 is converted in peripheral tissues to T_3. Both T_3 and T_4 bind to thyroid-binding proteins, primarily thyroid-binding globulin (TBG). The free, unbound form of T_3 and T_4 is biologically active. T_4 inhibits hypothalamic TRH and pituitary TSH secretion. Thyroid hormone has an important role in growth and development, basal metabolic activity,

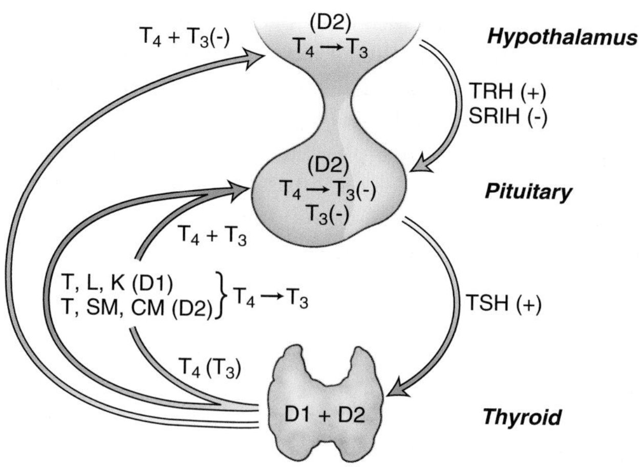

• **Figure 26-2** Interrelationships of the hypothalamic-pituitary-thyroid axis. *CM,* cardiac muscle; *D1,* type 12 iodothyronine deiodinase; *D2,* type 2 iodothyronine deiodinase; *K,* kidney; *L,* liver; *SM,* skeletal muscle; *SRIH,* somatotropin release-inhibiting factor; T_3, triiodothyronine; T_4, thyroxine; *TRH,* thyrotropin-releasing hormone; *TSH,* thyroid-stimulating hormone. (From Wilson JD, Foster DW, editors: *Williams textbook of endocrinology*, ed 8, Philadelphia, 1992, WB Saunders, p 169.)

oxygen consumption, brain development, and metabolism of lipids, carbohydrates, and proteins.

Hypothyroidism

Primary hypothyroidism (hypothyroidism caused by a problem in the thyroid gland itself) may be either congenital or acquired. Congenital hypothyroidism (CH) affects between 1 in 3000 and 4000 infants (Larson, 2013) with female infants more commonly affected. CH results from an abnormality in development of the thyroid gland during fetal life (dysgenesis or agenesis) or a problem with the ability of the thyroid to make thyroid hormone. Less frequently, CH may result from an abnormality at the level of the pituitary or hypothalamus (affecting 1 in 100,000 infants). CH is the most common cause of preventable mental retardation. Untreated CH leads to irreversible brain damage and variable degrees of growth failure, deafness, and neurologic abnormalities. Earlier detection of CH through improvements in newborn screening combined with more aggressive thyroid hormone replacement regimens (10 to 15 mcg/kg/day) at diagnosis have led to improved developmental outcomes for newborns with CH.

The most common cause of acquired hypothyroidism in children in the Western world is Hashimoto's thyroiditis, an autoimmune condition leading to destruction of the thyroid gland (Huang, 2013). Worldwide, iodine deficiency is the main cause of acquired primary hypothyroidism and has led to salt iodination as a public health measure in many countries. Hypothyroidism can also be due to a TSH deficiency that is secondary to pituitary disease or dysfunction of the hypothalamus (central hypothyroidism). Other causes of acquired hypothyroidism are listed in Box 26-8. Children with type 1 diabetes mellitus are at increased risk for hypothyroidism.

• BOX 26-8 Acquired Primary Hypothyroidism: Etiology

Chronic lymphocytic thyroiditis (Hashimoto's thyroiditis)
Drug induced (iodine, lithium, thioamides, resorcinol)
Thyroidectomy
I^{131} ablation
Infiltrative and storage disorders (histiocytosis X, cystinosis)
Subacute thyroiditis
Cranial/spinal radiation

Clinical Findings

History. Growth failure, goiter, delayed or arrested puberty, delayed dentition, weight gain, fatigue, dry skin, hyperlipidemia, decline in school performance, and menorrhagia can be present in the child with hypothyroidism. A family history of thyroid disease or other autoimmune conditions is frequently present. A past history of risk factors for hypopituitarism (e.g., CNS insult, frequent headaches, midline defects) is useful information when assessing the risk for TSH deficiency.

Physical Examination. The clinical manifestations of primary hypothyroidism vary with the age of the child:

- At birth the newborn may appear completely normal, thus the importance of newborn screening programs for early identification of hypothyroidism. The most common neonatal signs are prolonged jaundice, constipation, and umbilical hernia. Infants with CH may also have a large anterior and posterior fontanelle, macroglossia, decreased muscle tone, and be poor feeders. They may have respiratory distress and poor peripheral circulation with cool, cyanotic skin in the extremities.
- Older children who present with acquired hypothyroidism may exhibit delayed growth or subnormal growth velocity, goiter, weight gain, and delayed return of the deep tendon reflexes. Children with central hypothyroidism (thyroid deficiency secondary to pituitary or hypothalamus dysfunction) may show poor growth, increased weight for height, and features suggestive of hypopituitarism, such as midline facial or eye abnormalities.

Diagnostic Studies. For primary hypothyroidism:

- The diagnosis of CH is usually made in infancy, detected by newborn screening tests. Newborn screening programs test filter paper blood spots using one of two screening strategies: (1) a primary TSH/backup T_4 method or (2) a primary T_4/backup TSH method to identify newborns with either primary or central hypothyroidism. When a result is abnormal, the primary care provider or hospital of record is contacted to obtain a confirmatory free T_4 and TSH serum sample. A serum sample is also indicated if clinical features of CH are detected. Infants born with Down syndrome are at higher risk for CH with males and females equally affected.
- In older children, TSH is abnormally elevated, whereas the free T_4 is either within the normal range or low.

TABLE 26-2 Thyroid Hormone Dosing

Age	Levothyroxine Sodium (L-Thyroxine) (mcg/kg/day)
0-3 months	10-15
3-6 months	8-10
6-12 months	6-8
1-5 years	5-6
6-12 years	4-5
>12 years	2-3

Data from Huang SA: Autoimmune thyroid disease. In Radovick S, MacGillivray MH, editors: *Pediatric endocrinology: a practical clinical guide*, ed 2, New York, 2013, Humana Press.

For central hypothyroidism:
- Free serum T_4 is low with a normal TSH.

For children with TBG deficiency:
- Total T_4 will be low, but free T_4 and TSH will be normal. TBG level should then be measured to confirm TBG deficiency.

Management
TBG does not require treatment. Hypothyroidism is treated with replacement doses of levothyroxine sodium. The dose varies by age and weight (Table 26-2). Ongoing laboratory monitoring and follow up are also age-dependent. Because normal thyroid function in the first 3 years of life is critical for normal cognitive development, more frequent monitoring is necessary for young infants and young children. Thyroid function testing is recommended every 2 to 4 weeks after starting treatment and then every month after TSH has normalized until the infant is 6 months old. From 6 months to 3 years old, the child should be tested every 1 to 2 months. For older children, the American Academy of Pediatrics (AAP) recommends testing every 6 to 12 months until growth is complete (Levitsky and Straussman, 2012). In general, an elevated TSH (in primary hypothyroidism) or depression of the free T_4 (in central hypothyroidism) indicates the need to increase the dose of medication. Following an adjustment in thyroid hormone replacement, thyroid function testing should be repeated in 4 weeks to be sure that the new dose is adequate.

Hyperthyroidism
Hyperthyroidism occurs in childhood when the thyroid gland overproduces thyroid hormone or when a child is given too large a dose of thyroid hormone replacement. Graves' disease, an autoimmune condition, is the most common cause of hyperthyroidism (Huang, 2013). In this condition, thyroid-stimulating immunoglobulin binds to the TSH receptor, resulting in excessive thyroid hormone production. Infants born to women with a current or past history of Graves' disease sometimes present with neonatal Graves' disease, secondary to passage of antibody from mother to fetus. Neonatal Graves' disease is self-limiting with dissipation of maternal antibodies by about 3 months old. Some children with Hashimoto's thyroiditis will have a short (6 to 18 months) phase of hyperthyroidism (Hashimoto's thyrotoxicosis) at the onset of disease. Other causes of hyperthyroidism (e.g., autonomous thyroid nodules) are less common.

Clinical Findings
History. The history of a child with hyperthyroidism may include:
- Palpitations
- Tremor
- Increased appetite often accompanied by weight loss
- Fatigue
- Muscle weakness
- Emotional lability
- Poor concentration with decreased school performance
- Hyperdefecation
- Poor sleep

Physical Examination. Often observed findings in hyperthyroidism include:
- Goiter (almost 100%)
- An audible thyroid bruit may be present
- Tachycardia
- Wide pulse pressure
- Underweight for height
- Eyelid lag or exophthalmos (approximately 50% of children with Graves' disease have exophthalmos)
- A hyperfunctioning nodule in the thyroid may be present
- Warm, moist skin
- Tremor or hyperreflexia

Diagnostic Studies. The free T_4 and total T_4 levels will be elevated and the TSH suppressed below the sensitivity of the assay. Measuring a T_3 level is helpful in hyperthyroidism because it may be more dramatically elevated than the T_4 and be a better marker to monitor.

Management
Children with hyperthyroidism should be referred to a pediatric endocrinologist for discussion of treatment options (i.e., medical therapy using antithyroid drugs, subtotal thyroidectomy or radioiodine) and ongoing management (Huang, 2013).

Diabetes Mellitus

Diabetes is the third most common chronic disease in childhood. Diabetes mellitus is a group of conditions characterized by inadequate insulin secretion, insulin resistance, or both. These dynamics lead to defective metabolism of carbohydrate, protein, and fat and subsequent hyperglycemia. Diabetes (type 1 or 2) affects approximately 208,000 individuals 20 years old or younger in the United States (Centers for Disease Control and Prevention [CDC], 2014) which is approximately 2.2 per 1000 American youth younger

BOX 26-9 Types of Diabetes

Type 1
Type 2
Genetic defects in β-cell function:
- MODY syndrome
- Mitochondrial DNA mutations
- Wolfram syndrome (diabetes insipidus, diabetes mellitus, optic atrophy, deafness)
- Thiamine responsive

Drug or chemical induced:
- Glucocorticoids
- L-asparaginase
- Antirejection medications

Conditions affecting function of the exocrine pancreas:
- Cystic fibrosis
- Pancreatitis
- Trauma
- HUS

Infections:
- Congenital rubella
- CMV

Genetic syndromes with diabetes:
- Prader-Willi
- Turner
- Alström
- Down

Neonatal diabetes

CMV, Cytomegalovirus; *DNA,* deoxyribonucleic acid; *HUS,* hemolytic uremic syndrome; *MODY,* maturity-onset diabetes of youth.

than 20 years of age (Pettitt et al, 2014). In addition to the most familiar forms—type 1 (formerly called *insulin-dependent diabetes mellitus* or *juvenile-onset diabetes*) and type 2 (formerly called *non–insulin-dependent diabetes mellitus* or *adult-onset diabetes*)—there are others (Box 26-9). Among youth, the majority (87%) have type 1 diabetes, 10.5% have type 2 diabetes, and 2.5% have other types (Pettitt et al, 2014). New cases are more frequently diagnosed during the autumn and winter months. The incidence of both type 1 and type 2 diabetes is increasing dramatically in children in the United States and other countries throughout the world (Gregory et al, 2013). Table 26-3 shows the distinguishing features of type 1 and type 2 diabetes.

Type 1 Diabetes

Type 1 diabetes is caused by autoimmune destruction of pancreatic beta cells in the islets of Langerhans thought to be triggered by a preceding environmental event in genetically susceptible individuals. This destruction of beta cells results in an absolute deficiency in insulin secretion, reduced biologic effectiveness, or both. Normal metabolic function depends upon sufficient amounts of circulating insulin. Insulin deficiency results in uninhibited gluconeogenesis and a blockage in the use and storage of circulating glucose. High blood glucose levels, therefore, are a result of the defective metabolism of carbohydrate, protein, and fats.

TABLE 26-3 Comparison of Type 1 and Type 2 Diabetes in Youth

	Type 1 Diabetes	Type 2 Diabetes
Age at onset	All ages	≥10 years old
Gender	Equal distribution by gender	More frequent in females
Race/ethnicity	Most frequent in non-Hispanic whites May occur in all racial and ethnic groups	More frequent in African Americans, Asians, Native Americans, Hispanics
Obesity	Similar to the general population; not related to type 1 diabetes	>90%
Family history of diabetes	5% to 10% have first-degree relative affected	About 80% have first-degree relative affected
Insulin secretion	Very low	Low, normal, or high
Insulin sensitivity	Normal	Decreased
Onset	Acute, severe	Subtle to severe
Ketosis, DKA	Approximately ⅓ of new cases	Uncommon
Hypertension	Uncommon	Common
Acanthosis nigricans	Rare	Common
Polycystic ovary syndrome	Rare	Common
Islet autoimmunity	Present	Uncommon

DKA, Diabetic ketoacidosis.

Based on 2009 data from the SEARCH for Diabetes in Youth study, 6666 of 3.4 million youth were diagnosed with type 1 diabetes, and 558 of 1.7 million youth were diagnosed with type 2 diabetes in the United States (Dabelea et al, 2014). When these data are compared with those from 2001 (Writing Group for the SEARCH for Diabetes in Youth Study Group, 2007), a 21% increase in diabetes was seen over 8 years; the greatest increase was observed in youth diagnosed with type 1 diabetes. Females and males were shown to be affected in equal numbers. The prevalence of type 1 diabetes varied by race and ethnicity and was highest among non-Hispanic white youth (2.55 per 1000 children). Native American children had a much lower prevalence of type 1 diabetes (0.35 per 1000 children), and only 32% of diabetes among Native American children was type 1. Although children were most often diagnosed during the time of puberty, and onset of symptoms can present at any age, the highest age specific increase occurred in youth from the ages of 15 to 19 years old and older (from 2.42 to 3.22 per 1000 children) (Dabelea et al, 2014).

Clinical Findings

Although the onset of type 1 diabetes is gradual with destruction of pancreatic islet cells over time, children may become ill quite suddenly once symptoms manifest. As diabetes develops, the symptomatology reflects the decreasing degree of beta cell mass, increasing insulinopenia and hyperglycemia, and increasing ketoacids.

History. With type 1 diabetes, the child may have had a viral infection, cold, or flu; parents may notice increased urination and thirst during the recovery period, with additional signs and symptoms appearing over a period of days or weeks. The following early symptoms are often reported:

- Polydipsia
- Polyphagia
- Polyuria
- Nocturia
- Blurred vision
- Weight loss or poor weight gain
- Fatigue
- Lethargy
- Vaginal moniliasis

As ketoacids accumulate, the following history is reported:

- Abdominal pain
- Nausea, vomiting
- Fruity-smelling breath
- Weakness (caused by dehydration)
- Mental confusion
- Coma

Approximately 25% of children with new-onset type 1 diabetes present in diabetic ketoacidosis (DKA). Younger age, ethnic minority status, lower socioeconomic status, and lower parent education levels are risk factors for presenting in DKA at diabetes onset; children younger than 2 years old are at the highest risk (Gregory et al, 2013).

Physical Examination. Although children typically have polyuria, polydipsia, and weight loss, the physical examination of children with new-onset type 1 diabetes may be remarkably benign. Findings can range from benign to severe and can include:

- Dehydration (child may not look clinically dehydrated unless actively vomiting)
- Weight loss or slow weight gain
- Muscle wasting
- Tachycardia
- Slow, labored breathing (Kussmaul breathing) (if ketotic)
- Flushed cheeks and face (if ketotic)
- Fruity-smelling breath (if ketotic)
- Vaginal yeast, thrush, or other infection

Diagnostic Studies. Urine testing and blood glucose measurements are generally all that are required to make the diagnosis:

- Urine for glucose and ketones
- Metabolic screen for acid-base status to exclude DKA
- Hemoglobin A_{1c} (HbA_{1c}) 6.5% or greater (American Diabetes Association [ADA], 2014): Ehehalt and colleagues (2010) found that all children with HbA_{1c} greater than 6.35% were subsequently diagnosed with type 1 diabetes, despite lack of other symptoms.
- Blood glucose:
  - Fasting plasma glucose 126 mg/dL or greater
  - Random plasma glucose 200 mg/dL or greater
  - Postprandial (2 hours after eating) plasma glucose 200 mg/dL or greater
- Screen for the presence of pancreatic autoantibodies: This should be considered to confirm the diagnosis of type 1 diabetes particularly in those cases where there may be uncertainty regarding type (Chiang et al, 2014).
- Screen for concomitant associated autoimmune conditions: About 25% of children with type 1 diabetes have thyroid autoantibodies present at the time of diagnosis, which is predictive of thyroid dysfunction. Hypothyroidism is more common. Celiac disease occurs more frequently in children with diabetes (1% to 16%) compared to children without diabetes (0.3% to 1%) (Chiang et al, 2014).

Capillary blood samples, reagent sticks, and glucose meters should only be used for monitoring diabetes control and not for diagnosing diabetes mellitus.

Screening for Type 1 Diabetes in Family Members

When someone in the family develops type 1 diabetes, other family members may be at risk. Families concerned about risk to other family members should be directed to the Type 1 Diabetes TrialNet website (www.diabetestrialnet.org) where screening can be obtained from 18 clinical centers or TrialNet network medical offices/physicians as part of an international clinical study. Children younger than 18 years old who test negative for the presence of antibodies associated with type 1 diabetes can be retested each year to determine if risk has changed. If antibodies are present, information will be provided regarding eligibility for participation in a diabetes prevention study.

Differential Diagnosis

Type 1 diabetes must be distinguished from stress-induced hyperglycemia, which in some studies occurs in up to 4% of normal children during a serious illness. Thyroiditis and/or celiac disease may be present at initial diagnosis of type 1 diabetes.

Management

The treatment goals for children with type 1 diabetes are to achieve normal growth and development, optimal glycemic control, and positive psychosocial adjustment to diabetes while minimizing acute or chronic complications. In 2014, the American Diabetes Association published a comprehensive position paper regarding the treatment goals of type 1 diabetes across the lifespan. Rather than base the glycemic goal on age, the new standard is to maintain a uniform glycemic level of HbA_{1c} less than 7.5% for all youth (Chiang et al, 2014). HbA_{1c} closely correlates with average blood glucose concentrations over the previous 3 months.

Diabetes treatment and education approaches for children and adolescents with type 1 diabetes are well defined and supported by strong evidence from the Diabetes Control and Complications Trial, a multi-center randomized controlled trial that demonstrated that glycemic control through use of intensive insulin management prevents and/or delays development of microvascular complications of diabetes (Diabetes Control and Complications Trial Research Group, 1993, 1994). Each year, the American Diabetes Association publishes and makes available on their website standards of care for the management of diabetes in children (see Resources on the Evolve Website).

Management of new-onset type 1 diabetes involves determining the insulin regimen and dose best suited to the individual child, target range for blood glucose levels, and best methods to manage the child's diet. Children and families must learn how to inject insulin, monitor blood glucose levels, quantify the amount of carbohydrates in food, prevent hypoglycemia, manage diabetes during illness, and adjust insulin dose or carbohydrate intake for strenuous activities. Diabetes education should be structured based on the child's age and developmental tasks, family management priorities, and family health literacy status. Beginning on or around 6 years old, the child should be incorporated into the educational experience (Chiang et al, 2014). These children and families need ongoing access to certified pediatric diabetes educators, pediatric dieticians, and psychologists or social workers when necessary. Each component of the treatment regimen is discussed in the following sections.

Initial Management. All children with type 1 diabetes should be started on insulin at diagnosis. Children with ketoacidosis should be admitted to the hospital for IV insulin treatment, fluid replacement, and careful monitoring to prevent cerebral edema that, although rare, can cause significant morbidity or mortality.

Whenever possible, children should be referred for ongoing care provided at a children's diabetes center for initiation of insulin therapy and diabetes education. Traditionally, most children with new-onset type 1 diabetes were hospitalized to initiate insulin therapy. However, current practice in many diabetes centers is to routinely manage children with new-onset diabetes as an outpatient unless DKA is present. Outpatient management at initial diagnosis of type 1 diabetes has no disadvantages regarding glycemic control, complications, psychosocial factors, or total costs.

Insulin. Insulin therapy choices are many. The selection of an insulin regimen depends on the age of the child, family preferences and lifestyle, the family's social and educational resources, and the clinician's comfort level. All children require medical nutrition therapy (MNT) that must match the insulin schedule. The most frequently used insulin preparations are listed in Table 26-4. For general guidelines regarding insulin dosing, goals for glycemic control, and blood glucose target ranges by age group, see Table 26-5.

To achieve glycemic targets, most youth with type 1 diabetes should be treated with an intensive basal bolus insulin regimen using either multiple daily injections (a long-active insulin analog combined with short-acting insulin analog administered prior to eating a meal or snack), or continuous subcutaneous insulin infusion (CSII) using

TABLE 26-4 Types of Insulin Analogs

Insulin	Onset	Peak	Duration
Rapid Acting			
Aspart (NovoLog)	10-15 min	1/2-1 h	3-4 h
Lispro (Humalog)	10-15 min	1/2-1 h	3-4 h
Glulisine (Apidra)	10-15 min	1/2-1 h	3-4 h
Long Acting			
Detemir (Levemir)	Slowly	6-8 h	6-24 h
Glargine (Lantus)	120-180 min	No peak	20-24 h

TABLE 26-5 Insulin Dosages (units/kg/day) and Glycated Hemoglobin Goals*

Age	Total Daily Insulin (units /kg/day)	Percentage Total Dosage as Basal Insulin	Glycated Hemoglobin (HbA_{1C}) Goal	Blood Glucose Before Meals	Blood Glucose Bedtime/ Overnight
0-5 years old	0.6-0.7	25%-30%	<7.5%	90-130 mg/dL	90-150 mg/dL
6-12 years old	0.7-1.0	40%-50%	<7.5%	90-130 mg/dL	90-150 mg/dL
13-19 years old	1.0-1.2	40%-50%	<7.5%	90-130 mg/dL	90-150 mg/dL

Adapted from American Diabetes Association (ADA): Standards of medical care in diabetes—2014, *Diabetes Care* 37(Suppl 1):S14–S80, 2014; Chiang JL, Kirkman MS, Laffel LM, et al: Type 1 diabetes through the life span: a position statement of the American Diabetes Association, *Diabetes Care* 37(7):2034–2054, 2014.

*Blood glucose goals should be modified in children with frequent hypoglycemia or hypoglycemia unawareness.

an insulin pump based on patient and family preferences. Multiple daily injection regimens can be implemented using a long-acting insulin analog administered at breakfast (infants and toddlers) or bedtime (teens) to provide a steady background amount of insulin with boluses of short-acting insulin at meal and snack times. This regimen allows unreliable eaters to match their carbohydrate intake with insulin; children may be flexible with the timing of meals and snacks. However, this regimen requires a minimum of four injections per day. Families learn to use a carbohydrate-to-insulin ratio (to cover the carbohydrate content of the meal/snack) and a blood sugar correction formula (if the blood glucose is above the target range) to determine each quick-acting insulin dose.

The usual sites for insulin injection are the legs, arms, abdomen, hips, and buttocks. School-age children and adolescents can be encouraged to use their abdomen as a regular injection site. However, young children with minimal subcutaneous abdominal fat may have difficulty with this site. Rotation of injection sites is necessary to prevent lipohypertrophy and poor absorption of insulin. Many of the insulin analogs are available in pen delivery systems.

CSII via an insulin pump is particularly useful for delivering small basal doses of insulin and varying the dose of basal insulin delivered over the 24-hour period. The pump infuses short-acting insulin into the subcutaneous tissue through a small, flexible, soft cannula. The cannula is replaced in a new site by the wearer or the family every 2 or 3 days. The pump is programmed to deliver small amounts of basal insulin on a continuous basis with the ability to tailor basal insulin delivery to the child's physiologic requirements over the 24-hour period. Bolus insulin at meals and snacks is calculated to cover the amount of carbohydrate eaten. The amount of insulin delivered in a bolus is tailored to be determined by the user and may be adjusted for level of activity and blood glucose level at the time of the meal or snack. Insulin pumps are not "automatic," require more work and deeper understanding of diabetes than subcutaneous injections, and put the child at risk for ketosis if the infusion catheter kinks or becomes obstructed or if the pump malfunctions. Use of insulin pumps is considered safe and efficacious even when used with young children and has become a popular way to deliver insulin in children with type 1 diabetes (Maahs et al, 2010).

After insulin treatment has been started, children may enter a "honeymoon period" during which insulin doses decrease. Close follow up—often daily phone calls—after beginning insulin therapy is necessary to prevent hypoglycemic episodes. Generally, insulin dose adjustments are based on the blood glucose patterns over several days. In general, the insulin dose would be decreased if any unexplained severe hypoglycemic events occur.

Monitoring Blood Glucose Levels. Children and families are taught to self-monitor blood glucose (SMBG) before meals, at bedtime, and sometimes in the middle of the night. Blood glucose meters have benefited from continued advances in technology; many blood glucose meters provide results within 5 seconds and automatically store and categorize blood glucose values by time of day or relation to meals. The continuous glucose monitor (CGM) is different from a traditional glucose meter in that it requires placement of a sensor in subcutaneous tissue where a sensor, transmitter, and receiver measures and reports both real-time interstitial glucose levels and directional trending graphs every few minutes. Alarms warn of low and high blood glucose levels, using individually determined preset blood glucose ranges. Recent research indicates that use of the CGM is effective in lowering HbA_{1c} and decreasing hypoglycemic episodes (Larson and Pinsker, 2013; Poolsup et al, 2013) but that children and adolescents are less likely than adults to continue its use (Juvenile Diabetes Research Foundation Continuous Glucose Monitoring Study Group, 2010). This may be due to anxiety and perceived burden of using the device, although most studies show satisfaction and improved glucose control (Hommel et al, 2014).

Adjusting Insulin Dosages. Parents and teens can be educated to make adjustments in insulin based on blood glucose patterns. They analyze what time of day the blood glucose is consistently outside of the target range (either too low or too high) and adjust the insulin dose that most directly is related to the problematic blood glucose pattern. Usually, parents can safely make up to a 10% adjustment to the basal or bolus insulin dose. With practice and guidance, many families eventually feel comfortable adjusting the insulin dose independently; others may feel more comfortable conferring with their diabetes care provider.

Initial management of new-onset diabetes also includes:

- At diagnosis, screening for hypothyroidism by thyroid peroxidase and thyroglobulin antibodies testing; annual screening thereafter
- At diagnosis, screening for celiac disease by measuring tissue transglutaminase or anti-endomysial antibodies; screening thereafter if growth failure, abdominal symptoms, or failure to gain weight/weight loss are present

Ongoing Management. Children with type 1 diabetes should be seen every 3 to 4 months with the visit tailored by age and developmental stage and careful attention paid to diabetes management including:

- Home glucose monitoring results
- Frequency of hypoglycemia
- HbA_{1c}
- Physical activities
- Emotional adjustment to the disease
- Social issues, such as peer pressure
- Eating issues: Young women with diabetes have an increased incidence of eating disorders, such as "diabulemia" in which insulin dosage is decreased in order to lose weight (Callum and Lewis, 2014).
- A physical examination that focuses on:
  - Growth and weight gain
  - Blood pressure
  - Stage of puberty
  - Injection site assessment for lipodystrophy

- Clues for other autoimmune disease (thyroiditis and celiac disease)

Ongoing management of type 1 diabetes also includes the following referrals and monitoring:

- Referral for a dilated and comprehensive ophthalmologic examination 3 to 5 years after diabetes onset in children 10 years old and older: The examination should then be repeated annually.
- Annual screening for microalbuminuria with random spot urine sample for microalbumin to creatinine ratio in children who have had diabetes for more than 5 years and are 10 years old and older
- Annual screening for hypothyroidism
- Lipid screening: Diabetes, types 1 or 2, is a known risk factor for atherosclerosis and early cardiovascular disease. Guidelines for lipid screening and treatment of dyslipidemia are consistent with those of the National Heart, Lung, and Blood Institute Expert Panel (Expert Panel on Integrated Guidelines for Cardiovascular Health and Risk Reduction in Children and Adolescents, 2011) and the American Diabetes Association (2014) and apply to youth with either type 1 or type 2 diabetes. For children 2 years old and older with a family history of hypercholesterolemia or early cardiovascular event, a fasting lipid profile should be obtained shortly after diabetes diagnosis when glycemic control has been established. For those children with negative family history, the first lipid screening should begin at 10 years old. If lipids are abnormal, Expert Panel guidelines (2011) should be implemented with annual or more frequent monitoring as indicated. If low-density lipoprotein (LDL) cholesterol values are less than 100 mg/dL, lipid profiles may be repeated every 5 years (ADA, 2014).
- Appropriate referrals for psychological counseling and nutritional review
- Collaboration with school nurses, teachers, and administrators to ensure treatment regimens are followed in the school or day care setting
- Continued well child health supervision and appropriate immunizations (e.g., annual influenza vaccination)

Medical Nutrition Therapy. Nutrition is an essential component of diabetes management. Diets should be healthy and daily calories spread over three meals and snacks. Caloric requirements are based on the child's age, body weight, and activity level. Calories are distributed between protein (15%), carbohydrates (55%), and fat (less than 30% of caloric intake with less than 7% in the form of saturated fats) and account for food preferences, including those pertinent to culture and ethnicity. The meal plan for a child with diabetes should include the same healthy foods that clinicians recommend to all pediatric patients. The goal is to balance food intake with insulin dose and activity to maintain blood glucose levels within the target range and to prevent both hyperglycemic and hypoglycemic episodes.

A pediatric dietician is essential to provide ongoing guidance to the child and family. Various approaches to nutrition therapy are being used. Carbohydrate counting is an approach that allows greater flexibility for children using basal bolus insulin regimens. Children with diabetes can safely eat sugary treats on occasion by including those treats within their prescribed carbohydrate allotment. Low calorie (e.g., saccharin, aspartame, sucralose, and acesulfame potassium) and reduced calorie (e.g., sorbitol and xylitol) sweeteners are safe in moderation. Fad diets are discouraged (ADA, 2014). Monitoring intake when eating out can be a challenge. Dieticians may help families identify effective computer applications that can be used to determine appropriate intake.

Exercise. Exercise is encouraged in all children, including those with diabetes, to promote cardiovascular fitness, control weight, and enhance social interaction and self-esteem. Children and adolescents with type 1 diabetes should not be excluded from participation in sports activities, including competitive sports. Any restrictions placed on an individual would only be necessary when optimal glycemic control cannot be maintained or if complications or comorbidities are not compatible with the activity. Youth with diabetes should follow the same physical activity guidelines as all children—striving for 60 minutes of physical activity daily (ADA, 2014).

Control of the child's blood glucose level during exercise, especially rigorous exercise such as athletic competition, is a challenge. It requires ongoing blood glucose monitoring (before, during, and after exercise), careful planning of meals and carbohydrates, snacks around the time of exercise, and adjustment of insulin dosing to counterbalance the effect of exercise on blood glucose levels.

During physical exercise, the body's oxygen and energy demands increase greatly. In order to meet these energy needs, there is increased uptake of glucose into the tissues, and blood glucose levels fall. Skeletal muscle also relies on stores of glycogen, triglycerides, free fatty acids, and glucose production, largely from the liver. For athletes without diabetes, hormonal mediators maintain normal blood glucose levels even under high athletic conditions. In these individuals, exercise leads to decreased plasma insulin levels and increased glucagon that trigger hepatic glucose production. However, in youth with type 1 diabetes, this hormonal pathway is interrupted. Thus, if the level of insulin is too low, exercise can trigger release of high levels of glucose and ketone bodies, leading to hyperglycemia and eventually, if unchecked, to DKA. Conversely, if too much exogenous insulin is administered, the feedback loop for increased glucose mobilization is interrupted and hypoglycemia results.

Therefore, children and families are taught to either decrease the insulin dose or take extra carbohydrates prior to exercise to compensate for this effect. With greater use of basal bolus regimens by either multiple daily injections or CSII via insulin pumps, the preferred adjustment is to decrease insulin dose prior to exercise (Gregory et al, 2013). Because exercise may affect blood glucose levels for as long as 24 hours after exercise has occurred, parents need to be aware of the risk of nocturnal hypoglycemia on active days and monitor blood glucose levels more frequently.

It is generally recommended that athletes with type 1 diabetes have a medical team participating in their health care. This team ideally includes an endocrinologist and nutritionist who specialize in diabetes and are familiar with the energy requirements of the individual's sport. Depending on the level of athletic endeavor, a trainer may also be part of the team.

It is essential that coaches, trainers, or other athletic staff be aware of the young athlete's diabetes care plan and be trained in aspects of care. Specific recommendations are outlined in Box 13-7.

Complications

Morbidity and mortality in type 1 diabetes come from metabolic derangements and from long-term complications that affect the small and large blood vessels. Chronic high blood glucose levels have been shown to cause the long-term complications of microvascular disease (retinopathy, nephropathy, neuropathy, depression, and cognitive defects) and macrovascular disease (arterial obstruction with gangrene of extremities and ischemic heart disease). These complications can be prevented or their rate of progression slowed by improving glycemic control through use of intensive insulin regimens consisting of multiple daily injections or CSII. Screening for nephropathy, retinopathy, and neuropathy should begin when the youth with type 1 diabetes is 10 years old and has had diabetes for 3 to 5 years (Gregory et al, 2013).

Patient and Family Education

Providing families and children with information that helps them gain control of a very difficult disease is crucial. The National Diabetes Education Program offers education materials specifically targeted to both type 1 and type 2 diabetes (see Resources on the Evolve Website). Education of the child, family, and caregivers should include insulin therapy, self-monitoring of glucose, nutrition and meal planning (including carbohydrate counting), exercise, managing sick days, school issues, coping skills, and prevention of complications. Those with diabetes should always wear a form of medical identification. School personnel must be informed of the plan of care and must implement an individualized care plan for the child.

Type 2 Diabetes

The prevalence of type 2 diabetes in youth 10 to 19 years old is 0.46 per 1000 youth. Notably, the prevalence of type 2 diabetes has increased by approximately 30% over the period from 2001 to 2009. These estimates suggest that the number of youth diagnosed with type 2 diabetes will nearly quadruple by 2050 (Dabelea et al, 2014). Type 2 diabetes in youth accounts for up to 11% of all new total diabetes cases among children in the United States. Prevalence is highest among Native American youth; in 2009, 64% of all cases of diabetes were type 2 in this racial ethnic group. Type 2 diabetes is least common among non-Hispanic whites (Dabelea et al, 2014). The overall prevalence rates may be underreported, especially because children may have no symptoms or mild symptoms for a long period of time. Children usually are diagnosed during the teenage years, between 10 and 19 years old.

Clearly, type 2 diabetes in youth is a serious and growing public health problem. Type 2 diabetes begins with increased tissue resistance to insulin, resulting in hyperinsulinemia and hyperglycemia. Although pancreatic beta cells initially produce insulin, hyperglycemia creates an increased insulin demand; with increasing demand for insulin over time, the pancreas loses its ability to effectively secrete insulin. Autoimmune destruction of pancreatic beta cells does not typically occur. During puberty, GH secretion as part of the pubertal growth spurt further increases resistance to insulin action for those predisposed to type 2 diabetes. Adolescents with normally functioning pancreatic beta cells secrete additional insulin to compensate for this puberty-related effect. However, when beta cells do not function properly, metabolic decompensation begins and leads to a state of prediabetes (impaired fasting glucose and/or impaired glucose tolerance) with eventual progression to type 2 diabetes (Dileepan and Feldt, 2013).

Type 2 diabetes is strongly associated with environmental factors, such as obesity, sedentary lifestyles, and high-caloric lipid-rich foods. Children born to a mother with gestational diabetes, who are small for gestational age at birth (sign of intrauterine undernutrition), and those who are overweight and/or obese or have a family history of type 2 diabetes are at increased risk for type 2 diabetes (Dilleepan and Feldt, 2013).

Clinical Findings

Screening Guidelines. The symptoms of type 2 diabetes may be absent or subtle, so children at risk should be screened. The American Diabetes Association (2014) and American Academy of Pediatrics (Copeland et al, 2013) provide guidelines for screening children at risk:

- Screen if overweight (BMI is greater than 85th percentile for age and gender, or weight is greater than 120% of ideal weight), plus any two of following risk factors:
  - Family history of type 2 diabetes in first- or second-degree relative
  - Race/ethnicity (Native American, African American, Latino, Asian American, Pacific Islander)
  - Signs of insulin resistance or conditions associated with insulin resistance (e.g., acanthosis nigricans, polycystic ovary syndrome, hypertension, dyslipidemia)
  - Maternal history of diabetes or gestational diabetes during pregnancy with this child
- Screen every 3 years.
- Use fasting plasma glucose test following diagnostic criteria for diabetes discussed earlier.
- Use clinical judgment to screen for type 2 diabetes in high-risk patients who do not meet these guidelines.

History. The history of patients with type 2 diabetes may include:

- Polydipsia
- Polyphagia
- Polyuria
- Nocturia or bedwetting
- Blurred vision
- Obesity, especially central
- Report of a hyperpigmented, velvet-like rash in skin folds
- Frequent or slow-healing infections
- Fatigue
- History of premature adrenarche
- Symptoms of sleep apnea
- Family history of type 2 diabetes

Physical Examination. The physical examination should include assessment of height, weight, stage of pubertal development, and blood pressure. The following findings may be present:

- Dehydration
- Overweight (BMI greater than 85th percentile for age and gender) or obesity
- Weight loss (less common)
- Acanthosis nigricans noted in the axilla, base of the neck, groin, knuckles, and other skin folds
- Vaginal yeast, thrush, other infection
- Polycystic ovary syndrome symptoms (e.g., acne, hirsutism)
- Hypertension

Diagnostic Studies. Screening should be conducted in high-risk children without symptoms (see earlier Screening Guidelines) and should include (ADA, 2014):

- Urine for glucose and albumin (can be performed in the office)
- Children can have ketoacidosis if they have gone undiagnosed for a long time
- Fasting blood sample for blood glucose, HbA_{1c}, lipid panel, TSH and free T_4, and insulin level

Diagnosis is made if the following exist:

- Random plasma glucose concentration 200 mg/dL (11.1 mmol/L) or greater
- Fasting plasma glucose 126 mg/dL (7 mmol/L) or greater
- Postprandial (2 hours after eating) plasma glucose 200 mg/dL (11.1 mmol/L) or greater
- HbA_{1c} 6.5% or greater

Differential Diagnosis

Some obese children have type 1 diabetes and may be misdiagnosed as type 2. The presentation of type 1 diabetes can be of slower onset in older children and adults. Maturity-onset diabetes of youth (MODY) is a group of autosomal dominant, single gene disorders that may clinically resemble type 2 diabetes. MODY is characterized by impaired insulin secretion without significant defects in the action of insulin. To date, six genetic loci on different chromosomes have been identified as being related with MODY (ADA, 2014). On average, children with MODY are younger, less likely to be overweight or obese, and less likely to be from an ethnic minority group compared to children presenting with new-onset type 2 diabetes.

Management

Treatment of type 2 diabetes in youth remains in its infancy and currently lacks the strong evidence base of type 1 diabetes. The primary treatment for children and adolescents with type 2 diabetes is education and lifestyle modification, particularly improvement of nutritional practices and physical activity behaviors leading to weight loss. In the United States, however, fewer than 10% of children with type 2 diabetes are successful in achieving glycemic control with diet and exercise alone. If lifestyle changes are not successful in normalizing blood glucose levels, pharmacologic agents should be added to the treatment regimen.

As with type 1 diabetes, the treatment plan for children with type 2 diabetes must be individualized. The treatment goal is the normalization of blood glucose values:

- HbA_{1c} less than or equal to 7%
  - Daily self-monitoring by the child: If the child is treated with multiple insulin injections or continuous pump therapy, check levels three or more times each day; for those on less frequent insulin injections, oral medication or MNT alone, a daily check may be adequate.
  - Monitor every 3 months in clinic and intensify treatment if the goal is not met.
  - Monitor in clinic every 3 to 6 months if glycemic goal is met and maintained.
  - Occasional monitoring of post-prandial blood glucose levels (Copeland et al, 2013).
- LDL less than 100 mg/dL
- High-density lipoprotein (HDL) greater than 45 mg/dL
- Triglycerides less than 125 mg/dL

Successful control of the associated complications, such as hypertension and hyperlipidemia, is important.

Ongoing management strategies include the following:

- Annual dilated and comprehensive eye examination to monitor for microvascular changes (e.g., retinopathy, nephropathy)
- Annual urine test for microalbumin
- HbA_{1C} and plasma glucose levels monitored every 3 to 4 months for those whose therapy has changed or who are not meeting glycemic goals: Children who are meeting goals and have stable glycemic control can be monitored every 6 months.
- Follow up every 3 to 4 months on lifestyle, nutrition, and other complications of obesity, discussed in more detail later.

Lifestyle Changes: Nutrition and Exercise. When discovered early, type 2 diabetes may respond to lifestyle changes, such as alterations in diet and exercise. These changes must be comprehensive and family based. MNT is an important part of the treatment plan. Referral to a registered pediatric dietician is essential, with the goals of weight loss and regulating nutritional intake. A low-fat diet, self-monitoring of weight, and being physically active are important components of MNT. Successful weight management may consist of weight maintenance rather than weight loss depending on the child's age and BMI. Changes in family eating patterns can contribute to weight maintenance or loss that may normalize insulin levels. Nutrition counseling should be provided both at the time of diagnosis of type 2 diabetes and as part of ongoing clinical management and should be consistent with guidelines of the Academy of Nutrition and Dietetics (see Chapter 13).

Inactivity and the increasing obesity epidemic are directly related to the escalating incidence of type 2 diabetes in young people. Physical activity is not only one of the major type 2 diabetes prevention messages, but it is also a critical component in treatment. Youth with type 2 diabetes should be strongly encouraged to be physically active by participating in sports and regular exercise. Daily vigorous exercise (30 to 60 minutes a day) helps control weight and even modest weight loss has been shown to reduce insulin resistance (ADA, 2014).

Overweight or obese youth may initially be in poor physical condition with regard to sports endurance. Therefore, activity and exercise plans should allow for a gradual and safe buildup in intensity and length. A nutritionist can be helpful in ensuring adequate calories for performance needs as well as for safe weight loss. Overweight or obese adolescents may lack self-esteem or motivation to participate in school sports activities but may be willing to walk as a form of exercise. Use of pedometers has been effective in improving physical activity levels in adolescents, particularly when individualized behavioral goals are set (Philpott et al, 2010). Wireless applications to monitor activity, caloric expenditure, heart rate, and fitness are gaining popularity.

The benefits of regular physical exercise for youth with type 2 diabetes include increased insulin effectiveness due to improving insulin-receptor sensitivity, weight control, reduced risk of cardiovascular disease, reduced dyslipidemia risk, and improved self-confidence and self-esteem. Glycemic control during exercise is generally not difficult to maintain. In addition to weight loss, regular physical activity of moderate to strenuous level improves body composition; further, both aerobic and resistance training increase insulin sensitivity, thereby fostering improved glycemic control (Bremer, 2012). For adolescents who are taking oral hypoglycemic medication or insulin for type 2 diabetes, the benefits of improved insulin sensitivity through regular exercise participation may enable them to reduce medication.

Pharmacotherapy. Little research has been done on the use of hypoglycemic agents in children. The Treatment Options for Type 2 Diabetes in Adolescents and Youth (TODAY) study compared the effectiveness of three treatment options for type 2 diabetes in youth 10 to 17 years old: (1) metformin, (2) metformin plus rosiglitazone, and (3) metformin plus an intensive behavioral intervention. The study found that glycemic control (defined as HbA_{1c} greater than or equal to 8% for 6 months or need for ongoing insulin therapy) was not maintained for almost half of the study's subjects with any of the three treatments. Of the three treatment arms, rosiglitazone plus metformin was the most successful, yet 39% of subjects assigned to that group had treatment failure (TODAY Study Group, 2012). The implications for long-term health complications related to type 2 diabetes in youth are significant (Narasimhan and Weinstock, 2014).

Metformin is the only oral agent approved by the FDA for use in children with type 2 diabetes and, although rosiglitazone is used in combination with metformin in adults, the FDA has found insufficient evidence to approve it for pediatric use. Most children are begun on metformin in doses up to 1000 mg twice a day. Metformin rarely causes hypoglycemia, so blood glucose need only be checked before breakfast and 2 hours after dinner. Mild gastrointestinal side effects may occur with metformin use but are usually self-limiting. Metformin users can experience vitamin B_{12} deficiency probably secondary to malabsorption, especially with higher doses and longer use. Providers should counsel youth taking metformin to increase foods high in vitamin B_{12}; they should also have a high suspicion of vitamin B_{12} deficiency if clinical signs appear. Although there is no consensus on requiring laboratory testing, youth taking metformin, especially long-term users, should probably be assessed regularly for vitamin B_{12} deficits and high homocysteine levels (de Jager et al, 2010). Should the youth fail to respond to metformin, a combination of two oral agents may be employed (Table 26-6).

When a child or adolescent with type 2 diabetes has ketonuria or is in DKA, insulin therapy will be needed initially. These children need to be started on the same insulin regimen with home glucose monitoring and a precise food plan as those with type 1 diabetes. Typically, the insulin needs are higher than in children with type 1 diabetes because of insulin resistance. Following stabilization of blood glucose levels, it may be possible to gradually wean the insulin and begin metformin. Over time, the natural course of type 2 diabetes can result in the body's inability to produce sufficient endogenous insulin, making treatment with oral agents ineffective. If this occurs, insulin replacement using long- and/or short-acting insulin will be necessary.

Medication may also be needed to control hypertension (see Chapter 31) and dyslipidemia (discussed later in this chapter), which are two frequent comorbidities of type 2 diabetes in youth.

Complications

Complications of type 2 diabetes are similar to those of type 1 diabetes (micro- and macrovascular diseases). Nephropathy is a more common complication in those with type 2 than type 1 diabetes. Nonalcoholic fatty liver disease and eventual dependence upon insulin for control can occur.

Patient and Family Education

The same education needs apply to children with type 1 and type 2 diabetes: information about the nature of the disease;

TABLE 26-6 Medications Used in Treatment of Type 2 Diabetes Mellitus

Drug	Action/Comments
Biguanides* (metformin [Glucophage, Glucophage XR])	Decreases the amount of sugar produced by the liver; increases insulin sensitivity of the liver and muscles. No direct effect on β-cells in pancreas. Used as first-line monotherapy.
Sulfonylureas (glimepiride [Amaryl], glyburide [DiaBeta, Micronase, Glynase PresTab])	Stimulates β-cells to make more insulin; may make body tissue more sensitive to insulin. Side effects include weight gain, hypoglycemia; no effect on lipids; possible liver toxicity. Not approved for use in children. Used as second-line therapy in combination with thiazolidinediones
Thiazolidinediones (rosiglitazone [Avandia]†, pioglitazone [Actos])	Increases insulin sensitivity at the cellular level; improves glucose usage. Side effects include weight gain; unknown if may cause edema and congestive heart failure in children. Not approved for use in children.
Meglitinides (repaglinide [Prandin])	Stimulates β-cells; no known effect on insulin sensitivity.
Glucosidase inhibitors (acarbose [Precose], miglitol [Glyset])	Slows down the conversion of ingested carbohydrates to sugar in the intestine. Side effects primarily GI distress.
Incretins (exenatide [Byetta Prefilled Pen])‡	Increases postprandial insulin secretion.

GI, Gastrointestinal.
*Approved by the U.S. Food and Drug Administration (FDA) for use in children.
†FDA has issued safety warning for rosiglitazone (Avandia).
‡Administered as injection twice daily.

strategies and techniques to manage the physical disease (e.g., medication, insulin, nutrition, exercise); networks, support, and skills to cope with emotional and psychological issues; collaboration with school personnel; and wearing a form of medical identification. The National Diabetes Education Program is an invaluable resource for both providers and children and their families (see Resources on the Evolve Website).

Obesity

The prevalence of obesity has dramatically increased in children and adults around the world. Obesity in childhood is defined as a BMI greater than or equal to the 95th percentile for age. Approximately 17% of youth meet this definition (Ogden et al, 2014). A more detailed discussion of obesity is found in Chapter 13.

In most children, overweight and obesity are thought to be due to an imbalance between calories consumed and calories burned. From an endocrine perspective, the mechanisms of weight homeostasis are complex and involve hypothalamic hormones, hormones produced by adipocytes (e.g., leptin), and the gut (e.g., ghrelin). In most children, hormone deficiency or excess does not explain obesity. Although several "classic" hormonal imbalances (such as, hypothyroidism, cortisol excess, and GHD) may be associated with overweight or obesity, the child with these endocrine conditions is likely to be either of short stature or growing at a subnormal growth velocity. Several genetic conditions predispose children to being overweight (e.g., Prader-Willi syndrome). Developmental delay and dysmorphic features are key to identifying these conditions.

Diagnostic Studies

Children with a BMI greater than 85th percentile for age and gender should be screened for a number of conditions:

- Abnormalities in glucose tolerance with a fasting glucose and/or an oral glucose tolerance test
- Nonalcoholic steatohepatitis with liver enzyme tests of aspartate aminotransferase (AST) and alanine amino transferase (ALT)
- Dyslipidemia with a fasting lipid panel
- Thyroid function with a thyroid panel
- Sleep apnea by history of snoring, daytime somnolence
- Polycystic ovary syndrome with a free and total testosterone level (if symptomatic with irregular menses, acne, or hirsutism)
- Hypertension with a blood pressure measurement
- Orthopedic issues by history (e.g., slipped capital femoral epiphysis)
- Psychological issues by history (Some children with obesity suffer from low self-esteem, behavior problems, or depression.)

Management

Children with type 2 diabetes, polycystic ovary syndrome, or other metabolic or endocrine disorders associated with obesity should be followed in concert with a pediatric endocrinologist. Those with obesity alone are more effectively treated in the primary care office with nutritional counseling and ongoing support to achieve a more active lifestyle (Nieman and McKnight, 2010). In general, the goal is weight maintenance, not loss, in the overweight child without any of the aforementioned complications; it is expected that these children will eventually grow into their weight and achieve a BMI less than the 85th percentile. For children with an overweight-related complication, weight loss of 1 pound per month would be an appropriate goal; more rapid weight loss in children who have not yet reached their growth potential may be associated with slowing in linear growth.

Consensus is lacking as to the most effective way to manage obesity. Goals for reducing calories consumed and increasing daily exercise must be made within the context of each family; success is more likely to be achieved if the entire family participates in lifestyle changes. Providers must work closely with families to ensure consistent follow-up, to assess the effectiveness of interventions, and to modify the treatment strategy if necessary (see Chapter 10).

Posterior Pituitary Gland Disorders

Abnormal posterior pituitary function is uncommon in pediatrics. Children with inappropriately dilute urine for the clinical situation may only be identified when they develop hypernatremic dehydration, secondary enuresis, or polyuria. They may also be discovered in an evaluation of a child at risk for hypopituitarism. If a screening of first morning urine shows low specific gravity in the absence of urinary glucose, a pediatric endocrinologist should be consulted.

Introduction to Inborn Errors of Metabolism

Inborn errors of metabolism (IEM) encompass a wide range of inherited disorders with alterations of specific biochemical reactions. The term "inborn error of metabolism" was coined by Garrod in 1908 to describe the hereditary alteration in enzyme reactions that he observed in the first identified "inborn error," alkaptonuria, and use of the term has persisted.

Although individually rare, IEM have a collective incidence of approximately 1 in 700 to 800 live births (CDC, 2012), and all health care providers will likely encounter a child with an IEM at some point in their career. Clinical consequences for the affected individual vary from mild to severe. Early detection, accurate diagnosis, and rapid intervention are necessary to achieve favorable outcomes; prevent irreversible intellectual disability, physical disability, neurologic damage, or death; and reduce long-term financial burden and human suffering. This section discusses the classification and pathophysiology of IEM; overviews newborn screening, including common clinical presentations and emergency management of conditions found in the newborn period; and presents a brief overview of the diagnosis and treatment of a few more common disorders.

Classification of Inborn Errors of Metabolism

Classification of IEM presents a challenge because of the number and diversity of disorders. Proposed classification systems have suggested categorizing based on affected organ (e.g., neurologic or hepatic diseases), cellular organelle (e.g., mitochondrial or lysosomal disorders), age of presentation (e.g., neonatal or adult onset), large or small molecule diseases, or affected metabolic pathway (e.g., urea cycle defects [UCDs] or defects of amino acid metabolism) (Box 26-10).

Pathophysiology

Most metabolic disorders are caused by an inherited defect, generally of a single enzyme or its cofactor, resulting in altered function of a metabolic pathway. Autosomal recessive inheritance patterns are most common.

Figure 26-3 provides an overview of the major metabolic pathways. The majority of defects are caused by a single gene mutation encoding a specific enzyme whose function is to facilitate the conversion of various substances (substrates, [e.g., foodstuffs]) into others (metabolic products, [e.g., urea]). The block in the pathway variably leads to accumulation of substrate proximal to the block (e.g., lyosomal storage disorders); accumulation of toxic metabolites (e.g., galactose byproducts in galactosemia); deficiency of a product distal to the block (e.g., tyrosine in PKU); feedback inhibition or activation by the metabolite; or some combination thereof. Loss of enzyme function varies by degree, altering the clinical phenotype, the clinical course, and the response to treatment among individuals with the same diagnosis.

Assessment of Inborn Errors of Metabolism

IEM are rare but should be included in the differential diagnosis of any critically ill neonate, as well as infants, children, adolescents, and adults presenting with symptoms that are progressive or otherwise unexplained. The timing of symptom onset in relation to initiation of feedings can be an important clue. Infants with IEM commonly appear normal at birth with effects of the disease becoming apparent over the course of days to months. As substrates or toxic metabolites accumulate, such as in organic acidemias, nonspecific symptoms that may be indistinguishable from sepsis typically appear. Finding a cause of symptoms, however, does not necessarily rule out the possibility of an IEM (e.g., electrolyte abnormalities diagnosed as renal Fanconi syndrome may be caused by underlying cystinosis).

• BOX 26-10 Classification of Inborn Errors of Metabolism with Partial List of Disorders

Amino Acid Disorders

MSUD
PKU
Tyrosinemia
Homocystinuria

Organic Acidemias

Propionic acidemia
Methylmalonic acidemia

Urea Cycle Disorders

Ornithine transcarbamylase deficiency
Citrullinemia

Carbohydrate Disorders

Galactosemia
Glycogen storage disease
Hereditary fructose intolerance

Fatty Acid Oxidation Disorders

MCAD
VLCAD
LCHAD

Mitochondrial Disorders

Leigh disease
MNGIE syndrome
Pearson syndrome

Peroxisomal Disorders

Zellweger syndrome
Adrenoleukodystrophy
Infantile Refsum disease

Lysosomal Storage Disorders

Hurler syndrome
Fabry disease
Gaucher disease
Niemann-Pick disease

Purine and Pyrimidine Disorders

Lesch-Nyhan disease
Hereditary orotic aciduria

Metal Metabolism Disorder

Wilson disease

LCHAD, Long-chain 3-hydroxyacyl-coenzyme A dehydrogenase deficiency; *MCAD,* medium-chain acyl-coenzyme A dehydrogenase deficiency; *MNGIE,* mitochondrial neurogastrointestinal encephalopathy; *MSUD,* maple syrup urine disease; *PKU,* phenylketonuria; *VLCAD,* very long-chain acyl-coenzyme A dehydrogenase deficiency.

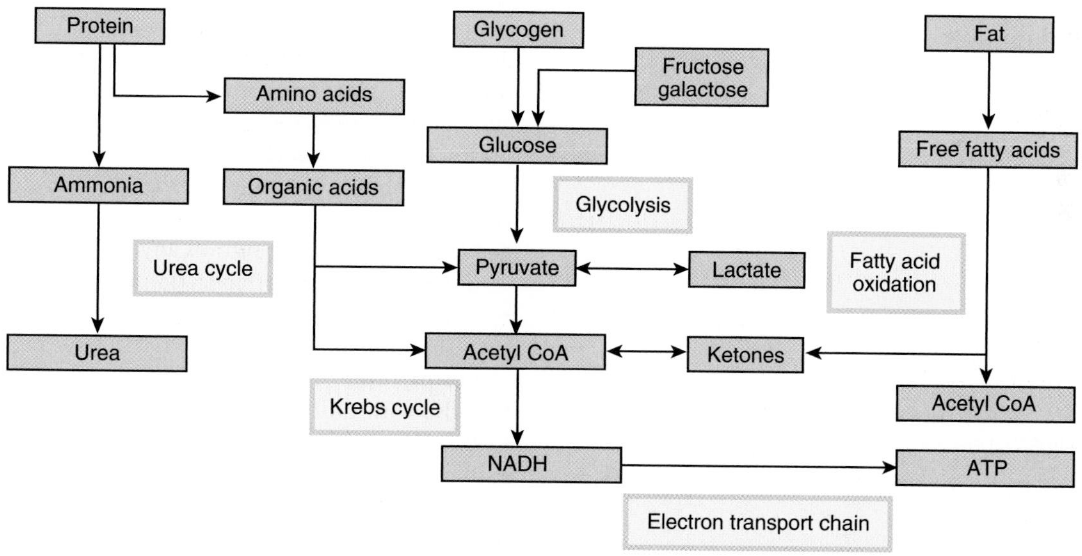

• Figure 26-3 Overview of major metabolic pathways. *Acetyl CoA,* Acetyl coenzyme A; *ATP,* adenosine triphosphate; *NADH,* nicotinamide adenine dinucleotide. (From Logan A: Metabolic disease. In Cheng A, Williams BA, Sivarajan VB, editors: *The hospital for sick children handbook of pediatrics*, ed 10, Toronto, 2004, Saunders Canada, p 474.)

Clinical Findings

History

A thorough family and individual history is important to identify possibilities of IEM. Details in a family and patient history that should raise suspicion include:

- Consanguinity
- Decompensation when ill greater than anticipated for the nature of the illness (commonly seen in acidosis)
- Developmental delay, psychomotor retardation, or loss of milestones
- Failure to thrive
- Family history of IEM
- Siblings with unexplained infant or neonatal death
- Symptoms concurrent with a change in diet
- Unusual odor (sweat, urine, or cerumen)

Physical Examination

A complete examination is essential, with attention to dysmorphia, muscle tone, ocular symptoms, organomegaly, and respiratory function. Box 26-11 provides an overview of symptoms suspicious for an inborn error at various ages.

• BOX 26-11 Signs/Symptoms Suggesting an Inborn Error of Metabolism in Children by Age

Neonates and Infants

Abnormal neurologic examination
Acidosis
Cardiomyopathy
Coagulopathy
Coarse facial features
Dysmorphic features
Hyperammonemia
Hypotonia or hypertonia
Jaundice
Metabolic acidosis
Neutropenia and/or thrombocytopenia
Ocular findings (retinitis pigmentosa, cherry red spots, cataracts or corneal clouding)
Organomegaly
Respiratory distress (apnea or tachypnea)
Seizures
Unexplained hypoglycemia
Vomiting
Xanthomas

Older Children and Adolescents (in Addition to Those of Neonates and Infants)

Ataxia
Dementia
Dystonia or chorea
Intellectual disability
Muscular weakness
Ophthalmoplegia
Progressive deterioration
Skeletal changes

Diagnostic Studies

Effective intervention for IEM depends on the ability to identify the disorder before the onset of symptoms. Screening for the presence of IEM allows the provider to identify the condition and, if possible, begin treatment before damage has occurred. Not all IEMs are amenable to treatment, however, and in some cases supportive or palliative care may be the only option. The capability to screen for IEM dates to the early 1960s when an inexpensive test for PKU using a small blood sample collected on a filter paper was developed (Guthrie and Susi, 1963). Four hundred thousand newborns in 29 states were part of a pilot study that confirmed the effectiveness of this test to detect PKU. As a result, states instituted screening programs for newborn infants, and today, virtually all of the millions of infants born each year in the United States are screened (see Chapter 39).

Technologic advances have allowed for screening a wide array of disorders, and the newborn screening test encompasses much more than screening for PKU. Laboratory studies are generally necessary in the diagnosis of IEM; however, determining what studies to perform may not always be straightforward. Testing for common (i.e., nonmetabolic) causes of presenting symptoms should not be sacrificed for metabolic testing, but it is not always wise to wait until all routine tests have been performed and the results known before submitting samples for metabolic disease testing. This additional step facilitates work-up should the patient be referred to a metabolic specialist. When the ill child has signs and symptoms of what could be an IEM, the primary care provider should consult immediately with a metabolic specialist, rather than wait for results of tests. For chronic presentations, after common etiologies are ruled out, refer to a metabolic specialist for testing beyond routine analysis.

Initial laboratory studies for the neonate with a suspected IEM include:

- Newborn screening test on any significantly ill neonate, unless proof of prior collection is obtained
- A second newborn screening test at 10 to 14 days of age if the ill neonate was discharged early (before 24 hours postpartum)
- CBC with differential
- Blood glucose
- Blood urea nitrogen (BUN) and creatinine
- ALT, AST, bilirubin
- Coagulation studies
- Blood gases
- Serum electrolytes with special attention to anion gap = $Na^+ - (Cl^- + HCO^-_3)$: Normal anion gap is between 8 to 12 mEq/L
- Plasma ammonia: Collected free flowing (no tourniquet, no heel stick, preferably no capillary tubes) immediately placed on ice and analyzed within 45 to 60 minutes
- Plasma lactate: Collected free flowing
- Creatine kinase
- Plasma quantitative amino acids; plasma acylcarnitine profile, and plasma carnitine levels

- Urinalysis
- Urine reducing substances, ketones (if acidotic and hypoglycemic), organic acids, and mucopolysaccharides and oligosaccharides if storage disease is suspected

Some labs offer a metabolic screening panel, typically on urine, but some labs prefer urine and blood. Metabolic panels vary between laboratories. Testing may also consist of biochemical or molecular (DNA) analysis obtained from blood. Other more invasive tests may be needed, including cerebral spinal fluid (lactate, amino acids, glucose) or biopsy from skin, liver, or muscle (enzyme assays). Additionally, for the child with chronic encephalopathy, consider an MRI and magnetic resonance spectroscopy (MRS) for brain imaging. Familiarity with the appropriate methods of specimen collection and handling (before and during shipment of the samples to the laboratory) is important, because inappropriate practices alter the quality of the sample, potentially leading to unreliable results and missed cases.

Management

Management of metabolic disorders varies depending on the specific condition, its severity, and whether it is an acute or chronic presentation. Caregivers of children with a known diagnosis of inborn errors (e.g., those that cause hyperammonemia) become very astute at early recognition of symptoms in their child and should be viewed as crucial partners in the health care team.

Metabolic Emergencies

Emergency management of many metabolic disorders requires hospital admission and specialist care. The goal of emergency management is twofold: (1) prevent catabolism and (2) remove toxic substrates or metabolites. Aggressive management is necessary to avert or reduce neurologic sequelae. This acute care management may require IV medications (including glucose to halt catabolism), diet restriction (e.g., no protein for 24 to 48 hours or until mental status is back to baseline), hemodialysis, or life support.

Stable Metabolic Disorders

The variability of IEM requires individual management tailored to the patient's specific diagnosis and phenotype. However, the following strategies provide several broad categories from which treatments are drawn:

- Control substrate accumulation:
  - Restrict dietary intake (e.g., restricting phenylalanine intake in PKU).
  - Control endogenous production of the substrate (e.g., give high-calorie, no-protein feeds during illness to prevent catabolism, which would release amino acids).
  - Accelerate removal of the substrate (e.g., administer sodium benzoate/phenylacetate in urea cycle disorders [UCDs] to increase elimination of waste nitrogen through an alternate pathway).
- Dietary supplementation:
  - Replace or supplement the diet with products that become deficient distal to the metabolic block or if the diet is medically restricted (e.g., arginine or citrulline in UCD).
- Vitamin and cofactor replacement:
  - Increase the supply of certain vitamins or medications (e.g., Sapropterin dihydrochloride) that act as cofactors to metabolic reactions to improve function of the residual enzyme activity. Vitamin replacement is also important with severely restricted diets.
- Enzyme replacement therapy (ERT):
  - ERT (an IV infusion of enzyme replacement given every 1 to 2 weeks) is becoming widely available in the clinical setting for lysosomal storage diseases.
- Bone marrow or organ transplant:
  - Stem cell transplantation using exogenous bone marrow or cord blood as a donor site is clinically available for some disorders, but it is in early stages of widespread clinical use (Prasad and Kurtzberg, 2010).
  - Organ transplant can essentially "cure" some metabolic diseases by transplanting an organ in which the mutant genes are expressed. Liver transplantation has shown success in some IEM (Moini et al, 2010).

Complications

Multiple complications such as renal failure, hypertension, spinal cord compression, and carpal tunnel syndrome may be seen with IEM, often necessitating a multidisciplinary management team.

Specific Metabolic Disorders of Children

Disorders of Carbohydrate Metabolism

This group of disorders is caused by the inability to metabolize the monosaccharides (glucose, galactose, and fructose) and the polysaccharide glycogen. Aberrant glycogen synthesis or disorders of gluconeogenesis also contribute to faulty carbohydrate metabolism.

Glycogen Storage Diseases

Glycogen is a glucose polymer stored in muscle and the liver, and deficiency of any enzyme involved in the metabolic pathway of glycogen can affect biosynthesis or degradation of glycogen in the organ in which the enzyme is expressed. This deficiency results in a variety of presentations of disease. Glucose-6-phosphatase or translocase deficiency (type I), debrancher enzyme deficiency (type III), and liver phosphorylase kinase deficiency (type IX) are the most common early childhood presentations. Overall frequency of all forms is 1:20,000 to 45,000 live births (Chen, 2011).

Clinical Findings. Signs and symptoms may include cardiomegaly, hepatosplenomegaly, hypoglycemic seizures, lactic acidosis, ketosis, hyperlipidemia, elevated transaminases, easy fatigability, hypotonia, and muscle weakness.

Diagnostic Studies. Enzyme assays and mutation analysis are available for essentially all identified forms of glycogen storage disease.

Management. Treatment varies depending on the specific defect. Types I, III, and IX all affect enzyme activity in the liver, which is responsible for homeostasis of plasma glucose. Treatment is aimed at maintaining normal blood glucose levels and may require continuous feedings through a gastrostomy tube, frequent feedings, and/or ingestion of uncooked cornstarch or Glycosade (long-acting cornstarch) slurry at regular intervals throughout the day. Parents and children must be aware of symptoms of low blood sugar, and home glucose monitoring is recommended (Chou et al, 2015).

Galactosemia

Galactosemia results from a disorder of galactose metabolism. The classic form of galactosemia is caused by deficient galactose-1-phosphate uridyltransferase (GALT) activity. Dietary galactose is most commonly ingested as lactose, the principle carbohydrate in human milk and commercial non-soy formulas. The metabolism of galactose undergoes many enzymatic reactions. A block at the level of the GALT enzyme results in accumulation of galactose-1-phosphate (gal-1-P) and other galactose derivatives, leading to the clinical symptoms (Berry, 2012). Incidence of the classic autosomal recessive form is estimated at 1 in 40,000 live births.

Clinical Findings. Infants with classic galactosemia appear normal at birth, but demonstrate clinical manifestations after milk feeding. Although galactosemia is typically discovered on newborn screening, neonates may show clinical signs before results of the screening are known. Therefore, galactosemia should remain in the differential diagnosis of any ill neonate. Clinical manifestations of severe, untreated galactosemia include poor weight gain, lethargy, jaundice, vomiting, coagulopathies, and *Escherichia coli* sepsis (Berry, 2012).

Diagnostic Studies. Urine reducing substances will be positive in recently fed (lactose containing formulas or breastmilk) infants. Measurement of GALT activity in red cells will be deficient, and liver enzymes and gal-1-P levels will be elevated.

Management. Treatment in classic galactosemia consists of eliminating dietary galactose. Ensure that the child is receiving appropriate calcium supplementation. Controversy surrounding appropriate treatment of variants (e.g., Duarte) continues with some centers recommending dietary restriction, some recommending no therapy, and others using soy formula during the first year.

Complications. Long-term complications of untreated galactosemia include cirrhosis, cataracts, and irreversible brain damage; death can occur. Despite treatment, many children with classic galactosemia develop speech/language impairment, and some develop impaired motor and cognitive function (Berry, 2012). Premature ovarian failure is also common (Fridovich-Keil et al, 2012).

Urea Cycle Disorders

A defect in any enzyme of the urea cycle results in hyperammonemia secondary to the body's inability to detoxify waste nitrogen through its normal conversion to urea. Ammonia is an end product of amino acid catabolism and is highly toxic to the CNS. Five enzymes are required for the conversion of ammonia to urea, and deficiency in any of these enzymes results in disease. Incidence of the disorder is approximately 1 : 95,000 births (Therrell et al, 2014).

Clinical Findings and Diagnostic Studies

In infants, symptoms related to the effects of hyperammonemia start after protein ingestion and include vomiting, lethargy, irritability, malaise, and potential seizures and coma. Older children may exhibit ataxia, confusion, agitation, irritability, and combativeness (Braissant, 2010). No specific findings are typically found with initial laboratory testing, however:

- Blood urea nitrogen may be low.
- Ammonia level above 100 mmol/L (or lower in older children) evokes concern (normal values are typically less than 35 mmol/L).
- Enzyme assays are available for diagnosis of most of the disorders.
- Genetic mutation analysis may confirm the diagnosis of some IEM disorders.

Management and Complications

Treatment of acute hyperammonemia is completed by acute care staff with the goal being to establish a source of glucose and rapidly decreasing ammonia levels. Principles of treatment of chronic UCD are very similar, but they also include limiting endogenous protein catabolism and dietary protein consumption under the supervision of a metabolic dietician. Despite appropriate treatment, children with UCD are vulnerable to metabolic decompensation, mild to moderate mental retardation, and premature death.

Amino Acid Metabolism Disorders: Aminoacidopathies and Organic Acidurias and Acidemias

More than 30 defects of amino acid metabolism are attributed to enzyme or cofactor defects. Although all of these disorders result from defects in amino acid metabolism, they are generally classified as aminoacidopathies or organic acidurias or acidemias, depending on whether amino acids or organic acids are detected in urine or plasma. The more common aminoacidopathies include PKU, maple syrup urine disease (MSUD), tyrosinemia types 1 and 2, and homocystinuria.

Phenylketonuria

Classic PKU is the most common form of PKU and results from deficiency of the enzyme phenylalanine hydroxylase, which converts phenylalanine to tyrosine. Untreated PKU leads to elevated phenylalanine concentrations in the blood and brain and results in CNS damage with profound mental retardation. The resulting lower level of tyrosine leads to impaired synthesis of other amines, including dopamine, norepinephrine, and melanin. More prevalent in Caucasians, PKU is an autosomal recessive disorder with an incidence of approximately 1 : 23,000 (Therrell et al, 2014).

Clinical Findings. No clinical manifestations are noted at birth, and the effects of high phenylalanine levels may not be apparent in the first few months, by which time, if untreated, irreversible brain damage has occurred. Children with more advanced, untreated disease tend to have lighter skin and hair than typical for their race and develop an eczematous rash and a musty or mousy odor related to build up of phenylacetate (Blau et al, 2010). PKU should be detected on newborn screening. Infants with classic PKU ingesting a normal diet will have serum phenylalanine levels greater than 1200 mmol/L on confirmatory testing for PKU, whereas others with milder hyperphenylalaninemia will have intermediate levels.

Differential Diagnosis. Biopterin is a cofactor for phenylalanine, tyrosine, and tryptophan hydroxylases. Children with biopterin defects may be detected on newborn screening but will continue to deteriorate despite usual dietary intervention for PKU. Testing blood and urine pterins and biopterin enzymes is recommended in any child with high phenylalanine levels because treatment for biopterin defects is different than PKU treatment.

Management. Treatment for PKU involves limiting the dietary intake of phenylalanine, with a goal of serum phenylalanine levels between 120 and 360 mmol/L in all patients (Vockley et al, 2014). Phenylalanine is an essential amino acid that cannot be eliminated entirely because patients need to receive enough to meet growth needs. To obtain the essential amino acids and to meet energy and other nutritional needs, the diet is supplemented with a medically modified formula, free of phenylalanine. Over the child's first few years of life, parents are educated on the phenylalanine content of foods; the child's phenylalanine level is frequently monitored; and a phenylalanine "allowance" is established based on the child's dietary tolerance. The current recommendation is "diet for life" to prevent long-term cognitive and neurologic sequelae. Medically modified low-phenylalanine food products are available online and in some stores, with insurance reimbursement in some states. Pregnant females with PKU must maintain very strict dietary restrictions to protect the fetus (Vockley et al, 2014). Consultation with or referral to a dietician is essential.

Classic Homocystinuria

Homocystinuria due to cystathionine synthase deficiency is the most common form of these disorders, with a prevalence of approximately 1:200,000 (Schulze et al, 2009). Discussion of homocystinuria caused by defects in vitamin metabolism and deficiency of methylenetetrahydrofolate reductase (MTHFR) is beyond the scope of this chapter.

Clinical Findings and Diagnostic Studies. Clinical manifestations are nonspecific and include failure to thrive and developmental delay. Plasma and urine amino acid testing is completed to evaluate concentrations of:

- Methionine: Elevated levels may be found on the newborn screening but values rise slowly, and high methionine levels may not be detected on specimens obtained from affected infants in the first few days after birth; a second newborn screening is necessary.
- Homocystine
- Total homocysteine

Management and Complications. Some children respond to vitamin B_6 therapy with frequent monitoring of plasma homocystine and methionine concentrations. If the child responds, treatment with vitamin B_6 is continued. Children who do not respond to vitamin B_6 are placed on a methionine-restricted diet with frequent monitoring of plasma amino acids and total plasma homocystine. Betaine is administered. Folate and vitamin B_{12} optimize conversion of homocystine to methionine (Schiff and Blom, 2012).

Treatment outcomes are variable, and these children are at high risk for metabolic stroke, although prognosis is good for those with the classical form of homocystinuria identified on newborn screening. Untreated patients develop ocular lens dislocation, progressive mental retardation, thromboembolic events, convulsions, and skeletal abnormalities resembling Marfan syndrome.

Disorders of Fatty Acid Oxidation

Medium-Chain Acyl-Coenzyme A Dehydrogenase Deficiency

Fatty acids are an important energy resource for the body, used during times of fasting and stress when glycogen stores become depleted. Defects can occur at any point in fatty acid transport or the mitochondrial beta-oxidation pathway, yielding more than 20 disorders in which individuals are unable to metabolize fatty acids. The more common fatty acid oxidation disorders are medium-chain acyl-coenzyme A dehydrogenase deficiency (MCAD), very long-chain acyl-coenzyme A dehydrogenase deficiency (VLCAD), and long-chain 3-hydroxyacyl-coenzyme A dehydrogenase deficiency (LCHAD). The incidence of all disorders ranges from 1:17,000 to 1:360,000. MCAD is quickly becoming one of the most common IEM identified in infants by newborn screening with an estimated incidence of 1:17,000 live births (Therrell et al, 2014).

Clinical Findings and Diagnostic Studies. Individuals with MCAD may be asymptomatic for a lifetime or have premature death. Fasting, stress, or illness may lead to hypoketotic hypoglycemia, hypotonia, muscle weakness, lethargy, and vomiting progressing to seizures, coma, encephalopathy, and death. Before newborn screening, up to 25% of patients died during their first episode, 50% were never symptomatic, and the overall prognosis for survivors was excellent, because fasting tolerance was found to improve with age (Bennett, 2010). Any increase in energy demand may tip the balance and result in a metabolic crisis as vital organs are deprived of fuel. Fatty acid oxidation disorders (all types) have been implicated as the cause of death in 5% of sudden unexpected deaths in infancy (Schulze et al, 2009).

Expanded newborn screening will identify the majority of fatty acid oxidation defects. Confirmatory tests for MCAD include:

- Plasma acylcarnitine profile
- Mutation analysis

Hypoglycemia or normoglycemia may be present during times of illness, and blood glucose monitoring is not a reliable measure of metabolic status in these children.

Management. Treatment varies and may include fasting avoidance and carnitine supplementation to correct secondary carnitine deficiency. For individuals with MCAD, avoidance of fasting is the mainstay of treatment. Infants should not fast for longer than 3 hours for the first 3 months. For each month of age, 1 hour of fasting can be added up to a maximum of 10 hours of fasting, which is likely to be safe until 2 years old. These guidelines do not apply during times of higher energy demand (Walter, 2009). Providers should maintain a low threshold for recommending IV glucose infusions during times of illness and fever when energy requirements increase. Monitor carnitine level and supplement with oral carnitine 50 to 100 mg/kg/day in divided doses if the free carnitine level is below the reference range (Schatz and Ensenauer, 2010).

Complications. The most serious consequence of this group of disorders is the inability to use fatty acids for energy production and lack of ketone production (burned for energy) during times of fasting, which may result in death.

Lysosomal Storage Disorders

Lysosomal storage disorders are caused by an accumulation (storage) of glycoproteins, glycolipids, or glycosaminoglycans (MPS) within lysosomes and various tissues, which leads to the various clinical presentations and symptoms. Incidence for all lysosomal storage disorders is 1:7700 live births. Symptoms vary depending on the site of storage and the specific disorder and may include hepatosplenomegaly, coarse facies, corneal clouding, developmental regression, intellectual disability, thrombocytopenia, bone pain, abnormal liver function studies, respiratory problems, hydrocephalus, and cardiomyopathy. Enzymatic assay and mutation analysis are available for most disorders. Initial diagnostic testing for mucopolysaccharidosis consists of screening urinary glycosaminoglycans (urine MPS screen) (Platt et al, 2012), but a normal screen does not rule out the diagnosis. Treatment varies from symptom management to ERT with varying degrees of success (Henley et al, 2014).

Dyslipidemia: Hypercholesterolemia and Hyperlipidemia

Dyslipidemias are disorders of lipoprotein metabolism, some of which lead to increased levels of total cholesterol and LDL cholesterol, a varied presentation of triglycerides, and/or decreased levels of HDL cholesterol.

Dyslipidemias can be acquired (secondary) or genetic (primary). Secondary hyperlipidemias result from exogenous factors, such as obesity, drugs (e.g., isotretinoin, oral contraceptives, antipsychotics), and alcohol; endocrine or metabolic disorders (e.g., hypothyroidism, diabetes); storage disease (e.g., glycogen storage disease); obstructive liver disease (e.g., biliary atresia); and other causes, such as anorexia nervosa.

Among primary dyslipidemia, familial hypercholesterolemia is most common; it is also the most commonly occurring congenital metabolic disorder (Goldberg et al, 2011). Familial hypercholesterolemia results from pathogenic mutation in the LDL receptor (most common), apolipoprotein B (ApoB), or protein convertase subtilisin/kexin type 9 (PCSK9) genes. These mutations compromise the receptor cells' ability to facilitate clearance of LDL cholesterol through the liver; as a result, LDL accumulates in the body. Triglycerides are usually normal. The two types of familial hypercholesterolemia are heterozygous, which is common (1:300 to 1:500), and homozygous, which is exceedingly rare (1:1,000,000). Homozygous hypercholesterolemia is characterized by extremely high LDL levels (e.g., 600 mg/dL or more) and a poor outcome if the patient does not have very aggressive early treatment; treatment may include LDL apheresis, new specific medications that have been developed, and possible liver transplant. Even with treatment, atherosclerotic vascular disease is common by 30 years old (Goldberg et al, 2011).

Clinical Findings

Hyperlipidemia does not typically present as a clinical illness in children. Although not all children with dyslipidemia will have cardiovascular problems as adults, screening of children at risk is important to identify those with hyperlipidemia and hypercholesterolemia and intervene in an effort to prevent problems from occurring later in life.

History. Risk factors for hypercholesterolemia and hyperlipidemia found in the history include (Daniels et al, 2011):

- Family history of premature heart disease (men ≥55 years old; women ≥65 years old)
- Increased age (men >30 years old; women >40 years old)
- Male sex
- Hypertension
- Diabetes mellitus
- Smoking
- Reduced HDL cholesterol concentration

Physical Examination. The child may have no clinical signs or symptoms or may have (Goldberg et al, 2011):

- Tendon xanthomas at any age (most common in finger extensor tendons and Achilles tendon)
- Arcus corneae (partial or complete) younger than 4 or 5 years old
- Tuberous xanthomas or xanthelasma

Diagnostic Studies. The clinical conditions of dyslipidemia can be determined by lipoprotein analysis. Universal screening for elevated serum cholesterol is recommended at 9 to 11 years old with a fasting lipid profile or non-fasting non-HDL cholesterol measurement. When the family history is positive for hypercholesterolemia or premature congenital heart disease (CHD), screening should be considered by 2 years old (Goldberg et al, 2011).

Precise genetic etiology is not needed for therapeutic decisions, although conditions with overlapping signs and laboratory derangements and with different treatment (e.g.,

• BOX 26-12 Guidelines for Cardiovascular Health and Risk Reduction in Children and Adolescents

- Infants should be exclusively breastfeed for the first 6 months.
- Try to maintain breastfeeding for 12 months.
- Transition to reduced fat (fat free to 2%) unflavored cow's milk at 12 months.
- Avoid/limit sugar-sweetened beverage intake; encourage water.
- Transition to table foods with total fat intake limited to 25% to 30% of daily kilocalories, saturated fat limited to 8% to 10% of daily kilocalories, and cholesterol to less than 300 mg per day.
- Encourage high dietary fiber intake from foods.
- Achieve 1 hour of moderate to vigorous physical activity every day.
- Limit daily leisure screen time to no more than 1 to 2 hours per day.
- Provide smoke-free home environment.
- Measure fasting lipid profile in pediatric patients (2 to 8 years old) with risk factors.
- Measure fasting lipid profile in all pediatric patients (9 to 11 years old) and then again at 17 to 21 years old.
- Identify children at risk for obesity. Provide focused education for family.
- Stop smoking.

Adapted from U. S. Department of Health and Human Services; National Institutes of Health; National Heart, Lung, and Blood Institute: *Expert panel on integrated guidelines for cardiovascular health and risk reduction in children and adolescents, summary report (NIH Publication No. 12-7486A)*, 2012. Available at: www.nhlbi.nih.gov/files/docs/peds_guidelines_sum.pdf. Accessed December 1, 2014.

cerebrotendinous xanthomatosis, sitosterolemia, and cholesterol ester storage disease) should be considered and ruled out if appropriate.

Management

Lifestyle Changes. Prevention and/or control of hypercholesterolemia through lifestyle changes is a primary intervention (Box 26-12). Dietary change has been the first step in treatment of children older than 2 years with hypercholesterolemia (LDL >130 mg/dL on screening tests) and, combined with other lifestyle changes, remains a mainstay of treatment—even if medications are added to the regimen. The National Lipid Association (NLA) encourages individuals to change lifestyle patterns as well as alter diet; educational materials related to this approach are available on the NLA website (see Resources on the Evolve Website). Many issues arise with dietary changes in children (e.g., increasing dietary fiber may "fill up" the child and increase the risk of poor nutrient intake), so consultation with a pediatric dietitian is essential to ensure that children receive adequate nutrition.

Pharmacotherapy. Drug therapy should be considered in children 8 years old or older who, after 6 to 12 months of therapy focused on diet and lifestyle changes, continue to have the following (Daniels et al, 2011):

- LDL concentration greater than 190 mg/dL *or*
- LDL concentration between 160 and 190 mg/dL *and* positive family history of premature CHD or a high-level risk factor or two moderate-level risk factors *or*
- LDL concentration between 130 and 159 mg/dL *and* at least two high-level risk factors or one high- and at least two moderate-level risk factors
  - High-level risk factors:
    - Hypertension requiring treatment
    - Current cigarette smoker
    - Obesity (BMI greater than 97 percentile)
    - Presence of high-risk conditions, such as diabetes mellitus, chronic kidney disease, Kawasaki disease with aneurysms
  - Moderate-level risk factors:
    - Hypertension not requiring treatment
    - Obesity (BMI 95 to 97 percentile)
    - HDL less than 40 mg/dL
    - Presence of moderate-risk conditions, such as chronic inflammatory disease (e.g., lupus, rheumatoid arthritis, human immunodeficiency virus infection, nephrotic syndrome, Kawasaki disease without current aneurysms)

If the child is taking antipsychotic medication, a consult with the behavioral health provider is necessary before beginning treatment, because some antipsychotic medications increase the risk of hyperlipidemia. Use of HMG-CoA reductase inhibitors (statins) can be considered if the child has severe hypercholesterolemia. The statins function by inhibiting the rate-limiting enzyme in the synthesis of cholesterol. Because of the side effects of drugs and the uncertainty about their long-term use in the pediatric population, children who need drug therapy should be referred to a specialized pediatric lipid center for treatment.

For a complete list of references, please visit http://evolve.elsevier.com/Burns/pediatric/.

27 Hematologic Disorders

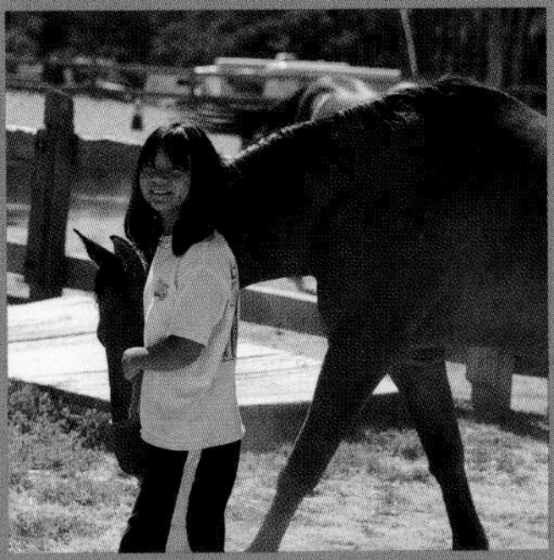

TEREA GIANNETTA AND VERONICA KANE

The hematologic system is a massive fluid organ that permeates the entire body, delivering nutrients and other vital elements throughout. Essential body functions carried out by blood include the transfer of respiratory gases, hemostasis, phagocytosis, and the provision of cellular and humoral agents to fight infection. Abnormalities of blood cells are seen in various disease states and alterations in nutrition, necessitating the use of diagnostic hematologic studies to differentiate common nutritional deficiencies with straightforward treatments from rare diseases with a genetic or chronic component. Extensive referral and multidisciplinary approaches are needed for these latter conditions. Because of the effect of impaired cellular nutrition on normal growth and development of sensitive systems in pediatrics, early diagnosis of blood disorders is vital to ensure the best possible prognosis.

Anatomy and Physiology

Blood is made of cellular components, each with specialized functions, and a fluid component called *plasma,* which serves as the transport medium. The cells that comprise whole blood are categorized as erythrocytes (red blood cells [RBCs]); leukocytes (white blood cells [WBCs]); and thrombocytes (platelets). Leukocytes are further differentiated into subtypes (lymphocytes, granulocytes, and monocytes). Abnormally high or low counts of any of the cell categories may indicate the presence of many conditions. Due to its sensitivity in screening for a variety of disorders, the complete blood count (CBC) is among the most performed studies and is commonly used in routine health screening. Plasma is the clear yellow fluid in which proteins (primarily albumins, globulins, and fibrinogen) are the major solutes. These plasma proteins maintain intravascular volume, contribute to the coagulation of blood, and are important in acid-base balance. Figure 27-1 shows the breakdown of all components of whole blood.

Blood formation in the human embryo begins in the yolk sac during the first several weeks of gestation. During the second trimester, blood is formed primarily in the fetal liver, spleen, and lymph nodes. In the last half of gestation, hematopoiesis shifts from the fetal liver and spleen to the bone marrow, where, by birth, most blood formation takes place. Most erythropoiesis occurs in the last month of gestation. The bone marrow produces erythrocytes, granulocytes, monocytes, and platelets and provides lymphocytes and lymphocytic precursors to the spleen, lymph nodes, and other lymphatic tissues.

Erythrocytes

Erythropoietin, produced primarily by renal glomerular epithelial cells, regulates erythrocyte (RBC) production. In response to a decrease in the number of circulating RBCs or a decrease in the oxygen pressure (Pao_2) of arterial blood, erythropoietin stimulates the bone marrow to convert certain stem cells to proerythroblasts. Substances essential for RBC formation include iron, vitamin B_{12}, folic acid, amino acids, and other nutrients.

The RBC matures through the following stages: proerythroblast, erythroblast, normoblast, reticulocyte, and erythrocyte. As cellular differentiation occurs, the nucleus present in the early forms of the cell is extruded and replaced by hemoglobin (Hgb). The RBC assumes its characteristic anucleated biconcave disk shape, which is easily distorted, thereby enabling it to pass through small capillaries and sinuses without being destroyed. The large surface-to-volume ratio of the semipermeable membrane facilitates rapid gas exchange.

The youngest RBCs are the reticulocytes. After release from the bone marrow, reticulocytes stay in circulation for about 1 to 2 days before becoming mature RBCs. The *reticulocyte count* is about 4% to 6% for the first 3 days of life, which reflects the relatively greater amount of erythropoiesis that occurs in the fetus. This increased reticulocyte count is followed by a sudden drop around 1 year of age from 0.5% to 1.5%, which remains the norm for the rest of life (Table 27-1). In cases of low RBC levels (such as, anemia or sudden blood loss), the effectiveness of the body's early response to treatment or progress of healing can be

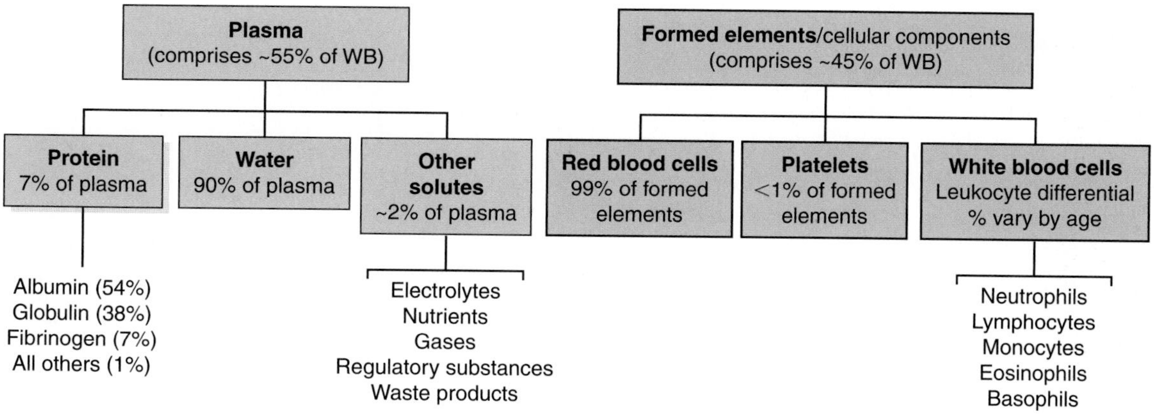

• **Figure 27-1** Composition of whole blood *(WB).*

measured via the reticulocyte count. A mature RBC survives about 120 days before it is destroyed through phagocytosis in the spleen, liver, or bone marrow. Table 27-2 presents an overview of the common clinical diagnostic blood tests, including those used to assess RBC functioning.

Hemoglobin

Hgb is the oxygen-carrying protein molecule in the RBC. Production of Hgb requires circulating iron, the synthesis of a protoporphyrin ring, and the production of globin. Each Hgb molecule is comprised of two pairs of polypeptide chains. The globin portion contains protein in a precise sequence of amino acids that is coded by genes located on chromosomes 11 and 16. Normal Hgb contains two alpha chains and two beta chains. These chains then attach to heme groups, large iron-containing disks, and porphyrin, a nitrogen-containing organic compound.

Each of the four iron atoms in the Hgb molecule combines reversibly with an atom of oxygen to form oxyhemoglobin. This reaction occurs when the oxygen concentration is relatively high, as in the lungs, where oxygen crosses the alveolocapillary membrane and saturates about 96% of the Hgb. The percentage of oxyhemoglobin is the arterial oxygen saturation (SaO_2), and it is measured through pulse oximetry or arterial blood gas determination. When the oxygen concentration is lower (as in the tissues), oxygen is released from Hgb to meet cellular demands.

Erythrocyte Development

Many dietary elements are essential to the developmental process of mature RBCs, including amino acids, carbohydrates, lipids, vitamin B_{12}, folate, vitamin C, and iron. Free Hgb, which is released during RBC lysis, is transported to the reticuloendothelial system by haptoglobin. The reticuloendothelial system is located in the spleen, liver, and bone marrow; and it is where the lysis substrates, iron, amino acids, carbohydrate, and lipids are reclaimed. Transferrin transports iron to the bone marrow and into the maturing RBC, where it is incorporated into the new heme molecule.

Structural Variations

Hgb molecules normally represent the majority of the body's Hgb and, in adult Hgb, are composed of two fundamental subunit chains, alpha (α) and beta (β). Equal numbers of each chain are essential for normal cell function. An imbalance of the chains damages and destroys RBCs thereby producing anemia.

Various forms of Hgb are found in the embryo, fetus, and adult, depending on changes in globin chain synthesis. At birth, approximately 70% of Hgb is made up of fetal hemoglobin (Hgb F), which is composed of two α-chains and two gamma (γ)-chains. By 12 months old, 95% of a person's Hgb typically consists of adult Hgb molecules (Hgb A), which are composed of two α- and two β-polypeptide chains attached to four heme groups. In the majority of individuals, Hgb F remains present at levels of less than 2%. Hgb A_2 is another type of adult Hgb but consists of two α- and two delta (δ)-chains. Hgb A_2 normally makes up about 2.5% of the total Hgb and may be increased in beta-thalassemia. Mutations occur whenever there are gene defects in either of the subunit chains resulting in Hgb variants. Any alteration of the amino acid sequencing on the chromosomes (11, 16) that code production of the beta globin chain results in one of over 600 identified variants of Hgb. Some abnormal hemoglobins are the result of amino acid substitutions. Although many mutations are innocuous, with indiscernible physiologic impact, other structural defects are devastating.

Among the most commonly occurring Hgb variants are Hgb S (sickle), Hgb C, Hgb E, persistence of Hgb F, and Hgb H. The incidence of these hemoglobins tends to peak within certain regional or racial populations. Atypical combinations of Hgb variants can occur, each with its own resulting condition or problems. *Hemoglobin electrophoresis,* which separates each Hgb out on a gel medium, is used to differentiate the Hgb variants from Hgb A, thus aiding in the diagnosis of specific hemoglobinopathies.

Diminished production of one of the two subunit chains results in disorders referred to as *thalassemias.* Thalassemias

TABLE 27-1 Hematologic Values and Normal Leukocyte Differential Count During Infancy and Childhood

	Hematologic Values											
	Hemoglobin (g/dL)		Hematocrit (%)		Reticulocytes (%)	Mean Corpuscular Volume (fL)	Leukocytes (WBC/mm³)		Neutrophils (%)		Lymphocytes (%)	Eosinophils (%)
Age	Mean	Range	Mean	Range	Mean	Lowest	Mean	Range	Mean	Range	Mean*	Mean
Cord blood	16.8	13.7-20.1	55	45-65	5	110	18,000	(9000-30,000)	61	(40-80)	31	2
2 weeks old	16.5	13-20	50	42-66	1		12,000	(5000-21,000)	40		63	3
3 months old	12	9.5-14.5	36	31-41	1		12,000	(6000-18,000)	30		48	2
6 months to 6 years old	12	10.5-14	37	33-42	1	70-74	10,000	(6000-18,000)	45		48	2
7 to 12 years old	13	11-16	38	34-40	1	76-80	8000	(4500-13,500)	55		38	2
Adult												
Female	14	12-16	42	37-47	1.6	80	7500	(5000-10,000)	55	(35-70)	35	3
Male	16	14-18	47	42-52		80						

Other Red Cell Indices

RDW: 0 to 3 days old, <18; 1 to 6 months old, <16.5; 7 months old to 2 years old, <16; 2 to 8 years old, <15; 13 to 18 years old, <14.5 MCHC: 1 to 2 weeks old, 28% to 38%; 1 to 6 months old, 30% to 36%; 7 months old to adult, 31% to 37%

	Normal Leukocyte Differential Count					
		Granulocytes			Agranulocytes	
Age	Segmented Neutrophils (%)	Band Neutrophils (%)	Eosinophils (%)	Basophils (%)	Lymphocytes (%)	Monocytes (%)
Birth	47 ± 15	14.1 ± 4	2.2	0.6	31 ± 5	5.8
6 months old	23	8.8	2.5	0.4	61	4.8
12 months old	23	8.1	2.6	0.4	61	4.8
2 years old	25	8	2.6	0.5	59	5
4 years old	34 ± 11	8 ± 3	2.8	0.6	50 ± 15	5
6 years old	43	8	2.7	0.6	42	4.7
8 years old	45	8	2.4	0.6	39	4.2
10 years old	46 ± 15	8 ± 3	2.4	0.5	38 ± 10	4.3
12 years old	47	8	2.5	0.5	38	4.4

	Platelets (Conventional Units)	
Age	Platelet (×10³/μL)	Mean Platelet Volume (fL)
All ages	150 to 450	6.5 to 10.0

Data from Kliegman RM, Behrman RE, Jenson HB, et al: editors: *Nelson textbook of pediatrics*, ed 18, Philadelphia, 2007, Saunders/Elsevier; Taketomo CK, Hodding JH, Kraus: *Pediatric dosage handbook*, ed 17, Hudson, OH, 2011, Lexi-Comp, p 1676; Wallach J: *Interpretation of diagnostic tests*, ed 8, Philadelphia, 2006, Lippincott Williams & Wilkins.

MCHC, Mean corpuscular hemoglobin concentration; *RDW*, red (blood cell) distribution width; *WBC*, white blood cell.

*Relatively wide range.

TABLE 27-2 **Clinical Diagnostic Interpretation**

Test	Description
Complete blood count (CBC)	Broad screening test for illnesses that cause alteration in RBC indices and WBC count
CBC with differential	Additionally assesses the amounts of the WBC subtypes present in a given sample of whole blood
CBC with peripheral smear	Additionally assesses the size and shapes of a sample of RBC
Red blood cell (RBC)	Increased with polycythemia vera and fluid loss—diarrhea, burns, dehydration Decreased with anemia
Hemoglobin (Hgb)	Iron-binding portion of RBC
Hematocrit (Hct)	Calculation of the percentage of RBC in a given volume of whole blood
Mean corpuscular volume (MCV)	Determines the volume of the average RBC in femtoliters; increased (macro) with B_{12}, folic acid deficiency, hypothyroid; decreased (micro) with iron deficiency, thalassemia, lead poisoning, anemia of chronic disease
Mean corpuscular hemoglobin concentration (MCHC)	Average amount of Hgb in red cells Used in determining type and severity of anemia Mirrors MCV
Mentzer Index = MCV/RBC	Differentiates between iron deficiency and thalassemia Ratio <13: Thalassemia Ratio >13: Iron deficiency, hemoglobinopathy
Red (blood cell) distribution width (RDW)	Increased RDW indicates mixed population of RBCs; immature RBCs are larger than mature, so increase is associated with anemias
Reticulocyte (Retic) count	A percentage of the circulating erythrocytes; this reflects the bone marrow production of new RBCs, reticulocytes, and their subsequent release into the bloodstream Important in assessing the body's response to an anemic state
Reticulocyte production index (RPI)	A calculation to more accurately reflect the reticulocyte production in the diagnosis of anemia because the absolute RBC count decreases in anemia; it indicates whether the bone marrow is responding and corrects for the degree of anemia RPI >3 associated with hemolysis or blood loss; <2 reflects decreased or ineffective production for the degree of anemia
Absolute neutrophil count (ANC)	Refers to the total number of neutrophil granulocytes present in the blood Normal value: ≥1500 cells/mm^3 Mild neutropenia: ≥1000 to <1500 cells/mm^3 Moderate neutropenia: ≥500 to <1000 cells/mm^3 Severe neutropenia: ≤500 cells/mm^3
Poikilocytosis	Refers to an increase in abnormal RBCs of any shape where they make up 10% or more of the total population
White blood cell (WBC)	May be increased with infections, inflammation, cancer, leukemia; decreased with some medications, some severe infections; bone marrow failure

are categorized into two types: alpha and beta, and they are named based on the affected chain. In the carrier state for alpha-thalassemia, there is one α-chain present, enabling the production of adequate amounts of Hgb with no symptoms in the carrier. In alpha-thalassemia the beta-globulin subunits cluster into groups of four in the absence of any α-chains with which to partner. These beta-tetramers are incapable of carrying oxygen, and the affected fetuses die in utero *(hydrops fetalis).* In beta-thalassemia major, the α-chains do not bind with each other but rather degrade in the absence of β-chains. Conversely, in beta-thalassemia minor, there are sufficient β-chains present to bind with the abundant α-chains to create functional Hgb molecules and a resultant asymptomatic mild microcytic anemia.

There are also altered states of Hgb, such as occurs with methemoglobin. In this condition, the ferrous form of iron oxidizes to the ferric state, causing the *heme* moiety to be incapable of carrying oxygen. If reduced Hgb (i.e., Hgb present in the blood that is not carrying oxygen) levels exceed 5 g/dL (i.e., 5 grams of Hgb per liter not transporting oxygen), serious tissue hypoxia and cyanosis can occur. Methemoglobinemia can be congenital or caused by exposure to certain drugs and chemicals.

Normal Values

Hgb increases with increased gestational age. Hgb levels in a term newborn range from 14 to 20 g/dL but may be 1 to 2 g/dL lower in very low birth weight infants. A physiologic drop to its lowest point occurs around 2 to 4 months old for term infants and at about 6 weeks old in premature infants. This drop represents a physiologic anemia caused by the shortened survival of fetal RBCs and the rapid expansion of blood volume during this period. A decrease in Hgb can also develop secondary to a decrease in RBC production, blood loss, or increased RBC destruction. Due to the effect of these latter processes, oxygen transport to the tissues is adversely affected, and the individual can become clinically anemic as manifested by pallor, heart failure, or shock. Anemias may be categorized on the basis of the RBC size, which is indicated by the mean corpuscular volume (MCV) and microscopic appearance. RBC size also changes with age, and the normal developmental changes in the MCV should be recognized as well. Examination of the peripheral smear may reveal changes in the RBC appearance that will help to narrow diagnostic categories. Table 27-1 summarizes the RBC indices.

Antigenic Properties of Red Blood Cells

Red cells are classified into different types according to the presence of antigens on the cell membrane. The antigenicity is genetically determined and represents contributions from both parents. The most common antigens are designated A, B, and Rh. A person inherits either A or B antigen (type A or B blood), both antigens (type AB blood, which is the universal recipient), or neither antigen (type O blood, which is the universal donor) (Fig. 27-2). In the United States, the overwhelming majority of Caucasians and African Americans are Rh-positive. Clinically, these distinctions become important when blood transfusions are necessary or in the assessment for maternal-fetal blood incompatibilities. The International Society for Blood Transfusion recognizes more than 20 blood group systems (including Rh and ABO).

Leukocytes

Leukocytes, or WBCs, are larger and fewer in number than erythrocytes. Normally about 5000 to 10,000 leukocytes are contained in a microliter of blood. The primary function of WBCs is protection of the body from invasion by foreign organisms and distribution of antibodies and other immune response components. When levels reach critical low and high values for leukocytes, there are great risks to the child. A WBC count of less than 500/mm^3 places the patient at risk for a fatal infection. However, a WBC count greater than 30,000/mm^3 indicates massive infection or a serious disease, such as leukemia.

Five distinct types of WBCs can be grouped into two broad classifications: (1) granulocytes (also known as *polymorphonuclear [PMN] leukocytes,* or *polys*) and (2) agranulocytes. Granulocytes contain large granules and horseshoe-shaped nuclei that become segmented and are connected by thin strands (Table 27-3). With Wright stain the cytoplasm stains blue or pink. Granulocytes are further divided into neutrophils; eosinophils, which absorb the acid dye eosin; and basophils, which absorb a basic dye. Agranulocytes include lymphocytes (also known as *immunocytes*) and monocytes.

Granular Leukocytes (Polymorphonuclear Leukocytes, Polys)

Neutrophils, Basophils, and Eosinophils

In children, granulocytes comprise 40% to 70% of all WBCs. The morphology of the developing *neutrophil* takes on various features and forms as they mature in the bone marrow through the following stages: stem cells, myeloblasts, promyelocytes, myelocytes, metamyelocytes, band forms, and, finally, mature segmented neutrophils. This maturational process takes approximately 6 to 11 days.

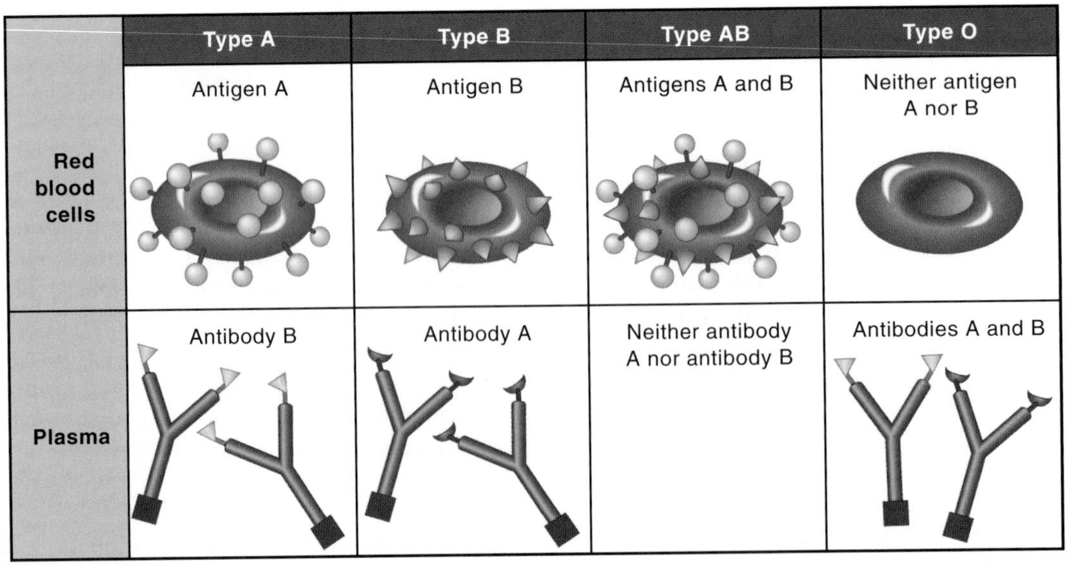

Type A
Type B
Type AB
Type O
Antigen A
Antigen B
Antigens A and B
Neither antigen A nor B
Red blood cells
Antibody B
Antibody A
Neither antibody A nor antibody B
Antibodies A and B
Plasma

• **Figure 27-2** Red cell antigenicity. (From Patton K: *Anatomy & physiology*, ed 7, St. Louis, 2010, Mosby/Elsevier.)

TABLE 27-3 Overview of Leukocytes

Cell Type	Characteristics	Diagram
Granulocytes (Polymorphonuclear Leukocytes, Polys)		
Neutrophils	Have small, fine, light pink or lilac acidophilic granules when stained and a segmented, irregularly lobed, purple nucleus.	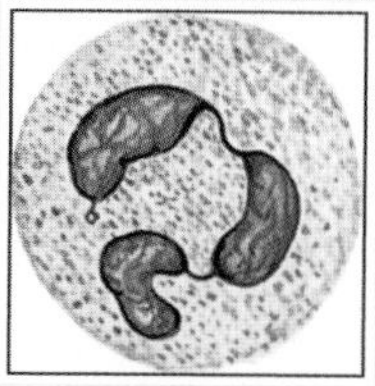
Eosinophils	Have large round granules that contain red-staining basic mucopolysaccharides and multilobed purple-blue nuclei.	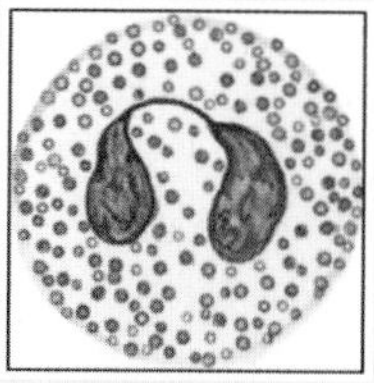
Basophils	Coarse blue granules conceal the segmented nucleus. Granules contain histamine, heparin, and acid mucopolysaccharides.	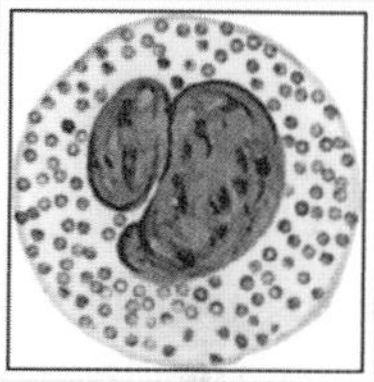
Agranulocytes		
Lymphocytes	Small cells with a large, round, deep-staining, single-lobed nucleus and very little cytoplasm. The cytoplasm is slightly basophilic and stains pale blue.	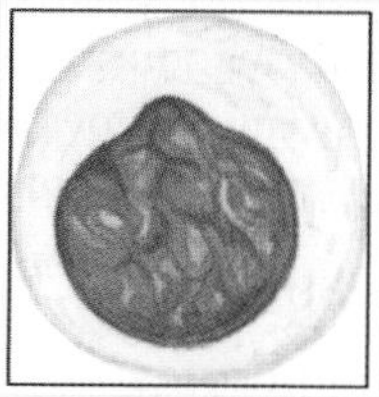
Monocytes	Large cells with a prominent, multi-shaped nucleus that sometimes is kidney shaped. Chromatin in the nucleus looks like lace, with small particles linked together like strands. The gray-blue cytoplasm is filled with many fine lysozymes that stain pink with Wright stain.	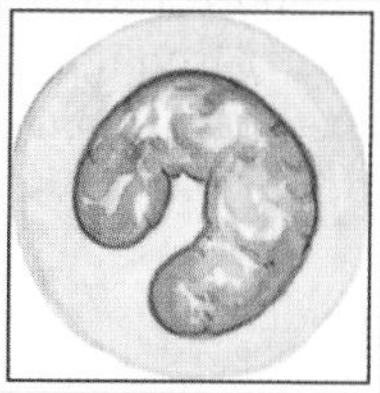

Once a neutrophil is released into the bloodstream, it circulates for about 6 to 9 hours before entering the tissues, where the major function of PMN leukocytes is phagocytosis of harmful particles and cells, particularly bacterial organisms. Thus neutrophils are the primary WBC involved in fighting bacterial infections.

A frequency distribution of the types of WBCs is obtained by the differential count, and quantitative alterations within the categories are important diagnostically (Table 27-4). A relative increase in the number of circulating immature neutrophils (band forms, metamyelocytes, and myelocytes) is referred to as a "shift to the left," which is a phrase derived from how the differential count used to be tabulated on written forms. This phenomenon is indicative of an inflammatory process or the body's immunologic response to an acute bacterial infection. The phrase "shift to the right" indicates an increase in the total lymphocyte count.

Basophils, which account for less than 1% of circulating leukocytes, are closely related to tissue mast cells. Both cells react immediately in the face of a hypersensitivity reaction by granules releasing heparin and histamine into the bloodstream during systemic allergic reactions. Renal disease, rare carcinomas, and medications (such as, estrogen and antithyroid agents) are among the reasons for increased basophils.

Eosinophils (1% to 2% WBCs) have two main functions: (1) to immediately release histamine in hypersensitivity reactions and (2) to destroy parasites. Other causes of

TABLE 27-4 White Blood Cell Differential and Key Characteristics

Major Division of White Blood Cells	Differential	Description
Granulocytes (50% to 75%)	Neutrophils	Primary defense against bacterial infection and mediating stress Elevated with bacterial or inflammatory disorders
	Bands (<1%)	Immature neutrophils put out by the bone marrow
	Eosinophils (2% to 4%)	Associated with antigen-antibody response; elevated with exposure to allergens or inflammation of skin, parasites
	Basophils (1% to 2%)	Phagocytes: Contain heparin, histamines, and serotonin Increased in leukemia, chronic inflammation, hypersensitivity to food, radiation therapy Mast cells
Nongranulocytes (30% to 40%)	Lymphocytes (25% to 35%)	Primary components of the immune system Elevated with viral infections, leukemia, radiation exposure; decreased with diseases affecting the immune system
	Monocytes (<2%)	Elevated in infections and inflammation, leukemia; decreased with some bone marrow injury, leukemias

eosinophilia include connective tissue and collagen vascular diseases, immunodeficiencies, and neoplasms, such as carcinoma, lymphoma, and Hodgkin lymphoma. Eosinophils contain receptor sites for immunoglobulin E (IgE), levels of which are elevated in people with allergies; they also prevent clot formation in the microcirculation. Eosinophils found in the mucosa of the gastrointestinal (GI) tract and in the lungs are weakly phagocytic.

Agranulocytes—Leukocytes

Lymphocytes

Lymphocytes (or immunocytes) comprise 25% to 35% of WBCs. Although not phagocytic, they protect the body against specific antigens. They originate in the bone marrow but differentiate in lymphoid tissues, such as the spleen, liver, thymus, lymph nodes, and intestines. Thymus-dependent lymphocytes, or T cells, are part of the cell-mediated immune response in which cytotoxic agents and macrophages are synthesized. B-cell lymphocytes are precursors of the humoral immune response whereby the cells are transformed into plasma cells that release immunoglobulins or antibodies into the bloodstream. Lymphocytes are an important defense component.

Monocytes

Monocytes, which contain a large lobulated nucleus, are relatively immature cells that circulate for about 8 hours before migrating to tissues where they assume their mature form as macrophages. They constitute 4% to 6% of WBCs with the absolute monocyte count of 0.1 to 0.9×10^9/L. After briefly circulating in the peripheral vascular system, monocytes migrate to the tissue to mature and become part of the monocyte/histiocyte/immune cell system. Fixed and mobile macrophages are located primarily in the liver, spleen, lymph nodes, and GI tract; and they make up the mononuclear phagocyte system. Like granulocytes, which are the first line of defense against microbe invasion, their primary function is phagocytosis of bacteria and cellular debris. Monocyte elevation occurs in collagen vascular disease, Hodgkin lymphoma, non-Hodgkin lymphoma (NHL), chronic infections (such as tuberculosis), and syphilis.

Platelet Cells and Coagulation Factors

The smallest cellular components in blood are the platelets, or thrombocytes, which are essential to hemostasis and clot formation. Circulating platelets are fragments of megakaryocytes, which are precursor cells that form in the bone marrow. The normal platelet count ranges from 150,000 to 450,000 cells/mm^3. When a blood vessel is injured (or in the presence of intrinsic damage to the blood), platelets adhere to the inner surface of the vessel and form a hemostatic plug. As platelets degrade, a series of at least 13 clotting factors or proteolytic enzymes are released that bring about the clotting process in a cascading sequence of successive reactions. These clotting factors are listed in Table 27-5.

The basic reactions that occur in the sequential process of blood coagulation are as follows: factor X activates and prothrombin (factor II) converts to thrombin, which then catalyzes the conversion of fibrinogen (factor I) to fibrin. Fibrin provides the matrix in which blood cells aggregate to form a clot. A deficiency of any of the proteins in the pathway leads to a clotting disorder. In particular, if factor VIII is deficient (as in classic hemophilia A) or the number of platelets is inadequate (thrombocytopenia), activation of factor X is impaired. Figure 27-3 illustrates the entire coagulation cascade. Age-specific coagulation values exist for each aspect of the coagulation process and should be referenced for proper assessment and treatment management.

TABLE 27-5 Blood Coagulation Factors

Factor (International Nomenclature)	Common Synonyms
I	Fibrinogen
II	Prothrombin*
III	Tissue thromboplastin, thrombokinase
V	Proaccelerin, labile factor, accelerator globulin
VII	Proconvertin,* stable factor
VIII	Antihemophilic globulin (AHG), antihemophilic factor (AHF), antihemophilic factor A
IX	Plasma thromboplastin component (PTC), Christmas factor,* antihemophilic factor B
X	Stuart-Prower factor, Stuart factor*
XI	Plasma thromboplastin antecedent (PTA), antihemophilic factor C
XII	Hageman factor, contact factor, antihemophilic factor
XIII	Fibrin-stabilizing factor (FSF), plasma transglutaminase
Kininogen	Fitzgerald factor
Prekallikrein	Fletcher factor

*Vitamin K dependent.

Pathophysiology

Hematologic problems are generally classified as disorders of RBC function, WBC function, and platelet and coagulation function. These three broad categories are further divided into disorders of blood cell production, maturation, or destruction. Although most RBC disorders result in a decreased quantity of cells or cell abnormalities, it is important not to forget the congenital, though rare, proliferative disorder, primary polycythemia (polycythemia rubra vera). This entity is a myeloproliferative disorder. Children usually have hepatosplenomegaly, neurologic and cardiovascular symptoms caused by erythrocytosis, diarrhea, and pruritus due to histamine release related to granulocytosis, and thrombosis or hemorrhage from thrombocytosis. Knowledge of these pathophysiologic classifications gives the pediatric provider a rationale for routine screening and useful algorithms to guide further clinical investigation.

Assessment of Disorders of Erythrocytes

History

A comprehensive history and physical examination are essential to unravel the mystery behind suspected hematologic disorders. Many hematologic processes have genetic bases. In order to discern inheritable disorders, it is necessary to identify the child's ethnicity and race(s), plus obtain a detailed family medical history. Certain disorders occur with greater frequency in individuals of certain races or whose ancestors were from specific geographic regions. One example of this phenomenon is sickle cell anemia (SCA), which is the most common genetic disease identified in state-mandated newborn screening programs. In the United States, it occurs in black or African Americans at a rate of approximately 1:500 births and in Hispanics at a rate of 1:36,000 births. Sickle cell trait occurs in approximately one in 12 black or African Americans (Centers for Disease Control and Prevention [CDC], 2015). Recording all family health data in a genogram provides visual clues to patterns of heritability and assists with narrowing the diagnostic possibilities. The provider should obtain information about family members with a history of any of the following:

- Genetically based disorders (include, but are not exclusive to, sickle cell or thalassemia disease or trait)
- Anemia
- Jaundice
- Splenomegaly
- Gallbladder disease
- Lead exposure
- Bleeding tendencies
- Drug and toxin exposure
- Bone marrow failure
- Chronic illnesses

Maternal history is significant in young children and should include:

- Pregnancy and delivery
- Gestational drug ingestion
- Anemia during pregnancy
- Transfusion
- Pica, eating nonfood product

A comprehensive review of a child's medical history and a review of systems are fundamental. Particular attention should focus on:

- Prematurity (especially if anemia detected in infancy)
- Environmental exposures (lead, cadmium, pesticides, toxic waste, and so on)
- Any chronic illnesses
- Growth changes or weight loss, unexplained
- Persistent pallor and/or adenopathy
- Evidence of endocrinopathy
- Jaundice episodes (including in the newborn period)
- Extremity pain, with or without swelling
- Prolonged or unusual blood loss (particularly from mucous membranes)
- Unexplained petechiae, easy bruising
- Behavioral changes: Irritable, quiet, restless, subdued
- GI disorders: Liver disease, abdominal pain, changes in stool patterns
- Bone fractures
- Changes in stool characteristics indicating GI bleeding
- Lack of energy, fatigue

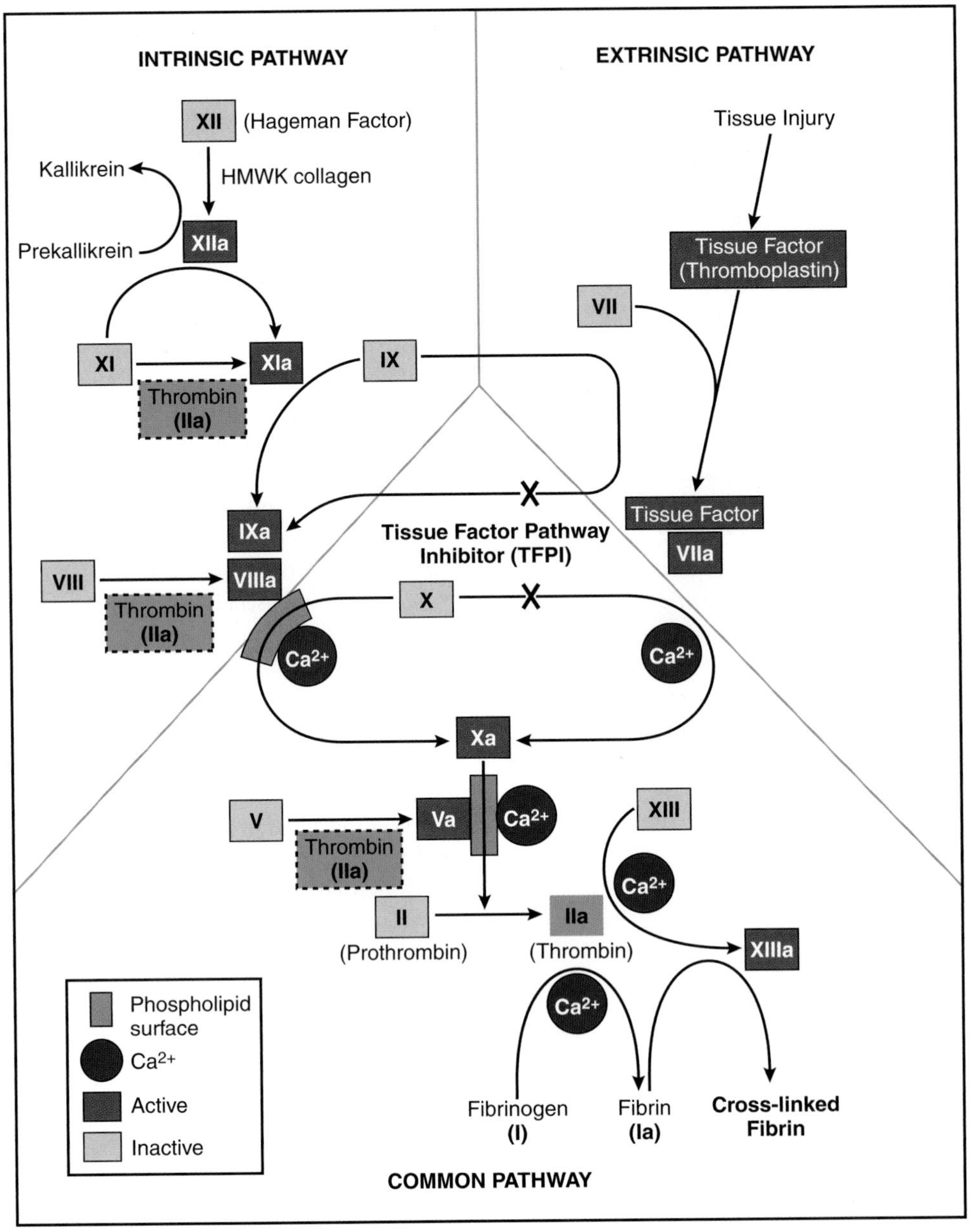

• **Figure 27-3** The classical coagulation cascade. Note the common link between the intrinsic and extrinsic pathways at the level of factor IX activation. *HMWK,* High-molecular-weight kininogen. The inhibitory anticoagulant pathways are not shown. (From Kumar V, Abbas A, Fausto N, et al: *Robbins basic pathology*, ed 8, Philadelphia, 2007, Elsevier.)

- Recent acute infections or drug exposure
- International travel and immunization history

The nutritional history of the child (and of the breastfeeding mother) should include the following:

- Dietary intake of iron sources, quantities and types of milk, and meat
- Type and dosing of vitamin supplements, include possibility of excessive ingestion
- A 24-hour dietary recall
- Any history of pica, protracted mouthing behaviors (particularly when iron deficiency or plumbism is suspected)

Newborn screening panel results need to be reviewed. In most states, routine screening of newborn heel stick blood is done to detect genetic and metabolic disorders, such as sickle cell disease, sickle cell trait, and other hemoglobinopathies. The primary care provider (PCP) should validate home address and phone while doing newborn rounds to ensure that the newborn screening results are reported to the office in a timely manner and there is correct information to contact the family if abnormal results are noted. The PCP also needs to verify and document the infant's results in the medical record. In the United States, sickle cell disease is the most common genetic disease identified through the state-mandated screening programs. It exceeds the incidence of hypothyroidism, cystic fibrosis, and hyperphenylalaninemia. (More information about newborn screening can be found at www.cdc.gov/ncbddd/newbornscreening/index.html.)

Physical Examination

The physical examination of the child should be comprehensive and include vital signs and growth documentation. The following positive signs are particularly important to identify due to their association with specific problems:

- Pallor (especially of the conjunctivae, buccal mucosa, and palmar creases)
- Jaundice (indicates a hemolytic process)
- Petechiae (indicates multiple cell involvement)
- Retinal hemorrhages (hemolytic disorders)
- Excessive bruising, multiple stages of healing (coagulopathy)
- Bleeding from mucous membranes (coagulopathy)
- Lymphadenopathy (infection, malignancy)
- Frontal bossing and/or prominent maxilla (secondary to bone marrow expansion in thalassemia major)
- Joint or extremity pain (sickle cell, leukemia)
- Heart murmurs (may be heard with anemias), signs of congestive heart failure, or tachycardia (acute process with poor compensation)
- Hepatomegaly or splenomegaly (splenomegaly—associated with hemolytic processes, malignancy, acute infection; hypersplenism due to portal hypertension)
- Congenital anomalies that are associated with hematologic disorders

Pancytopenia

Pancytopenia is marked by a decrease in all three formed elements of the blood—erythrocytes, leukocytes, and platelets. A child usually presents with clinical findings of infection or bleeding rather than anemia because of the longer lifespan of RBCs compared with platelets and WBCs. As such, it is not a single disease but results from a combination of disease processes. Pancytopenia is caused by one of three processes:

- Production failure (intrinsic bone marrow disease, as occurs in aplastic anemia)
- Sequestration (as occurs with hypersplenism)
- Increased peripheral destruction of mature cells (as occurs in certain infections and with known medications) (Zitelli and Davis, 2012)

The child should be referred to a pediatric hematologist for treatment focused at correcting the underlying mechanism, such as hematopoietic stem cell transplantation (failure of production), splenectomy, or other treatments aimed at reducing peripheral destruction of cells or sequestration.

Erythrocyte Disorders

Anemia

Classification of the Anemias

Anemia is a reduction in circulating RBCs s and results from a reduction in RBC production, abnormalities of the RBC itself, shortened RBC lifespan, RBC destruction, or acute or chronic loss of circulating RBCs. Various anemias are more common in specific races and geographic populations, such as SCA and glucose-6-phosphate dehydrogenase (G6PD) deficiency in people of African and Mediterranean decent. Nutritional deficiencies and toxic ingestions play integral roles in the incidence of anemias (i.e., folic acid deficiency, B_{12} deficiency, iron deficiency anemia [IDA], and lead poisoning). Anemia affects many systems, because it causes stress on the cardiovascular and respiratory systems. This may manifest as decreased exercise tolerance, fatigue, shortness of breath, or congestive heart failure. However, the majority of children and adolescents with anemia are asymptomatic.

RBCs may be described by the cell size, shape, or color (e.g., hypochromic, microcytic; macrocytic; normochromic, normocytic). The use of this standardized nomenclature facilitates the diagnostic process by distinguishing the various anemias (Table 27-6). For instance, IDA is microcytic (small cell) and hypochromic (pale), whereas aplastic anemia is macrocytic (large), and anemia from malignancies and chronic illness tends to be normocytic. To narrow the diagnostic possibilities, anemia can be classified on the basis of their MCV and reticulocyte count (Fig. 27-4).

In toddlers and young children, approximately 90% of anemias are caused by either IDA, lead poisoning (also called *plumbism*), infection, or hemoglobinopathy. The first two of these problems result from a reduction in available Hgb for nutrient transport within the RBC. This reduction of circulating Hgb results in small, pale RBCs (microcytic, hypochromic) with decreased oxygen-carrying potential. Inadequate RBC production can be either acquired or constitutional, resulting in such anemias as aplastic anemia, red cell aplasia, and transient erythroblastopenia of childhood (TEC). Table 27-7 outlines the history, physical findings, and laboratory diagnosis and treatment of the common RBC anemias in infants and children.

Another classification system defines anemias into three categories by the type of problem with RBC production (Fig. 27-5). *Hypoproliferative anemias* result from a failure in erythrocyte marrow production. These anemias tend to be normocytic-normochromic with a reticulocyte count less than 2, giving the semblance of the body not responding to the anemia. Among the causes for the hypoproliferative anemias are iron deficiency, marrow damage, decreased stimulation of the marrow (as in renal disease), inflammation, and metabolic disorders. *Maturational anemias*, in which there is a defect in nuclear maturation, are caused by nutritional disturbances, such as deficiencies in folic acid and vitamin B_{12} and exposure to chemotherapeutic agents. In chronic illnesses, there may be a decrease in red cell survival time, the bone marrow response or impaired iron transport. Such an effect is often seen in chronic inflammatory illnesses, chronic infections, renal and liver disease, endocrine disorders, and malignant neoplastic diseases. In the third category increased cell destruction produces *hemolytic anemias*. The hemolysis may be caused by defects in the red cell membrane, hereditary hemoglobinopathies (as

TABLE 27-6 Acute Anemia in Childhood and Adolescence

Classification	History	Physical Findings	Screening Tests	Diagnostic Studies	Treatment
I. Microcytic					
Iron deficiency anemia (IDA)	Infant and toddler Excessive cow's milk ingestion Poor solid food intake	Waxy, sallow appearance of skin	Hgb: 8-11 g/dL (moderate); <7 g/dL (severe) MCV: <60 fL Reticulocyte count: ↓ to sl ↑	Serum Fe: ↓ TIBC: ↑ % Saturation: ↓	Ferrous sulfate, 3 to 6 mg/kg/day of elemental iron Discontinue cow's milk Limit formula to <24 oz/day and encourage solid food
Homozygous thalassemia (Cooley anemia)	Infant and toddler Growth failure Ethnic background consistent	Hepatosplenomegaly Frontal bossing	MCV: 50-60 fL	Hgb: var ↓	Hypertransfusion program; chelation therapy if iron overload, hematopoietic stem cell transplantation
II. Macrocytic					
Diamond-Blackfan anemia Megaloblastic anemia	(See III: Normocytic) Variable, depending on etiology	Variable, depending on etiology	Hgb: var ↓ MCV: ↑ Reticulocyte count: ↓ Platelets and WBC: ↓ Hypersegmented polys	Bone marrow: Megaloblastic Vitamin B_{12} level: nl to ↓ Folate Others	Variable, depending on etiology (e.g., folic acid, vitamin B_{12}, transfusion)
III. Normocytic					
A. Production Defect					
Diamond-Blackfan anemia	Age of onset: 65% <6 months old 90% <1 year old Insidious onset	25% with physical abnormalities	Hgb: <8 g/dL MCV: ↑ in 30% (100% after treatment) Reticulocyte count: <1%	Bone marrow: Erythroid hypoplasia and lymphocytosis Hgb F: ↑ RBCi antigen: ↑	Prednisone: 2 mg/kg/day and may be tapered gradually
Transient erythroblastopenia of childhood (TEC)	1 to 3 years old Viral illness in preceding 3 months	None	Hgb: 3-9 g/dL MCV: normal Reticulocyte count: <1%	Bone marrow: Erythroid hypoplasia	Supportive
Aplastic anemia	Bleeding Infection	Petechiae, purpura Infection Multiple anomalies possible with Fanconi anemia	Hgb: var ↓ MCV: ↑ in Fanconi anemia Reticulocyte count: ↓ Platelets and WBC: ↓	Bone marrow: Hypoplasia of all hematopoietic elements	Variable
B. Hemolytic					
Autoimmune hemolytic anemia	Jaundice GI symptoms Dark, red urine	Icterus Hepatosplenomegaly	Hgb: var ↓ Reticulocyte count: ↑ (occ ↓) Smear: Microspherocytes	Direct Coombs test: Positive	Corticosteroids: Prednisone or intravenous equivalent: 2 to 6 mg/kg/day Transfusion indicated
Hemolytic-uremic syndrome	Infant and toddler Viral prodrome GI bleeding in 20% Sudden pallor, purpura CNS symptoms	Purpura Hypotension CNS abnormalities	Hgb: 7-8 g/dL Reticulocyte count: ↑ Platelets: ↓ Smear: Microangiopathy	None Renal tests: Failure	Supportive: Early dialysis? Plasma infusion/exchange? Antiplatelet drugs
C. Blood loss					
Splenic sequestration crisis of sickle cell (SS) disease (internal blood loss)	SS disease: 5 months to 2 years old Hgb SC or S-thalassemia: All ages Sudden weakness, dyspnea, abdominal distention Shock	Hypotension Massive splenomegaly	Hgb: <4 g/dL Reticulocyte count: ↑ Smear: Sickle cells	None	Plasma expanders: Whole or reconstituted blood

Adapted from Burg F, Ingelfinger J, Polin, R, et al: editors: *Current pediatric therapy*, ed 18, Philadelphia, 2006, Saunders.

CNS, Central nervous system; *Fe,* iron; *GI,* gastrointestinal; *Hgb,* hemoglobin; *Hgb F,* fetal hemoglobin; *MCV,* mean corpuscular volume; *RBCi,* red blood cell i antigen; *TIBC,* total iron-binding capacity; *WBC,* white blood cell.
nl, Normal; *var,* variably; *occ,* occasionally; *sl,* slightly; *?,* questionable use.

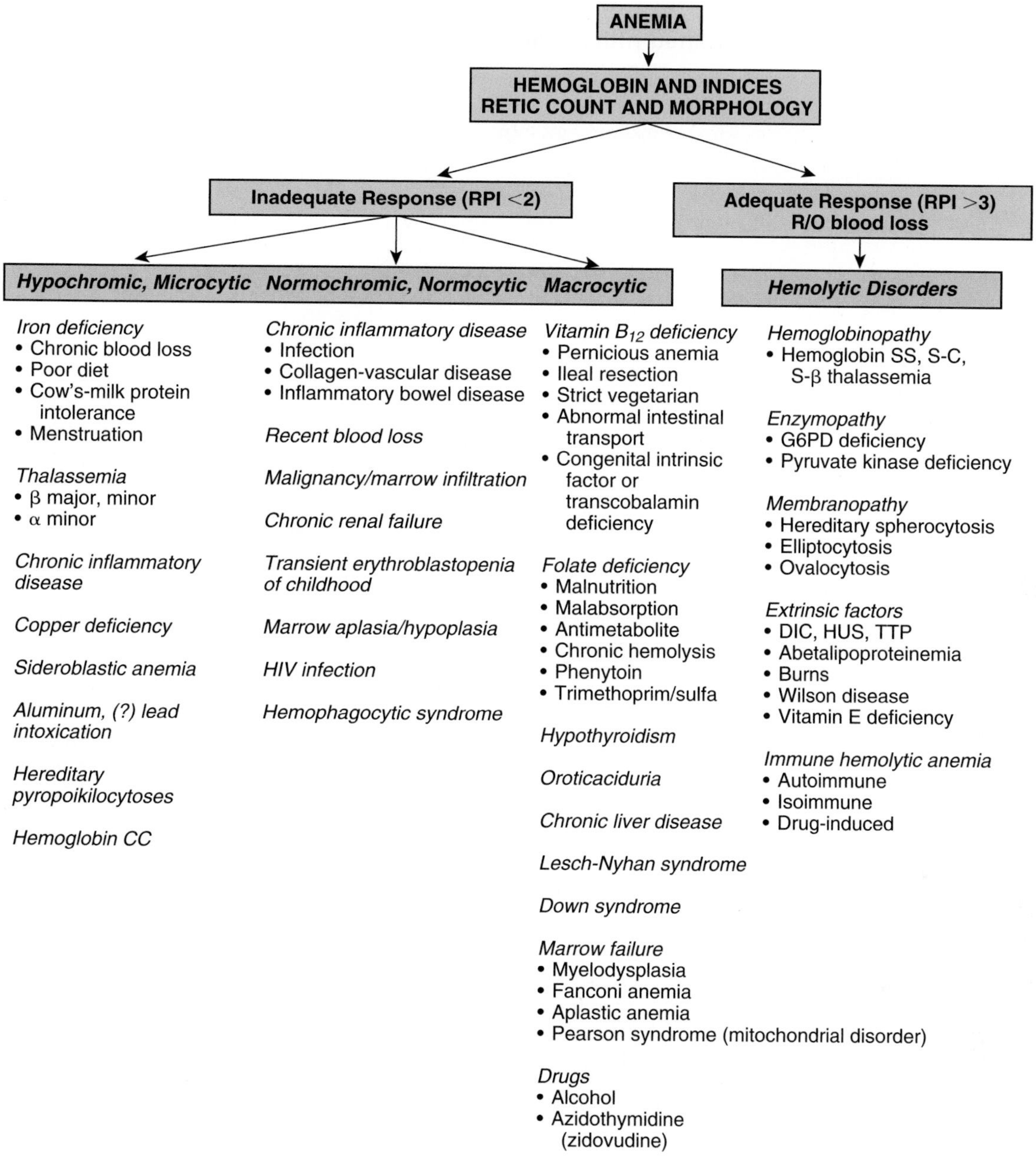

• **Figure 27-4** Use of the complete blood count (CBC), reticulocyte count, and blood smear in the diagnosis of anemia. *DIC,* Disseminated intravascular coagulation; *G6PD,* glucose-6-phosphate dehydrogenase; *HIV,* human immunodeficiency virus; *HUS,* hemolytic-uremic syndrome; *R/O,* rule out; *RPI,* reticulocyte production index; *TTP,* thrombotic thrombocytopenic purpura. (From Scott J: Hematology. In Kliegman RM, Marcdante K, Jenson H, et al, editors: *Nelson essentials of pediatrics*, ed 5, Philadelphia, 2006, Saunders.)

in SCA), or congenital enzyme defects. Among these syndromes are hereditary spherocytosis (HS) and G6PD deficiency.

Epidemiology

Despite a steady decline in the United States, anemia continues to be a major health problem here and, to an even greater extent, internationally. Iron deficiency is the most common cause of anemia, even as cases steadily decline when nutritional practices improve. The thalassemias are a group of inherited disorders that cause a significant number of pediatric anemias. One of the most common single gene disorders in the world is alpha-thalassemia. This genetic disorder affects up to 40% of the population in the China and Southeast Asia and 5% to 10% in the Mediterranean region. Historically the disease was rare in the United States; however, the incidence is increasing with the surge in Asian immigration. Alpha-thalassemia mutations affect approximately 5% of the world's population from asymptomatic states to in utero demise (Vichinsky, 2013). Hgb H disease

TABLE 27-7 Red Blood Cell Disorders Associated with Anemia in Infants and Children

	Clinical Presentation			
Disease	**History**	**Physical Findings**	**Laboratory Diagnosis**	**Treatment**
Iron deficiency	Fatigue Irritability Excess milk intake	Pallor or none	RBC hypochromic, microcytic MCV ↓ Serum iron ↓ TIBC ↑ Percentage of saturation ↓ Ferritin ↓ Blood in stool or urine Ratio of MCV/RBC >13	Correct diet Eliminate source of bleeding Ferrous SO_4 up to 6 mg/kg/day of elemental iron
Alpha- and beta-thalassemia trait	None Pallor Family history	None Pallor	RBC hypochromic, microcytic MCV ↓↓ Basophilic stippling (beta-thalassemia trait)↑ Hgb A_2 (beta-thalassemia trait) Ratio of MCV/RBC <13	None for child Test both parents Genetic counseling Avoid iron therapy
Hereditary spherocytosis (HS)	None Family history History of neonatal jaundice	Pallor, jaundice Splenomegaly	Spherocytosis Coombs test negative Reticulocyte percentage ↑ Osmotic fragility increased MCHC ↑	No splenectomy if Hgb >10 g/dL and reticulocyte <10% Folic acid (0.5 mg daily <5 years old; 1 mg daily >5 years old) Splenectomy; immunizations for pneumococcus, *Haemophilus influenzae*, and meningococcus; penicillin prophylaxis
Chronic inflammation	Depends on the cause of the inflammation and the severity of anemia (fatigue to symptoms of congestive heart failure)	Depends on the cause of the inflammation and the severity of anemia (pallor to signs of congestive heart failure)	Nonspecific tests: Erythrocyte sedimentation rate Acute-phase reactants: C-reactive protein, fibrinogen, haptoglobin Serum ferritin Serum iron, TIBC, percentage of iron saturation Bone marrow iron stores Bone marrow sideroblasts	Treat underlying disease or condition Treat anemia
Lead intoxication	Pica—ingestion of nonfood substances, especially those containing lead Neurobehavioral problems (e.g., irritability, poor appetite, inattention, hyperactivity) Neurodevelopmental delay (e.g., learning problems to severe cognitive dysfunction)	Poor speech Visuomotor integration problems Encephalopathy, neuropathy, cerebral edema if severe poisoning	Basophilic stippling Erythrocyte protoporphyrin blood lead	Eliminate source of lead in the child's environment Diet rich in iron and calcium Iron supplementation, 4-6 mg/kg/day to reduce further absorption of lead Chelation therapy based on lead levels and symptoms (use Centers for Disease Control and Prevention guidelines)

Adapted from Segel G, Hirsh M, Feig S: Managing anemia in a pediatric office practice: part 1, *Pediatr Rev* 23:75–83, 2002.
Hgb, Hemoglobin; *MCHC,* mean corpuscular hemoglobin concentration; *MCV,* mean corpuscular volume; *RBC,* red blood cell; *TIBC,* total iron-binding capacity.

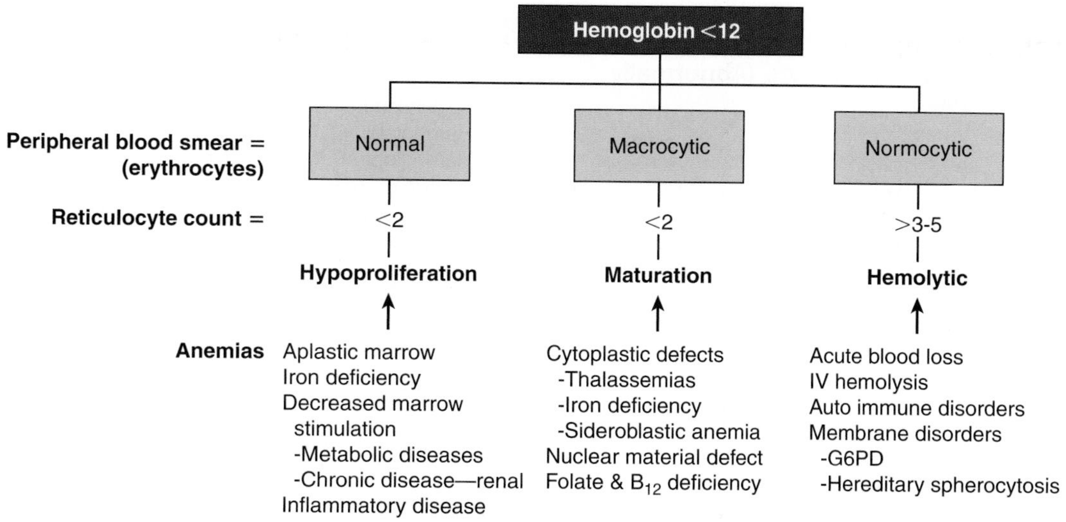

• **Figure 27-5** Classification of anemia by underlying erythrocyte disorder. *G6PD,* Glucose-6-phosphate dehydrogenase; *IV,* intravenous. (Adapted from Hillman RS, Ault KA, Rinder HM: *Hematology in clinical practice*, ed 4, New York, 2005, McGraw-Hill.)

occurs when an individual has only one working gene for alpha-globin. Beta-thalassemia manifests with greater numbers in Mediterranean, northern African, and Indian peoples, whereas SCA is highest among African populations; and all are rare in persons of northern European ancestry.

Workup for Anemia

Anemia may be suspected on the basis of clinical judgment, but is often detected though hematocrit (Hct) and Hgb screening. Understanding which tests to order and how to interpret laboratory data are integral to analyzing the information communicated by the hematopoietic system (see Tables 27-1 and 27-2). Laboratory norms vary slightly with the individual lab, so evaluate the child's results in accordance with local lab norms. Therefore, be sure to understand if the local lab uses pediatric normal reference ranges. If they are only using adult normed references, then the "flagged" level may be within an expected pediatric range and needs to be verified through an age appropriate reference.

The initial laboratory evaluation of suspected anemia includes the following:

- CBC with RBC indices and morphology
- Reticulocyte count
- Peripheral smear to examine the morphologic characteristics and staining properties of the RBC

A standardized vocabulary is used to describe the characteristics of erythrocytes that enable the provider to differentiate and categorize the disorders. The language of morphology is summarized in Box 27-1 with examples of associated disorders.

Following an abnormal screening for Hgb or Hct, further diagnostic studies may be indicated to delineate the type of acute anemia. The PCP may wish to consider ordering serum iron (Fe), free erythrocyte protoporphyrin (FEP), total iron-binding capacity (TIBC), serum ferritin, and the red (blood cell) distribution width (RDW) if that was not included in the CBC. Table 27-8 presents a summary of how these laboratory findings help to differentiate the microcytic anemias.

Microcytic Anemia

By far the most common of the anemias in children, microcytic anemia, often results from a defect in Hgb (from inadequate availability or usage of a substrate) or globin synthesis (as in inherited hemoglobinopathy). Chronic inflammation, plumbism (i.e., lead poisoning), and iron deficiency result in decreased iron delivery to the marrow. In the thalassemias, globin chain synthesis is defective; and although rare in children, in sideroblastic anemias, the heme synthesis malfunctions. In addition to obtaining a CBC, key laboratory tests for the microcytic anemias include TIBC and Fe to differentiate IDA from the rest of the possible disorders. If the anemias of chronic illness and iron deficiency are ruled out or if there is treatment failure, an Hgb electrophoresis with a quantitative Hgb A_2 and Hgb F can diagnose hemoglobinopathy, such as thalassemia. Bone marrow aspiration with iron staining is used to diagnose sideroblastic anemia, but this disorder is rare in children. Table 27-8 compares the microcytic anemias laboratory findings.

Iron Deficiency Anemia

IDA is the most common nutritional disorder and hematologic condition in the world. Approximately 3% to 7% of children at age 1 year suffer from iron deficiency (Powers and Buchanan, 2014). Nine percent of adolescent girls develop iron deficiency and 2% to 3% between the ages of 12 and 19 years old develop anemia primarily due to rapid growth, heavy menses, and nutritionally inadequate diets

• BOX 27-1 Erythrocyte Morphology

Macrocytic Erythrocyte/Megalocyte (Abnormally Large Red Blood Cells)

- Pernicious anemia
- Lack of vitamin B_{12} and folic acid
- Megaloblastic anemia and liver disease

Schistocyte (Fragmented Cell, Helmet Cell)

- Microangiopathic hemolytic anemia
- Disseminated intravascular coagulation (DIC)
- Thrombotic microangiopathies
- Thrombocytopenic purpura
- Glomerulonephritis
- Hemolytic-uremic syndrome
- Giant hemangioma

Anisocytosis (Unequally Sized Red Blood Cell)

- Iron deficiency
- Sideroblastic anemia
- Vitamin A deficiency
- Kwashiorkor
- Hemoglobin H disease
- Hemoglobin Bart's
- Folate and vitamin B_{12} deficiency

Sideroblasts*

- Myelodysplastic syndrome
- Acute myelogenous leukemia
- Sideroblastic anemia

Membrane Abnormalities

- Acanthocytes or spur/spike cells
- Codocyte cells or target cells
- Echinocytes and burr cells
- Elliptocytes and ovalocytes
- Spherocytes

Target Cells†

- Thalassemia
- Hemoglobin C
- Hemoglobin S (sickle cell anemia [SCA])
- Iron deficiency
- Postsplenectomy
- Liver disease (obstructive)

Elliptocyte-Ovalocyte

- Hereditary spherocytosis (HS)
- Thalassemia
- Iron deficiency
- Myelophthisic anemia
- Megaloblastic anemias
- Posttransfusion

Sickle Cells

- Sickle cell disease
- Hgb SC
- Hgb S thalassemia
- Parasites
- Malaria, babesiosis

Acanthocytes (Spur Cell)

- Postsplenectomy
- Cirrhosis
- Pyruvate kinase deficiency
- Uremia
- Infantile pyknocytosis

Dacryocytes—Teardrop

- Extramedullary hematopoiesis
- Myelophthisic anemia
- Severe hemolytic anemia
- Erythroleukemia

*Erythroid precursor, ringed red blood cell (RBC) body has iron available but cannot incorporate it into hemoglobin.
†Abnormal hypochromic RBCs that have a bull's-eye appearance.

TABLE 27-8 Microcytic Anemias

Diagnosis	Mean Corpuscular Volume	Red Blood Count Number	Red Blood Cell Distribution Width	Ferritin	Total Iron-Binding Capacity
Iron deficiency anemia (IDA)	Low or normal	Low	High (>14%)	Low	High
Thalassemia trait	Low	Normal to high	Normal (<14%)	Normal	Normal
Viral suppression or chronic depression	Normal or low	Low	Normal	High	Low
Lead poisoning	Low or normal	Low	Normal to high	Normal to high	Normal

From Burg F, Ingelfinger J, Polin R, et al: editors: *Current pediatric therapy*, ed 18, Philadelphia, 2006, Saunders.

(Abrams, 2014). The incidence of IDA among children in the United States has been declining slightly during the past four decades, although the prevalence remains high among children living at or below poverty level and in black and Hispanic children. Other risk factors include childhood obesity and a history of prematurity or low birth weight (Mahoney, 2015). Iron deficiency correlates with rapid increases in body size and blood volume during the first 2 years, along with diets low in iron, such as occurs with an overuse of goat's or cow's milk. The deficient iron intake is also associated with prolonged bottle-feeding.

Dietary iron is absorbed throughout the intestine but especially in the duodenum. Malabsorption of iron occurs in diseases that affect this segment of the intestine, such as celiac disease, Crohn disease, giardiasis, or resection of the proximal small intestine. Disorders causing GI blood loss such as inflammatory bowel disease, cow's milk–induced colitis, or chronic use of aspirin or nonsteroidal anti-inflammatory drugs (NSAIDs) also deplete iron stores and contribute to iron deficiency (Mahoney, 2015).

Anemia (Hgb level <11 g/dL) is neither a sensitive nor a specific screen for iron deficiency because about two thirds of iron-deficient children are not anemic. Conversely, the detection of anemia is not specific to iron deficiency, because two thirds of anemic children have another cause for their anemia. The minimum laboratory screening for iron deficiency is the Hgb level. Often, the simplest and most cost-effective measurement is a CBC, which includes the Hgb, Hct, MCV, and RDW. A ferritin level may also be helpful because this indicates body stores of iron, but it must be interpreted carefully because ferritin is an acute phase reactant and may be increased with inflammatory conditions (Mahoney, 2015). The American Academy of Pediatrics (AAP) Committee on Nutrition recommends universal Hgb screening for anemia at 12 months old (Baker and Greer, 2010). This screening should include an assessment of risk factors for iron deficiency and IDA (Box 27-2).

Screening Hgb can be performed on children younger than 1 year old when risk factors warrant it. Menstruating females may also require screening for IDA due to the monthly blood loss, rapid growth, and potentially inadequate diet. When screening for IDA or any other routine health screening recommendation, remember that screening is not just a one-time test; the effectiveness of treatment must be determined through follow-up testing. Thus after the routine 12-month Hgb/Hct testing, risk assessment for anemia should be performed at all preventive pediatric health care visits with follow-up blood testing if positive. If children are at risk for IDA, a repeat Hgb/Hct should be performed as often as indicated.

• BOX 27-2 Risk Factors for Iron Deficiency Anemia

- History of prematurity or low birth weight
- Exposure to lead
- Exclusive breastfeeding beyond 6 months without iron supplementation
- Weaning to whole cow's milk without iron source
- Feeding problems
- Special health care needs
- Prolonged bottle use
- Low socioeconomic status
- Excessive or prolonged intake of cow's milk
- Obesity
- Hispanic or Asian descent
- Adolescent female, excessive menstrual bleeding

Effects of Iron Deficiency

Many studies demonstrate that iron-deficient states in the first few years of life are associated with subsequent cognitive deficits well into adulthood, although direct causality is difficult to prove. Further complicating the picture of causality is that lead poisoning is often a comorbid condition to IDA. The presence of low levels of iron facilitates intestinal absorption of lead. Lead poisoning and iron deficiency have significant effects on the developing brain. Due to these factors, lead screening is an integral part of pediatric primary care. Early in the child's life, there is critical and rapid brain development; the brain grows to 95% of its adult size by 2 years old. Nutritional deficits that result in IDA or plumbism can cause lasting damage, perhaps manifesting as diminished reading and math computational ability. A child at risk for lead exposure should typically have blood drawn to determine the level of lead at 9 to 12 months old and again at 24 months old. Additional screening should be done at 15 and 30 months old based on at-risk status. Local health departments determine the prevalence of lead poisoning in their area and issue guidelines related to blood lead screenings for targeted children in their catchment areas (Simon et al, 2014). If the initial blood lead level is 10 mcg/dL or greater on a single visit, it is a concern for public health purposes. The United States has made great strides in reducing lead toxicity through the elimination of tetraethyl leaded gasoline, banning lead-containing solder to seal food and beverage cans, and a federal rule to limit the amount of lead allowed in paint intended for household use. An estimated 99% of lead-poisoned children are identified through screening procedures rather than through clinical recognition.

Clinical Findings

History

Conduct a detailed history for hematologic disorders mentioned at the beginning of this chapter, but keep in mind that even children with moderate to severe anemia may be asymptomatic. Some key elements to remember are:

- Infants and toddlers may be irritable and restless, but this only occurs with Hgb less than 8 g/dL and is often noticed in retrospect—after treatment. Pica (appetite for nonfood items such as paper, dirt, and clay) and pagophagia (the desire to ingest ice) may be present and is common and specific for the iron-deficient state.

- Anorexia has been reported with Hgb levels less than 8 g/dL.
- Developmental delays (mental and motor areas) and social-emotional behavioral disturbances that may be irreversible have been reported in infants and young children; adolescents may experience cognitive impairment (Mahoney, 2015).

Physical Examination

In mild to moderate iron deficiency, few symptoms are seen, but all systems must be methodically assessed. The child may appear normal, or pallor may be present. Rarely, in anemias that develop slowly, the physical examination may reveal tachycardia or systolic murmurs and signs of congestive heart failure. If symptoms of severe anemia exist, the examination should include stool guaiac testing.

Diagnostic Studies

The two most commonly used screening tests for IDA are Hgb and Hct, with Hgb being the more direct and sensitive marker of anemia compared with Hct measurements. IDA is frequently identified in routine screenings of Hgb level via capillary sampling. Excessive squeezing of the finger for capillary sample may produce inaccurate results (lower Hct), so proper technique is essential. Venous sampling is the most reliable indicator. IDA is likely if there is a low Hgb level for age (in the range of 8 to 11 g/dL), a history of low iron intake, and no concern about other possible causes for the anemia or the possibility of another hemoglobinopathy. Table 27-9 provides laboratory cutoff values for anemia. If the age of the child and the dietary patterns are consistent with IDA and there is microcytic anemia (Hgb >9 g/dL), many clinicians begin a trial of iron supplementation for 4 to 6 weeks without further diagnostic testing and then follow the child's Hgb and reticulocyte counts. The RDW is the earliest marker of iron deficiency. Serum ferritin is low with iron deficiency (Powers and Buchanan, 2014).

Mild to moderate IDA is characterized by Hgb levels of 7 to 10 g/dL. Levels less than 4 g/dL necessitate consultation with a hematologist; and levels of 7 or less should be carefully evaluated as to whether the child needs referral to hematology. If treatment with oral iron supplements is effective, follow-up Hgb in 1 month should reveal a minimum 1 to 2 g/dL improvement, but the reticulocyte count will increase to greater than 3% in 48 to 96 hours (Lerner and Sills, 2011).

There is a high comorbidity between IDA and lead poisoning (Pb >10 mcg/dL) because lead molecules block iron from binding to protoporphyrin by inhibiting essential mitochondrial membrane function and interfering with enzymes. In low iron states, the lack of iron results in an accumulation of erythrocyte protoporphyrin in blood.

The typical profile for IDA is:

- Microcytic, hypochromic RBCs on CBC
- Low or normal MCV; low to normal RBC number
- High RDW (>14%)
- Low ferritin
- High TIBC
- Mentzer Index greater than 13 (IDA more likely)

Clinical Pearl

Chelating medications for lead toxicity will also pull out iron, so iron supplements, if needed, should be given when the child is not on oral chelators.

Differential Diagnosis

Iron deficiency should be differentiated from other microcytic, hypochromic anemias, such as lead poisoning, thalassemia minor, anemia of chronic disease, and hereditary sideroblastic anemia (see Fig. 27-4). In lead poisoning, the FEP may be more than 200 mcg/dL, and basophilic

TABLE 27-9 Age- and Gender-Specific Laboratory Cutoff Values for Anemia

Age (Years)	Hemoglobin Concentration (g/dL)	Hematocrit (%)	Mean Corpuscular Volume (fL)
1 to <2	<11	32.9	<77
2 to <5	<11.1	33	<79
5 to <8	<11.5	33.5	<80
8 to <12	<11.9	35.4	<80
12 to <15, male	<12.5	37.3	<85
15 to <18, male	<13.3	39.7	<85
12 to <15, female	<11.8	35.7	<85
15 to <18, female	<12	35.9	<85

From Burg F, Ingelfinger J, Polin R, et al: editors: *Gellis and Kagan's current pediatric therapy*, ed 17, Philadelphia, 2002, Saunders.

stippling may be seen on the RBCs in the peripheral smear. Beta-thalassemia is indicated by elevations in Hgb A_2 on electrophoresis and Mentzer Index less than 13.

If there is no response to iron therapy within 1 month and there is confidence that the iron supplements are being given correctly, a more extensive workup should include a CBC with differential, platelet count, RBC indices, and reticulocyte count. A peripheral blood smear should also be examined to assess the number and morphology of RBCs, WBCs, and platelets. The differential diagnosis for anemia can then be determined on the basis of whether RBC production is adequate or inadequate, and whether the cells are microcytic, normocytic, or macrocytic (see Fig. 27-4).

Other causes of anemia, such as blood loss with occult rectal bleeding, should be considered in children with a low Hgb level on screening who eat a normal diet with adequate servings of iron-rich foods. Additional investigation is warranted in children younger than 6 months old or older than 18 months old or who demonstrate no response to treatment after 2 to 4 weeks. For those children with low Hgb/Hct who do not have a history suspicious for IDA, the investigation must expand to include less common sources for the anemia. Findings of severe anemia or atypical hematologic results require consultation and further investigation. Pairing the classification of the cells with the clinical findings, red cell indices, and additional diagnostic studies enables the provider to determine the appropriate treatment plan.

Management

Treatment for IDA consists of iron supplementation, typically as ferrous sulfate (3 to 6 mg/kg/day of elemental iron in two to three divided doses or 3 mg/kg/day in one or two divided doses for mild or moderate IDA) (Lerner and Sills, 2011). The child's Hgb/Hct and reticulocyte count should be reassessed in 4 weeks following initiation of treatment. If there is an adequate response to treatment with supplemental iron, a diagnosis of IDA is confirmed. Responses to treatment with iron supplementation are important diagnostically and therapeutically. Peripheral reticulocytosis may be seen after the first 4 days of treatment, and Hgb should return to a normal level within 4 to 6 weeks. If a therapeutic response is observed (Hgb increase of >1 g/dL or >3% increase in Hct), iron supplementation should continue for 2 to 3 months to normalize Hgb, then continue for 2 to 4 months to replace depleted iron stores. Hematologic and iron status should be rechecked 6 months after iron supplements are stopped to determine resolution of the anemia and adequacy of iron stores (Lerner and Sills, 2011; Mahoney, 2015).

Iron Requirements

Full-term infants accumulate almost 80% of their iron stores during the last trimester of pregnancy. Maternal conditions such as anemia, maternal hypertension with intrauterine growth retardation, or even gestational diabetes can contribute to less iron transferred to the fetus. In the case of preterm births, the decreased iron stores are depleted rapidly as the infants experience rapid postnatal growth. They also have a smaller total blood volume at birth, increased loss through phlebotomy, and poor GI absorption. The use of erythropoietin to prevent and treat anemia of prematurity also increases the risk of iron deficiency (Mahoney, 2015). Thus, preterm (<37 weeks' gestation) breastfed infants require an oral supplement of elemental iron at 2 mg/kg/day after 2 weeks of age through 12 months old (Baker and Greer, 2010; Mahoney, 2015).

Breast milk provides an average iron content of 1.0 mg/L to 0.3 mg/L with a high bioavailability. Because there is large variation in the iron content in human milk, the content of maternal milk may not always provide for the needs of the growing infant. It is recommended that the exclusively breastfed term infant receive elemental iron supplementation of 1 mg/kg/day (15 mg maximum) beginning at 4 months old and continuing until iron containing complementary foods are introduced and taken in adequate quantities (Mahoney, 2015). This same iron supplementation recommendation holds for the partially breastfed infants who receive more than one-half of their daily feeding as human milk (Baker and Greer, 2010). Formula-fed infants receive sufficient iron intake of 12 mg/dL in standard infant formulas. Whole milk should be avoided until after 12 months old.

IOM-calculated iron recommendations increase dramatically to 11 mg/day between 7 and 12 months old based on cells sloughing and demands of increasing body mass. As the rate of growth decreases in toddlerhood, so too does the nutritional requirement of iron, down to 7 mg/day between 1 and 3 years old. Iron deficiency becomes more prevalent during these ages as well, reaching 6.6% to 15.2% depending on ethnicity and socioeconomic status, although the occurrence of IDA is 0.9% to 4.4%. Despite these seemingly low levels of incidence, IDA accounts for more than 40% of the anemias of toddlerhood. Liquid supplementation for this age group is appropriate until 36 months old. Chewable multivitamins can be used for children older than 3 years old, but the supplement formulation must be evaluated for adequate replacement.

Complications

Adherence issues and alternative diagnoses should be explored if there is no response to iron supplementation. Dietary counseling is critical and families may need support with making necessary changes. Iron-deficient states can exist in the absence of anemia as a precursor to IDA and require intervention. A more extensive determination of the child's iron status is obtained by measuring serum iron, iron-binding capacity, and the venous lead level. Stool guaiac should be checked for occult blood loss. Children with extremely low Hgb, hypotension, or signs of congestive heart failure should be referred to a pediatric hematologist and may need hospitalization. Laboratory results that also indicate referral are neutropenia, thrombocytopenia, nucleated RBCs, or immature myeloid elements. When disorders of erythrocytes, platelets, and leukocytes are found, a bone marrow disorder is probable.

Patient and Family Education

Parents or caretakers should be counseled to increase iron-rich food sources in their child's diet. Exclusively breastfed term infants should be started on iron supplementation at 4 months old and pureed meats added to the child's diet after 6 months old. Whole cow's milk should be avoided in infants younger than 12 months old due to its low iron content and possibility of insensible GI blood loss. After 12 months old, cow's milk ingestion should be limited to 24 ounces per day. Goat's milk should not be the sole diet for the child, not only due to lack of iron but also its lack of folic acid. For preterm infants, supplementation with oral iron drops should begin no later than 1 month old. Education for children taking iron supplements includes advising parents to avoid giving iron with meals or milk, that vitamin C juice enhances absorption, and that the child's stools will probably turn black. Foods containing soy can inhibit the absorption of iron. Any dental staining associated with taking iron can be removed with dental cleaning. Parents should also be cautioned to keep the medication safely out of reach to prevent accidental ingestion.

There are some helpful tips to give parents related to increasing iron in their young child's diet and supplemental iron administration. Commercial cereal (such as, Kix) can be given as a dry food snack and ¾ cup a day will give approximately 8 mg of iron. This low sugar, corn-based food is great for toddlers who may spit out iron drops. Mixing the iron drops with a teaspoon of chocolate or strawberry syrup may also help get toddlers to take their medications. The smell of the syrup masks the odd metallic odor of the drops; and most children are not familiar with the taste of these syrups, so they do not know there is a medication mixed within them.

Thalassemias

The thalassemias are hereditary, hypochromic anemias associated with the absence or decreased synthesis of the normal Hgb polypeptide chains—usually the α- and β-globin chains—and a relative excess of the other chains. The protein abnormality results in hemoglobinopathies whose names are based on the altered globulin chain. The possibility of thalassemia increases if the onset of anemia and symptoms is prior to 3 to 6 months of age and there is a family history of anemia, miscarriage, jaundice, gallstones, anemia, or splenomegaly.

Categorizing the thalassemias is less straightforward than with many anemias, because although the heterozygous disease is hypochromic and microcytic, the homozygous diseases are also hemolytic. There is anemia and increased erythropoiesis. The erythropoiesis results in bone marrow expansion, but the pathogenesis of this is not fully understood. Focal osteomalacia and delayed bone maturation are at least partially explained by suboptimal blood transfusions and iron overload. Furthermore, the marrow expansion results in frontal bossing and hyperplasia of the maxillary bones leading to typical facies (DeBaun et al, 2011).

Alpha-Thalassemias

The alpha-thalassemias are composed of several variant hemoglobins that are responsible for the various presentations. Current nomenclature often refers to the subtypes by including indication of the number of gene deletions of α-globin, with severity of symptoms increasing with more deletions. Three gene deletions result in severe, even fatal, manifestation of disease. Two gene deletions present with hypochromia; the absence of gene deletions causes mild anemia and often erythrocytosis. A single globin gene deletion is clinically insignificant (DeBaun et al, 2011).

There are two manifestations of the disease expression of alpha-thalassemia. The homozygous Hgb type, hemoglobin Bart's (or Hgb H) with four γ-chains, results in *hydrops fetalis* and is incompatible with life because of severe anemia. Homozygous Hgb H disease can also present as a microcytic, hypochromic anemia that most often manifests as a hemolytic anemia, hepatosplenomegaly, and mild jaundice, and sometimes includes thalassemia-like bone changes. During times of physiologic stress the child may require RBC transfusion.

There are two different carrier states of alpha-thalassemia. In alpha-thalassemia trait, the child exhibits microcytosis and hypochromia but has normal percentages of Hgb A_2 and Hgb F. The other trait state is referred to as a *silent carrier state,* but can have either a silent hematologic phenotype or present with microcytic hypochromia and some erythropoiesis.

Management

Hgb H disease exacerbations may necessitate occasional transfusion during hemolytic or aplastic crises. No treatment is indicated for the carrier trait expressions of disease, and the microcytosis seen in these expressions require that serum iron studies should be done before starting any iron supplements. Those carrying the alpha-thalassemia trait alleles require careful genetic counseling, because there are complex patterns of inheritance that could affect the phenotype of their offspring (Benz, 2015a).

Beta-Thalassemia Minor/Minima

Beta-thalassemia minor and minima disease, also known as *trait,* is associated with a mild, hypochromic, microcytic anemia in which Hgb levels are 2 to 3 g/dL below normal, and the MCV averages 65 fL. These children need to be monitored for iron accumulation but are otherwise asymptomatic. The disease may be confused with iron deficiency or lead poisoning and can be differentiated by measuring serum iron or lead levels, transferrin saturation, or serum ferritin levels (see Table 27-6). It is particularly important to correctly diagnose this condition in order to avoid unnecessary administration of iron supplements, which do not improve the Hgb and could result in iron overload. The primary diagnostic feature is increased Hgb A_2 (>3.5%) on electrophoresis (Benz, 2015a).

Clinical Findings

Clinically most individuals with thalassemia trait are asymptomatic, although mild pallor and splenomegaly may be found. A Hgb of 9.5 to 11 g/dL, Hct less than 30%, and a MCV of less than 75 fL/cell are commonly seen in thalassemia minor. The MCV/RBC count per milliliter is less than 13 (the Mentzer Index). In contrast, the Mentzer Index of iron deficiency is usually greater than 13; however, some sources use 13.5 as the indicator for IDA (Benz, 2015a). The degree of anemia may be exacerbated in concurrent illness or pregnancy.

Management

No specific treatment is known for beta-thalassemia minor. Primary emphasis should be on education of all family members and genetic testing, and counseling should be offered.

Beta-Thalassemia, Intermedia

This variant of thalassemia is the result of various mutations that cause a disorder with a clinical severity that spans from the mild symptoms of the beta-thalassemia trait to the severe manifestations of beta-thalassemia major. Classification is typically based on the severity of the symptoms and the type of treatment necessary rather than by the specific genotype. Diagnosis and management are clinically based with a goal toward maintaining a satisfactory Hgb of at least 6 to 7 g/dL without the regular need for RBC transfusions. Transfusions alleviate thalassemic features, but there is controversy whether these children should receive transfusions. This decision needs to be balanced against the future need for chelation if there is iron overload from repeated transfusions (DeBaun et al, 2011).

Beta-Thalassemia Major

Homozygous forms are thalassemia intermedia and thalassemia major. Homozygous beta-thalassemia major (or Cooley anemia) is associated with severe anemia resulting from decreased or absent production of Hgb A and hemolysis caused by the precipitation of excess α-chains in the RBCs.

Clinical Findings

Affected infants usually become symptomatic in the first year of life and have pallor, failure to thrive, hepatosplenomegaly, and a severe anemia with an average Hgb of 6 g/dL and low MCV (60 to 70 fL). RBC morphology reveals significant microcytosis, poikilocytosis, hypochromia, target cells, and nucleated RBCs. Hgb A_2 and Hgb F levels are elevated.

Management

Proper management of the child requires collaboration with a pediatric hematologist. Standards of care for thalassemia patients should be followed (Vichinsky and Levine, 2012). RBC transfusions are usually necessary every 2 to 4 weeks to maintain a pre-transfusion Hgb level between 9.5 and 10.5 g/dL as the goal. To help with future crossmatching, the provider should obtain a complete typing of the patient's erythrocyte profile before the first transfusion (phenotyping). This helps decrease difficulties with subsequent transfusions. Splenectomy may be indicated as well. Hematopoietic stem cell transplantation is the only curative modality for beta-thalassemia major. This has been most successful in children younger than 15 years old without excessive iron overload and hepatosplenomegaly, who have sibling-matched human leukocyte antigen (HLA) allogeneic hematopoietic transplantation (Benz, 2015b; DeBaun et al, 2011). Gene therapy is being investigated and holds promise for those with this major disorder.

Iron chelation is necessary to treat the hyperferric state produced by repeated transfusions and prevent complications primarily of the heart, liver, and endocrine system. Iron overload can develop even without the use of blood transfusions because of the increased iron absorption associated with high rates of erythropoiesis and red cell destruction. Monitoring for iron stores should be done on a regular basis (Benz, 2015a). Chronic iron chelation therapy is necessary in order to remove the excess iron that results from the frequent transfusions.

Indications for chelation occur when the serum ferritin concentrations are excessive (variably stated as >300, >400, or >1000 mcg/L) and/or imaging with magnetic resonance imaging (MRI) T_2 suggest the presence of iron loading in the critical organs, such as the liver (>3 mg of iron per gram of dry weight) and the heart (Benz, 2015b). Deferoxamine is administered parenterally or subcutaneously usually via a pump overnight. It is time consuming and is associated with pain. Subcutaneously infused medications have been replaced by oral chelators. Deferasirox is an oral agent, taken once daily, at a dose of 20 to 30 mg/kg/day; it stabilizes the ferritin levels, thus achieving a negative iron balance (DeBaun et al, 2011). Iron excretion through chelation is further aided by the ingestion of vitamin C. The iron is excreted through the kidneys, so hydration and monitoring of renal status is vital.

Complications

If the condition is left untreated, bone marrow expansion causes the characteristic facies with frontal bossing and maxillary overgrowth. Other complications of disease and treatment include osteopenia, thrombolytic symptoms, cardiopulmonary problems, asplenia secondary to splenectomy, cholelithiasis, and extramedullary hematopoiesis.

The medications used to chelate iron have additional side effects. Deferasirox, the daily oral agent, commonly produces headache, nausea, vomiting, joint pain, and fatigue. It has a black box warning of GI hemorrhage, as well as kidney and liver failure. Deferoxamine has risks associated with intravenous medication administration (infection) and vision and hearing loss. Additionally there are the inherent risks and complications of transfusion, including transfusion reaction, fever, and, though rare, hepatitis or human immunodeficiency virus (HIV) infection.

The disease, its complications, and treatments are painful for the child and monopolize a large portion of the children's and families' lives. Families need not only professional support and education but also interaction with other families affected by this disorder, such as found at the Thalassemia Support Foundation or Cooley's Anemia Foundation.

Megaloblastic Anemias

Megaloblastic anemias are characterized by oval macrocytes and hypersegmented PMN leukocytes in the peripheral blood and megaloblasts in the bone marrow. Relatively rare, megaloblastic anemias are due primarily to a lack of folic acid, vitamin B_{12}, or both. These two substances function as coenzymes in nuclear protein synthesis. Megaloblastic anemias may develop if the diet lacks these two substances or if the gastric intrinsic factor necessary for the absorption of vitamin B_{12} is absent.

Clinical Findings

History

Suspicion of megaloblastic anemia should be high if there is any history of young infants who are being fed a diet of powdered cow's milk products or goat's milk. These are deficient in folic acid and vitamin B_{12}. Of equal concern are older children who have strict vegetarian diets and those with signs of severe nutritional deficiencies, absorption problems, or tapeworm infestations. Children with folic acid deficiency tend to have irritability, inadequate weight gain, and chronic diarrhea.

Physical Examination

Physical findings relate to the severity of the anemia but commonly include:

- Weakness, pallor
- Beefy-red, smooth, sore mouth and tongue

Diagnostic Studies

The following results may be seen:

- Elevated MCV (>100 fL) and decreased reticulocyte count
- Blood smear showing nucleated RBCs and macro-ovalocytes with anisocytosis and poikilocytosis
- Normal white cell count and platelet count, but possibly decreased in more severe cases
- Large and hypersegmented neutrophils
- Thrombocytopenia or possible large platelets
- In suspected folic acid deficiency—RBC folate level is decreased, iron and B_{12} levels tend to be normal or elevated (Schrier, 2015)

Management

Management of folic acid deficiency and juvenile pernicious anemia (caused by a lack of vitamin B_{12}) is typically best done in consultation with a pediatric hematologist. Treatment is dietary supplementation and correction of the underlying disorder (e.g., infection) if possible.

In folic acid deficiency confirmed by measurement of the RBC folate level, folic acid may be administered in a dose of 1 to 5 mg/day and continued for 1 to 4 months or until a complete hematologic recovery has occurred. This is followed by maintenance therapy with a multivitamin containing 0.2 mg of folate. Prolonged use of high-dose folic acid should be avoided (Schrier, 2015). In vitamin B_{12} deficiency (levels <200 pg/mL), a prompt hematologic response is usually seen after parenteral (either intramuscular or deep subcutaneous) administration of vitamin B_{12}. Treatment with 1 mg of vitamin B_{12} daily for at least 1 week, followed by 1 mg every week for 4 weeks, and then 1 mg monthly if the disorder persists and no underlying cause identified and eliminated. A maintenance dose of a 1 mg intramuscular injection of vitamin B_{12} is administered monthly throughout the patient's life. Nasal and oral formulations are available but have shown variability of absorption and have not been well studied. They also require greater patient compliance (Schrier, 2015).

Normocytic Anemias

Anemias that have an RBC size within the normal value range are termed *normocytic.* Normocytic anemias tend to coincide with chronic illness, B_{12} deficiency, traumatic blood loss, or pregnancy. They are not common in children. Final determination of the etiology extends beyond blood cell indices and includes further chemistry laboratory tests, such as blood urea nitrogen (BUN), creatinine, serum glutamic-oxaloacetic transaminase (SGOT), alkaline phosphatase, bilirubin, erythrocyte sedimentation rate, urinalysis, and thyroid profile.

Transient Erythroblastopenia of Childhood

Idiopathic or transient erythroblastopenia of childhood, or TEC, is a benign disorder of unknown cause that occurs in children during the first few years of life, usually after 1 year old. It is characterized by anemia, reticulocytopenia, and erythroid hypoplasia of the bone marrow. The cause of this transient suppression of erythropoiesis with resultant decreased RBC production is not clear, although it frequently follows a viral infection. Thus viral and immunologic mechanisms are suspected, but no specific virus has been implicated. TEC is associated with temporary failure of erythropoiesis caused by probable viral suppression or as a result of an IgG, IgM or cell-mediated autoimmune response (van den Akker et al, 2014).

Clinical Findings

History

TEC occurs mainly in previously healthy children between 6 months old and 3 years old. The child may have a history of a preceding infection.

Physical Examination

Patients have symptoms of anemia, typically a gradually increasing pallor. Parents may report noticing decreased energy levels or fatigue in their child. Pallor and fatigue develop over a course of days or weeks and are often associated with viral symptoms, such as fever, malaise, lethargy, abdominal pain, or upper respiratory symptoms. Jaundice may be noted, especially if the child has a preexisting hemoglobinopathy (Huang et al, 2014).

Diagnostic Studies

The following are seen in TEC:

- Anemia (in which the Hgb content may be as low as 2.5 g/dL or only slightly decreased but is generally around 6 to 8 g/dL)
- Markedly low reticulocyte count
- MCV is characteristically normal for age
- WBC count usually normal, but some degree of neutropenia can occur in up to 20%
- Platelet count is normal or elevated
- High serum iron level reflecting decreased utilization
- Bone marrow aspiration results indicating erythroid hypoplasia

Differential Diagnosis

The syndrome can be differentiated from congenital hypoplastic anemia (Diamond-Blackfan syndrome) by the normal size of the RBCs (MCV less than 80 fL). Approximately 50% of children with Diamond-Blackfan syndrome have dysmorphic features (e.g., short stature, congenital heart disease, and mental retardation), whereas children with TEC have a normal physical examination. The peak incidence of TEC coincides with that of IDA, but the differences in MCV should help differentiate between these diagnoses (van den Akker et al, 2014).

Management

TEC is self-limited, with recovery taking place 1 to 2 months after diagnosis. No specific treatment is indicated, although transfusions may be required for severe anemia. A referral to a hematologist may be needed.

Hemolytic Anemia

Hemolytic anemias are caused by premature destruction of RBCs and increase marrow production of reticulocytes. They can be classified as either hereditary or acquired and should be suspected in cases of an elevated reticulocyte count in the absence of bleeding or heparin therapy. In particular, the hereditary and congenital anemias manifest in infancy and early childhood. They may be due to a variety of hemoglobinopathies or to defects in the red cell membrane. Determining the etiology of hemolysis necessitates careful history taking, including family medical history, child's medical history, diet, medication intake, and environmental exposures. Confirmation of the diagnosis comes from Hgb electrophoresis, Heinz body stain, and osmotic fragility test.

Sickle Cell Anemia and Trait

Sickle cell disease describes a group of complex, chronic disorders characterized by hemolysis, unpredictable acute complications that may become life threatening, and the possible development of chronic organ damage. Children who have homozygous inheritance have SCA or disease (Hgb SS). Their bodies do not form the normal Hgb A molecule, but rather synthesize hemoglobin S (Hgb S), which carries the amino acid valine instead of glutamic acid. Because of this change, Hgb S tends to polymerize or come out of solution at low Pao_2, low pH, low temperature, and low osmolality. This process collapses the RBC, giving it a "sickled" shape, and produces a chronic hemolytic anemia. The new shape is rigid and clogs small blood vessels, producing ischemia, pain, and other vaso-occlusive problems.

Sickle cell disease has an autosomal recessive inheritance pattern. It is found most often in people of African descent, but it is also detected among ethnic groups from the Mediterranean, the Caribbean, Central and South America, and India. Due to migration, it now occurs worldwide. Sickle trait occurs in 8% of African Americans. This incidence exceeds that of most other serious genetic disorders in children, including cystic fibrosis and hemophilia; only alpha-thalassemia is more common. Routine neonatal screening identifies most infants with sickle cell disease born in the United States, because it is mandated in all states and the District of Columbia. It is still important to do a careful family medical history because many adults do not realize they are carriers.

Clinical Findings

The symptoms of sickle cell disease are multisystem, necessitating vigilant care to minimize occurrence of crises and complications. Common symptoms include:

- Fatigue and anemia
- Pain crises
- Dactylitis (swelling and inflammation of the hands and/or feet) and arthritis
- Bacterial infections
- Lung and heart injury
- Leg ulcers
- Priapism
- Splenic sequestration (sudden pooling of blood in the spleen) and liver congestion

- Aseptic necrosis and bone infarcts (death of portions of bone)
- Eye damage
- Abdominal pain

Children with sickle cell trait who are heterozygous (Hgb A + Hgb S) for the gene essentially have a benign clinical course. Their RBCs contain only 30% to 40% Hgb S, and sickling does not occur under most conditions. It is only in rare instances of hypoxia, such as in shock, while flying in unpressurized aircraft, or traveling to high elevations, that signs of vaso-occlusion can occur. However, the presence of sickle cell trait has been implicated as a causative factor in the sudden deaths of young military recruits, college football players, and some teens. Extreme exercise, typically to exhaustion, dehydration, and relative hypoxia (altitude) are major confounding factors (Harris et al, 2012).

Physical Examination

SCA symptoms typically begin to emerge in the second 6 months of life as the amount of Hgb S increases and Hgb F declines. Subsequently, painful, vaso-occlusive crises occur. Due to the multisystem nature of complications these children need prompt, detailed evaluation and intervention. After 5 years old, splenomegaly usually disappears because of autoinfarction of the organ. Rates of height and weight gain usually slow after 7 years old, and puberty may be delayed 3 to 4 years.

Diagnostic Studies

The following laboratory results are seen in sickle cell disease:

- Hct of 20% to 29%
- Hgb 6 to 10 g/dL (severe)
- Reticulocyte count elevated: 5% to 15%
- Normal to increased WBC and platelet count
- MCV greater than 80 fL; mean corpuscular hemoglobin concentration (MCHC) greater than 37 mg/dL
- Hgb electrophoresis (after infancy), isoelectric focusing or high performance of liquid chromatography showing a predominance of Hgb S and no Hgb A.
- Morphology: Irreversibly sickled cells or chronic elliptocytes, Howell-Jolly bodies, nucleated RBCs

Hgb electrophoresis results in a newborn with sickle cell trait will be Hgb FAS, and Hgb FS for a child with either SCA or sickle beta-zero thalassemia (SBO). Normal results of Hgb electrophoresis are Hgb FA.

Differential Diagnosis

Chronic hemolytic anemia should be included in the differential diagnosis. Other syndromes characterized by hemolytic anemia and vaso-occlusion are Hgb SC disease, SCA, and a combination of Hgb S with alpha- or beta-thalassemia. These diseases may be differentiated through electrophoresis and family testing if necessary. Hgb SC disease is typically less severe than Hgb SS; the course of sickle cell beta-thalassemia can be severe or mild depending on the amount of beta-globin; sickle cell alpha-thalassemia is associated with milder anemia (Vichinsky, 2015). Prenatal genetic testing is available in instances of high suspicion; otherwise mandated newborn screening will render the diagnosis in most cases before symptoms present.

Management

Management of the child with SCA is complicated and should be done in consultation with a pediatric hematologist. Remarkable progress in the care of children with SCA can be directly attributed to the development of standards of care and anticipatory guidance. The National Institutes of Health (NIH) has an expert panel that developed evidenced-based guidelines, "The Management of Sickle Cell Disease" (NIH, 2002). The National Heart, Lung, and Blood Institute continues its work to develop and disseminate evidence-based clinical practice guidelines for the management of SCA.

Children with sickle cell disease still need regular primary care services and coordination of consultative services and information. Growth is closely monitored, immunizations need to be done on time, parents require support, and communication with specialty services should be coordinated, such as an annual ophthalmologic examination by a retinal specialist. Care is comprehensive, spanning normal well-child issues through acute crises and hospitalization. Some of the key aspects of care for the child with SCA are as follows:

- Hydration, illness prevention, and pain management are fundamental aspects of disease management. NSAIDs or acetaminophen may be adequate for mild to moderate pain, but narcotics should be used when these are not adequate for management. (As with anyone taking narcotics, abuse and addiction issues must be considered.)
- CBC and reticulocyte count are monitored every few months.
- All the usual immunizations of childhood are to be administered on time including 13-valent pneumococcal conjugate (four doses at appropriate intervals) and 23-valent pneumococcal polysaccharide vaccines (first does at or after 24 months of age) with a second dose of PPSV23 given 3 years after the first dose. The conjugate Hib and meningococcus vaccine (HibMenCY) is recommended for infants with sickle cell disease at 2, 4, 6, and 12 to 15 months of age and booster doses of MCV4 every 5 years thereafter. An annual flu vaccination is essential (Rogers, 2015).
- Invasive bacterial infection is the leading cause of death in young children with SCA. Penicillin V prophylaxis (125 mg orally, twice daily) is initiated by 2 months old. At 3 years old, increase the dose to 250 mg orally twice a day, and continue at least until the fifth birthday or until the child has received two doses of PPSV23 (Rogers, 2015).
- Folic acid supplementation at 1 mg/day is typically given to adults to prevent folate deficiency due to hemolysis. It is not standard therapy for children unless a folic acid

deficiency is suspected and should be individualized for each patient (Al-Yassin et al, 2012; Rogers, 2015).

- Aggressive treatment of infections and maintenance of hydration and body temperature are used to prevent hypoxia and acidosis; volume replacement may be necessary to prevent circulatory collapse.
- Treatment of coexisting medical problems associated with lower oxygen saturations, such as asthma and obstructive sleep apnea.
- In children with severe SCA, hydroxyurea is used to reduce the number of painful crises and incidences of acute chest syndrome (a leading cause of death in adolescents with SCA). It is a preventive medication and not effective during the acute crisis. Hydroxyurea use is associated with a lower need of blood transfusions and fewer hospital visits by reducing the frequency and severity of painful events and acute chest syndrome episodes. It increases Hgb F levels within cells, which decreases Hgb S levels, increases RBC water content, and alters adhesion of RBCs to endothelium. There is some early evidence suggesting it helps improve growth and preserves organ function. The results of two studies suggested that hydroxyurea may be given safely to children as young as 8 months old, although it is not approved for this age group (Rogers, 2015). Despite these benefits, side effects do occur, including increased risk for serious infection. As always, the practitioner must carefully weigh all risks and benefits before integrating this medication into the treatment plan.
- Annual stroke prevention screening of major intracranial vessels with transcranial Doppler ultrasound evaluation is planned for 2- to 16-year-old children or as long as their bone windows allow meaningful evaluation. A reading of greater than 200 cm/sec time-averaged mean maximal velocity indicates high risk for stroke and an indication to start transfusion programs to maintain Hgb S levels less than 30% (Rogers, 2015).

Children with sickle cell disease are usually co-managed by specialists in hematology and their PCP. Emergency admission or referral is necessary in the presence of the following:

- Fever (to rule out sepsis) greater than 101°F (38.3°C)
- Pneumonia, chest pain, or other pulmonary symptoms (acute chest syndrome)
- Sequestration crisis (splenomegaly with decreased Hgb or Hct)
- Aplastic crisis (decreased Hct and reticulocyte count)
- Severe painful crisis
- Unusual headache, visual disturbances
- Priapism

Consultation is also necessary for the chronic sequelae of persistent bone pain or leg ulcers, pregnancy, and contraception. Stem cell transplantation may be a consideration in children with significant disease and is curative in some persons. Gene therapy is under investigation and may be available in the future. New medications are under investigation as well.

Complications

Because of functional asplenia, the greatest concern is febrile illness indicating infection and possible sepsis. In view of the serious threat of pneumococcal sepsis in children younger than 5 years old, all complaints of fever, poor feeding, lethargy, and irritability should be clinically evaluated. The consequences of hemolysis may include chronic anemia, jaundice, cholelithiasis, and delayed growth and sexual maturation. Vaso-occlusion and tissue ischemia may result in acute and chronic injury to virtually every organ system, with stroke being a major concern.

Patient and Family Education

The parents of children with SCA need a great deal of support in raising a child with a genetically transmitted chronic disease. Clear patterns of communication should be established between the family and the provider using a partnership model. Initial education includes the genetics and pathophysiology of the disease and the importance of regular health maintenance visits. Discussion should emphasize the need for early evaluation and treatment of febrile illness, acute splenic sequestration, aplastic crisis, and acute chest syndrome. Parents can be taught to palpate their child's spleen. Any downward displacement or enlargement of the spleen below the left costal margin should be evaluated by a health care professional and blood counts monitored for increasing anemia. As the child grows, the family should be educated about other potential clinical complications, such as stroke, enuresis, priapism, cholelithiasis, delayed puberty, retinopathy, avascular necrosis of the hip and shoulder, and leg ulcers (Rogers, 2015).

Preventive care measures also include the following:

- Timely administration of routine immunizations, including pneumococcal and meningococcal vaccines, and yearly influenza vaccine
- Prophylactic antibiotics
- Genetic counseling for those with sickle cell trait
- Support groups
- Educating adolescents with the trait about their status and the risk of disease transmission
- Hematopoietic stem cell transplant (the only intervention that can cure sickle cell disease with strict inclusion criteria identified for transplant eligibility)
- Gene therapy (under investigation)

Hereditary Spherocytosis

HS is a hemolytic anemia characterized by a deficiency or abnormality of the RBC membrane protein spectrin, which reduces the RBC surface area. The RBC membranes assume a more spherical shape. Hence RBCs are more likely to be sequestered and prematurely destroyed in the spleen. HS causes mild chronic hemolysis to severe transfusion-dependent anemia. HS occurs in 1 in 5000 persons of mainly northern European ancestry.

Clinical Findings

Jaundice usually appears in the newborn period, and it may be difficult to differentiate HS from hyperbilirubinemia caused by ABO incompatibility. After 2 years of age, splenomegaly is usually present. Chronic fatigue, malaise, and abdominal pain may also be noted.

Diagnostic Studies

Laboratory findings in HS include the following:

- Chronic anemia: Hgb is 6 to 10 g/dL.
- Reticulocyte count ranges from 5% to 20%.
- On peripheral smear, a small proportion of the RBCs is spherocytic and smaller than normal and lacks the central pallor of the usual biconcave disk-shaped cell.
- Osmotic fragility of the cells is increased, as is the rate of autohemolysis of incubated blood.
- Prenatal and carrier testing for sequence analysis of the entire coding region has limited laboratory availability.

Management

The treatment of choice for children with severe HS requiring multiple transfusions is splenectomy (with removal of the gallbladder), which usually produces a clinical cure. It should be deferred until after 6 years of age because of the increased risk of encapsulated bacterial infection before that age. Risks associated with splenectomy are postsplenectomy sepsis, penicillin-resistant pneumococci infection, pulmonary hypertension, and ischemic heart disease and stroke seen in HS patients (Bolton-Maggs et al, 2012). Pneumococcal and meningococcal vaccines should be given before splenectomy.

After splenectomy, prophylactic penicillin therapy (younger than 5 years old: 125 mg orally twice a day; older than 5 years old: 250 mg orally twice a day) through adulthood is recommended; prophylaxis after 5 years old is individualized depending on a history of prior pneumococcal disease and having recommended pneumococcal vaccine. Because of increased hemolysis, children with HS and active hemolysis should receive 1 mg of folic acid daily until splenectomy especially if the reticulocyte count is more than 3%. Splenectomy is an effective strategy to eliminate most of the hemolysis associated with HS (Bolton-Maggs et al, 2012).

Complications

Aplastic crises (often indicated by fever, fatigue, abdominal pain, and jaundice) associated with parvovirus and other viral infections are the most serious complications during childhood. Febrile illnesses should be vigorously treated. A child who is postsplenectomy and has a temperature greater than 101.5° F (>38.5° C) without an obvious source of infection should be hospitalized and treated with intravenous antibiotics until blood cultures prove to be negative (Panepinto and Scott, 2011). Gallstone formation can occur as a result of chronic hemolysis, and ultrasounds should be performed annually, before splenectomy, and for increased abdominal symptoms (Segel, 2011).

Glucose-6-Phosphate Dehydrogenase Deficiency

A drug-induced hemolytic anemia can be caused by genetic deficiency of the G6PD enzyme in the RBC. Symptoms are generally associated with infections or exposure to oxidant metabolites of certain drugs that cause precipitation of Hgb, injury to the red cells, and rapid hemolysis. The *G6PD* gene is found on the X chromosome. G6PD deficiency is transmitted as an X-linked recessive trait. In the United States, about 13% of African American males and 1% to 2% of African American females are affected. It may also occur in a more severe form in Greeks, Italians, Arabs, Southeast Asians, and Chinese with the incidence ranging from 5% to 40% (Segel and Hackney, 2011).

Clinical Findings

History

Patients generally have a history of recent infection (particularly hepatitis) or oxidant drug ingestion—specifically, aspirin-containing antipyretics, sulfonamides, antimalarials, antihelmintics, naphtha quinolones—and fava beans. The degree of hemolysis is dependent on the amount of the drug ingested and the extent of enzyme deficiency.

Physical Examination

The patient may have pallor and jaundice if there is chronic hemolysis, or have jaundice, pallor, lethargy, irritability, headache, and red or dark clear urine after drug ingestion.

Diagnostic Studies

Several dye reduction tests provide the diagnosis. Screening tests available to measure a deficiency of G6PD should be used in high-risk groups. Only a few states include G6PD in their routine newborn screening panel. These tests measure G6PD enzyme activity in the RBC. After a hemolytic crisis, however, screening may produce a false-negative result because the younger blood cells that remain after hemolysis may show normal enzymatic activity. This is thought to be associated with higher G6PD activity taking place in reticulocytes. The enzyme assay should be obtained 2 to 3 months after an episode (Segel and Hackney, 2011).

Management

No specific treatment is available. RBC transfusion and supportive therapy may be indicated in cases of severe anemia. Keeping the child well hydrated and monitoring for renal failure are important during hemolytic crisis.

Patient and Family Education

Patients should avoid the offending foods and drugs—the most common being fava beans, foods containing menthol and sulfites, aspirin, sulfonamide antibiotics, and antimalarials.

Platelet and Coagulation Disorders

Platelet disorders should be ruled out in children before undergoing extensive surgery and in children with petechiae, frequent nosebleeds, mucous membrane bleeding, or excessive bleeding from minor trauma. Evaluation of these complaints includes a family history of bleeding or platelet disorders and a history of drug or toxin exposure. Initial laboratory studies should include a CBC, platelet count, prothrombin time (PT), and activated partial thromboplastin time (aPTT). The diagnoses that may be differentiated with these tests are idiopathic thrombocytopenic purpura (ITP), hemophilia, von Willebrand disease, and leukemia. The coagulation cascade (see Fig. 27-3) provides a mechanism for understanding the interconnectedness of all the factors involved in coagulation.

Overview of Diagnostic Studies

- Platelet count (normal range is 150,000 to 450,000/mm^3)
- Platelet function tests, such as platelet function analyzer (PFA)
- PT (normal range is 11.5 to 14 seconds)
- aPTT is the method used to determine partial thromboplastin time (PTT) and is commonly still referred to as the PTT (normal range is 25 to 40 seconds)
- Specific coagulation factor assays determine which clotting factors are absent

The PT and aPTT measure all of the clotting factors except factor XIII. If the platelet count is normal, and either the aPTT or PT is prolonged, or both, then a coagulation factor deficiency is possible. The typical laboratory findings of hemophilia are normal PT and PFA and an abnormal aPTT.

If the PT and aPTT are elevated in association with thrombocytopenia, the probable diagnosis is disseminated intravascular coagulation (DIC), which is a syndrome secondary to an underlying disorder, such as sepsis, malignancy, toxins, or liver failure. In DIC, there is a systemic activation of the coagulation process. Extensive, ongoing activation of coagulation results in the depletion of platelets and coagulation factors, which then leads to bleeding and thrombosis.

Immune or Idiopathic Thrombocytopenic Purpura

Immune or idiopathic thrombocytopenic purpura (ITP) is the most common of the thrombocytopenic purpuras in childhood and is believed to be an autoimmune response in which circulating platelets are destroyed. It usually occurs after viral illnesses. In many cases, the cause is autoimmune. Most cases occur between 1 and 4 years old. The vast majority of cases resolve within 6 months, even without treatment. If ITP lasts longer than 12 months, it is termed *chronic ITP*, and a careful reevaluation for associated disorders should be done. These include leukemia, medications (e.g., quinine, heparin), lupus erythematosus, cirrhosis, HIV, hepatitis C, congenital causes (such as, x-linked thrombocytopenia), autosomal macrothrombocytopenia, Wiskott-Aldrich syndrome (WAS), and von Willebrand factor (vWF) deficiency.

Clinical Findings

ITP is essentially a clinical diagnosis and not established by a single diagnostic test, although most symptoms do not develop until the platelet count is less than 20,000/mm^3. It is characterized by the following:

- Acute onset of petechiae, purpura, and bleeding in an otherwise healthy child; the bruising or bleeding may be most prominent over the legs
- A recent viral illness 1 to 4 weeks before onset is common
- Hemorrhage of the mucous membranes, particularly the gums and lips
- Nosebleeds that can be severe and difficult to control
- Menorrhagia in an adolescent female
- Liver, spleen, and lymph nodes are not generally enlarged
- Bone pain and pallor are rare

Diagnostic Studies

Laboratory findings in ITP include:

- Low platelet count (<150,000/mm^3) with an otherwise normal CBC
- Severe thrombocytopenia with the platelet count less than 20,000/mm^3 is common and platelet size is normal or increased
- Normal PT and aPTT
- Megathrombocytes on the peripheral smear
- Normal WBC and RBC counts
- Hgb may be decreased if there is a history of significant nose or menstrual bleeding but the MVC remains normal

Differential Diagnosis

If the smear shows fragmented RBCs, BUN and creatinine levels should be measured to rule out hemolytic-uremic syndrome. If the PT and aPTT are elevated with thrombocytopenia, DIC is a possibility, and cultures should be taken to identify sources of infection. A prolonged PT and aPTT with a normal platelet count suggest a coagulation factor deficiency. If the syndrome is complicated by prolonged thrombocytopenia, neutropenia, anemia, bone pain, or congenital anomalies, the child should be referred to a hematologist for possible bone marrow aspiration to rule out acute lymphoblastic leukemia (ALL) and other disorders. In a *sick, febrile child* with isolated thrombocytopenia, petechiae, or purpura, the major diagnosis to consider first is meningococcemia. These children should also be referred, hospitalized, and treated for presumed sepsis.

Management

The prognosis with ITP is excellent, with spontaneous recovery in the majority of pediatric cases within the first

6 months. Most cases can be managed on an outpatient basis without any specific therapy. If the platelet count is greater than 20,000/mm^3 and no bleeding is observed, children and parents should be advised to avoid contact sports, aspirin and NSAID ingestion, and any other herbal or pharmacologic agents that interfere with platelet function, and to notify the practitioner of any excessive bleeding. Epistaxis can be treated with local measures. In severe cases (platelets <20,000/mm^3) a short course of corticosteroid therapy may reduce severity in the initial phases. Whether bone marrow evaluation is done to rule out other causes of acute thrombocytopenia, such as ALL, before initiating steroid treatment is controversial. Intravenous immunoglobulin (IVIG) is also given to children with active severe bleeding and who have contraindications for steroid use; WinRho (Anti-D) is given intravenously with the dose depending on Hgb level; Rh(D) immune globulin is useful only in Rh-positive individuals. Splenectomy, immunosuppressives, and anti-CD20 antibody are options for those children with refractory or chronic ITP. New agents that stimulate thrombopoiesis, such as romiplostim and eltrombopag, have been approved by the U.S. Food and Drug Administration for use in adults with chronic ITP, but there are no data regarding safety or efficacy in children (Scott and Montgomery, 2011). Guidelines for immune thrombocytopenia are available through "The American Society of Hematology 2011 Evidence-Based Practice Guideline for Immune Thrombocytopenia" (Neunert et al, 2011).

Complications

The most serious complication is intracranial hemorrhage, which occurs in less than 1% of cases. Complaints of significant headache necessitate a careful neurologic evaluation.

Hemophilia A and B and von Willebrand Disease

Inherited coagulation deficiencies are described according to the absent coagulation factor. Most result in abnormal bleeding. Hemophilia results from a deficiency of factor VIII (hemophilia A) or factor IX (hemophilia B). In hemophilia A and B, absence or deficiency of the coagulation factor results in prolonged bleeding either spontaneously from small vessels or as a result of trauma. A rough guide to gauge the severity of hemophilia is the percentage of function of the factor levels with 100% (100 units/dL) equal to the function of factor found in 1 mL of normal plasma. The clotting factor levels with percentage of factor activity associated with severity of bleeding are as follows: less than 1 unit/dL (<1%), severe; between 1 and 5 units/dL (1% to 5%), moderate; and more than 5 units/dL (>5%), mild.

In plasma, factor VIII binds with vWF, which is a specific circulatory protein and acts as a carrier protein. Von Willebrand disease (also known as *vascular hemophilia*) is a heterogeneous group of hereditary bleeding disorders caused by a quantitative or qualitative abnormality of vWF protein (Table 27-10). In type I, the protein is quantitatively reduced; in type II, it is qualitatively abnormal; and it is absent in type III.

Because the genes for the coagulation factors are sex linked (carried on the X chromosome) and recessive, hemophilia A and B affect primarily males. Females are generally only carriers of the disorder. About 1 in 5000 males is affected with hemophilia; and approximately 85% have hemophilia A and 10% to 15% have hemophilia B. Von Willebrand disease occurs in both sexes with an incidence of 1 in 100 individuals. It is the most common inherited bleeding disorder and is associated with either a qualitative or quantitative defect in vWF. The primary sites of bleeding differ depending on whether the problem is hemophilia A or B or von Willebrand disease. The fibrin/clotting cascade is available in Figure 27-3 for review.

Clinical Findings

The following are seen in hemophilia:

- A positive family history in the vast majority of cases
- Excessive bruising
- Prolonged bleeding from mucous membranes after minor lacerations, immunizations, circumcision, or during menstruation (menorrhagia)
- Hemarthrosis characterized by pain and swelling in the elbows, knees, and ankles
- A greatly prolonged aPTT
- A specific assay for factor VIII or IX activity confirms the diagnosis

Clinical findings associated with von Willebrand disease include the following:

- Mucous membrane bleeding (epistaxis, menorrhagia), easy bruising, and excessive posttraumatic or postsurgical bleeding
- History of ecchymosis of trunk, upper arms, and thighs
- Factor VIII clotting activity usually decreased
- vWF antigen usually decreased
- Decreased vWF
- Normal platelet count but isolated decreased platelet count associated with type 2B (Montgomery and Scott, 2011)

Management

Treatment of hemophilia consists of prevention of trauma and replacement therapy to increase factor VIII or factor IX activity in plasma. Plasma-derived and recombinant factor concentrates are available for replacement, with recombinant factor preferred. Hemarthrosis is the leading type of significant local bleeding. Local measures include the application of cold and pressure to affected, painful joints. As with all bleeding disorders, aspirin and NSAIDs should be avoided. Anticipatory guidance should be directed at avoiding high-risk behaviors and contact sports and wearing a bike helmet. Physical therapy may be needed to assist with decreased mobility caused by hemarthrosis and joint scarring. Psychosocial intervention may be needed to help families avoid overprotectiveness or permissiveness.

TABLE 27-10 Comparisons of Hemophilia A, Hemophilia B, and von Willebrand Disease

	Hemophilia A	Hemophilia B	von Willebrand Disease
Inheritance Factor deficiency	X-linked Factor VIII	X-linked Factor IX	Autosomal dominant vWF and VIIIC
Bleeding site(s)	Muscle, joint, surgical	Muscle, joint, surgical	Mucous membranes, skin, surgical, menstrual
Prothrombin time (PT)	Normal	Normal	Normal
Activated partial thromboplastin time (aPTT)	Prolonged	Prolonged	Prolonged or normal
Bleeding time	Normal	Normal	Prolonged or normal
Factor VIII coagulant activity (VIIIC)	Low	Normal	Low or normal
von Willebrand factor antigen (vWF: Ag)	Normal	Normal	Low
von Willebrand factor activity (vWF: Act)	Normal	Normal	Low
Factor IX	Normal	Low	Normal
Ristocetin-induced	Normal	Normal	Normal, low, or increased at low-dose ristocetin
Platelet aggregation	Normal	Normal	Normal
Treatment	DDAVP* or recombinant VIII	Recombinant IX	DDAVP* or vWF concentrate

From Scott J: Hematology. In Kliegman R, Marcdante K, Jenson H, et al: editors: *Nelson essentials of pediatrics*, ed 5, Philadelphia, 2006, Saunders, p 718.
*Desmopressin (DDAVP) for mild to moderate hemophilia A or type I von Willebrand disease.

Ideally most children with hemophilia should be enrolled in a comprehensive hemophilia treatment center (HTC) to facilitate a collaborative, interdisciplinary approach to management. The PCP should remain central to the care of the child. Immunizations should be given either subcutaneously with a 26-gauge needle or intramuscularly with a 23-gauge needle, followed by firm pressure, without rubbing, and ice at the site for several minutes (National Hemophilia Foundation, 2001). Iron replacement may also be necessary in children with severe bleeding disorders.

Von Willebrand disease is treated depending on the type and severity of the bleeding. The treatment for von Willebrand disease is desmopressin (DDAVP) and factor VIII-vWF concentrates. Local measures to control bleeding may also be part of the treatment plan. Adjunctive therapy (e.g., estrogen and/or aminocaproic acid) depends on the type of von Willebrand disease (type 1, 2A, 2B, 2M, 2N, or 3), which is determined by the level of qualitative or quantitative factor deficiency. The use of aminocaproic acid, an antifibrinolytic agent, is sometimes recommended for dental extraction and nosebleeds (Montgomery and Scott, 2011).

Most patients are now given lifelong prophylaxis to prevent spontaneous bleeding and preserve joints. The National Hemophilia Foundation recommends that prophylaxis therapy be considered optimal treatment for children with severe hemophilia and is usually initiated with the first joint bleed. This is often in the first year of life as mobility increases. A written treatment plan tailoring replacement product dosage based on the location of the bleed should be in the chart and given to the parents to carry with them. The child should wear a medical alert bracelet or necklace.

Complications

In patients with hemophilia A and B, bleeding occurs particularly in closed areas, such as the joints, when coagulation factor levels decrease. Brain hemorrhage can be a serious consequence of head trauma. Continued hemorrhage results in anemia and eventually hypovolemic shock. The National Hemophilia Foundation publishes recommendations supported by the Medical and Scientific Advisory Council (MASAC) and their recommendations are available through the National Hemophilia Foundation website (www.hemophilia.org). Guidelines are available as the "2012 Clinical Practice Guidelines on the Evaluation and Management of von Willebrand Disease" through the National Heart, Lung, and Blood Institute.

Thrombophilia

Thrombophilia refers to the increased ability to form blood clots and may result from either acquired and/or inherited risks factors. Thrombotic events (venous thromboembolism [VTE] and stroke) are rare in healthy children, 0.07 out of 100,000, but have been increasingly recognized in tertiary pediatric centers (Raffini, 2015). The advances in treating critically ill children, coupled with the increased awareness of inherited factors, improved imaging to identify thrombosis, and the prothrombotic lifestyle choices in society today have led to families seeking testing in healthy children. Screening for inherited thrombophilia in children with VTE is controversial, but the testing of healthy children who have a family history of thrombosis or thrombophilia is even more controversial (Raffini, 2015).

The most common inherited thrombophilias are:

- Factor V Leiden mutation
- Prothrombin 20210 mutation
- Antithrombin deficiency
- Protein C deficiency
- Protein S deficiency

Also to be considered are factors that may be either inherited or acquired and are helpful to identify patients who have multiple prothrombotic risk factors and may need testing:

- Antiphospholipid antibodies
- Elevated fasting homocysteine levels
- Elevated factor VIII (Raffini, 2015; Silvey and Carpenter, 2013)

Pediatric patients who have two or more inherited thrombophilia traits have been shown to be at increased risk for VTE (Chan and Monagle, 2012). The most common risk factor is the presence of a central (indwelling) venous catheter (CVC), but other factors include surgery, trauma, use of oral contraceptives, immobilization, infection, systemic lupus erythematosus, structural venous anomalies, and cancer (Chan and Monagle, 2012; Raffini, 2015).

Those with potential benefits from screening and testing are children with a strong family history of thrombophilia, such as a VTE in a first-degree relative younger than 40 years old. Identifying these children has the benefit of counseling adolescent females considering oral contraceptives, targeted thromboprophylaxis in high-risk situations (femur fracture in an obese teen who also has inherited thrombophilia), and educating patients about signs and symptoms of VTE, which could lead to earlier diagnosis. Counseling also should revolve around lifestyle modifications including avoiding sedentary lifestyle, overweight or obesity, and smoking (Raffini, 2015).

The American College of Chest Physicians has developed evidenced-based guidelines and recommendations for neonates and children and recommends referral to pediatric hematologists (Monagle et al, 2012). Testing for children who have had a stroke is common but should be done when the child is recovered, because some factors levels may be affected by acute episode-specific events (such as sepsis, asphyxia, dehydration, and central venous line infection).

Clinical Pearl

A careful family and patient history is the best way to determine if there is an increased risk for adolescent females starting hormone therapy.

White Blood Cell Disorders

White Blood Cell Count

The WBC count is used as an indicator of infection or illness; the percentages of the different types of cells also provide useful diagnostic information. The WBC count is automated and is a routine part of the CBC. The WBC differential is obtained on a smear of blood one cell layer thick, usually with a Wright stain procedure that contains both basic and acidic dyes. The absolute neutrophil count (ANC) is calculated from the results of the differential: If WBCs = 3600/mm^3, percentage of segmented neutrophils = 20, percentage of band neutrophils = 5, lymphocytes = 60, monocytes = 10, and eosinophils = 5, then ANC = 3600 × 0.25 (sum of % segs and bands) = 900.

White Blood Cell Dysfunction

The WBC count and differential are useful diagnostic guides in the management of a variety of childhood illnesses. The normal range of granulocyte and lymphocyte counts varies throughout childhood. Leukocytosis is an increase in the number of circulating leukocytes, primarily with a neutrophilic response particularly to bacterial infections (Box 27-3). A relative increase in the number of circulating immature neutrophils ("left shift") is a defensive mechanism in response to an inflammatory process or acute bacterial infection. Multiple WBC indices abnormalities should raise suspicion of a malignant disorder.

Alterations of Granulocytes

Neutropenia (measured as the ANC) is defined as a decrease in the number of circulating neutrophils and bands (ANC) in the peripheral blood to fewer than 1500 cells/mm^3 for children older than 1 year and to fewer than 1000 cells/mm^3 in infants between 2 weeks and 1 year old. There are some racial differences in neutrophil counts with some African American children having slightly lower counts than white children. Neutropenia is classified as mild (ANC

• BOX 27-3 Key Characteristics of Leukocytosis

- *Definition:* Elevated total WBCs due to an increase in one of five types of WBCs:
  - Neutrophilic leukocytosis
  - Lymphocytic leukocytosis
  - Eosinophilic leukocytosis
  - Monocytic leukocytosis
  - Basophilic leukocytosis
- Differential count
  - Percentages: Always add up to 100%
  - Left-sided shift: Granulocytes >75% of WBC
  - Right-sided shift: Nongranulocytes >40% of WBC

WBC, White blood cell.

of 1000 to 1500 cells/mm^3), moderate (ANC of 500 to 1000 cells/mm^3), or severe (ANC <500 cells/mm^3).

Neutropenia results from decreased cellular production (as in various hematologic diseases, infections, drug-induced states, and nutritional deficiencies), increased peripheral destruction (as in autoimmune disorders), or peripheral pooling (as in bacterial infections, hemodialysis, and cardiopulmonary bypass). Most cases of neutropenia are discovered during evaluation of the WBC count in a child with an acute febrile illness, and the most common infectious causes are hepatitis A and B, respiratory syncytial virus, influenza A and B, Epstein-Barr virus, and cytomegalovirus. General management of neutropenic patients includes careful identification and prompt treatment of any suspected or proven infections.

Neutropenia is frequently seen in preterm infants and those with intrauterine growth retardation. Because the neutrophil storage pool in newborn infants is only 20% to 30% of that of adults, it is easily depleted under stressful conditions, such as infection with resultant sepsis. Isoimmune neonatal neutropenia is a transient process resulting from transplacental transfer of maternal antibodies to fetal neutrophil antigens. Antineutrophil antibodies can be detected in maternal and infant serum.

The largest group of neutropenic patients includes children who are receiving chemotherapy. They are at risk for developing severe life-threatening bacterial infections, depending on the degree and duration of neutropenia. Despite improvements in supportive care and treatment with granulocyte colony–stimulating factor (G-CSF), bacterial and fungal infections remain a major cause for morbidity and mortality in these patients.

Qualitative abnormalities of granulocytes are usually related to defects of phagocytosis. Although individually rare, these defects may be genetic or acquired. Malnutrition, sepsis, diabetes, and leukemia are acquired disorders related to defects in leukocyte function, particularly phagocytosis and microbicidal activity. Granulomatous diseases are relatively rare disorders of granulocytes, particularly neutrophils, in which the enzymes necessary for bactericidal activity are lacking. Such diseases result in severe, recurrent infections of the skin, lymph nodes, lungs, liver, and bone.

Lymphocytosis

Lymphocytosis is produced by viral illnesses, including mumps, measles (rubeola), rubella, varicella, mononucleosis, and hepatitis. Pertussis and chronic lymphocytic leukemia also elevate the lymphocyte count. An increase in the number of atypical lymphocytes is evident in infectious mononucleosis, cytomegalic inclusion disease, and toxoplasmosis.

Cancer

Childhood cancer is uncommon and often presents with symptoms of a benign illness. The signs and symptoms are variable and nonspecific and can include continued, unexplained weight loss; headaches (typically early morning); swelling or persistent pain in bones, joints, back, or legs; lumps or masses; excessive bruising, bleeding, or rash; constant infections; persistent nausea or vomiting without nausea; persistent tiredness; vision changes; and/or recurrent or persistent fevers with no known etiology (Bass, 2014). Pediatric cancers differ significantly from adult malignancies in both prognosis and tumor site. Cancer among children younger than 19 years old represents 1% of all new cancers diagnosed in the United States. The most common types in children, birth to 14 years old, are ALL 26%, brain and central nervous system (CNS) tumors (21%), neuroblastoma (7%), and NHL (6%). Hodgkin lymphoma (15%), thyroid carcinoma (11%), brain and CNS tumors (10%), and testicular germ cell tumors (8%) are the most common cancers diagnosed in adolescents (Ward et al, 2014).

Cancer incidence, mortality and survival rates vary by race and ethnicity, but childhood and adolescent cancer incidence is not consistently higher among populations with lower economic status (Ward et al, 2014). In contrast to adult cancers, only a small percentage of all childhood cancers have a known preventable cause. Ionizing radiation is a well-recognized risk factor, and health care providers are encouraged to limit the use of computed tomography (CT) scans in children and pregnant women to those situations with a defined clinical indication and to use the lowest possible radiation dose. Numerous epidemiologic studies have investigated potential environmental causes of childhood cancer, but there have been few strong or consistent associations found (Ward et al, 2014).

Leukemia refers to a group of malignant diseases with qualitative and quantitative changes in circulating leukocytes characterized by diffuse, abnormal growth of leukocytic precursors in the bone marrow. This uncontrolled increase in immature WBCs suppresses normal hematopoietic stem cells and leads to anemia and thrombocytopenia. Life-threatening infections occur because of a decrease in the function of circulating WBCs. Leukemias are further classified according to the course of the illness and the types of cells and tissues involved.

Malignant lymphomas, as in Hodgkin lymphoma, are solid neoplasms that are lymphocytic in origin. Lymphocytes are the only WBCs involved—the malignant process occurs during their maturation or storage in bone marrow. They are associated with lymphadenopathy and tumor development in the liver, spleen, thymus, bone marrow, and submucosa of the GI and respiratory tracts. As in leukemia, immune deficiencies develop and are followed by infection. Most lymphoid neoplasms are of B-cell origin, with T-cell tumors making up the remainder. Hodgkin lymphoma is set apart from NHLs by the presence of the malignant Hodgkin and Reed-Sternberg (HRS) giant cells in the neoplastic tissue. Also, in classical Hodgkin lymphoma, within the involved nodes the HRS cells account for less than 3% of the total cellular mass of the affected lymph nodes, thus the non-neoplastic inflammatory cells usually greatly outnumber the tumor cells (Knecht et al, 2013).

Leukemias

The leukemias represent a group of malignant hematologic diseases in which normal bone marrow elements are replaced by abnormal, poorly differentiated lymphocytes known as *blast cells*. Genetic abnormalities in the hematopoietic cells take over and result in unregulated clonal proliferation of malignant cells. Leukemias are classified according to cell type involvement (i.e., lymphocytic or nonlymphocytic) and by cellular differentiation. ALL is characterized by preponderantly undifferentiated WBCs.

The leukemias are the most common form of childhood cancer. They account for approximately 26% of pediatric malignancies in children younger than 15 years old. ALL accounts for about 80% of childhood leukemia cases, with a peak incidence between 2 and 6 years old, and 56% of leukemia cases in adolescents. Acute myeloid leukemia (AML) is less common in children than ALL and accounts for about 15% of leukemia cases in children and 31% of the cases in adolescents (Ward et al, 2014).

Clinical Findings

Most of the clinical signs and symptoms of leukemia are related to leukemic replacement of the bone marrow and the absence of blood cell precursors. The child may be anemic, pale, listless, irritable, or chronically tired and have the following:

- A history of repeated infections, fever, weight loss
- Bleeding episodes characterized by epistaxis, petechiae, and hematomas
- Lymphadenopathy and hepatosplenomegaly
- Bone and joint pain

CNS symptoms, such as headache, vomiting, or lethargy, are rare at the time of diagnosis but can present due to an intracranial or spinal mass (Horton and Steuber, 2015a). All these symptoms may be vague or nonspecific; providers need to maintain a high index of suspicion for cancer.

Diagnostic Studies

The following are used to diagnose leukemia:

- CBC with differential WBC, platelet, and reticulocyte counts. Thrombocytopenia and anemia are present in most cases. WBC count may be elevated, normal, or low with varying levels of neutropenia.
- Peripheral smear may demonstrate malignant cells.
- Bone marrow examination shows an infiltration of blast cells replacing normal elements of the marrow (Horton and Steuber, 2015a).
- Chromosomal and genetic abnormalities are found in most children with ALL. The genetic alterations in their leukemic blast cells may include changes in the number of chromosomes and their structure with recurrent translocations and deletions which provide important prognostic information (Horton and Steuber, 2015a).

Further classification regarding cell type, morphologic characteristics, and cell surface markers is generally made at the cancer treatment center to which the child is referred.

Management

Approximately 90% of children diagnosed with ALL can now be cured; children are considered cured after 10 years in remission. Key genetic features are critical factors in the management plan. The treatment program for most types of acute leukemia involves 4 to 6 weeks of induction phase (usually with vincristine, prednisone, and L-asparaginase), with the goal of inducing a complete remission and restoring normal hematopoiesis. This is followed by a consolidation phase of therapy lasting several months, and then a maintenance phase of therapy for 2 to 3 years. Chemotherapy, CNS therapy (cranial irradiation, which is now reserved only for a high-risk child—those with CNS disease or high WBC counts at diagnosis), or intrathecal administration of chemotherapy, and systemic administration of corticosteroids are the key interventions. The use of cranial irradiation as part of therapy is decreasing. For children with ALL who relapse, the need for allogeneic stem cell transplantation is not considered until the second complete remission. However, children with certain chromosomal rearrangements or those who are not in remission by the end of the first induction phases are considered high risk for relapse and need to consider transplantation sooner. Minimal residual disease measurement is part of the current protocol treatment to determine the end-of-leukemic induction burden and ALL outcome (Horton and Steuber, 2015b; Ward et al, 2014).

For those with AML, the treatment consists of induction chemotherapy, CNS prophylaxis, and postremission therapy. Allogeneic stem cell transplantation from an HLA-matched sibling or parent is considered in the first complete remission for children with high-risk disease (Ward et al, 2014).

Long-term sequelae of cancer therapy for ALL have been identified in research studies and include effects on cognition, neuropsychological functioning, and growth deficiencies and an increased risk for second malignancies, such as AML or lymphoma (Ward et al, 2014). CNS irradiation has been linked to learning disabilities and impaired IQ, especially in children younger than 5 years old who also received intrathecal therapy. As a result, cranial radiation dosages have been reduced, and earlier neuropsychological testing is recommended. Other documented potential late effects of ALL treatment include congestive heart failure, avascular necrosis, and osteoporosis (Ward et al, 2014). Late effects associated with common childhood cancers are further discussed at the end of this chapter.

The role of the PCP is crucial to facilitate proper referrals and effective interdisciplinary communication and to assist the family in their coping and adaptation processes. Regular health supervision visits are also important and should not be overlooked. Immunizations should be given as appropriate depending on the stage of treatment and the child should be monitored for failed remission or metastasis (CNS and testicles are common sites) and late effects.

Lymphomas

Non-Hodgkin Lymphoma

The NHLs are a diverse group of solid tumors of the lymphatic tissues that form from malignant proliferation of T cells, B cells, or indeterminate lymphocyte cells. Different classification systems have been used to categorize these tumors. In pediatrics, the common types of NHL are small noncleaved cell lymphoma (Burkitt and non-Burkitt subtypes, B-cell origin), lymphoblastic lymphoma, and diffuse large B-cell lymphoma (Ward et al, 2014). NHLs account for 6% of all pediatric cancers (Kupfer, 2015; Ward et al, 2014).

Each year in the United States, approximately 500 children and 400 teens are diagnosed with NHL. The subtypes most common in pediatrics include Burkitt lymphoma (19%), diffuse large B-cell lymphoma (22%), lymphoblastic lymphoma (20%), and anaplastic large-cell lymphoma (10%). Incidence rates of most subtypes of NHL are higher in boys than in girls, but the incidence and subtype distribution vary throughout the world (Johnston, 2014; Ward et al, 2014). NHL occurs most frequently in children during the second decade of life and infrequently in children younger than 3 years old. It is the most frequent malignancy in children with acquired immunodeficiency syndrome and is also associated with Epstein-Barr and cytomegalovirus infections.

Clinical Findings

The most common site of origin is in the lymphoid structures of the intestinal tract. The most common manifestations in children are (1) acute abdomen, including abdominal pain, distention, fullness, and constipation and (2) nontender lymph node enlargement. Histologic differences account for varying disease sites; lymphoblastic NHLs often present as intrathoracic tumors; in contrast, small noncleaved cell lymphomas commonly present as abdominal tumors. Other sites include the CNS and the bone marrow. Initial presentation is often with advanced disease of stage III or IV in approximately 70% of the patients (Waxman et al, 2011). Duration of symptoms before a diagnosis is made is typically 1 month or less, and a common presentation is enlarging, nontender lymphadenopathy or symptoms indicating compression of surrounding tissue and structures. Three clinical manifestations that may present as emergencies are superior or inferior vena cava obstruction, acute paraplegias due to spinal cord or CNS compression, and tumor lysis syndrome (Termuhlen and Gross, 2015).

Diagnostic Studies

Diagnostic studies are ordered depending on the location of the lymphoma and symptoms. They include CBC with differential, but this may be normal at diagnosis, liver function tests, lactate dehydrogenase (LDH), uric acid, and electrolyte levels. Unexplained anemia, thrombocytopenia, or leukopenia can be due to bone marrow infiltration; and elevated electrolytes and LDH may indicate rapidly proliferating tumors and tumor lysis syndromes. Imaging studies such as chest radiograph, ultrasound, CT or MRI scan, or positron emission tomography (PET) of the area in question may demonstrate masses and/or lymphadenopathy in the neck, chest, or abdomen. Staging the extent of the disease is mandatory before beginning treatment and may include gallium and/or bone scan, bone marrow aspirates and biopsies, and lumbar puncture with CNS fluid analysis (Termuhlen and Gross, 2015).

Management

Optimal therapy involves a multidisciplinary approach from the time of diagnosis. Because of rapid developments in treatment and the importance of careful histologic evaluation, these children should be referred to a comprehensive pediatric oncology center for care.

Lymphomas are sensitive to chemotherapy. Unlike adults, radiation therapy is not commonly used in pediatric care. The prognosis has improved dramatically with an estimated 5-year survival rate of over 85% (Termuhlen and Gross, 2015; Ward et al, 2014).

Hodgkin Lymphoma

Like the NHLs, Hodgkin lymphoma is a malignancy of the reticuloendothelial and lymphatic systems and involves B cells. It usually originates in a cervical lymph node and spreads to other lymph node regions and, if left untreated, to organ systems, including liver, spleen, bone, bone marrow, and brain. Unlike the NHL, involvement of the bone marrow and CNS is rare. Clinical and pathologic staging of the disease is usually done by specialists according to the Ann Arbor Staging Criteria (Termuhlen and Gross, 2015). Hodgkin lymphoma represents 6% of the childhood cancers. It is rare in children younger than 15 years old (5.5 cases per million per year). The NIH National Cancer Institute estimated incidence of Hodgkin lymphoma in the United States in adolescents (15 to 19 years old) is 29 cases per million per year. Clusters of cases in families suggest a genetic predisposition, but this association may include shared environments and exposure to viruses as well as inherited immunodeficiency states (McClain and Kamdar, 2015).

Clinical Findings

The most common manifestations of Hodgkin lymphoma include the following:

- Painless enlargement of the lymph nodes, usually in the cervical area; the nodes may feel rubbery and firm, are often matted together, and are nontender to palpation
- Chronic cough if the trachea is compressed by a large mediastinal mass
- Fever, decreased appetite, weight loss of 10% or more of total body weight within 6 months of diagnosis, and drenching night sweats are systemic symptoms, classified as B symptoms, and are important for staging (McClain and Kamdar, 2015)

Diagnostic Studies

Hematologic findings are often normal but may include the following:

- Anemia
- Elevated or depressed leukocytes or platelets
- Elevated sedimentation rate and C-reactive protein; serum copper and ferritin level
- Abnormal liver function test results
- Urinalysis may have proteinuria
- Imaging studies: Chest radiography, ultrasound, CT, MRI, and PET

Management

The child should receive treatment at a comprehensive pediatric oncology center in collaboration with the PCP. The diagnosis is confirmed by histologic examination of an excised lymph node, followed by bone marrow studies to determine the extent of the disease. Multiple treatment agents allow different mechanisms of action to avoid overlapping toxicities. Optimal results are obtained through irradiation, chemotherapy with numerous agents, or a combination of both. Data from 2003 to 2009 indicated a 97% relative survival rate for children 0 to 19 years old (Ward et al, 2014). Infertility is problematic for those receiving high doses of alkylators; sperm banking is discussed as an option for males before starting therapy. Approximately 75% of children who survive Hodgkin lymphoma have chronic medical conditions. They may develop secondary malignancy 30 years later, typically thyroid, breast, nonmelanoma skin cancers, and NHL and acute leukemia. Therefore, lifelong monitoring is necessary through a comprehensive pediatric oncology center where long-term complications can be anticipated, monitored, and treated (McClain and Kamdar, 2015). Current guidelines recommend annual MRI as an adjunct to mammography for women who were treated for Hodgkin lymphoma (Ward et al, 2014).

Late Effects of Childhood Cancers

Estimates are given that 1 in 530 young adults between 20 and 39 years old is a long-term cancer survivor (Ward et al, 2014). Any adverse effect that does not resolve after completion of therapy or a problem that develops after completion of therapy is labeled as a late effect of childhood cancer. Late effects can be attributed to radiation therapy, chemotherapy, or a combination of both and can occur later during puberty or with aging. Common problems have been identified, and pediatric survivors of cancer need to be monitored for these issues. Problems need to be identified early and promptly addressed. They can include the following:

- Short stature from cranial irradiation and intensive chemotherapy
- Precocious puberty after cranial irradiation and hypothyroidism with neck or mantle radiation therapy
- Avascular necrosis of the bone caused by high-dose steroid therapy—more pronounced in young children—and with local irradiation
- Osteoporosis from cranial irradiation, glucocorticoids, and antimetabolites
- Leukoencephalopathy resulting from cranial irradiation, methotrexate, glucocorticoids
- Peripheral neuropathy and hearing loss from cisplatin
- Cognitive dysfunction, stroke, and seizures from intrathecal chemotherapy, certain systemic chemotherapy agents, and radiation: Cranial radiation effects are dose dependent and more deleterious on young developing brains.
- Vision, auditory, and skeletal changes from head and neck radiation
- Obesity and gonadal dysfunction resulting from a neuroendocrine effect
- Potential alterations in pubertal development and gonadal function if given high-dose alkylating agents, especially in puberty and to girls
- Cardiomyopathy and arrhythmias if given anthracyclines: Children given these drugs need to be educated just before their teen years about avoiding alcohol, which increases the likelihood of cardiotoxicity, and cautioned about cigarette smoking.
- Pericardial effusion, constrictive pericarditis, or late coronary artery disease from radiation therapy that includes all or part of the heart (e.g., used in treatment for some Hodgkin lymphoma cases)
- Pneumonitis and pulmonary fibrosis from chest and thorax radiation and with chemotherapy agents, such as bleomycin and carmustine
- Malignant glioma associated with cranial irradiation and sarcomas associated with musculoskeletal radiation
- Secondary leukemias (usually AML) associated with therapy with alkylating agents and epipodophyllotoxins; secondary solid tumors are associated with radiation therapy
- Glomerular or tubular injury, renal insufficiency with heavy metals (e.g., cisplatin)
- Infertility and early menopause with alkylator therapy
- Cystitis or bladder dysfunction with cyclophosphamide
- Delayed recovery of normal immune function (may need readministration of immunization)
- Psychosocial effects associated with chronic illness (e.g., less likely to go to college, marry, and be employed)
- Cancer relapse
- Possibility of hepatitis C virus infection if the individual had a blood transfusion before 1992
- Bone marrow transplant recipients can experience unique late effects associated with treatment and require monitoring; medical insurance coverage may also be problematic in later years

The Children's Oncology Group (COG), a National Cancer Institute–supported clinical trials group, cares for more than 90% of children and adolescents diagnosed with cancer in the United States. Monitoring programs for childhood cancer survivors provides a rich source of data to guide cancer treatment and its follow-up. All survivors of childhood cancers need regular health care supervision from a provider who is aware of their prior treatment modalities and knowledgeable of late effects, aware of their risk of occurrence, and comfortable with risk-based monitoring for such problems. COG published the survivorship guidelines in 2007, and those are available at www.survivorshipguidelines.org. Healthy lifestyles and dietary practices, and avoidance of sun, alcohol, recreational drug use, and tobacco should always be stressed (Ward et al, 2014).

If a neoplasm of some sort is suspected by the PCP, a phone call to the nearest comprehensive pediatric oncology/hematology center will facilitate the child being seen quickly and prevents a delay in diagnosis by waiting for insurance authorization. Staff in these centers can obtain authorization quickly based on clinical findings. The PCP needs to maintain a relationship and follow the child for well-child care when the disease process is stabilized. In addition, watchful monitoring for late effects is often done in partnership with specialists. Bass (2014) recommends that PCPs initiate the following survivor care plan as part of coordinated care: (1) secure basic information on the type of cancer, stage, location, and histology; (2) treatments (i.e., chemotherapy, radiation, surgery); (3) list of potential or at-risk late effects and monitoring needs; (4) any psychological issues; and (5) preventive strategies (e.g., immunizations, exercise, diet). The NIH National Cancer Institute has excellent materials for health professionals, parents, and children about childhood cancer (www.cancer.gov/types/childhood-cancers). This resource provides up-to-date information about changes in treatment therapy and long-term effects.

For a complete list of references, please visit http://evolve.elsevier.com/Burns/pediatric/.

28

Neurologic Disorders

RUTH K. ROSENBLUM AND CATHERINE G. BLOSSER

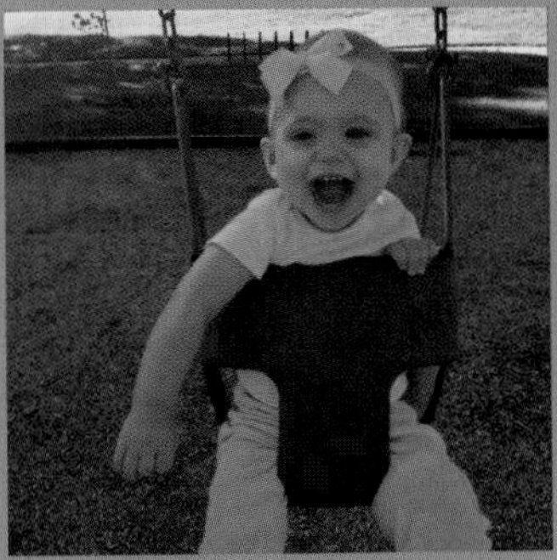

Central nervous system (CNS) problems can affect many systems and present in a variety of ways and degrees. No other body system has as much influence on a child's overall development. The challenge for health care providers is to be able to screen and identify neurologic problems, know when to appropriately refer to specialists, be able to monitor the general health of the patient and provide routine preventive care, serve as a case manager based on school and health care issues, help coordinate resources, and support families with children who have neurologic deficits as they deal with the challenges of grief and long-term care.

Anatomy and Physiology

Anatomy

Briefly, the nervous system is divided into two parts: the CNS and the peripheral nervous system (PNS). The CNS consists of the brain and spinal cord. The PNS is made up of a network of afferent nerves and sense organs, which send information to the brain, and the efferent nerves, which send information out to the body for responses. Descending tracts from the brain to the gray matter of the spinal cord include the extrapyramidal tract, which conveys information from the cerebellum to the motor cells of the anterior column, and the pyramidal tract, which is the main motor pathway from the cerebral cortex to the spinal nerves and carries messages for voluntary movement. Most pyramidal tract fibers cross in the medulla, so the left half of the brain controls the right side of the body and vice versa. The anatomic units of the brain and their functions are listed in Table 28-1 and shown in Figs. 28-1 and 28-2.

Autonomic Nervous System

The visceral activities of the body (i.e., blood vessels, glandular secretions, gastrointestinal tract, and cardiac muscle) are controlled by the autonomic nervous system (ANS). The ANS is comprised of the sympathetic system and the parasympathetic system, which are principally under the control of the hypothalamus. When the hypothalamus receives information from the cortical centers (e.g., visual, auditory, and olfactory) and sensory stimuli from the various parts of the body (e.g., organs and glands), it functions as a "switchboard" between the two systems. Generally, both systems supply the same organs, glands, and smooth muscles. The sympathetic system begins in the thoracolumbar area of the spinal cord and extends distally; its function is often referred to as the "fight-or-flight" reaction. It is most active when an individual is physically or mentally stressed. The parasympathetic system begins in the medulla and midbrain with relays to the thalamus and higher centers. Enervation results in slowed activity, a decreased metabolic rate, and the conservation of energy; this system is active when an individual is mentally or physically relaxed. The principal sympathetic system neurotransmitters are epinephrine and norepinephrine. The parasympathetic fibers produce acetylcholine. The two systems function in balance—one excites and the other inhibits (Box 28-1). The enteric system is a component of the ANS, but it does not play a role specifically in neurology. This system consists of a meshwork of nerve fibers that innervate the digestive system.

Physiology

Nerve impulses are transmitted along a nerve fiber through changes in polarization of the membrane, during which electrical activity is produced. Certain chemicals diffuse across the synapses between nerves and end organs. There are approximately 50 substances that act as neurotransmitters in the brain. The main categories of neurotransmitters are acetylcholine (a primary transmitter released by neurons projecting through the cerebral cortex and limbic system), amino acids (e.g., glutamate, aspartate, glycine, gamma-aminobutyric acid [GABA]), biogenic amines (e.g., norepinephrine, dopamine, serotonin, histamine), and the largest family, neuropeptides (e.g., endorphins, angiotension II, melatonin, oxytocin, and many others). All of the neurotransmitters play an important role in either excitation or inhibition of neurons.

TABLE 28-1 **Anatomic Units of the Nervous System and Functions**

Anatomic Unit	Functions
I. Central nervous system	
A. Brain	
1. Forebrain—cerebrum	
a. Cortex (gray matter)	Posterior—motor skills
(1) Frontal area	Anterior—decision-making, emotions, memory, judgment, ethics, abstract thinking Broca area—speech
(2) Parietal area	Sensory integration, language, reading, writing, pattern recognition
(3) Temporal area	Memory storage, auditory processing, olfaction, limbic system in deep temporal lobe—arousal
(4) Occipital area	Visual processing
b. Diencephalon	
(1) Thalamus	Receives and sorts sensory input, modulates motor impulses from cortex
(2) Hypothalamus	Integrates autonomic functions
2. Midbrain	Connects brain with cerebellum, pons, medulla
3. Hindbrain	
a. Pons	Bridges cerebellum, medulla, midbrain; cranial nerves (CN V, CN VI, CN VIII) arise here
b. Medulla	Proximal end of spinal cord; contains reticular system—arousal; CN IX to CN XII arise here
c. Cerebellum	Coordination and movement; balance; smooth movements
B. Cranial nerves	Sensory and motor components; olfaction; vision; hearing; facial, tongue, pharyngeal, eye, shoulder movements
II. Spinal cord	
A. Dorsal roots	Afferent sensory fibers
B. Ventral roots	Efferent motor fibers
III. Protective layers	
A. Meninges	Protection of delicate nervous tissues
B. Ventricles	
C. Cerebrospinal fluid	

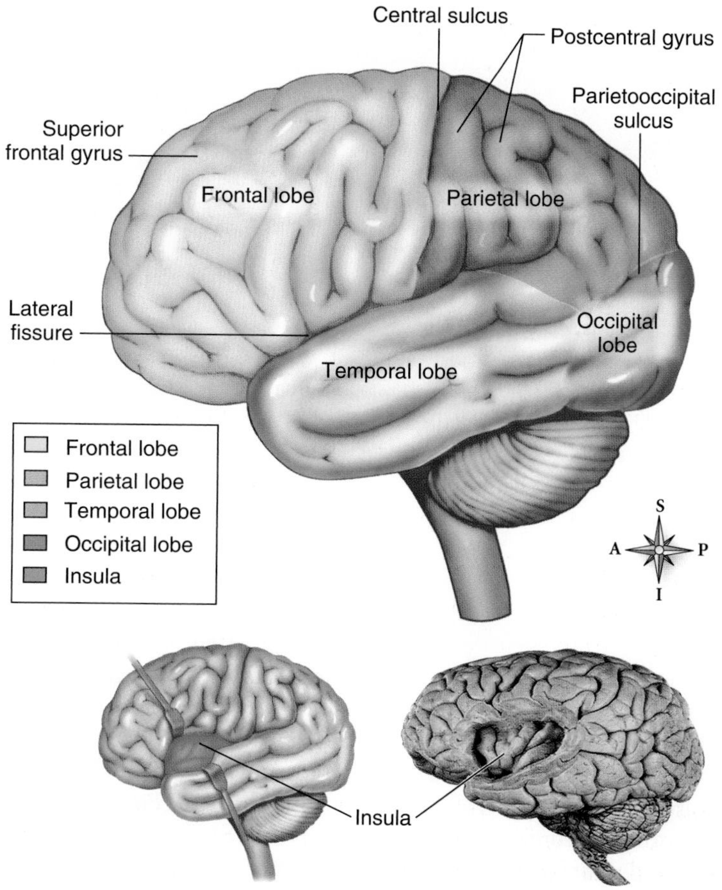

• **Figure 28-1** Lobes and functional areas of the cerebrum. (From Patton K: *Anatomy & physiology*, ed 9, St Louis, 2015, Mosby/Elsevier.)

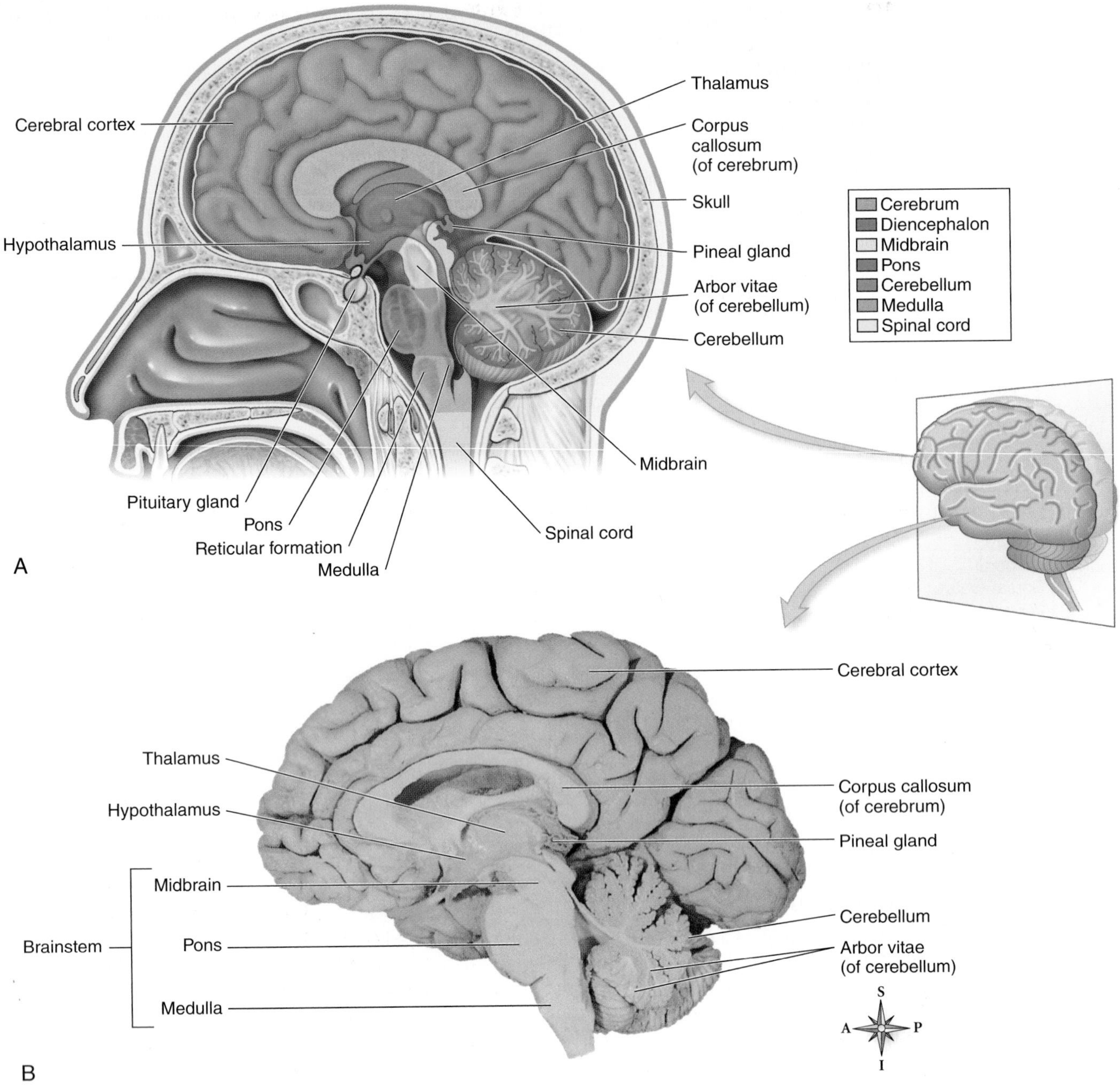

• **Figure 28-2** Midsagittal section of the brain showing the major portions of the diencephalon, brainstem, and cerebellum. (From Patton K: *Anatomy & physiology*, ed 9, St Louis, 2015, Mosby/Elsevier.)

Pathophysiology and Defense Mechanisms

The nervous system is intimately related to the functioning of the entire body; problems in any part of the system can have neurologic implications. Examples include uncontrolled firing of cerebral neurons (seizures), the inability of cerebral neurons to fire or the inability of the CNS to process stimuli and respond accordingly (coma), or the inability of peripheral nerves to respond to or receive signals through the pyramidal system of afferent and efferent nerves (paralysis). Other problems occur when special areas of the nervous system or individual nerves are damaged. Neurotransmitters may include dopamine, serotonin, and glutamate. When neurotransmitters do not work properly, problems may ensue. Examples include depression (serotonin) and attention-deficit/hyperactivity disorder (ADHD) in children and Parkinson disease in adults (dopamine). Many CNS disorders have interactive genetic, immunologic, and infectious factors that are probably causative (e.g.,

• BOX 28-1 Autonomic Nervous System: Parasympathetic and Sympathetic Functions

Parasympathetic System

Pupil constriction
Increased watery saliva
Lacrimal gland vasodilation
Coronary vessel vasoconstriction
Bronchial muscle constriction
Stomach peristalsis
Colon peristalsis
Genitalia vasodilation
Urinary bladder constriction
Skin vessel dilation

Sympathetic System

Pupil dilation
Increased viscous/thick saliva
Coronary vessel vasodilation
Bronchial muscle relaxation
Stomach constriction
Adrenaline secretion
Colon relaxation
Sphincter relaxation
Sphincter constriction
Genitalia vasoconstriction
Urinary bladder relaxation
Skin vessel constriction

multiple sclerosis [MS] and cerebral palsy [CP]). Other causative factors include:

- Systemic problems: The brain is extremely sensitive to changes in physiology anywhere in the body. Thus, any metabolic change, whether from external or internal factors (autoimmune, inflammatory, and/or infectious causes), may affect the CNS. Examples include delirium from toxins, diabetic coma, meningitis, epilepsy, ataxias, and chorea.
- Neurodegenerative disorders: Neurodegenerative disorders result from a loss of structure or function of neurons in the brain or spine, including death of neurons. Many neurodegenerative diseases are caused by genetic mutations (e.g., MS and Rett syndrome).
- Genetic problems: Many medical disorders have a genetic component that directly affects the nervous system. Some of the single-gene defects may have direct neurologic effects (such as, neurofibromatosis), whereas others, typically inborn errors of metabolism, can have indirect effects via the abnormal metabolites released (e.g., phenylketonuria). Other examples of disorders with a genetic component include Down and Rett syndromes.
- Structural defects: Because the CNS is structurally complex, there are many opportunities for defects to occur in utero. Examples of such defects include hydrocephaly, anencephaly, and spina bifida.
- Trauma: Head and spinal cord injuries occur frequently and can have long-term, serious consequences for the child. Recovery from head trauma can be lengthy and require a long rehabilitation time. Even then, return to baseline does not always occur. Peripheral nerves can regenerate somewhat if conditions are optimal. In the spinal cord, the axons of injured neurons cannot regrow within the cord, but they can grow in peripheral nerves outside the cord. In this case, if the cut ends are reconnected with special attention to the myelin sheath, regeneration of the injured nerve begins at the proximal end of the neuron soon after injury.
- Tumors and cancer: Benign or malignant tumors evolve when there is a problem with cellular division, which can cause unrestricted growth. Problems with the body's immune system can also lead to such tumors.

Assessment of the Nervous System

Assessment of the nervous system requires a careful history from the child and family and a detailed physical examination. The examiner needs to determine if a neurologic disorder exists and, if so, the disorder's location and the patterns of impairment. For children with complex or severe neurologic problems, social, environmental, developmental, and family issues need thorough exploration. Historical information from children older than 3 years old and from one or more family members provides the most accurate picture. Imaging or laboratory studies may be required. See Chapter 4 for guidelines on neurodevelopmental assessments of children.

History

History of Present Illness

- Onset: When did the first symptoms appear? Was the onset insidious or sudden? Was it associated with an injury or other event, such as an illness, surgery, poisoning, ingestion, or recent exacerbating event? If yes, describe the event. Was the onset accompanied by any constitutional symptoms? How has the disorder evolved?
- Pain and/or headache: Location and character, path of radiation, severity, extent of disability produced, effect of various activities or stimuli (including light and sound sensitivity), aggravating or alleviating factors (e.g., changes in position or worse in the morning versus the evening or from day to nighttime), effects of previous treatment, and/or presence of pain or discomfort in other parts of the body. Morning awakening with headaches, vomiting, double vision, and/or balance problems require immediate referral.
- Sensory deficits: Changes in hearing, vision, taste, or smell; loss of pain sensation; vertigo; dizziness; numbness; and/or tingling.
- Injury: How, when (time and date), why, where? Mechanism or manner in which the injury was produced: accidental or nonaccidental? Immediate treatment provided? If past injury, at what age did the injury occur?
- Reflexive responses: Vomiting, coughing, primitive reflexes, tics, and/or clonus.

- Behavioral changes: Irritability, stupor, changes in appetite, lack of attention, random activity, emotional lability, and/or changes in school performance.
- Motor and balance changes: Ataxia, spasticity, and/or increased or decreased tone.

Medical History

- Prenatal history: Maternal and paternal ages, alcohol, drug ingestion (including environmental toxins, such as fish contaminated with mercury and workplace exposures), radiation exposure, nutrition, prenatal care, injuries, hyperthermia, smoking, human immunodeficiency virus (HIV) or other infectious disease exposure, maternal illness, bleeding, toxemia, diabetes, previous abortions and stillbirths
- Birth history and neonatal course: Place of birth, complications, labor and delivery, resuscitation, trauma, congenital anomalies, feeding history (reflux, colic, frequent formula changes), jaundice, convulsions, infection, gestational age, sleep disturbances, multiple birth (Prematurity, low birth weight, and infants who are small for gestational age face particular challenges regarding future development.)
- Injuries or infections: Meningitis, encephalitis, head injuries, frequent musculoskeletal injuries (These can suggest coordination disturbance or impulsive behavior.)
- Cardiovascular or respiratory disorders
- Environmental exposure to toxins (e.g., lead exposure)
- Metabolic disorders: Diabetes mellitus, thyroid disease (Hypoglycemia causes confusion, convulsion, and/or loss of consciousness. Hyperglycemia causes lethargy and coma. Hyperthyroidism causes tremor. Hypothyroidism causes weakness and coma.)
- Past neurologic disease and tests: Tics, hydrocephaly, genetic screening or imaging studies done, electroencephalograms (EEGs), history of seizures—type, description, frequency, onset, medications
- Psychiatric disorders: Hallucinations, delusions, illusions
- Drug ingestion: Lead poisoning, dietary/herbal supplements, pharmaceuticals, maternal drug use while pregnant
- Urinary tract disease: Uremic syndrome manifests with confusion, convulsions, coma
- Physical growth

Family Disease History

- Family members with similar symptoms and features or genetic disorders; obtain a pedigree
- Consanguinity
- Migraine history
- Intellectual functioning of family members

Developmental History

Review achievement plateau or loss of skills in all developmental milestone categories—language, gross motor skills, fine motor skills, social skills, and cognitive skills—and school performance. The Ages & Stages and the World-Class Instructional Design and Assessment (WIDA)-ACCESS Placement Test (W-APT) are useful assessment guides.

Functional Health

Inquire about the effects of symptoms on all areas of health promotion and safety, nutrition, elimination, activity, communication, role relationships, values and beliefs, sexuality, sleep, family coping and resilience (management style), and stress tolerance, temperament, and self-concept. Masten (2014) describes resilience as the capacity of a dynamic system to adapt successfully to disturbances that threaten system function, viability, or development. Neurobiology, epigenetics, and developmental timing may play a role in resilience (or the ability to rebound) in children. Resilience in children ranges from the micro (how they function in their day-to-day lives) to the macro (their response to global threats and surprises). Developmental science will continue to explore this phenomenon in the coming years.

Social Context

Inquire about the family composition (including critical family events, such as additions or losses of family members); home, neighborhood, and school environment; culture and ethnicity; other stressors; strengths; resources; child care; financial issues (socioeconomic status, poverty); identified social supports (e.g., family, friends, health professionals); and community agencies involved with the family and child. Additionally, if it is a military family, query if trauma has occurred or if a family member is deployed for a long period of time.

Review All Systems

Review all systems plus:

- Allergies, immunizations, hearing, vision, dental, skin integrity, behavior, nutritional status, and eating disorders
- Medications (over-the-counter and prescription drugs) and recreational drug use
- Other health conditions, treatments, providers, or resources involved with patient

Physical Examination

The following should be noted:

- Growth pattern, including height, weight, body mass index (BMI), and head circumference
- Abnormalities of the skin (café au lait macules, angiomas, neurofibromas, ash leaf spots, or other pigmentation changes)
- Anomalies (e.g., unusual facies, shape and number of digits, low-set ears, symmetry of body)
- Cardiovascular system (including blood pressure)
- Musculoskeletal system: Gowers sign, calf muscle hypertrophy, and muscular function
- Hearing
- Vision: Eye problems, including cataract, corneal clouding, cherry-red spot, change of visual function

- Tanner stage
- Hepatomegaly/splenomegaly

Specifics of the Neurologic Examination

The neurologic examination moves from the highest level of functioning to the lowest. Cerebral function is tested first; then cranial nerves, motor function, and sensory function; and finally reflexes. The neonate's neurologic functioning is largely subcortical. Therefore, the examination is more limited than in an older infant or child. In infants and children, watching them carefully while collecting the history and actively playing with them in an age-appropriate manner provide a great deal of neurologic information. A tennis ball, some small toys (e.g., a small car), a bell, and something that attracts attention (e.g., a pinwheel) are useful throughout the examination.

Behavior and Mental Status

Test the following cortical functions:

- Responsiveness
- Judgment
- Language and speech (receptive, expressive, written); speech flow, voice quality, organization of thoughts
- Memory
- General knowledge
- Ability to relate to others: Parents versus strangers
- Mood and affect

Cranial Nerve Function

The majority of the neurologic examination to test for cranial nerve function assesses cranial nerve (CN) II through CN XII because CN I (the olfactory) is difficult to assess in children and is not functional until the infant is 5 to 7 months old. Vision (CN II) is indicated by blinking in response to a bright light. In the neonate, CN III, CN IV, and CN VI can be tested by assessing the ability to track through the visual fields. Facial grimaces test for CN V and CN VII. Hearing (CN VIII) can be tested with a small bell, finger rub, or snap. The gag reflex tests CN IX and CN X.

Motor Examination

Gait, posture, coordination, balance, strength, symmetry, quality of movement, and tone are aspects of the motor examination. Information can be gained from questioning the parent, because it is often difficult to elicit the needed information about these skills in the time and environment given for the examination.

- Muscle strength and size: Look at muscle size, contour, and symmetry. Have the child stand from a lying position. Look for Gowers sign (i.e., a child using the arms to push off from bent knees and gradually climbing the body and straightening up, which is common in children with muscular dystrophy). Ask the child to move extremities against resistance and to grip your fingers hard. The presence of muscular hypertrophy or hypotrophy should be noted.
- Muscle tone: Muscle tone might be considered the resting strength of the muscle. Is the trunk control and/or extremities floppy, rigid, or somewhat stiff when the child is resting or active? How difficult is it to move body parts passively? Tone may be increased or decreased all over or differ between the legs and the trunk and arms. Additionally, symmetry of muscle tone, bulk, and power should be noted.
- Fine motor coordination: Fine motor coordination is tested by having the child pick up small pieces, write, stack blocks, copy pictures, turn book pages, put puzzles together, or do other hand activities. In older children, assessment of their handwriting appropriateness for age should be observed.
- Involuntary movements: Tremors are fine involuntary movements. *Chorea* or *choreiform movements* are large, irregular jerking and writhing movements. *Athetoid movements* are slow writhing movements, especially of the hands and feet. *Dystonia* is an uncontrolled change in tone with movement and a tendency to hyperextend the joints.
- Reflexes: When a reflex is abnormal, the question is: Why? Did the impulse not go through, or did the child have a problem in the ability to move responsively because of problems in efferent signals or muscle tissue contractility? (See the Reflexes section that follows.)
- Posture: *In an infant, assessing posture and muscle tone is fundamental.* Motor testing should include observation for symmetry of movements, consistent fisting of the hands, opisthotonos, scissoring, abnormal tone, and tremors. The infant's cry can be an indicator of several diseases (e.g., it is high pitched with increased intracranial pressure, it resembles mewing in cri du chat syndrome, and it is hoarse with hypothyroidism).

Sensory Examination

Examine for pain sensation and stereognosis. The accuracy of interpretation of this part of the examination is always limited in infants and young children. Use a light pinprick to check for mild pain sensation.

Reflexes

- Deep tendon reflexes include the biceps, brachioradialis, triceps, patellar, and Achilles jerk reflex.
- Superficial reflexes include the upper abdominal, lower abdominal, cremasteric, gluteal, and plantar.
- Primitive reflexes include sucking, rooting, asymmetric tonic neck, grasp, trunk incurvation, stepping, and others found in Table 28-2. These primitive reflexes can be absent or decreased in a satiated or sleepy infant. Tendon reflexes can be tested in an older child. In older children and adults, a Babinski sign is an important sign of upper motor neuron disease.

Cranium Examination

The neurologic examination should always include measurement of head circumference until the child is 2 years

TABLE 28-2 Primitive Reflexes

Reflex	Age Appears	Age Disappears	How to Elicit	Response	Notes
Newborn Reflexes					
Rooting	Birth	3-4 months	Head midline, stroke perioral area	Infant opens mouth and turns head to stimulated side	Absence indicates CNS disease or severely depressed infant; sleeping infant may not respond
Sucking	Birth	3-4 months	Place nipple or finger 3-4 cm into mouth	Suck should be strong: Push finger up and back; note rate	Absence indicates CNS depression; satiated or sleeping baby may not respond well
Asymmetric tonic neck reflex (ATNR)	Birth	4-6 months	With baby supine, turn head to one side; hold 15 seconds	Arm and leg extend on facial side; arm and leg on other side flex	Obligatory response when child cannot get out of position is abnormal; persistence beyond 4-6 months indicates CNS lesion (e.g., CP)
Palmar grasp	Birth	3-6 months	Place finger into infant's palm and press against palm	Infant flexes all fingers around examiner's finger	Grasp should be strong and symmetric
Trunk incurvation (Galant)	Birth	2 months	Suspend baby prone; stroke 2-3 cm from spine with fingernail	Baby flexes toward stimulus	Asymmetry is significant; tests for spinal cord lesions; should not persist after 6 months
Stepping	Birth	6-8 weeks	Infant is held as though weight bearing with feet on surface	Infant steps along, raising one foot at a time	Tests brainstem, spinal column; absence indicates paralysis or depressed baby
Moro	Birth	4 months	Present loud noise or allow infant's head to drop slightly	Arms spread and fingers extend and then flex; then arms come toward each other; cry is possible	Asymmetry indicates paralysis or fractured clavicle, absence indicates brainstem problem, usually severe; persistence also abnormal
Crossed extension	0-4 months		Passively extend one leg and press knee to table; prick sole of that foot with pin	Other leg should slightly extend and adduct	
Plantar grasp	Birth	8-10 months	Place finger firmly against base of toes	Toes should curl down	Tests S1-S2 spinal nerves; lessens by 8 months, suspect any asymmetry
Later Reflexes					
Landau	3 months	15 months to 2 years	Suspend infant prone by supporting abdomen	Infant should lift both head and legs	Abnormal if arm tone increased with internal rotation, arm held at side, or arm does not lift as noted
Neck righting	6 months	2 years	With infant supine, turn head to one side	Infant's trunk rotates in direction of head	Absent or decreased can indicate spasticity; can also rotate trunk and then look for head to follow; tests midbrain
Parachute	6-8 months	Never	Suspend infant prone and lower quickly toward table	Infant should extend arms, hands, fingers	Response should be symmetric and "protective"

CNS, Central nervous system; *CP,* cerebral palsy.

old (The American Academy of Pediatrics *Bright Futures*) or until 36 months old per the Centers for Disease Control and Prevention (CDC) and if it appears abnormally large or small in an older child. Inspect the skull for symmetry and shape. Auscultation over the skull or above the eyes may reveal a cranial bruit. Percussion of the skull can give a sound resembling a cracked pot when the sutures are separated, as with increased intracranial pressure. The anterior fontanelle should normally be slightly depressed with very faintly perceived pulsations.

Autonomic Nervous System

Alterations in blood pressure, sweating, or body temperature can be indicators of ANS problems.

Meningeal Signs

Evidence of meningeal irritation, such as with meningitis, includes positive Kernig and Brudzinski signs. A Kernig sign is positive if resistance and head or neck pain are elicited when the patient bends over from the waist and touches fingers to toes. In an infant, the Kernig sign can be tested by extending the leg at the knee with the infant lying supine. A positive sign can be as subtle as facial grimacing. A positive Brudzinski sign is evidenced by the patient spontaneously flexing the hip and knees after the examiner passively flexes the neck.

Diagnostic Studies

- Radiographs have relatively little diagnostic value for the neurologic system since the advent of computed tomography (CT) and magnetic resonance imaging (MRI). CT scans display differences in density of the intracranial tissues and structures. CT scans are no longer in favor as a routine study; rather this imaging study should be ordered with caution due to radiation exposure. MRI provides additional information related to aneurysms (e.g., hemorrhages, calcifications, and abscesses), brain structure, and the cellular activity of various parts of the neurologic system (e.g., tumors, CNS, spinal cord, and malformations). There may be a medical need to order more specific tests, such as a magnetic resonance angiogram (used to detect blood vessel stenosis and aneurysms) or functional magnetic resonance imaging (fMRI; used to detect subtle metabolic changes in the brain that indicate how certain parts of the brain are working), or a positron emission tomography (PET) scan to assess blood flow, oxygen use, and sugar (glucose) metabolism. A neurologic consultant can advise when these would be necessary.
- Laboratory studies provide indicators of systemic disease, infection, or inflammation. They are especially important for children receiving medication for seizures. Drug levels, liver function, and blood studies may need to be monitored routinely.
- Lumbar puncture provides information about metabolism, infections, and trauma.
- The EEG provides information about the electrical activity of the CNS, which is important in assessing function rather than structure.
- Ultrasonography can be useful in infants to evaluate brain tissue.
- Other studies can include polysomnography (helps assess narcolepsy, apnea of infancy, certain movement disorders, nocturnal seizures, and obstructive sleep apnea, which may contribute to headaches or other neurologic symptoms), electromyography (EMG; tests muscle activity), nerve conduction studies, evoked responses (brainstem—auditory, somatosensory, and visual); electronystagmography (measures eye movements to assess vertigo and post-concussion syndrome); and cerebral arteriography (visualizes cerebral blood vessels to evaluate vascular anomalies and tumors). Children needing such studies would typically need to be referred to a neurologist.

Management Strategies Involving Anticipatory Guidance

Neurologic Development

Families are sometimes concerned about problems that providers believe are within normal limits. No neurology referral is necessary in these situations. The family needs to understand the anticipated pattern of neurologic development, including timelines and markers that they can use to monitor their child's development. Misperceptions about the implications of minor variations must be dealt with, and the family should always be given the opportunity to return for further assessment or discussion if concerns remain. The temperament of the child and the child's learned social behavior versus pathologic symptoms may need to be addressed (e.g., breath holding versus seizures).

Educational Needs

Many neurologic problems in children affect learning, although neurologic problems are not synonymous with intellectual disability. Sensory problems affect the child's ability to receive the input necessary for learning. Motor problems may affect both the child's ability to interact with the environment and the ability to communicate or indicate understanding. Management strategies should always include the educational needs of the child. Special infant or preschool early intervention educational programs can assist the child to learn by using the most appropriate learning modalities. Teachers often need assistance in understanding the limitations and strengths of the child. Parents need to be encouraged to develop close communication with the educational staff because this relationship is mutually beneficial for optimizing the learning experience of the child (see Chapter 20).

Referrals for Other Key Assessments

Many neurologic conditions are genetic in origin. Genetic implications are best communicated through formal genetics counseling; feelings of parental guilt need to be addressed. See Chapter 41 for guidance. Physical therapy can be useful to help restore or maintain function or to teach new motor skills. The physical therapist should be accustomed to dealing with children. Physical therapy services are often combined with occupational and speech therapy to promote maximal development. Early intervention programs offer such assistance in many states and are generally free to qualifying patients. Should any services be denied, families should be advised to inquire about the appeal process in their state. Federal funding is available in most states for therapy programs for children from birth through 2 years old. Referral for social services is another key intervention. Children and families with children that experience multiple handicapping conditions frequently have ongoing issues of coping, monitoring, and management of medical and financial resources. Medical social workers, public health nurses, and case managers can provide invaluable assistance for these families for continuity and coordination of care.

Medications

A variety of medications are used to control the effects of neurologic problems. These may include antiepileptic drugs (AEDs), mood stabilizers, and antidepressants. Most require time for the effects to become apparent, need dosage adjustments, and are affected by the metabolism of the individual child. Periodic measurement of blood levels is often needed. Side effects of medications need to be weighed against their beneficial effects. Many require tapering of dosages when treatment with the medication is to be discontinued.

Specific Neurologic Problems of Children

Neurodegenerative Disorders

Neurodegenerative disorders occur when the gray or white matter of the brain is affected. These are believed to be the result of biochemical or metabolic dysfunctions (in turn caused by genetic, immune-mediated demyelination or by unknown etiologies) that lead to anatomic or functional insults to major portions of the brain. These insults can affect the basal ganglia, cerebellum, brainstem, spinal cord, peripheral and cranial nerves, or cerebrum. Such insults can also follow infections or an altered immune state.

Gray matter diseases involve neurons, and their onset is heralded by seizures, a decrease in cognitive functioning, and visual changes. Gray matter disorders that are exceedingly rare include Menkes syndrome (also called *kinky hair syndrome*), progressive infantile poliodystrophy, neuronal ceroid-lipofuscinoses, and Rett syndrome, which is discussed later in the chapter. White matter diseases are characterized by demyelination and are evidenced by decreasing motor skills, ataxia, and spasticity. Such disorders include Schilder disease, acute disseminating encephalomyelitis, acute hemorrhagic leukoencephalitis, and MS (discussed later). The diagnosis is based on age of onset, clinical features (signs and symptoms), genetic transmission, and chemical and chromosomal studies. It also must be determined if the episodes of disability are single (monophasic) or polyphasic (relapses close to initial onset of symptoms with similar areas of involvement as in MS).

In the case of inflammatory demyelination, separate events are determined by whether or not they occur more than 30 days apart and involve separate white matter pathways. In an initial acute demyelinating event, it may be difficult to determine a diagnosis; the extent of motor, visual, and neurologic involvement needs to be determined in all events. If a demyelinating event is suspected, the child should be referred to a neurologist (preferably pediatric) for a comprehensive evaluation and diagnosis.

Rett Syndrome

A mutation in the X-linked, methyl-CpG-binding protein 2 (MECP2) gene occurs in 80% of females with classic Rett syndrome features (Neul et al, 2010). This gene contains instructions for protein synthesis of methyl cytosine–binding protein. MECP2 is abundant in the brain. When not disabled by mutation, it silences certain genes that control motion and emotion. This neurodevelopmental disorder was previously thought to affect only females and to be lethal to males. Defects in MECP2 also occur in patients with autism, schizophrenia, learning disabilities, and neonatal encephalopathy (National Institute of Neurological Disorders and Stroke [NINDS], 2015a). Most females with Rett syndrome represent de novo mutations. However, MECP2 mutations alone are not sufficient to make a Rett diagnosis, because they may not be present in all cases. Therefore the diagnosis of Rett remains clinical (Neul et al, 2010). Deoxyribonucleic acid (DNA) tests for the presence of mutations in MECP2 and are typically found in 95% of children meeting consensus criteria for Rett syndrome (Cuddapah et al, 2014). This is likely attributed to the possibility that some affected children inherit only a part of the gene that is affected, which is undetected with current laboratory testing. In addition, MECP2 mutation type has been linked to disease severity.

Rather than cause brain degeneration, Rett syndrome arrests maturation of certain areas of the brain. The child is typically female with an onset of symptoms at 5 to 18 months old. The developmental milestones of those affected plateau, and the child's intellectual development remains at the level of plateau. CNS irritability and withdrawal develop, and then these children begin to lose skills, including partial or complete loss of purposeful hand skills and partial or complete loss of acquired spoken language. They develop bruxism, gait abnormalities, and stereotypic hand movements, such as hand wringing/squeezing, clapping/tapping, hand-mouthing or biting and handwashing/rubbing automatisms. Disorganized breathing and apnea followed by hyperpnea occur, as well as impaired sleep and peripheral vasomotor abnormalities (Neul et al, 2010). Seizures, scoliosis, and spastic paraparesis and quadriparesis are late developments in the syndrome.

Physical, occupational, and speech therapies and seizure management are important to preserve functional abilities. As with all neurodevelopmental problems, families need significant support and social services. Life expectancy varies depending on complicating factors. Differential diagnoses include CP, autism, psychosis, and other neurodegenerative diseases.

Multiple Sclerosis

MS is a chronic, relapsing disorder of the CNS that involves demyelination of the brain, spinal cord, and optic nerves. It is rare to observe symptoms of MS before a child is 10 years old (0.2% to 2% of all cases). The median age of disease onset of pediatric cases is 14 years old, with the median age at diagnosis age 15 (range of 11 to 19 years old) (Boesen et al, 2014). Two to three times as many females as males are affected. It is widely believed that MS is an autoimmune inflammatory neurodegenerative disorder of the CNS. Macrophages, activated T-lymphocytes, and other destructive molecules are stimulated by yet not fully understood events. These inflammatory cells cause both CNS demyelination and axon damage within the white brain matter, including the optic nerve. Research is focused on environmental (including geography and living north of 40 degrees latitude), infectious, toxic, immunologic, hormonal, or genetic causes. No specific virus has been isolated, although the most likely agent seems to be the Epstein-Barr virus. Some scientists propose that it is multifactorial (National Multiple Sclerosis Society, n.d.a). Children are noted to have acute exacerbations three times as frequently as adults. Therefore it is imperative to explore and research disease modifying therapies for children in addition to symptomatic interventions to improve quality of life (Yeh and Weinstock-Guttman, 2012).

Overall, the clinical course is variable. The disease is typified by two phases: (1) initial relapse and remittance and (2) secondary progression. The episodes of focal neurologic dysfunction can last weeks or months, followed by partial or complete recovery. Frequent relapses early in the disease process may lead to a more rapid progression to irreversible disability. However, once irreversible disability begins, the rate of progression is independent of the frequency of relapses. The relapsing–remitting type accounts for 99% of pediatric MS cases (Yeh and Weinstock-Guttman, 2012).

It is recognized that focal inflammation of the brain is active, even during the remission phase, and that there seems to be a point of no return for the brain's coping mechanism. This coping mechanism appears to allow for a degree of adaptation for different types of mechanisms of inflammation that originate from outside the CNS, from target-determined changes in immune cells and microglial activation, and from the accumulation of cortical gray matter lesions.

Clinical Findings

Most symptoms seen in children are the same as for all other ages. However, seizures and mental status changes (lethargy) are seen in children but are not typically seen in adults with MS. A diagnosis of pediatric MS can be given after two episodes of demyelinating events, lasting longer than 24 hours, separated by more than 30 days, involving a distinct CNS region(s) and with no other plausible diagnosis (Ness, 2011). Symptoms include the following (Boesen et al, 2014):

- Unilateral weakness or ataxia or other cerebellar symptoms (frequent presenting symptom)
- Symptoms that last more than 24 hours
- Headache (may be severe, prolonged, generalized)
- Motor symptoms, such as vague paresthesias of lower extremities, distal portions of hands and feet, and face
- Visual disturbance (diplopia, blurred vision, or sudden loss of vision as a result of optic neuritis)
- Vertigo, dysarthria, and sphincter disturbances are uncommon. Neurogenic bladder may present in acute transverse myelitis.
- Repeated episodes are frequently preceded by fever, nausea and vomiting, and lethargy; they may occur within months or years of each other.

Diagnostic Studies. Diagnostic studies are typically ordered by the neurologist and include:

- Neuroimaging: An MRI (gadolinium enhanced) early in the course of the disease can be important in predicting the clinical future. In children, demyelination of white matter presents as well defined and perpendicular to the corpus callosum. Evidence of disturbance of the blood-brain barrier is thought to be a better predictor than the number of T2 white matter lesions for developing inflammatory MS lesions and atrophy. Gray matter lesions are believed to play a role but are undetectable using current imaging.
- Later in the course of the disease, nonconventional neuroimaging techniques (magnetization transfer imaging and imaging for whole brain atrophy) are more useful than the gadolinium-enhanced MRI for tracking the progression of disability. However, many locations do not have this technology available and will continue to use traditional MRI methods.
- Other studies may include a lumbar puncture (may show oligoclonal bands) and visual-evoked responses.

Differential Diagnosis

Because of the frequency of other childhood conditions and disorders that have similar presentations and symptoms, determining a diagnosis of MS in a child may be challenging. However, a diagnosis of MS can be considered during the initial episode of a neurologic dysfunction that affects a certain region of the body and occurs over a limited period of time. Brain tumor, focal encephalitis, nonviral infections with focal cerebritis or abscess formation, cerebrovascular diseases, leukodystrophies, and systemic vasculitis, mitochondrial, vitamin B_{12} deficiency (with macrocytic anemia), and spinal cord symptoms should be considered in the differential diagnosis after initial presentation.

Management

Disease-modifying therapies are currently the standard method of prevention of disability in children with MS (Yeh and Weinstock-Guttman, 2012). First-line therapies include corticosteroids, intravenous immunoglobulin (IVIG), and plasmapheresis. Intravenous methylprednisone results in a faster resolution of visual disturbances and is a widely used treatment for the pediatric population. IVIG is postulated to work by binding to circulating antibodies and preventing them from entering the CNS. Other treatments used are immunomodulatory therapies (interferon-beta 1 α or interferon-beta 1 β and glatiramer acetate treatments), which may reduce the frequency of contrast-enhancing lesions (Ness, 2011). Second-line treatments include monoclonal antibodies (such as, natalizumab [Tysabri]), immunosuppressive toxic agents (such as, mitoxantrone [Novantrone]), and monoclonal antibodies (including rituximab [Rituxan]). Cyclophosphamide (Note: there is a risk of secondary neoplasms and infertility) and various newer oral agents should also be considered (Yeh and Weinstock-Guttman, 2012).

Treatment decisions are not dependent on MRI alone. Tools to monitor subtle changes in abilities are often used, such as the McDonald criteria for MS (Hawkes and Giovannoni, 2010). The McDonald criteria and spinal MRI data provide an early diagnosis in almost 90% of cases (Reinhardt et al, 2014). Continuing research is targeting a variety of the mechanisms and processes of the disease to prevent and treat relapses, alter disease progression, and discover neuroprotective factors. Symptomatic treatment involves exercises—resistance, aerobic, and stretching—and routines that promote agility and speed.

Nondegenerative Disorders

Benign Paroxysmal Vertigo

Benign paroxysmal vertigo (BPV) may be incorrectly diagnosed as epilepsy due to the rotatory to-and-fro vertigo, headache, and sensitivity to light and noise (Langhagen et al, 2013). It is the most common cause of episodic vertigo in children aged 2 to 6 years old. BPV is associated with a family history of migraine and development of more typical migraines later in life (Langhagen et al, 2013). The history may include rapid onset of an attack (vertigo, disequilibrium, and nausea) that lasts seconds to minutes, daily attacks that occur in clusters over several days and then may not recur for weeks or months, and a possible history of motion sickness. Symptoms are likely to have resolved by the time the child is examined. BPV is not associated with hearing loss, tinnitus, or loss of consciousness. The physical examination findings consist of:

- Acute unsteadiness: The child may fall or refuse to walk or sit; the child may grab on to a parent or object for steadiness.
- Nystagmus may be present within but not between attacks; again, no loss of consciousness, tinnitus, or hearing loss is associated with BPV events (Robertson, 2015).
- Vomiting and nausea may be present and be quite prominent.
- Appearance of child is frightened and/or pale.
- Child may be lethargic or drowsy; some children may sleep and return to normal activities on awakening.
- Neurologic examination is essentially negative except for abnormal vestibular function.

Because the symptoms of BPV can mimic symptoms of cranial neuropathy associated with a tumor, brain MRI will generally be ordered to assess for tumor (posterior fossa abnormalities). MRI would be essential if abnormalities in the neurologic examination are found between episodes.

One possible diagnostic study involves ice water caloric testing to detect abnormal vestibular function. However, this test is rarely done due to the intense discomfort that it produces. The clusters of attacks may be managed with diphenhydramine, 5 mg/kg/24 hours divided into three to four doses (maximum 300 mg/24 hours) by mouth, intramuscularly or intravenously. Once a diagnosis is made, parental reassurance is key. Children may be inappropriately diagnosed as having epilepsy and started on anticonvulsants; attacks will not respond to such drugs. They may go on to develop migraine headaches.

Cerebral Palsy

The term *cerebral palsy* encompasses a wide variety of nonreversible disorders of movement and posture that originate in the developing fetal or infant brain, often from an unknown cause (Ketelaar et al, 2014). CP is a chronic, nonprogressive disorder that impairs control of movement by damaging motor areas in the brain. Symptoms appear within the first few years of life. Depending on the area affected and the extent of damage, children with CP can also have disturbances in sensation, perception, cognition, communication, and behavior. In addition, epilepsy and musculoskeletal problems exacerbated by the motor impairment are often present (Ketelaar et al, 2014). The degree of brain injury is very individual, and the degree of impairment may not be directly associated with the degree of injury. There are three major types of CP: (1) spastic, (2) athetoid (or dyskinetic), and (3) ataxic. Spastic CP is characterized by muscle stiffening, causing muscle tightness. Athetoid affects the muscles that enable smooth, coordinated movement and maintain body posture; without this control, movement becomes involuntary and purposeless. The ataxic type affects balance and coordination. Children may exhibit varying degrees of involvement and severity; capabilities may improve over time depending on the degree of involvement and treatment. Table 28-3 lists more terms that describe CP.

TABLE 28-3 Terms Used to Describe Cerebral Palsy

Term	Description	Associated Impairments
Movement Type		
Spastic	Inability of a muscle to relax	Often evident after 4-6 months; retarded speech; convergent strabismus; toe-walking; flexed elbows; delayed walking until 18-24 months; one third have seizures
Athetoid	Inability to control muscle movement (continuous, writhing movements)	Infant has difficult feeding as a result of tongue thrust, is initially hypotonic with head lag; increasing tone with rigidity over time; speech delay
Ataxic	Problems with balance and coordination	Tremors
Body Part Involved		
Diplegic	Affects both legs more than both arms	Most have limited use of legs; can walk often with aids; walk typically "scissor-like" with knees bent in and crisscross over each other
Hemiplegic	Affects one side of the body (upper extremity is usually affected more than the lower extremity)	Often not detected at birth; right side often more affected than left; 50% develop seizures; growth arrest of affected limb(s); individuals usually able to walk
Tetraplegic/ quadriplegic	Affects all four extremities, trunk and head	Affects upper extremities more than lower; 50% with grand mal seizures; IQ impairment can be severe; most unable to walk or stand
Specific Problems with Movement or Function		
Dystonia	Involuntary, slow, sustained muscle contraction	Abnormal posture, writhing motion of arms, legs, trunk
Choreic	Disorganized tone	Uncontrollable jerky movements of toes and fingers
Tremor	Involuntary, rhythmic movements of opposing muscles; can affect extremities, head, face, vocal cords, trunk	
Ballismus	Violent, jerky movements; may affect only one side of body	
Rigidity	Stiffness	

IQ, Intelligence quotient.

CP was once believed to be caused only by birth complications (neonatal or perinatal asphyxia or trauma); however, current thinking and decades of study, including that by the Collaborative Perinatal Project (1959-1974), continue to demonstrate that labor and delivery are not major contributors to the occurrence of CP or most other neurodevelopmental disorders. The etiology is unknown in a large percentage of cases. Small for gestational age, low birth weight (less than 1000 g), or preterm babies (less than 37 weeks of gestation), and multiple births are at greater risk for CP. Complicated labor and delivery, breech presentation, Apgar score of less than 3 at 10 minutes or more; traumatic delivery; microcephaly; exposure to maternal infection (evidenced by chorioamnionitis, inflamed placental membranes, umbilical cord inflammation, foul-smelling amniotic fluid, maternal temperature greater than 100.4° F [38° C] during labor, or urinary tract infection [UTI]); maternal vaginal bleeding (between the sixth and ninth months of pregnancy); severe proteinuria late in pregnancy; maternal hyperthyroidism, intellectual disability, and seizures; intracranial hemorrhage; toxemia; preeclampsia; antepartal hemorrhage; postmaturity; fetal distress; maternal stroke; coagulation in the fetus or newborn; and neonatal seizures are considered risk factors.

Other etiologies may include intrauterine drug exposure (e.g., alcohol, cocaine, tobacco, crack cocaine), intrauterine infections (e.g., cytomegalovirus, toxoplasmosis, rubella), and congenital brain malformations. In the United States, it is estimated that children who acquire CP postnatally account for 10% to 15% of those with the disorder (CDC, 2015). In such cases, the cause can be attributed to meningitis, encephalitis, head trauma (e.g., secondary to shaken baby syndrome, also known as nonaccidental trauma), or other nonaccidental trauma, car accidents, falls, and near drowning.

The prevalence is 2 to 3.6 per 1000 live births across many studies (Ketelaar et al, 2014). Antenatal steroids and cesarean deliveries may decrease neurodevelopmental impairment, sepsis, and postnatal steroid use in extremely low birth weight infants.

Clinical Findings

History. The history should include prenatal and natal history and assessment for the presence of associated comorbid, developmental, and functional health problems.

- Prenatal/natal history of risk factors as listed previously
- Seizures
- Hearing and vision or ocular problems, such as strabismus, nystagmus, and optic atrophy
- Change in growth parameters, especially decreased head circumference
- Early head injury or meningitis
- Muscle tone: It can be hypotonic before 6 months old and then become hypertonic, as evidenced by unusual posture or favoring one side.
- Developmental milestones: They may be delayed but should still be attained depending on the extent of CP; persistent primitive reflexes are common (e.g., Moro and tonic neck). Hand preference before 1 year old is highly suspect.
- Functional health problems such as:
  - Feeding history of regurgitating through the nose, inability to coordinate suck and swallow, inability to advance the diet to textured foods—oral-motor coordination problems
  - Irritability or depressed affect (including unusual sleepiness) as a neonate
  - Difficulty with movement, cuddliness, grasp and release, self-feeding, and head control to look around; inability to change position per developmental level
  - Persistent primitive reflexes
  - Communication problems, either in language or speech proficiency

Physical Examination

- Skin: Dermatologic signs of syndromes, such as café au lait spots associated with neurofibromatosis, may be present.
- Orthopedic examination: Scoliosis, contractures, and dislocated hip(s) may be present after they have had months or years to develop.
- Neurologic examination: The following may be seen:
  - Deep tendon reflexes increased
  - Tone increased: Although tone is occasionally decreased; hypotonia before 6 months old is common. Tone may also be mixed.
  - Minimal muscle atrophy
  - No fasciculations
  - Persistent primitive reflexes (e.g., tonic neck and Moro after 6 months old)
  - Delayed reflexes (e.g., parachute reflex remains absent after 9 to 10 months old; side-protective reflexes remain absent after 5 months old)
  - Asymmetric movements
  - Preferred handedness before 1 to 2 years old
  - Abnormalities of head size, such as hydrocephaly, macrocephaly, or microcephaly
- Vision and hearing: Visual refractive errors occur in 50% of children; strabismus is found in 33%. Hearing problems may have resulted from the initial brain insult.
- Development: Assess gross motor, fine motor, language, and personal social skills. Motor milestones are commonly delayed. Note quality of movements (e.g., smoothness of gait, grasping, and clarity of speech).
- Feeding: Note a reversed swallow wave; uncoordinated suck and swallow, which may cause reflux and respiratory problems; decreased tone of the lips, tongue, and cheeks; increased gag reflex; involuntary tongue and lip movements; increased sensitivity to food stimuli; poor occlusion; and delayed inhibition of the suck reflex.
- Evaluate the diet, height, weight, and BMI for adequate nutrition.

Diagnostic Studies

- Imaging studies: A CT scan can be obtained to identify brain malformations. However, these are generally not present with CP. An MRI will aid the visualization of structures and abnormalities that are nearer to bony structures.
- Chromosomal and metabolic studies: These studies can be done to identify genetic disorders, especially single-gene defects.
- Lumbar puncture if sepsis is suspected.

Differential Diagnosis

The first and main requirement is to differentiate central from peripheral disorders. CP is always central and is characterized by brisk deep tendon reflexes. Many other conditions can have CP motor involvement features. These conditions include organic causes, such as sepsis from intrauterine infections, fetal alcohol syndrome, hydrocephalus, tumors, agenesis of the corpus callosum or other brain malformations, Tay-Sachs disease, phenylketonuria, Lesch-Nyhan syndrome, spinal cord injury, hypothyroidism, muscle diseases, seizures, and many genetic and metabolic disorders (e.g., cerebral folate deficiency), or acquired causes, such as a severe traumatic brain injury.

Management

The management of children with CP described here can serve as a model for the management of children with a variety of neurologic problems:

- *Referral of suspected cases:* Children with CP should be evaluated and cared for at centers that provide interdisciplinary health care professionals, including a developmental pediatrician, gastroenterologist, orthopedist, neurologist, nurse or nurse practitioner, speech pathologist, physical and occupational therapists, education consultant and psychologist, and social worker. Care may also involve an ophthalmologist, feeding clinic and nutritionist services, and genetics counseling.
- *Family education about the diagnosis:* Families need to understand the diagnosis and its nonprogressive but

ongoing characteristics and possible complications. They need to understand that the extent of brain damage is not always related to the level of disability; no one can predict what the future for a given child will be. Children who receive special services—physical therapy, occupational therapy, speech therapy, and other interventions—have better outcomes than children who do not. United Cerebral Palsy has educational materials and a variety of services available.

- *Family support:* Generally, families grieve when given the diagnosis of CP and need support during this time. Support groups or opportunities to meet other families with affected children are often helpful. The emotional needs of siblings must not be overlooked. The social worker can be very helpful to families trying to cope with complex health problems.
- *Financial resources:* CP services are long term and expensive and adaptive equipment, such as leg braces and wheelchairs, need periodic maintenance and replacement. Many children will be eligible for Supplemental Security Income or state program benefits for the severely handicapped. Respite care may be available. The Individuals with Disabilities Education Act of 1997 (IDEA) requires children with disabilities to be assessed for and instructed in the use of assistive devices along with appropriate referrals to regional centers. Medical social workers and public health nurses can be very helpful in connecting families to appropriate services.
- *Nutrition:* Children with CP often have inadequate nutrition because of their oral-motor coordination problems. Additionally, children with athetosis may need as much as 50% to 100% more calories to support their constant writhing movements. Children with spasticity, on the other hand, may need fewer calories because of their decreased movements. Occasionally, the problems are so severe that a gastrostomy is needed, sometimes with fundoplication to prevent reflux and aspiration. Special positioning, feeding therapy, and special feeding devices can help. High nutrient density is a key to providing a nutritious diet (i.e., getting more nutrients into the same volume of food) (also see Chapter 10). Feeding clinics are often helpful.
- *Elimination:* Constipation is common because of lack of exercise, inadequate fluid and fiber intake, medications, poor positioning, low abdominal muscle tone, and other factors. Stool softeners, such as docusate sodium, may help. Laxatives, such as senna concentrate or milk of magnesia may be useful but should not be used long term. Osmotic agents may also be used (e.g., polyethylene glycol). Bladder control and urinary retention are also problems in CP; these children are at risk for UTIs. Most children achieve bladder control between 3 and 10 years old. For some, toilet training may be difficult, especially for those with intellectual disability.
- *Dentistry:* Orofacial muscle tone can contribute to malocclusion. Problems with oral mobility make daily dental hygiene difficult, leading to gum disease. The side effects of some seizure medications can include swollen gums and tooth decay. A careful dental care program is necessary.
- *Drooling:* Inability to manage oral secretions results in drooling. Social isolation, wet clothing, skin excoriation, malodorous breath, discomfort, choking, gagging, and aspiration can make these oral secretions a serious problem. The anticholinergic, glycopyrrolate, is approved for use in those 3 to 16 years old with chronic excessive drooling from neurologic conditions. Oral dosage is 20 mcg/kg/dose three times a day initially with increases of 20 mcg/kg dose every 5 to 7 days if needed; maximum dosage is 100 mcg/kg/dose three times daily not exceeding 1500 to 3000 mcg/dose. Oral solutions should be given 1 hour before or 2 hours after meals. Side effects may be problematic (e.g., dry mouth, vomiting, constipation, flushing, urinary retention, and nasal congestion). Clinical improvement resulting in a reduction in drooling has been demonstrated. Surgical intervention is a last resort and commonly involves removing the submandibular gland or nerves, or cutting or rerouting the salivary duct.
- *Respiratory:* Positioning problems, an increase in gastroesophageal reflux disorder, and difficulty in clearing secretions place children with CP at higher risk for respiratory problems, notably pneumonias (especially from aspiration). The duration of respiratory symptoms with upper respiratory infections (URIs) may be increased in these children because they may have sleep-related obstruction or other positioning difficulties, which slow respiratory return to baseline. A tracheotomy may be necessary in severe cases of upper airway obstruction or difficulty. Suctioning equipment may be required.
- *Skin:* The skin in sedentary children is more likely to break down and cause a pressure ulcer(s). There is an increased incidence of skin latex allergies with CP.
- *Movement and mobility:* Positioning and seating, standing, transportation, bathing, dressing, and mobility for play and getting to school are important to assess and manage. Occupational and physical therapists are essential to these aspects of care, and families need their help incorporating various strategies into their homes and lifestyles. The goals of therapy are to improve physical conditioning and gain maximal independence in mobility, fine motor activities, self-care, and communication by promoting efficient movement patterns, inhibiting primitive reflexes, and achieving isolated extremity movements. Bracing, postural support and seating systems, adaptive devices, and early intervention programs beginning in infancy are important. Open-front walkers, quadrupedal canes, gait poles, wheelchairs, and motorized wheelchairs are beneficial in helping children explore their environment more efficiently. Although the condition is not progressive in terms of the brain lesion, contractures, scoliosis, dislocated hips, and other deformities can develop if the child is allowed to maintain in abnormal positions for long periods; range-of-motion

exercises are a long-term need. Orthopedic care may be necessary. A recent longitudinal study (Ketelaar et al, 2014) provides an evidence base for prognosis in daily mobility and self-care skills. A developmental trajectory classification system was employed. These evidence-based trajectories are helpful when discussing expectations and long-term goals with patients and families.

- *Medications:* Antispasmodic medications (baclofen, tizanidine, diazepam, and dantrolene) may be used to minimize contractures and spasticity. They are appropriate for children needing only a mild decrease in their muscle tone or in those with widespread spasticity. For optimal results, dosages often need to be high, and side effects can result (drowsiness, upset stomach, high blood pressure, and possible liver damage with chronic use).
  - Botulinum toxin A injections are used to eliminate pain, minimize contractures, delay or prevent surgery, and maximize function (Quality Standards Subcommittee of the American Academy of Neurology and the Practice Committee of the Child Neurology Society et al, 2010). Although botulinum toxin A has become standard treatment in pediatrics, it is used off-label (NINDS, 2015b). Its use is dependent on the recommendation of—and after a thorough evaluation by—a pediatric physiatrist, pediatric neurologist, or pediatric orthopedic surgeon, and after input of therapists and family. It is injected directly into muscles (sometimes guided by an electromyogram or electrical stimulation). The child may experience mild flulike symptoms and transient worsening of spasticity; for this reason, injections are best followed by physical and occupational therapies that help strengthen the antagonist and agonist muscles (NINDS, 2015b). The dosage administered depends on which muscles are being selected and muscle size. Results are generally seen within 5 to 7 days and last 3 to 4 months. The toxin has been safely used in infants older than 1 month. Resistance can occur because neutralizing antibodies can develop. Therefore, only the smallest possible effective dose must be used, and at least 3 months must lapse between injections. Injection of botulinum toxin into salivary glands is also being used to reduce severity of drooling. Contraindications include diffuse hypertonia, myasthenia gravis (MG), motor neuron disease, injection into an infected muscle, caution in pregnancy (fetal complications have been seen in animal studies), and caution when it is coadministered with an aminoglycoside or another agent that interferes with neuromuscular transmission (toxin effect can be increased) (Quality Standards Subcommittee of the American Academy of Neurology and the Practice Committee of the Child Neurology Society et al, 2010). The numerous side effects should be thoroughly understood by care providers.
- *Communication:* With the combined problems of lack of oral-motor control and the high incidence of intellectual disability, communication can be a problem. Speech therapy may be of assistance; augmentative devices, such as computers with voices, can allow for language development and communication of needs even without oral speech. Hearing deficits need to be identified and managed by an audiologist.
- *Vision:* Visual acuity, eye tracking, and binocularity are key factors to be assessed by a pediatric ophthalmologist.
- *Osteopenia:* Individuals with CP are at risk of bone density loss secondary to their inability to ambulate and place weight on their bones. Some medical providers prescribe bisphosphonates off-label to children (NINDS, 2015b). Monitoring of calcium and vitamin D should be strongly considered and supplemental vitamin D prescribed if vitamin D levels are low.
- *Pain:* Spastic muscles, strain on compensatory muscles, and frequent or irregularly occurring muscle spasms can cause chronic and acute pain. Diazepam, gabapentin, and complementary therapies (distraction, biofeedback, relaxation, and therapeutic massage) can help (NINDS, 2015b).
- *Special education:* Early intervention programs and specialized educational programs through school systems are often beneficial.
- *Other treatments:* Surgery is used to release contractures or to sever overactivated nerves (called a *selective dorsal root rhizotomy*). Selective dorsal root rhizotomy (of spinal nerves) plus intrathecal baclofen decrease spasticity and increase range of motion of affected limbs. Intrathecal baclofen uses an implantable pump to deliver the drug, a muscle relaxant. The pump is programmable with an electronic telemetry wand. Pumps have been successfully implanted in children as young as 3 years of age; this treatment has small but significant risks of complications. It is most efficacious in children who have some motor movement control and who have few muscles to treat that are not fixed or rigid (NINDS, 2015b). As an added benefit, it overcomes the problem of CNS adverse effects associated with administration of large oral doses. Intense physical therapy is an instrumental adjunct treatment.
  - Strength training can help with balance and weakness. Functional electrical stimulation (involves insertion of a microscopic wireless device into specific muscles or nerves) has been used to activate and strengthen muscles in the hand, shoulder, and ankle. It should be regarded as experimental in CP and is used only as an alternative treatment if other treatments fail to relax muscles or relieve pain (NINDS, 2015b).

Complications

An Autism and Developmental Disabilities Monitoring (ADDM) Network study noted approximately 41% of children with CP had epilepsy and 7% had co-occurring autism spectrum disorder, with nonspastic CP having an 18% association with ASD (Christensen et al, 2014). Children who

• BOX 28-2 Problems Associated with Cerebral Palsy

Cognitive

Learning disabilities
Intellectual disability

Seizure Disorders

Various types of seizures

Language and Speech Disorders

Articulation
Vocal strength and quality
Language processing

Vision

Refractive errors
Strabismus
Amblyopia
Cataracts
Retinopathy of prematurity
Cortical blindness
Homonymous hemianopsia (hemiplegia)

Hearing

Conductive
Sensorineural

Other Sensory

Tactile hypersensitivity or hyposensitivity
Dyspraxia
Balance and movement problems
Proprioception difficulties
Stereognosis

Motor

Prolonged primitive reflexes
Absence of protective reflexes
Delayed motor milestones
Hip subluxation and dislocation
Scoliosis
Contractures

Feeding and Eating Problems

Chewing, sucking, and swallowing deficits
Drooling
Hypoxemia
Fatigue
Underweight and overweight
Gastroesophageal reflux
Aspiration

Bowel

Constipation
Encopresis

Urinary

Bladder control
Urinary retention
Urinary tract infections

Dental

Malocclusions
Enamel deficits and caries
Gum hyperplasia (with phenytoin)

Pulmonary

Respiratory infections
Pneumonia

Skin

Pressure ulcers
Latex allergy

Behavioral and Emotional

Behavioral disorders
Attention-deficit disorder, with and without hyperactivity
Self-injurious behaviors
Depression
Autism
Growth failure
Other

receive no intervention have poorer functional abilities; they make less progress developmentally and are at risk for unnecessary contractures and deformities. Box 28-2 lists associated problems seen in CP.

Prevention and Screening

The incidence of CP can be decreased to some extent through good prenatal care. Recent research is centered on several processes believed to play a causative role in CP. These research endeavors include identifying genes that may be associated with abnormal neuronal migration, evaluating the role that excessive amounts of glutamate in the brain play in over excitation and death of neurons, investigating whether synthetic neuroprotective substances can be developed (neurotrophins) and given to an infant after stroke or hypoxia, and continuing to evaluate the relationship between elevations in interferons or other inflammatory cytokines that result from maternal infection and interrupt normal fetal brain development. Also, RH incompatibility during pregnancy may cause CP in the child if not treated (NINDS, 2015b). During the 28th week of pregnancy, immunoglobulin (RhoGAM) can be administered to the mother to prevent CP in this situation.

Bell Palsy

Bell palsy is a sudden, acute unilateral paralysis or weakening of any facet of the facial nerve without sensory loss. There is edema of CN VII and venous congestion in areas of the nerve canal. A viral etiology is suspected but the exact mechanism or etiology of Bell palsy remains unknown (Baugh et al, 2013). It can occur in infants and all other ages. Onset is rapid and can progress to maximal intensity within hours. Symptoms may last for 1 to 9 weeks (average 2 to 4 weeks) with spontaneous remission and recovery.

Clinical Findings

History. The child may initially experience localized pain or tingling in one ear and then experience sagging on one side of the face with the eyelid completely or partially closed. The history usually reveals a URI within the previous 2 weeks or exposure to cold temperature.

Physical Examination. A neurologic assessment of all facial nerve functions may be difficult in children and is not critical to make an accurate diagnosis. The clinician should note the following:

- Unilateral motor changes in the forehead, cheek, and perioral area; face muscles pull to the normal side when the child makes facial expressions
- Normal blood pressure
- Dribbling liquids from the weak side; eating and drinking are more difficult
- Hypersensitivity to loud noises
- Eyelid fails to close on the affected side, and complete blinking may be absent; exposure keratitis may be present
- Lacrimation, taste (50% of patients); anterior two thirds of tongue), and salivation may be impaired
- No limb weakness
- Any skin lesions to suggest herpes on the affected side of the face (would indicate active viral infection of the nerve or its motor neurons)

Diagnostic Studies. It is widely accepted that diagnostic testing is not indicated unless the patient fails to improve over a 6-week period or other neurologic symptoms occur.

Differential Diagnosis

Included in the differential diagnosis are Guillain-Barré syndrome (usually includes an additional symptom of absent tendon reflexes of limbs), hypertension, congenital absence of the depressor angularis oris muscle, infection, trauma (the use of forceps during delivery can cause a facial nerve compression neuropathy that spontaneously resolves within a few days to weeks), Melkersson syndrome (involves recurrent facial palsies with swollen lips, tongue, cheeks, or eyelids), Möbius syndrome, acute otitis media, poliomyelitis, histiocytosis X, varicella, facial nerve tumors, neurofibroma, infiltration of facial nerves with leukemic cells, rhabdomyosarcoma of the middle ear, and brainstem infarcts.

Management

If eyelid closure is incomplete, prescribe methylcellulose eye drops or ocular lubricant to the affected eye several times daily and patch the eye if the child plays outdoors, during active play, and when sleeping. The American Academy of Neurology and the American Academy of Otolaryngology agree that steroids should be used in newly diagnosed patients (oral prednisone is dosed at 1 mg/kg/day for 1 week, then tapered for 1 week; start within the first 3 to 5 days) (Schwartz et al, 2014). Worster and colleagues (2010) and the aforementioned organizations acknowledge lack of strong evidence for the efficacy of combined steroid and antiretroviral therapy. However, they also state that the possibility exists of some small benefit with combined therapy.

Complications

Approximately 85% of children recover spontaneously without facial weakness (Sarnat, 2011). If recovery is incomplete, lack of salivation in response to food, lack of lacrimation, facial contractures, and tics may occur.

Epilepsy and Seizure Disorders

Seizures are due to the misfiring of the cortical neurons of the brain. Convulsive seizures occur when misfiring causes episodes of involuntary contraction of voluntary muscles. Fig. 28-3 summarizes the types of seizures. When seizures are recurrent, unrelated to fever, and unprovoked, the disorder is called *epilepsy*. Seizures represent either brain dysfunction or significant underlying disorders. A child may demonstrate characteristics of more than one type of seizure. Different types of seizures arise from disorders in various locations throughout the brain. Seizures can result from a variety of genetic, symptomatic, or idiopathic conditions. More than 30,000 genes are expressed in the brain, and approximately 20% of individuals with epilepsy have a genetic etiology. Several familial epilepsies have been identified. These include benign neonatal convulsions, juvenile myoclonic epilepsy, and progressive myoclonic epilepsy (Camfield and Camfield, 2009).

Clinical Findings

History. Historical questioning should include the following:

- Description of the seizure: Focal or generalized, loss of consciousness, aura, length of postictal sleep or confusion, duration of the episode, associated illness, and incontinence
- Any underlying medical diagnosis (e.g., diabetes, renal disease, cardiovascular disorder)
- Previous CNS infection or birth trauma
- Intrauterine infection, trauma, bleeding
- Toxic exposure or drug use
- Anticonvulsant medication stopped abruptly or doses missed, or change to generic from brand or vice versa
- Recent head injury
- Family history of seizures
- Any noted missed milestones

Physical Examination. The following should be determined on physical examination:

- Focal abnormalities, weakness
- Presence of seizure activity during the examination
- Hypertension (for renal disease)
- Systemic disease
- Cardiovascular disorder
- Neurocutaneous disease, café au lait spots of neurofibromatosis, ash leaf spots or adenoma sebaceum of tuberous sclerosis, facial hemangioma of Sturge-Weber syndrome
- Signs of head trauma
- Transillumination of the skull in infants

ILAE Proposal for Revised Terminology for Organization of Seizures and Epilepsies 2010

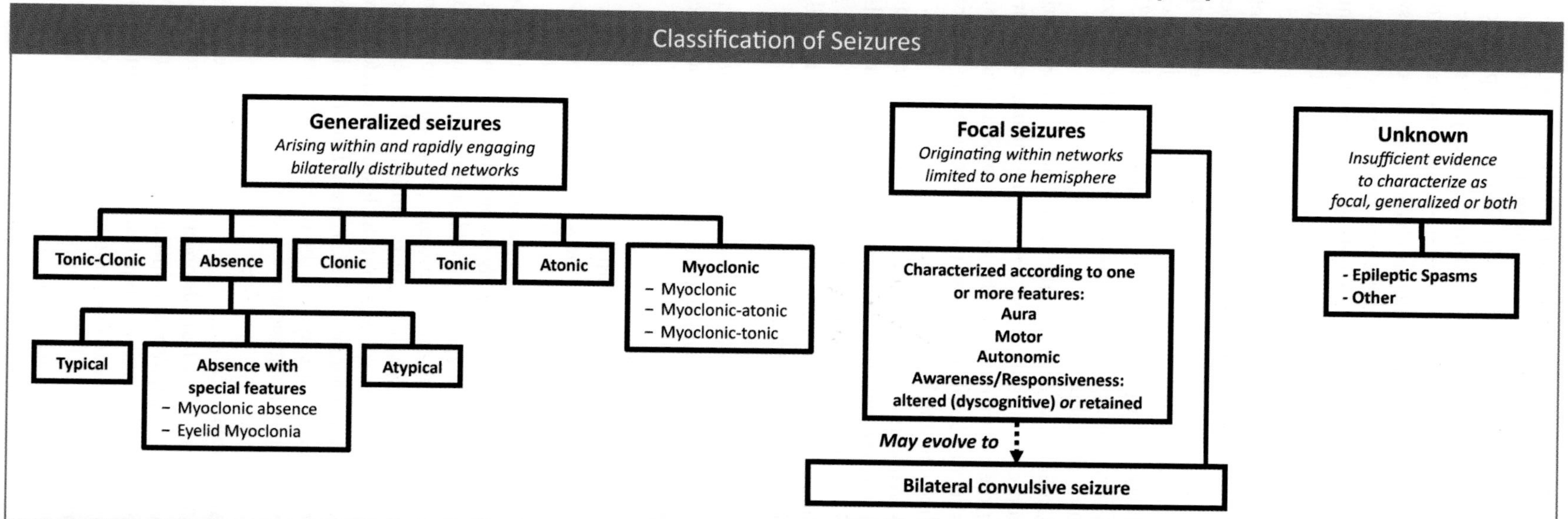

Changes in terminology and concepts

Etiology

New Term and Concept	Examples	Old Term and Concept
Genetic: *genetic defect directly contributes to the epilepsy and seizures are the core symptom of the disorder*	*Channelopathies, Glut1 deficiency, etc.*	**Idiopathic:** *presumed genetic*
Structural-metabolic: *caused by a structural or metabolic disorder of the brain*	*Tuberous sclerosis, cortical malformations, etc.*	**Symptomatic:** *secondary to a known or presumed disorder of the brain*
Unknown: *the cause is unknown and might be genetic, structural or metabolic*		**Cryptogenic:** *presumed symptomatic*

Terminology

Terminology	Terms no longer recommended
Self-limited: *tendency to resolve spontaneously with time* **Pharmacoresponsive:** *highly likely to be controlled with medication*	**Benign** **Catastrophic**
Focal seizures: *seizure semiology described according to specific subjective (auras), motor, autonomic, and dyscognitive features*	**Complex partial** **Simple partial**
Evolving to a bilateral convulsive seizure: *eg. tonic, clonic, tonic-clonic*	**Secondarily generalized**

References: 1.Berg AT et al. Revised terminology and concepts for organization of seizures and epilepsies: report of the ILAE Commission on Classification and Terminology, 2005-2009. *Epilepsia* 2010;51:676-685. 2.Berg AT, Cross JH. *Lancet* 2010:9;459-61. 3.Blume WT et al. Glossary of descriptive terminology for ictal semiology: Report of the ILAE task force on classification and terminology. *Epilepsia* 2001:42;1212-1218.

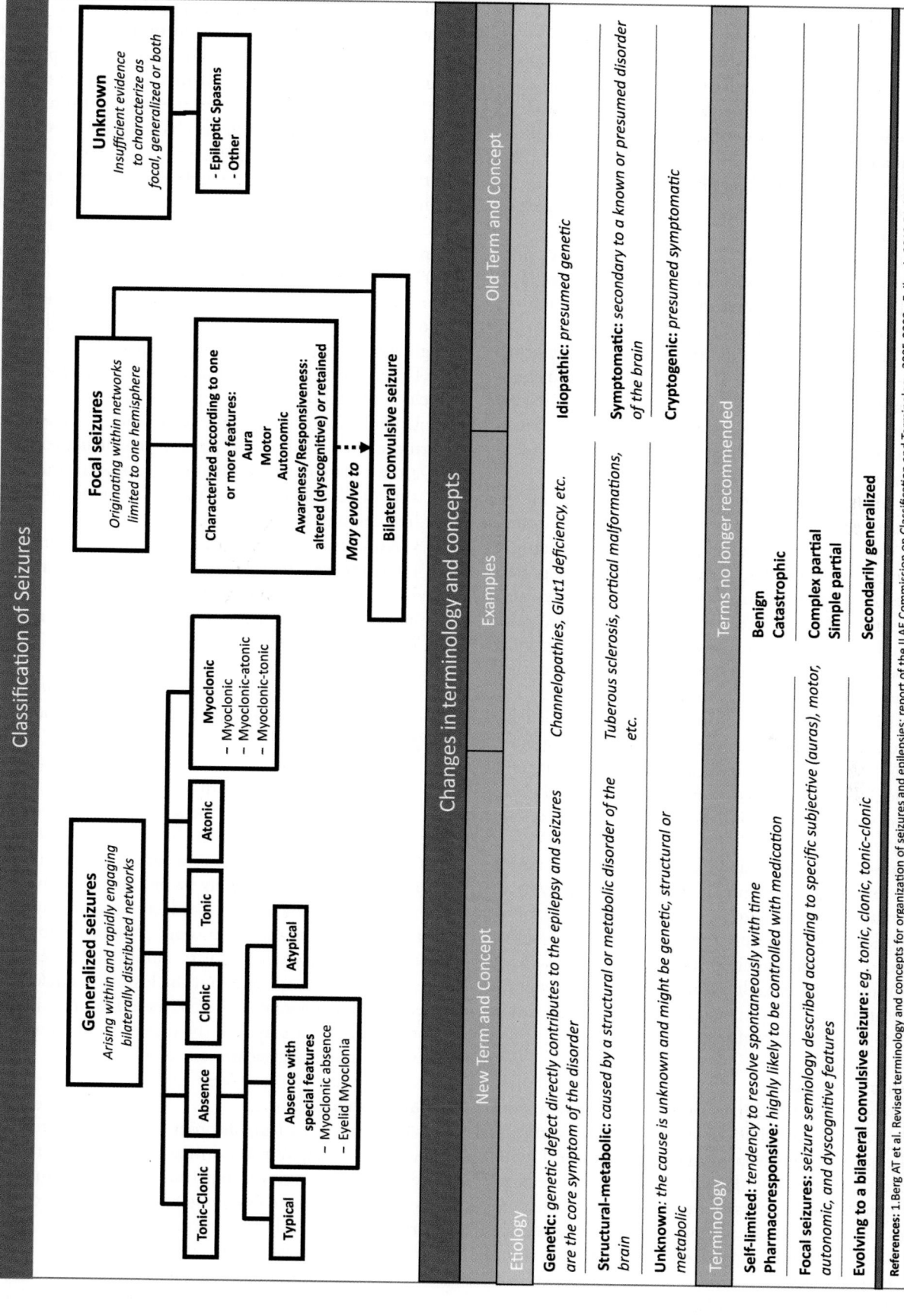

• **Figure 28-3** Classifications of seizures. ILAE, International League Against Epilepsy. (Reprinted with permission from International League Against Epilepsy (ILAE), available at www.ilae.org/Commission/Class/documents/ILAE%20HandoutV10.pdf.)

Diagnostic Studies. These are the typical diagnostic test recommendations:

- Complete blood count (CBC) (including platelets, liver function tests [LFTs])—useful for diagnostic purposes or as a baseline before anticonvulsant therapy is started.
- Metabolic screen may be considered later in the workup, not initially.
- Blood glucose—standard in all patients.
- Urine and serum toxicology—only if illicit drug exposure is suspected.
- Lumbar puncture—only if child is younger than 6 months; child of any age with persistent changes in mental status or failure to return to baseline functioning; patients with meningeal signs.
- EEG—standard in all children after first nonfebrile seizure. An abnormal EEG supports the seizure diagnosis. However, a normal EEG when the child is not seizing does not rule out a seizure disorder. Video electroencephalogram over 1 to 6 days is another option to identify seizure activity.
- MRI—imaging studies are not routinely indicated if the initial seizure is followed by a normal neurologic examination and return to baseline mental status. Imaging is recommended: (1) if the patient demonstrates cognitive changes after several hours and postictal focal dysfunction (signs of increased intracranial pressure, such as found with tumors, abscesses, strokes, or vascular malformations); (2) if the seizure lasted more than 15 minutes; (3) in infants younger than 6 months old; and (4) if any new onset of focal neurologic deficit has occurred. An MRI is now the preferred imaging study over CT scans because of its increased sensitivity and because of the risk of increased radiation with CT. MRI may be ordered if EEG shows focal locus of seizure activity.
- CT scan—used only in cases of marked cognitive, motor, or neurologic dysfunction of unknown etiology (e.g., head injury, brain infection or tumor, abscesses); abnormal EEGs; or focal seizure symptoms that may or may not evolve into a generalized seizure.
- Polysomnography (simultaneous EEG, electromyogram, electrocardiogram [ECG], and electrooculogram) can be useful to assess nocturnal seizures.

Differential Diagnosis

Consider breath-holding, inattentive staring, benign shudders, self-gratification behavior, tantrums, cyclic vomiting, BPV, syncope, migraine headaches, gastroesophageal reflux, night terrors, conversion disorder, nonepileptic seizures, metabolic problems, tumors or other CNS problems, or a cardiovascular problem. Vertigo has been confused with epilepsy. Tics (involuntary, spasmodic, nonrhythmic, repetitive movements) are stereotypic but not associated with impaired consciousness and at times can be suppressed by the patient.

Nonepileptic Seizures. A nonepileptic seizure (formerly referred to as a "pseudoseizure") may be difficult to distinguish from true seizures, even after direct observation. It is the most common manifestation of a conversion disorder in children (Reilly et al, 2013). Suspect nonepileptic seizures in a child with a documented underlying seizure disorder who has gained more recent control; up to one third of patients who exhibit this also have coexisting epilepsy. In such cases, the nonepileptic seizures serve as attention-getting behaviors for the child who misses the attention gained before control. Nonepileptic seizures also may be seen in adolescents; more often in girls than in boys (3 : 1). Stress and anxiety, especially within the family, are found in 50% of cases. The most common precipitating factors would appear to be school-related difficulties and interpersonal conflict within the child's family; these children are at high risk for depression and anxiety (Reilly et al, 2013).

Distinguishing characteristics of nonepileptic seizures include the following:

- Unilaterally or bilaterally coordinated motor activity more like thrashing and jerking (scissor-like movements) rather than characteristic tonic-clonic movements; no aura or complaints of malaise; heart palpitations; feeling like choking before seizure onset
- Occur only before a witness; occur at home; do not interrupt play, may occur at school, witnessed
- Normally reactive pupils to light
- Are situation specific and have a gradual onset
- No associated tongue biting or injury
- Have an abrupt recovery—no postictal state
- Discomfort, distress expressed; sometimes ataxia, fumbling; consciousness may be impaired, but the patient is not unconscious
- No incontinence
- No EEG changes, even during episodes

Treatment for nonepileptic seizures involves developing alternative gains to seizure behavior. Most children stop after the diagnosis is made and interventions are in place. A referral for counseling may be indicated in a multifaceted approach of therapy and medications for psychological illness, depending on the etiology. Assess previous somatic complaints, stress factors, peers, family, and illness modeled in the home. If suspected, but the history is unclear, a video electroencephalogram (VEEG) should be considered. No anticonvulsants are used in the case of children who do not have an underlying seizure disorder.

Management

Referral. If a seizure disorder is suspected, refer to a neurologist for diagnosis and initiation of treatment. AEDs are usually prescribed, especially after a second seizure. Delaying treatment does not affect ultimate control, but early diagnosis and intervention can often reduce the disabilities and risks associated with the condition.

Management of Stable Patients with Diagnosed Seizure Disorders. The primary care provider (PCP) can monitor stable children with seizures, including continuing the prescription for their anticonvulsant(s), monitoring drug levels, and performing case management. Approximately one third

TABLE 28-4 Antiepileptic Drug Therapy for Children: Seizure Type and Epilepsy Syndrome*

Seizure Type or Epilepsy Syndrome	First-Line Monotherapy for Initial Onset	Adjunctive Therapy	Comments
Partial-onset seizures	Oxcarbazepine	Carbamazepine, lamotrigine, levetiracetam, phenobarbital, topiramate, valproic acid, vigabatrin	Adjunct therapy may be needed.
Generalized tonic-clonic seizures	Valproic acid (drug of first choice), lamotrigine, carbamazepine, topiramate	Levetiracetam, phenobarbital, phenytoin, clobazam	Adjunct therapy may be needed.
Absence seizures	Ethosuximide (drug of first choice) or valproic acid, lamotrigine	Clobazam	Other AEDs may worsen seizures. There are two types: • Childhood—onset 5 to 6 years old; remission 10 to 12 years old • Juvenile—onset 10 to 12 years old; usually lifelong
Juvenile myoclonic epilepsy	Valproate (drug of first choice), lamotrigine, levetiracetam, topiramate, zonisamide	Clobazam, clonazepam	Other AEDs may worsen seizures (including lamotrigine).
Lennox-Gastaut syndrome	Valproic acid, clobazam, rufinamide	Lamotrigine, topiramate	Typically requires multidrug therapy; seizures are difficult to control Rufinamide associated with life-threatening events, including first-degree heart block.
Benign epilepsy of childhood with centrotemporal spikes	Valproic acid (drug of choice if needed)	Gabapentin,	Medication may not be required.
Infantile spasms	ACTH	Corticosteroids, vigabatrin, clobazam	Vigabatrin has access and prescribing restrictions. Onset in newborn-infant; no remission.
Neonatal seizures	Phenobarbital	Phenytoin	No treatment guidelines for treatment exist.

Data from Mikati MM: Seizures in childhood. Kliegman RM, Stanton BF, St. Geme JW, et al, editors: *Nelson textbook of pediatrics*, ed 19, Philadelphia, 2011, Elsevier/Saunders, pp 2013–2038.
ACTH, Adrenocorticotropic hormone; *AED,* antiepileptic drug.
*See an appropriate pharmacology reference for dosing, therapeutic drug levels, and necessary laboratory testing.

of children who have a history of cognitive or motor impairments will have a recurrent unprovoked seizure within 1 year.

Drug Monitoring. All providers working with patients receiving anticonvulsants should be familiar with the common drugs (Tables 28-4 and 28-5; Box 28-3) and their major side effects. Evaluating and investigating compliance issues are also components of the monitoring role. If possible, start with one drug with the fewest side effects and describe how the drug works with the child and parent, with an explanation of side effects. Key points for drug monitoring include:

- Some children with epilepsy can be controlled with subtherapeutic blood levels.
- Some children can be free of side effects at levels beyond the therapeutic range.
- Phenytoin saturates the enzyme system; therefore, even a small increase in dosage can cause a marked increase in blood levels. Phenytoin is rarely used due to the advent of newer medications.
- Half-lives and steady state concentrations can vary when new AEDs are introduced or when other non-AEDs are being taken (e.g., antibiotics, antipyretics). Half-lives are longer with the introduction to a new drug; steady concentrations (and elimination) of the drug are achieved at five half-lives.
- If gastrointestinal side effects occur, decreasing the dosage and increasing the frequency of administration may help;

TABLE 28-5 Additional Considerations in Antiepileptic Drug Selection

Consideration	Comments
Child-related	Age, gender, concurrent medication, and comorbidity; ability to swallow
Medication-related	Adverse effects of medication (nuisance to irreversible damage) pharmacokinetics, taste, need for laboratory monitoring (therapeutic levels and liver and hematologic testing); formulation of drug (e.g., pill or capsule); teratogenesis of the drug (adolescent female on AED)
Special setting use of diazepam (Diastat)	Diazepam (Diastat), rectal gel: Used in school and home settings for emergency treatment of refractory seizures in children (≥ 2 years old). Place child on side; gently place the lubricated rectal tip into the rectum, snug against the rectal opening; push plunger with medication over 3 seconds; leave in place for 3 seconds before removing plunger; and then hold buttock cheeks together for a count of three. Requires careful respiratory monitoring. Its use in school settings requires a written protocol. If Diastat AcuDial syringe used, set to correct dose before insertion. Consult drug textbook for pediatric dosage.
Other	Insurance coverage; ability to pay for medication; availability of medication; compliance (e.g., frequency of medication administration)

Data from Taketomo CK, Hodding JH, Kraus DM: *Pediatric dosage handbook*, ed 21, Hudson, OH, 2014, Lexi-Comp.
AED, Antiepileptic drug.

• BOX 28-3 Antiepileptic Drug (Therapeutic Level)

Carbamazepine: 3-12 mg/L
Clobazam: 60-200 μg/L
Clonazepam: 25-85 μg/L
Ethosuximide: 40-100 mg/L
Gabapentin: 2-20 mg/L
Lamotrigine: 1-15 mg/L
Levetiracetam: 6-20 mg/L
Oxcarbazepine: 13-28 mg/L
Phenobarbital: 10-40 mg/L
Phenytoin: 5-20 mg/L
Rufinamide: Monitor by neurologist for life-threatening adverse events
Topiramate: 2-25 mg/L
Valproic acid: 50-100 mg/L
Vigabatrin: Prescribing and access restrictions; monitor by neurologist
Zonisamide: 10-40 mg/L

try changing to an enteric-coated pill or taking the medication after eating.

- Administer AED no more frequently than twice daily or daily for better adherence.
- The first signs of toxicity usually include sedation, changes in behavior, and changes in cognition and balance; other drug toxicities may cause decreases in memory and attention span or interpersonal relationship difficulties. It is important to note that some children may exhibit these changes and have drug levels within the normal range.
- Metabolites of the drugs can cause hypersensitivity side effects.
- Monitor routine drug levels based on the clinical picture with trough levels (random drug levels are rarely helpful).
- Some herbal products interfere with seizure control.

Antiepileptic Medication Withdrawal. After 2 years or longer without seizures, most pediatric neurologists will consider gradually withdrawing anticonvulsant therapy after obtaining an EEG. Patients with histories of benign epilepsy with rolandic spikes or with idiopathic generalized seizures are more likely to be successfully withdrawn. Those with complex partial seizures and juvenile myoclonic seizures are more likely to have a recurrence once medication has been withdrawn. Anticonvulsant medication withdrawal should occur over a span of several months, because abrupt weaning can cause withdrawal seizures (particularly with phenobarbital and benzodiazepines) or status epilepticus (SE). Children with intellectual disability, CP, focal motor deficits, age of onset younger than 2 years, symptomatic seizures, and abnormal EEGs may not be appropriate candidates for weaning. Weaning is supervised closely, with one anticonvulsant medication removed at a time. An EEG during drug withdrawal of valproate is recommended for children with primary generalized epilepsy (Mikati, 2011). Of children who have been seizure-free for 2 years and have low risk factors, most remain seizure-free without anticonvulsant medication. If seizures do recur, most relapses do so within the first 6 months of weaning. Children whose seizures recur within 2 to 3 months after AED therapy is discontinued typically will need to have their AEDs restarted to treat seizure relapse (Mikati, 2011). If the onset of seizures occurred during a time of anoxia, head injury, meningitis, or encephalitis, the AED treatment can be stopped after recovery from the condition is complete. The child can always be restarted should there be a recurrence.

Ketogenic Diet. The ketogenic diet is useful in young children with all types of seizures, particularly those with refractory epilepsy from a variety of causes, including infantile spasms and Lennox-Gastaut syndrome (Selter et al, 2015). The diet is considered when the side effects of anticonvulsant medications are intolerable or when allergies preclude their administration. The ideal child is between

2 and 5 years old because the desired steady state of ketosis is easier to maintain. The diet is stringent and requires utmost vigilance to the ratios of calories, protein, fat, carbohydrates, vitamins, and minerals. It is best managed under very tight control with medical and dietetic leadership. Side effects usually involve abdominal pain and diarrhea. A prescreening process, including psychological testing to determine the child's and family's emotional functioning, coping, and problem-solving abilities, is recommended. A dietitian should screen the child for nutrition and growth status. The family should be interviewed for understanding of and education about the protocol. The diet is usually started while the child is admitted to the hospital, where metabolic and neurologic states can be monitored. Many centers now use the modified Atkins diet, a variation of the original ketogenic diet, due to its somewhat less restrictive nature. This diet is generally effective and well tolerated in children with drug-refractory epilepsy and has sometimes even shown greater improvement in seizure reduction than the original ketogenic diet (Sharma et al, 2013).

Surgery. Surgical interventions have been successful in helping some children with complex partial seizures; however, selection of appropriate children must be done with great care. *Focal resection* surgery is used only in children whose epileptic focus is localized, who have failed to respond to AEDs, and whose development has been assessed over time. Seizure-free rates after resection vary depending on the type of resective surgery and underlying seizure disorder. *Hemispherectomy* or *inter-hemispherectomy* can be curative. Side effects of the surgery include hemiparesis, incontinence, stuttering, and poor hand coordination. *Temporal lobotomies* are an option for treating intractable partial complex seizures localized to the temporal area; side effects are aphasia and superior quadrant visual loss. Slightly more than 50% of candidates achieve freedom from seizures. *Callosotomy* and *vagus nerve stimulation (VNS)*, as palliative surgeries, are options for children with multiple regions of hemispheric involvement that result in intractable seizures. In VNS, a programmed device—"pacemaker of the brain"—is implanted in the anterior chest wall. A wire wraps around the left vagus nerve and sends regular, mild pulses of electrical energy to the brain via the nerve. A patient with an aura can stimulate the device to prevent a seizure. For those without an aura, the device is set on specific parameters given the child's seizure pattern. With VNS, seizures and side effects can be better controlled. Children, as well as adults, are good candidates.

Counseling. Older children and parents need to understand the diagnosis, treatment (including specifics of the prescribed antiepileptic medications), necessary follow-up, and long-term prognosis. Laws vary from state to state regarding driving, but generally a teenager who has been seizure-free for 6 months and has demonstrated consistent medication compliance should be allowed to drive. Some states may require a 2-year period of time. One study revealed that fatal car crashes attributed to seizures were rare versus those caused by other medical conditions (Tiamkao et al, 2009). Many antiseizure medications are teratogenic; therefore, contraception and thorough patient and family education is essential for sexually active females.

Children with epilepsy may experience social stigmas and problems with self-esteem. Other mental health problems may also occur in these children as they try to cope with a chronic disease. Parents are encouraged to treat children as normally as possible and seek appropriate support groups.

Safety. Uncontrolled seizures can present safety hazards for an unsupervised child. The child and family need to consider situations that the child will be in and be sure that someone knows what to do if a seizure occurs, including school personnel. Safety helmets worn at all times are sometimes warranted if falls and head injury occur frequently. Swimming alone is never recommended, but swimming, contact sports, and climbing are to be allowed if the child is well controlled and there is constant supervision during these activities.

Immunizations. The decision to give pertussis vaccine to children with neurologic seizures or other neurologic conditions needs to be made on an individual basis. The CDC recommends deferring diphtheria-tetanus-acellular pertussis (DTaP) until a child's neurologic status is clarified and stabilized from a known progressive neurologic disorder, such as infantile spasms, uncontrolled epilepsy, or progressive encephalopathy. In children who have experienced encephalopathy (e.g., coma, decreased level of consciousness, or prolonged seizures), not attributable to another identifiable cause, within 7 days of administration of a previous dose of DTP, DTaP, or Tdap, theses vaccines are contraindicated (CDC, 2011).

Vaccine safety is constantly being investigated. Of note, in a large study examining data from 1997 to 2006, Huang and colleagues (2010) did not observe an increased risk for seizures among children 6 to 23 months old who received the DTaP. Furthermore, they found a negative association between all seizures and DTaP, supporting the absence of increased risk.

Complications

Status epilepticus (SE) are seizures that may be continuous, or frequent, without recovery between episodes. *Nonconvulsive SE* is characterized by continuous abnormal EEG activity without tonic-clonic activity. *Convulsive SE* typically involves tonic-clonic activity in two or more seizures between which there is no recovery of consciousness or a prolonged single seizure lasting more than 30 minutes. A child who has generalized tonic-clonic seizures and who is in SE may be at increased risk for morbidity and mortality due to lack of oxygenation, decreased cerebral perfusion, metabolic acidosis, hypoglycemia, hyperkalemia, lactic acidosis, increased temperature, and increased intracranial pressure. Such an occurrence needs to be handled as a medical emergency. SE can be triggered by an acute brain infection, progressive neurologic disease, medication failure or noncompliance, or, rarely, a febrile seizure in an otherwise healthy child without other risk factors. However, most cases of SE occur in children with underlying neurologic deficits. It is difficult to diagnose SE in children with absence of or complex partial seizures because the children may just appear confused. Adverse outcomes can include behavioral problems, acquired intellectual disability, and focal motor deficits. Diazepam rectal gel is recommended for use by health care providers, parents, and caregivers (including school personnel) in children older than 2 years old who have a seizure lasting more than 5 minutes. It is administered once and takes effect in 5 to 15 minutes. Its use has decreased emergency department (ED) visits by 67%; it is safe at higher than recommended doses; and it has less than a 1% incidence of respiratory depression. The most common side effect is somnolence. It is available in a premeasured portable syringe and dosed according to age and weight. The use of intranasal midazolam is also effective in controlling acute seizures (Humphries and Eiland, 2013).

Febrile Seizures

Febrile seizures are the most common type of seizures in children. They are brief, generalized, clonic or tonic-clonic in nature, and can be either simple or complex. A concurrent illness is present with rapid fever rise to at least more than 102.2° F (39° C), but the fever is not necessarily that high at the time of the seizure. It is conjectured that these seizures may be related to peak temperature reached during the febrile episode. Minimal postictal confusion is associated with febrile seizures. Simple febrile seizures last less than 15 minutes and may recur during the same febrile illness period. Complex febrile seizures last longer than 15 minutes, can recur on the same day, and can have focal attributes (even during the postictal phase). Febrile SE is uncommon, rarely stops spontaneously, is fairly resistant to medications, and can persist for a long period of time. Most children in febrile SE require one or more medications to end the seizure. A report found that reducing the time from seizure onset to anticonvulsant medication administration was key to reducing the seizure duration during an episode (Seinfeld et al, 2014).

The etiology of febrile seizures is unclear and by definition excludes seizures that are caused by intracranial illness or are related to an underlying CNS problem. The risk is higher in children with a family medical history for febrile seizures or in those with predisposing factors (e.g., neonatal intensive care unit [NICU] stay more than 30 days, developmental delay, day care attendance).

The age range associated with febrile seizures is 6 months to 60 months. Male gender is a minor risk factor as is a lower sodium level. Approximately 2% to 5% of neurologically healthy infants and young children experience at least one simple febrile seizure with about 30% of this group experiencing a second episode (Mikati, 2011).

Clinical Findings

History. Include the following:

- Description of seizure duration, type (generalized or focal), frequency in 24 hours
- Relationship of the seizure to a febrile episode and level of temperature
- Any abnormal neurologic findings noted before the seizure (is not consistent with a febrile seizure)
- Family history of afebrile or febrile seizures
- Maternal smoking in the perinatal period
- Prematurity or neonatal hospitalizations for more than 28 days
- Parents' perception of development of child

Physical Examination. The physical examination is the same as that described earlier for seizures.

Diagnostic Studies. Diagnostic studies include the following:

- A lumbar puncture may be done in infants younger than 12 months old and who may also have used an antibiotic prior to seizure onset, and/or in those who have signs of meningeal irritation.
- Blood glucose in all children.
- CBC, calcium, electrolytes, and urinalysis are optional but frequently included.
- EEG if neurologic signs are present or seizure was atypical.
- MRI for complex febrile seizure features or if any doubt exists about the diagnosis.

Differential Diagnosis

Consider sepsis, meningitis, metabolic or toxic encephalopathies, hypoglycemia, anoxia, trauma, tumor, and hemorrhage. Febrile delirium and febrile shivering can be confused with seizures. Breath-holding spells can mimic febrile seizures; however, the former are always related to crying or tantrums. Febrile seizures come at unpredictable times during sleep, eating, play, or other generally calm times and are related to the onset of an illness. Epileptic seizures occur without concurrent illness and at unpredictable times.

Management

- Protect the airway, breathing, and circulation if the seizure is still occurring. Place the child in a side-lying position to prevent aspiration or airway obstruction.
- Do not put anything into the child's mouth during the seizure.
- Time the duration of the seizure and observe whether it is focal or generalized.
- Reduce the fever with acetaminophen or ibuprofen (oral or suppository) after the seizure has stopped, although the use of antipyretics will not necessarily prevent another febrile seizure.
- The child should be seen shortly after the seizure. Advise transport to an emergency center if the seizure lasts more than 10 minutes.
- Most medical providers agree that anticonvulsants are not recommended for febrile seizures, but they may be considered if the child has abnormal neurologic findings or developmental delays; the initial seizure was complex febrile, *and* there is a family history of afebrile seizures;

or if the child has recurrent, prolonged simple febrile seizures.

Prophylaxis for Recurrent Febrile Seizures

Prolonged anticonvulsant prophylaxis is not recommended. In the rare instance that prophylaxis is indicated, diazepam by mouth 0.33 mg/kg every 8 hours (1 mg/kg/24 hours) can be given over the course of the febrile illness (usually for 2 to 3 days). Another approach is to use rectal diazepam in a gel form (dosed at 0.5 mg/kg for children 2 to 5 years of age) at the time of a seizure; this will prevent recurrence for approximately 12 hours. Side effects of diazepam include transient ataxia, lethargy, and irritability that can be decreased by adjusting the dosage.

Antipyretics can reduce the discomfort associated with a fever but do not alter the risk of having another febrile seizure. The thought as to why antipyretics are not helpful as prophylactic agents involves the mechanism implicated in a simple febrile seizure which likely takes place when the temperature is either rising or falling (Mikati, 2011).

Education

The family should receive information about febrile seizures, their risks, and their management. Education should include information explaining the febrile seizure, reassurance that no long-term consequences are associated with febrile seizures, information that febrile seizures recur in some children and that nothing can be done to prevent the seizures, and first-aid information in case another seizure occurs at some time. The decision to use prophylaxis is up to the parents and the PCP on a case-by-case basis. A follow-up phone call after the event is useful.

Complications

Death or persisting motor deficits do not occur in patients with febrile seizures. No indication has been found that intellect or learning is impaired. An affected child has an increased risk for the development of epilepsy (less than 5%) if the seizure is prolonged and focal; if the child has repeated seizures with the same febrile episode; or if the child has had a prior neurologic deficit, a family history of epilepsy, or both. Two thirds of children who have had one simple febrile seizure will have no more. The younger the age at onset (younger than 18 months old) of the first febrile seizure, the lower the temperature threshold that is needed to cause the child to seize and the more likely the child is to have a recurrence.

Brachial Palsy

A stretch injury of the brachial plexus in neonates can occur during a difficult vaginal delivery; such injury has also been reported following cesarean births. Injury involves the upper cervical nerve roots C5 and C6 (Erb-Duchenne palsy) and the lower cervical nerve roots C7, C8, and T1 (Klumpke palsy). The injuries are attributed to traction of the involved nerves (with mild effect) to more serious complete nerve root avulsion from the spinal cord. Partial diaphragmatic paralysis can result because innervation comes from C3, C4, and C5.

Neonatal risk factors for plexus injuries include high birth weight, shoulder dystocia, a lengthy labor, breech delivery, maternal gestational diabetes, and forceps or vacuum extraction. The incidence is approximately 3 per 1000 live births for Erb palsy. Klumpke palsy is rare (about 0.5% of plexus palsies) and is believed to be caused by delivering the head before the upper arm in a breech baby whose arms are extended. Recent findings have noted that shoulder dystocia occurs in 1.4% of all deliveries and 0.7% of vaginal births, is higher in diabetic mothers, and in newborns delivered via vacuum or forceps (Hansen and Chauhan, 2014). Brachial plexus injuries can also occur to children restrained with a seatbelt during an automobile accident.

Clinical Findings

Physical Examination. Typically, soon after birth, the infant is found to have asymmetric active range of motion of the arms. On further evaluation the following may be determined:

- Erb palsy: "Waiter's tip" positioning of the arm (shoulder adduction and internal rotation with wrist flexion); there may be some sensory impairment; ability to fist is a favorable sign for a good outcome.
- Klumpke palsy: Paralyzed hand and forearm with good shoulder and elbow function.
- Total plexus avulsion: Completely flaccid upper extremity.
- The neonatal physical examination should include a careful evaluation of the Moro reflex (for symmetry), respiratory effort, evidence of Horner syndrome (ptosis, myosis [pupillary contraction], anhidrosis [absence of sweat]), and the neuromuscular function of the involved extremity. After the neonatal period, examine for posterior shoulder dislocation (would present as markedly limited external rotation) or bony deformity of the glenoid.

Diagnostic Studies. If nerve root avulsion is suspected, high-resolution CT myelography, fast spin-echo MRI, and EMG and nerve conduction studies can be used to evaluate the injury.

Differential Diagnosis

Consider ipsilateral clavicle fracture (with resultant pain that can explain the immobility of the extremity) and Horner syndrome (also presents with ptosis, myosis, and anhidrosis in addition to avulsion of the T1 nerve root).

Management

Gentle range-of-motion exercises by parents and scheduled follow-up appointments to note progress by the PCP are routine. A referral to physical therapy may be indicated. Surgical exploration and repair of neurolysis and nerve grafting may be undertaken in those with nerve root avulsion. Outcomes and comparisons between treatment modalities have been inconclusive. Older children with permanent functional limitations may be candidates for corrective shoulder surgery.

Prognosis

The majority of brachial plexus palsies (80% to 95%) spontaneously resolve over several weeks to several months. By the third month, recovery of biceps function (active motion against gravity) is evidenced. Should wrist, thumb, and finger extension occur by this time, a complete recovery can be expected. In those with nerve root avulsions, early intervention is crucial to achieve some functional recovery.

Guillain-Barré Syndrome

Guillain-Barré syndrome is an immune-mediated polyneuropathy that mainly affects peripheral nerves and is characterized by progressive weakness and diminished or absent reflexes (Walling and Dickson, 2013). The paralysis follows a respiratory (notably *Mycoplasma pneumoniae*) or gastrointestinal (notably *Campylobacter jejuni* or *Helicobacter pylori*) viral infection by approximately 10 days. Infection with Epstein-Barr virus has also been implicated, linked to a milder form of Guillain-Barré syndrome. Case reports exist of Guillain-Barré syndrome development after various immunizations; however, the risk of Guillain-Barré syndrome is not increased with immunizations. The 2009 influenza pandemic may have increased the incidence to 2 cases per 1 million doses, mainly in elderly, not children (Walling and Dickson, 2013). Most patients have acute demyelinating neuropathy. Known variants include acute motor axonal degeneration (as evidenced by ophthalmoparesis, ataxia, and areflexia) and acute sensory neuropathy.

Clinical Findings

History. The following are reported:

- Nonspecific viral infection (gastrointestinal or respiratory) occurring within recent past
- Weakness or neurologic changes in sensory, motor, or visual systems: Onset is gradual, progressing in an ascending order (known as *Landry ascending paralysis*), starting in the lower extremities and progressing to the bulbar muscles over days or weeks; maximum weakness reached within 2 to 3 weeks.
- Fever

Physical Examination

- Tenderness and pain in muscles with palpation
- Irritability
- Inability or refusal to walk due to flaccid tetraplegia or quadriplegia
- Paresthesia may or may not be present
- Respiratory insufficiency
- Dysphagia, facial weakness
- Extraocular muscle involvement rare; papilledema and visual acuity changes may be seen
- Miller-Fisher syndrome may be seen (acute external ophthalmoplegia, ataxia, areflexia)
- Signs of viral meningitis or meningoencephalitis
- Urinary retention or incontinence (20% of cases and is usually transient in nature)
- Blood pressure and cardiac rate changes, including bradycardia, postural hypotension, asystole

Diagnostic Studies

- Cerebrospinal fluid (CSF) studies: Elevated CSF protein (usually greater than twice upper limit of normal); normal glucose, no pleocytosis (fewer than 10 white blood cells [WBCs]/mm^3)
- Negative blood cultures; viral cultures rarely conclusive
- Normal or mildly elevated creatine kinase (CK) level; antiganglioside antibodies (against GM1, GD1) may be elevated in axonal neuropathy form of the disease
- Decreased motor nerve conduction velocities; slowed sensory nerve conduction
- EMG: Shows acute denervation of muscle

Differential Diagnosis

Bickerstaff brainstem encephalitis, meningitis, meningoencephalitis, spinal muscle atrophy, HIV, metabolic diseases, and West Nile virus are included in the differential diagnoses.

Management

Hospitalization is paramount for observation and for handling complications of respiratory muscle paralysis. IVIG for 5 days is standard protocol. Plasmapheresis and/or immunosuppressive drugs may be used in cases unresponsive to IVIG. Care is supportive (respiratory, prevention of decubitus, treatment of secondary bacterial infection). Rehabilitative therapy should begin early. Children with GMS may have neuropathic and nociceptive pain, which may be severe. Nonsteroidal anti-inflammatory drugs may not provide adequate relief, and opioids may exacerbate autonomic symptoms. Chronic pain must be addressed during treatment and rehabilitation therapy.

Complications

Chronic varieties of Guillain-Barré can occur, as evidenced by recurrence or lack of improvement of symptoms over months or years. Children may have relapses. Unresolved weakness, flaccid tetraplegia or quadriplegia, and bulbar and respiratory muscle compromise may linger or remain and last longer than 2 months. This is then considered chronic inflammatory demyelinating radiculopathy.

Headaches

Headaches of all types are one of the most common reasons parents seek medical care for their children (Raieli et al, 2010). They are common during childhood, increasing in frequency and incidence during adolescence. Headaches fall into two classifications—acute and chronic. Box 28-4 lists the more common types found in these classifications. A person may experience different types of headaches, and migraines may be particularly difficult to diagnose because they can be expressed differently and incompletely during childhood.

• BOX 28-4 Most Common Types of Primary Headaches Seen in Primary Care Settings

Diagnostic Criteria Based on History

Pediatric Migraine Headache

A. More than five attacks fulfilling features of B through D
B. Duration: 2 to 72 hours
C. At least two of the following features:
   1. Bilateral or unilateral (commonly bilateral in young children; unilateral pain usually emerges in late adolescence or early adult life)
      a. Usually frontal/temporal
      b. Occipital is unusual and should be carefully evaluated (occipital headache in children whether unilateral or bilateral is rare and calls for diagnostic caution; many cases are attributable to structural lesions)
   2. Pulsating quality
   3. Moderate to severe intensity aggravated by routine physical activity
   4. At least one of the following:
      a. Nausea and/or vomiting
      b. Photophobia and phonophobia (can infer from behavior)
   5. Not attributed to another disorder

Infrequent Episodic Tension Type Headache

A. At least 10 episodes occurring on <1 day per month on average (<12 days per year) and fulfilling criteria B through D
B. Headache lasting from 30 minutes to 7 days
C. Headache has at least two of the following characteristics:
   1. Bilateral location
   2. Pressing/tightening (non-pulsating) quality
   3. Mild or moderate intensity
   4. Not aggravated by routine physical activity, such as walking or climbing stairs
D. Both of the following:
   1. No nausea or vomiting (anorexia may occur)
   2. No more than one of photophobia or phonophobia
E. Not attributed to another ICHD-3 diagnosis

Chronic Tension Headache

A. Headache occurring on ≥15 days per month on average for >3 months (≥180 days per year) and fulfilling criteria B through D
B. Headache lasts hours to days or may be continuous
C. Headache has at least two of the following characteristics:
   1. Bilateral location
   2. Pressing/tightening (non-pulsating) quality
   3. Mild or moderate intensity
   4. Not aggravated by routine physical activity such as walking or climbing stairs
D. Both of the following:
   1. No more than one of photophobia, phonophobia, or mild nausea
   2. Neither moderate or severe nausea nor vomiting
E. Not attributed to another ICHD-3 diagnosis

Adapted from Headache Classification Committee of the International Headache Society (IHS): The international classification of headache disorders, 3rd edition (beta version), *Cephalalgia* 33(9):644–645, 660–661, 2013.
ICHD-3, International Classification of Headache Disorders, 3rd edition.

The exact physiologic mechanism and etiology for many headaches have not been conclusively determined. Headache pain occurs when pain-sensitive intracranial structures are activated. Such structures include the arteries of the circle of Willis and some of their branches, meningeal arteries, large veins and dural venous sinuses, and part of the dura near blood vessels. Muscles around the head, neck, scalp, eyes, jaw, teeth, sinuses, and the external carotid artery and its branches are pain sensitive structures external to the skull. Stimulation of these structures results in more localized pain that is carried by CN V, CN VII, CN IX, and CN X. In contrast, intracranial stimulation refers pain imprecisely (e.g., occipital lobe tumor).

Studies indicate that 40% of children will experience a headache by 7 years old and 75% by 15 years old (Rubin et al, 2010). Prevalence rates for migraine headaches are reported to be: age 3 (3% to 8%), age 5 (19.5%), age 7 (37% to 51%), and 7 to 15 years old (57% to 82%). Before 10 years old, the incidence is higher in males than females. During teenage years, females have a higher headache incidence. The mean age at onset of migraine is 7.2 years old for males and 10.9 years old for females (Lewis et al, 2004).

The provider must discern between symptoms that suggest that a headache is primary (e.g., tension-type, cluster, migraine type) or due to a secondary cause (e.g., tumor, hydrocephaly, infection, intoxication [lead, carbon monoxide], idiopathic intracranial hypertension, increased intracranial pressure). Key historical questions and a thorough workup are mandatory in order to exclude secondary headache etiology. In the absence of findings suggestive of a secondary headache, a more certain diagnosis of a primary headache disorder can be made. The International Headache Society (IHS) provides succinct clinical criteria (available at www.ihs-classification.org/en/) to help the provider evaluate, delineate between, and classify primary headaches (e.g., including migraines with or without aura and migraine subtypes) and secondary headaches.

Clinical Findings

History. Headache diaries may be used to gather history and track symptoms over time. Some useful ones are available for downloading at www.achenet.org/resources/headache_diaries/. Important questions to ask the child and parent(s) include:

- Duration: Recent severe onset is worrisome.
- Frequency and triggers: Children with recurrent, low-intensity headaches, with no neurologic changes, and who recover completely between episodes are unlikely to have serious intracranial etiology. Triggers can include ovulation or menstruation, exercise, food or odors, and stress. Other triggers can include chocolate, processed meats, aged cheeses, nuts, altered amounts of caffeine intake, dairy products, shellfish, and some dried fruits. Consistent findings such as perimenstrual exacerbation, food triggers, and a stable pattern to the headache with intervals of wellness over a long time period are reassuring symptoms that suggest a primary headache.

In most cases, a specific trigger or etiology is not ever identified.

- Location: Occipital or consistently localized headaches can indicate underlying pathology. Facial pain might be sinusitis. Ocular motor imbalance can produce a dull periorbital discomfort, whereas temporomandibular joint pain tends to localize around the periauricular or temporal areas.
- Quality and severity of pain: Sharp, throbbing, or pounding pain is vascular (migraine). Dull and constant pain may be tension or organic. Severity can be assessed by asking about limitations to activities and missed school days, although there are other factors that contribute to missed school and limited activities. How many "different kinds of headaches" are experienced?
- Age of onset: Progression of the headaches over time and longest period of time without symptoms.
- Home management and medication dosages, including dosage and self-management activities.
- Associated symptoms can include nausea, vomiting, visual changes, dizziness, paresthesia, neck/shoulder pain, back pain, otalgia, abdominal pain, hypersomnia, food cravings, confusion, ataxia, pallor, photophobia, and phonophobia. Changes in gait, personality, vision, mentation, or behavior that do not occur at the same time as the headache are worrisome and merit further evaluation with referral. There are some precursor symptoms and conditions that can indicate a predisposition to migraines. These include cyclic vomiting (see Chapter 33), abdominal migraine (see Chapter 33), and BPV. Alone, they do not warrant extensive or expensive workups unless the diagnosis is unclear. These conditions may evolve into migraine without aura in later childhood (Hershey, 2011; Lewis et al, 2008a).
- Head trauma: If associated with headache, a subdural hematoma or postconcussive syndrome must be considered.
- Psychologic symptoms: Evaluate for the presence of depression, school stressors, or concerns about family functioning. Additional things to consider include bullying or peer issues at school, "over programming" and family expectations, and meal, hydration, and sleep status.
- Family history: Some children with headache, especially migraine, have a family history of headaches.

Distinguishing Features of Headache Types

- Migraine and migraine with aura: These can be differentiated by the presence or absence of aura symptoms (Table 28-6). Characteristics of migraines include nausea, abdominal pain, vomiting, unilateral pain, pulsating pain, relief with sleep, an aura, visual changes such as dark or blind spots, and a history of a family member (usually on the maternal side) with migraine without aura. Dizziness and motion sickness may be described. Infants and toddlers may present with irritability, sleepiness, and pallor. In preadolescents, common migraine symptoms are more likely. Nausea and vomiting might not occur, and the pain can be more frontal. Lethargy and sleep can follow. Visual changes are rare, and the pain quality is variable. Times between headaches are pain free.
- Abdominal migraine: This is rare and is a somewhat controversial diagnosis; symptoms include midline pain, nausea, and vomiting with minimal or no headache.

TABLE 28-6 Pediatric and Adolescent Migraine: With or Without Aura

Classic Migraine With Aura	Common Migraine Without Aura
Aura usually visual with sparkling lights or colored lines, visual hallucinations, blindness, hemianopia, blurred vision, or micropsia. Less common auras of sensory symptoms or focal motor deficits	No aura
Represent about one-third of children with migraines	Represent about two-thirds of children with migraines
Prodrome may precede headache up to 24 hours characterized by irritability, elation/sadness, talkativeness/social withdrawal, food craving/anorexia, water retention, sleep disturbance	Also has similar prodrome features but more pronounced
Severe, unilateral often throbbing headache follows aura >30 minutes later; lasts 5-20 minutes; may generalize About 5% of children with classic migraine do not have headache with their auras	Headache in young children: Commonly bilateral, orbital, or frontotemporal; pain may radiate to face, occiput, neck Headache throbbing or pulsating; typically lasts <4 hours but can last up to 72 hours; moderate or severe intensity
	Activity aggravates and sleeps relives headache Nausea or vomiting or both Sensitivity to light, sound, and movement

Adapted from Robertson WC: Migraine in children, Medscape (website) updated 2015, available at http://emedicine.medscape.com/article/1179268-overview#aw2aab6b3. Accessed October 3, 2015.

Such symptoms can also be suggestive of complex partial seizures.

- Muscle contraction or tension headaches: The pain is dull and bifrontal or occipital, with nausea and vomiting occurring only rarely; there is no prodrome. Tension headaches can last for days or weeks but generally do not interfere with activities. In children, it can be difficult to differentiate migraine and tension-type headaches. Psychosocial stress seems to be a major factor in tension and chronic daily headaches in both children and adolescents.
- Secondary headaches (or those headaches that have a pathologic process): Key historical markers are sudden onset of hyperacute or increasing pain severity or accompanying neurologic signs. These require prompt referral. Box 28-5 presents red flag warnings of a pathologic process indicating immediate referral. Presenting symptoms of these headaches include the following (Lewis et al, 2008b; Sprague-McRae et al, 2009):
  - Headache pain that is worse in the morning on awakening and standing up, and then fades; increases in frequency and severity over a period of only a few weeks; persistent and unilateral
  - Pain that wakens the child from sleep
  - Vomiting but not nausea; vomiting may relieve the headache
  - Visual disturbances, diplopia, edema of the optic disc (papilledema)
  - Increased pain with straining, sneezing, coughing, defecation, or changes in position
  - Occipital region and neck pain
  - Educational, mental, personality, or behavioral alterations; irritability

• BOX 28-5 Red Flags Warnings Suggestive of Intracranial Structural Pathology

Infants

Full anterior fontanelle
Open metopic and coronal sutures
Poor growth
Impaired upward gaze
Abnormal head growth
Shrill cry
Lethargy
Vomiting

Children

Headache described as severe, excruciating of recent onset, unlike any previously experienced headache, no period of normal functioning between episodes, *or* persistent and unilateral
Papilledema or abnormal eye movements (or one or both eyes suddenly turn in)
Ataxia, hemiparesis, or abnormal deep tendon reflexes
Cranial bruits
Personality changes

- Seizures
- Unsteadiness or dramati
- Fever
- Family history of neuro tumors, neurofibromatosi
- Child has a history of a meningitis, hydrocephaly,

Physical Examination. A com logic examination is in order:

- Blood pressure, supine and standing with 2-minute interval between them
- Height and weight
- Head circumference (all children)
- Eyes: Palpate for tenderness; check discs for papilledema, movements
- Ears: Patency of canals, normal tympanic membranes
- Neck: Palpate muscles; check range of motion for nuchal rigidity
- Sinuses (frontal and maxillary)
- Teeth (percuss, inspect)
- Temporomandibular joints (mouth and jaw): Palpate and check range of motion
- Thyroid gland
- Bones and muscles of skull: Palpate for tenderness; listen for cranial bruits; check range of motion of cervical spine
- Extremities: Tandem gait
- Nerves: Palpate supraorbital, trochlear, occipital nerves; assess CN IX to CN XII
- Reflexes: Pronator drift test (Romberg)
- Vision screen

Diagnostic Studies. Imaging studies are rarely indicated unless the history suggests intracranial pressure (see Box 28-5); there is a sudden onset, increased severity, or change in headache pattern; the neurologic examination is abnormal; or when a complaint of "dizziness" fits the criteria listed in Table 28-7. CTs are generally out of favor due to radiation. MRI is the first-line treatment unless extremely urgent and it cannot be obtained immediately. If abnormal, an MRI should be done. An EEG should be obtained if the history and physical examination suggest a seizure process.

TABLE 28-7 How to Proceed When the Complaint Is Dizziness

Complaint of Dizziness	Studies Indicated
Lightheaded	None
Double vision (posterior fossa location)	MRI
Sensation of whirling motion of oneself or of room or objects (vertigo)	MRI
Confusion	MRI, EEG, comprehensive metabolic screen

EEG, Electroencephalogram; *MRI,* magnetic resonance imaging.

tory of external trauma, such as from a motor dent, cervical and spinal x-rays should be ordered.

erential Diagnosis

he differential diagnosis consists of sinusitis, trigeminal neuralgia, pseudotumor cerebri, sleep disorder, hyperthyroidism, hypertension, cyclic vomiting, abdominal migraine, BPV, and temporomandibular joint dysfunction. Brain tumors, abscesses, hematomas, and arteriovenous malformations in children are generally associated with ataxia, papilledema, intellectual changes, or behavioral changes. These processes are termed *space occupying lesions* because they crowd out other intracranial structures, precipitating edema and interfering with the normal actions of CSF and vessels. Infants may initially accommodate well to the increase in intracranial pressure because of the ability of their cranial sutures to expand. Visual acuity is rarely a cause of headaches. Determining the correct headache classification or entity is also part of the differential diagnosis. These and other causes of headaches in children are outlined in (Table 28-8).

Management

For nonorganic headaches, there may be no known etiology (e.g., no tumor, aneurysm, or metabolic or structural cause). The child and parents should be taught pain and stress management techniques; nonsteroidal anti-inflammatory drugs are the first-line pharmaceutical for acute treatment. There can be significant loss of school attendance as a result of headaches, but attendance should be mandatory. A quiet

TABLE 28-8 Additional Causes of Headaches in Children

Cause	Characteristics
Drugs	
Cocaine	Migraine-like pain in patient with no history of migraine headaches
Marijuana	Frontal, mild
Analgesics, methylphenidate, oral contraceptives, steroids, and cardiovascular agents	Pain follows administration (of drug) or withdrawal (typical of analgesics)
Food additives (nitrites and/or monosodium glutamate are common)	Pain occurs only in individual genetically sensitive; pain is diffuse, throbbing after ingestion
Physiologic	
Vasculitis	Uncommon in children; can occur as part of a collagen-vascular disease, such as systemic lupus erythematosus
Chronic hypertension	Low-grade occipital pain on awakening or frontal during day
Eyestrain	Dull, aching pain behind eyes relieved when eyes are closed; caused by muscular fatigue during prolonged ocular convergence; not a refractive error
Temporomandibular joint (TMJ) syndrome	>8 years old; pain on one side of face and vertex of TMJ; may be a history of jaw injury
Whiplash and neck injury	Pain dull, aching in neck, shoulders, upper arms with poor neck rotation; no nausea or vomiting; caused by muscles contracted to "splint" area of dysfunction in cervical joint areas or soft tissue
Following partial or generalized seizure	Diffuse pain
Infectious illness (viral or bacterial): meningitis, sinusitis, pharyngitis, upper respiratory infection; fever	Pain may be nonspecific
Dental disease	Uncommon
Malfunctioning shunt or hydrocephalus	History of ventriculoperitoneal, ventriculopleural, or ventriculoatrial shunt
Toxins—carbon monoxide, lead	Dull, aching pain
Tumor, brain abscess, subarachnoid or intracranial hemorrhage	Progressive worsening; can be severe; worst in early morning and with lying down (brain tumors); occipital location
Exertional	Sharp and occurs after exercise
Posttraumatic head injury	Pain can be severe when associated with epidural hematoma; if not associated with epidural hematoma, can start within hours up to weeks following injury

rest period may be allowed at school if needed, and school nurses can be helpful in developing a plan for this. If the child remains home, activities should be restricted to bed and all homework completed. The child should be returned to school if the pain improves during the school day. Minimize attention to the headache. Relaxation exercises or biofeedback training can be helpful. Trigger factors should be avoided, if possible.

The goals of treating acute-onset migraines include:
- Abortive therapy
- Reducing frequency, severity, and length of treatment
- Reducing impairment
- Improving overall quality of life
- Avoiding escalation of medications
- Optimizing self-care abilities of the patient and family
- Using beneficial and cost-effective treatment
- Minimizing medication side effects

Many of the newer medications for migraines (e.g., triptans) have not been adequately tested for safety and efficacy in children and adolescents, with the exception of sumatriptan and zolmitriptan (refer to Table 28-9 for treatment options). Lewis (2009) recommends treating throughout the school year and then gradually curtailing daily agents during the summer months. An alternative for younger children is to use shorter courses of preventive medications (6 to 8 weeks) followed by gradual weaning. All individuals with migraines benefit from regular sleep, exercise, moderate caffeine intake, and adequate hydration. Medications should be taken as soon as possible after the onset of the headache; should be taken in the prescribed dosage; should be available at home, school, or work; and the overuse of analgesics is to be avoided (more than three doses per week).

Prophylactic therapy is considered when migraines cause a child to miss school regularly and when the child suffers severe migraine headaches two to four times a month or tension or migraine three to four times per week with a clear sense of functional disability. The aim of prophylactic treatment is to reduce headache severity, frequency, or both (El-Chammas et al, 2013). Medication classifications to consider include beta-blockers, antidepressants, anticonvulsants that treat headaches also, or calcium channel blockers.

The use of magnesium oxide, CoQ10, and riboflavin as dietary supplements is gaining popularity in practice due to tolerance, cost, and ease of use. However, the evidence in favor of these modalities is limited, and further research is warranted (Orr and Venkateswaran, 2014).

Refer all patients with organic (structural) headaches. Parents seek medical attention for pain relief for their child, in addition to reassurance that there are no intracranial processes occurring (brain tumors). Each child with headaches requires an individually tailored strategy that may include pharmacologic and nonpharmacologic modalities.

Complications

School absence and depression are known complications.

Head Injury

Traumatic brain injury (TBI) involves tissue damage to the brain and its surrounding structures, and injury can range from mild to severe. Most TBIs occur secondary to acceleration-deceleration or rotational forces, and long-term sequelae are much more likely in children with developing brains. Head injuries can be either open or closed. Open head trauma produces more focal injuries. Closed head trauma causes more multifocal or diffuse damage. Primary effects are from the initial injury and are related to mechanical forces that tear connections within the brain and cause contusions where the brain hits the skull surfaces (e.g., shaken baby syndrome). Axons to distant areas, fibers in the corpus callosum connecting the two hemispheres, or both can be torn. Contusions and hemorrhage can occur. Secondary effects of the trauma, such as hypoxia, ischemia, hypotension, brain swelling, hemorrhage, contusion, and seizures, can affect recovery.

TBI is a common cause of trauma in pediatrics, resulting in almost 2200 deaths, 35,000 hospitalizations, and 474,000 ED visits annually in the United States for children 0 to 14 years old. Approximately 2 to 5 million children sustain head traumas of varying intensities each year in the United States when all ages during childhood and adolescence are considered. Common causes of ED-treated TBI include falls, sports-related injuries, motor vehicle accidents, violence and assaults, and being struck by or against objects (Faul et al, 2010). Boys experience head injury twice as frequently as girls. Children with impulse control issues may experience more head trauma. Children who survive their injuries can have significant long-term disability.

The most common causes of head trauma differ according to age. Infants and toddlers are more likely to obtain head trauma from falls and nonaccidental trauma. Children 0 to 4 years old and 15 to 24 years old have the highest risk of TBI. Young children receive head injuries from falls and pedestrian and bicycle accidents, whereas adolescents receive TBI from motor vehicle accidents, sports-related injuries, and assaults (CDC, 2015; Su, 2013).

Young children are particularly vulnerable to mild traumatic brain injury (MTBI), also known as *concussion.* The CDC defines MTBI as a complex pathologic brain process that results from primary or secondary forces on the head that disrupt brain processes and functioning. MTBI results in physical, cognitive, emotional, and sleep symptoms (CDC, 2015; Halstead and Walter, 2010) (Table 28-10).

Table 28-11 identifies the key characteristics that are used in the classification system of mild, moderate, and severe head injury. Various types of head injuries can result in pathologic conditions: skull fracture, concussion, posttraumatic seizure, cerebral contusion, epidural hematoma, subdural hematoma, cerebral edema, and penetrating injury. Children can also experience subtle symptoms of TBI that may not appear until days or weeks after the injury.

TABLE 28-9 **Therapies for Pediatric Migraine**

Drug	Dosage	Side Effects and Comments
Treatment for Acute Migraine		
Medications (These Should Be Tried First in Acute Management.)		
Acetaminophen (gel capsule)*	10-15 mg/kg PO every 4 hours up to 500 mg every 4 hours	Acetaminophen has faster onset of action than ibuprofen. Used for mild to moderate pain.
Ibuprofen*	7.5-10 mg/kg/dose PO every 6-8 hours; maximum daily dose of ≤2400 mg	Ibuprofen showed greater headache resolution than acetaminophen (rebound headache can occur). Use at onset of attack. Take with food.
Naproxen sodium	Children >2 years old: 5-7 mg/kg PO every 8-12 hours Adolescents: 200 mg PO every 8-12 hours, take 400 mg as initial dose (maximum 1000 mg/24 hours)	Safe and effective.
Dimenhydrinate	2-5 years old: 12.5-25 mg PO every 6-8 hours (maximum 75 mg/24 hours) 6-12 years old: 25-50 mg PO every 6-8 hours (maximum 150 mg/24 hours) >12 years old: 50-100 mg PO every 4-6 hours (maximum 400 mg/24 hours)	Use when vomiting is a major symptom.
Ondansetron (Zofran)	For pediatric patients 4-11 years old, the dosage is one 4-mg Zofran tablet, *or* one 4-mg Zofran ODT tablet, *or* 5 mL (1 teaspoonful equivalent to 4 mg of ondansetron) of Zofran oral solution given three times a day	For vomiting associated with headaches.
Migraine-Specific Abortive Acute Medications*†		
Sumatriptan*	Consider for children >12 years old when there is no response to analgesics Nasal spray*: 5 mg/spray; 5-20 mg each nostril once (may repeat every 2 hours if headache unresolved; maximum dosage 40 mg/24 hours) Subcutaneous (self-administered): 3-6 mg single dose Oral: 25-100 mg once (may be repeated every 2 hours; maximum 200 mg/24 hours); available in tablets: 25, 50, or 100 mg	Triptans are all FDA approved for those ≥18 years old; they are regarded safe, and well tolerated in children ≥12 years old; efficacy rates for the triptans *(except for sumatriptan nasal spray and oral zolmitriptan)* are essentially the same as for placebos; they may prolong an aura. If the first dose is given in the outpatient setting, the patient should be monitored for 1 hour. • When compared with placebo, nasal sumatriptan significantly reduces headache • Inadequate data to support use of subcutaneous sumatriptan use in children; do not use in basilar-type and hemiplegic migraine or in those with cardiovascular disease, uncontrolled hypertension, or who have used MAOI in prior 2 weeks. Has been used off-label in children <12 years old who have not responded to typical analgesic regimens.
Rizatriptan	≥18 years old: 5-10 mg PO repeated every 2 hours prn (maximum 30 mg/24 hours) (ODT available)	Studies limited in children; one study found no difference in symptom relief between drug and placebo; side effects well tolerated.
Almotriptan	≥12 years old: 6.25-12.5 mg PO once, repeat once in 2 hours prn (maximum 25 mg/24 hours)	

TABLE 28-9 Therapies for Pediatric Migraine—cont'd

Drug	Dosage	Side Effects and Comments
Prophylaxis Treatment (Maintain use for at least 4 to 6 months and then wean slowly.)		
Antidepressants		
Amitriptyline	0.25 mg/kg/day PO at bedtime; may increase dose by 0.25 mg/kg/day every 2 weeks; maximum dosage 1 mg/kg/day	Migraine prophylaxis is off-label use. Not assessed in controlled studies but is one of the most widely used agents. Efficacy in 50% to 80% of children. Adverse effects: Somnolence, dry mouth, dysrhythmia; order an ECG if dosage exceeds 25 mg/day. Use with caution in children younger than 12 years old.
Anticonvulsants		
Divalproex sodium	Dosage depends on preparation and age—consult pharmacology text.	Open-label trials only done: Showed 50% reduction in headache frequency in children 7-16 years old. Adverse effects: Weight gain, heartburn, hair loss, dizziness. Not for use in children younger than 2 years old.
Topiramate	Adolescent/adult immediate release oral preparation: Initially 25 mg once daily (in evening); may increase weekly by 25 mg daily up to 100 mg daily divided in two equal doses.	Gaining wide acceptance for efficacy; well-designed study showed benefit at 50 mg twice daily dosing with more than 80% of patients showing >50% improvement after 8 weeks of treatment. Adverse effects: Weight loss, episodes of paresthesia, cognitive slowing, loss of appetite, dizziness, irritability; monitor any change in school/cognitive performance. Indicated in epilepsy for children as young as 2 years old.
Anti-Serotonergic Agents		
Cyproheptadine	Age <2 years old: Not recommended ≥3 and adolescents: 0.2-0.4 mg/kg/day divided in two equal doses; maximum daily dose 0.5 mg/day	Used more in toddlers because weight gain (due to appetite stimulation) and somnolence are primary adverse effects in older children; sedation more problematic at doses higher than 4-8 mg/24 hours. In children ages 3-12 years old, drug was effective in migraine prophylaxis in up to 83% of patients, per retrospective study.
Antihypertensives		
Propranol	≤35 kg: 10-20 mg three times a day >35 kg: 20-40 mg three times a day Adults: 80 mg/day divided every 6-8 hours with a maximum of 160-240 mg/day in divided doses every 6-8 hours	May take up to several weeks to a month to be effective. May lower blood pressure or cause depressive adverse effects or exercise-induced asthma. 71% of children 7-16 years old had complete remission using 60-120 mg/day in a double-blind control trial; other trials failed to show any improvement in headache frequency. Do not use in children with history of asthma; use with caution in children with depression.

Data from Chawla J: Migraine headache medication, Medscape (website), 2015, available at http://emedicine.medscape.com/article/1142556-medication#2. Accessed October 4, 2015; Hershey AD: Migraine. In Kliegman RM, Stanton BF, St. Geme JW, et al, editors: *Nelson textbook of pediatrics*, ed 19, Philadelphia, 2011, Saunders/Elsevier, pp 2040–2045; Taketomo CK, Hodding JH, Kraus DM: *Pediatric & neonatal dosage handbook*, ed 21, Hudson, OH, 2014, Lexi-Comp.

5-HT, 5-hydroxtryptamine; *ECG,* electrocardiogram; *FDA,* U.S. Food and Drug Administration; *MAOI,* monoamine oxidase inhibitor; *ODT,* orally disintegrating tablet: *PO, per os* (by mouth, orally); *prn, pro re nata* (when necessary).

*Recommended as most effective treatment for acute migraine in children and adolescents.

†Selected list of triptans: $5\text{-}HT_1$-receptor agonists.

Indications for use: Moderately severe to severe migraines.

Common side effects: Asthenia, nausea/vomiting, dizziness, somnolence, chest, throat, or jaw tightness/discomfort, worsening of head pain (often transient). Avoid if risk factors of cardiovascular disease.

TABLE 28-10 Mild Traumatic Brain Injury (Concussion) Symptoms

Physical	Cognitive	Emotional	Sleep
Headache	Confusion	Abnormal irritability	Drowsiness
Nausea/vomiting	Altered concentration	Feelings of sadness or being "emotional"	Insomnia or hypersomnia
Difficulty with balance	Mental torpor	Abnormal feelings of being nervous	Difficulty falling asleep
Changes in vision	Altered memory		
Dizziness	Forgetfulness (especially conversations or recent events)		
Light or sound sensitivity	Needs to repeat or slowly answer questions		
Paresthesias			
Feelings of being dazed or stunned			

Adapted from Centers for Disease Control and Prevention (CDC): Heads up: facts for physicians about mild traumatic brain injury (MTBI), available at www.cdc.gov/concussion/headsup/pdf/Facts_for_Physicians_booklet-a.pdf. Accessed September 22, 2014; Halstead ME, Walter KD, the Council on Sports Medicine and Fitness: Clinical report—sport-related concussion in children and adolescents, *Pediatrics* 126(3):597–615, 2010.

TABLE 28-11 Classification of Head Injuries Based on Key Characteristics

Classification	Glasgow Coma Scale*	Neurologic Focal Deficit†	Loss of Consciousness	Other Neurologic Findings
Mild	13-15	No	No or brief loss (<30 minutes)	May have linear skull fractures
Moderate	9-12	Focal signs	Variable loss	May have depressed skull fracture or intracranial hematoma
Severe	≤8	Focal signs	Prolonged loss	Often have depressed skull fractures and intracranial hematoma

*Either initial or subsequent scores.
†Neurologic focal deficit (e.g., hemiparesis, reflex asymmetry, Babinski sign, abnormal cranial nerve findings).

This discussion of head injury is limited to minor traumatic brain injuries, and indications of impending CNS compromise are presented.

Clinical Findings

History. Symptoms of TBI can mimic those of other medical conditions, thus making the diagnosis challenging. It is recommended that providers use an evidence-based assessment tool like the CDC's Acute Concussion Evaluation (ACE) tool (available at www.cdc.gov/headsup/pdfs/providers/ace-a.pdf).

The following information should be obtained:

- History of how injury occurred; if injury involved a fall, the height from which the child fell needs to be determined. Specifically, providers should ascertain injury cause, body part affected, forces, and circumstances.
- Loss of or alteration in consciousness or memory, confusion, irritability, inappropriate behavior, repetitive questioning
- Presence of vomiting and frequency
- Presence of headache, description of the headache pain
- Presence of blurred vision, diplopia, or other vision problem
- Numbness or loss of sensation, loss of balance, or difficulty walking
- Specify symptoms occurring at the time of injury and interval changes

Because sports-related head injuries are common in children and teens, prescreening using standardized neuropsychologic testing is encouraged for all student athletes as a baseline measure. Assessments are then completed at various intervals after an injury has occurred to assess for cognitive deficits.

Nonaccidental trauma should be strongly suspected when a head injury is present in a child without a history of a fall or with a history of a fall from a relatively low height of less than 4 feet. It is also recommended that a skeletal survey be obtained in children younger than 3 years old when inflicted head injuries are suspected, because younger children are at higher risk for skeletal trauma as well. With concerns about radiation exposure, there are data suggesting that skeletal surveys may be modified to limit radiation exposure (Bregstein et al, 2014).

Physical Examination. Check vital signs (temperature, blood pressure, pulse, and respiration) and compare findings with normal parameters expected for children of varying ages. Changes in vital signs can indicate shock or intracranial hypertension. Perform a thorough physical examination (including a careful oral examination) and a careful neurologic examination including level of consciousness, mental status, motor function (both gross and fine motor), sensory function, cranial nerve functioning, and reflexes. Be alert to any signs of CNS involvement. Evaluation of mental status can be based on the Glasgow Coma Scale (GCS) (Table 28-12) that has traditionally been used to measure the severity of head injury. Modification to the GCS for pediatrics has resulted in the implementation of the Pediatric GCS scoring system (Menkes and Ellenbogen, 2009). However, such predictive scales of outcome should not be the sole determinant of patient management. See Table 28-13 for a useful head injury acuity assessment guideline.

TABLE 28-12 Glasgow Coma Scale

Category	Best Response	Score*
Eye opening (E)	Spontaneous	4
	To speech (command)	3
	To pain	2
	None	1
Motor (M)	Obeys (command)	6
	Localizes	5
	Withdraws	4
	Abnormal flexion	3
	Extensor response	2
	None	1
Verbal (V)	Oriented	5
	Confused conversation	4
	Inappropriate words	3
	Incomprehensible sounds	2
	None	1

From Coulter DL: Head trauma. In Finberg LL, editor: *Saunders manual of pediatric practice*, Philadelphia, 1998, Saunders, pp 883–885.
*Total score (E + M + V): maximum 15; minimum 3.

TABLE 28-13 Head Injury Acuity Risk Assessment

Characteristic	Mild/Low Risk	Moderate/Moderate Risk	Major/High Risk
Length of time patient was unconscious or had posttraumatic amnesia	<1 hour	1-24 hour	>24 hours
Glasgow Coma Scale score	13-15	9-12	3-8
Symptom	Usually alert in the ED with headache, dizziness, lethargy, irritability; withdrawn, may or may not be labile	Occasional brain swelling and hematomas, brief LOC, seizure, vomiting, headache, concentration, problem-solving and memory problems; symptoms can last for several months	Impaired level of consciousness, focal neurologic findings, skull injuries Approximately 50% mortality rate
Sequelae	Repeated "minor" damage (e.g., head trauma with sports) can result in change in neuropsychology (attention, arousal, and information processing) ADHD-like symptoms, decreased attention span, emotional changes, sleep disturbances, memory problems, headache, language deficits can result	Same as for "mild" with concentration, problem-solving and memory problems; symptoms can last for several months	Seizures, hemiparesis, aphasia, cognitive problems, behavior changes Anxiety, attention problems (concentration, problem-solving and memory problems; ADHD-like symptoms); symptoms can last for several months

Data from Menkes JH, Ellenbogen MD: Traumatic brain and spinal injuries in children. In Maria BL, editor: *Current management in child neurology*, ed 4, Hamilton, Ontario, 2009, BC Decker, pp 624–637.
ADHD, Attention-deficit/hyperactivity disorder; *ED,* emergency department; *LOC,* loss of consciousness.

Always remember to examine the entire child for other signs of trauma, such as neck injury, internal abdominal injuries, or bone fractures. Periorbital hemorrhage ("raccoon-eyes"), ecchymosis behind the ear (Battle sign), blood behind the eardrum, and bleeding from the ears or nose indicate a basilar skull fracture.

Diagnostic Studies. The severity of the head trauma dictates the need for investigative studies. All children with moderate (GCS 9 to 12) and severe (GCS 3 to 8) acute trauma should have a cranial CT scan. In addition, the need for skull radiographs and other views is determined by the severity of the head trauma. Schutzman (2010) recommends including plain radiographs (cervical spine and a series of skull views) with significant head injury, loss of consciousness, focal neurologic signs (GCS 3 to 8), and further neurologic imaging studies. Indications for obtaining a CT scan include any of the following:

- Penetrating trauma
- Altered level of consciousness (excessive irritability or lethargy)
- History of loss of consciousness (exceeding 1 minute)
- Amnesia about the injury
- Focal neurologic signs or deficit
- Depressed skull fracture or signs of basilar injury
- Seizures
- Persistent vomiting
- History of coagulopathy

CT is the preferred imaging technique for emergency situations, because it can be obtained rapidly, and the child can be monitored easily during the study. Skull fractures are better visualized on skull radiographs. Acute hemorrhage is detected more easily by CT (without contrast) than by MRI. If CT is ordered after several days (3 or more days past injury), it should be done both with contrast (to pick up extravasated blood) and without. CT can demonstrate brain edema, midline displacements, hydrocephalus, loss of brain tissue, and most skull fractures. Although CT itself is a safe procedure, some healthy children require sedation or anesthesia (with some risk), so the benefits gained from CT should be carefully weighed against the possible harm of sedating or anesthetizing a child. In addition, CT scans obtained for asymptomatic children may show incidental findings that lead to subsequent unnecessary medical or surgical interventions. There are current concerns regarding the amount of radiation in a CT; however, it remains the imaging of choice for closed head injuries.

CT scans, MRI, or skull radiographs are generally not indicated for mild or minor closed head trauma without focal neurologic signs or loss of consciousness.

Differential Diagnosis

History of a head injury is the key to diagnosis. Differentiating minor head trauma that will resolve on its own from more extensive brain injury is problematic at times. Head trauma may cause injuries of the scalp, skull, dentition, and intracranial contents. Remember that these injuries may occur alone or in combination (Schutzman, 2010). Children with intracranial lesions after minor closed head injury are not easily distinguishable clinically from the large majority with no intracranial injury. Children with mild nonspecific signs such as headache, vomiting, or lethargy after minor closed head injury may be more likely to have intracranial lesions than children without such signs. However, these clinical signs are of limited predictive value, and most children with headache, lethargy, or vomiting after minor closed head injury do not have demonstrable intracranial injury. In addition, some children with intracranial injury do not have any such signs or symptoms, showing a normal neurologic assessment. Because of these findings, some experts recommend a liberal policy on the ordering of cranial CT scans following any head trauma; however, there are drawbacks to routine CT scanning (see prior discussion).

Management

Management issues related to only mild and moderate head injuries are discussed in this chapter. The level of consciousness is a key determinant of the child's prognosis. Prompt identification of a deteriorating level of consciousness and quick medical and/or surgical intervention are essential components of the management plan. See Chapter 13 for return-to-play guidelines after head injury/concussions.

Management of the Child with Minor Closed Head Injury and No Loss of Consciousness. Observation in the clinic, office, ED, or home, under the care of a competent caregiver, who understands what signs and symptoms to watch for, is able to closely and reliably monitor, and can quickly bring the child back for treatment or access emergency medical services if necessary, is recommended for children with minor closed head injury and no loss of consciousness. Observation implies regular monitoring by a competent adult who would be able to recognize abnormalities and seek appropriate assistance.

Management of the Child with Minor Closed Head Injury and Brief Loss of Consciousness. For children with minor closed head injury and brief loss of consciousness (several minutes) and no other neurologic or physical deficits reported or detected on examination, observation in the office, clinic, ED, hospital, or home, when under the care of a competent caregiver may be used to evaluate such a child. However, CT scanning along with observation is also accepted. If the provider is not assured that the child will be closely and reliably monitored at home, hospitalization is indicated.

Management of the Child with Moderate Head Injury or Worrisome Symptoms. Children with moderate head injuries (GCS 9 to 12) may require admission or prolonged observation in the ED until their mental status stabilizes; children with severe head injuries (GCS less than 8 or coma and physical findings) need immediate hospital admission and consultation with a neurologist and critical care team. Children with any of the following should be hospitalized:

- Changing vital signs
- Seizures

- Altered mental status
- Slurred speech
- Prolonged unconsciousness (greater than 30 seconds)
- Persisting memory deficit or focal neurologic signs
- Depressed or basilar skull fractures
- Persistent headache (particularly with stiff neck)
- Recurrent vomiting or unexplained fever
- Unexplained injury (suspected child abuse)
- CT scan or MRI findings that are worrisome

A child with a skull fracture or transient neurologic findings whose level of consciousness is normal may be admitted for overnight observation.

Complications

Initial complications of head injury can include concussion, posttraumatic seizures, cerebral contusion, epidural hematoma, subdural hematoma, intracerebral hematoma, subarachnoid hemorrhage, acute brain swelling, and penetrating injuries. Second impact syndrome is a concern and discussed in the next section. Intracranial lesions, particularly epidural hematomas, are life threatening and have significant complications. Features indicative of serious injury include loss of consciousness (longer than 1 minute), persistent vomiting, depressed level of consciousness, seizures, unequal pupil size, severe headache, and GCS less than 15.

Posttrauma Sequelae and Post-Concussion Syndrome. Minor head injury without neurologic changes generally has no resulting physical deficit. However, subtle cognitive deficits may be present for weeks to months. TBI severity is correlated with a risk for psychiatric conditions and long-term neurologic deficits (Stippler, 2012). After severe injury, cognitive function changes generally will not improve after 12 months, but speech and motor difficulties may continue to improve for up to several years. A neuropsychological evaluation may be helpful to plan appropriate educational and behavioral management.

Children (2 to 6 years old) may be more impaired than adolescents, with secondary to immature brain development and general vulnerability. However, children and adolescents are more likely to show improvement in cognitive and social skills than adults who suffered the same degree of head trauma. Such improvement may evolve steadily over several years. Matsumoto and colleagues (2013) found that posttraumatic epilepsy was present in up to 40% of children who had experienced a TBI.

Typical postconcussive syndrome in adolescents is manifested by headache, dizziness, irritability, and impaired ability to concentrate. In younger children, it is manifested as aggression, disobedience, behavioral regression, inattention, and anxiety. Sleep-related issues also occur. Cognitive and physical brain rest are the essential components of the management plan. The treatment plan must be communicated to school personnel—teachers and coaches (see Chapter 13)—and should identify a gradual/step-wise return to school with modifications outlined related to academics and school and sport activities being allowed or restricted. Neuropsychological testing may be indicated as one assessment component for selective cases of concussion. Such testing can provide an objective measure of brain-behavior relationships.

Patient and Parent Education

Give caregivers written patient education materials and make every effort to ensure that they understand the instructions about observing the child and indications for immediate follow-up and will comply with them. Salient points to cover in a pediatric head injury information sheet include instructions about when to contact the health care provider or take the child to an ED. Indications for such actions are the following:

- Increased drowsiness, sleepiness, inability to wake up, unconsciousness
- Vomiting more than twice
- Neck pain
- Watery or bloody drainage from ear or nose
- Seizures, "fits," or fainting
- Unusual irritability, personality change, confusion, or any unusual behavior
- Headache that gets worse or lasts more than a day
- Unequal pupils
- Trouble with vision (blurred), hearing, or speech
- Trouble with walking (e.g., clumsiness or stumbling) or weakness of any muscle of arms, legs, or face

In addition, parents or caregivers should be given the following specific instructions:

- Wake child every 2 to 4 hours for the first 24 hours after injury; child should wake easily and be able to stay awake for a few minutes.
- Make sure child is moving his or her arms and legs normally.
- Give only acetaminophen, if needed, for headache or relief of soft tissue pain.

Parents should also be informed that sometimes symptoms from head trauma occur days, weeks, or months after the initial trauma. Long-term complications may include cognitive difficulties, concentration problems, sleep issues, and irritability. Although this may not be pertinent immediately, it may become more important after days or weeks.

Neurologic sequelae following mild head injury in children often improve or resolve within 9 to 12 months. These sequelae include the following:

- Headache
- Vertigo or dizziness
- Difficulty concentrating or loss of memory
- Depression, fatigue
- Poor school performance and neurobehavioral problems

Eisenberg and colleagues (2014) found the following sequence of events:

- Headache is prevalent immediately after a head injury
- Emotional symptoms may develop later during the recovery
- Cognitive symptoms span the entire injury spectrum

Prevention

- Wear helmets when using bicycles, skateboards, scooters, motorcycles, inline skates, snowboarding, ski racing, and when appropriate for sports participation. The proper fitting of helmets is important.
- Protect children from falls in the home or from playground equipment. Discourage the purchase of residential trampolines.
- Use appropriate seat restraints when riding in motor vehicles.

Disturbances of Head Growth

Macrocephaly

Macrocephaly is defined as a head circumference more than two standard deviations above the mean for age and gender or one that increases too rapidly. "Large" heads may be genetic and only of statistical significance; the provider's initial evaluation should be to measure both parents' head circumferences. Macrocephaly can also be attributed to hydrocephaly, megalencephaly (enlarged brain), subdural hematoma, tumor, thickening of the skull, or other problems. Benign familial macrocephaly may occur as a part of, or be related to, a genetic syndrome (anatomic or metabolic), such as Sotos syndrome (cerebral gigantism) or neurofibromatosis type 1. Infants with anatomic megalencephaly have macrocephaly at birth, but those with a metabolic etiology are normocephalic at birth. In cases of excessive volumes of CSF, the fluid may be located within the brain (in the ventricular cavities) or outside the brain, in the subarachnoid spaces.

A CT scan can be diagnostic with consultation or referral if abnormal. A CT interpretation of benign enlargement of the subarachnoid spaces (BESS) generally requires no further treatment. The subarachnoid enlargement resolves by school age, although the macrocephaly remains. This finding is found more often in boys, and there is a family history of macrocephaly in most cases (Weerakkody and Di Muzio, n.d.).

Hydrocephaly

See Chapter 39 for the discussion on congenital hydrocephalus.

Microcephaly

Microcephaly is defined as a head circumference two standard deviations below the mean for age and sex, or a head in which the growth decelerates from the normal pattern. On examination the skull appears to be normally shaped; palpation may reveal some overlapping bones along the suture lines. This disorder can result from conditions in which the brain never formed correctly because of genetic or chromosomal abnormalities. Disease processes that interfere with normal brain growth can also be causative (these infants have normal head circumferences at birth). Brain damage that occurs prenatally may or may not always be evident initially in the newborn; a decreasing or plateauing head circumference curve may start to occur after the infant reaches 3 to 6 months of age.

Commonly, microcephalic children have delayed developmental milestones and neurologic problems. Management of microcephaly is supportive, may involve an interdisciplinary team, and is directed toward management of the resulting deficits. Protein-calorie malnutrition, craniosynostosis, and hypopituitarism are treatable causes of microcephaly. Referral to a neurologist should be made for diagnostic purposes.

Craniosynostosis

Skull malformations may be due to primary or secondary causes. Congenital (or "true" or "primary") craniosynostosis involves early closure or absence of one or more cranial sutures. Syndromic craniosynostosis accounts for about 25% of craniosynostosis cases and is associated with more than 180 familial syndromes (Greenwood et al, 2014). Growth along the remaining open suture lines produces progressive skull deformity in one or more directions. The skull is flat over the closed suture(s). Increased intracranial pressure may result as the brain tries to grow within the confined space, but this does not always occur. Primary craniosynostosis occurs in 1 per 2000 to 2500 births (Greenwood et al, 2014), is ethnically neutral, and can vary in type and prominence between genders. The sagittal suture is most commonly fused (referred to as *scaphocephaly* or *dolichocephaly*), is found in 1 in 5000 births, and accounts for 40% to 55% of all cases (Greenwood et al, 2014). Figure 28-4 illustrates the different descriptions for skull deformities seen.

Secondary synostosis results when outside forces put pressure on the growing cranium, causing the skull to become misshapen (referred to as *deformational plagiocephaly*). Secondary synostosis is most commonly seen with premature infants (termed *deformational scaphocephaly*), after shunting an infant with hydrocephaly, in children who have microcephaly and aberrant positioning in utero, during birth, or perinatally because of torticollis or positioning traditions. The success of the Back to Sleep campaign has resulted in an increase of infants with secondary (or pressure-related) occipital flattening. Such occipital deformity is not accompanied by compensatory suture line growth that would be seen with a primary lambdoidal synostosis.

Clinical Findings

Physical Examination. Monitor cranial symmetry for the first year. This is best done by looking down at the top of the head, noting the position of the ears and cheekbones. Typically, a deformational plagiocephaly will form a parallelogram characterized by unilateral occipital flattening and contralateral occipital bossing, ipsilateral ear displacement anteriorly, and associated parietal bossing and cheekbone prominence on the side of the occipital flattening. In contrast, the deformity of lambdoidal craniosynostosis does not assume a parallelogram shape, may be present at birth, has less frontal asymmetry than positional plagiocephaly, the ear ipsilateral to the occipital flattening is posterior and displaced inferiorly to the contralateral ear; the deformity may

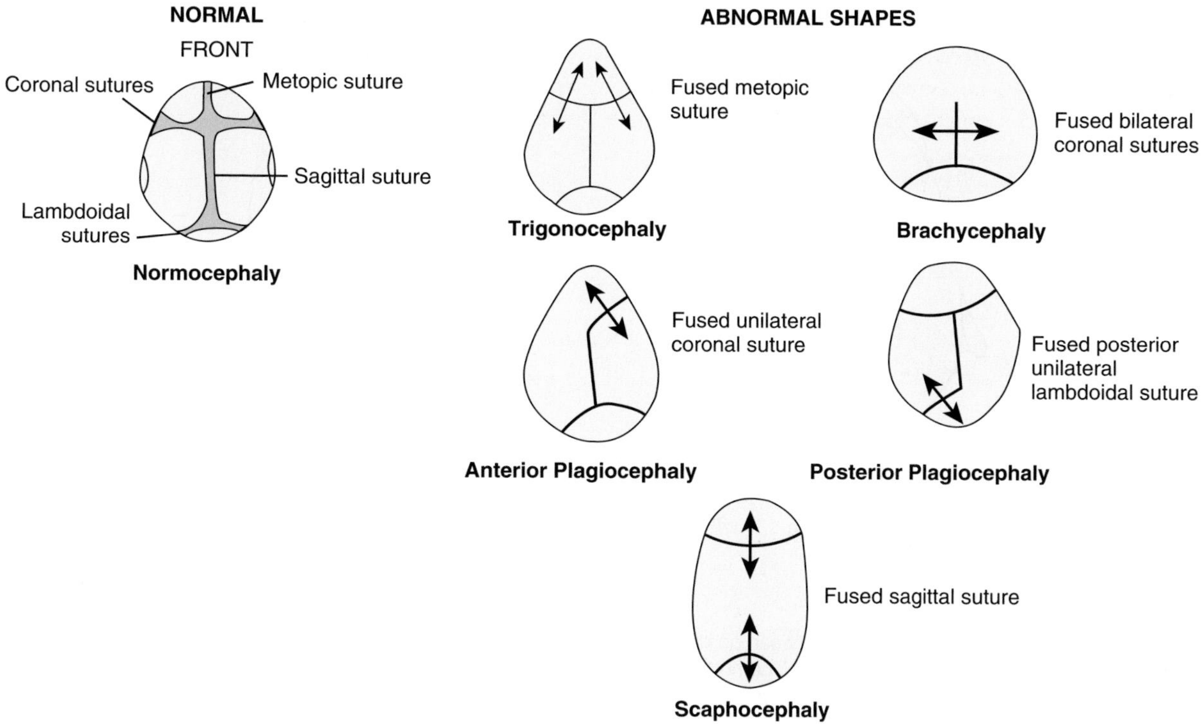

• **Figure 28-4** Characteristics of skull deformities seen with craniosynostosis. (Adapted from Cohen MM Jr: Craniosynostosis update 1987, *Am J Med Genet Suppl* 4:99–148, 1988.)

become more severe over time. Figure 28-5 compares these two deformities.

Symmetry of neck rotation should also be included in the examination to rule out torticollis. Infants with torticollis typically have some limitation of neck rotation away from the side of their occipital flattening.

Diagnostic Studies. A CT scan is standard for a skull shape deformity. Deformational plagiocephaly does not require imaging studies in most situations when the history and physical examination are diagnostic. Consider further neuroimaging with MRI if the neurologic examination is abnormal.

Differential Diagnosis. In about 5% of young infants, the frontal metopic suture may normally be prominent. This prominence is not clinically significant, does not signify craniosynostosis, and does not require intervention.

Management. If craniosynostosis is suspected, refer the child to an experienced pediatric neurosurgeon or craniofacial plastic surgeon. Treatment is often surgical, but in some cases reassurance, repositioning, exercises for any associated torticollis, and clinical follow-up are sufficient. If the condition is genetic, management needs to be planned according to the problems associated with the syndrome. Genetic counseling is important.

PCPs can anticipate concern about deformational plagiocephaly by counseling parents at the newborn visit to: (1) lay infant down in the Back to Sleep position for sleep, alternating positions (i.e., left and right occiputs); (2) when awake and observed, place infants prone for "tummy time" or in a side position to reduce the flattening; (3) during feedings have parents avoid holding an infant in a manner that puts pressure on the flattened part of the skull; and (4) have infants spend minimal time in car seats or other upright devices that maintain supine positioning. Improvement should occur over a 2- to 3-month period if interventions are instituted early. Throughout the first year, emphasize tummy time. Monitor head shape during all well-child visits. The majority of positional plagiocephalies are self-limited; sometimes physical therapy is indicated in recalcitrant cases (e.g., with torticollis).

For positional plagiocephaly, orthotic cranial molding helmet therapy may be prescribed when repositioning and exercises are not successful. The helmet is individually engineered to allow growth where needed and restrict it where the head is prominent; it needs to be worn for 23 hours a day for 4 to 6 months, can lead to odor and skin breakdown, is costly, and may not be covered by health insurance (Taub and Pierce, 2011).

Central Nervous System Infections

All the infections of the CNS have similar symptoms. These infections can be manifested acutely (over 1 to 24 hours) or chronically (over 1 to 7 days or more). Bacteria, viruses, fungi, spirochetes, protozoa, and parasites can all cause CNS infection. The meninges, superficial cortical structures, blood vessels, and brain parenchyma can be involved. The most common microbes are:

- Infants: The most common pathogen is *Escherichia coli* (42%), followed by group B *Streptococcus* (23%). Streptococcus pneumoniae is more likely in older infants. Listeria has not been identified at all (Biondi et al, 2013).

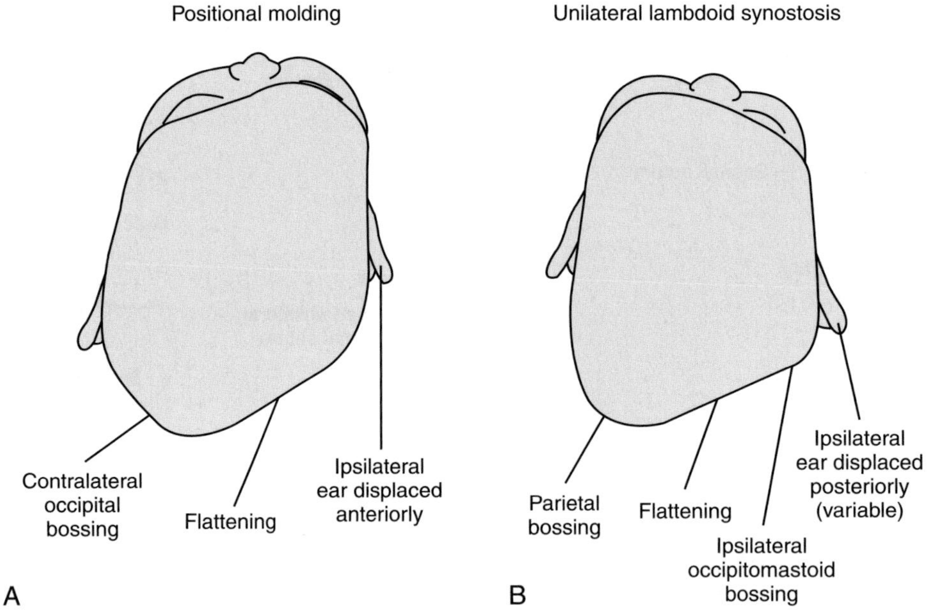

• **Figure 28-5** Differences between positional molding **(A)** and unilambdoid synostosis **(B).** (From Gruss JS, Ellenbogen RG, Whelan MF: Lambdoid synostosis and posterior plagiocephaly. In Lin KY, Ogle RC, Jane JA, editors: *Craniofacial surgery: science and surgical technique*, Philadelphia, 2002, Saunders.)

- Children: Bacterial infections—*Haemophilus influenzae* type B, *Neisseria meningitidis*, and *Streptococcus pneumoniae* are the most common. In those with immune deficiencies *Pseudomonas aeruginosa, Staphylococcus aureus,* coagulase-negative staphylococci, *Salmonella* spp. and *Listeria monocytogenes* can be implicated.

Clinical Findings

History. The following may be reported:

- Upper respiratory tract or gastrointestinal symptoms accompanied by fever
- Increasing lethargy and irritability
- Recent head injury or neurosurgical procedure
- Immunodeficiency diseases

Physical Examination. Findings on physical examination include the following:

- Systemic signs, including fever, malaise, and/or impaired heart, lung, or kidney function
- CNS signs, including headache; stiff neck and spine; nausea and vomiting; fever or hypothermia; changes in mental status, ranging from irritability to lethargy or coma; seizures; and focal or sensory deficits in cranial nerves, notably CN III, CN IV, and CN VI
- Presence of Kernig or Brudzinski signs of meningeal irritation (may be absent in a young infant)
- Bulging fontanelle and increasing head circumference in a young infant
- Papilledema—a late finding in older children or adolescents
- Cranial nerve palsies

By age, the most common findings are as follows:

- From 0 to 3 months old: Fever, hypothermia, lethargy, irritability, poor feeding, apnea, focal seizures, enteric or respiratory symptoms, nuchal rigidity, and a bulging fontanelle (infrequent)
- From 3 months to 5 years old: Petechial rash, localized CNS signs as described earlier
- From 6 to 18 years old: Petechial rash, CN VII palsy (Lyme disease), sinusitis symptoms, localized CNS signs

Diagnostic Studies. Blood cultures, CBC with differential, urinalysis, chemistry panel, and lumbar puncture for CSF studies are done. Enterovirus meningitis and herpes simplex virus rapid tests are available. EEGs, CT or MRI scan, and brain biopsy may be needed.

Management and Complications

The PCP needs to refer all children with potential CNS infection as rapidly as possible. Hypovolemia, hypoglycemia, hyponatremia, acidosis, septic shock, increased intracranial pressure, and other complications can occur quickly and need aggressive management. Hearing loss can occur in all forms of meningitis, and all children with meningitis merit postinfection auditory evaluation. Blindness, hydrocephaly, CP, seizures, and developmental delays can also occur depending on the type of organism involved. Outcomes are typically based on the type of infectious agent and severity of initial infection, age of patient (the younger, the worse the outcome), length of symptoms before the diagnosis and initiation of treatment, and antibiotic and dosage.

The Hypotonic Infant

When supported with a hand under the chest, the normal infant will hold the back straight or nearly so, the arms flexed and slightly abducted at the elbows, and the head slightly up at less than 45 degrees. The "floppy" infant will droop over the hand. A hypotonic infant is alert but has depressed spontaneous movements, which should arouse suspicion. By history, movement may have been abnormal in utero. Other symptoms seen in a range of known causes include seizures, failure to react to pain, muscle wasting, absent reflexes, tongue fasciculation, and unilateral muscular movement defects. Etiologies usually focus on a metabolic or CNS dysfunction or a systemic illness. Most conditions involving the CNS are serious and lasting; others may be transitory, such as brachial plexus nerve palsy after birth or congenital myasthenia gravis.

Hypotonic infants can increase their tone over the first year of life and then demonstrate spastic CP. A baby can have low tone but still not lack strength when actively moving. The infant may also be weak, which means that its maximal effort lacks strength. Floppy infants with brisk reflexes almost certainly have a CNS disorder. All hypotonic babies need to be referred to specialists, including a geneticist. The diagnostic tool of choice is the MRI; sometimes muscle biopsies or various neurophysiologic studies are used. Many conditions of floppy infant syndrome do not respond well to treatment; rehabilitation can help maximize function.

Reye Syndrome

Reye syndrome is an encephalopathy process often associated with a viral infection. Infrequently, cases are seen with varicella or nonspecific respiratory infections, notably *H. influenzae* type B. A decline in incidence has been associated with the decreased use of salicylates and possibly to improvements in the diagnosis of underlying inborn errors of metabolism. The use of the term *Reye-like* has been advocated among experts in the field (du Toit-Prinsloo et al, 2014).

Unless treated, the clinical course in Reye syndrome proceeds in predictable stages after the initial prodromal symptoms of the illness: severe vomiting progresses to irrational behavior; to stupor and coma; to apnea, fixed pupils, and decorticate posturing with increasing brain edema; and then to death. Management involves immediate referral with admission to a hospital for supportive care. About 70% of patients survive, some with severe neurologic sequelae. Infants are more severely affected than older children.

Tethered Cord

The spinal cord is attached to the base of the brain and free at the caudal end, allowing for freedom of movement during growth, activities, and skeletal changes (including such abnormalities as scoliotic curves). With a tethered cord, however, the caudal end is fixed by a ropelike filum terminale at or below the L2 level. This can cause abnormal stretching and damage to nerve cells, fibers, and blood vessels. Eventually, symptoms of neurologic deterioration occur. It is often associated with a congenital spinal anomaly, such as spina bifida (90%), but tethering can also result from bony protrusions, tough membranous bands, lipomas, tumors, cysts, scarring, and trauma in the area of the cauda equina.

Not all tethering leads to clinical symptoms. If symptoms do occur, they manifest as functional deficits to nerves that emanate from the area of the cauda equina. Common findings or complaints include asymmetry of leg or foot growth and muscle wasting in an infant, leg weakness, incontinence of bladder and bowel (or worsening of such), back or leg pain (especially with flexion or extension), groin or genitorectal pain, loss of reflexes and sensation in the legs, scoliosis, or deformity of the legs or hips (NINDS, 2012). Symptoms are not necessarily evident in infancy but can be manifested in early childhood to adulthood. The following skin changes are often seen in individuals later diagnosed with tethered cord or other spinal abnormalities: dimples above the gluteal cleft or within the cleft (dimples at the coccyx are generally benign), spinal hair tufts, a deviated gluteal fold, spinal fatty deposits, midline birthmarks, and sacral sinuses or tracts (Fig. 28-6).

If a provider is suspicious of a tethered cord, an MRI of the spine is the gold standard for viewing the parenchymal anatomy. A referral to a pediatric neurosurgeon is also indicated. Surgery is usually the treatment of choice and can halt and prevent further neurologic dysfunction. If a child has reached full skeletal height with minimal symptoms, monitoring is all that is often done. Be watchful for re-tethering in children who have had surgery for tethered cord; this can occur as the child gets older. A child with a history of repaired spina bifida needs to be closely monitored for early symptoms of tethered cord.

Arnold-Chiari Malformation

Arnold-Chiari malformations consist of two types of uncommon congenital spinal cord anomalies whose sequelae are usually not evident until late childhood or into adulthood. Type I malformation involves the downward elongation (herniation) of the caudal end of the cerebellar vermis through the foramen magnum. Type II malformation is present in 0.5 to 1 per 1000 of children with spina bifida myelomeningocele. The herniation can lead to brainstem and upper cervical cord compression that may ultimately cause necrosis of both structures. The etiology is believed to be secondary to disruption of the process of neural tube closure (Wallingford et al, 2013). The symptoms of a malformation may not be readily apparent. Type I malformation can cause headache, neck pain, atrophy and decreased reflexes in the lower extremities, sensory losses, and scoliosis. Any child with myelomeningocele should be suspected of having type II malformation. Type II malformation involves the same herniation as type I plus an alteration in the shape and development of the medulla. Further symptoms of type II may include hydrocephaly, respiratory distress, syncope, poor feeding, vomiting, dysphagia, tongue paralysis, and cardiopulmonary failure. Epilepsy is not related. Diagnosis is made by MRI and the condition may inadvertently be found at the time of an MRI for a possibly unrelated reason (e.g., headache). Management strategies are not always successful; surgery to relieve the compression or a ventriculoperitoneal shunt may

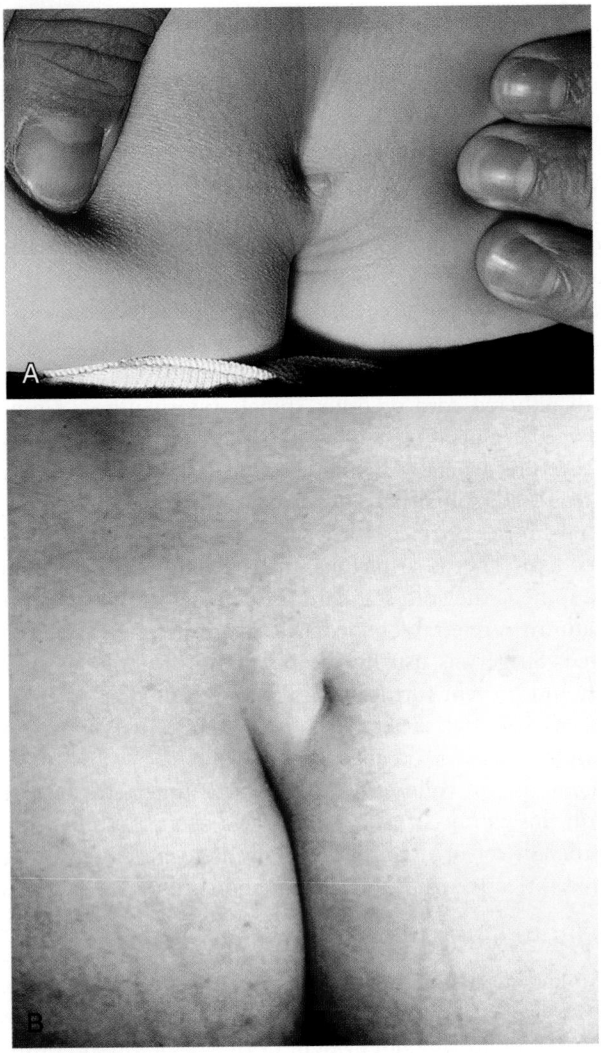

• **Figure 28-6 A,** Deep sacral dimple above the gluteal crease. Most sacral dimples that fall within the gluteal crease are normal. Dimples that are deep, large (>0.5 cm), located in the superior portion or above the gluteal crease (>2.5 cm from the anal verge), or that are associated with a deviated gluteal crease or other cutaneous markers should be radiologically imaged. **B,** Buttocks of teenage boy with tethered cord secondary to lipomeningocele. Note sacral dimple and deviation of gluteal fold to the left.

be tried in symptomatic cases. Older children may benefit from a cervical laminectomy to relieve compression as the child grows. Due to the risk of brainstem herniation, a lumbar puncture (LP) should never be attempted in a child with an Arnold-Chiari malformation. Always consult with neurosurgery prior to LP when this is present.

Myelomeningocele

Failure during embryogenesis of the vertebrae, skull, meninges, brain, or spinal cord to be encapsulated by the lamina of the vertebrae along the dorsal midline of the body is referred to as a *dysraphic defect.* Therefore, the posterior neural tube and the vertebral column are not closed. *Myelomeningocele* refers to the protrusion of both the spinal cord nerve roots *(myelo)* and the three layers of membranes *(meninges)* that cover the spinal cord and brain through this spinal defect. The protruding dural sac may contain only the meninges (10% to 20% of cases) or both meninges and nerve roots (the remaining cases). The term *spina bifida cystica* is often used interchangeably with myelomeningocele. When the vertebral arches fail to close, but there is no subsequent herniation of cord or meninges, the term *spina bifida occulta* is used. Most cases of spina bifida cystica occur in the thoracolumbar area (90%). Meningoceles may also protrude through the skull and may or may not be covered with skin. Such a cranial meningocele consists only of a CSF-filled meningeal sac; no nerve roots are involved, and therefore no neurologic deficits exist. However, there may be brain malformation under the mass that does have neurologic consequences. Encephaloceles or cephaloceles refer to cranial lesions that contain a meningocele sac plus cerebral cortex, cerebellum, or portions of brainstem that protrude from fissures in the occipital (most common), frontal, or nasal cavity areas of the skull.

Closure of the neural tube usually occurs during the third and fourth weeks of gestation. Genetic and environmental factors are believed to play a causative role in the failure of the closure to occur. Current CDC estimates show that neural tube defects account for 1 in 2000 births in the United States, and significantly more in China, Latin America, and other areas of the developing world (Wallingford et al, 2013). A lack of sufficient levels of folic acid and vitamin A increases the incidence of neural tube defects. All women of childbearing age are encouraged to take 0.4 mg/day of folic acid. A woman wishing to conceive, or who has had a prior pregnancy that resulted in a neural tube defect, should take 4 mg/day for 4 weeks before conception and through the first trimester (CDC et al, 2009). Intake of certain drugs and toxins is associated with neural tube defects; they include folic acid antagonists (trimethoprim, carbamazepine, phenytoin, phenobarbital, and primidone), retinoic acid derivatives (e.g., vitamin A, a paradox given that insufficient levels also cause the defect), valproic acid, and alcohol. A multitude of genetic and environmental risk factors have been proposed with no specific cause cited (Wallingford et al, 2013).

The rate of affected pregnancies with neural tube defects dramatically dropped after the mandatory fortification of cereal grains with folic acid. Since 2004, the incidence has leveled off to about 3000 affected pregnancies in the United States rather than continue to decline. The incidence worldwide is approximately 300,000 births (CDC, 2010), or 20/100,000 live births in the United States and Canada (Young et al, 2013). There is speculation that this leveling may be due to overall decreases in serum folate, red blood cell (RBC) folate concentrations in nonpregnant women, and to some non-folate risk factors yet to be identified (CDC, 2007, 2015). Proposed explanations for the decline in serum folate include increasing obesity rates (obese individuals metabolize folate differently), low-carbohydrate diet trends (which requires the elimination of breads, cereals, and other products that contain the mandatory fortified folic acid-enriched flour), the popularity of whole-grain breads (which have lower natural folate levels), the reduction in the mean folate content of certain enriched breads, and maternal diabetes (CDC, 2007).

A maternal serum test showing an increase in the concentration of alpha-fetoprotein is diagnostic; if elevated, an ultrasound and amniocentesis are performed (alpha-fetoprotein is the primary plasma protein found within the fetus and in the amniotic fluid and is elevated if there is a defect in the skin of the fetus). Cranial ultrasounds should be done to look for hydrocephaly and cephaloceles (and in turn the Arnold-Chiari type II malformation). It is preferable that these infants be delivered by cesarean section.

The *MTHFR* gene is critical in providing instructions for making an enzyme called *methylenetetrahydrofolate reductase.* This enzyme is critical in B-vitamin folate (also called *folic acid* or *vitamin* B_9) chemical reactions. *MTHFR* mutations are associated with neural tube defects. It is also a possible risk factor for preeclampsia and cancer among others. Testing for this gene mutation is available and used with women with certain risk factors (Yaliwal and Desai, 2012).

Clinical Findings

- Poor intake of folic acid, exposure to known toxins, or no known risk factors
- Saclike cyst containing meninges and spinal fluid covered by a thin layer of partially epithelialized skin; 75% found in the lumbosacral area
- Flaccid paralysis of lower extremities
- Absence of deep tendon reflexes
- Lack of response to touch and pain
- Constant urinary dribbling

Other physical anomalies can accompany myelomeningocele including cleft lip and palate, omphalocele, diaphragmatic hernia, tracheoesophageal fistula, congenital heart disease, bladder exstrophy, and imperforate anus.

Management and Complications

In the neonatal period, serial cranial ultrasounds are conducted to watch for the development of hydrocephaly if this condition has not shown up prenatally. Surgical resection and closure of the involved neural tube structures are done within a week after birth; often shunting for hydrocephaly is also required. If surgery is not done during that time, death may result in the first year from meningitis or sepsis. Intrauterine surgery has also been successful in closing the defect and preventing exposure of the neural tube to amniotic fluid and possible postnatal infection. If the defect occurs in a high spinal region or there is clinical hydrocephalus at birth, survival is also compromised. Multidisciplinary supportive management is indicated.

The PCP's role includes delivering well-child care, assessing and treating acute illnesses (especially UTIs and constipation), monitoring shunt function, checking for skin breakdown, and communicating with and often coordinating services between myriad specialists who will be involved (e.g., orthopedists, ophthalmologists [strabismus is common], neurologists, nephrologists, physical therapists, social workers, and geneticists).

Genitourinary management entails teaching parents (and eventually the child) how to regularly catheterize a neurogenic bladder. Periodic urine cultures, assessing renal function (with serum electrolytes, creatinine), and, depending on the child's course, ordering appropriate imaging studies (renal scans, intravenous pyelograms [IVPs], ultrasounds) fit within the PCP's role. In addition, the PCP needs to be alert to the onset of symptoms indicative of Arnold-Chiari type II malformation and tethered cord, and watch for seizures (15% incidence), learning difficulties, and ADHD. Bowel training can help control stool incontinence. Young and colleagues (2013) found that age and level of lesion were the best predictors for youths regarding what to expect regarding their quality of life over time.

Prognosis

With aggressive early treatment, survival rates can be as high as 85% to 90%; deaths more commonly occur before 4 years of age. Normal intelligence is seen in 70% of survivors, but they experience more learning and seizure problems. Continence can sometimes be achieved with an artificial urinary sphincter or bladder augmentation when the child is older. Functional mobility depends on the level and degree of the defect and on the intact function of the iliopsoas muscle. A child with a defect in the sacral and lumbosacral area almost certainly will be able to achieve functional ambulation; those with a higher defect may have variable function with mobility aids.

Prevention

Folic acid supplementation (400 mcg/day) with a daily multivitamin is helpful in preventing neural tube defects and should be taken by all females of childbearing age. Prenatal vitamins have at least 400 mcg/vitamin; however, additional folic acid supplementation (4000 mcg) is recommended for those women who have had a child with a neural tube defect (CDC, 2015).

Myasthenia Gravis

MG is an autoimmune disorder that produces an immune-mediated neuromuscular blockade or neuromuscular junction disorder. It originates when circulating receptor-binding antibodies decrease the number of available acetylcholine receptors (AChRs) on the postsynaptic muscle membrane or motor endplate, leaving the motor endplate less responsive than normal.

MG is nonhereditary in most cases; however, three rare presynaptic congenital forms exist. Symptoms of congenital MG start at or close after birth and persist. Myasthenic mothers may have infants with a transient neonatal myasthenic syndrome as a result of the transfer of placental anti-AChR antibodies. Once the infant's own receptors regenerate and reinsert into synaptic membranes, the symptoms resolve. Children with MG can also experience other autoimmune diseases (e.g., systemic lupus erythematosus, thyroiditis, rheumatoid arthritis, and/or diabetes mellitus).

MG affects approximately 40 per 1 million population; about one fifth of these develop symptoms before 20 years of age. The nonhereditary form of MG can occur any time after birth, although onset before 1 year old is rare. There is no racial or geographic predilection.

Clinical Findings

Physical Examination. The key findings of this disorder include:

- Ptosis and some degree of extraocular muscle weakness (usually the first symptom): Older children may complain of double vision; younger children may endeavor to hold their eyelids open with their fingers. The ocular signs may be asymmetric.
- Dysphagia: Infants commonly have feeding problems; older children fatigue when chewing. There may be slurred speech and a snarling appearance when trying to smile.
- Muscular weakness of neck flexor muscles (infants), limb-girdle and distal muscles of the hands: Ten percent of patients have limb weakness as the initial symptom. Symptoms do not include muscle fasciculations, myalgias, or sensory symptoms. Other times, the weakness may be so mild as to only occur after exercise.
- Rapid muscular fatigue as evidenced by inability to:
  - Hold an upward gaze for 30 to 90 seconds
  - Sustain a chin to chest position while supine
  - Maintain arm abduction for more than 1 to 2 minutes
  - Sustain rapid hand-fisting movements for long periods of time

Twelve percent of infants born to mothers with MG develop symptoms within 72 hours of birth—respiratory insufficiency, dysphagia, hypotonia, weakness, poor spontaneous motor activity, weak cry, poor sucking, choking, expressionless face, and absent Moro reflex. Symptoms generally resolve within 12 weeks. With congenital MG, symptoms are permanent, there is no remission, and these children do not experience myasthenic crises.

Diagnostic Studies

- A short-acting cholinesterase inhibitor (edrophonium chloride) is given as a clinical test; it should cause spontaneous improvement in the ptosis and ophthalmoplegia within seconds; other muscles should fatigue less rapidly.
- An EMG is more diagnostic than a muscle biopsy.
- Estimation of the number of AChRs per endplate and in vitro endplate function studies are also possible. An assay of plasma antibodies to AChRs is often inconclusive; only one third of adolescents and an occasional prepubertal child exhibit these antibodies.
- Other tests can include serologic antinuclear antibodies and immune complexes; thyroid profile; CK level (normal with MG); chest x-ray (any enlarged thymus needs to be followed up with a tomography or CT scan of the anterior mediastinum); ECG (should be normal); muscle biopsy may be considered.

Differential Diagnosis

Hypothyroidism (caused by Hashimoto thyroiditis), polymyalgia rheumatica, MS, progressive external ophthalmoplegia, Guillain-Barré syndrome, Möbius syndrome, congenital ptosis, congenital myopathies, myotonic dystrophy, and glycogen-storage disease are in the differential.

Management

MG (including neonatal MG) is treated with anticholinesterase therapy (pyridostigmine), because it is longer acting and produces less severe side effects than neostigmine. In one study, pyridostigmine improved 100% of generalized cases of MG and 88% of ocular cases (VanderPluym et al, 2013). The initial dosage is age and weight dependent and is then titrated upward until the patient responds, side effects are controlled, or until increases are no longer effective. Corticosteroids, cytotoxic agents (azathioprine and cyclosporine), or thymectomy may also be considered, especially if symptoms are severely debilitating (bulbar or respiratory involvement). Corticosteroids should be administered on an alternate-day regimen. Plasmapheresis and IVIG are alternative treatments and limited in scope.

Complications

Complications include growth retardation from steroids and possible immunodeficiency in adulthood after thymectomy. Long-term therapy with anticholinergics may lead to cholinergic crises that present similarly to myasthenic crises.

For a complete list of references, please visit http://evolve.elsevier.com/Burns/pediatric/.

29 Eye Disorders

TERI MOSER WOO

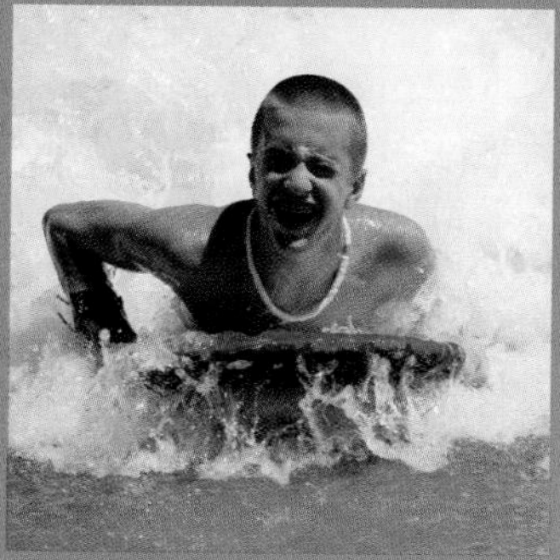

Ophthalmic diseases occur most often in the very young or elderly, with the exception of eye trauma, refractive errors, and other select disorders (e.g., retinoblastoma). Infants and children are particularly susceptible to permanent central visual loss (amblyopia), opacities (congenital cataracts), refractive errors not associated with amblyopia, strabismus (ocular misalignment), and other conditions that interfere with visual acuity (ptosis, anisometropia). With early detection and correction these conditions do not lead to permanent loss in the mature central visual system of the older child or adult (American Association for Pediatric Ophthalmology and Strabismus [AAPOS] and American Academy of Ophthalmology [AAO], 2013). When caring for children with eye problems, priorities include promoting optimal growth and development of the ocular structures and maximizing visual acuity. To this end, primary care providers (PCPs) seek to promote good vision and health, detect abnormalities, treat those conditions that fall within their scope of practice, refer patients with conditions requiring an ophthalmologist's expertise, and provide education and reassurance to parents and children. Care of blind or visually impaired children is discussed in Chapter 20.

Standards for Visual Screening and Care

Standards and guidelines for visual screening and eye care in children are set by a number of agencies and professional groups. Pediatric-focused objectives related to vision in the proposed U.S. Department of Health and Human Services (HHS) Healthy People 2020 (2014) propose to:

- Increase the proportion of preschool children (5 years old and younger) who receive vision screening.
- Reduce blindness and visual impairment in children and adolescents (17 years old and younger).
- Reduce uncorrected visual impairment due to refractive errors.
- Increase the use of personal protective eyewear in recreational activities and hazardous situations around the home.

The U.S. Preventive Services Task Force (USPSTF) recommendations for vision screening for children 1 to 5 years old (2011) notes that screening tests have reasonable accuracy in identifying strabismus, amblyopia, and refractive errors in children 3 to 5 years old. Providers should be alert for signs of ocular misalignment when examining infants and children. Treating strabismus and amblyopia early greatly reduces long-term amblyopia and improves visual acuity.

The American Academy of Pediatrics (AAP), American Association of Certified Orthoptists, American Association for Pediatric Ophthalmology and Strabismus (AAPOS), and the American Academy of Ophthalmology (AAO) jointly recommend that well-child examinations should include ocular history, vision assessment, external inspection of the eyes (including pupils and red light reflex), lids, and ocular mobility (Committee on Practice and Ambulatory Medicine et al, 2003). This also includes an evaluation of fixation and following (binocularly and monocularly) starting at birth, with patched visual acuity screening starting at 3 years old (Tables 29-1, 29-2, and 29-3). If the child is uncooperative, retesting should occur 6 months later. Inability to fix and follow after 3 months old warrants a referral to a pediatric ophthalmologist or an eye specialist trained to treat pediatric patients. Subsequent testing should occur at 4, 5, 6, 8, 10, 12, 15, and 18 years old. A subjective historical assessment should occur during visits at all other ages. Children who are difficult to screen after two attempts or who demonstrate any other eye abnormality should undergo photoscreening techniques to detect amblyopia, media opacities, and treatable ocular disease processes with referral to an ophthalmologist considered.

For high-risk children, the AAO (2012a) recommends that asymptomatic children have a comprehensive examination by an ophthalmologist if they have any of the following:

- Health or developmental problems that make screening by the primary care clinician difficult or inaccurate (e.g., retinopathy of prematurity [ROP], or diagnostic

TABLE 29-1 Normal Visual Developmental Milestones

Age	Milestone
Birth to 2 weeks old	Infant sees and responds to change in illumination; refuses to reopen eyes after exposure to bright light; increasing alertness to objects; fixes on contrasts (e.g., black and white); jerky movements; pupillary reaction present.
By 2 to 4 weeks old	Infant fixes and follows on an object, though sporadically.
By 3 to 4 months old	Infant recognizes parent's smile; looks from near to far and focuses close again; beginning development of depth perception; follows 180-degree arc; reaches toward toy; few exodeviations; esotropia abnormal.
By 4 months old	Color vision near that of an adult; tears are present.
By 6 to 10 months old	Infant fixes on and follows toy in all directions; movements smooth.
By 12 months old	Vision is close to fully developed.

TABLE 29-2 Visual Acuity Norms (Snellen Equivalents)

Age	Forced-Choice Preferential Looking (FPL)	Age Visual-Evoked Potential (VEP)
Birth	20/400	20/800
2 months old	20/400	
4 months old	20/200	20/600
6 months old	20/150	20/400
12 months old	20/50	20/20
18 to 24 months old	20/25 or 20/20	
5 years old	20/25 or 20/20	

Adapted from Eustis HS, Guthrie ME: Postnatal development. In Wright KW, Spiegel PH, editors: *Pediatric ophthalmology and strabismus*, New York, 2003, Springer; Stout A: Pediatric eye examination. In Wright KW, Spiegel PH, editors: *Pediatric ophthalmology and strabismus*, New York, 2003, Springer.

evaluation of a complex disease with ophthalmologic manifestations)

- A family history of conditions that cause or are associated with eye or vision problems (e.g., retinoblastoma, significant hyperopia, strabismus [particularly accommodative esotropia], amblyopia, congenital cataract, or glaucoma)
- Multiple health problems, systemic disease, or the use of medications that are known to be associated with eye disease and vision abnormalities (e.g., neurodegenerative disease, juvenile rheumatoid arthritis, systemic steroid therapy, systemic syndromes with ocular manifestations, or developmental delay with visual system manifestations)

Development, Physiology, and Pathophysiology of the Eye

Development of the Ocular Structures

At 21 days of gestation ocular tissue is visible on each side of the head. By the end of the eighth week of pregnancy the eyelids are completely formed, and the upper and lower lids fuse to seal the eye while it develops. At 16 weeks of gestation, the eyes are fully anterior. By the seventh month of pregnancy, the fetus can open its eyes. Development of the eye as a visual organ is not complete at birth, yet newborns have the ability to fix their gaze, follow an object to midline, and react to a change in the intensity of light. Over the first 2 to 3 months of extrauterine life, the ability to focus at any range develops as the eyes become coordinated horizontally and vertically. By 3 months old, infants can follow moving objects; and by 4 months old, they can indicate visual recognition of familiar objects. The shape and contour of the eyeball changes, and visual acuity and binocularity gradually increase with age. The volume of the orbits doubles by the time the child is 1 year old and almost doubles again by 6 to 8 years old. Eye growth is completed at 10 to 13 years old. The corneal dimension, however, changes minimally from full-term newborn to adulthood.

During early childhood the visual pathways that ensure central vision are developing. The brain must receive equally clear, bilaterally focused images at the same time for this development to occur. The adult visual field is obtained by 10 years old. The visual pathways are amenable to the greatest corrective influences (e.g., adequate treatment of amblyopia) until 7 to 8 years old. Research has demonstrated that the visual system of teens and adults with amblyopia might still retain substantial plasticity (Olitsky et al, 2011).

Anatomy and Physiology of the Eye

The eyeball consists of three layers of tissue: the fibrous tunic, the vascular tunic, and the inner tunic or retina. The fibrous tunic consists of the sclera and the cornea. The vascular tunic, the middle layer, is composed of the choroid, the ciliary body, and the iris (Fig. 29-1). All the structures of the eye are dedicated to accurate and efficient functioning of the innermost layer of the eyeball, the retina. The optic disc consists only of nerve fibers (no rods or cones), so no visual images are formed here. Thus, it is referred to as the *blind spot.*

The inside of the eyeball consists of the anterior and posterior cavities (see Fig. 29-1). The anterior cavity is

TABLE 29-3 Recommended Ages and Methods for Pediatric Eye Evaluation Screening

Recommended Age	Method	Indications for Referral to an Ophthalmologist
Newborn to 3 months old	Ocular history Red reflex Inspection	 Abnormal or asymmetric Structural abnormality
3 to 6 months old (approximately)	Ocular history Fix and follow Red reflex Inspection	 Failure to fix and follow in a cooperative infant Abnormal or asymmetric Structural abnormality
6 to 12 months old and until child is able to cooperate for verbal visual acuity	Ocular history Fix and follow with each eye Alternate occlusion Corneal light reflex Red reflex Inspection Photoscreening	 Failure to fix and follow Failure to object equally to covering each eye Asymmetric Abnormal or asymmetric Structural abnormality Abnormal finding
3 years old and older and every 1 to 2 years after 5 years old	Ocular history Visual acuity* (monocular)	 36 to 47 months old: 20/50 or worse 48 to 59 months old: 20/40 or worse >5 years old: 20/30 or worse, or two lines of difference between the eyes 36 to 47 months old: Must correctly identify the majority of the optotypes on the 20/50 line to pass 48 to 59 months old: Must correctly identify the majority of the optotypes on the 20/40 line to pass
	Corneal light reflex/cover-uncover reflex Red reflex Inspection Photoscreening or autorefraction Attempt ophthalmoscopy	Asymmetric/ocular refixation movements Abnormal or asymmetric Structural abnormality Abnormal findings

Derived from American Academy of Pediatrics (AAP) Committee on Practice and Ambulatory Medicine and Section on Ophthalmology, American Association of Certified Orthoptists, American Association of Pediatric Ophthalmology and Strabismus, American Academy of Ophthalmology (AAO): Eye examination in infants, children, and young adults by pediatricians: policy statement, *Pediatrics* 111(4):902–907, 2003; and American Association of Pediatric Ophthalmology and Strabismus (2014) Vision screening recommendations.

*Pictures (Lea Hyvärinen [LH/LEA] symbols or Allen cards for 2- to 4-year-olds); "tumbling E" or HOTV for ≥4-year-olds; or vision-testing machines.

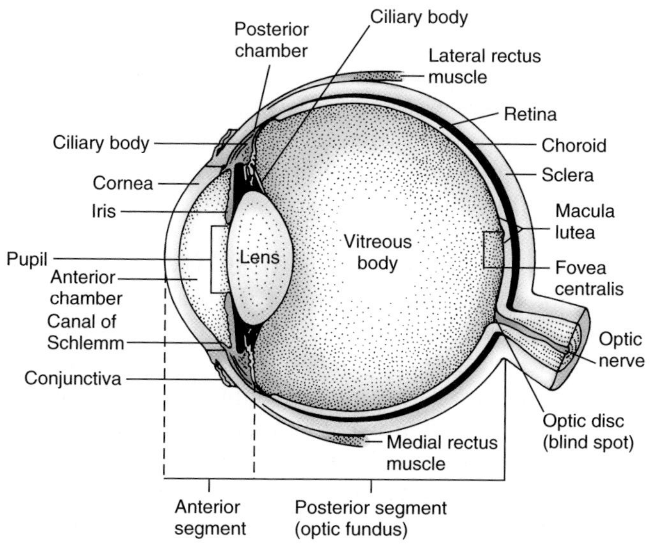

• **Figure 29-1** Anatomy of the eye. (From Ignatavicius D, Workman L: *Medical-surgical nursing: patient-centered collaborative care*, ed 8, Philadelphia, 2016, Saunders/Elsevier.)

divided into anterior and posterior chambers. The anterior chamber lies between the cornea and the iris. The posterior chamber lies between the iris and the suspensory ligament. Aqueous humor circulates throughout these chambers to maintain intraocular pressure (IOP) and link the circulatory system with the avascular lens and cornea. The other cavity within the eyeball, the posterior cavity, lies between the lens and the retina. The gelatinous vitreous humor found in this cavity contributes to the maintenance of IOP and holds the retina in place. The lens, which separates the cavities, hangs by the suspensory ligament. Six muscles guide movement of the globe. Four rectus muscles (superior, inferior, lateral, and medial) move the eyeball up, down, in, and out, respectively. Two oblique muscles (superior and inferior) rotate the eyeball on its axis. Cranial nerve (CN) III (oculomotor), CN IV (trochlear), and CN VI (abducens) innervate these muscles.

The focusing of light rays involves four basic processes: (1) refraction of light rays, (2) accommodation of the lens, (3) constriction of the pupil, and (4) convergence of the

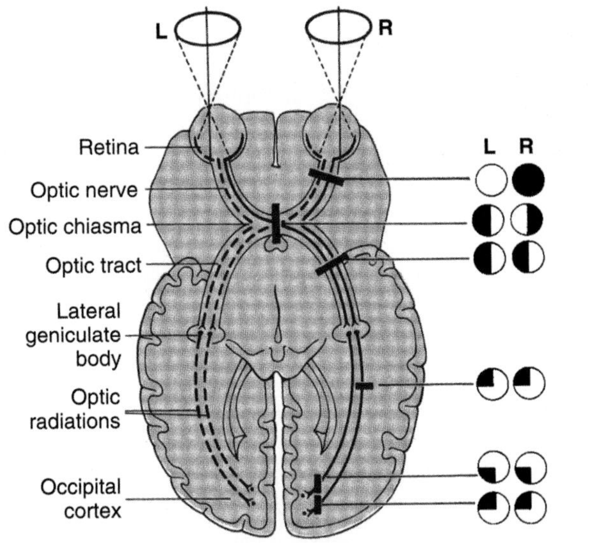

• **Figure 29-2** Visual pathway. On the right are diagrams of the visual fields with areas of blindness darkened to show the effects of injuries in various locations. (From Patton K, Thibodeau G: *Anatomy and physiology,* ed 9, St Louis, 2016, Mosby/Elsevier.)

eyes. *Refraction* is the bending of light rays as they pass from one transparent medium (air) to another (cornea or lens). The lens modifies the degree of refraction to create the sharpest image on the retina. *Accommodation* is the ability of the lens to focus on close objects by increasing its curvature. The normal eye refracts light rays from an object 20 feet away to focus a clear image onto the retina; hence the fraction 20/20 is used to denote the accepted standard of normal vision. The circular muscle fibers of the iris, which contract in response to light, cause constriction of the pupil. Regulating the light entering the eye can also facilitate production of a precise image. To maintain single binocular vision, close objects require the eyes to rotate medially so that the light rays from the object hit the same points on both retinas. This rotation is called *convergence.* A normal neonate demonstrates disconjugate fixation, but convergence and accommodation normally develop by 3 to 4 months old, with parallel alignment by 5 to 6 months old without nystagmus or strabismus. Jerky eye movements can be seen until 2 months old, after which time smooth tracking movements are expected.

After an image is formed on the retina, light impulses are converted into nerve impulses and transmitted to the visual centers located in the occipital lobes of the cerebral cortex. Lesions in various places along the neural tracts from the eye to the cortex cause different types of loss of visual fields (Fig. 29-2).

Pathophysiology of the Eyes

Potential problems with the eyes or visual system can take the form of specific disorders, infections, or injuries to the eye. The most common disorders of the eye interfering with vision are refractive errors (myopia, hyperopia, astigmatism, and anisometropia). Less common disorders include strabismus, amblyopia, ptosis, nystagmus, cataracts, glaucoma, ROP, and retinoblastoma. Infections and injuries may be relatively minor and superficial or critical and involve deep tissues of the eye. Certain systemic diseases (e.g., juvenile rheumatoid arthritis) and medications (e.g., steroids) can also affect the eyes and warrant extra assessment measures.

Assessment

Assessment of the eye, as with all body systems, requires a thoughtful history, careful physical examination, and certain specialized screening tests.

History

- General medical history, including birth weight; pertinent prenatal, perinatal, postnatal factors (e.g., prematurity, infections); past hospitalizations and surgery; general health and development
- Family medical history of ocular problems (including eye surgeries), such as glaucoma, blindness, poor vision, difficulty walking in dim light, photophobia, use of thick glasses, lazy eye, strabismus, nystagmus, leukokoria, retinoblastoma, congenital cataracts
- History of chronic systemic disease in patient or family (e.g., inflammatory bowel disease; connective tissue disorders; cardiac defects of Marfan syndrome; midfacial hypoplasia; abnormalities of teeth, umbilical cord, or urinary tract; neurologic or skin anomalies; developmental delay; mental retardation; diabetes; sickle cell hemoglobinopathies; Tay-Sachs disease; tuberculosis)
- Presence of allergies and specific allergens
- Current medications (e.g., steroids); past or present substance abuse
- Child's ocular history, which includes:
  - Date (and results) of the last vision screening and prior eye problems or diseases, including diagnoses and treatments
  - If history of eye injury: Unilateral or bilateral injury? Were there visual changes or photophobia? What treatment was received?
  - Prescription and use of eyeglasses or contact lenses: Does the child have glasses that were prescribed? Are they used? If not, why?
  - Use of sunglasses with ultraviolet (UV) protection or protective eyewear for sports activities
- Symptoms or indications of eye dysfunction or disease:
  - Older children may report visual loss or change in vision, such as blurring, diplopia, spots, and halos. Younger children may be observed to have problems with fixing or focusing (holding objects up close to see), tracking, squinting, head tilt, eye-hand coordination, grasp, gait, balance, behavior, and changes in the ability to maintain eye contact; eyelid droop
  - Photophobia may present as irritability, shielding, or rubbing of the eyes

- Swollen eyelids, pruritus, excessive tearing or discharge, erythema, burning, eye fatigue, strabismus
- Constant blinking, chronic bulbar conjunctival injection

Physical Examination

The physical examination can be challenging, depending on the child's age. The components need to be done quickly to accommodate the child's short attention span. Knowledge of visual developmental milestones is essential in assessing a child's visual capabilities (see Table 29-1).

- Gross inspection should be made of the external structures with a penlight (lids, bulbar and palpebral conjunctiva, cornea, lacrimal structures, and the size, symmetry, and reactivity of the pupils), orbits, eye muscle balance, and mobility.
- The red reflex is tested in all ages. It needs to be assessed for color, intensity, and clarity (opacities or white spots). A rule of thumb is that if the examiner cannot see into the eye (e.g., absent red light reflex), the patient cannot see out.
- In children older than 5 years old, funduscopic examination allows for visualization of the retina, choroid, fovea, macula, optic disc and cup, and entry and exit of the vessels and nerves.
- Examination of the eye is sometimes facilitated by using a cotton-tipped applicator to evert the eyelid. Eyelid eversion is accomplished by having the patient look down while the examiner grasps the lashes with the thumb and index finger, places the applicator in the middle of the lid, pulls the eyelid down and out, and everts it over the applicator.
- Growth parameters (especially head growth and shape) and the head and neck or other structures should be examined if a systemic condition is suspected.

Screening Tests

Conducting Screening Tests

Fatigue, hunger, anxiety, and environmental distractions can interfere with vision testing. Testing should always precede the administration of immunizations or any procedure that might cause discomfort. While testing, observe children for behavior indicating that they are having difficulty, such as straining, squinting, excessive blinking, head tilting or shaking, or thrusting the trunk or head forward. The tendency to peek out from behind the eye shield may or may not reflect difficulty; the child may do so out of a desire to be successful and please the tester. The examiner should resist the tendency to correct a mistake or give the child nonverbal clues that can influence the results. Three-year-old children who have difficulty performing any of the vision tests in the PCP's office should be tested again within 6 months; those unable to perform when older than 4 years of age should be retested in 1 month. A child who is uncooperative on the second attempt should be referred for a formal examination (AAPOS and AAO, 2013).

Red Reflex

The red reflex should be tested at every well examination, including the initial newborn examination. Performing an adequate red reflex test (Bruckner test) allows the clinician to detect the presence of asymmetric refractive errors, strabismic deviations, and abnormalities in the ocular media (e.g., cataracts, corneal abnormalities, retinoblastoma). Disease processes involving the cornea, lens, vitreous, or retina block the light from entering or exiting the pupil and result in an abnormal red reflex. The recommended technique follows:

- Darken the examination room, it is easier to detect more subtle asymmetries between the red reflexes.
- Stand an arm-length away from the infant or child and use the ophthalmoscope light set at 0 or +1 to illuminate the face.
- Look at both pupils simultaneously and separately. In children with fair skin pigmentation, the red reflex is bright red-orange; in those with darker pigmentation, the red reflex is dark red-brown.
- The red reflexes should be symmetric; any asymmetry, dark or white spots, opacities, or leukokoria (white pupillary reflex) requires prompt referral to an ophthalmologist.

Visual Acuity Testing

Visual acuity screening (see Tables 29-2 and 29-3), for both near and distance vision, should be performed on all children during routine physical examinations when problems with visual acuity are suspected and/or when eye trauma occurs. Children who are not reading at grade level after 5 years old should also have formal visual acuity screening (AAPOS, 2014f). If the child wears eyeglasses or contact lenses, visual acuity measurement must be obtained using corrective devices.

Color Vision Testing

The human retina contains 6 million red and green cones and approximately 1 million blue cones. Alterations in color vision occur when the normal photopigments in the photoreceptor cones are replaced with different ones. Color ranges are then interpreted or perceived differently.

Red-green color deficiency is an X-linked inherited disorder or may indicate optic nerve disease. Inherited color deficiencies are more common in males and affect up to 8% of males and 5% of females (Olitsky et al, 2011). Color vision deficiency may also be acquired. A patient with acquired deficiency may have had normal color vision and then experienced color changes and losses. Diabetes, infections, optic neuritis, and toxins are systemic conditions that can lead to such losses. Blue-yellow deficiency is the most common type of acquired color deficiency.

Significant color blindness can affect school performance, have safety implications if the child is unable able to distinguish traffic or vehicle brake lights, and affect career choices. Color vision is tested by using the Richmond

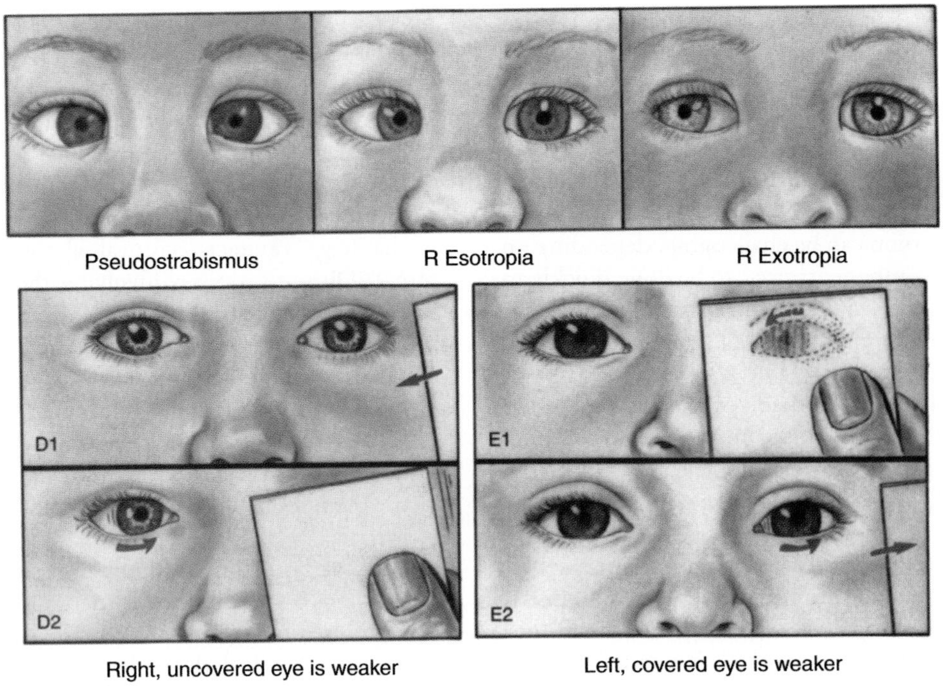

• **Figure 29-3** Extra ocular muscle function testing (corneal light reflex and cover test). (From Jarvis C: *Physical examination and health assessment*, ed 2, Philadelphia, 1996, Saunders.)

pseudoisochromatic plates (formerly Hardy-Rand-Rittler plates) or Ishihara plates. Children 3 to 4 years old are usually able to comply with testing directions, but the test does not routinely need to be administered (parents may request testing when their child is young and makes errors when asked to identify colors). In a child who is truly color deficient, the colors are not misnamed.

Peripheral Vision Testing

Examination of peripheral visual fields provides information about retinal function, the neuronal visual pathway to the brain, and the function of CN II (optic nerve). In an infant, assessment is limited to a rough estimate of peripheral visual fields by watching the child's response to a familiar object (e.g., bottle, toy) or a threatening gesture as it is brought into each of the four quadrants. In children mature enough to cooperate, peripheral visual fields can be measured by confrontation or by finger counting. Peripheral visual fields should be approximately 50 degrees upward, 70 degrees downward, 60 degrees medially (toward the nose), and 90 degrees laterally.

Testing for Ocular Mobility and Alignment

The Hirschberg test (also called the *corneal light reflex*) evaluates extra ocular muscle function by projecting a small light source onto the cornea of the eye with the child looking straight ahead. A normal test reveals the reflected light as a small white dot symmetrically located in the same position of each eye (often slightly nasal of center). The cover-uncover test and the alternating cover test should be performed with the child fixating straight ahead, first on a near point object and then on a far point object about 20 feet away (Fig. 29-3). The process is sometimes aided by asking the child questions about the object (e.g., "How many cows do you see?" in a picture that has been placed for this purpose on the wall). During the alternating cover test, the examiner rapidly covers and uncovers the eye while shifting between the two eyes. Any orbital movement is an indication of misalignment.

Assessment of Visual Loss

If significant visual disturbance is suspected, the following functional vision assessments should be performed, and the child referred immediately to an ophthalmologist:

- Shine a penlight into the eye from a lateral position and turn the light off and on several times to assess light perception. If the child can identify when the light is on or off, vision is described as "LP" (light perception).
- Move a hand back and forth with periodic cessation 12 inches from the child's face. Indication of search and recognition is documented as "H/M at 1 ft" (hand motion).
- Ask the child to count the number of fingers (C/F) seen when one, two, or three fingers are held up 12 inches from the child's face. If the child is correct, document the vision as "C/F at 1 ft."

Diagnostic Studies

Photoscreening and Autorefractors

Photoscreeners and autorefractors may be used to screen for optical and physical abnormalities of the eyes (Miller et al, 2012). Photoscreeners can assess the red light reflex and refractive error and screen for amblyopia. Autorefractors may be used to determine the refractive error of each eye. (Medial opacities and refractive errors can be discerned using instrument-based screening in preverbal or developmentally delayed children.) Instrument-based vision screening has had extensive validation and is a reliable, alternative method for visual screening in children 6 months to 3 years old who are not able to use vision charts (Miller et al, 2012).

Laboratory and Imaging Studies

Cultures and Gram stain of eye discharge are done if identification of infection or particular organisms would be helpful in guiding management. Ultrasound (not to be used in cases of a suspected ruptured globe), computed tomography (CT), or magnetic resonance imaging (MRI) is sometimes useful in determining a diagnosis of orbital cellulitis, trauma, or tumor, or in substantiating a concern about the central nervous system (CNS). An MRI should not be used in the case of a suspected intraocular metal foreign body.

Fluorescein Staining

Fluorescein staining may be used to determine the extent of damage to the corneal or conjunctival epithelium as a result of trauma, infection, or exposure to a foreign body. After applying fluorescein examine the cornea with a cobalt blue filter light; any injury will take up the fluorescein stain and appear as a greenish area. Too much of the stain will cloud the entire cornea.

Management Strategies

Referral for Ophthalmologic and Specialty Management

See Table 29-4 for guidance on when to refer for a more comprehensive examination. Although any child with eye pathologic conditions should be referred to an ophthalmologist, optometrists can be a valuable resource in caring for children with refractive errors or certain common eye conditions (e.g., corneal abrasions, foreign bodies). PCPs should acquaint themselves with the statutory guidelines for scope of practice and prescription privileges as designated by the state boards of optometry within their state to optimize referral possibilities.

Ophthalmologic or optometric management of potential or present central vision deficiencies may include the following strategies.

Occlusion

Patching, occlusive contact lens (a last resort method), optical penalization (overplusses the lens on the sound eye), or pharmacologic penalization with 0.5% or 1% atropine (not used in infants) may be used to treat strabismus and improve or prevent amblyopia by blocking vision in the sound eye.

TABLE 29-4 Indications for a Comprehensive Pediatric Medical Eye Evaluation

Indication	Specific Examples
Risk factors (general health problems, systemic disease, or use of medications that are known to be associated with eye disease and visual abnormalities)	Prematurity (birth weight less than 1500 g or gestational age 30 weeks or less) Retinopathy of prematurity Intrauterine growth retardation Perinatal complications (evaluation at birth and at 6 months old) Neurologic disorders or neurodevelopmental delay (at diagnosis) Juvenile idiopathic arthritis (at diagnosis) Thyroid disease Cleft palate or other craniofacial abnormalities Diabetes mellitus (5 years old after onset) Systemic syndromes with known ocular manifestations (at 6 months old or at diagnosis) Chronic systemic corticosteroid therapy or other medications known to cause eye disease Suspected child abuse
A family history of conditions that cause or are associated with eye or vision problems	Retinoblastoma Childhood cataract Childhood glaucoma Retinal dystrophy/degeneration Strabismus Amblyopia Eyeglasses in early childhood Sickle cell anemia Systemic syndromes with known ocular manifestations Any history of childhood blindness not due to trauma in a parent or sibling
Signs or symptoms of eye problems by history or observations by family members*	Defective ocular fixation or visual interactions Abnormal light reflex (including both the corneal light reflections and the red fundus reflection) Abnormal or irregular pupils Large and/or cloudy eyes Drooping eyelid Lumps or swelling around the eyes Ocular alignment or movement abnormality Nystagmus Persistent tearing, ocular discharge Persistent or recurrent redness Persistent light sensitivity Squinting/eye closure Persistent head tilt Learning disabilities or dyslexia

From American Academy of Ophthalmology (AAO): *Pediatric eye evaluations PPP—2012, ONE Network* (website), 2012a. Available at www.aao.org/preferred-practice-pattern/pediatric-eye-evaluations-ppp–september-2012. Accessed October 22, 2014.

*Headache is not included because it is rarely caused by eye problems in children. This complaint should first be evaluated by the primary care physician.

Corrective Lenses

In children, eyeglasses are used to correct refractive errors. Gas-permeable or soft contact lenses can be successfully worn by children as young as 8 years old (Roach, 2012). Silsoft silicon polymer lenses may be used in aphakic infants and can be worn 24 hours a day for as long as a week (Roach, 2012). Keratorefractive (laser-assisted in situ keratomileusis [LASIK]) surgery is undergoing worldwide research for its applicability in children with low to moderate myopia, severe anisometropia, bilateral high ametropia, and refractive amblyopia; however, its use remains controversial. The AAO discourages LASIK surgery in individuals younger than 18 years old and provides guidelines regarding suitable candidates for the procedure (AAO, 2013c). LASIK and photo refractive keratectomy (PRK) lasers are not approved by the U.S. Food and Drug Administration (FDA) for use under 21 years old (AAO, 2013c). General guidelines for glasses and contact lenses can be found in Box 29-1. Glasses must be changed frequently in children because of head growth. Because the child may be reluctant to wear eyeglasses that hurt or pinch, parents should assess the fit of the eyeglasses on a monthly basis and watch for behavior that indicates discomfort in a preverbal child (e.g., constantly removing glasses, rubbing at the frames or face).

Contact lenses (includes daily wear [hard lenses] and soft, extended and/or disposable wear lenses), in addition to the cosmetic benefit, can provide better refractive error correction than eyeglasses, thereby enhancing visual acuity and the total corrected field of vision. Studies have also shown that their use improves how children feel about their appearance, athletic abilities, and what friends think of them (Jones-Jordan et al, 2010). Eye health can be promoted by reinforcing instructions regarding proper contact lens care and reminding the patient that contact lenses should not be worn when the eye is inflamed or topical ophthalmic medications are being used. The Centers for Disease Control and Prevention (CDC) has recommendations for parents considering contact lenses for their children (CDC, 2014a).

"Plano" (noncorrective, decorative, or theatrical contact lenses used for cosmetic purposes) are available for purchase from nonvision care resources. Severe eye injuries (including blindness) result when people bypass the usual regulatory safeguards (proper fit, adequate instruction on use, and hygiene). Such cases prompted the AAO to sponsor legislation that required the FDA to regulate the lenses as medical devices. The law requires that these types of lenses be properly fitted and dispensed by prescription only from a qualified eye care professional. Another type of plano lens includes those with light-filtering tints. These block or enhance certain colors and are designed for sports use by tennis players, golfers, baseball players, spectators, trapshooters, and skiers. Regardless of federal regulations, over-the-counter decorative contact lenses are still illegally sold on the market (CDC, 2014b). The AAO provides information regarding risks of nonprescription contacts, including corneal abrasions and ulcers, infection, and scarring leading to blindness (Dang, 2014).

• BOX 29-1 Recommendations for Use of Corrective Lenses

Eyeglasses

Polycarbonate lenses are lightweight, strong, and shatterproof; scratch-resistant coating is recommended.
Silicone nose pads with nonskid surfaces prevent glasses from slipping.
Comfort cables secure frames by wrapping around the child's ears and are available for children 1 to 4 years old. Straps are recommended for infants younger than 1 year old and allow them to roll and lie down.
Flexible hinges allow outward bending for easy removal by the child.
Match the frame to the child's facial shape and features to encourage compliance; if old enough, allow the child to choose the frames.
To encourage compliance with infants and children, do not fight them when they remove glasses; be persistent, replace the glasses, and provide distraction. Parents may need to set the glasses aside for a few hours before trying again. Seek counsel from the prescribing provider for further help.
Tinted lenses can be used for photosensitivity; ultraviolet (UV) light filters are helpful with aphakia (absence of lens), congenital absence of iris, and albinism.
Do not place the glasses down with lenses in contact with hard surfaces.
Clean glasses daily with liquid soap and a soft cloth. (Do not use paper products.)

Contact Lenses

Contact lenses are appropriate for children 8 years old and older; children need to be able to demonstrate ability to manage lens hygiene, including insertion and removal.
Contact lenses are helpful for an aphakic child who would otherwise need very thick glasses that distort images.
Wear protective outer eyewear for sports.
Do not wear contact lenses if one or both eyes are inflamed or when using topical ophthalmic medications. Children with recurrent conjunctival or corneal infections, inadequate tears, severe allergies, or excessive exposure to dust or smoke should not wear contact lenses.
Omit wearing extended-wear contact lenses (usually worn overnight) for 1 night a week in order to perform lens hygiene procedures.

Ophthalmic Medications

Caution and precision must be exercised when administering ocular medications to children, because their smaller body mass and faster metabolism may potentiate the action of the drugs and result in adverse ocular and systemic side effects. Topical ophthalmic medications, such as antibiotics, mydriatics, and corticosteroids, are frequently found in ointment or solution vehicles. These topical agents are primarily used for treating disorders affecting the anterior segment of the eye. Solubility is one of several factors that influence the absorption of topical ophthalmic medications. Those that are water soluble (e.g., anesthetics, steroids, and alkaloids) penetrate the corneal epithelium easily. Fat-soluble preparations (e.g., most antibiotics) do not penetrate the epithelium of the cornea unless it is inflamed.

Topical Antibiotics

Prescription of topical antibiotics is ideally based on empirical evidence of infection. The best choice of a topical antibiotic is one that is not often prescribed for problems in other body systems. Topical ophthalmologic preparations, such as fluoroquinolones, sulfacetamide, and trimethoprim/polymyxin B, are effective and rarely produce a hypersensitivity reaction. Topical penicillins, on the other hand, are to be avoided. The pros and cons of these antibiotics are addressed in later sections of this chapter. Ophthalmic ointments may be preferred over solutions for use in children, especially infants, because they last longer, do not sting, do not need to be given as often, and are less likely to be absorbed into the lacrimal passage.

Ophthalmic Corticosteroids

Although ophthalmic corticosteroids are effective in the treatment of ocular inflammation and traumatic iritis (excluding ocular allergy), a patient with a condition severe enough to warrant consideration of corticosteroid use should be referred to an ophthalmologist. Steroids are associated with numerous complications, such as an increased incidence of herpes simplex keratitis and corneal ulcers, fungal keratitis, corneal perforation and intraocular sepsis, glaucoma, slowed healing of corneal abrasions and wounds, increased IOP, cataract formation, and permanent loss of sight. A child receiving long-term ophthalmologic steroids should be assessed frequently for signs of adrenal suppression or other side effects. Encourage parents to keep scheduled tonometry appointments at 2- to 3-month intervals.

Other Topical Preparations

Topical decongestants or antihistamines or a combination of the two, mast cell stabilizers, and nonsteroidal anti-inflammatory drugs (NSAIDs) are used in treating various ophthalmologic conditions. Over-the-counter vasoconstrictors or vasoconstrictor-antihistamine preparations can be tried first for mild allergic conjunctivitis. Cycloplegic agents are used for iritis.

Systemic Medications

In ocular infections involving the posterior segment and the orbit, systemic antibiotic preparations are necessary. A combination of topical and systemic antibiotics can also be used. In general, these conditions warrant referral to an ophthalmologist. Systemic drugs may also cause damage to the eyes (Table 29-5).

Eye Injury Prevention

Ocular trauma accounts for one third of all cases of acquired blindness in children. Male-to-female trauma incidence ratio is 4 : 1, with males 11 to 15 years old outnumbering all other age groups. Ninety percent of the injuries could be prevented by using protective eyewear (AAO, 2013b). The majority of the injuries are the result of sports-related accidents (50% of all eye injuries), toy darts, sticks, stones, BB shot, paintball sports, other projectiles, and alpine skiing (AAO, 2013a, 2013b). Other causes include battered child syndrome (40% have ocular findings), birth trauma, fingers/fists/other body parts in the eye, fireworks (firecrackers, sparklers, rockets), and airbags (though the injury is less than that suffered in cars without airbags or when the airbags failed to deploy). Slightly more than 44% of eye injuries occur in the home (AAO, 2013b). The areas most affected by superficial trauma include the cornea (50%), conjunctiva (49%), and sclera; the most serious eye injuries involve the cornea, iris, lens, and optic nerve and may result from anterior chamber hyphema, vitreous hemorrhage, or retinal tear or detachment (AAO, 2013b).

Prevent Blindness (2013b) recommends parental supervision and child education regarding eye injury prevention as essential to minimize eye injuries. Prevention includes fundamental concepts, such as instructing the child:

- Not run with or throw sharp objects
- Use protective eyewear when hammering, using power tools or lawnmowers, or participating in a sport where there is a higher risk of ocular injury (see list under Sports Protection)
- Use orthodontic headwear that breaks away if force is applied
- Not shine laser pointers in eyes
- Use eye wash fountains when indicated

Parents need to be instructed to:

- Store harmful chemicals and sharp objects out of the reach of small children
- Limit and supervise the use of BB guns, air rifles, paintball devices, darts, and fireworks.

Sunglasses

Ultraviolet A (UVA) and ultraviolet B (UVB) radiation from the sun can damage the lens and retina of the eye and cause cataracts and other conditions harmful to vision later in life (e.g., macular degeneration). Sunlight has more UVA than UVB, but UVB is more damaging. Sunglasses should be used to minimize such damage by absorbing these light wavelengths, even if wearing UV-treated contact lenses. It is never too early to start wearing sunglasses. Wearing a hat with a wide (3-inch) brim only reduces the UV rays that reach the eyes by half (Prevent Blindness, 2013a).

Sunglasses that have large-framed wraparound lenses with side shields provide the best protection. They should provide 99% to 100% protection from the UVA and UVB short waves (Prevent Blindness, 2013a). The lens and frame should be constructed of nonbreakable plastic or polycarbonate. The protection comes from the chemical coating on top of, or incorporated into, the lenses. Gray, brown, and green colors are sufficient for general purposes and lead to minimal color distortion. Darker colors or polarized lenses

TABLE 29-5 Systemic Drugs, Herbs, and Nutritional Supplements that Can Cause Ocular Side Effects

Drug	Ocular Side Effects	Intervention
Corticosteroids (prednisone at dosage of 15 mg/day for ≥1 year)	Cataracts, increased IOP	Monitor with ophthalmologic examinations.
Digoxin at moderately toxic ranges	Snowy, flickering, yellow vision	Resolves when drug is administered in correct range.
Isoniazid in greater than recommended dosages	Loss in color vision, decreased visual acuity, and visual field changes	Effects are reversible only if discovered early. Ophthalmologic examination is indicated before treatment and every 6 months; any changes warrant stopping isoniazid and referring to an ophthalmologist.
Isotretinoin	Pseudotumor cerebri (after initiating treatment) with resultant blurred vision, visual field loss, and varying visual acuity changes, including optic neuritis, dry eye, decreased night vision, and transitory myopia	Monitor for symptoms. Annual eye examination recommended while on isotretinoin.
Minocycline hydrochloride	Pseudotumor cerebri and orthostatic blackouts, evidenced by blurred vision, visual field loss, varying visual acuity changes, diplopia; scleral pigmentation	Monitor for symptoms; scleral pigmentation may not resolve.
Phenytoin and carbamazepine	Blood levels in moderately toxic ranges can produce diplopia, blurred vision, nystagmus; sensitivity to glare	Resolve when therapeutic doses are within normal ranges.
Topiramate	Acute angle closure glaucoma; mydriasis; ocular pain; decreased visual acuity (myopia)	Onset of symptoms within 3 to 14 days after medication started. Stop medication. Treatment may include cycloplegics, hyperosmotic therapy, and topical antiglaucoma medications.
Quetiapine	Cataracts	Monitor with ophthalmologic examinations.
Oral contraceptives (estrogen and/or progesterone)	Optic neuritis, pseudotumor cerebri, dry eyes	Monitor.
Fluoxetine/SSRIs	Dry eye, blurred vision, mydriasis, photophobia, diplopia, conjunctivitis, and ptosis	Monitor.
Herbs		
Canthaxanthin (taken to produce artificial suntan; food coloring)	Decreased visual acuity; retinopathy	
Cassava (with prolonged usage)	Decreased visual acuity; retinopathy	Contains natural cyanide, so it is important that this plant is processed correctly.
Datura (may be used by those with asthma, influenza, coughs)	Mydriasis	
Ginkgo biloba	Retrobulbar and retinal hemorrhage; hyphema	
Licorice	Decreased visual acuity	
Vitamin A	Intracranial hypertension	

Data from Anderson AC: Ocular toxicology. In Shannon MW, Borron SW, Burns MJ, editors: *Haddad and Winchester's clinical management of poisoning and drug overdose*, ed 4, Philadelphia, 2007, Saunders; Reed B, Hua L: *Potential ocular side effects of select systemic drugs*, 2010. Available at http://commons.pacificu.edu/cgi/viewcontent.cgi?article=1002&context=coofac. Accessed November 2, 2014; Trobe J: *The physician's guide to eye care*, San Francisco, 2001, The Foundation of the American Academy of Ophthalmology; Gurwood AS, American Optometric Association (AOA): *Optometric clinical practice recommendations for monitoring ocular toxicity of selected medications*. Available at www.aoa.org/documents/optometrists/Ocular-Toxicity.pdf. Accessed October 20, 2015.

IOP, Intraocular pressure; *SSRI*, selective serotonin reuptake inhibitor.

alone do not offer the protection that is needed unless they specifically state otherwise. Sunglasses that are for fashion purposes or that do not list the UV protective wave spectrum should be avoided. Lenses should only be purchased if they carry the American National Standards Institute (ANSI) label or American Optometric Association (AOA) notation. ANSI communicates their standards by labeling their lenses Z80.3 and "general purpose," "special purpose" (for snow and water sports), and "cosmetic use" (lowest protection) (Bishop et al, 2009). In addition to the requisite UVA and UVB protection, the AOA recommends purchasing only lenses that state that they screen out 75% to 90% of visible light, are gray (for best color perception), and cause no distortion in vision (AOA, n.d.).

Sports Protection

Protective glasses or goggles are mandatory for all functionally one-eyed individuals (with best corrected vision worse than 20/40 in the poorer-seeing eye) or for any athlete who has had eye surgery or trauma or whose ophthalmologist recommends eye protection (AAO, 2013b; Prevent Blindness, 2013b). Additionally, these children or adolescents should not participate in boxing or full-contact martial arts. Caution is also recommended in these individuals if they choose to wrestle, even though there is a low rate of reported injury.

Eye protection is recommended for any child or adolescent participating in sports that have a high eye injury rate, specifically hockey, fencing, boxing, full-contact martial arts, racquetball, lacrosse, squash, basketball, baseball, tennis, badminton, soccer, volleyball, water polo, fishing, golf, field hockey, paintball games, pool activities, and football. Specific protective eyewear is available; however, there are no standards for eyewear in these sports.

Protective eyewear should be properly fitted and selected specifically for the sport. A complete list of recommended eyewear for each sport is available online from the AAO website (www.aao.org). The list serves as a useful handout for parents. A headband or wraparound earpieces should be used to secure the glasses (AAO, 2013b). Sports eye guards should have protective lenses designed to stay in place or pop outward in case of a blow to the eye (Prevent Blindness, 2013b). Athletes who need prescription eyewear can either choose polycarbonate lenses in a sports frame that is rated for the specific sport, wear polycarbonate contact lenses plus the appropriate protective eyewear, or wear an attached over-the-glasses eye guard that also meets sport specifications. Younger children who do not fit into manufactured protective eyewear may be fitted with 3-mm polycarbonate lenses though adequate protection cannot be guaranteed and perhaps another choice of sport should be discussed.

Laser Pointers

Lasers are rated on a scale of I to IV, with class I lasers used in laser printers and class IV used in research lasers. The FDA strengthened its message to manufacturers regarding the labeling and safety of laser pointers in 2009 and to consumers in 2014, stating class IIIa lasers may be used as pointers, but class IIIb (laser light shows, industrial lasers) and class IV lasers should not be used (FDA, 2014). Lasers traditionally available to the public had a maximum output of from 1 to 5 milliwatts (mW). Although harmless when used as intended by lecturers, potential injury from direct, intentional, prolonged exposure to the retina is of concern if the pointers are used as toys. There are case reports of children and adolescents buying high-powered lasers from the Internet (with outputs ranging from 150 to 700 mW) and suffering permanent retinal injury and vision loss after playing with them (Wyrsch et al, 2010). The AAO recommends that laser devices not be made available as toys to children and adolescents (AAO, 2013a).

Computer Use

The aging eye can develop "computer vision syndrome" leading to eyestrain, headaches, blurred vision, dry eyes, and neck and shoulder pain (AOA, 2014). Children's eyes have more flexibility of the lens allowing them to adapt to different visual environments without eye strain (AAPOS, 2014b). The AAPOS issued a policy statement indicating there is no evidence that the use of computer, phone, or video screens increases the incidence of visual problems (AAPOS, 2014b).

Vision Therapy, Lenses, and Prisms

Vision therapy, lenses, and prisms are controversial methods of treatment claimed by some to be effective therapy for those with learning disabilities and dyslexia. These interventions consist of (1) visual training, including muscle exercises, ocular pursuit, tracking exercises, or "training" glasses (with or without bifocals or prisms); (2) neurologic organizational training (laterality training, crawling, balance board, perceptual training); and (3) wearing of colored lenses.

In a joint statement, the AAP and other organizations state that there is insufficient evidence to support the contention that vision abnormalities cause disabilities, including dyslexia (AAP et al, 2008). Therefore, vision therapy "to improve visual function by training is misdirected" (AAP et al, 2008, p 8). The joint statement further notes that the literature supporting vision therapy is "poorly validated," anecdotal, and consists of poorly controlled studies. Recommendations regarding vision care for children with learning disabilities include the following (AAP et al, 2014):

- PCPs should perform periodic eye and vision screening for all children according to national standards and refer those who do not pass screening to ophthalmologists.
- Children with a suspected or diagnosed learning disability in which vision is felt to play a role by parents, educators, or physicians should be referred to an ophthalmologist.
- Ophthalmologists should identify and treat any significant ocular or visual disorder present.

- PCPs should recommend only evidence-based treatments and educational accommodations to school districts.
- Diagnostic and treatment approaches for dyslexia that lack scientific evidence of efficacy (such as, behavioral vision therapy, eye muscle exercises, or colored filters and lenses) are not endorsed or recommended.

When counseling parents who inquire about vision therapy, the clinician should be aware of the pressure that parents may be under from optometrists who may be advocating vision therapy for learning disabilities and the divergent opinions held by educators and the ophthalmologic community about this modality of treatment. Managing a child with academic difficulties requires a multidisciplinary approach involving education and psychological and other medical specialists. Screening for ocular defects early is a routine part of primary care practice, and defects should be referred to the appropriate specialist.

Visual Disorders

Refractive Errors and Amblyopia

Alterations in the refractive power of the eye include myopia, hyperopia, astigmatism, accommodation, and anisometropia. In a normal eye, light from a distant object focuses directly on the retina. When variations in axial length of the eyeball or curvature of the cornea or lens exist, light focuses in front of or behind the retina. This abnormal focusing produces an alteration in the refractive power of the eye that results in a visual acuity deficit. Box 29-2 provides more complete definitions.

Genetic and heritable conditions account for approximately half of the children with visual impairment in the United States. Cortical visual impairment, ROP, and optic nerve hypoplasia are the most prevalent conditions in preschool children. Amblyopia is usually a unilateral deficit in which there is defective development of the visual pathways needed to attain central vision. Clear focused images fail to reach the brain and result in reduced or permanent loss of vision. The condition is labeled (or typed) according to the structural or refractive problem that is causing the poor visual image to reach the brain: *deprivational,* or obstruction of vision (e.g., caused by ptosis, cataract, nystagmus), *strabismic* (caused by strabismus or lazy eye), or *refractive* (myopia, hyperopia, astigmatism, anisometropia).

Refractive errors are the most common visual disorders seen in children. Approximately 30% of preadolescent children have significant refractive errors. Myopia may be present at birth, but it is more likely to develop between 6 and 9 years old with increased prevalence after the adolescent growth spurt (Coats and Paysse, 2014a). Mild hyperopia is normal in a young child but should decrease rapidly between 7 and 14 years old. Amblyopia affects approximately 1% to 4% of children in the general population (Coats and Paysse, 2014b).

Definitions of varying degrees of visual impairment include:

- Legal blindness: Best corrected distance acuity in the better eye is less than 20/200, a visual field restriction in the better eye of less than 20 degrees, or both.
- Low vision: Corrected acuity is in the 20/70 to 20/200 range; these individuals generally meet requirements for special education.

Clinical Findings

- Squinting
- Fatigue
- Headaches (rare)
- Pain in or around eyes
- Dizziness
- Mild nausea
- Developmental delay
- Tendency to cover or close one eye when concentrating
- Family history of refractive errors, strabismus, or amblyopia

Management

- Refer to an ophthalmologist or optometrist for prescription corrective lenses. School-age children and teenagers should participate in the selection of frames; contact lenses may be considered. Extended-wear contact lenses may be prescribed in unilateral aphakia, severe anisometropia, corneal scarring with irregular astigmatism, and keratoconus.
- Once a refractive error has been determined or if a child is wearing glasses, an annual refraction and evaluation is recommended.
- Unilateral visual occlusion may be necessary, and occasionally surgery may be necessary.
- Support and reassurance according to the child's developmental level are needed during the period of adjustment to contact lenses or eyeglasses. Infants and toddlers

• BOX 29-2 Descriptive Terms for Refractive Errors

Myopia, or nearsightedness, exists when the axial length of the eye is increased in relation to the eye's optical power. As a result, light from a distant object is focused in front of the retina rather than directly on it. A myopic child sees close objects clearly, but distant objects are blurry.

Hyperopia, or farsightedness, exists when the visual image is focused behind the retina. As a result, distant objects are seen clearly, but close objects are blurry.

Astigmatism exists when the curvature of the cornea or the lens is uneven; thus the retina cannot appropriately focus light from an object regardless of the distance, which makes vision blurry close up and far away. Rarely, astigmatism can be caused by an alteration in the corneal sphere caused by a soft tissue mass on the inner aspect of the eyelid, such as a chalazion or hemangioma.

Anisometropia is a different refractive error in each eye. It may consist of any combination of refractive errors discussed earlier, or it may occur with aphakia.

need distraction with consistent replacement of glasses once removed. Verbal children may be aided by the use of positive reinforcement, such as sticker charts.
- Untreated or insufficiently treated amblyopia in young childhood results in irreversible and lifelong visual loss.

Strabismus

Strabismus is a defect in ocular alignment, or the position of the eyes in relation to each other; it is commonly called *lazy eye*. In strabismus, the visual axes are not parallel because the muscles of the eyes are not coordinated; when one eye is directed straight ahead, the other deviates. As a result, one or both eyes appear crossed. In children, strabismus may be manifested as a phoria or a tropia (Box 29-3). Pseudostrabismus is present when the sclera between the cornea and the inner canthus is obscured by closely placed eyes, a flat nasal bridge, or prominent epicanthal folds (see Fig. 29-3). In children older than 7 to 9 years old who have acquired tropia, double vision occurs. In those younger than 6 to 7 years old, cortical suppression of vision in the deviated eye results, which stops the diplopia but leads to amblyopia. Exo-deviations may be constant or intermittent—the intermittent type occurs more often. Both types of strabismus may be hereditary or the result of various eye diseases (e.g., neuroblastoma), trauma, systemic or neurologic dysfunction that paralyzes the extra ocular muscles, uncorrected hyperopia, craniofacial abnormalities, accommodation and accommodative convergence (Coats, 2014). Esotropia can also be seen in those with a history of prematurity, low birth weight, cerebral palsy, hydrocephalus, and maternal substance or tobacco use (AAO, 2012; Coats, 2014).

The incidence of ocular misalignments is approximately 1% to 6%, and each type varies by population (e.g., there are more exo-deviations in Japan and more eso-deviations in Ireland). Accommodative esotropia is most visible when the child is looking at a near object, occurs between 1 and 8 years old (average between 2 and 3 years old), and is seen in children with a history of acquired intermittent or constant crossing (AAO, 2012).

• BOX 29-3 Descriptive Terms for Strabismus

A **phoria** is an intermittent deviation in ocular alignment that is held latent by sensory fusion. The child can maintain alignment on an object.

A **tropia** is a consistent or intermittent deviation in ocular alignment. A child with a tropia is unable to maintain alignment on an object of fixation.

Phorias and tropias are classified according to the pattern of deviation seen:

- *Hyper-* (up) and *hypo-* (down) are used to classify vertical strabismus.
- *Exo-* (away from the nose) and *eso-* (toward the nose) describe horizontal deviations.
- *Cyclo-* describes a rotational or torsional deviation.

Variable alignment is common in the newborn. Most have straight eyes; up to 70% can exhibit transient exotropia, which should resolve by 6 months old, and 0.5% to 2% have esotropia. Up to 25% of esotropia that occurs between 3 and 6 months old resolves over time (AAO, 2012). Congenital esotropia is ascribed to an infant with an onset younger than 6 months old who did not have a deviation as a newborn. Accommodative esotropia is an inward deviation caused by high hyperopia (AAO, 2012).

Clinical Findings

- Intermittent exotropia in normal children 6 months to 4 years old who are ill or tired or when they are exposed to bright light or with sudden changes from close to distant vision. It is more often seen when the child is looking with distant fixation.
- When only one eye is affected, the child always fixates with the unaffected eye.
- When both eyes are affected, the eye that looks straight at any given time is the fixating eye.
- The angle of deviation may be inconsistent in all fields of gaze, actually changing in some forms of strabismus.
- Persistent squinting, head tilting, face turning, overpointing, awkwardness, marked decreased visual acuity in one eye, or nystagmus may be seen.
- Cataracts, retinoblastoma, anisometropia, and severe refractive errors are found infrequently.

Diagnostic Techniques

The corneal light reflection technique and the cover-uncover and alternating cover tests are used to screen for strabismus. Asymmetry of light reflection on the cornea is indicative of a deviation in ocular alignment. The cover-uncover test is used to detect tropias, whereas the alternating cover test detects phorias (see Fig. 29-3). The photoscreener can also be used to detect strabismus.

Management

- Any ocular misalignment seen after 4 months old is considered suspicious, and the child should be referred. Hypertropia or hypotropia, exotropia, acquired esotropia or exotropia, cyclovertical deviation, or any fixed deviation is an indication for referral as soon as it is first observed.
- The unaffected ("good") eye is occluded (using an adhesive bandage eyepatch, an occlusive contact lens, or an overplussed lens), which forces the child to use the deviating eye. Patching for 2 hours per day is as successful as patching 6 hours a day (DeSantis, 2014). Surgical alignment of the eyes may be necessary, but this does not preclude additional amblyopia therapy.
- Corrective lenses alone improve amblyopia in 27% of patients (DeSantis, 2014). Assessment for amblyopia should be done at every visit, even after straightening the eyes, because changes in alignment can occur through the fifth year.

- The ocular status of an affected child's siblings is monitored.
- Ophthalmologists may use local botulinum toxin injection with certain deviations.

Although response to treatment is more rapid in younger children, age should not be used as the deciding factor for referring a child with amblyopia. Typically change is minimal in children over 12 years old, but there have been reports of improvement with treatment even into adulthood (AAO, 2012).

Complications

Amblyopia (secondary visual loss) occurs in 30% to 50% of children with strabismus (Coats, 2014). Uncorrected strabismus can have a negative effect on self-esteem.

Blepharoptosis

Blepharoptosis or ptosis is drooping of the upper eyelids affecting one or both eyes. It can be congenital or acquired, secondary to trauma or inflammation. Congenital ptosis is caused by striated muscle fibers of the levator muscle being replaced by fibrous tissue. It can be transmitted as an autosomal dominant trait. Other possible etiologies include trauma to CN III during the birthing process, trauma to the eyelid or neck, chronic inflammation (particularly of the anterior segment of the eye), or a neurologic disorder (myasthenia gravis, botulism, muscular dystrophy). Parents may remark that one eye appears smaller. In severe cases, children may have a chin-up head position or adapt by raising their brow.

Management

- Refer to an ophthalmologist. If vision is compromised, surgery is performed in an effort to prevent amblyopia and developmental delay. Surgical correction depends on the degree of levator muscle compromise (AAO, 2012).
- Correct any underlying systemic disease.
- Evaluate for anisometropia (unequal refractive errors in each eye), anisocoria, and decrease in pupillary light reflex.

Nystagmus

Nystagmus is the presence of involuntary, rhythmic movements that may be pendular oscillations or jerky drifts of one or both eyes. Movement is horizontal, vertical, rotary, or mixed, and is classified as congenital or acquired. Congenital nystagmus is present between 6 weeks and 3 months old; acquired nystagmus occurs at a later age (AAPOS, 2014d). Nystagmus can occur in association with albinism, high refractive errors, CNS abnormalities, tumors, postinfection (e.g., coxsackievirus B, cytomegalovirus [CMV], *Haemophilus influenzae* meningitis), various diseases of the inner ear and the retina, middle ear trauma, visual loss before 2 years old, and pharmacologic toxicity. The child may have a birth history of prematurity, intraventricular hemorrhage, intrauterine psychogenic drug exposure, developmental delays, hydrocephaly, or be an infant of a mother with gestational diabetes. Nystagmus can be inherited, sometimes with a strong family history.

Clinical Findings

The clinician should closely observe the nystagmus and note as much as possible about the type of movement (up, down, sideways), frequency (number of oscillations per a time unit), distance of movement, field(s) of gaze within which the nystagmus is evident (e.g., field of gaze straight ahead, left, or up), and any compensatory head or neck postures of the child. The movements may be constant or varied, depending on the direction of gaze and head position. Latent nystagmus only manifests when one eye is covered (Coats, 2014). Oscillation of the newborn's eyes is common and exists for a short time during the neonatal period. Involuntary oscillation (opsoclonus) that persists or occurs beyond the initial weeks of life indicates a pathologic condition.

Management and Prognosis

Management consists of treating any underlying systemic disorder and referring the patient to an ophthalmologist. Any acquired nystagmus is most worrisome and requires prompt evaluation. Prognosis is varied, with sometimes only a slightly decreased acuity (20/50 or better) and other times severe disability (20/200) (AAPOS, 2014d).

Cataracts

Cataract, a partial or complete opacity of the lens affecting one or both eyes, is the most common cause of an abnormal pupillary reflex (Fig. 29-4). Some cataracts are considered clinically significant, others insignificant. They are categorized as congenital or acquired, and most commonly are

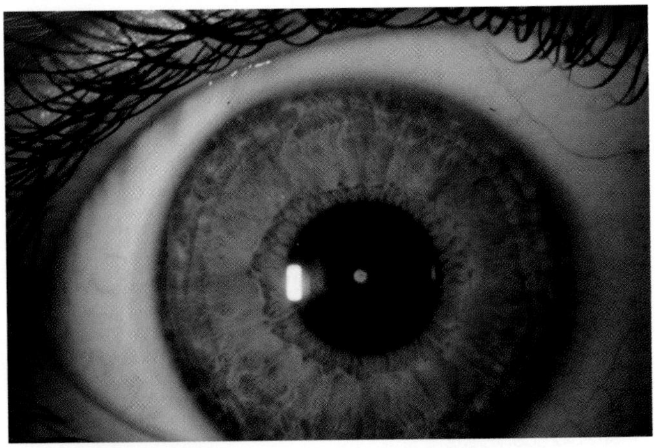

• **Figure 29-4** Anterior polar cataract. A small anterior polar cataract generally results in minimal visual deprivation, but is commonly associated with anisometropic amblyopia. (From Hoyt CS, Taylor D: *Pediatric ophthalmology and strabismus*, ed 4, Philadelphia, 2013, Elsevier/Saunders.)

isolated findings, not associated with other abnormalities (AAPOS, 2014a).

Cataracts may occur spontaneously or be genetic (e.g., Down syndrome, albinism). If there is a family history of cataracts, present in multiple family members, a referral to a geneticist is indicated. Cataracts can be the result of infection (e.g., congenital rubella, CMV, toxoplasmosis), trauma to the eye (including physical abuse, airbag deployment), metabolic disease (e.g., galactosemia, hypocalcemia), long-term use of systemic corticosteroids or ocular corticosteroid drops, prematurity, CNS anomalies (e.g., craniosynostosis, cranial defects), and demyelinating sclerosis and ataxia-telangiectasia. They may also be seen in children who have other ocular abnormalities, such as strabismus or pendular nystagmus, and in children with diabetes mellitus, atopic dermatitis, or Marfan syndrome.

The incidence of cataracts is approximately 3 out of 10,000 children, with a variable incidence worldwide (AAPOS, 2014a). Incidence rates vary between industrialized nations (lower) and undeveloped countries (believed to be higher) (Bashour et al, 2014).

Clinical Findings

- A history of maternal prenatal infection, drug exposure, or hypocalcemia may be elicited.
- Cataract appears as an opacity on the lens—unilateral or bilateral.
- Visual acuity deficits vary.
- A pale red reflex in people of color should not be confused with a cataract.

Management

Management depends on the size, density, and location of the cataract. Often congenital or infantile cataracts can be monitored over several years for a progression that could produce amblyopia; some types of cataracts do not progress. Surgical removal of the lens optically clears the visual axis. The resultant aphakic refractive error can be corrected with a permanent intraocular implant, the use of a contact lens, or glasses, although lenses are often very thick causing magnification and limitation of visual fields. Ophthalmic surgeons may insert an intraocular lens into the posterior chamber to partially correct aphakia, with residual refractive error corrected with spectacles.

Complications

Complications include amblyopia, which can be a particular challenge to treat; residual anisometropia; aniseikonia (unequal ocular image between eyes); or intraocular competition. Complications of surgery include infection, retinal detachment, glaucoma, displacement of the intraocular lens, or development of cloudiness.

Prognosis and Prevention

The ultimate degree of visual function depends on the cataract type, age at time of surgery, underlying disease(s), age of onset and duration, and presence of amblyopia or other ocular abnormalities. If the cataract is dense and present at birth, outcomes are better if removed within the first few weeks of life or before 2 months old. Visual outcomes are variable, with poorer results seen with congenital unilateral cataracts than with congenital incomplete bilateral cataracts. Children with histories of cataract surgery may exhibit later inflammatory sequelae, glaucoma, retinal detachment, secondary membranes, and orbital architectural distortions. Use of UV protectant sunglasses is essential in the prevention of cataract formation.

Glaucoma

Glaucoma is a disturbance in the circulation of aqueous fluid that results in an increase in IOP and subsequent damage to the optic nerve. It can be classified according to age at the time of its appearance and type of structural abnormality or other associated conditions. Congenital glaucoma is present at birth; infantile glaucoma develops in the first 1 to 2 years of life; juvenile glaucoma occurs after age 3. Most glaucoma has no identifiable cause and is considered primary. Secondary glaucoma is associated with another condition. Primary glaucoma occurs because of a congenital abnormality of the structures that drain the aqueous humor. Fortunately, it is rare and generally caught early. The incidence is approximately 1 in 10,000 live births in the United States (AAPOS, 2014c; Glaucoma Foundation, 2010).

Ten percent of cases are present at birth, and 80% are diagnosed by 12 months old. About 10% of primary cases are hereditary, and research is identifying gene mutations linked to glaucoma (AAPOS, 2014c; Glaucoma Foundation, 2010). It is also seen in association with dominantly inherited conditions, such as neurofibromatosis or aniridia; diffuse facial nevus flammeus (port-wine stain); Sturge-Weber, Marfan, Hurler, or Pierre Robin syndromes; intraocular hemorrhage; or intraocular tumor. There is a higher incidence in children with a history of cataract removal.

Secondary or juvenile glaucoma occurs when the drainage network for aqueous humor becomes obstructed after ocular infection, trauma, systemic disease, or long-term corticosteroid use.

Clinical Findings

Parents may report that something is unusual about their child's eyes. This occurs more often in unilateral glaucoma when the orbital size discrepancy is more noticeable. The clinician should then note the following symptoms of infantile glaucoma:

- "Classic triad" of tearing, photophobia, and excessive blinking or blepharospasm caused by irritation (only 30% of patients manifest this triad)
- Infants may turn away from light
- Hazy corneas
- Corneal edema

Corneal and ocular enlargements are common in infants and young children. Bulbar conjunctival erythema and visual impairment may occur. If the condition is bilateral, parents may not notice any difference in the size of the corneas.

Symptoms of secondary glaucoma include the following:
- Extreme pain, vomiting
- Blurred or lost vision
- Tunnel vision
- Pupillary dilation
- Erythema (often in only one eye)
- Change in configuration of optic nerve cupping with asymmetry between the eyes and loss of vision over time

Management

Early diagnosis is important. The goal is normalization of IOP and prevention of optic nerve damage along with correction of associated refractive errors and prevention of amblyopia.
- Prompt recognitions and referral to an ophthalmologist. Primary treatment is surgery as early as possible (often multiple surgeries are required). Medications may be used as part of the medical management; drug therapy may be difficult as a result of its prolonged nature, drug side effects, and adverse system effects.
- Parent and patient education must emphasize the importance of medication compliance and discourage excessive physical or emotional stress and straining during defecation.
- A medical identification tag should be worn at all times.
- Follow-up is for life, often every 3 to 6 months.
- Ophthalmoscopic examination (including tonometry) is needed for every member of the family.

Complications and Prognosis

Myopia, amblyopia, and strabismus are not uncommon in these children. Additionally, permanent vision loss secondary to stretching of the cornea and sclera with resultant scarring and glaucomatous optic nerve damage can also occur. Eighty percent to 90% of infants who receive prompt surgery and long-term monitoring will do well, but blindness occurs in 2% to 15% of childhood patients (Glaucoma Foundation, 2010).

Retinopathy of Prematurity

ROP is a multifactorial retinal vascular pathologic disease primarily caused by early gestational age with low birth weight. It involves the abnormal growth of the retinal vessels in incompletely vascularized retinas of premature infants. Previously ROP was called *retrolental fibroplasia*. An international classification system provides guidance for understanding this disease and for predicting outcome. ROP is classified according to the distance to which the vascularization has progressed away from the optic nerve (zone I, II, or III), severity of inflammatory changes (stage), duration (clock hours), extent of disease, presence of plus disease (degree of large vessel engorgement and tortuosity), scarring patterns, prethreshold and threshold ROP (a clinical subclassification system), and presence of Rush disease (rapidly progressing ROP, especially posterior retina) (Jordan, 2014).

Developing retinal vessels grow outward from the optic nerve. The immature and incompletely vascularized retina is in a state of hypoxia, which stimulates the production of vascular endothelial growth factor (VEGF). Requisite levels of VEGF are needed to maintain the integrity of and stimulate retinal vessel growth. Exposure to supplemental oxygen presents an additional risk factor. Higher oxygen concentrations produce lower VEGF levels and result in slowed vessel growth. Over several weeks, an avascular retina becomes ischemic, and, in turn, stimulates renewed VEGF production. The increase in VEGF stimulates vessel growth but not necessarily in an ordered manner. Multiple studies have established a target oxygen saturation of 90% to 95% to lower the risk of ROP and have the lowest patient morbidity and mortality (Jordan, 2014). ROP occurs primarily in premature infants born at or less than 28 weeks of gestation or weighing less than 1500 g. The overall incidence of ROP in all newborns is 0.14% (Jordan, 2014) with incidence inversely proportional to weight. The risk in infants under 1250 g is approximately 50% (Bashour et al, 2014). Other risk factors for ROP in premature infants include poor weight gain, dopamine-resistant hypotension, white race, hyperglycemia, insulin treatment, corticosteroid treatment, and insufficient intake of docosahexaenoic acid (Jordan, 2014). Hypoxia, hemolytic disease, necrotizing enterocolitis, maternal preeclampsia, breast milk, and adequate intake of lipids and calories may protect against developing ROP (Jordan, 2014).

Clinical Findings

ROP is initially diagnosed by a pediatric ophthalmologist while the infant is in the nursery (at 32 to 44 weeks postconception). Once the baby is discharged, the following may be seen:
- Leukokoria (white fibrovascular tissue in the retrolental space), glaucoma, cataracts
- Pupillary rigidity
- Vitreous haziness, hemorrhage
- Retinal and iris changes
- Pallor of optic nerve
- Strabismus
- Cataracts
- Detached retinas (often with secondary glaucoma, entropion, and eye infections)

An infant (especially if full or near term) not previously diagnosed with ROP with detached retinas or leukokoria needs an ophthalmologic evaluation to rule out genetic disorders (e.g., Norrie syndrome, familial exudative vitreoretinopathy [X-linked recessive]).

Management

ROP progresses at variable rates. Initial ophthalmologic examinations should be done on all infants born at less than 30 weeks' gestation or weighing 1500 g or less or those born at more than 1500 g or 29 to 34 weeks with an unstable course during hospitalization (Jordan, 2014). Examinations should occur at 31 to 32 weeks of postconceptual or postmenstrual age or 4 to 6 weeks of chronologic age; any vitreoretinal sequelae need to be followed throughout life (Jordan, 2014). The PCP's role in managing ROP is to ensure that all infants fitting these criteria (even in those whose ROP resolved or who did not have ROP) receive the initial and follow-up ophthalmologic examinations (within 2 weeks or less after discharge) by a specialist experienced in examining preterm infants. The PCP further needs to:

- Discuss with parents the implications of their child's disease.
- Monitor for late sequelae or ROP progression (e.g., strabismus, pseudostrabismus, amblyopia, myopia, anisometropia, leukokoria, and cataracts).
- Assist children who have sequelae to maximize their potential by referring to early intervention services for low-vision children, to low-vision community support services, and to family support groups.
- Refer all children for yearly ophthalmologic follow-up if ROP required any treatment (even if ROP has resolved completely); less frequent follow-up is needed if no treatment was needed.

Cryosurgery or laser photocoagulation is used to arrest the progression of abnormally growing blood vessels; laser is treatment of choice (Jordan, 2014). Off-label use of the intravitreal VEGF inhibitor bevacizumab (Avastin) has been used successfully in treatment of zone I stage 3 ROP and may be used in conjunction with laser treatment (Jordan, 2014).

Complications

Complications can arise secondary to ROP or the treatment. Retinal detachment, strabismus, amblyopia, cataracts, serious myopia, nystagmus, astigmatism, anisometropia, uveitis, hyphema, macular burns, occlusion of the central retinal artery, glaucoma, and cicatrix (residual retinal scars) leading to later vision loss are possible (Jordan, 2014).

Prevention

Minimizing or preventing ROP can be accomplished by decreasing the occurrence of premature births and closely monitoring the oxygen needed to keep oxygen saturation at 90% to 95%.

Retinoblastoma

Retinoblastoma is an intraocular tumor that develops in the retina. Although it is rare, this malignant tumor of the retina is the most common tumor in childhood (3% to 4% of cancers in children younger than 15 years old) (National Cancer Institute, 2014; U.S. National Library of Medicine [NLM], 2009). Approximately 300 children per year are diagnosed in the United States and Canada, and 6000 children worldwide (AAPOS, 2014e). Age-adjusted incidence is 1 in 14,000 to 18,000 live births with two-thirds diagnosed before 2 years old, and 95% diagnosed before 5 years old (National Cancer Institute, 2014). A single or multiple tumors may be found in one or both eyes. Most children have unilateral tumors, but one in three will have bilateral tumors (NLM, 2014).

Hereditary and nonhereditary forms occur, and carrier and prenatal diagnosis is possible. Mutation of the *RB1* gene occurs in hereditary retinoblastoma (40%) and is known as *germinal retinoblastoma.* A small percentage have deletion on the q14 band of chromosome 13, and these children often have intellectual disability, slow growth, and distinctive facial features (prominent eyebrow, short nose and broad nasal bridge, ear abnormalities). All bilateral disease is considered hereditary, whereas only 15% of unilateral is non-germinal (nonhereditary). Retinoblastoma occurs 60% of the time and is usually unilateral (National Cancer Institute, 2014; NLM, 2009). There is some evidence that human papillomavirus (HPV) contributes to retinoblastoma development in children in developing countries, with HPV 16 and HPV 18 both contributing to the development of retinoblastoma in children in India (Anand et al, 2011; Shetty et al, 2012).

The diagnosis of retinoblastoma in developing countries can be delayed and the care suboptimal due to poor education, lower socioeconomic conditions, and inadequate access to health care. The extra ocular spread of retinoblastoma due to delayed diagnosis makes the possibility of death a real concern in developing countries.

Clinical Findings

- Positive family history
- Strabismus is the most common finding.
- Unilateral or bilateral white pupil (leukokoria), described often as an intermittent "glow, glint, gleam, or glare" by parents, usually in low-light settings or noted in photographs taken with a flash also called *cat's eye reflex*
- Decreased visual acuity
- Abnormal red reflex, nystagmus, glaucoma, orbital cellulitis and photophobia (causes pain), hyphema, hypopyon (pus in anterior chamber of eye), or signs of global rupture possible

Diagnosis is made via CT scan with contrast and/or echography and/or MRI. Other tests may include fundus photography, fluorescein angiography, ocular ultrasonography, or fine-needle aspiration.

Management

Refer the patient to an ophthalmologist for diagnosis and management by a multidisciplinary team. An international classification system for intraocular retinoblastoma lists the criteria of tumors based on their size, location, number, and degree of invasiveness or seeding. Depending on the diagnosis, treatment may involve external beam radiation, cryotherapy, laser photocoagulation, episcleral plaque brachytherapy, or systemic chemotherapy. Early detection and advances in treatment have led to less enucleation and less use of external beam radiation, preserving sight. In those with advanced tumors requiring enucleation, the hydroxyapatite implant provides excellent cosmetic appearance and acceptable motility of the implant. Siblings and parents should receive a referral for examination of the fundi and genetic testing and counseling.

Frequent follow-up (every 2 to 4 months for at least 28 months or until 5 years old if heritable form) to assess treatment and monitor for recurrence is important. Close to half of children will develop new or recurrent ocular tumors that require further treatment.

Complications and Prognosis

Retinoblastoma has a high cure rate (95%) with unilateral retinoblastoma having the best prognosis (AAPOS, 2014e). Children with germinal retinoblastoma have increased risk of other cancers outside the eye. These subsequent neoplasms are the most common cause of death, contributing to more than 50% of deaths for children with bilateral disease. Most commonly these are pinealoma, osteosarcoma, cancers of the soft tissues, and melanoma (National Cancer Institute, 2014; NLM, 2009). Those who survive are at high risk for cataracts, vitreous hemorrhage, neovascular glaucoma, lacrimal duct or gland injury, impaired orbit bone growth, radiation retinopathy, optic neuropathy, or bone marrow suppression. Late effects of retinoblastoma therapy include diminished orbital growth, visual-field deficits, and hearing loss.

Infections

Conjunctivitis

An estimated 6 million cases of bacterial conjunctivitis occur in the United States annually, at an estimated cost of $377 million to $857 million (Azari and Barney, 2013). Conjunctivitis is an inflammation of the palpebral and occasionally the bulbar conjunctiva (Fig. 29-5). It is the most frequently seen ocular disorder in pediatric practice. In pediatric patients, bacteria are the most common cause of infection (50% to 75%) most commonly from December to April. Pathogens include *H. influenzae, Streptococcus pneumoniae,* and *Moraxella* species with both gram-negative and gram-positive organisms implicated (Azari and Barney, 2013).

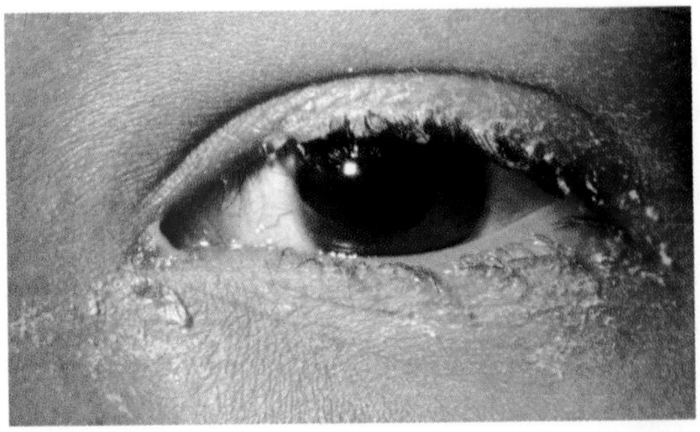

• **Figure 29-5** Bacterial conjunctivitis. (From Palay DA, Krachmer JH: *Primary care ophthalmology*, ed 2, Philadelphia, 2005, Mosby.)

Conjunctivitis also occurs as a viral or fungal infection or as a response to allergens or chemical irritants. Bacterial conjunctivitis is often unilateral, whereas viral conjunctivitis is most often bilateral. Unilateral disease can also suggest a toxic, chemical, mechanical, or lacrimal cause. Blockage of the tear drainage system (e.g., from meibomianitis or blepharitis), injury, foreign body, abrasion or ulcers, keratitis, iritis, herpes simplex virus (HSV), and infantile glaucoma are other known causes. Patient age is a major indicator of etiology (Table 29-6).

Conjunctivitis in the Newborn (Ophthalmia Neonatorum)

Conjunctivitis in the newborn, also known as *ophthalmia neonatorum* or *neonatal blennorrhea,* is a form of conjunctivitis that occurs in the first month of life. In most states, conjunctivitis of the newborn is a reportable infectious disease. It occurs in 0.3% to 11% of newborns. A common cause is chemical conjunctivitis from the prophylactic instillation of silver nitrate at birth, which is one reason the product is no longer recommended. *Chlamydia trachomatis* is the most common cause of ophthalmia neonatorum, and 50% of newborns with a mother positive for *C. trachomatis* at the time of delivery will contract the disease (AAP, 2012a). Various bacteria account for 30% to 50% of cases *(Staphylococcus, Streptococcus, Pseudomonas, H. influenzae, Escherichia coli, Corynebacterium* species, *Moraxella catarrhalis, Klebsiella pneumoniae, Pseudomonas aeruginosa). Neisseria gonorrhoeae* and HSV are also seen (AAP, 2012a). Gonococcal conjunctivitis is the most serious cause of ophthalmia neonatorum owing to concerns of the bacteria causing blindness (AAP, 2012a).

Clinical Findings

History and Physical Examination.

- Chemical conjunctivitis usually occurs in the first 24 to 72 hours of life.
- Septic conjunctivitis caused by:
  - Bacteria usually occurs from 5 to 14 days of life.
  - *C. trachomatis* usually begins between 5 to 14 days of life; it can also occur in newborns born via cesarean section with intact membranes.
  - *N. gonorrhoeae* usually appears in the first 3 to 5 days of life (up to 29 days).
  - HSV presents at birth or in the first 4 weeks of life.

Symptoms most commonly seen include the following:

- Chemical-induced conjunctivitis frequently manifests as nonpurulent discharge and edematous bulbar and palpebral conjunctiva.
- *C. trachomatis* specifically causes moderate eyelid swelling and palpebral or bulbar conjunctival injection and moderate thick, purulent discharge.
- *N. gonorrhoeae* specifically causes acute conjunctival inflammation, lid edema, erythema, and excessive, purulent discharge.
- Bacteria present with conjunctival erythema, purulent discharge.

TABLE 29-6 Types of Conjunctivitis

Type	Incidence/Etiology	Clinical Findings	Diagnosis	Management*
Ophthalmia neonatorum	Neonates: *Chlamydia trachomatis, Staphylococcus aureus, Neisseria gonorrhoeae,* HSV (silver nitrate reaction occurs in 10% of neonates)	Erythema, chemosis, purulent exudate with *N. gonorrhoeae*; clear to mucoid exudate with chlamydia	Culture (ELISA, PCR), Gram stain, R/O *N. gonorrhoeae,* chlamydia	Saline irrigation to eyes until exudate gone; follow with erythromycin ointment For *N. gonorrhoeae:* ceftriaxone or IM or IV For chlamydia: erythromycin or possibly azithromycin PO For HSV: antivirals IV or PO
Bacterial conjunctivitis	In neonates 5 to 14 days old, preschoolers, and sexually active teens: *Haemophilus influenzae* (nontypeable), *Streptococcus pneumoniae, S. aureus, N. gonorrhoeae*	Erythema, chemosis, itching, burning, mucopurulent exudate, matter in eyelashes; ↑ in winter	Cultures (required in neonate); Gram stain (optional); chocolate agar (for *N. gonorrhoeae*) R/O pharyngitis, *N. gonorrhoeae*, AOM, URI, seborrhea	Neonates: Erythromycin 0.5% ophthalmic ointment ≥1 year old: Fourth-generation fluoroquinolone For concurrent AOM: Treat accordingly for AOM Warm soaks to eyes three times a day until clear No sharing towels, pillows No school until treatment begins
Chronic bacterial conjunctivitis (unresponsive conjunctivitis previously treated as bacterial in etiology)	School-age children and teens: Bacteria, viruses, *C. trachomatis*	Same as above; foreign body sensation	Cultures, Gram stain; R/O dacryostenosis, blepharitis, corneal ulcers, trachoma	Depends on prior treatment, laboratory results, and differential diagnoses Review compliance and prior drug choices of conjunctivitis treatment Consult with ophthalmologist
Inclusion conjunctivitis	Neonates 5 to 14 days old and sexually active teens: *C. trachomatis*	Erythema, chemosis, clear or mucoid exudate, palpebral follicles	Cultures (ELISA, PCR), R/O sexual activity	Neonates: Erythromycin or azithromycin PO Adolescents: Doxycycline, azithromycin, EES, erythromycin base, levofloxacin PO
Viral conjunctivitis	Adenovirus 3, 4, 7; HSV, herpes zoster, varicella	Erythema, chemosis, tearing (bilateral); HSV and herpes zoster: unilateral with photophobia, fever; zoster: nose lesion; spring and fall	Cultures, R/O corneal infiltration	Refer to ophthalmologist if HSV or photophobia present Cool compresses three or four times a day
Allergic and vernal conjunctivitis	Atopy sufferers, seasonal	Stringy, mucoid exudate, swollen eyelids and conjunctivae, itching (key finding), tearing, palpebral follicles, headache, rhinitis	Eosinophils in conjunctival scrapings	Naphazoline/pheniramine, naphazoline/antazoline ophthalmic solution (see text) Mast cell stabilizer (see text) Refer to allergist if needed

AOM, Acute otitis media; *EES,* erythromycin ethylsuccinate; *ELISA,* enzyme-linked immunosorbent assay; *HSV,* herpes simplex virus; *IM,* intramuscular; *IV,* intravenous; *PCR,* polymerase chain reaction; *PO,* (by mouth, orally); *R/O,* rule out; *URI,* upper respiratory infection.
*See text for dosages.

- HSV specifically causes mild conjunctivitis, erythema, corneal opacity, serosanguineous discharge, and vesicular rash on eyelids and is often unilateral.

There may be a maternal history of vaginal infection during pregnancy or current sexually transmitted infection (STI).

Diagnostic Studies. Swabs and scrapings must be done. Gram and Giemsa staining, direct immunofluorescent monoclonal antibody staining, cultures, enzyme-linked immunosorbent assay (ELISA), or polymerase chain reaction (PCR) testing can be used. Any infant younger than 2 weeks old should be tested for gonorrhea. A culture for gonorrhea (on chocolate agar or Thayer-Martin medium) or aggressive scraping for a Gram stain is used for diagnosis. (Do not just sample the purulent discharge.) If gonorrhea is suspected, also check for *C. trachomatis.*

Management

- Irrigate the eyes with sterile normal saline until clear of exudate.
- Gonococcal conjunctivitis: In the newborn, gonococcal conjunctivitis requires intramuscular (IM) ceftriaxone given once (AAP, 2012b). If there are extra ocular manifestations, a 7-day course of IM or IV ceftriaxone is warranted. Ceftriaxone is not given to neonates with hyperbilirubinemia; cefotaxime is an alternative (AAP, 2012b). Ocular morbidity (corneal infection with possible scarring or perforation) can result if infection is missed.
- Nongonococcal conjunctivitis: A topical ophthalmic antibiotic preparation, such as erythromycin 0.5% ointment or moxifloxacin, is indicated (AAP, 2012c). The eyes should be cleansed with water or saline applied to cotton balls before instilling the ointment into the lower conjunctival sac.
- Herpes simplex conjunctivitis: Immediate referral for hospitalization and topical and systemic antivirals are needed. Spread of virus to the CNS, mouth, and skin is of concern.
- *Chlamydia:* Assess for systemic infection (pharyngitis, ear infection, pneumonia). Chlamydial conjunctivitis is treated with systemic erythromycin (AAP, 2012c). A short course of azithromycin may also be effective (AAP, 2012c). Topical treatment is not indicated because it does not lower the risk for a subsequent pneumonia caused by *Chlamydia* (see Inclusion Conjunctivitis in the next section).
- Chemical-induced conjunctivitis resolves spontaneously within 3 to 4 days without specific treatment.
- Mothers and their sexual partners should receive treatment if gonococcal and/or chlamydial infections occur in their newborns.

Prevention

To prevent ophthalmia neonatorum, the CDC and the USPSTF recommend prophylactic administration of antibiotic eye medication within 1 hour of vaginal delivery or delivery via cesarean (CDC, 2011; USPSTF, 2011). The recommended antibiotic is erythromycin ointment 0.5% (0.25- to 0.5-inch strip to each eye). Prophylaxis is required by law in most states and territories to prevent gonococcal conjunctivitis in the newborn. However, prophylaxis does not prevent neonatal chlamydial conjunctivitis or extra ocular infection. It should be determined at the time of the first visit whether infants born at home have received this prophylaxis.

Inclusion Conjunctivitis (Chlamydia)

Inclusion conjunctivitis is usually caused by one of eight known strains of *C. trachomatis* and is most often seen in a neonate or sexually active adolescent. Neonates usually demonstrate symptoms within the first 5 to 14 days of life (to 6 weeks), whereas *N. gonorrhoeae* symptoms are usually detected earlier. Nasopharyngeal infection with *C. trachomatis* is found in 50% of infants with inclusion conjunctivitis, whereas 54% of men and 74% of women have genital chlamydial infection (Azari and Barney, 2013).

Clinical Findings

History and Physical Examination.

- Maternal history of an STI or a history of a sexual partner with an STI
- Conjunctival erythema and mild to severe mucopurulent to bloody discharge, usually bilateral
- Follicular reaction (large, round elevations) in the conjunctiva of the lower eyelids; conjunctiva may bleed if stroked
- Associated cervicitis, urethritis, or rectal infection

Infants may have symptoms suggestive of chlamydial pneumonia at 1 to 3 months old.

Diagnostic Studies. Definitive diagnosis of *Chlamydia* can be made by isolating the organism by tissue culture and by performing a nucleic acid amplification test (NAAT) (AAP, 2012c). Conjunctival scrapings for Giemsa staining are indicated. Scrapings must contain epithelial cells because *Chlamydia* is an obligate intracellular organism (AAP, 2012c). Other nonculture tests for *Chlamydia* include direct fluorescent antibody (DFA) and enzyme immunoassay (EIA). A specimen should also be gathered appropriately to test for gonorrhea because of the comorbidity of these two organisms. Ocular morbidity can result if gonorrhea is missed (refer to Chapter 32 for guidance on pneumonia caused by *C. trachomatis*).

Management

Systemic therapy is required for treatment of conjunctivitis caused by *C. trachomatis* due to high incidence of concurrent nasopharynx, lung, and genital tract infections in infants and genital infections in adolescents (Azari and Barney, 2013). Treatment options have expanded from the traditional use of oral erythromycin ethylsuccinate (EES) to other macrolides, azithromycin, and clarithromycin. There is an increased incidence of idiopathic hypertrophic pyloric stenosis (IHPS) in infants younger than 6 weeks old following systemic EES. However, this has not altered the recommendation of EES as the preferred treatment. The risk of using azithromycin and clarithromycin has not been fully established, although there have been reports of IHPS after the use of azithromycin (AAP, 2012c). Medical providers who treat newborns with EES should discuss the signs and potential risks of developing IHPS with parents.

Treatment recommendations include:

- A 14-day course of oral EES. Sometimes a second 14-day course is required because the failure rate with EES is 10% to 20%. EES may be repeated, or oral azithromycin is also found effective (AAP, 2012c). Providers are encouraged to use systemic EES with caution; if no other

alternatives are viable, they need to have a high index of suspicion for the development of IHPS.
- Trimethoprim-sulfamethoxazole (TMP-SMX is an alternative systemic treatment after the neonatal period (AAP, 2012a), and azithromycin and clarithromycin have been used, although they are not FDA approved in this age group.
- Doxycycline, adeletezithromycin, ofloxacin, or levofloxacin can be used in young adults.
- Topical ointment (erythromycin, moxifloxacin) is sometimes recommended despite systemic drug treatment; the AAP notes that such concurrent treatment is unnecessary and ineffective (AAP, 2012c).
- Mothers of infants with *C. trachomatis* conjunctivitis, partners of such mothers, and partners of sexually active adolescents also need examinations and treatment for 2 weeks with tetracycline or erythromycin.

Complications

Complications include chlamydial pneumonia (5% to 20% of infants will develop pneumonia if their mother has a chlamydial infection at delivery), nasopharyngeal colonization (in up to 50% of infants treated for inclusion conjunctivitis), or gastroenteritis in infants (AAP, 2012c). Complications may occur 6 to 8 weeks following the conjunctivitis.

Bacterial Conjunctivitis

Acute bacterial conjunctivitis (commonly called *pinkeye*) is a contagious and easily spread disease. *H. influenzae* is the most common organism isolated in children who are younger than 7 years old (Azari and Barney, 2013). *S. pneumoniae, M. catarrhalis,* and adenovirus are also common pathogens. It is most common in the winter and in toddlers and preschoolers (see Fig. 29-5).

Clinical Findings

- Erythema of one or both eyes, usually starting unilaterally and becoming bilateral (key finding)
- Yellow-green purulent discharge (key finding)
- Encrusted and matted eyelids on awakening (key finding)
- Burning, stinging, or itching of the eyes and a feeling of a foreign body
- Photophobia
- Petechiae on bulbar conjunctiva
- Symptoms of upper respiratory infection, otitis media, or acute pharyngitis
- Vision screen should be normal and documented in the patient's record

Diagnostic Studies. Routine culture testing is *not necessary*. Gram stain and culture can be done if the conjunctivitis is chronic, recurrent, or difficult to treat. An in-office rapid antigen test with high sensitivity and specificity for adenovirus is available and may be warranted to decrease inappropriate prescribing of antibiotics for viral conjunctivitis.

Differential Diagnosis. Bacterial conjunctivitis requires consideration of nasolacrimal duct obstruction in infants, ear infection, Kawasaki syndrome, foreign body, corneal abrasion, uveitis, herpetic conjunctivitis, poor compliance, or wrong choice of drug. Cultures or scrapings are appropriate for unresolved infection.

Management

Bacterial conjunctivitis is considered a self-limited disease (unless caused by gonorrhea or *Chlamydia*) that usually resolves within 8 to 10 days. However, because both gram-negative and gram-positive organisms have been implicated, children who receive topical antibiotics demonstrate faster clinical improvement, can return to day care or school faster, and cause less parental work loss. The common practice of prescribing antibiotics for conjunctivitis, however, has led to an increasing rate of drug resistance. It is imperative that providers make their diagnosis judiciously and then treat with an effective drug that is more likely to be tolerated and taken as directed. For this reason, older children and teens may be treated conservatively without using antibiotics. This prevents the overuse of antibiotics and takes into consideration the self-limited nature of this disease.

Choose broad-spectrum coverage that has the lowest resistance rate, greatest compliance, and best penetration of tissues. The cost of ophthalmic antibiotics varies significantly. If patients have a large copayment for brand-name drugs or if they lack paid drug coverage, cost should be factored in when prescribing for this self-limited disease.

Parents can be instructed to put pressure over the lacrimal duct when instilling the medication to prevent drainage into the nasolacrimal system. If improvement is not seen in 3 days after treatment is initiated, refer to or consult as appropriate with an ophthalmologist. Contacts should not be worn during conjunctivitis treatment. Disposable lenses should be discarded and permanent contacts sterilized before reinserting.

For uncomplicated bacterial conjunctivitis, treatment includes (Azari and Barney, 2013):
- Sodium sulfacetamide 10% ophthalmic solution or ointment; not effective against *H. influenzae;* stings; can cause allergic reactions (including Stevens-Johnson syndrome).
- Trimethoprim sulfate plus polymyxin B sulfate ophthalmic solution for 5 to 7 days.
- Erythromycin 0.5% ophthalmic ointment is recommended for patients with sulfa allergy and for infants for 7 days.
- Azithromycin drops for children older than 12 months for 5 days.
- Fluoroquinolone ophthalmic drops including besifloxacin, ciprofloxacin, gatifloxacin, levofloxacin, moxifloxacin, or ofloxacin may be prescribed for children older than 12 months for 5 to 7 days (regimens vary by medication).

The aminoglycosides (neomycin, tobramycin, gentamicin) are to be avoided because of possible hypersensitization, severe allergic reactions, and increasing resistance.

Conjunctivitis-Otitis Syndrome. This syndrome is usually caused by *H. influenzae*. Treat for the otitis media (see Chapter 30). Concurrent use of a topical antibiotic is not necessary.

Patient Education

If only one eye is involved, it is likely that the infection will spread within a day or two to involve both eyes. The patient (or parent) is instructed to do the following:

- Cleanse the eyelashes several times a day with a weak solution of no-tears shampoo and warm water. The importance of wiping from the inner canthus outward and using a different cloth or cotton ball for each eye should be emphasized.
- Use warm soaks three or four times a day to relieve itching and burning.
- Instill the prescribed ophthalmic solution or ointment into the lower conjunctival sac. A moistened cotton swab may be used to facilitate instillation of ointments. Dosing while the child is sleeping greatly increases compliance and, therefore, effectiveness.
- Wash hands frequently and avoid shared linens to limit spread of the infection.

Also treat seborrheic dermatitis on the scalp and face if present (refer to Chapter 37 for treatment recommendations). Day care center exclusion policies vary. (Some allow return once the treatment is started, while others allow return only after completing 1 to 2 days of treatment.) Improvement in the child's condition should be seen within 48 hours. If medication compliance is not in question and improvement is not seen within 72 hours of administration, the parent should be instructed to return so that a smear of the exudate can be taken for culture and sensitivity testing.

Complications

If the infection proves recalcitrant to treatment, eye pain is present, vision is blurred, or ophthalmoscopic examination reveals a bulging iris and a contracted, fixed pupil, suspect more serious inflammation of the uveal tract (iritis, cyclitis, or choroiditis). Refer immediately to an ophthalmologist to avoid ocular morbidity.

Viral Conjunctivitis

Viral conjunctivitis is usually caused by an adenovirus but can also be caused by herpes simplex, herpes zoster, enterovirus, molluscum contagiosum, or varicella virus. It is more common in children older than 6 years old and in the spring and fall (see Table 29-6). In-office testing is available for adenovirus, which can cause up to 80% of acute conjunctivitis cases (Azari and Barney, 2013).

Clinical Findings

- Tearing and profuse clear, watery discharge (key findings)
- Fever, headache, anorexia, malaise, upper respiratory symptoms (pharyngitis-conjunctivitis-fever triad with adenovirus [key findings])
- Pharyngitis with enlarged preauricular nodes (key findings)
- Itchy, red, and swollen conjunctiva
- Hyperemia and swollen eyelids
- Photophobia with measles or varicella rashes
- Herpetic vesicles on the eyelid margins and eyelashes (marginal blepharitis) or on the conjunctiva and cornea (keratoconjunctivitis)

Management

- Good hygiene is essential. Viral conjunctivitis is self-limited and should resolve in 7 to 14 days. Conjunctivitis is often difficult to distinguish from keratitis. If there is any question about diagnosis, refer for ophthalmologic assessment.
- Warm or cold compresses and artificial tears can be used.
- Prophylaxis with antibiotics is not recommended.
- Antihistamine or vasoconstrictive ophthalmic solutions may be used for symptomatic relief.
- If HSV infection is suspected, immediate referral to an ophthalmologist is indicated. Topical corticosteroids should be avoided because they may worsen the course.
- Molluscum on the eyelid margins requires referral for excision.

Conjunctivitis-Pharyngitis Syndrome. This syndrome is more likely to be caused by adenovirus than by a bacterium. Treat accordingly.

Complications

Involvement of deeper layers of the cornea (keratitis) can occur and must be differentiated from conjunctivitis. Scarring of the cornea resulting in blindness is a significant complication of HSV infection. If in any doubt, refer to an ophthalmologist for a slit-lamp examination.

Allergic Conjunctivitis

Allergic conjunctivitis usually occurs in childhood but can occur after adolescence (Fig. 29-6). Four types of allergic conjunctivitis have been identified:

- Hay fever–associated conjunctivitis is characterized by mild injection and swelling and is associated with exposing the eyes to environmental allergens (dust, grass, molds, animal dander) and may be associated with generalized allergic reaction including nasal congestion.
- Vernal conjunctivitis is more severe, with peak incidence in 10- to 12-year-olds, occurs in boys at twice the

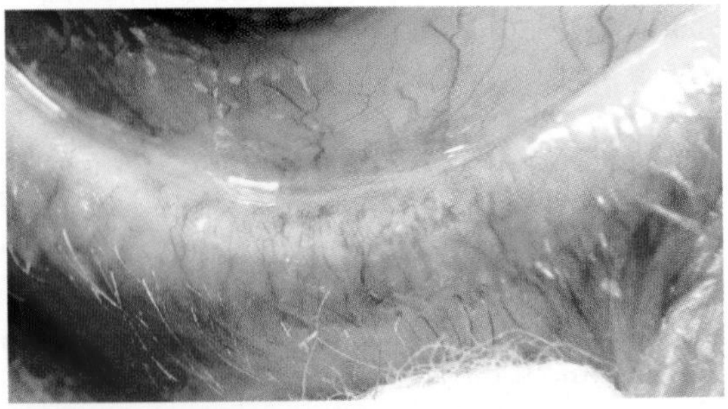

• **Figure 29-6** Allergic conjunctivitis. (From Palay DA, Krachmer JH: *Primary care ophthalmology*, ed 2, Philadelphia, 2005, Mosby.)

rate of girls, and has an increased prevalence in warm weather.

- Atopic keratoconjunctivitis occurs in those with atopic dermatitis and/or asthma, affecting the lower tarsal conjunctiva, usually occurring in late adolescence, and is notable for significant (beyond that seen in allergic conjunctivitis) itching, burning, and tearing that is often chronic.
- Giant papillary conjunctivitis occurs most often in contact lens wearers, occurring 10 times more frequently in those wearing soft contacts than hard contacts.

Seasonal allergens (notably grass pollens and ragweed) cause 90% of allergic conjunctivitis in the United States (Azari and Barney, 2013). Rhinitis, eczema, and asthma may be associated conditions. The incidence is up to 40% of the general population and is experienced by approximately 32% of atopic children (Azari and Barney, 2013).

Clinical Findings

- Severe itching and tearing (key findings)
- Family history of atopy or seasonal allergies
- Rhinitis, eczema, asthma
- Acute attacks precipitated by allergens (e.g., pollen, animals, molds, dust, dust mites, occasionally food)
- Redness and swelling of the conjunctiva or eyelid (or both)
- Follicular reaction of the conjunctiva
- Stringy, mucoid discharge
- Bilateral involvement most common
- Cobblestone papillary hypertrophy in the tarsal conjunctiva
- Vision screening should be normal; document in patient's record

Diagnostic Studies. Conjunctival or nasal smears (using Wright stain) reveal numerous eosinophils.

Management

- Prevention is best; avoid allergens.
- For mild cases, saline solution or artificial tears are administered along with cool compresses. Refrigerated eye drops are more soothing.
- Topical decongestants, oral or topical antihistamines, topical mast cell stabilizers, or topical NSAIDs may be used (Azari and Barney, 2013). The decongestants do not decrease the allergic response, but do relieve erythema, injection, and lid edema. Prescribed agents can provide quicker, more long-term relief with fewer side effects than over-the-counter agents. Vasoconstrictors should be avoided because of rebound hyperemia (Azari and Barney, 2013). Patients may be treated with systemic antihistamines (fexofenadine, loratadine, or cetirizine) if systemic symptoms are present (see Chapter 25 for management of allergies).
  - Topical decongestants like naphazoline hydrochloride ophthalmic solution
  - A combination antihistamine-decongestant is more effective than either agent alone; naphazoline hydrochloride plus antazoline ophthalmic solution can be used sparingly to reduce ocular congestion, irritation, and itching.
- Topical mast cell stabilizers may be helpful for maintenance therapy, chronic allergies, or vernal conjunctivitis.
  - Cromolyn sodium 4% on a regular basis
  - Nedocromil sodium 2% or lodoxamide tromethamine 0.1%.
- Topical olopatadine hydrochloride 0.1% is a mast cell stabilizer combined with an antihistamine for children older than 3 years old.
  - Topical NSAIDs, like ketorolac tromethamine 0.5%, provide relief of itching and burning though it often stings when applied.
- The ophthalmic histamine 1 (H_1) blockers ketotifen or levocabastine can be prescribed for allergic conjunctivitis and ocular pruritus.
- Topical steroids should not be used because of possible side effects (increased IOP, potential for viral infection, contraindication with herpes, potential to cause cataracts, and poor corneal healing). An ophthalmologist should be consulted if a patient's condition warrants considering topical corticosteroids.
- Refer to an allergist for allergen immunotherapy when rhinitis is present because therapy can lead to better control without the need for medication.
- Refer to an ophthalmologist if unresponsive to treatment or if the following is present: corneal abrasions, impaired vision, need for corticosteroids, severe keratoconjunctivitis, or atypical manifestations.
- Maintain a high threshold of suspicion for herpes-induced blepharitis or atopic keratoconjunctivitis if pain is present.

Complications

Some forms of allergic conjunctivitis (e.g., vernal conjunctivitis) can lead to corneal ulceration, scarring and vision loss, corneal degeneration, and changes in the corneal curvature.

Blepharitis

Blepharitis is an acute or chronic inflammation of the eyelash follicles or meibomian sebaceous glands of the eyelids (or both). It is usually bilateral. There may be a history of contact lens wear or physical contact with another symptomatic person. It is commonly caused by contaminated makeup or contact lens solution. Poor hygiene, tear deficiency, rosacea, and seborrheic dermatitis of the scalp and face are also possible etiologic factors. The ulcerative form of blepharitis is usually caused by *S. aureus*. Nonulcerative blepharitis is occasionally seen in children with psoriasis, seborrhea, eczema, allergies, lice infestation, or in children with trisomy 21.

Clinical Findings

- Swelling and erythema of the eyelid margins and palpebral conjunctiva

- Flaky, scaly debris over eyelid margins on awakening; presence of lice
- Gritty, burning feeling in eyes
- Mild bulbar conjunctival injection
- Ulcerative form: Hard scales at the base of the lashes (if the crust is removed, ulceration is seen at the hair follicles, the lashes fall out, and an associated conjunctivitis is present)

Differential Diagnosis

Pediculosis of the eyelashes.

Management

Explain to the patient that this may be chronic or relapsing. Instructions for the patient include:

- Scrub the eyelashes and eyelids with a cotton-tipped applicator containing a weak (50%) solution of no-tears shampoo to maintain proper hygiene and debride the scales.
- Use warm compresses for 5 to 10 minutes at a time two to four times a day and wipe away lid debris.
- At times antistaphylococcal antibiotic (e.g., erythromycin 0.5% ophthalmic ointment) is used until symptoms subside and for at least 1 week thereafter. Ointment is preferable to eye drops because of increased duration of contact with the ocular tissue. Azithromycin 1% ophthalmic solution for 4 weeks may also be used (Shtein, 2014).
- Treat associated seborrhea, psoriasis, eczema, or allergies as indicated.
- Remove contact lenses and wear eyeglasses for the duration of the treatment period. Sterilize or clean lenses before reinserting.
- Purchase new eye makeup; minimize use of mascara and eyeliner.
- Use artificial tears for patients with inadequate tear pools.

Chronic staphylococcal blepharitis and meibomian keratoconjunctivitis respond to oral erythromycin. Doxycycline, tetracycline, or minocycline can be used chronically in children older than 8 years old.

Hordeolum

Commonly called a *stye,* hordeolum is an infection of either the sebaceous glands (Zeis or Molls glands), the eyelids (external hordeolum), or the meibomian glands of the eyelid (internal hordeolum). The causative organism is *S. aureus* or, rarely, *P. aeruginosa.*

Clinical Findings

A tender, swollen red furuncle is seen. In an external hordeolum, the swelling is generally smaller, superficial, and located along the lid margin. An internal hordeolum is larger and may point through the skin or conjunctival surface. The patient complains of a foreign body sensation. An internal hordeolum on the palpebral conjunctiva can be inspected by rolling back the eyelid (Fig. 29-7).

Differential Diagnosis

If the hordeolum does not resolve, consider cellulitis of the lid or orbit, sebaceous cell cancer, or pyogenic granuloma.

Management

- Rupture often occurs spontaneously when the furuncle becomes large and a point develops. Removal of an eyelash near the furuncle frequently promotes rupture.
- Warm, moist compresses three or four times daily, 10 to 15 minutes each time, facilitate the process of rupturing. Hygiene for the eye can be maintained by scrubbing the eyelashes and eyelids with a cotton-tipped applicator containing a weak (50%) solution of no-tears shampoo once or twice a day.
- At times antistaphylococcal ointment (e.g., 0.5% erythromycin) is effective treatment.
- Steroids are not indicated.
- Refer to an ophthalmologist for incision and drainage if the hordeolum does not rupture on its own after coming to a point or for multiple or recurrent hordeolum.

Chalazion

Chalazion is a chronic sterile inflammation of the eyelid resulting from a lipogranuloma of the meibomian glands that line the posterior margins of the eyelids (see Fig. 29-7). It is deeper in the eyelid tissue than a hordeolum and may result from an internal hordeolum or retained lipid granular secretions.

Clinical Findings

Initially, mild erythema and slight swelling of the involved eyelid are seen. After a few days the inflammation resolves, and a slow growing, round, nonpigmented, painless (key finding) mass remains. It may persist for a long time and is a commonly acquired lid lesion seen in children (see Fig. 29-7).

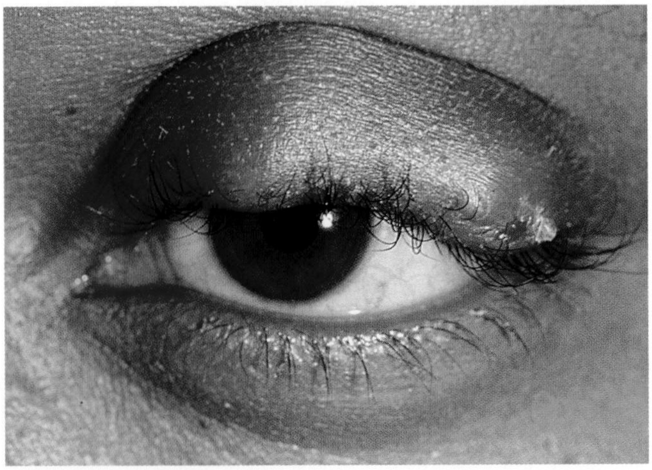

• **Figure 29-7** Chalazion and external hordeolum. (From Neff AG, Carter KD: Benign eyelid lesions. In Yanoff M, Duker JS: *Ophthalmology*, ed 4, Philadelphia, 2014, Elsevier/Saunders, Fig. 12.9-22, *A*.)

Management

- Acute lesions are treated with hot compresses.
- Refer to an ophthalmologist for surgical incision or topical intralesional corticosteroid injections if the condition is unresolved or if the lesion causes cosmetic concerns. A chalazion can distort vision by causing astigmatism as a result of pressure on the orbit.

Complications

Recurrence is common. Fragile, vascular granulation tissue called *pyogenic granuloma* that enlarges and bleeds rapidly can occur if a chalazion breaks through the conjunctival surface.

Nasolacrimal Duct Conditions: Dacryostenosis and Dacryocystitis

Nasolacrimal duct obstruction, or dacryostenosis, is an abnormal obstruction (imperforate valve of Hasner) of the nasolacrimal duct that prevents tears from flowing into an opening in the nasal mucosa. Dacryocystitis is an inflammation of the involved nasolacrimal duct; infection can result (Fig. 29-8). Nasolacrimal duct obstruction is fairly common in neonates (up to 6% of live births) (Örge and Boente, 2014). It is thought to be due to a membrane at birth that covers the nasolacrimal duct, which then fails to break down quickly. It may also occur at any age secondary to trauma to the duct or to a chronic duct obstruction complicated by an upper respiratory infection. The condition is also found more frequently in those with craniofacial disorders and Down syndrome. Congenital failure of the duct to canalize may be unilateral or bilateral, and clinical signs appear 2 to 6 weeks after birth when tear production develops. Duct blockage usually resolves spontaneously in 56% to 66% of infants by 6 months old and 96% of infants by 12 months old (Örge and Boente, 2014). Bacterial overgrowth may occur resulting in excessive mucus production.

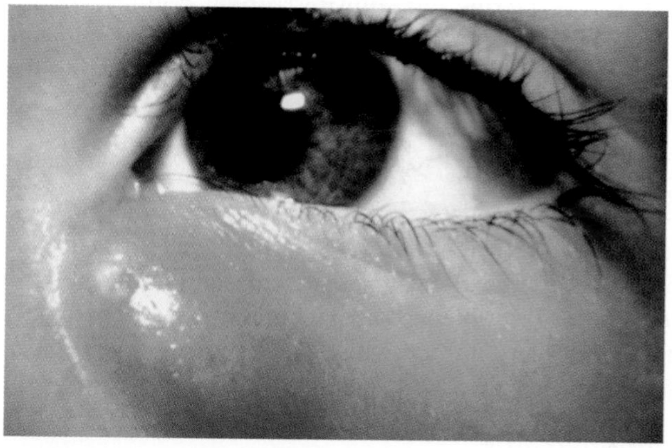

• **Figure 29-8** Dacryocystitis. (From Sharma R, Brunette DD: Ophthalmology. In Marx JA, Hockberger RS, Walls RM: *Rosen's emergency medicine*, ed 8, Philadelphia, 2014, Elsevier, Fig. 71-20.)

Clinical Findings

- Continuous or intermittent tearing, stickiness, and mucoid discharge at the inner canthus that can become purulent with possible expression of purulent material
- Blepharitis in lids and lashes
- Occasional nasal obstruction and drainage
- Expression of thin mucopurulent exudate from the punctum lacrimale
- Tenderness and swelling over the lacrimal duct (can be exquisite) (see Fig. 29-8)
- Eyelids stuck shut on awakening
- Edema and erythema of the tear sac (most prominent in the triangular area just below the medial canthus)
- Excoriation and thickening of the periorbital skin
- Conjunctival injection
- Fever
- Mucocele of inner canthal tendon (unusual; presents as a bluish mass)

Diagnostic Studies

- Fluorescein dye, instilled bilaterally in the inferior conjunctival sac and checked in 2 and 5 minutes with a cobalt blue light source, will disappear if duct is patent.
- A white blood cell (WBC) count (elevated) and cultures are obtained from the expressed exudate if the inflammation is severe.

Differential Diagnosis

Punctual or canalicular atresia, conjunctivitis, foreign body, corneal abrasion, congenital glaucoma, dacryocele, intraocular inflammation, and nasal mucosal edema are differential diagnoses (Örge and Boente, 2014).

Management

The treatment goals are to minimize stagnation in the tear duct and prevent infection.

- Daily massage of the lacrimal sac may be performed to facilitate canalization of the duct. The technique involves placing a clean finger over the medial canthus and pressing in a posterior direction until the fingertip enters the space behind the inferior bony orbital ridge. Gentle pressure applied in a downward and medial direction transmits hydrostatic force through the nasolacrimal duct to the obstruction (Fig. 29-9). This technique should be performed about 10 times, two or three times a day. The eyelid should be cleaned with plain water after massage (Örge and Boente, 2014).
- Bacterial conjunctivitis or excessive mucopurulent exudate is most commonly *S. pneumoniae* (35%) or *H. influenzae* (20%) and may be treated with erythromycin ophthalmic ointment, tobramycin ophthalmic, or the fluoroquinolones (moxifloxacin, ciprofloxacin, ofloxacin, norfloxacin) for 1 to 3 weeks with massage and frequent cleansing of secretions (Paysse et al, 2014). The duct may open spontaneously with resolution of the bacterial infection.

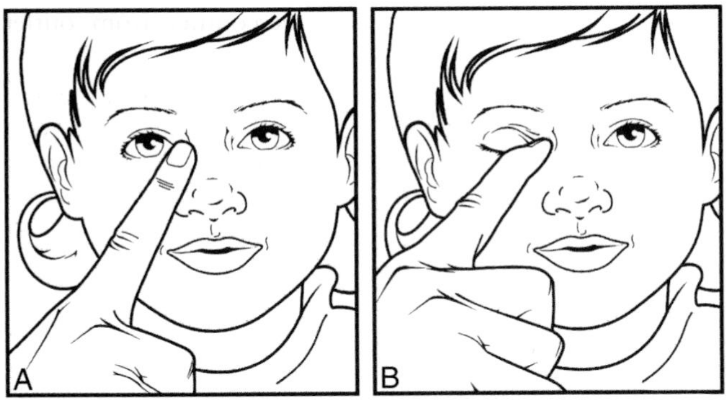

• **Figure 29-9** Technique to clear nasolacrimal duct obstruction. **A,** Incorrect technique. **B,** Correct technique. The finger is pushing behind the bone, "in and up." Note that the fingertip is not visible in the proper technique.

- Saline drops into the nose, followed by aspiration before feeding and at bedtime, help relieve any concurrent nasal congestion.

If the mucopurulent exudate persists for 1 to 2 weeks despite the aforementioned interventions, the infant or child needs a referral to an ophthalmologist regardless of age. Some ophthalmologists may probe the duct in an infant as early as 6 months old, whereas others wait until 9 to 12 months old. Early in-office probing is less expensive and does not require anesthesia, but it does require a skilled ophthalmologist (Örge and Boente, 2014). If probing fails to alleviate the problem (which is unusual), surgery may be required for placement of a tube stent or for a dacryocystorhinostomy (DCR). Dacryocystitis may be acute or chronic and is evidenced by erythematous swelling below the medial canthal area. Treatment of dacryocystitis is warm compresses and oral or parenteral antibiotics (Örge and Boente, 2014). When fever, marked erythema, swelling, tenderness, and toxic appearance occur, hospitalization is indicated for parenteral antibiotics. Periorbital or orbital cellulitis is a complication of chronic dacryocystitis.

Periorbital Cellulitis

Periorbital cellulitis, or inflammation of the tissues surrounding the involved eye, is often associated with trauma or focal infection near the eye, eyelid abscess, or sinusitis (Gappy et al, 2014). Periorbital cellulitis may also be called *preseptal cellulitis* (Fig. 29-10). It is predominantly an infection in children, spread from the upper respiratory tract or middle ear.

It is most commonly seen in children up to 6 years old. It can also occur with infected lacerations, abrasions, insect stings or bites, impetigo, or a foreign body where the infection is spread via venous or lymphatic channels. It may also be secondary to paranasal sinusitis (Gappy et al, 2014). The etiology is often unknown, but the bacteria most commonly responsible for periorbital cellulitis are streptococcal organisms, *S. aureus,* and, until the introduction of the *Haemophilus influenzae* type B (Hib) vaccine, Hib (Gappy et al, 2014). Community acquired methicillin-resistant *Staphylococcus aureus* (MRSA) has been reported as a cause of periorbital cellulitis and appears to be on the rise (Gappy et al, 2014).

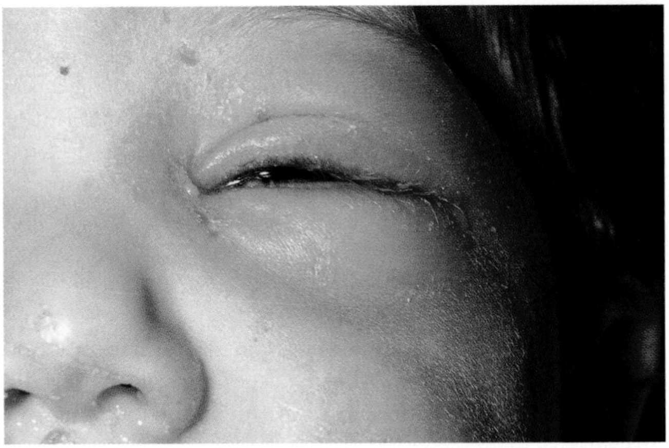

• **Figure 29-10** Preseptal cellulitis due to *Haemophilus influenzae* in a 6-month-old infant. (From Hoyt C, Taylor D: *Pediatric ophthalmology and strabismus*, ed 4, Philadelphia, 2013, Elsevier/Saunders.)

Clinical Findings

- Acute febrile illness (temperature higher than 102.2° F [39° C] if associated with bacteremia)
- Swelling and erythema of tissues surrounding the eye; upper lid affected more often than the lower lid
- Deep red eyelid (color is purple-blue with *H. influenzae* infection)
- Symptoms of bacteremia or sinusitis (headache, decreased vision)
- Orbital discomfort or pain, proptosis, or paralysis of extra ocular muscles

Diagnostic Studies

Depending on the severity and speed of progression of the cellulitis, the following are useful:

- Complete blood count (CBC) with differential (WBC count usually greater than 15,000 if bacteremic)
- Blood cultures and culture of purulent wounds near the eye
- Lumbar puncture (infants younger than 1 year old)
- CT scan to rule out sinusitis, orbital cellulitis, or subperiosteal abscess
- Visual acuity, extra ocular movement, and pupillary reaction testing

Differential Diagnosis

Conjunctivitis (bilateral conjunctival inflammation), cavernous sinus thrombosis, and orbital cellulitis (proptosis, limited extra ocular movement, and reduced visual acuity) are the differential diagnoses in children; in neonates, consider conjunctivitis, dacryocystitis, and ruptured dacryocystocele.

Management

- Management must be made on a case-by-case basis. Referral to an ophthalmologist is needed when proptosis, ophthalmoplegia, or changes in visual acuity occur; these conditions are suggestive of orbital cellulitis. Moderate to severe cases of cellulitis, a child younger than 1 year old, a poor response to outpatient management, or a purulent wound near the eyelid require hospitalization and intravenous administration of antibiotics followed by a 10-day course of oral antibiotics (Gappy et al, 2014).

The child may be managed as an outpatient if the child is older than 1 year old, the cellulitis is mild, the orbit is not involved (full eye movements are present, no pain with eye movement, visual changes, or ptosis), and the child exhibits no symptoms of systemic bacterial sepsis.

Outpatient management consists of:

- Oral antibiotics to complete 7- to 14-day course. Amoxicillin (high-dose), amoxicillin with clavulanic acid, and cefixime are first-line choices for treatment.
- If MRSA is suspected, treat with clindamycin or a combination regimen of TMP-SMX *plus* amoxicillin *or* cefpodoxime *or* cefdinir (Gappy et al, 2014).
- Warm soaks to the periorbital area every 2 to 4 hours for 15 minutes may provide comfort and speed healing.
- If a rapid clinical response is not seen, further evaluation and treatment should be done. The parent is advised to call immediately if there is any change in condition.
- Reexamine the patient in 24 hours. Failure to improve in 24 hours indicates a need for hospitalization and parenteral antibiotics, usually ceftriaxone. The child is monitored daily until blood cultures are negative for 48 hours or clinical improvement is seen.

Complications

Complications include orbital cellulitis or extension of the infection into the orbit, subperiosteal or orbital abscess, optic neuritis, retinal vein thrombosis, panophthalmitis, meningitis, epidural and subdural abscesses, and cavernous sinus thrombosis.

Keratitis and Corneal Ulcers

Inflammation of the cornea (keratitis) can cause a dramatic alteration in visual acuity and can progress to corneal ulceration and blindness. It is a medical emergency and requires prompt referral to an ophthalmologist. A corneal ulcer begins as a well-defined infiltration at the center or edge of the cornea and subsequently suppurates and forms an ulcer that may penetrate deep into the corneal tissue or spread to involve the width of the cornea. Involvement is usually unilateral. The causative agents include viruses (HSV-1, varicella-zoster, hepatitis C), bacteria (*H. influenzae, Moraxella, S. aureus, S. pneumoniae, Pseudomonas, N. gonorrhoeae,* Enterobacteriaceae [including *Klebsiella, Enterobacter, Serratia,* and *Proteus*]), fungi (rare), and protozoa. Less common causes include an allergic reaction, conjunctivitis, systemic infections, toxic chemicals, and the use of corticosteroids. The use of improperly fitted decorative contact lenses, popular with teenagers, has also been implicated; these lenses are often purchased over-the-counter from outlet stores (CDC, 2014b).

The most common risk factor for keratitis is trauma (which can also result from wearing extended-wear contact lenses or having poor contact lens hygiene). Age (younger than 30 and older than 50 years old), gender (males more than females [secondary to increased ocular trauma]), smoking, and low socioeconomic status, with vitamin A deficiency are high risk factors.

Clinical Findings

Symptoms vary in intensity according to the depth and extent of ulceration. The following are reported or seen:

- Exposure to an infected individual
- History of illness, eye trauma, extended contact lens wear, foreign body, or history of recent antibiotic treatment for conjunctivitis that was unresponsive
- White lesions on cornea
- Vesicles on the skin or eyelids and herpes lesions elsewhere on the body
- Severe pain, sensation of a foreign body ("gritty"), and photophobia
- Tearing, erythema, and spasms of the eyelid
- Inflamed eye
- Blurred vision
- Occasional corneal opacification
- Area staining green with a fluorescein strip (if herpes, a dendritic ulcer is seen)

Management

When a corneal ulcer is suspected, the child should be referred immediately for a slit-lamp examination. Delay can result in loss of vision in the eye. Do not attempt to treat. Visual acuity outcome is good when these ulcers are treated aggressively with the appropriate agent.

- Steroids should never be used.
- Treatment with antivirals, such as trifluridine or vidarabine, may be used to speed healing in herpes simplex infections.
- Complications include corneal opacification, scarring, and loss of vision can if treatment is delayed.

Inflammation of the Uveal Tract

Inflammation of the uveal tract (iris, ciliary body, choroids) and other ocular structures is often called *uveitis* (Fig. 29-11). The inflammation may be anterior (affecting the iris, ciliary body, or both) or posterior (affecting the choroid). Adjacent ocular structures can also be involved, including the retina, vitreous, sclera, lens, and optic nerve. The inflammation may be acute or chronic. In the United States, 2% to 13% of patients with uveitis are children; prevalence in children with juvenile idiopathic arthritis (JIA) is 4% to 38% (Wentworth et al, 2014). Many processes have been implicated, broadly divided into infectious and noninfectious. Known etiologies include viral or bacterial infections, ocular trauma, and infection elsewhere in the

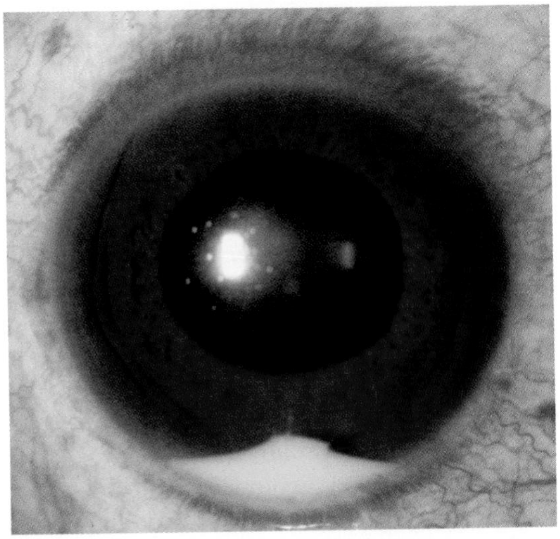

• **Figure 29-11** Uveitis. (From Palay DA, Krachmer JH: *Primary care ophthalmology*, ed 2, Philadelphia, 2005, Mosby.)

eye. Other causes include allergy, malignancy, and systemic diseases, such as JIA, inflammatory bowel, Kawasaki syndrome, herpes simplex, tuberculosis, Lyme disease, CMV, toxoplasmosis, syphilis, acquired immune deficiency syndrome (AIDS), ulcerative colitis, rubella retinitis, and Stevens-Johnson syndrome (Wentworth et al, 2014).

Clinical Findings

- Acute onset of pain (key finding)
- Red eye, photophobia, and blurred or decreased vision (key findings)
- Excessive tearing and eyelid edema
- Conjunctival erythema
- Circumcorneal injection
- Hypopyon (pus layer in the bottom of the anterior chamber) (see Fig. 29-11)
- Cloudy appearance of the eye with a bulging iris and a contracted, irregular, or fixed pupil (see Fig. 29-11)
- If chronic, there may be no ocular pain, photophobia, redness, or tearing
- May be a history of prior viral infection, joint pain, trauma, gastrointestinal problems

Management

Evaluate and treat any underlying systemic disease. Refer the patient to an ophthalmologist; definitive diagnosis is made by slit-lamp examination. The prognosis is improved with early treatment. Cycloplegics and topical or systemic corticosteroids (depending on the cause of the inflammation) are often used in treatment. Cycloplegic-mydriatics are used regularly to prevent posterior synechiae (adhesions of iris to lens and cornea); NSAIDs may be used as adjunct treatment.

Complications

Anterior and posterior synechiae, changes in IOP, corneal edema, various degrees of visual impairment, papillary scarring, retinal detachment, glaucoma, enucleation, and cataracts are possible complications.

Trachoma

Trachoma is a chronic infectious disease of the eye characterized by follicular keratoconjunctivitis with neovascularization of the cornea. It is contagious, often spread from eye to eye by flies. Though rare in the United States, it is the second leading cause of blindness in the world, with over 80 million people infected worldwide. It is caused by one of the two *C. trachomatis* biovars that exist in the world; it is endemic in Africa, the Middle East, Asia, the Pacific Islands, and in the Aboriginal population in Australia (Wright and Taylor, 2014).

Clinical Findings

Clinical findings include inflammation, pain, photophobia, excessive tearing, granulation follicles (large white or pale yellow follicles 0.5 to 2 mm on the upper tarsal conjunctiva), and, in adults, eventual entropion—inversion of the eyelid leading to corneal trauma, scarring, and blindness. In endemic areas, diagnosis is made by clinical presentation, although cultures may be done to confirm diagnosis.

Management

Consult with an ophthalmologist because trachoma treatment is difficult and recommendations vary. The World Health Organization (WHO) recommends mass antibiotic treatment within a region when the prevalence of trachoma in children is greater than 10%. Trachoma may be treated with a single dose of azithromycin. Other options include a topical tetracycline antibiotic ointment twice daily for 6 weeks. Topical azithromycin drops may be as effective as oral azithromycin (Wright and Taylor, 2014). Steroids are contraindicated.

Trachoma is spread by close personal contact, so education reinforcing the need for frequent hand washing and careful cleansing of the eyes and discouraging sharing of towels and handkerchiefs is important. The WHO and the CDC have set a goal of eliminating trachoma by 2020 through a public health campaign known as *S.A.F.E.: **S**urgery to correct advanced disease, **A**ntibiotics to treat active disease, **F**acial cleanliness, and **E**nvironmental improvements in water and sanitation.*

The Injured Eye

Corneal Abrasion

Damage to or loss of the epithelial cells of the cornea in the form of a corneal abrasion or tear is relatively common. Scratches from forceps delivery, paper, brushes, fingernails, contact lens overuse, improperly fitted cosmetic contact lenses, airbag deployment, plants, or foreign body in the conjunctival sac are often responsible.

Clinical Findings

- Evidence and sensation of a foreign body
- Severe pain and photophobia
- Tearing and blepharospasm
- Decreased vision
- Conjunctival erythema

On examination, disrupted tear film over the corneal epithelium is seen with a penlight.

Fluorescein staining with superficial uptake is indicative of a minor corneal abrasion. If the fluorescein staining goes deeply into the cornea, subepithelial corneal damage (e.g., corneal ulceration or corneal tear) is possible. Vertical striations on the cornea suggest a foreign body embedded under the eyelid.

Management

- Refer severe corneal injuries or possible subepithelial damage to an ophthalmologist. Refer those who wear contact lenses with an abrasion to an ophthalmologist to rule out bacterial corneal infection (a prophylactic topical antibiotic [e.g., gentamicin or ciprofloxacin] may be prescribed in these circumstances to cover *Pseudomonas*).
- If no symptoms of corneal infection, use topical antibiotics (0.5% erythromycin or Polysporin drops or ointment [preferred as more lubricating]) four times daily (Jacobs, 2014). The use of a patch does not improve healing or decrease pain and a poorly applied patch may cause a corneal abrasion. An abrasion generally heals in 24 to 48 hours. Advise the patient to return daily for follow-up evaluation or refer for slit-lamp examination within 24 to 36 hours. If responding, continue the ointment for 2 to 3 days. If no improvement is seen after 24 to 48 hours or if symptoms worsen, refer to an ophthalmologist.
- Use elbow restraints for the infant to ensure that the eye is not rubbed or further irritated.
- Oral analgesics or ophthalmologic NSAIDs (e.g., ketorolac 0.5%) may be used to ease the discomfort. Do not use topical anesthetics, because they are toxic to the epithelium.

Foreign Body

A superficial foreign body in the eye is usually lodged on the surface of the eye or superficially in the cornea. It rarely results in serious trauma but may penetrate the globe (intraocular) with more serious consequences. Foreign bodies commonly occur in younger children during play and in older children during sports; they can include dirt, dust, metallic particles, or alkaline products from the deployment of an airbag.

Clinical Findings

Be sure to include in the history if the individual was working on a metal-on-metal activity. The following may be noted:

- Pain and foreign body sensation
- Foreign body visible in the conjunctival sac
- Tearing
- Inflammation
- Irregular or peaked pupil
- Photophobia
- Opaque lens
- Perforating wound to the cornea or iris

Fluorescein staining may be useful if no foreign body is visualized.

Diagnostic Studies

Ultrasonography or CT scan may be needed, depending on the foreign body and its location. An MRI is contraindicated.

Management

- Never remove an intraocular foreign body (including a metal object or fragment) and never remove a foreign body if the history indicates that a projectile object was possibly involved in the injury or patient has had LASIK procedure. Refer immediately to an ophthalmologist.
- View the upper bulbar conjunctiva by having the patient look down while the upper lid is pulled away from the globe and the upper recess illuminated. Evert the eyelid to visualize the superior tarsal conjunctiva.
- Use of a topical anesthetic facilitates patient cooperation.
- If not visualized but suspected, remove an extra ocular foreign body via irrigation with sterile saline or sterile eye irrigant.
- If the object is visualized, either irrigate or gently lift object away with a moistened cotton-tipped swab (after instillation of topical anesthetic). The latter technique should be used only for cooperative individuals and for small foreign bodies in order to avoid further trauma to the epithelial surface.
- If any difficulty is encountered, stop all efforts, and refer the patient immediately to an ophthalmologist. Treat with antibiotic ointment (erythromycin four times a day) until seen by ophthalmologist (Jacobs, 2014).
- After removing any extra ocular object, instill fluorescein stain and inspect the cornea with cobalt-blue light to look for green staining or lines; check visual acuity. Follow guidelines for managing a corneal abrasion.
- Reschedule the patient in 24 hours or refer to an ophthalmologist for follow-up.
- In the case of an airbag deployment (talc, cornstarch, and/or baking soda are released), irrigate the eyes with sterile saline or sterile eye irrigant and carefully examine the eye(s) for further evidence of trauma.

Complications

Sympathetic ophthalmia, chronic siderosis, or a uveitis of the injured eye can occur any time from 10 days to many years after a penetrating injury of the globe.

Burns

Burns to the eyes and surrounding tissues can be thermal (caused by exposure to steam, flame, intense heat [e.g., touching cornea with a curling iron], cinders, or cigarettes), chemical (e.g., cleaning agents, fertilizers, pesticides, battery fluid, or laboratory products), or induced by UV light (e.g., from bright snow, laser pointers, or a sunlamp). The amount of damage to the eye is directly related to the length of exposure and the nature of the source of the burn (Solano, 2013). Chemical burns are true emergencies because of the progressive damage that can occur. Alkaline solutions are especially damaging. Burns on the eyelids are classified and treated the same as burns elsewhere on the body.

Clinical Findings

- Pale or necrosed appearance of the surrounding skin and eyelids
- Opacity of corneal tissue
- Visual impairment (decreased acuity)
- Initial exquisite pain or delayed complaints of pain (e.g., in UV burns, pain emerges about 6 hours after exposure)
- Photophobia
- Tearing within 12 hours of exposure
- Swollen corneas
- Fluorescein stain revealing pinpoint uptake

Management

- Instill a topical anesthetic if available.
- Chemical burns require immediate, ongoing, copious irrigation (Solano, 2013). With the eyelids held apart, instill a steady, gentle solution of tepid water, saline, or Ringer irrigation for 20 to 30 minutes or until the pH of the tear film is 7.3 to 7.7. The pH should be rechecked after 30 minutes to ensure it maintains this level. Refer to an ophthalmologist after irrigation to determine the extent of the damage. Do not patch the eye; allow tearing to continue to cleanse the eye. Cool compresses applied to the surrounding skin may be comforting. Hospitalization may be needed for sedation and analgesia.
- Thermal burns may be treated the same way as corneal abrasions
- UV burns are treated by using topical antibiotic prophylaxis, patches, and analgesics. Healing should occur in 1 to 2 days.

Lacerations of the Orbit

Lacerations from injuries cause perforation of the cornea and lead to uveal prolapse. They are described as to whether they are of the anterior segment (cornea, anterior chamber, iris, lens) or posterior segment (sclera, retina, vitreous).

Clinical Findings

The clinical findings (only a few of the more obvious are mentioned here) depend on which segment is involved.

- Anterior segment: irregular pupil (retracted or peaked), iris prolapse
- Posterior segment: poor red light reflex, decreased vision, black tissue or fluid seen under the conjunctiva

Management

Apply an eye shield (can be made from a cup) to protect the eye. Refer the patient immediately to an ophthalmologist to rule out damage to the globe and surrounding structures.

Traumatic Hyphema

A hyphema is an accumulation of visible blood or blood products in the anterior chamber of the eye and is the result of blunt trauma to the globe without penetration or perforation. This condition is most often caused by balls, fists or fingers, elbows, rocks, exploding airbags, and sticks. High risk sports associated with hyphema include baseball, hockey, racquetball and squash, with the stick or racket often responsible for the injury (Andreoli and Gardiner, 2014). It may also occur in infants with birth trauma or in patients with retinoblastoma, abnormal iris vessels (rubeosis), leukemia, juvenile xanthogranuloma of the iris, or abnormal hematologic profiles, such as sickle cell trait or disease, or secondary to child abuse.

Clinical Findings

Vision, pupil motility, the lids and adnexa, the cornea and anterior segment, and the red light reflex should be assessed. An open globe must be excluded before any examination that would increase IOP (Andreoli and Gardiner, 2014). The following may be noted:

- History of traumatic eye injury
- Somnolence (often associated with intracranial trauma)
- Blood appearing as a dark red fluid level between the cornea and iris on gross examination or as a hazy-appearing iris
- Inability to detect a bilateral red light reflex
- Pain, photophobia, and tearing
- Visual acuity changes and impaired vision (light perception and hand motion perception)
- Abnormal pupillary reflex

Management

The goals of treatment include resolving the hyphema, making the patient comfortable, and preventing complications. There is a risk of recurrent bleeding. The following steps should be taken:

- Refer the patient immediately to an ophthalmologist. A slit-lamp examination is indicated.
- Restrict oral intake until the child has been seen by an ophthalmologist.
- Place a perforated eye shield (not a patch) over the eye; avoid pressure to prevent reinjury.
- If a hematologic disorder is detected, ensure quick intervention and close follow-up.

The following steps are commonly recognized for treatment of a traumatic hyphema:

- Outpatient management is acceptable for those with a small hyphema (grade I): Elevate the head of the bed to

30 degrees. Child should wear a Fox eye shield; maintain bed rest with bathroom privileges for 5 days; participate in no strenuous activities for 10 days; have daily eye examinations to check for blood staining and IOP. Cycloplegic agents may be used (Andreoli and Gardiner, 2014).
- Children should be hospitalized with a hyphema of grade II or III, those with sickle cell, if there is an increase in IOP, or if there is a question about compliance with outpatient treatment.
- Acetaminophen is the analgesic of choice; avoid aspirin and NSAIDs because they may add to the risk of a rebleed. Sedatives may be necessary in pediatric patients.
- Surgery may be necessary to remove the trapped blood from the chamber for the following reasons: (1) if it is causing an increase in IOP; (2) in sickle cell patients, to prevent corneal blood staining; (3) if the hyphema remains without some clearing in the first 4 days; or (4) if a clot is pressing against the corneal epithelium.
- After hospital discharge, the child should be followed closely by an ophthalmologist because long-term monitoring is necessary to detect possible traumatic cataract, retinal detachment, or glaucoma.

Complications

A second hemorrhage can occur within 3 to 5 days of the first, increasing the risk of glaucoma, amblyopia, or corneal blood staining that can result in permanent visual loss. This rebleed occurs in 7% to 38% of all cases. The larger the hyphema, the more likely the child is to rebleed. Patients with abnormal hematologic profiles (e.g., sickle cell hemoglobinopathies) are more likely to have visual loss because of optic atrophy (Andreoli and Gardiner, 2014).

Success in treatment is determined by the recovery of visual acuity. A small grade I hyphema will lead to permanent visual loss (worse than 20/50) in less than 10% of cases. When less than a third of the anterior chamber is filled with blood, approximately 80% regain acuity of 20/40 or better. When more than half (but less than total) of the chamber is filled, this same visual acuity is regained in about 60%. However, only 35% of those with total hyphema will have this return in acuity. Patients should be followed by an ophthalmologist due to elevated risk of developing glaucoma (Andreoli and Gardiner, 2014).

Retinal Detachment

Retinal detachment is detachment of the neurosensory retina from its retinal pigment epithelium base within the globe. It is rare in children, so suspicion should be high for traumatic causes (e.g., child abuse), a congenital abnormality or syndrome (aphakia, cataracts, Ehlers-Danlos, Stickler, Marfan, Norrie syndromes), or specific disease (ROP, viral retinitis, retinoblastoma, or various retinopathies) (Wenick and Barañano, 2012). Some detachments may not be diagnosed for months or years after a blunt trauma injury due to the support of the vitreous (Wenick and Barañano, 2012). Children who have had cataract surgery are at increased risk of retinal detachment, with an overall 20-year risk of 7%, with a median time of 9.1 years after surgery (Haargaard et al, 2014). There may be concurrent ocular disease or a family history of retinal detachment.

Clinical Findings

- Blurry vision that becomes progressively worse
- Dark cloud in one visual field, flashing lights, or a "shower of floaters"
- Darkening of retinal vessels on funduscopic examination
- Gray elevation at the site of detachment

Management

Instruct the patient not to eat and refer to an ophthalmologist for evaluation emergently.

Orbital Hematoma and Contusion of the Globe

This condition is usually the result of a blow to the globe. The degree of damage depends on the energy of the object hitting the globe. Such injuries commonly occur as a result of sports activities, motor vehicle accidents, assault, BB gun accidents, or airbag deployment.

Clinical Findings

- Milky white appearance of the retina
- Visual acuity changes
- Severe bruising of the eyelids and periorbital tissues
- Lens dislocation
- Retinal detachment or edema
- Vitreous, retinal, or choroid hemorrhage
- Rupture of the eyeball

Management

Refer the patient immediately to an ophthalmologist. A closed head injury, damage to the skull, and facial bone fractures need to be ruled out via CT scan, MRI, or ultrasound radiography. Occasionally cryopexy or laser photocoagulation surgery is needed for contusions of the globe.

Complications

Possible complications include permanent visual loss, retinal necrosis, subretinal hemorrhage, and retinal or macular holes.

Orbital Fractures

An orbital fracture is a fracture of the walls of the orbit secondary to blunt trauma to the orbital rim or eye(s). The orbital floor is thin and subject to fracture. The inferior rectus muscle may become caught in the fracture site. The usual cause of an orbital fracture is a blow or blunt trauma to the orbit (e.g., ball, fist, motor vehicle accident [hitting the dashboard], or fall).

Clinical Findings

- Pain, diplopia
- Numbness below orbit
- Ecchymosis of the lids, nosebleed, trouble chewing
- Limited ocular movement (especially upward) and weakness in downward movement
- Globe displacement with a sunken-eye appearance or a protruding eye
- Bony discontinuity or "step-off"
- Subcutaneous emphysema in surrounding tissues and edema
- Enophthalmos (recession of the eyeball within the orbit)
- Corneal laceration
- Irregular pupil
- Hyphema or absent red light reflex

Diagnostic Studies

Plain film radiography and CT scan are the best imaging modalities. A CT is preformed if the patient has evidence of fracture upon examination, limited extra ocular motility, decreased visual acuity, pain or inability to perform an accurate examination (Neuman and Bachur, 2014).

Management

- An orbital fracture is an ophthalmologic emergency requiring immediate intervention and referral. Diagnostic studies are performed to rule out injury to the skull and cranial contents. Open reduction may be necessary if any of the orbital bones are displaced or to rule out displacement of the globe or enophthalmos.
- Ice the injury for 48 hours, and have the patient sleep with the head of bed elevated (Neuman and Bachur, 2014). Antibiotic prophylaxis to cover nasal pathogens is recommended if the patient has an orbital fracture into the sinus (Neuman and Bachur, 2014).
- Nasal decongestants may also be used.

Pterygium

A pterygium is a fibrovascular mass of thickened bulbar conjunctiva that extends beyond the limbus onto the cornea. Elastic and hyaline degenerative changes occur. The lesion is usually triangular and more commonly found on the nasal side of the orbit. It is caused by irritation of the bulbar conjunctiva from sunlight, wind, dust, fumes, or airborne allergens; it can also be hereditary. Growth rates of the lesions vary. A pinguecula may precede the pterygium, which occurs as a yellow-white, slightly raised mass on the bulbar conjunctiva. The lesion is usually painless, may itch, and may be accompanied by occasional complaints of blurred vision if the lesion enlarges.

Because a pterygium is uncommon in children, the clinician needs to consider other causes: papillomas, dermoids, keratoacanthomas, an epithelial inclusion or a dermoid cyst, or a rare malignancy. Treatment involves protecting against irritants (use of goggles or sunglasses, or topical lubricants, such as artificial tears) and using mild vasoconstrictors or short-term steroids for inflammation. Surgical removal may be needed if the pterygium impedes vision. Recurrence after surgical removal, restricted ocular mobility (especially with abduction), and diplopia may be complications.

Subconjunctival Hemorrhage

Subconjunctival hemorrhage is splotchy bulbar conjunctival redness that spontaneously occurs or is secondary to increased intrathoracic pressure (from coughing, sneezing, straining, or trauma) that results in the bursting of conjunctival vessels. It is commonly found in neonates as a benign occurrence to a vaginal delivery. The hemorrhages are painless and usually spontaneously resolve within 2 to 3 weeks. No treatment is indicated unless there is pain, vision loss, or photophobia, which indicate a referral to an ophthalmologist. Spontaneous hemorrhages can (rarely) occur with hypertension, diabetes mellitus, and blood dyscrasias, or can be a sign of a ruptured globe if there is a history of trauma (Sharma and Brunette, 2010).

Eyelid Contusion ("Black Eye")

An eyelid contusion is usually a result of blunt injury to the eye and surrounding tissues. The result is bruising, swelling, and often an impressive appearance ("black eye"). If the child complains of increased pain or swelling, decrease in visual acuity, double vision, flashing lights or "floaters," or develops a bilateral "raccoon eyes" appearance, an ophthalmologic evaluation is needed to rule out a more serious eye injury (e.g., ruptured globe, basilar skull fracture, detached retina, hyphema). Examine all eye structures before excessive swelling sets in. Treatment consists of elevating the head and intermittent ice compresses for 48 hours. A CT scan may be warranted (Sharma and Brunette, 2010).

Deformities of the Eyelids

Entropion

Entropion is a condition in which the eyelids invert so that the cilia or epithelium rubs against the corneal surface, causing abrasion or irritation. The upper and lower eyelids may be involved. There is a rare congenital form. Examination reveals evidence of lid laxity. Pain or irritation and photophobia are typical symptoms. Complications include corneal scarring and corneal infections. Management involves surgical intervention.

Ectropion

Ectropion is a rare condition in which the eyelid margins evert. The condition may be congenital, seen after infection, or secondary to scarring after trauma, radiation, or prior surgery. It can be confused with euryblepharon.

Management involves lubrication for mild cases; surgery is indicated for chronic or symptomatic cases.

Euryblepharon

Euryblepharon appears as a wide palpebral fissure with the appearance of a sagging half of the lower eyelid (temporal side) or a pulling away of the lid from the orbit. It can have a genetic etiology (e.g., Down syndrome), be associated with other ocular anomalies (e.g., congenital cleft lip, strabismus, congenital ptosis), or be seen in association with nonocular anomalies (e.g., hypospadias, inguinal hernias, dental anomalies). It is often confused with ectropion. It is usually a mild cosmetic condition that the child may outgrow. No treatment is indicated unless chronic tearing or exposure keratitis occurs; in such cases, reconstruction can be done.

For a complete list of references, please visit http://evolve.elsevier.com/Burns/pediatric/.

30

Ear Disorders

ANN M. PETERSEN-SMITH

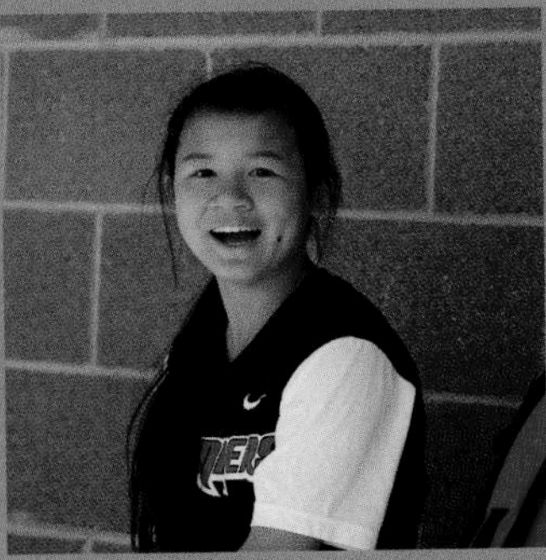

The ear serves two functions—hearing and equilibrium. The ear includes both external and inner ear structures. Malfunction of any of the ear structures can have an impact on the ear itself, as well as the surrounding tissues. Additionally, ear dysfunction can cause global problems that have lifelong effects. Adequate hearing is important for speech and language acquisition, academic performance, and socialization. Pediatric primary care providers must have an understanding of normal ear anatomy and physiology and be able to confidently identify, assess, and diagnose ear disorders in children. The cognitive-perceptual effects and long-term management of hearing loss is discussed in Chapter 20.

Standards for Hearing Screening

The Joint Committee on Infant Hearing (2007), the U.S. Preventive Services Task Force (USPSTF) (2008), and the National Institute on Deafness and Other Communication Disorders (NIDCD) (2010) advocate for universal detection of hearing loss before a child is 1 month old. These organizations also recommend follow-up of abnormal newborn hearing screening by 3 months old and appropriate family-centered intervention by 6 months old. A USPSTF review cited that children identified by universal newborn hearing screening had better language outcomes at school age than those not screened; and they had earlier referral, diagnosis, and management than those identified by other means (USPSTF, 2008). The National Center for Hearing Assessment and Management (NCHAM) reports that the detection and treatment of hearing loss at birth saves $400,000 in special education costs by the time the child finishes high school (NCHAM, 2011).

Screening of newborns or infants can be done by using evoked otoacoustic emission (EOAE) testing or automated auditory brainstem response (ABR). All American states and territories and the District of Columbia have established Early Hearing Detection and Intervention (EHDI) programs. In addition, various locations in Canada and Europe offer newborn hearing screening programs (Centers for Disease Control and Prevention [CDC], 2015). Unfortunately, programs vary greatly with some states continuing to allow a parental exemption. The United States government approved the Early Hearing Detection and Intervention Act of 2010, which mandates monitoring the effectiveness of statewide programs and systems for hearing screening of newborns and infants, prompt evaluation and diagnosis, appropriate education, and medical interventions and development of efficient models to ensure that identified newborns and infants receive follow-up from a qualified health care provider. Further, a sufficient number of trained professionals should be available to meet the screening, evaluation, and early intervention needs of children (Early Hearing Detection and Intervention Act of 2010, 2010). In addition to newborn screening, the American Academy of Pediatrics (AAP) Bright Futures guidelines recommend pure-tone audiometry at 3, 4, 5, 6, 8, 10, 12, 15, and 18 years of age, with subjective assessment at other ages (AAP, 2014). According to the Executive Summary of The Joint Commission on Infant Hearing, infants who pass newborn screening but have other risk factors for hearing loss should have at least one diagnostic audiology assessment by 24 to 30 months of age (AAP, The Joint Committee on Infant Hearing, 2007). More frequent hearing, speech-language, and communication screenings are indicated for children at high risk for hearing loss, including those with persistent or recurrent acute otitis media (AOM), middle ear effusion (MEE), and those with chronic exposure to loud noises.

Development, Anatomy, and Physiology

Development of the ear begins during the third week of gestation and is complete by the third month of embryonic life. Insult to the fetus during this time can cause irreparable damage to the ear and negatively affect hearing. Ear development occurs at the same time as kidney development, so malformation or dysfunction in one system should alert the health care provider to problems in the other.

The external ear is responsible for transmission of sound waves from outside the ear to the middle ear and for clearance of debris. The canal contains glands that secrete sweat, sebum, and cerumen that help lubricate the hair follicles and aid in the removal of debris. Patency of the ear canal is imperative for proper functioning.

The tympanic cavity constitutes the middle ear. The tympanic membrane (TM) is at the proximal end of the external auditory canal (EAC) and separates the external ear from the middle ear. The middle ear is a small chamber in the temporal bone that contains the ossicles—the malleus, incus, and stapes—which function to transmit sound waves from the EAC to the inner ear. The malleus lies against the TM, which vibrates when sound waves hit it. The stapes rests against the oval window, and its vibration causes the oval window to stimulate the fluids of the inner ear.

The eustachian tube has three physiologic functions with respect to the middle ear: (1) ventilation of the middle ear to equalize air pressure in the middle ear with atmospheric pressure and to replace oxygen that has been absorbed; (2) protection from nasopharyngeal sound, pressure, and secretions; and (3) drainage of secretions from the middle ear into the nasopharynx.

The inner ear functions to transmit sound and aid in balance. Vibrations of the TM, ossicles, and oval window set the inner ear fluids in motion. The fluid sound waves reach the cochlea, wherein lies the organ of Corti, which contains the hearing receptor hair cells. The hair cells transmit impulses to the auditory nerve (cranial nerve VIII), which transmits stimuli to the auditory cortex of the temporal lobe in the brain. The equilibrium receptors lie in the semicircular canals and vestibule of the inner ear. The semicircular canals respond to changes in direction of movement. The vestibule contains receptors essential to the maintenance of equilibrium.

Pathophysiology and Defense Mechanisms

The processes that negatively affect the ear are usually localized; however, pathologic ear conditions can be related to systemic dysfunction or disorders. Common localized pathologic conditions include viral, bacterial, or fungal infections in the inner, middle, and outer ear; foreign bodies in the ear; and trauma. Neurologic dysfunction, poor immunologic competence, and congenital anomalies are common disorders that can affect the ear and its functions. External influences, such as excessive noise in the environment, can cause irreparable damage to the ear's hearing function.

Debris formed by keratinizing cells in the ear is lubricated and extruded by the cilia in the EAC. Maintenance of an acidic pH in the ear canal prevents the growth of pathogenic bacteria. Additionally the surface lining of the external ear is water resistant and has ample blood and lymph supplies. These characteristics and the antibacterial properties of cerumen help protect against invading microorganisms. In comparison with the distal end of the EAC, the proximal end has fewer hair fibers, a thinner epithelial layer, and more nerve fibers that cause great discomfort when touched. This sensitivity to pain serves a protective function by deterring the insertion of foreign bodies into the ear, thus preventing damage to the middle ear.

The inner ear is also well protected inasmuch as the structures for both hearing and equilibrium are set deep within the skull.

Assessment

History

The history of a patient with an ear disorder should include the following:

- Craniofacial abnormalities (e.g., cleft lip or palate) or syndromes associated with craniofacial anomalies (Down syndrome)
- Prematurity
- Ear conditions (e.g., central nervous system [CNS] infections, otitis media, trauma)
- Pain (onset, location, quality, duration, alleviating or aggravating factors)
- Associated symptoms, such as fever, vomiting and diarrhea, nasal congestion, or other symptoms of upper respiratory infection
- Itching or discharge
- Tinnitus or hearing loss
- Exposure to risk factors: Environmental tobacco smoke (ETS), bottle propping, pacifier use, child care, noise, swimming
- Diabetes mellitus
- Family history of ear dysfunction or presence or history of, kidney malformation
- Box 20-15 lists for Red Flags of Hearing Loss

Physical Examination

The physical examination includes the following:

- Inspection of the external ear structures for symmetry, skin abnormalities, or discharge. The inner and outer canthi of the eye should form a straight line with the superior portion of the pinna. If the pinna inserts below this line, the ear is considered low-set, which can be associated with renal disorders and a number of genetic/congenital syndromes.
- Assessment of developmental milestones for speech and hearing-impaired children (see Table 20-10).
- Palpation and rotation of the external ear for tenderness and inflammation: Push on the tragus and apply pressure to the mastoid process.
- Otoscopic examination, which is best accomplished in a young child at the end of the physical examination with the child on an examining table or seated on the parent's lap. Pulling the ear downward, outward, and backward can enhance visualization of the EAC and TM in infants and small children. In older children and adolescents,

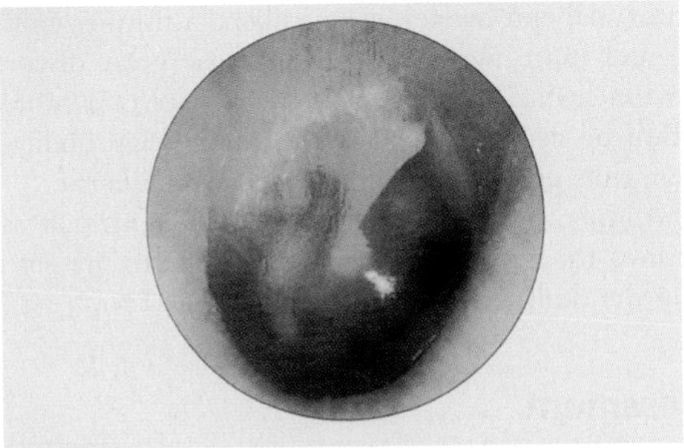

• **Figure 30-1** Normal tympanic membrane. (Photograph courtesy Sylvan Stool, MD, The Children's Hospital, Denver, CO.)

the ear is lifted upward and backward, slightly away from the head. Examine the EAC for redness, edema, or discharge. Assess all 360 degrees of the TM, the bony processes, and the cone of light (Fig. 30-1). Look for air-fluid level or bubbles behind the tympanic membrane.

Note any retraction, bulging, perforation, fibrosis, redness, or other alteration in color. Assess TM mobility using pneumatic otoscopy, tympanometry, or acoustic reflectometry.

Common Diagnostic Studies

- **Evoked otoacoustic emission** (EOAE) testing is the method of hearing screening used for universal newborn screening. The normal-hearing ear has the ability to emit detectable sounds called *spontaneous otoacoustic emissions.* The normal ear also emits these sounds when given a stimulus (EOAE) and provides evidence that the outer hair cells of the cochlea are functioning appropriately and hearing is likely to be intact. EOAE is efficient, highly sensitive, and easy to perform in a quiet, cooperative child, which makes it conducive for use in newborns. However, the EOAE does not quantify hearing deficit and may not identify auditory nerve dysfunction; ambient room noise and an uncooperative child may interfere with the test and provide unreliable results. The EOAE and ABR technologies result in highly acceptable levels of hearing sensitivity and specificity at relatively low cost.
- **Auditory brainstem response** (ABR) measures the initiation of sound-induced electrical signals in the cochlea and the functioning of the peripheral auditory system and neurologic pathways related to hearing. Although it is not a direct measure of hearing, ABR allows for inferences to be made about hearing thresholds. The ABR is useful in identifying hearing loss in a young infant or in children unable to cooperate with EOAE or audiometry. Occasionally sedation is required. Neurologic abnormalities may make interpretation of an ABR impossible. Automated ABR is available as a screening device.
- **Audiometry**, useful in assessing hearing loss in older children, measures the hearing threshold via bone or air conduction, or both, in decibels (dBs) at varying frequencies (Tables 30-1 and 30-2). For comparison, 20 dB is about as loud as a whisper, 40 dB is normal speaking loudness, and 90 dB produces pain. The frequencies of normal speaking range from 250 to 4000 Hz. Hearing loss, especially in the higher frequencies (2000 to 6000 Hz), can cause significant problems in understanding speech. A screening audiogram that tests each ear at 20 dB and frequencies of 500, 1000, 2000, and 4000 Hz is a useful assessment tool in office pediatrics. If a more detailed audiogram is needed, a qualified audiologist should perform it.
- **Pneumatic otoscopy** helps assess TM mobility. A good seal with the speculum and otoscope is required before insufflation of air into the ear canal. Brisk movement of the membrane should be seen; altered mobility suggests MEE or possible perforation.
- **Tympanometry** evaluates the function of the middle ear by assessing the movement of the TM by applying from –400 to +100 mm H_2O pressure to the ear canal. Movement of the TM is translated into a graph called a *tympanogram* (Fig. 30-2). The type A tympanogram has a compliance peak between ±100 mm H_2O and reflects a normal TM. The type B tympanogram generally has no peak or a flattened wave and suggests effusion, perforation, or the presence of a pressure-equalizing tube (Fig. 30-3). The type C tympanogram has a sharp peak between –100 and –200 mm H_2O and reflects negative ear pressure. Tympanograms are helpful when otitis media with effusion is persistent or a question remains regarding the results of physical examination of the eardrum. Tympanograms are of little use in children younger than 7 months old because their ear canals are hypercompliant in response to pressure from the tympanometer.
- **Acoustic reflectometry** is used to detect an MEE by directing a sound of varying frequency toward the TM and measuring the intensity of reflected sound. The fluid-filled middle ear space restricts vibration of the eardrum, so sound is intensified when returning to the device. Unfortunately the reflectometer cannot distinguish if an MEE is serous or suppurative. Acoustic reflectometry is less accurate than pneumatic otoscopy.
- **Tympanocentesis**, aspiration of the middle ear fluid, is helpful for the relief of pain and identification of persistent infecting organisms. It is rarely done in clinical pediatrics and is considered outside the scope of practice of the primary care provider.

Laboratory tests of blood and urine are rarely indicated unless questions remain regarding perinatal infection, systemic illness, or concomitant kidney dysfunction. Exudate from AOM with perforation may be cultured.

Genetic testing may be useful in determining if the hearing loss is inherited. According to the CDC (2015), 50% to 60% of all cases of congenital deafness are genetic. Twenty-five percent of hearing loss in newborns is due to environmental causes, such as maternal infection during

TABLE 30-1 Audiologic Tests for Infants and Young Children

Test	Characteristics	Age Range	Advantages	Disadvantages
Behavioral observation audiometry (BOA)	Behavioral test: Responses to noisemakers or calibrated sounds are observed	0 to 5 months	Low cost	Insensitive to unilateral or less than severe hearing loss; highly subject to observer bias; child tires rapidly when subjected to repeated stimuli
Visual reinforced audiometry (VRA)	Behavioral test: Child is given an animated toy for turning to sounds	5 to 24 months	Low cost; child responds at softer levels and for longer periods compared with BOA	Insensitive to unilateral loss (unless earphones used); need two examiners to reduce bias
Play audiometry	Behavioral test: Child is trained to respond to tones by playing game	2 to 5 years	Low cost; can detect unilateral and mild hearing loss	Requires cooperation of child
Screening audiometry	Behavioral test: Child raises hand or responds verbally to tones at fixed levels (20 to 25 dB)	4 years and older	Can be performed by trained paraprofessional in most children 4 years and older; can detect unilateral and mild hearing loss	Further tests required if failed
Otoacoustic emission (OAE)	Physiologic test: Response of inner ear to brief clicks or tones is measured with specialized instrument	Any	Child's response not needed; takes less than 2 minutes if child is quiet; can be performed by a trained paraprofessional; low cost; can detect unilateral and mild hearing loss	Cannot tell type or degree of loss; further tests required if failed
Auditory brainstem response (ABR) audiometry	Physiologic test: Averaged number of responses of brainstem to brief tones or clicks	Any	Child's response not needed; can detect unilateral and mild loss; can determine degree and slope of loss (with tone bursts and bone conduction testing)	Requires audiologist and equipment to administer and interpret; expensive; requires sedation beyond about 6 months old

TABLE 30-2 Evaluation of Audiometric Results

Average Threshold at 500 to 2000 Hz (Decibels)	Description	Significance
−10 to +15	Normal	
16 to 25	Slight loss (minimal)	Difficulty hearing faint speech, slight verbal deficit
26 to 40	Mild loss	Auditory learning dysfunction, language, or speech problems
41 to 55	Moderate loss	Trouble hearing conversational speech; may miss 50% of class discussion
56 to 70	Moderately severe loss	
71 to 90	Severe loss	Educational retardation, learning disability, limited vocabulary
90+	Profound loss	

A normal tympanogram is depicted below. Four features of the tympanogram can be used to evaluate the ear under test:

1. **Static admittance (Peak Y_a)** is a measure of the height of the tympanometric peak. Given appropriate norms, static admittance is a useful indicator of middle ear disease.
2. **Equivalent ear canal volume (+200 Vea)** is the admittance value determined with an ear canal air pressure of +200 d_aP_a (dekapascals). An abnormally high equivalent ear canal volume suggests the presence of a tympanic membrane perforation, or a patent tympanostomy tube.
3. **Tympanometric peak pressure (TPP)** is the position of the tympanometric peak on the pressure axis. TPP is an imprecise measure of the middle ear pressure. By itself, TPP is not an accurate indicator of middle ear disease.
4. **Tympanometric gradient (GR) or tympanometric width** is a measure of the width of the tympanometric peak. Defined as the pressure interval required for a 50% reduction of peak eardrum admittance, tympanometric width is a good indicator of the presence of **middle ear effusion**.

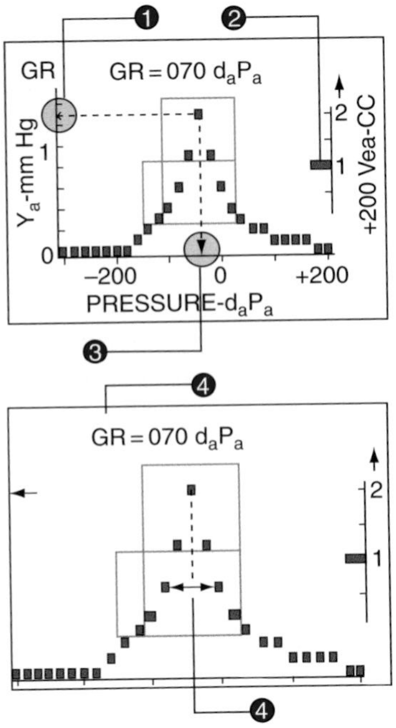

• **Figure 30-2** A normal tympanogram.

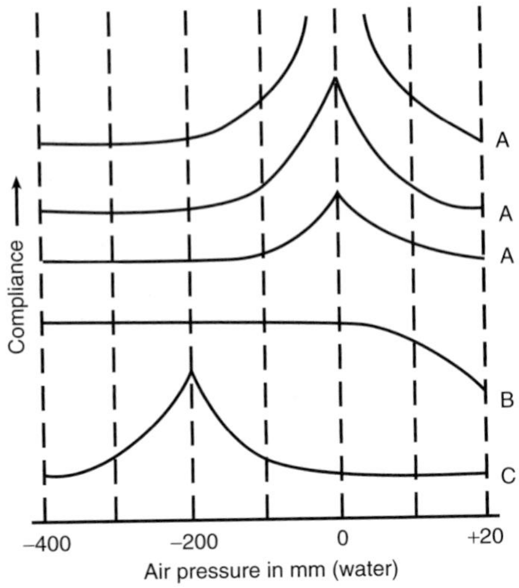

• **Figure 30-3** Five types of tympanogram curves. Generally an *A curve* indicates a normal tympanic membrane (TM), a *B curve* is abnormal, a *C curve* may be abnormal, and a *D curve* indicates hypermobility. An A_s *curve* may be normal in infants.

pregnancy or complications at the time of delivery. A combination of genetics and environmental factors may cause the hearing loss. Seventy percent of genetic mutations that cause hearing loss are not associated with a syndrome. Mutations of the GJB2 gene have been identified as causing about 40% of genetic hearing loss in children without a syndrome (CDC, 2015).

Management Strategies

Medications

In 2013, Lieberthal and colleagues, on behalf of the AAP, published an evidence-based practice guideline as a revision of the 2004 guidelines. The focus of the guideline is the appropriate diagnosis and treatment of AOM. The major tenants of the guideline are accurate diagnosis of AOM, pain management, initial observation versus antibiotic treatment, appropriate antibiotic choice, and preventive measures and plan if there is a recurrence of AOM. The definition of AOM included rapid onset of otalgia, MEE confirmed with pneumatic otoscopy or tympanogram, and signs of middle ear inflammation. Treatment strategies for AOM are based on the presence of the three diagnostic criteria for AOM plus the severity of the illness (duration, degree of fever, and severity of ear pain). Some patients require immediate treatment with antibiotics and others may only need watchful waiting and close follow-up. Prophylactic antibiotics are never recommended in the treatment of chronic or recurrent AOM (Lieberthal et al, 2013).

Pain management is the cornerstone of treatment for ear maladies. Antibiotics may take 48 to 72 hours to help reduce pain caused by middle ear inflammation. Antipyretics and analgesics are useful in treating fever and discomfort. Medicated otic drops for pain relief can be used as long as the TM is intact. Otic preparations must be administered appropriately to help ensure successful treatment. These medications should be warmed before instilling the drops, the tragus should be pumped a few times after instillation of the drops, and the affected ear should remain up for at least 2 to 3 minutes after the procedure is complete.

The removal of impacted cerumen is essential when excessive cerumen impedes examination of the ear or alters hearing and can be accomplished by mechanical removal or by using ceruminolytics with or without irrigation. Acidic eardrops help maintain an environment in the EAC that prevents the growth of fungi and bacteria.

Education and Counseling

Education and counseling of the patient and family regarding the watchful waiting concept, management of prolonged effusion in the ear, the prevention of additional problems, and the treatment course are key counseling points. Areas of particular importance include avoiding passive smoke exposure, breastfeeding during the first 6 months of life, avoiding bottle propping, minimizing exposure to other children with minor acute illnesses, decreasing exposure to loud noises, receiving an annual influenza vaccine for all children 6 months or older, and completing the pneumococcal conjugate vaccine (PCV13) vaccination series for children younger than 2 years old.

Removal of Cerumen

Removal of cerumen is only indicated when visualization of the EAC and TM is necessary. Cerumen in the ear canal can be removed mechanically, with gentle irrigation, by using a ceruminolytic, or more likely with a combination (Loveman et al, 2011). Loveman and colleagues found that there was no superior ceruminolytics, and the best results occurred when the ear was irrigated with water following the instillation of a ceruminolytic agent. Common ceruminolytics include docusate sodium, mineral oil, olive oil, or baking soda mixed with water. Irrigation is accomplished by using a bulb syringe or "water jet" (on low setting). Water-based ceruminolytics disintegrate the wax, whereas oil-based products soften the wax. Irrigation should not be attempted if the TM is possibly perforated or pressure-equalizing tubes are in place. Providers and parents prefer the irrigation technique to manual removal of cerumen (Loveman et al, 2011).

Mechanical cerumen removal (curettage) requires skill and the use of a cerumen spoon. Blunt plastic ear curettes may be less traumatic than the metal variety. Always carefully explain the procedure to parents and inform them that the ear canal is extremely sensitive and fragile and bleeds easily when touched. This may prevent an adverse parent reaction when there is blood on the curette or in the ear canal.

Follow-Up and Referral

The need for follow-up for ear disorders depends on the age of the child, the severity of illness, the diagnosis, the treatment plan, and the response to treatment. Young infants with a severe infection, children with continuing fever or pain, and those given a prescription to use if needed should have phone follow-up within a few days (Lieberthal et al, 2013). Infants and toddlers with more severe illness should be seen again if there is not complete resolution of symptoms. Older children with milder disease need no follow-up.

An otolaryngology referral is indicated for unusual ear conditions, congenital malformation of the head and neck structures, craniofacial anomalies, sensory dysfunction involving hearing or speech, when appropriate therapy for otitis media has failed, or if ongoing effusion or infection persists. Immediate myringotomy (and/or pressure-equalizing tube insertion) is indicated when there is severe, refractory pain; hyperpyrexia; facial paralysis; mastoiditis; labyrinthitis; CNS infection; or immunologic compromise. Referral to an audiologist is necessary if the ear pathology is prolonged or when the child's ability to hear is questioned. Speech and language evaluations are imperative to resolve questions about whether the child's verbal development is delayed because of persistent or recurring ear problems. Chapter 32 addresses criteria for tonsillectomy and adenoidectomy.

Pressure-Equalizing Tubes

Clinical practice guidelines recommend referral to an otolaryngologist for pressure-equalizing tube insertion only if the child has recurrent AOM three times in 6 months or four times in 1 year with at least one episode in the past 6 months (Lieberthal et al, 2013). Children with craniofacial abnormalities may need pressure-equalizing tubes in order to maximize hearing and speech acquisition.

Placing pressure-equalizing tubes takes less than 15 minutes and is usually done using general anesthesia. The child is usually discharged after about 1 hour and is treated with antibiotic otic drops for several days. Children with persistent hearing loss after pressure-equalizing tube placement should be further evaluated. The examiner can establish that the tube is functioning properly if the tube spans the eardrum, the lumen is unobstructed, and no MEE is present. If appropriate functioning of the tube cannot be established, pneumatic otoscopy or tympanometry may be useful. A flat (type B) tympanogram with large-volume measurements confirms appropriate function of the tube. A normal (type A) tympanogram suggests a clogged or extruded tube. The use of ototopical antibiotic/corticosteroid drops for 5 to 7 days can occasionally clear a clogged pressure-equalizing tube. If the child can taste the drops or complains of stinging, the drops are most likely reaching the middle ear space, which indicates a functioning tube.

A child with pressure-equalizing tubes does not need to take precautions during bathing, showering, or surface swimming (Wilcox and Darrow, 2014). Earplugs should be used if the child is diving or dunking the head below water level. Diving and head dunking in any water allows water into the middle ear space, leaving a moist environment where bacteria can grow.

Viral myringitis or early AOM without otorrhea in a child with pressure-equalizing tubes will most likely resolve spontaneously because of increased middle ear ventilation. Tympanostomy tube otorrhea (TTO) usually occurs when a child with tubes has an upper respiratory infection and has drainage coming from the tubes. TTO usually involves the same bacterial pathogens seen in AOM. Combination antibiotic and corticosteroid otic drops are the preferred

TABLE 30-3 Commonly Used Topical Preparations for Otitis Externa and Analgesia

Product Name (Manufacturer)	Antibiotic	Steroid	Acid	Comments
Analgesic				
Antipyrine/benzocaine/ u-polycosanol (Auralgan) Antipyrine/benzocaine (Aurodex)	None	None	None	Benzocaine in a glycerin and propylene base Used for ear pain Not to be used if TM integrity unsure
Antibiotics (Not Ototoxic)				
Ciprodex (Alcon)	Ciprofloxacin	Dexamethasone		Use ≥6 months old Contains steroid
Floxin Otic (Daiichi Pharmaceutical)	Ofloxacin	None	Acetic and boric	Does not contain steroid
Vasocidin ophthalmic (Ciba Vision Ophthalmics)	Sulfacetamide sodium	Prednisolone sodium phosphate		No documented ototoxicity with either agent Excellent broad-spectrum coverage Contains steroid
Antibiotics (Ototoxic)				
Cortisporin Otic Susp Pediotic (King Pharmaceutical)	Polymyxin B and neomycin	Hydrocortisone	Hydrochloric acid	May be painful on instillation Neomycin may cause cutaneous irritation Not to be used if TM integrity unknown
Cipro HC Otic (Alcon Labs)	Ciprofloxacin	Hydrocortisone	Glacial acetic acid	Use ≥1 year old Contraindicated with TM perforation
Cleansing and Antipruritic Agent (Ototoxic)				
Domeboro Otic (Bayer Pharmaceutical Division)	None	None	Acetic acid	Excellent choice for cleansing of the EAC Aluminum acetate helps to prevent itching Not to be used if TM integrity is unknown

EAC, External auditory canal; *TM*, tympanic membrane.

treatment for TTO (van Dongen et al, 2014). Otic medications are listed in Table 30-3.

Many pressure-equalizing tubes fall out while they are still useful. If the tube is extruded and there are persistent ear complaints, or if it remains in the TM for more than 2 or 3 years, the child should see the otolaryngologist (Rosenfeld et al, 2013). Complications of pressure-equalizing tubes include otorrhea, otitis externa (OE), granuloma, cholesteatoma, tube obstruction, persistent TM perforation, and tympanosclerosis. Bacterial biofilms can form on implanted prostheses, including pressure-equalizing tubes, and tend to be resistant to systemic antibiotics.

Prevention of Noise-Induced Hearing Loss

Noise is a common cause of sensorineural hearing loss (SNHL) in children, and the pattern of damage depends on the frequency, intensity, and duration of the noise. Any structure in the ear can be permanently damaged by noise 140 dB or more. (See Chapter 42 for discussion of this environmental hazard and a list of risky noise sources.)

Specific Ear Problems in Children

Otitis Externa

Otitis externa (OE), commonly called *swimmer's ear,* is a diffuse inflammation of the EAC and can involve the pinna or TM. Inflammation is evidenced as (1) simple infection with edema, discharge, and erythema; (2) furuncles or small abscesses that form in hair follicles; or (3) impetigo or infection of the superficial layers of the epidermis. OE can also be classified as mycotic otitis externa, caused by fungus, or as chronic external otitis, a diffuse low-grade infection of the EAC. Severe infection or systemic infection can be seen in children who have diabetes mellitus, are immunocompromised, or have received head and neck irradiation.

OE results when the protective barriers in the EAC are damaged by mechanical or chemical mechanisms. OE is most frequently caused by retained moisture in the EAC, which changes the usually acidic environment to a neutral or basic environment, thereby promoting bacterial or fungal growth. Chlorine in swimming pools adds to the problem because it kills the normal ear flora, allowing the growth of pathogens. Regular cleaning of the EAC removes cerumen, which is an important barrier to water and infection. Soapy deposits, alkaline drops, debris from skin conditions, local trauma, sweating, allergy, stress, and hearing aids can also be responsible for causing OE (Rosenfeld et al, 2014).

OE is most often caused by *Pseudomonas aeruginosa* and *Staphylococcus aureus,* but it is not uncommon for the infection to be polymicrobial. Furunculosis of the external canal is generally caused by *S. aureus* and *Streptococcus pyogenes.* Otomycosis is caused by *Aspergillus* or *Candida* and can be the result of systemic or topical antibiotics or steroids. Otomycosis is also more common in children with diabetes mellitus or immune dysfunction and in these cases is most commonly caused by *Aspergillus niger, Escherichia coli,* or *Klebsiella pneumonia. Group B streptococci* are a more common cause in neonates.

Long-standing ear drainage may suggest a foreign body, chronic middle ear pathology (such as, a cholesteatoma), or granulomatous tissue. Bloody drainage may indicate trauma, severe otitis media, or granulation tissue. Chronic or recurrent OE may result from eczema, seborrhea, or psoriasis. Eczematous dermatitis, moist vesicles, and pustules are seen in acute infection, whereas crusting is more consistent with chronic infection.

Clinical Findings

History

The following can be found:

- Itching and irritation
- Pain that seems disproportionate to what is seen on examination
- Pressure and fullness in ear and occasionally hearing loss that can be conductive or sensorineural
- Rare hearing loss and otorrhea or systemic complaints and symptoms
- Sagging of the superior canal, periauricular edema, and preauricular and postauricular lymphadenopathy with more severe disease

  Extension to the surrounding soft tissue results in the obstruction of the canal with or without cellulitis.

Physical Examination

Findings on physical examination can include the following:

- Pain, often quite severe, with movement of the tragus (when pushed) or pinna (when pulled) or on attempts to examine the ear with an otoscope
- Swollen EAC with debris, making visualization of the TM difficult or impossible
- Rare otorrhea
- Occasional regional lymphadenopathy
- Tragal tenderness with a red, raised area of induration that can be deep and diffuse or superficial and pointing, which is characteristic of furunculosis
- Red, crusty, or pustular spreading lesions
- Pruritus associated with thick otorrhea that can be black, gray, blue-green, yellow, or white, and black spots over the TM are indicative of mycotic infection
- Dry-appearing canal with some atrophy or thinning of the canal and virtually no cerumen visible with chronic OE
- Presence of pressure-equalizing tube or perforation of TM

Diagnostic Studies

Culturing the discharge from the ear is not customary but may be indicated if clinical improvement is not seen during or after treatment, severe pain persists, the child is a neonate, the child is immunocompromised, or chronic or recurrent OE is suspected. Culturing requires a swab premoistened with sterile nonbacteriostatic saline or water.

Differential Diagnosis

AOM with perforation, TTO, chronic suppurative otitis media (CSOM), necrotizing OE, cholesteatoma, mastoiditis, posterior auricular lymphadenopathy, dental infection, and eczema are all possible differential diagnoses.

Management

The following steps outline the management of OE:

- Eardrops are the mainstay of therapy for OE (see Table 30-3). Eardrops containing acetic acid or antibiotic with and without corticosteroid drops are the treatment of choice for OE. Symptoms should be markedly improved within 7 days, but resolution of the infection may take up to 2 weeks. Drops should be used until all symptoms have resolved. Ototoxic drugs should not be used if there is a risk of TM perforation.
  - Antibiotic agents should be chosen based on efficacy, resistance patterns, low incidence of adverse effects, cost, and likelihood of compliance. Neomycin, polymyxin, or hydrocortisone drops should not be used if the TM is not intact, because these drugs are known to cause damage to the cochlea (Rosenfeld et al, 2014).
  - The quinolone products are effective against *Pseudomonas, S. aureus,* and *Streptococcus pneumoniae,* which may be a factor if the OE is a complication of AOM.
- Systemic antibiotics should not be used unless there is extension of infection beyond the ear or host factors that require more systemic treatment (severe OE, systemic illness, fever, lymphadenitis, or failed topical treatment).
- Treatment for OE must include thorough parent education regarding the instillation of otic drops so that they are effective in eradicating infection. The drops should be administered with the child lying down with the affected ear upward. Drops should run into the EAC until it is filled. Move the pinna in a to-and-fro movement or pump the tragus to remove any trapped air and ensure filling (Rosenfeld et al, 2014). The child should remain lying down for 3 to 5 minutes, leaving the ear open to the air.

- If the infection is severe and not improving in the first 5 to 7 days, aural irrigation with water, saline, or hydrogen peroxide may be tried, or refer to the otolaryngologist for débridement and suction.
- If significant swelling is present, inserting a wick into the EAC is helpful. A wick made of compressed cellulose, hydrogel polymer (Merocel XL), or gauze (0.25 inch) usually works well. The tip of the wick is lubricated with water or saline just before insertion into the ear. Once in place, the wick should be impregnated with antibiotics for as long as it remains in the auditory canal. (This may require reapplication of drops every 2 to 3 hours.) Wicks are usually removed after several days. The wick will fall out when the swelling has subsided, and treatment with direct application of drops to the ear canal should continue for the entire course.
- Avoid cleaning, manipulating, and getting water into the ear. Swimming is prohibited during acute infection.
- Administer analgesics for pain. Narcotic analgesics may be necessary for severe pain but are only indicated for short-term use.
- Débridement with a cotton-tipped applicator, self-made cotton wick, or calcium alginate swabs is indicated once the inflammatory process has subsided and can enhance the effectiveness of the ototopical antibiotic drops. Lance a furuncle that is superficial and pointed with a 14-gauge needle. If it is deep and diffuse, a heating pad or warm oil-based drops can speed resolution.
- If impetigo is present, clear the canal by using water or an antiseptic solution followed by a warm-water rinse. Apply an antibiotic ointment (mupirocin) twice a day for 5 to 7 days. There is increasing resistance to mupirocin, and retapamulin might be necessary in children over 9 months of age (Bangert et al, 2012; Drucker, 2012). The child should avoid touching the ear. Fingernails should be short, and hands should be cleansed with soap and water. Systemic antibiotics are generally unnecessary.
- Fungal OE is uncommon in primary OE. Fungal OE is more likely related to chronic OE or following treatment with topical and/or systemic antibiotics. *Aspergillus* and *Candida* species are most commonly seen in mycotic OE (Rosenfeld et al, 2014). Treatment consists of antifungal solutions, such as clotrimazole-miconazole, nystatin, or other antifungal agents, including gentian violet and thimerosal 1 : 1000.
- The canal should be cleansed with a 5% boric acid in ethanol solution prior to antifungal solution.

If the child is not improved within 72 hours (relief of otalgia, itching, and fullness), recheck to confirm diagnosis. Lack of improvement may be due to obstructed ear canal, foreign body, poor adherence, or contact sensitivity among other things. A follow-up visit may be necessary after 1 to 2 weeks for reevaluation of the OE and removal of debris. If symptoms are worsening or there is no improvement in a week, a referral to an otolaryngologist or dermatologist is indicated.

Complications

Infection of surrounding tissues with impetigo, irritated furunculosis, and malignant OE with progression and necrosis caused by *Pseudomonas* are possible complications. Involvement of the parotid gland, mastoid bone, and infratemporal fossa is rare (Rosenfeld et al, 2014).

Prevention

The patient should be instructed to do the following:

- Avoid water in the ear canals.
- Use well-fitting earplugs for swimming especially in "dirty water."
- Use alcohol vinegar otic mix (two parts rubbing alcohol, one part white vinegar, and one part distilled water) 3 to 5 drops daily, especially after swimming or bathing, to prevent the recurrence of OE (Waitzman, 2015).
- Use a blow dryer on warm setting to dry the EAC.
- Avoid persistent scratching or cleaning of the external canal.
- Avoid prolonged use of ceruminolytic agents.

Foreign Body in the Ear Canal

A foreign body in the external ear canal is a problem frequently seen by pediatric health care providers, in emergency departments, and by otolaryngologists worldwide.

Foreign bodies are usually placed or thrown into the ear canal by the child or other children. Insects can also be found in the canal. Leaves and other plant materials can be intentionally inserted into the EAC as a form of native remedy (Shafi et al, 2010).

Clinical Findings

History

The history can include the following:

- Child reports putting something into the ear or having something thrown at him or her
- Complaints of itching, buzzing, fullness, or an object in the ear
- Persistent cough or hiccups
- Unilateral otalgia and otorrhea
- Asymptomatic

Physical Examination

A foreign body is visible with the naked eye or by otoscopic examination.

Management

Adequate visualization in a cooperative patient and a skilled provider with the appropriate equipment are the keys to successfully removing a foreign body in the EAC. It is critical that the object be removed on the first attempt, because the success rate is markedly decreased after the first attempt. A provider has one attempt to remove the object and if the object is not successfully removed, then a referral to an ear, nose, and throat (ENT) specialist is recommended.

Foreign bodies in the lateral one third of the ear canal are the easiest to remove. Foreign bodies in the medial two thirds of the ear canal are more difficult to remove, because the canal is narrower, is lined with bone, is quite vascular, and is exquisitely sensitive. Occasionally, straightening the ear canal by pulling on the pinna and gently shaking the patient's head will cause the foreign body to fall out.

- Disk batteries must be removed emergently.
- Spherical objects are the most difficult to remove and should be referred to an otolaryngologist.
- Soft, irregularly shaped objects are generally graspable with a bayonet forceps, alligator forceps, or curved hook.
- Round or breakable objects can be removed using a wire loop, a curette, or right-angle hook that is slowly advanced beyond the object and withdrawn carefully.
- If the object is made of iron, nickel, or cobalt, try using a magnet to retrieve it.
- Insects in the ear canal should be suffocated with mineral oil, and the child should be referred for otomicroscopic removal.
- Irrigation can only be done if the TM is intact and should be done using fluid at body temperature and a commercial irrigator or 60-mL syringe with an angiocatheter on the end (Stoner and Dulaurier, 2013).
  - Irrigation may push the object farther into the ear canal.
  - Do not irrigate if the object is a disk battery, the TM is not intact, or the object is made of organic material (corn, peas, and so on).
- Refer the patient to an otolaryngologist if the object cannot be extracted on the first attempt, the object cannot be removed without causing further damage or worsening pain, the child is unable to cooperate, the foreign body has a higher likelihood of failure (in the medial third of the ear canal, spherical shape, vegetable matter, and so on), or the object has been in the EAC more than 24 hours or is lying on the TM (Conover, 2013).
- Ear blocks (regional anesthesia) are not recommended.
- Consider conscious sedation if the clinical setting is appropriate.
- Once the object is removed, topical antibiotic drops with steroid are recommended for any drainage, potential for infection due to trauma of removal, and to decrease inflammation.

Complications

Infection, perforation of the TM, and damage to the ossicles are possible if the object is not removed.

Acute Otitis Media

AOM is an acute infection of the middle ear (Fig. 30-4). The AAP Clinical Practice Guideline requires the presence of the following three components to diagnose AOM (Lieberthal et al, 2013):

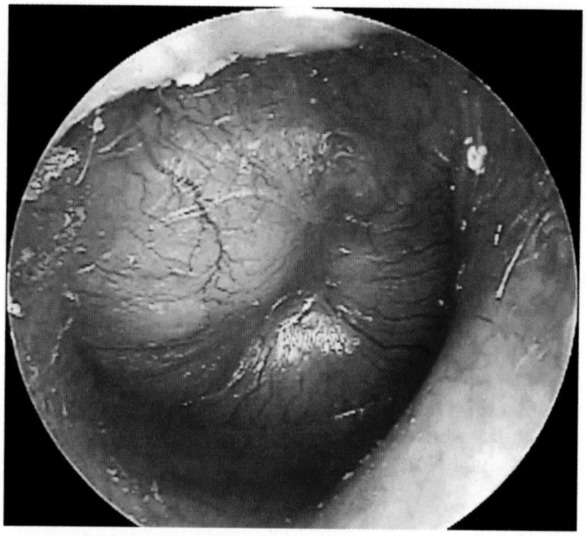

• **Figure 30-4** Acute otitis media of the right ear.

TABLE 30-4 Types of Acute Otitis Media

Type	Characteristics
AOM	Suppurative effusion of the middle ear
Bullous myringitis	AOM in which bullae form between the inner and middle layers of the TM and bulge outward
Persistent AOM	AOM that has not resolved when antibiotic therapy has been completed or AOM recurs within days of treatment
Recurrent AOM	Three separate bouts of AOM within a 6-month period or four within a 12-month period; often a positive family history of otitis media and other ENT disease

AOM, Acute otitis media; *ENT,* ear, nose, and throat; *TM,* tympanic membrane.

- Recent, abrupt onset of signs and symptoms of middle ear inflammation and effusion (ear pain, irritability, otorrhea, and/or fever)
- MEE as confirmed by bulging TM, limited or absent mobility by pneumatic otoscopy, air-fluid level behind TM, and/or otorrhea
- Signs and symptoms of middle ear inflammation as confirmed by distinct erythema of the TM or onset of ear pain (holding, tugging, rubbing of the ear in a nonverbal manner)

Characteristics of different types of AOM are defined in Table 30-4. AOM often follows eustachian tube dysfunction (ETD). Common causes of ETD include upper respiratory infections, allergies, and ETS. ETD leads to

• BOX 30-1 Risk Factors for Otitis Media, Chronic Otitis Media, or Otitis Media with Effusion

Genetic susceptibility/sibling with history of otitis media
Native Americans and Native Alaskans
Non-Hispanic Caucasian
Prematurity
Younger than 2 years of age
Unimmunized
Day care attendance
Sharing a bedroom
Breastfeeding for less than 6 months
Parental smoking and other ETS exposure
Environmental pollution exposure
Overweight or obese
Feeding in supine position
Autumn season
Male gender
Early onset otitis media
Bilateral OME
Lower socioeconomic status

ETS, Environmental tobacco smoke; *OME,* otitis media with effusion.

• BOX 30-2 Risk Factors for Hearing Loss Caused by Otitis Media with Effusion

Bilateral OME for 4 months or longer
If two or more present:
- OME present for longer than 8 weeks
- Speech development slower than peers
- Speech less clear than previously
- Child decreases amount of talking
- Child less responsive to name and other familiar sounds
- Child says "Huh?" or "What?" frequently
- Child sits close to TV or wants volume louder
- Child has difficulty learning (reading, spelling)
- Child is hyperactive or overly inattentive

OME, Otitis media with effusion.

functional eustachian tube obstruction and inflammation that decreases the protective ciliary action in the eustachian tube. When the eustachian tube is obstructed, negative pressure develops as air is absorbed in the middle ear (see Fig. 30-4). The negative pressure pulls fluid from the mucosal lining and causes an accumulation of sterile fluid. Bacteria pulled in from the eustachian tube lead to the accumulation of purulent fluid. Young children have shorter, more horizontal and more flaccid eustachian tubes that are easily disrupted by viruses, which predisposes them to AOM. Respiratory syncytial virus and influenza are two of the viruses most responsible for the increase in the incidence of AOM seen from January to April. Other risk factors associated with AOM are listed in Boxes 30-1 and 30-2.

S. pneumoniae, nontypeable *Haemophilus influenzae, Moraxella catarrhalis,* and *S. pyogenes* (group A streptococci) are the most common infecting organisms in AOM (Conover, 2013). *S. pneumoniae* continues to be the most common bacteria responsible for AOM. The strains of *S. pneumoniae* in the heptavalent pneumococcal conjugate vaccine (PCV7) have virtually disappeared from the middle ear fluid of children with AOM (Lieberthal et al, 2013). With the introduction of the 13-valent *S. pneumoniae* vaccine, the bacteriology of the middle ear is likely to continue to evolve. Bullous myringitis is almost always caused by *S. pneumonia.* Nontypeable *H. influenza* remains a common cause of AOM. It is the most common cause of bilateral otitis media, severe inflammation of the TM, and otitis-conjunctivitis syndrome. *M. catarrhalis* obtained from the nasopharynx has become increasingly more beta-lactamase positive, but the high rate of clinical resolution in children with AOM from *M. catarrhalis* makes amoxicillin a good choice for initial therapy (Lieberthal et al, 2013). *M. catarrhalis* rarely causes invasive disease. *S. pyogenes* is responsible for AOM in older children, is responsible for more TM ruptures, and is more likely to cause mastoiditis.

Although a virus is usually the initial causative factor in AOM, strict diagnostic criteria, careful specimen handling, and sensitive microbiologic techniques have shown that the majority of AOM is caused by bacteria or bacteria and virus together (Lieberthal et al, 2013).

Clinical Findings

History

Rapid onset of signs and symptoms:
- Ear pain with possible ear pulling in the infant; may interfere with activity and/or sleep
- Irritability in an infant or toddler
- Otorrhea
- Fever

Other key factors or symptoms:
- Prematurity
- Craniofacial anomalies or congenital syndromes associated with craniofacial anomalies
- Exposure to risk factors
- Disrupted sleep or inability to sleep
- Lethargy, dizziness, tinnitus, and unsteady gait
- Diarrhea and vomiting
- Sudden hearing loss
- Stuffy nose, rhinorrhea, and sneezing
- Rare facial palsy and ataxia

Physical Examination

- Presence of MEE, confirmed by pneumatic otoscopy, tympanometry, or acoustic reflectometry, as evidenced by:
  - Bulging TM (see Fig. 30-4)
  - Decreased translucency of TM
  - Absent or decreased mobility of the TM
  - Air-fluid level behind the TM
  - Otorrhea

- Signs and symptoms of middle ear inflammation indicated by either:
  - Erythema of the TM (Amber is usually seen in otitis media with effusion [OME]; white or yellow may be seen in either AOM or OME [Shaikh et al, 2010].)
  or
  - Distinct otalgia that interferes with normal activity or sleep
- In addition, the following TM findings may be present:
  - Increased vascularity with obscured or absent landmarks (see Fig. 30-4).
  - Red, yellow, or purple TM (Redness alone should not be used to diagnose AOM, especially in a crying child.)
  - Thin-walled, sagging bullae filled with straw-colored fluid seen with bullous myringitis

Diagnostic Studies

Pneumatic otoscopy is the simplest and most efficient way to diagnose AOM. Tympanometry reflects effusion (type B pattern). Tympanocentesis to identify the infecting organism is helpful in the treatment of infants younger than 2 months old. In older infants and children, tympanocentesis is rarely done and is useful only if the patient is toxic or immunocompromised or in the presence of resistant infection or acute pain from bullous myringitis. If a tympanocentesis is warranted, refer the patient to an otolaryngologist for this procedure.

Differential Diagnosis

OME, mastoiditis, dental abscess, sinusitis, lymphadenitis, parotitis, peritonsillar abscess, trauma, ETD, impacted teeth, temporomandibular joint dysfunction, and immune deficiency are differential diagnoses. Any infant 2 months old or younger with AOM should be evaluated for fever without focus and not just treated for an ear infection.

Management

Many changes have been made in the treatment of AOM because of the increasing rate of antibiotic-resistant bacteria related to the injudicious use of antibiotics. Ample evidence has been presented that symptom management may be all that is required in children with MEE without other symptoms of AOM (Lieberthal et al, 2013). Treatment guidelines are decided based on the child's age, illness severity, and the certainty of diagnosis. Table 30-5 shows the recommendation for the diagnosis and subsequent treatment of AOM.

1. Pain management is the first principle of treatment.
   - Weight-appropriate doses of ibuprofen or acetaminophen should be encouraged to decrease discomfort and fever.
   - Topical analgesics, such as benzocaine or antipyrine/benzocaine otic preparations, can be added to systemic pain management if the TM is known to be intact. Topical analgesics should not be used alone.
   - Distraction, oil application, or external use of heat or cold may be of some use.

TABLE 30-5 Treatment Guidelines for Acute Otitis Media

Diagnosis	Treat
Any child with moderate/severe bulging TM with otorrhea not associated with AOM	Yes
Any child with mild bulging of the TM with recent (<48 hours) onset pain (holding, tugging, and so on) or intensely erythematous TM	Yes
Babies ≥6 months of age with severe signs of AOM (fever >102.2° F [39° C], otalgia for ≥48 hours)	Yes
Any child 6 to 23 months old with acute bilateral otitis media without severe symptoms, without fever, and sick less than 48 hours	Yes
Young children with unilateral AOM without severe symptoms and fever <102.2° F [39° C]	Provide prescription and/or wait Close follow-up
Children ≥24 months old without severe symptoms	Provide prescription and/or wait Close follow-up
Children not treated and no improvement in 48 to 72 hours	See the patient again Clinician discretion whether or not to treat

From Lieberthal AS, Carroll AE, Chonmaitree T, et al: The diagnosis and management of acute otitis media, *Pediatrics* 131(3):e964–e999, 2013. Adapted from Clinical Practice Guidelines.
AOM, Acute otitis media; *TM,* tympanic membrane.

2. Antibiotics are also effective. (Table 30-6 lists dosage recommendations.)
   - Amoxicillin remains the first-line antibiotic for AOM if there has not been a previous treated AOM in the previous 30 days, there is no conjunctivitis, and no penicillin allergy (Lieberthal et al, 2013). *Beta-lactam* coverage (amoxicillin/clavulanate, third-generation cephalosporin) is recommended when the child has been treated with amoxicillin in the previous 30 days, there is an allergy to penicillin, and the child has concurrent conjunctivitis or has recurrent otitis that has not responded to amoxicillin. If there is a documented hypersensitivity reaction to amoxicillin, the following antibiotics are acceptable, follow the non-type 1 hypersensitivity and type 1 hypersensitivity recommendations in Table 30-6:
     - Ceftriaxone may be effective for the vomiting child, the child unable to tolerate oral medications, or the child who has failed amoxicillin/clavulanate.

TABLE 30-6 Medications Used to Treat Acute Otitis Media

Drug	Dosage	Comments
Amoxicillin	80 to 90 mg/kg/day divided twice a day	First choice unless allergy
Amoxicillin-clavulanate	80 to 90 mg/kg/day divided twice a day	Clavulanate <10 mg/kg/day Good beta-lactamase coverage Costly and more likely to cause diarrhea
Azithromycin	10 mg/kg/day on day 1 (maximum dose 500 mg/day) then 5 mg/kg/day on days 2 to 5 given daily (maximum dose 250 mg/day)	Children older than 6 months need 5-day treatment course Macrolide primarily used because of penicillin allergy Should not be used as first-line treatment
Cefdinir	14 mg/kg/day daily or divided twice a day	Broad-spectrum Third-generation cephalosporin Causes red stool
Cefixime	8 mg/kg daily or divided twice a day	Broad-spectrum Third-generation cephalosporin Reduced efficacy against *Streptococcus pneumoniae*
Cefpodoxime	10 mg/kg/day daily divided twice a day	Broad spectrum of coverage Third-generation cephalosporin
Ceftibuten	9 mg/kg/day given daily	Children older than 6 months Third-generation cephalosporin Active against beta-lactamase Reduced efficacy against *S. pneumoniae*
Ceftriaxone	50 mg/kg/day IM 1 to 3 doses over 5 days	Costly Third-generation cephalosporin
Cefuroxime	30 mg/kg/day divided twice a day 125 mg every 12 hours if younger than 2 years old 250 mg every 12 hours if 2 to 12 years old 250 to 500 mg every 12 hours if older than 12 years old	Broad spectrum of coverage Costly Most potent second-generation cephalosporin Poor taste
Clarithromycin	15 mg/kg/day divided twice a day	Children older than 6 months need 5-day treatment course Macrolide Primarily used with type I penicillin allergy Should not be used as first-line treatment
Clindamycin	30 to 40 mg/kg/day given divided three times a day	Should not be used unless culture and sensitivities are done

Data from Taketomo CK, Hodding JH, Kraus DM: *Pediatric dosage handbook*, ed 21, Hudson, OH, 2014, Lexi-Comp.
IM, Intramuscular.

- Clindamycin may be considered for ceftriaxone failure but *should only* be used if susceptibilities are known.
- Prophylactic antibiotics for chronic or recurrent AOM are *not* recommended.

3. Observation or "watchful waiting" for 48 to 72 hours (see Table 30-5) allows the patient to improve without antibiotic treatment. Pain relief should be provided, and a means of follow-up must be in place. Options for follow-up include:
   - Parent-initiated visit or phone call for worsening or no improvement
   - Scheduled follow-up appointment
   - Routine follow-up phone call
   - Given a prescription to be started if the child's symptoms do not improve or if they worsen in 48 to 72 hours (Table 30-7)
   - Communication with the parent, reevaluation, and the ability to obtain medication must be in place.
4. Recommendations for follow-up include:
   - After 48 to 72 hours if a child has not showed improvement in ear symptomatology, the child should be seen to confirm or exclude the presence of AOM. If the initial management option was an antibacterial agent, the agent should be changed.

TABLE 30-7 Recommended Antibiotics to Treat Acute Otitis Media

Initial Antibiotic Treatment at Diagnosis		Clinically Defined Treatment Failure After 48 to 72 Hours of Observation		Clinically Defined Treatment Failure After Initial Treatment with Antibiotic	
Recommended	**Alternate for Penicillin Allergy**	**Recommended**	**Alternate for Penicillin Allergy**	**Recommended**	**Alternate for Penicillin Allergy**
Amoxicillin	Non-Type 1: Cefdinir Type 1: Azithromycin	Amoxicillin	Non-Type 1: Cefdinir Type 1: Azithromycin	Amoxicillin-clavulanate	Non-Type 1: Ceftriaxone Type 1: Clindamycin
Amoxicillin-clavulanate	Ceftriaxone	Amoxicillin-clavulanate	Ceftriaxone	Ceftriaxone	Tympanocentesis Treat to sensitivities

Management of Persistent and Recurrent Acute Otitis Media

- Persistent AOM occurs when antibiotic therapy has been completed and evidence of AOM is still present or AOM recurs within days of treatment. Retreatment with a broader-spectrum antibiotic is suggested.
- Persistent MEE is common after resolution of acute symptoms and should not be seen as a need for continuing antibiotics (see Otitis Media with Effusion section).
- Recurrent AOM is present when more than three distinct and well-documented bouts of AOM have occurred in 6 months or four or more episodes have occurred in 12 months.

An otolaryngology referral is indicated when appropriate therapy for otitis media has failed. Myringotomy or placement of pressure-equalizing tubes can help relieve discomfort, reduce time with OME, improve hearing, and decrease the likelihood of further infection (Wallace et al, 2014). Indications for tympanostomy and the insertion of pressure-equalizing tubes were discussed earlier.

Other Issues in Treating Acute Otitis Media

- The pediatric provider is encouraged to keep current on updated recommendations for the treatment of AOM because of the rapid changes in resistance patterns and newly developed treatments.
- Decongestants and antihistamines are not helpful in the treatment of AOM.
- Antimicrobial ototopical drops (ofloxacin or ciprofloxacin) or ophthalmic drops (tobramycin or gentamicin) are indicated if the TM is perforated (Fig. 30-5), the child has otorrhea, or the child has patent, draining pressure-equalizing tubes.
- Xylitol, a sugar found in fruits and the bark of birch trees, has bacteriostatic effects against *S. pneumoniae* and interferes with bacterial adhesion to mucous membranes. It appears to have some suppressive effects in preventing ear infections. Xylitol is available in an oral solution, lozenges, and chewing gum. The lozenges and chewing gum are more effective than the oral solution. Children younger than 2 years old cannot have chewing gum or lozenges. Xylitol must be given three to five times a day on a regular basis to be effective.

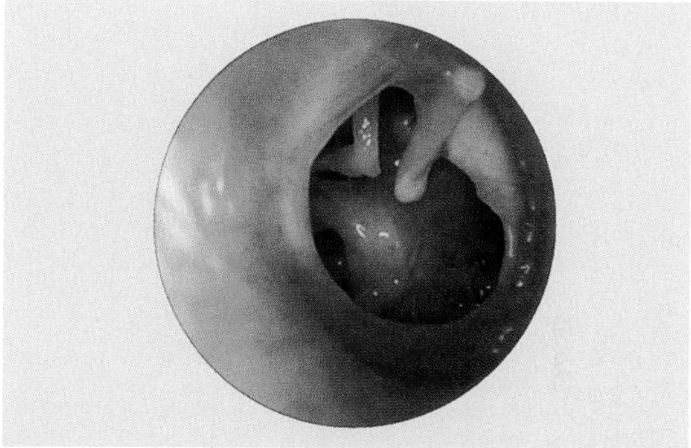

• **Figure 30-5** Perforated tympanic membrane (TM). (Photograph courtesy Sylvan Stool, MD, The Children's Hospital, Denver, CO.)

- There is no safe or effective herbal treatment for the treatment of AOM or OME.

Complications

Persistent AOM, persistent OME, TM perforation (Fig. 30-6), OE, mastoiditis, cholesteatoma, tympanosclerosis (Fig. 30-7), hearing loss of 25 to 30 dB for several months, ossicle necrosis, pseudotumor cerebri, cerebral thrombophlebitis, and facial paralysis are possible complications.

Prevention and Education

The following interventions, shown to be helpful in preventing AOM, should be encouraged:

- Exclusive breastfeeding until at least 6 months of age seems to be protective against AOM
- Avoid bottle propping, feeding infants lying down, and passive smoke exposure
- Avoid the use of pacifiers: Although the relationship cannot be fully explained, multiple studies have shown that pacifier use increases the incidence of AOM (Lieberthal et al, 2013).
- Pneumococcal vaccine; specifically PCV13, which contains subtype 19A
- Annual influenza vaccine may help prevent otitis media

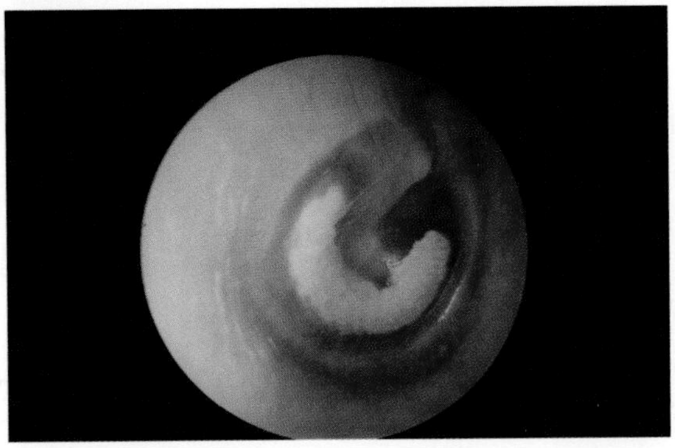

• **Figure 30-6** Tympanosclerosis of the right ear. (Photo courtesy Sylvan Stool, MD, The Children's Hospital, Denver, CO.)

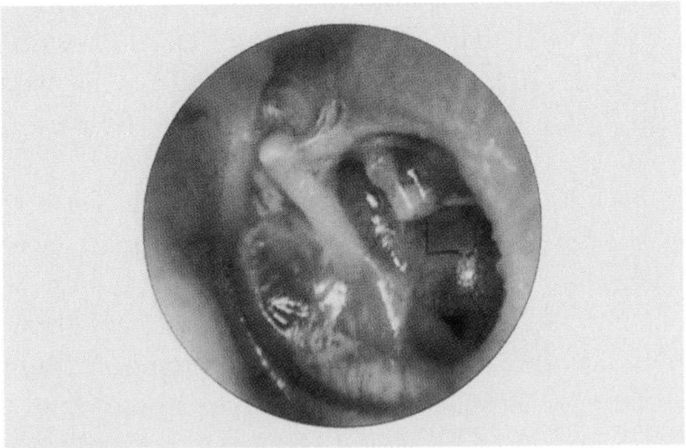

• **Figure 30-7** Left ear with posterior retraction (Photo courtesy Sylvan Stool, MD, The Children's Hospital, Denver, CO.)

- Xylitol liquid or chewing gum as tolerated
- Choose licensed day care facilities with fewer children
- Educate regarding the problem of drug-resistant bacteria and the need to avoid the use of antibiotics unless absolutely necessary; if antibiotics are used, the child needs to complete the entire course of the prescription and follow up if symptoms do not resolve

Otitis Media with Effusion

The diagnosis of OME is made when there is evidence of MEE without signs or symptoms of acute ear infection (Figs. 30-7 and 30-8). MEE decreases the mobility of the TM and interferes with sound conduction.

OME can occur spontaneously with ETD caused by an inflammatory process after AOM, viral illness, anatomic abnormalities, barotrauma, allergies, or a combination of these conditions. ETD changes the middle ear mucosa in the following sequence: (1) the mucosa becomes secretory with increased mucus production, (2) the mucus becomes viscous as the mucosa absorbs water, and (3) fluid becomes stuck behind the TM. Bacterial biofilms may explain the persistence of OME. Biofilms are mixed microorganisms enclosed in a polymeric matrix that adhere to surfaces, such as the middle ear mucosa.

Risk factors for chronic OME are listed in Box 30-2.

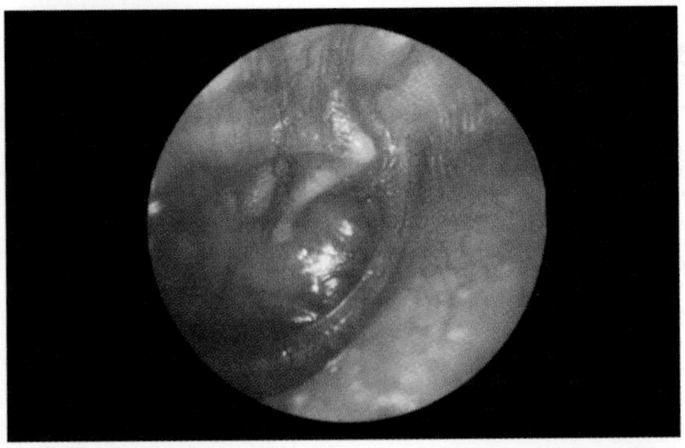

• **Figure 30-8** Severely retracted, opaque right tympanic membrane in otitis media with effusion. (From Bluestone CD, Klein JO: *Otitis media in infants and children*, ed 2, Philadelphia, 1995, Saunders.)

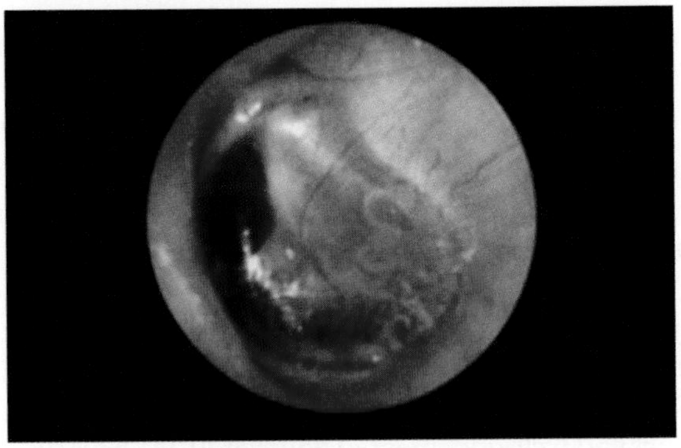

• **Figure 30-9** Serous effusion.

Clinical Findings

History

The following features may be noted in the affected child:

- Often asymptomatic and afebrile
- Intermittent complaints of mild ear pain
- Fullness in the ear ("popping" or the feeling of "talking in a barrel")
- Complaint of hearing loss in older children
- Dizziness or impaired balance
- Chronic vomiting with failure to thrive, which can be related to chronic OME

Physical Examination

Pneumatic otoscopy reveals decreased TM mobility. An abnormal-appearing TM, often described as dull, varying from bulging and opaque with no visible landmarks to retracted and translucent with visible landmarks and an air-fluid level or bubble, may be seen (Fig. 30-9). Head and neck structures should be examined for abnormalities.

Diagnostic Studies

The tympanogram is flat-type B. The audiogram can show hearing loss of 15 to 31 dB.

Differential Diagnosis

Differential diagnoses include AOM, all causes of hearing loss and anatomic abnormalities, and persistent unilateral OME can indicate nasopharyngeal carcinoma.

Management

Recommendations for management of OME in children 2 months to 12 years old has remained the same as in the clinical practice guidelines from 2004 (Rosenfeld et al, 2004):

1. A 3-month period of watchful waiting
2. Documenting in the medical record at each visit the presence and duration of effusion, whether it is unilateral or bilateral, and any associated symptoms
3. Checking hearing tests
4. Identifying children at risk for speech, language, or learning problems
   - At-risk children are defined as having developmental delays because of sensory, physical, cognitive, or behavioral factors (e.g., hearing loss independent of OME, speech or language delays, pervasive or other developmental disorders, syndromes or craniofacial disorders, blindness, and/or cleft palate). These children should be promptly referred for hearing, speech, and language evaluation.
5. Referral, rationale, expectations, and decision-making process
   - These should be communicated to the parent when referral to an otolaryngologist is made. Duration of effusion, reason for referral, and any relevant information should be communicated to the otolaryngologist.
6. Bilateral myringotomy with insertion of tympanostomy tubes as discussed earlier in the chapter

There are other considerations the clinician should be aware of. There is no evidence that decongestants, antibiotics, and nasal steroids are of any benefit in the management of OME (Conover, 2013; Lieberthal et al, 2013). Antihistamines might be of some benefit if the OME is associated with allergies (Conover, 2013). Tonsillectomy or adenoidectomy alone should not be used to treat OME. The use of complementary and alternative medicine as an exclusive treatment for OME lacks scientific evidence documenting efficacy and the uncertain balance of harm and benefit (see Chapter 43). Complications include recurrent AOM and hearing loss that may be temporary conductive or, over time, permanent high-frequency SNHL.

Prevention and Education

- Stress the importance of follow-up until the TM and hearing are normal. Advise parents of the length of time (weeks to months) required for resolution of OME.
- Remind parents of their important role in language development of their child. Conversation and parent interaction through reading and play, along with affirmative sounds and gestures, are the most important factors in language development and school readiness.
- Strategies for maximizing hearing for the child:
  - Face the child, and get within 3 feet before speaking.
  - Enunciate clearly; speak slower and louder.
  - Use visual clues, and repeat as necessary.
  - Turn off competing background noise (music, radio, television).
  - Request preferential seating in the classroom.

Perforated Tympanic Membrane

Perforated TMs are most commonly associated with AOM. Perforation occurs in approximately 30% of children with a middle ear infection (Conover, 2013). Children with a perforation are more likely to have had otitis media in the past.

The pain associated with the AOM generally improves immensely once the rupture has occurred and there is usually profuse otorrhea. The fluid that drains from the ruptured TM usually contains the same virus and bacteria as that associated with TTO. In older children with ruptured TM, the most common bacteria are *P. aeruginosa* and *S. aureus* (Conover, 2013). Most ruptures are completely healed in 1 month.

Traumatic TM perforations are caused by blows to the ear, blasts (fireworks), improper attempts at ear cleaning, and children putting things in their ears. Perforating the TM is not necessarily painful, and most children will present with acute onset of bleeding from the ear. Traumatic perforations are less likely to heal spontaneously than those caused by infections. These perforations are generally not painful but can be prone to infection and hearing loss.

Clinical Findings

History, Physical Examination, and Diagnostic Studies

- The child may have no symptoms at all. With perforation the child may feel immediately better. Children may present with whistling sounds during sneezing or nose blowing, or hearing loss.
- TM perforation should be evident on otoscopic examination. Profuse otorrhea from the perforation may decrease visibility of the TM (see Fig. 30-5).
- Tympanogram will be flat. Hearing test should be performed once the acute infection is cleared or the traumatic perforation has had a chance to heal.

Differential Diagnosis

Some possibilities are AOM, TTO, or nonaccidental trauma (boxed ears).

Management

The goal of therapy with a TM perforation is to control the otorrhea and watchful waiting to ensure healing of the perforation.

Medications

Some eardrops may cause ototoxicity and should be avoided (gentamycin, neomycin, and tobramycin). See Table 30-2 for ototopical medications. If the perforation was caused by an AOM, treat the ear with otic drops and the ear infection as outlined in the Acute Otitis Media section (Conover, 2013). There is no evidence that medicated eardrops improve healing of traumatic perforations (Conover, 2013).

Other Treatment Considerations

- Perforation makes the ear more susceptible to infection if water enters the EAC. Thus, having a TM perforation is an absolute contraindication to swimming, getting water into the ears when shampooing, and irrigation for cerumen removal (Howard, 2015).
- It is recommended that there be no instrumentation in the ear for at least 2 weeks after the traumatic perforation.
- Small perforations are not usually repaired unless there is a quality of life issue. Perforations caused by acute infection will heal within a month. Primary care follow-up is important to make sure there are no sequelae from the perforation.
- Referral to the otolaryngologist should not be done for at least 3 months. Otolaryngologists generally wait 3 to 6 months to discuss the option to repair the perforation.

Cholesteatoma

Cholesteatoma is usually the result of a chronic ear infection and involves the formation of an epidermal inclusion cyst of the middle ear or mastoid consisting of desquamated debris from the keratinizing, squamous epithelial lining of the middle ear (Fig. 30-10). As the cholesteatoma grows in size, it can destroy the surrounding structures. Infection, hearing loss, dizziness, and facial muscle paralysis are rare complications (Conover, 2013).

Cholesteatomas can be congenital, primary acquired, or secondary acquired. Varied theories explaining their formation include an inflammatory process, perforation of the TM, and failure of desquamated tissue to clear from the middle ear. The incidence rate is unknown.

Clinical Findings

History and Physical Examination

The history may be negative with congenital cholesteatomas. The history with an acquired cholesteatoma might include:

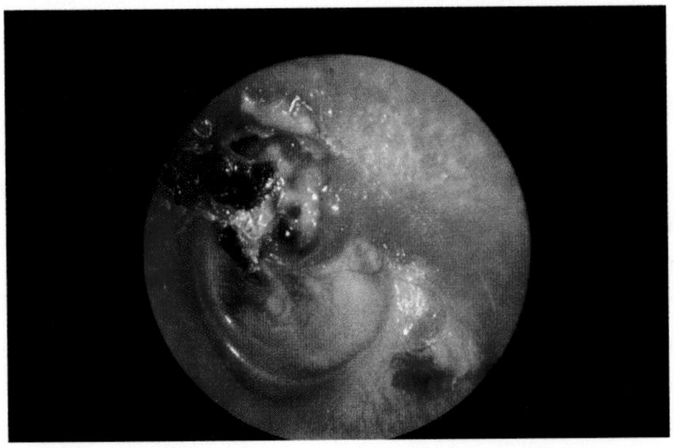

• **Figure 30-10** Cholesteatoma of the left ear. (Photograph courtesy Sylvan Stool, MD, The Children's Hospital, Denver, CO.)

- Chronic otitis media with malodorous purulent otorrhea
- Vertigo and hearing loss
- History or presence of pressure-equalizing tube
- A pearly white lesion is present on or behind the TM. Aural polyps are considered cholesteatomas unless proven otherwise. Congenital cholesteatomas are often in the most anteroinferior position of the TM (see Fig. 30-10).

Differential Diagnosis

Tympanosclerosis, debris from chronic OME, malignant rhabdomyosarcoma, and aural polyps are some of the differential diagnoses.

Management and Complications

Accurate diagnosis and immediate referral to an otolaryngologist for surgical excision are needed. Make sure to examine siblings of children with cholesteatoma. Complications include irreversible structural damage, permanent bone damage, facial nerve palsy, hearing loss, and intracranial infection, especially in untreated cases.

Mastoiditis

Mastoiditis is a suppurative infection of the mastoid cells. It is most common in children younger than 2 years old. Mastoiditis may accompany AOM. The mucoperiosteal lining of the mastoid air cells becomes inflamed, with subsequent progressive swelling and obstruction caused by drainage from the mastoid. Common invasive organisms identified include *S. pneumoniae, H. influenzae, M. catarrhalis, S. aureus, S. pyogenes,* and *Mycobacterium tuberculosis* (rare). Gram-negative *E. coli, Proteus,* and *Pseudomonas* are more common in chronic mastoiditis, more virulent infections, and young infants. Antibiotic treatment for AOM does not safeguard against and may actually mask mastoiditis with a normal TM. Intracranial complications of mastoiditis are common and may develop despite treatment.

The exact incidence of mastoiditis is unknown but has been described as low since the introduction of antibiotics. It is most common in children from infancy to adolescence with a peak between 6 and 13 months of age; gender distribution is equal. Although uncommon, it is potentially life-threatening. It is important to note that the watchful waiting and "prescriptions to be used as needed" approach to AOM and OME have not increased the incidence of acute mastoiditis (Ho et al, 2008).

Clinical Findings

History, Physical Examination, and Diagnostic Studies

- Concurrent or recurrent AOM
- Fever and otalgia
- Persistent otitis media unresponsive to antibiotic therapy
- Postauricular swelling: Infants may have swelling above the ear, displacing the pinna inferiorly or laterally. Older

children have swelling that pushes the earlobe superiorly and laterally.
- Computed tomography (CT) or magnetic resonance imaging (MRI) can provide definitive anatomical information. (May be done by ENT after referral.)
- Tympanocentesis with culture and Gram stain help identify offending organism.

Differential Diagnosis

Include other causes of postauricular inflammation or swelling such as lymphadenopathy, periauricular cellulitis, perichondritis of auricle, mumps, or tumors of the mastoid bone.

Management

Urgent ENT referral is imperative. Hospitalization, intravenous antibiotics, myringotomy, and pressure-equalizing tube placement are necessary.

If no abscess or CNS involvement is noted, there often is a 48-hour period of observation with broad-spectrum antibiotics before considering mastoidectomy as an intervention.

Prevention

The PCV13 has reduced the incidence of mastoiditis caused by *S. pneumoniae.*

Sensorineural and Conductive Hearing Loss

Hearing loss is defined as bilateral pure-tone hearing loss of 40 dB or more at frequencies of 500, 1000, and 2000 Hz in the better ear. Three types of hearing loss are recognized: sensorineural, conductive, or mixed. Either or both ears may be involved.

SNHL is most commonly associated with dysfunction of or damage to the cochlea (inner ear) and less often associated with damage to the auditory nerve (cranial nerve VIII). SNHL that is related to the auditory nerve is usually labeled *auditory neuropathy* or *auditory dyssynchrony,* neither of which is amenable to treatment with hearing aids but may respond to cochlear implants. SNHL can be congenital or acquired, mild or severe, and is permanent. This chapter only addresses the medical issues of assessment and initial intervention for recent hearing loss. The child living with impaired hearing has many issues of daily living, communication, audiologic care, speech, development, and education, which are addressed in Chapter 20.

Conductive hearing loss (CHL), either congenital or acquired, implies a problem in the outer or middle ear, and results from blocked transmission of sound waves from the EAC to the inner ear (e.g., AOM, OME). The cochlea functions normally. Bone conduction is usually normal with decreased air conduction. CHL is usually in the range of 20 to 60 dB. MEEs result in an average hearing loss of 27 to 31 dB.

Mixed hearing loss involves a combination of SNHL and CHL. Abnormalities are identified in outer, middle, and inner ear spaces. Central hearing loss occurs when the nerves or nuclei of the CNS, either in the pathways to the brain or the brain, are damaged or impaired.

SNHL and CHL can be associated with craniofacial anomalies (e.g., aural atresia, cleft lip or cleft palate, external ear deformity without atresia, dysmorphic facies without external ear deformity), genetic aberrations or congenital deformities (e.g., white forelock, café au lait spots, family history of SNHL, metabolic abnormalities), or environmental exposure (e.g., ototoxic drugs, bacterial or viral meningitis, other infectious diseases, loud noises, head trauma).

SNHL can occur when hair cells in the cochlea are injured by exposure to excessive noise over a variable period. SNHL can also come from prenatal and perinatal exposure (e.g., intrauterine infections, toxic chemicals, erythroblastosis fetalis). Seventy percent of genetic hearing loss is nonsyndromic (Moody Antonio, 2014). More than 300 genetic conditions that have deafness as one component have been identified. There are now more than 100 chromosomal loci and 65 genes associated with hearing loss (Alford et al, 2014).

CHL can also be congenital or acquired. Congenital causes include aural stenosis or atresia and ossicle malformations. Acquired CHL can be caused by AOM, OME, foreign bodies in the ear canal, cerumen impaction, TM perforation, cholesteatoma, ossicular discontinuity, collapsing ear canals, otosclerosis, and tympanosclerosis.

The overall prevalence of congenital deafness is estimated to be one to three in 1000 births, 1.1 per 1000 children 3 to 10 years old, and 14.9% of children 6 to 19 years old (CDC, 2015).

Clinical Findings

History

Hearing loss is often a "silent disease." Careful consideration and attention to identified risk factors are essential in identifying hearing loss in children.

The risk factors for SNHL in newborns include the following:
- Birth weight less than 1500 g
- Severe depression at birth (e.g., Apgar score of 0 to 3 at 5 minutes, failure to initiate a response by 10 minutes, or hypotonia at up to 2 hours old)
- Neonatal intensive care unit admission for 2 days or longer
- Prolonged mechanical ventilation for greater than 10 days
- Persistent pulmonary hypertension
- Long QT syndrome (usually profound hearing loss)
- Congenital infections, such as toxoplasmosis, bacterial meningitis, syphilis, rubella, cytomegalovirus, and herpes
- Metabolic disorders, such as phenylketonuria (PKU) and galactosemia
- Endocrine disorders, such as adrenal hyperplasia and hypothyroidism
- Craniofacial anomalies, including morphologic abnormalities of the pinna and ear canal
- Genetic syndromes, such as sickle cell disease, Usher syndrome, neurofibromatosis, Waardenburg syndrome,

osteopetrosis, or findings associated with other genetic syndromes known to include hearing loss
- Hyperbilirubinemia requiring exchange transfusion or causing kernicterus
- Family history of hereditary childhood SNHL
- Ototoxic drug exposure

The risk factors for hearing loss in children 1 month to 3 years old include the following (AAP Joint Committee on Infant Hearing, 2007):
- All of the above plus:
  - Parental or caregiver concern regarding hearing, speech, language, or developmental delay; parents tend to be about 12 months ahead of care providers in identifying hearing loss in children (Harlor and Bower, 2009)
  - Kidney malformation
  - Neurodegenerative disorders (such as, Hunter syndrome) or sensorimotor neuropathies (such as, Friedreich ataxia and Charcot-Marie-Tooth disease)
  - Head trauma with loss of consciousness or skull fracture
  - Bacterial meningitis
  - Ototoxic medication exposure
  - Diabetes mellitus
  - Recurrent or persistent OME for at least 3 months

Other risk factors or indicators for hearing loss are found in Box 20-15 and include the following:
- Failure to learn to speak at the appropriate age or failure to respond to auditory stimuli; speech that sounds like baby talk or is monotone and difficult to understand; avoidance of speaking
- Failed school screening audiogram; decreased note taking; seeming to misunderstand, ignore, confuse, or miss what is being said
- Aggression, increased physical complaints, difficulty in school and social situations
- Environmental exposure to firecrackers, toy cap pistols, firearms, loud music, loud television, squeaking toys, and machines (e.g., snowmobiles, farm equipment, lawn mowers)
- History of head or neck irradiation

Physical Examination
The following may be found in children with SNHL and CHL:
- Abnormal hearing screening during routine newborn or well-child care visits or other office visits: For children younger than 6 months old, an ABR test is recommended. Behavioral testing using a conditioned response or an ABR is appropriate for children older than 6 months.
- Physical examination: A complete physical examination with special attention to the eyes, skin, and skeletal and nervous systems is needed.
- Ears: Preauricular pits, auricular malformation or appendage, abnormal TM integrity, or impaired mobility with pneumatic otoscopy.
- Eyes: Cataracts, corneal opacities, coloboma, blindness, nystagmus, exophthalmos, night blindness, heterochromia iridis, or blue sclerae (associated with genetic disorders that can cause SNHL).
- Craniofacial anomalies or genetic stigmata associated with SNHL

Diagnostic Studies
EOAE and ABR are the diagnostic tests used for newborn hearing screening. After that period of time, audiometry is the preferred hearing testing of choice. If the cause of the hearing impairment is evident (cholesteatoma, ossicle malformation, otitis media), the diagnostic workup is limited. If the cause of the hearing loss is not readily apparent, consider the following diagnostic tests:
- Urinalysis, serum blood urea nitrogen, and creatinine to rule out renal disease
- Complete blood count, thyroid function tests, sickle cell screen
- Toxoplasmosis, other agents, rubella, cytomegalovirus, herpes simplex (TORCH) screen in newborns
- Genetic testing
- Electrocardiogram (ECG) (long QT syndrome)
- Ophthalmologic examination
- CT as indicated to rule out inner ear malformation

Differential Diagnosis
Cerumen impaction, OME, and CSOM with perforation of TM are differential diagnoses for conductive loss. Consider tumor with sensorineural loss. For the child with significant hearing loss, comorbidities may exist, including developmental and communication problems, family disruptions, depression, genetic disorders, and others.

Mixed SNHL with CHL and central hearing loss are included in the differential diagnosis.

Management
The following should occur for any child with suspected hearing loss:
- Evaluate and treat AOM and OME if present (see the Acute Otitis Media and Otitis Media with Effusion sections).
- Screen for hearing loss if bilateral MEE is present for 3 months or longer and refer for surgical intervention as indicated.
- If suspected hearing loss, refer to an audiologist and otolaryngologist for full evaluation as soon as possible. Include information about the patient's symptoms, history or physical findings, and any known diagnosis associated with hearing loss in the referral.
- Treat known medically related conditions (diabetes, hypothyroidism).
- Refer families for genetic counseling if the problem is inheritable.
- Encourage the use of amplification devices as appropriate. They may be personal (e.g., hearing aids) or group (e.g., teacher microphone).

- Cochlear implants with an external speech processor are sometimes used for profound SNHL. If implants are in place, it is imperative that the child's immunizations be up to date, specifically the PCV13.
- Recommend special school and teaching strategies, such as front-of-room placement and facing the child when speaking.
- Ensure a family-centered approach in making decisions regarding interventions for the child (e.g., Individuals with Disabilities Education Act [IDEA]).
- If hearing loss is an ongoing issue, refer to Chapter 20 for management of children with hearing loss.

Complications

Significant hearing loss impedes speech, language, cognitive development, and social interaction skills.

Prevention

- Provide good prenatal care.
- Provide Rho(D) immune globulin to prevent erythroblastosis fetalis in susceptible women.
- Treat prenatal and perinatal infections promptly.
- Avoid ototoxic drug use.
- Immunize against measles, mumps, rubella, varicella, *H. influenzae* type B, *S. pneumoniae,* influenza, and other diseases that can cause SNHL through CNS damage.
- Recommend avoidance of environmental factors associated with hearing loss.

For a complete list of references, please visit http://evolve.elsevier.com/Burns/pediatric/.

31 Cardiovascular Disorders

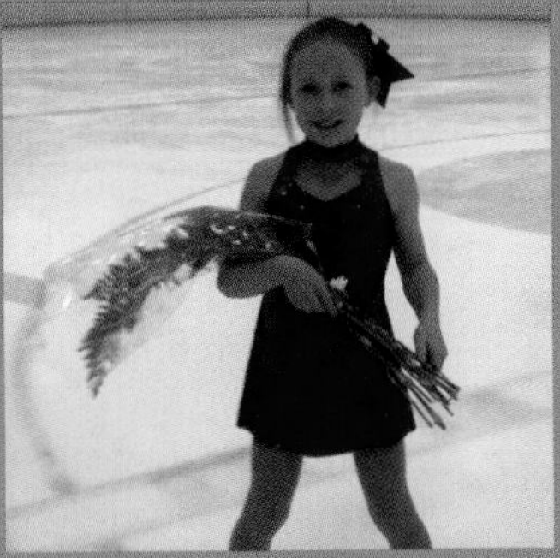

JULIE MARTCHENKE AND MARY RUMMELL

Most cardiovascular problems in the pediatric population are due to congenital heart disease (CHD), which affects nearly 1% of all live births—or about 40,000 babies per year. Greater numbers of these children are surviving to adulthood, increasing the total population of adults and children with CHD. CHD is the leading cause of morbidity and mortality within the first year of life in children with congenital malformations (Centers for Disease Control and Prevention [CDC], 2014).

The primary care provider (PCP) must maintain a high index of suspicion regarding any signs or symptoms of cardiovascular disease in young children. Many congenital heart defects may be recognized by a detailed fetal ultrasound and known before delivery. Critical congenital heart defects may also be detected in the immediate post delivery period by using pulse-oximetry screening (Oster et al, 2013). Early identification significantly decreases the morbidity and mortality associated with cyanotic and ductal dependent structural heart defects (Kemper et al, 2011).

This chapter presents information on both congenital and acquired heart disease in the pediatric population. A thorough discussion of the examination and assessment of the cardiac system is included, as well as guidance for screening, identifying, and managing specific cardiovascular disorders during the course of delivering primary health care.

Anatomy and Physiology

Fetal Circulation

Knowledge of fetal circulation is essential for understanding the circulatory changes that occur in the newborn at delivery (Fig. 31-1). Fetal circulation has four unique features that differ from postnatal circulation:

- Oxygenation of the blood occurs in the placenta, not the lungs.
- Fetal pulmonary vascular resistance is high, and systemic vascular resistance is low (high pressure on the right side of the heart, low pressure on the left side).
- The foramen ovale, the opening in the septum between the two atria, permits a portion of the blood to flow from the right atrium directly to the left atrium.
- A patent ductus arteriosus (PDA) provides a connection between the pulmonary artery and the aorta that allows blood to flow from the pulmonary artery to the aorta and bypass the fetal lungs.

Oxygen from the maternal uterine arteries is diffused into the fetal circulation via the placenta. The placenta delivers oxygenated blood through the umbilical vein to the fetus by diverting blood through the liver to the inferior vena cava (IVC) by the ductus venosus. When this well-oxygenated blood reaches the right atrium, it flows preferentially toward the atrial septum, through the foramen ovale, and into the left atrium. Oxygenated blood then flows into the left ventricle and out the aorta. Approximately two thirds of the blood from the aorta flows toward the head and neck to ensure that the fetal brain constantly receives well-oxygenated blood.

Venous blood returns from the head and upper extremities via the superior vena cava (SVC) to the right atrium. This blood preferentially flows toward the tricuspid valve into the right ventricle. From the right ventricle, the blood enters the pulmonary artery. Because pulmonary vascular resistance is high and systemic resistance is low, most blood in the pulmonary artery flows through the ductus arteriosus into the descending aorta to supply oxygen and nutrients to the trunk and lower extremities. Only a small amount of blood flows into the pulmonary circuit to perfuse the lungs.

The fetal circulation is best described as two parallel circuits, with the left ventricle supplying blood to the upper extremities and the right ventricle serving the lower extremities and the placenta. At the time of transition to extrauterine life, these separate blood flow circuits become a serial circuit.

Neonatal Circulation

A number of complex events occur at birth that rapidly shift the fetal circulation toward the neonatal circulation pattern. Clamping of the umbilical cord, with subsequent removal of the placenta as the oxygenating organ, causes an immediate circulatory change requiring the lungs to be the new mechanism of oxygenation. Clamping the cord

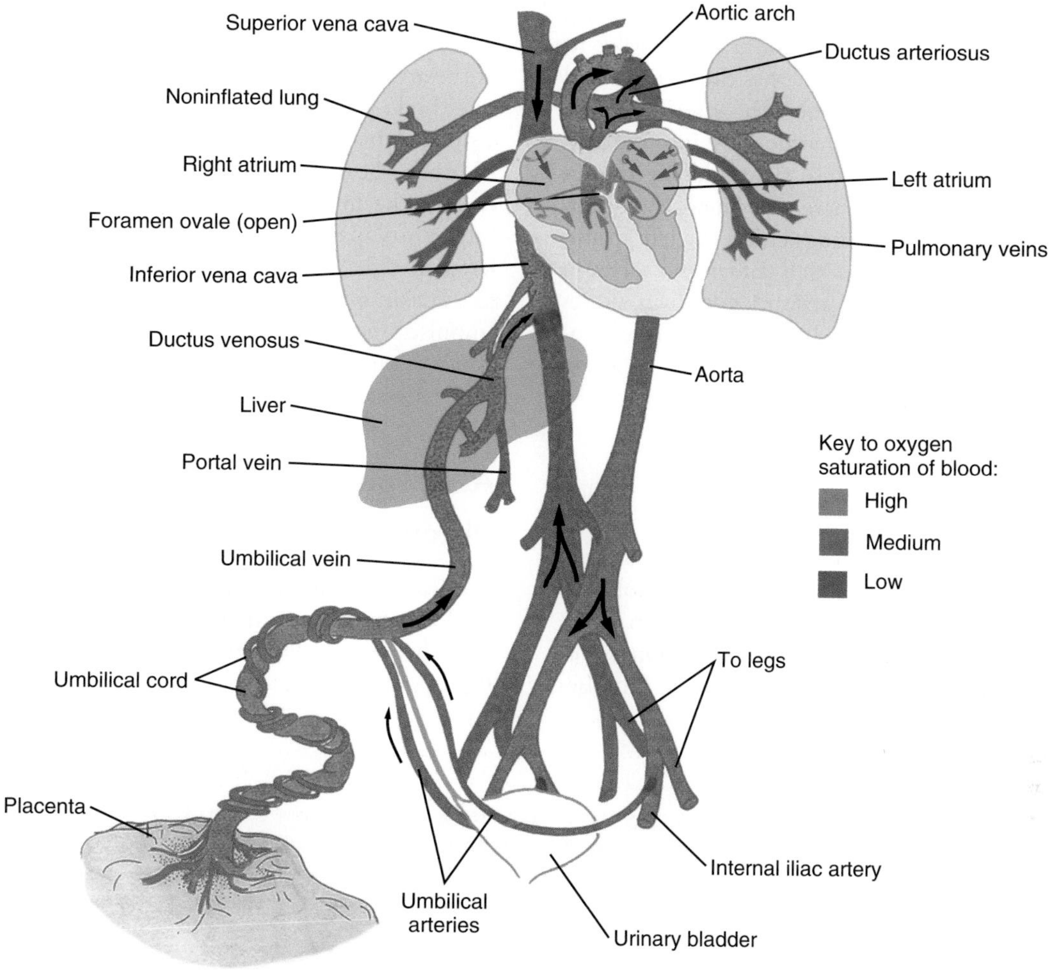

• **Figure 31-1** Fetal circulation. (From Murray S, McKinney E: *Foundations of maternal-newborn and women's health nursing,* ed 6, Philadelphia, 2014, Saunders/Elsevier.)

also causes an increase in systemic vascular resistance (systemic blood pressure [BP]). With the first breath, mechanical inflation of the lungs and an increase in oxygen saturation bring about a dramatic fall in pulmonary vascular resistance and, consequently, increase pulmonary blood flow. The increased oxygen saturation begins the process of constricting the ductus arteriosus. As the pressures within the heart become relatively higher on the left side and lower on the right, the foramen ovale closes. Functional closure of the ductus arteriosus and foramen ovale usually occurs within the first hours to days of life, and a serial circuit forms out of the once-parallel pulmonary and systemic circulation.

The transition toward complete anatomic closure, or obliteration of fetal structures by tissue growth or constriction, is more gradual. Pulmonary vascular resistance drops gradually over the first 6 to 8 weeks of life, which can protect the pulmonary circulation against volume overload in some congenital heart anomalies. If not noted earlier, shunt murmurs or symptoms of congestive heart failure (CHF) gradually become apparent as the infant approaches 8 weeks old. At this time, pulmonary vascular resistance has dropped and shunting to the pulmonary bed increases.

Conditions that cause persistence of fetal shunts allow unoxygenated blood to flow from the right side of the heart to the left. Any murmur or cyanosis in a newborn should be carefully monitored and evaluated to detect cardiac abnormalities.

Normal Cardiac Structure and Function

The heart is a muscular four-chambered organ located in the mediastinum, the space in the chest between the lungs. The four chambers are divided into two larger muscular pumping chambers, the ventricles, and two smaller receiving chambers, the atria. The heart has one-way valves that open and close in response to pressure changes within the heart, thus controlling blood flow from chamber to chamber. Desaturated systemic blood returns to the right atrium by way of the inferior and superior venae cavae. The blood passes from the right atrium through the tricuspid valve to the right ventricle. The tricuspid value has three cusps held in place by the chordate tendineae. The right ventricle pumps the blood through the pulmonic valve into the pulmonary artery, which bifurcates into right and left arteries to allow flow into both lungs. Here, the blood is oxygenated. Blood returning from the lungs enters the left atrium by way of the pulmonary veins (which contain no valves to allow easy blood flow into the atrium) and then passes through the mitral valve into the left ventricle. The high-pressured left ventricle pumps the blood through the aortic valve into the aorta to provide oxygenated blood for the systemic circulation.

Conduction System

Myocardial contraction is stimulated by electrical depolarization along the conduction tract within the heart. Depolarization begins at the sinoatrial (SA) node, which is high in the wall of the right atrium. This node acts as the pacemaker of the heart by regularly beginning the depolarizing impulses of each heartbeat. The wave of depolarization travels from the SA node throughout the atria and produces contraction of the atrial muscle. The impulses reach the atrioventricular (AV) node, which is located in the lower portion of the right atrium at the junction of the atrium and ventricle. From the AV node, the depolarization wave passes through the bundle of His, the fibers extending from the AV node along the intraventricular septum. Depolarization spreads through the left and right branches of the bundle of His and through the Purkinje fibers extending into the ventricular muscle. Impulses then spread throughout the ventricles and cause contraction. The electrocardiogram (ECG) demonstrates this pattern of changing electrical impulses.

Assessment of the Cardiovascular System

History

Cardiac evaluation includes review of the family, maternal, fetal, neonatal, and infant medical history, in addition to growth and development (Box 31-1 lists risk factors for CHD).

• BOX 31-1 Risk Factors Suggestive of Congenital Heart Disease

Perinatal Risk Factors

Maternal infections and exposures (CMV, rubella, other viral syndromes)
Maternal use of tobacco, alcohol, street drugs, retinoic acid, hydantoins, lithium, valproates, ibuprofen, naproxen, ACE inhibitors, tricyclic antidepressants, sulfonamides, sulfasalazines
Maternal chronic disease (CHD, lupus, insulin-dependent diabetes, phenylketonuria)
Maternal age at child's birth (increase in chromosomal abnormalities after 40 years old)
Maternal pregnancy history (excessive weight gain, gestational diabetes)

Neonatal Risk Factors

Fetal or newborn distress (aspiration, hypoxia, cyanosis)
Prematurity (increased incidence of CHD in premature infants)
Presence of associated anomalies (genetic or chromosomal abnormalities or syndromes)
Neonatal infections (GBS)
Birthweight (term infants, <2500 g; SGA, less than two standard deviations from the mean for gestational age)

Newborn Risk Factors

Murmur at birth or early infancy
Hypertension (at birth or beyond)
Feeding difficulty (shortness of breath, easily fatigued, diaphoresis, poor intake)
Cyanosis (increase with crying, feeding, exertion)
Tachypnea (persistent, with crying, feeding)

Toddler, School-Age, and Teenage Risk Factors

Deviation from individual's normal growth and development
Deviation from an activity level appropriate for chronologic age (unable to keep up with peers; unable to run or ride bike)
Frequent respiratory tract infections (pneumonia, URIs that last longer than normal)
Prior murmurs, blue spells
Documented GABHS infection
Hypertension (documented on a minimum of three separate visits)
Chest pain with exertion
Shortness of breath with exertion (beyond normal peers)
Syncope or dizziness (especially associated with noted heart rate change)
Tachycardia or bradycardia (fluttering in chest, racing heart)

Family History Risk Factors

CHD (especially siblings, parents, first-degree relatives)
Sudden death or premature myocardial infarction (before 50 years old; includes any deaths by drowning)
Hypertension
Rheumatic fever
Genetic syndromes
Hypercholesterolemia

Data from Richards A, Garg V: Genetics of congenital heart disease, *Curr Cardiology Rev* 6:91–97, 2010; Sayasathid J, Sukonpan K, Somboonna N: Epidemiology and etiology of congenital heart diseases. In Syamasundar P, editor: *Congenital heart disease: selected aspects,* 2011. Available at www.intechopen.com/books/congenital-heart-disease-selected-aspects/epidemiology-and-etiology-of-congenital-heart-diseases. Accessed November 17, 2014.
ACE, Angiotensin-converting enzyme; *CHD,* congenital heart disease; *CMV,* cytomegalovirus; *GABHS,* group A beta-hemolytic streptococci; *GBS,* group B streptococcus; *SGA,* small for gestational age; *URI,* upper respiratory infection.

Physical Examination

Physical assessment of a child with suspected CHD should be adapted to the age of the child. Be flexible, yet thorough, in any evaluation and include all aspects of the physical examination in an order that best suits the comfort and needs of the infant, child, or adolescent.

Vital Signs

Heart rate, respiratory rate, and BP vary considerably throughout childhood.

- Heart rate (Table 31-1): Heart rates should always be obtained by auscultation. Assessment should include rate and rhythm variations. An increased heart rate can be caused by excitement, anxiety, hyperthyroidism, heart disease, anemia, or fever. Irregularity may be caused by a normal sinus arrhythmia (the normal variation in heart rate that occurs with inhalation and exhalation; it is more common in children than adults).
- Pulses: Pulses should be palpated in the upper and lower extremities and evaluated for character (strength) and variation between the different sites. A bounding pulse may indicate a PDA or aortic insufficiency. Weak or "thready" pulses may indicate CHF or an obstructive lesion, such as severe aortic stenosis. Strong brachial pulses in conjunction with weak or absent femoral pulses may indicate coarctation of the aorta.
- Blood pressure (BP): The National Heart, Lung, and Blood Institute (NHLBI), National High Blood Pressure Education Program recommends measuring BP annually beginning at 3 years old and during every health care episode. Providers should manually auscultate BP on children 3 years old or older and when found to have elevated levels exceeding the 90% percentile on an oscillometric (automatic) device. (These readings can vary widely and differ between devices and need to be calibrated periodically to maintain accuracy.) Auscultation remains the preferred method; BP tables are based upon this technique (NHLBI, 2012). If the index of suspicion of heart disease is high, providers should check BPs in younger children. It is important to always use a BP cuff that is appropriate for the child's size. For arm pressure, the width of the cuff should be two thirds the length of the upper arm measured from the axilla to the antecubital space. A cuff that is too narrow, too wide, or does not fit around a chubby arm may cause an erroneous reading. Cuff sizes of 3, 5, 7, 12, and 18 cm should be on hand in order to accommodate the array of pediatric sizes. Initial evaluation should compare the pressure in all four extremities. Pressure in all extremities should be equal, with pressure in the legs being slightly higher (10 to 20 mm Hg) in a child who walks. Lower extremity pressure is measured with the stethoscope placed over the popliteal artery. The NHLBI publishes norms for BP by gender, age, and height; they are found in Tables 31-2 and 31-3. Hypertension is discussed later in this chapter.
- Respiratory rate: Evaluation of the respiratory system includes the respiratory rate, assessment of effort, and breath sounds in all five lobes of the lungs. It is important to evaluate the respiratory rate in a quiet infant or child. A respiratory rate greater than 40 in a young child or 60 in a newborn who is quiet, resting, and afebrile warrants further evaluation. An infant with CHD may be happily tachypneic and not show significant signs of grunting, intercostal retractions, nasal flaring, or tracheal tug (up and down movement of the trachea with each inspiration).
- Oxygen saturation: Oxygen saturation is considered to be an essential vital sign in a cardiac assessment. It is important to obtain oxygen saturations in newborns or children suspected of having a cardiac condition since cyanosis is not always readily perceptible. A joint statement by the American Academy of Pediatrics (AAP) and the American Heart Association (AHA) recommends that pulse oximetry screening be automatically done for all newborns (Kemper et al, 2011).

General Appearance and Growth Parameters

The PCP should observe an infant while obtaining the history and before proceeding with the complete physical examination. General nutritional state, respiratory effort,

TABLE 31-1 Normal Heart Rates in Infants and Children

Age	Resting (Awake)	Resting (Asleep)	Exercise/Fever
Newborn	100-180 bpm	80-160 bpm	Up to 220 bpm
1 week to 3 months old	100-220 bpm	80-200 bpm	Up to 220 bpm
3 months to 2 years old	80-150 bpm	70-120 bpm	Up to 220 bpm
2 to 10 years old	70-100 bpm	60-90 bpm	195-215 bpm
10 to 20 years old	55-90 bpm	50-90 bpm	195-215 bpm

bpm, Beats per minute.

TABLE 31-2 Blood Pressure Levels in the 90th and 95th Percentiles for Girls 1 to 17 Years Old by Percentiles of Height

Age	→ Height Percentiles*	Systolic BP (mm Hg)							Diastolic BP (mm Hg)						
	BP†	5%	10%	25%	50%	75%	90%	95%	5%	10%	25%	50%	75%	90%	95%
1	90th	97	97	98	100	101	102	103	52	53	53	54	55	55	56
	95th	100	101	103	104	105	106	107	56	57	57	58	59	59	60
2	90th	98	99	100	101	103	104	105	57	58	58	59	60	61	61
	95th	102	103	104	105	107	108	109	61	62	62	63	63	65	65
3	90th	100	100	102	103	104	106	106	61	62	62	63	64	64	65
	95th	104	104	105	107	108	109	110	65	66	66	67	68	68	69
4	90th	101	102	103	104	106	107	108	64	64	65	66	67	67	68
	95th	105	106	107	108	110	111	112	68	68	69	70	71	71	72
5	90th	103	103	105	106	107	109	109	66	67	67	68	69	69	70
	95th	107	107	108	110	111	112	113	70	71	71	72	73	73	74
6	90th	104	105	106	108	109	110	111	68	68	69	70	70	71	72
	95th	108	109	110	111	113	114	115	72	72	73	74	74	75	76
7	90th	106	107	108	109	111	112	113	69	70	70	71	72	72	73
	95th	110	111	112	113	115	116	116	73	74	74	75	76	76	77
8	90th	108	109	110	111	113	114	114	71	71	71	72	73	74	74
	95th	112	112	114	115	116	118	118	75	75	75	76	77	78	78
9	90th	110	110	112	113	114	116	116	71	72	72	73	74	75	75
	95th	114	114	115	117	118	119	120	76	76	76	77	78	79	79
10	90th	112	112	114	115	116	118	118	73	73	73	74	75	76	76
	95th	116	116	117	119	120	121	122	77	77	77	78	79	80	80
11	90th	114	114	116	117	118	119	120	74	74	74	75	76	77	77
	95th	118	118	119	121	122	123	124	78	78	78	79	80	81	81
12	90th	116	116	117	119	120	121	122	75	75	75	76	77	78	78
	95th	119	120	121	123	124	125	126	79	79	79	80	81	82	82
13	90th	117	118	119	121	122	123	124	76	76	76	77	78	79	79
	95th	121	122	123	124	126	127	128	80	80	80	81	82	83	83
14	90th	119	120	121	122	124	125	125	77	77	77	78	79	80	80
	95th	123	123	125	126	127	129	129	81	81	81	82	83	84	84
15	90th	120	121	122	123	125	126	127	78	78	79	79	80	81	81
	95th	124	125	126	127	129	130	131	82	82	82	83	84	85	85
16	90th	121	122	123	124	126	127	128	78	78	79	80	81	81	82
	95th	125	126	127	128	130	131	132	82	82	83	84	85	85	86
17	90th	122	122	123	125	126	127	128	78	79	79	80	81	81	82
	95th	125	126	127	129	130	131	132	82	83	83	84	85	85	86

From National Heart, Lung, and Blood Institute, National High Blood Pressure Education Program Working Group on High Blood Pressure in Children and Adolescents (NIH-NHBPEP): *The fourth report on the diagnosis, evaluation, and treatment of high blood pressure in children and adolescents* (1996, revised 2005). Available at www.nhlbi.nih.gov/health/prof/heart/hbp/hbp_ped.pdf. Accessed October 22, 2014.

*Height percentile determined by standard growth curves.

†BP (blood pressure) percentile determined by a single measurement.

TABLE 31-3 Blood Pressure Levels in the 90th and 95th Percentiles for Boys 1 to 17 Years Old by Percentiles of Height

	→ Height	Systolic BP (mm Hg)							Diastolic BP (mm Hg)						
Age	Percentiles*	5%	10%	25%	50%	75%	90%	95%	5%	10%	25%	50%	75%	90%	95%
	BP†														
1	90th	94	95	97	99	100	102	103	49	50	51	52	53	53	54
	95th	98	99	101	103	104	106	106	54	54	55	56	57	58	58
2	90th	97	99	100	102	104	105	106	54	55	56	57	58	58	59
	95th	101	102	104	106	108	109	110	59	59	60	61	62	63	63
3	90th	100	101	103	105	107	108	109	59	59	60	61	62	63	63
	95th	104	105	107	109	110	112	113	63	63	64	65	66	67	67
4	90th	102	103	105	107	109	110	111	62	63	64	65	66	66	67
	95th	106	107	109	111	112	114	115	66	67	68	69	70	71	71
5	90th	104	105	106	108	110	111	112	65	66	67	68	69	69	70
	95th	108	109	110	112	114	115	116	69	70	71	72	73	74	74
6	90th	105	106	108	110	111	113	113	68	68	69	70	71	72	72
	95th	109	110	112	114	115	117	117	72	72	73	74	75	76	76
7	90th	106	107	109	111	113	114	115	70	70	71	72	73	74	74
	95th	110	111	113	115	117	118	119	74	74	75	76	77	78	78
8	90th	107	109	110	112	114	115	116	71	72	72	73	74	75	76
	95th	111	112	114	116	118	119	120	75	76	77	78	79	79	80
9	90th	109	110	112	114	115	117	118	72	73	74	75	76	76	77
	95th	113	114	116	118	119	121	121	76	77	78	79	80	81	81
10	90th	111	112	114	115	117	119	119	73	73	74	75	76	77	78
	95th	115	116	117	119	121	122	123	77	78	79	80	81	81	82
11	90th	113	114	115	117	119	120	121	74	74	75	76	77	78	78
	95th	117	118	119	121	123	124	125	78	78	79	80	81	82	82
12	90th	115	116	118	120	121	123	123	74	75	75	76	77	78	79
	95th	119	120	122	123	125	127	127	78	79	80	81	82	82	83
13	90th	117	118	120	122	124	125	126	75	75	76	77	78	79	79
	95th	121	122	124	126	128	129	130	79	79	80	81	82	83	83
14	90th	120	121	123	125	126	128	128	75	76	77	78	79	79	80
	95th	124	125	127	128	130	132	132	80	80	81	82	83	84	84
15	90th	122	124	125	127	129	130	131	76	77	78	79	80	80	81
	95th	126	128	129	131	133	134	135	81	81	82	83	84	85	85
16	90th	125	126	128	130	131	133	134	78	78	79	80	81	82	82
	95th	129	130	132	134	135	137	137	82	83	83	84	85	86	87
17	90th	127	128	130	132	134	135	136	80	80	81	82	83	84	84
	95th	131	132	134	136	138	139	140	84	85	86	87	87	88	89

From National Heart, Lung, and Blood Institute, National High Blood Pressure Education Program Working Group on High Blood Pressure in Children and Adolescents (NHBPEP): *The fourth report on the diagnosis, evaluation, and treatment of high blood pressure in children and adolescents* (1996, revised 2005). Available at www.nhlbi.nih.gov/health/prof/heart/hbp/hbp_ped.pdf. Accessed October 22, 2014.

*Height percentile determined by standard growth curves.

†BP (blood pressure) percentile determined by a single measurement.

color, physical abnormalities, and distress or discomfort level should be observed.

- Look for the presence of unusual facial characteristics (e.g., malformed ears, wide-spaced eyes, noticeable anomalies) or extracardiac anomalies (e.g., cleft lip or palate, polydactyly, microcephaly) that may be associated with a syndrome or chromosomal abnormalities. Children may have obvious stigmata, such as those seen with Down syndrome, Marfan syndrome (unusually tall with an arm span wider than the head-to-toe height), Turner syndrome (webbed neck, prominent ears), or fetal alcohol spectrum disorder (microcephaly and pinched facies), all of which are associated with CHD.
- Overall skin color should be assessed for signs of mottling or central cyanosis while the infant is at rest. Cyanosis caused by heart disease is recognized as a pale blue or ruddy red color of the mucous membranes (lips, tongue, and nailbeds). The tongue is the best indicator because it lacks pigmentation and is abundantly served by the vascular system. Peripheral cyanosis or acrocyanosis, a blueness or pallor noted around the mouth and on the hands or feet, can be a normal variant, especially if it intensifies when the infant is cold. Clubbing of the fingers and toes may be seen in children with long-standing cyanosis.
- Note any wheezing, nasal flaring, retractions, prominent neck veins, or head bobbing with respirations.
- Note any peripheral or periorbital edema. Edema or puffiness around the eyes may be evident in an infant with CHF even in the absence of peripheral edema of the hands or feet. True pitting edema of the feet is an unusual finding in an infant with CHF.
- At each assessment, measure and plot height and weight on standardized charts, including Down syndrome and Turner syndrome charts as appropriate. Although many children with CHD fall within the normal height, weight, and development ranges, a large number of infants and children with heart disease experience poor weight gain, less than normal linear growth, and delays in achieving developmental milestones.

Palpation

Palpate all five areas of the chest: the aortic, pulmonic, tricuspid, and mitral areas, and Erb's point (Fig. 31-2). Chest palpation is best accomplished by using the open palm of the hand near the base of the fingers. The hand should be gently moved across the chest to assess abnormal precordial activity, including pulsations, lifts, heaves, or thrills, and to determine the location of the apical impulse. The apical impulse is used to determine the size of the heart and is the most lateral point at which cardiac activity can be palpated. In infants and children, the impulse is normally palpated at the apex of the heart in the fourth intercostal space just to the left of the midclavicular line. At approximately 7 years old, the point shifts to the fifth intercostal space. Cardiomegaly causes the apical impulse to shift laterally or downward.

- Thrills are a palpable vibration caused by turbulent blood flow through abnormal structures or defects in the heart. The turbulent flow may be due to valvular narrowing or stenosis or defects, such as a ventricular septal defect (VSD).

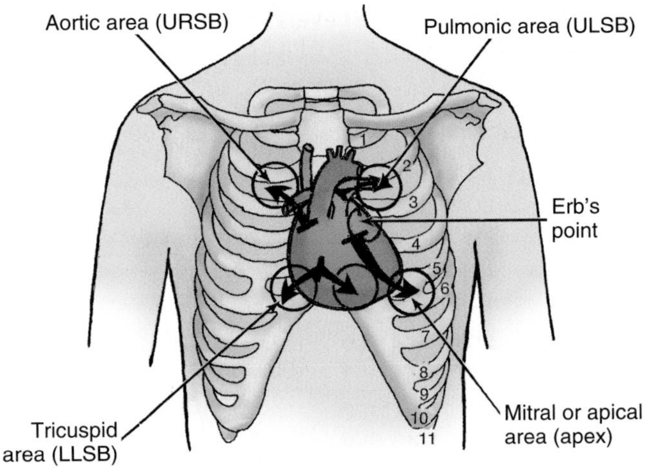

• **Figure 31-2** Direction of heart sounds for clicks and murmurs (auscultatory areas circled) with associated cardiac conditions. *Upper right sternal border* (URSB): aortic valve clicks of aortic stenosis, venous hum. *Upper left sternal border* (ULSB): Pulmonary valve clicks of pulmonary stenosis, pulmonary flow murmurs, ASD, PDA, venous hum. *Lower left sternal border* (LLSB): VSDs, Still's murmur, tricuspid valve regurgitation, hypertrophic cardiomyopathy, subaortic stenosis. *Apex:* aortic or mitral valve clicks, mitral valve regurgitation. *Erb's point:* aortic ejection click or aortic stenosis, or dilated aortic root. (From Hockenberry M, Wilson D: *Nursing care of infants and children,* ed 10, St. Louis, 2015, Mosby/Elsevier.)

- Assess peripheral pulses (radial, brachial, carotid, dorsalis pedis, and posterior tibial) for amplitude and intensity. In coarctation of the aorta, there may be decreased or absent femoral pulses and impulse lag if the radial pulse is palpated simultaneously. A fast pulse rate may indicate arrhythmia or CHF.
- The liver and spleen should be assessed for enlargement. Hepatomegaly is an important finding. Infants may have a palpable liver edge as a normal finding.
- The back should be examined for scoliosis, a finding that may be associated with CHD.

Auscultation of Heart Sounds

- Ascultate the heart in the same manner for every child by beginning at the base or apex of the heart. Ideally, assess heart sounds in a quiet environment when the child is cooperative.
- Four individual heart sounds can be heard: S_1, S_2, S_3, and S_4. S_1 and S_2 represent normal heart sounds, whereas the presence of S_3 or S_4 may indicate cardiac enlargement or volume overload.
- At each area of examination, the provider should accurately identify the first (S_1) and second (S_2) heart sounds.
- S_1 has the following characteristics:
  - It is heard in the beginning of systole and indicates closure of AV valves (mitral and tricuspid). It is the "lubb" of the lubb-dupp.
  - Often detected as a single sound. Even though the left side of the heart reacts slightly before the right side,

the closure of the two values occurs so closely together that a single sound may be heard.
- It may be differentiated from early systolic clicks by the low frequency of the sound (clicks have a higher frequency). It is best heard with the diaphragm of the stethoscope.
- It is usually loudest at the apex.
- It is synchronous with the apical and carotid pulses.

- S_2 has the following characteristics:
  - It is composed of the aortic (A_2) and pulmonic (P_2) components and marks the end of systole and onset of diastole. It is the "dupp" of lubb-dupp.
  - S_2 is normally split with inspiration in children because pulmonic valve closure lags behind aortic valve closure. S_2 becomes single with expiration. The intensity of splitting of S_2 is one of the most important parts of the cardiac examination.
  - S_2 is best assessed at the upper left sternal border in the pulmonic area.
  - Pulmonary hypertension causes early closure of P_2 and accentuation of S_2, which may sound like a loud, single second heart sound.
  - Absence of one of the semilunar valves (as in pulmonary atresia) causes single S_2.
  - Wide splitting of S_2 without becoming a single sound on expiration may indicate increased pulmonary flow (typical of atrial septal defect [ASD]).
- S_3 and S_4 have the following characteristics:
  - S_3 is associated with rapid ventricular filling; it may be heard in a quiet infant or child with a rapid heart rate.
  - S_3 "gallop" is best heard at the apex with the bell of the stethoscope during early diastole. When combined with S_1 and S_2, it gives the impression of the word "Kentucky." S_3 is easier to appreciate when the child is in the left lateral decubitus position.
  - S_4 is always pathologic; it represents increased force of atrial contraction and ventricular distention.
  - S_4 "gallop" sounds like the word "Tennessee." It is best heard in late diastole just before S_1.
  - S_4 is low-pitched and is best heard at the apex with the bell of the stethoscope.
- Clicks: Ejection clicks are heard early in systole, immediately after S_1 and may sound like a split first heart sound. Pulmonic ejection clicks are high in frequency, vary with respiration, and disappear with inspiration. An aortic ejection click, heard best at Erb's point, is constant in intensity with a sound of a "snap" or a "click." Nonejection clicks are heard best in midsystole, or midway between S_1 and S_2 in the cardiac cycle at the apex. These clicks are best heard in those who are leaning forward or standing, may disappear with inspiration, and are due to mitral valve prolapse. Fig. 31-2 describes cardiac conditions associated with each of these clicks.

Murmurs

Up to 80% of children may be found to have an innocent or "functional" murmur at some time during childhood, especially beginning at 3 to 4 years old (Park, 2014). These are caused by normal blood flow through normal cardiac structures rather than by turbulent blood flow caused by a defect or abnormal cardiac structures. All murmurs may be intensified by factors that increase cardiac output (e.g., anemia, fever, exercise). It is important to remember that significant heart defects may *not* have a murmur because there may not be turbulent blood flow (e.g., a large septal defect or nonrestrictive patent ductus) (Park, 2014). Fig. 31-2 shows ascultatory areas for different murmurs.

Criteria for Describing a Heart Murmur

Every murmur is assessed according to the criteria listed in Table 31-4. These are further illustrated in Fig. 31-3. Characteristics of pathologic murmurs needing referral are listed in Box 31-2. The presence of a murmur causes great anxiety for a family awaiting a diagnosis. All murmurs should have a second opinion from a pediatric colleague or pediatric cardiologist if the diagnosis is uncertain or there is a suspicion of heart disease.

TABLE 31-4 Describing a Heart Murmur

Heart Murmur	Description
Grade or intensity: Does not necessarily indicate severity of the problem May be altered with positional change from supine to sitting	Grade I: Barely audible; heard faintly after a period of attentive listening Grade II: Soft but easily audible Grade III: Moderately loud; no thrill Grade IV: Loud, present over widespread area; thrill present Grade V: Loud, audible with stethoscope barely on the chest; precordial thrill present Grade VI: Heard without stethoscope (rare)
Timing with cardiac cycle	Systolic Diastolic Continuous
Location on chest where murmur is loudest	Aortic or pulmonic listening areas, URSB, ULSB, Erb's point, LLSB, apex
Radiations or transmission to other locations	To back To apex To carotids
Quality	Musical Harsh blowing
Duration	Point of onset and length of time systole and diastole murmurs last (e.g., "early systole, heard throughout cardiac cycle")
Pitch	Low Middle High

LLSB, Left lower sternal border; *ULSB*, upper left sternal border; *URSB*, upper right sternal border.

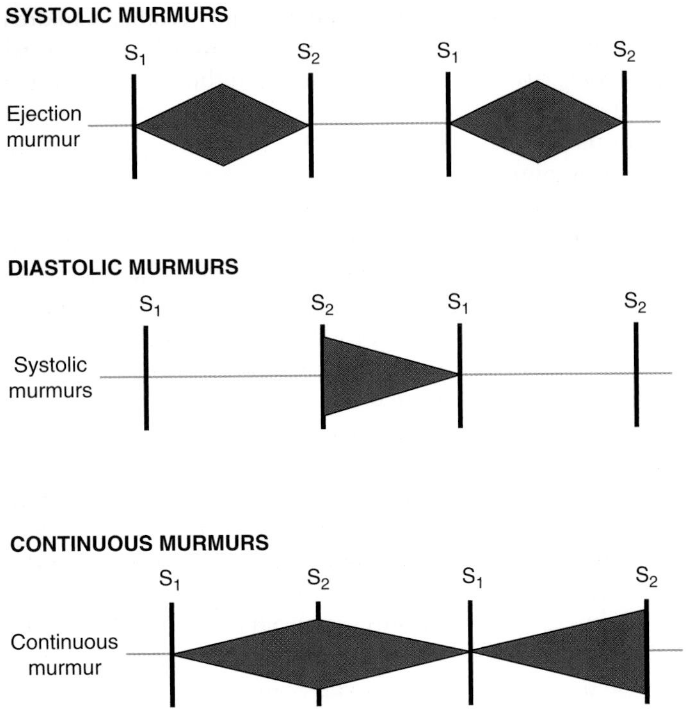

Systolic murmurs

- Comprise most murmurs heard and occur between S_1 and S_2.
- Are either regurgitation murmurs (e.g., the holosystolic murmur of a VSD that begins with S_1 and continues throughout systole) or ejection murmur caused by flow of blood through narrowed or stenotic areas (e.g., AS).
- Best heard at second left or right intercostal space (ICS)
- Begin with or after S_1 and end with or before S_2.
- Include all innocent and physiologic murmurs.

Diastolic murmurs

- Typically occur between S_2 and before or at S_1.
- Always indicate cardiac pathology.
- Murmur that starts with S_2 and has a decrescendo quality is most commonly due to aortic or pulmonic regurgitation.
- Mid-diastolic "rumble," a short low-pitched rumble heard best at the apex, is commonly due to atrioventricular valve stenosis or increased flow across a nonstenotic valve, such as seen with a large VSD or PDA.

Continuous murmurs

- Start at S_1 and go completely through systole and diastole.
- Most common cause is PDA.
- These murmurs need to be differentiated from the coexistence of separate systolic and diastolic murmurs and venous hums.

• **Figure 31-3** Timing of heart murmurs. *AS,* Aortic stenosis; *PDA,* patent ductus arteriosus; *VSD,* ventricular septal defect. (Cassidy SC, Allen HD, Phillips JR: History and physical examination. In Allen HD, Driscoll DJ, Shaddy RE, et al, editors: *Moss and Adams' heart disease in infants, children, and adolescents including the fetus and young adult,* ed 8, Philadelphia, 2013, Lippincott Williams & Wilkins, Figure 5-1, p 89.)

Innocent or Functional Murmurs

Functional or innocent cardiac murmurs are common in children and can be evident in newborns. Table 31-5 describes common types of innocent murmurs; Box 31-2 describes the characteristics of an innocent murmur. Families and older children with innocent murmurs should be reassured that there is no cardiac pathology. They should be informed that this murmur may come and go and may be louder at times of fever, anxiety, pain, or exercise, and that activities do not need to be limited or any special precautions taken.

Common Diagnostic Studies

If the PCP intends to refer for a cardiology consult, performing any of the following routine diagnostic studies is not cost-effective. The cardiology consultant is able to determine with greater discrimination which, if any, tests should be ordered (Park, 2014).

- Chest radiograph: Radiography provides the following information: cardiac size and size of specific chambers and great vessels, cardiac contour, status of pulmonary blood flow, and status of the lungs and other surrounding tissue (Fig. 31-4).
- Electrocardiogram (ECG): The ECG monitors the electrical activity of the heart from different locations and in different planes of the body and gives information about forces of ventricular contraction, hypertrophy, chamber dilation, and rhythm.
- Echocardiogram: Echocardiography uses reflected sound waves to identify intracardiac structures and their motion. The types of recordings include two-dimensional, M-mode, contrast, Doppler, and tissue Doppler studies (Fig. 31-5). Fetal echocardiography can diagnose CHD as early as 16 to 18 weeks' gestation (high-frequency transvaginal echocardiography as early as 10 weeks' gestation), as well as arrhythmias and hemodynamic changes (Park, 2014).
- Complete blood count (CBC): CBC rules out severe anemia or polycythemia as a cause of a murmur.

Other diagnostic studies may include the following:

- Cardiac catheterization: This provides information about cardiac output, vascular resistance, and the response of the heart to exercise and medications; heart anatomy is outlined.
- Hyperoxia test: Supplementation of 100% oxygen results in "pinking" and increased arterial oxygen saturation when the disease is primarily pulmonary; minimal or no color improvement indicates that the disease is cardiac. More commonly, simple pulse oximetry saturations are used to evaluate for cyanosis.
- Magnetic resonance imaging (MRI): This technique yields an image of the heart structures and information about chamber volumes and function.

• BOX 31-2 Auscultatory Findings—Innocent versus Pathologic Murmur

Innocent Murmur

Usually grade I to III/VI in intensity and localized
Changes with position (sitting to lying)
May vary in loudness or presence from visit to visit
May increase in loudness (intensity) with fever, anemia, exercise, or anxiety
Musical or vibratory in quality, sometimes blowing
Systolic in timing (except for venous hum, which is continuous), peaking in first half of systole
Duration is short
Best heard in LLSB or pulmonic area (except for venous hum)
Rarely transmitted
May disappear with Valsalva maneuver, position, or gentle jugular pressure
Vital signs: Normal
ECG: Normal
General health status: Good

Possible Pathologic Murmur*

A murmur in a child with a syndrome associated with CHD (e.g., trisomy 21)
Any diastolic murmur
Any systolic murmur associated with a thrill
Pansystolic murmurs
Continuous murmurs that cannot be suppressed
Systolic clicks
Opening snaps
Fixed splitting of the second heart sound not associated with bundle branch block
An accentuated S_2
S_4 gallops
Not positional
Grade III/VI or higher
Harsh quality

CHD, Congenital heart disease; *ECG,* electrocardiogram; *LLSB,* left lower sternal border.
*Refer to a pediatric cardiologist.

- Exercise testing: A graded treadmill or bicycle ergometer is used to determine cardiac output (myocardial blood flow and rhythm) response to exercise for endurance and capacity measurement.

Primary Health Care Management Strategies

The goals of primary health care for a child with cardiovascular disease include the following:

- Adequate nutritional intake and optimal growth: Depending on the child's condition, the diet may need modification to provide maximum calories or limit various types of foods. The young infant with CHF may need 24, 27, or 30 kilocalories per ounce of formula or fortified breast milk. The child may also need a nasogastric or gastric tube to obtain adequate calories because of an inadequate suck or fatigue with feeding. Children with cyanotic conditions may initially have adequate weight gain. The PCP should refer to a nutritionist if available for assistance with complex diets. (See Chapter 10 for further information on altered patterns of nutrition.)
- Optimal psychosocial development and functioning: Discuss with the family the need to treat the child as normally as possible. Direct parents to support groups that provide informational and emotional support for all family members. Poor sibling bonding and unexpressed fears and anger in young siblings toward an infant with a severe or chronic disease can affect their relationships and family dynamics for many years. A multicenter prospective study concluded that psychological functioning and quality of life of children and adolescents with serious congenital heart defects decreased significantly as the number of cardiac interventions increased (Knowles et al, 2014).
- Preventive vaccines: Live virus vaccines should be delayed until 6 months after cardiopulmonary bypass and exposure to red blood cells and plasma (CDC, 2011). This most often affects 1-year-old infants who are due for varicella and measles, mumps, and rubella vaccines. Other vaccines can be given on a regular schedule. The AAP now recommends provision of respiratory syncytial virus (RSV) prophylaxis for infants younger than 1 year old who have cyanotic or complicated CHD, especially those with CHF or pulmonary hypertension (AAP Committee on Infectious Diseases and AAP Bronchiolitis Guidelines Committee, 2014). Anyone older than 19 years old spending time with infants needs to have the Tdap vaccine, even if they have had a prior tetanus booster (Td).
- Prevention of avoidable complications: Emphasize prevention of respiratory infections through good hand washing and avoiding contact (if possible) with others with upper respiratory infection (URI) symptoms. Vaccination against seasonal influenza is prudent for infants and family members/caregivers, per CDC guidelines.
- Prevention of infective endocarditis (IE): Although uncommon in children, IE (also called *subacute bacterial endocarditis [SBE]*) is associated with significant morbidity and mortality rates and warrants primary prevention whenever indicated. Standards for prophylaxis against SBE for children undergoing dental procedures are available in Box 31-3 and Table 31-6. A high index of suspicion for IE should be maintained if any unusual clinical findings (e.g., petechiae, fever) are present after any procedure (Wilson et al, 2008). Children with CHD appear to have more severe gingival inflammatory conditions, with a concomitant increase in *Haemophilus* species, *Actinobacillus actinomycetemcomitans, Cardiobacterium hominis, Eikenella corrodens,* and *Kingella* species (HACEK) and other microbes known to cause endocarditis, compared with other children (Steelman et al,

TABLE 31-5 Common Innocent Murmurs*

	Stills	Pulmonary Flow Murmur of Childhood	Pulmonary Flow Murmur of Infancy	Venous Hum
Other names	Innocent Vibratory Functional Physiologic "Head start" murmur	Flow murmur	Peripheral pulmonary stenosis	
Description	Midsystolic, louder in supine position or with inspiration	Early systolic to midsystolic; decreases or disappears with standing; increases with cardiac output or in supine position	Short, midsystolic ejection murmur	Constant swishing sound, disappears with head turning, compression of jugular vein(s), or supine position; varies with respirations
Age	Any age, but most common between 2 and 6 years old	Any age, but more commonly heard in thin-chested adolescents between 8 and 14 years old	Common during newborn period, especially in preterm infants	Any age, but commonly between 2 and 8 years old
Best heard	Midpoint, left lower/apex and midsternal border; does not radiate	Pulmonary outflow area; radiates to lung fields	Murmur radiates from left upper sternal border to both axilla and back, usually gone by 6 months old	In upright position, left and right upper chest below clavicles
Quality	Short, vibratory, musical, "twangy string," medium-pitched	Soft, blowing with normally split S_2; no click or thrill	Soft with middle to high pitch	Soft, high pitch; does not radiate
Intensity	Grades II (rarely III)	Grades I to II	Grades I to II	Grades II to III
Differential diagnosis	Small VSD, IHSS	ASD, pulmonic stenosis	Supravalvular pulmonic stenosis or aortic stenosis	PDA

Adapted from Cassidy SC, Allen HD, Phillips JR: History and physical examination. In Allen HD, Driscoll DJ, Shaddy RE, et al, editors: *Moss and Adams' heart disease in infants, children, and adolescents including the fetus and young adult,* ed 8, Philadelphia, 2013, Lippincott Williams & Wilkins, pp 82–92; Bernstein D: Evaluation of the cardiovascular system. In Kliegman RM, Stanton BF, Schor NF, et al: *Nelson textbook of pediatrics,* ed 19, Philadelphia, 2011, Saunders, pp 1529–1536.
ASD, Atrial septal defect; *IHSS,* idiopathic hypertrophic subaortic stenosis; *PDA,* patent ductus arteriosis; *VSD,* ventricular septal defect.
*Note: Innocent murmurs typically increase with cardiac output (excitement, fever, anemia).

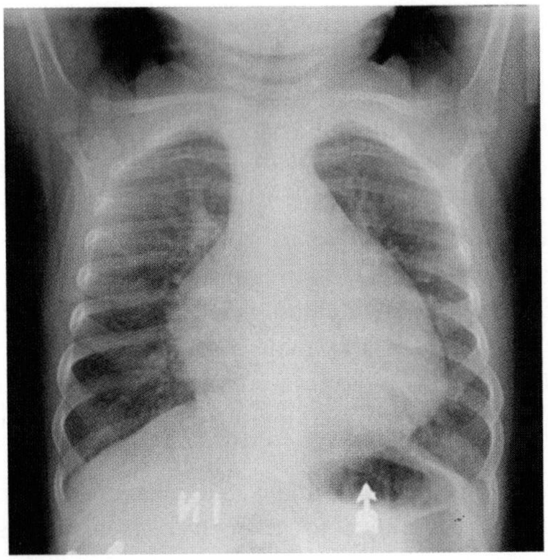

• **Figure 31-4** Chest radiogram of a 3-month-old with ventricular septal defect (VSD) and congestive heart failure (CHF). Cardiomegaly with increased pulmonary vascular markings from pulmonary venous congestion is visible.

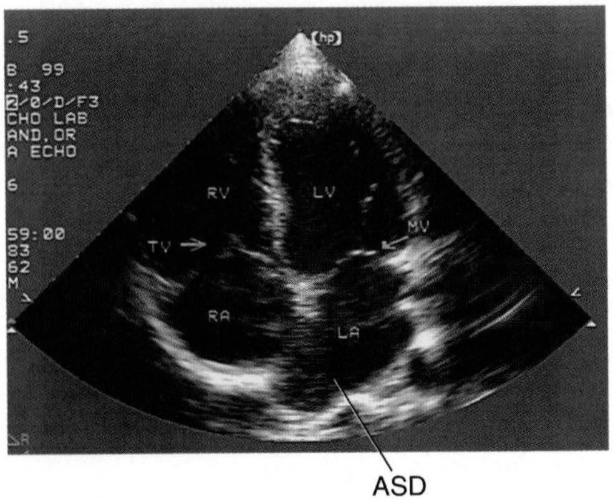

• **Figure 31-5** Echocardiogram of a 2-year-old with an atrial septal defect *(ASD).*

• BOX 31-3 Cardiac Conditions Associated with the Highest Risk of Endocarditis: Prophylaxis for Dental Procedures Recommended

- Prosthetic cardiac valve(s) or prosthetic material used for cardiac valve repair
- Previous infective endocarditis
- Congenital heart disease (CHD)
  - Unrepaired cyanotic CHD including palliative shunts and conduits
  - Completely repaired CHD with prosthetic material or device(s) by surgery or interventional catheterization, for 6 months after repair (due to the endothelialization of prosthetic material within that period)
  - Repaired CHD with residual defects (e.g., residual VSD) at the site or adjacent to the site of a prosthetic patch or device
- Cardiac transplantation recipients who have valve disease

Data from Nishimura RA, Carabello BA, Faxon DP, et al: ACC/AHA 2008 guidelines update on valvular heart disease; focused update on infective endocarditis, *Circulation* 52(8):676–685, 2008; Wilson W, Taubert KA, Gewitz M, et al: AHA guideline: prevention of infective endocarditis, *Circulation* 116:1736–1754, 2007.

2003). The reason for this is not clear. Good dental hygiene is extremely important for these children, and parents have shown poor knowledge about the risk of IE in children with CHD (Suma et al, 2011).

- Optimal fitness: Parents and children should be counseled on the importance of daily physical activity and limiting sedentary behavior. The initial goal is to develop habitual physical activity, including all types of physical movement, not just organized exercise designed to increase fitness. Certain children, such as those with ventricular arrhythmias, need complete activity restrictions (see Chapter 13, Table 13-6 for the parameters for sports participation for children with various forms of cardiac diseases or conditions). Children who have motor skill delays, which may be due to perioperative morbidity, tend to have more sedentary lifestyles and may need encouragement to be more active.
  - Prior to discussing physical activity, assessment of the child should include a detailed history looking for exertional symptoms, such as angina, excessive dyspnea, palpitations, dizziness, and syncope (see Chapter 13, Box 13-3 for the 14-element cardiovascular screening checklist for congenital and genetic heart disease).
  - The assessment of capacity for physical activity should also include current behavior, current motor

TABLE 31-6 Prophylactic Regimens for Dental Procedures*

Route	Agent	Regimen†
Able to take oral medication	Amoxicillin	Adults: 2 g PO; children: 50 mg/kg PO (maximum 2 g)
Unable to take oral medication	Ampicillin or‡ Cefazolin or ceftriaxone	Adults: 2 g IM or IV; children: 50 mg/kg IM or IV (maximum 2 g) Adults: 1 g IM or IV; children: 50 mg/kg IM or IV (maximum 1 g)
If penicillin allergic, oral	Clindamycin or‡ Cephalexin or Azithromycin or clarithromycin	Adults: 600 mg PO; children: 20 mg/kg PO (maximum 600 mg) Adults: 2 g PO; children: 50 mg/kg PO (maximum 2 g) Adults: 500 mg PO; children: 15 mg/kg PO (maximum 500 mg)
Penicillin allergic and unable to take oral medication	Clindamycin or‡ Cefazolin or ceftriaxone	Adults: 600 mg IM or IV; children: 20 mg/kg IM or IV (maximum 600 mg) Adults: 1 g IM or IV; children: 50 mg/kg IM or IV (maximum 1 g)

Data from Nishimura RA, Carabello BA, Faxon DP, et al: ACC 2008 guideline update on valvular heart disease: focused update on infective endocarditis, *Circulation* 118:887–896, 2008.

IM, Intramuscular; *IV,* intravenous; *PO, per os* (by mouth, orally).

*Antibiotic regimens are procedure specific; refer to the American Heart Association reference (Wilson et al, 2008) for nondental prophylaxis recommendations.

†Administer 30 to 60 minutes prior to the procedure.

‡Or other first- or second-generation oral cephalosporin in equivalent adult or pediatric dosage. Cephalosporins should not be used if there is a history of anaphylaxis, angioedema, or urticaria with penicillins.

skills (and expected skill development that will be required), motivation, anticipated time to be spent in the physical activity, and the type of activity. Reassure the parents that the child generally "self-limits" activity according to ability. If the child can comfortably talk during the activity, he/she will automatically limit their activity intensity to a desirable 60% to 80% of maximum (Longmuir et al, 2013). The cardiology provider should be consulted regarding exercise limitations before entrance into sports or any activities that require strenuous physical exertion.

- Optimal neurodevelopmental adaptation to school and life tasks: Children who require heart surgery in the first year of life can have significant neurodevelopmental impairment (Knowles et al, 2014). Those undergoing a first operation after 1 year generally have subtle or no impairment. Risk factors that predict worse neurodevelopmental outcomes include genetic syndromes, low birth weight, single ventricle physiology, low socioeconomic status, low maternal education, need for cardiopulmonary resuscitation, duration of mechanical ventilation, duration of intensive care unit (ICU) stay, gestational age at surgery, and preoperative intubation. Only a few of these are amenable to modification in the surgical period. However, early recognition of and intervention for developmental and cognitive delays lead to improved neurodevelopmental outcomes (Tabbutt et al, 2012). Although mean intelligence scores are generally within the average range, many of these children have difficulties with visuospatial tasks, fine motor functions, higher order language skills, memory, and/or attention. They may be impaired in their ability to coordinate lower-order skills or to perform higher-order tasks. Assessment tools to assist in neurodevelopment may be found in Additional Resources on the Evolve site.

Referral

If a PCP suspects cardiac disease or is unsure about findings, it is best to refer the patient to a pediatric cardiologist if available. Findings suggestive of cardiac disease are the presence of oxygen saturation less than 95%, symptoms of CHF, a pathologic murmur, or a murmur that is difficult to differentiate in the presence of poor growth and development. A murmur alone in a child who is otherwise doing well should be referred to a pediatric cardiologist for further evaluation in a timely but not urgent time frame. Newborns should be evaluated within 1 or 2 days of noticeable signs or immediately (change in breathing patterns, increased irritability and poor feeding, and/or cyanosis), depending on the severity of their symptoms. An older child with dizziness, chest pain with exertion, arrhythmia, dyspnea, syncope, signs of CHF, or abnormal vital signs should also be referred as soon as possible (Cassidy et al, 2013).

Some defects, such as small VSDs or bicuspid aortic valves, escape early detection and may cause no disability to a child. However, they pose a risk for bacterial endocarditis and should be identified.

Genetic Testing

A referral for genetic testing should be done in children who have, in addition to CHD, other congenital anomalies, dysmorphic features, neurocognitive deficits, growth retardation, mothers with multiple miscarriages, or siblings with congenital defects. Comparative genomic hybridization array testing is now widely available and allows for more specific and detailed detection of small structural variations of deoxyribonucleic acid (DNA) sequences indicating anomalies (Richards and Garg, 2010).

Family Support

Families need the support of the PCP to help them understand the diagnosis, to cope with the short- and long-term consequences, and to advocate for them within the referral system, which may be an overwhelming experience. Because of the stress involved in initial diagnosis, many parents do not absorb all of the information presented and may need multiple opportunities to ask questions and learn about the diagnosis.

Parents and their designated support people should clearly understand the diagnosis and have diagrams of the defect and general information to take away with them for future reference. Should medication be necessary, parents should understand the reason for the drug and the regimen for administration and side effects. They should understand the signs and symptoms of deterioration (e.g., CHF) and have clear information regarding how to proceed should symptoms develop. Infant and child cardiopulmonary resuscitation certification is critical for anyone caring for a child with a heart condition.

Congenital Heart Disease: General Information

When CHD is diagnosed in an infant or child, parents may incorrectly assume that they are somehow responsible for the child's defect. Health care professionals must be clear about what is and what is not known about CHD to help allay needless worry and guilt.

CHD is caused by an alteration in development of or failure of the embryonic heart to progress beyond an early developmental stage. This alteration occurs in the 2nd to 8th weeks of gestation due to genetic, environmental, or multifactorial influences. Most cases of CHD have no identifiable cause. With the publication of the human genome and advances in molecular techniques, more genetic factors have been identified as playing a possible role in CHD. This is increasingly important as more children with CHD survive to their own childbearing years.

Two percent to 4% of CHD is caused by teratogens, maternal conditions, or environmental influences. Drugs or teratogens linked to CHD include lithium, retinoic acid, antiepileptics, ibuprofen and naproxen, angiotensin-converting enzyme (ACE) inhibitors, tricyclic antidepressants, sulfonamides, sulfasalazine, tobacco, alcohol, cocaine, and marijuana. Environmental exposures to organic solvents, pesticides, and air pollution have also been implicated in CHD. Exposure to these agents during the vulnerable period (2 to 8 weeks of gestation) is best avoided, although often women do not know they are pregnant this early in gestation. Maternal illnesses (such as, diabetes mellitus, connective tissue disorders, phenylketonuria, rubella, and febrile illnesses—especially influenza) have also been implicated with CHD (van der Bom et al, 2011) (see Box 31-1).

Many genes have etiologic roles in the development of human CHD. Most infants born with CHD do not have other birth defects, but CHD does occur in association with other anomalies or syndromes in 25% to 40% of cases. Children with an abnormal chromosomal number (aneuploidy) account for a significant percentage of these children (Richards and Garg, 2010). Table 31-7 lists the most common known genetic syndromes, aneuploidies, single

TABLE 31-7 Congenital Malformation Syndromes Associated with Selected Congenital Heart Disease

Disorders	Resultant Heart Defect(s)/Occurrence
Syndromes with Aneuploidy (Abnormal Chromosome Number) or Microdeletion (≈10% of Congenital Heart Disease)	
Trisomy 21 (Down syndrome)	AV septal defect, VSD, ASD, PDA, TOF (50%)
Trisomy 18 (Edwards syndrome)	VSD, ASD, PDA, COA, bicuspid aortic or pulmonary valve (99%)
Trisomy 13 (Patau syndrome)	VSD, PDA, dextrocardia (90%)
Monosomy X (Turner syndrome)	Bicuspid aortic valve, COA (35%), pulmonic stenosis
Klinefelter variant (XXXXY)	PDA, ASD (15%)
22q11.2 deletion (DiGeorge syndrome)	Interrupted aortic arch, truncus arteriosus, TOF, perimembranous VSD, aortic arch anomalies
7q11.23 deletion (Williams syndrome)	Pulmonic stenosis, supravalvular aortic stenosis
Syndromes with Congenital Heart Disease from Single Gene Defects	
Marfan syndrome (FBN1, TGFBR1, TGFBR2)	Mitral valve prolapse, aortic root dilation
Noonan syndrome (PTPN11)	Valvular pulmonic stenosis, HCM
Costello syndrome (HRAS)	Pulmonary stenosis, HCM, conduction abnormalities
Alagille syndrome (JAG1, NOTCH2)	Pulmonic stenosis, TOF, ASD, peripheral pulmonic stenosis
Heterotaxy syndrome (ZIC3, CFC1)	DILV, DORV, d-TGA, AVSD
CHARGE (CHD7, SEMA3E)	Truncus arteriosus, interrupted aortic arch
Jacobsen (11q23 deletion)	HLHS, COA
Holt-Oram syndrome (TBX5)	ASD, VSD
Cri du chat syndrome (5p)	VSD, PDA, ASD (25%)
Neurofibromatosis	Pulmonic stenosis, COA
Leopard syndrome (PTPN11, RAF 1)	Pulmonic stenosis, conduction abnormalities
Nonhereditary Syndromes (Fetal Exposure)	
Fetal alcohol syndrome	VSD, PDA, ASD, TOF (25% to 30%)
Fetal hydantoin syndrome	Pulmonic stenosis, aortic stenosis, COA, PDA, VSD, ASD (<5%)
Fetal trimethadione syndrome	TGA, VSD, TOF (15% to 30%)
Infant of diabetic mother	TGA, VSD, COA (3% to 5%); cardiomyopathy (10% to 20%)

Data from Richards A, Garg V: Genetics of congenital heart disease, *Curr Cardiol Rev* 6:91–97, 2010; van der Bom T, Zomer C, et al: The changing epidemiology of congenital heart disease, *Nat Rev Cardiol* 8(1):50–60, 2011.

ASD, Atrial septal defect; *AV,* atrioventricular; *COA,* coarctation of the aorta; *DILV,* double inlet left ventricle; *DORV,* double outlet right ventricle; *d-TGA,* dextro-transposition of the great arteries; *HCM,* hypertrophic cardiomyopathy; *HLHS,* hypoplastic left heart syndrome; *PDA,* patent ductus arteriosis; *TGA,* transposition of the great arteries; *TOF,* tetralogy of Fallot; *VSD,* ventricular septal defect.

gene defects, and microdeletions associated with heart disease. (See Additional Resources on the Evolve site for information on genetic tests and specific genetic defects or syndromes.)

Specific Congenital Heart Diseases

Congestive Heart Failure

CHF refers to a progressive clinical and pathophysiologic syndrome found in many children with heart problems. The symptoms vary with age of the child and the root cardiac problem (Box 31-4). Besides functional changes, CHF is marked by changes in neurohormonal and molecular changes within the heart.

CHF in children can be caused by congenital malformations leading to volume overload (such as, a large VSD) or pressure overload (such as, aortic stenosis) or more complex heart disease. CHF can also occur in children with structurally normal hearts due to cardiomyopathy or secondary to arrhythmias, ischemia, toxins, or infections (Table 31-8). CHF is estimated to affect 12,000 to 35,000 children each year (Simpson and Canter, 2012).

The largest group of infants and children with CHF are those with excessive left to right shunting through unrepaired congenital defects. CHF is somewhat of a misnomer in these cases, because the myocardium generally responds quite well to the challenge of excessive blood volume for a long time, and cardiac output remains adequate. However, the compensatory response to this excessive workload for the lungs and some heart chambers includes electrolyte and fluid imbalances and neurohormonal changes. Children with heart failure from systolic or diastolic cardiac dysfunction caused by infections, obstruction, or arrhythmias also need treatment to ameliorate fluid and electrolyte imbalances, increase contractility, and decrease cardiac afterload.

Depending on the underlying pathophysiology, elevated neurohormonal and inflammatory mediators (aldosterone, norepinephrine, natriuretic peptides, tumor necrosis factor, and renin) circulate in children with CHF. Large-scale studies in adult populations show the value of blocking some of the chronic neurohormonal changes in CHF with agents, such as aldosterone inhibitors, angiotensin inhibitors, and sympathetic inhibitors (beta-blockers). Various studies show that the use of neurohormonal agents is more complex in children than adults. Whether a given neurohormonal agent benefits or harms depends on the underlying cause of CHF (CHD, infection, or other) as well as the degree of heart failure (Simpson and Canter, 2012).

The traditional heart failure therapies (i.e., diuretics, inotropes, and afterload reducers) are still used in many cases, although further elucidation of the neurohormonal responses in children with the different conditions listed in Table 31-7 may change this. Pulmonary vasodilators (such as, sildenafil) have been shown to be helpful in single ventricle heart failure. Monitoring B natriuretic peptides (amino acid polypeptides secreted by the *ventricles* in

• BOX 31-4 Signs and Symptoms of Congestive Heart Failure

Infants

- Tachypnea
- Tachycardia
- Rales or wheezing
- Cardiomegaly and hepatomegaly
- Periorbital edema
- Poor feeding/tires easily when feeding
- Poor weight gain
- Diaphoresis

Children and Teens

- Tachypnea
- Tachycardia
- Rales or wheezing
- Cardiomegaly and hepatomegaly
- Orthopnea
- Shortness of breath or dyspnea with exertion
- Peripheral edema
- Poor growth and development

TABLE 31-8 Conditions Associated with Congestive Heart Failure in Children

Age	Condition
Premature infant	Patent ductus arteriosus (PDA)
Birth to 1 week old	Hypoplastic left heart syndrome (HLHS) Coarctation of the aorta (COA) Critical aortic stenosis Interrupted aortic arch Arteriovenous malformations Tachycardia Cardiomyopathy
1 week to 3 months old	Ventricular septal defect (VSD) Truncus arteriosus Atrioventricular (AV) canal (endocardial cushion defect) Total anomalous pulmonary venous return Coarctation Tachycardia PDA Aortic stenosis Tricuspid atresia
Older than 1 year	Bacterial endocarditis Rheumatic fever Myocarditis

response to stretching) in the management of CHF may be helpful in bi-ventricular heart failure but is not recommended in single ventricle disease (Simpson and Canter, 2012). Future approaches to heart failure that are being studied include agents to decrease or block myocardial fibrosis, myocardial cell regeneration, and use of stem cell and microRNA to facilitate remodeling of the heart (Burns et al, 2014).

Left-to-Right Shunting Congenital Heart Disease (Acyanotic)

Pulmonary overflow lesions have communication between the two sides of the heart through which extra blood shunts from the high-pressure, oxygenated left side of the heart to the low-pressure, deoxygenated right side of the heart. The result is an increase in pulmonary blood flow. These lesions are acyanotic in nature. Fig. 31-6 lists the various left-to-right versus right-to-left shunting disorders.

Atrial Septal Defect

An atrial septal defect (ASD) is a defect or hole in the atrial septum. Of the four types of ASD, the most common involves the midseptum in the area of the foramen ovale and is called an *ostium secundum-type defect* (Fig. 31-7). Defects of the sinus venosus type are high in the atrial septum, near the entry of the SVC, or low near the IVC, and are frequently associated with anomalous pulmonary venous return. A primum ASD is in the lower portion of the septum and is most often seen in children with Down syndrome. The rarest form of ASD is an unroofed coronary sinus. The incidence is 5% to 10% of all CHDs with a female to male ratio of 2:1 (Park, 2014). Usually ASDs occur spontaneously; however, there are a few identified genetic mutations that cause familial ASDs (Park, 2014).

Clinical Findings

History. The child is often completely asymptomatic and may fatigue easily or have exertional dyspnea, be somewhat thin, and have a history of frequent upper respiratory tract infections or pneumonia. Symptoms may become more common in late adolescence or early adulthood.

Physical Examination.

- Typically a murmur may not be noticed until the child is 2 to 3 years old.
- Possible mild left anterior chest bulge or palpable lift at the left sternal border.
- S_1 is normal or split, with accentuation of the tricuspid valve closure sound.
- S_2 is often split widely and is relatively fixed.
- A grade I to III/VI, widely radiating, medium-pitched, not harsh systolic crescendo-decrescendo murmur is heard best at the pulmonic area. This murmur is not due to flow across the atrial septum, but it is due to increased flow across the pulmonary valve.

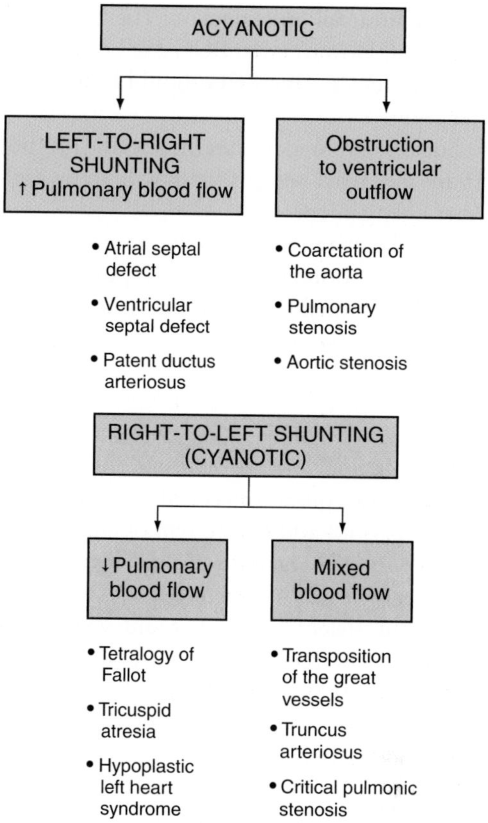

• **Figure 31-6** Classification of congenital heart disease (CHD).

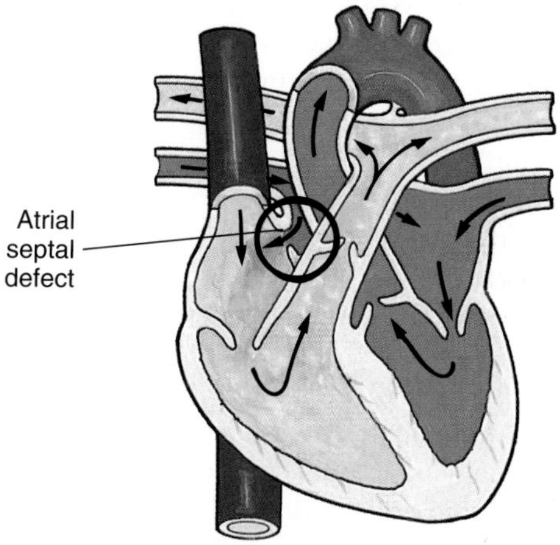

• **Figure 31-7** Atrial septal defect (ASD). (From Hockenberry M, Wilson D: *Nursing care of infants and children,* ed 10, St. Louis, 2015, Mosby/Elsevier.)

Diagnostic Studies.

- Chest radiography may reveal cardiac enlargement, especially of the right atrium and right ventricle. The main pulmonary artery may be dilated and pulmonary vascular markings increased.
- The ECG shows right axis deviation with right atrial enlargement. Lead V_1 usually shows a right bundle branch block with an rSR′ pattern. P wave may be tall

showing right atrial enlargement. The PR interval may be prolonged. However, the ECG can be normal in small left-to-right defects. The ECG should be assessed for AV prolongation.
- The echocardiogram identifies the specific location of the defect in the atrial septum and will show right-sided chamber enlargement.
- Cardiac catheterization is rarely necessary unless the diagnosis is in doubt, the site of pulmonary venous return is questionable, or when a device closure is planned (Park, 2014).

Management

- Small defects found in infancy may close spontaneously.
- Larger defects require intervention, usually after the child is 1 year old and before school entry or when the defect is identified in an older child. Most ASDs can now be closed in the cardiac catheterization lab with a closure device. If the defect is large or unfavorable to device closure, cardiac surgery is indicated. Surgical mortality rate is less than 0.5% (Park, 2014).
- SBE prophylaxis (see Table 31-6) precautions are necessary only in the first 6 months after cardiac surgery or device closure (81 mg of aspirin daily for 6 months may be prescribed after device closure).
- Long-term outcome is excellent after ASD repair. However, there is a small incidence of atrial arrhythmias in teenagers and adults (Sachdeva, 2013).
- Left untreated, with time ASDs can result in right ventricular enlargement, fibrosis, and failure; although rare in children, paradoxical emboli can occur (a thrombus transverses the intracardiac defect and enters the systemic circulation).
- Some with uncorrected ASDs develop severe irreversible pulmonary hypertension that is disabling and life-shortening.
- Exercise restriction is unnecessary (Park, 2014).

Ventricular Septal Defect

A VSD is a hole or defect in one of the areas of the ventricular septum and accounts for between 20% and 30% of all CHDs (Rubio and Lewin, 2013). There are four types of VSDs: perimembranous, supracristal (occurs in the outflow part of the right ventricle above crista supraventricularis), inlet, and muscular. The most common type is the perimembranous VSD (Fig. 31-8). VSDs are associated with many congenital defects, but 95% demonstrate no chromosomal anomaly (see Table 31-7). Approximately 30% to 50% of these defects are small; the vast majority of these close by 4 years old (Park, 2014).

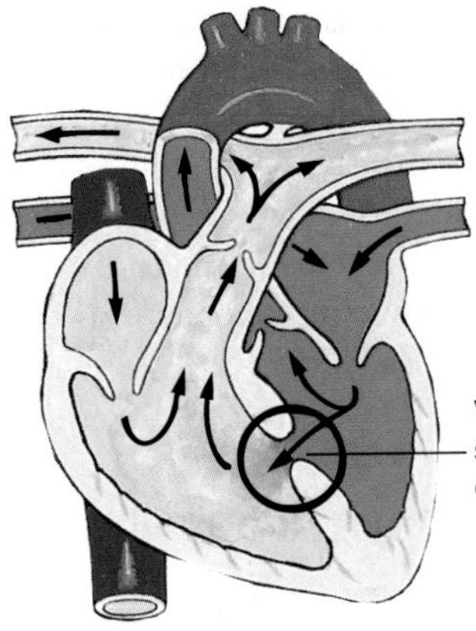

• **Figure 31-8** Ventricular septal defect (VSD). (From Hockenberry M, Wilson D: *Nursing care of infants and children,* ed 10, St. Louis, 2015, Mosby/Elsevier.)

Clinical Findings

History.

- A murmur is often not heard immediately after birth. When pulmonary vascular resistance falls (normally at 2 to 8 weeks old), more blood is shunted across the VSD from left ventricle to right ventricle and hence to the pulmonary circulation. This causes a classic loud murmur. Early signs and symptoms of CHF may also begin at this time.
- Parents may note signs and symptoms of CHF (see Box 31-4).
- Small defects may be completely asymptomatic at birth, appearing by 6 months old.

Physical Examination.

- Small VSD
  - Harsh, high-pitched, grade II to IV/VI holosystolic murmur at left lower sternal border (LLSB)
  - All other findings within normal limits
- Large VSD
  - Low-pitched, grade II to V/VI holosystolic murmur at LLSB
  - VSD murmur that becomes higher pitched over time indicates that the defect is becoming smaller
  - Diastolic rumble at the apex
  - Thrill along the left sternal border
  - Signs of progressing CHF after the first weeks of life
  - S_3 or S_4 gallop if CHF is present

Diagnostic Studies.

- Chest radiography findings vary depending on the shunt's size. Children with small shunts have a normal heart size and pulmonary vascular markings that are just beyond the upper limits of normal. Those with large shunts have cardiac enlargement involving both left and right ventricles and left atrium, as well as pulmonary vascular markings that are significantly increased (see Fig. 31-4).
- The ECG is normal with small defects and may show left ventricular hypertrophy (LVH) or biventricular hypertrophy (BVH) with large shunts.
- Echocardiography provides visualization of defects and pinpoints the exact anatomic location. In "pinhole" VSDs, a murmur may be present; however, a defect may not be visualized on the echocardiogram.

- Cardiac catheterization is rarely necessary except when there is a question of elevated pulmonary vascular resistance or when the VSD can be closed in the catheterization laboratory (Park, 2014).

Management

- Infants with small defects and no symptoms of CHF are monitored every 6 months throughout the first year of life and then biannually to assess for closure of the VSD. Some defects may never close and cause no difficulty. SBE prophylaxis is not recommended.
- Larger defects with signs of CHF are managed as follows:
  - Lanoxin, diuretics, ACE inhibitors, and beta-blocker dosages are prescribed, as needed, by the pediatric cardiologist.
  - Nutritional intake and weight gain must be monitored in infants and children. It is also important to teach families to fortify an infant's calories to 24, 27, or 30 kcal/oz, as needed. Arrange for enteric nutritional support via nasogastric tube for young infants struggling to meet their caloric needs.
  - Families must be taught the signs and symptoms of developing or progressing CHF.
  - Surgery or device closure is performed if no improvement is seen over weeks or months; the long-term outcome is excellent after repair (Park, 2014).
  - SBE prophylaxis precautions are necessary for 6 months after surgery (see Box 31-3 and Table 31-6).

Atrioventricular Septal Defect (Atrioventricular Canal Defect or Endocardial Cushion Defect)

The endocardial cushion is a central cardiac structure that includes the septal portions of the mitral and tricuspid valves and the lower portion of the atrial septum and upper portion of the ventricular septum. Variable portions of the endocardial cushion are absent. Complete AV septal defect implies the absence of this cushion, leading to a primum ASD, a single AV valve (composed of leaflets of the intended mitral and tricuspid valves), and an inlet VSD. There may also be partial, transitional, and intermediate defects with less profound abnormalities and usually less severe symptoms (Fig. 31-9). These complete or partial AV canal defects account for 4% to 5% of all CHDs; trisomy 21 (Down) syndrome children with CHD have a 45% incidence of AV canal defects (Cetta et al, 2013).

Clinical Findings

History. Children with only a primum ASD (partial AV canal) may not manifest symptoms. In infants with complete AV canal defects, parents may note signs and symptoms of CHF (see Box 31-4); recurrent pneumonia is common.

Physical Examination.

- Partial AV canal (primum ASD) findings are the same as those with secundum ASD. There may also be a soft blowing murmur of mitral regurgitation in the apex and/or infrascapular area.

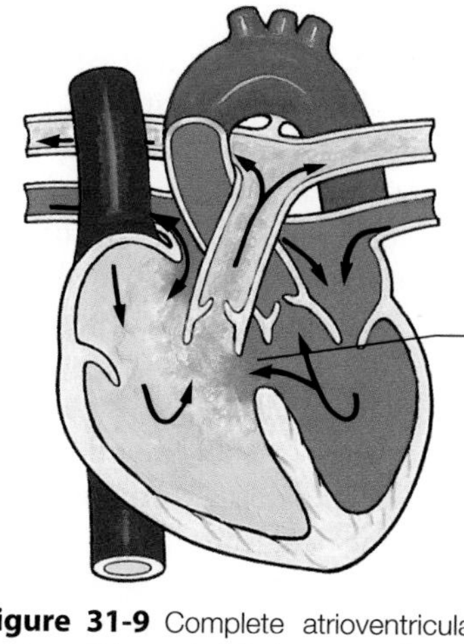

• **Figure 31-9** Complete atrioventricular (AV) septal defect (also known as AV canal defect or complete endocardial cushion defect). (From Hockenberry M, Wilson D: *Nursing care of infants and children*, ed 10, St. Louis, 2015, Mosby/Elsevier.)

- Complete AV canal defect findings:
  - Low-pitched, grade II to V/VI holosystolic murmur at LLSB. A murmur may not be evident at birth but increases in loudness at 2 to 8 weeks after pulmonary vascular resistance falls.
  - Diastolic rumble at the apex; thrill along the left sternal border.
  - Signs of progressing CHF after the first weeks of life; S_3 or S_4 gallop if CHF is present.
  - Some infants, particularly those with trisomy 21, maintain neonatal high pulmonary vascular resistance and do not show signs of CHF. Instead they may manifest signs of pulmonary hypertension with loud single S_2, precordial heave, minimal murmur, and desaturation with agitation or effort (Park, 2014).

Diagnostic Studies.

- Chest radiography findings vary depending on the size of the shunt. Children with small shunts have a normal heart size and pulmonary vascular markings just beyond the upper limits of normal. Those with large shunts (complete AV canal defect) have cardiac enlargement involving both the left and right ventricles and left atrium, as well as increased pulmonary vascular markings (see Fig. 31-4).
- The ECG usually shows superior axis between −40 and −160 degrees. Right ventricular hypertrophy is usually present, and left- or bi-ventricular hypertrophy in large shunts may be present. In 50% of children, the PR interval is prolonged.
- Echocardiography (two-dimensional, Doppler, or transesophageal) provides visualization of the size of ASD and VSD defects, size and other characteristics of the AV valve(s), and relative sizes of the ventricles.
- Cardiac catheterization may be performed if there is a question of elevated pulmonary vascular resistance or discrepancy in ventricular size.

Management

- Children with a partial AV canal defect that consists of a primum ASD and possibly a cleft mitral valve are monitored every 3 to 6 months throughout the first year of life and then biannually until the defect is closed surgically during toddler or preschool years. They usually do not have signs of CHF but may gain weight slowly. They rarely manifest difficulty with pulmonary hypertension after surgery.
- Infants with a complete AV canal defect usually need surgical correction before they reach 6 months of life. Infants who desaturate or develop CHF should see a cardiologist to determine surgical timing. Medical management before surgery may include:
  - Digoxin, diuretics, ACE inhibitors, and beta-blockers.
  - Monitoring nutritional intake and weight and fortifying breast milk or infant formulas; enteric nutritional support via nasogastric tube may be needed.
  - Educating families on the signs and symptoms of developing or progressing CHF.

Surgical repair consists of closure of the defect and reconstruction of the common AV valve into separate tricuspid and mitral valves. Residual mitral and/or tricuspid insufficiency is common after surgery. Surgical mortality is between 3% and 10% for those with complete AV defects and 3% for those with partial defects (Park, 2014); SBE prophylaxis precautions are necessary for only 6 months.

Patent Ductus Arteriosus

Normal functional closure of the ductus arteriosus occurs in the first 12 to 72 hours after birth. Permanent sealing occurs in 2 to 3 weeks. The ductus arteriosus may remain patent in some infants and leave a connection between the aorta and the pulmonary artery. As pulmonary vascular resistance falls, aortic blood is shunted into the pulmonary artery and recirculates through the lungs (Fig. 31-10). The incidence is 5% to 10% of all CHDs with a female to male ratio of 3:1 (Park, 2014). The frequency of a PDA increases with decreasing gestational age of premature infants; it is as high as 45% to 80% in very young infants less than 1750 g (Park, 2014). This condition occurs with many congenital malformation syndromes (see Table 31-7).

Clinical Findings

History. The infant or child may be asymptomatic if the PDA is small. Increasing signs of CHF may appear in the first weeks of life in larger PDAs. PDA usually is evident by 3 months old.

Physical Examination.

- In the immediate postnatal period, the murmur is soft, systolic, and heard along the left sternal border, under the left clavicle, and in the back.
- After the first weeks of life, a typical grade II to V/VI, harsh, rumbling, continuous "machinery murmur" is heard in the left infraclavicular fossa and pulmonic area with a thrill at the base.
- Physical findings of CHF may be present with a large shunt.

Diagnostic Studies.

- Chest radiographic findings: With a small to moderate shunt, the heart is not enlarged; with larger shunts, both the left atrium and left ventricle can show enlargement. Pulmonary vascular markings may be increased.
- ECG: Large shunts show LVH; QRS axis is normal or rightward.
- Echocardiogram: Demonstrates the patent ductus and usually enlargement of the left atrium.

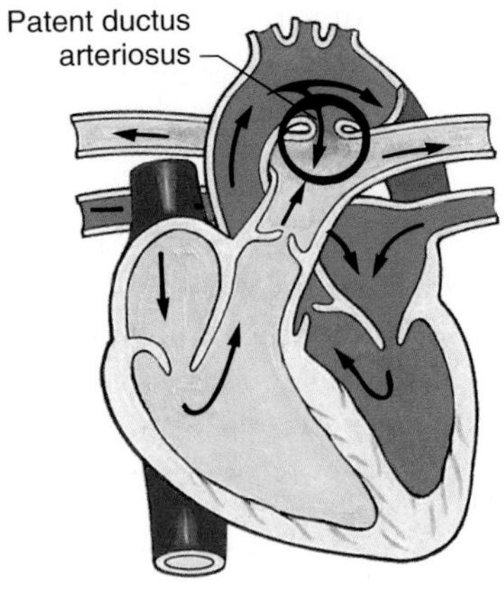

• **Figure 31-10** Patent ductus arteriosus (PDA). (From Hockenberry M, Wilson D: *Nursing care of infants and children,* ed 10, St. Louis, 2015, Mosby/Elsevier.)

Management

- Indomethacin or ibuprofen may be given to preterm infants to effect closure when there is significant left-to-right shunt. It is contraindicated and ineffective in term or older infants (Park, 2014).
- An asymptomatic infant with a small left-to-right shunt from a PDA is followed for spontaneous closure or device closure in the catheterization laboratory, preferably before 1 year old. Infants with large shunts or pulmonary hypertension should have their PDA surgically closed within the first few months of life to prevent the development of progressive pulmonary vascular obstruction. Surgical ligation of the ductus is a low-risk procedure because cardiopulmonary bypass is not necessary (Park, 2014).
- Interventional cardiologists now close many PDAs in children older than 8 months old by inserting coils or closure plugs into the shunt in the cardiac catheterization laboratory.
- Families should be reassured that their child will live an active, normal life.
- SBE prophylaxis precautions are recommended for the 6-month period after the surgical or device closure.

Right-to-Left Shunting Congenital Heart Disease (Cyanotic)

Cyanotic CHD represents 10% to 18% of all congenital heart lesions (Park, 2014). Cardiac cyanosis is due to obstruction of pulmonary blood flow or mixing of oxygenated and unoxygenated blood. Visible cyanosis occurs when oxygen saturation in blood reaches around 85%. Cyanosis is more readily apparent with polycythemia and less readily apparent with anemia or the presence of fetal hemoglobin. Polycythemia is a compensatory mechanism to increase the oxygen-carrying capacity in cyanotic patients; however, it increases the risk for cerebral thromboses (Park, 2014).The most common heart conditions causing cyanosis in the immediate newborn period are listed in Fig. 31-6.

Transposition of the Great Arteries

Dextro-transposition of the great arteries (d-TGA) results from incomplete septation and migration of the truncus arteriosus during fetal development. In d-TGA, the aorta arises from the right ventricle and the pulmonary artery arises from the left ventricle. The aorta receives the deoxygenated systemic venous blood and returns it to the systemic arteries. The pulmonary artery receives oxygenated pulmonary venous blood and returns it to the pulmonary circulation (Fig. 31-11). There may be a number of comorbid heart malformations with d-TGA—most commonly VSD, PDA, and coronary artery defects. The incidence is 5% to7% of all CHDs with a male to female ratio of 3 : 1 (Park, 2014).

Clinical Findings

History.

- Cyanosis is immediately evident by 1 hour of birth (52%) or within the first day after birth (92%). Because d-TGA allows mixing of oxygenated and unoxygenated blood, occasionally less cyanotic infants may present as late as 3 months old.

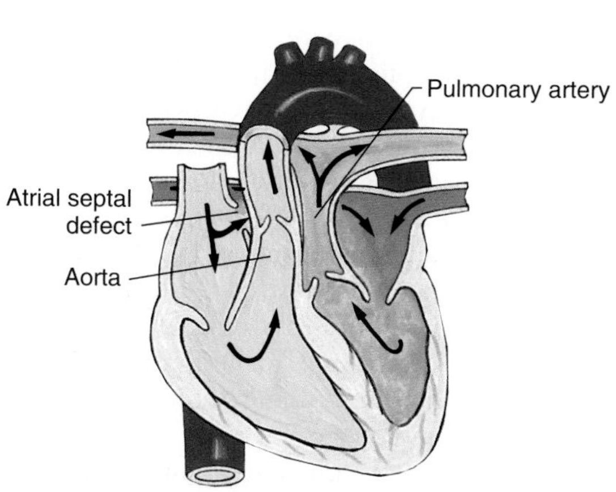

• **Figure 31-11** Complete transposition of the great vessels. (Modified from Hockenberry M, Wilson D: *Nursing care of infants and children,* ed 10, St. Louis, 2015, Mosby/Elsevier.)

- CHF symptoms may be present.
- Affected infants are often large for gestational age with retardation of growth and development after the neonatal period.

Physical Examination. Infants may have no murmur at birth or may have a murmur characteristic of associated lesions, such as VSD, ASD, or PDA. The S_2 is loud and single because of the anatomic placement of the great arteries.

Diagnostic Studies.

- Chest radiography and ECG findings may be normal in the early newborn period, or the heart may appear egg shaped.
- ECG findings show right axis deviation and right ventricular hypertrophy.
- Echocardiography shows the pulmonary artery arising from the left ventricle and the aorta arising from the right.

Management

- Immediate referral to a pediatric cardiac center is necessary. Correction of electrolyte and acid-base imbalance may be necessary.
- Intravenous prostaglandin E_1 (PGE_1) is given to delay closure or reopen the ductus arteriosus.
- A balloon atrial septostomy may be performed in the catheterization laboratory to promote mixing of oxygenated and unoxygenated blood in the atria.
- The arterial switch (Jatene procedure) is usually performed in the first few days of life. If this is not possible, a number of other operations may be performed, such as the Nakaidoh, Damus-Kaye-Stansel or réparation à l'étage ventriculaire (REV) procedures.
- Children are monitored closely throughout life with annual echocardiogram follow-up.
- SBE prophylaxis precautions are indicated for life.

Prognosis

Without treatment, there is a 50% mortality rate in the first month of life and 90% by the first year. Operative mortality is from 5% to 17%; there are excellent long-term results after surgery (Tabbutt et al, 2012). However, close monitoring for long-term patency and growth of the coronary arteries is warranted. Neopulmonic stenosis and neoaortic regurgitation may occur after the arterial switch. Refer any patient with a history of arterial or atrial switch to a pediatric cardiologist, especially with a history of palpitations, syncope, and/or shortness of breath with exertion.

Tetralogy of Fallot

Tetralogy of Fallot (TOF; also referred to as TET) is a combination of four anatomic cardiac defects resulting in right ventricular outflow tract obstruction: (1) pulmonary valve stenosis, (2) right ventricular hypertrophy, (3) VSD, and (4) an aorta that overrides the ventricular septum (Fig. 31-12). It is the most common cyanotic cardiac lesion

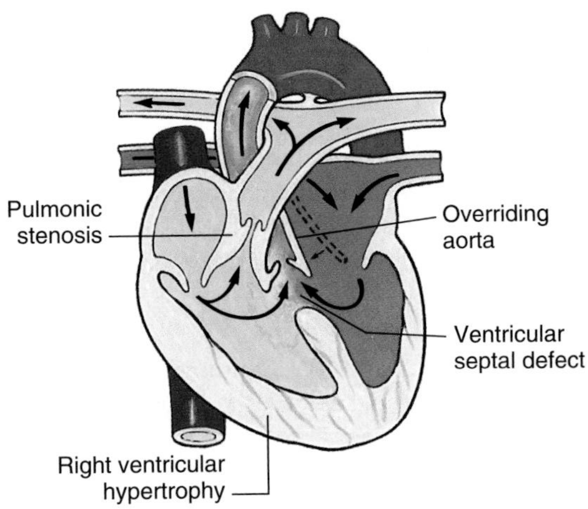

• **Figure 31-12** Tetralogy of Fallot (TOF). (From Hockenberry M, Wilson D: *Nursing care of infants and children,* ed 10, St. Louis, 2015, Mosby/Elsevier.)

(5% to 10% of all CHDs), occurs slightly more in males, and has a spectrum of severity (Park, 2014). The most severe forms involve non-patent pulmonary valve and artery atresia. This is referred to as *TOF pulmonary atresia,* and these infants are quite cyanotic as newborns. In the mildest form, "pink TETs," the infant may not display signs of cyanosis because the valvular stenosis is mild, and their symptoms may be similar to a large VSD. However, in most cases of TOF, right-to-left shunting across the VSD and cyanosis increase over the first months of life. This is a result of increasing obstruction in the right ventricular outflow tract. Children with chromosome 22q11.2 deletion syndrome or Down syndrome have a higher risk of this defect.

Clinical Findings

History. The severity of symptoms with TOF depends on the degree of right ventricular outflow obstruction. Symptoms include:

- Cyanosis in cases with mild right ventricular outflow obstruction, cyanosis may be so slight that it is not initially evident, or it may be present at birth (with severe obstruction). Cyanosis is usually present by 6 months old.
- Dyspnea and cyanosis (including hypercyanotic episodes, or "TET spells") increase by 2 to 4 months old, especially with crying, feeding, and/or defecation. The infant may have a history of poor weight gain.

Physical Examination. The following findings may be evident:

- Cyanosis of the mucous membranes and dyspnea
- A grade III to V/VI, harsh systolic ejection murmur at the left mid- to upper sternal border (VSD murmur and symptoms of a large VSD). There may be a palpable thrill and a holosystolic murmur at the LLSB.
- Sternal lift secondary to right ventricular hypertrophy.

Diagnostic Studies.

- Chest radiography may show a boot-shaped heart with decreased pulmonary vascular markings.
- ECG shows right ventricular hypertrophy and right axis deviation and may show a conduction delay in V_1.
- An echocardiogram shows the extent of the pulmonary obstruction and demonstrates the anatomy of the overriding aorta and VSD.
- Pulse oximetry values decrease over time, with resultant increase in hemoglobin and hematocrit values.
- Cardiac catheterization may be performed, in the most severe forms, to delineate pulmonary artery anatomy.

Management

- In neonates with severe pulmonary obstruction, the ductus arteriosus is maintained or reopened with PGE_1 until more definitive repair or palliation is possible.
- For hypercyanotic episodes, the child should be cradled in a knee-chest position, soothed, and given oxygen and perhaps morphine sulfate subcutaneously until the spell subsides. The knee-chest maneuver increases systemic resistance, decreases right-to-left shunting, and increases pulmonary blood flow, hopefully alleviating symptoms. Immediate intervention is required for infants who are "spelling," especially if the previously mentioned maneuvers do not end the spell. Most children are surgically repaired before hypercyanotic spells begin.
- Complete repair with open-heart surgery is usually performed in infancy.
- Lifelong cardiology follow-up for pulmonic regurgitation or late arrhythmias is required. Recent studies indicate that progressive right ventricular dilation leads to increasing QRS duration on ECG. QRS duration of 180 ms significantly increases the risk of ventricular tachycardia and sudden death. A cardiology consult is indicated before clearing for sports participation (Park, 2014).
- SBE prophylaxis is indicated before surgery and usually for 6 months after repair.

Tricuspid Atresia, Hypoplastic Left Heart Syndrome, and Other Single Ventricle Defects

Tricuspid atresia, pulmonary atresia/intact ventricular septum, and hypoplastic left heart syndrome (HLHS) are the most common types of single ventricle defects. In most cases, there is functionally only one ventricle of either right or left morphology that must do the work of pumping blood to both the systemic and pulmonary circulations. Oxygenated and deoxygenated blood mix in this ventricle, and the child is cyanotic. Most of these children require palliative cardiac procedures to survive.

Tricuspid atresia results in a small right ventricle without access from the right atrium. Blood returning from the systemic circulation must pass over an ASD to the left atrium and then left ventricle before being pumped to either the lungs or the body (Fig. 31-13). TGA also occurs in 50% of these patients. Less than 3% of all children with CHD have tricuspid atresia; its etiology is unknown (Epstein, 2013).

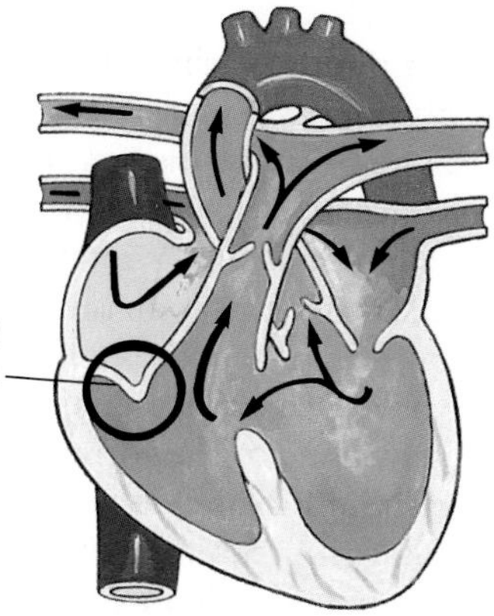

• **Figure 31-13** Tricuspid atresia. (Modified from Hockenberry M, Wilson D: *Nursing care of infants and children,* ed 10, St. Louis, 2015, Mosby/Elsevier.)

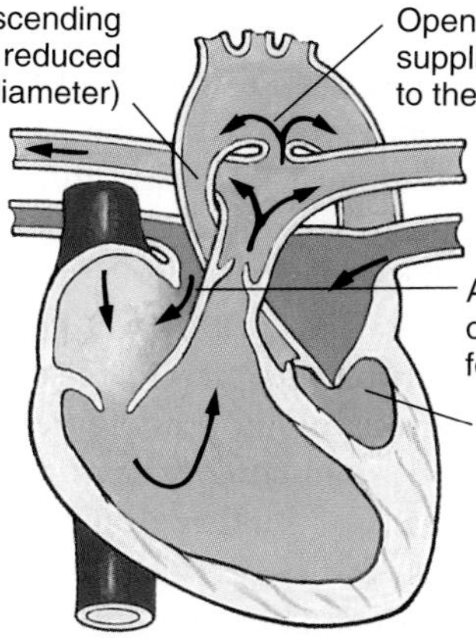

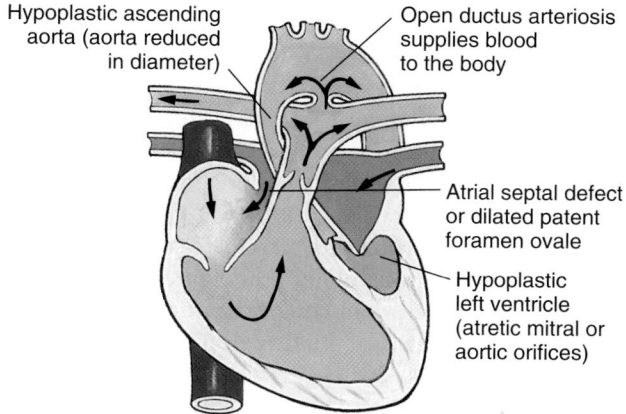

• **Figure 31-14** Hypoplastic left heart syndrome (HLHS). (Modified from Hockenberry M, Wilson D: *Nursing care of infants and children,* ed 10, St. Louis, 2015, Mosby/Elsevier.)

HLHS occurs in less than 4% of congenital heart defects (Tweddell et al, 2013). Intrauterine stenosis of either the mitral or aortic valves or both, results in a small left ventricle and hypoplasia of the ascending aorta and arch (Fig. 31-14). The cause is unknown although it is linked to some genetic syndromes, such as Jacobsen syndrome and Turner syndrome in 10% of cases. Central nervous system abnormalities have also been associated with HLHS in 10% to 29% of cases (Park, 2014).

Clinical Findings

History. Cyanosis occurs soon after birth with increased respiratory rate, fatigue with the effort of crying, or feeding with subsequent poor weight gain. This often progresses to cardiorespiratory shock as the ductus arteriosus closes.

Physical Examination.

- A grade I to III/VI early systolic murmur may be present; usually a single S_2 is heard.
- Cyanosis is generally evident as soon as the ductus arteriosus closes.
- Hepatomegaly (may or may not be present)

Diagnostic Studies.

- Heart size on chest radiography is generally normal initially. Cardiomegaly and decreased pulmonary blood flow occur over time.
- ECG findings depend on the type of single ventricle disease but are always abnormal for age. Right ventricular forces are diminished in tricuspid atresia.
- Two-dimensional echocardiography is diagnostic and shows the specifics of the anatomy.

Management

- Intravenous PGE_1 may be indicated in newborns. Most children are initially palliated with aortopulmonary shunts or other procedures depending on their anatomy. At 4 to 6 months old, palliation is continued with a bidirectional anastomosis of the SVC to the pulmonary artery. The third stage of palliation (Fontan procedure) occurs at 2 to 4 years old; the IVC is connected to the pulmonary artery. Some children are considered for cardiac transplantation early in life if their anatomy is not amenable to the Fontan pathway, or heart function and pulmonary vascular resistance do not allow completion of palliative staging (Park, 2014).
- Families require support throughout the child's life. Frequent surgeries and hospitalizations can interfere with normal social development. Early recognition and intervention for developmental delays are important.
- SBE prophylaxis is recommended while the child remains cyanotic (see Box 31-3 and Table 31-6).

Complications

Complications include development of collateral arterial and venous vessels, protein-losing enteropathy, arrhythmias, thromboembolic events including strokes, and many others. A decrease in exercise tolerance throughout life can be expected, in addition to left or right ventricular dysfunction. There may be fewer complications with surgical palliation at earlier ages. For those with severe long-term complications, heart transplantation can be an option.

Obstructive Cardiac Lesions

Aortic Stenosis and Insufficiency

Aortic stenosis or narrowing may occur at the aortic valvular, subvalvular, or supravalvular level. Valvular stenosis is the most common form (Fig. 31-15). The stenotic aortic valve is usually bicuspid rather than tricuspid. Stenosis causes increased pressure load on the left ventricle leading to LVH and, ultimately, ventricular failure. The imbalance between increased myocardial oxygen demand of hypertrophied myocardium and coronary blood supply may lead to ischemia and fatal ventricular arrhythmias. The bicuspid aortic valve generally becomes more stenotic and often regurgitant (insufficient) over time. Some infants are born with critical aortic stenosis and require urgent intervention, usually a balloon valvuloplasty early in life. Children with only a congenital bicuspid aortic valve and no stenosis or

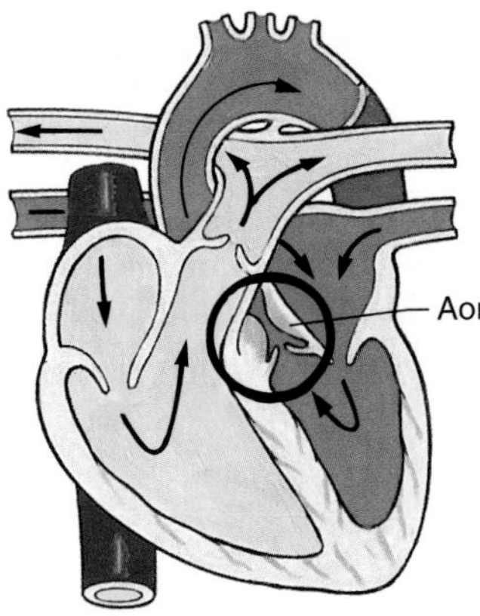

• **Figure 31-15** Aortic stenosis. (From Hockenberry M, Wilson D: *Nursing care of infants and children,* ed 10, St. Louis, 2015, Mosby/Elsevier.)

regurgitation are at risk of developing symptoms by adolescence. Aortic stenosis occurs in 3% to 8% of all CHDs with a male to female ratio of approximately 4 : 1 (Schneider and Moore, 2013).Thirty percent of females with Turner syndrome have obstruction at some level of the left heart outflow tract (Richards and Garg, 2010).

Clinical Findings

History.

- Growth and development may be normal.
- Activity intolerance, fatigue, chest pain (angina pectoris), or syncope can develop or increase with age.
- CHF, low cardiac output, and shock may be evident in newborns with severe aortic stenosis.
- Sudden death, presumably due to arrhythmias, can occur with increasing severity of stenosis and exertion.

Physical Examination.

- BP may reveal a narrow pulse pressure. The apical impulse may be pronounced with moderate to severe stenosis.
- A grade III to IV/VI, loud, harsh systolic crescendo-decrescendo murmur is best heard at the upper right sternal border with radiation to the neck, LLSB, and apex.
- With a valvular lesion, a faint, early systolic click at the LLSB may be heard.
- With aortic insufficiency, an early diastolic blowing murmur is heard at the LLSB to apex.
- In the most severe lesions, S_2 is single or closely split; S_3 or S_4 heart sounds may also be heard.
- A thrill may be present at the suprasternal notch.

Diagnostic Studies.

- Chest radiographs are usually normal or may show LVH. Adults frequently develop radiographic evidence of calcification on the aortic valve over time.
- ECG can be normal or reveal LVH and inverted T-waves.
- A 24-hour Holter monitor or 30-day event monitor demonstrates ventricular arrhythmia.
- Echocardiogram is the diagnostic examination of choice.

Management

- The type and timing of treatment depends on the severity of the obstruction.
- Balloon valvuloplasty of the stenotic valve is the initial palliative treatment in the newborn. However, the aortic valve generally needs further intervention.
- In older children, surgical division of fused valve commissures may relieve stenosis but often valve replacement is necessary for severe aortic stenosis and/or insufficiency. Unfortunately, none of the current replacement options are ideal or enduring for children. Mechanical valves are prothrombotic and require anticoagulation with warfarin. Heterograph and homograft valves have limited durability in the aortic position, and the Ross procedure requires placement of the homograft in the pulmonic position, leading to future replacements of that valve as it becomes stenosed.
- Children with subaortic stenosis require surgical resection when the gradient is greater than 35 mm Hg.
- Patients with supravalvar aortic stenosis require resection of the narrowed area with patch material.
- Children with mild aortic stenosis can participate in all sports but should have annual cardiac examinations. Those with moderate aortic stenosis should choose low-intensity sports (such as, golf, bowling, table tennis, or softball) as guided by their cardiologist. Children with severe aortic stenosis or moderate aortic stenosis with symptoms should avoid competitive or intensive sports because of the risk of sudden death from ventricular arrhythmias (Park, 2014) (see Chapter 13, Table 13-6).
- Any aortic root dilation (commonly seen with bicuspid or stenotic aortic valves) may require intervention to prevent aortic dissection.
- SBE prophylaxis is necessary for 6 months after surgery.
- Anticoagulation is necessary with mechanical valve replacement (Park, 2014).

Pulmonic Stenosis

Normally the pulmonary valve opens to allow the flow of blood from the right ventricle into the pulmonary artery. In pulmonic stenosis, there is narrowing at the subpulmonic, valvular, or supravalvular area. Right-sided pressure is increased as the ventricle pumps against the obstruction. Right ventricular hypertrophy occurs as a result of this increased load. Pulmonary stenosis can also occur in the main and/or branch pulmonary arterial system. Mild pulmonic stenosis is usually identified on routine examination. Many also develop poststenotic dilation of the pulmonary artery. Isolated pulmonic stenosis occurs in 8% to 12% of all CHDs (Park, 2014). (See Table 31-7 for associated congenital malformation syndromes.)

Clinical Findings

History.

- The child is usually asymptomatic, with a murmur noted on routine physical examination in the newborn to school-age child.

- Exertional dyspnea and fatigue are noticeable as stenosis progresses.
- Cyanosis from right-to-left shunting over the foramen ovale may be evident with critical pulmonic stenosis in the newborn.
- Growth and development are usually normal except in cases of Turner or Noonan syndrome in which short stature is common (Park, 2014).

Physical Examination.

- A grade II to IV/VI, harsh, mid- to late systolic ejection murmur is heard at the upper left sternal border over the pulmonic region with transmission along the left sternal border, neck and back, and into both lung fields.
- An intermittent systolic ejection click may be evident in the pulmonic area that decreases with inspiration and increases with expiration.
- Cyanosis and symptoms of right-sided CHF can occur in severe pulmonic stenosis in the newborn.

Diagnostic Studies.

- Chest radiographs may be within normal limits in infants or show prominent main pulmonary artery segments. Right-sided cardiac enlargement and decreased peripheral pulmonary vascular markings may be evident if heart failure develops.
- ECG may be normal with mild stenosis; with moderate to severe pulmonic stenosis, right axis deviation and right ventricular hypertrophy occur.
- Echocardiograms confirm the diagnosis, identifying the gradient and monitoring progression of the stenosis.
- Cardiac catheterization may be used to delineate location of the main and branch pulmonary artery stenosis.

Management

- Balloon valvuloplasty in neonates and older children with stenosis greater than 50 mm Hg are performed. If unsuccessful, surgical valvuloplasty or replacement may be indicated. Stents and balloons are also used for branch stenosis.
- With mild stenosis, families must be encouraged to treat their children normally and not limit their activity. Moderate stenosis can progress to severe narrowing during periods of rapid growth, such as during infancy or adolescence (Park, 2014).
- SBE prophylaxis is not considered necessary except in the 6-month postoperative period or if prosthetic material is used (see Box 31-3).

Coarctation of the Aorta

Coarctation of the aorta (COA) is a narrowing of a small or long segment of the aorta (Fig. 31-16). Coarctation may occur as a single defect caused by a disturbance in the development of the aorta or may be secondary to constriction of the ductus arteriosus. The severity of the coarctation, its location, and the degree of obstruction determine the clinical presentation. Systolic and diastolic hypertension exists in vessels proximal to the narrowing, whereas hypotension is present in vessels below the narrowing. COA accounts for 6% to 8% of all congenital heart defects and occurs slightly more in males (Beckman, 2013). The incidence in females with Turner syndrome is close to 30%; it is also commonly associated with a bicuspid aortic valve in greater than 50% of cases (Park, 2014).

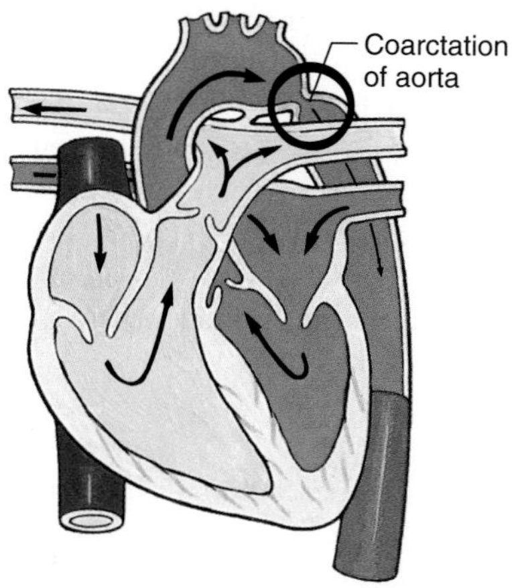

• **Figure 31-16** Coarctation of the aorta (COA). (From Hockenberry M, Wilson D: *Nursing care of infants and children,* ed 10, St. Louis, 2015, Mosby/Elsevier.)

Clinical Findings

History. In newborns, COA is not always apparent until the ductus closes and decreases blood flow to the lower body. Severe coarctation in infants is apparent in the first 6 weeks; symptoms include tachypnea, poor feeding, and possibly cool lower extremities. In children 3 to 5 years old, coarctation may go unnoticed until hypertension or a murmur is detected. Retrospectively, children with coarctation may have had complaints of leg pain with exercise or headaches.

Physical Examination.

- Upper extremity hypertension with lower extremity hypotension are present, although milder cases may cause only a minimal discrepancy between upper and lower extremity BPs. In severe cases, poor lower extremity perfusion may be noticed with lower body mottling or pallor.
- Delayed timing and absent or weak arterial and other distal arterial pulses may occur.
- Bounding brachial, radial, and carotid pulses may occur.
- Signs of CHF may be evident.
- A systolic ejection murmur may be detected in the left infraclavicular region with transmission to the back.
- A ventricular heave at the apex may be palpated.
- A gallop rhythm may occur in infants with CHF.

Diagnostic Studies.

- Chest radiography may reveal a normal or slightly enlarged heart and normal to increased pulmonary vascular markings; rib notching may be seen.
- ECG findings depend on the severity of the lesion and the age of the child. In infants, right ventricular

hypertrophy may be seen; in older children, LVH develops secondary to hypertension.
- Echocardiography is helpful in confirming the diagnosis and locating the constricted aortic segment. It may also show associated cardiac abnormalities. In newborns with a PDA diagnosis by echocardiogram can be challenging.
- MRI can define the location, severity, and anatomy of the aortic arch.

Management
- In critical neonatal coarctation, PGE_1 is used to maintain or reopen the ductus.
- If possible, surgical resection of the constricted area and anastomosis of the upper and lower portions of the aorta is performed. Restenosis is more likely to occur if repair was before 1 year old (Park, 2014). Cardiologists may dilate or stent the coarcted area in recoarctation or mild coarctation. Other procedures, including bypass grafting, may be necessary with unusually long coarcted segments. Surgical mortality is rare. Some centers choose balloon valvuloplasty or stent procedures for initial coarctation management (Park, 2014).
- In older children with long-standing hypertension, antihypertensive medication may be required for several months after repair. Long-term prognosis is excellent unless there are associated intracardiac defects. BP should be monitored postoperatively for recoarctation.
- Children with previous coarctation repairs may participate in any competitive sport if residual BP gradient between arm and legs is less than 20 mm Hg and peak systolic BP is normal at rest and with exercise. However, during the first year after surgery, high-intensity static exercises, such as weight lifting and wrestling, should be avoided (Park, 2014).
- Lifelong follow-up is necessary due to risk of recoarctation, residual hypertension, and often associated bicuspid aortic valve.
- SBE prophylaxis is no longer considered necessary except in the 6-month postoperative period or if prosthetic material is used (see Box 31-3).

Long-Term Complications for Children and Young Adults with Congenital Heart Disease: Transitioning to Adult Care

As children grow into adulthood, they are vulnerable to a host of long-term complications depending on their particular disease, repair, and residual lesions. Because of the success of pediatric cardiac surgery, 90% of children born with CHD live to adulthood. As a result, there are now more adults with CHD than children. The adult CHD population exceeds 1 million individuals in the United States (20,000 reach adolescence each year) and 1.2 million in Europe (Zaidi and Daniels, 2013; Zomer et al, 2013).

Not all surgeries performed during childhood are corrective. Many surgeries are palliative or incompletely corrective with residual problems. Thus, these individuals continue to require close supervision to assess their cardiac function and need for further interventions.

However, Fernandes and colleagues (2013) found that only a small percentage of adults with CHD actually received the follow-up care that was advised; 42% had more than a 3-year gap in their care with the first gap occurring between adolescence and adulthood. Zomer and colleagues (2013) found that 70% were either lost to follow-up or had lapses in care after failing to breach the transition to adult cardiology. The most common reasons for returning to specialty care included a recommendation from a health care provider due to new symptoms. Late adolescent patients should, therefore, be transitioned to adult congenital heart specialists in order to maintain continuity of care and prevent long-term complications.

The particular problems faced by the adolescents or adults with CHD are beyond the scope of this text. However, there are some key points in the evaluation of an older child, adolescent, or young adult with CHD worth mentioning (Zaidi and Daniels, 2013):
- Left-sided lesions: Those with a history of bicuspid aortic valves, subaortic stenosis, aortic valve stenosis, coarctation, or aortic aneurysm may worsen over time and present with significant stenosis or regurgitation. Symptoms include exercise intolerance, dyspnea on exertion, or atypical chest pain. Problems include arrhythmias, sudden death, endocarditis, syncope, and angina.
- Left-to-right shunt lesions: Repaired or unrepaired atrial or VSDs, AV septal defect, aortopulmonary window (a hole between the aorta and the pulmonary artery), or coronary sinus fistulas may be hemodynamically significant and lead to elevated pulmonary vascular resistance and Eisenmenger syndrome (right to left shunting through a lesion due to elevated pulmonary vascular resistance). Symptoms may include arrhythmias, dyspnea on exertion, unexplained deterioration of left ventricular function, and/or left ventricular dilation.
- Chronic cyanosis: In addition to left-to-right shunt lesions causing Eisenmenger syndrome, chronic cyanosis can also result from defects causing right ventricular outflow obstruction, baffle leaks (can occur after certain surgical procedures to correct TGA), or palliation for a single ventricle. Chronic hypoxia to vital organs, hyperviscosity, and hematologic problems (e.g., thrombocytopenia, erythrocytosis, thromboemboli, iron deficiency, and bleeding) can result.
- Valvar problems: Besides aortic stenosis, other long-term valve abnormalities can include mitral valve prolapse (causes mitral regurgitation) and/or pulmonary valve stenosis or regurgitation (more frequent in those with repaired TOF). Adolescents, particularly girls, should be examined for mitral value prolapse and mitral regurgitation due to the risk of arrhythmias and sudden death.

- Ventricular failure: Ventricular failure can occur via many different pathways depending on the underlying disease and previous interventions. Prolonged aortic or pulmonic valvar stenosis or regurgitation is a common mechanism for failure. In single ventricle patients, the development of systemic venous collateral vessels or arteriovenous pulmonary fistulas can increase ventricular volumes. Over time, these hemodynamic problems can lead to chronic cyanosis, myocardial ischemia, poor ventricular compliance, and serious ventricular arrhythmias. Management of each problem is challenging; ultimately, a heart transplant may be required.
- Arrhythmias and heart blocks: The risk of sudden cardiac death (SCD) is the most significant complication facing the adult with CHD. Congenital diagnoses at greatest risk for subsequent SCD include coarctation of the aorta, TOF, aortic stenosis, d-TGA with aortic stenosis, and TGA. Single ventricle patients with a Fontan procedure are also at increased risk for arrhythmias. Rhythm disturbances can occur as a result of long-standing cyanosis, the aforementioned chamber dilation, increased atrial pressures, dysfunction of the sinus node, and extensive fibrotic suture lines. Management is complex. Although episodes of palpitations or chest pain may bring those with CHD into care, they need to be referred to cardiology specialists.

Sudden Cardiac Death

The PCP has a responsibility to screen for causes of SCD whenever performing a sports physical examination or assessing a complaint of chest pain, syncope, or palpitations. This can be a daunting challenge, because none of the most common causes of SCD are easily diagnosed by history or examination. In the United States, the incidence of SCD (excludes sudden infant death syndrome) in children is 2.3 to 4.4/100,000 per year. The most frequent cause of exercise-related SCD is cardiomyopathy, especially hypertrophic cardiomyopathy (HCM), and to a far lesser extent, arrhythmogenic right ventricular cardiomyopathy (Chandra et al, 2013). Both are inherited, structural, abnormalities of the myocardium, and both result in ventricular arrhythmias leading to death.

Other congenital structural abnormalities that can cause sudden death include coronary artery anomalies, aortic dissection/rupture (usually seen in children with Marfan syndrome), mitral valve prolapse, and aortic stenosis. Congenital, electrical cardiac abnormalities can also cause SCD, including Wolff-Parkinson-White syndrome, congenital long QT syndromes, and Brugada syndrome (discussed later in the Cardiac Arrhythmias section).

Sudden death from acquired cardiac abnormalities include commotio cordis from blunt, nonpenetrating trauma to the midchest (e.g., blow by a baseball or other object), myocarditis, performance-enhancing drugs, and premature coronary artery disease (usually due to familial hypercholesterolemia). Commotio cordis triggers ventricular fibrillation and SCD as a result of the blow during the timing of the T-wave in the cardiac cycle.

Clinical Findings

Hypertrophic and arrhythmogenic right ventricular cardiomyopathy present with a history of syncope and a family history of either of these conditions. Most individuals are asymptomatic, and arrhythmogenic right ventricular cardiomyopathy is more likely to occur in males beginning around 15 years old. There may be other reports of shortness of breath with activity, palpitations, dizziness/lightheadedness, fatigue, and chest pain/pressure with or without activity.

On the physical examination, HCM may include a dynamic murmur (late systolic ejection) and forceful apex beat. Arrhythmias and shortness of breath with exertion may be found with both conditions.

Diagnostic Studies

- Hypertropic cardiomyopathy: Abnormal ECG (greater than 90% have an abnormal resting ECG), sustained or nonsustained ventricular tachycardia on Holter or 30-day event monitor, severe LVH on echocardiogram, and an attenuated BP response to exercise.
- Arrhythmogenic right ventricular cardiomyopathy: Changes seen with resting/ambulatory ECG and on echocardiographic and cardiac MRI studies.

Management

Refer all children to a pediatric cardiology provider for evaluation and diagnosis who have a family history of SCD; inheritable cardiomyopathies; Marfan syndrome; chest pain of concern; syncope; acquired cardiac disease, such as Kawasaki disease; and those with known CHD, cardiac rhythm disturbances, or palpitations. See Chapter 13, Box 13-3 for a cardiovascular screening checklist to use during the pre-participation physical examination for sports.

Acquired Heart Disease

Chest Pain

Chest pain in children is a common complaint but represents a serious cardiovascular problem in only 5% or less of cases. Although children of all ages can have chest pain, it is the young adolescent who most frequently presents to the emergency department and PCP with this complaint (Park, 2014).The first goal of chest pain evaluation is to rule out cardiac causes, which are also the main concern of most children and their parents. Table 31-9 lists possible cardiac causes of chest pain, history, and examination findings. It is important to understand these conditions to safely rule them out and then look for more likely musculoskeletal and respiratory causes. A careful history and a thorough physical

TABLE 31-9 **Cardiac Causes of Chest Pain and Associated Findings**

Condition	History	Physical Exam	Electrocardiogram	Chest Radiograph
Abnormal coronaries due to Kawasaki disease or other coronary artery disease	Previous history consistent with disease; typical exercise anginal pain	Usually normal; continuous murmur or possible fistulae	ST segment elevation +/– myocardial infarction findings	Normal
Cocaine abuse	History of substance abuse	Hypertension; tachycardia	ST elevation +/–	Normal
Pericarditis and myocarditis	History of URI +/– sharp chest pain	Friction rub; muffled heart sounds	Low QRS voltages; ST segment shift	Cardiomegaly
Postpericardiotomy syndrome	Recent heart surgery; pain positional	Muffled heart sounds; rub	ST segment elevation	Cardiomegaly
Arrhythmia	May have history of Wolff-Parkinson-White or long-QT syndrome	Normal to irregular heart rate	Preexcitation, long QT, or normal QT	Normal
Aortic stenosis (severe)	History of aortic stenosis	Loud SEM at USB radiating to neck	LVH with or without strain	Prominent ascending aorta and aortic knob
Pulmonary stenosis (severe)	History of pulmonary stenosis	Loud SEM at ULSB	RVH with or without strain	Prominent PA segment
Hypertrophic cardiomyopathy (HCM)	Positive family history (in ⅓ of patients)	Variable murmur	LVH; deep Q/small R or QS in LPLs	Mild cardiomegaly
Mitral valve prolapse	Positive family history	Midsystolic click; thin; thoracic skeletal abnormalities	Inverted T waves in aVF	Normal except skeletal anomalies
Eisenmenger syndrome (untreated or untreatable congenital heart disease [CHD])	History of congenital heart disease	Cyanosis, clubbing, loud S_2	Right ventricular hypertrophy	Prominent PA; normal heart size

Adapted from Park M: *Park's pediatric cardiology for practitioners*, ed 6, Philadelphia, 2014, Mosby/Elsevier.
LPL, Lateral precordial leads; *LVH*, left ventricular hypertrophy; *PA*, pulmonary artery; *RVH*, right ventricular hypertrophy; *SEM*, systolic ejection murmur; *ULSB*, upper left sternal border; *URI*, upper respiratory infection; *USB*, upper sternal border.

examination are especially important in assessing this complaint. The provider may need to order ECG, chest radiograph, and other laboratory studies if indicated (Park, 2014).

The most frequent cause of chest pain is musculoskeletal that originates in the chest wall or chest cage, is benign, and rarely requires any treatment. Chest wall pain, particularly with exercise, may indicate exercise-induced bronchospasm, but rarely indicates cardiac disease. Chronic chest pain that is vague and occurs over many months in a variety of circumstances, particularly around stressful events, may be psychogenic (anxiety or hyperventilation). Chest pain associated with syncope, exertional dyspnea, or irregularities in heart rhythm needs careful evaluation for a cardiac cause. Usually children or adolescents, who have pain of cardiac origin, describe a specific history with details that are consistent from event to event (Park, 2014).

Clinical Findings

History

Inquire about the following:

- Past medical history or family history of sudden death (including drownings), heart disease or condition, asthma, eczema, Marfan syndrome, sickle cell disease
- Past sports activities, including friendly wrestling at home

- Previous trauma or muscle strains
- Characteristics of the chest pain:
  - Relationship of pain to exercise; any syncope, exertional dyspnea, or wheezing
  - Any burning, substernal pain that worsens with reclining or with spicy foods (gastrointestinal etiology)
  - Pain that is sharp or stabbing, lasting several seconds to minutes, located over the midsternum or inframipple area, and occurring with nonexertion or deep inspirations (more likely musculoskeletal in origin)
  - Pain that awakens the patient (more likely organic)
  - Any other associated symptoms, such as fever, nausea, vomiting, headaches, or choking episodes
  - Any recent, major stressful events
- Medication, tobacco, or other drug use, including oral contraceptives (embolism)

Physical Examination

A complete chest (lungs and heart) and abdominal examination should be performed. Key findings to focus on include the presence of the following:

- Cardiac murmur, rubs, or clicks
- Point tenderness of one or more costochondral joints exaggerated with physical activity or deep inspirations (suggests costochondritis or Tietze syndrome [if associated with warmth, swelling, or tenderness over costochondral junction]): Use the middle fingertip to palpate each costochondral and chondrosternal junction for tenderness to avoid missing this finding. Tenderness and swelling may also be found in pectoral and shoulder carriage muscles due to overuse by excessive weight-lifting or excessive electronic game playing.
- Irregular heart rhythm (cardiac disease)
- Rales, wheezing, tachypnea, decreased breath sounds (pulmonary disease)

Diagnostic Studies

In most cases, only the history and physical are necessary to make the diagnosis; other tests are not indicated unless the following problems are suspected:

- Febrile, cardiac, or pulmonary condition: Obtain a chest radiograph.
- Exercise-induced asthma: Perform a pulmonary function test with exercise.
- Rhythm disturbance: Order a 24-hour Holter or 30-day event monitor or stress test (or both).
- Signs of CHD, pericarditis, or myocarditis: Order an ECG and perhaps a chest radiograph.

Differential Diagnosis

Those of musculoskeletal origin include costochondritis, Tietze syndrome, idiopathic chest pain, precordial catch syndrome, slipping-rib syndrome, hypersensitive xiphoid syndrome, trauma, and muscle strain; they are usually responsive to nonsteroidal anti-inflammatory drug (NSAID) treatment and rest. Esophagitis, esophageal foreign body ingestion, and exercise-induced bronchospasm are additional differential diagnoses (see Chapters 25 and 33 for discussions about these disorders).

Management

When chest pain has no clear etiology, the child appears well, and all aspects of the evaluation are normal, reassurance may be the most important treatment. Refer any child to a pediatric cardiology with chest pain that worsens with exercise or that suggests angina, who has positive findings on examination, ECG, or chest radiograph, or who has a concerning personal or family history.

Hypertension

Normal BP in chilcren and adolescents is defined as systolic and diastolic BP below the 90th percentile for age, sex, and height. *Hypertension* in children is defined as a systolic or diastolic (or both) BP in the 95th or higher percentile for age, sex, and height on at least three separate occasions. Adolescents with BP levels of 120/80 mm Hg or above (using the auscultatory method) are considered hypertensive even if they are below the 95th percentile. High-normal, or pre-hypertensive, BP in children and adolescents is defined as average systolic or diastolic BP in the 90th percentile or higher but less than the 95th percentile. Stage 1 hypertension is BP that is between the 95th and 99th percentiles for age, sex, and height. Stage 2 hypertension is BP 5 mm Hg or greater above the 99th percentile (NHLBI, 2012).

Hypertension is a significant problem affecting 2% to 13% of children and adolescents (Feber and Ahmed, 2010). Increasingly, children are found to have high BP associated with obesity, sedentary lifestyles, and stress. Secondary hypertension is more commonly seen in children younger than 6 years old (at significant or severe hypertension levels). The primary cause of secondary, severe hypertension is renovascular or parenchymal renal diseases. Other causes include coarctation of aorta, endocrine disorders, genetic disorders such as Williams syndrome, neurofibromatosis and tuberous sclerosis, drugs, and central nervous system tumors. The onset of primary hypertension is more likely to occur after 10 years old. Neonates with hypertension are generally severely ill with neurologic, cardiac, and renal symptoms.

Clinical Findings

The goal of the clinical history and physical examination is to assess whether hypertension is primary or secondary to renal disease or other causes. If secondary hypertension is ruled out, then the evaluation must focus on comorbidities of primary hypertension. With either secondary or primary hypertension, the PCP must assess for signs of end-organ damage from prolonged hypertension.

History

Inquire about:

- Neonatal history of prolonged mechanical ventilation, umbilical catheterization, prematurity, or small for gestational age at birth. Poor maternal nutrition and high

stress appear to have an epigenetic effect on the embryo, making hypertension more likely for the child (Cowley et al, 2012).
- Cause of any prior hospitalizations
- Trauma
- Diet, physical activities, and other habits (e.g., smoking, drinking, substance abuse)
- Sleep history, particularly symptoms of sleep apnea
- Medications taken, including oral contraceptives, cold medications, steroids, and diet aids
- Chronic illness, especially renal disease, past history of urinary tract infections, diabetes, or seizures
- Headache, chest pain, dyspnea, muscle weakness, palpitations, abdominal pain, facial palsy, decreased vision, excessive sweating
- Family history of a first-degree relative with myocardial infarction (especially before 50 years old), stroke, hypertension, diabetes, hyperlipidemia, SCD, polycystic kidney disease, neurofibromatosis, pheochromocytoma, or obesity

Physical Examination

Note the following:
- Body habitus, especially overweight (body mass index [BMI]); poor growth (height, weight); signs of metabolic syndrome
- Dysmorphic features
- Edema, pallor, flushing, or skin lesions suggestive of tuberous sclerosis, systemic lupus erythematosus, neurofibromatosis
- Upper and lower extremity central pulses; absent, diminished, or pounding pulses in all extremities
- Fundi abnormalities, enlarged thyroid gland, abdominal mass, flank bruit; decreased visual acuity, facial palsy
- Elevated BP on at least three separate occasions

Diagnostic Studies

- Laboratory evaluation of stage 1 or 2 HTN should focus on searching for causes of secondary hypertension, comorbidities of primary hypertension, and target organ damage of either primary or secondary hypertension. The search for secondary causes of hypertension needs to be individualized based upon age, history, physical examination, and extent of BP elevation. Because the majority of children have renal or renovascular causes for BP elevation, initial laboratory studies should include tests for renal function and plasma renin levels.
- Children younger than 10 years old with stage 2 hypertension require more aggressive laboratory evaluation compared with older children with stage 1 hypertension and obesity. CBC, erythrocyte sedimentation rate (ESR), C-reactive protein (CRP), urinalysis and culture, electrolytes, blood urea nitrogen, creatinine and plasma renin levels, renal nuclear medicine scans, and renal ultrasound are screening studies for the most common secondary causes of hypertension.
- If renal vascular disease is suspected, the workup is best managed by a nephrologist because newer technologies, such as MRI and spiral computed tomography (CT), are replacing angiography.
- Additional organ assessments include echocardiography for LVH and coarctation of the aorta and a thorough ophthalmologic examination.

Management

Figs. 31-17 and 31-18 show algorithms that categorize and manage children with high BP.
- BP measurements should be done annually on all children 3 years and older, with baseline and serial measurements documented carefully in the child's record. Standardized BP norms are available (see Tables 31-2 and 31-3).
- Prehypertension: At least two follow-up BP measurements should be taken within 1 to 2 months of the initial reading to determine whether a high reading is a single, isolated event. If subsequent readings fall below the 95th percentile, the child should continue with routine BP checks during annual visits.
- Hypertension secondary to overweight, can be as serious as hypertension secondary to other organic disease and should be treated as such. For those with high-normal BP without any indication of organic disease, treatment should consist of nonpharmacologic intervention—diet, exercise, and weight management. Caloric restriction with exercise is more effective than caloric restriction alone (NHLBI, 2012). Recommendations should include the following:
  - Dietary intervention to control or reduce overweight is covered in Chapter 10 and in guidelines provided by NHLBI (2012). High sodium foods and sodium supplements should be eliminated.
  - Increase physical exercise and sports participation to 30 to 60 minutes a day balanced with relaxation techniques. Aerobic, not static or isometric exercise, is recommended. (See Chapter 13 and Table 13-8 for information on sports activities, readiness, conditioning strategies, and management for youth with hypertension.)
  - Avoid smoking, caffeine, alcoholic beverages, and illicit drug consumption.
- If the BP elevation is persistent, referral should be made to a nephrologist or cardiologist who has experience using antihypertensive agents in children. Children with confirmed BP equal to or greater than the 99th percentile should have immediate referral (NHLBI, 2012).
- The goal is to reduce systolic or diastolic BP below the 95th percentile. If a concurrent condition exists, the goal becomes reducing BP to the 90th percentile.
- Medication management starts with a single drug (usually an ACE inhibitor, angiotensin-receptor blocker [ARB], beta-blocker, calcium channel blocker, or diuretic) at the lowest recommended dose and advanced

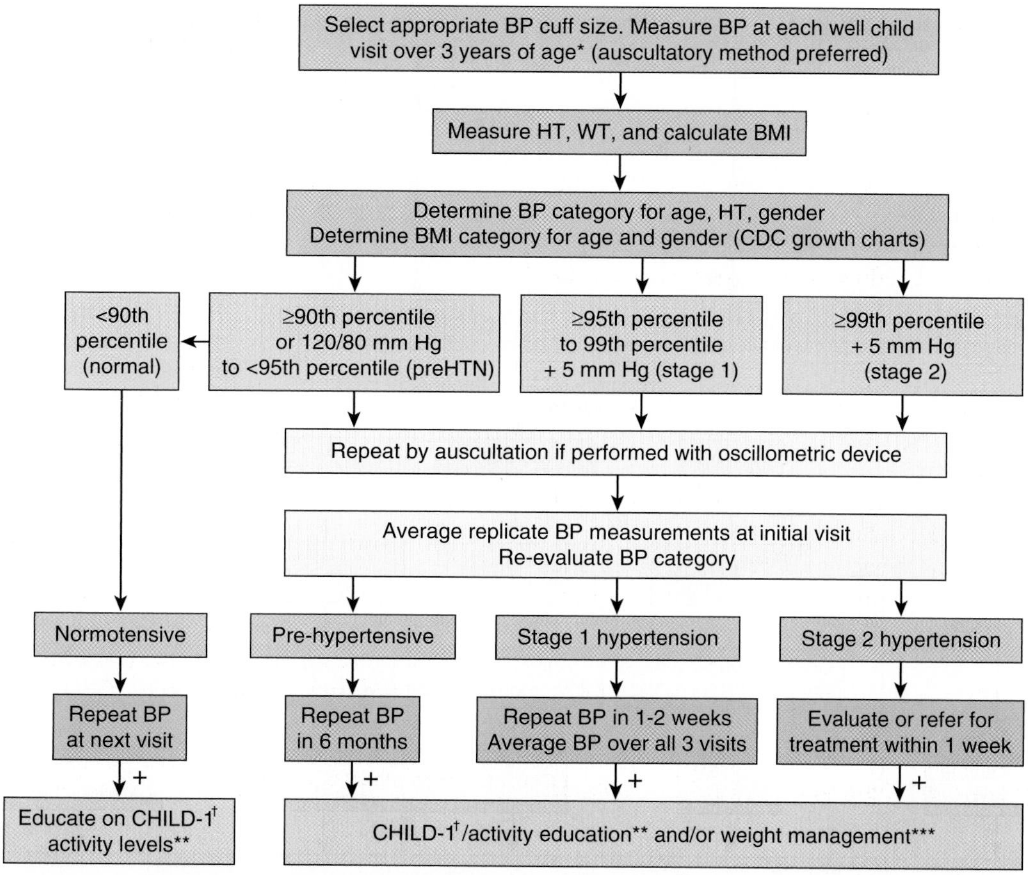

• **Figure 31-17** Blood pressure *(BP)* measurement and categorization algorithm. *BMI,* Body mass index; *CDC,* Centers of Disease Control and Prevention; *HT,* height; *WT,* weight. *See Tables 31-2 and 31-3. †Cardiovascular health integrated lifestyle diet *(CHILD-1)* recommended (see Section 5, "Nutrition and Diet" in the NHLBI reference for these nutrition and diet recommendations). **See Section 6, "Physical Activity" in the NHLBI reference for physical activity recommendations. ***See Section 10, "Overweight and Obesity" in the NHLBI reference for discussion regarding overweight and obesity. (From National Heart, Lung, and Blood Institute (NHLBI): *Expert panel on integrated guidelines for cardiovascular health and risk reduction in children and adolescents: full report,* 2012. Available at www.nhlbi.nih.gov/files/docs/guidelines/peds_guidelines_full.pdf. Accessed November 3, 2014, Fig. 8-1, p 84.)

until the desired BP is reached. If maximum dose or adverse side effects are reached, a second medication should be added. Step-down therapy may be possible for overweight children who lose weight and achieve BP goals. Studies of antihypertensives in children indicate racial differences may exist in the medication effect of ACE inhibitors; ARBs and beta-blockers were not studied. Side effect profiles are similar to those found in adults (NHLBI, 2012). Medication recommendations are in Table 31-10.

Complications

Long-term BP elevation leads to an increase in left ventricular mass, increased carotid intimal medial thickness, and coronary artery calcification, especially if combined with overweight, lipid and lipoprotein abnormalities, and tobacco use. There are some indications of cognitive impairments in children with hypertension as well (Feber and Ahmed, 2010). Yearly echocardiograms are recommended to evaluate LVH.

Patient and Family Education

Because much of hypertension is related to lifestyle, prevention through optimal health promotion and maintenance is essential. Regular health maintenance, including evaluation of BP and health education regarding risk factors, is critical. Counseling should emphasize both behavioral modification and parental involvement. Decreasing BMI and increasing aerobic fitness have been shown to reduce elevations in age-related BP. Specific preventive measures include the following:

- Good nutrition with a decrease in dietary fat and sodium
- Prevention of overweight with diet and aerobic exercise for at least 30 minutes daily
- Stress management
- Avoidance of caffeine, tobacco use, and prescription or over-the-counter medications that can exacerbate high BP (e.g., cold medications with ephedrine or phenylephrine, steroids)
- Monitoring BP if oral contraceptives are used

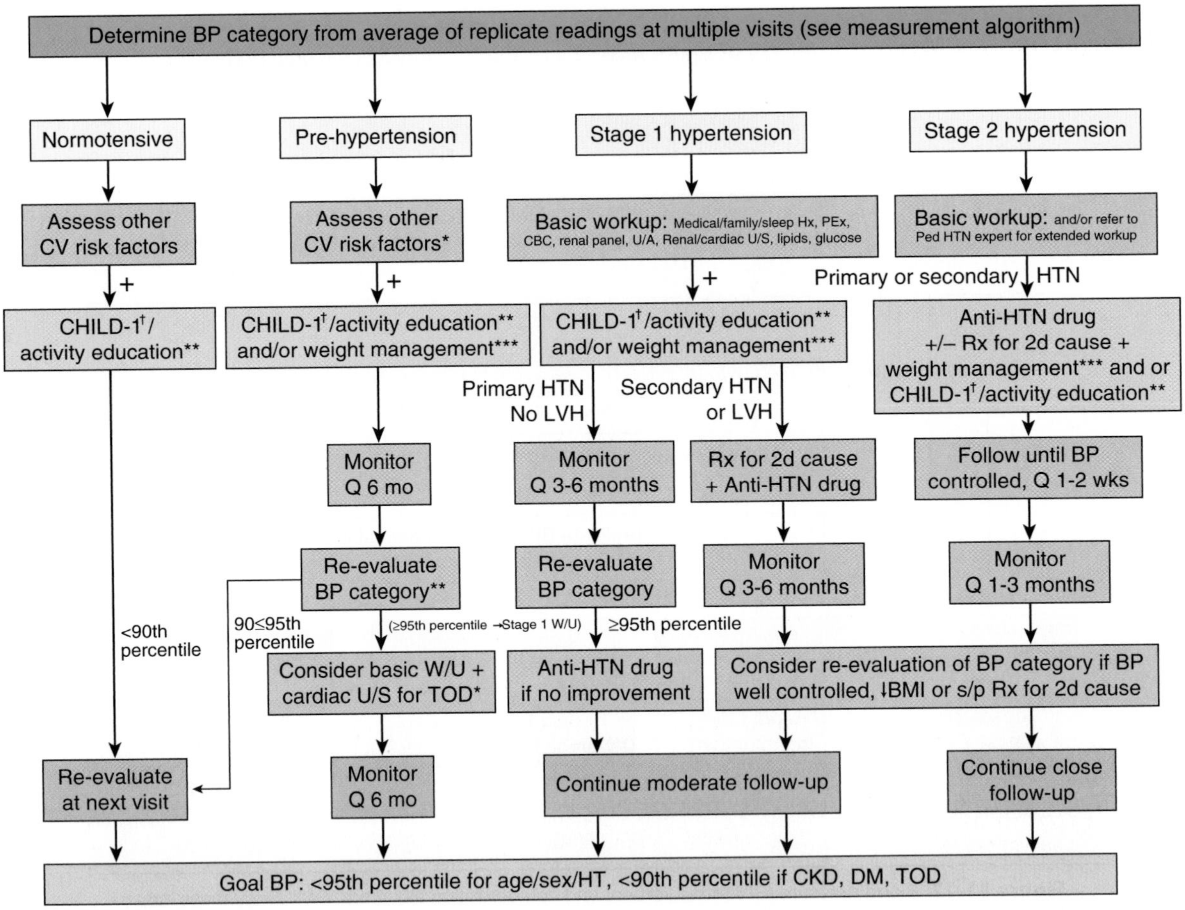

• **Figure 31-18** Blood pressure *(BP)* management by category algorithm. *2d,* Secondary; *Anti-HTN,* antihypertensive; *BMI,* body mass index; *CBC,* complete blood count; *CKD,* chronic kidney disease; *CV,* cardiovascular; *DM,* diabetes mellitus; *HT,* height; *HTN,* hypertension; *Hx,* history; *LVH,* left ventricular hypertrophy; *Ped,* pediatric; *PEx,* physical examination; *Q,* every; *Rx,* prescription; *s/p,* status post; *TOD,* target organ damage; *U/A,* urinalysis; *U/S,* ultrasound; *W/U,* workup. *W/U for TOD/ LVH if obese or (+) for other CV risk factors. †Cardiovascular health integrated lifestyle diet *(CHILD-1)* (see Section 5, "Nutrition and Diet" in the NHLBI reference). **Activity education (see Section 6, "Physical Activity" in the NHLBI reference). ***Weight management for overweight and obesity (see Section 10, "Overweight and Obesity" in the NHLBI reference). (From National Heart, Lung, and Blood Institute (NHLBI): *Expert panel on integrated guidelines for cardiovascular health and risk reduction in children and adolescents: full report,* 2012. Available at www.nhlbi.nih.gov/files/docs/guidelines/peds_guidelines_full.pdf. Accessed November 3, 2014, Fig. 8-2, p 84.)

Infective Endocarditis

Infective endocarditis (IE; also known as *subacute bacterial endocarditis [SBE]*) is a condition in which a bacterial or fungal infection invades endocardial surfaces of the heart. Turbulence caused by stenotic cardiac valves, previous surgical repairs, or high-velocity jets (from blood flowing under force through a structural heart defect) traumatizes cardiac endothelium and leads to thrombogenesis. Clumps of platelets and fibrin provide a nidus for circulating bacteria or rarely fungi. The bacteria or fungi multiply, shielded from circulating white cells by the platelet-fibrin matrix. These vegetations cause further damage by destroying nearby valve tissue and extending to surrounding endothelium.

Infection can occur in any age group (Gewitz and Taubert, 2013). The incidence of IE has increased as more children with CHD are surviving due to improved treatments, especially surgical interventions. In developing countries where there is a high prevalence of rheumatic heart disease (RHD), there is a concurrent increase in IE because RHD-damaged valves are extremely vulnerable to IE.

Gram-positive cocci cause 80% of cases of IE in children. *Staphylococcus aureus* is the most common causative organism, followed by *Streptococcus viridans* (Bor et al, 2013). A group of gram-negative bacilli referred to as *HACEK* (***H**aemophilus* species [*H. parainfluenzae, H. aphrophilus,* and *H. paraphrophilus], **A**ctinobacillus actinomycetemcomitans, **C**ardiobacterium hominis, **E**ikenella corrodens,* and ***K**ingella* species) are less commonly implicated.

Children with CHD appear to have more severe gingival inflammatory conditions, increased plaque accumulation, and more HACEK microbes, which lead to endocarditis.

TABLE 31-10 Antihypertensive Medications for Children

Class	Drugs	Initial Dose, Maximum Dose, and Dosing Interval	Comments
Angiotensin-converting enzyme (ACE) inhibitors	Captopril	0.3 to 0.5 mg/kg/dose; maximum dose: 6 mg/kg/day or 450 mg/day; divided tid	ACE inhibitors are contraindicated in pregnancy. Check serum potassium and creatinine periodically. All can be compounded into a suspension.
	Enalapril	0.08 mg/kg/day up to 5 mg/day; maximum dose: 0.6 mg/kg/day up to 40 mg; qd to bid divided dosing	
	Lisinopril	0.07 mg/kg/day up to 5 mg/day; maximum dose: 0.6 mg/kg/day up to 40 mg/day; qd dosing	
	Benazepril	0.2 mg/kg/day up to 10 mg/day; maximum dose: 0.6 mg/kg/day up to 40 mg/day; qd dosing	
	Quinapril	5 to 10 mg/ day; maximum dose: 80 mg/ day; qd dosing	
Alpha- and beta-blocker	Labetalol	1 to 3 mg/kg/day; maximum dose: 10 to 12 mg/kg/day up to 1,200 mg/day; divided bid	
Beta-adrenergic antagonist	Propranolol	1 to 2 mg/kg/day; maximum dose: 4 mg/kg/day up to 640 mg/day; divided bid or tid	Asthma, heart failure, and insulin-dependent diabetes are contraindications.
	Metoprolol	Children over 6 years old: 1 mg/kg/day or 12.5 to 50 mg/day: maximum dose: 2 mg/kg/day up to 200 mg/day; divided bid	Monitor heart rate for excessive bradycardia.
	Atenolol	0.5 to 1 mg/kg/day; maximum dose: 2 mg/kg/day up to 100 mg/day; qd or divided bid	Athletic performance may be impaired.
Angiotensin-receptor blocker (ARB)	Losartan	0.7 mg/kg/day up to 50 mg/day; maximum dose: 1.4 mg/kg/day up to 100 mg/day; qd or divided bid	Check serum potassium and creatinine periodically.
	Valsartan	0.4 mg/kg/day or 5 to 10 mg/day; maximum dose: 3.4 mg/kg/day or 40 to 80 mg/day; qd dosing	
Calcium channel blocker	Amlodipine	Children 6 to 17 years old: 2.5 mg/day; maximum dose: 5 mg/day; qd dosing	Amlodipine and isradipine can be compounded into a suspension.
	Felodipine	2.5 mg/day; maximum dose: 10 mg/day; qd dosing	
	Extended-release nifedipine	0.25 to 0.5 mg/kg/day; maximum dose: 3 mg/kg/day up to 120 mg/day; qd or divided bid	
Central-adrenergic agonists	Clonidine	Children 12 years old and older: 0.2 mg/day; maximum dose: 2.4 mg/day; divided bid	May cause dry mouth or sedation. Sudden cessation can cause rebound.
Direct vasodilators	Hydralazine	0.75 mg/kg/day; maximum dose: 7.5 mg/kg/day up to 200 mg/day; divided qid	Fluid retention and tachycardia commonly occur. Hydralazine can cause lupus-like syndrome in some patients.

Continued

TABLE 31-10 Antihypertensive Medications for Children—cont'd

Class	Drugs	Initial Dose, Maximum Dose, and Dosing Interval	Comments
Diuretics	Chlorthalidone	0.3 mg/kg/day; maximum dose: 2 mg/kg/day up to 50 mg/day; qd dosing	Patients on diuretics should have electrolytes monitored. Potassium-sparing diuretics (spironolactone, triamterene, amiloride) can cause hyperkalemia, especially when given with ACE inhibitor or ARB. Chlorthalidone may cause azotemia in patients with renal disease.
	Furosemide	0.5 to 2.0 mg/kg/dose; maximum dose: 6 mg/kg/day; dosed qd or divided bid	
	Hydrochlorothiazide (HCTZ)	1 mg/kg/day; maximum dose: 3 mg/kg/day up to 50 mg/day; dosed qd	
	Spironolactone	1 mg/kg/day, maximum dose: 3.3 mg/kg/day up to 100 mg/day; dosed qd or divided bid	

From U.S. Department Health and Human Services Department (USDHHS), National Heart, Lung, and Blood Institute (NHLBI), Expert Panel on Integrated Guidelines for Cardiovascular Health and Risk Reduction in Children and Adolescents: *Expert panel on integrated guidelines for cardiovascular health and risk reduction in children and adolescents: summary report,* 2012. Available at www.nhlbi.nih,gov/files/docs/guidelines/peds_guidelines_full.pdf. Accessed November 3, 2014.

bid, bis in die (twice a day); *qid, quater in die* (four times a day); *qd, quaque die* (every day/once daily); *tid, ter in die* (three times a day).

Lexicomp (fee based) is also an excellent reference for drug dosing and dosage forms for these medications (see Additional Resources on the Evolve site).

Fungal endocarditis is the most severe form with alarming mortality especially in immunocompromised children and neonates; fortunately it rarely occurs (Gewitz and Taubert, 2013).

Clinical Findings

History and Physical Examination

- History of underlying structural cardiac abnormality(ies) (e.g., CHD or acute rheumatic fever [rarely in those without structural heart disease]) in those who have had palliative surgery for cyanotic heart disease, those with prosthetic aortic valve replacements, or who have indwelling catheters and devices. (These may also be used for oncology or neonatology purposes.)
- Ask about any dental procedures or oral surgery that may have caused gingival or mucosal bleeding even if months in the past; intravenous drug use.
- Acute manifestations: Short duration of illness, high fever (greater than 102.2° F [39° C]), myalgias, night sweats, arthralgias, headache, general malaise, decreased appetite, increase in intensity of preexisting murmur or new onset of murmur
- Subacute manifestations: Low-grade or relapsing fever, progressive nonspecific symptoms (e.g., myalgias, arthralgias, headache, and general malaise)
- Neonates: Symptoms may range from relatively few to systemic hypotension, respiratory distress or other generalized signs of sepsis, and neurologic findings
- Evidence of dental caries and/or periodontal or gingival disease
- Embolization symptoms: Hematuria, acute onset of respiratory distress, splenomegaly, neurologic changes (stroke, brain abscesses, hemorrhage, meningitis), petechiae (in conjunctiva, buccal mucosa, palatal area, nailbeds, palms, and soles). The classical findings—Janeway lesions (flat, nontender lesions on palms and soles), Osler nodes (small raised lesions on pad of fingers and toes), Roth spots (retinal hemorrhages with a central white spot), and splinter hemorrhages—occur rarely in children.

Diagnostic Studies

- The diagnosis is based on clinical findings and results of blood cultures. A persistent low-grade fever in a child with known cardiac abnormalities should be evaluated immediately with three sets of blood cultures over 24 hours from different sites before the administration of empirical antibiotic therapy. When three cultures are positive for the same organism, IE must be considered and treatment instituted. Greater than 90% of those without prior antibiotic treatment will have a positive blood culture (Park, 2014).
- The ESR, CRP, and white blood cell (WBC) count are elevated in the acute stage; anemia may be evidenced.
- Two-dimensional echocardiography (main modality for detecting infection).

Differential Diagnosis

The differential diagnoses include postoperative fever, collagen vascular diseases, and childhood cancers.

Management and Complications

All children with suspected IE should be hospitalized and referred to pediatric cardiology. Treatment should begin as soon as IE is suspected in order to decrease the subsequent morbidity and mortality associated with untreated bacteremia. High doses of appropriate antibiotics are given intravenously for 4 to 6 weeks.

IE carries high morbidity and mortality rates and can lead to destruction of heart valves or disseminated sepsis.

Septic and thrombotic emboli from bacterial or fungal vegetations can cause abscesses and ischemic damage to distant areas, such as the brain, abdominal viscera, and extremities.

Patient and Family Education

For children with high-risk cardiac conditions (previous endocarditis; unrepaired or palliated cyanotic CHD; prosthetic or bioprosthetic valve, shunt, or conduit; repaired CHD with residual defects adjacent to the site of the prosthetic patch or device; and heart transplant recipients), prophylactic antibiotic therapy is given before all dental procedures involving manipulation of gingival tissue. Endocarditis prophylaxis is also recommended for 6 months after heart surgery for all congenital heart patients (see Box 31-3 and Table 31-6). Maintaining good oral hygiene is requisite.

Myocarditis and Cardiomyopathy

Myocarditis is a rare inflammatory illness of the muscular walls of the heart. It may go unrecognized in children whose inflammatory process resolves spontaneously, or it may progress to fulminant disease resulting in chronic cardiomyopathy or even death. Myocarditis is often caused by viral infections, most commonly adenoviruses, coxsackievirus A and B, parvovirus B19, echoviruses, and poliovirus. Influenza, cytomegalovirus (CMV), varicella, mumps, human immunodeficiency virus (HIV), RSV, and rubella are other viral causes. Nonviral infections (fungal, bacterial, protozoal, and rickettsial), various medications, autoimmune or inflammatory disorders (e.g., acute rheumatic fever, systemic lupus erythematosus), toxic reactions to infectious agents, or other disorders (e.g., Kawasaki disease) may also be causative factors; however, the etiology is often unknown. Myocarditis may occur in epidemics, usually in infants in association with coxsackievirus B. In Central and South America, myocarditis is commonly caused by Chagas disease, a protozoal infection with *Typanosoma cruzi* (Canter and Simpson, 2014).

The inflammatory process in the myocardium leads to dilation of all cardiac chambers, especially the left ventricle, which results in poor function and stretching of mitral annulus with regurgitation. The healing process may lead to replacement of myofibers with fibroblasts and scar formation. Scarring decreases elasticity and performance and creates the substrate for ventricular arrhythmias. Myocarditis causes approximately 9% of sudden death in young athletes (Canter and Simpson, 2014).

Clinical Findings

History

As the interstitial inflammation process progresses, cardiac function decreases and symptoms of CHF become evident. The following history is characteristic:

- Infants (may be manifesting intrauterine exposure): Fever, irritability or listlessness, episodes of pallor, diaphoresis; tachypnea or respiratory distress; poor appetite and vomiting
- Children and adolescents: Recent flulike or gastrointestinal viral illness (10 to 14 days previously); lethargy, low-grade fever, pallor; decreased appetite and abdominal pain; exercise intolerance, rashes, palpitations, respiratory distress (late finding)

Physical Examination

- Pallor, mild cyanosis, skin cool and mottled with poor perfusion (in infants)
- Rapid, labored respirations, grunting, decreased pulse oximetry reading
- Tachycardia, gallop rhythm, muffled heart sounds, apical systolic murmur, weak pulses
- Hepatomegaly, jugular venous distention (older children and adolescents)

Diagnostic Studies

Refer children with symptoms suggestive of myocarditis to a pediatric cardiologist. Diagnostic testing usually involves chest radiography, ECG, two-dimensional echocardiography, MRI, CBC, ESR, CRP, cardiac and liver enzymes, B-type natriuretic peptide, viral titers, blood cultures, metabolic studies (e.g., thyroid and carnitine), and viral cultures or polymerase chain reaction (PCR) from the myocardial tissue (Canter and Simpson, 2014).

Differential Diagnosis

Sepsis, asthma, recurrent vomiting, and chronic viral illness are in the differential diagnosis.

Management

Treatment is supportive with bed rest and medications, such as diuretics, ACE inhibitors, and carvedilol. Occasionally, anti-coagulation and anti-arrhythmia medications may be used. Digitalis and NSAIDs are not recommended due to studies showing deleterious impact in mice. New modes of therapies, including the use of immunomodulators and antiviral therapy, are under investigation (Canter and Simpson, 2014). Severe cases may require mechanical ventilation and inotropic support. Recovery often takes 2 to 3 months; follow-up is lifelong.

Complications and Prognosis

Pericardial effusion and pericarditis can occur concurrently. Scarring of the myocardium can be a complication and cause persistent heart failure and ventricular arrhythmias. Cardiac transplantation may be necessary in some children with myocarditis or cardiomyopathy. However, approximately 50% of children go on to complete recovery (Canter and Simpson, 2014).

Pericarditis

Pericarditis refers to an inflammation or other abnormality of the pericardium, the sac that surrounds the heart. Excess fluid accumulates in the pericardial space and causes the normally compliant pericardium to distend. As intrapericardial pressure increases, the heart becomes compressed and its ability to fill is limited. Pericarditis may be seen in those without a history of cardiac disease. Viral infection (especially with coxsackievirus and adenovirus) is the most common cause of pericarditis in infants and children. Other etiologic agents include infections (tuberculosis, other bacteria), trauma, hypersensitivity to medication (isoniazid [INH], hydralazine), collagen-vascular and connective tissue diseases (acute rheumatic fever, juvenile rheumatoid arthritis, and systemic lupus erythematosus), Kawasaki disease, postsurgical complications, and complications of systemic infection. Bacterial pericarditis is most common in children younger than 2 years old (Johnson and Cetta, 2013). It is a serious illness that may have rapidly fatal consequences if not diagnosed and treated in a timely manner. The following findings should alert the provider to refer the patient to a pediatric cardiologist:

- History of precordial or substernal chest pain altered by respiration, coughing, or position (may not be found in small children); lethargy, loss of appetite, abdominal pain; fever, irritability; tachycardia; viral illness 10 to 14 days before onset of symptoms
- Physical examination findings: Distended neck veins; tachycardia, pericardial friction rub (an early sign heard best along the left sternal border with the child leaning forward) or muffled heart sounds (if the effusion is large); Kussmaul sign (slow, deep respirations); pulsus paradoxus, a decrease in BP of greater than 10 mm Hg during inspiration when in a supine position; hepatomegaly
- ECG can show diffuse ST segment elevation (80%), PR depression, and T-wave inversion
- Chest x-ray may show enlargement of cardiac silhouette
- Echocardiogram shows relative quantities of pericardial fluid and compression of cavities if large effusion is seen

Pericarditis requires inpatient management. Cardiac tamponade can occur with large or rapid effusions. There is a relapse rate of 15% if the causative agent was viral. Most children recover fully within 3 to 4 weeks (Park, 2014). Myocarditis is the main differential diagnosis.

Heart Conduction Disturbances

Cardiac Arrhythmias

Arrhythmias can manifest as a primary disorder or as a consequence of cardiac or other systemic disorders. The following arrhythmias (see Table 31-1 for normal heart rates) may be noted:

- Sinus arrhythmia—variable heart rate that increases with inspiration and decreases with expiration. This is a normal finding in children.
- Bradycardia or slow heart rate for age:
  - Sinus bradycardia is the most common cause of bradycardia in children and may be due to hypoxia, acidosis, increased intracranial pressure, abdominal distention, hypothermia, or hypoglycemia. It may also be caused by drugs, such as beta-blockers or digoxin. Slowing may be due to increased vagal tone or cardiac conditioning (e.g., athletes).
  - Complete AV block can either be congenital, as seen in infants of mothers with autoimmune diseases, such as SLE, or may be acquired after cardiac surgery. Certain rare cardiac defects, such as levo- or L-looped transposition of the great arteries (L-TGA) and heterotaxy, are also associated with complete heart block. The hemodynamic effect of a slow heart rate depends on how slow it is (Park, 2014).
- Tachycardias:
  - Sinus tachycardia is caused by predisposing factors that increase cardiac output, including fever, anxiety, infection, drug exposure, dehydration, pain, hyperthyroidism, or anemia among many others. Treatment is directed at the underlying disorder.
  - Supraventricular tachycardias (SVTs) are the most common pathologic tachycardias in children.
  - AV reentrant tachycardia is the most common SVT. In AV reentrant tachycardia, there is an additional (accessory) pathway for impulse transmission from atria to ventricles besides the normal AV node. Less commonly this may be through a dual AV node (nodal reentrant AV tachycardia). AV reentrant tachycardias often first present in infants younger than 4 months old and again in young adolescents (Park, 2014).
- Long QT syndrome–induced ventricular tachycardia: Long-QT syndrome is linked to 13 different genes. The clinical manifestation is delayed repolarization (the long-QT interval). Genetic prolongation of the QT segment increases the susceptibility to further drug-induced long-QT interval. Such drugs include antiarrhythmics (such as, amiodarone and sotalol), psychotic drugs (such as, haloperidol and ziprasidone), and antibiotics (such as, ciprofloxacin, clarithromycin, and erythromycin). A list of medications that prolong QT is available at www.sads.org.uk/drugs_to_avoid.htm.
- Premature atrial contraction (PAC): This arrhythmia occurs in children and adults. The PAC depolarization may or may not be conducted through the AV node. PACs in a child with an otherwise normal heart is usually benign. It is not unusual to see multiple PACs on the ECG of a newborn.
- Premature ventricular contraction (PVC): PVCs are premature QRS complexes with a prolonged duration or morphologic difference from the preceding QRS. Occasional PVCs are also seen in otherwise normal infants and children. PVCs that are uniform in appearance, which means that they have the same QRS complex appearance every time, are usually of no consequence.

Clinical Findings

- Slow or fast heart rate; rhythm—regular, irregular, or regularly irregular
- Long-QT syndrome: The child may be asymptomatic until experiencing syncope or sudden death from a torsade de pointe ventricular tachycardia. Family history may include syncope, sudden death, or known long-QT syndrome. Congenital deafness is an additional family characteristic in one type of long-QT syndrome.

Diagnostic Studies

- Supraventricular tachycardia (SVT): Wolff-Parkinson-White is one subtype of AV reentrant tachycardia in which there are markers on the resting (non SVT) ECG that indicate an accessory pathway. These markers are delta waves, short PR interval, and prolonged QRS duration. Diagnosis is usually made when capturing SVT on ECG, Holter monitor, or other device. A QT interval corrected for the heart rate (QTc) of greater than 0.44 second in males and 0.46 second in females is worthy of investigation (Park, 2014).
- Long-QT syndrome: 12-lead ECG (shows a long-QT interval); genetic testing

Management and Complications

- SVT: Vagal maneuvers, intravenous adenosine, or if necessary, synchronized cardioversion. Long-term management involves prevention of recurrence with beta-blockade or, in the absence of Wolff-Parkinson-White, digoxin. Radio frequency ablation of accessory pathway is attempted if medical therapy fails and the child is old enough for the procedure.
- Long-QT syndrome: If long-QT syndrome is suspected, the child should be referred to a pediatric electrophysiologist. Treatment options include beta-blockers and placement of an implantable defibrillator.

These children are at risk of SCD from ventricular fibrillation secondary to rapid conduction of atrial arrhythmias (Chandra et al, 2013).

Syncope

Syncope is a transient loss of consciousness due to a decrease in cerebral blood flow; recovery is relatively prompt. Most syncope or near syncope in children is benign, unlike in older adults where cardiac causes are predominant. In assessing a syncopal episode, the provider must distinguish between a simple fainting event versus one that is a red flag for a serious cardiovascular or other medical condition.

Simple, or common, fainting occurs in approximately 15% of children from 8 to 18 years old. The relatively high incidence of syncope contrasts with a low incidence of aborted and cardiac-related sudden death in the pediatric and young adult population (Park, 2014).

Syncope related to cardiac causes can occur as a result of obstruction to left ventricular filling (e.g., mitral stenosis), obstruction to left ventricular ejection (e.g., aortic stenosis), or ineffective contraction along with an underlying structural, functional, or electrical heart disturbance. Syncope can also be due to primary pulmonary hypertension, which is an often clinically silent disease until severe symptoms are present. Syncope due to a cardiac cause often comes without prodromal symptoms or may be associated with palpitation or chest pain (angina).

In contrast, non-cardiac syncope (also called *neurocardiogenic syncope [NCS]*, or simple fainting) is neurally mediated and involves systemic vasodilation, vagally-induced bradycardia, and hypotension which result in decreased cerebral blood flow and fainting. NCS includes different overlapping subtypes, such as vasovagal syncope, cardioinhibitory syncope, pallid breath-holding spells (or reflex anoxic seizures), vasodepressor syncope, postural orthostatic tachycardia syndrome, or others. Ninety-five percent of syncope is vasodepressive or vasovagal. The incidence of simple fainting in female adolescents supersedes that of males (Park, 2014).

Additional causes of syncope include neurologic (headache, seizure, transient ischemic attack), psychiatric (depression, panic attack, conversion reaction), and metabolic (drugs, carbon monoxide, electrolyte imbalance/problems). Toddlers may faint with breath-holding spells, most commonly between 6 months and 3 years old. Many of these cases resolve by 5 years old and the majority by 8 years old (after this time, they are usually classified as convulsive syncope) (Park, 2014).

Clinical Findings

History

A thorough history that focuses on triggers and presyncopal symptoms is the most critical "test" of syncopal causation (Table 31-11). Key history elements to review include:

- Triggering factor, such as exercise, pain, or an emotional event (e.g., anxiety, panic)
- Prior incident(s) of syncope or fainting (e.g., venipuncture, seeing blood, experiencing an injury)
- Associated injury, clonic-tonic movements, or vertigo
- Associated chest pain, palpitations, tachycardia, or bradycardia
- Family history of sudden death before age 40, congenital deafness, long-QT syndrome, cardiomyopathy, and/or recurrent adolescent or toddler syncope that was outgrown
- Possibility of pregnancy or the use of drugs; list all medications taken (including diet supplements, herbs, other botanicals, energy drinks)
- History of exercise-induced bronchospasms, respiratory distress, or other concomitant medical disorder
- Known psychological stress or stressors at home or school or in social environments
- Standing for any length of time prior to the episode (indicates orthostasis); history of "head rushes" when standing up

TABLE 31-11 Relative Frequency of Premonitory Symptoms and Residual Findings with Common Neurally Mediated Syncope versus More Serious Cardiac Syncope

	Neurally Mediated	Cardiac Syncope
Symptoms		
Premonitory symptoms	+++	±
Lightheadedness	+++	+/±
Palpitations	+	++
Occurs while upright	+++	+
Occurs while sitting	+/±	+
Emotional trigger	++	++
Exercise trigger	+	++
Residual Findings		
Pallor	+++	+/±
Incontinence	–	+
Disorientation	–	+
Fatigue	++	±
Diaphoresis	++	±
Injury	+	++

From Newburger JW, Alexander ME, Fulton DR: Innocent murmurs, syncope, and chest pain. In Keane JF, Lock JE, Fyler DC, editors: *Nadas' pediatric cardiology,* ed 2, Philadelphia, 2006, Saunders. Reprinted with permission.

+++, Very common (>50%); ++, common (>20%); +, not rare (>≈5%); ±, uncommon (<5%); –, rare (<≈1%).

- In a hot environment, sweating, dehydration; hunger
- Nausea, constriction of visual fields ("world going dark") prior to episode
- Any postepisode symptoms, such as dizziness, pallor, clammy feeling, exhaustion, headache
- History of otherwise being well, active, with minimal medical issues
- Arousal after fainting within 1 to 2 minutes; recovery to full baseline state may have taken more than 1 hour (Many patients, though awake and alert, may not totally feel "like themselves" for a while.)
- Stiffening, jerking motions during unconsciousness (tonic-clonic muscular contractions of face [including fixed upward deviation of eyes], trunk, and extremities mimicking epilepsy occurs in approximately 50% of individuals experiencing a syncopal episode)
- Other activities prior to episode: hair grooming, coughing, micturition, neck stretching

Physical Examination

A detailed neurologic examination is needed if the syncopal episode suggests a seizure disorder. A cardiovascular examination is especially important. In most cases, the physical examination is completely normal.

Diagnostic Studies

The majority of individuals with cardiac syncope are identified either by a history of associated presyncopal symptoms with exercise, abnormal ECG, family history of arrhythmia, or abnormal physical examination. The diagnosis of neurally mediated syncope can confidently be made based on history, normal examination, and normal ECG. The diagnostic workup to distinguish between the two consists of:

- Orthostatic vital signs: More than a 30 mm Hg drop in BP after standing for 5 to 10 minutes, or a baseline systolic pressure of less than 80 mm Hg in an adolescent.
- Hemoglobin, if anemia is suspected: CBC, random glucose, and glucose tolerance tests have low yields and are not recommended routine tests for syncope.
- 12-lead ECG, looking for LVH, Wolff-Parkinson-White syndrome, AV and interventricular conduction defects, electrical myopathies (e.g., long-QT syndrome): If ECG results are borderline or family history is highly suggestive of cardiac etiology, ECGs on siblings and parents may be useful. Twenty-four-hour Holter monitoring and portable 30-day event monitoring can be useful.
- Echocardiography: Can be useful when history, physical, ECG, or family history suggests cardiac disease or cardiac syncope.
- Tilt table testing is not recommended for use in primary care due to poor reliability.
- Treadmill exercise testing may be used in cases of exercise-related syncope.

Management and Differential Diagnosis

If cardiac syncope is suspected, a referral to a pediatric cardiologist for further evaluation is paramount; restrict the child from sports participation until then. For neurally mediated syncope, education is key (cause, prevention, and how to abort a syncopal event). Prevention involves ensuring good hydration (along with decreasing caffeine and increasing sodium intake) and initiating antigravity techniques at the onset of presyncopal sensations (isometric leg or arm contractions; squatting or lying down; possibly using compression socks). The individual should rest for 5 to 10 minutes either supine or with legs up if prodromal symptoms occur or after a fainting. Concomitant cognitive-behavioral therapy is indicated if the episodes are psychogenic in etiology (Park, 2014).

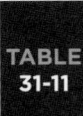

In refractory cases, pharmacologic management by cardiology specialists may play a role, although this should not be the first-line treatment. These therapies may involve the use of volume enhancement (fludrocortisone); limiting excessive catecholamine drive (using beta-blockers, such as atenolol); vagolytic agents (disopyramide); and/or selective serotonin reuptake inhibitors (SSRIs). If drug therapy is used, the typical duration is for 1 year followed by weaning. Pacemaker implantation has been used in rare cases.

Differential diagnoses include migraine with confusion or stupor, seizures, hypoglycemia, hysteria, hyperventilation, vertigo, carbon monoxide poisoning, electrolyte imbalance, drugs, and cardiovascular disease including underlying arrhythmia.

For a complete list of references, please visit http://evolve.elsevier.com/Burns/pediatric/.

32 Respiratory Disorders

RITA MARIE JOHN

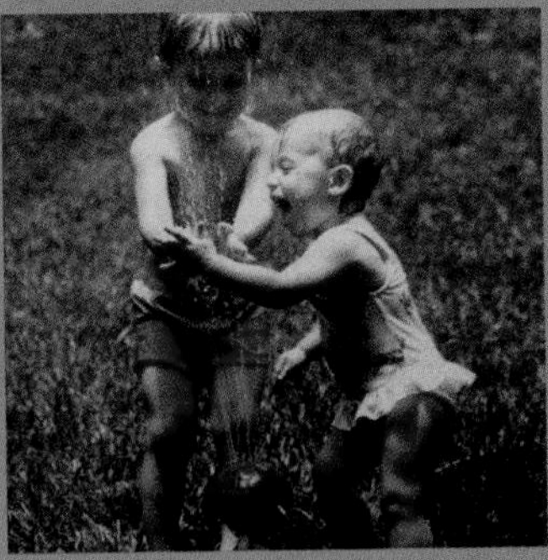

Respiratory problems are a leading cause of illness in children and a major reason for health care visits. Viral upper respiratory infections (URIs), pharyngitis, and otitis media are common diagnoses. Parents seek health care to confirm the appropriate management of upper respiratory disorders for the common cold, otitis media, rhinosinusitis, and tonsillopharyngitis. This leads to overprescribing of antibiotics by some practitioners (Hersh et al, 2013). Parents seeking to relieve their child's upper respiratory tract symptoms may use a variety of over-the-counter (OTC) cold medications, leading to overdosages of antipyretics and decongestants (Fashner et al, 2012). In contrast, a child with a lower respiratory tract disorder (e.g., asthma or bacterial pneumonia) can experience a potentially life-threatening illness that demands prompt attention. Providers need to ask key questions about the history of the respiratory symptoms; do a systematic and complete examination of the upper and lower airways; and, if indicated, order specific laboratory tests and radiographic examinations. This helps determine an accurate diagnosis and develop a successful treatment plan. When children have complicated problems, they should be referred with baseline information to the appropriate medical specialist for additional studies and treatment.

Anatomy and Physiology

Upper Respiratory Tract

The upper respiratory tract includes the nostrils, nasopharynx, larynx, upper part of the trachea, eustachian tubes, and sinuses. Air is warmed and humidified as it travels through the nasal passages, and coarse nasal hairs filter out particles. The nasal passages are lined with lysozymes, secretory immunoglobulin A (IgA), and immunoglobulin G (IgG) in nasal mucosa to defend against microbial invasion. The nasal mucosa is continuous and similar to the sinus mucosa except that the nasal mucosa is thicker with more glands. A blanket of mucus covers the surface epithelium of the nasal and sinus mucosa.

The mucosal lining of the sinuses is composed of pseudostratified, ciliated columnar epithelium interspersed with mucus producing goblet cells (Rose et al, 2013). The mucociliary action of the paranasal epithelium moves secretions from the sinuses to the nasal cavity. The frontal, maxillary, and anterior parts of the ethmoid sinuses drain to the middle meatus of the nose, whereas the sphenoid and posterior parts of the ethmoid sinuses drain to the superior meatus of the nose. Secretions need to be able to move through patent ostia into the nose. The quality of secretions and normally functioning cilia are key factors in the movement of secretions into the nose. Inflammation of nasal mucosa frequently causes edema and disruption of the sinus secretions. If there is significant swelling of the ostia due to a URI or allergic inflammation, or mechanical or local obstruction, ostial obstruction results and obstruction of the sinus secretions occurs. Cilia movement and mucus flow allow the sinuses to be free of pathogens.

The maxillary sinuses are present by the second trimester of gestation but are not fully pneumatized until a child is about 4 years old. Ethmoid sinuses develop by the fourth month of gestation and form the thin lateral walls of the orbit of the eye. They are pneumatized at birth and can be visualized on plain radiographs when the child is 1 to 2 years old. The sphenoid sinuses start to form in the first 2 years of life but remain rudimentary until age 6, which is when they become visible on radiographs. By 12 years old, they reach their permanent size, but not shape. As a result, the nasal cavity and paranasal sinuses reach adult proportion by age 12 (Cherry and Shapiro, 2009). The sinuses become clinically significant sites of infection at the following ages:

- Maxillary and ethmoid sinuses: As early as late infancy
- Sphenoid sinuses: Around 3 and 4 years old
- Frontal sinuses: Around 6 to 10 years old

The epiglottis deflects swallowed material toward the esophagus to protect the larynx. The vocal cords form a V-shaped opening known as the *glottis.* The subglottic space is beneath the vocal cords, and its walls converge toward the cricoid ring to form a complete ring of cartilage around the larynx. In children younger than 2 to 3 years old, the cricoid ring is the narrowest part of the airway; in older children and adults, the glottis is narrowest. The rings of tracheal cartilage support the trachea and the mainstem bronchi.

The trachea and airways of the infant and young child are more compliant than those of an adult. Hyperextension of the neck can constrict the airway of infants. Consequently, changes in intrapleural pressure lead to greater changes in an infant's or young child's airway compared with the effect that such changes would exert on adult airways, thereby causing an increased risk of airway collapse. Similarly, increased chest wall compliance in young infants makes them more vulnerable to adverse events, and their respiratory muscles cannot effectively handle sustained, intense respiratory workload that occurs during severe pulmonary illnesses.

Lower Respiratory Tract

The lower respiratory tract passages begin at the trachea and include the right and left lungs that branch out to smaller airways—first the bronchi, then the bronchioles, and end at the alveoli. The right lung has three lobes—upper, middle, and lower—with the upper and middle being separated by a minor fissure. The left lung has two lobes—upper and lower—separated by a major fissure. The upper left lobe has an area called the *lingula* that corresponds to the right middle lobe. The right mainstem bronchus is shorter and wider than the left bronchus. It forms a smaller angle away from the trachea than the left bronchus does. This anatomic variation explains why foreign bodies (FBs) usually lodge in the right mainstem bronchus. Although the body surface and the number of respiratory airways and alveoli increase tenfold from birth to adult life, the tissue available for gas exchange increases approximately twentyfold. The newborn's chest is cylindrically shaped and has relatively horizontal ribs, which limits the infant's ability to expand his or her chest. Because there is greater transverse growth in the lower part of the chest wall, the shape of the chest changes during the first few years of life. This differential growth results in the ribs being positioned lower anteriorly than posteriorly. The change in positioning of the ribs adds rigidity to the thorax of older children.

The diaphragm is the main muscle of respiration, and the intercostal, sternocleidomastoid, spinal, neck, and abdominal muscles are accessory muscles that can be used to increase effort. Normal exhalation occurs from elastic recoil of the lung.

Primitive airways appear at approximately week 4 of gestation. At about week 16 of gestation, the number of bronchial branches equals that in adults. Subsequent growth continues by increasing the length of the respiratory tract. During weeks 16 to 26 of gestation, vascularization of the future respiratory portion of the lung occurs. Cartilage, glands, and muscles of the airways and type II alveolar cells are formed by week 28. Type II cells allow the fetus to produce a phospholipid called *surfactant.* The airways continue to grow, and terminal sac formation occurs. At approximately week 36, the terminal sacs divide, and alveoli are formed. Approximately 50 million primitive alveoli are present at birth.

After birth, the alveolar ducts branch out from the respiratory bronchioles. Alveoli continue to form and number 100 to 200 million in older children and 200 to 600 million in adolescents. The alveolar sacs continue to increase in size. The adult lung contains approximately 300 million alveoli.

Other structures important for gas exchange and pulmonary function are present at birth and include cartilage, mucus glands, goblet cells, and ciliated cells of the conducting airways. The airways above the bronchioles are lined with ciliated pseudostratified columnar cells as well as goblet cells. Mucus is produced from the mucus glands that line the respiratory tract. The cilia play a critical role of sweeping mucus and debris toward the upper respiratory tract. Smooth muscle is also present; therefore, even very young infants can have bronchospasm. Beyond the bronchioles there is a thin layer of surfactant that reduces surface tension and prevents airway collapse.

Airway resistance is higher in newborns and young children than in adults. The airways of young infants and children are easily obstructed by inflammation, FBs, or mucous. The maximal inspiratory pressure generated by an infant is equal to that of an adult. However, the chest wall and supporting structures are softer and more flexible, so chest wall retraction is greatest in young infants. The chest wall of a newborn is highly compliant.

Pathophysiology Involved in Airway Disease

All lung disorders cause some form of airway obstruction. Narrowing of the airway lumen results from one or more of the following:

- Presence of intraluminal material (e.g., secretions, tumors, or foreign matter)
- Mural thickening (e.g., edema or hypertrophy of the glands or mucosa)
- Contraction of smooth muscle (e.g., spasm)
- Extrinsic compression

These factors rarely occur in isolation. They cause pulmonary malfunction by impairing tracheobronchial hygiene and impeding normal airflow. Severe airway obstruction can occur in infants or young children from very small blockages because of their airway size.

Obstructive Processes

Airway obstruction is the underlying etiology for the most common forms of pediatric lung diseases. The two major types of airway obstruction are complete and partial. In complete obstruction, neither airflow nor drainage of secretions occurs. Such occlusion leads to lobar atelectasis after the residual gas diffuses into the pulmonary circulation. In partial airway obstruction, airflow and secretion drainage occur but are impaired. Partial obstruction can be further divided into two separate classifications. The first consists of a bypass valve obstruction caused by narrowing of the lumen; a wheeze may be produced. Although resistance to flow is increased, air can still flow in during inspiration and out during expiration. The second is a check-valve or ball-valve obstruction; air entry is possible, but during expiration the lumen is completely occluded so that escape of air is impossible. Bronchial FBs and emphysema are associated with bypass, check-valve, or ball-valve obstructions that result in overinflation of lung airways.

Airway obstruction that occurs above the level of the secondary bronchi generally interferes more with inspiration than expiration. If the obstruction is complete and above the bifurcation of the trachea, asphyxia and death can result. Partial obstruction may result in severe dyspnea, stridor (a harsh high-pitched inspiratory sound), and subcostal retractions. Coughing removes nonfixed, high airway obstruction. Poor inspiratory airflow limits the coughing effectiveness. The sound produced by coughing may indicate the level of airway obstruction and assists in making a diagnosis. Obstructions next to the larynx produce a cough that sounds croupy or barking. Obstructions in the trachea or major bronchi produce a brassy sound.

Lower airway obstructions result from peripheral lesions that are usually diffuse in location and involve bronchioles smaller than 3 mm. The usual mechanism of narrowing is spasm, accumulation of secretions, edema of the mucous membrane, extrinsic compression, or any combination of these factors. Complete airway obstruction causes atelectasis. A large percentage of the lung volume needs to be involved before symptoms become apparent; small atelectatic changes do not produce obvious clinical manifestations.

The primary clinical manifestation of lower airway obstruction occurs during expiration. Wheezing is the principal sound patients make if the obstruction allows enough air to pass through the narrowed lumen. Chest excursion diminishes, and the expiratory phase prolongs. Increased airway resistance during exhalation results in overinflation of the lungs, which in turn eventually increases the anteroposterior diameter of the chest. Chronic overinflation results in a "barrel chest" typically noted in a child with chronic lung disease, such as cystic fibrosis (CF) or emphysema. The accumulation of fluids and inflammation in the lower airways usually results in a repetitive hacking, ineffectual cough. On physical examination, percussing an overinflated chest elicits hyperresonance.

Symptoms worsen as the obstruction increases. The body attempts to compensate by using accessory muscles to assist in breathing. Dyspnea can result and may include orthopnea and exercise intolerance. Cyanosis appears as the oxygen saturation drops below 85% and is an ominous sign. Mild obstruction is marked by reduced respiratory rate and increased tidal volume; severe obstruction is characterized by increased respiratory rate, increased retractions with the use of accessory muscles, anxiety, and cyanosis.

Fine crackles (formerly called *rales*) are intermittent, nonmusical, short, explosive, clicking, or rattling sounds, best heard on mid- to late inspiration and occasionally on expiration. These sounds are gravity dependent, not transmitted to the mouth, and are unaffected by cough. They are heard in pneumonia and interstitial lung disease (Bohadana et al, 2014). These sounds are caused by airways suddenly opening after having been previously closed. The gas pressure between the compartments equalizes and creates the crackling sound. Coarse crackles are also nonmusical and are short and explosive, but these are heard on early inspiration and throughout expiration. They are intermittent bubbling or brief popping sounds that are longer in duration than fine crackles. Course crackles may be affected by cough and are more common during inspiration. They may indicate intermittent airway opening and may be related to secretions (Bohadana et al, 2014).

Restrictive Processes

Restrictive disease is less common in pediatric patients and is characterized by decreased lung compliance with relatively normal flow rates. Examples of causative factors include neuromuscular weakness, lobar pneumonia, pleural effusion or masses, severe pectus excavatum, or abdominal distention. Key findings of restrictive lung disease are rapid respiratory rate and decreased tidal volume/capacity (Carter and Marshall, 2011).

Defense Systems

The respiratory defense system includes mechanical and biologic processes. Mechanical defenses include:

- Filtering of particles
- Warming and humidifying of inspired air
- Clearing of airway through mucociliary and coughing actions
- Spasm and breathing changes

Approximately 75% of inspired air is warmed as it passes through the nose, paranasal sinuses, pharynx, larynx, and upper portion of the trachea. Final warming and humidifying of the airstream take place in the trachea and large bronchi. Heat and moisture are removed during the expiratory phase of respiration. The nose has a large surface area on which particles larger than 5 mm are trapped and filtered to prevent them from entering the lower airways. The trachea and bronchioles are lined with various defensive cells and mucus glands. Goblet cells secrete the mucous layer that lies on the tip of cilia. Particles entering the conducting airway are quickly cleared by the mucociliary defenses. Coughing is a reflex mechanism that has three phases: (1) inspiratory, (2) compressive, and (3) expiratory. Through forceful expiration FBs and other materials can be removed from the airways; coughing propels particles. Young infants and children cannot effectively expectorate mucus, so they swallow it. Loss of the cough reflex leads to aspiration and pneumonia. Temporary breathing cessation, reflex shallow breathing, laryngospasm, and even bronchospasm are compensatory efforts aimed at stopping foreign matter from further entry into the lower respiratory tract.

However, these respiratory efforts offer limited protection and have significant drawbacks.

Biologic processes that protect the respiratory system include:

- Phagocytosis
- Absorption of noxious gases in the vasculature of the upper airway
- Absorption of particles by the lymph system

Phagocytosis, aided by the secretory IgA plus interferon, lysozyme, and lactoferrin, is the principal antimicrobial defense. Particles reaching the alveoli can be phagocytized by alveolar macrophages and polymorphonuclear (PMN) cells, cleared from the lung by the mucociliary system, or carried by lymphocytes into regional nodes or the blood. These particles can take days to months to clear.

The respiratory defense system is at risk for compromise from numerous environmental factors. Damage to epithelial cells is caused by a variety of substances and gases, such as sulfur, nitrogen dioxide, ozone, chlorine, ammonia, and cigarette smoke. Hypothermia, hyperthermia, morphine, codeine, and hypothyroidism can adversely alter mucociliary defenses. Dry air from mouth breathing during periods of nasal obstruction, tracheostomy placement, or inadequately humidified oxygen therapy results in dryness of the mucous membrane and slowing of the cilia beat. Cold air is also irritating to the lower airways.

Phagocytic ability is also reduced by many substances, including ethanol ingestion and cigarette smoke. Hypoxemia, starvation, chilling, corticosteroids, increased oxygen, narcotics, and some anesthetic gases also impair phagocytosis. Recent acute viral infections can reduce antibacterial killing capacity. Damage from infection and chemical irritants may or may not be reversible.

Recurrent respiratory infections in children merit investigation for immunodeficiency or other underlying diseases, such as primary ciliary dyskinesia or CF. The mnemonic SPUR (Bush, 2009) can help determine which children need further workup:

Severe infection
Persistent infection and poor recovery
Unusual organisms
Recurrent infection

Immunodeficiencies should be considered if the child has four or more new ear infections in a year, two or more serious sinus infections, two or more pneumonias in a year, persistent oral candidiasis, failure to thrive, two or more deep seeded skin abscesses, 2 or more months on antibiotics without improvement, and/or the need for intravenous (IV) antibiotics to clear infections. Also consider immunodeficiencies if there is a family history of immunodeficiency or two or more deep skin infections (Modell et al, 2014).

Assessment of the Respiratory System

The history provides valuable information about the causes, progression, and potential complications of a child's respiratory condition. The physical examination and diagnostic testing allow the provider to determine the extent of respiratory distress.

History

History of the present illness can be assessed using the mnemonic PQRST:

- **P**romoting, preventing, precipitating, palliating factors
  - *Contacts:* Are any family members or close contacts (e.g., day care, school) ill with similar signs and symptoms?
  - *Prevention:* Do you give your child any medications or supplements (include any herbs, botanicals, or vitamins) to try to prevent a cold? What are your hand washing practices? Do you encourage fluids when your child has a URI? Are the child's immunizations up to date?
  - *Progression:* Are the respiratory signs or symptoms increasing in severity, lessening, or about the same? Is the child easily fatigued, less active, having trouble sleeping, or working harder to breathe?
  - *Treatment:* Have any OTC, prescription drugs, herbs, supplements, or botanicals been used? Have any other treatment modalities been used, including folk cures or home remedies?
- **Q**uality or quantity
  - How severe are the symptoms? Is the illness interfering with school attendance or play? Are breathing problems affecting the child's ability to sleep and eat?
- **R**egion or radiation
  - Does the child complain of chest pain?
- **S**everity, setting, simultaneous symptoms or similar illnesses in the past
  - *Key signs and symptoms:* Has the child had symptoms or signs of a daytime or nighttime cough, fever, vomiting, malaise, rhinorrhea, sore throat, lesions in the mouth, retractions, cyanosis, dyspnea, or increased respiratory effort? Table 32-1 lists key characteristics and causes of cough.
  - *Associated symptoms:* Has there been a decrease in appetite or feeding? Any rashes, headaches, or abdominal pain?
  - *Similar illnesses in the past:* Does the child have a history of respiratory tract infections, allergies, or asthma? How many similar infections has the child had (e.g., croup, pneumonia, rhinosinusitis, streptococcal tonsillopharyngitis, or frequent colds)?
- **T**emporal factors
  - When did the illness begin?
  - Was the onset acute or insidious or proceeded by the common cold?
  - How long has it lasted? How has it changed over time?
- Family history
  - Do others in the family have a history of allergies or asthma?

TABLE 32-1 Key Characteristics of Cough, Common Causes, and Questions to Ask in a Pediatric History

Key Characteristics to Consider	Description and Questions to Ask
Age factor	Infants have a weak, nonproductive cough.
Quality	Staccato-like (*Chlamydia trachomatis* in infants); barking or brassy (croup, tracheomalacia, habit cough); paroxysmal or inspiratory whoop (pertussis or parapertussis); honking (psychogenic). Is the cough wet or dry?
Duration	*Acute* (most causes are infectious and last less than 2 weeks), *subacute* (cough lasts from 2 to 4 weeks); *recurrent* (associated with allergies and asthma), or *chronic* (lasting greater than 4 to 8 weeks [e.g., CF, asthma]). Is the cough continuous or intermittent?
Productivity	Mucus producing or nonproductive?
Timing	During the day, night (associated with asthma), or both?
Effect on parent and child	Are parents frustrated with the cough? Is it causing them to lose sleep and work time? Are they concerned that the child may have something serious?
Associated symptoms	Fever: May indicate bacterial infection (pneumonia). Rhinorrhea, sneezing, wheezing, atopic dermatitis: Associated with asthma and allergic rhinitis. Malaise, sneezing, watery nasal discharge, mild sore throat, no or low fever, not ill appearing: Typical of URI. Tachypnea: Pneumonia or bronchiolitis in infants (infants may not have a cough).
Exposure to infection or travel	Has the child been out of the country (tuberculosis)? Is there a member of the household being treated for "bronchitis" or another cough illness?
Causes	
Congenital anomalies	Tracheoesophageal fistula, vascular ring, laryngeal cleft, vocal cord paralysis, pulmonary malformations, tracheobronchomalacia, congenital heart disease
Infectious agent	Viral (RSV, adenovirus, parainfluenza, HIV, metapneumovirus, human bocavirus), bacterial (tuberculosis, pertussis, *Streptococcus pneumoniae*), fungal, and atypical bacteria (*C.* and *M. pneumoniae*)
Allergic condition	Allergic rhinitis, asthma
Other	FB aspiration, gastroesophageal reflux, psychogenic cough, environmental triggers (air pollution, tobacco smoke, wood smoke, glue sniffing, volatile chemicals), CF, drug induced, tumor, congestive heart failure

Adapted from Chang AB: Cough, *Pediatr Clin North Am* 56(1):19–31, 2009; Cherry JD: Croup (laryngitis, laryngotracheitis, spasmodic croup, laryngotracheobronchitis, bacterial tracheitis, and laryngotracheobronchopneumonitis). In Cherry J, Kaplan S, Demmler-Harrison G, et al, editors: *Feigin & Cherry's textbook of pediatric infectious diseases*, ed 6, vol 1, Philadelphia, 2009, Saunders/Elsevier, pp 254–268.
CF, Cystic fibrosis; *FB*, foreign body; *HIV*, human immunodeficiency virus; *RSV*, respiratory syncytial virus; *URI*, upper respiratory infection.

    - Is there any family history of immunodeficiency, ear-nose-throat, or respiratory problems?
    - Does anyone in the family have genetic diseases, such as CF or alpha 1-antitrypsin deficiency?
    - Are other family members ill?
- Review of systems
    - Note any infections, constitutional diseases, or congenital problems that might have a respiratory component.
- Environment
    - Does anyone in the family or in the day care setting smoke? Does the child live or attend school in an urban or industrial area subject to air pollution (e.g., near a major highway, industrial plant, or bus terminal)? Has the child or a family contact traveled recently and where?

Physical Examination

When determining respiratory distress, think about the total presentation and not just individual isolated findings. Consider the anxiety level, respiratory rate and rhythm, use of accessory muscles, color, breath sounds, grunting, and pulse oximetry results. Information pertinent to the physical examination of a child with suspected respiratory disease includes the following:

- Measurement of vital signs and observation of general appearance:
    - A normal respiratory rate is age dependent and, if elevated, is a key indicator of lower respiratory involvement.
    - The level of anxiety, nasal flaring, and position of comfort are useful indicators of respiratory distress.

Changes in skin color may be subtle or obvious, depending on the level of deoxygenation. Grunting is a sign of small airway disease.

- Inspection of:
  - Nose: Look for rhinorrhea—clear, mucoid, mucopurulent; FBs, erosion, polyps, lesions, bleeding, septal position, and color of the mucous membrane.
  - Throat, pharynx, and tonsils: Look for lesions, vesicles, exudate, enlargement of any structure, or other abnormalities. If epiglottitis is a consideration, do not inspect the mouth or attempt to elicit a gag reflex (see discussion later in this chapter).
  - Chest: Look at the depth, ease, symmetry, and rhythm of respiration. These are key indicators of lower respiratory tract involvement. The use of accessory muscles and the presence of retractions should be noted. A prolonged expiratory phase is associated with respiratory obstruction in the lower airways.
- Palpation or percussion of:
  - Chest: Percuss for signs of dullness or hyperresonance caused by consolidation, fluid, or air trapping.
- Auscultation of the chest:
  - Upper tract: Pathology frequently causes noisy breathing, snoring, stridor, and musical or wheezing tracheal breath sounds and can be a source of referred breath sounds (Bohadana et al, 2014).
  - Lower tract: Pathology is suggested by fine crackles, coarse crackles, rhonchus, pleural friction rub, wheezing, and bronchial breath sounds (Bohadana et al, 2014).

Diagnostic Studies

Diagnostic procedures used to evaluate respiratory illness in children managed as outpatients include the following:

- Monitoring oxygenation by pulse oximetry:
  - Pulse oximetry can be used to continuously measure pulse rate and peripheral oxygen saturation in arterial blood. The oxyhemoglobin saturation percentage (Spo_2) is digitally displayed. Results generally correlate well with simultaneous arterial oxygen saturation (Sao_2). With anoxia, there is a rise in organic phosphate content within the red blood cells (RBCs) resulting in more oxygen (O_2) available to tissues. People living at higher elevations suffer from chronic hypoxia. When first arriving at a high elevation, many individuals experience a transient mountain sickness with symptoms that include headache, insomnia, irritability, breathlessness, nausea, and vomiting. This phenomenon lasts approximately 1 week before acclimatization begins. The affected person begins to increase production of RBCs. Finally, a functional nonpathologic right ventricular hypertrophy takes place. These effects last as long as the person remains at high elevation. Severe altitude sickness can lead to cerebral and pulmonary edema and can be life-threatening.
  - Blood gas studies can help the provider assess possible respiratory collapse and are used in acute care settings. A rising partial arterial pressure of carbon dioxide ($Paco_2$) is an ominous sign.
- Radiographic imaging in respiratory disease may be efficacious in certain circumstances. Such imaging can include radiographs, ultrasonography, magnetic resonance imaging (MRI), and computed tomography (CT) of the sinuses, soft tissues of the neck, and chest. Abnormalities of the nasal mucosa, such as thickening, may reflect inflammation. Unless there is chronic or complicated rhinosinusitis, imaging in acute rhinosinusitis (ARS) is not indicated, because uncomplicated URIs can cause abnormalities of the paranasal sinuses (Brook, 2013). Chest radiographs should be done in both posteroanterior and lateral positions, because lesions may only be seen in one of the two views. Other pulmonary studies may be ordered by the medical specialists to whom the child is referred. Pulmonary function tests are discussed in Chapter 25 in the section on asthma.
- Other specialized tests, including sweat testing, cultures, and blood work, are addressed under the specific illness.
- Children who have unusual signs and symptoms should be referred to a pulmonary specialist at which time further diagnostic procedures might be performed. Fluoroscopy is useful in the evaluation of stridor and abnormal movement of the diaphragm. Endoscopy (bronchoscopy and laryngoscopy), bronchoalveolar lavage, percutaneous tap, lung biopsy, and microbiology studies can be helpful if used appropriately. Contrast studies (e.g., barium esophagogram) are useful for patients with recurrent pneumonia, persistent cough, tracheal ring, or suspected fistulas. Other imaging studies that might be needed to assess these children include bronchograms (useful in delineating the smaller airways), pulmonary arteriograms (evaluation of the pulmonary vasculature), and radionuclide studies (evaluation of the pulmonary capillary bed).

Basic Respiratory Management Strategies

General Measures

There are several essential and basic measures related to the prevention of respiratory illnesses that should be emphasized. They include avoidance of smoke or exposure to secondhand smoke, good hand washing practices, and immunization coverage for age.

Children who are significantly ill or have unusual manifestations need referral to or consultation with a pediatrician or pediatric subspecialist. For those children with mild or moderate respiratory illnesses, the following general management measures are applicable and include the following:

- *Fluid:* Hydration is important to keep mucous membranes and secretions moist. Intake of fluids should be encouraged, and parents of young children should be given guidelines regarding the type, amount, and frequency of fluids and feedings that their child should take.

- *Oxygen administration:* The use of supplemental oxygen is important to help relieve hypoxemia in most children who have acute respiratory distress. Depression of the respiratory drive is possible with supplemental oxygen administration if the central nervous system (CNS) chemoreceptors are blunted by hypercapnia. However, children at risk for blunting are those with issues related to chronic hypercapnia and are generally easily recognized, because they tend to have chronic severe respiratory diseases, such as CF and bronchopulmonary dysplasia. In acute situations, administer oxygen using an appropriately sized mask or a high-flow oxygen source held near the child's face if a mask frightens the child. The safe, acceptable range of oxygen saturation is 92% to 95%; higher levels may lead to oxygen toxicity (Ambalavanan, 2014; Chin, 2010; Robinson and Van Asperen, 2009). Children seen in primary care settings who require supplemental oxygen may need to be transported to an acute care hospital setting via emergency medical services for evaluation and stabilization (see the Bronchiolitis section about the use of oxygen in the home setting).
- *Humidification:* A cold-mist vaporizer helps provide moisture to the nares and oropharynx in a dry environment during a common cold, but the vaporizer must be cleaned daily so that it will not become a source of infection.
- *Bulb syringe:* Because infants are obligate nose breathers, parents should be instructed in use of the nasal bulb syringe to relieve obstruction of the infant's nares with mucus. Use the bulb syringe gently and intermittently, because improper use can cause irritation, inflammation, and respiratory obstruction from tissue damage. Providing parents with written instructions about suctioning the infant's nose with a bulb syringe is advantageous.
- *Normal saline nose drops, nasal rinses, or spray:* Use before feedings and when mucus is thick or crusted. Follow by suctioning the nares with a bulb syringe. Saline nasal rinses are widely available commercially and are helpful for older children and adolescents (Box 32-1).

BOX 32-1 Parental Education for At-Home Care of the Child with a Respiratory Tract Infection

General Management Issues to Discuss

Fluid: Give guidelines on type, amount, and frequency of fluids child should take.

Humidification: For acute laryngotracheitis, take the child out into the cold night air or open a freezer door. In dry climates, humidifiers help in common colds; instruct about cleaning of nebulizers and humidifiers (see the following bullet about care of nebulizers and humidifiers).

Bulb syringe: Instruct to use the bulb syringe gently and intermittently for suctioning the nares.

Normal saline nose drops or spray: Use before feedings and when mucus is thick or crusted. Follow by suctioning nares with bulb syringe.

Good hand washing and avoidance of exposure to smoke or secondhand smoke

Other Educational Topics to Cover

- Indications for immediate reevaluation of child:
  - Signs and symptoms of respiratory distress
  - Other indicators of worsening of illness (e.g., toxic appearance, malaise, feeding difficulty)
- Give information on when to expect improvement in the child's symptoms and what to do if symptoms do not improve as expected.
- Clear instructions about medications: Give instructions regarding how much medication to give, when to give it, what side effects to watch for, how long to give the medication, and the necessity of completing the course of antibiotics.
- Infection control information if needed: Give information regarding hand washing and disposal of infected secretions; the CDC has excellent written and video education materials available on hand washing at www.cdc.gov/Features/HandWashing.
- Care of nebulizers and humidifiers: To prevent the growth of organisms, nebulizers and humidifiers should be cleaned daily with soapy water, rinsed thoroughly, soaked for one half hour in a solution of one part vinegar to two or three parts distilled water, and then air-dried. Control III disinfectant is a commercial product that can be substituted for vinegar; however, it is expensive.
- Give instructions regarding next return visit.

CDC, Centers for Disease Control and Prevention.

Medications

The following pharmacologic agents may be needed to treat various respiratory illnesses:

- *Antibiotics:* Specific agents are discussed in the section on individual illnesses. If an antibiotic is prescribed, the drug should be taken until completed.
- *Analgesics and antipyretics:* Acetaminophen and ibuprofen may be prescribed for relief of pain or fever.
- *Decongestant, antihistamines, and cough medicine:* The use of decongestants, antihistamines, and cough medicine does not shorten the course of a disease. Antihistamines and decongestants can provide relief of nasal symptoms. However, due to the risk of overdosage and unsupervised ingestions, the use of decongestants, antihistamines, and or cough medication is not recommended for children younger than 6 years old because of their potential for harm and little evidence of efficacy (Ballengee and Turner, 2014; Pappas and Hendley, 2011). A total of 123 deaths have been attributed to the use of these medications, and poison control centers continue to report calls related to OTC cold medications (Pappas and Hendley, 2011).
- *Expectorants:* Water is one of the most effective expectorants. OTC agents provide some symptomatic relief, but do not shorten the course of respiratory illnesses. Do not use OTC agents in children younger than 6 years old (Ballengee and Turner, 2014).

- *Cough medication:* Cough suppressant medications should be prescribed judiciously because coughing is a protective mechanism to clear secretions. In review of evidence-based guidelines for the intervention in pediatric cough, the only cough medication recommended in a child older than 1 year old was buckwheat honey. However, the study results may be the result of a placebo effect (Paul et al, 2007).
- *Zinc and vitamin C:* The use of zinc is not recommended in children due to potential side effects and questionable efficacy. Similarly, studies investigating the effect of large dosages of vitamin C in either the prevention or treatment of the common cold have demonstrated little to no benefit with their use (Ballengee and Turner, 2014).
- *Probiotics:* The use of probiotics is being explored as a possible option for prevention of common cold illnesses in young children (Ballengee and Turner, 2014).

Patient and Parent Education

Frequent hand washing and avoiding touching the eyes and nose can help prevent the spread of infection. Always educate about the dangers related to exposure to smoke and secondhand smoke exposure and the need to avoid this respiratory trigger. Teach the child and other family members how to cough/sneeze into sleeve, disposal of tissues, and use of hand sanitizers, because these are measures that may decrease the spread of infectious agents. Parents should be educated about assessment and management of changes in the child's condition. Significant educational issues are identified in Box 32-1.

Indications for Tonsillectomy and Adenoidectomy

Current guidelines for tonsillectomy and adenoidectomy clearly define the indications for tonsillectomy (Belderbos et al, 2011). They include having more than seven episodes of throat infections in the past year, or more than five episodes of throat infection in the past 2 years or at least three episodes per year for the past 3 years. The definition of throat infections includes a temperature of higher than 100.9° F (38.3° C), cervical lymphadenopathy with tonsillar exudate, or a positive group A beta-hemolytic streptococci (GABHS) culture or if antibiotics had been administered in suspected or proved cases of GABHS. Studies have shown that tonsillectomy helps reduce the recurrent sore throats for 2 years (Belderbos et al, 2011). Recurrent peritonsillar abscesses and periodic fever with aphthous ulcers and adenopathy (PFAPA) may be indications for a tonsillectomy. Correction of obstructive sleep apnea (diagnosed with a positive polysomnography) may improve the patient's quality of life and is considered another indication for a tonsillectomy.

Adenoidectomy can also be considered if appropriate medical treatment fails to correct obstructive adenoidal hypertrophy, recurrent or chronic otitis media (after tympanostomy tube placement has been tried), and chronic unresponsive rhinosinusitis. Adenoidectomy may be considered in children with obstructive sleep apnea, because some attention deficit and hyperactivity behaviors may be due to interrupted sleep rather than a misdiagnosis of attention deficit hyperactivity disorder. The morbidity and mortality rates connected with adenoidectomy are not as high as with tonsillectomy.

Upper Respiratory Tract Disorders

The Common Cold

The common cold is a frequent problem seen in pediatric practice, and parents often seek information from their child's primary health care provider as to whether their child's symptoms represent a typical URI or indicate the beginning or advancing signs of a more serious illness. Young children have on average 6 to 10 URIs, or colds, per year. The typical course of these illnesses is an initial low-grade fever with clear rhinitis changing by day 3 to purulent discharge and to a slow resolution with clear nasal discharge by day 10 (Wald et al, 2013). Viruses cause most common colds, with 50% resulting from infection by the more than 100 serotypes of rhinoviruses. Parainfluenza viruses, respiratory syncytial virus (RSV), coronavirus, and human metapneumovirus are also common agents (Cherry and Nieves, 2009; Schuster and Williams, 2013). Other agents that occasionally cause cold symptoms include adenovirus, enterovirus, influenza viruses, reoviruses, and human bocavirus. Day care and preschool attendance are associated with an increased number of common colds in young children and their spread to school-age children in the family. The acquisition of a common cold virus occurs via inoculation of the nose and possibly the conjunctiva. Colds can be spread through direct inhalation of virus from a sneeze, nasal blowing, or inoculation via fingers from nasal secretions or fomites. Mental stress, lack of sleep, high basal levels of catecholamines, infrequent exercise, smoking, and low vitamin C intake are risk factors for colds in adults, but these have not been studied in children (Cherry and Nieves, 2009).

Pathophysiology

The viral infection of the nasopharyngeal mucosa initiates a host response that produces the symptoms of a cold. Once the cold viral is deposited on the nasal mucosa, it attaches to cell receptors and enters the cells. Potent cytokines including interleukin (IL)-8 attract large number of PMN cells. As a result, vascular permeability increases, causing the leak of plasma proteins into nasal secretions. Bradykinins cause the pharyngitis and rhinitis. The presence of PMN, rather than bacterial colonization, changes the color of nasal mucus, with yellow-green mucus due to PMN enzymatic activity and yellow mucus being caused by the simple presence of PMN. With rhinovirus, there is an increase in bradykinins and albumin in the nasal secretions but no increase in histamines. Rhinovirus and coronaviruses do not cause destruction of the nasal epithelium, but adenovirus and influenza have a significant destructive effect on the respiratory epithelium (Pappas and Hendley, 2011).

Clinical Findings

Symptoms of a viral cold include nasal congestion, cough, sneezing, rhinorrhea, fever, hoarseness, and pharyngitis (Fashner et al, 2012). Sleep disturbances do occur with URIs, but vomiting and diarrhea are uncommon. The symptoms should decrease at the end of 10 days.

History

The following may be reported:

- Gradual onset
- Prominent nasal symptoms of rhinorrhea (key finding)
- Sore throat and dysphagia
- Mild cough and poor sleep
- Low-grade fever especially in younger children
- After a variable period of 1 to 3 days, nasal secretions are thicker and more purulent, leading to nasal excoriation

Physical Examination

Virus-specific findings include:

- Conjunctiva: Mild injection
- Nose: Red nasal mucosa with secretions of varying colors depending on the degree of nasal mucosa destruction and PMN activity
- Throat: Mild erythema
- Lymph: Anterior cervical lymphadenopathy with freely movable nodes less than 2 cm
- Chest: Clear to auscultation and without adventitious sounds

Diagnostic Studies

A throat culture should not be done if there are nasal symptoms with complaints of throat pain. However, if the diagnosis of common cold is in doubt, a rapid antigen detection test (RADT), often called a *rapid strep test,* should be done with a throat culture if the RADT is negative (Shulman et al, 2012).

Differential Diagnosis

The most common differentials are allergic rhinitis, rhinosinusitis, and adenoiditis (Table 32-2).

Management

Only supportive care is needed for a viral URI. See the Basic Respiratory Management Strategies section and see Box 32-1 for guidance regarding the use of decongestants, antihistamines, and cough medications. Antibiotics are not appropriate treatment. The child should receive symptomatic relief for fever, pain, and nasal congestion using normal saline and an antipyretic. Although topically applied menthol may improve nighttime cough, there is a risk of chemical irritation and accidental ingestion, causing CNS and gastrointestinal (GI) side effects. Fluid intake should be encouraged.

Complications

Common colds are self-limiting, but secondary bacterial infections including otitis media, pneumonia, and sinusitis can occur along with secondary wheezing.

Pharyngitis, Tonsillitis, and Tonsillopharyngitis

Pharyngitis is an inflammation of the mucosa lining the structures of the throat, including the tonsils, pharynx, uvula, soft palate, and nasopharynx. It can be due to infectious agents or noninfectious causes, such as smoke or other air irritants. The illness is generally acute and involves an inflammatory response, including erythema, exudate, or ulceration.

The etiology could include a number of viruses and bacteria. If there are nasal symptoms, it is called *nasopharyngitis,* but if there are no nasal symptoms, the disease is called *pharyngitis* or *tonsillopharyngitis.* Most cases of pharyngitis are caused by viruses (Gereige and Cunill-De Sautu, 2011). Adenovirus is the most common cause of nasopharyngitis (Cherry, 2009c). Other viruses include Epstein-Barr virus (EBV), herpes simplex virus (HSV), cytomegalovirus (CMV), enterovirus, influenza virus, parainfluenza, and human immunodeficiency virus (HIV). The viral organisms generally present with upper nasal symptoms. The common bacterial etiology is GABHS in children between 5 and 11 years old, whereas 40% of reported cases of gonococcal infections occur in females 15 to 19 years old. Other organisms include *Corynebacterium diphtheriae, Arcanobacterium haemolyticum, Neisseria gonorrhoeae,* group C and group G streptococci, *Chlamydia trachomatis, Francisella tularensis,* and *Mycoplasma pneumonia* (Gereige and Cunill-De Sautu, 2011).

Acute Viral Pharyngitis, Tonsillitis, or Tonsillopharyngitis

Adenoviruses are more likely to cause pharyngitis as a prominent symptom. Other viruses (e.g., rhinovirus) are associated with pharyngitis as a minor symptom and rhinorrhea or cough as predominant features. The enterovirus (coxsackievirus, echovirus), herpesvirus, and EBV are also common. Viral infections occur year-round, but adenovirus presenting as pharyngoconjunctival fever occurs in outbreaks during the summer due to contaminated swimming pools (Gereige and Cunill-De Sautu, 2011). It is helpful to know what agents are currently infecting children in the community. However, when a patient only has a sore throat, it is difficult to differentiate viral from bacterial causes. Hoarseness, cough, coryza, conjunctivitis, and diarrhea are classic features of a viral infection (Gereige and Cunill-De Sautu, 2011).

TABLE 32-2 Differentiations of Common Upper Respiratory Infections in Children

Site of Infection	Symptoms	Duration of Symptoms	Etiologic Agent	Management	Duration of Treatment	Comments
The common cold (viral URI)	Malaise, sneezing, watery nasal discharge, mild sore throat, may have a fever, not ill appearing	0-10 days	Adenovirus, rhinovirus, RSV, parainfluenza, adenovirus	No antibiotics; symptomatic treatment (e.g., saline nose drops, increased fluids); for infants, bulb-syringe the nose before meals and bedtime; for older children, use a humidifier	0-10 days (as long as symptoms last)	If lasts longer than 10-14 days, consider other diagnosis (e.g., rhinosinusitis).
Acute rhinosinusitis (ARS)	Persistent nasal symptoms for more than 10 days with URI, nasal drainage (purulent or discolored), cough Acute presentation with high fever, purulent rhinitis	10-30 days	*Streptococcus pneumoniae, Moraxella catarrhalis,* nontypable *Haemophilus influenzae*	Amoxicillin, or amoxicillin-clavulanic acid	10 days	By 7 days, should be asymptomatic; change antibiotics 48-72 hours after start of treatment if no response.
Subacute rhinosinusitis	Same as above but persistent for at least 30 days	30-84 days	Same as above; may be beta-lactamase producing	Amoxicillin-clavulanic acid		If initial acute infection did not clear, need to switch antibiotics.
Chronic/recurrent rhinosinusitis	Malaise, easy fatigability, unilateral or bilateral nasal discharge, postnasal discharge, nasal obstruction if middle turbinate significantly obstructed	Recurrent >10 to <28 days but symptom free for at least 10 days in between bouts Chronic >84 days	Same as above plus alpha-hemolytic streptococci and *Staphylococcus aureus*	Amoxicillin-clavulanic, azithromycin, staph coverage	3-6 weeks	May need endoscopic sinus surgery if CRS does not respond to prolonged medical management; investigate differential diagnoses or underlying issues (e.g., allergic rhinitis).

CRS, Chronic rhinosinusitis; *RSV,* respiratory syncytial virus; *URI,* upper respiratory infection.

Clinical Findings

History

The following may be reported:

- Pain
- Myalgia and arthralgia
- Fever
- Sore throat and dysphagia
- Rhinitis, cough, hoarseness, stomatitis, stridor and conjunctivitis, nonspecific rash, or diarrhea points to a viral cause (Gereige and Cunill-De Sautu, 2011)
- Acute onset of sore throat with headache, nausea, vomiting, and abdominal pain in the winter and early spring points to GABHS (Gereige and Cunill-De Sautu, 2011)

Physical Examination

Common findings include:

- Erythema of the tonsils and the pharynx
- Reactive cervical lymphadenopathy

Virus-specific physical findings include the following:

- EBV can produce exudate on the tonsils, soft palate petechiae, and diffuse adenopathy.
- Adenovirus can cause a follicular pattern on the pharynx (Cherry, 2009c).
- Enterovirus can produce vesicles or ulcers on the tonsillar pillars and posterior fauces; coryza, vomiting, or diarrhea may be present.
- Herpesvirus produces ulcers anteriorly and marked adenopathy.
- Parainfluenza and RSVs cause more lower respiratory tract disease (e.g., croup, pneumonia, and bronchiolitis) with their typical respiratory signs of stridor, rales, or wheezing.
- Influenza usually is associated with a cough, fever, and multiple systemic complaints.

Diagnostic Studies

A RADT and/or culture should be performed in children older than 3 years old with pharyngitis, because it is difficult to distinguish viral and streptococcal infections by history and physical examination. The incidence of GABHS is rare in children younger than 3 years; however, if there is a child in the household with a positive test for GABHS, children younger than 3 years can be tested (Shulman et al, 2012). In children and adolescents, negative RADT should be backed up by a throat culture, but positive tests do not need a backup due to high specificity of RADT testing (Gereige and Cunill-De Sautu, 2011; Shulman et al, 2012). This careful screening avoids the use of unnecessary antibiotics. Most viral causes of pharyngitis are benign, and other diagnostic studies are not usually used.

Management

For viral infection, only supportive care is needed, including fever and sore throat pain relief with acetaminophen or ibuprofen. Adequate fluid intake should be encouraged.

Acute Bacterial Pharyngitis and Tonsillitis

The most common bacterial cause of pharyngitis and tonsillitis in children and adolescents is GABHS, which accounts for about 15% to 30% of infections in children with acute sore throat and fever. Group C and group G streptococci can cause pharyngitis, but antibiotic treatment does not prevent its only nonsuppurative complication, glomerulonephritis (Shulman et al, 2012). *A. haemolyticum* is more common in adolescents but is difficult to culture, because the organism grows slowly (Martin, 2010). *N. gonorrhoeae* is a cause of adolescent pharyngitis if the patient engages in oral sex. *M. pneumoniae* and *Chlamydophila pneumoniae* are associated with cough along with pharyngitis. *C. diphtheriae* is an extremely rare cause of pharyngitis in the United States. See the GABHS discussion in Chapter 24.

Clinical Findings

History

The following characterize GABHS infection:

- Most commonly found in 5- to 13-year-old children; infrequent in children younger than 3 years old
- Abrupt onset without nasal symptoms
- Constitutional symptoms, such as arthralgia, myalgia, headache
- Moderate to high fever, malaise, prominent sore throat, dysphagia
- Nausea, abdominal discomfort, vomiting, headache
- Presentation in late winter or early spring
- Lack of a cough or nasal symptoms, along with an exudative, erythematous pharyngitis with a follicular pattern and typical historical findings point to GABHS

Physical Examination

The following may be seen in GABHS:

- Petechiae on soft palate and pharynx, swollen beefy-red uvula, red enlarged tonsillopharyngeal tissue
- Tonsillopharyngeal exudate that is yellow, blood-tinged (frequently)
- Tender and enlarged anterior cervical lymph nodes
- Bad breath
- Stigmata of scarlet fever may be seen—scarlatiniform rash, strawberry tongue, circumoral pallor
- Other bacterial infections may present with similar clinical findings:
  - *A. haemolyticum* causes an exudative pharyngitis with marked erythema and a pruritic, fine, scarlatiniform rash (Martin, 2010)
  - Adolescents and young adults with pharyngitis caused by *A. haemolyticum* may present with a scarlatiniform rash similar to scarlet fever
- Variable presentation; may have mild pharyngeal erythema without tonsillar exudate or cervical adenopathy

Diagnostic Studies

It is important to use RADT for patients with clinical features consistent with GABHS to increase the yield of positive tests and avoid false-positive tests on patients who are carriers of streptococcus and do not need treatment. A RADT has a high specificity but variable sensitivity; therefore, a positive test indicates that a symptomatic person has strep infection and should be treated. However, a negative test does not mean that streptococcal infection is not present (Shulman et al, 2012). It is important not to do a strep test unless the patient has signs and symptoms, because a positive rapid strep test or a positive throat culture can identify a carrier state.

Anti-streptococcal antibody titers, such as anti-streptolysin O (ASO) and anti-deoxyribonuclease B tests (anti-DNase B), are not useful in the diagnosis of acute pharyngitis, because the titers remain elevated for months after an acute infection. Anti-streptolysin O (ASO) is the most common test used to document past GABHS infection. ASO and anti-DNase B testing involves documenting antibody titers in response to streptolysin O or deoxyribonuclease B, respectively (Shulman et al, 2012). These two tests are often done together. The ASO titer rises 1 week postinfection and peaks 3 to 6 weeks after infection. Measurement of anti-streptococcal antibody titers is useful in the diagnosis of the nonsuppurative complications of GABHS, such as rheumatic fever or acute glomerulonephritis. The anti-DNase B test rises 1 to 2 weeks after infection, peaks 6 to 8 weeks following infection, and remains elevated for months even in the face of a mild infection with GABHS. As a result, these tests should not be used to diagnosis acute GABHS infection in a patient.

Rare bacterial causes of pharyngitis that need treatment with antibiotics include *C. diphtheriae* and *N. gonorrhoeae*. Adolescents who have oral to genital sex with individuals who have *N. gonorrhoeae* of the genital region can develop pharyngitis from *N. gonorrhoeae. A. haemolyticum* is found in adolescents and young adults with a sore throat, and they may have a scarlatiniform rash similar to scarlet fever. These specimens need to be sent out for a culture with specific instructions to evaluate for these organisms.

If infectious mononucleosis is suspected in a child, a complete blood count (CBC) can identify a lymphocytosis with atypical lymphocytes. This is a nonspecific test, because reactive (atypical) lymphocytes can occur in EBV, acquired CMV, viral hepatitis, rubella, roseola, and mumps (Jensen, 2011). Heterophile antibody testing can be helpful in school-age children and adolescents after the first week of infection but may yield a false negative in preschool and younger children (Gereige and Cunill-De Sautu, 2011). EBV-specific antibody testing is used to confirm acute or past infection. The presence of EBV immunoglobulin M (IgM), EBV IgG, and the late response (3 to 4 months) of antibodies to Epstein-Barr nuclear antigens (anti-EBNA) helps to confirm the diagnosis of EBV. The presence of IgM antibody to the viral capsid antigen is the specific serologic test for EBV infection and generally confirms the diagnosis of acute infection; however, its presence is time sensitive (Jensen, 2011).

Management

Antibiotics should only be used in a symptomatic child with GABHS when the RADT or throat culture is positive due to increasing antibiotic resistance associated with overuse (Shulman et al, 2012). The goal of antibiotic therapy is to shorten the course and severity of illness, prevent the spread of illness to others, and prevent the development of suppurative and nonsuppurative complications. The use of beta-lactam antibiotics during an acute CMV or EBV infection causes a diffuse, morbilliform skin eruption (Schleiss, 2012) and should not be prescribed. It is important to treat these children within 9 days to prevent the nonsuppurative complication of rheumatic fever (Shulman et al, 2012). The management plan includes the following:

- Antimicrobial therapy is based on positive tests results in a symptomatic patient (Shulman et al, 2012):
  - Penicillins (drugs of choice due to cost, efficacy, and infrequent adverse reactions):
    - Penicillin V potassium: Children (27 kg): 250 mg twice daily or three times daily; children (greater than 27 kg), adolescents, and adults: 500 mg twice daily or three times daily for 10 days; can do 250 mg four times a day with teens (Taketomo et al, 2014)
    - Amoxicillin suspension is more palatable (efficacy seems equal to penicillin): 50 mg/kg once daily (maximum dose = 1000 mg); alternate: 25 mg/kg (maximum dose = 500 mg) twice daily for 10 days
    - Benzathine penicillin G intramuscular (IM): 600,000 units as a single dose if less than 27 kg; 1.2 million units as a single dose for larger children and adults
  - If allergic to penicillin:
    - Pen Cephalexin: 20 mg/kg/dose twice daily (maximum dose = 500 mg/dose) for 10 days but should be avoided in patients with moderate hypersensitivity reaction to penicillin.
    - Cefadroxil: 30 mg/kg/day divided twice daily (maximum daily dose = 2 gms/day) for 10 days but should be avoided with moderate hypersensitivity reaction to penicillin.
    - Clindamycin: 7 mg/kg/dose three times daily (maximum dose = 300 mg/dose) for 10 days.
    - Azithromycin: 12 mg/kg once a day to a maximum of 500 mg. It should be noted that macrolide resistance is variable in the United States (Shulman et al, 2012).
    - Clarithromycin: 7.5 mg/kg/dose to a maximum of 250 mg twice per day for 10 days.
- Supportive care: Antipyretics, fluids, and rest.
- Use of corticosteroids is not indicated (Shulman et al, 2012).
- Repeat culture is not generally needed except in situations where it is necessary to ensure eradication of the organism.
- Continued symptoms of streptococcal pharyngitis and a positive culture for streptococcus may represent an actual

treatment failure or a new infection with a different serologic type of streptococcus.

- Noncompliance with pharmacologic therapy can explain treatment failure, and in these instances, an injection of benzathine penicillin is recommended.
- Fomites, such as bathroom cups, toothbrushes, or orthodontic devices, may harbor GABHS and should be cleaned or discarded.
- Children can return to school when they are afebrile and have been taking antibiotics for at least 24 hours.
- Streptococcal treatment guidelines may include tonsillectomy as an intervention for recurrent GABHS; note that tonsillectomy should only be considered for the rare child who fails to improve over time despite good compliance (Shulman et al, 2012). This recommendation is different from the guidelines issued for tonsillectomy discussed earlier (Belderbos et al, 2011).
- Treatment of chronic symptomatic carriage of GABHS:
  - Clindamycin: 20 to 30 mg/kg/day in three doses (maximum dose = 300 mg/dose) for 10 days
  - Amoxicillin-clavulanic acid: 40 mg/kg/day in three doses (maximum daily dose = 2000 mg/day) for 10 days
  - Penicillin V: 50 mg/kg/day in four doses for 10 days (maximum dose = 2000 mg/day) with the use of rifampin: 20 mg/kg/day in one dose (maximum dose = 600 mg/day) during the last 4 days of treatment
  - Benzathine penicillin G: 600,000 units for less than 27 kg and 1,200,000 units for 27 kg or greater; rifampin: 20 mg/kg/day in two doses (maximum dose = 600 mg/day)
  - If clinical relapse occurs, a second course of antibiotic is indicated, as discussed earlier. If recurrent infection is a problem, culturing of the family for the chronic carrier state is advised.

Complications

Major nonsuppurative late complications caused by GABHS are rheumatic fever, poststreptococcal reactive arthritis, and acute glomerulonephritis. Suppurative complications include cervical adenitis, rhinosinusitis, otitis media, pneumonia, mastoiditis, and retropharyngeal or peritonsillar abscess. Retropharyngeal abscess is more common in children younger than 6 years old, whereas peritonsillar abscess is more common from the ages of 20 to 40 years old (Gereige and Cunill-De Saut, 2011). Recurrent GABHS tonsillopharyngitis can also be a problem. Sydenham chorea is linked to GABHS infection. Pediatric autoimmune neuropsychiatric disorder syndrome (PANDAS) is characterized by various movement disorders, including tics, hyperactivity, paroxysmal and stereotypic motor movement, and psychiatric symptoms (e.g., obsessions and compulsions) and is associated with prior GABHS infection. There are five clinical criteria to diagnosis PANDAS. The child must have an (1) obsessive-compulsive disorder and/or other tic disorders; (2) onset of the disease must be prepubertal (3 years old to pubertal onset); (3) abrupt onset with a symptom course that is relapsing and remitting; (4) clear association with GABHS infection; and (5) neurologic abnormalities, such as motor hyperactivity or adventitious movements associated with exacerbations (Esposito et al, 2014). Due to the difficulties in establishing the temporal relationship between GABHS infection and the onset of neuropsychiatric symptoms and the lack of improvement with antibiotic therapy, it has been suggested that the diagnosis be changed to pediatric acute neuropsychiatric symptoms (PA6NS). This would require a complete history and examination confirming the sudden acute onset of neuropsychiatric symptoms with therapies based on treatment of the symptoms (Swedo et al, 2012).

Rhinosinusitis

Inflammation and edema of the mucous membranes lining the sinuses cause obstruction and set up an ideal situation for bacteria to invade the sinus cavities. The maxillary and anterior ethmoid sinuses are most frequently involved in children because they are present at birth, but only the ethmoidal sinuses are pneumatized. (Refer to Pathophysiology Involved in Airway Disease earlier in this chapter.)

Rhinosinusitis can be divided into acute or chronic designations. *Acute rhinosinusitis (ARS)* involves inflamed mucosal lining of the nasal passages and paranasal sinuses lasting as long as 4 weeks. *Chronic rhinosinusitis (CRS)* symptoms must persist for 12 weeks or longer (Brook, 2013). It is estimated that 5% to 10% of URIs are complicated by sinusitis (Wald et al, 2013).

The common bacterial organisms responsible for ARS include *Streptococcus pneumoniae,* nontypable *Haemophilus influenzae, Moraxella catarrhalis,* and, less often, *Staphylococcus aureus* (Brook, 2013). The common bacteria responsible for CRS are similar to ARS. They include *S. pneumonia, M. catarrhalis,* and nontypable *H. influenza.* Chronic sinusitis may be supported by bacterial exotoxins and biofilm formation. Biofilms are a common mode of bacterial growth, resulting in multicellular communities joined together by a self-produced extracellular matrix. They decrease the efficacy of antimicrobials by a hundredfold, allowing bacterial growth in the nose and sinuses (Rose et al, 2013).

Predisposing factors for CRS include a preceding viral, bacterial, and/or fungal infection; environmental irritants; allergies; anatomic problems, including septal deviation, nasal polyps, trauma, FB, or abnormality of the ostiomeatal complex; gastroesophageal reflux; cigarette smoking; CF; primary ciliary dyskinesia, and immunodeficiencies (Brook, 2013; Rose et al, 2013). Persistent swelling of the sinonasal mucosa impairs sinus drainage.

The presence of antibiotic-resistant organisms is associated with prior antibiotic therapy. The role of viruses in rhinosinusitis is not clear. Children with immunodeficiency disorders or CF are predisposed to infections with *Aspergillus* and *Zygomycetes.*

Clinical Findings

The duration of symptoms determines the classification of rhinosinusitis as described earlier. The history of acute sinusitis is different from an uncomplicated URI. The latter may present with a thick, yellow discharge on the third or fourth day (peaking by day 6) with no or low-grade fever followed by improvement. The history of sinusitis is either acute with high fever and purulent nasal discharge or a "double sickening" in which the child experiences worsening of symptoms after initial symptoms of recovering from the URI (Wald et al, 2013). Headache, bad breath, fatigue, and decreased appetite are nonspecific symptoms and therefore not helpful in the diagnosis. CRS is also associated with intractable wheezing in children with asthma (Cherry and Shapiro, 2009).

Major criteria suggestive of acute bacterial sinusitis include facial pain, facial or nasal congestion or fullness, nasal discharge, purulence or discolored postnasal drip, hyposmia or anosmia, fever, and/or purulence on intranasal examination.

Minor criteria include headache, fever, halitosis, fatigue, dental pain, cough, and ear pain, pressure, or fullness (Brook, 2013). Transillumination and percussion of the sinuses are not recommended (Wald et al, 2013).

Diagnostic Studies

Imaging studies are not needed in sinusitis, because MRI, CT, and plain radiographs are likely to be positive for sinusitis if the patient has a cold. However, if these studies are negative for sinusitis, the child does not have sinusitis. If the child is suspected of having an orbital or CNS extension of sinusitis, then contrast-enhanced CT or MRI with contrast is needed. However, both studies are complementary when the diagnosis is in doubt (Wald et al, 2013).

Differential Diagnosis

Viral URI, allergic rhinitis, and other causes of headache are the differential diagnoses. Remember that sinusitis may exacerbate asthma. Ethmoiditis can occur after a child is 6 months old, in contrast to frontal rhinosinusitis, which is first seen around 10 years old.

Management

The health provider must be cautious to not overdiagnose rhinosinusitis and subsequently indiscriminately use antibiotics (DeMuri and Wald, 2010). Chronic or recurrent rhinosinusitis may result in referral to an otolaryngologist and/or allergist.

To aid the clinician in decision making about when to treat, the American Academy of Pediatrics (AAP) developed clinical guidelines for the treatment of ARS based upon three different clinical presentations (Wald et al, 2013):

- The child with an URI with persistent nasal discharge or daytime cough lasting for more than 10 days without clinical improvement
- The child with a URI who develops a worsening or new onset of fever, nasal discharge, or daytime cough after initial improvement
- The child with a fever higher than 102.2° F (39° C) with purulent nasal discharge for at least 3 days who also has sinusitis

Severe onset or a worsening course requires oral antibiotics. If the child has a persistent illness suggestive of rhinosinusitis, antibiotics can be given or a watchful waiting for 3 days can be offered. Symptomatic pain relief with acetaminophen or ibuprofen has been shown to be helpful. The sinusitis guidelines suggest treatment with amoxicillin with or without clavulanate as a first-line treatment (Wald et al, 2013). Treatment length varies from 10 to 28 days. An alternative to this is to continue treatment for 7 days after the patient is completely free of any signs or symptoms. After starting treatment with antibiotics or watchful waiting, reassessment is needed after 72 hours.

Treatment considerations include the following:

- Amoxicillin at a standard dose of 45 mg/kg/day divided in two doses is the first-line treatment in communities with low incidence of nonsusceptible *S. pneumoniae.* In communities with more than 10% of resistant *S. pneumonia,* amoxicillin should be used at 80 to 90 mg/kg/day divided every 12 hours (maximum dose: 1000 mg/dose).
- In patients younger than 2 years old, day care attendees, recent antimicrobial use, or in patients with moderate to severe illness, amoxicillin-clavulanate at 80 to 90 mg/day of amoxicillin component divided every 12 hours with a maximum of 2 g per dose should be prescribed.
- In vomiting children, a single dose of 50 mg/kg of ceftriaxone can be given either IV or IM.

In patients with allergy to amoxicillin, the type of allergic reaction determines the antibiotic:

- If the child has a serious type 1 immediate or accelerated reaction, the cephalosporins cannot be used. However, if they have a non-type 1 hypersensitivity reaction, they can safely be treated with one of the third-generation, cephalosporin antibiotics—cefdinir, cefpodoxime, or cefuroxime.

The management of CRS is more complicated because bacteria are generally only one of other contributing factors. Referral to an otolaryngologist is often needed. Children with complications or signs of invasive infection should be referred to the appropriate medical specialist. Surgical drainage by an otolaryngologist, treatment of allergies and control of allergic rhinitis by an allergist, or both may be necessary.

Additional management considerations include the following:

- *Decongestants and antihistamines:* There is no randomized controlled trial (RCT) to support the use of topical decongestants (Wald et al, 2013). Similarly, there are no data to support the use of either topical or oral antihistamines as an adjuvant therapy. See Chapter 25 for information on the use of decongestants and antihistamines.

- *Topical corticosteroids:* The data for the use of topical corticosteroid in children are plagued with methodological problems; thus, a clear recommendation for topical corticosteroid use in children cannot be made.
- *Saline irrigation:* The use of buffered isotonic saline into the nasal cavity by squeeze bottle or neti pot (in late childhood and adolescence) may be helpful, but the clinical guidelines do not support or negate the use of saline (Wald et al, 2013). Nasal saline can be used by patients to help thin secretions.
- *Analgesics:* Comfort measures include the use of acetaminophen and ibuprofen for severe pain. Adequate hydration is important.
- Diving is contraindicated with rhinosinusitis.

Complications

Orbital extension, inflammation, and infection from an ethmoid sinusitis in a child younger than 5 years old are the most common complications with sinusitis (Wald et al, 2013). Orbital cellulitis secondary to ethmoiditis is a serious, life-threatening complication that is a medical emergency. It is manifested by swelling and erythema of the eyelids, proptosis, decreased extraocular movements, and altered vision. Other orbital complications include periorbital or preseptal inflammation involving only the eyelid as well as orbital cellulitis.

CNS inflammation and infection is another possible complication of sinusitis. Intracranial complications include Pott's puffy tumor, epidural abscess, subperiosteal abscess, brain abscess, venous thrombosis, and meningitis. The child with Pott's puffy tumor has osteomyelitis of the frontal bone, and a neurosurgical consult should be obtained.

An infectious disease and otolaryngology consult is important in all patients with complications (Wald et al, 2013).

Prevention

Prevention of sinusitis includes good allergy management, management of gastroesophageal reflux, influenza vaccine, and relief of nasal airway obstruction.

Diphtheria

Diphtheria is a rare infection of the respiratory tract caused by toxigenic strains of gram-positive *C. diphtheriae* or, less commonly, *Corynebacterium ulcerans.* The toxigenic strains produce two exotoxins—enzymatically active A domain and binding B domain. The binding B domain promotes entry of A into the cell. The bacterium has four biotypes (mitis, intermedius, belfanti, and gravis) that can be toxigenic or nontoxigenic. The ability of a strain of *C. diphtheriae* to produce toxin is related to bacteriophage infection of the bacterium, not to colony type.

Humans are the only reservoir, and the organism is spread by respiratory droplets as well as contact with skin lesions. There have been no cases in the United States since 2003 (AAP, 2012). The bacteria can be shed for 2 to 6 weeks in an untreated patient. Disease may be mild or asymptomatic in partially or fully immunized individuals and severe if unimmunized. With toxin production, the primary infection can become lethal.

Although rare, fomites can act as a vehicle of transmission; and raw milk and milk products can transmit *C. diphtheriae.* Asymptomatic carriers can transmit the organism. The incubation period averages from 2 to 7 days but occasionally can be longer (AAP, 2012). The incidence of respiratory diphtheria is greater in the fall and the winter, but skin infections are more common in the summer. Endemic areas include Africa, Latin America, Asia, and the Middle East. In developing countries, a diphtheria-like illness caused by *C. ulcerans* is emerging (AAP, 2012).

Clinical Findings

History

Infection is associated with a history of low-grade fever and gradual onset of symptoms over 1 to 2 days with bacterial shedding for 2 to 6 weeks if untreated. Fully immunized individuals can carry the bacteria asymptomatically and may present with a mild sore throat (AAP, 2012).

Primary Infection

- Low-grade fever
- Grayish, adherent pseudomembrane found in either the nasopharynx, pharynx, or trachea
- Bloody nasal discharge (with membranous pharyngitis is highly suggestive of diphtheria) (AAP, 2012)
- Sore throat, serosanguineous or seropurulent nasal discharge, hoarseness, cough
- Cutaneous lesions (nonhealing ulcers with dirty gray membrane or colonization of preexisting dermatoses) infected with diphtheria (seen less often)
- Extensive neck swelling with cervical lymphadenitis, causing airway obstruction (due to membranous obstruction of the upper airway)
- Possible otic and/or conjunctival infection findings

Clinical indications of toxin production include the following: myocarditis and electrocardiographic changes, respiratory compromise, cranial nerve and local neuropathies, and peripheral neuritis.

Diagnostic Studies

A confirmatory diagnosis is based on a positive culture of *C. diphtheriae.* Specimens should be obtained from the nose, throat, any skin lesions, and either beneath the membrane or from a portion of the membrane. Because a special culture medium is needed, the lab needs to be notified if *C. diphtheriae* is suspected. Toxigenicity tests are performed if *C. diphtheriae* is confirmed. Culture results take 8 to 48 hours; however, treatment begins when diphtheria is suspected (AAP, 2012). Do not wait for laboratory confirmation. Results of the CBC may be normal or show a slight leukocytosis and thrombocytopenia.

Differential Diagnosis

Acute streptococcal pharyngitis and infectious mononucleosis are included in the differential diagnosis of pharyngeal diphtheria. A nasal FB or purulent rhinosinusitis can resemble nasal diphtheria; epiglottitis, laryngeal diphtheria, and viral croup can also cause obstruction.

Management

Children with diphtheria require hospitalization. Treatment consists of the following:

- *Antitoxin administration (hyperimmune equine antiserum):* A single dose needs to be administered if there is a high index of suspicion prior to a positive culture result (AAP, 2015). Allergic reaction to the serum occurs in 5% to 20%, so a scratch test should be performed prior to administration. IV immunoglobulin has not been approved for use.
- *Antimicrobial therapy:* Erythromycin given orally or parenterally for 14 days, penicillin G for 14 days either IM or IV, or penicillin G procaine IM for 14 days. This is not a substitute for antitoxin administration.
- Supportive care for respiratory, cardiac, and neurologic complications as appropriate.
- Standard and droplet precautions until two cultures are negative.
- Immunization after recovery because disease does not necessarily confer immunity.
- Monitoring and antimicrobial prophylaxis of contacts regardless of immunization status.
- Care for respiratory, cardiac, and neurologic complications.

Complications and Prevention

Peripheral neuropathy, myocarditis, acute tubular necrosis, and respiratory collapse can occur with severe disease. Universal immunization against diphtheria with regular booster injections is the only effective method of control. Infection can occur in immunized or partially immunized children, but the disease severity is greatly diminished in these individuals. Disease generally occurs in nonimmunized children; the frequency of severe life-threatening complications in this group is high. Care of a child exposed to diphtheria is individualized and based on immunization status, likelihood of follow-up, and compliance with antimicrobial therapy. The AAP Committee on Infectious Diseases' *Red Book* (2012) lists specific guidelines that should be followed for the care of exposed children.

Pertussis

Classic pertussis is either a primary disease or reinfection. Pertussis is caused by a gram-negative bacillus, *Bordetella pertussis,* of which there are six species. The most common types are *B. pertussis* and *B. parapertussis* (*B. parapertussis* causes a mild pertussis-like illness). *B. bronchiseptica* infrequently causes respiratory infection, and *B. holmesii* causes bacteremia. The last three bacteria are not affected by the vaccine. This infection is also known as *whooping cough* because of the high-pitched inspiratory whoop following spasms of coughing.

B. pertussis produces a variety of components that are highly antigenic as well as biologically active. These include pertussis toxin (PT), adenylate cyclase toxin, dermonecrotic toxin, fimbriae, filamentous hemagglutinin, pertactin, and autotransporters. Pertactin, filamentous hemagglutinin, and fimbriae allow for bacterial adhesion, whereas PT inactivates the signaling pathways of the immune system, leading to a delay in recruitment of neutrophils. PT also causes the lymphocytosis and leukocytosis seen in the disease, as well as an activation of pancreatic beta cells leading to hypoglycemia. The *B. pertussis* irritates and inflames the ciliated epithelium lining, leading to tissue necrosis with epithelial cell damage from macrophages and reactive lymphoid hyperplasia (Snyder and Fisher, 2012).

Transmission of these gram-negative pleomorphic bacilli is by aerosol droplet from coughing or from close contact with infected individuals. Contaminated droplets are inhaled and adhere to the ciliated epithelium of the nasopharynx. The incubation period is usually 7 to 10 days but can range from 5 to 21 days (AAP, 2015). Children are most contagious during the catarrhal stage and the first 2 weeks after the cough onset (AAP, 2012). The usual source of *B. pertussis* infection in infants is an unrecognized infection in an adult family member with a cough. The highest incidence of mortality occurs in infants less than 1 month old (Cherry and Heininger, 2009).

The classic cough of pertussis lasts 6 to 10 weeks, but in 50% of adolescents it can last longer than 10 weeks. In infants under 6 months, there may be a short catarrhal stage and no whoop but a prolonged recovery period (AAP, 2012). Table 32-3 shows the stages of pertussis with accompanying symptoms. The cough is an attempt to dislodge plugs of necrotic bronchial epithelial tissue and thick mucus.

Outbreaks of pertussis are increasing despite vaccination of adolescents and adults (Chiappini et al, 2013). Older children and adults are the likely vector of pertussis, because their disease may be mild or atypical in course (AAP, 2015). Up to 80% of household contacts acquire the disease from an index case due to waning immunization immunity and unrecognized disease. See Chapter 24 for information about the vaccine.

Clinical Findings

Manifestations of this disease vary by age group, stage of disease, immunization status, and the presence of transplacentally acquired antibodies (Cherry and Heininger, 2009). There is the classic illness and an asymptomatic infection. The latter occurs in patients who are vaccinated or as a primary illness in those who are not vaccinated. Characteristics of the classic disease in infants and young children are found in Table 32-3.

Specific findings in infants younger than 6 months old are generally severe, particularly in neonates, and include:

- Apnea (common) often with seizures caused by hypoxemia
- Cough without an inspiratory whoop
- Tachypnea

TABLE 32-3 Stages of Pertussis

Stage of Pertussis	Length of Time	Manifestation
Catarrhal	1-2 weeks	Nonspecific complaints URI similar to common cold Mild but worsening cough, coryza, sneezing, and low-grade fever (to 101° F [38.3° C])
Paroxysmal	2 to 4 weeks	Fever is absent or minimal Persistent staccato or rapid firing cough, paroxysmal cough ending with an inspiratory whoop Paroxysms can be several times per hour with vomiting at the end Cyanosis, sweating, prostration, and exhaustion after coughing Sleep is disturbed
Convalescent	3 weeks to 6 months	Symptoms wane over a variable period that can last months Waning of paroxysmal coughing episodes

Data from Snyder J, Fisher D: Pertussis in childhood, *Pediatr Rev* 33(9):412–420, 2012.
URI, Upper respiratory infection.

- Poor feeding
- Leukocytosis with a marked lymphocytosis (in the presence of persistent cough illness points to *B. pertussis*)

Findings in children and adolescent may resemble the clinical course illustrated in Table 32-3 (Snyder and Fisher, 2012).

Diagnostic Studies

Although culturing for *B. pertussis* is considered the gold standard for pertussis (it is 100% specific), it should be noted that it is 12% to 60% sensitive, leading to missed diagnosis. It is difficult to do, because it requires collection from the nasopharynx with a Dacron or calcium alginate fiber-tipped swab placed immediately into a special transport medium. It is best done in the first 2 weeks post cough onset. Culture can be negative if the person has been ill for 2 weeks or more, has previously been vaccinated, or if antibiotics have been started (AAP, 2015). The organism is found most frequently during the catarrhal or early paroxysmal stage. Polymerase chain reaction (PCR) is increasingly popular due to its improved sensitivity (70% to 99%) and specificity (86% to 100%), as well as rapid result. PCR testing is done using a Dacron swab or nasal wash from the nasopharynx. However, the U.S. Food and Drug Administration (FDA) has not licensed any PCR tests or commercial kit for diagnostic use (AAP, 2012).

The commercial tests using IgG to PT have not been FDA established, and IgM antibodies lack sensitivity and specificity (AAP, 2012). An increasing titer or a single IgG anti-PT has been used for diagnosis (AAP, 2012). As previously mentioned, leukocytosis and lymphocytosis are common findings in infants and young children, but they are rare in adolescents (AAP, 2012).

Differential Diagnosis

In the classic form of the disease, the diagnosis is clear due to the paroxysmal cough (Mueller et al, 2013). RSV can present with apnea. In infants, *C. trachomatis* is a differential diagnosis but tends to present with an interstitial pattern on chest x-ray (Snyder and Fisher, 2012). *B. parapertussis, C. pneumonia,* and *M. pneumonia* can cause a prolonged course in older children and adolescents. Adenoviruses, bocaviruses, and other viral agents can present with a cough illness. Gastroesophageal reflux, CF, asthma, and FBs should be included in the differential diagnosis.

Management

Treatment consists of the following:

- Treatment with antimicrobial agents in the macrolide class is the treatment of choice. However, because the development of pyloric stenosis is linked with the administration of erythromycin in infants younger than 1 month, its use is discouraged in this age group (AAP, 2015).
- Antibiotic treatment choices include (AAP, 2012; Taketomo et al, 2014):
  - Azithromycin: 10 mg/kg in a single dose for 5 days is given to infants from 1 to 6 months of age.
  - Azithromycin: 5-day treatment for infants older than 6 months of age, children, and adolescents, a single dose of 10 mg/kg/day (maximum dose of 500 mg) on day 1, then a single dose of 5 mg/kg/day (maximum dose of 250 mg) on days 2 to 5.
  - Clarithromycin: For infants, children, and adolescents, 15 mg/kg/day in two divided doses for 7 days with a maximum dose of 1 g/day.
  - Erythromycin: Used in all age groups except for infants younger than 1 month old; for infants 1 to 5 months: 10 mg/kg/dose, four times per day for 14 days; infants 6 months or older and children: 10 mg/kg/dose, four times per day for 7 to 14 days, with a maximum dose of 2 g/day; and adolescents: 500 mg four times a day for 7 to 14 days.
  - Trimethoprim (TMP)-sulfamethoxazole (SMX): Can be used as an alternative in infants older than 2 months who cannot tolerate macrolides at a dose of TMP 8 mg/kg/day and SMX 40 mg/kg/day in divided doses every 12 hours (maximum single dose 160 mg TMP).

- Antimicrobial therapy given in the paroxysmal stage does not alter the course of pertussis, but does limit the spreading of the organism (AAP, 2012).
- Corticosteroids should not be used.
- Use of albuterol and other beta 2-adrenergic medications is not supported by controlled, prospective studies (Bocka, 2014).

Care of Exposed Children

Chemoprophylaxis is recommended for household and close contacts irrespective of immunization status. Early chemoprophylaxis in a household contact can limit secondary transmission. The value of chemoprophylaxis is limited after 21 days has elapsed but should be considered in high-risk household contacts (young infant, pregnant woman, or person who is in contact with infants) (AAP, 2012):

- Immunization coverage with diphtheria-tetanus-acellular pertussis (DTaP) or Tdap depending on age group needs to be reviewed and updated.
- Students and staff in schools need to be monitored for any respiratory symptoms with exclusion and evaluation for anyone with a cough illness.
- Close monitoring of respiratory symptoms for 21 days after last contact with an infected individual.

Complications

The complication rate is higher in infants younger than 6 months old with a 1% mortality reported (Snyder and Fisher, 2012). Complications of pertussis include apnea in young infants, secondary bacterial pneumonia, seizures, encephalopathy, epistaxis, subconjunctival hemorrhage, syncope, sleep disturbances, rib fracture, incontinence, and death (AAP, 2012; Snyder and Fisher, 2012). Activation of tuberculosis is associated with pertussis infection.

Prevention

The concept of "cocooning" around the infant is designed to protect the infants from dangerous or unwanted environmental hazards (Grizas et al, 2012; Healy et al, 2011). The recommendations of this strategy include targeting adult immunization by immunizing adults around the infant, including caretakers, grandparents over 65 years old, fathers, and mothers who were not immunized in the last trimester. In addition, all adolescents 11 to 18 years old should receive the Tdap vaccine. The infrastructure within maternity units as to immunization coverage has to be changed if "cocooning" can take place in hospitals (Grizas et al, 2012).

In addition, the recommended guidelines for the initial series of DTaP vaccines and booster doses should be followed. Remember that just one DTaP immunization can reduce the severity of symptoms in an infant infected with pertussis. See Chapter 24 for a discussion regarding this vaccine. The clinician needs to be mindful of valid contraindications to receiving pertussis vaccine. Immunity following either natural pertussis infection or illness or vaccination is *not* long lasting. Immunity wanes over time, and the vaccine does not confer active immunity. Pertussis in older children, adolescents, and adults is a mild, often unrecognized disease that if transmitted to an unimmunized infant can result in life-threatening illness. Universal immunization of children younger than 7 years old and adolescents is crucial to control this disease.

Recurrent Epistaxis

Recurrent epistaxis is common in children, with an incidence of 30% in children from birth to 5 years old, 56% in school-age children 6 to 10 years old, and 64% in adolescents (Siddiq and Grainger, 2015). It is even higher for families living in dry climates or during the winter months when artificial heating is used. The cause is often benign and typically related to mechanical trauma to the area (e.g., nose-picking), and thus it is generally self-limiting. Other factors that can cause mucosal irritation resulting in bleeding include coagulopathies, allergies, neoplasms (e.g., rhabdomyosarcoma), polyps, hemangiomas, chronic rhinitis, URI, FB, chronic use of topical nasal sprays containing corticosteroids or antihistamine decongestants, and viral or bacterial infections of nasal tissue. In adolescents, epistaxis may result from the use of recreational drugs, such as cocaine.

The bleeding originates from the anterior portion of the nasal septum, called *Little area* where a plexus of vessels (called *Kiesselbach plexus*) meet under the thin nasal mucosa. The blood supply of the Kiesselbach area comes from the external carotid through the external maxillary artery. Posterior nosebleeds are far more common in older adult patients. A coagulopathy, generally von Willebrand disease or platelet aggregation disorders, can manifest as recurrent epistaxis, but a careful history will reveal signs of mucocutaneous bleeding beyond epistaxis that includes easy bruisability and menorrhagia (Cooper and Takemoto, 2014).

Clinical Findings

History

The following may be reported:

- Recent nasal trauma, including nose-picking
- Allergies or a recent URI
- Unexpected bruising or bleeding from other sites
- Frequent nosebleeds (unilateral or bilateral)
- Tarry stools (the result of swallowed blood)

The provider should always ask about a family history of excessive bleeding episodes or bleeding disorders. In addition, topical nasal medication use, including topical steroid spray, nasal decongestants, or in the case of the teen, cocaine or other inhaled recreational drugs should be explored.

Physical Examination

Nares visualization using the otoscope without a tip may reveal fresh or old clots, nasal masses, FB, polyps, and/or raw, red Little area (Patel et al, 2014; Siddiq and Grainger, 2015). The nasal mucosa on the medial surface of the anterior septum may be dry, cracked, excoriated, or scabbed. Signs of nasal allergy including allergic shiners,

Dennie-Morgan lines, adenoidal facies, and pale boggy mucosa should be assessed.

Diagnostic Studies

A baseline hematocrit may be indicated in severe or chronic epistaxis. It can reveal iron deficiency anemia secondary to the bleeding. Unless the history points to a coagulopathy or the nosebleeds are recurrent and refractory to treatment, coagulation studies are not indicated (Siddiq and Grainger, 2015).

If a coagulopathy is suspected, order a CBC, platelet count, prothrombin time, and activated partial thromboplastin time (aPTT). If the labs are normal but the diagnosis is strongly suspected, further workup for von Willebrand disease will be needed (Cooper and Takemoto, 2014).

Differential Diagnosis

Differential diagnoses as to causes of epistaxis include tumors, long-standing nasal FB, congenital bleeding disorders, idiopathic thrombocytopenia purpura (ITP), vasculitis, nasal hemangioma, hereditary hemorrhagic telangiectasia, and allergic rhinitis (Siddiq and Grainger, 2015). A bleeding disorder is characterized by epistaxis that is severe, prolonged, and recurrent. Nonaccidental injury or coagulopathy should be considered in children younger than 2 years of age with spontaneous epistaxis. If epistaxis is associated with a traumatic injury, evaluate for the presence of a nasal fracture and/or septal hematoma. A nasal neoplasm may present with facial swelling, pain, nasal obstruction, eustachian tube dysfunction with effusion, and cranial neuropathies with severe epistaxis. Wegener granulomatosis, a small vessel vasculitis, can present in adolescents with nasal bleeding (Siddiq and Grainger, 2015).

Management

There is a lack of studies regarding the optimal management for epistaxis (Qureishi and Burton, 2012). The following steps are recommended (Haddad, 2011a; Manes, 2010; Siddiq and Grainger, 2015):

- Have the child sit upright and lean forward to prevent swallowing the blood.
- Apply direct pressure at the nasal ala (pinch the nares together at the bony structure) for 10 to 15 minutes. Have the parent watch the time, because perceptions of time are subjective.
- Packing and topical vasoconstrictor drugs are occasionally needed.
- Use a bedside humidifier to moisten the air in dry climates or in winter with forced-air heating. Normal saline nose sprays can add moisture to dry nasal mucosa.
- Apply topical antibiotic to the site of the septal scab for 2 weeks to reduce nasal colonization with *S. aureus* crusting and inflammation.
- Barrier agents like petroleum jelly have not been shown to be effective.
- Topical agents, such as Nosebleeds QR, are hydrophilic polymers that form an artificial scab when they come into contact with blood. These can be applied via a swab to the Kiesselbach plexus. Local applications of a solution of oxymetazoline or Neo-Synephrine (0.25 1%) can also be used.
- Silver nitrate sticks can be used to cauterize exposed vessels if bleeding persists; however, the site must be easily accessible, visible, and not bleeding briskly. It has a high failure rate and is associated with nasal septum atrophy.
- Nasal packing with absorbable oxycellulose material can be used if bleeding continues or the site cannot be localized, but the patients should be referred to an ear, nose, and throat (ENT) specialist for further evaluation and management.
- Treat the underlying cause of the problem (e.g., trauma from nose-picking, dry air, and/or topical nasal sprays).
- Teach parents to leave blood scabs alone, because removal may precipitate further bleeding.

Prevention

Preventive measures include instructions on a good nasal regimen to keep the nasal mucosa moist, such as vaporizer use and normal saline nose drops or sprays. If the child uses nasal corticosteroids, make sure that the child directs the spray laterally rather than toward the septum. This reduces epistaxis related to nasal spray (Siddiq and Grainger, 2015).

Nasal Foreign Body

Young children tend to insert all types of FBs into a body orifice. Nasal FBs can be noted immediately by the parent or lie undetected until classic symptoms appear.

Clinical Findings

History

A persistent or recurrent unilateral purulent nasal discharge is reported. Foul odor, epistaxis, nasal obstruction, and mouth breathing are less commonly reported symptoms (Haddad, 2011b). Young children will often deny inserting a FB.

Physical Examination

The classic symptom of a nasal FB is unilateral, purulent, foul-smelling nasal discharge. If the FB is embedded in granulation tissue or mucosa, it may take on the appearance of a nasal mass. Other symptoms include mouth breathing, epistaxis, and nasal obstruction.

Differential Diagnosis

Nasal polyps, purulent rhinitis, adenoiditis, rhinosinusitis, and nasal tumors are conditions that cause bilateral or unilateral discharge.

Management

Management involves the following (Haddad, 2011b):

- Detection of an FB in the nasal cavity, which establishes the diagnosis.

- Removal of the nasal FB, depending on its location, its composition, and the skill of the practitioner. Alligator forceps, suction with narrow tips, and cotton-tipped applicators with collodion with or without topical vasoconstrictor drugs (to reduce swelling) can be used. Other techniques include using a hook or curette to roll the object out. A 5-French catheter with a balloon can be advanced past the FB; inflate the balloon before removing the catheter and (it is hoped) the object with it.
- Good lighting (use a headlight) is essential, as is immobilization of the young child via papoose board.
- Elevate the child's head and suction blood and secretions.
- Otolaryngology referral is merited for young children who cannot cooperate or when the FB is extremely difficult or dangerous to remove, such as paper clips or staples. Providers must remember that the FB can be forced deeper into the nose if the practitioner is inexperienced at nasal FB removal.

Extrathoracic Airway Disorders

Croup (Laryngotracheitis and Spasmodic Croup)

Croup is an acute, inflammatory disease of the larynx, trachea, and bronchi that clinically presents with a brassy cough that sounds like a bark and is associated with varying degrees of inspiratory stridor, hoarseness, and respiratory distress. Croup (laryngotracheitis and spasmodic croup) causes disease in children younger than 6 years old. The most common form of croup is typically termed *laryngotracheitis*. A viral infection of the glottic region extending into the subglottic region is called *laryngotracheobronchitis (LTB)*, which is the term reserved for the more severe form of croup. It is an extension of laryngotracheitis occurring 5 to 7 days into the disease and is associated with bacterial superinfection (Roosevelt, 2011).

Human parainfluenza types 1 and 2 (less so) are the most common viral agents responsible for fall outbreaks in children 1 to 6 years old, typically in odd numbered years. Other causative agents include other human parainfluenza types (notably HPIV-3), influenza A and B, human coronavirus HL-63, coxsackieviruses, echoviruses, metapneumovirus, adenoviruses, RSV, and rhinovirus (Mejias and Ramilo, 2012).

Viral croup is most common in children between 6 and 36 months old (60% are younger than 24 months), and it occurs most often in fall and winter. HPIV-3 is endemic in children younger than 6 months old and occurs in the spring and summer months, less commonly in the autumn if other parainfluenzae viruses are absent (Fox and Christenson, 2014). The incubation period is 2 to 4 days with viral shedding for up to 1 week before the onset of the disease (can shed up to 3 to 4 weeks with HPIV-3) (Mejias and Ramilo, 2012). See Chapter 24 for more discussion about human parainfluenza viruses. Males are affected more often than females. Recurrent croup and recurrent laryngitis can develop in children until they are 6 years old. A positive family history has been noted in a small percentage of children in whom croup develops. Croup lasts approximately 5 days. With growth, the child's laryngeal tracheal airway is less vulnerable to the effects of viral infections and less susceptible to obstruction.

Clinical Findings

Clinical manifestations depend on the infectious agent responsible for the croup and the extent of the upper airway involvement.

History

The history typically includes the following:

- URI prodromal symptoms (rhinorrhea, conjunctivitis, or both) are sometimes present before stridor
- Acute onset of a hoarse, barking-like cough
- Mild to severe laryngeal obstruction
- Mild to severe inspiratory stridor with dyspnea
- Gradual onset of symptoms (2 to 3 days)
- Symptoms worse at night (Fox and Christenson, 2014)
- May or may not have sore throat
- Duration is generally 3 to 5 days for viral croup
- The presence of fever without reoccurrence differentiates it from spasmodic croup (Fox and Christenson, 2014)

Physical Examination

The following can be seen:

- Slight dyspnea, tachypnea, and retractions
- Mild, brassy, or barking cough (harsh sounding)
- Stridor—a high-pitched, harsh sound from turbulent airflow that is generally inspiratory, but may be biphasic
- Temperature is typically low grade, but may be elevated to 104° F (40° C)
- If visualized on examination of the mouth, the epiglottis will appear normal
- Substernal and chest wall retraction in severe cases
- Prolonged inspiration
- Wheezing and rales may be heard if there is additional lower airway involvement

Diagnostic Studies

Croup is a clinical diagnosis. Radiography of the soft tissues of the neck and chest displays a classic pattern of subglottic narrowing ("steeple sign") on posteroanterior views but is usually not done unless there is a question about the diagnosis. Microbiology cultures of the pharynx can be helpful in selected cases that have atypical presentations with severe fever, toxic presentations, and severe inspiratory stridor because this presentation is more typical of bacterial tracheitis.

Differential Diagnosis

Differential diagnoses include acute epiglottitis; acute spasmodic croup (no signs of infection); FB aspiration; retropharyngeal abscess; extrinsic compression from tumors, trauma, or congenital malformations; angioedema (anaphylaxis) or early asthmatic attack; bacterial tracheitis, infectious mononucleosis; and psychogenic stridor (Roosevelt, 2011).

Croup is different from bacterial tracheitis, which is a bacterial infection of the trachea that occurs rarely and results in inflammatory cell infiltration of the larynx, trachea, and bronchi causing epithelial lining sloughing and mucopurulent membranes (Rajan, 2012). Bacterial tracheitis is a rapidly progressive disease of children 3 weeks to 16 years old accompanied by high fever. The most common ages are between 5 to 7 years old; it is associated with airway obstruction (Roosevelt, 2011). Staphylococcus is the most common organism, but *M. catarrhalis*, nontypable *H. influenzae,* and, less commonly, anaerobic organisms cause this disease (Roosevelt, 2011). Unlike viral croup, bacterial croup results in thick pus within the trachea and lower airways. These patients do not respond to the standard croup treatment and get clinically worse.

Table 32-4 differentiates acute laryngotracheitis from other common causes of stridor.

Management

Therapy depends on the cause, severity, and location of the disease. The aim of therapy is to provide adequate respiratory exchange. Table 32-5 shows management of the patient based on the degree of severity of croup.

- *Humidified air:* A Cochrane review showed no evidence that inhalation of humidified air improved the outcome in croup scores in children with mild to moderate croup (Moore and Little, 2006). There is no evidence that the use of steam or cold humidification is harmful. However, cold air can be helpful. For a child with LTB, taking the child out into the cold night air or putting them by an opened freezer door may be beneficial. Often a ride in a car at night with the windows down accomplishes the same result. There is no evidence for the use of steam or humidification in croup. Occasionally, vomiting relieves the bronchospasm.
- *Nebulized epinephrine:* Nebulized epinephrine has shown benefit in treatment of croup (Bjornson et al, 2013).
- *Corticosteroids:* Corticosteroids decrease inflammation and cell damage without prolonging the viral shedding duration. In patients with croup, dexamethasone, oral or IM (0.6 mg/kg) or nebulized budesonide is beneficial, decreasing return visits and resulting in shorter hospital stay (Russell et al, 2011). IM dexamethasone can be used in a vomiting child. The rate of oral absorption equals that of IM therapy (Cherry, 2009a). The use of these agents should be limited to 1 to 2 days to avoid immunosuppression and the possibility of secondary bacterial infection. Dexamethasone has been shown to reduce inflammatory edema and to prevent destruction of ciliated epithelium (Cherry, 2009a). Antibiotics are not indicated.
- *Cold medications:* Cough and cold medicines are not indicated in croup.
- *Bronchodilators:* If bronchospasm is also suspected, the use of bronchodilators in the usual doses prescribed for relief of asthma (as discussed in Chapter 25) may be advantageous.
- *Oxygen*: Blow-by oxygen is only used if the oxygen saturation falls below 92%.
- *Other modalities:* In severe croup, a helium-oxygen mixture known as *heliox* can be used.

Indications for Hospitalization

Children in distress with respiratory rates between 70 and 90 breaths per minute or exhibiting stridor at rest should be hospitalized. A child with a temperature higher than 102.2° F (39° C) should be carefully evaluated; hospitalization may be necessary if other worrisome symptoms are present. Racemic epinephrine by aerosol may help but should be used in conjunction with corticosteroids to limit rebound swelling (dexamethasone 0.5 to 2 mg/kg/dose every 8 hours IV). Hydration is important (Fox and Christenson, 2014). IV fluids may be needed in patients who cannot tolerate feedings.

Complications

Increasing obstruction of the airways causes continuous stridor, nasal flaring, and suprasternal, infrasternal, and intercostal retractions. With further obstruction, air hunger and restlessness occur and are quickly followed by hypoxia, weakness, decreased air exchange, decreased stridor, increased pulse rate, and eventual death from hypoventilation. Anything that taxes the child's respiratory efforts, such as crying or feeding, causes more respiratory distress. Examination of the nasopharynx with a tongue depressor may result in sudden respiratory compromise. Severely ill children should be evaluated for acute epiglottitis or bacterial tracheitis. Viral pneumonia complicates about 1% to 2% of croup cases.

Acute Spasmodic Croup

Although some people feel that spasmodic croup is the same as croup because there are viral causes for both, others feel they are different. Spasmodic croup is the onset of croup in the early morning hours as a result of laryngopharyngeal reflux accompanied by transient laryngospasm and laryngeal edema (Roosevelt, 2011). The etiologic agents are similar to those in laryngotracheitis (Roosevelt, 2011), but the condition occurs in families with a history of croup. Spasmodic croup presents with minimal coryza and acute onset of nighttime croup in a child that is well or a child with very mild cold symptoms. There is no fever, no pharyngitis, and a normal epiglottis. The episode is usually milder and of short duration, but symptoms may be recurrent. The treatment plan is the same as indicated for acute

TABLE 32-4 Differentiating Common Respiratory Diseases That Can Cause Stridor or Similar Signs

Characteristic	Acute Laryngotracheitis	Epiglottitis	Laryngotracheobronchitis	Diphtheria	Foreign Body
Peak age	3 to 36 months old	1 to 5 years old	3 months to 36 months old	Any age/unimmunized	Toddlers
Onset	Gradual, acute onset at night	Rapid	Acute	Gradual onset over 1-2 days	Acute symptoms or gradual onset
Common findings	URI, seal-bark cough, mild to moderate dyspnea, symptoms worse at night	Sore throat, dysphagia, anxiety with inspiratory distress without significant stridor, drooling, muffled speech, looks toxic, tripod position	Hoarseness with barking cough, inspiratory stridor and toxic presentation with purulent sputum	Membranous nasopharyngitis, obstructive laryngotracheitis with local infection presenting as sore throat, nasal discharge, hoarseness	Coughing and/or choking episode, dyspnea, wheezing, cyanosis, signs and symptoms of secondary infection
Respiratory efforts	Rate generally <50	Marked distress	Marked distress	Minor to significant signs and symptoms of obstruction	Minor to significant distress
Fever	Common—low grade	High (ranges from 101.8° to 104° F [38.8° to 40° C])	High (102.2° F [39° C])	Low grade	Normal to low grade
CBC	Generally normal	High, left shift	High, left shift	Normal to slight leukocytosis, decreased thrombocyte count	Normal unless secondary infection
Organism(s)	Usually viral: parainfluenza, adenovirus, RSV	Usually HIB	Usually *Staphylococcus aureus*	*Corynebacterium diphtheria*	
Specific laboratory tests	None	None	None	Positive culture	None
Radiographic view with findings	Lateral or AP of neck/ subglottic narrowing	Lateral of neck/thumb sign	Lateral of neck/subglottic narrowing	Signs of obstruction in severe cases	May see localized hyperinflation, mediastinal shift, atelectasis
Treatment	Humidification, corticosteroids in selected cases	Hospitalization, cephalosporin, corticosteroids	Hospitalization, staphylococcus coverage	Hospitalization, erythromycin/ penicillin, antitoxin	FB removal, treatment of secondary infection or bronchospasm
Intubation	Rare	Usually necessary	Frequently necessary	May be necessary	Endoscopy to remove FB
Prevention	None	Immunization—HIB	None	Immunization—DTaP	Education on child-proofing home and monitoring child

AP, Anteroposterior; *CBC*, complete blood count; *DTaP*, diphtheria-tetanus-acellular pertussis; *FB*, foreign body; *HIB*, *Haemophilus influenzae* type B; *RSV*, respiratory syncytial virus; *URI*, upper respiratory infection.

TABLE 32-5 Croup Severity and Treatment Based on Severity

Symptoms and Treatment	Mild	Moderate	Severe	Impending Respiratory Failure
Symptoms	Occasional croupy cough No retractions No chest wall retractions	Frequent croupy cough Audible stridor and suprasternal and sternal retractions at rest No agitation	Frequent croupy cough Tachypnea Prominent inspiratory and occasional expiratory stridor Agitation and distress	Audible stridor at rest Sternal retractions Lethargy Decreased level of consciousness with dusky color
Treatment				
Education of parent	X	X	X	X
Corticosteroid	X	X	X	X
Nebulized epinephrine			X	X
Blow-by oxygen			X	X until intubation
Intubation				X

Data from Alberta Clinical Practice Guidelines Working Group: *Guidelines for diagnosis and management of croup*, Canada, 2003; Alberta, ON.

LTB. Spasmodic croup tends to respond well to exposure to cool air.

Epiglottitis

Epiglottitis (supraglottitis) is characterized by inflammation of the epiglottis, the aryepiglottic folds, and the ventricular bands at the base of the epiglottis. The causative organism is *Haemophilus influenzae* type B (HIB). It occurs usually in children between 1 and 5 years old with 25% of cases in children younger than 2 years old. The disease is 4 to 10 times higher in Navajo Native Americans and Alaska Natives (Cherry, 2009b). Since the introduction of the HIB vaccine, there has been a drastic decline in the number of children with invasive infections caused by this organism; fortunately, epiglottitis is now a rare event. The following organisms have been implicated as causes of supraglottitis: *S. pneumoniae, S. aureus, H. parainfluenzae,* group A, B, C, and G streptococcus, and *Bacillus* spp.

Clinical Findings

History

There is an abrupt onset of fever, severe sore throat, dyspnea, inspiratory distress without stridor, and drooling. The child looks acutely ill and toxic.

Physical Examination

Findings include the following:

- Inspiratory and sometimes expiratory stridor
- Drooling, aphonia (muffled voice), and high fever
- Rapidly progressive respiratory obstruction and prostration
- Flaring of the ala nasi and retraction of the supraclavicular, intercostal, and subcostal spaces
- Child assumes a position of hyperextension of the neck

In older children, one may find:

- Complaints of sore throat and dysphagia
- Stridor, irritability, restlessness, and brassy cough (uncommon)
- Airway obstruction follows within 2 to 24 hours; the child sits up with arms back, trunk forward, neck hyperextended, and chin thrust forward (tripod position)
- A rare, unusual finding is that of just a hoarse cough and a cherry-red epiglottis

Diagnostic Studies

Blood cultures should be ordered. If the possibility of epiglottitis is thought to be remote in a patient with croup, a lateral neck radiograph may be obtained before the physical examination is undertaken. Absence of the "thumb" sign on the radiograph rules out the condition. A health care professional capable of supporting the airway and skilled in intubation must accompany the child to the radiology department and back.

Management

The time from the onset of symptoms until death may be only a matter of hours. Acute epiglottitis is a pediatric otolaryngologic emergency because of the risk of sudden airway obstruction. The goal of therapy is to establish an airway and appropriately start antimicrobials. If epiglottitis is suspected, do not examine the throat. Do not place the child in the supine position, and immediately transport the child to the hospital via emergency medical services. The child should be examined in the operating room by an otolaryngologist or an emergency department physician skilled in performing an emergency tracheostomy. An airway must be established, either a nasotracheal airway or a tracheostomy. The diagnosis is confirmed in the operating room by depressing the tongue to view the swollen cherry-red epiglottis. An expert in establishing an airway needs to be present because there is a risk of reflex laryngospasm, with acute and complete airway obstruction.

Begin the following treatments:

- Establish an airway, preferably by nasotracheal intubation (Cherry, 2009b).
- Administer IV broad-spectrum antibiotics to cover *H. influenzae.*
- Administer oxygen and respiratory support.

The acute infection rarely lasts more than 48 to 72 hours. However, idiopathic pulmonary edema can follow (in up to 9% of patients) after the establishment of an airway due to the changes in pulmonary microvascular pressure subsequent to relieving the obstruction. As improvement occurs, the child can be extubated, but antibiotic therapy should be continued for 10 days. Children heal completely. Untreated or undertreated patients have a significant mortality rate. Remember that the time from the onset of symptoms to death can be a matter of hours. If *H. influenzae* is identified as the causative agent, rifampin prophylaxis (20 mg/kg in a single dose [maximum, 600 mg] for 4 days for infants and children and 600 mg once a day for adults for 4 days) should be given to all household contacts of the patient whose household has:

- At least one child younger than 4 years old who is unimmunized or incompletely immunized
- Children less than 12 months old who have not received the primary series of HIB vaccine
- Immunocompromised children (AAP, 2012; Cherry, 2009b)

In addition, if there are two cases of invasive HIB disease in a day care center or nursery within 60 days, all members of the nursery need to receive prophylaxis (AAP, 2012).

Complications

The complications from epiglottis involve systemic spread of the organism causing the epiglottis and include cervical lymphadenitis, pneumonia, otitis media, or less commonly septic arthritis or meningitis (Roosevelt, 2011).

Prevention

Routine immunization against HIB, the leading cause of epiglottitis, is the primary means of prevention. Hand washing is also an effective method of preventing spread of infection. See the prior discussion regarding rifampin prophylaxis.

Intrathoracic Airway Disorders

Bronchiolitis

Bronchiolitis is also called *infectious asthma, asthmatic bronchitis, wheezy bronchitis,* or *virus-induced asthma.* Bronchiolitis is a disease that causes inflammation, necrosis, and edema of the respiratory epithelial cells in the lining of small airways, as well as copious mucus production (Ralston et al, 2014). Bronchiolitis is characterized by the insidious onset of URI symptoms over 2 to 3 days that progresses to lower respiratory symptoms that last as long as 10 days (Da Dalt et al, 2013). It is a communicable disease found primarily in infancy to 2 years old (Teshome et al, 2013) that accounts for 10% of visits to a primary provider the first 2 years of life (Schroeder and Mansbach, 2014). Bronchiolitis is a common diagnosis used for an infant seen with wheezing for the very first time and is the leading cause of hospitalizations for infants. The most common age for severe disease occurs in infants between 2 to 3 months due to the natural postnatal nadir in maternal immunoglobulins received via the placenta during the last trimester (Da Dalt et al, 2013). More than 80% of the cases of bronchiolitis occur in infants younger than 1 year of age with a male-to-female ratio of 1.5 : 1 (Welliver, 2009). In mild cases, symptoms can last for 1 to 3 days. In severe cases, cyanosis, air hunger, retractions, and nasal flaring with symptoms of severe respiratory distress within a few hours may be seen. Apnea can occur with a wide range of prevalence reported (Ralston et al, 2014) and may require mechanical ventilation.

Newer understanding of the pathophysiology in bronchiolitis points to airway obstruction as a result of epithelial and inflammatory cellular debris due to infiltration of the virus into the small bronchiole epithelium and alveolar epithelial cells (AEC), types I and II. Membranous pneumatoceles, or AEC type I, are dominant and cover 96% of the respiratory tree. Their role is in gas exchange, whereas AEC type II are important to surfactant production (Chuquimia et al, 2013). It is a disease of the small bronchioles that are 2 mm in size. There is a sparing of basal cells in the bronchiole. The main lesion is epithelial necrosis, which leads to a dense plugging of the bronchial lining. This results in increased airway resistance, atelectasis, hyperinflation, and increased mucus production (Teshome et al, 2013).

Bronchiolitis is a viral illness predominantly caused by RSV, especially in outbreaks (Da Dalt et al, 2013; Welliver, 2009). Recent data suggest that up to 30% of infants with severe bronchiolitis are co-infected with two or more viruses (Mansbach et al, 2012). In descending order after RSV, rhinovirus, parainfluenza, adenovirus, and mycoplasma are causes (Teshome et al, 2013). Metapneumovirus was discovered in 2001 and is a cause of bronchiolitis 7% of the time. Human bocavirus is a common co-infecting virus with RSV and is found up to 80% of the time (Teshome et al, 2013). RSV-specific immunoglobulin E (IgE), eosinophils, and chemokines may play a role in the pathogenesis of bronchiolitis (Welliver, 2009). Adenovirus and RSV can cause long-term complications. The incubation period for RSV is 2 to 8 days and typically occurs from November through March with virtually no outbreaks in the summer (Teshome et al, 2013; Welliver, 2009). Fever tends to be higher with adenovirus versus RSV (Teshome et al, 2013).

Respiratory viruses are spread by close contact with infected respiratory secretions or fomites and can live on surfaces for up to 30 minutes (Teshome et al, 2013). The most frequent mode of transmission is hand carriage of contaminated secretion. The source of infection is an older child or adult family member with a "mild" URI. Older children and adults have larger airways and tolerate the swelling associated with this infection better than infants do. Most cases of bronchiolitis resolve completely, but recurrence of infection is common, and symptoms tend to be mild.

Infants who are at higher risk of severe RSV include children with major chronic pulmonary disease, such as CF, neuromuscular disorders, or bronchopulmonary dysplasia; premature birth before 35 weeks of gestational age; and infants with significant hemodynamically difficulties due to congenital heart disease (Teshome et al, 2013). Other risk factors for severe RSV disease are male gender, crowded household, lack of breastfeeding, smoke exposure, day care attendance, having siblings, birth during the winter months, and immunodeficiency (Da Dalt et al, 2013).

Clinical Findings

History

The following are reported:

- Initial presentation: Typically the illness begins with URI symptoms of cough, coryza, and rhinorrhea and progresses over 3 to 7 days (Smith, 2011).
- Gradual development of respiratory distress marked by noisy, raspy breathing with audible expiratory wheezing.
- Low-grade to moderate fever up to 102°F (38.9°C).
- Decrease in appetite.
- No prodrome in some infants; rather they have apnea as the initial symptom.
- Usually the patient's course is the worst by 48 to 72 hours after the wheezing starts and then the patient starts to improve. If the child has a bacterial illness, the child will continue to worsen with a high fever.

Physical Examination

Findings include the following:

- Upper respiratory findings
  - Coryza
  - Mild conjunctivitis in 33% (Welliver, 2009)
  - Pharyngitis
  - Otitis media in up to 15% (Welliver, 2009)
- Lower respiratory findings (Teshome et al, 2013)
  - Tachypnea (approximately 40 to 80 breaths per minute)
  - Substernal and/or intercostal retractions
  - Heterophonous expiratory wheezing
  - Fine or coarse crackles may be heard throughout the breathing cycle
  - Varying signs of respiratory distress and pulmonary involvement (e.g., nasal flaring, grunting, retractions, cyanosis, prolonged expiration)
  - Abdominal distention
  - Palpable liver and spleen, pushed down by hyperinflated lungs and a flattened diaphragm

Diagnostic Studies

A diagnosis of bronchiolitis should be based on the history and physical examination (Ralston et al, 2014). Overuse of diagnostic testing persists in clinical practice despite available guidelines on the diagnosis and management of bronchiolitis (Librizzi et al, 2014; Ralston et al, 2014; Turner et al, 2014). The routine use of chest radiographs in previously healthy infants with mild RSV bronchiolitis is not indicated. Evidence-based guidelines from the AAP and the Scottish Intercollegiate Guidelines Network (SIGN) are strongly against routine chest radiography, including those in previously healthy infants with mild RSV bronchiolitis (Ralston et al, 2014; SIGN, 2006). In severe illness, a chest x-ray may be ordered to rule out pneumonia or pneumothorax, but its use must be weighed against the dangers of radiation exposure. The findings of chest radiography can vary, and even with severe illness the x-ray can be clear with a flattened diaphragm and an increase in anteroposterior diameter. Areas of atelectasis can appear like a pneumonitis, but true pneumonia is uncommon (early bacterial pneumonia can be difficult to detect and cannot be ruled out by radiographs).

Routine virologic testing is not recommended. In selected situations (hospitalization or if an infant has received monthly palivizumab [Synagis]), enzyme-linked immunosorbent assays or fluorescent antibody techniques to look for RSV are the diagnostic procedures of choice in most laboratories. Viral culture of nasal washings can be done in severe cases to confirm RSV, parainfluenza viruses, influenza viruses, and adenoviruses. PCR is helpful in deciding about isolation of cohorts with the same infection in the hospital setting. The cost of the diagnostic viral testing may outweigh the clinical usefulness of knowing which virus is infecting the patient.

Hematologic testing is not recommended in the latest guidelines. If a CBC is done for another reason, a mild leukocytosis may be seen with 12,000 to 16,000/mm^3. Routine laboratory tests are usually not required to confirm the diagnosis, because they lack specificity. However, young infants pose a diagnostic dilemma, because they are at greater risk of a serious bacterial infection (SBI) and, therefore, blood cultures and CBC with differential are done with a higher rate of antibiotic use in infants who had these blood tests (Librizzi et al, 2014). Urine cultures actually have a higher rate of positive results in the young febrile infant (up to 2.3% in a bronchiolitis study conducted by Librizzi and colleagues).

Differential Diagnosis

The diagnosis of bronchiolitis can be confused with asthma, but there are some differences that may be helpful. Asthma is an acute process due to airway hyperreactivity and inflammation, whereas the onset of bronchiolitis is insidious. The response to the usual asthma therapies of beta agonist and steroids is poor in infants with bronchiolitis. In contrast, certain viral illnesses in young children can induce wheezing that will respond to a β-agonist with good results.

FB aspiration is discussed in greater detail later in this chapter, but this is usually a toddler with a history of choking who then develops focal areas of wheezing. Although children with congestive heart failure can wheeze, they also show symptoms of sweating and the signs of failure to thrive with a murmur and an S_4 gallop rhythm. Other differentials include airway irritants, gastroesophageal reflux, pneumonia, allergic pneumonitis, vascular rings, lung cysts, and lobar emphysema (Teshome et al, 2013; Welliver, 2009).

Management

Evidence-based guidelines published by the AAP no longer support a trial of bronchodilators as an option for infants and children with bronchiolitis because of the risk associated with its use and the lack of evidence of an effect (Ralston et al, 2014; Schroeder and Mansbach, 2014). The use of epinephrine is also not recommended for infants and children. Administration of nebulized hypertonic saline to infants in the emergency department is not recommended; however, nebulized hypertonic saline can be administered to infants and children diagnosed with bronchiolitis and hospitalized. Systemic corticosteroids should *not* be administered in the treatment of bronchiolitis in infants; chest physiotherapy is contraindicated in infants and children. Antibiotics have no place in the treatment of a viral disease (such as, bronchiolitis), unless there is a concomitant bacterial infection or strong suspicion. Most infants with mild signs of respiratory distress can be treated as outpatients if their oxygen level is within a normal range (Ralston et al, 2014; Schroeder and Mansbach, 2014):

- Supportive care consists of adequate hydration and use of antipyretics.
- The need for supplemental oxygen administration is based on oxyhemoglobin saturation levels. If an infant's or child's oxyhemoglobin level is greater than 90%, the decision to administer oxygen is left up to the provider (Ralston et al, 2014).
- Transcutaneous oxygen saturation monitoring (continuous pulse oximetry) is also an individual provider's choice (Ralston et al, 2014).
- Fluid intake is strongly recommended to prevent dehydration.
- Nasal suctioning to clear the upper nasal passages is recommended.

The inpatient management of bronchiolitis may include using heated, humidified, high-flow oxygen via nasal canula. The mechanism of action is to improve mucous ciliary clearance and avoid nasal dryness. The high flow delivers positive airway pressure to keep the alveoli open and reduce ventilation perfusion mismatch and small airway microatelectasis (Da Dalt et al, 2013). This method needs more research but is being regularly used in the inpatient basis (Schroeder and Mansbach, 2014; Teshome et al, 2013).

Hypertonic saline (3%) is being used to treat bronchiolitis in hospitalized infants and children. The mechanism of action is due to decreasing mucus viscosity, thus improving airway clearance. It is not recommended for outpatient use and does not reduce hospital admission in patients being treated in the emergency department. However, its use does reduce length of hospital stay (Da Dalt et al, 2013; Zhang et al, 2008). Research on this method is ongoing.

The use of deep airway suctioning is avoided, though continuing to keep the nasal airway clear on a regular basis may improve airflow. This intervention is intuitive and does not need a randomized trial to show its benefit (Schroeder and Mansbach, 2014).

As stated previously, there is no evidence for the routine use of antibiotics, β-agonist, or corticosteroids. Ribavirin is no longer recommended routinely and is presently only used in infants with severe illness due to underlying immunodeficiency, chronic lung disease, or hemodynamically unstable cardiac conditions (Da Dalt et al, 2013). Although leukotriene levels are high in bronchiolitis, the use of antileukotriene inhibitors has not been adequately studied and, thus, is not recommended. A recent review showed an increased risk of bronchiolitis with low cord blood vitamin D level (Belderbos et al, 2011). At present, there is no evidence to show any pharmacologic therapy is clearly superior.

Parents caring for infants and children at home need to understand:

- The management of rhinitis (use of saline drops and suctioning of nares)
- Indications for the use of antipyretics
- The use of home oxygen
- Signs of increasing respiratory distress or dehydration that call for hospitalization
- Guidelines for feeding an infant with signs of mild respiratory distress (amount of fluid needed per 24 hours; smaller, more frequent feedings; monitoring of the respiratory rate; and guarding against vomiting)
- Education that infants and children with bronchiolitis typically have symptoms for 2 to 3 weeks

Infants younger than 2 months old and older infants with signs of severe respiratory distress should be hospitalized. Signs that suggest increasing respiratory distress include the following (Smith, 2011):

- Progressive stridor or stridor at rest
- Apnea
- Increasing respiratory rate (sleeping rate of greater than 50 to 60 breaths per minute)
- Restlessness, pallor, or cyanosis
- Hypoxia recorded by either blood gas (partial pressure of oxygen [P_{O_2}] less than 60 mm Hg) or pulse oximetry (less than 92% on room air)
- Rising partial pressure of carbon dioxide (P_{CO_2}) (recorded by blood gas)
- Inability to tolerate oral feedings
- Depressed sensorium

- Presence of chronic cardiovascular or immunodeficiency disease
- Parent unable to manage at home for any reason

In-hospital management focuses on supportive care, focusing on suctioning of nares, humidified supplemental oxygen, and elevation of the child to a sitting position at a 30- to 40-degree angle. IV hydration (or in infants nasogastric hydration) is needed when respiratory distress interferes with nursing or bottle feeding.

Occasionally a hospitalized child is not able to be quickly weaned back to room air. Home management of these infants requiring oxygen is sometimes difficult and may require a team approach, including involvement of a pediatric health care provider and home care nursing visits. Strict outpatient follow-up is mandatory for as long as the child is receiving home oxygen.

Complications

The first 48 to 72 hours after the onset of cough are the most critical. Apneic spells are common in infants. The child is ill-appearing and toxic but gradually improves. The fatality rate associated with bronchiolitis is about 1% to 2%. Infants younger than 12 weeks old and those with underlying cardiorespiratory or immunodeficiency are at risk for severe disease.

Prolonged apnea, uncompensated respiratory acidosis, and profound dehydration secondary to loss of water from tachypnea and an inability to drink are the factors leading to death in young infants with bronchiolitis. In some children, bronchiolitis can cause minor pulmonary function problems and a tendency for bronchial hyperreactivity that lasts for years. RSV bronchiolitis has been associated with the development of asthma, but its role in the causality of asthma is still debated. Recurrent episodes of wheezing can be seen during childhood in patients with a history of bronchiolitis. This persists into adolescence with 10% of the children still wheezing. However, this figure may not be different from the general population (Welliver, 2009).

Prevention

Palivizumab (Synagis) is an RSV-specific monoclonal antibody used to provide some protection from severe RSV infection for high-risk infants (see Chapter 24 for guidelines). Educate caregivers about decreasing exposure to and transmission of RSV, especially those with high-risk infants. Advice should include limiting exposure to child care centers whenever possible; use of alcohol-based hand sanitizers if available or hand washing if the alcohol-based hand sanitizer is not available (Ralston et al, 2014); avoiding tobacco smoke exposure; and scheduling RSV prophylaxis vaccination, when indicated.

Foreign Body Aspiration

The symptoms and physical findings associated with aspiration of an FB depend on the nature of the material aspirated, plus the location and degree of the obstruction. The cough reflex protects the lower airways, and most aspirated material is immediately expelled with coughing. Onset of a sudden episode of coughing without a prodrome or signs of respiratory infection should make the provider suspicious of FB aspiration.

Objects that are either too large to be eliminated by the mucociliary system or cannot be expelled by coughing eventually lead to some form of respiratory symptomatology. Obviously a large FB occluding the upper airway can cause suffocation. A small object in the lower respiratory tree may not produce symptoms for days to weeks. Obstruction results from either the FB itself or edema associated with its presence. Hot dogs are one of the most common causes of fatal aspiration. Although toddlers commonly aspirate FBs, aspiration occurs in children of all ages.

Laryngeal Foreign Body

Clinical Findings

History. A rapid onset of hoarseness and the development of a chronic croupy cough with aphonia are reported. Be suspicious of an FB aspiration in children with sudden episode of cough, unilateral wheezing, and or recurrent pneumonia.

Physical Examination. The child can present with cough, unilateral wheezing, clinical signs of pneumonia, hemoptysis, dyspnea, and cyanosis.

Diagnostic Studies. Expiratory or lateral decubitus chest radiographs should be ordered. Because most FBs are not radiopaque, radiographs may not be useful in the diagnosis. However, if a chest radiograph does not reveal an FB but shows local emphysema—an area that does not inflate or deflate—suspect FB aspiration (Carter and Marshall, 2011). If the history suggests FB aspiration, bronchoscopy must be undertaken. Direct laryngoscopy might reveal the presence of foreign matter.

Tracheal Foreign Body

Clinically the child has a history of a brassy cough, hoarseness, dyspnea, and possibly cyanosis. The most characteristic signs of tracheal FB aspiration are the homophonic wheeze and the audible slap and palpable thud sound produced by the momentary expiratory effect of the FB at the subglottic level.

Bronchial Foreign Body

Most objects are aspirated into the right lung. A careful medical history may reveal a forgotten episode of choking.

Clinical Findings

History. An initial episode of coughing, gagging, and choking is described. Some objects are inhaled with no choking (e.g., a spear of grass). Blood-streaked sputum may be expectorated, but hemoptysis rarely occurs as an early symptom. On rare occasions hemoptysis does occur as an initial symptom months or years after the aspiration event took place. Children aspirating a metallic object often complain of a "metallic taste" in their mouths.

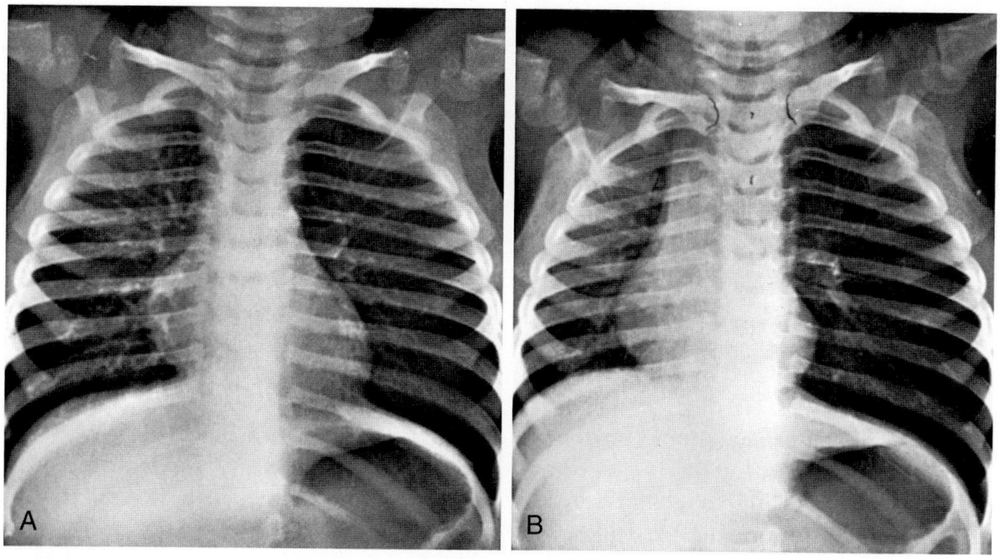

• **Figure 32-1** **A**, Normal inspiratory chest radiograph in a toddler with a peanut fragment in the left main bronchus. **B**, Expiratory radiograph of the same child showing the classic obstructive emphysema (air trapping) on the involved (left) side. Air leaves the normal right side, allowing the lung to deflate. The medium shifts toward the unobstructed side. (From Hollinger LD: Foreign bodies of the airway. In Kliegman RM, Stanton BF, St. Geme JW, et al, editors: *Nelson textbook of pediatrics*, ed 19, Philadelphia, 2011, Saunders/Elsevier, p 1453.)

Physical Examination. The initial clinical findings are similar to those seen in either tracheal or laryngeal FB aspiration. If the object is nonobstructive and nonirritating, few or no initial symptoms may be seen. The child may have limited chest expansion, decreased vocal fremitus, atelectasis, or emphysema-like changes with resulting hyporesonance or hyperresonance. Diminished breath sounds are often found. A small object can act as a bypass valve, and homophonic wheezes can be heard. Crackles, rhonchi, and wheezes can be present if air movement is adequate. If the acute episode is missed or not appreciated, a latent period of mild "wheezing" or cough may be evident.

Diagnostic Studies. Clinical suspicion is the clue to this diagnosis. Inspiratory and forced expiratory chest radiographs and chest fluoroscopy are useful in identifying radiolucent FBs (Fig. 32-1).

Management

The patient should be referred to a pulmonary specialist for bronchoscopy. If the object is removed via bronchoscopy before permanent damage occurs, recovery is usually complete. Secondary lung infections and bronchospasms should be treated as suggested in the section on management of pneumonia in this chapter and asthma in Chapter 25.

Complications

If the FB is vegetable matter, vegetal or arachidic bronchitis can occur. This severe condition can be characterized by sepsis-like fever, dyspnea, and cough. If the material has been there for a long time, suppuration can occur. Lobar pneumonia, intractable wheezing, status asthmaticus can develop. Emphysema or atelectasis can also occur as the result of a large obstruction caused by a bronchial FB.

Prevention. Anticipatory education regarding prevention of FB aspiration should be part of well-child supervision guidance. Parents should be cautioned about high-risk foods (e.g., whole carrots, nuts, popcorn, and hot dogs). Young children need to be supervised closely as they put small objects into their mouths as well as when they cry, shout, run, and play with food or other objects in their mouths.

Bronchitis

Acute bronchitis is defined as a nonspecific inflammation of the bronchioles and can be classified as *acute* or *chronic*. The common viral agents implicated in bronchitis are influenza virus, RSV, adenovirus, and parainfluenza virus. Other viral agents include rhinovirus, enterovirus, human metapneumovirus, human bocavirus, and the newer human coronavirus. *S. pneumoniae, B. pertussis,* and *H. influenzae* are the most commonly cultured bacterial organisms. *M. pneumoniae* and *C. pneumoniae* are also causative agents. *Pseudomonas aeruginosa* is the common agent in children with CF. The incidence of the disease peaks in midwinter and declines by midsummer with an increase in the fall. The entire episode seldom lasts more than 2 to 3 weeks.

Acute bronchitis is usually preceded by a viral infection (Goodman, 2011). It is associated with inflammation of the large airways, including the trachea and the large- and medium-sized bronchi. There is associated destruction of the ciliated epithelium by the causative agent. This illness is associated with pharyngitis as well as rhinitis. Although a virus is the most common cause of acute bronchitis, weakened tissue can succumb to a secondary bacterial infection.

Chronic bronchitis is characterized by a productive cough lasting for more than 3 months and is well defined clinically in adults. In children, this condition per se is ill defined, because it is usually a symptom of another chronic disorder, such as allergies, asthma, CF, and/or cigarette smoke (Goodman, 2011). A chronic cough should provoke a search for another condition (Kaslovsky and Sadof, 2013).

Clinical Findings

History

The usual course of illness can be divided into three phases (Goodman, 2011):

1. A phase where upper respiratory symptoms predominate, lasting 3 to 4 days
2. The development of a dry, hacking cough for several days with production of a sputum due to leukocyte infiltration
3. Recovery with decreasing cough symptoms

The following are reported:

- A dry, hacking, unproductive cough that begins a few days after the onset of rhinitis and fever.
- Complaints of low substernal discomfort or burning chest pain aggravated by coughing.
- Initially the cough is dry, harsh, and sometimes brassy in younger children. However, as it progresses, the cough becomes productive, and because younger children swallow the sputum, vomiting and gagging can occur.
- A family history of asthma, CF, atopy, infections as well as a history of environmental irritants, such as tobacco smoke and pollution, should be obtained.
- A history of prematurity, gastroesophageal reflux, or exposure to infection due to day care should be elicited.
- The nature of the cough, timing, previous history of cough and responses to therapy, wheezing or stridor should be obtained.
- Check for tobacco or marijuana use in teenagers.

Physical Examination

Findings can vary and include the following:

- Variable rhinitis
- Low-grade or no fever
- Signs of nasopharyngeal infection and conjunctivitis
- Coarse breath sounds, rhonchi, and coarse, changing rales

Diagnostic Studies

Chest x-ray is not routinely done unless the child is worsening or there is a suspicion of an FB.

Differential Diagnosis

Pertussis should be considered in patients with a cough lasting 2 to 3 weeks, because it is found in 10% of patients with a new onset of a chronic cough. Children with recurrent acute bronchitis must be evaluated for underlying pathologic conditions. Respiratory tract anomalies, FB aspiration, bronchiectasis, immunodeficiency, allergy, rhinosinusitis, anatomic problems (e.g., gastroesophageal reflux and tracheoesophageal fistulas), tonsillitis, exposure to air pollutants, adenoiditis, and CF must be considered in the differential diagnosis. In chronic bronchitis, primary ciliary dyskinesia, CF, FB, congenital anomalies, reflux, aspiration, asthma, allergies, autoimmune diseases, immune deficiency, and bacteria pathogens (e.g., *B. pertussis, M. pneumoniae,* and *C. pneumoniae*) should be considered.

Management

For acute bronchitis, no specific therapy is known, and most patients require none. Care is primarily supportive.

- *Analgesia:* Use for pain.
- *Hydration:* Intake of fluids to avoid dehydration (helps to thin mucus generally in 5 to 10 days, and the cough decreases).
- *Antiviral/antibiotics:* If influenza A is the likely etiologic agent and there are underlying pulmonary diseases, antiviral therapy should be used. Because most cases of acute bronchitis are from viral sources, antibiotics are not indicated. If *M. pneumoniae* or *C. pneumoniae* is suspected, macrolides can be used.
- *Cough suppressants:* There is no evidence to support the use of cough suppressants. Antihistamines should not be used because of their excessive drying effect; these agents tend to prolong the symptoms.
- *Bronchodilators:* There is no evidence to support the use of inhaled β-agonists, unless there is obstruction and wheezing at the onset of illness. If there is a suspicion of asthma, then a trial of bronchodilators can be used (Kaslovsky and Sadof, 2013).

For chronic bronchitis, treatment depends on whether an underlying cause is found. Bronchodilators, cromolyn sodium, corticosteroids, and anticholinergic agents are used for the treatment of chronic cough associated with asthma or underlying chronic lung disease. If reflux is the cause, underlying treatment of the reflux is indicated. Avoidance of tobacco smoke, dust exposure, and air pollution is important.

Complications

In normal, healthy children, the condition is not serious; however, malaise continues for another week or so after the cough lessens. In undernourished or chronically ill children, otitis, rhinosinusitis, and pneumonia are common.

Valley Fever (Coccidioidomycosis)

Coccidioides is a fungal spore that can cause a primary pulmonary infection when these spores are inhaled. The clinical presentation can be asymptomatic or self-limited in 60% of children (AAP, 2012). However, symptomatic infection occurs and presents as an acute illness that looks similar to pneumonia or influenza. It also can be associated with erythema multiforme and erythema nodosum. Chronic pulmonary infections are rare, and disseminated lesions occur with bone, joint, and CNS disease occurring. Infants and young children are more likely to develop dissemination. Coccidioides species are found in the southwestern United States, as well as Mexico, Central America, and South America. A single infection gives lifelong immunity. The incubation period ranges from 7 to 28 days but is usually between 10 to 15 days. Person-to-person transmission only occurs in congenital infection or in patients with draining skin lesions.

There has been an increasing incidence of this disease in the southwestern United States; with this infection, 75% of those infected miss work or school and 40% are hospitalized (CDC, 2013). The increasing incidence of Coccidioides is likely due to environmental factors, such as drought (which may cause an increase in spore dispersal) and the increase in construction. There is marked underreporting of the disease because of the voluntary nature of reporting and undertesting by providers who fail to consider coccidioidomycosis in the differential of an influenza-like illness.

Clinical Findings in Infants and Children

The clinical findings are similar to influenza in most symptomatic patients.

History

- Fatigue
- Weight loss
- Cough and headache
- Malaise myalgia
- Chest pain (with pulmonary infection)
- Bone pain (with osteomyelitis) (Ho et al, 2014)
- Neck stiffness (with meningitis)

Physical Examination

- Fever
- Crackles (with respiratory infection)
- Cutaneous abnormalities, including erythema multiforme and erythema nodosum

Diagnostic Studies

Serologic tests provide key information. The response of IgM detected by immunodiffusion and enzyme immunoassay (EIA) tests is helpful in establishing the diagnosis. In primary infection, the IgM can be found in the first and third weeks. Complement fixation tests, immunodiffusion, and EIA tests evaluating IgG response are used, but complement fixation tests and immunodiffusion are more specific. Persistent titers of 1 : 16 or greater occur with severe disease that is likely disseminated. The spherules of Coccidioides species can be seen under a microscope when infected body fluids are used.

Differential Diagnosis

The differential diagnoses include a variety of respiratory conditions, such as pneumonias from other organisms, bronchitis, and influenza.

Management

Although the treatment with antifungal for pulmonary disease is controversial and deserves further exploration, treatment for high-risk children who are immune suppressed is recommended. Children at high risk for disease include those with T lymphocyte–mediated immunity, African and Filipino ancestry, infants younger than 1 year old, and those with underlying cardiopulmonary disease and diabetes, as well as pregnant women in their third trimester. Donor organ transmission has occurred. Treatment with fluconazole or itraconazole for 3 to 6 months is recommended for those with severe primary infection. Patients with severe infection include those with complement fixation titers of 1:16 or greater, weight loss of greater than 10%, symptoms for more than 2 months, and severe malaise or inability to carry out normal activities, which may require treatment with fluconazole or itraconazole on an outpatient basis.

Indications for Hospitalization

Patients with disseminated disease involving the CNS not responding to high-dose oral fluconazole may require IV amphotericin B. In addition, if the patient has severe pulmonary involvement and low oxygen level, hospitalization may be necessary for oxygen and fluids.

Prevention

Immunocompromised patients should avoid activities that might expose them to aerosolized spores in dust-laden areas in the southwestern United States, Mexico, Central America, and South America. Control of dust in construction sites, archaeological digs, or in locations where there is soil disturbances is considered a way of prevention (AAP, 2012).

Nonbacterial and Bacterial Pneumonia

Pneumonia is a lower respiratory tract infection associated with fever and respiratory symptoms involving the parenchyma of the lung (Gereige and Laufer, 2013). It can be lobar, interstitial, or bronchopneumonia. Lobar pneumonia involves infection of the alveolar space that results in consolidation; it is described as "typical" pneumonia. Atypical pneumonia describes patterns of consolidation that are not localized. In interstitial pneumonia, cellular infiltrates attack the interstitium, which makes up the walls of the alveoli, the alveolar sacs and ducts, and the bronchioles; this type of pneumonia is typical of acute viral infections but may also be a chronic process. Viral infection affects the lung defenses by altering normal secretions, inhibiting phagocytosis, modifying the normal bacterial flora, and disrupting the epithelial layer. Many childhood viruses set the stage for secondary bacterial infection. Children with immunologic problems or chronic illnesses are prone to primary bacterial pneumonia and experience recurrent pneumonias or fail to clear the initial infection completely. Bronchial pneumonia is associated with bacterial infection with multiple areas of consolidation involving one or more pulmonary lobules. *Pneumonitis* is a general term used to describe lung inflammation that may or may not be associated with consolidation. Community-acquired pneumonia is acquired in the community as opposed to hospital-acquired or nosocomial pneumonia.

In neonates, the risk factors for early onset pneumonia include prolonged rupture of membranes, maternal amnionitis, premature delivery, fetal tachycardia, or maternal intrapartum fever. The risk factors for late onset pneumonia include having anomalies of the airway, severe underlying disease, prolonged hospitalization, neurologic impairment, or nosocomial infection from poor hand washing or overcrowding. Risk factors for childhood pneumonia include male gender, coming from a lower socioeconomic class, poor nutrition, lack of breastfeeding, exposure to cigarette smoke (either passive or active), alcohol use, drug use, having underlying cardiopulmonary disease or neuromuscular disease, gastroesophageal reflux, tracheoesophageal fistula, or congenital and acquired immunodeficiency (Gereige and Laufer, 2013).

Bacterial pneumonia occurs as a primary infection caused by organisms that spread from the nasopharynx or as a secondary complication of a viral pneumonia (Bradley et al, 2011). Primary bacterial pneumonia is less common in childhood than secondary bacterial infection after a viral infection. *S. pneumoniae* is the leading cause of bacterial pneumonia in all age groups except newborns (Gereige and Laufer, 2013). Certain bacterial pneumonias have a specific pattern of disease: *S. pneumoniae* causes a lobar pneumonia, whereas community-associated methicillin-resistant *Staphylococcus aureus* (MRSA) is associated with empyema and necrosis. It has been associated with influenza A; this virus may enhance the transmission of *S. aureus* (Geriege and Laufer, 2013). The identification of the infecting organism is difficult and, particularly in young children, leads to overuse of antibiotics.

Viral pneumonia is the most common pulmonary infection, especially in children younger than 2 years old, and can result in serious illness in a young infant (Bradley et al, 2011). It often involves both the conducting airways and the alveoli. Viral infection affects the lung defenses by altering normal secretions, inhibiting phagocytosis, modifying the normal bacterial flora, and disrupting the epithelial layer. Many childhood viruses set the stage for secondary bacterial infection. Children with immunologic problems or chronic illnesses are prone to primary bacterial pneumonia and experience recurrent pneumonias or fail to clear the initial infection completely. The onset of viral pneumonia is gradual over a 1- to 2-day period of coryza, respiratory congestion, fever, cough, and increasing fretfulness (Boyer, 2009).

Atypical bacterial pneumonia is caused by *M. pneumoniae, Chlamydophila (*formerly *Chlamydia) pneumoniae,* and *C. trachomatis* and is called *walking pneumonia. M. pneumonia* (or primary atypical pneumonia) is the most common cause of pneumonia in children older than 5 years through the young adult years. *M. pneumoniae,* an organism without a cell wall, is transmitted from one symptomatic patient to another by droplet spread. The incubation period is 2 to 3 weeks, and asymptomatic carriage after infection can last for weeks. Wheezing in a child over 5 years of age without a history of wheezing may point to an atypical pneumonia. This disease is usually mild and self-limited.

C. trachomatis pneumonia is a characteristic pneumonia resulting from the transmission of *C. trachomatis* from the infected genital tract of the mother to the infant. It does not become apparent until the infant is 2 to 19 weeks old. Due to prenatal screening, the incidence of *C. trachomatis* infection of the newborn has decreased but should be considered in a mother with inadequate or no prenatal care. *C. trachomatis* is an organism that has many subtypes within the species. Approximately 50% of infants born to infected mothers acquire this infection, but only 5% to 20% of these infants develop *C. trachomatis* pneumonia with a typical onset between 1 and 3 months of age.

Age influences the clinical manifestations of pneumonia and differing infectious agents cause different presentations and symptoms. Table 32-6 differentiates the various forms of pneumonia commonly found in infants, children, and adolescents. Table 32-7 shows the most common infecting organisms associated with pneumonia by age. Treatment is often empirical and varies with age.

Conjugated vaccines, such as Prevnar 13 and HIB vaccine, have decreased the incidence of these bacteria. The introduction of Prevnar 13 has decreased the incidence of pneumococcal pneumonia. Pneumococcal pneumonia occurs most commonly in the late winter and early spring after the cycle of viral URIs. Asymptomatic carriers play a more important role in dissemination of disease than sick contacts. Children younger than 4 years old suffer the highest attack rate.

Clinical Findings in Infants and Young Children

The hallmark of pneumonia is fever and cough in all age groups. Tachypnea and increased work of breathing may precede coughing. Cough, hypoxia, nasal flaring, rales, retractions, and rhonchus lung sounds are specific but not as sensitive for pneumonia. Viral pneumonia tends to have an insidious onset that is associated with more wheezing than what is typically noted with bacterial pneumonia. In contrast, lobar pneumonia (caused by pneumococcal pneumonia) typically presents with fever, cough, and decreased breath sounds in the area of the pneumonia. However, the child may present with a mixture of symptoms. Pneumonia can cause referred symptoms, such as abdominal pain, which may be present in a child with a diaphragmatic pneumonia or radiating neck pain that may be associated with upper lobe pneumonias. Irritation of the pleura causes the chest pain in children with pneumonia.

History

The following may be reported (Bradley et al, 2011; Gereige and Laufer, 2013; Iroh Tam, 2013):

- Neonate
  - History of group B streptococcal or *C. trachomatis* infection in the mother

TABLE 32-6 Differentiating Various Forms of Pneumonia in Infants, Young Children, and Adolescents

Characteristic	Bacterial	Viral	*Mycoplasma pneumonia* and *Chlamydophila pneumonia*	*Chlamydia trachomatis*
Common age	All ages	All ages	>5 years old	2 to 19 weeks old (typically 1 to 3 months old)
Onset	Acute; gradual	Acute; gradual	Slow	Gradual
Clinical findings	Depends on age; starts with URI, cough, dyspnea, tachypnea, rales, decreased breath sounds, grunting, retractions, toxic look; potential progression to severe respiratory distress	Depends on age; cough, coryza, hoarseness, crackles, wheezing, stridor	Persistent cough, malaise, headache	Tachypnea, staccato cough, crackles, wheezing rare, 50% have signs or history of conjunctivitis
Fever	Acute onset of fever (≥102.2° F [≥39° C])	Present (less prominent)	>102.2° F (>39° C)	Afebrile
CBC	WBCs often elevated >15,000/mcl	Normal or slight elevation of WBC	Normal	Eosinophilia in 75% of cases
Organism(s)	90% caused by *Streptococcus pneumoniae*	RSV, parainfluenza, influenza	*M. pneumoniae* *C. pneumoniae*	*C. trachomatis*
Radiographic findings	Lobar consolidation	Transient lobar infiltrates	Varies, interstitial infiltrates	Hyperinflation, infiltrates
Treatment	Depends on bacteria and age of child; amoxicillin, penicillin, methicillin, cefuroxime, gentamicin, vancomycin	Supportive care	Erythromycin Azithromycin Clarithromycin	Erythromycin

CBC, Complete blood count; *RSV*, respiratory syncytial virus; *URI*, upper respiratory infection; *WBC*, white blood cell.

  - Prenatal drug use or lack of prenatal care as risk factors for SBI in the neonate
  - With *C. trachomatis,* the infant is typically afebrile; prior, concurrent, or no history of inclusion conjunctivitis reported
- Infant
  - Slower onset of respiratory symptoms, cough, wheezing, or stridor with less prominent fever suggests viral pneumonia (bacterial pneumonia is less likely in a wheezing child)
  - Determine mother's HIV status or infant's exposure to tuberculosis
- Child and adolescent
  - Get immunization history and travel history of the family
  - Tuberculosis status
  - Evaluate sick contacts at home
  - Evaluate for possible FB aspiration
  - Initial history of a mild URI for a few days—similar for both bacterial and viral
  - Abrupt high fever with temperatures greater than 103.3° F (39.6° C), chills, cough, and dyspnea suggest bacterial pneumonia
  - Other manifestations include restlessness, shaking chills, apprehension, shortness of breath, malaise, and pleuritic chest pain; irritation of the pleura causes chest pain

Physical Examination

The health care provider needs to pay close attention to the general appearance, looking at the work of breathing, assessing for hypoxia, and evaluating tachypnea, which is considered to be the most valuable sign for ruling out pneumonia.

Early onset pneumonia in the neonate presents within the first 3 days of life with:

- Respiratory distress, apnea, tachycardia, poor perfusion
- Tachycardia
- No fever, or fever only with subtle or no physical findings

Typical findings seen in all types of pneumonia include:

- Nasal flaring, grunting, retractions
- Tachypnea (may be the only clue), generally more than 60 breaths per minute in infants younger than 2 months old, more than 50 breaths per minute in children 2 to

TABLE 32-7 Age Variants in Pneumonia Microorganisms

Age	Viral Organisms	Bacterial Organisms
Neonatal	Cytomegalovirus (CMV)	More common Group B streptococci Gram-negative enteric bacteria *Listeria* *Chlamydia trachomatis* Uncommon organisms *Streptococcus pneumoniae* Group D streptococcus Anaerobes
Infants	Most common Respiratory syncytial virus (RSV) Parainfluenza Influenza Adenoviruses Metapneumovirus	Less common *S. pneumoniae* *Haemophilus influenzae* *Mycoplasma pneumonia* *Mycobacterium tuberculosis* *Bordetella pertussis* *Pneumocystis jiroveci*
Preschool children	Most common RSV Parainfluenza Influenza Adenoviruses Metapneumovirus Bocavirus role is not clear	Less common *S. pneumoniae* *H. influenzae* *M. pneumoniae* *M. tuberculosis* *Chlamydophila pneumoniae*
School-age children	Respiratory viruses as above	*M. pneumoniae* *C. pneumoniae* *S. pneumoniae* *M. tuberculosis*

Adapted from Ranganathan SC, Sonnappa S: Pneumonia and other respiratory infections, *Pediatr Clin North Am* 56(1):140, 2009.

11 months old, or more than 40 breaths per minute at rest in children 1 to 5 years old

- Tachycardia, air hunger, and cyanosis are significant findings
- Fine crackles, dullness, diminished breath sounds
- To encourage preschoolers and school-age children to breathe deeply, ask them to blow crumbled papers off your hands or use a phone application that allows them to "blow up a balloon"

In bacterial pneumonia:

- Fever, hypoxia, lethargy
- Splinting the affected side to minimize pleuritic pain or lying on the side in a fetal position helps compensate for decreased air exchange and improves ventilation
- Tachypnea and retractions
- Progression to delirium, circumoral cyanosis, and posturing
- Presence of a pleural effusion and signs of congestive heart failure
- Abdominal distention, downward displacement of the liver or spleen

In viral pneumonia:

- Wheezing
- Downward displacement of the liver or spleen

In primary atypical bacterial pneumonia (*C. trachomatis*):

- *C. trachomatis* pneumonia characterized by repetitive, staccato cough with tachypnea, cervical adenopathy, crackles, and rarely wheezing
- Conjunctivitis is associated with *C. trachomatis* in infants (Iroh Tam, 2013)

Diagnostic Studies

A chest x-ray should not be routinely performed in children with pneumonia (Bradley et al, 2011). However, a chest x-ray is recommended for any child older than 3 months who fails to improve after 72 hours on the standard treatment or who is being admitted. Follow-up films are not needed in patients who have an uneventful recovery.

Blood cultures should not be routinely used in outpatient setting unless the child fails to improve or deteriorates on antibiotic therapy. Blood cultures should be done on children who are admitted with moderate to severe pneumonia. Sputum cultures can be used in hospitalized children who can produce sputum. Urine antigen detection tests for *S. pneumonia* are not recommended, because the false-positive rate is high.

Rapid tests for influenza and other respiratory viruses are helpful, whereas a CBC is not recommended in outpatient settings but may be helpful in inpatient settings. Acute phase reactants do not differentiate between viral and bacterial pneumonia and are not recommended for fully immunized children who are being treated as an outpatient. These tests may be useful for more seriously ill patients. Testing for *M. pneumonia* when the clinician is suspicious of that organism as the cause of the pneumonia can be helpful in selected situations but is not required in children with classic presentations.

Differential Diagnosis

The child's age and characteristic signs and symptoms as discussed previously can help distinguish between a viral and a bacterial pneumonia. The differential diagnoses to consider with pneumonia include bronchiolitis, congestive heart failure, acute bronchiectasis, FB aspiration, pulmonary abscess, parasitic pneumonia, and endotracheal tuberculosis. Right lower lobe pneumonia can present with abdominal pain and be confused with appendicitis. Right upper lobe pneumonia can often closely resemble meningitis.

Management

Most otherwise healthy children can be managed as outpatients. Guidelines for admission are identified in Box 32-2.

• BOX 32-2 Criteria for Hospital Admission for Pneumonia

Neonate to 3 Months Old

- Fever
- Poor oral intake with signs of dehydration
- Pulmonary complications noted on radiographs—abscess, empyema, pneumatocele

Infants and Children Older Than 3 Months

- Hypoxemia with oxygen less than 90%
- Tachypnea: >60 breaths/min in infants younger than 2 months old; >50 breaths/min in children 2 to 11 months old; or >40 breaths/min at rest in children 1 to 5 years old
- Respiratory rate >70 breaths/min in infants or older children >50 breaths/min indicates more severe community-acquired pneumonia
- Grunting, dyspnea, or apnea
- Poor feeding with tachycardia and signs of dehydration (slow capillary refill of >2 seconds) in infants
- Severe respiratory distress
- Oxygen saturation <90% with the need for supplemental oxygen (pulse oximetry reading or arterial blood gas)
- Toxic appearance
- Failure to respond to appropriate oral antibiotic

All Age Groups

- Social issues at home that indicate parent or caretaker cannot appropriately monitor and/or care for the child

Neonates must always be admitted to the hospital if diagnosed with pneumonia regardless of infecting pathogen. Young infants may also need hospitalization unless *C. trachomatis* is suspected.

All children with pneumonia require supportive care with antipyretics, hydration, and rest. Antibiotics should be reserved for those with suspected bacterial infection only. Serious infections may require hospitalization for respiratory therapy, including humidified oxygen, pulmonary therapy, and/or intubation.

Guidelines for outpatient and inpatient treatment of bacterial pneumonia by age and certain specific pathogens are as follows (Bradley et al, 2011):

- *Outpatient antibiotic treatment*: Oral antibiotics are considered safe for most children older than 3 months with pneumonia (Bradley et al, 2011; Taketomo et al, 2014).
  - *2 months to 3 months old:* If chlamydia is suspected, treat with oral azithromycin for 5 days or erythromycin base or ethyl succinate for 14 days (AAP, 2012). Admission may be needed depending on clinical presentation.
  - *3 months to 18 years old:* Amoxicillin 90 mg/kg/day, divided every 12 hours for 10 days (maximum daily dose: 4000 mg/day).
  - If *C. pneumonia* or *M. pneumonia* (community-acquired) is suspected, azithromycin is an appropriate choice. Azithromycin 10 mg/kg/day once on day 1 (maximum dose = 500 mg) and then 5 mg/kg daily for the next 4 days (maximum dose = 250 mg).
  - For influenza, oseltamivir (Tamiflu) is recommended; zanamivir (Relenza) can be used in children older than 7 years.
- *Inpatient treatment:* Testing to identify the pathogen is important for selection of appropriate antimicrobial therapy.
  - *Neonate:* Ampicillin and cefotaxime, ceftriaxone, or gentamicin.
  - Ampicillin or penicillin G in a fully-immunized infant or school-age child with community-acquired pneumonia unless there is a high incidence of *S. pneumoniae.*
  - Empiric therapy with a third-generation cephalosporin (ceftriaxone or cefotaxime) if there are high rates of penicillin-resistant *S. pneumoniae.*
  - The addition of macrolide to a beta-lactam therapy, if *M. pneumonia* and *C. pneumonia* are present or considered likely to be present.
  - Vancomycin or clindamycin in addition to beta-lactam therapy if *S. aureus* is strongly considered, keeping in mind that community-acquired MRSA may require more than 10 days of therapy (Bradley et al, 2011).

Parental education about medication administration, hydration, fever control, and worrisome signs and symptoms is important. In addition, the child should be seen for follow-up at the conclusion of antibiotic treatment or sooner if there is no improvement or worsening of symptoms. Children with recurrent pneumonias should be referred for further pulmonary evaluation.

Prognosis

By the second to third day of treatment, auscultation should reveal a change in respiratory sounds as the infection begins to consolidate. Increased fremitus, tubular breath sounds, and the disappearance of crackles may be noted. Most children have an uneventful recovery, but it is important to inform parents that their child's cough can last for several weeks. Routine rechecks with chest x-rays are not recommended. If pneumonia recurs or persists for longer than 1 month, the child needs further evaluation for underlying immunodeficiency disease.

Complications

Complications associated with community-acquired pneumonia can involve other systems and include meningitis, CNS abscess, endocarditis, pericarditis, osteomyelitis, and/or septic arthritis. Pulmonary complications include empyema (which is more common in staphylococcal and GABHS infections), pneumothorax, bronchopleural fistula, and/or lung abscess. Scarring of the airways and lung tissue can cause dilated bronchi, which results in bronchiectasis. *M. pneumoniae* can spread to the blood, CNS, heart, skin, or joints. A child with sickle cell disease and pneumonia caused by *M. pneumoniae* has more severe pulmonary disease than the average child does.

Prevention

Identify and treat pregnant women with *C. trachomatis*. Universal vaccination against influenza, HIB, and pneumococcal infection is essential. Current guidelines limit the use of palivizumab (Synagis) prophylaxis (see Chapter 24).

TABLE 32-8 Cystic Fibrosis Transmembrane Conductance Regulator Mutation Classes

Class of Defect	Abnormalities of Cystic Fibrosis Transmembrane Conductance Regulator Synthesis, Structure, and Function
I	No functional CFTR protein made due to defective or absent biosynthesis
II	CFTR defect in trafficking as a result of mutation of protein variants that are improperly processed to the apical cell membrane Delta-508 is a class II mutation
III	Affects CFTR channel regulation that impairs the chloride conduction through the channel Ivacaftor (Kalydeco) is the medication that improves chloride conductivity
IV	Defects in channel conducting with a decreased amount of CFTR with decreased in function of the apical cell membrane
V	Decreased amount of fully active CFTR
VI	Stability of CFTR at the cell surface is decreased

CFTR, Cystic fibrosis transmembrane conductance regulator.

Cystic Fibrosis

CF is a multisystem genetic disorder manifested by chronic obstructive pulmonary disease (COPD), GI disturbances, and exocrine dysfunction. Over the past decade, the life expectancy for individuals with CF has increased to 41.1 years (Paranjape and Mogayzel, 2014). Newer therapies that target the genetic defect may further increase the lifespan of the patient with CF (Milla, 2013). CF occurs in approximately 1 in 3000 white births. Although not common, its occurrence rate is 1 in 15,000 African American, 1 in 13,500 Hispanic, and 1 in 35,000 Asian descent births (Paranjape and Mogayzel, 2014).

This autosomal recessive genetic disorder involves mutation of the cystic fibrosis transmembrane conductance regulator (CFTR) protein, which is expressed in epithelial cells and blood cells. The gene is on chromosome 7, but more than 1900 CFTR mutations have been identified and are categorized into six distinct classes, although the functional importance of only a few of those mutations is known. CFTR functions in sodium transport through the epithelial sodium channel, regulates the adenosine triphosphate (ATP) channels, and is involved in bicarbonate chloride exchange. The CFTR gene defect causes defective ion transport, airway surface liquid depletion, and defective mucociliary clearance (Paranjape and Mogayzel, 2014). Table 32-8 shows the different types of mutations.

The most common defect, found in 70% of cases, is a deletion of phenylalanine in position 508 (D508) (Paranjape and Mogayzel, 2014). Polymorphism in non-CFTR genes may explain the difference in the manifestations of the genetic change within different families. Ultimately, the mucus obstruction that results causes inflammation and infection. This failure to conduct ions across the epithelial cell membranes leads to problems in the lungs, biliary tree, pancreas, intestines, vas deferens, and sweat glands. This results in mucus thickening and target organ damage in the lungs and exocrine glands. In the lung, there is airway depletion, which leads to ciliary collapse and decreased mucociliary transport. Ultimately, the mucous obstruction causes chronic inflammation and infection, and bacterial colonization in trapped mucous secretions (Mogayzel et al, 2013). In the exocrine system, the pancreas, liver, and intestinal tract viscid secretions lead to malabsorption of fat and proteins as a result of pancreatic insufficiency.

Clinical Findings

CF is a multisystem progressive illness with varying levels of severity. Table 32-9 outlines clinical manifestations

TABLE 32-9 Clinical Manifestations of Cystic Fibrosis: from Neonatal Period to Adolescence

Stage of Childhood	Clinical Manifestations
Fetal ultrasound	Hyperechoic bowel is suggestive of meconium ileus and is present in 10% of fetuses with CF
Neonatal period	Meconium ileus, delayed meconium passage, meconium plug Prolonged jaundice Intestinal atresia Edema, hypoproteinemia, and acrodermatitis enteropathica due to malabsorption Hemorrhagic disease of newborn due to vitamin K deficiency
Infancy	Cough Colonization with bacteria in mucus Bacterial pneumonia Failure to thrive Hypoproteinemia Abdominal distention Cholestasis Rectal prolapse Steatorrhea DIOS Hemolytic anemia
Childhood	Respiratory manifestations: Chronic recurrent infection of sinuses and respiratory tract/polyps/poorly controlled asthma Bronchiectasis Digital clubbing GI manifestations: Poor weight gain and growth Steatorrhea Chronic constipation Rectal prolapse DIOS Idiopathic pancreatitis/liver disease
Adolescence	ABPA Chronic pansinusitis Nasal polyposis Bronchiectasis/hemoptysis Idiopathic pancreatitis Osteoporosis Diabetes

Adapted from O'Sullivan B, Freedman SD: Cystic fibrosis, *Lancet* 373:1891–1904, 2009; Paranjape SM, Mogayzel PJ: Cystic fibrosis, *Pediatr Rev* 35(5):194–205, 2014.

ABPA, Allergic bronchopulmonary aspergillosis; *CF*, cystic fibrosis; *DIOS*, distal intestinal obstruction syndrome; *GI*, gastrointestinal.

seen in children at various ages. They may include the following:

- *Pulmonary:* CF is a major cause of severe chronic lung disease in children. The lungs of children with CF are normal at birth but become inflamed with chronic airway infection within a short time following birth. The respiratory epithelium exhibits marked impermeability to chloride and excessive sodium reabsorption. Mucus is viscous, and dehydration of the airway secretions occurs, leading to dysfunctional mucociliary transport, airway obstruction, and chronic infections. Pulmonary system manifestations run the clinical spectrum from chronic, dry, frequent cough and sputum production to respiratory failure. Bronchitis, bronchiolitis, bronchiectasis, and pneumonia occur frequently. Bronchospasm resembling acute or chronic asthma may be present. The airways become colonized with *S. aureus, H. influenzae,* and, finally, *P. aeruginosa. Burkholderia cepacia* is a slower-growing organism found in children with CF. Infection can present in infancy. Pulmonary disease usually becomes progressive and leads to cor pulmonale, respiratory failure, and death by adulthood. Other respiratory problems associated with CF include recurrent ARS, nasal polyps, and allergic bronchopulmonary aspergillosis (ABPA), which starts by childhood and continues into adulthood. Digital clubbing is common.
- *GI tract and nutrition:* During infancy, meconium ileus, pancreatic insufficiency, and rectal prolapse can be manifestations of CF. Meconium ileus develops in up to 15% of newborns born with CF. A meconium ileus syndrome equivalent can also develop in older patients, with desiccated fecal material causing GI obstruction. Eighty-five percent of affected children have failure to thrive because of pancreatic enzyme insufficiency. Edema with hypoproteinemia may also be present. These children have thick fat-laden stools (steatorrhea), poor muscle mass, and delayed maturation. Infants with CF who are fed soy-based formulas do very poorly, and severe hypoproteinemia and anasarca quickly result. During childhood, intussusception, hepatic steatosis, biliary fibrosis, and rectal prolapse can occur. Childhood problems continue into adulthood. Clinically apparent cirrhosis occurs in 15% of patients with subsequent risk of portal hypertension. Adenocarcinoma of the digestive tract can occur. Other GI problems associated with CF include volvulus, duodenal inflammation, gastroesophageal reflux, bile reflux, fibrosing colonopathy, and poor fat absorption that lead to vitamin A, K, E, and D deficiencies with resulting anemia, neuropathy, night blindness, osteoporosis, and bleeding disorders. Distal intestinal obstructive syndrome (DIOS) occurs when viscous fecal matter causes blockage in the distal intestine and presents with abdominal pain and distention with pain. This occurs as a result of poor fat absorption, pancreatic insufficiency, and dehydration.
- *Hepatobiliary tract:* Biliary cirrhosis occurs in 2% to 3% of children with CF and is characterized by jaundice, ascites, hematemesis from esophageal varices, and splenomegaly. Hepatic steatosis is also a known complication of CF. Adolescent patients may experience biliary colic and cholelithiasis.
- *Endocrine:* Recurrent acute pancreatitis is not uncommon. Cystic fibrosis–related diabetes (CFRD) with relative insulin deficiency develops as the patient ages due

to autolysis of the pancreas as the pancreas body becomes fatty. CF patients need annual blood glucose screening, because up to 30% of patients develop CFRD by adulthood (Paranjape and Mogayzel, 2014).

- *Musculoskeletal:* Vitamin D deficiency may result in osteoporosis when bone reabsorption exceeds bone formation.
- *Reproductive:* Affected children have delayed sexual development. The vas deferens is nonfunctional and atrophied due to CFTR dysfunction, leading to azoospermia and male sterility. The incidence of inguinal hernia, hydrocele, and undescended testes is also high. Females experience secondary amenorrhea, cervicitis, and decreased fertility. A pregnancy is usually carried to term if pulmonary function is not severely compromised.
- *Sweat glands:* Excessive salt loss can lead to hypochloremic alkalosis, especially in warm weather or after gastroenteritis. Children with CF often taste salty because of elevated amounts of sodium chloride (NaCl) lost in endogenous sweat. Dehydration and heat exhaustion are concerns.

Diagnostic Studies

The diagnosis of CF is made on the basis of clinical features and laboratory findings. The gold standard for diagnosis is the pilocarpine iontophoresis sweat test (Nicholson, 2013; Wagener et al, 2012). The child must have one of more of the clinical features of CF before ordering this test, which include chronic sinopulmonary disease, GI and nutritional abnormalities, salt loss syndrome, chronic metabolic alkalosis, or male urogenital abnormalities, resulting in obstructive azoospermia (Paranjape and Mogayzel, 2014). The results of the sweat test are determined differently depending on age.

The diagnosis of CF can be made in patients with clinical features of the disease under the following guidelines:

- The concentration of sweat chloride is greater than 60 mmol/L.
- The concentration of sweat chloride is in the intermediate range of 30 to 59 mmol/L for infants younger than 6 months old or in the range of 40 to 59 mmol/L for older individuals.
- The child has two disease-causing CFTR mutations (Wagener et al, 2012).

Sweat tests should be done at a laboratory that regularly deals with children and routinely does these tests. Sodium chloride concentration goes up with age but a concentration greater than 60 mmol/L is still a diagnostic level. A result of greater than 60 mEq/L of chloride on two specimens is in the diagnostic range for CF. Children with hypoproteinemia may elicit false-negative sweat test results.

The second test is genetic analysis for the CFTR mutation. Commercial labs evaluate for the common mutations of the CFTR gene; however, complete sequencing of the gene is also available (Paranjape and Mogayzel, 2014). A limited number of CF centers also test for nasal potential difference measurement. Newborn screening is now done in all 50 states by state labs that may measure immunoreactive trypsinogen (IRT) in the newborn's blood. The lab will either perform two IRT measurements (IRT/IRT) or test for CFTR mutation if the IRT is elevated (IRT/CFTR). If the IRT is elevated or the child has one CFTR mutation, the infant's primary provider is notified and the child is referred for sweat testing. There are false-negative screens, so if an infant has symptoms and signs of CF, a sweat test should be performed.

Other diagnostic testing is indicated depending on secondary complications of CF. Glycosylated hemoglobin levels may be elevated in older children because of impaired pancreatic functioning. Pulmonary function tests are used to follow the clinical course.

Management

Children with CF have complicated treatment regimens and should be monitored by a multidisciplinary team at a CF-accredited center. The major aim of pulmonary disease treatment is to optimize lung functioning, prevent disease progression, and avoid complications. The treatment of CF-related lung disease requires control of airway infections, clearance of airway secretions, and decreasing inflammation in the lung. Pulmonary, nutritional, physical, and pharmacologic (antibiotic and anti-inflammatory) therapy and psychological counseling must be individualized for each child at each stage of the illness.

- Pulmonary
  - To promote airway clearance, inhaled dornase alfa (recombinant human deoxyribonuclease) selectively cleaves the DNA and reduces the mucus viscosity. Hypertonic saline works by drawing water into secretions and is used to thin secretions to allow removal of them. The use of postural drainage, active cycle of breathing, autogenic drainage, percussion, positive expiratory pressure, exercise, and high-frequency chest wall oscillation are done twice a day to facilitate secretion removal (Mogayzel et al, 2013).
  - The use of ivacaftor (Kalydeco; a medication that is a CFTR potentiator) is limited to patients who carry at least one G551D mutation (Paranjape and Mogayzel, 2014).
  - To reduce chronic airway inflammation, high-dose ibuprofen and oral azithromycin dosed three times a week are used. Patients must be screened for atypical mycobacterial infection before starting long-term azithromycin. Although high-dose ibuprofen decreases neutrophil migration in children from 6 to 17 years old, the therapy is not widely used due to risk of GI bleeding and frequent drug blood level measurements. Hemoptysis can be scant (less than 5 mL), moderate (5 to 240 mL), or massive (greater than 240 mL) and is associated with advancing lung disease as well as vitamin K deficiency. It results from the hypertrophy and proliferation of the bronchial arteries rupturing

into the airways as a result of the disease process. The management includes antibiotic therapy, cessation of the anti-inflammatory drugs and limiting therapies for airway clearance (Hurt and Simmonds, 2012).
    - Pneumothorax presents as acute onset of chest pain and dyspnea and is confirmed by chest x-ray. Smaller pneumothoraces are managed by observation and discontinuation of positive pressure. Surgical or chemical pleurodesis is used in recurrent large pneumothoraces.
    - Lung transplantation is a viable therapy for selected patients who have terminal lung disease.
- Gastrointestinal
    - Patients with CF have an 85% rate of pancreatic insufficiency. This leads to bulky, malodorous stools resulting in failure to thrive. Replacement with enzymes in the dosage ranges of 2000 to 2500 units/kg of lipase to a maximum of 10,000 units/kg/day. Higher dosing of lipase can lead to fibrosing colonopathy in a small number of patients.
    - Fat malabsorption causes deficiency of vitamins A, D, E, and K; therefore, replacement must be started along with serum monitoring of the levels annually. Vitamin D deficiency can occur, resulting in osteopenia, osteoporosis, or rickets.
    - Cystic fibrosis liver disease (CFLD) is diagnosed when there are at least two of the following: (1) hepatomegaly and/or splenomegaly, (2) liver function tests abnormalities on three tests in a 12-month period, (3) portal hypertension or abnormal liver echotexture on ultrasound, and (4) cirrhosis on liver tissue biopsy. Treatment with ursodeoxycholic acid is recommended (Debray et al, 2011).
    - DIOS is managed using osmotic laxatives to promote lower bowel clearance. The use of sodium meglumine diatrizoate (Gastrografin) enemas can be used for a near complete obstruction by an experienced radiologist.
- Endocrine disorder
    - CFRD is the result of the fatty infiltration and destruction off the islet cells due to the thick viscous secretions in the pancreas. Microvascular complication of diabetes including renal disease, retinopathy, and neuropathy are associated with hyperglycemia. Ketoacidosis is rare. At age 10, an oral glucose tolerance test is done annually to screen for CFRD. Hemoglobin A_{1C} is not recommended because it underestimates overall glycemic control.
    - Insulin is used to treat CFRD.

Pectus Deformity

A pectus excavatum (PE) is when the lower ribs and lower sternum bow inward on the anterior chest wall. Mechanical forces, genetics, or cartilaginous and collagen defects are linked to PE. In fact, 40% of children with PE have family members with a pectus deformity, 6% have muscular and connective tissue disorders, such as Duchenne and infantile muscular dystrophy, Werdnig-Hoffman disease, and Marfan, Ehler-Danlos, and Kippel-Feil syndromes, and 40% to 65% have scoliosis. PE is identified at birth in one third of patients and will develop in early childhood and become more prominent during adolescence in the remaining patients (Dean et al, 2012).

The etiology of PE is not clear; however, risk factors include family members with PE, the muscular and connective tissue disorders listed earlier, or spinal muscular atrophy type 1 (Jaroszewski et al, 2010). The deformity can interfere with respiratory function, and lung volumes, although often normal, are decreased. The chest has a smaller anteroposterior diameter, and this can lead to a decrease in cardiac stroke volume and output. When it is severe, the heart can be compressed, or displaced to the left causing the great vessel to rotate. In addition, there is an additional risk of cardiac dysrhythmias due to lower oxygen supply to the heart.

Pectus carinatum is much less common than pectus excavatum. It also progresses during puberty. In pectus carinatum, there is a bowing out of the sternum (also called "pigeon chest"). Although this shape may be cosmetically unattractive, there are fewer complaints about shortness of breath, chest pain, or dyspnea.

Clinical Findings

The degree of chest concavity determines the clinical manifestations (Jaroszewski et al, 2010). Mild deformities of the chest are well tolerated, whereas more severe deformities may require intervention. Feeling of inferiority, depression, and insecurities occur as a result of teasing or body image disturbances (Habelt et al, 2011; Ji et al, 2011).

The parent may note a depression (excavatum) or bowing out (pectus carinatum) of the sternum. Exercise intolerance, easy fatigability, wheezing, chest tightness, chest pain, palpitations, or dizziness may be reported. The finding in pectus deformities include:

- Posterior depression of the sternum and costal cartilage (PE)
- More protuberant abdomen due to the narrowed chest (PE)
- Anterior bowing of the sternum (pectus carinatum)

Diagnostic studies include chest radiography, chest CT (controversial due to exposure to radiation), exercise testing if substantial PE deformity is present, and echocardiogram and pulmonary function studies as suggested by the symptomatology.

Management

PE can affect cardiac and pulmonary function. If the excavatum deformity is significant, surgical repair may be indicated. The indications for surgery are based on the degree of psychological and physical impairment rather than the severity of the pectus carinatum or PE. It is important to do routine broad-based psychological screens for children with PE or pectus carinatum (Ji et al, 2011). Many children want to look normal, and this may dictate surgery (Krasopoulos and Goldstraw, 2011). The health care provider needs to evaluate for possible genetic etiology of PE and make appropriate referrals to geneticists. The Nuss procedure or the highly modified Ravitch technique is the surgical approach used for correction. The timing of the surgery is usually at the start of puberty.

For a complete list of references, please visit http://evolve.elsevier.com/Burns/pediatric/.

33 Gastrointestinal Disorders

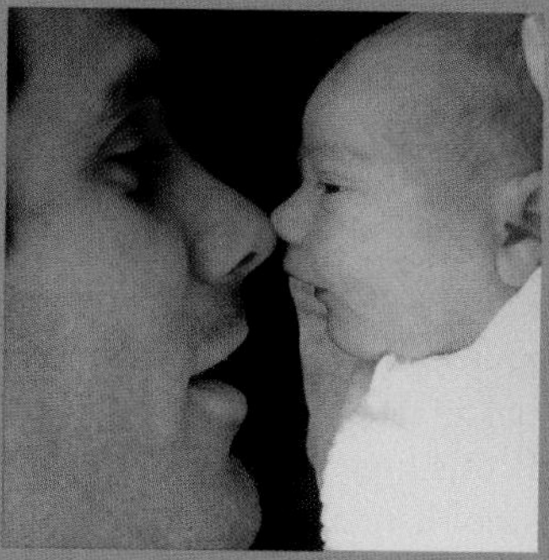

ELIZABETH E. WILLER, BELINDA JAMES-PETERSEN, AND ANN M. PETERSEN-SMITH

The gastrointestinal (GI) system, also known as the *digestive system,* is essential for lifelong health. This system provides the nutrients that give the body's cells the energy needed to function. Sustained operation and maintenance of this system are essential for normal growth and development and for the effective functioning of other organ systems.

The pediatric primary care provider plays an integral role in the care of children with GI dysfunction. A thorough understanding of the anatomy, physiology, and common disorders of the GI system is needed to appropriately assess and treat pediatric GI problems. This chapter focuses on pathologic GI disorders commonly seen in children. Other problems of the GI system, such as obesity, anorexia, bulimia, encopresis, and constipation, are discussed in Chapters 10, 12, and 19.

Anatomy and Physiology

The GI system begins to develop during the third week of gestation. The primitive gut is initially formed and then divides into the foregut, midgut, and hindgut. The structures further develop in an intricate and complex fashion to become the digestive tract and accessory organs.

The GI tract extends from the mouth to the anus. It includes the organs of digestion and accessory organs, such as the liver, pancreas, and gallbladder. The system provides the following functions: ingestion of food, movement of food from the mouth toward the rectum, mechanical dissolution of food, chemical dissolution of food, absorption of nutrients, and expulsion of waste products. The mouth serves as the site for ingestion, chewing, and mixing of food with saliva. The tongue senses the texture and taste of foods, which initiates salivation and the release of gastric juices in the stomach. The esophagus transports food from the mouth to the stomach by *peristalsis,* the sequential contraction and relaxation of the musculature in the esophagus. The upper esophageal sphincter prevents air from being swallowed while breathing. The lower esophageal sphincter (LES) prevents food from being regurgitated from the stomach, which is important because intraabdominal pressure exceeds intrathoracic and atmospheric pressures. The stomach serves as a reservoir for ingested foods. It secretes digestive juices, mixes food with the gastric fluids, and propels the liquid material into the small intestine. The small intestine's primary function is absorption of nutrients (carbohydrates, fats, proteins, minerals, and vitamins) into the systemic circulation. Absorption occurs through villi, which cover the mucosal folds and serve as the functional unit of the intestine. Each villus contains an artery, a vein, and a lymph vessel that transport nutrients from the intestine into the systemic circulation. The villi are covered with enterocytes, whose major role is the digestion of carbohydrates and proteins. Enterocytes secrete proteins and enzymes known as *brush border enzymes,* which assist in digestion.

Carbohydrates must be converted to monosaccharides before their absorption is possible. This process begins in the mouth, where the salivary enzyme amylase breaks down complex starches into disaccharides. The brush border enzymes in the small intestine convert disaccharides into monosaccharides (sucrose to glucose and fructose, lactose to glucose and galactose, and maltose to glucose). When this process is hindered, disaccharides remain osmotically active and can cause diarrhea.

Fat absorption, which occurs mainly in the jejunum, is accomplished through the addition of lipases secreted by the pancreas. Lipases break down fats into particles that are easily absorbed by the villi. Fats then rely on the lymphatic system for absorption.

Proteins are converted to amino acids by pancreatic enzymes. The resulting amino acids are further divided into smaller amino acid particles that are absorbed via the brush border into the systemic circulation. After appropriate absorption of nutrients, the small intestine is left with the initial fecal liquid. This liquid is then propelled by peristalsis into the large intestine. The large intestine removes water from the fecal liquid and allows for short-term storage. The fecal mass, which consists of waste products, bacteria, intestinal secretions, and shed cells, is pushed into the sigmoid colon.

Entry of feces into the rectum stimulates the defecation reflex. This reflex stretches the rectal wall, relaxes the internal anal sphincter, and thereby creates the need to defecate. If this urge is ignored, further fluid resorption occurs as the stool is retained, resulting in an increase in stool mass and dryness. Excessive stretching of the colon from the hard, dry stool bolus can lead to decreased peristalsis, further complicating the retention of stool.

Pathophysiology

The GI tract can be affected by illness, injury, or other problems that prevent it from functioning normally. Dysfunction can be localized or systemic. Categories of dysfunction include disorders of motility; infection; malabsorption syndromes; impairment of digestion, absorption, and nutrition; congenital malformations and genetic syndromes; metabolic disorders; behavioral problems; injuries and trauma; and food intolerances, such as lactose and gluten intolerance due to absence of essential enzymes.

Assessment

History

The history assesses the following:

- Symptom analysis: How long? How bad? What makes it better? What makes it worse? Interventions attempted? Impact on activities of daily living?
- Heartburn, belching and flatulence, vomiting
- Nutritional patterns:
  - Feeding habits and nutrition history or current diet (what, when, how often, what tolerated)
  - Thirst level (increased or decreased)
  - Changes in appetite
  - Food intolerance or allergy (what foods, symptoms, treatment)
- Elimination patterns: Bowel habits (frequency, times per week, consistency, associated pain, the need for medications or enemas)
  - Constipation and diarrhea (patient's definition of each, how often they occur, treatment tried)
- Presence of pain (onset, location, type, quality, aggravating and alleviating factors)
  - *Epigastric* pain usually indicates pain from the liver, pancreas, biliary tree, stomach, and upper part of the small bowel (duodenum).
  - *Periumbilical* pain is generated from the distal end of the small intestine, cecum, appendix, and ascending colon.
  - *Colonic* visceral pain is lower abdominal pain that can be dull, diffuse, cramping, or burning.
  - *Suprapubic* discomfort indicates distal intestine, urinary tract, and pelvic organ dysfunction.
  - *Referred* pain is a diagnostic challenge. For example, because of convergent nerve pathways, inflammation of the diaphragm can generate pain that is perceived as shoulder or lower neck pain. When visceral pain is overwhelming, referred pain occurs.
  - *Acute* continuous pain is more indicative of an acute process.
- Family history of any GI disease (e.g., gallbladder disease, ulcers, or allergy to any food product)
- Past medical history related to the GI system (e.g., illnesses, surgeries, anatomic problems, such as cleft lip or palate, esophageal atresia)
- Review of systems: Apnea or asthma that may be caused by gastroesophageal reflux (GER), concerns/symptoms of cardiac insufficiency, other autoimmune symptoms (e.g., rashes)

Physical Examination

When assessing a suspected GI problem, a head-to-toe physical examination is indicated.

- Plot growth parameters, including weight for height, to establish proportionality of the patient and exclude certain growth aberrations from the diagnosis.
- Determine body mass index (BMI). The BMI is one of the first indicators used to assess body fat and is a common method of tracking weight problems and obesity in children 2 years old and older (see Chapter 10 for more details).
- Determine hydration status (skin turgor, mucous membranes, peripheral pulses, tears, capillary filling).
- Inspect the abdomen for visible peristalsis, rashes, lesions, asymmetry, masses, enlarged organs, and pulsations.
- Auscultate for frequency of bowel sounds (normal is 5 to 20 per minute).
- Percuss for density and to measure organs.
- Palpate both lightly and deeply.
- Assess peritoneal irritation:
  - Have the patient walk standing straight up or cough.
  - Have the patient stand on tiptoes and fall onto the heels or jump.
  - Palpate for rebound tenderness and a positive Rovsing sign (palpation in the left iliac fossa produces pain in the right iliac fossa).
  - Check for the obturator sign: A supine patient flexes the right thigh at the hip with the knee bent and internally rotates the hip. The sign is positive when it induces abdominal pain.
  - Check for the psoas sign: The patient lies on the left side and extends and then flexes the right leg at the hip. A positive sign is one that induces abdominal pain.
- Perform a rectal examination when intraabdominal, pelvic, or perirectal disease is suspected (the newborn

examination should routinely assess for anal stenosis). Include external inspection and internal palpation for masses, stool, or irregularities. The index finger is typically used because of its increased sensitivity; however, in infants and young children, use the fifth finger. Insert a gloved, lubricated finger into the rectum. Place the other hand on the abdomen for a bimanual examination. Young pediatric patients should be supine with their feet held together and knees and hips flexed, putting their legs over their abdomen. Adolescent males can be lying on their side or standing with the hips flexed and the upper part of the body on the examination table. Adolescent females can be lying on their side or, if a concurrent pelvic examination is to be done, in the lithotomy position.
- Perform a gynecologic examination if a pathologic pelvic condition is suspected (see Chapter 36).

Common Diagnostic Studies

Laboratory tests are performed as indicated:
- Urinalysis (UA) and urine culture
- Complete blood count (CBC) with differential
- Serum chemistry screen, liver profile, lipid profile, erythrocyte sedimentation rate (ESR), C-reactive protein (CRP), thyroid function
- Stool examination for ova and parasites (O&P), culture, blood, white blood cells (WBCs), pH, reducing substances
- Fecal fat collection for 72 hours to rule out fat malabsorption
- Pregnancy test
- Urine tests for gonorrhea or chlamydia, Papanicolaou (Pap) smear and vaginal cultures and/or smears if pelvic or gynecologic pathologic condition is suspected

Imaging of the abdomen may include the following (Clayton, 2010):
- Radiography
  - Abdominal x-ray, as the preliminary study; available, less expensive, with lower radiation
  - Upper and lower GI series with fluoroscopy demonstrate anatomy and function
  - Air contrast enema (diagnose and treat intussusceptions)
  - Bone age (to assess suspected growth abnormalities)
  - Chest radiographs (to rule out pneumonia)
- Ultrasound—no ionizing radiation, noninvasive, relatively inexpensive (especially for pyloric stenosis, intussusceptions, appendicitis, cholelithiasis, trauma)
- Computed tomography (CT) scan—used only after other imaging studies; quick, but invasive, increased radiation, possible sedation (helpful in nephrolithiasis, appendicitis [the gold standard], intraabdominal masses, pancreatitis)
- Magnetic resonance imaging (MRI)—noninvasive and no ionizing radiation; more costly, sedation may be required (useful in a wide range of disorders)
- Nuclear medicine (scintigraphy)—provide functional and quantifiable data (especially with biliary disease, GER, and Meckel diverticulum)

Specialized tests may also be considered:
- Barium swallow
- Duodenal aspirate to identify existing infection
- Esophageal pH probe to establish gastroesophageal reflux disease (GERD), with a pH of less than 4 representing a reflux episode
- Capsule endoscopy
- Breath hydrogen test if lactose intolerance is suspected
- Sweat chloride test if cystic fibrosis (CF) is suspected (see Chapter 32)

Management Strategies

Medications

Many common medications are used to treat GI disorders:
- Antibiotics, antifungals, or anthelmintics for bacterial, fungal, or parasitic infections
- Antiemetics for nausea or vomiting
- Antidiarrheals occasionally for persistent diarrhea or diarrhea associated with chronic disease but never for acute diarrheal diseases, because toxins need to be excreted from the body
- Stool softeners, laxatives, and cathartics for acute treatment and long-term management of constipation and encopresis (see Chapter 12)
- Medications that alter GI motility or tone to treat GERD
- Oral steroids, parenteral steroids, and other immunosuppressants in the treatment of inflammatory bowel disease (IBD)
- Pain medication and antispasmodics in selected acute and chronic GI conditions
- Medications that alter gastric acidity to treat GERD and ulcer disease
- Iron supplementation as supportive therapy for chronic disease

Probiotics and Prebiotics

Prebiotics are non-digestible dietary fibers and fructooligosaccharides (carbohydrate molecules made up of a relatively small number of simple sugars) acquired from food that are used as an energy source by certain beneficial bacteria that naturally live in the intestines. Prebiotics are sometimes known as *fermentable fiber.* Probiotics, on the other hand, are the beneficial bacteria themselves. By acting as a food source, prebiotics give the probiotic bacteria a chance to exert their influence. The concept of prebiotics was introduced in 1995 by Gibson and Roberfoid as an alternative approach to the modulation of the gut microbiota. The role of prebiotics in the treatment of disease is controversial, and more studies are needed to determine their usefulness. Preliminary evidence shows that prebiotics may have a role in improving antibiotic-associated diarrhea, traveler's diarrhea, and gastroenteritis; normalizing bowel function; improving colitis; reducing irritable bowel problems; aiding calcium absorption; and boosting the immune system. Some common prebiotics include oligosaccharides and inulin (found in 36,000 plants).

Probiotics are live microbial food supplements or components of bacteria with demonstrated beneficial effects for the host. The phenomenon of eating probiotic products started 100 years ago, when the first reports showed beneficial effects of probiotic bacteria on human health. Several mechanisms have been proposed to explain the actions of probiotics. In most cases, it is likely that more than one mechanism is at work simultaneously. To be most effective, a probiotic species must be able to survive passage through the acidic environment of the stomach and grow in and colonize the intestine, even in the presence of antibiotics. Probiotics are presumed to promote healing of the intestinal mucosa by reducing gut permeability and by enhancing local intestinal immune responses, as well as by reconstituting the intestinal flora.

Probiotics are often regulated as dietary supplements rather than as pharmaceuticals or biologic products. Thus there is usually no requirement to demonstrate safety, purity, or potency before marketing probiotics. This could lead to significant inconsistencies between the stated and actual contents of probiotic preparations. In the United States, dietary supplements generally do not require premarket review and approval by the U.S. Food and Drug Administration (FDA).

A large number of organisms are being used in clinical practice for a variety of purposes. Most of the identified benefits of probiotics relate to GI conditions, including irritable bowel syndrome (IBS), infectious diarrhea, antibiotic-related diarrhea, and traveler's diarrhea. The most widely used and thoroughly researched organisms are *Lactobacillus, Bifidobacterium,* and *Saccharomyces;* however, the mechanism of action of probiotics remains unclear. *Lactobacillus* promotes healthy bacterial flora in the digestive tract and is widely used to manage and prevent antibiotic-associated diarrhea, traveler's diarrhea, and infectious diarrhea. There is also some research that suggests specific strains of *Lactobacillus* may help relieve infantile colic. *Bifidobacterium* is widely associated with the management of abdominal bloating, flatus, and abdominal pain, which are all symptoms of IBS. *Saccharomyces* have been shown to be effective in the treatment and management of antibiotic-associated and infectious diarrhea.

Some of the most common uses of probiotics in the treatment of digestive disease include:

- IBS: A recurrent disorder of GI functioning that involves the small and large intestines with disturbances of intestinal/bowel motor function and sensation (International Foundation for Functional Gastrointestinal Disorders [IFFGD], 2014). Specific probiotics have a role in the management of some IBS symptoms and can also be used as an adjunct to conventional treatment (Hungin et al, 2013). A definitive therapeutic role remains unproven and further research is needed in order to define the benefits of probiotics in treating IBS.
- Infectious diarrhea: This can be caused by infectious agents, such as viruses, bacteria, and/or parasites. Rehydration is a key element in the treatment of diarrhea. There is some clinical evidence that specific probiotic strains may have a therapeutic benefit when given early in the course of the acute illness as adjunct therapy with rehydration. Particular probiotic strains have been found to shorten the course of rotavirus-associated diarrhea (Grandy et al, 2010).
- Antibiotic-associated diarrhea (AAD): AAD results when the number of healthy microorganisms in the gut decreases as a result of antibiotics given to treat infections. *Clostridium difficile* is the most common bacteria found in AAD. Based on the most recent clinical trials research, probiotics may be helpful in preventing AAD but are not commonly recommended as routine treatment as their feasibility and efficacy have not yet been fully established. Probiotics may be considered in persons with a known increased risk of *C. difficile* (previous infection) as adjunct therapy with the antibiotic treatment regimen (Hickson, 2011).
- Colic: *Colic* is defined as crying for no apparent reason that lasts for 3 hours or more per day and occurs on 3 days or more per week in an otherwise healthy infant younger than 3 months of age. In recent years, small clinical studies have shown some promise in managing infantile colic with administration of certain probiotic strains *(Lactobacillus);* however, research is contradictory at this point and other studies (Sung et al, 2014) report no improvement in colic behaviors with administration of the probiotic.

Nutrition and Activity

Nutrition is essential for the growth and development of every individual (child/adult).

A nutritional plan that meets the recommended daily needs should be encouraged to promote normal GI function, growth, and development. A large number of GI-related illnesses and disorders require a specific diet as part of disease management. Adequate nutrition, therefore, is pivotal to effectively treat a wide variety of acute and chronic GI dysfunctions. Some GI disorders that require alteration in dietary intake as adjunct therapy for disease management include constipation, celiac disease, failure to thrive (FTT), IBS, GER, IBD, eosinophilic esophagitis (EoE), pancreatitis, and liver disease. Consultation with a registered dietician is important to help design an adequate nutritional plan for a child with a chronic GI disorder.

Age-appropriate activity should be encouraged on a regular basis to help maintain normal GI function. Some GI maladies require short-term rest, but generally the system functions better when activity is regular and consistent.

Counseling and Education

It is important to spend time assessing and planning for the unique needs of a child with a GI disorder. The practitioner is responsible for assisting the child and family with information and resources (see Additional Resources at the end of this chapter) that will increase their knowledge of the GI disorder, its course, treatment, and prognosis.

Upper Gastrointestinal Tract Disorders

Dysphagia

Dysphagia, or difficulty swallowing, may be caused by a variety of disorders. Younger children may be unable to swallow, and older children can have awareness that something is wrong with their swallowing ability or may complain of something stuck in their throat (globus). The physiology of swallowing is complex with oral, pharyngeal, and esophageal phases. The *oral phase* refers to ingestion, mastication, and the propulsion of food to the back of the mouth as a bolus. The *pharyngeal phase* includes the swallowing and transfer of food from the pharynx to the esophagus. Airway closure is critical during the pharyngeal phase, and the child needs to have intact motor and sensory pharyngeal protective mechanisms to prevent aspiration. The *esophageal phase* allows food to pass into the stomach.

Dysphagia may occur as a result of a structural defect, neurologic, allergic, or motor disorders, or mucosal injury. Structural defects make it more difficult to swallow solids than liquids. Common structural defects include esophageal narrowing (stricture, web, or tumor) or extrinsic obstruction (vascular ring). Nonstructural causes arise from motility disorders of the oropharynx or esophagus and are uncommon in children. Prematurity and neurologic impairment from disorders (such as, cerebral palsy or muscular dystrophy) can be causes of dysphagia. Mucosal injury most commonly occurs from GERD, EoE, or gastritis, but can also be due to caustic ingestion or medication. The number of children with swallowing difficulties has escalated, because the advances in technology have increased the survival of children with special health care needs.

Clinical Findings

History

- Progressive dysfunction
- Persistent drooling or cough
- Discomfort with swallowing or a sense of food getting stuck
- Picky eating (e.g., a child who prefers liquids to solids) or food refusal
- Heartburn, halitosis, chest pain

Physical Examination

- Observe the infant or child feeding, paying special attention to the adequacy of the child's oral motor skills and safety of swallowing.
- Perform a complete physical examination, paying particular attention to mouth, throat, and neck.

Diagnostic Studies

Diagnostic tests may include:

- Lateral neck films
- Barium swallow (usually the initial procedure because it is especially effective in detecting esophageal narrowing)
- Fiberoptic endoscopy evaluation of swallowing
- Videofluoroscopy swallowing study
- Manometry (gold standard for diagnosing motor disorders)
- MRI (for structural abnormalities)
- Electromyography

Differential Diagnosis

Obstructive and compressive lesions usually cause trouble only with solids. Physiologic dysfunction is usually associated with systemic disease, and the patient has trouble with both liquids and solids. A dysfunctional feeding relationship between child and feeder can manifest as dysphagia.

Management

Difficulty with swallowing requires evaluating associated cognitive, developmental, and behavioral issues. A multidisciplinary approach is recommended to provide a comprehensive, cost-effective evaluation and consistent care for the child and family. Health professionals from otolaryngology, gastroenterology, nutrition, occupational therapy, psychology, and speech-language pathology may be involved.

Vomiting and Dehydration

Vomiting is the forceful emptying of gastric contents coordinated by the medullary vomiting center and/or the chemoreceptor trigger zone of the brain. It is differentiated from regurgitation, which is a passive reflux of gastric contents into the oral pharynx. It can be caused by GI or extraintestinal disorders that are either acute or chronic. Vomiting can be classified as projectile (often arising from the central nervous system [CNS]) or non-projectile (often seen in GER), and bilious, bloody, nonbilious, or nonbloody.

The age of the child helps to formulate an appropriate list of potential diagnoses:

- Newborn or young infant—infectious process, congenital GI anomaly, CNS abnormality, or inborn errors of metabolism
- Infants and young children—gastroenteritis, GERD, milk/soy protein allergies, pyloric stenosis or obstructive lesion, inborn errors of metabolism, intussusception, child abuse, intracranial mass lesion
- Older children and adolescents—gastroenteritis, systemic illness, CNS (cyclic vomiting syndrome [CVS], abdominal migraine, meningitis, brain tumor), intussusception, rumination, superior mesenteric artery syndrome, pregnancy

Dehydration is the loss of water and extracellular fluid. *Volume depletion* or *hypovolemia* (loss of extracellular fluid) and dehydration are used interchangeably. Dehydration is classified as mild (less than 3% weight loss when compared with recent current weight in older children and 5% in infants), moderate (6% in older children and 10% in infants), or severe (9% or greater in older children and 15% or greater in infants) (Thomas, 2015).

Vomiting is one of the most common symptoms in childhood. Nonbilious vomit is generally caused by infection, inflammation, and metabolic, neurologic, or psychological problems. An obstructive lesion generally causes bilious vomiting. Bloody vomit accompanies active bleeding in the upper GI tract (gastritis, peptic ulcer disease [PUD]).

Following is a list of potential causes of vomiting by site of origin:

- Oropharynx: Cleft palate and laryngopharyngeal cleft
- Upper GI: Congenital stricture, foreign body, gastritis and/or esophagitis, gastric web, pyloric stenosis, tracheoesophageal fistula, vascular ring, PUD
- Small intestine: Annular pancreas, choledochal cyst, intestinal atresias and stenosis, intestinal malrotation with volvulus, intestinal pseudo-obstruction
- Colon: Hirschsprung disease, intussusception, meconium ileus, necrotizing enterocolitis, fecal impaction
- Hepatobiliary or pancreatic dysfunction
- Infections: Bacterial enteritis, otitis media, sepsis, urinary tract infection (UTI), viral gastroenteritis (VGE), hepatitis
- Neurologic: Congenital anatomic malformation, gray and white matter degenerative disorders, hydrocephalus, kernicterus, brain tumors, migraine headache, head trauma
- Other: Cow's-milk protein (CMP) allergy (intolerance), inborn errors of metabolism, maternal drug exposure and/or withdrawal, toxic ingestions, appendicitis, cyclic vomiting, pneumonia, drug or alcohol ingestion, eating disorders, pregnancy

Dehydration

Dehydration is overwhelmingly the result of an infectious process, primarily viral, that often causes diarrhea. Children are at increased risk due to their higher surface area–to-volume ratios, higher rate of insensible loss, and in younger children the inability to communicate or actively replenish losses. Depending on the cause of dehydration, water and salts (primarily sodium chloride) may be lost in physiologic proportion or disparately, producing one of three types of dehydration: isonatremic (isotonic), hypernatremic (hypertonic), or hyponatremic (hypotonic). When dehydration is caused by simple diarrhea, homeostatic mechanisms can usually maintain sodium concentrations in the serum, resulting in isonatremia. When vomiting occurs with diarrhea and water intake is less, there is greater water loss than salt loss, potentially resulting in hypernatremic dehydration. When there is massive stool loss of water and salt and only water is ingested, there is a large salt loss, potentially resulting in hyponatremia.

Clinical Findings

History

The vomiting history should assess the following:

- Symptoms with the onset of vomiting; duration of vomiting, quality and quantity, presence of blood or bile, odor, precipitating event; pain; relationship of vomiting to meals, activities, or time of day (Vomiting early in the morning is indicative of increased intracranial pressure.)
- Recent exposure to illness, injury, or stress; recent travel (including camping); swimming activities; possibility of poisoning or bad food
- Medications currently being taken (including over-the-counter, herbal, cultural, and homeopathic remedies)
- Presence of associated symptoms: Diarrhea, fever, ear pain, UTI symptoms, vision changes, cough, headache, seizures, high-pitched cry, polydipsia, polyuria, polyphagia, anorexia
- Past history of illnesses, surgeries, or hospitalizations
- Family history of GI disease or fetal or neonatal deaths (metabolic syndrome, congenital anomaly)

The dehydration history should assess the following:

- Mental status and thirst
- Parental concern regarding decreased tearing or urination, or depressed fontanelle in infants

Physical Examination

- Growth parameters and vital signs
- Neurologic examination: Nuchal rigidity, decreased level of consciousness, and behavioral changes, which can include irritability or lethargy. Sensorium remains intact until there is greater than 6% weight loss as a result of dehydration. Hypotension is a late manifestation of dehydration.
- Abdominal examination: Inspect for distention, abdominal scars from previous surgery (may be associated with obstruction and/or adhesions), or visible peristaltic waves. Auscultate bowel sounds (i.e., increased with gastroenteritis, decreased with obstruction, absent with ileus or peritonitis). Palpate the abdomen for pain and/or rebound tenderness. Assess abdominal organs (liver and spleen size, masses). Perform a rectal examination as indicated.
- Respiratory examination: Tachypnea, decreased oxygen saturation, stridor
- Assessment of dehydration (Table 33-1)
    - One of the most useful clinical signs of hydration is capillary refill time (CRT). Normal CRT is less than 2 seconds. CRT, skin turgor, and tachypnea, considered together, are most helpful in determining dehydration (Guarino et al, 2014).
    - A clinical dehydration scale (CDS) is a predictive tool regarding length of stay and need for intravenous (IV) fluids (Guarino et al, 2014). The four parameters used for assessment are general appearance, eyes

TABLE 33-1 Stages of Dehydration

	Stages of Dehydration		
Symptoms	Minimal or None (<3% Loss of Body Weight)	Mild to Moderate (3% to 9% Loss of Body Weight)	Severe (>9% Loss of Body Weight)
Mental status	Well; alert	Normal, fatigued or restless, irritable	Apathetic, lethargic, unconscious
Thirst	Drinks normally; might refuse liquids	Thirsty; eager to drink	Drinks poorly; unable to drink
Heart rate	Normal	Normal to increased	Tachycardic; bradycardic in severe cases
Quality of pulses	Normal	Normal to decreased	Weak, thready, or impalpable
Breathing	Normal	Normal; fast	Deep
Eyes	Normal	Slightly sunken	Deeply sunken
Tears	Present	Decreased	Absent
Mouth and tongue	Moist	Dry	Parched
Skinfold	Instant recoil	Recoil in <2 seconds	Recoil in >2 seconds
Capillary refill	Normal	Prolonged	Prolonged; minimal
Extremities	Warm	Cool	Cold; mottled; cyanotic
Urine output	Normal to decreased	Decreased	Minimal

From Centers for Disease Control and Prevention (CDC): *Guidelines for the management of acute diarrhea after a disater*, 2014. Available at http://emergency.cdc.gov/disasters/disease/diarrheaguidelines.asp. Accessed February 2, 2015.

(sunken or not), moistness of mucous membranes, and presence of tears.

Diagnostic Studies

Diagnostic studies are performed as indicated by the probable diagnosis:

- Laboratory studies:
  - CBC with differential, blood culture
  - Electrolytes, including blood urea nitrogen (BUN) and creatinine, glucose, and liver function tests
    - Serum sodium less than 130 (hyponatremic) or greater than 150 (hypernatremic)
  - CRP and ESR
  - Serum lactate, organic acids, ammonia for metabolic disorders (may only be abnormal during episodes of vomiting)
  - UA and urine culture
  - Toxicology screen
  - Stool for culture and occult blood, leukocytes, parasites, fat, pH, reducing substances
  - Rapid strep test and/or throat culture
  - Pregnancy test
- Imaging;
  - Abdominal radiographs (suspected obstruction or foreign body ingestion, organomegaly, or a palpable mass)
  - Chest radiograph (suspected pneumonia)
  - Ultrasound (abscesses, masses, stenoses, cysts, appendicitis, pyloric stenosis)
  - Barium swallow or enema (malrotation, pyloric stenosis, GER, masses)
  - CT scan or MRI to diagnose masses, inflammation, herniations, perforations, and obstructions
- Other studies
  - Endoscopy (obstruction, hemorrhage, infection, collect biopsies)
  - Esophageal pH probe analysis, scintiscan
  - Electroencephalogram (EEG)

Differential Diagnosis

See Table 33-2.

Management

Vomiting

- Identify and alleviate the cause as soon as possible.
- Antiemetics (not recommended in acute gastroenteritis or when cause is unknown) may at times be warranted. Newer medications, such as 5-HT_3 receptor antagonists (ondansetron or granisetron) do not have adverse effects on the CNS and may be indicated in children and their use encouraged (Freedman et al, 2014).
- Refer to specialist for persistent vomiting, recurrent vomiting, or vomiting associated with significant underlying process.

TABLE 33-2 Differential Diagnosis of Vomiting in Infants and Children

Infant	Child	Adolescent
Common Conditions		
Gastroenteritis	Gastroenteritis	Gastroenteritis
GERD	GERD	GERD
Overfeeding	Gastritis	Gastritis
Anatomic obstruction: Pyloric stenosis, malrotation with intermittent volvulus, intestinal duplication, Hirschsprung disease, antral/duodenal web, foreign body, or incarcerated hernia	Toxic ingestion: Lead, iron, or vitamins A and D	Toxic ingestion
Systemic infection: UTI, pneumonia, hepatitis	Systemic infection: UTI or pyelonephritis; pneumonia; hepatitis	Systemic infection
Pertussis syndrome	Pertussis syndrome	Pertussis syndrome
Otitis media	Otitis media, sinusitis Appendicitis, small bowel obstruction Migraine Medication: Ipecac, digoxin, theophylline, and so on	Sinusitis Appendicitis, small bowel obstruction, IBD Migraine Medication: Ipecac abuse/bulimia Pregnancy, PID

Rare Conditions

- Other gastrointestinal disorders: achalasia, gastroparesis, peptic ulcer, food allergy or pancreatitis
- Neurologic: Hydrocephalus, subdural hematoma, intracranial hemorrhage or mass, infant migraine, Chiari malformation, or meningitis
- Metabolic/endocrine: Galactosemia, hereditary fructose intolerance, urea cycle defects or amino and organic acidemias, congenital adrenal hyperplasia
- Renal: Obstructive uropathy or renal insufficiency
- Cardiac: Congestive heart failure or vascular ring
- Others: Pediatric falsification disorder (Munchausen syndrome by proxy), child neglect or abuse, CVS, or autonomic dysfunction

Adapted from Blanchard S, Czinn S: Peptic ulcer disease in children. In Kliegman RM, Behrman RE, Jenson HB, et al: *Nelson textbook of pediatrics,* ed 18, Philadelphia, 2011, Saunders, pp 1572–1574; Vandenplas Y, Rudolph C, Di Lorenzo C, et al: Pediatric gastroesophageal reflux clinical practice guidelines: joint recommendations of the North American Society for Pediatric Gastroenterology, Hepatology, and Nutrition (NASPGHAN) and the European Society for Pediatric Gastroenterology, Hepatology, and Nutrition (ESPGHAN), *J Pediatr Gastroenterol Nutr* 49(4):498–547, 2009. Used with permission of Lippincott Williams & Wilkins.

CVS, Cyclic vomiting syndrome; *GERD,* gastroesophageal reflux disease; *IBD,* inflammatory bowel disease; *PID,* pelvic inflammatory disease, *UTI,* urinary tract infection.

Dehydration

- Determine the degree of dehydration.
  - If minimal, mild, or moderate, oral rehydration solution (ORS) with 70 to 90 mEq/L sodium, 25 g/L glucose, 20 mEq/L potassium, 30 mEq/L base (in the form of citrate, acetate, or lactate) with a defined osmolarity of 240 to 300 mOsm/L is recommended.
  - If severe, immediate and aggressive intervention is needed (e.g., IV fluids).
- Pediatric subcutaneous rehydration using recombinant human hyaluronidase is an alternate method, effective when used in children with mild to moderate dehydration who require parenteral therapy (Spandorfer et al, 2012)

Initial rehydration, maintenance of fluids, and replacement of ongoing losses are stages of treatment (Table 33-3). Physiologically sodium and glucose are coupled in transport across the intestinal brush border into systemic circulation to maximize rehydration. Administration of oral fluid should be in frequent, small (5 mL or less) amounts. Larger amounts may be given as tolerated. Plain water, juices, soda, milk, and sports drinks should be avoided, because these liquids are hyperosmolar and do not provide appropriate replacement of sugars and electrolytes. A pediatric emergency department using ORS in children with moderate dehydration showed not only successful rehydration but also a decreased length of stay, less staff use, and more satisfied parents (Bell, 2010). Palatability of ORS does not affect

TABLE 33-3 Treatment Based on Stages and Management of Dehydration

Degree of Dehydration	Rehydration Therapy	Maintenance	Replacement of Ongoing Losses
Minimal or none	Not applicable	0-10 kg: 100 mL/kg/24 h 10-20 kg: 1000 mL + 50 mL/kg for each kg over 10 kg >20 kg: 1500 mL + 20 mL/kg for each kg over 20 kg	<10 kg body weight: 60-120 mL ORS for each diarrheal stool or vomiting episode >10 kg body weight: 120-240 mL ORS for each diarrheal stool or vomiting episode
Mild to moderate	ORS: 50-100 mL/kg body weight over 3 to 4 hours or 10-20 mL/kg/h	Same	Same
Severe	Lactated Ringer solution or normal saline* intravenously in boluses of 20 mL/kg body weight until perfusion and mental status improve, then administer 100 mL/kg body weight ORS over 4 hours or 5% dextrose in ½ normal saline intravenously at twice the maintenance fluid rates	Same	Same: If unable to drink, administer through nasogastric tube or administer 5% dextrose in ¼ normal saline with 20 mEq/L potassium chloride intravenously

Nutrition

- Continue breastfeeding.
- Lactose-containing formulas are usually well tolerated. If lactose malabsorption appears clinically substantial, lactose-free formulas can be used.
- Return to regular milk in smaller amounts more often.
- Resume age-appropriate normal diet after initial rehydration, including adequate caloric intake for maintenance.
- Complex carbohydrates, fresh fruits, lean meats, yogurt, and vegetables are all recommended.
- Avoid fatty foods and foods high in simple sugars.
- Avoid carbonated drinks or commercial juices.

Adapted from Thomas EY: Fluid and electrolytes. In Engorn B, Flerage J: *The Harriet Lane handbook: a manual for pediatric house officer,* ed 20, Philadelphia, 2015, Elsevier.
ORS, Oral rehydration solution.
*In severe dehydrating diarrhea, normal saline is less effective for treatment because it contains no bicarbonate or potassium. Use normal saline only if Ringer lactate solution is not available, and supplement with ORS as soon as the patient can drink. Plain glucose in water is ineffective and should not be used.

the quantity consumed. Homemade solute ions can be used when premade ORS is not available (see rehydrate.org). Refeeding should resume as quickly as possible, because the gut needs nutrition to facilitate mucosal repair following injury.

- Antiemetics: A single dose of an oral disintegrating tablet of ondansetron (2 mg for children 8 to 15 kg, 4 mg for children 15 to 30 kg, and 8 mg for more than 30 kg) reduces vomiting (Freedman et al, 2014).
- Treat fever and monitor urine output.
- Refer if the child has a toxic appearance, severe dehydration, projectile vomiting, abnormal examination, vomiting for greater than 12 hours, or vomiting of blood, bile, or fecal matter, or significantly decreased urine output.

Complications

Dehydration, fluid and electrolyte imbalance, aspiration pneumonia, hemorrhage, or a tear of the esophagus are possible.

Patient and Family Education

Providing written information to the parent about care that is needed during all stages of oral rehydration therapy is helpful. Also include information about signs that indicate the child is worse or not responding to treatment in the expected time frame.

Cyclic Vomiting Syndrome

CVS is characterized by recurrent, discrete, self-limited episodes of vomiting between which are completely symptom-free periods. CVS is often associated with abdominal migraines (discussed later in chapter). During episodes there is intense nausea and unremitting vomiting (a median of six times per hour at peak) often with bilious emesis (83%) and severe abdominal pain (80%) (Li et al, 2008). Accompanying symptoms include pallor, listlessness, anorexia, nausea, retching, abdominal pain, headache, and photophobia. The periods of vomiting may last hours or even days; the symptom-free periods may last for weeks or even years. Consensus statements for CVS have been established for diagnosis (see Li et al, 2008).

Although the typical child with CVS is healthy up to 90% of the time, there are substantial morbidity and medical costs when episodes occur because of missed days of school (average 24 days per child), high rate of IV rehydration, the cost of laboratory and imaging studies, endoscopic procedures, emergency department visits, and missed work by a parent (Li et al, 2008).

The etiology of CVS is unknown, but there is a link with headaches. It has also been associated with mitochondrial, endocrine, allergy, and metabolic disorders. Cyclic vomiting may occur any time between infancy and young adulthood, with presentation of symptoms around 3 years old and diagnosed between 7 to 10 years old. Girls are affected more often than boys (60:40), as are Caucasian, elementary school–age children. Affected individuals tend to have mothers and maternal grandmothers who have a higher incidence of migraine headaches, depression, anxiety, IBS, and hypothyroidism (Boles, 2011; Li et al, 2008). CVS is often a precursor of later classic migraines.

Clinical Findings

History

- Red flags have been identified (Box 33-1)
- Family history positive for migraine headache is common
- A prodromal period (some combination of pallor, anorexia, nausea, abdominal pain, or lethargy) and/or a recovery period (from ill to playing again) that is brief
- Episodes that begin and end abruptly
- Episodes more likely to occur early in the morning (3:00 to 4:00 AM) or on awakening
- An identifiable trigger is commonly seen in children—physical stress (infection, lack of sleep, menstrual periods) or psychological stress (birthdays, holidays, school-related), or food products (e.g., chocolate, cheese, monosodium glutamate)
- Intense nausea not relieved by vomiting
- Headache, motion sickness, photophobia, phonophobia, or vertigo may occur

• BOX 33-1 Red Flags of Cyclic Vomiting Syndrome

- Abdominal signs (e.g., bilious vomiting, abdominal tenderness, and/or severe abdominal pain, hematemesis)
- Triggering events (e.g., fasting, high-protein meal, or intercurrent illness)
- Abnormal neurologic examination (e.g., severely altered mental status, abnormal eye movements, papilledema, motor asymmetry, and/or gait abnormality [ataxia])
- Progressively worsening episodes or conversion to a continuous or chronic pattern

Physical Examination

Physical examination is normal, although children with CVS appear substantially more ill than children with VGE. If any red flags are present, further workup is indicated.

Diagnostic Studies

Screening labs during a vomiting episode help exclude other diagnoses:

- Electrolytes including HCO_3
- Upper GI radiographs (to exclude malrotation)
- Abdominal ultrasound in refractory cases (rule out transient hydronephrosis)
- If hyponatremic or hypoglycemic, rule out Addison disease and fatty acid oxidation

Differential Diagnosis

CVS is a diagnosis of exclusion. Severe GI symptoms can indicate hydronephrosis, cholelithiasis, pancreatic disease, or ureteropelvic junction. CVS precipitated by concurrent illness, fasting, or high-protein meals can indicate a metabolic disorder. An abnormal neurologic examination is suggestive of increased intracranial pressure. Approximately 10% of children with CVS-like history have a specific underlying disorder. Although uncommon, Munchausen by proxy syndrome has been known to mimic CVS in a child given ipecac (Li et al, 2008).

Management

There is no definite treatment proven to be effective in managing CVS, but some empiric treatments have shown some benefit in case-by-case series. Treatment regimens are often guided by patient and family history, physical examination, and diagnostic and laboratory test results. If there are no findings suggestive of another disorder, a trial of therapy is targeted at prophylaxis during the well phase and at acute and supportive measures during the three phases of the episode—prodrome, vomiting, and recovery. Consideration of the child's clinical course, frequency and severity of attacks, and resultant morbidity directs the treatment plan.

Well Phase: Prevention and Prophylaxis

- Lifestyle changes (up to 70% respond with decreased episode frequency) (Li et al, 2008) (Box 33-2).
- Daily prophylactic therapy if abortive therapy fails consistently or episodes are frequent and/or severe (Box 33-3). Doses can be titrated every 1 to 4 weeks to achieve therapeutic dose for at least two CVS cycles. Phenobarbital and supplements (L-carnitine and coenzyme Q10) have also been used (Boles, 2011).

Episode: Acute Interventions

- Supportive measures include early intervention (within 2 to 4 hours of onset of symptoms), dark, quiet environment, and replacement of fluids, electrolytes, and calories. If anxiety is a trigger, relaxation exercises are reported as helpful.

• BOX 33-2 Lifestyle Changes for Cyclic Vomiting Syndrome

1. Keep a journal of potential precipitating factors in order to identify triggers (75% of children can be helped by this alone).
   - Recognize the role of excitement as a trigger (e.g., downplay big events) to avoid excessive energy output.
   - Avoid trigger foods (chocolate, cheese, monosodium glutamate, hot dogs, aspartame, antigenic foods).
2. Provide supplemental carbohydrate for fasting-induced episodes or high-energy demand times (e.g., fruit juices or other sugar-containing drinks, snacks between meals, before exertion, or at bedtime).
3. Maintain healthy lifestyle.
   - Regular aerobic exercise, avoiding overexercising.
   - Regular meal schedules; don't skip meals.
   - Maintain good sleep hygiene.
   - Maintain good hydration.
   - Avoidance or moderation in consumption of caffeine.

• BOX 33-3 Prophylactic Medication for Cyclic Vomiting Syndrome

Children 5 Years Old or Younger

- Cyproheptadine (first choice): 0.25 to 0.5 mg/kg/day divided bid or tid. Maximum dosage *2–6 yr:* 12 mg/24 hr; *7–14 yr:* 16 mg/24 hr; *Adult:* 0.5 mg/kg/24 hr or 32 mg/24 hr
- Propranolol (second choice): 0.25 to 1 mg/kg/day, most often 10 mg bid to tid; *<35 kg:* 10–20 mg PO tid; *≥35 kg:* 20–40 mg PO tid. *Adult:* 80 mg/24 hr ÷ q6–8 hr PO; increase dose by 20–40 mg/dose q3–4 wk PRN. Usual effective dose range: 160–240 mg/24 hr. Taper when discontinuing; monitor resting heart rate

Children Older than 5 Years Old

- Amitriptyline (first choice): 0.1 to 0.25 mg/kg at bedtime, increase weekly by 0.1–0.25 until maximum dose of 2 mg/kg/24 hr or 75 mg/24 hr. For doses >1 mg/kg/24 hr, divide daily dose bid and monitor electrocardiogram (ECG). Monitor ECG before starting and 10 days after peak dose. *Adult:* Initial 10–25 mg/dose qhs PO; reported range of 10–400 mg/24 hr
- Propranolol (second choice): see above

- Pharmacologic: Administer abortive therapy as early as possible.
  - Antimigraine (triptans) in children older than 12 years of age with infrequent and/or mild episodes (less than one per month); sumatriptan 20 mg intranasally at onset is contraindicated if basilar artery migraine or a migraine with at least two of the following brainstem symptoms: dysarthria, vertigo, tinnitus, hypacusis, diplopia, ataxia, or decreased level of consciousness.
  - Antiemetic (5-HT_3 receptor antagonist): Ondansetron 0.3 to 0.4 mg/kg/dose IV every 4 to 6 hours (up to 16 mg) and no more than 3 doses in 24 hours.
  - Sedatives for unrelenting nausea and vomiting to induce sleep: Lorazepam (with ondansetron) is considered most effective, but chlorpromazine with diphenhydramine can be used.
  - Analgesic: Ketorolac 0.5 mg/kg IV every 6 hours (maximum dose 30 mg; maximum daily dose 120 mg for no longer than 3 to 5 days) with ranitidine for severe midline abdominal pain; morphine or hydromorphone can be added.
  - Treatment of specific symptoms can include histamine 2 receptor antagonists (H2RAs) or proton pump inhibitors (PPIs) for epigastric/dyspeptic pain, antidiarrheals for diarrhea, short-acting angiotensin-converting enzyme (ACE) inhibitors for hypertension, and/or anxiolytic medication for anxiety (panic) triggers.
- Complementary modalities (e.g., biofeedback, massage, imagery) have also been used (see Chapter 43 under Headaches).

Referral

Referral is recommended if red flag symptoms occur or if the child fails to respond to appropriate acute treatment and/or prophylaxis. (Response is defined as at least a 50% reduction in episode frequency and/or severity of vomiting during attacks over a 2-month period of therapy.)

Complications

Dehydration, electrolyte derangement, metabolic acidosis, hematemesis, and weight loss can be complications of an acute episode. Ongoing esophagitis may require acid suppression. Frequent or prolonged episodes may lead to growth failure. Abdominal epilepsy is an uncommon cause of cyclic vomiting; an EEG is useful in evaluation and anticonvulsants can be helpful in treatment.

Patient and Family Education

Work with families using their knowledge of the child to determine individual triggers and develop a plan of care for all stages.

Abdominal Migraine

Abdominal migraine is thought to be part of a continuum with migraine and CVS (see earlier section). It typically occurs in children rather than adults. The diagnosis is often difficult to determine during the first episode but becomes evident with cyclic episodes. The diagnostic criteria for abdominal migraine (also known as *Rome III diagnostic criteria for abdominal migraine*) must include *all* of the following (Dafer, 2012; Gelfand, 2013):

- Paroxysmal episodes of intense, acute periumbilical (midabdominal) pain that lasts from 1 to 72 hours
- Intervening periods of usual health lasting weeks to months
- Pain that interferes with normal activities

- Pain associated with two or more of the following: nausea, vomiting, anorexia, headache, photophobia, or pallor
- No evidence of an inflammatory, anatomic, metabolic, or neoplastic process that explains the symptoms
- These criteria need to be present two or more times in the preceding 12 months

Family migraine history is common (Dafer, 2012). Abnormal visual-evoked responses, hypothalamic-pituitary-adrenal axis abnormalities, and autonomic dysfunction are possible mechanisms. Abdominal migraine affects 1% to 4% of children, and it is considered one of the common reasons for recurrent abdominal pain in childhood. It tends to be more common in girls than boys (3:2), with a mean onset at 7 years old and a peak at 10 to 12 years old (Gelfand, 2013; Pacheva and Ivanov, 2013).

Clinical Findings

History

- Rome criteria for abdominal migraine (see prior description)
- Family history of migraine or motion sickness
- History of motion sickness
- Most episodes last hours to days with a 1-hour minimum
- Aura not frequently experienced
- Headache complaints typically absent or minimal
- May have prodrome symptoms of fatigue and drowsiness

Physical Examination

- Normal physical examination; normal growth curves and BMI
- Absence of alarm signals

Diagnostic Studies

There are no laboratory markers for abdominal migraine. EEG is not necessary unless other symptoms are present, such as seizure and episodes of confusion (Dafer, 2012). During the first or worst episodes appropriate laboratory and neurologic studies may be needed to exclude other serious conditions or diseases (Dafer, 2012).

Differential Diagnosis

The diagnosis is often difficult to determine during the first episode. Obstructive GI and renal processes, biliary tract disease, recurrent pancreatitis, familial Mediterranean fever, and metabolic disorders, such as porphyria, should be ruled out. Cyclic vomiting is thought to be a severe variant of abdominal migraine (Gelfand, 2013).

Management

- Identify and avoid triggers: Caffeine, nitrates, and amine-containing foods; excessive emotional stress; travel; prolonged fasting; altered sleep; flickering or glaring lights.
- Sleep often relieves symptoms; antiemetics may abort an attack (Dafer, 2012).
- Abdominal migraine should respond to migraine prophylactic therapy (cyproheptadine, amitriptyline, topiramate). A positive response helps confirm diagnosis.

Prognosis

The child may develop migraine headaches later in life (Dafer, 2012).

Gastroesophageal Reflux Disease

Gastroesophageal reflux refers to the passage of gastric contents into the esophagus from the stomach through the LES. It is a normal physiologic process that occurs several times a day in healthy infants, children, and adults. "GERD is present when the reflux causes troublesome symptoms and or complications" (Vandenplas et al, 2009, p 499). GERD is the most common esophageal disorder in children (Khan and Orenstein, 2011b).

The etiology of GERD is unclear and probably multifactorial. Inappropriate relaxation of the LES with failure to prevent gastric acid reflux into the esophagus, prolonged esophageal clearance of the gastric refluxate, and impaired esophageal mucosal barrier function are the likely causes of most GERD (Loots et al, 2014). LES function usually is influenced by intraabdominal pressure, hormones, neurologic control, and age. Young infants have increased intraabdominal pressure because of their inability to sit upright. They can also regurgitate when they cough, cry, or strain. In healthy infants, regurgitation is highest in the first month of life (73%) and decreases to 50% by the fifth month of life. During the first 2 months of life, 20% of infants regurgitate more than four times per day. After 1 year old, less than 4% of infants regurgitate daily and nearly all resolve by 2 years old. Weight gain is less in infants who regurgitate more than four times per day and breastfed babies regurgitate less than formula-fed babies (Khan and Orenstein, 2011b).

Alterations in swallowing, pharyngeal coordination, esophageal motility, and delayed gastric emptying are also potential factors related to GERD. Increased muscle tone, chronic supine positioning, and altered GI motility exacerbate GERD. *Helicobacter pylori* has been associated with GERD. Children with *H. pylori* are about six times more likely to develop GERD than non–*H. pylori*-positive children. *H. pylori* has not been found in infants younger than 1 year old (Polat and Polat, 2012).

The American Academy of Otolaryngology—Head and Neck Surgery (AAO-HNS) states that 10% of infants younger than 1 year old with regurgitation develop significant complications (GERD) (AAO-HNS, 2011). Risk factors include prematurity, neurologic impairment, obesity, CF, hiatal hernia, and family history of GERD.

Clinical Findings

Common signs and symptoms by age that should lead the clinician to suspect GERD are found in Table 33-4;

TABLE 33-4 Symptoms and Signs that May Be Associated with Gastroesophageal Reflux

Symptoms and Signs that Vary by Age	Symptoms for All Children	Signs for All Children
Infancy: Regurgitation; signs of esophagitis (irritability, arching, choking, gagging, feeding aversion); FTT. Usually symptoms resolve between 12 and 24 months of age. Obstructive apnea, stridor, lower airway disease by which reflux complicates a primary airway disease (e.g., bronchopulmonary dysplasia). Otitis media, sinusitis, lymphoid hyperplasia, hoarseness, vocal cord nodules, laryngeal edema. *Child and adolescent*: Regurgitation during preschool years, complaints of abdominal and chest pain, neck contortions (arching, turning of head), asthma, sinusitis, laryngitis	Recurrent regurgitation with/without vomiting Ruminative behavior Heartburn or chest pain Hematemesis Dysphagia, odynophagia Respiratory disorders, such as wheezing, stridor, cough, hoarseness, persistent throat clearing or cough Halitosis	Esophagitis Esophageal stricture Barrett esophagus Laryngeal/pharyngeal inflammation Recurrent pneumonia Anemia Dental erosion Apnea spells Apparent life-threatening events Weight loss or poor weight gain

Adapted from Vandenplas Y, Rudolph C, Di Lorenzo C, et al: Pediatric gastroesophageal reflux clinical practice guidelines: joint recommendations of the North American Society for Pediatric Gastroenterology, Hepatology, and Nutrition (NASPGHAN) and the European Society for Pediatric Gastroenterology, Hepatology, and Nutrition (ESPGHAN), *J Pediatr Gastroenterol Nutr* 49(4):498–547, 2009, p 519.
FTT, Failure to thrive.

although, according to the guidelines, there is no symptom or symptom complex that is diagnostic of GERD or predicts response to therapy. In older children and adolescents, history and physical examination may be sufficient to diagnose GERD. The most common symptom is "heartburn." Recurrent regurgitation with or without vomiting, weight loss or poor weight gain, ruminative behavior, hematemesis, dysphagia, and respiratory disorders such as, wheezing, stridor, cough, apnea, hoarseness, and recurrent pneumonia are also associated with GERD.

History

Box 33-4 summarizes the history for GERD that should be collected according to the national guidelines. Warning signs that merit urgent investigation of vomiting are found in Box 33-5.

Physical Examination

- Review of height, weight, and head circumference
- Signs of FTT
- Torticollis: Neck arching
- Hoarseness
- Anemia
- Tooth erosion resulting from destruction of enamel by gastric acids caused by frequent vomiting
- Rash, recurrent diarrhea, persistent vomiting, or early-morning vomiting (symptoms of other primary disease with GERD as a secondary problem)

Diagnostic Studies

In most infants with vomiting and in older children with regurgitation and heartburn, a history and physical examination are sufficient to reliably diagnose GERD, recognize

• BOX 33-4 History for the Child with Suspected Gastroesophageal Reflux Disease

Feeding and Dietary History

- Amount/frequency (overfeeding)
- Preparation of formula
- Observe the child during a feeding (clinician)
- Recent changes in feeding type or technique
- Position during feeding, burping technique and frequency

Behavior during Feeding

- Choking, gagging, coughing, arching, discomfort, refusal

Pattern of Vomiting

- Frequency and amount, pain, forceful
- Blood or bile
- Associated fever, lethargy, diarrhea

Medical History

- Prematurity and newborn screen results
- Growth and development, previous weight and height gain (growth charts)
- Past surgery, hospitalizations
- Recurrent illnesses, especially croup, pneumonia, asthma
- Symptoms of hoarseness, fussiness, hiccups, apnea
- Other chronic conditions
- Medications: Current, recent, prescription, nonprescription

Family Psychosocial History

- Sources of stress and/or postpartum depression
- Maternal or paternal drug use

Family Medical History

- Significant illnesses
- Family history of gastrointestinal (GI) disorders
- Family history of atopy

• BOX 33-5 Warning Signals Requiring Urgent Investigation in Infants with Regurgitation or Vomiting

- Bilious vomiting
- Gastrointestinal (GI) bleeding, hematemesis, hematochezia
- Consistently forceful vomiting or onset of vomiting after 6 months old
- Failure to thrive (FTT)
- Recurrent respiratory infections
- Feeding problems (uncoordinated swallow, choking or cough associated with feeding)
- Diarrhea or constipation
- Fever and/or lethargy
- Hepatosplenomegaly
- Bulging fontanelles, macrocephaly, or microcephaly
- Seizures
- Abdominal tenderness or distension
- Documented or suspected genetic/metabolic syndrome

complications, and initiate treatment. An empiric trial of acid suppression with a PPI for 4 weeks may be used as a diagnostic test in older children and adolescents but is not recommended in infants and young children.

Nonradiologic diagnostic tests as indicated:

- CBC with differential to rule out anemia and infection
- UA and urine culture
- Stool for occult blood
- Testing for *H. pylori*

The following specialized tests may be obtained following consultation with a physician or a pediatric gastroenterologist.

- Esophageal pH monitoring has been the gold standard to diagnose reflux. However, the presence of reflux may not correlate with the severity of illness, and some gastric contents may not be acidic. Transnasal pH placement may be uncomfortable, decrease appetite and activity, and thus underestimate the true incidence of reflux episodes. Typically, patients are asked to discontinue H2 blockers for 72 hours before the test and PPIs for 1 week before the study.
- Multichannel intraluminal impedance (MII) measures episodes of reflux independent of the pH of the fluid. It is especially useful for making a diagnosis in children with respiratory events related to reflux, because it can measure multiple indices, such as heart rate, oxygenation, sleep state, and apnea episodes. It can also measure the height of refluxed material and the content and direction of the reflux (liquid, air, or both). It is preferred by many gastroenterologists because it can measure acid and nonacid reflux (50% of reflux in infants is nonacidic). Cost, time to interpret results, and lack of consensus about norms for frequency or length of nonacidic reflux events are disadvantages to this study (Vandenplas et al, 2009).
- Wireless pH monitoring is also available. A pH probe is placed transorally, temporarily attached to the esophageal mucosa where it is programmed to record events for 48 hours. The capsule typically sloughs in about 5 days. Failure to attach, chest pain, feeling of foreign body, and premature detachment are negative aspects of this technology.
- Endoscopy to obtain a biopsy can help determine severity of reflux esophagitis. It can rule out esophagitis and other pathologic conditions if deemed necessary. It may also be used to re-dilate strictures.
- Barium upper GI series should only be used if obstruction or an anatomic abnormality of the upper GI tract is suspected.
- Radionuclide scan with scintiscan and esophageal and gastric ultrasonography studies are not recommended for routine evaluation of GERD.
- Gastric emptying scan can be used to evaluate for delayed gastric motility associated with GER.
- A video swallow study may be necessary if recurrent respiratory infection, persistent cough, or feeding refusal (or difficulty) is present to evaluate for effective esophageal swallow and to rule out aspiration.

Differential Diagnosis

The clinician should also consider other causes of vomiting as found in Table 33-2.

Management

See Figures 33-1, 33-2, and 33-3, and Table 33-5.

Pharmacologic

Acid-suppression agents are the mainstays of treatment. These pharmacologic agents include H2RAs, PPIs, and buffering agents (Table 33-6).

PPIs are superior to H2RAs in relieving symptoms and promoting mucosal healing and do not result in tolerance as do H2RAs. However H2RAs and buffering agents have a rapid onset of action and are useful in on-demand treatment (Vandenplas et al, 2009).

There is insufficient evidence to justify the routine use of prokinetic agents such as cisapride, metoclopramide, domperidone, bethanechol, erythromycin, or baclofen for GERD. Because safe and convenient alternatives are available that are more acceptable to patients, chronic antacid therapy is generally not recommended for patients with GERD (Vandenplas et al, 2009).

Nutrition

Feeding techniques, volumes, and frequency of feeding should be normalized. A trial of extensively hydrolyzed protein formula may be used for 2 to 4 weeks in formula-fed infants with vomiting. Thickening agents for formula (1 tablespoon rice cereal/ounce formula) reduce regurgitation but not significantly (Hegar et al, 2008). An increase in caloric density may be necessary in infants with FTT (poor weight gain or weight loss). In older children and adolescents, there is no evidence to support specific dietary restrictions to decrease symptoms; however, avoiding eating

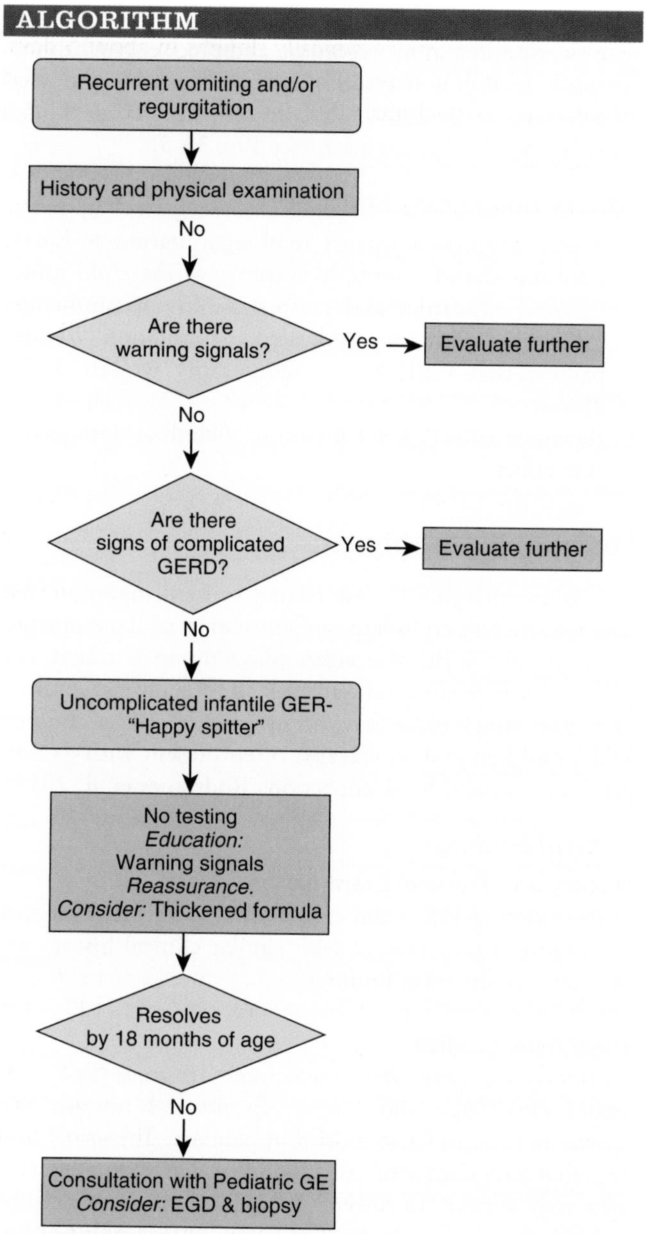

• **Figure 33-1** Approach to the infant with recurrent regurgitation and vomiting. *EGD,* Esophagogastroduodenoscopy; *GE,* gastroenterologist; *GER,* gastroesophageal reflux; *GERD,* gastroesophageal reflux disease. (From Vandenplas Y, Rudolph C, Di Lorenzo C, et al: Pediatric gastroesophageal reflux clinical practice guidelines: joint recommendations of the North American Society for Pediatric Gastroenterology, Hepatology, and Nutrition [NASPGHAN] and the European Society for Pediatric Gastroenterology, Hepatology, and Nutrition [ESPGHAN], *J Pediatr Gastroenterol Nutr* 49[4]:498–547, 2009.)

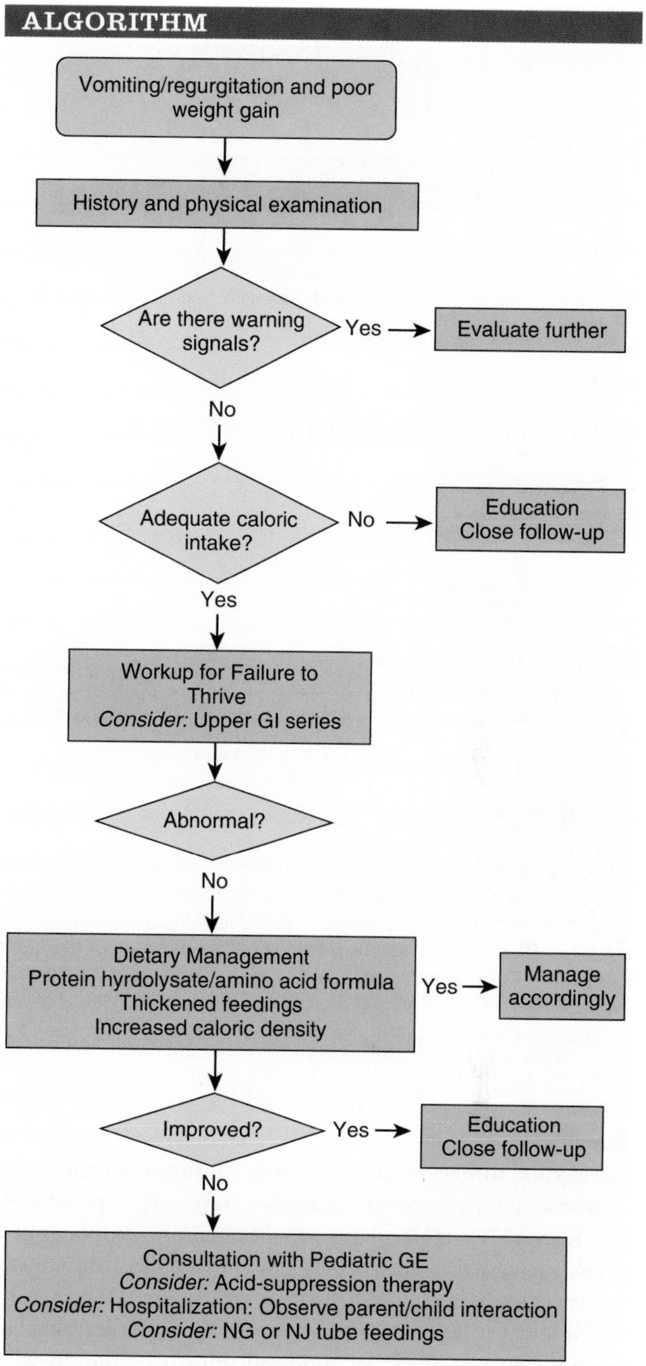

• **Figure 33-2** Approach to the infant with recurrent regurgitation and weight loss. *GE,* Gastroenterologist; *GI,* gastrointestinal; *NG,* nasogastric; *NJ,* nasojejunal. (From Vandenplas Y, Rudolph C, Di Lorenzo C, et al: Pediatric gastroesophageal reflux clinical practice guidelines: joint recommendations of the North American Society for Pediatric Gastroenterology, Hepatology, and Nutrition [NASPGHAN] and the European Society for Pediatric Gastroenterology, Hepatology, and Nutrition [ESPGHAN], *J Pediatr Gastroenterol Nutr* 49[4]:498–547, 2009.)

less than 2 hours before bedtime may be helpful. Obesity is related to GERD, so weight management could be helpful.

Lifestyle

Because prone positioning is associated with increased risk of sudden infant death syndrome (SIDS), supine positioning during sleep in infants is recommended. Positioning infants upright may worsen reflux. There may be some benefit in older children to left-side positioning during sleep or elevation of the head of the bed (elevate the head of the bed and don't add pillows because it may increase abdominal flexion and compression).

ALGORITHM

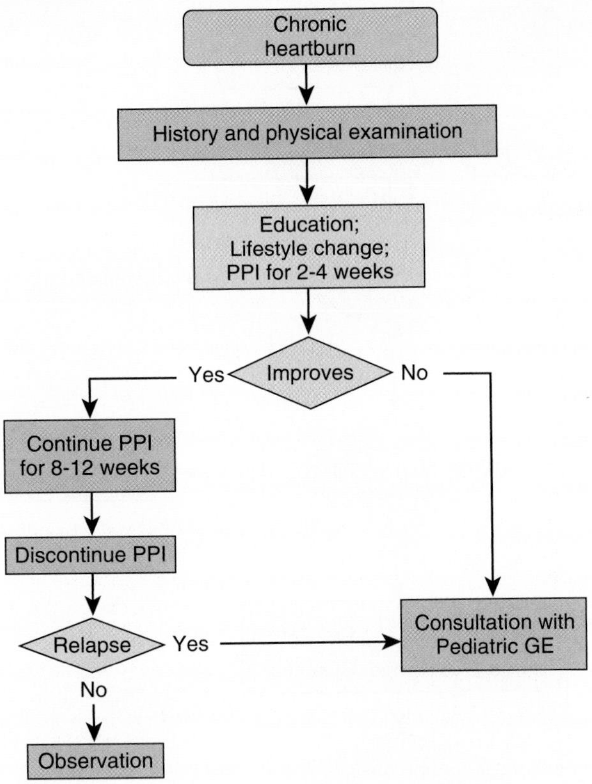

• **Figure 33-3** Approach to the older child or adolescent with heartburn. *GE,* Gastroenterologist; *PPI,* proton pump inhibitor. (From Vandenplas Y, Rudolph C, Di Lorenzo C, et al: Pediatric gastroesophageal reflux clinical practice guidelines: joint recommendations of the North American Society for Pediatric Gastroenterology, Hepatology, and Nutrition [NASPGHAN] and the European Society for Pediatric Gastroenterology, Hepatology, and Nutrition [ESPGHAN], *J Pediatr Gastroenterol Nutr* 49[4]:498–547, 2009.)

Surgical

Antireflux surgery strategies, such as fundoplication, are used for management of cases that have not responded to less invasive strategies, have life-threatening complications, or will have long-term dependence on medical therapy in which compliance or patient preference precludes ongoing use. However, the surgery is not necessarily curative. For example, in one study of fundoplication in children with cystic fibrosis (CF), 12% had repeat surgery, 48% had recurrent GERD symptoms, and only 28% discontinued GERD medications (Vandenplas et al, 2009). Now that PPI therapy is so successful, fundoplication may become less common (Khan and Orenstein, 2011b).

Complications

Complications include chronic cough, FTT, irritability, and malnutrition. Esophageal injury secondary to reflux results in bleeding, stricture formation, and Barrett esophagus. GERD is circumstantially associated with significant asthma, recurrent pneumonia, or laryngeal disorders. In the majority of infants with apnea or apparent life-threatening event, GERD is not the cause. However, in the rare case where a relationship is suspected, pH monitoring in combination with polysomnographic recording and precise, synchronous symptom recording may aid in establishing cause and effect (Vandenplas et al, 2009). Red flags in infants are bilious vomiting and/or hematemesis (see Box 33-5).

Patient and Family Education

- Assure parents of infants that regurgitation is usually self-limited and symptoms improve as the child grows. Parental education and reassurance are recommended for infants with uncomplicated regurgitation. Remind parents that GERD may temporarily worsen during illness.
- Review medication information, including dosages and side effects.

Eosinophilic Esophagitis

EoE is an emerging disease related to food ingestion. It is characterized by an isolated inflammation of the esophagus by a specific WBC the eosinophil. Young children may present with feeding refusal or FTT. Recurrent vomiting and abdominal pain may occur in school-age children. Older children and adolescents often present with dysphagia, choking, and food impaction (Rodrigues et al, 2013).

Clinical Findings

History and Physical Examination

Differentiating EoE from GERD may be difficult because both entities may present with similar clinical history and physical examination findings.

Diagnostic Studies

Currently the only way to accurately diagnose EoE is by upper endoscopy and biopsy. Esophageal mucosa may appear normal in up to a third of patients. The visual findings that have been associated with EoE are when the esophagus may appear "furrowed," "ring-like," or show multiple "white plaques or exudate" (Dellon, 2012; Schuval and Gold, 2013).

Management

Objectives of EoE therapy include improvement in histology and quality of life, reduction in clinical symptoms, and prevention of complications (such as, food impactions) or long-term sequelae (such as, strictures or small caliber esophagus). Current treatment modalities include dietary modification and pharmacotherapy.

Three dietary strategies include elemental diet administration, empiric dietary elimination, and targeted food elimination. Use of an elemental diet consisting of an amino acid-based formula remains the most effective and accepted dietary intervention for EoE in infants. For older children, many clinicians will recommend initially initiating the six-food (milk, soy, egg, wheat, peanut/tree nuts, and fish/shellfish) elimination diet and then an immediate referral to a pediatric allergist for identification and targeted food

TABLE 33-5 Management Strategies for Infants and Children with Gastroesophageal Reflux

Population	Diagnostic Tests	Management Strategies
Infant with uncomplicated recurrent regurgitation (GER)	None needed	Provide parental education and reassurance. In formula-fed babies, a thickened formula may reduce over-regurgitation and vomiting but does not reduce the reflux itself.
Infants with recurrent vomiting and poor weight gain (GERD)	Diet history, UA, CBC, serum electrolytes, BUN, serum creatinine Other tests as indicated	For breastfed infants, continue to breastfeed. For formula-fed babies, 2-week trial of extensively hydrolyzed formula or amino acid–based formula to exclude CMA. Increase caloric density. Thicken formula if needed. Educate regarding formula intake needed to sustain normal weight gain. Refer to pediatric gastroenterologist if management fails to improve symptoms and weight gain.
Infants with unexplained crying and/or distressed behavior	Evaluate for CMA, neurologic disorders, constipation, infection (especially UTIs)	Empiric trial with extensively hydrolyzed protein formula or amino acid–based formula. No evidence to support the empiric use of acid suppression for the treatment of irritable infants. However, if irritability persists and no condition other than GERD remains, then continued support of parents with the anticipation of improvement over time; workup to establish the relationship of reflux to feeding or to diagnose esophagitis; or trial of antisecretory therapy, although there is a potential risk for adverse effects. Clinical improvement following empiric therapy may result in spontaneous symptom resolution or placebo response.
Child older than 18 months old with chronic regurgitation or vomiting	Consider diagnosis other than GERD; testing may include upper GI endoscopy, esophageal pH/MII, and barium upper GI series	Treatment depends on diagnosis.
Heartburn in older children and adolescents	No further studies needed if problem is episodic and not severe	On-demand therapy with buffering agents, sodium alginate, or H2RA may be used for occasional symptoms. For chronic heartburn, lifestyle changes, such as diet change, weight loss, smoking avoidance, sleeping position, no late-night eating, and a 2-week trial with a PPI may help. PPI can be continued for up to 3 months if symptoms resolve. Persistent heartburn after that time should be referred to a pediatric gastroenterologist.
Reflux esophagitis—endoscopically diagnosed	No further studies needed	PPI for 3 months is initial therapy. Trial of tapering the dose and then withdrawal of PPI. Chronic relapsing esophagitis may be the diagnosis if PPI cannot be withdrawn and may involve long-term therapy with PPI or antireflux surgery.

Adapted from Vandenplas Y, Rudolph C, Di Lorenzo C, et al: Pediatric gastroesophageal reflux clinical practice guidelines: joint recommendations of the North American Society for Pediatric Gastroenterology, Hepatology, and Nutrition (NASPGHAN) and the European Society for Pediatric Gastroenterology, Hepatology, and Nutrition (ESPGHAN), *J Pediatr Gastroenterol Nutr* 49(4):498–547, 2009.

BUN, Blood urea nitrogen; *CBC,* complete blood count; *CMA,* cow's-milk allergy; *GER,* gastroesophageal reflux; *GERD,* gastroesophageal reflux disease; *GI,* gastrointestinal; *H2RA,* histamine 2 receptor antagonist; *MII,* multichannel intraluminal impedance; *PPI,* proton pump inhibitor; *UA,* urinalysis; *UTI,* urinary tract infection.

elimination, based on the allergy testing (Dellon, 2012; Wechsler et al, 2014).

Treatment of EoE usually consists of PPIs and topical swallowed corticosteroids (fluticasone, propionate, budesonide, and ciclesonide) for 12 weeks. However, currently there is no medication specifically approved by the FDA for the disease.

Peptic Ulcer Disease

PUD consists of a group of gastric and duodenal disorders ranging from gastritis to ulceration. With duodenal ulcers, mucosal defects penetrate the duodenal mucosa and submucosa. Gastric ulcers result from mucosal defects that penetrate the gastric mucosa and submucosa. Peptic ulcers

TABLE 33-6 Common Medications Used to Treat Gastroesophageal Reflux Disease

Medication	Pediatric Dosage
Histamine 2 Receptor Antagonists	
Cimetidine	Infants: 10-20 mg/kg/day divided doses every 6 to 12 hours Children: 20-40 mg/kg/day in divided doses every 6 hours Adult dose: 300 mg/dose PO qid **OR** 400 mg/dose PO bid **OR** 800 mg/dose PO qhs
Famotidine (Pepcid)	Infants: 1 to 3 months old: 0.5 mg/kg/dose once daily for up to 8 weeks Infants >3 months old to 1 year old: 0.5 mg/kg/dose twice daily for up to 8 weeks Children and adolescents: Initially 0.25 mg/kg/dose every 12 hours (maximum dose: 20 mg/dose)
Nizatidine (Axid)	Infants 6 months old to children 11 years old: 5-10 mg/kg/day divided twice daily Children 12 years+: 150 mg once daily
Ranitidine (Zantac)	Infants >1 month, children, and adolescents <16 years old: 4-8 mg/kg/day divided twice daily (maximum dose: 300 mg) Adolescents >16 years old: 150 mg twice daily or 300 mg once HS
Proton Pump Inhibitors	
Lansoprazole (Prevacid)	Children 1 to 11 years old: <30 kg: 15 mg once daily for up to 12 weeks >30 kg: 30 mg once daily for up to 12 weeks
Omeprazole (Prilosec)	Children > 1 year: 5 to 10 kg: 5 mg once daily for up to 12 weeks 10 to 20 kg: 10 mg once daily for up to 12 weeks >20 kg: 20 mg once daily for up to 12 weeks
Rabeprazole (Aciphex)	Children 1 to 11 years old: <15 kg: 5 mg once daily for <12 weeks >15 kg: 10 mg once daily for <12 weeks Adult dose: 20 mg once daily for <12 weeks
Pantoprazole (Protonix)	Infants and children <5 years old: 1.2 mg/kg/day once daily for 4 weeks Children 5 to 11 years old: 20-40 mg once daily for up to 8 weeks Children and adolescents 12 to 16 years old: 20 or 40 mg once daily for up to 8 weeks
Esomeprazole (Nexium)	Infants: 3 to 5 kg: 2.5 mg once daily for up to 8 weeks 5 to 7.5 kg: 5 mg once daily for up to 8 weeks >7.5 kg: 10 mg once daily for up to 8 weeks Children 1 to 11 years old: <20 kg 10 mg once daily for up to 8 weeks >20 kg: 10-20 mg once daily for up to 8 weeks Children >12 years old: 20-40 mg once daily for up to 8 weeks Contents of capsule may be mixed with 1 tablespoon of applesauce for easier swallowing, if needed.
Cytoprotective Agent	
Sucralfate (Carafate)	40-80 mg/kg/day divided every 6 hours Adult dose 250 mg divided every 6 hours Take on an empty stomach 1 hour before meal and HS

Data from Engorn B, Flerage J: *The Harriet Lane handbook: a manual for pediatric house officer,* ed 20, Philadelphia, 2015, Elsevier; Khan S, Orenstein S: Gastroesophageal reflux disease. In Kliegman RM, Stanton BF, St. Geme JW, et al: *Nelson textbook of pediatrics,* ed 19, Philadelphia, 2011, Elsevier; Lightdale JR, Gremse DA, Section on Gastroenterology, Hepatology, and Nutrition: Gastroesophageal reflux: management guidance for the pediatrician, *Pediatrics* 131(5):e1684–e1685, 2013.

are different in children compared with adults in clinical presentation, as well as in prevalence rates, types of ulcer disease, and complications (Blanchard and Czinn, 2011).

PUD is classified as primary or secondary. Most *primary ulcers* are duodenal, have no underlying cause, and tend to be chronic with resulting granulation tissue and fibrosis. They tend to recur. They are more common in adolescents and rare in children. *Secondary ulcers* are more often gastric, generally more acute, and associated with known ulcerogenic events. Severe erosive gastropathy can result in bleeding ulcers or gastric perforations, more commonly in the stomach than duodenum. Head trauma, severe burns, use of corticosteroids, and nonsteroidal anti-inflammatory drugs (NSAIDs) are associated with secondary ulcers. Aspirin or NSAIDs cause mucosal injury by direct injury or inhibiting cyclooxygenase and prostaglandin formation. Chronic therapy with these medicines causes gastric mucosal damage but is not associated with ulcer formation. Stress ulceration usually occurs within 24 hours of critical illness and may occur in 25% of critically ill children in intensive care units. Preterm and term infants in neonatal intensive care units (NICUs) can also develop gastric mucosal lesions with bleeding or perforation. *Idiopathic ulcers* are found in *H. pylori*–negative children who have no history of taking NSAIDs; 20% of pediatric duodenal ulcers are of this type. A strong familial predisposition for PUD has been noted, and most children with duodenal ulcers have a positive family medical history, which is a key finding. There is no evidence that diet plays a role in the formation of ulcers. Smoking can cause duodenal ulcers and slows the rate of healing (Blanchard and Czinn, 2011).

Peptic ulcers result from an imbalance between protective and aggressive factors. *Protective factors* include the water-insoluble mucous gel lining, local production of bicarbonate, regulation of gastric acid, and adequate mucosal blood flow. *Aggressive factors* include the acid-pepsin environment, infection with *H. pylori,* and mucosal ischemia. Colonization rates with *H. pylori* in the United States and Europe are less than 10%; there are much higher rates in less-developed countries. Colonization likely occurs during the first years of life, but the infection often remains asymptomatic with low-grade inflammation or no mucosal changes. Peptic ulcers in children are much less related to *H. pylori* infection than they were in past years, because the incidence of *H. pylori* in the general population is decreasing as living conditions have improved (Koletzko et al, 2011). PUD has an estimated frequency of five to seven cases in 2500 hospital admissions. Zollinger-Ellison syndrome (ZES) is a rare syndrome involving refractory severe PUD caused by gastric hypersecretion due to the autonomous secretion of gastrin by a neuroendocrine tumor (Blanchard and Czinn, 2011).

Clinical Findings

The most common symptom of PUD is vague, dull abdominal pain; however, the presenting symptoms vary depending on the age of the child. Hematemesis or melena is reported in up to 50% of patients. Neonates can present with gastric perforation. Infants usually present with feeding difficulty, vomiting, crying episodes, hematemesis, or melena. Epigastric pain and nausea are reported more often by school-age children and adolescents. The classic adult symptom of PUD, pain alleviated by ingestion of food, is present in only a minority of children. Most children presenting with epigastric or periumbilical pain do not have PUD, but rather functional bowel disorder, IBS, or functional dyspepsia. They rarely present with acute abdominal pain with ulceration from perforation or symptoms of pancreatitis from a posterior penetrating ulcer (Blanchard and Czinn, 2011).

History

- Asymptomatic or symptoms wax and wane. Remissions may last from weeks to months.
- Pain with eating, dyspepsia; can awaken from sleep.
- GI tract bleeding may be a presenting symptom.
- Infants: Poor feeding, GI bleeding, vomiting, intestinal perforation, slow growth; history of prematurity or time in NICU.
- Toddlers and preschoolers: Poorly localized abdominal pain, vomiting, GI bleeding. May worsen after eating; irritability; anorexia.
- School-age children and adolescents: Poorly localized epigastric or right lower quadrant (RLQ) pain. Pain is often described as dull, aching, and lasting from minutes to hours. Nocturnal pain is common in older children. Relief from antacids is reported by less than 33% of children. If the pain awakens the child, worsens with food, and is relieved by fasting, this may help distinguish GI pathology from psychogenic pathology, although these symptoms are infrequently described in children. Recurrent vomiting may occur.
- GI bleeding may lead to iron deficiency anemia with symptoms of fatigue, headache, dyspnea, and malaise.
- Family history of PUD.
- Predisposing factors: Alcohol, smoking, aspirin, NSAIDs, corticosteroids, emotional stress, serious systemic disease, sepsis, hypotension, respiratory failure, multiple traumatic injuries, and extensive burns.
- ZES presents with severe peptic ulceration, kidney stones, watery diarrhea, or malabsorption (fasting serum gastrin level greater than 200 pg/mL and baseline gastric acid hypersecretion at more than 15 mEq/hr).

Physical Examination

A careful physical examination should be performed; however, there may be no physical findings. The physical examination should include the following:

- Height, weight, head circumference, BMI, and percentiles
- Vital signs
- General observation of the appearance of the child
- Assessment of perfusion: Mental status, heart rate, pulses, capillary refill, pallor
- Assessment of hydration: Mucous membranes and skin turgor
- Careful mouth inspection for ulcers (associated with Crohn disease) and dental enamel erosion (associated with GERD)
- Lung examination for wheezing (associated with GERD)
- Abdominal examination for tenderness and hepatosplenomegaly

- Rectal examination (to assess perirectal disease)
- Pelvic examination in sexually active female patients with pain
- Testicles and inguinal examination in male patients

Diagnostic Studies

Endoscopy with mucosal biopsy is the diagnostic test of choice, and validates *H. pylori* infection. However, if a child has mild PUD, minimal laboratory studies are needed. Diagnostic studies to consider include the following.

Laboratory Studies

- Initially (red flags for systemic disease): CBC (anemia is associated with chronic infection with *H. pylori* or acute or chronic blood loss due to ulcer perforation into the abdominal cavity), albumin (low), and ESR (high). May also consider stool for guaiac and *H. pylori* (especially in children).
- If child is unstable, severe, or has chronic, recurrent symptoms, or serious complications consider also iron studies; *H. pylori* serology (most useful in teenagers, only helpful in children if negative due to high false-positive rate); prothrombin time and activated partial thromboplastin time (aPTT; useful to identify coagulopathy); electrolyte, BUN, creatinine levels (to assess volume depletion); arterial blood gases (acidosis); UA (hydration, infection, or stones); serum gastrin and gastrin-releasing peptide levels (in patients with refractory ulcers to exclude ZES). *Note:* PPIs must be discontinued 2 weeks before gastrin level measurement. Type and cross-match for blood may also be done.

Imaging Studies

- Abdominal or chest x-ray for perforation
- Upper GI series helps diagnosis in about 70% of children (sensitivity higher for duodenal ulcers). A fibrinous clot in the ulcer may lead to false-negative findings. Barium studies have false-positive rates as high as 30% to 40%. Gastric outlet obstructions often due to pyloric lesions can be identified.
- Angiography is sometimes done if there is a massive bleed and endoscopy cannot be performed.

Procedures

- Esophagogastroduodenoscopy (EGD) is the procedure of choice in children for detecting PUD, because it allows direct visualization of mucosa, localization of source of bleeding, and collection of biopsy specimens. It is also used therapeutically for acute bleeding.

Studies to Detect Helicobacter Pylori

- Histologic examination and culture biopsies obtained via endoscopy are the gold standard for detecting acute infection, but this is an invasive procedure that requires anesthesia. It is appropriate for persistent or recurrent infection or severe symptoms.
- C-urea breath test is the noninvasive diagnostic test of choice; it can distinguish between past and present infection. It is sensitive to children older than 2 years of age, but requires special equipment. It should be performed off acid suppression to avoid false-negative results.
- Stool monoclonal antibody test distinguishes between past and present infection. It is reliable for evaluating response to therapy if symptoms persist and should be performed off acid suppression (4 weeks) to avoid false-negative results.
- Serum immunoglobulin G (IgG) antibody titer. A positive result (greater than 500 units) only means exposure to the disease. This test should neither be the sole basis for starting therapy nor used to test for eradication. It is good for initial screening in the workup of epigastric pain/dyspepsia.

Differential Diagnosis

All other causes of abdominal pain, especially GERD, IBS, GI bleeding, cholelithiasis, cholecystitis, pancreatitis, lactose intolerance, hyperkalemia, and hypercalcemia, are in the differential.

Management

- The goals of treatment include ulcer healing, elimination of the primary cause, relief of symptoms, and prevention of complications.
- Medications:
  - H2RAs or PPIs are first-line therapy (see Table 33-6). PPIs have the best effect if given before a meal.
  - Antacids: Any liquid preparation, 0.5 mL/kg, given between 1 and 3 hours after eating and before bed.
  - *Eradication therapy* for *H. pylori* is indicated for children with a duodenal or gastric ulcer identified by endoscopy and histopathology. *Empiric therapy* for suspected *H. pylori* is not recommended. There is increasing antibiotic resistance to *H. pylori.* Therapy is not indicated for gastritis without PUD, recurrent abdominal pain, or for children with asymptomatic PUD or with a family member with PUD. See Table 33-7 for treatment guidelines when *H. pylori* is confirmed. Compliance with the treatment regimen is the single most important determinant of eradication. Eradication rates are more than 90%. The test of cure can either be the stool antigen test or the urea breath test.
- Referral to a gastroenterologist should occur if there is:
  - Lack of improvement or inability to wean off medications
  - History of hematemesis, melena, occult blood in stools, anemia, and/or weight loss
- Idiopathic ulcers: The preferred treatment is acid suppression with either H2RAs or PPIs. Patients should be followed closely and, if symptoms recur, acid suppression restarted. PPIs are preferred for maintenance in children older than 1 year of age.

TABLE 33-7 Recommended Eradication Therapies for *Helicobacter Pylori* Disease in Children

Medications	Dosage
Option 1 (Three Drugs)	
Amoxicillin	50 mg/kg/day up to 1 g twice daily
Clarithromycin	15 mg/kg/day up to 500 mg twice daily
Omeprazole	1 mg/kg/day up to 20 mg twice daily
Option 2 (Three Drugs)	
Amoxicillin	50 mg/kg/day up to 1 g twice daily
Metronidazole	20 mg/kg/day up to 500 mg twice daily
Omeprazole	1-2 mg/kg/day up to 20 mg twice daily
Option 3 (Three Drugs; 8 Years Old or Older)	
Bismuth sub salicylate	8 to 12 years old: 8 mg/kg/day times a day
Amoxicillin	50 mg/kg/day up to 1 g twice daily
Metronidazole	20 mg/kg/day divided up to 500 mg twice daily
Option 4 (Sequential Therapy)	
	Omeprazole and amoxicillin for 5 days then omeprazole, clarithromycin, and metronidazole for 5 days at dosages above

From Koletzko S, Jones NL, Goodman KJ: Evidence-based guidelines from ESPGHAN and NASPGHAN for *Helicobacter pylori* infection in children, *J Pediatr Gastroenterol Nutr* 53(2):230–243, 2011.

- ZES: PPIs are the mainstay of treatment and must be started promptly (Blanchard and Czinn, 2011).

Complications

Acute hemorrhage, chronic blood loss, penetration of the ulcer into the abdominal cavity, or adjacent organs may produce shock, anemia, peritonitis, or pancreatitis. Obstruction can occur if inflammation and edema are extensive. Hemorrhage occurs in 15% to 20% of patients, and perforation occurs in less than 5%. Recurrence, gastric outlet obstruction, gastric adenocarcinoma, and gastric lymphoma are other possible complications. The highest rates of mortality are found in young infants with secondary stress ulcers in which GI bleeding or hemorrhage occur, sometimes catastrophically (Blanchard and Czinn, 2011).

Patient and Family Education

Treatment success depends on the child completing the drug regimen. PUD in children is being actively studied, and clinicians must be aware of ongoing changes. With the introduction of H2RAs and PPIs and the recognition that *H. pylori* can be treated, the incidence of complications has decreased dramatically.

Lower Gastrointestinal Tract Disorders

Infantile Colic

Infantile colic is characterized by persistent crying in infants younger than 3 months old. The average infant cries for 2 to 3 hours per day. In contrast, an infant with colic usually cries for more than 4 hours per day. In 1954, Wessel and colleagues established the original criteria known as *the rule of threes:* beginning at 1 to 2 weeks of life, periods of crying for 3 or more hours per day, 3 or more days per week, lasting for 3 or more weeks. Illingsworth (1985) described colicky infants as having attacks of screaming in the evening with classic motor features that included flushed face, furrowed brow, and clenched fists, with legs drawn up and a piercing high-pitched scream.

No specific cause of colic has been identified, and multiple independent causes are felt to contribute, with both physical and psychosocial factors playing a role. Organic causes for excessive crying account for less than 5% of infants. Differences in functional biomarkers, such as breath hydrogen production in response to lactose-containing milk, intestinal permeability changes, circulating gut hormones, food intolerance, gut microflora, and inflammatory markers may or may not indicate pathology. One study describes aberrant intestinal microflora and inflammation the effects on gut motor function and gas production by coliform bacteria *Escherichia coli* (Savino et al, 2010). Another study reports that the microbiota diversity in fecal matter was only present in those infants without colic (de Weerth et al, 2013). As a result, recommendations regarding probiotic supplementation are varied.

Psychosocial factors that may play a role in the intensity of colic include the perception of a stressful pregnancy, negative childbirth experience, unsatisfying interactions among family members, and overstimulation. The parents' inability to accurately interpret and respond to the infant's cries may contribute to colic. The stress created by a crying baby contributes to ineffective parental communication and interventions, family dysfunction, parental anxiety, and fatigue. In a study by Megel and colleagues (2011) mothers with infants who cry persistently had a sense of loss, not only of her competence as a mother but also of the infant she brought home from the hospital. Until the colic resolved, the mothers went through cycles of "searching" for the feeling of being a "good" mother.

Carey's study on colic (1972) described colicky babies as having a low sensory threshold. Keefe (1988) suggested the term *irritable infant syndrome* "characterized by excessive crying, increased activity, and difficulty falling asleep" (p 76) and attributed symptoms to the infant's inability to regulate state. More recent studies do not support the notion that colic is a manifestation of a child with "difficult temperament," but it is more likely just a manifestation of the spectrum of variation of typical behavioral development and physical maturation, although new research suggests a possible link between colic and migraines (Deshpande, 2014; Gelfand et al, 2015). The fact that colic tends to go away completely by 4 months of age may support this notion.

The incidence of colic varies greatly depending on the definition used. Studies using the Wessel definition tend to cite an incidence of about 20% of infants. However, other studies range as high as 40% (Deshpande, 2014; Megel et al, 2011; Savino et al, 2010).

Clinical Findings

History

- Infant is younger than 3 months old and cries 3 hours or more a day for 3 days or more per week
- Demands frequent feeding and is often fussy while feeding
- Has excessive gas
- Is inconsolable or is comforted for short periods only
- Is "tense" or "tight" and keeps legs stiff and fists clenched tightly
- Red flags in the history indicating a potential organic cause for crying include apnea, cyanosis, struggling to breathe; excessive spitting or vomiting; and stool retention

Physical Examination

If possible, see the family during a crying time. A thorough examination must be completed to rule out other pathologic conditions and should include the following:

- Body temperature and evaluation of growth parameters
- Full body examination to look for signs of trauma or abuse
- Abdominal examination for distention, masses, tenderness, and bowel sounds
- Stool for blood or mucus

Diagnostic Studies

If the child is gaining weight and has a normal examination, no other laboratory tests are indicated.

Differential Diagnosis

All other causes of abdominal pain are in the differential diagnosis. UTI, other infection, corneal abrasion, or traumatic injury are also included.

Management

No treatment is totally effective for infantile colic. The goal of treatment is to manage the situation until the colic resolves itself. Parents and providers who are flexible, creative, and persistent in seeking solutions are most likely to be successful. Recommendations for providers include the following (Megel et al, 2011):

- Rule out potential physiologic causes of crying.
- Review strategies already used and offer other suggestions (Box 33-6).
- Allow the mother to talk about effects on herself and other family members.

• BOX 33-6 Management Strategies for Infantile Colic

Nutritional

- Elimination of certain foods from the diet of breastfeeding mothers may prove beneficial: cow's-milk products, eggs, peanuts, tree nuts, wheat, soy, and fish (Iacovou et al, 2012).
- Hydrolyzed formula may show some effectiveness.

Parent Education and Support

- Affirm the baby's good health and reinforce the parents' efforts to comfort their infant.
- Acknowledge the importance of the concern. Allow parents to express feelings of anger, guilt, and frustration.
- Help parents distinguish infant cries and understand typical infant crying, crying associated with illness, and infant state.
- Encourage parents to take time off by seeking help from family or friends.
- Repeat information, because parents are often sleep deprived and anxious.
- Meet the infant's needs: Feed, sleep, hold, suck, and stimulate.
- Reduce stimulation (quiet, dark, motionless) and avoid the overtired state (nap within 1 to 2 hours of wakefulness).
- Promote regularity and predictability of feeding and sleeping.
- Keep a diary of baby's fussing, crying, and sleeping; analyze to develop a clear daily routine and identify patterns that may be addressed by behavioral intervention (e.g., attunement, self-soothing).

Soothing Techniques

- Encourage sucking at breast, fist, fingers, or pacifier.
- Provide rhythmic activities: Rock, swing, jogger, bouncing, walking, and dancing.
- Swaddling reduces crying, improves sleep, and shortens periods of distress.
- Provide "white" noise: Lullabies, shushing, nature-recorded sounds, heartbeat or womb-recorded sounds, and hair dryer or vacuum cleaner sounds.
- Kangaroo care (skin-to-skin) contact may be beneficial.
- Car rides, crib vibrators, infant massage, and increased holding (front carrier) may be beneficial (Patterson, 2013).

Complementary Therapies*

- Probiotics have shown improvement in episodes and length of crying.
- Herbal teas (chamomile, vervain, licorice, fennel, and lemon balm) may reduce crying.
- Gripe water (mixture of herbs and herb oils) is touted to provide relief from flatulence and indigestion, but is not entirely without risk. Parents need to avoid products that contain alcohol or are made outside the United States.
- Sucrose solutions may offer some analgesic effect for single procedure in newborn infants (Harrison et al, 2010).
- Chiropractic, osteopathic, and massage interventions have also been used.
- Homeopathic remedies are considered benign because they are low concentration. However, one study of a homeopathic remedy, Gali-col Baby, showed an association between an apparent life-threatening event and use of this remedy in infants (Aviner et al, 2010).

*See also Chapter 43.

- Acknowledge the challenges of the situation and the mother's efforts to help.
- Follow up by phone call or visit.

Complications

Stress created by a crying baby can contribute to parental feelings of hostility, anger, and guilt, ultimately leading to poor parent-child interaction. Early termination of breastfeeding, postpartum depression, shaken baby syndrome, unnecessary treatment for GERD, postpartum resumption of cigarette smoking, and SIDS have a relationship to an infant's excessive crying. Parents may self-impose isolation because they do not want to burden others with the crying infant, may fear being perceived as an inadequate parent, and/or fear the infant's safety in the hands of a sitter (Megel et al, 2011). Parents may respond by physically or emotionally abusing their infant.

Patient and Family Education

Given the risk for child abuse, the National Center for Shaken Baby Syndrome "Period of PURPLE Crying" campaign (**P**eak, **U**npredictability of crying bouts, **R**esistance to soothing, **P**ain-like expression, **L**ong crying bouts, and **E**vening clustering) has materials to educate parents about the characteristics of early (first 3 months of life) crying. If abuse or neglect has occurred or the family appears to be at significant risk, reporting to the local child abuse intervention center or hotline is required and the parents need significant help.

Foreign Body Ingestion

Most foreign body ingestions are not serious; objects pass through the gut without consequence. Most swallowed items are radiopaque; coins and small toy objects are the most commonly ingested items. Food impactions are less common in children than adults. Most ingestions of foreign bodies occur in children between 6 months and 3 years of age (80%) and more than 125,000 ingestions occur annually in patients younger than 19 years old (Sandoval, 2013). Teens may have psychiatric problems or engage in risk-taking behaviors leading to foreign body ingestion. Disk battery ingestions have increased dramatically in the past few years and are very serious (Litovitz et al, 2010).

Esophageal Foreign Bodies

Esophageal foreign bodies lodge at three spots most commonly—at the thoracic inlet where skeletal muscle changes to smooth muscle (between the clavicles at about C6) (70%), at the mid-esophagus where the aortic arch and carina overlap the esophagus (15%), or at the LES (15%). Pointed objects or small objects, such as pills or small button batteries, may lodge anywhere along the slightly moist esophageal mucosa. Up to 30% of children with foreign bodies lodged in the esophagus are asymptomatic (Khan and Orenstein, 2011a). Common symptoms include an initial episode of choking, gagging, and coughing. Excessive salivation; dysphagia; food refusal; emesis/hematemesis; or pain in the neck, throat, or sternal notch areas may follow. Respiratory symptoms such as stridor, wheezing, cyanosis, or dyspnea may occur if the esophageal body impinges on the larynx or tracheal wall. Cervical swelling, erythema, or subcutaneous crepitations may indicate perforation of the oropharynx or proximal esophagus (Khan and Orenstein, 2011a; Sandoval, 2013). Drooling or pooling of secretions may be related to an esophageal foreign body or abrasion of the esophagus as a result of swallowing the object. Disk batteries cause a liquefactive necrosis, electrical discharge leading to low-voltage burns, and pressure necrosis. Some patients have documented severe erosion or ulceration in as little as 2 hours after ingestion (Kimball et al, 2010). Emergency endoscopic removal is essential. Children who have swallowed lithium batteries greater than or equal to 20 mm diameter are at greatest risk of problems due to battery ingestion.

Abdominal Foreign Bodies

Most ingested objects that reach the stomach pass through the remainder of the GI tract without difficulty (Kelsen and Liacouras, 2011). Items greater than 5 cm in diameter or 2 cm in thickness tend to lodge in the stomach and need to be retrieved. Thin objects longer than 10 cm may not make the duodenal sweep turn and also need to be retrieved. In infants and toddlers, objects greater than 3 cm in length or 20 mm in diameter may not pass through the pyloric sphincter. Open safety pins or other pointed objects, such as needles or thumbtacks, also should be retrieved.

Perforation after ingestion occurs in only 1% of ingestions. Perforation occurs near physiologic sphincters, areas of angulation, congenital malformations of the gut, or near areas of previous bowel surgery. Coins made with nickel have been reported to interact with gastric acid to cause stomach ulceration (Sandoval, 2013). Abdominal distention or pain, vomiting, hematochezia, and unexplained fever are symptoms related to ingestions lodging in the stomach or intestinal areas. Items that pose a greater risk include multiple small magnets that may cling together across the bowel wall, leading to pressure necrosis; items containing lead; and batteries, which usually do not cause problems but might lead to symptoms if there is leakage of alkali or mercury from battery degradation. Lithium toxicity has been reported. Nickel in coins can lead to allergic symptoms in children with a nickel allergy.

Rectal Foreign Bodies

Children sometimes put items into their rectum. Small blunt objects usually will pass spontaneously, but large or sharp objects should be retrieved after sedation to relax the anal sphincter.

Clinical Findings

History, Physical Examination, and Laboratory Studies

Specific physical findings are unusual. Abrasions, streaks of blood, or edema of the hypopharynx may occasionally indicate a foreign body. Laboratory studies are usually not helpful, although they may be useful to identify potential infection.

Imaging Studies

Most foreign bodies are radiopaque. A single frontal radiograph that includes the neck, chest, and entire abdomen is usually sufficient to locate the object. Subsequent radiographs may be useful to more fully evaluate the patient. Esophageal objects should be precisely located with frontal and lateral chest radiographs and to make sure that there are not two objects closely aligned. Coins in the esophagus are usually seen on the frontal view, whereas tracheal coins are more often seen from the side view (Sandoval, 2013). Having the child ingest a small amount of dilute contrast material may help locate radiolucent objects. Endoscopy may be needed and also allows removal of the object.

Management

Most objects do not require special care. Patients who are drooling may require suction.

Esophageal Foreign Bodies

Objects in the esophagus should generally be considered impacted. Removal is mandatory except for blunt objects that have been in place less than 24 hours. Disk batteries and sharp objects should be removed without waiting. Endoscopy is the method of choice for removal except that experienced gastroenterology practitioners may use a Foley catheter to pull the object up or a bougienage method to push the object into the stomach. Only experienced clinicians working with healthy children who ingested an item less than 24 hours previously should try these methods. They are preceded by a radiograph to be sure the item has not moved in the immediate period before the procedure and followed by another radiograph to be sure there are not any retained parts or complications, such as a pneumomediastinum.

Stomach/Lower Gastrointestinal Tract Foreign Bodies

Most foreign bodies that reach the stomach may be left to pass through the system, usually within 2 to 3 days. Very sharp items may perforate the bowel and should be removed endoscopically from the stomach or surgically from the intestine. Button batteries in the stomach or intestine may be left to pass but should be removed if the family has not identified the battery in the stool after 2 to 3 days. It should be removed endoscopically from the stomach at that time or watched with repeat radiographs to be sure it is progressing through the tract if it is in the intestine. Items may not pass through the gut if the child has a bowel abnormality or has had bowel surgery. Use of laxatives is not necessary. Inducing vomiting may lead to aspiration.

Complications

Systemic reactions from allergy or toxic response to massive ingestion can occur. Retained foreign bodies may cause erosion, abrasion, local scarring, obstruction, abscess, FTT, perforation, pneumomediastinum, pneumonia, or other respiratory disease. Complications from the removal process can occur. Traumatic epiglottitis can occur from trauma during swallowing or a finger sweep trying to dislodge the item.

Appendicitis

Appendicitis is inflammation of the appendix that leads to distention and ischemia that can result in necrosis, perforation, and peritonitis or abscess formation. Although a classic presentation is easy to discern, appendicitis can mimic many other intraabdominal conditions, making diagnosis tricky.

Following a closed-loop obstruction of the appendiceal lumen by a fecalith, lymphoid tissue, tumor, parasite, foreign body, or inspissated CF secretions, the appendix becomes distended, experiences increased bacterial overgrowth, and becomes subject to ischemia and necrosis. Peritoneal inflammation around the infected appendix causes the characteristic symptoms. There is about a 36- to 72-hour maximum window from the onset of pain to the rupture of the gangrenous appendix. Rupture results in the release of inflammatory fluid and bacteria into the abdominal cavity, resulting in infection of the peritoneum with resultant generalized peritonitis. The infected fluid may be walled off by the omentum and loops of small bowel with resultant abscess formation and localized pain (Minkes, 2014).

The average age of appendicitis in children is 6 to 10 years old, with a male-to-female ratio of approximately 2:1. It is rare in infancy. The incidence is 4 cases per 1000 children. Perforation is most common in younger children (under 5 years old) and is complicated by the fact that appendicitis is less common in this age group and that the ability of very young children (younger than 5 years) to communicate location and type of pain is not yet well developed (Minkes, 2014). Thus it is challenging at times to make a timely diagnosis.

Clinical Findings

History

- The most reliable information is gained from the sequence of symptoms (Minkes, 2014):
  - Pain: Initially poorly defined periumbilical pain (earliest sign); acute onset of severe pain is not typical of acute appendicitis. A shifting of pain to the RLQ may occur after a few hours and becomes more intense, continuous, and localized.
  - Nausea and vomiting: Typically occurs after pain; however, in retrocecal appendicitis, this may be reversed. In gastroenteritis, vomiting precedes the pain.
  - Anorexia occurs (although up to 50% of children state that they are hungry).
  - Stool is low volume with mucus; diarrhea is atypical but can occur (gastroenteritis has high-volume, watery stools).

- Fever is neither sensitive nor specific for appendicitis; many children present as afebrile or with low-grade fever. High fever may be associated with perforation.
- A scoring system may be helpful (Kharbanda et al, 2005). A score of 5 or less is highly sensitive in the exclusion of the diagnosis of appendicitis:
  - Nausea (2 points)
  - Focal RLQ pain (2 points)
  - Migration of pain (1 point)
  - Difficulty walking (1 point)
  - Rebound tenderness and/or pain with percussion (2 points)
  - Absolute neutrophil count more than 6.75 × 103/µL (6 points)
- The process evolves over 12 hours, with the potential for infants and young children to become sick much more quickly.
- Following perforation, symptoms lessen, with less vomiting, fever greater than 101° F (38.3° C), and the most comfortable position being on the side with the legs flexed.
- Infants demonstrate irritability, pain with movement, and flexed hips.
- The child may become quiet because crying and movement hurt.

Physical Examination

A complete physical examination is necessary. Reexamination may be needed in 4 to 6 hours.

- Presence of involuntary guarding, RLQ rebound tenderness, maximal pain over McBurney point (1.5 to 2 inches in from the right anterior superior iliac crest on a line toward the umbilicus) on abdominal examination (most reliable finding); percussion is best method for eliciting rebound tenderness.
- Heel-drop jarring test (on toes for 15 seconds, dropping down forcefully on heels); inability to stand straight or climb stairs; winces when getting off examination table or riding in a car over bumps; child most comfortable with bent knees.
- Positive psoas sign or obturator sign (or both).
- Rovsing sign (pressure deep in left lower quadrant with sudden release elicits RLQ pain) strongly suggests peritoneal irritation (Minkes, 2014).
- Tenderness and possibly a mass (abscess) on the right side on rectal examination.

Diagnostic Studies

The following may be noted with appendicitis (Minkes, 2014):

- CBC with differential may show an increased WBC count (greater than 10,000) with an increased neutrophil count. This occurs in 70% to 90% of those with acute appendicitis. However, an elevated WBC count may be neither sensitive nor specific in the clinical diagnosis of appendicitis; during the first 24 hours of symptoms it is often within a normal range.
- Amylase, lipase, and liver enzymes help to differentiate liver, gallbladder, or pancreatic issues.
- UA can show small numbers of WBCs (less than 20) and red blood cells (RBCs) (less than 20 per high-power field).
- Examination of stool may demonstrate blood and pus (rare finding).
- Abdominal radiographs can show a fecalith, especially if rupture has occurred.
- Ultrasound demonstrates enlargement of the appendix and changes in its wall, increased field around the appendix, or an abscess. Ultrasound has excellent specificity, but it has only fair sensitivity and is operator dependent.
- CT scan with contrast has the highest accuracy, especially in adolescents. CT scan compared with ultrasound has higher sensitivity and specificity, is not operator dependent, and may be more cost effective in preventing an unnecessary appendectomy. An appendiceal diameter of greater than 6 mm is considered diagnostic (in both ultrasound and CT scan).
- A beta-human chorionic gonadotropin (β-hCG) test to rule out pregnancy or ectopic pregnancy.

Differential Diagnosis

The differential diagnosis includes vomiting and gastroenteritis (fever and crampy abdominal pain with vomiting, diarrhea, or both), constipation, UTI (fever, chills, and urinary symptoms), pregnancy, pelvic inflammatory disease (PID) or organ pathologic condition, pneumonia, duodenal ulcer (gnawing and burning pain), intestinal obstruction (crampy pain), peritonitis (worse pain when jumping or coughing), and intussusception (child younger than 2 years old with a right upper quadrant [RUQ] mass) (Fig. 33-4).

Management

- A surgical consultation for an appendectomy is needed. Administering opioid narcotics for pain before surgical consultation effectively reduces acute abdominal pain, does not impede the diagnostic process, and does not lead to an inappropriate increased use of CT scanning preoperatively. IV and preoperative antibiotics are given if perforation is suspected.
- Open appendectomy (OA) or laparoscopic appendectomy (LA) is indicated in nonperforated appendicitis. The management of perforated appendicitis is controversial, including surgical intervention. Urgent appendectomy may not be indicated in cases of perforated appendicitis. Instead, surgeons may choose to perform appendectomy once fluid resuscitation and antibiotics have been administered. This nonoperative approach is utilized as long as the child's clinical condition improves with antibiotic treatment. An appendectomy may be performed 8 to 12 weeks after recovery.
- Patients should be seen for follow-up 2 to 4 weeks after surgery. If appetite, bowel function, energy, and activity level are normal; no pain or fever is present; findings on physical examination are normal; and the wound is well healed, the child can resume unrestricted activity. If at

ALGORITHM

Differential Diagnosis

Accidental injury
Accidental ingestion
Anaphylactoid purpura
Appendicitis
Child abuse
Constipation
Ectopic pregnancy
Food intolerance
Gastroenteritis
Hemolytic uremic syndrome
Mechanical obstruction
Mononucleosis
Pneumonia
Renal stones
Sickle cell anemia
Tortion of ovary or testicle
Trauma
Urinary tract infection
Viral syndrome

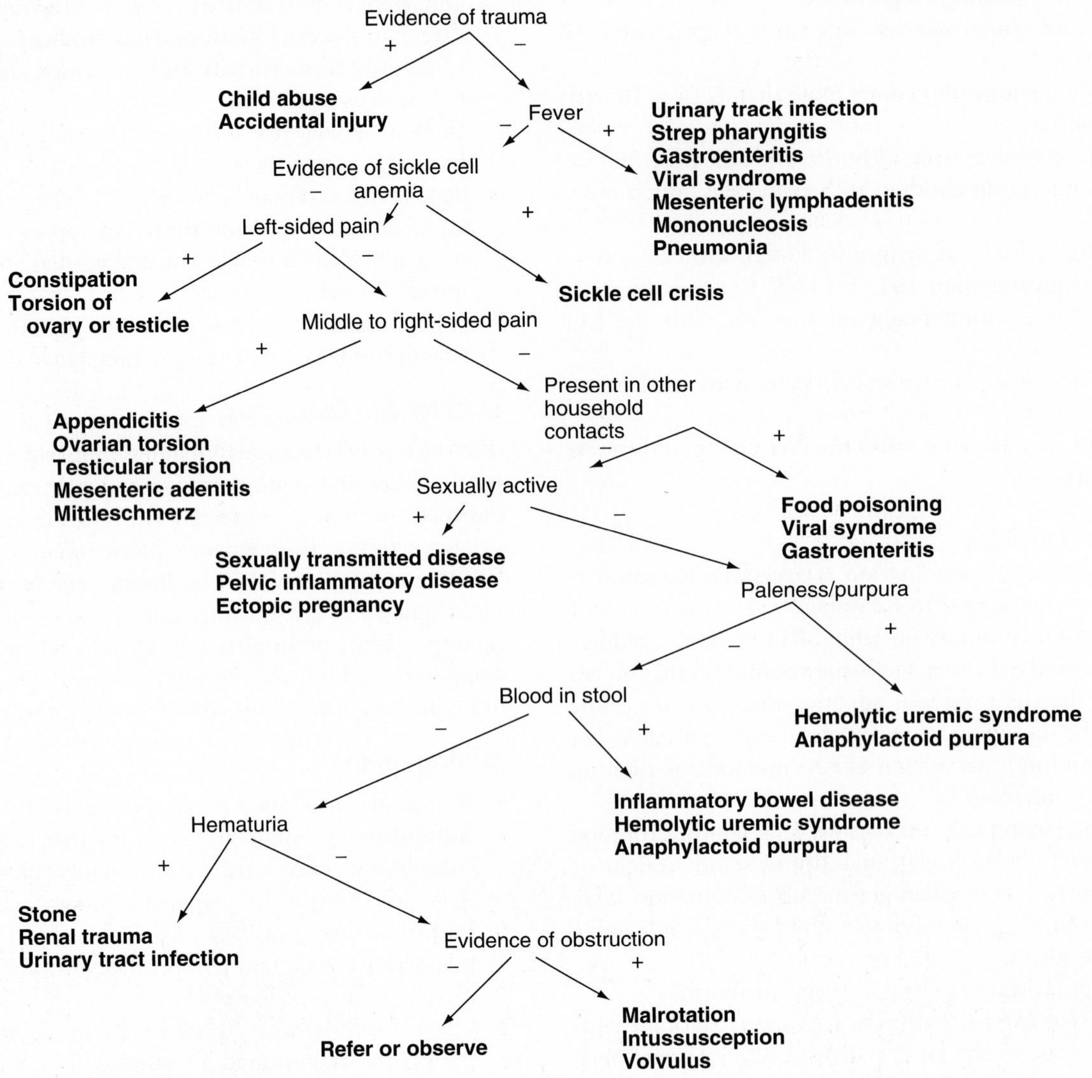

• **Figure 33-4** Decision tree for differential diagnosis of acute abdominal pain. (From Schwartz MW, Curry TA, Sargent J, editors: *Pediatric primary care: a problem-oriented approach*, ed 3, St. Louis, 1997, Mosby.)

the 2- to 4-week follow-up the child has signs of delayed infection, abnormal bowel function, or unexplained weight loss, refer back to the surgeon.

Complications

Perforation, peritonitis, pelvic abscess, ileus, obstruction, sepsis, shock, and death can occur.

Intussusception

Intussusception involves a section of intestine being pulled antegrade into adjacent intestine with the proximal bowel trapped in the distal segment. The invagination of bowel begins proximal to the ileocecal valve and is usually ileocolic, but it can be ileoileal or colocolic. Intussusception is thought to be the most frequent reason for intestinal obstruction in children. Intussusception most commonly occurs between 5 and 10 months of age and is also the most common cause of intestinal obstruction in children 3 months to 6 years old; 80% of the cases occur before 2 years of age. In younger infants, intussusception is generally idiopathic and responds to nonoperative approaches. In some children, there is a known medical predisposing factor, such as polyps, Meckel diverticulum, Henoch-Schönlein purpura, constipation, lymphomas, lipomas, parasites, rotavirus, adenovirus, and foreign bodies. Intussusception may also be a complication of CF. Children older than 3 years are more likely to have a lead point caused by polyps, lymphoma, Meckel diverticulum, or Henoch-Schönlein purpura; therefore, a cause must be investigated. The currently approved rotavirus vaccines have not been associated with an increased risk of intussusception (Kennedy and Liacouras, 2011).

Clinical Findings

History

- The classic triad for intussusception, intermittent colicky (crampy) abdominal pain, vomiting, and bloody mucous stools, are present in fewer than 15% of cases (Kennedy and Liacouras, 2011):
  - Paroxysmal, episodic abdominal pain with vomiting every 5 to 30 minutes. Vomiting is nonbilious initially. Some children do not have any pain.
  - Screaming with drawing up of the legs with periods of calm, sleeping, or lethargy between episodes.
  - Stool, possibly diarrhea in nature, with blood ("currant jelly").
- A history of a URI is common.
- Lethargy is a common presenting symptom.
- Fever may or may not be present; can be a late sign of transmural gangrene and infarction.
- Severe prostration is possible.

Physical Examination

- Observe the baby's appearance and behavior over a period of time; often the child appears glassy-eyed and groggy between episodes, almost as if sedated.
- A sausage-like mass may be felt in the RUQ of the abdomen with emptiness in the RLQ (Dance sign); observe the infant when quiet between spasms.
- The abdomen is often distended and tender to palpation.
- Grossly bloody or guaiac-positive stools.

Diagnostic Studies

- An abdominal flat-plate radiograph can appear normal, especially early in the course and reveal intussusceptions in only about 60% of cases (Fig. 33-5). A plain radiograph may show sparse or no intestinal gas or stool in the ascending colon with air-fluid levels and distension in the small bowel only.
- Abdominal ultrasound is very accurate in detecting intussusception and is the test of choice (Ross and LeLeiko, 2010). It shows "target sign" and the "pseudo kidney" sign and can also be used to evaluate resolution following air contrast enema.
- An air contrast enema is both diagnostic and a treatment modality.

Differential Diagnosis

The differential diagnosis includes incarcerated hernia, testicular torsion, acute gastroenteritis, appendicitis, colic, and intestinal obstruction.

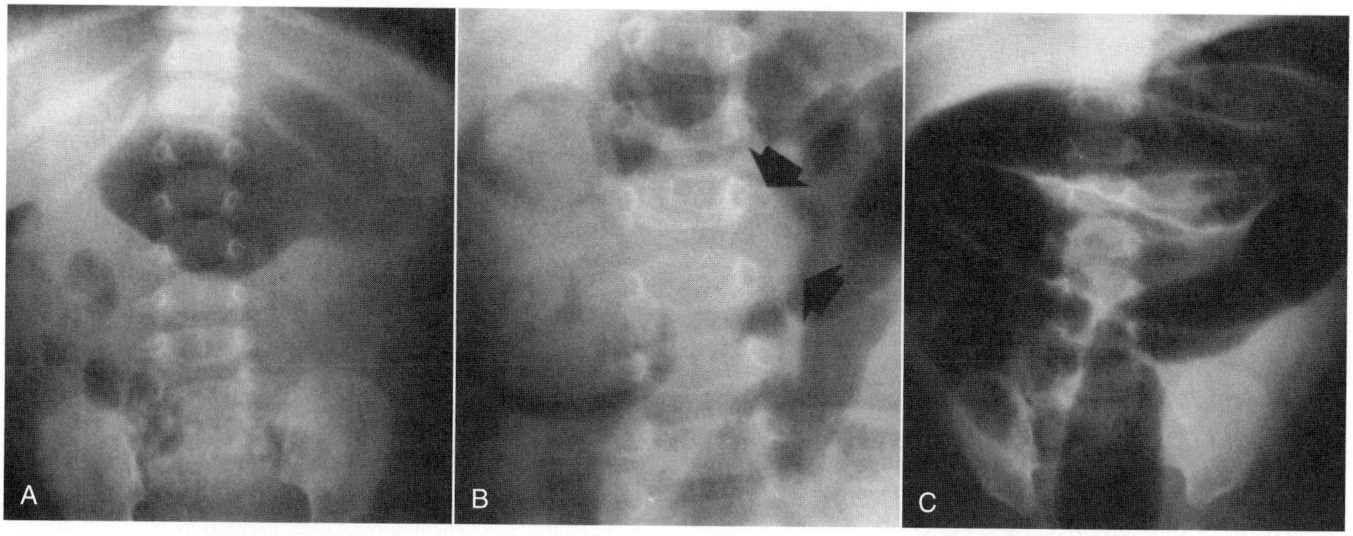

• **Figure 33-5** Intussusception. **A,** Plain abdominal radiograph demonstrating a gas-filled stomach and relatively little gas in the distal end of the bowel. This baby had typical clinical features of intussusception and a palpable upper abdominal mass. Therefore, an enema with air was performed. **B,** The intussusception *(arrows)* is outlined by air. **C,** Reduction is proved by air refluxing into loops of small bowel. (From Burg FD, Ingelfinger JR, Wald ER, editors: *Gellis and Kagan's current pediatric therapy*, ed 15, Philadelphia, 1999, Saunders.)

Management

- Emergency management and consultation with a pediatric radiologist and a pediatric surgeon is recommended.
- Rehydration and stabilization of fluid status; gastric decompression.
- Radiologic reduction using a therapeutic air contrast enema under fluoroscopy is the gold standard.
- Surgery is necessary if perforation, peritonitis, or hypovolemic shock is suspected or radiologic reduction fails.
- IV antibiotics are often administered to cover potential intestinal perforation.
- A period of observation following radiologic reduction is recommended (12 to 18 hours); clear discharge instructions to return with any recurrence of symptoms are required, and close phone follow-up for up to 72 hours is prudent.

Complications

Swelling, hemorrhage, incarceration, and necrosis of the bowel requiring bowel resection may occur. Perforation, sepsis, shock, and re-intussusception (reported to typically be less than 10%, usually within 72 hours of radiologic reduction but can occur up to 36 months later) can all occur. Recurrence is associated with the lead points described earlier.

Childhood Functional Abdominal Pain and Functional Abdominal Pain Syndrome

Children who have recurrent abdominal pain with no specific organic etiology are said to have functional abdominal pain (FAP), which is also known as *recurrent abdominal pain* and is often a puzzling problem for providers. FAP is much more common than organic reasons for abdominal pain. The Rome III criteria are used as the diagnostic standards (Rasquin et al, 2006; Rutten et al, 2014). These criteria include:

- FAP: The following must occur at least once per week for at least 2 months before diagnosis:
  - Episodic or continuous abdominal pain
  - Insufficient criteria for other functional GI disorders
  - No evidence of an inflammatory, anatomic, metabolic, or neoplastic process to explain symptoms
- Functional abdominal pain syndrome (FAPS): One or more of the following must occur at least once per week for at least 2 months before diagnosis and include childhood FAP criteria at least 25% of the time:
  - Some loss of daily functioning
  - Additional somatic symptoms, such as headache, limb pain, or difficulty sleeping

FAP is a fairly common pediatric complaint. The cause of the pain remains unclear, but the pain is genuine. There is no evidence of visceral hypersensitivity in the rectum (Rasquin et al, 2006; Rutten et al, 2014) as occurs with IBS. Affected children have an involuntary predisposition for the development of physiologic pain (e.g., a family history of FAP). Temperament and personality can make the child more vulnerable to environmental stressors (often minor) that precipitate the sensation of pain. Children who are perfectionists and have a tendency toward anxiety are more likely to experience FAP. Stress at school, home, with friends, or because of a novel social situation may be associated with FAP symptoms (Bishop and Ebach, 2015). Positive and negative reinforcement can modify the pain.

Approximately 15% to 35% of children worldwide have recurrent abdominal pain with about one third of those having no specific organic disorder (Gottsegen, 2010). FAP is the most common pain complaint of preschoolers and accounts for 2% of pediatric visits (Scheffer, 2011). The peak incidence of FAP occurs between 7 and 12 years old (Bishop and Ebach, 2015).

Clinical Findings

History

- A complete review of systems
- Parental history of FAP
- A careful psychosocial history (home, school, parents, friends); secondary gains from symptoms and lack of coping skills; endeavor to determine the degree of functional impairment
- Existence of associated symptoms, such as headache, joint pain, anorexia, vomiting, nausea, excessive gas, and altered bowel pattern
- Comorbidity of anxiety and/or depression (in children or adults), behavioral problems, a negative life event
- Identification of alarm symptoms or red flags (Box 33-7); there is an association between these symptoms and an

BOX 33-7 Alarm Symptoms for Functional Abdominal Pain

Red Flags on History

- Localization of the pain away from the umbilicus, especially right or left upper quadrant
- Pain associated with a change in bowel habits, particularly chronic, severe diarrhea; constipation; or nocturnal bowel movements
- Pain associated with night wakening
- Repetitive, significant emesis, especially if bilious
- Constitutional symptoms, such as recurrent fever, loss of appetite or energy
- Recurrent abdominal pain occurring in a child younger than 4 years old
- Blood in stool or emesis

Red Flags on Physical Examination

- Unexplained fever
- Unintentional loss of weight or decline in height velocity
- Organomegaly
- Localized abdominal tenderness, particularly removed from the umbilicus
- Perirectal abnormalities (e.g., fissures, ulceration, or skin tags)
- Joint swelling, redness, heat, or discoloration
- Ventral hernias of the abdominal wall

organic cause to the chronic pain (Bishop and Ebach, 2015; Gottsegen, 2010)
- Presence of Rome criteria for FAP or FAPS (see prior description)
- Report of abdominal pain often accompanied by a dramatic reaction (clutching abdomen, doubling over, or throwing self to ground)
- Determination that symptoms may be worse in the morning, preventing the child from going to school and resulting in school avoidance
- Report that pain medications do not alleviate pain
- Illicit drug use
- Sexual activity or abuse and possibility of pregnancy

Physical Examination

Following initial examination, reexamination should be done during an acute episode and with each subsequent visit. The physical examination is usually normal, but should include:
- Weight, height, and BMI plotted on growth curves
- Vital signs (temperature, heart rate, respiratory rate, blood pressure)
- Abdominal examination: Presence of pain, rebound tenderness, masses
- Perianal and rectal examination
- Complete neurologic examination
- Pelvic examination as indicated
- Examination of skin and joints
- Alarm symptoms (see Box 33-7)

Diagnostic Studies

There are two different approaches the clinician can consider:
- In their discussion of the application of the Rome III criteria, Rasquin and colleagues (2006) recommend that any testing be reserved for the presence of alarm symptoms or specific symptoms of organic disease. In these situations, testing includes:
  - CBC, ESR, CRP, UA, and urine culture if FAPS is suspected. If indicated, a biochemical profile (liver and kidney function); stool for O&P and culture; and breath hydrogen testing may be useful.
  - Other tests to consider in addition to the above are stool for *H. pylori* antigen and serum IgA, IgG, tissue transglutaminase (tTG) antibody to rule out celiac disease.
  - Ultrasound, endoscopy with or without biopsy, and esophageal pH monitoring as indicated by alarm symptoms.
- After performing a complete history and physical examination, Bishop and Ebach, (2015) suggest the following *initial* approach for ordering diagnostic studies to evaluate FAP:
  - CBC, ESR, amylase, lipase, UA, and abdominal ultrasound (liver, bile ducts, gallbladder, pancreas, kidneys, ureters).
  - A 3-day trial of a lactose-free diet.
  - If results are negative and there are no red flags, further testing is not needed.
  - Fecal calprotectin assay can also be a good initial test in a child with recurrent abdominal pain and changes in stool habits (Diamante et al, 2010).

Follow-up evaluation with additional and more invasive GI or other testing should be considered if there are positive results noted in the initial diagnostic testing, symptoms progress, or warning signs develop. These may include such testing as CT, endoscopy, celiac disease serology, and/or colonoscopy.

Differential Diagnosis

There is no evidence that the presence of the associated symptoms, a negative life event, or the presence of anxiety or depression can help distinguish between organic and FAP. Figure 33-6 outlines a decision tree for differential diagnosis of chronic abdominal pain. The following are included in the differential diagnosis: all organic causes of abdominal pain, including urinary tract, GI tract (IBS, celiac disease, intestinal malformations), and extraabdominal causes; malabsorption syndromes (usually with diarrhea, belching, flatulence, and bloating); lactose intolerance; constipation; small intestine bowel overgrowth (SIBO); abdominal pain associated with depression (usually includes social isolation, decreased activity and attention span, difficulty sleeping, and irritability); and school avoidance (usually associated with severe pain and anxiety on weekday mornings only).

Management

- Establish a therapeutic parent-child-practitioner relationship to improve patient satisfaction, adherence to treatment, symptom reduction, and other outcomes.
- Explain the brain-gut interaction and that biobehavioral methods are the most effective evidence-based treatments of FAP (Gottsegen, 2010).
- Use medications judiciously. H_2 blockers should not be used unless dyspepsia is present.
- Early in the visit, discuss the possibility with the child and parent that the pain can be functional (inorganic). Assure them that the symptoms are real and will be addressed.
- Encourage return to school and normalization of lifestyle. Limit attention given for pain episodes.
- Consider the use of complementary and alternative medicine (CAM) approaches (see Chapter 43). If certain dietary practices seem to cause pain, a more bland diet may be helpful (e.g., a lactose-free diet with documented lactose intolerance). Avoiding sorbitol and fructose may be useful if malabsorption is considered a contributing factor. There is a lack of high-quality evidence that dietary intervention (fiber supplements, lactose-free diets, or lactobacillus supplementation) is an effective strategy in managing FAP in children (Huertas-Ceballos et al, 2009). A mind-body approach is often useful, combining relaxation, behavioral management, stress coping

ALGORITHM

Differential Diagnosis

Bacterial enteritis	Functional pain	Tumor
Collagen vascular disease	Inflammatory bowel disease	Ureteropelvic obstruction
Constipation	Lactase deficiency	Urinary tract infection
Enteritis	Pancreatitis	

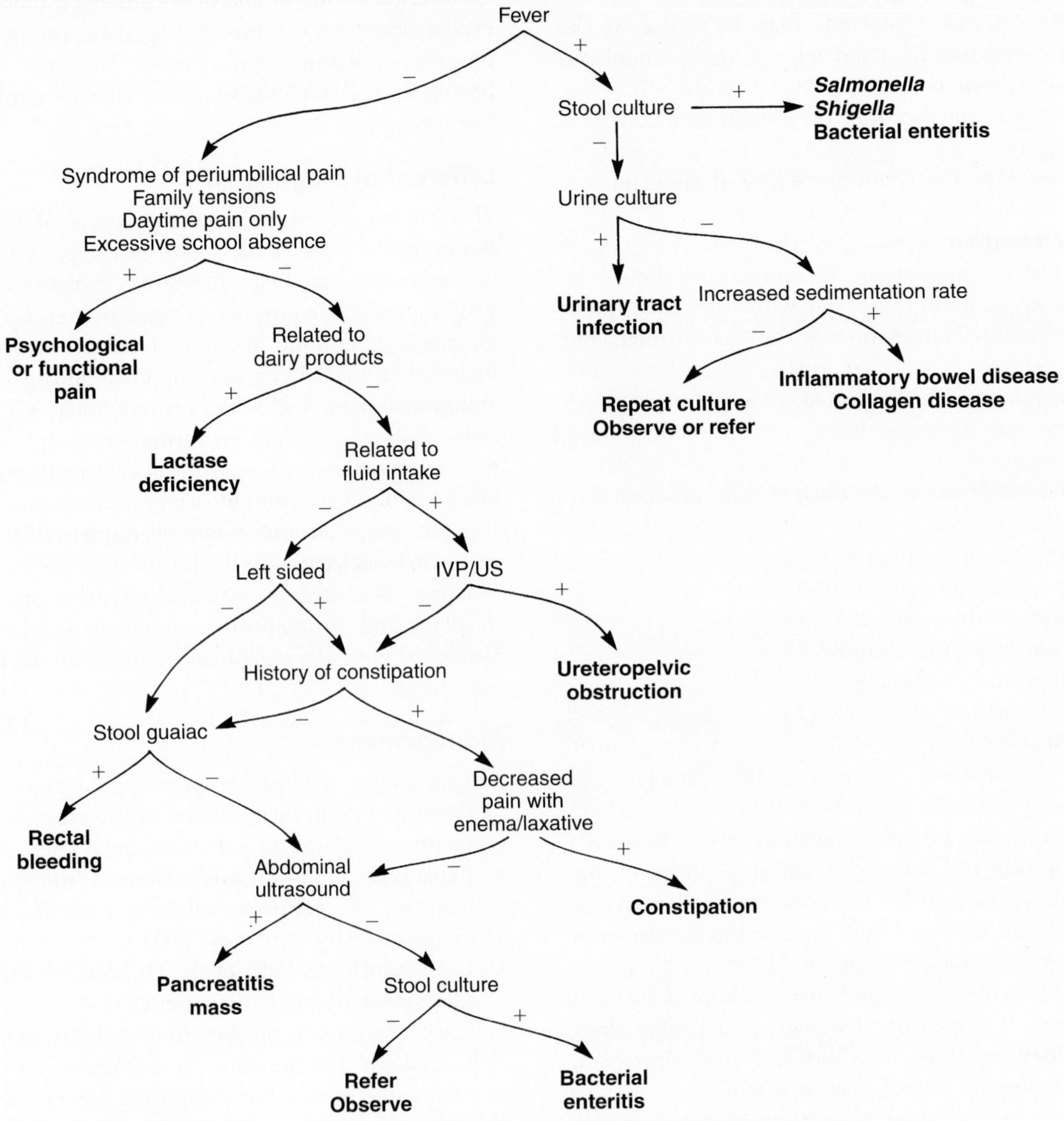

• **Figure 33-6** Decision tree for the differential diagnosis of chronic abdominal pain. *IVP/US,* Intravenous pyelogram/ultrasound. (From Schwartz MW, Curry TA, Sargent J, et al, editors: *Pediatric primary care: a problem-oriented approach*, ed 3, St. Louis, 1997, Mosby.)

training, meditation, and biofeedback. Acupuncture, massage, and hypnosis have also been shown to help with chronic abdominal pain.

- Consider SIBO as a diagnosis which also has dietary interventions in addition to antibiotics.
- Explore psychological triggers and use management strategies for the pain. Discuss how stressful events and emotional issues might affect the pain. Suggest distraction to shift attention from abdominal pain to other activities; attending school is a good distraction. Biofeedback provides evidence to the child that he or she can change muscle tension, skin temperature, and relaxation. Relaxation and guided imagery decrease abdominal pain.
- Identify, treat, and refer for any significant psychological issues. Psychotherapy and family therapy may be of some benefit. Cognitive behavioral therapy has also been helpful for all forms of FAP (Gottsegen, 2010). Using a biopsychosocial approach is especially helpful for FAPS. Refer for psychological dysfunction (maladaptive behavior, conversion reaction, depression, anxiety).

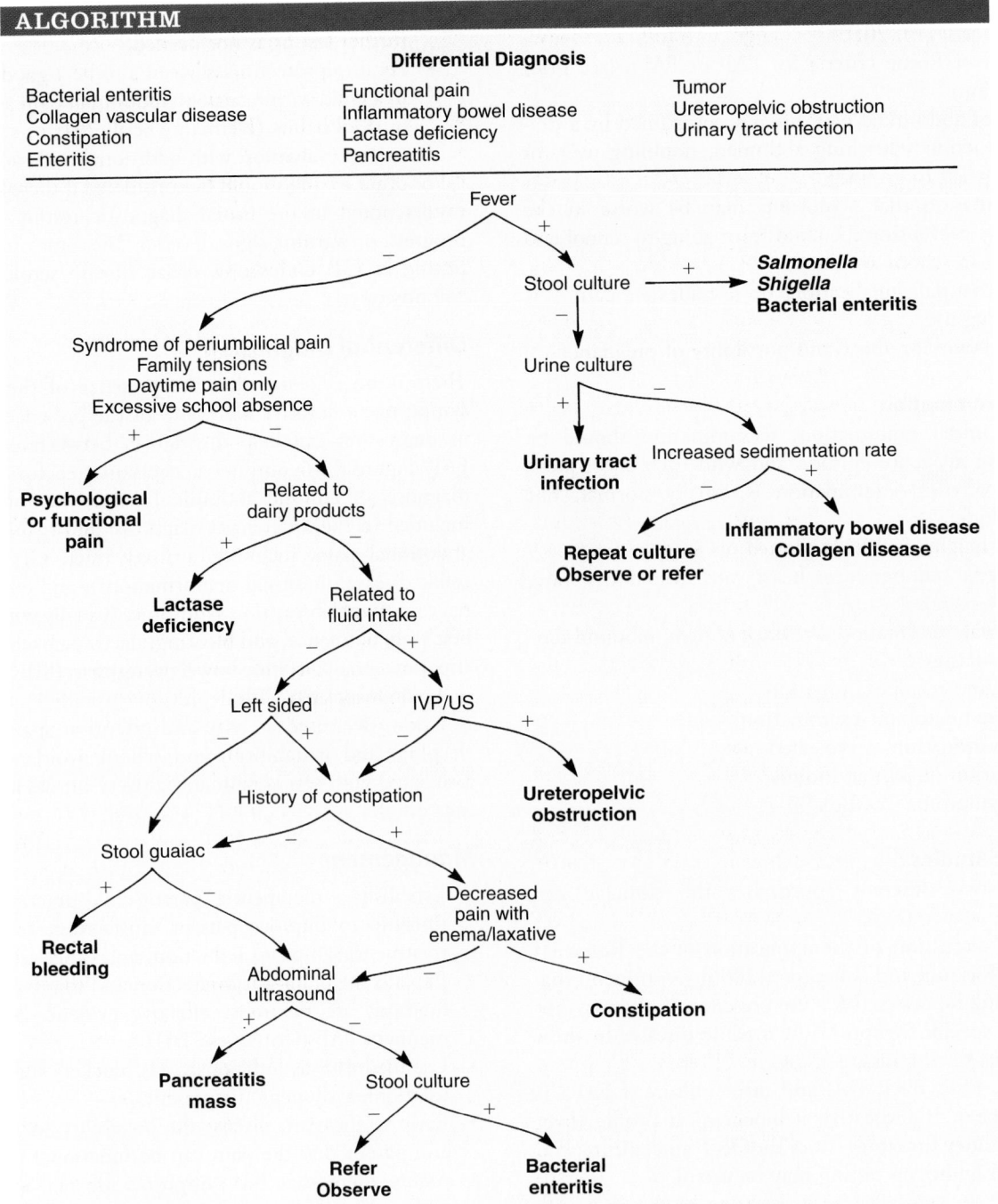

- Discuss alarm symptoms (see Box 33-7) so that the parents and child can identify changes in status and illness.
- Establish regular follow-up.

Prognosis and Complications

FAP can be a lifelong and chronic condition. Although one third of cases resolve within 2 months of diagnosis, one third has a long-term course with similar complaints in adulthood. The final third of cases has chronic complaints of pain (often headache) instead of abdominal pain that continue through adulthood (Walker et al, 2010). Male gender, onset of FAP before 6 years old, a delay in diagnosis greater than 6 months, and a family history of somatic pain, as first reported by Apley and Naisch (1958), are factors still predictive of a poor long-term prognosis.

Irritable Bowel Syndrome

IBS is defined as chronic or FAP with altered bowel habits and bloating that is not explained by structural or biochemical abnormalities (El-Baba, 2014). It is considered a functional GI disorder. The criteria for IBS (also known as *IBS Rome III diagnostic criteria*) must include *all* of the following at least once per week for at least 2 months before diagnosis:

- Abdominal discomfort (an uncomfortable sensation not described as pain) or pain associated with two or more of the following at least 25% of the time:
  - Improved with defecation
  - Onset associated with a change in frequency of stool
  - Onset associated with a change in form (appearance) of stool
- No evidence of an inflammatory, anatomic, metabolic, or neoplastic process that explains the child's symptoms

IBS is the most common cause of FAP in children in the Western world. The exact etiology of IBS remains to be determined. There is some debate on whether it is caused by hereditary or environmental factors. Infection, inflammation, visceral hypersensitivity, allergy, and disordered gut motility may also be involved. There is a strong familial trend, and finding a genetic link is currently being investigated (Rutten et al, 2014). Psychological comorbidity (somatic symptoms, anxiety, and depression) has also been reported. It is estimated that 10% to 15% of older children and adolescents suffer from IBS (El-Baba, 2014; Sandhu and Paul, 2014).

Clinical Findings

History

- Rome criteria symptoms for IBS (see prior description)
- Abnormal stool frequency (four or more stools per day and two or fewer stools per week)
- Abnormal stool form (lumpy/hard or loose/watery or alternating constipation and diarrhea)
- Abnormal stool passage (straining, urgency, or feeling incomplete evacuation)
- Passage of mucus
- Bloating or feeling of abdominal distention
- Dyspepsia (present in 30% of pediatric patients)
- Potential triggering events and psychosocial factors
- Family history of IBS
- Psychosocial history
- Nutrition history: Fiber and water intake, excessive sorbitol or fructose intake

Physical Examination

- Normal physical examination; normal growth curves and BMI
- Absence of alarm signals

Diagnostic Studies

There are no specific laboratory markers for IBS.

Differential Diagnosis

See FAP for differential diagnosis. Consider SIBO.

Management

- Confirm and explain diagnosis.
- The goal is to modify severity of symptoms. Identify and develop strategies to deal with triggering events and psychosocial factors.
- Antidepressants and serotonergic agents have not been widely used in children.
- Treatment goals should be to improve the quality of life. This includes ensuring pain is minimized and stool consistency and frequency is normalized. The following therapeutic interventions have been used in children with IBS:
  - Dietary interventions (fiber supplement; fermentable oligo-di-monosaccharides and polyol [FODMAP] diet) (Magge and Lembo, 2012). Avoid trigger foods known to exacerbate pain episodes: caffeine; sorbitol; fatty food; large meals; gas-producing foods, such as carbonated beverages, lactose (with lactose intolerance), and cruciferous vegetables (Hayes et al, 2014).
  - Probiotics lactobacillus and bifidobacteria are commonly used.
  - Drug therapy (peppermint oil, tegaserod, antispasmodic agents, antidiarrheal agents, antibiotics, and amitriptyline) or selective serotonin reuptake inhibitors (SSRIs) are sometimes used.
  - Biopsychosocial therapy for IBS includes hypnotherapy, cognitive behavioral therapy, yoga, and acupuncture (Sandhu and Paul, 2014).

Malabsorption Syndromes: Celiac Disease, Lactose Intolerance, Cow's-Milk Protein Intolerance or Allergy

Malabsorption syndromes can be caused by many different genetic, congenital, and acquired conditions and usually lead to an initial decrease in weight followed by a deceleration in height velocity. This section discusses celiac disease, lactose intolerance, and cow's-milk protein intolerance (CMPI).

Celiac disease is an immune-mediated systemic disorder triggered by dietary exposure to wheat gluten and related proteins in barley and rye. It is characterized by the presence of a variable combination of gluten-dependent clinical manifestations, celiac disease–specific antibodies, HLA-DQ2.5 or HLA-DQ8 haplotypes, and enteropathy. This disease frequently co-occurs with other autoimmune diseases: diabetes mellitus type 1, autoimmune thyroiditis, autoimmune liver disease, IgA nephropathy, and juvenile chronic arthritis (Mubarak et al, 2012). A number of conditions or variables may contribute to the development of celiac disease. It is suggested that demographic changes, such as immigration from developing to developed countries, increase exposure to gluten and an increased incidence of celiac disease follows (Scanlon and Murray, 2011). Celiac disease is greater among infants born by cesarean section; the development of enteric homeostasis in the newborn period may be altered, increasing susceptibility (Decker et al, 2010). Parent reported gastroenteritis occurring at the time gluten was introduced into the child's diet does not appear to be associated with celiac disease (Welander et al, 2010). Celiac disease has a worldwide distribution with overall prevalence of 1% (Mustalahti et al, 2010). The most typical presentation occurs between 6 months and 2 years old.

Lactose intolerance is a clinical syndrome characterized by abdominal pain, diarrhea, nausea, flatulence, and bloating after the ingestion of lactose-containing foods. The symptoms are caused when lactose, a disaccharide (glucose and galactose) found exclusively in mammalian milk, is not absorbed in the gut. It is usually secondary to a deficiency of the lactose enzyme. Increased lactose draws fluid and electrolytes into the intestine, resulting in an osmotic diarrhea. Intestinal bacteria also metabolize excess lactose in the gut, creating methane, carbon dioxide, and hydrogen gases that lead to bloating and flatulence (Misselwitz et al, 2013). Four types of lactase deficiency have been noted:

- Primary lactase deficiency, also known as *lactase non-persistence,* is the most common cause of lactose intolerance. It develops in most children after weaning and at varying ages and is more common in various ethnic groups. The prevalence of primary lactase deficiency has not been established in the United States, although it is found more often in Hispanic, African American, Ashkenazi Jewish, Asian, and Native American populations than in Caucasian European Americans.
- Secondary lactase deficiency results from small bowel injury (e.g., gastroenteritis, chemotherapy, chronic diarrhea) and is more common in infancy.
- Congenital lactase deficiency is an extremely rare congenital absence of lactase, but if it is left untreated, it can be fatal in early infancy.
- Developmental lactase deficiency describes the lactase deficiency that occurs in preterm infants born before 34 weeks because of the immaturity of the intestinal tract.

CMPI and *cow's-milk allergy (CMA)* can have similar clinical pictures; however, the body's immune response differs in each of these conditions. CMPI is a nonallergic hypersensitivity to CMP, whereas CMA is antigen mediated. Most CMA is immunoglobulin E (IgE) mediated, an expression of atopy in which eczema, allergic rhinitis, and/or asthma may also be seen. Some cases of CMA are probably cell-mediated, presenting with primarily GI symptoms (Fiocchi et al, 2010).

CMA typically develops in the neonatal period, peaks in infancy, and tends to remit during childhood. Approximately 2% to 5% of infants have CMA diagnosed by food challenge and elimination diet (Fiocchi et al, 2010). IgE-mediated CMA decreased from about 4% in 2-year-olds to less than 1% in 10-year-olds. Up to 80% of children with CMA develop tolerance within 3 to 4 years of diagnosis (Sommanus et al, 2013).

Clinical Findings

General History for Malabsorption Syndromes

Careful medical and family medical histories are very important in the evaluation of a malabsorption syndrome and are often the key to the diagnosis. In addition, a complete dietary history is needed to distinguish between undernutrition and malabsorption. Important historical findings include:

- Past surgical and trauma history
- Growth failure (a common symptom of nutritional deficiency and malabsorption)
- Delayed puberty can coexist with malabsorption.
- A voracious appetite or particular food avoidance is present in small children with malabsorption syndromes
- Chronic diarrhea with frequent, large, foul-smelling, pale stools
- Excessive flatus with abdominal distention
- Pallor, fatigue, hair and dermatologic abnormalities, digital clubbing, dizziness, cheilosis, glossitis, peripheral neuropathy (symptoms of vitamin deficiency seen with malabsorption)

Disease-Specific History

In addition to the list in the earlier section, the following may stand out.

Celiac Disease.

- Chronic or intermittent diarrhea, persistent or unexplained GI symptoms (e.g., nausea and vomiting), sudden or unexpected weight loss, and prolonged fatigue

Lactose Intolerance.

- Abdominal pain, diarrhea, nausea, flatulence, and bloating often related to the amount of lactose ingested

Cow's-Milk Protein Intolerance and Cow's-Milk Allergy.

- Family history of allergy and/or atopy

General Physical Examination

- Growth parameters and percentiles (weight, height, BMI, head circumference)

- Skinfold thickness and lean body mass
- Examination for delayed growth and puberty, including Tanner staging

Disease-Specific Physical Examination

Celiac Disease.

- Impaired growth, FTT, unexplained iron deficiency anemia, abdominal distention, bloating or cramping pain
- May have no symptoms at all despite evidence of small bowel changes; maintain a high suspicion for celiac disease in children with metabolic bone disease (such as rickets or osteomalacia), low-trauma fractures, or those with dental enamel defects. An estimated 85% to 90% of individuals with celiac disease are undiagnosed (NICE, 2010).

Lactose Intolerance.

- Abdominal distention

Cow's-Milk Protein Intolerance and Cow's-Milk Allergy. Symptoms may be immediate or late onset (Fiocchi et al, 2010):

- Immediate
  - Anaphylaxis (rare) but can be life threatening
  - GI: Lip or tongue swelling, oral pruritus, nausea, vomiting
  - Skin: Urticaria, rash, flushing, angioedema
  - Respiratory: Nasal pruritus, sneezing, rhinitis, congestion, wheezing, dyspnea, chest tightness
- Late onset (1 hour to several days after ingestion of CMP)
  - Typically, non–IgE-mediated allergic reaction
  - Symptoms are mostly GI: Varied, including nausea, vomiting, abdominal pain, diarrhea, bloody stool, GERD-like symptoms, pyloric stenosis, malabsorption, FTT, IBD
  - Can see skin reaction (with both IgE- and non–IgE-mediated allergy); eczema
  - Respiratory: Heiner syndrome is very rare

Diagnostic Studies

- Stool assessment for occult blood, WBCs, and culture; liquid stool for pH and reducing substances; 72-hour fecal fat collection or Sudan stain for stool fat
- Spot stool testing for alpha 1-antitrypsin level to establish the diagnosis of protein-losing enteropathy
- Sweat chloride test (in the presence of steatorrhea to evaluate for CF)
- Stool for O&P: Giardiasis is a common intestinal infection causing malabsorption. See later discussion for symptoms suggestive of infestation.
- CBC with differential, mean corpuscular hemoglobin concentration (MCHC), iron, folic acid, and ferritin
- Serum calcium, phosphorus, magnesium, alkaline phosphatase, serum protein, liver function tests, vitamin D and its metabolites, vitamins A, B_{12}, E, and K
- Human immunodeficiency virus (HIV) testing (for symptoms of FTT and chronic diarrhea)
- Small bowel biopsy helps identify diseases of the small bowel mucosa and obtain material for culture and sensitivity
- Plain abdominal radiographs and barium contrast studies as indicated
- Abdominal ultrasound can detect masses and stones in the hepatobiliary system
- Retrograde studies of the pancreas and biliary tree if indicated
- Bone age

Specific Tests for Celiac Disease

- Serologic testing should be done if there is clinical suspicion of celiac disease, the child has an associated disorder, or there is a first-degree relative with celiac disease. Gluten should be eaten in more than one meal every day for 6 weeks prior to testing. Recommended serologic tests include IgA tissue transglutaminase antibody (tTGA) and IgA endomysial antibody (EMA) because of their high sensitivity and specificity (Guandalini et al, 2014; Tran, 2014). EMA is more expensive and less accurate in children younger than 2 years old (Gelfand, 2013).
- Home blood testing is not recommended (NICE, 2010).
- If serologic testing is positive, refer for endoscopy with biopsy for a definitive diagnosis, although colonoscopy may not be necessary if the tTGA level is greater than 100 units/mL (Mubarak et al, 2011).
- Careful follow-up of growth parameters, tTGA testing after 6 months of gluten-free diet (GFD), and then yearly (Hill et al, 2005).
- Bone density testing (bone problems may be first symptom of celiac disease).

Specific Tests for Lactose Intolerance

- Lactose hydrogen breath test is the gold standard. Children should not be taking antibiotics at the time of the study, because the intestinal bacteria that act on lactose may be diminished.
- Trial of a lactose-free diet for 2 weeks, being aware of hidden sources of lactose. Symptoms should disappear with the diet and reappear when lactose is reintroduced.
- Bone density if calcium deficiency is suspected (lactose is necessary for calcium absorption into bone, and lactose-free diets can predispose to osteoporosis).
- If secondary cause of lactose intolerance is suspected, continue workup for all other causes of malabsorption.

Cow's-Milk Protein Intolerance and Cow's-Milk Allergy

- Elimination diet followed by a double-blind placebo-controlled oral food challenge in an allergist's office is test of choice for CMA.
- Skin patch test for allergies may be performed.
- Serum IgE antibodies testing may be performed.
- Diagnosis of CMPI is made when there is clinical improvement on CMP-free diet.

Differential Diagnosis

Organic and inorganic FTT, colic, short stature, chronic diarrhea, CF, immunodeficiency, cholestatic liver disease, GERD, SIBO, and IBD are included in the differential diagnoses.

Management

Celiac Disease

- A strict GFD for life is currently the only effective treatment for celiac disease. The standard for being gluten-free is a limit of 20 ppm of gluten (Hill et al, 2005). Adding pure oats to a GFD can improve palatability and increase fiber and vitamin B intake without causing a systemic or autoantibody response (Mubarak et al, 2012; Scanlon and Murray, 2011).
- Alternative treatments are being explored, including enzyme therapy, developing genetically engineered grains, inhibiting tTGA in the intestine, and correcting intestinal barrier defects (particularly increased permeability).
- A lactose-free diet for young children may be helpful. This is generally not the case in adolescents and adults unless they are lactose intolerant (Hill et al, 2005).

Lactose Intolerance

- Test to ensure that the individual actually has lactose intolerance.
- Reduce exposure to lactose:
  - Avoid lactose-containing milk and other dairy products, including goat's milk.
  - Use lactose-free dairy products (e.g., milk prehydrolyzed with lactase).
  - Use alternate milk sources (soy, rice, and so on).
- Use oral lactase supplements.
- Ensure adequate intake of calcium and vitamin D from other food products.
- Most individuals with primary lactase deficiency can ingest dairy products in small to moderate amounts, especially if taken with other foods.

Cow's-Milk Protein Intolerance and Cow's-Milk Allergy

Take the following precautions for infants and young children (Fiocchi et al, 2010):

- Breastfeed.
- Restrict milk and milk products from the diet of breastfeeding mothers.
- If formula fed, use extensively hydrolyzed formula initially. Partially hydrolyzed formula is *not* appropriate for infants with CMA.
- Use amino-acid formula for infants who demonstrate severe allergy (e.g., prior history of anaphylaxis) or who do not respond to extensively hydrolyzed formula.
- Extensively hydrolyzed soy formula is appropriate for infants after 6 months old only; before 6 months old, infants fed soy formula are at risk for nutritional deficit.
- Avoid use of other mammals' milk (e.g., sheep, goat, camel) due to risk of cross-allergic reaction.
- After 2 years old, formula is not appropriate, but ensure daily dietary intake of 600 to 800 mg of calcium.
- Probiotics may be helpful in creating tolerance, but more clinical research is needed.
- Have EpiPen if anaphylaxis is a concern.
- Monitor growth and development carefully.
- Refer to an allergist or gastroenterologist if symptoms are severe; immunotherapy is not recommended.
- Annual reevaluation of sensitivity, preferably an oral food challenge under medical supervision.

Complications and Prognosis

Celiac Disease

Growth failure is the primary complication of celiac disease. With delayed diagnosis or inadequate treatment, there is risk for fractures and osteoporosis (due to reduced bone mineral density), lymphoma, autoimmune diseases (e.g., type 1 diabetes, thyroid disorders), primary biliary cirrhosis, and primary sclerosing cholangitis. Sensory peripheral neuropathy may be related to gluten sensitivity (Hadjivassiliou et al, 2010). Celiac crisis consisting of abdominal distention, explosive watery diarrhea, dehydration with hypoproteinemia, electrolyte imbalance, hypotensive shock, and lethargy, although rare, can be the first indication of celiac disease. Prognosis is improved with lifelong GFD.

Lactose Intolerance

Unabsorbed lactose does not cause clinical intestinal damage despite clinical symptoms. Bone density loss may occur if there is inadequate calcium and vitamin D. Other conditions misdiagnosed as lactose intolerance may worsen.

Cow's-Milk Protein Intolerance and Cow's-Milk Allergy

CMPI usually resolves by 1 to 3 years old; when there are only GI symptoms, CMPI resolves completely. CMA cannot be reversed, and there is a high likelihood of other food allergies. Complications include rickets, poor growth, and FTT.

Polyps

Intestinal polyps in children may be benign or present a risk for subsequent cancer or other conditions (e.g., anemia). *Solitary polyps,* often called *juvenile polyps,* are the most frequently seen (90%) polyps in children (Lee et al, 2010). They are most often found in preschool-age children (4 to 5 years old), are usually located in the rectosigmoid area, have an incidence of about 2% in children younger than 10 years old, and are considered to present negligible or no risk for malignancy (Manfredi, 2010). Polyps are also found in familial adenomatous polyposis, juvenile polyposis syndrome (JPS), phosphatase and tensin homolog (PTEN) hamartoma tumor syndrome, and Peutz-Jeghers syndrome (PJS), all of which are autosomal dominant conditions with variable penetrance.

Clinical Findings

History

- May be asymptomatic. A careful family history is imperative to identify children at risk for polyposis.
- Painless, bright red rectal bleeding (hematochezia). Usually the blood coats or is mixed in with the stool. Bleeding can be daily, intermittent, or infrequent. Large volume blood loss is extremely rare.
- Familial adenomatous polyposis: Nonspecific complaints, diarrhea, constipation, or changes in bowel habits

Physical Examination

- Anorectal examination to find polyp or other source of rectal bleeding
- Pallor and edema caused by anemia and hypoproteinemia from GI hemorrhage and protein-losing enteropathy indicate a heavy polyp burden
- Extraintestinal symptoms of familial adenomatous polyposis include ophthalmologic changes (may see hypertrophy of retinal pigment); dental anomalies (supernumerary or unerupted teeth); osteomas of skull, jaw or extremities; and multiple lipomas

Diagnostic Studies

- CBC with differential and ESR, CRP, prothrombin time, and partial thromboplastin time
- Fecal occult blood test, even if blood appears to be present
- Stool culture for bacterial pathogens and O&P
- Colonoscopy to the terminal ileum with biopsy evaluation is the diagnostic test of choice
- Upper endoscopy if there is concern for gastric or duodenal polyps; small-bowel video capsule endoscopy may be used
- Barium contrast of upper intestine

Management

- Refer to a pediatric gastroenterologist for management and follow-up screening.
- Treatment involves resection of the polyp(s), usually with diagnostic or surveillance screening. If multiple polyps are present, bowel resection (colectomy) is common. For familial adenomatous polyposis, colectomy is standard therapy.
- Children with one or two juvenile colonic polyps at diagnosis usually need no further follow-up.
- Follow-up is required if:
  - There is a family history of polyps (i.e., all children are at risk for polyposis).
  - The child has three or more polyps on colonoscopy.
  - Polyps are found outside the colon.
  - Extraintestinal symptoms are present.
- Follow-up varies by condition, severity, and pediatric specialist provider. Genetic testing to determine presence of gene mutation is usually done at 8 to 10 years old.
- Ophthalmologic evaluation may be recommended.
- Genetic counseling may be recommended.

Complications

Children with polyps are at risk for colorectal, gastric, duodenal, pancreatic, and extraintestinal cancer as adults (usually appearing in the fourth decade of life or later). Psychological issues related to having a hereditary condition with uncertain long-term outcomes (i.e., high risk for malignancies) can cause family problems.

Anal Fissure

Anal fissures are small tears in the anal mucosa. The usual cause of an anal fissure is passage of frequent or hard stools. Anal stenosis and other trauma can also be causative factors. Anal fissures are the most common cause of rectal bleeding in all pediatric groups.

Clinical Findings

History

- Crying with bowel movement
- Bright red streaks of blood in the stool or diaper
- Withholding of stool

Physical Examination

With the patient in the knee-chest position and the anus slightly everted, small tears in the anal mucosa can be visible. An otoscope with a large speculum is needed if the external fissures are not readily visible. A digital anal examination with the fifth finger rules out anal stenosis.

Differential Diagnosis

Other sources of lower intestinal hemorrhage, such as infection, formula intolerance, necrotizing enterocolitis, intussusception, juvenile polyps, hemolytic-uremic syndrome, Henoch-Schönlein purpura, irritable bowel disease, and vascular lesions are included in the differential diagnosis. Sexual abuse should be considered in children with large, irregular, or multiple fissures.

Management

- Treat the cause (see Chapter 12).
- Local wound care should include sitz baths twice a day and application of 0.5% hydrocortisone cream or K-Y jelly to the anus.

Complications

Recurrence is common. Constipation causes a fissure, which leads to a stool withholding-encopresis–painful stooling cycle.

Patient and Family Education

Preventive measures include avoiding constipation, encouraging regular toileting habits, and avoiding the use of laxatives and enemas.

Inflammatory Bowel Disease

IBD is thought to be a dysregulated immune response of intestinal mucosa to microbes in genetically susceptible individuals. Defects may be present in both the barrier function of intestinal epithelium and the immune system (Xu et al, 2014). Three primary types of IBD are recognized: (1) Crohn disease, (2) ulcerative colitis, (3) and unclassified IBD. See Table 33-8 for features contrasting Crohn disease and ulcerative colitis. Symptoms of IBD in children can be difficult to interpret and a definitive diagnosis between Crohn disease and ulcerative colitis may be elusive, especially in early, active disease. Numerous contacts with health care providers may be necessary to establish a diagnosis, and the initial diagnosis may change as the disease progresses (da Silva et al, 2014). Several indices are used to assess and classify IBD; the Crohn Disease Activity Index (CDAI) and the Pediatric Ulcerative Colitis Activity Index (PUCAI) rate the severity of disease (Surti et al, 2013). The Paris classification, a modification of the Montreal classification, identifies the location of the disease in children (Levine et al, 2011), and the Cardiff-Hughes classification gives guidelines on diagnosis and scoring of perianal disease (de Zoeten et al, 2013).

The incidence of IBD appears to be increasing worldwide, especially the incidence of Crohn disease and pediatric-onset IBD (Benchimol et al, 2011). IBD can occur at any age, with a peak onset between 15 and 30 years. Up to 25% of cases are in children and adolescents, and 4% are found in children younger than 5 years old. IBD in infants is extremely rare. In contrast to adults, children diagnosed with IBD are more likely to have Crohn disease than ulcerative colitis, to have more severe or extensive disease (both Crohn disease and ulcerative colitis), more vague symptoms, more extraintestinal symptoms (e.g., arthralgia), and more relapses (Billiet and Vermeire, 2014; Rufo et al, 2012).

Crohn Disease

Crohn disease is a chronic disease with dysregulated inflammation and cytokine production in the intestinal tract.

TABLE 33-8 Features of Crohn Disease and Ulcerative Colitis

Feature	Crohn Disease	Ulcerative Colitis
Age at onset	10 to 20 years old	10 to 20 years old
Area of bowel affected	Can affect any part of the GI system; often in terminal ileum or colon; may be small bowel only; small bowel and cecum; small bowel and colon; or colon only; occasionally isolated perianal disease	Affects colon and rectum; entire colon may be inflamed (pancolitis); may have subtotal colitis or "ileal backwash" (i.e., superficial inflammation of ileum proximal to splenic flexure); may be left-sided (distal to splenic flexure); may have proctitis (limited to rectum or distal 15 cm)
Distribution	Segmental; disease-free "skip" areas common	Continuous distal to proximal
Endoscopic, radiographic, or biopsy findings	Noncaseating granulomas located in the inflamed mucosa; cobblestone appearance of bowel wall; linear/serpiginous ulcers and transverse fissures; fixation and separation of loops; small bowel strictures/stenoses; bowel or perianal fistulas; perianal abscesses or large (>5 mm) skin tags	Superficial inflammation of mucosa; friable tissue with exudates and granularity; loss of vascular pattern; small perianal skin tags (<5 mm)
Intestinal symptoms	Abdominal pain, diarrhea, anorexia, weight loss	Abdominal pain with or around time of stooling, bloody diarrhea, urgency, and tenesmus
Extraintestinal manifestations: Seen more often in Crohn disease than ulcerative colitis; similar types for both conditions	Ophthalmologic conditions (uveitis, iritis, conjunctivitis) more likely in Crohn disease	Primary sclerosing cholangitis more likely in ulcerative colitis

Data from da Silva B, Lyra A, Rocha R, et al: Epidemiology, demographic characteristics and prognostic predictors of ulcerative colitis, *World J Gastroenterol* 20(28):9458–9467, 2014; Day AS, Ledder O, Leach ST, et al: Crohn and colitis in children and adolescents, *World J Gastroenterol* 18(41):5862–5869, 2012; Dotson JL, Hyams JS, Markowitz J, et al: Extraintestinal manifestations of pediatric inflammatory bowel disease and their relation to disease type and severity, *J Pediatr Gastroenterol Nutr* 51(2):140–145, 2010.
GI, Gastrointestinal.

Any part of the GI tract can be involved, although the terminal ileum and colon are most commonly affected. Esophageal disease, often without upper GI symptoms, has been found in about 20% of all Crohn disease cases, and perianal disease is common (Ammoury and Pfefferkorn, 2011; Day et al, 2012). Inflammation is usually transmural, affecting the entire wall of the intestine, creating fissures and fistulas. Unaffected areas of intestine are called *skip areas.*

The exact cause is unknown, although it is likely due to environmental exposure that triggers an abnormal immune reaction in a genetically susceptible individual. Crohn disease peaks in late adolescence and early adulthood, then again in middle adulthood (50 to 70 years); 25% to 40% of cases are diagnosed in childhood and adolescence. The Centers for Disease Control and Prevention (CDC) estimates the worldwide incidence rate for Crohn disease is between 0.1 and 16 per 100,000 individuals; prevalence rate is about 400 per 100,000 (CDC, 2014). It is more common in Caucasians, and males and females are affected about equally, except in esophageal disease, which is more common in boys than girls (Ammoury and Pfefferkorn, 2011). Siblings are more likely to have Crohn disease than is the general population. Approximately 10% to 15% of cases are re-diagnosed as ulcerative colitis within the first year of illness (da Silva et al, 2014).

Clinical Findings

History

- Fever, usually low grade, of unknown etiology
- Weight loss (average of 5 to 7 kg)
- Delayed growth velocity, short stature, delayed bone age
- Arthralgias and/or arthritis in large joints, occasional joint destruction
- Obstructive symptoms associated with meals, bloating, early satiety
- Pain in the umbilical region and RLQ; may awaken at night
- Anorexia
- Malabsorption and lactose intolerance
- Diarrhea (with or without blood or mucus) and pain with stooling
- Jaundice
- Oral aphthous ulcers, especially during exacerbations of the illness
- Use of tobacco
- Positive family history

Physical Examination

- Carefully measure growth parameters (height, weight, and BMI).
- Perform an abdominal examination while observing for RLQ tenderness and a mass.
- Perianal skin tags, deep anal fissures, and perianal fistulas strongly suggest Crohn disease.
- Clubbing of digits may be present.
- Erythema nodosum is common.

Diagnostic Studies

The following are ordered as needed:

- Inflammatory markers: ESR, CRP
- Nutritional labs: Albumin, total protein (consider iron panel, calcium, zinc, alkaline phosphatase, folate, vitamin B_{12})
- Other blood tests: CBC with differential (consider liver enzymes—aspartate aminotransferase [AST], alanine amino transferase [ALT], total bilirubin, gamma-glutamyltransferase [GGT]; amylase; lipase)
- Stool: Routine culture, O&P, *C. difficile* (with recent antibiotic use), blood, WBCs, and fecal alpha 1-antitrypsin; fecal calprotectin assay (good initial test in a child with recurrent abdominal pain and changes in stool habits) (Diamante et al, 2010)
- Radiologic studies: Bone age (usually delayed by 2 years), bone density, abdominal plain films, upper GI series with small bowel follow-through, abdominal CT with contrast
- Ileocolonoscopy is a first step to assess for Crohn disease. Other endoscopic studies include small bowel capsule endoscopy (SBCE), push enteroscopy, single- or double-balloon enteroscopy, inter-operative enteroscopy or spiral enteroscopy. Esophageal endoscopy is recommended in children diagnosed with Crohn disease who have perianal disease (Ammoury and Pfefferkorn, 2011).
- Screen for tuberculosis (TB) if child is at risk (see Chapter 24 for risk criteria). Biologic agents used in Crohn disease therapy can activate latent TB (Naser et al, 2014).

Differential Diagnosis

Rheumatoid arthritis, systemic lupus erythematosus, hypopituitarism, acute appendicitis, peptic ulcer, intestinal obstruction, intestinal lymphoma, anorexia, chronic granulomatous disease, sarcoidosis, and growth failure are included in the differential diagnosis. Abdominal TB and Hermansky-Pudlak syndrome are rare conditions with Crohn-like symptoms (Damen et al, 2010).

Management

The goals of therapy are to (1) control the disease; (2) prevent relapses; and (3) achieve normal nutrition, growth, and lifestyle. Treatment is pharmacologic, nutritional, surgical, and psychosocial. The following management steps are taken:

- Refer to a pediatric gastroenterologist for colonoscopy, endoscopy, more definitive diagnosis, consultation, and follow-up care.
- In the United States, corticosteroid management is most common. In Europe, exclusive enteral nutrition (EEN) had been used as first-line therapy. Currently, it is indicated for patients who are malnourished or at risk of becoming malnourished and who have an inadequate or unsafe oral intake (Mallon and Suskind, 2010).
- Medications:
    - Corticosteroids (e.g., prednisone, budesonide) are used orally, rectally, or intravenously for acute

inflammation of mild to moderate disease. They are not intended for use in remission.
  - 5-aminosalicylates (balsalazide, sulfasalazine, olsalazine, and mesalamine) are used orally or rectally for mild disease to control inflammation.
  - Immunomodulator agents are used (azathioprine, 6-mercaptopurine, methotrexate, and cyclosporine) for severe small or large bowel disease, steroid-dependent or refractory disease, severe fistula, and growth failure.
  - Biologic agents (e.g., infliximab, a chimeric, anti-tumor necrosis factor alpha [anti-TNF-α] antibody) for steroid-dependent or refractory disease, perirectal fistula, and maintenance of remission, can be given alone or in combination with immunomodulators. One IV infusion of infliximab has been shown to induce remission in Crohn disease. Greater mucosal healing follows treatment with immunomodulators and biologic agents than with corticosteroids and improved growth is seen with early anti-TNF-α treatment (Puthoor and de Zoeten, 2013).
  - Antibiotics are used for acute infections (ampicillin, gentamicin, clindamycin, ciprofloxacin, or metronidazole).
  - Adjunctive therapy, including growth hormone prior to or at the time of puberty, enhances optimal growth (Vortia et al, 2011).
- Severe disease can require hospitalization, total parenteral nutrition, a nasogastric tube for decompression, or surgery. Studies indicate that 15% to 20% of children require surgery within 2 years of diagnosis and most patients eventually require surgery. Surgery before puberty has been shown to improve growth, though there is a high relapse rate (55%), and surgery does not cure the disease (Pacilli et al, 2011).
- Monitor growth and pubertal changes.
- An ophthalmologic examination is needed to rule out underlying ophthalmologic manifestations of the disease.
- Refer for nutritional counseling during remission, to prevent or correct malnutrition, and to maintain and promote growth. See Chapter 10 for specific nutritional recommendations.
- Encourage participation in social activities, such as support and fitness groups (e.g., Team Challenge, a fund-raising running event for Crohn disease and colitis), and Crohn disease camps. Refer for psychosocial and family therapy as indicated.

Complications

Intestinal obstruction with scarring and strictures is the major complication of Crohn disease. Growth failure (especially linear growth) is extremely common. Fistula and abscesses can occur, but perforation and hemorrhage are rare. Primary sclerosing cholangitis, pancreatitis, pericarditis, arthritis, peripheral neuropathy, and an increased risk of lymphoma and colon cancer are other complications of Crohn disease (Peyrin-Biroulet et al, 2011). Treatment with corticosteroids or immunosuppressive drugs increases the risk for opportunistic infections and inadequate response to immunizations (Lu and Bousvaros, 2014). Care must be taken with long-term use of biologics in children because of a risk of infection or malignancy. The child and family are at risk for social functioning difficulties, anxiety, depression, somatization disorders, and school difficulties.

Prevention and Prognosis

Follow recommended therapy to prevent sequelae. Crohn disease is progressive and without cure, although about 55% of individuals are in remission at any one time and only about 1% of individuals experience continuous active disease. Child-onset disease tends to be more severe and requires more immunosuppressive treatment than adult-onset disease (Pigneur et al, 2010).

Ulcerative Colitis

Ulcerative colitis is a chronic disease that is characterized by diffuse inflammation of the rectal and colonic mucosa. Ulcerative colitis involves the rectum in 95% of cases and may be extended continuously and circumferentially to more proximal parts of the large intestine (da Silva et al, 2014). Pediatric patients, especially those younger than 10 years old, may appear to have no lesions in the rectum, and can lead to a misdiagnosis of Crohn disease.

The cause is unknown, but the disease has a multifactorial basis (i.e., heredity, diet, environment, immunologic alterations, and ineffective mucosal integrity). The annual incidence rate in the United States is 10 to 12 cases per 100,000, and the overall prevalence rate is 37 to 238 cases per 100,000 individuals. The incidence of ulcerative colitis has increased worldwide over recent decades, especially in developing nations. Although ulcerative colitis is less common in children, recent studies have shown that the number of cases has increased in pediatric patient and adolescents (da Silva et al, 2014).

Clinical Findings

History

- Fever
- Weight loss (average of 4 kg)
- Delayed growth and sexual maturation
- Arthritis and/or arthralgias of the large joints
- Anorexia
- Diarrhea
- Lower abdominal cramping, left lower quadrant pain
- Pain increased before stooling and passing flatus
- Stool with bright red blood and mucus
- Nocturnal stooling
- Oral aphthous ulcers
- Skin lesions (erythema nodosum, pyoderma gangrenosum, and diffuse papulonecrotic eruptions)

Physical Examination

- Carefully measure growth parameters (weight, height, and BMI) and perform a complete physical examination. Abdominal examination can reveal rebound tenderness if the disease is severe.

Diagnostic Studies

- CBC with differential, iron-binding capacity, total protein, albumin, ESR, CRP: Children with low WBC counts and normal to near-normal hematocrit levels are more likely to have a mild course and are at lower risk for colectomy (Moore et al, 2011).
- Stool for WBCs, blood, and culture (bloody diarrhea with negative stool culture characteristic of ulcerative colitis)
- Bone age (usually delayed up to 2 years)
- Colonoscopy (diffuse mucosal inflammation)
- Perinuclear neutrophil cytoplasmic antigen (positive in 60% to 70% of cases)
- Fecal calprotectin assay: Good initial test in a child with recurrent abdominal pain and changes in stool habits (Diamante et al, 2010).

Differential Diagnosis

Shigella, Salmonella, Yersinia, Campylobacter, E. coli, C. difficile, IBS, self-limited colitis, and Crohn disease are in the differential diagnosis.

Management

The goals of therapy are to (1) control the disease; (2) prevent relapses; and (3) achieve normal nutrition, growth, and lifestyle. Treatment is pharmacologic, nutritional, surgical, and psychosocial. Management involves the following:

- Refer for colonoscopy, biopsy, definitive diagnosis, consultation, and close follow-up care.
- Pharmacologic treatment options: Treatment for ulcerative colitis can become quite complex and requires an individualized approach. Patients with mild-to-moderate disease can usually be managed in the outpatient setting, whereas severe ulcerative colitis warrants inpatient care.
  - Mild to moderate ulcerative colitis: Topical mesalamine, oral 5-aminosalicylates, or topical steroids with topical mesalamine as a superior first-line agent.
  - Moderate-to-severe ulcerative colitis: Systemic steroids, such as oral prednisone 40 to 60 mg/day for 1 to 2 weeks until clinical response is established followed by a steroid taper by 5 to 10 mg/week depending on disease severity and response. Once at a 20 mg/day dose, tapering of a patient's dose proceeds at 2.5 mg/week.
  - Thiopurines: Azathioprine and 6-mercaptopurine have limited utility in the acute setting. Adverse effects include fever, rash, nausea, diarrhea, arthralgia, thrombocytopenia, leukopenia, infection, pancreatitis, hepatitis, non-Hodgkin lymphoma, and hepatosplenic T-cell lymphoma.
  - Biologic agents (infliximab, adalimumab, golimumab) for induction of remission and maintenance in steroid-refractory and moderate to severe disease (Marchioni Beery and Kane, 2014).
  - Hydrocortisone rectal preparation for tenesmus.
  - Cyclosporin monotherapy is as effective as or more effective than corticosteroids for initial treatment of fulminating disease.
  - Probiotics (e.g., VSL#3, *Saccharomyces boulardii*) may provide benefits when used with other therapies in mild to moderately active disease.
  - Curcumin (active ingredient in turmeric) may assist in maintenance of inactive disease.
  - Iron supplementation to correct anemia; multivitamin.
- Nutrition (see Chapter 10 for nutritional recommendations):
  - Diet: High in protein and carbohydrates, normal amount of fat, and decreased roughage. Omega-3 fatty acids (in contrast to omega-6 fatty acids) have an anti-inflammatory effect on the bowel, though there is not enough evidence currently to recommend their use for treatment of ulcerative colitis (Turner et al, 2011).
  - Lactose is poorly tolerated.
  - Parenteral or enteral nutritional supplements (60 to 70 cal/kg/day) may be used.
  - Refer for nutritional therapy to prevent or correct malnutrition and maintain and promote growth.
- Monitor growth.
- Surgery may be indicated (complete proctocolectomy with permanent ileostomy is curative).
- Refer for ophthalmologic examination to rule out ophthalmologic manifestations of the disease.
- Refer for psychosocial therapy as indicated. Depressive disorders are common.
- Assess immunization status and ensure child is up to date; there is controversy regarding immunizing with live vaccines (e.g., varicella) (Campins et al, 2013; Carrera et al, 2013; Lu et al, 2014).

Complications

Complications can include growth failure, toxic megacolon, intestinal perforation, liver disease, sepsis, cancer of the colon (a long-term sequela—1% to 2% per year after 10 years of disease), arthritis, uveitis, malnutrition, as well as behavioral and emotional problems similar to those of children with celiac disease.

Prevention and Prognosis

Follow the recommended therapy to optimize remission, maintain inactive disease state, and prevent complications. Prognosis is good for patients with mild disease and those who respond quickly to initial therapy. Those with untreated or poorly treated disease are at increased risk for colectomy and colon cancer. In one study of children who had colectomy, 73% reported pouchitis (inflammation of the ileal pouch), and 56% required a second surgery, but overall quality of life, BMI, and number of offspring were equal to that of control subjects (da Silva et al, 2014).

Failure to Thrive

FTT is a broad term referring to a symptom of a lack of weight gain proportional to age as determined by standardized growth charts. The diagnosis is based on a child's weight but the definition varies in the literature. It is also called *growth deficiency, growth delay, protein energy malnutrition, faltering weight,* and *faltering growth.* FTT should be considered if any of the criteria in Box 33-8 are found. The pathway to FTT is based on "disruptions in the complex system of biological, psychosocial, and environmental factors contributing to a child's growth and development" (Jaffe, 2011). FTT in early childhood reflects general undernutrition (Cole and Lanham, 2011).

FTT has three basic causes: (1) inadequate caloric intake, (2) inadequate caloric absorption, and (3) excessive caloric expenditure. The most common cause is nutritional deficiency without an underlying medical condition (greater than 80%) (Cole and Lanham, 2011). Generally the prevalence rates are thought to be around 5% to 10% in the United States. Children living in poverty and/or from developing countries with higher rates of malnutrition and/or HIV infection are more likely to have FTT. Rates may be increasing, because more preterm infants are surviving (Cole and Lanham, 2011).

Onset between 2 weeks and 4 months is more often associated with congenital disorders, serious somatic illness, and with deviant mother-infant interactions. Onset between 4 and 8 months in otherwise healthy children is more clearly associated with feeding problems (Olsen et al, 2010). In chronic cases, weight for height may appear to be normal because of concurrent reductions in velocity. The length of time over which weight loss is experienced in order to be considered FTT has not been determined (Cole and Lanham, 2011).

• BOX 33-8 Criteria that Define Failure to Thrive

- Weight less than 80% of median weight for length
- Weight for length less than 80% of ideal weight
- Weight for length less than the 10th percentile
- Body mass index (BMI) for chronologic age less than 5th percentile
- Weight for chronologic age and sex less than 5th percentile or more than two standard deviations below the mean
- Length for chronologic age and sex less than fifth percentile
- Weight deceleration crossing more than two major percentile lines on age and population appropriate growth chart
- Height, head circumference, and developmental skills may be affected

Clinical Findings and Risk Factors

Clinical findings include poor weight gain associated with poor intake, vomiting, food refusal, food fixation, abnormal feeding practices, presence of anticipatory gagging, irritability, chronic physical problems in any body system, or psychosocial problems. Inborn errors of metabolism should be suspected with history of acute, severe, and potentially life-threatening symptoms, liver dysfunction, recurrent vomiting, neurologic symptoms, cardiomyopathy, impairment of vision or hearing, renal symptoms, dysmorphic features, organomegaly, and/or high anion gap acidosis, lactic acidosis, or hypoketotic hypoglycemia. In more severe cases, height, head circumference, and developmental progress may also be affected.

Yoo and colleagues (2013) studied the predictive value of a set of predefined symptoms and signs that might point toward "nonorganic" versus "organic" etiologies for FTT. They found that the presence of vivacity, food restriction, and/or feeding rituals and poor appetite were more predictive of nonorganic (or inadequate caloric intake) and that vomiting, diarrhea, irregular bowel movements, and abdominal distention were more typical symptoms of organic (or malabsorption/excessive expenditure of calories). Vomiting and abdominal distention were noted to be of particular significance. Yoo and colleagues' review (2013) also noted that infants hospitalized for FTT predictably related to social encounters and objects differently, depending on what their eventual causative deficiency proved to be. Infants with organic causes were more likely to prefer close, personal interactions (i.e., with touching/holding) than those later diagnosed as having a nonorganic deficiency due to psychosocial factors (preferred distant social encounters and relating to inanimate objects).

Therefore, a thoughtful approach to the history (medical, developmental-behavioral, nutritional, and social), physical examination, and limited laboratory evaluation of children with FTT can be more predictive than relying on a battery of laboratory tests or empiric hospitalization. The following should be included in the assessment.

History

General parental concerns about the child's weight and growth need to be addressed. Look for conditions that would negatively affect the child's growth potential, increase the caloric needs, decrease the availability or use of calories, or affect the child's ability to feed or willingness to feed or factors that might affect the parent's ability or interest in feeding the child.

Prenatal.

- Maternal health including chronic illness, such as diabetes mellitus, HIV, CMV, infection; maternal habits, such as nutrition, alcohol, cigarette use
- Obstetric complications, such as toxemia, hemorrhage, multiple pregnancies

Perinatal.
- Birthweight, Apgar scores, complications, length of stay in the hospital, congenital anomalies, neurologic insults, newborn screening results, weight for gestational age

Neonatal.
- Intraventricular hemorrhage, seizures, hypoxia, extreme hyperbilirubinemia, infection

Postnatal Health.
- Hospitalizations, medications, surgeries, accidents, illnesses
- Serious or recurrent infections
- Recurrent symptoms, such as vomiting, diarrhea, wheezing, snoring
- Chronic health condition (Table 33-9)
- Collection and interpretation of growth data, percentiles, BMI, height for weight over time
- Stooling and voiding history: Diarrhea, constipation, vomiting, poor urine stream
- Careful review of systems

Developmental Trajectory and Temperamental Style.
- Developmental and behavioral history

Family and Psychosocial History.
- Social and family factors: Family composition, caregiving environment, day care, family support, poverty, parent-child relationship, parenting attitudes, typical day
- Family health history: Size and growth, developmental disabilities, inherited diseases that may affect growth and development

Physical Examination
- Weight, height, BMI, and head circumference (in those younger than 2 years old) plotted on standardized growth curves and percentiles, including weight-for-height graphs (include past and present growth parameters)
- Skinfold measurements: Loss of subcutaneous fat; general wasting (more common in developing countries; seen with malignancy, HIV, cerebral palsy, inflammatory diseases)
- Vital signs (temperature, pulse, respiratory rate, blood pressure)
- Hydration status
- Presence of dysmorphic features
- Skin, hair, nails, and mucous membranes: Scaling skin (seen with zinc deficiency); rough or hard skin (with hypothyroidism); edema (with protein deficiency); alopecia (with hypervitaminosis, kwashiorkor, or syphilis); hair color/texture changes (with zinc deficiency, Menkes kinky hair disease); spoon-shaped nails (with iron deficiency or GI diseases); cyanosis (with heart disease); and labial fissures (with vitamin deficiency)
- Evidence of abuse or neglect: Unexplained burns or skin lesions; fractures; retinal hemorrhages; unwashed skin; diaper rash; untreated impetigo; uncut and dirty fingernails; unwashed clothing
- Oral findings: Dental caries, tonsillar hypertrophy, submucous cleft palate, or tongue enlargement (may require oral-motor function studies, including lip/tongue/swallowing assessment)
- Respiratory compromise (with CF, bronchopulmonary dysplasia)
- Cardiovascular examination for congenital heart disease

TABLE 33-9 Major Causes of Failure to Thrive

System	Cause
Gastrointestinal	GER, Crohn disease, pyloric stenosis, cleft palate or cleft lip, lactose intolerance, Hirschsprung disease, CMPI, hepatitis, cirrhosis, pancreatic insufficiency, biliary disease, IBD, malabsorption, alkaline foods
Cardiac	Cardiac diseases leading to congestive heart failure
Renal	UTI, renal tubular acidosis, diabetes insipidus, chronic kidney disease
Pulmonary	Asthma, bronchopulmonary dysplasia, CF, anatomic abnormalities of the upper airway; obstructive sleep apnea; recurrently infected adenoids and tonsils
Endocrine and metabolic	Hypothyroidism, diabetes mellitus, adrenal insufficiency or excess, parathyroid disorders, pituitary disorders, growth hormone deficiency; inborn errors of metabolism
Neurologic	Mental retardation, cerebral hemorrhage, degenerative disorders, cerebral palsy
Infectious	Parasitic or bacterial infections of the GI tract, TB, HIV
Congenital	Many genetic abnormalities
Malignancy and autoimmune disorders	Many cancers of childhood, collagen-vascular disease, juvenile idiopathic rheumatoid arthritis
Nutritional	Lack of calories, lack of micronutrients including vitamin A, zinc, iron
Hematologic	Sickle cell disease and others
Prenatal	Small for gestational age, perinatal infection
Psychosocial	Depression, anorexia nervosa, bulimia, maternal depression, child abuse or neglect, ADHD, autism, chronic pain
Environmental toxins	Heavy metal poisoning; other toxins

ADHD, Attention-deficit/hyperactivity disorder; *CF,* cystic fibrosis; *CMPI,* cow's-milk protein intolerance; *GER,* gastroesophageal reflux; *HIV,* human immunodeficiency virus; *TB,* tuberculosis; *UTI,* urinary tract infection.

- Abdominal: Lymphadenopathy, hepatosplenomegaly, masses, distention (with malignancy, inborn errors of metabolism, and immunodeficiency)
- Endocrine: Thyroid enlargement, precocious or ambiguous sexual development
- Neuromuscular tone and strength, cranial nerves for swallowing (cerebral palsy)
- Hypertonicity/hyperreflexia for cerebral palsy

Diagnostic Studies

- Feeding assessment: Nutritional and feeding history for calorie, protein, micronutrient intake.
  - Quality of food for age and ability to suck, chew, and swallow
  - Social nature of the feeding event and family eating patterns (meals and child feeding)
  - Feeding history: Caloric intake; feeding behavior; feeding cues; cues to hunger and satiety; progression to solids; frequency of feedings; amount taken per feeding; preparation of formula (over dilution)
  - Twenty-four-hour diet recall for infants, 3-day diet history for older children eating solid foods
  - Parental understanding of nutrition and feeding of children
- Developmental assessment
- Laboratory and imaging studies as delineated in Table 33-10

Differential Diagnosis

See Tables 33-9 and 33-10.

Management

Management is often best addressed by an interdisciplinary team that includes pediatrics (with specialty consultants for specific medical conditions), nutrition (may include lactation specialist), mental health, other community resources

TABLE 33-10 Evaluation Studies for Failure to Thrive

Generic Cause	Associated Conditions	Physical Findings	Diagnostic Evaluation
Inadequate caloric intake	Poor food intake Chronic illness Inappropriate type/volume of feeding Anorexia, bulimia Food not available, parental withholding Poverty, neglect	Signs of neglect or abuse Minimal subcutaneous fat Protuberant abdomen	Complete dietary history Complete psychosocial evaluation Basic metabolic profile, vitamin D (calcidiol), lead, zinc, iron screening, albumin for protein status in severe FTT
Inadequate caloric absorption	GI causes (malabsorption, chronic vomiting, pancreatic insufficiency, celiac disease, chronic reflux, IBD) Chronic renal disease, CF, inborn errors of metabolism, infestations	Dysmorphism suggestive of chronic disease, organomegaly, skin/mucosal changes	CBC/ESR, basic metabolic profile, serum electrolytes (include total CO_2 to rule out renal tubular acidosis), UA and urine culture, sweat test, stool studies for fat, reducing substances, O&P, and culture Review of newborn metabolic screening tests Extremity radiographs if indicated (e.g., rickets)
Excessive caloric expenditure	Hyperthyroidism, chronic disease (cardiac, renal, endocrine, hepatic), malignancy	Dysmorphisms, skin dysmorphology, cardiac findings, abdominal mass or lymphadenopathy, hepatosplenomegaly	TSH, CBC/ESR, serum protein, albumin, alkaline phosphatase, BUN, creatinine, liver function tests Chest radiograph Renal ultrasound and voiding cystourethrography
Growth failure	Genetic, familial short stature, small for gestational age, hypothyroidism	Short stature, dysmorphisms, decreasing height growth with symmetric weight to height	Thyroid studies, HIV screening Karyotype (especially in small girls for Turner syndrome) Bone age Developmental testing Growth hormone (expensive, often done later in workup)

Data from Cole SZ, Lanham JS: Failure to thrive: an update, *Am Fam Physician* 83(7):829–834, 2011; Jeong SJ: Nutritional approach to failure to thrive, *Korean J Pediatr* 54(7):277–281, 2011; Nutzenadel W: Failure to thrive in childhood, *Dtsch Arztebl Int* 108(38):642–649, 2011.

BUN, Blood urea nitrogen; *CBC,* complete blood count; *CF,* cystic fibrosis; *ESR,* erythrocyte sedimentation rate; *FTT,* failure to thrive; *GI,* gastrointestinal; *HIV,* human immunodeficiency virus; *IBD,* inflammatory bowel disease; *O&P,* ova and parasites; *TSH,* thyroid-stimulating hormone; *UA,* urinalysis.

(e.g., Women, Infants, and Children [WIC] program, food stamps, Medicaid, housing authorities), and social work personnel. Community nurse home visits can aid in observations (mealtime behaviors, such as food refusal, spitting, food throwing, oral retention), assessment, and support.

- Manage treatable causes with prompt attention to urgent, life-threatening medical conditions.
- Restore nutritional intake and appropriate intake patterns.
- Provide nutritional rehabilitation: Vitamin supplementation with iron, zinc, and minerals; calorically enriched formula and foods (up to 150 cal/kg/day for infants less than 6 months old). In older infants and toddlers, solids should be offered before liquids, and they should not be force fed. See Chapter 10 for further information related to nutrition for FTT. The expected normal weight gain by age should be:
  - Birth to 3 months old: 25 to 30 g/day
  - 3 to 6 months old: 15 to 20 g/day
  - 6 to 12 months old: 10 to 15 g/day
  - 12 months old and older: 5 to 10 g/day
- Provide parent education and support and improve parent-child interaction.
- Treat underlying chronic condition.
- Make referrals as needed including feeding clinics.
- Evaluate for normal weight gain every 1 to 3 weeks. Catch-up growth can occur rapidly but can take up to 2 weeks before growth occurs with more involved cases. One must be careful to not overshoot the mark, resulting in overweight.
- Hospitalize for evaluation and intervention to protect from abuse when intentional etiology is suspected, to avoid further starvation and sequelae, to manage extreme child-parent interaction problems, to provide care when outpatient management is not feasible or practical, and to provide more intensive care after failure of outpatient management.

Prognosis

The goal of nutrition management is to achieve symmetry of weight and height and genetic growth potential. Nutritional effects of chronic conditions may persist if not treated with the primary condition. Outcomes are variable depending on the underlying condition and severity.

Most children achieve expected growth and development. However, because brain growth occurs maximally in the first 6 months of life, nutritional insufficiency in an infant can severely affect long-term development and social/emotional health. Subtle neurodevelopmental abnormalities, the home environment, and the quality of nurturing by caregivers can affect outcomes. Many studies document that FTT can result in long-term detrimental effects—short stature, lower cognitive functioning, poorer academic functioning, and increased risk for adult diseases, such as cardiovascular disease, obesity, hypertension, and diabetes (Jaffe, 2011; Jeong, 2011).

Lower Gastrointestinal Tract Infections and Infestations

Acute and chronic diarrhea results from alterations in the normal functioning of the intestinal system. The altered intestinal mechanisms that result in diarrhea vary; briefly, diarrhea can occur as a result of:

- Nonabsorbable solutes in the GI tract, when fluids exceed the transport capacity, or when water-soluble nutrients are not absorbed (osmotic diarrhea). Such nutrient malabsorption and/or excessive fluid intake account for most chronic diarrhea; dumping syndrome, lactase deficiency, overfeeding, and malabsorption syndromes are causative conditions (Guarino et al, 2012; Lee et al, 2012).
- Invasion, inflammation, and/or release of toxins by bacteria or viruses (such as in traveler's diarrhea) that decrease absorption and increase secretion and transportation of electrolytes and water from mucosal crypt cells in the small intestine into the bowel lumen (secretory diarrhea). As an example, viruses injure the absorptive mature mucosal surface cells, thereby altering the release of disaccharides and preventing the conversion of carbohydrates to monosaccharides necessary for normal absorption. Congenital disorders, mucosal disorders, and tumors can also lead to secretory diarrhea.
- Mutations in the ion transport proteins, such as chloride-bicarbonate exchange.
- Alterations in the anatomy of the intestinal surface or functional ability due to inflammation or surgical procedures (e.g., short bowel syndrome, celiac disease, IBS) with a subsequent loss of fluids, electrolytes, macronutrients and micronutrients, and normal peristalsis.
- A change in intestinal motility, either increased or decreased (e.g., irritable bowel, bacterial overgrowth due to stasis [pseudo obstruction], toddler's diarrhea).
- Altered immune function.

Acute Diarrhea

The term *acute gastroenteritis* was formerly used to describe acute diarrhea, but this term is technically a misnomer because the etiology of diarrhea does not technically involve the stomach (Guandalini and Assiri, 2014). With acute diarrhea, there is a disruption of the normal intestinal net absorptive versus secretory mechanisms of fluids and electrolytes, resulting in excessive loss of fluid into the intestinal lumen. This can lead to dehydration, electrolyte imbalance, and in severe cases, death in those also malnourished. In children younger than 2 years old, this translates to a daily stool volume of more than 10 mL/kg (this definition excludes the normal breastfeeding stooling of five or six stools per day). In children older than 2 years old, diarrheal stooling is described as occurring four or more times in 24 hours. The duration can last up to 14 days.

Viruses can injure the absorptive surface of mature villous cells, which reduces the amount of fluid absorbed. Some can release a viral enterotoxin (e.g., rotavirus). A loss of water and electrolytes ensues, and there can be volumes of watery diarrhea, even if the child is not being fed. Bacterial and parasitic agents can adhere and/or translocate, causing noninflammatory diarrhea. Bacteria can also damage the anatomy and functional ability of the intestinal mucosa by direct invasion. Some bacteria release endotoxins, whereas others release cytotoxins that result in the excretion of fluid, protein, and cells into the intestinal lumen and an inflammatory response in some cases. Abnormal peristalsis for any reason can result in acute diarrhea. The enteric pathogens are spread through the fecal-oral route and by ingestion of contaminated food or water.

Worldwide, the burden of acute diarrhea is huge, resulting in 3 to 5 billion cases and nearly 2 billion deaths (20% of total child deaths) in children younger than 5 years old (particularly vulnerable) (Bell, 2010; Guandalini and Assiri, 2014; Norman et al, 2010). Developing countries also see their share of the burden of this disease (approximately 10%), attributable to poor water, sanitation, and hygiene (Norman et al, 2010). Globally, females have higher rates of *Campylobacter* species infections and hemolytic uremic syndrome; otherwise the incidence of cases shows no gender preference. Nontyphoidal *Salmonella, Shigella, Campylobacter, E. coli* organisms (bacteria); rotavirus, norovirus, enteric adenovirus (viruses); and *Giardia, Cryptosporidium*, and *Strongyloides* (parasites) cause most disease (Ahmed Bhutta, 2011). *Shigella, E. coli, Giardia lamblia, Cryptosporidium parvum,* and *Entamoeba histolytica* are particularly infectious in small amounts. The term "dysentery" is used to indicate infection with specific species of *Shigella* and *Salmonella* (e.g., *Shigella dysenteriae*).

In the United States, those most vulnerable include Native Americans and Native Alaskans, where remote residential locations or living on reservations compomises sanitation and safe water supplies, and where severe rotavirus diarrhea occurs. About 200,000 hospitalizations in the United States occur annually due to diarrheal illness with 300 deaths (Bell, 2010). The most common viral pathogens are noroviruses and rotavirus, followed by adenoviruses and astroviruses. Food-borne bacterial or parasitic diarrheal diseases are most commonly due to *Salmonella* and *Campylobacter* species, followed by *Shigella, Cryptosporidium, E. coli* O157:H7, *Yersinia, Listeria, Vibrio* (*Vibrio cholerae* and other species), and *Cyclospora* species. *C. difficile* has been associated with pseudomembranous colitis and diarrhea after the use of antibiotics, but it is not the causative agent in most antibiotic-associated diarrhea in children in the United States (Ahmed Bhutta, 2011).

Tables 33-11 and 33-14 discuss the characteristics of diarrheal diseases caused by bacteria, viruses, and parasites that a primary care provider is more likely to encounter and needs to differentiate. Infections due to *Cryptosporidium, E. coli* O157:H7, *Giardia, Listeria, Salmonella, Shigella,* and *V. cholerae* are required to be reported to the CDC. The enteric pathogens encountered more in day care settings include rotavirus, astrovirus, calicivirus, *Campylobacter, Shigella, Giardia*, and *Cryptosporidium* species (Guandalini and Assisri, 2014).

Nausea and vomiting are not good indicators of the severity of a condition; however, the absence of or low-grade fever, mild to moderate periumbilical pain, and watery diarrhea are more typically associated with less serious bacterial infection and suggest small intestine involvement (Ahmed Bhutta, 2011). The following are more indicative of potentially serious infection in the upper intestine:

- Food-borne illness suspected
- Bloody diarrhea, weight loss, dehydration, severe abdominal pain, and fever
- Diarrhea lasting several days with more than three stools per day
- Neurologic involvement on physical examination

Clinical Findings

History

- Pattern of diarrhea: Onset, number of stools, volume, frequency
- Appearance of stool: Odor, mucoid, and/or bloody
- Associated symptoms: Abdominal pain, nausea, vomiting, or fever
- Number of wet diapers in the past 24 hours and approximate time of last void
- Dietary consumption: Changes in diet that might correlate with increased stooling; ingestion (and when) of raw or poorly cooked foods (e.g., raw or undercooked eggs, meat, shellfish, fish, poultry), unpasteurized or under-pasteurized milk or juices, home-canned foods, fresh produce (fruits/vegetables), soft cheeses, deli meats
- If given, response to oral rehydration therapy
- Food allergies
- Family members or close friends with similar illness or other GI diseases
- Day care, school attendance, recreational swimming exposure (even if chlorinated): Illness patterns and contacts at these locations; walking in soil without shoes
- Travel history: Foreign or coastal areas; camping or travel where untreated water might have been consumed
- Attendance at picnics or other outings where food was consumed
- Most recent weight and previous growth pattern
- Medications: Antibiotics, laxatives, antacids, opiates (withdrawal), vitamins (toxicity)
- Pica (metals, plants)
- Chemotherapy
- Recent surgeries (abdominal)

Physical Examination

- Complete a physical examination including vital signs and assessment of behavior/mental status changes
- Assess for dehydration (see Table 33-1)

Text continued on p. 881

TABLE 33-11 **Diarrheal Illnesses Due to Common Bacterial or Viral Pathogens**

Etiology	Incubation Period	Signs and Symptoms	Duration of Illness	Route of Transmission	Laboratory Testing	Treatment and Complications*
Campylobacter jejuni	2 to 5 days, but can be longer	Diarrhea (foul smelling), cramps, fever, nausea and vomiting; diarrhea may be bloody in neonates Occurs in warm weather months	2 to 10 days	Raw and undercooked poultry, unpasteurized milk, contaminated water; low inoculum dose produces infection	Routine stool culture; *Campylobacter* requires special media and incubation temperature; positive gross blood, leukocytes; CBC: ↑ WBCs	Rehydration is the mainstay. Azithromycin and erythromycin shorten the duration of the illness when given early, and usually eradicates the organism from stool within 2 to 3 days.
Clostridium difficile	Unknown	Variety of symptoms and severity are seen: mild to explosive diarrhea, bloody stools, abdominal pain, fever, nausea, vomiting Mild to moderate illness is characterized by watery diarrhea, low-grade fever, and mild abdominal pain	During or after several weeks of antibiotic use; can occur without being associated with such treatment	Acquired from the environment or from stool of other colonized or infected people by the fecal-oral route	Stool cultures; enzyme immunoassay for toxin A, or A and B; positive gross blood, leukocytes; CBC: ↑ WBCs; ESR normal	Discontinue current antibiotic (any antibiotic, but notably ampicillin, clindamycin, second- and third-generation cephalosporins). Fluids and electrolyte replacement are usually sufficient. If antibiotic is still needed or illness is severe, treat with oral metronidazole (drug of choice in children) or vancomycin for 7 to 10 days. Supplement with probiotics. Lactobacillus GG, *Saccharomyces boulardii* are recommended (Jones, 2010; Shane, 2010). Complications include pseudomembranous colitis, toxic megacolon, colonic perforation, relapse, intractable proctitis, death in debilitated children.

Continued

TABLE 33-11 Diarrheal Illnesses Due to Common Bacterial or Viral Pathogens—cont'd

Etiology	Incubation Period	Signs and Symptoms	Duration of Illness	Route of Transmission	Laboratory Testing	Treatment and Complications*
Enterohemorrhagic *Escherichia coli* (EHEC) including *E. coli* O157:H7 and other Shiga toxin–producing *E. coli* (STEC)	1 to 8 days	Severe diarrhea that is often bloody, abdominal pain and vomiting Usually little or no fever More common in children <4 years old	5 to 10 days	Undercooked beef, especially hamburger, unpasteurized milk and juice, raw fruits, vegetables (e.g., sprouts, spinach, lettuce), salami (rarely) Contaminated water; petting zoos	Stool culture; *E. coli* O157:H7 requires special media to grow. If *E. coli* O157:H7 is suspected, specific testing must be requested. Shiga toxin testing may be done using commercial kits; positive isolates should be forwarded to public health laboratories for confirmation and serotyping. Stool grossly positive for blood.	Supportive care: Monitor CBC, platelets, and kidney function closely. *E. coli* O157:H7 infection is also associated with HUS, which can cause lifelong complications. Studies indicate that antibiotics may promote the development of HUS.
Enterotoxigenic *E. coli* (ETEC) and enteroadherent *E. coli* (frequent cause of traveler's diarrhea)	1 to 3 days	Watery diarrhea, abdominal cramps, some vomiting; often cause of mild traveler's diarrhea	3 to >7 days	Water or food contaminated with human feces	Stool culture. ETEC requires special laboratory techniques for identification. If suspected, must request specific testing.	Supportive care: Antibiotics are rarely needed except in severe cases. Recommended antibiotics include TMP-SMX and quinolones. See www.cdc.gov/travel.
Listeria monocytogenes	Variable, ranging from 1 day to more than 3 weeks	Rare, but serious Fever, muscle aches, and nausea or diarrhea Pregnant women may have mild flulike illness, and infection can lead to premature delivery or stillbirth Older adults or immunocompromised patients may have bacteremia or meningitis Infants infected from mother at risk for sepsis or meningitis	Variable	Thrives in salty and acidic conditions, such as fresh soft cheeses, ready-to-eat deli meats, hot dogs; also unpasteurized milk, inadequately pasteurized milk; multiplies at low temperatures, even in properly refrigerated foods	Blood or cerebrospinal fluid cultures. Asymptomatic fecal carriage occurs; therefore, stool culture usually not helpful. Antibody to listeriolysin O may be helpful to identify outbreak retrospectively.	Initial therapy with IV ampicillin and an aminoglycoside usually gentamicin, recommended for severe infections.

Adenovirus, enteric	3 to 10 days	Children >4 years old	Variable	Fecal-oral, throughout year; can remain viable on inanimate objects	Stool specimen for adenovirus antigen via rapid commercial immunoassay techniques or per electron microscopy	Supportive care: Monitor intake and hydration status Preventive care: Good hand washing and diapering precaution
Norovirus	12 to 48 hours	Abrupt-onset watery diarrhea, nausea, vomiting, abdominal cramps	24 to 60 hours Often associated with closed venues (child care centers, cruise ships)	Fecal-oral; contaminated food (ice, shellfish, ready-to-eat foods [e.g., salads, bakery products], or water)	No commercial assay available; CDC can support laboratory evaluation or state and local health department laboratories can perform RT-PCR assays.	Supportive care: May need to treat dehydration and/or electrolyte imbalance. Preventive care: Hand hygiene, clean surfaces and food preparation areas; no swimming in recreational venues for 2 weeks after symptoms resolve.
Rotavirus	1 to 3 days; prevalent during cooler months in temperate climates	Acute-onset fever, vomiting, and watery diarrhea occur 2 to 4 days later in children <5 years old, especially those between 3 to 24 months old	3 to 8 days	Fecal-oral; viable on inanimate objects; rarely contaminated water or food	Enzyme immunoassay and latex agglutination assays for group A rotavirus antigen; virus can be found by electron microscopy and specific nucleic acid amplification methods.	Supportive care: May need to correct dehydration and electrolyte imbalances. Oral IG has been used in those immunocompromised. Preventive care: Rotavirus vaccine; hygiene and diapering precautions in day care facilities.
Salmonella spp.	1 to 3 days	Diarrhea, fever, abdominal cramps, rebound tenderness, vomiting. *S. typhi* and *S. paratyphi* produce typhoid with insidious onset characterized by fever, headache, constipation, malaise, chills, and myalgia; diarrhea is uncommon, and vomiting is not usually severe	4 to 7 days	Contaminated eggs, poultry, unpasteurized milk or juice, cheese, contaminated raw fruits and vegetables (alfalfa sprouts, melons) *S. typhi* epidemics are often related to fecal contamination of water supplies or street-vended foods	Routine stool cultures; positive leukocytes and gross blood. CBC: WBC can be slightly ↑ with left shift, ↓, or normal.	Supportive care: *Only* consider antibiotics (other than for *S. typhi* or *S. paratyphi*) for infants <3 months old, those with chronic GI disease, malignant neoplasm, hemoglobinopathies, HIV, other immunosuppressive illnesses or therapies. If indicated, consider ampicillin or amoxicillin, azithromycin, or TMP-SMX; if resistance shown to any of those, use IM ceftriaxone, cefotaxime; or azithromycin or quinolones. A vaccine exists for *S. typhi* in certain cases.

Continued

TABLE 33-11 Diarrheal Illnesses Due to Common Bacterial or Viral Pathogens—cont'd

Etiology	Incubation Period	Signs and Symptoms	Duration of Illness	Route of Transmission	Laboratory Testing	Treatment and Complications*
Shigella spp.	Varies from 1 to 7 days, but typically is 1 to 3 days	Abdominal cramps, fever, and diarrhea; Stools may contain blood and mucus Seen most commonly in those 6 months old to 3 years old	4 to 7 days	Food or water contaminated with human fecal material Usually person-to-person spread, fecal-oral transmission Ready-to-eat foods touched by infected food workers (e.g., raw vegetables, salads, sandwiches)	Routine stool cultures; gross blood, leukocytes. CBC: normal or slightly ↑ WBCs with left shift	Supportive care: If antibiotics indicated (severe disease, dysentery, immunocompromised), test first for susceptibility. Oral ampicillin (amoxicillin less so) or TMP-SMX recommended in the United States; for organism resistance, use IM ceftriaxone for 2 to 5 days; PO ciprofloxacin; azithromycin (oral cephalosporins not useful). If child is at risk of malnutrition, supplement with vitamin A (200,000 international units). No swimming in recreational pools/slides for 1 week after symptoms resolve.
Yersinia enterocolytica and *Y. pseudotuberculosis*	Typically 4 to 6 days with a range of 1 to 14 days	Appendicitis-like symptoms (diarrhea and vomiting, fever, and RLQ pain) occur primarily in older children and young adults May have a scarlatiniform rash or erythema nodosum with *Y. pseudotuberculosis* Seen in all ages	1 to 3 weeks, usually self-limiting	Undercooked pork, unpasteurized milk, tofu, contaminated water Infection has occurred in infants whose caregivers handled chitterlings	Stool, vomitus, or blood culture. *Yersinia* requires special medium to grow. If suspected, must request specific testing. Serology is available in research and reference laboratories.	Supportive care: If septicemia or other invasive disease occurs, antibiotic therapy with gentamicin or cefotaxime (doxycycline and ciprofloxacin also effective) after susceptibility testing is done.

Adapted from Department of Health and Human Services, Centers for Disease Control and Prevention (CDC): Diagnosis and management of food borne illnesses: a primer for physicians and other health professionals, *MMWR Morb Mortal Wkly Rep* 53(RR04):7–9, 2004. Additional information from Mezoff EA, Cohen MB: *Clostridium difficile* infection. In Kliegman RM, Behrman RE, Jenson HB, et al: *Nelson textbook of pediatrics,* ed 19, Philadelphia, 2011, Elsevier, p 994; Red book: *2012 report of the committee on infectious diseases,* ed 29, Elk Grove Village, IL, 2012, American Academy of Pediatrics.

CBC, Complete blood count; *CDC,* Centers for Disease Control and Prevention; *ESR,* erythrocyte sedimentation rate; *GI,* gastrointestinal; *HIV,* human immunodeficiency virus; *HUS,* hemolytic uremic syndrome; *IG,* immunoglobulin; *IM,* intramuscular; *IV,* intravenous; *RLQ,* right lower quadrant; *RT-PCR,* reverse transcription-polymerase chain reaction; *TMP-SMX,* trimethoprim-sulfamethoxazole; *WBC,* white blood cell.

*See Table 33-12 for dosages.

Diagnostic Studies

Diagnostic studies are ordered if the symptoms (discussed earlier) of more serious infection are present. Some specific diagnostic findings associated with the more common infectious diarrheal illness are found in Table 33-11. Molecular diagnostic tests (e.g., polymerase chain reaction [PCR]) have greatly improved the ability to diagnose diarrheal illness due to bacteria. The following tests may be ordered:

- Stool examination (color, consistency, blood, mucus, pus, odor, volume): In endemic areas, microscopy examination for parasites (e.g., *G. lamblia* and *E. histolytica*).
- Stool: pH (less than 5.5 suggests carbohydrate intolerance typically seen in viral infections), leukocytes (suggest bacterial invasion), reducing substances (viral infections), and occult blood. Normal stool: pH greater than 5.5, carbohydrate negative.
- Stool cultures should be considered early in the course of illness for bloody or prolonged diarrhea; in the presence of leukocytes; if clinical signs of colitis are present; for suspected food-borne illness outbreaks (especially with *E. coli* O157:H7); in the immunocompromised; or after recent travel abroad.
- Electrolytes, if indicated, to evaluate degree of dehydration and for more serious signs and symptoms of infectious disease.
- CBC, as indicated for serious infectious disease.

Differential Diagnosis

Diarrhea from viral etiology and antibiotic use are the most common causes of diarrhea in all age groups. Systemic infection is a common cause in infants and children, and food poisoning is a common cause in children and adolescents. Overfeeding should also be considered in infants. Rare causes of acute diarrhea in infants include primary disaccharidase deficiency, Hirschsprung toxic colitis, adrenogenital syndrome, and neonate opiate withdrawal; toxic ingestion in children; and hyperthyroidism in adolescents.

Management

The foundation of all treatment of acute diarrhea is fourfold:

- Restore and maintain hydration and correct/maintain electrolyte and acid-base balance. Oral rehydration with an oral electrolyte solution should be attempted when dehydration is assessed between 3% and 9%. Administer parenteral hydration if necessary for the following: impaired circulation and possible shock, weight less than 4 to 5 kg or a child younger than 3 months old, intractable diarrhea, lethargy, anatomic anomalies, or failure to gain weight or continued weight loss despite oral fluids (see Table 33-3).
- Maintain nutrition. Resume early refeeding because contents of the bowel stimulate the growth of enterocytes and help facilitate mucosal repair following injury (see Table 33-3).
- Prescribe antibiotics prudently. Antibiotics are recommended for acute diarrhea caused by *G. lamblia, V. cholerae,* and *Shigella* species and can be considered for infections caused by enteropathogenic *E. coli* (if infection prolonged), enteroinvasive *E. coli, Yersinia* for those with sickle cell disease, and *Salmonella* in young infants with fever or positive blood culture findings (Guandalini and Assiri, 2014) (see Tables 33-11 and 33-12). Children with HIV at risk for acute diarrhea may benefit from cotrimoxazole and vitamin A (Humphreys et al, 2010).
- Treat any related conditions, such as sepsis and cardiovascular collapse.

Some adjunct medications and treatments have received wider use in countries outside of the United States and show efficacy in some studies. Some of these include:

- Antidiarrheals (antimotility agents or adsorbents) are not generally recommended (Bell, 2010). However, a review of literature demonstrated that loperamide in children older than 3 years old is safe and decreases the duration and frequency of diarrhea compared with placebo. Children younger than 3 years old and those who are malnourished, those with moderate or severe dehydration, those who are systemically ill, or those who have bloody diarrhea should not be treated with this drug (Li et al, 2008). Some over-the-counter products intended for diarrhea contain salicylates (e.g., Pepto-Bismol), and there is concern for Reye syndrome.
- Probiotics: *Lactobacillus casei* strain GG or *S. boulardii* (a yeast) given early in a viral diarrheal illness or antibiotic-associated diarrhea can both treat diarrhea (decrease duration by about 25 hours) (Allen et al, 2010) and ameliorate the risk of antibiotic-associated diarrhea (Johnston et al, 2007). Exact doses are undetermined, but Jones (2010) cites studies suggesting at least more than 5 billion colony-forming units (CFUs) per day.
- Dioctahedral smectite, adsorbent clay, is used in many countries to protect the intestinal mucosa by absorbing viruses, bacteria, and bacterial toxins; there are few reported side effects. Studies have shown that smectite can reduce the duration of diarrhea (Piescik-Lech et al, 2013). Its use is not routinely recommended in the United States.
- Oral enteric peppermint oil capsules have been studied for use with diarrhea, cramping, and bloating, especially when related to IBS. It may produce smooth muscle relaxation, slow food transit through the intestines, and help with general symptom relief; its efficacy is still debated. Essential peppermint oil *(Mentha piperita)* aromatherapy can be used for abdominal pain and relaxation (Wall et al, 2014). See Chapter 43 for complementary medicine therapies for diarrhea.
- Zinc is commonly prescribed to shorten the duration of acute diarrhea in children from developing countries. Patel and colleagues (2010) found that zinc was efficacious for diarrhea caused by *Klebsiella,* not necessarily for *E. coli* or parasitic infections, and was detrimental when used in infections caused by rotavirus. The optimal dose of zinc has not been established and variations may account for varying efficacy. Zinc supplementation

TABLE 33-12 Antibiotics More Commonly Used for Diarrheal Infections

Drug	Dosage	Indication
Amoxicillin	25-50 mg divided in three doses, PO, for 7 to 10 days (maximum daily dose 1.5 g)	*Salmonella, Shigella*
Ampicillin	50-100 mg/kg/day divided into four doses for 5 to 10 days (maximum daily dose 4 g)	*Salmonella, Shigella*
Azithromycin	10 mg/kg/day first day, then 5 mg/kg/day days 2 to 5, PO (up to maximum daily dose of 500 mg on day 1; 250 mg on days 2 to 5)	*Clostridium jejuni, Escherichia coli* O157:H7
Cefotaxime	IM: 75-100 mg in three or four doses	*Salmonella*
Ceftriaxone	IM: 50-75 mg in one or two doses, maximum single dose 1000 mg	*Salmonella, Shigella*
Ciprofloxacin (in pediatric patients, not routinely first-line therapy)	>18 years old: 20-30 mg/kg/day divided into two divided doses, PO (maximum daily dose 1.5 g) for 5 to 10 days for *E. coli*. Same dosage divided in two doses and treated for 7 to 10 days for *Salmonella* and *Shigella;* for 5 to 7 days for *Campylobacter*	*E. coli* O157:H7, *Listeria, Shigella, Salmonella, Campylobacter*
Doxycycline	<8 years old: 2 mg/kg/dose every 12 hours for 3 days >8 years old: 2-4 mg/kg/day in one or two doses, PO for 7 to 10 days (maximum daily dose 200 mg)	*Yersinia enterocolitis*
Erythromycin	30-50 mg/kg/day in two to four divided doses PO for 5 to 7 days (maximum daily dose 2 g)	*C. jejuni*
Metronidazole	Amebiasis: 30-50 mg/kg/day in three divided doses for 7 to 10 days *Clostridium difficile:* 30 mg/kg/day in four divided doses for 7 to 14 days Giardiasis: 15 mg/kg/day three times a day for 5 to 7 days	*C. difficile* (first-line drug), *Entamoeba histolytica, Giardia lamblia, C. jejuni, E. coli* O157:H7
Tetracycline	>8 years old: 25-50 mg/kg/day in four divided doses PO for 7 to 10 days (maximum dose 3 g)	*Y. enterocolitis*
Trimethoprim-sulfamethoxazole (TMP-SMX)	Cyclosporiasis: 10 mg/kg/day in two divided doses for 7 to 10 days Shigellosis: Not recommended	*Y. enterocolitis, Salmonella, Shigella, E. coli* O157:H7, *Cyclospora cayetanensis*
Vancomycin	40 mg/kg/day in four divided doses PO for 7 to 10 days (maximum 500 mg daily dose)	*C. difficile*

Data from Ahmed Bhutta Z: Acute gastroenteritis in children. In Kliegman RM, Behrman RE, Jenson HB, et al: *Nelson textbook of pediatrics,* ed 18, Philadelphia, 2011; Schleiss MR, Chen SF: Principles of antiparasitic therapy. In Kliegman RM, Behrman RE, Jenson HB, et al: *Nelson textbook of pediatrics,* ed 19, Philadelphia, 2011; Red book: *2012 report of the committee on infectious diseases,* ed 29, Elk Grove Village, IL, 2012, American Academy of Pediatrics.

might have limited effect if the child is not zinc deficient (Patro et al, 2010). It is added to ORS solutions (along with prebiotics) in many developing countries (Passariello et al, 2011).

Complications

See Table 33-11 for complications associated with some common pathogens.

Prevention

Preventive measures include the following:

- Good hand washing by all individuals (including children and all care providers), especially when handling food: Liquid soap and paper towels are recommended at day care centers. Use of non-water alcohol hand sanitizers with an ethanol content of at least 60% has also shown efficacy to reduce GI illnesses (CDC, 2011).
- Good sanitation and appropriate removal of soiled clothing and diapers: The diapering area should be cleaned after changing each child at day care centers.
- Avoid contaminated sources; meat should be properly cooked.
- Promote exclusive breastfeeding for the first 6 months of life to promote passive immunity and guard against exposure to contaminated food and water.
- Promote appropriate supplemental nutrition starting at 6 months (breastfeeding should continue through the

first year or longer in developing countries), food handling, and storage.
- In developing countries, consider addition of vitamin A and zinc in cases of malnutrition.
- With *Shigella,* culture all symptomatic contacts and treat those with positive stool cultures.
- Avoid unnecessary antibiotic usage.
- Promote well-functioning sewage system in developing countries (including latrines, septic tanks, dry-composting toilets), which can cut diarrheal illness by up to 30% (Norman et al, 2010).
- Promote rotavirus vaccine for all children worldwide.

Chronic Diarrhea

Chronic diarrhea is defined as loose stools of less than 10 mL/kg/day in infants and less than 200 g/24 hours in older children (Lee et al, 2012). The terms *persistent* or *prolonged diarrhea* have also been used when describing a state of chronic diarrhea; these generally refer to a continuing diarrheal illness that started as acute diarrhea and is affecting growth. Diarrhea that is chronic is the result of intraluminal factors (that influence digestion) or mucosal factors (that influence digestion and transport of nutrients across the mucosa); either factor affects the normal cellular mechanisms of the GI tract. Because "persistent" diarrhea is generally associated with an acute diarrheal onset, it is surmised that there is either persistent infectious colonization with an enteric pathogen or impaired healing and return to the normal intestinal processes/structure. Table 33-13 lists the most common causes of chronic diarrhea by age group. Infants and children have difficulty absorbing volumes of liquid larger than 200 mL/kg/day; an excess can cause diarrhea, which is not an uncommon finding in toddlers ("toddler's diarrhea").

Clinical Findings

History

- Occurrence of three or more watery stools per day for more than 2 weeks; 10 watery/runny stools per day that often contain undigested food particles is more typical of "toddler's diarrhea"
- Presence of red flags:
  - Hematochezia or melena
  - Persistent fever
  - Weight loss or growth arrest
  - Anemia
- Dietary history (including amount of fruit juices or high-carbohydrate fluids ingested per day)
- Stool consistency, blood, mucus, pus, particles of food
- Stool incontinence
- Exposure to illness (including day care; contact with pets/other animals)
- Teething
- Prior treatments for diarrhea (any dietary manipulation, drug, or home treatments)
- Recent travel

TABLE 33-13 Common Causes of Chronic Diarrhea Seen in Children

Age	Conditions
0 to 6 months old	• Carbohydrate malabsorption (acquired, congenital) (e.g., CMPI) • Protein hypersensitivity • Excessive intake of formula or other fluid (water, juice [especially those containing sorbitol/fructose], high-carbohydrate liquids) • Postenteritis • Infections • CF or other fat absorption conditions • Neuroblastoma (rare) • Immunodeficiency (e.g., HIV/AIDS and others) • Lymphangiectasia (rare) • Hirschsprung disease • Neonatal or infant enteropathies (rare) • Radiation treatments
7 to 24 months old	First eight bulleted conditions listed above plus: • Chronic nonspecific diarrhea • Small-bowel overgrowth • Celiac disease • Graft-versus-host enteropathy • Autoimmune enteropathy • Radiation treatments
>24 months old	• Excessive intake of fruit juice/ high-carbohydrate drinks • Infections • Small-bowel bacterial overgrowth • Celiac disease • Munchausen syndrome by proxy • Grant-versus-host enteropathy • Carbohydrate malabsorption • IBS • Adult-type hypolactasia • Encopresis • IBD (e.g., Crohn disease) • Excessive use of laxatives • Radiation treatments • Acquired lactase deficiency in older children, primarily of African, Asian, or Middle Eastern descent • Perforated appendix

Data from Guarino A, LoVecchio A, Berni Canani R: Chronic diarrhea in children, *Best Pract Res Clin Gastroenterol* 26(5):649–661, 2012; Lee KS, Kang DS, Yu J, et al: How to do in persistent diarrhea of children? Concepts and treatments of chronic diarrhea, *Pediatr Gastroenterol Hepatol Nutr* 15(4):229–236, 2012.

AIDS, Acquired immune deficiency syndrome; *CF,* cystic fibrosis; *CMPI,* cow's-milk protein intolerance; *HIV,* human immunodeficiency virus; *IBD,* inflammatory bowel disease; *IBS,* irritable bowel syndrome.

Physical Examination

Look for physical findings associated with the underlying pathologic condition:
- Assessment of hydration status
- Weight and height measurements; any weight loss

- Growth retardation
- Skin and hair condition, color of skin and conjunctivae
- Vital signs (heart rate and blood pressure)
- Palpation of the thyroid for enlargement
- Increased heart rate
- Respiratory symptoms
- Clubbing of fingers
- Abdominal examination
- Rectal examination (skin tags, impaction, tenderness)

Diagnostic Studies

- Stool: Culture, O&P (best done on three specimens collected on separate days), pH, reducing substances, occult blood, leukocytes, fat and fecal elastase (to evaluate for pancreatic insufficiency) (Normal stool pH greater than 5.5 indicates negative carbohydrate.)
- CBC with differential, electrolytes, and albumin
- UA and culture in young children

The following are ordered as indicated by the history, physical examination, and consideration of differential diagnoses:

- ESR, CRP
- Hormonal studies to assess for secretory tumors (vasoactive intestinal peptide, gastrin, secretin, urine assay for 5-hydroxytryptamine [5-HT])
- Breath hydrogen test for lactose or sucrose intolerance (difficult to assess in infants)
- Viral serologies, such as HIV or CMV
- Sweat chloride test
- Endoscopy, barium studies

Differential Diagnosis

See Table 33-13.

Management

- Treat the underlying cause.
- Chronic nonspecific diarrhea (toddler's diarrhea): Normalize the diet; remove offending foods and fluids; eliminate sorbitol and fructose-containing fluids; reduce fluid intake to no greater than 90 mL/kg/24 hours (give half of fluid as milk [whole or 2%]); increase fat to 35% to 40% of the diet; and increase fiber to bulk up stools.
- Treat carbohydrate malabsorption by decreasing lactose or sucrose; add lactase or sacrosidase as indicated by particular carbohydrate intolerance.
- Post-gastroenteritis malabsorption syndrome (evidenced in infants with weight loss and fat globules in the stool) can be given a predigested formula (e.g., Pregestimil or Alimentum), if tolerated, for 3 to 4 weeks (elemental formula can be used if those are not tolerated). Refer the following patients to a gastroenterologist: Newborns with diarrhea in first hours of life; patients with growth delay or failure or abnormal physical findings (anorexia, abdominal pain, chronic bloating, vomiting, or weakness); or those with severe illness.

Complications

Malnutrition, growth failure, and cognitive/developmental impairments (found more in developing countries) can occur.

Intestinal Parasites

Various protozoa and helminths can invade the GI tract and cause disease. In developed countries, such infestations are usually by protozoa. Endemic areas of developing countries are subject to more significant morbidity and mortality from parasitic infestations. All can multiply within the human body, are associated with diarrheal symptoms, and are spread by fecal contamination due to poor water and sewage disposal practices. Cysts of these parasites are often resistant to chlorine.

Helminths are worms; nematodes (roundworms), cestodes (tapeworms), and trematodes (flatworms) that most commonly reside in the human intestines but do not multiply there. Fecal-oral contact with eggs or cysts excreted from the initial vector via ingestion of contaminated food or water is one route of infestation. Some helminths (hookworms and whipworms) release larvae into the soil; humans become infected when they walk barefoot on contaminated soil and the skin is penetrated by the larvae. These larvae then travel to the lungs and intestines. Eggs can also be excreted in the stool; poor sanitary disposal of human waste into soils affords the further potential for ingestion via contamination of food and water. They are found worldwide, principally in tropical and subtropical developing countries. In industrialized countries, infestation is found in those who travel to endemic areas, in the immunocompromised, and immigrants from endemic areas. Their insidious nature causes chronic health and nutritional problems that can impair physical and mental growth of children. *Enterobius vermicularis* (pinworm), *Ascaris lumbricoides* (roundworm), and *Taenia* (tapeworm) are some of the more common intestinal parasites that affect the pediatric population (Harhay et al, 2010).

Clinical Findings, Management, and Differential Diagnosis

See Tables 33-14 and 33-15 for clinical findings and management. The differential diagnosis includes all other causes of infectious and noninfectious diarrhea.

Patient and Family Education

Most parasitic infestations can be prevented by good hand washing and good sanitation. The following preventive measures are recommended:

- Travelers to developing countries need to eat only foods that can be peeled or have been cooked. Ice, "washed" foods, and tap water can be contaminated. Bottled or treated water is advised for drinking and brushing teeth. Shoes should be worn when walking on potentially contaminated soil.

TABLE 33-14 **Intestinal Illnesses Due to More Common Parasites (Protozoa and Helminths)**

Etiology	Incubation Period	Signs and Symptoms	Duration of Illness	Route of Transmission	Laboratory Testing	Treatment*
Cryptosporidium parvum	3 to 14 days	Diarrhea (usually watery), stomach cramps, upset stomach, bloating, slight fever, anorexia, weight loss, flatulence, nausea, vomiting, fatigue	Self-limiting, usually lasts 6 to 14 days	Fecal-oral route; from uncooked food or food contaminated by an ill food handler after cooking; drinking water (collects on water filters and membranes that cannot be disinfected); reservoirs include cattle, sheep, goats, birds, reptiles, young animals	Request specific testing of the stool for *Cryptosporidium* using antigen-detection tests. May need to examine water or food.	Supportive care, self-limited. If severe, or individual immunocompromised consider paromomycin for 7 days. For children 1 to 11 years old, consider nitazoxanide for 3 days.
Cyclospora cayetanensis	Usually 7 days, but can range from 2 to 14 days	Diarrhea (usually watery), loss of appetite, substantial loss of weight, stomach cramps, nausea, vomiting, fatigue, myalgia, low-grade fevers	May remit and relapse over weeks to months	Fecal-oral from sewage or nontreated water; food (various types of fresh produce [imported berries, lettuce])	Request specific examination of the stool for *Cyclospora*. May need to examine water or food.	TMP-SMX for 7 to 10 days.
Entamoeba histolytica	Commonly 2 to 4 weeks (known to also range from days, months, to years); fecal-oral transmission	Can be asymptomatic with nonspecific complaints of diarrhea, lower abdominal pain In invasive disease (amebic colitis) symptoms of increasing diarrhea, bloody diarrhea, lower abdominal pain, tenesmus, weight loss progress over a 1- to 3-week period; occasional fever Advanced disease hepatomegaly, liver tenderness	Weeks to years, depending on response to treatment; no drug is completely effective	Spread by fecal-oral route	Stool examination for trophozoites or cysts; PCR, isoenzyme analysis, monoclonal antibody–based antigen; enzyme immunoassay; ultrasounds and CT scans to identify suspected liver abscess or other extraintestinal infection.	Asymptomatic cyst excreters: Luminal amebicide (iodoquinol, paromomycin, diloxanide). Mild to moderate or severe involvement/liver abscesses: metronidazole or tinidazole followed by luminal amebicide. Follow-up stool examination after treatment. Perform stool examinations on household members or other suspected contacts. Do not treat with corticosteroids or antimotility drugs. Complications include liver abscess, ameboma.

Continued

TABLE 33-14 Intestinal Illnesses Due to More Common Parasites (Protozoa and Helminths)—cont'd

Etiology	Incubation Period	Signs and Symptoms	Duration of Illness	Route of Transmission	Laboratory Testing	Treatment*
Giardia intestinalis	3 weeks	Can include bouts of watery diarrhea; abdominal pain, greasy, foul-smelling stools; bloody diarrhea (rare); flatulence; abdominal distention; anorexia; weight loss; FTT; anemia; asymptomatic infection common	Pending effective treatment	Fecal-oral or contaminated food or water. Water can be contaminated by *Giardia* from dogs, cats, beavers, and other animals.	Stool specimens for trophozoites or cysts using staining methods; antigens using enzyme immunoassay; PCR techniques. Increased sensitivity by obtaining three or more specimens every other day and by rapid examination of stool (can be placed in a fixative).	Correct for any dehydration or electrolyte imbalance. Tinidazole, metronidazole, nitazoxanide drugs of choice. Albendazole, mebendazole effective also in children with fewer side effects. Consult for those immunocompromised. Contact local health departments in cases of outbreaks. Infected individuals should not use recreational water sources for swimming until 2 weeks after symptoms resolve. Filtration, boiling, chemical disinfection may be required for drinking water. Some infections are self-limited and treatment is not required. Dehydration and electrolyte abnormalities can occur and should be corrected. Complications: Debilitating disease leading to malabsorption; anorexia; weight loss; FTT.
Ancylostoma duodenale (hookworm)	5 to 8 weeks for eggs to appear in feces; 4 to 12 weeks for onset of symptoms	Often asymptomatic or stinging/burning sensation in feet followed by pruritus, papulovesicular rash (lasting up to 2 weeks), pharyngeal itching, hoarseness, nausea, vomiting As migrates through lungs: Mild cough, pneumonitis Chronic infestation: Anemia, edema, growth delays, slowed development and cognition in children	5 year unless treated	Larvae in feces-contaminated soil penetrate skin (travel to lungs and settle in the intestines) or are directly ingested from contaminated food or water, including human milk.	CBC shows hypochromic microcytic anemia, eosinophilia; hypoproteinemia. Stool microscopic examination for ova.	Albendazole, pyrantel pamoate; repeat stool examination in 2 weeks recommended. Iron and nutritional supplementation if indicated; severe cases require blood transfusions. Complications: Delayed growth, developmental/mental status delays in children.

Enterobius vermicularis (pinworm)	1 to 2 months, or longer from ingestion to migration to perianal area	Perirectal and/or vaginal pruritus; nervous irritability, hyperactivity, insomnia; urethritis, vaginitis, salpingitis, and pelvic peritonitis have been reported	Reinfection common in children	Ingested eggs from soil, water contamination, or direct fecal-oral route from fomites on bedding, clothing, toys, baths; person-to-person. Female lays eggs in perianal area and dies; ingested eggs hatch, become larvae in small intestine and migrate to rectum.	1 cm long white, threadlike worms can be visualized at anus during night after child has been asleep for 2 to 3 hours. Microscopic examination: Use transparent adhesive tape applied to anus to collect any eggs or pinworms present on three consecutive nights or mornings before child arises. Direct stool examination usually not productive.	Mebendazole, pyrantel pamoate or albendazole and repeated in 2 weeks; also treat family members; vaginitis is self-limiting. Easily spread among family members, in day care settings, and institutions (up to 50% infestation rates in these populations). Preventive: Morning baths, change bedding, hand hygiene, clip fingernails, avoid scratching perianal region, avoid nail biting. Day care precautions include hand hygiene, proper handling of underwear and diapers.
Ascaris lumbricoides (roundworm)	8 weeks from egg ingestion to adult egg-laying capacity	Weight loss, malnutrition; worms can be seen in vomitus and stools; can cause cough, fever, chest discomfort if pass through lungs (not a common occurrence) Children can have large worm burdens Stressful conditions (fever, illness) and some anthelmintic drugs can cause adults to migrate	12 to 18 months without treatment	Fecal-oral from ingestion of eggs from contaminated food (fruit, vegetables) or soil (where incubation occurs; adult worms live in small intestine and eggs are excreted in feces). Larvae migrate from intestines via portal blood to liver and lungs, ascend through tracheobronchial tree to pharynx, to intestines again to develop into adults. Found in areas where human feces are used for fertilizer.	Stool/vomitus/nares: Worms seen via microscopy. CBC: Marked eosinophilia. Have laboratory check for all concurrent worm infestations in order to treat all worms appropriately.	Albendazole, mebendazole, ivermectin; surgical intervention if necessary. Complications: Impaired nutritional status of children and growth; bowel or biliary obstruction, peritonitis, obstruction of common bile duct (biliary colic, cholangitis, pancreatitis); Löffler syndrome due to allergic response as larvae migrate to the lungs. Reinfection common. Globally, most common human intestinal nematode.
Taenia (tapeworm) (*T. saginata* [beef]; *T. solium* [pork])	2 to 3 months after larvae ingested to feces excretion	Worm(s) may be seen in perianal region May be asymptomatic or have abdominal pain, nausea, diarrhea, excessive appetite	Several years before cysticercosis symptoms evident	Fecal-oral from ingestion of water or food contaminated with eggs or from ingested cysts or larvae in inadequately cooked pork or beef.	Stool microscopy: ova seen.	Praziquantel, niclosamide, nitazoxanide. Complications: Systemic cysticercosis from *T. solium* (viscera, brain, muscle invasion with possible seizures).
Trichuris trichiura (whipworm)	12 weeks	Asymptomatic unless infestation is heavy; abdominal pain, tenesmus, bloody diarrhea with mucus; can mimic IBD; growth retardation		Fecal-oral from contaminated soil (where eggs incubate), water, and/or food (embeds in mucosal lining of large intestines). Not spread person to person.	Stool microscopy or concentration techniques.	Mebendazole, albendazole, ivermectin for 3 days; can reexamine stools after 2 weeks to ensure resolution. Complications: Chronic colitis, rectal prolapse, compromised nutritional status, growth retardation.

CBC, Complete blood count; *CT,* computed tomography; *FTT,* failure to thrive; *IBD,* inflammatory bowel disease; *PCR,* polymerase chain reaction; *TMP-SMX,* trimethoprim-sulfamethoxazole.
*See Table 33-15 for dosages.

TABLE 33-15 Medications for Treatment of Parasite Infestations*

Drug	Dosage
Albendazole (Albenza): Take with food. The tablet may be crushed or chewed and swallowed with a drink of water.	*Ascariasis:* 1 year old: 200 mg once; >2 years old: 400 mg once *Taenia solium:* 15 mg/kg/day in 2 doses × 8 to 30 days; can be repeated as necessary (maximum 400 mg per dose)
Mebendazole (Vermox): Tablet may be crushed, mixed with food, swallowed whole, or chewed.	*Pinworms:* 100 mg once; may need to repeat in 2 weeks *Whipworms, roundworms, and hookworms:* 100 mg twice daily for 3 days *Toxocariasis:* 100-200 mg twice daily for 5 days
Diloxanide furoate (Furamide): Give with meals.	20 mg/kg/day in 3 doses × 10 days (maximum 500 mg per dose)
Ivermectin (Stromectal): Take on an empty stomach.	All ages: 150-200 mcg/kg/dose once
Iodoquinol (Yodoxin): Administer after meals, tablets may be crushed and mixed with applesauce or chocolate syrup.	30-40 mg/kg/day in 3 doses × 20 days (maximum 2 g) Adults: 650 mg three times daily × 20 days
Metronidazole (Flagyl)	35-50 mg/kg/day in 3 doses × 7 to 10 days (maximum 500-750 mg per dose) *Giardia lamblia:* 15 mg/kg/day in 3 doses × 5 days (maximum 250 mg per dose)
Nitazoxanide (Alinia): Administer with food, shake suspension well prior to use.	1 to 3 years old: 100 mg in 2 doses × 3 days 4 to 11 years old: 200 mg in 2 doses × 3 days 11 years old to adult: 500 mg twice daily × 3 days
Paromomycin (Humatin): Administer with or without meals, protect from moisture.	25-35 mg/kg/day in 3 doses × 7 days
Praziquantel (Biltricide): Administer tablets with water during meals; do not chew due to bitter taste.	*Tapeworm:* 5-10 mg/kg once *Liver Fluke:* Up to 75 mg/kg in 3 doses in 1 day
Pyrantel pamoate (Pamix, Pin-X): Over the counter. May be mixed with milk or fruit juice. Shake suspension well.	11 mg/kg daily (maximum 1 g) × 3 days Use with caution in children <2 years old
Tinidazole (Tindamax)	*Giardia lamblia:* 50 mg/kg once (maximum 2 g)

Data from Schleiss MR, Chen SF: Principles of antiparasitic therapy. In Kliegman RM, Behrman RE, Jenson HB, et al: *Nelson textbook of pediatrics,* ed 19, Philadelphia, 2011, Elsevier.

*Medication choices and dosages are dependent upon child's condition at diagnosis and parasite. Consult CDC or latest recommendations for treatment regimes.

- *G. lamblia:* Encourage good hand hygiene. Prevent contamination of water sources. Treat questionable water with iodine, boiling for 20 minutes, or use commercial filters to filter contaminated water. Exclude symptomatic children and staff from school and day care until asymptomatic.
- *E. vermicularis:* Avoid scratching. Wash sheets and clothing in hot water and detergent.
- *A. lumbricoides:* Appropriate food preparation is necessary to prevent infection. When human feces are used for fertilizer, thoroughly cook or soak fruit and vegetables in diluted iodine solution before consuming. Periodic, empiric treatment of children may prevent nutritional and cognitive deficits in endemic areas.
- *Taenia:* Avoid raw or undercooked beef or pork.

Congenital Gastrointestinal Conditions

These are discussed in Chapter 40 with other perinatal concerns.

For a complete list of references, please visit http://evolve.elsevier.com/Burns/pediatric/.

34

Dental and Oral Disorders

DONALD L. CHI, PETER M. MILGROM, OHNMAR K. TUT, MARY ANN DRAYE, AND MICHELE E. ACKER

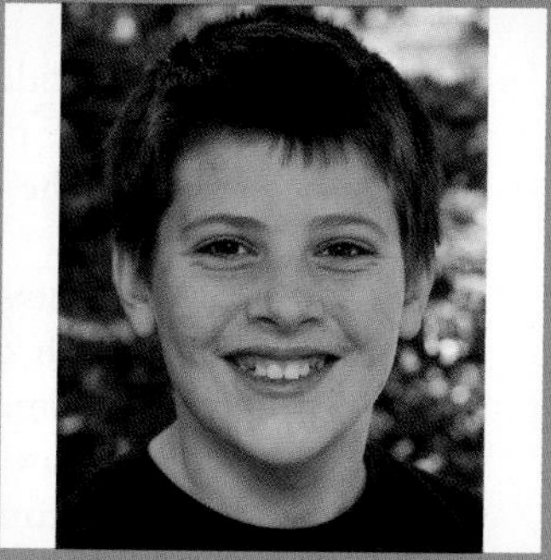

The mouth serves many functions, including speech and digestion, and is richly endowed with special systems that serve complex needs. It is increasingly recognized as a barometer of health and well-being throughout life. For this reason, good oral health is essential for normal growth and development. Oral samples (e.g., saliva, gingival crevicular fluid, oral swabs, dental plaque, and volatiles) are replacing serum and blood as vehicles for noninvasive diagnostic tests for systemic diseases. Many of these tests are already on the market (Malamud and Rodriguez-Chavez, 2011).

In children, infections caused by bacteria, viruses, and fungi cause tooth decay (dental caries), gum disease (gingivitis and periodontitis), cold sores (herpes labialis), canker sores (aphthous ulcers), and thrush (candidiasis). Moreover, inherited and congenital conditions result in impairments and cosmetic defects that have serious effects on children as they grow and develop. Lifestyle choices such as frequent intake of sugary foods and beverages, irregular oral hygiene, tobacco and drug use, and oral piercings create challenges for maintaining optimal oral health.

Meeting the oral health care needs of children requires involvement of primary care providers (PCPs). Most socioeconomically vulnerable children see PCPs regularly for preventive care (Chi et al, 2013a), which gives PCPs a critical role as part of the oral health team to help prevent oral disease, identify and minimize the effects of oral disease, and provide guidance to parents and children about oral health. Studies have shown that physician assistants, nurse practitioners, and dentists recognize the importance of performing an oral examination during medical visits but lack confidence in their ability to do so (Danielson et al, 2006; Hallas and Shelley, 2009; Pierce et al, 2002).

This chapter offers information and practical answers for PCPs to ensure they have basic examination competencies; are able to distinguish between normal and abnormal structures, pathology, and common oral diseases; feel competent to educate regarding oral health; prescribe and apply preventive treatment (e.g., fluoride varnish); and know when to refer to dentists.

Standards and Guidelines for Dental Care in the United States

Healthy People 2020 identifies oral health as a priority. There are 17 objectives that address the prevention and control of oral and craniofacial disease, conditions, injuries, and improvements in accessing preventive dental services and care.

In 2010, the U.S. Department of Health and Human Services (USDHHS) launched a cross-agency initiative to improve oral health nationwide among children with Medicaid and the Children's Health Insurance Program (CHIP). Referred to as the *New Oral Health Initiative* (NOHI), it sets short-term and long-term goal attainment (including those identified in Healthy People 2020) and calls for increasing accountability, expanding research and data collection, emphasizing disease prevention and oral health promotion (including addressing health literacy and cultural competence), and reducing health disparities. Additionally, NOHI expands the dental health care team by promoting "dental care" or "oral health care" by dental practitioners (dentists and dental hygienists, dental therapists, community dental health practitioners under the supervision of a dentist) as well as by non-dental professionals (e.g., PCPs). It also includes a provision to reimburse PCPs for preventive dental services (e.g., oral examinations, risk assessment, fluoride varnish) (Institute of Medicine [IOM] and National Research Council [NRC], 2011).

Provisions in the Affordable Care Act of 2010 (ACA) address coverage and access (including insurance benefits for children), prevention, oral health infrastructure and surveillance, the dental health workforce, cost-sharing restrictions, public health grants that may include oral health initiatives, and a requirement to review dental provider reimbursement rates.

The U.S. Preventive Services Task Force (USPSTF) has issued two recommendations for preventing caries in children from birth to 5 years old—PCPs should (1) prescribe oral fluoride supplementation starting at 6 months old if the water supply is fluoride deficient, and (2) apply sodium fluoride varnish to the primary teeth of all infants and children beginning at the onset of primary tooth eruption (USPSTF, 2014).

The American Academy of Pediatric Dentistry (AAPD) recommends that health care providers encourage parents to establish a "dental home" for their children no later than 12 months old. For those with higher risk factors, referral to a dentist should be considered as early as 6 months old or at the eruption of the first primary tooth (AAPD, Council on Clinical Affairs, 2015a).

Access to Dental Care in the United States

Numerous studies report considerable disparities in oral health and access to care with the greatest burden experienced by low-income, racial/ethnic minority children in households with low parental education (IOM and NRC, 2011). Approximately 18% of children 2 to 17 years old in the United States did not have at least one dental visit in 2012. This represents about a 3% improvement in visits since 2010 (USDHHS, 2014). Although Medicaid-enrolled children have better access to dental care than uninsured children, they continue to exhibit low dental utilization rates (less than 50%); those 2 to 5 years old have the poorest attendance (USDHHS and Agency for Healthcare Research and Quality [AHRQ], 2013). Contributing factors to these lower rates include dentists' unwillingness to accept Medicaid insurance because of low reimbursement rates and the maldistribution of dentists across the nation (Mahat et al, 2014; PEW Charitable Trust, 2014). Low preventive dental care utilization rates can result in a cycle of emergency dental care with less comprehensive treatment, pain, and more symptom-driven care.

Normal Growth and Development

The Teeth

The structures of the mouth include the mucosa (buccal and gingival), palate, salivary glands, frenula, tongue, and teeth. Primary and permanent teeth have similar anatomy, differing primarily in the size and external shape of each tooth, which includes the crown, neck (where the crown meets the root), and root (encased in mandibular and maxillary bone; a small opening at the apex allows blood vessels and nerves to pass into the tooth). There are three layers: the outer enamel (of hard crystal), dentin (softer than enamel), and pulp (inner most layer containing nerves and blood vessels).

Pattern of Tooth Eruption

The first primary tooth (also called *baby tooth, milk tooth,* or *deciduous tooth*) may be present at birth. Normally the eruption of primary teeth begins with the anterior primary teeth, occurs during the first 6 to 8 months of life, and ends at about 30 to 36 months old with the maxillary second molars. The sequence of eruption and the timing of eruption for each tooth are similar for both genders. Variability in child age at emergence of individual teeth is small, with a standard deviation of 2 to 3 months. In most children, the 20 primary teeth (10 per arch) erupt in a period spanning about 2 years. Each of the 20 primary teeth has a designated letter (A through T) (Fig. 34-1). Tooth lettering begins at the second molar (tooth A) in the child's upper right quadrant, proceeds to the upper left quadrant (tooth J), continues down to the lower left quadrant (tooth K), and ends with the lower right mandibular second molar (tooth T).

The permanent teeth begin erupting as children reach school age (about 6 years old) and the jaws grow. There are a total of 32 permanent teeth. Permanent dentition eruption begins with the mandibular central incisors and ends with the maxillary third molars (also called *wisdom teeth*). The primary teeth are shed or exfoliated as the permanent teeth erupt. The shedding and replacement of the primary molars by permanent premolars is usually complete around the fifth grade or by 12 years old. This period, when both primary and permanent teeth are present, is called *mixed dentition.* The total period of permanent teeth eruption (except for the third molars) spans about 6 years in most children. Some children have congenitally missing teeth (hypodontia) and others may present with extra teeth (hyperdontia).

In general, the variability in permanent dentition eruption times is much greater than the variability observed in the primary dentition, with standard deviation of 8 to 18 months (about five times greater than in the primary dentition). The sequence of permanent tooth eruption is almost identical for both sexes. However, teeth generally

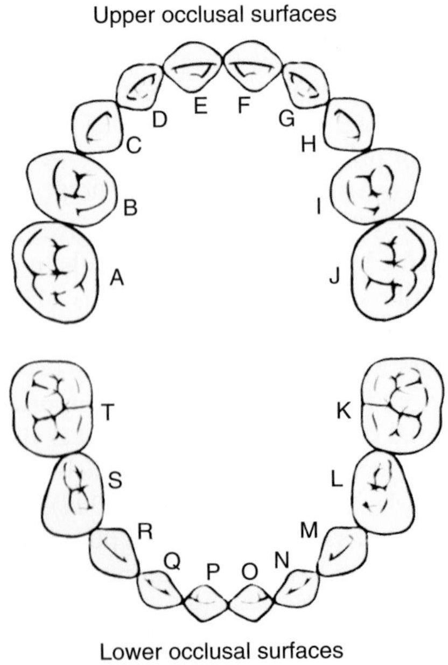

• **Figure 34-1** Lettering of primary teeth. **A,** Upper occlusal surfaces. **B,** Lower occlusal surfaces. (Courtesy Jaemi Yoo, University of Washington School of Dentistry RIDE. Used with permission.)

erupt approximately 6 months earlier in girls than in boys. The tooth eruption patterns are listed in Table 34-1.

Teething

Often, teeth erupt through the gums without causing any symptoms. However, parents may report their child having local symptoms, such as redness and swelling in the oral mucosa overlying the erupting tooth. These symptoms appear a few days before clinical eruption. The parent may also report signs of irritation, drooling, food refusal, sleeplessness, and sometimes, slight fever. Teething is not the cause of systemic health problems (e.g., diarrhea, high fever, vomiting, cough) in young children (U.S. National Library of Medicine, 2012). The recommended treatment for teething discomfort is to offer a cold rubber teething ring or a wet, chilled washcloth for gumming, massaging the gums, or allowing infants over 6 months old to chew on a chilled hard food under supervision (e.g., peeled cucumber or carrot). Oral acetaminophen can also help with the discomfort. Frozen objects (including those with a liquid component) should not be used due to added trauma to the gums and/or potential for poisoning.

A great number of folk remedies are used, especially in communities without good access to medical care (Smitherman et al, 2005). Rubbing whiskey on the gums or tying a penny on a string around the child's neck (creates a potential risk of strangulation) are discouraged, as is using a honey-coated pacifier, which could cause tooth decay or introduce botulism. At least one case of methemoglobinemia has been reported in a 6-year-old after the use of Baby Orajel for a toothache (symptoms of cyanosis, vomiting, lethargy, and tachycardia) (U.S. Food and Drug Administration [FDA], 2012). Thus, use of topical anesthetics (e.g., benzocaine) is discouraged. Topical application of salicylates (aspirin) can cause burns and should not be used.

TABLE 34-1 Calcification, Crown Completion, and Eruption

Tooth	Age of Eruption
Primary Dentition	
Maxillary	
Central incisor	7½ months old
Lateral incisor	8 months old
Canine	16 to 20 months old
First molar	12 to 16 months old
Second molar	20 to 30 months old
Mandibular	
Central incisor	6½ months old
Lateral incisor	7 months old
Canine	16 to 20 months old
First molar	12 to 16 months old
Second molar	20 to 30 months old
Permanent Dentition	
Maxillary	
Central incisor	7 to 8 years old
Lateral incisor	8 to 9 years old
Canine	11 to 12 years old
First premolar	10 to 11 years old
Second premolar	10 to 12 years old
First molar	6 to 7 years old
Second molar	12 to 13 years old
Third molar	17 to 21 years old
Mandibular	
Central incisor	6 to 7 years old
Lateral incisor	7 to 8 years old
Canine	9 to 10 years old
First premolar	10 to 12 years old
Second premolar	11 to 12 years old
First molar	6 to 7 years old
Second molar	11 to 13 years old
Third molar	17 to 21 years old

Adapted from Logan WHG, Kronfeld R: Development of the human jaws and surrounding structures from birth to age fifteen years, *J Am Dent Assoc* 20:379, 1993.

Performing the Oral Examination

An oral examination should be systematic. During the examination, take the opportunity to point out normal development (e.g., erupted teeth, eruption patterns) and abnormalities (e.g., bloody or inflamed gums, tooth decay) to the parent.

An infant's teeth and oral tissues are easily examined by placing the child on his or her back on an examining table with the head toward the end of the table. Have the parent immobilize the child's legs and hands. Stand at the head of the table and use a tongue blade or toothbrush as a mouth prop. Use a penlight and intraoral mirror for optimal visualization. Tip the head back to see the upper teeth. This table approach is also useful for looking at the teeth of older children. Trying to examine the mouth and teeth with the child sitting in the parent's lap is not recommended, because the provider has to bend over to see the upper teeth and the crying and movement of the child makes visibility very poor.

An alternative for examining a small child is the knee-to-knee approach favored by many dentists. In this approach, the provider and parent sit across from each other knee-to-knee. The parent holds the child facing him or her and then lowers the child's head into the provider's lap. The child's legs are wrapped around the parent's waist. Again the parent immobilizes the child's hands and legs. It is important to explain to the parent before the examination that small children may cry during the examination, but the examination is brief and the crying will stop as soon as the examination is completed.

Clinical Findings

Oral Mucosa

The soft mucosal tissues are examined before the teeth and should include an assessment of the tonsils for size and the presence of inflammation or exudate. Start the examination with the inside of the lips and continue to the buccal mucosa, including the mucosal surfaces that connect and surround each tooth. Inspect the palate directly by tipping the child's head backward. Examine the dorsal and ventral mucosal surfaces of the tongue and floor of the mouth by retracting the tongue with a tongue blade, a dental mirror, or by holding the tongue with cotton gauze. Note ulcerations, changes in color and surface texture, swelling, or fistulae of any of these tissues.

When examining the gums, give special attention to any gingival swelling or retraction. Healthy gums should not bleed when brushed. In racial or ethnic minority children, the gums may exhibit hyperpigmentation, which is normal. Note the presence and attachment of frenula, with special emphasis on the possible complicating effects of the maxillary labial frenum and lingual frenulum on breastfeeding. It may be helpful to ask breastfeeding mothers if the child seems to have difficulties latching onto the breast. Any of these factors may warrant a referral to a lactation counselor or pediatric dentist for further assessment and treatment.

Saliva

Note the quantity and quality of the saliva. Thick or ropy saliva or a dry mouth may be abnormal. Decreased salivary flow and changes in sensation in the area of the facial nerve can result from infection or tumor in the parotid space or facial musculature, or can be a side effect of dehydration or medications that cause xerostomia (dry mouth).

Teeth

Cleaning the teeth with a toothbrush and then drying them with gauze is best for visualizing and detecting early tooth decay. Note any surface roughness or loss of surface continuity. Retract or lift the lips away so that the teeth can be examined systematically, beginning with tooth A and moving around to the left, ending with tooth J. Examine the lingual surfaces of the upper teeth and the biting surfaces in the same systematic manner before repeating this examination on the lower teeth K through T. The number and types of teeth erupted, discoloration, irregularities, and asymmetries should be noted.

Variations in number, morphology, color, and surface structure should be noted. Primary teeth may be malformed or have incompletely formed, chalky, or pitted enamel due to other systematic conditions, such as ectodermal dysplasia. In the case of traumatically injured teeth, the color and translucency of the injured tooth or teeth may be altered (slight color changes are often found as one of the first signs of intrapulpal damage after trauma and may lead to an abscessed tooth).

Aberrations in Primary Tooth Eruption and Gums

Natal and Neonatal Teeth

The prevalence of natal or neonatal teeth is estimated to be 1 out of 2000 to 3000 births and is equally common in boys and girls. The teeth usually erupt in pairs. Natal and neonatal teeth occur in about 50 different syndromes, of which about 10 are associated with chromosomal aberrations. More than 90% of these prematurely erupting teeth are mandibular central incisors with normal shape and color. Supernumerary teeth may be abnormal in shape and color and only loosely attached to the gingiva. Natal or neonatal teeth can lead to gingivitis, self-mutilation of the tongue, and trauma to the mother during breastfeeding. However, they should only be extracted if they are loose enough to involve risk of aspiration, sublingual ulceration, or if feeding is severely disturbed. Most will develop normally with normal root structure (Khandelwal et al, 2013).

Delayed Tooth Eruption

Delayed tooth eruption can result from either systemic or local factors. These include prematurity, low birth weight, genetic syndromes (e.g., Down and Turner syndromes), a low protein diet, hereditary gingival fibromatosis, adjacent supernumeraries, dental tissue tumors (odontomas), and children born to mothers with severe iodine deficiency. In general, children with chronic health conditions with delays in both physical and dental development experience delayed but otherwise normal tooth eruption. Very low-birth-weight infants may present with enamel defects on primary teeth that may increase the dental caries risk (Nelson et al, 2013).

Preeruption Cysts

When a tooth starts erupting through the gingival tissue, a blood-filled cyst may precede it. Alarmed parents may report a purple, reddish, black, or blue bump or bruise in their child's mouth. If the enlargement is on the alveolar ridge, reassurance is all that is required. The symptom will resolve as the tooth erupts (Fig. 34-2).

Congenital Epulis

Congenital epulis is a fibrous, pedunculated, soft-tissue enlargement that occurs on the maxillary alveolar ridge at birth (Fig. 34-3). This condition is more common in female babies. It typically regresses with time, but large lesions should be excised.

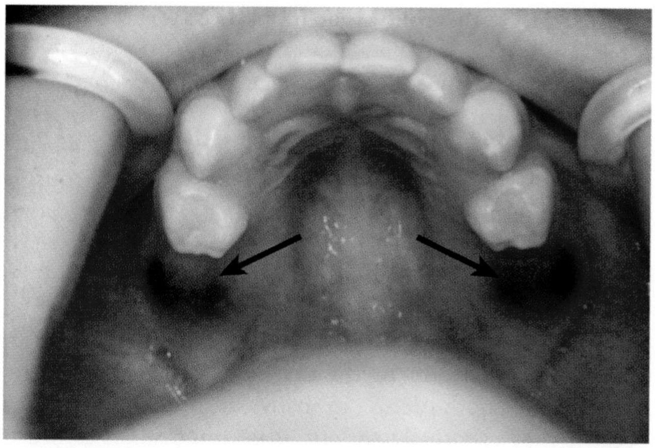

• **Figure 34-2** Preeruption cyst. Eruption hematomas *(arrows)* have developed before the eruption of the second primary molars. (From McDonald RE, Avery DR, Dean JA: *Dentistry for the child and adolescent*, ed 8, 2004, Mosby, p 182.)

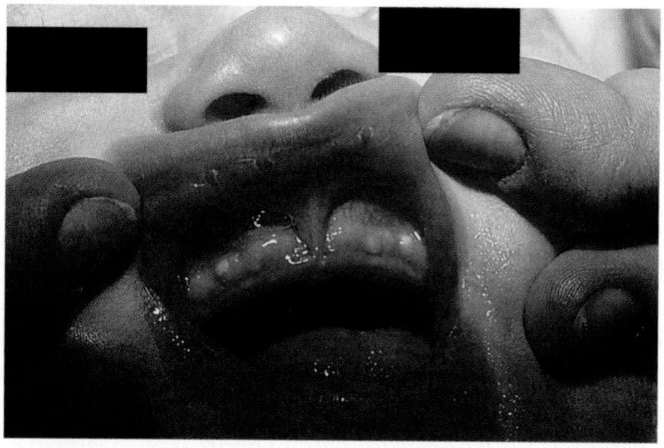

• **Figure 34-4** Bohn nodule. (From Eichenfield LF, Frieden IJ, Esterly NB: *Neonatal dermatology*, ed 2, Philadelphia, 2008, Mosby/Elsevier.)

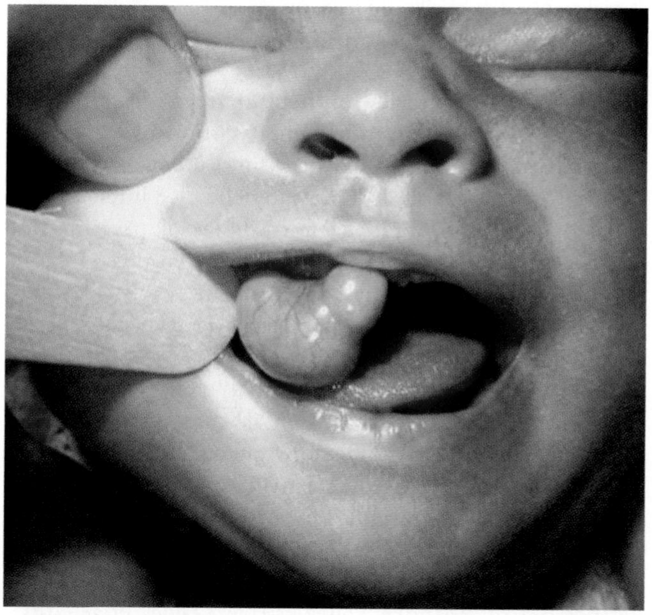

• **Figure 34-3** Congenital epulis. (From McDonald RE, Avery DR, Hartsfield JK Jr: *Dentistry for the child and adolescent*, ed 8, 2011, Elsevier, Figure 8-5, p 131.)

Bohn Nodules

Bohn nodules are present at birth and appear as firm nonpainful nodules on the buccal surface of the alveolar ridge (Fig. 34-4). They are remnants of dental lamina connecting the developing tooth bud to the epithelium of the oral cavity. No treatment is required because they will resolve spontaneously. If they appear in the midline of the palate, they are referred to as *Epstein pearls.*

Professional Dental Care

Fear of the Dentist

Parents' and caregivers' own fear of the dentist can have a negative effect on the oral health of children. Studies confirm the significant relationship between parental and child dental fear, particularly in children 8 years old and younger (Themessi-Huber et al, 2010). As many as one in five adults in North America report fear of the dentist; this is consistent with the 20% of children younger than 13 years old found to have dental phobia (Baier et al, 2004; Smith and Heaton, 2003). Many of the parents of children with whom PCPs interact may have this fear and consequently avoid dental visits themselves.

Early and consistent primary prevention is the best way to avoid the development of fear and avoidance. Allowing tooth decay to go untreated until a child is school age results in extensive restorative intervention, which can be a traumatic experience for any child. Dental restorative care is the only area of medicine in which children are expected to endure invasive surgical procedures while they are awake. Hospitalizing children and performing oral rehabilitation under general anesthesia is a costly treatment option and may be associated with health risks (Hays and Deshpande, 2013). Moreover, many children experience recurrence of dental disease within 6 months because such aggressive surgical treatment does not prevent relapse (Graves et al, 2004).

Choosing a Dentist

The choice of a dentist is critical, especially for children who have had negative experiences with dentists. Many general dentists are highly skilled at working with children, so the absence of a pediatric dentist is not a barrier. A dentist new to the child should be told about any prior dental experiences. Parents should be counseled to choose a dentist known to work well with children. Parents should be encouraged to ensure that their child has had a good night's sleep and is fed before a visit. The child's teeth should be brushed before the dental visit.

Visit preparation should focus on helping the child develop coping skills and ways to gain control. Children gain control when the dentist briefly explains procedures and allows them to signal any discomfort. An example of a coping skill is relaxation breathing. Finding a dentist who tells stories and riddles, sings to the children, or otherwise distracts them (e.g., with videos, music, or games) is particularly effective. Directed guidance strategies—specific kinds of direction followed by praise—are also very effective in managing children's behaviors. For fearful children, structured rehearsals are encouraged, where dental procedures are broken into small steps, and coping strategies are taught. Dentists and parents who rely solely on authoritarian approaches or who are permissive are likely to fail with a fearful child.

Parents should be cautious about dentists with laser-based or other electronic diagnostic devices. These devices are often marketed to dentists as being capable of detecting "invisible" cavities and are being misused to justify unnecessary fillings. The standard method of examination of the teeth is visual, using strong light and transillumination (shining light through the tooth) without using sharp probes, which can damage teeth and transfer potential pathogenic bacteria from one groove or surface to another. Most tooth decay in permanent teeth in children occurs on the biting surface, and x-rays are of limited diagnostic value in such cases. Parents should be urged to seek second opinions whenever large amounts of treatment are recommended.

The First Dental Visit

The child's first dental visit should occur before the child's first birthday (12 months old) or within 6 months of the first tooth eruption. This allows a dentist to establish an ongoing relationship with the parent and child (dental home), provide education and anticipatory guidance, and deliver preventive care, such as topical fluoride. Establishment of a dental home gives parents a familiar place to take their child for dental checkups and emergencies (e.g., trauma, dislodged filling, or dental pain).

The first dental visit commonly involves a cleaning, dental examination, and topical fluoride treatment. For children younger than 3 years old, the caregiver may be asked to help the dentist position the child. Encourage parents to inquire if they are allowed in the treatment area with their child prior to their making the first dental appointment; they should choose an alternative dentist if such an exclusionary policy is disagreeable to them or the child.

Dental Health Education

Dental health education is a crucial preventive strategy. Tailoring health education messages and instruction to an individual's capacity to "obtain, process, and understand" reflects a health literacy approach to oral health education. Low parental health literacy is most often associated with early childhood caries, low income, and inadequate maternal education (Miller et al, 2010). Low reading literacy, combined with low health literacy, is of particular concern given the role a parent plays as decision-maker for a child.

A review of dental education materials for parents found readability levels ranging from the 2nd- to 9th-grade level. Government materials required an average lower literacy level (4th grade) versus those issued by commercial sources (8th grade) or industry (7th grade) (Henrickson et al, 2006). The advice given in published materials often is inconsistent (e.g., amount of toothpaste to use can be described as "pea-sized," but photos often show a long ribbon of toothpaste on the toothbrush). In addition, there are many oral health myths that should be dispelled by PCPs (e.g., tooth decay in baby teeth isn't important because they eventually fall out, it is "impossible" to brush children's teeth, fluoride is unsafe, or pregnant women shouldn't see the dentist). A good source of reference material is www.medlineplus.gov.

Preventive Intervention and Management Strategies

A recent systematic review of literature regarding the effectiveness of using motivational intervention techniques to change dental hygiene behaviors found inconclusive effectiveness (Cascaes et al, 2014). Many effective interventions have involved collaborative efforts between primary care clinics, preschool, Head Start classrooms, Women, Infants, and Children (WIC) clinics, and/or in-home visits by staff. These efforts reinforced proper brushing techniques; gave parents a chance to practice; provided no-spill cups, toothpaste, toothbrushes, and educational pamphlets; applied fluoride varnish; facilitated dental care access; and/or sponsored dental fairs. Demonstrated benefits of these efforts included improved oral hygiene knowledge, nutrition, toothbrushing skills, fluoride varnish applications, utilization of dental homes, and oral hygiene, as well as decreased caries and gingivitis (Child Health Investment Partnership of Roanoke Valley, 2013; Davies et al, 2005; Kwan et al, 2005).

Other studies have shown that young Medicaid-enrolled children with a greater number of well-child visits between 1 to 3 years old were significantly more likely to have earlier first dental visits (Chi et al, 2013b). However, the number of well-baby visits before 1 year old was not related to the timing of the child's first dental visit. These findings indicate that PCPs should introduce oral health-related education and anticipatory guidance during early well-baby visits (e.g., 1 month, 2 months, 4 months, and 6 months) to ensure that children have their first visit to the dentist by 12 months old.

Beil and Rozier (2010) found that children 2 to 5 years old who received a recommendation by a PCP to see a dentist were more likely to have a dental examination, whereas children from 6 to 11 years old who received a recommendation showed no increase. This supports the efficacy of the recommendation that PCPs refer children at an early age.

Bacterial Diseases of the Mouth

Tooth Decay (Cavities, Dental Caries, or Baby Bottle Tooth Decay)

Dental caries is the most common chronic disease of children and is more common that asthma in childhood. The rates of untreated caries vary by age, averaging 14.4% in those 3 to 5 years old, 17% in those 6 to 9 years old, and 11.4% in those 13 to 15 years old. Black teens have more untreated caries than white teens (USDHHS and AHRQ, 2013). Tooth decay is a bacterial disease that can result in irreversible damage and potential loss of teeth. The decay is caused by acid demineralization of the tooth subsurface enamel. The acid is produced by an alpha hemolytic streptococcus (mutans streptococci) bacteria, in older literature referred to as *Streptococcus mutans,* after metabolism of carbohydrates in the diet. Unless neutralized and buffered by saliva or remineralized with fluorides, the demineralization process will lead to cavitation. Active cavities are also frequently infected with lactobacilli. The bacterial species are part of the biofilm adherent to the teeth. The bacteria are usually transmitted when saliva is shared between the child, caregivers, or other children (see Preventing Person-to-Person Spread of Caries-Causing Bacteria). Infection and colonization peak around the time of the eruption of the primary teeth, but may occur before that.

In infants, the carbohydrates may be present in the form of prolonged exposure to formula or breast milk, especially if the infant is allowed to sleep with the nipple in his or her mouth. Before and after weaning, carbohydrates may also come from milk sweetened with honey or sugar or from juices in baby bottles or no-spill training cups, especially when given at bedtime, naptime, or when a child is allowed to "graze" on sweet fluids throughout the day. In older children, the source of the carbohydrates is from sugar-sweetened beverages (e.g., Tang, Kool-Aid, sports drinks, and soda). This frequent carbohydrate exposure keeps the pH of mouth fluid near the tooth surface below 5 and results in an environment conducive to demineralization. The neutralization process does not have enough time to increase the mouth pH to a level that would allow remineralization. In children undergoing chemotherapy or radiation to the head and neck and/or who are immunocompromised, normal salivary flow and salivary buffering of acids is disrupted. Cavities result. See Box 34-1 for a list of risk factors for dental caries.

Clinical Findings

- Early caries lesions: These appear as horizontal bright white or brown lines or spots along the upper central gum line or gingival margin, more commonly in populations using baby bottles because the cavity-causing fluids pool in these areas of the mouth. In cultures where bottle use, especially at night or naptime, is less common the damage may occur in back teeth first as a function of other dietary patterns. When white lesions occur, the dentin is initially damaged. Then, as the lesion progresses, the hard enamel breaks, and a clinical cavity is evident (Fig. 34-5). Baby teeth are important for chewing food, serve an esthetic function, and hold space in the mouth so that the permanent teeth can erupt properly. Therefore, it is critical to prevent cavities and intervene early in any decay.
- Advanced tooth decay: This appears as cavitations (holes) in the teeth. Nearly all cavities in permanent teeth in children in the United States begin on the biting surface of the molars. The initial lesion appears as a pinhole

• BOX 34-1 Factors That Increase a Child's Risk for Developing Dental Caries

Health and Personal History

Extra health care need associated with poor motor coordination or cooperation
Xerostomia
No dental home
Previous history of tooth decay
Braces or orthodontic appliances
Child's parent or sibling has tooth decay
Low socioeconomic status
Frequent exposure to fermentable carbohydrates (e.g., snacking more than three times per day)
No exposure to topical fluoride

Clinical Evaluation

Visible plaque on teeth
Gingivitis (red, swollen gums)
Demineralized enamel (white spot lesions on teeth)
Enamel defects (e.g., hypercalcification, deep pits and fissures)

Supplemental Findings

Radiographic evidence of enamel caries
High levels of mutans streptococci

Adapted from American Academy of Pediatric Dentistry (AAPD), Council on Clinical Affairs: *Policy on use of a caries-risk assessment tool (CAT) for infants, children, and adolescents*, 2002, revised 2014. Available at www.aapd.org/media/Policies_Guidelines/G_CariesRiskAssessment.pdf. Accessed September 18, 2014.

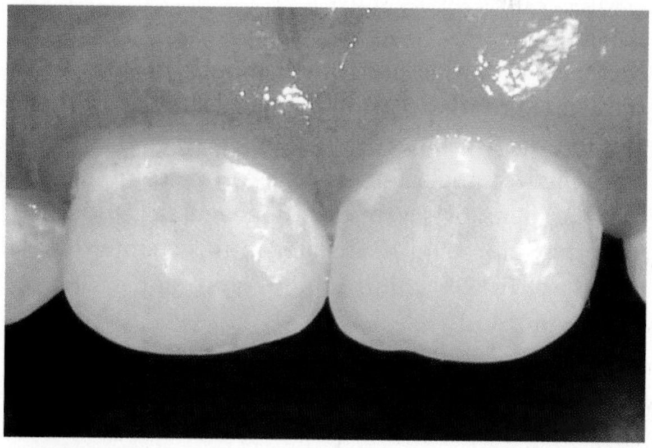

• Figure 34-5 White spots. (From Cameron AC, Widmer RP, editors: *Handbook of pediatric dentistry*, ed 2, London, 2003, Mosby/Elsevier.)

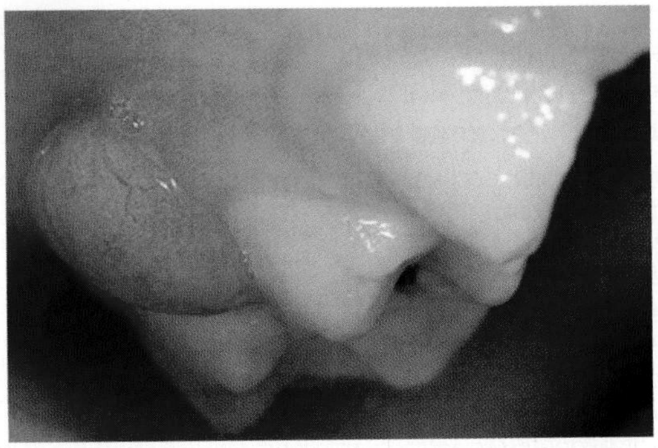

• **Figure 34-6** Abscess. (Courtesy Donald L. Chi, DDS, PhD, Associate Professor, Department of Oral Health Science, University of Washington School of Dentistry.)

surrounded by a white, opaque halo. As the lesion enlarges greater damage to the enamel becomes apparent. Lesions typically appear about 1 year after the eruption of the tooth and frequently begin while the tooth is still erupting.

- Sensitivity: Cavities can be hot, cold, or sweet sensitive.
- Localized dental or facial pain: Lesions that progress can begin to hurt all the time or may hurt intermittently, disrupting normal activity, sleeping, and eating.
- Abscesses on the gums due to bacterial invasion of the pulpal tissue (Fig. 34-6)
- Gingival inflammation with swelling and erythema
- Possible lymphadenopathy
- Possible fever
- Methamphetamine use ("meth mouth"): This can cause accelerated tooth decay on the facial surfaces of the teeth and between the teeth. In later stages, the teeth are blackened, stained, and appear to be crumbling. There may be signs of severe grinding and dry mouth. (See Chlorhexidine Oral Rinse later in this chapter regarding the use of 0.12% chlorhexidine gluconate oral rinse for this condition.)
- Cavities may spontaneously arrest: This is thought to occur when cavities are exposed to saliva high in fluoride or when the diet changes (such as, after weaning). Arrested caries appear as open cavities that are black or dark brown. If the child has such open cavities, is asymptomatic, the teeth are primary teeth, and access to dental care is problematic, these teeth can be left alone and allowed to shed normally. The discoloration also may be the result of previous topical treatment by a dentist with diamine silver fluoride or silver nitrate in an attempt to arrest and prevent caries.

Management and Prevention Strategies

Active Decay

When tooth decay is present, subsequent dental visits may involve arresting the decay or more extensive restorative treatment by topically treating the decayed surfaces with 38% diamine silver fluoride (side effect is black staining of the carious lesion) (Fung et al, 2013).This treatment is used internationally and was approved by the U.S. Food and Drug Administration (FDA) for caries treatment in mid-2014. In high-risk communities with poor access to dentists, PCPs can be trained in applying this treatment (Chi, 2014a). Larger cavities in primary teeth can be repaired with plastic fillings or with steel or plastic crowns. Teeth with deep cavities and draining abscesses are generally extracted.

A decision to repair teeth or remove them depends on the extent of damage and the length of time until the tooth would be normally exfoliated. Retention of primary molars is important, because they hold space to allow the normal eruption of permanent successors. Young children may need to be sedated or receive treatment under a general anesthetic to meet extensive treatment needs, making tooth decay arrest with topical treatment—at least until they get older—a noteworthy option.

Cavities in permanent teeth are also repaired with either silver amalgam or tooth-colored acrylic (plastic) composite resin fillings. About half of a silver amalgam filling is composed of liquid mercury, a binder for the other amalgam components (silver, copper, and other metals). Although mercury releases low levels of vapor, the FDA, based on scientific evidence, considers silver amalgams safe for adults and children. The mercury levels from amalgams have been determined by the Environmental Protection Agency (EPA) and the Centers for Disease Control and Prevention (CDC) to be below the lowest levels associated with brain and kidney toxicity. They are also considered safe for use in pregnant and lactating women and children younger than 6 years old (FDA, 2014). However, amalgams are less commonly used now in primary teeth, having been replaced by composite fillings. The longevity of the composite fillings is very much shorter than silver fillings, except when small and when not applied to high-stress chewing areas. Severe cavities resulting in abscess formation in permanent teeth are treated with root canal therapy (called a pulpotomy in children; the infected neurovascular bundle is removed and replaced with an inert filling material). Permanent molars either need to be capped (with a crown) after root canal therapy or treated with large amalgam fillings.

Remineralizing topical pastes are used by some dentists to prevent, reverse, or arrest white or brown tooth decay lesions. Limited data suggest that these pastes may be effective in some cases (high-caries risk, xerostomia, orthodontics, post-bleaching, oncology, pediatric, and high plaque/special needs) (Chan et al, 2013; Robertson et al, 2011).

Pit and fissure (occlusal) plastic sealants are effective in preventing tooth decay in high-risk children (Ney et al, 2014). High-risk children are those who have experienced a lot of primary teeth decay and/or have poor oral hygiene or diets with lots of refined carbohydrates and soft drinks. Sealants are polymerizing resin or glass ionomer coatings placed on the biting surfaces of primary molars at 2 to 3 years old and permanent molars at about 6 to 7 years old and 13 to 14 years old (Fig. 34-7). One study showed a 60% decrease in caries in posterior teeth in children 6

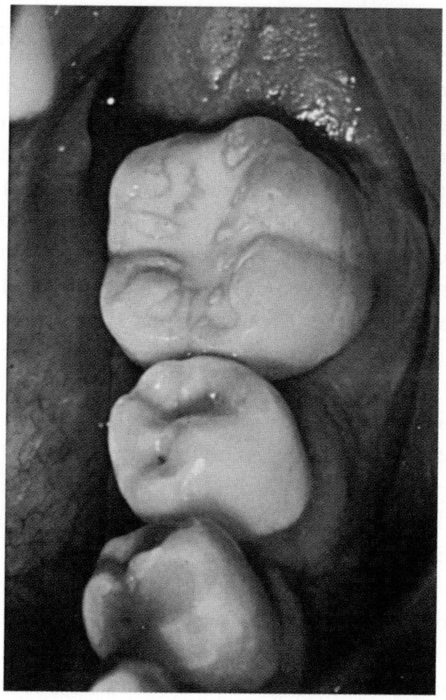

• **Figure 34-7** Sealant. (From Pinkham JR: *Pediatric dentistry: infancy through adolescence*, ed 4, St. Louis, 2005, Saunders, p 537.)

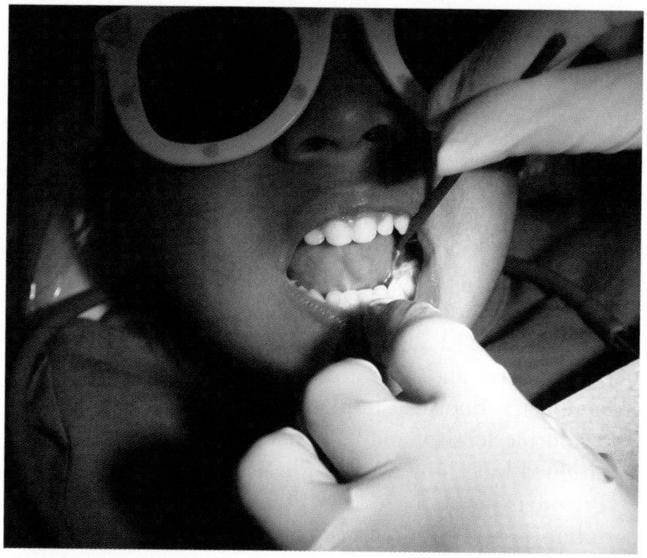

• **Figure 34-8** Applying fluoride varnish. (Courtesy Peter Milgrom, DDS.)

through 17 years old when sealants were used (Gooch et al, 2009). Some grade schools are replacing their voluntary school-based fluoride programs with a coordinated community sealant program.

Preventing Person-to-Person Spread of Caries-Causing Bacteria. Eating utensils should not be shared between caregivers and children, especially if the caregiver has untreated cavities in the mouth. Parents should not use their own saliva to clean pacifiers or bottles, and children should be discouraged from sharing beverages using the same cup. Dental visits are especially important for pregnant women because of the association between untreated cavities in the mother and future development of cavities in the child. Pregnant women can safely receive all diagnostic, preventive (including radiograph), and restorative dental treatment during pregnancy.

Fluoride Varnish

Early white spot lesions in primary and permanent teeth can be remineralized using topical fluoride varnish. Fluoride varnish is the agent of choice for young children and has been shown to be more effective than the fluoride gels that are still widely used in the United States. Fluoride gels are difficult to apply in preschool children and are not recommended because of the risk of acute toxicity. In many states, PCPs are permitted to apply fluoride and are reimbursed by insurance plans, including the ACA, Medicaid, and CHIP programs. Typically the 5% neutral sodium fluoride varnish (NaFV; 22,500 ppm of fluoride) or 1.23% acidulated phosphate fluoride (APF: 12,300 ppm fluoride) preparations are used for children. All of the 5% varnishes are essentially similar, varying in flavor or color. Twice-yearly applications have been shown to reduce tooth decay by about one third; more frequent applications may be needed in high-risk children (every 3 to 6 months). If the level of risk is uncertain, treating the child as high risk is efficacious until more objective assessment over time is ascertained (AAPD, Council on Clinical Affairs, 2014a). One study suggested that four treatments given at the same time as well-child visits before 24 months reduced tooth decay in high-risk children (Holve, 2008). Plasma fluoride levels following applications of varnish are low and are not associated with toxicity or fluorosis.

To apply fluoride varnish:

1. Dispense approximately 0.25 mL of fluoride varnish into a small well. Prepackaged individual-dose systems come with their own well that is filled with varnish. To avoid risk of over exposure, use only the size package recommended for the age of the child.
2. Lightly dry the teeth with air or gauze to remove moisture.
3. While keeping the teeth isolated from further moisture contamination, paint the varnish onto the teeth with a brush or another type of applicator (Fig. 34-8). Only a light coat is required, and applying more than necessary increases toxicity risk. The varnish sets on contact with the slightly moist teeth.

A short training video on the technique for applying varnish is available from the National Maternal and Child Oral Health Resource Center (see Additional Resources on the Evolve website). Health assistants within primary care clinics can also be trained to apply the varnish.

A recent study showed that topical fluoride varnish refusal by parents for their children is associated with their refusal of immunizations (Chi, 2014b). PCPs are in a good position to have discussions with concerned parents about the safety of fluoride varnish, as well as other sources of topical fluoride (drinking water, toothpastes) important in cavity prevention.

Fluoride in Water, Infant Formulas, and Fluoride Supplementation

The most effective preventive measure against dental caries is optimizing community water fluoridation levels to no more than 0.7 milligrams of fluoride per liter of water (0.7 part per million). Close to 75% of the population in the United States have access to publically fluoridated water (CDC, 2012, 2013). Children who consume fluoride-deficient water and who are at risk for caries will benefit from dietary fluoride supplementation (USPSTF, 2014). The fluoride level of public water supplies can usually be ascertained by calling the local health department.

Providers should be aware of the status of fluoride in the community and routinely ask new families about fluoride in their water source. If the child is on a private water supply (e.g., well water), the naturally-occurring fluoride level should be tested before prescribing fluoride supplements. To prevent potential overdoses, no prescription should be written for more than a total of 120 mg of fluoride. See Table 34-2 for adjusting the dose of fluoride supplements in relation to that found in the community/well water supply.

Although some bottled waters marketed in the United States contain an optimal concentration of fluoride, most contain less than 0.3 ppm fluoride. In the United States, current FDA regulations require that fluoride be listed on the bottled water or infant formula label only if fluoride is added during processing, but the concentration does not have to be stated. A child who uses bottled water with a low fluoride concentration instead of fluoridated community water may need fluoride supplementation. On the other hand, powdered infant formulas reconstituted with fluoridated water may pose an increased risk of fluorosis because of the prolonged accumulative effect of fluoride on enamel development. Therefore, health care providers and dentists need to help parents ascertain an infant's fluoride exposure.

Fluorosis. A complication of too much systemic fluoride exposure during the years of enamel development is fluorosis. Surveys show that there has been an increase in all levels of fluorosis that range from very mild to moderate-severe (see Fig. 34-9). Children 6 to 11 years old have rates of 33%, whereas those 12 to 15 years old have rates of about 41%. In the 12- to 15-year-olds, the rate represents about an 18% increase since the mid-1980s (Beltrán-Aguilar et al, 2010). Recognizing that children may be overexposed to fluoride is the reason for the USDHHS optimal community water fluoridation level recommendation.

In most cases, the fluorosis appears as white specks or streaks that are largely unnoticeable. The advisability of introducing fluoridated toothpaste for very young children should be based on the risk of tooth decay. When caries risk is high (e.g., if the mother or siblings have tooth decay, or child has poor hygiene and diet), the benefit outweighs the risk of mild or moderate fluorosis (AAPD, Council on Clinical Affairs, 2014a). Parents should administer the toothpaste at the recommended amount.

TABLE 34-2 Recommended* Fluoride Supplementation Based on Drinking Water Fluoride Concentration

	Fluoride Ion Level in Drinking Water (ppm)†		
Age	<0.3 ppm	0.3 to 0.6 ppm	>0.6 ppm
Birth to 6 months old	None	None	None
6 months old to 3 years old	0.25 mg/day‡	None	None
3 to 6 years old	0.50 mg/day	0.25 mg/day	None
6 to 16 years old	1 mg/day	0.50 mg/day	None

From American Academy of Pediatric Dentistry (AAPD), Council on Scientific Affairs: *Guideline on fluoride therapy*, 2014 available at www.aapd.org/media/Policies_Guidelines/G_FluorideTherapy.pdf. Accessed December 5, 2015.

*Take all sources of fluoride into consideration—from water (including bottled) and amount and frequency of fluoridated toothpaste used in brushing.

†Optimal concentration of fluoride in water supply in mg/L or parts per million (ppm).

‡2.2 mg sodium fluoride contains 1 mg fluoride ion.

Toothbrushing

Parents should be taught to clean a child's teeth with a small toothbrush as soon as teeth erupt, using the "lift the lip" method. They should check monthly to see if dental problems are beginning, looking closely for the signs of demineralization. A demonstration by the PCP during a well-child

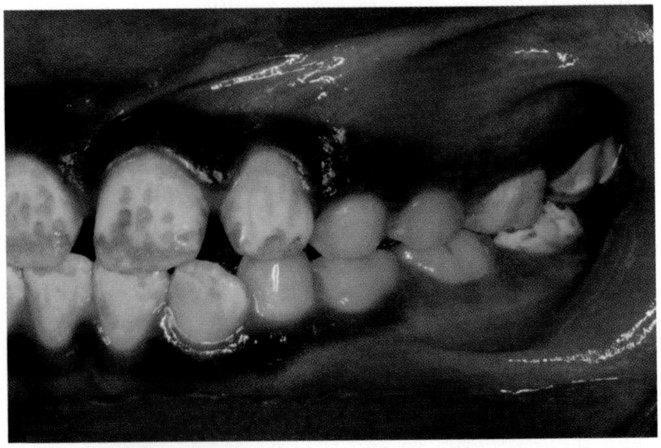

• **Figure 34-9** Fluorosis. (From Neville BW, Damm DD, Allen CM, et al: Abnormalities of teeth. In Neville BW, Damm DD, Allen CM, et al: *Oral and maxillofacial pathology*, ed 4, Philadelphia, 2016, Elsevier.)

visit is ideal. The technique involves having a parent lift the child's upper lip and use a soft toothbrush to cleanse each tooth surface. By making this an enjoyable, daily routine activity, the child will become comfortable and any resistance should decrease. It may be easier to brush a child's teeth if the child lies on the floor, on a couch with the child's head in the parent's lap, or using the knee-to-knee technique. A second adult can help by holding the hands and feet if necessary. Brushing in the bathroom standing up is more difficult. Toothbrush songs and timers help in teaching children and parents how long to brush. The type of toothbrush, manual or electric, is not clinically relevant. Small, soft brushes are widely available; large-handled brushes are available for those with physical disabilities.

Toothpaste

Fluoridated toothpaste works by creating a reservoir of fluoride in the fluid layer of the plaque and in the saliva that is available to remineralize or repair teeth that are being damaged by bacterial acids. All fluoridated toothpastes sold in the United States are similar. The PCP should know the fluoride content level in the community drinking water, other sources of fluoride the child might be consuming (including bottled water, reconstituted infant formulas made with fluoridated water, liquids given in day care or school, soda, juice, prepared foods, and toothpaste [especially if swallowed]), and risk factors for tooth decay prior to recommending the use of fluoride toothpaste in all children (AAPD, Council on Clinical Affairs, 2014a).

Parents should be encouraged to choose a toothpaste with a sweet flavor. Strongly flavored toothpastes and those containing whitening or bleaching agents are contraindicated. A small amount of toothpaste (a smear or "rice-sized" for children under 3 years old and about "pea-sized" for children 3 years old and older) should be used. The child should not rinse after brushing. Swallowing these small amounts of toothpaste twice daily is not harmful. However, the amount of toothpaste used should be controlled by an adult because children can swallow a large amount of what is brushed on; this added systemic intake of fluoride can lead to an increased risk of enamel fluorosis prior to complete enamel maturation. In children at very high risk for tooth decay, parents should begin brushing teeth with fluoridated toothpaste with the eruption of the first tooth at 6 to 9 months old. Toothpastes and fluoride supplements should be stored out of reach of younger children. If a child ingests a large dose of fluoride, the caregiver should contact 911 immediately.

Diet

Dietary advice is essential to parents. Sugar-sweetened beverages with energy-containing sweeteners, such as fruit juice concentrates, sucrose, or high-fructose corn syrup, are primary source of sugars in Western diets. Greater than half of American children between 2 and 19 years old consume sugar-sweetened beverages (soft drinks, fruit drinks, sports drinks) on any given day (Lasater et al, 2011; Ogden et al, 2011). Approximately 60% to 80% of all sugar-sweetened beverage calories are consumed in the home. Children younger than 6 years old consume an average of 15.5 ounces or 176 kcal from sugar-sweetened beverages on a typical day, representing approximately 10% of their total energy intake. This is more than twice the national dietary guideline (U.S. Department of Agriculture [USDA], 2010). Children on the lower socioeconomic scale—those at greatest risk for tooth decay—drink more fruit drinks than children with higher-income parents (Han and Powell, 2013). Intake of sugar-sweetened beverages by children should be limited to no more than 4 ounces per day and restricted to mealtimes. Because juices contain high concentrations of sugar, diluting juice with water will not prevent tooth decay.

Baby bottles should only be filled with milk, formula, or water, and the child weaned from a bottle at 12 months old. Nursing mothers should not allow their infants to sleep attached to the nipple. Bottles should never be propped during naps or sleep. Some WIC centers in the United States distribute no-spill training cups to promote appropriate eating behaviors and prevent tooth decay. However, personnel may not be aware of the potential danger of the cups themselves if sugar-sweetened beverages are available ad lib. It is ideal for parents to set established snack and meal times and avoid allowing their child to graze on foods all day. Use of vitamins containing table sugar (sucrose) and/or gummy vitamins that are sticky should be discouraged.

Xylitol-Containing Products

Xylitol, a naturally occurring sugar, is endorsed by the AAPD as a non-carcinogenic sugar substitute. The AAPD acknowledges that studies are inclusive for demonstrating short-term and long-term reductions in caries. More research is indicated to more clearly demonstrate optimal dosage and frequency and the most advantageous delivery vehicle (AAPD, Council on Clinical Affairs, 2015b). Xylitol's effect is topical (reduces the adhesiveness and overall numbers of bacteria). Sources of xylitol include chewing gum, mints, chewable tablets, lozenges, toothpastes, and mouthwashes. The act of chewing gum may account for some of the effectiveness in preventing decay, although chewing gum is not appropriate for preschoolers because of the risk of choking (AAPD, 2015b). If used, the product should contain at least 50% xylitol and be the first ingredient listed on the label. Gum is chewed for about 5 minutes or until the sweetness disappears, four to five times daily. Side effects are rare and usually limited to abdominal cramping. More risk of severe abdominal pain and diarrhea occur if xylitol is used concurrently with sorbitol. Studies are also inconclusive showing a decrease in caries in children whose mothers used xylitol chewing gum in an effort to reduce or postpone the maternal transmission of bacterial colonization by mutans streptococci (AAPD, 2015b).

Xylitol syrups have been shown to reduce cavities in young preschoolers. Children who received at least 8 g per day of xylitol in syrup divided into two or three doses and applied topically to the teeth by a caregiver had significantly fewer decayed teeth than children in the control group (Milgrom et al, 2009). Xylitol toothpastes are not effective at reducing tooth decay and should not be recommended to parents (Chi et al, 2014).

Topical Iodine

Polyvinylpyrrolidone (PVP) iodine (10% PVP-I or povidone-iodine [betadine solution]) can be painted on the teeth before the application of fluoride varnish for an additive effect to depress the tooth decay-causing mutans streptococci in high-risk children (Tut and Milgrom, 2010). Application of topical iodine alone at 3-month intervals over 12 months has been shown to cause a significant reduction in the growth of flora (Simratvir et al, 2010). The teeth are dried with cotton gauze or air, the povidone iodine is painted onto the teeth and gums with a cotton-tip applicator, and then immediately wiped off with gauze or rinsed with air and water.

Chlorhexidine Oral Rinse

Chlorhexidine gluconate oral rinse (0.12%) provides antimicrobial activity if used consistently. After rinsing, 30% of the chlorhexidine gluconate remains in the oral cavity and is released into the oral fluids. Studies show it is not effective in caries prevention in children (Rethman et al, 2011), but it has an important role as part of a treatment program for "meth mouth," aphthous ulcers, pyogenic granuloma, gingival hyperplasia, infected oral piercings, and children with special health care needs (these are discussed later in this chapter).

Instructions for the chlorhexidine gluconate mouth rinse are as follows: Half a capful (0.5 fl oz, undiluted) swished in the mouth for 30 seconds twice daily and then spit out. Individuals should not swallow the rinse, rinse the mouth afterward, or eat for 30 minutes. It is necessary to use it at least 60% of the time to have any clinical effect. Side effects include staining of teeth and restorations (can be removed by having the teeth professionally cleaned) and tongue; calculus formation above the gum line; and an aftertaste that may change taste perception temporarily. Pregnant and nursing mothers should use the product only if clearly needed. Safety of its use has not been established in children younger than 18 years old.

Managing Toothache or Tooth Sensitivity

If tooth decay has resulted in pain and a draining tract, analgesics, warm-water or saline rinses, and a bland diet are recommended. In the presence of cellulitis and fever, antibiotic therapy is appropriate; follow-up dental treatment is needed. Ideally, the child should have an emergency dental visit to receive treatment (not an emergency department visit) as soon as possible. Penicillin is the drug of choice. In the case of penicillin allergy, azithromycin or clindamycin are alternatives. Amoxicillin-clavulanic acid (dose using the amoxicillin component) can also be used, as well as cefoxitin.

Abscesses. Permanent teeth may be sensitive to hot and cold for many weeks after fillings are placed. Some teeth may develop abscesses after fillings are placed in them. Abscesses may appear as swelling on the buccal or palatal gingival mucosa and frequently present with purulent drainage. A child with an abscessed tooth may not always report pain or sensitivity. Untreated abscesses may develop into life-threatening bony facial space infections, requiring surgical drainage and parenteral antibiotic treatment. They require urgent dental referral. If a dentist or oral surgeon is not immediately available for drainage and the abscess is uncomplicated, antibiotics (see prior section, Toothache) and pain medication are appropriate interventions prior to further consult (Idzik and Krauss, 2013) (see Fig. 34-6).

"Meth Mouth"

Methamphetamine users should be encouraged to seek drug treatment. Any dental intervention will fail without control of the underlying condition. Encourage the patient to drink lots of water and switch to artificially sweetened drinks. Over-the-counter fluoride mouth rinse, remineralizing solutions, xylitol chewing gum, and prescription chlorhexidine gluconate mouth rinse 0.12% may be recommended (discussed previously).

Periodontal Diseases

Gingivitis

Gingivitis is marked by the presence of gingival inflammation without noticeable loss of bone or clinical attachment of structures that help anchor the teeth. This condition is caused by plaque and is present in some degree in nearly all children and adolescents. It may be associated with different subgingival microflora than found in adult gingivitis; the hormonal fluctuations inherent in puberty may also be a determinant of altered inflammatory response to plaque in this age group (AAPD, Council on Clinical Affairs, 2015c).

The gingiva will present with localized or generalized bleeding when brushed or flossed. The teeth will be covered in varying degrees of plaque and calculus secondary to poor or irregular hygiene. The teeth will not be loose. The treatment is consists of brushing and flossing. It can take several days for the gingiva to respond to the improved hygiene. Gingivitis is reversible.

Aggressive Periodontitis

Aggressive periodontitis is a bacterial infection of the gums and bone with phagocyte abnormalities and hyperresponsive macrophages. It results in rapid loss of periodontal attachment and supporting bone around the primary or permanent teeth. The primary infection is by *Actinobacillus* and *Bacteroides* species in younger children and by *Treponema* species and other gram-negative rods in older children. The disease may be localized or generalized (varies by age), depending on the location of the loss of attachment and which teeth are affected and age. Aggressive periodontitis is the most common type of periodontitis in children

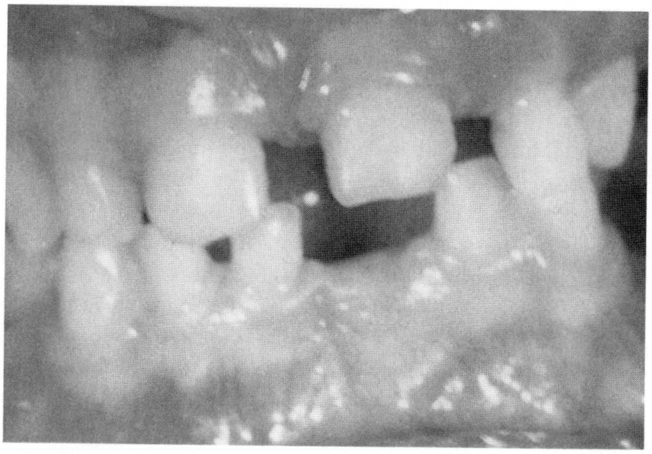

• **Figure 34-10** Prepubertal periodonditis in a 4½ year old girl. Loosening, migration, and spontaneous loss of the primary teeth occurred. (From McDonald RL, Avery DR, Weddell JA, et al: Gingivitis and periodontal disease. In McDonald RL, Avery DR, Hartsfield JK Jr, editors: *Dentistry for the child and adolescent*, ed 8, 2011, Elsevier, Fig 20-21A, p 382.)

and adolescents. The incidence is about 0.2% to 0.5% in children and adolescents, especially those 12 years old and older. African American children are at greater risk (AAPD, American Academy of Periodontology—Research, Science and Therapy Committee, 2004).

This infection either involves the surrounding gums and bone around primary incisors and molars (localized) or all teeth (generalized). The teeth may become loose, but in the localized form there is generally no inflammatory response, suppuration, or fever (Fig. 34-10).

All children with suspected periodontitis should be referred to a dentist or periodontist for local débridement (deep cleanings) and systemic antibiotics (tetracyclines [age appropriate] or metronidazole in combination with amoxicillin). For children with a familial history of gum disease, frequent dental examinations and radiographs during the peri-pubertal period are essential. Individuals should be counseled to avoid tobacco products, which increase the risk.

The major complication of gum disease is loss of bone and tooth attachment, resulting in the loss of teeth. Studies are ongoing to fully explore a possible causal relationship between untreated periodontal disease during pregnancy and later preeclampsia or premature labor (Gomes-Filho et al, 2010; Jeffcoat et al, 2011).

Periodontitis as a Manifestation of Systemic Disease (Prepubertal Periodontitis)

Periodontitis can occur between 4 and 5 years old and is associated with a number of systemic childhood diseases, including Papillon-Lefevre disease, Down syndrome, hypophosphatasia, leukocyte adherence deficiency, agranulocytosis, and cyclic neutropenia. It is a rare disease that typically manifests with the eruption of the primary tooth up to 5 years old. There are localized and generalized forms, both of which can result in loose teeth secondary to bone and attachment loss. Refer the child to a dentist or periodontist.

Necrotizing Periodontal Disease

This is an aggressive bacterial disease resulting in damage to the gum tissue between the teeth. The gum tissues harbor high levels of spirochetes, and invasion of the tissues has been demonstrated. Predisposing factors are viral infections (including human immunodeficiency virus [HIV] and other systemic diseases), malnutrition, emotional stress, and lack of sleep. The incidence in North America is less than 1% of children and adolescents; the prevalence is greater in those age groups from Africa, Asia, or South America (Tinanoff, 2011a). Children have severe gingival pain and fever. The triangular area of gums between the teeth is ulcerated and necrotic and covered with a gray film. There may be a fetid mouth odor. Careful oral hygiene and a bland diet are recommended. Address the predisposing conditions. As with all suspected periodontal conditions, individuals should be referred to a dentist or periodontist. Loss of teeth is a complication.

Pyogenic Granuloma

Pyogenic granuloma is an inflammatory hyperplasia that is usually caused by low-grade localized infection, trauma, or hormonal factors. It is usually a small exophytic (outward growing) lesion that is smooth or lobulated and sometimes hemorrhagic. It typically occurs on the gingival, lips, tongue, buccal mucosa, and hard plate. The surface color ranges from pink to red to deep purple, depending on how long the lesion has been present in the oral cavity. Pyogenic granulomas can occur after 4 years of age but are more common in pregnant women. Possible treatments include improved oral hygiene, 0.12% chlorhexidine gluconate rinses, surgical excision, cryosurgery, or intralesional injections of corticosteroids. If hygiene or chlorhexidine does not resolve the problem, the child should be referred.

Viral Diseases of the Mouth

Herpes Stomatitis

Herpes gingivostomatitis is a viral disease that results in oral and circumoral ulcers and is usually caused by herpes simplex virus type 1 (HSV-1) (Fig. 34-11). It most commonly affects children 6 months old to 5 years old as an initial infection. The classic signs and symptoms of HSV-1 orolabial infection occur in only 10% to 30% of children (Prober, 2012). The clinical findings are described in Chapter 37.

Lesions heal without treatment in 7 to 14 days. Supportive therapy is appropriate, such as cold liquids and analgesics. Topical treatment with an equal mixture of diphenhydramine and Maalox may provide symptomatic relief. Antimicrobials are not appropriate. Remove the child from day care or school during the drooling phase of the

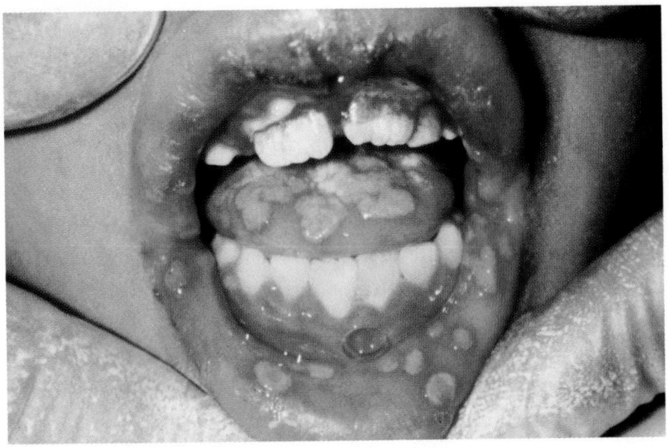

• **Figure 34-11** Herpes stomatitis in an infant.

illness. Encourage parents to clean the teeth with a soft toothbrush or cloth. Oral acyclovir is recommended to reduce the degree and length of symptoms if initiated within 3 days of the onset of the initial episode. Topical antiviral agents are ineffective (Prober, 2012).

Children with herpes are at risk for dehydration. Parents should be instructed to watch for signs and symptoms and seek medical care in such an event. Careful hand washing should be recommended to the child and the caregivers to prevent autoinoculation or transmission of infection to the eyes. An urgent referral to ophthalmology is needed if ocular spread is suspected.

Herpes stomatitis/labialis may be confused with aphthous ulcers (canker sores), ulcerative gingivitis, hand-foot-and-mouth disease, trauma, herpangina, or chemical burns. Rare conditions that may also cause lesions are neutrophil defects, systemic lupus, Behçet syndrome, and Crohn disease.

Idiopathic Oral Conditions

Ankyloglossia ("Tongue-Tie")

Ankyloglossia or "tongue-tie" is caused by a short lingual frenum that hinders tongue movement. The frenum may lengthen as the child gets older. Usually no treatment is needed. If the extent of the ankyloglossia is severe, breastfeeding may be difficult and a minor surgical incision is likely to help improve feeding. If speech is affected later in life, a referral for a surgical correction is indicated.

Aphthous Ulcers

This is a condition of recurrent, painful oral ulcers (also known as *canker sores*). The etiology is not well understood. Infectious agents, such as *Helicobacter pylori,* HSV-1, and measles, have been implicated in the etiology. Alterations of cell-mediated immunity may be associated with the disease. Emotional and physical stress, local trauma (orthodontic braces, toothbrush abrasion), hormonal factors, genetics, food hypersensitivity, and sodium lauryl sulfate in toothpaste have been implicated. Vitamin and mineral deficiencies also can cause recurrent oral aphthae, particularly deficiencies in several B vitamins (1, 2, 6, and 12), iron, folic acid, and zinc. Aphthous ulcers are reported to develop in 20% of the population, typically starting in childhood or adolescence (Weiss et al, 2010). There are three forms: minor (the most common), major, and herpetiform.

Single or multiple small, shallow mucosal lesions are present on alveolar or buccal mucosa, tongue, soft palate, or the floor of the mouth. The ulcers are surrounded with an erythematous halo and covered by gray, yellow, or white plaques. Minor lesions are less than 10 mm in diameter. Major lesions (also called *Sutton's disease*) are generally more than 1 cm in diameter. These lesions may take up to 30 days or more to heal and leave residual scarring. Herpetiform lesions are multiple, clustered, 1 to 2 mm that may coalesce; healing should be complete in about 7 to 10 days. Some individuals may complain of prodromal symptoms, such as tingling or burning. Consider HSV-1 infection as the differential diagnosis. The lesions may be seen with inflammatory bowel disease, Behçet disease, gluten-sensitive enteropathy, sweet syndrome, HIV infection, and neutropenia.

The goal of treatment is to decrease the ulcers, relieve pain, and reduce frequency of occurrence. Minor lesions generally resolve spontaneously in 10 to 14 days and heal without treatment or scarring. A bland diet and oral analgesics may be appropriate. Vitamin or mineral replacement may prevent recurrence if history suggests a deficiency. Over-the-counter treatments, such as triamcinolone hexacetonide in Orabase paste, fluocinonide gel covered by Orabase paste, or amlexanox 5% oral paste, may be applied four times per day for 3 to 4 days for pain relief and to promote healing. A mild mouthwash, such as sodium bicarbonate dissolved in warm water, may provide comfort. Chlorhexidine gluconate mouthwash (0.12%) can reduce the severity of an episode. Thalidomide has been used in severe cases associated with HIV infection (Weiss et al, 2010). Consider additional diagnostic testing should the symptoms and history suggest an infectious agent or gastrointestinal etiology. There are complementary therapies as well (see Chapter 43). Maintaining good oral hygiene is essential.

Benign Migratory Glossitis

Also known as *geographic tongue* or *erythema migrans,* benign migratory glossitis (BMG) usually presents as asymptomatic, yellowish-white, circular or serpentine-bordered lesions with atrophic red centers varying in intensity. They appear on the anterior two thirds of the dorsum of the tongue (Fig. 34-12). The lesions may heal and reappear on other areas of the tongue. The etiology is unknown. Approximately 1% to 2.5% of the population is affected, with children and young adults affected more than older individuals (Rozzolo and Sedrak, 2009). Females seem to be

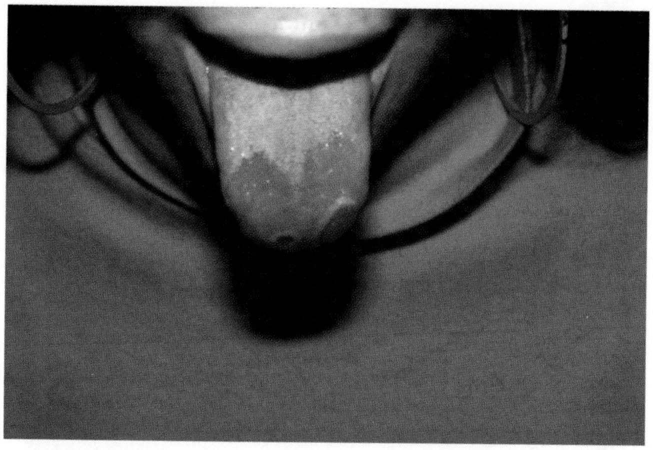

• **Figure 34-12** Benign migratory glossitis (BMG), or geographic tongue. (From Morelli JG: Disorders of the mucous membranes. In Kliegman RM, Stanton BF, St. Geme JW, et al, editors: *Nelson textbook of pediatrics*, ed 19, Philadelphia, 2011, Saunders/Elsevier, p 2298, Fig. 656-4.)

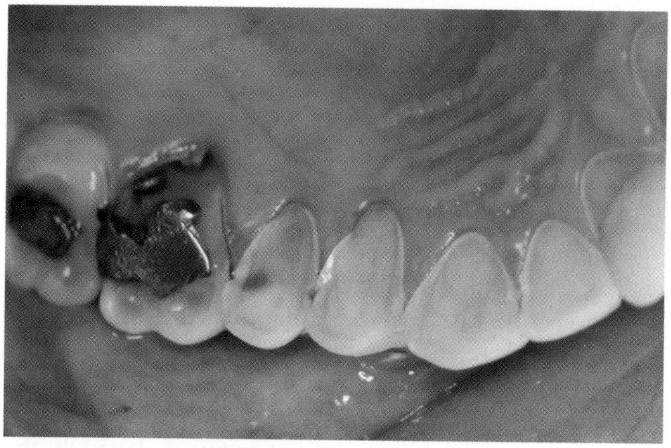

• **Figure 34-13** Dental erosion from bulimia. (From Neville BW, Damm DD, Allen CM, et al, editors: *Oral and maxillofacial pathology*, ed 2, St. Louis, 2002, Saunders/Elsevier.)

affected twice as often as males (Weiss et al, 2010). Occasionally one may experience pain, especially when eating hot or spicy foods. Proposed risk factors for BMG include immunologic factors, hormonal changes, use of oral contraceptives, diabetes mellitus, and stress. Diagnosis is made by appearance; patients can be reassured that the lesions are benign and do not generally require treatment. If treatment is indicated for pain, topical steroids, zinc supplements, and topical anesthetic rinses have been used with varying success (Weiss et al, 2010).

Bruxism/Grinding

Bruxism is a condition of excessive grinding of the teeth. Carra and colleagues (2011) found a prevalence rate of 15% for sleep-related bruxism and slightly over 12% for wake-time tooth clenching in children and adolescents seeking orthodontic treatment. Children 12 years old or younger were more likely to report sleep-related bruxism, whereas those 13 years old or older experienced more wake-time tooth clenching. Underlying stressors may be a contributing factor. An increase in bruxism has also been found in children exposed to high or moderate amounts of second-hand smoke (Montaldo et al, 2012).

Primary teeth show marked wear, and parents report that their child grinds his or her teeth during sleep. There may also be an orthodontic problem that needs attention. Carra and colleagues (2011) found that both children with sleep-related bruxism and wake-time tooth clenching complained of jaw muscle fatigue. Those with wake-time tooth clenching had more headaches and loud breathing during sleep, whereas those with sleep-related bruxism reported more temporomandibular joint (TMJ) clicking and sleep and behavioral issues.

No treatment is required for most grinding and tooth wear. The use of plastic night guards rarely eliminates grinding. Behavioral methods, such as relaxation training for stress management and other self-management skills, including control of gum chewing, have been shown to be effective in helping to manage facial muscle pain and headache. Parents should be told that tooth grinding is not associated with any damage to permanent dentition.

Dental Erosion

Dental erosion is a chemical process that leads to irreversible acid demineralization of tooth structure. Acids that cause dental erosion can be classified as intrinsic or extrinsic. Intrinsic acids include stomach acid introduced into the oral cavity by diagnosed or silent gastroesophageal reflux disorder (GERD), bulimia nervosa, and vomiting. Extrinsic acids include acidic beverages, methamphetamines, citrus fruits (e.g., sucking on lemons), and medications (e.g., chewable vitamin C tablets). Factors that can aggravate dental erosion include xerostomia (dry mouth) secondary to decreased salivary flow, medications that interfere with saliva composition or production (e.g., clonidine), dental attrition, possibly the use of the mood-altering drug ecstasy, and dental abrasion. Children and adolescents with bulimia frequently present with dental erosion. Children with asthma have greater amounts of dental erosion than other children. This may be due to increased gastroesophageal reflux in those with asthma, to acidic long-term medications, or to an increased consumption of erosive beverages taken to counteract the drying effect of inhalers (Hosey and Welbury, 2005). Prevalence rates vary by age, country, and study evaluation criteria; the mean rate in children is about 34% (Ren, 2011).

Clinical manifestations of dental erosion include smooth, cupped-out teeth on chewing surfaces; fillings that are raised above the normal level of the tooth; overly shiny silver fillings; enamel cuffing along the gums; and tooth hypersensitivity. Individuals with bulemia usually have very smooth lingual surfaces of the permanent teeth (Fig. 34-13).

Those with mild to moderate dental erosion may report tooth hypersensitivity.

The differential diagnosis includes abrasion caused by gritty substances (coarse toothpaste or toothbrushes with hard bristles) and attrition caused by mechanical forces (tooth grinding [bruxism] or brushing too hard). Also consider tooth decay.

Early detection, diagnosis, and treatment of dental erosion are critical. Hot and cold sensitivity can be managed by the use of "sensitive teeth" fluoridated toothpastes or topical fluoride treatments applied by the dentist. Treatment and/or referral for suspected cases of GERD or bulimia are warranted. Dietary counseling may be appropriate. Unless the erosion is deep, fillings are not required. Typically the problem can be managed by identifying and eliminating the etiologic agent. Over-the-counter products, such as soft toothbrushes, low-abrasive fluoridated toothpaste, and fluoride rinses, are helpful. Severe dental erosion can lead to dental nerve (pulp) exposures, which can necessitate root canal treatment.

Diastema

Spacing issues also affect the dentition. A space between any neighboring two teeth is referred to as a *diastema.* During the mixed dentition stage, when both primary and permanent teeth are present, a midline space between the upper front teeth is normal. If the teeth are not otherwise crowded or malaligned, these spaces usually close by the time the permanent maxillary canines fully erupt, and referral is not needed. Diastemas caused by missing incisors or midline supernumerary tooth or teeth will persist in the permanent dentition stage and require referral.

Another cause of a diastema is a prominent labial frenum, which is the tissue connecting the upper lip to the area of the gums between the front upper teeth. Sometimes the frenum is large and appears to be causing space between the front teeth. Generally the space closes as the jaws grow, and referral is not needed. Unnecessary or premature excision can result in scarring. A prominent labial frenum attachment during infancy that interferes with breastfeeding or persists in the permanent dentition stage may require excision (Kotlow, 2013) (Fig. 34-14).

Gingival Hyperplasia

Gingival hyperplasia is a fibrous enlargement of gingival tissue around the teeth. The enlargement is typically caused by drugs (phenytoin, cyclosporine, nifedipine), hormones, chronic inflammation, leukemia, or heredity. It can be idiopathic. The gingival tissue can be normal, red-blue, or lighter than the surrounding tissue. It may be spongy or firm and dense. The tissue is generally not inflamed, and patients are asymptomatic. Treatment consists of improved oral hygiene and 0.12% chlorhexidine gluconate mouth rinse. In cases in which the overgrowth interferes with chewing, gingivectomy is required.

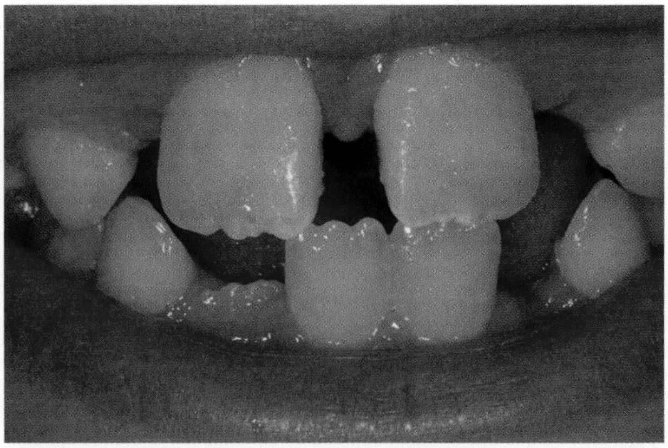

• **Figure 34-14** Diastema: labial frenum. (Courtesy Donald L. Chi, DDS, PhD, Associate Professor, Department of Oral Health Science, University of Washington School of Dentistry.)

Halitosis

Halitosis is oral malodor or bad breath. It is primarily associated with poor oral hygiene. It is more common in individuals who are mouth breathers, who suffer from postnasal drip or dry mouth, or who use tobacco products. Encourage proper oral hygiene, including regular brushing (including the tongue), flossing, and dental visits. Provide reassurance and encourage patients to avoid sugar-containing breath mints and other candies that might cause tooth decay or erosion; artificially sweetened gum or mints may be helpful. Individuals who have not had their teeth cleaned or an oral examination within the past 6 months should be referred to a dentist. For those with oral dryness, there are bioactive enzyme mouthwashes and lozenges available over the counter. The individual may also need to be evaluated for systemic disease, sleep apnea, and other airway-related conditions.

Malocclusion

Dental occlusion is the way the maxillary and the mandibular teeth articulate. From birth to adulthood and beyond, dental occlusion undergoes significant changes. Malocclusions have their basis in hereditary or genetic and/or environmental factors. Environmental factors include the premature loss of teeth due to trauma, caries, ectopic eruptions, or other causes before the end of active growth stages (e.g., non-nutritive sucking); these losses can lead to overcrowding problems (Agarwal et al, 2013).

Malocclusion rates vary among races and geographic regions of the world. Globally, Southeast Asian populations have the greatest degree of severe malocclusion; East Indian populations have the least (Hardy et al, 2012). In the United States, an estimated 57% to 59% of children younger than 18 years old need orthodontic treatment for malocclusions; in the United Kingdom the estimate is 66% of children at 12 years old. Severe problems related to occlusion and crowding occur in 15% to 20% of children in the United States and 33% in the United Kingdom (Mitchell,

2007; Proffit et al, 1998). In the United States, ethnic minorities and the uninsured and underinsured have higher levels of need.

The most common malocclusions that may require early diagnosis and interception include an anterior or posterior crossbite or an open bite. Retention of a primary tooth beyond the normal period can deflect the eruption of the permanent successor and lead to a crossbite. An anterior crossbite is due to crowding where one or more teeth are either behind or in front of the teeth in the opposing jaw while the others are in good alignment. With a posterior crossbite, one or more of the upper teeth is inside the opposing lower tooth. With an anterior open bite, the front teeth do not touch together when the back teeth are biting. Children with this problem may have a habit of passing their tongues through the space and can have problems speaking or chewing.

Primary dental health education and improved caries prevention globally by health care providers and dentists can affect the number of children who develop malocclusion because of the premature loss of primary teeth largely due to decayed teeth. Malocclusion has an important effect on the function and aesthetics of the entire dentition, and it can have a lifelong effect on the self-esteem of a child or an adolescent. A dentist or orthodontist can readily treat most crossbites in the permanent dentition. A persistent open bite in a school-age or older child is difficult to correct and requires referral to an orthodontist. The role of orthodontic treatment is irrelevant if improved dental health care and access is unattainable (Agarwal et al, 2013).

Mucocele

A mucocele is a salivary gland lesion caused by a blockage of a salivary gland duct. It is most common on the lower lip and has the appearance of a fluid-filled vesicle or a fluctuant nodule with the overlying mucosa normal in color. The patient should be referred to an oral surgeon for surgical excision of the involved accessory salivary gland (Fig. 34-15).

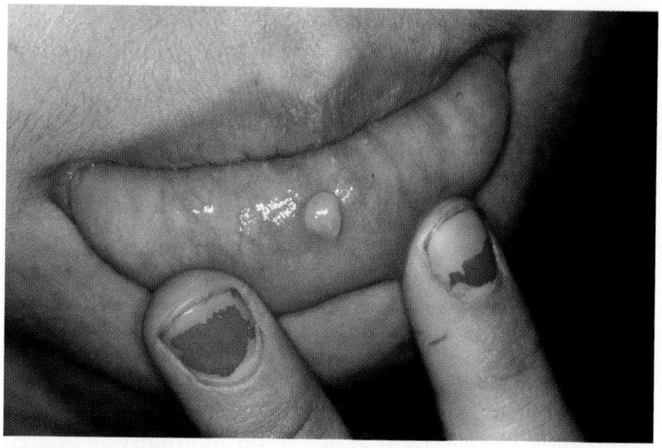

• **Figure 34-15** Mucocele. (From Morelli JG: Disorders of the mucous membranes. In Kliegman RM, Stanton BF, St. Geme JW, et al, editors: *Nelson textbook of pediatrics*, ed 19, Philadelphia, 2011, Saunders/Elsevier, p 2298, Fig. 656-2.)

Non-Nutritive Sucking

Non-nutritive sucking is normal at some point during infancy and includes sucking a digit (finger or thumb) or pacifier. The habit usually disappears between 1 and 3½ years old. The incidence of pacifier use ranges from 40% to 1% from 1 to 5 years old; for digits, the incidence is 31% to 12% between 1 and 4 years old. By 7 and 8 years old, 4% of children may still be sucking on a digit to some extent (Bishara et al, 2006). Breastfeeding and pacifiers do not normally cause lasting effects on occlusion (de Holanda et al, 2009).

In early stages of the mixed dentition period when both primary and permanent teeth are present, a child may have a temporary open bite, usually either a result of the still incomplete eruption of the incisors or a result of mechanical interference from a persistent finger habit. Thumb and finger sucking or long-term use of a pacifier that is not discontinued by the time the permanent teeth erupt may result in an anterior open bite. The upper front teeth will tip and push out. Self-correction of malocclusion becomes more unlikely at this point (Jyoti and Pavanalakshmi, 2014). Tongue habits exacerbate the open bite.

PCPs need to address non-nutritive sucking with parents of school-age children who continue to engage in this habit. In an older child, the key factor in extinguishing non-nutritive sucking is the child's desire to quit. For these children, an orthodontic appliance (e.g., crib, modified quad helix) can be placed on the teeth to remind the child not to suck. These appliances can make the bite worse if a child is not ready to quit, because the child can finds ways to suck around the appliance. Alternative behavioral therapy (e.g., positive reinforcement, comfort approaches) may be suggested (Tseng and Biagioli, 2009).

Pericoronitis Associated with Partially Erupted Wisdom Teeth

This condition is due to a partially erupted lower wisdom tooth with a tissue flap covering part of the crown. A foreign body, such as a piece of food, is forced under the flap, causing a localized infection. In some cases, upper wisdom teeth will erupt with the crown rubbing against the buccal mucosa and cause pain. The problem is common in college-age students. Partially erupted wisdom teeth can create an environment in which the distal surface of the second molar becomes decayed, because it cannot be cleaned. The gum tissue partially covering the tooth is inflamed and painful and fever may be present. The tissue flap may show trauma from biting. Aggressive periodontal diseases and severe tooth decay may have similar clinical presentations.

PCPs may recommend irrigation of the area with sterile water or saline, prescribe analgesics, and start amoxicillin if the individual is febrile. Not all wisdom teeth need to be removed. Wisdom teeth do not cause other teeth to become crooked. Most teeth that are fully covered in bone do not need to be removed and carry no significant risk. Similarly, if there is space for the erupting teeth, there is no reason to remove them. It is appropriate to wait for the teeth to fully erupt as much as they can. Waiting maximizes the chance that they will not need to be removed and minimizes injuries associated with the surgery. Impacted teeth, unerupted teeth with cysts, and upper teeth that have erupted toward the buccal mucosa should be examined and assessed for surgical removal.

Removal of wisdom teeth always requires a risk-benefit calculation, because there is significant morbidity associated with the surgery. Temporary or permanent nerve damage is possible as is TMJ disorder (Huang et al, 2014). A common complication of wisdom tooth surgery is alveolar osteitis or dry socket. This painful condition is associated with the loss of the normal clot in the healing socket that exposes bone. Smoking and the use of oral contraceptives are risk factors. Pretreatment rinsing with 0.12% chlorhexidine gluconate mouth rinse reduces the risk of complications. Treatment at the time of surgery with a nonsteroidal anti-inflammatory may reduce the extent of swelling postoperatively. Pain and foul taste in the mouth are the main symptoms, beginning 4 to 5 days after surgery. The individual should be referred back to his or her dentist.

Ranula

A ranula is a cyst filled with mucin from a ruptured salivary gland. It is associated with a major salivary gland in the sublingual area and is caused by lip or cheek biting. A common clinical problem occurring at any age, including infancy, a ranula is evidenced by a large, soft, mucus-containing swelling in the floor of the mouth. The cyst should be excised by an oral surgeon (Fig. 34-16).

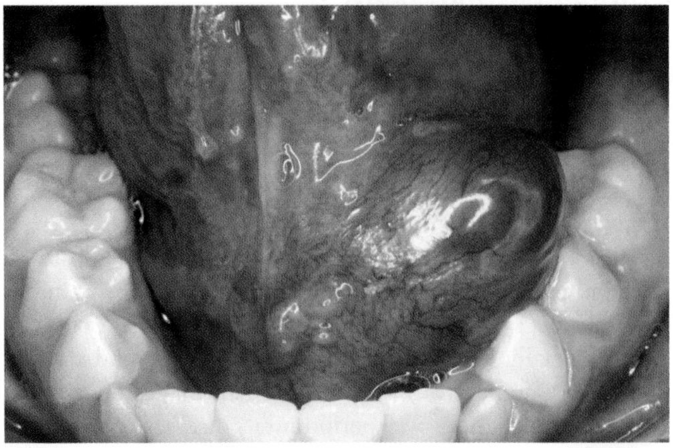

• **Figure 34-16** Ranula of the floor of the mouth. (From Neville BW, Damm DD, Allen CM, et al, editors: *Oral and maxillofacial pathology*, ed 2, St. Louis, 2002, Saunders/Elsevier.)

Temporomandibular Joint Disorder

TMJ disorder includes chronic facial pain and mandibular dysfunction. In the past, this disorder was evaluated strictly based on the physical state of the jaws or bite. This led to a great many inappropriate, ineffective, and even dangerous treatments. Results of the Orofacial Pain Prospective Evaluation and Risk Assessment (OPPERA) study conclude that besides sociodemographic factors, psychological distress, pain sensitivity, autonomic responses, and clinical variables, there is a strong genetic component to the development and experience of TMJ disorder (Fillingim et al, 2011). The condition is best evaluated within the context of a biopsychosocial model rather than purely on a functional level. Adaptive behaviors to the perceived discomfort or pain include being anxious, depressed, avoiding social interaction, developing other physical symptoms (e.g., migraines, tension headaches, back pain, ulcers, colitis), or by seeking pharmacologic relief. Studies suggest that the onset of most TMJ disorders increases with age with greater occurrence during adolescence. Prevalence rates range from 4.2% to 25% in those 5 to 19 years old. Females have significantly higher rates (correlated to onset of puberty) than males (AAPD, Clinical Affairs Committee, Temporomandibular Joint Problems in Children Subcommittee, 2015d). Third molar removal is associated with TMJ disorder (Huang et al, 2014).

Clinical Findings and Differential Diagnosis

Clinical symptoms may include self-reported facial (face, neck, temples, or jaw) pain once or more times per week associated with limitation in normal ability to open the mouth wide or with chewing; jaw locking; painful clicking, popping, or grating in jaw joint; and/or change in occlusion.

On examination, the facial muscles are tender to palpation, often unilaterally, but there is usually no swelling or skin bruising. The individual will be afebrile. Tooth pain, if present, is nonspecific. There may be a deviation to the painful side when the mouth is opened. Pain, particularly in the chewing muscles and/or jaw joint, is the most common symptom.

The differential diagnoses include infection of the face, ear, or teeth; traumatic injury (fracture of the jaw); myositis; sinusitis; headaches; dislocation of the jaw; neoplasm; arthritis; collagen diseases (systemic lupus erythematosus [SLE]); congenital and developmental anomalies of the joint (rare); and capsulitis.

Management

Viewed as a biopsychosocial problem, surgical interventions (particularly changes to the teeth), are inappropriate. Conservative treatment should always be the first course of treatment. Invasive, irreversible approaches have not proven effective (surgery, orthodontics, jaw implants) (National Institutes of Dental and Craniofacial Research [NIDCR] and National Institutes of Health [NIH], 2013). Treatment recommendations include avoiding extreme jaw movements, soft diet, muscle relaxation and gentle stretching exercises, application of ice packs, analgesics, and anti-inflammatory medication. A short-term, removable plastic splint (goes over the upper or lower teeth) may be fitted by a dentist to see if pain relief is achieved. Evidence does not support the supposition that chewing gum, bad bite, or orthodontic care cause TMJ disorder, but chewing gum may exacerbate it (NIDCR and NIH, 2013). Botox is currently being studied to see if it might be a useful treatment for chronic TMJ disorder; it is not FDA approved. Individuals who do not respond to the basic recommendations need referral to specialized centers where teams of dentists and psychologists work together. Diagnosis involves assessment of physical findings and both axis I and II dimensions of the mental state. Chronic headaches, otalgia, tinnitus, and lost time from work, school, or activities may result from TMJ.

Traumatic Injuries to Oral Structures

Injuries to the face usually result in trauma to the soft tissues of the mouth, teeth, or jaws. Such trauma is one of the most common presentations of young children to dentists. Dental injuries occur secondary to falls, motor vehicle accidents, violence, abuse, contact with hard objects, and sporting activities. Fewer traumas are presently seen from supervised, organized sports because most children wear mouth guards; nevertheless, a disproportionate amount of trauma results from leisure activities, such as skateboarding, swimming, and other noncontact sports. Upper incisors are particularly vulnerable to dental injuries particularly in those with protruding upper teeth (overjet bite) (AAPD, Council on Clinical Affairs, 2013). In addition, a child who has received local anesthesia for dental treatment may accidentally injure himself or herself by biting the inside of the cheek, tongue, or lip.

Age is a significant consideration in trauma to teeth. Most injuries cluster in three age groups: 1 to 3 years old (due to falls or child abuse), 7 to 10 years old (due to bicycle and playground accidents), and 16 to 18 years old (from sports injuries, fights, and vehicular accidents) (Tinanoff, 2011b). Males have dental injuries more frequently than females. Having cerebral palsy is another risk factor. It is important to rule out physical abuse because the orofacial region is commonly traumatized during such episodes. (See Chapter 17 for signs of physical abuse in the head area.)

Clinical Findings

History

Because a dental injury may become the subject of litigation, a thorough history and examination is mandatory. When possible, an injury should be photographed. Determine the following:

- When and how did the trauma occur?
- Were there any other injuries?
- Have there been any injuries in the past?
- Is there any concern for the safety of this child and family?
- Is there any history of physical abuse, drug or alcohol use in the family?
- Are any problems occurring as a result of the trauma?
- Is tetanus immunization current (within the last 5 years)? This question is especially important with soil-contaminated wounds or with complete displacement of a tooth from its socket. (See Chapter 24 for tetanus prophylaxis treatment.)
- For children presenting with trauma to the inside of the cheek, tongue, or lip, did the child recently receive local anesthetic for dental treatment?

Physical Examination

Blunt trauma tends to cause greater damage to soft tissues and supporting structures, whereas high-velocity or sharp injuries cause luxation and fractures of the teeth. Children with sports-related injuries can have teeth that are avulsed, fractured, or loosened/displaced from its normal position (luxated, intruded, or extruded). The examination should include:

- Soft tissue: Palpate the jaws and the rest of the facial skeleton to determine if a fracture is possible.
- Skin: Look for extraoral lacerations and facial wounds.
- Intraoral mucosa: Look for wounds, swelling, and bruising of the oral mucosa, gingiva, tongue, cheeks, and/or palate.
- Teeth: Look for the following:
  - Displaced, loose, missing, fractured teeth
  - Root fracture: Caused by injury to the tooth root
  - Bite problems: Check for abnormalities in occlusion
  - Pulp exposure: Bleeding from the broken stump of the tooth itself
  - Color change: The whole tooth turning dark from internal bleeding when the tooth is intact
  - Jaw movement: Deviation to one side or pain and limitation on opening

Management and Complications

Most minor injuries to the oral soft tissues do not require suturing unless bleeding is a problem. Wound care should consist of irrigating the area with sterile saline and prescribing water-based 0.12% chlorhexidine gluconate mouth rinse for 2 to 3 minutes twice daily. Avoid alcohol-based rinses because use of these rinses may be painful. If it is determined that a child self-injured the inside of the cheek, tongue, or lip after receiving local anesthesia for dental treatment, the child should be referred back to the dentist. Children with avulsed and fractured teeth, those unable to bite normally, and those with jaw injuries should be referred to a dentist promptly in order to avoid tooth abscesses, dental pain, and problems with the eruption of permanent teeth.

- Tooth avulsion: Avulsed primary teeth should not be replanted. If permanent teeth are knocked out, timing is important, and the following instructions can be provided over the phone. The child should be referred to a dentist at the same time:

- Replant an avulsed permanent, clean tooth immediately. If the tooth is dirty, rinse it gently under cold running water (for less than 10 seconds), and then replant it (Andersson et al, 2012). Do not rub the root surface. If the tooth can be replanted, have the child bite gently on a handkerchief or clean cloth to keep the tooth in place; the dentist will be able to ensure that the tooth is in the right position and stabilized. Antibiotics will be prescribed by the dentist for 7 days (doxycyline or Pen VK are standard, depending upon age and drug allergies). If unable to immediately replant the tooth, place the tooth in transport media; ViaSpan or Hanks Balanced Sat Solution are preferred. If those are not available, store the tooth in cold milk, physiologic saline, or saliva (the youth's buccal vestibule can be used for this purpose) to prevent dehydration. The prognosis for successful replantation decreases with time. A tooth that is allowed to dehydrate will not be viable after 1 hour. However, it is worth having a dentist evaluate anyway because there are some interventions that can be taken for a tooth that has been out longer than 60 minutes (AAPD, Council on Clinical Affairs, 2011). The dentist should also x-ray to rule out an alveolar fracture and for placement of a flexible plastic splint to maintain proper tooth position. A follow-up dental visit is also indicated within 7 to 10 days of reimplantation.
- Tooth fracture: If possible, have the child keep the pieces of permanent incisors and place them in saline or water to prevent drying. Sometimes the dentist can temporarily repair the tooth if the fragment is large enough. Tooth fractures with bleeding from the stump are emergencies. Simple fractures not involving the pulp or nerve tissue are not emergencies but still may be repaired.

The provider should be alert to the possibility of a closed head or neck injury if severe trauma is reported. See Chapter 13 and Chapter 28 for a discussion of traumatic head injuries and return-to-play policies. If child abuse is suspected, call the child abuse hotline.

Trauma compromises a previously healthy dentition and affects self-esteem and quality of life. In some cases, the traumatized tooth may be asymptomatic and appear to be clinically normal. This tooth can subsequently become darker or can become spontaneously symptomatic, with the child reporting cold sensitivity, pain on chewing, or unprovoked pain.

Patient and Family Education

It is important to identify and educate children who are at high risk for dental trauma–related injuries. Children and teenagers who participate in sports should be encouraged to wear mouth guards and helmets. Parents and coaches should also encourage youths to remove all intraoral piercings (e.g., tongue and lip rings or studs) while engaging in sports.

Parents, coaches, and physical education teachers should be alerted to the importance of including ViaSpan or Hanks Balanced Salt Solution in first-aid kits to manage tooth avulsions. Caregivers with children who are learning to walk should be instructed on how to childproof their homes. To prevent head/dental trauma in motor vehicle accidents, it is important that children be properly placed in car and booster seats (see Chapter 40).

Lifestyle Choices that Affect Dental Health

Piercings and Intraoral Tattoos

Adolescents may have studs and other piercings in the tongue and lower lip, or tattoos on the buccal mucosa of the lips. Tissue around tongue studs may be infected as evidenced by inflammation, swelling, and pain. The inflammation and pain may be an allergic response to the metals in the studs or piercings, particularly to nickel. There also may be gum recession or fractures of the lower anterior teeth from metal studs that habitually click against the teeth. Tongues, especially just after stud insertion, can become swollen.

The mouth heals quickly, and the inflammatory response should be resolved within 8 to 10 days without treatment. Swelling beyond this period suggests infection or an allergic response. Infection should be treated with 0.12% chlorhexidine gluconate mouthwash twice per day for at least 1 week and a broad-spectrum systemic antibiotic, such as penicillin or clindamycin (Jasper et al, 2013). If mouth tissue is infected, the ornament should be removed, at least temporarily. If an allergic reaction to nickel is suspected, advise changing to gold or silver. Devices that cause chronic allergic reactions should be removed permanently. Ensure vaccinations are current for tetanus and hepatitis B. Deep neck infection, airway obstruction, bleeding, nerve damage, tooth fracture, systemic infections, and hepatitis have been noted. Adolescents contemplating or who have oral piercings should be counseled about:

- The potential for acquiring an infectious disease
- Using only regulated practitioners
- Ensuring that only sterile equipment and noble metals are used
- Completing a hepatitis B vaccination series before seeking piercing
- The potential damage to the teeth and gums
- Removing studs and piercings during sports

Smokeless Tobacco and Betel Nut Use

Smokeless tobacco is a highly addictive substance that is held in the oral cavity, allowing nicotine to enter the bloodstream, and can be detrimental to oral health. Fewer than 9% of all teenagers nationwide report using smokeless tobacco; its use is more prevalent among rural youth. Popular cultural events (e.g., baseball) and heroes (e.g., rodeo riders and baseball players) make the habit "look cool." Its popularity has also been attributed to intensive promotion and flavors, being viewed as a way to lose weight, and a way to get nicotine without having to frequent restricted smoking areas (Muscari, 2010).

Betel nut (areca) is the fourth most commonly used drug in the world, is carcinogenic, and is legal in the United States. Betel nut may be crushed and chewed alone or combined with tobacco and held in the cheek like smokeless tobacco. Nearly 70% of adolescents in the Federated States of Micronesia use betel nut at least once per month, which is a growing concern for the mainland United States because of high rates of migration from the Pacific Islands (Milgrom et al, 2013).

PCPs should examine the posterior buccal vestibule of the lower jaw and the anterior buccal vestibule of the upper jaw. These are the areas where smokeless tobacco and betel nut are commonly held in the mouth. The intraoral findings include leukoplakia (matted white plaques on the soft tissues of the oral cavity) and or erythroplakia (matted red plaques), gingivitis and gum recession (particularly in the lower jaw), periodontitis, stained teeth, halitosis, and tooth decay (associated with tobacco products that have added sweeteners).

Individuals who use tobacco products and/or betel nut should be assessed for willingness to undergo tobacco cessation treatments. See Chapter 8 for a discussion of an effective strategy to use with adolescents. Active family involvement in the lives of children can help prevent the start of smokeless tobacco use. If children have relatives who use tobacco products, PCPs may need to focus tobacco cessation efforts on these family members. Complications include lip and oral cancer, gingivitis, gum recession, periodontitis, and stained teeth. There is little study to date on the oral effects of electronic cigarettes (e-cigarettes).

Tooth Whitening (Bleaching)

The desire for "whiter and brighter" smiles has resulted in increased demand for tooth whitening. Tooth whitening may be indicated for permanent teeth discolored or stained by trauma, fluorosis, tetracycline consumed during tooth development, or colored foods and beverages. Adolescents can be particularly self-conscience of discoloration. There have been few published studies on the use of these bleaching agents with children and adolescents. A pretreatment evaluation by a dentist is recommended prior to bleaching to determine the etiology of the discoloration and any contraindications to the bleaching. The AAPD recommends the judicious use of these products, particularly in a child with mixed primary and permanent teeth.

Tooth whitening can involve the use of over-the-counter kits, in-office treatment, or take-home bleaching trays that are customized by a dentist. The in-office tooth whitening process involves repeated short-term exposure of teeth to carbamide peroxide (typically in the range of 10% to 38%) until desired results are achieved. Over-the-counter kits include lower concentration carbamide peroxide in trays or hydrogen peroxide in strips. Most are used for 2-week periods. There are also numerous gels, rinses, gums, toothpastes, and paint-on films. Higher concentrations of hydrogen peroxide are more effective than lower concentrations. Up to 66% of those using bleaching agents can experience hypersensitive teeth and soft tissue/gum irritation, usually in the initial bleaching stages (AAPD, Council on Clinical Affairs, 2014b). Teeth will generally return to their normal sensation, gum status, and color if treatments are not repeated.

Health providers can remind parents and caregivers that permanent teeth are naturally darker than primary teeth and in most cases do not need whitening. Unless there are major esthetic concerns that could affect a child's psychosocial development, tooth whitening should not be undertaken until all permanent teeth have fully erupted. This measure will also prevent shade mismatching that can occur when teeth are whitened during the mixed dentition stage.

Dental Care of Children with Special Health Care Needs

Children with chronic disease or with congenital or acquired physical, intellectual, or developmental disabilities require extra preventive strategies and individualized dental appointments based upon their particular needs and conditions. At-risk children include those with neuropsychological conditions (e.g., intellectual and developmental disability, autism spectrum disorder); sensory challenges (e.g., blindness, visual impairment, deafness, and hearing impairments); musculoskeletal or other structural difficulties (e.g., osteogenesis imperfecta, cerebral palsy, spina bifida, cleft lip/palate, paralysis); and chronic diseases (e.g., asthma, cardiovascular disorders, cystic fibrosis, chronic renal failure, diabetes mellitus, bleeding disorders, malignant disease, and epilepsy). Low birth weight can be associated with structural tooth defects, which can lead to increased risk for tooth decay. Some individuals have a higher incidence of oral disease either because of a systemic problem itself or because of the secondary effects on tooth development, diet, medications, or the inability of caretakers to clean or maintain the teeth. Risks include:

- Diet: A number of conditions, such as congenital heart disease, facial clefts, esophageal defects, generalized hypotonia, muscular dysfunction, or intellectual and developmental disability involve feeding problems. A child's sucking or chewing problems may lead to meals lasting for an hour or more. Liquid, soft, and high cavity-causing sugary foods are common. Food is often retained in the mouth for a long time before it is swallowed.
- Elimination: Many children with extra needs experience chronic constipation or diarrhea. Sweet remedies, such as dried fruits or sodas and juices, are often used to cure such conditions. Frequent intake of beverages is often recommended for children on medication to prevent

• BOX 34-2 Classes and Examples of Drugs Associated with Decreased Salivation and Xerostomia

Analgesics: NSAIDs, narcotic analgesics
Antidepressants: Fluoxetine, amitriptyline
Antiemetics: Promethazine, metoclopramide
Antihistamines: Diphenhydramine, promethazine
Antihypertensives: Beta-blockers, diuretics, ACE inhibitors
Antipsychotics: Clozapine, chlorpromazine, risperidone

ACE, Angiotensin-converting enzyme; *NSAID*, nonsteroidal anti-inflammatory drug.

kidney failure. To increase hydration, parents often resort to sugar-containing drinks.

- Medications: Long-term use of sweetened medicines or syrups can also present a hazard to dental health. Box 34-2 lists the classes of drugs that may reduce salivation and thereby increase susceptibility to caries. Phenytoin commonly causes gingival hyperplasia.
- Cognition: In some children, problems may relate to an inability to understand the meaning behind oral hygiene procedures.
- Muscular function: Hypotonia may influence salivation and cause drooling or chewing problems. Impaired manual dexterity may make it difficult for children to perform preventive oral hygiene routines. Hyperfunction may result in extensive tooth wear as a result of grinding of teeth. Children with feeding tubes face many difficulties.

Management Strategies

The ability of parents to follow recommendations and assume long-term responsibility for preventive dental care varies with the difficulties presented by the child's condition. Therefore, recommendations for professional checkups and preventive services, such as fluoride treatments, should be individualized. If hygiene is poor, preventive treatments need to be provided more often. Health care providers are advised to frequently ask about the status of dental visits and whether routine oral hygiene is both taught to the child and actively supervised in the home and school. In addition, the following topics should be covered:

- Diet: For children with reduced salivary secretion or impaired self-cleaning mechanisms of the oral cavity, parents or caretakers must be especially attentive to the diet. Restrictions in cavity-causing foods are necessary to prevent tooth decay. If sweetened medicinal syrups cannot be replaced by sugar-free alternatives, these medications should be taken at mealtime. Rinsing the mouth and teeth with water after a meal may help if brushing is not feasible. Water or artificially sweetened beverages should be recommended for drinks between meals.
- Topical fluorides: A child with reduced salivary secretion, impaired muscular function, or with a cavity-causing diet may need an intense fluoride program in addition to careful oral hygiene. PCPs can apply 5% sodium fluoride topical varnish or prescribe a fluoride rinse, gel, or high-fluoride (1.1% sodium fluoride) toothpaste for home use. Carefully monitor the teeth of these patients and make prompt referrals when problems are noted.
- Topical iodine: The teeth and gums can be painted with topical PVP-iodine once every 4 to 6 months. As previously discussed, there is evidence that topical 10% povidone-iodine suppresses tooth decay-causing flora without major changes in the overall flora (Tut and Milgrom, 2010). Children who have had major dental treatment because of extensive dental caries are obvious candidates for repeated iodine treatments. Iodine can be painted on the teeth at the same visit in which fluoride varnish is applied with the iodine wiped off with gauze before applying the varnish. PCPs can do this treatment if dental services are lacking.
- Chemical plaque control: When oral hygiene is difficult to perform, chemical plaque control with a 0.12% chlorhexidine gluconate mouth rinse is recommended. Such rinses can be used daily. They are also recommended for use in children with hemophilia, cardiac disease, or immunodeficiency 7 to 10 days prior to dental procedures in order to minimize bleeding or bacteremia. Chlorhexidine is available with a prescription.

For a complete list of references, please visit http://evolve.elsevier.com/Burns/pediatric/.

35 Genitourinary Disorders

NAN M. GAYLORD

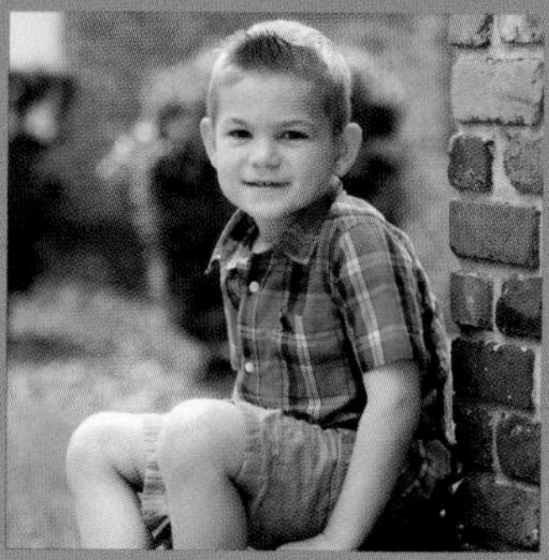

The genitourinary system is responsible for maintaining an optimal environment for metabolism, including regulation of water and electrolytes (sodium, potassium, chloride, calcium, phosphate, and magnesium); excretion of waste products (urea, creatinine, poisons, and drugs); acid-base regulation; and hormonal secretion (vitamin D, renin, erythropoietin, and prostaglandins). The male system has both reproductive and excretory functions. Genitourinary problems in children and adolescents range from commonly occurring easily treated diseases to significant congenital or acquired conditions. Pediatric primary care providers play a significant role in working with children, adolescents, and families to identify problems, manage disorders, maintain optimal function, and provide education and support related to genitourinary function. First-line assessment and management, provision of continuity of care, and referral to and collaboration with pediatric urologists and nephrologists are important components of patient management.

Discussion of related functional health problems—enuresis and dysfunctional voiding—is included in Chapter 12.

Standards of Care

The American Academy of Pediatrics (AAP) and the *Bright Futures Practice Guidelines* in their Recommendations for Pediatric Primary Care Prevention do not recommend screening for asymptomatic bacteremia or chronic kidney disease with a urine dipstick or complete urinalysis (UA) at any age (AAP Committee on Practice and Ambulatory Care, 2014).

Hypertension in infants and young children is usually secondary to another disease process; most commonly it is renal in origin. Older school-age children and adolescents may present with primary hypertension due to the increase in our rates of obesity, however, influence of the genitourinary system is considered. Blood pressure (BP) screening is recommended in the AAP/Bright Futures Recommendations for Pediatric Primary Care Prevention at every preventive health care visit beginning at 3 years old (AAP Committee on Practice and Ambulatory Care, 2014). The management and treatment of hypertension is discussed in Chapter 31.

Anatomy and Physiology

The renal system is composed of two kidneys, two ureters, a bladder, and a urethra. The kidneys are positioned posteriorly on the abdominal wall. The main structures of the kidney are the cortex, the medulla, and the collecting system. The renal medulla and nephrons are present at birth, but the peripheral tubules are small and immature. By adolescence, the kidneys are of adult size and weight. The ureters are muscular tubes that convey urine from the kidneys to the bladder by peristaltic contractions. The bladder is a muscular reservoir to collect the urine. It lies close to the anterior abdominal wall in early childhood. With growth, it descends into the pelvis and changes shape from cylindrical to pyramidal. As the bladder nears its capacity, nerve signals are transmitted to the brain to indicate that urination is required. When urination occurs, the sphincter between the bladder and urethra opens and contractions of the bladder create pressure to force urine out the urethral meatus. The male urethra is significantly longer than the female's because it leaves the bladder in the lower pelvis, passes through the prostate with openings for the release of bulbourethral gland fluids and semen during sexual activity, and extends the full length of the penile shaft. The urethral meatus is normally located on the tip of the glans in the male. In the female, the urethra descends from the bladder and exits the body inside the labia minora, midline, just posterior to the clitoris.

Physiologically the kidneys serve to filter, clear, reabsorb, and secrete substances essential to the body's metabolism. The urinary system begins forming and excreting urine at 3 months of gestational age. Glomerular filtration and renal blood flow begin to increase at birth and become stable by 1 to 2 years old. In infants, total extracellular fluid volume is significantly greater than that of adults, and fluid composition tends to have a lower bicarbonate concentration. Normal urine excretion is 1.5 to 3 mL/kg/hr. The kidneys mature throughout infancy, although all measurable variables of kidney function approach adult values between 6 and 12 months old.

Pathophysiology and Defense Mechanisms

Problems in the urinary system can occur at any point in the system from the kidneys to the urethral meatus. If the kidneys and ureters are involved, the disease is considered to be in the upper tract; if the problem is in the bladder, urethra, or meatus, it is considered a disease of the lower urinary tract. These differentiations can be difficult because frequently disease in one part of the system affects the entire system. Additionally, disease can present silently or be noticeably problematic at any age. The main mechanisms of disorders are classified as follows: infection, inflammatory response, congenital malformation or condition, and abnormalities acquired from injury, infection, or malfunction within the system.

The urinary tract is normally a sterile system. The mucosal lining of the bladder serves as the first line of defense and inhibits bacterial growth and adherence. The acid pH of the urine also protects the urinary system by inhibiting bacterial growth. Finally, the actual flow of urine out of the bladder provides mechanical defense by its flushing action. If these defenses are compromised, the body initiates an inflammatory response within the urinary system.

Assessment of the Genitourinary System

History

- History of the present illness
  - Onset and pattern of symptoms
  - Fever
  - Abdominal pain
  - Flank pain
  - Preceding injury or illness, especially streptococcal infection
  - Vomiting
  - Voiding pattern: Stream force and direction, any dribbling or discharge
  - Color, odor, frequency, and volume of urine, dysuria, urgency; enuresis, or incontinence
  - Diarrhea or chronic constipation
  - Sexual activity or abuse
- Family history
  - Any familial history of renal disease, deafness, hypertension, structural abnormalities, or syndromes involving the genitourinary system
- Past history of urinary tract infection (UTI), hematuria, proteinuria, syndromes associated with genitourinary abnormality, or any other related finding

Physical Examination

- Growth parameters: Failure to thrive (FTT) can be associated with UTI, renal tubular acidosis (RTA), and chronic renal failure in infants. Unusual weight gain can be associated with nephrotic syndrome or acute renal failure
- BP: Often elevated with nephritis and nephrotic syndrome
- Edema, pallor, dehydration
- Ear position and formation: If low-set or abnormal, may have concurrent renal involvement
- Abdominal masses, ascites, flank or suprapubic tenderness
- Costovertebral tenderness
- External genitalia abnormalities
- Unusual facial features associated with syndromes that have renal disease

Diagnostic Studies

Diagnostic studies are ordered as indicated. The proper collection, transport, and storage of urine is essential to obtain accurate results. The normal composition of urine varies considerably during a 24-hour period. Most reference values are based on analysis of the first morning voided urine. This specimen is preferred because it has a more uniform volume and concentration, and its lower pH helps preserve the formed elements. Urine should be evaluated within 30 minutes and, if stored, kept refrigerated (below 39.2° F or 4° C). If kept overnight a special preservative (e.g., boric acid) is recommended (Quest Diagnostics, 2014).

The following should be noted on the UA:

- Physical characteristics: Color, clarity, odor, specific gravity, and osmolality are noted.
  - Specific gravity is a measure of hydration and renal concentration ability and varies from 1.003 to 1.030. A random first-voided urine specimen specific gravity of 1.023 or more indicates intact renal concentrating ability. Urine with a specific gravity greater than 1.020 is considered concentrated.
- Chemical characteristics: Urine dipsticks are among the waived tests by the Clinical Laboratory and Improvement Amendments of 1988 (CLIA), and they are widely used to determine pH, specific gravity, glucose, ketones, protein, bile pigments, hemoglobin, nitrites, and leukocyte esterase. For correct results, strips must remain in their original containers and not be exposed to moisture, light, cold, or heat until used. Urine must be fresh, warmed to room temperature if refrigerated, and read at correct time intervals for each test strip (Table 35-1). Urine pH can vary from 4.6 to 8 and is reflective of the body's ability to maintain acid-base balance.
  - A dipstick positive for blood indicates the presence of hemoglobin. Intact erythrocytes cause spotty changes on the dipstick, whereas free hemoglobin or myoglobin causes uniform changes of color.

TABLE 35-1 Chemical Characteristics of Urine

Constituent	Positives Indicate	Cause of False Positive	Cause of False Negative
Glucose	Metabolic problem (e.g., diabetes), recent high glucose intake, oral corticosteroids, galactosemia	Antibiotics, delay in reading, myoglobin, oxidizing contaminants	Ascorbic acid intake, ketones, high specific gravity
Ketones	Dehydration, starvation, missed breakfast, strenuous exercise, stress, fever, metabolic problems (e.g., diabetes)	Rare	If urine left standing, acetone evaporates
Protein	Renal disease, orthostatic proteinuria	Exercise, fever, dehydration, alkaline or concentrated urine (specific gravity >1.02), semisynthetic penicillin, oxidizing, cleansing agents	Dilute or acidic urine
Blood (hemoglobin)	If concurrent microscopic examination is negative for RBCs: Free hemoglobin secondary to chemicals, illness, or drugs; myoglobin secondary to burns, muscle trauma, physical child abuse, myositis, strenuous exercise If concurrent microscopic examination is positive for RBCs: External excoriation, renal problems	Menses, oxidizing cleansing agents, dilute urine	Ascorbic acid
Nitrite	Bacteria causing UTI	Rare	Common; urine should be in bladder at least 4 hours
Leukocyte esterase	Pyuria (WBCs in urine); inflammation from irritation or infection of vulva, vagina, or urethra; inflammation of bladder or kidneys with or without infection	Oxidizing agents	Immunocompromised
Urobilinogen	Hemolytic disease; hepatic disease	Rare	Rare
Bilirubin	Hepatic disease; biliary obstruction	Rare	Rare

RBC, Red blood cell; *UTI,* urinary tract infection; *WBC,* white blood cell.

- Leukocyte esterase indicates white blood cells (WBCs) in the urine and, if positive, warrants further investigation.
- Nitrites: The nitrite test on the dipstick is an indirect measure of bacteria in the urine. Common urinary pathogens contain enzymes that reduce nitrate in urine to nitrite. However, the urine must usually be in the bladder at least 4 hours to show accurate results. Leukocyte esterase and nitrite dipsticks are not reliable in children younger than 3 years old, so a negative dipstick does not rule out a UTI (Mori et al, 2010). A urine culture should be done on any urine sample positive for nitrites or leukocyte esterase, if the child has symptoms of UTI, if the risk criteria as described in the section about UTIs are met, or if the child has a high fever without a source. The combination of leukocyte esterase and nitrites is highly predictive of a positive urine culture. Urine that is negative for leukocyte esterase and nitrites can be used to reasonably rule out a UTI; however, a culture is still indicated for both negative and positive urine dipstick findings, especially if the urine had not been in the bladder at least 4 hours (Perkins et al, 2012).
- Microscopic examination of urine: Urine can be spun by centrifuge and the sediment examined, or it can be examined without being spun. When evaluating results, consideration must be given to which method of collection was used. Urine should be examined under the microscope for red blood cells (RBCs), WBCs, bacteria, casts, and crystals. Microscopic examination of a fresh specimen is essential if blood or protein is found on the dipstick or urinary tract symptoms are present.
  - RBCs: The number of RBCs per high-power field (HPF) that are thought to be abnormal varies. In general more than two to five per HPF (×40) in unspun urine or more than 2 to 10 per HPF

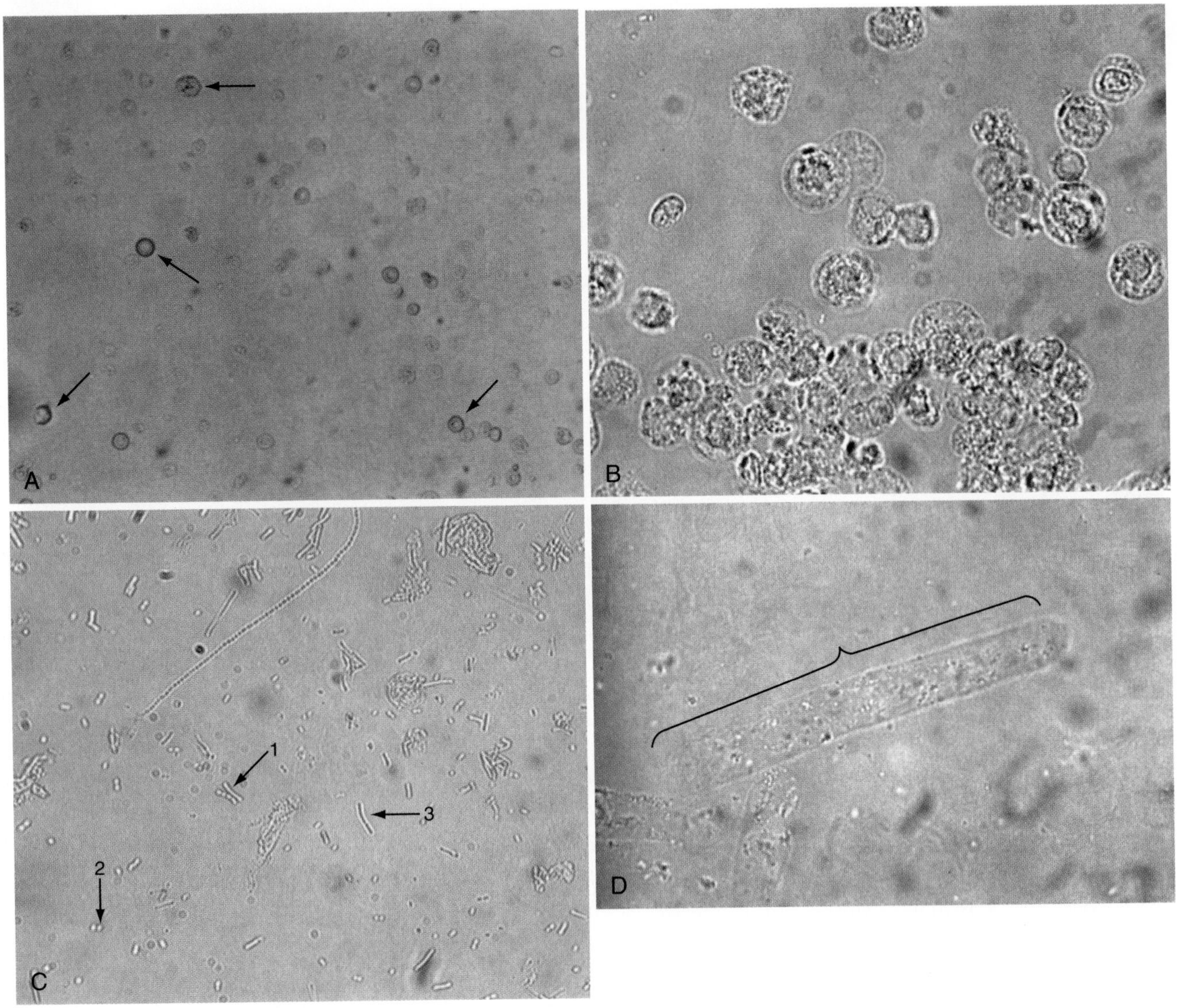

• **Figure 35-1** Findings in microscopic evaluation of urine. **A,** Red blood cells; **B,** white blood cells; **C,** bacteria; **D,** hyaline casts.

in spun urine is thought to be abnormal (Elder, 2011d) (Fig. 35-1). If cells are dysmorphic, the origin of the blood is most likely the kidney.

- WBCs: Fewer than two WBCs per HPF should be seen. More than 10 WBCs often indicates an infection (see Fig. 35-1).
- Bacteria: Leukocytes seen in unspun urine are associated with bacterial colony counts of greater than 100,000 (see Fig. 35-1).
- Casts: RBCs, hyaline, waxy, epithelial, leukocyte, or fatty casts are seen in various disease states (see Fig. 35-1).
- Crystals, if amorphous, are not unusual. Calcium oxalate, cystine, tyrosine, leucine, cholesterol, or sulfa crystals are abnormal.

Depending on the results of the UA and/or clinical symptoms, other tests may be indicated, including:

- Gram stain: A Gram stain of the urine can be helpful in identifying organisms when examining urine under the microscope. More than 10 WBCs per HPF and bacteria on the Gram stain are highly predictive of a UTI, and a urine culture should be performed.
- Urine culture and sensitivities: Culture remains the gold standard for diagnosing and treating UTIs. Urine should be cultured immediately but may be refrigerated for up to 24 hours before plating. Urine specimens unrefrigerated for 2 hours or more are subject to bacterial overgrowth, change in pH, and dissolution of RBC and WBC casts. Bacterial identification and sensitivities are recommended.
- A 24-hour urine collection: Collecting a 24-hour sample of urine is done to determine calcium excretion, the calcium-creatinine ratio, and quantification of protein.
- Blood work
  - Serum or blood urea nitrogen (BUN) estimates the urea concentration in serum or blood and is a measure of toxic metabolites that can cause uremic syndrome.

- Serum creatinine in combination with creatinine clearance is used to estimate the glomerular filtration rate (GFR) or kidney function.
- Serum electrolytes and acid-base status can detect renal tubular abnormalities.
- Serum procalcitonin level of more than 0.5 ng/mL is an accurate and reliable biologic marker for renal involvement during a febrile UTI, pyelonephritis, and renal scarring and may be useful in the clinical diagnosis and treatment of UTIs (Leroy et al, 2011).

- Ultrasonography of the renal system provides noninvasive structural information.
- Voiding urosonography (VUS) using a second-generation contrast agent is a safe, sensitive, and radiation-free method for detecting and grading vesicoureteral reflux (VUR) and has been shown to be superior to voiding cystourethrogram (VCUG) (Kis et al, 2010).
- Dimercaptosuccinic acid (DMSA) scanning is the most sensitive tool for detecting acute pyelonephritis and renal scarring and should be considered in a young child with febrile UTI (Elder, 2011d). Combined with renal ultrasound scanning, DMSA scanning has high sensitivity for detecting VUR. However, alone, the DMSA provides limited information regarding VUR (Elder, 2011e).
- Voiding cystourethrogram (VCUG): Indications for VCUG in a child with a UTI are limited to febrile UTIs after an abnormal ultrasound or DMSA scan or when there is a second febrile UTI (AAP Subcommittee on Urinary Tract Infection, Steering Committee on Quality Improvement and Management, 2011; Elder, 2011d).

Management Strategies

Education and Counseling

Education and counseling are essential components in the management of genitourinary tract disorders. Parents and children must be informed about the pathologic condition, etiology, treatment, prevention strategies, and prognosis with and without treatment. A plan of care that the family and care provider are comfortable with must be decided on and initiated. Urinary problems can begin in the neonatal period or occur any time during childhood or adolescence. They vary in severity, chronicity, and disability. The primary care provider must modify appropriate strategies for each individual situation.

Medication, Diet, and Activity

Depending on the diagnosis, medications can include antibiotics and steroids. Diet and activity may need to be modified in some chronic renal conditions. These modifications are usually carried out in consultation with appropriate specialists.

Referral

Referral to a pediatric urologist, nephrologist, or surgeon may be required. When a referral is made, the primary care provider retains the essential role of serving as case manager for the child and providing continuity of care over time. The primary care provider is often the one whom the family knows best and is most comfortable with when discussing concerns, potential plans, and long-term management.

Genitourinary Tract Disorders

Urinary Tract Infection and Pyelonephritis

There are three kinds of UTI in children: (1) asymptomatic bacteriuria, (2) cystitis, and (3) pyelonephritis. Young children may have limited or unusual symptoms; therefore, a high degree of suspicion must be maintained to diagnose UTI. Inflammation and infection can occur at any point in the urinary tract, so a UTI must be identified according to location. *Asymptomatic bacteriuria* is bacteria in the urine without other symptoms, is benign, and does not cause renal injury. *Cystitis* is an infection of the bladder that produces lower tract symptoms but does not cause fever or renal injury (Elder, 2011d). *Pyelonephritis* is the most severe type of UTI involving the renal parenchyma or kidneys and must be readily identified and treated because of the potential irreversible renal damage that can occur. Clinical signs thought to be consistent with pyelonephritis include fever, irritability, and vomiting in an infant, and urinary symptoms associated with fever, bacteriuria, vomiting, and renal tenderness in older children. UTIs are the most common cause of serious bacterial infection in infants younger than 24 months old with fever without a focus (Elder, 2011d). A *complicated UTI* is defined as a UTI with fever, toxicity, and dehydration or a UTI occurring in a child younger than 3 to 6 months old. The UTI may be classified based on its association with other structural or functional abnormality, such as VUR, obstruction, dysfunctional voiding, or pregnancy. Additionally, a UTI must be identified as a first occurrence, recurrent (within 2 weeks with the same organism or any reinfection with a different organism), or chronic (ongoing, unresolved, often caused by a structural abnormality or resistant organism). Finally, age and gender of the pediatric patient are important factors in determining the method of evaluation and the course of treatment.

The organism most commonly associated with UTI is *Escherichia coli* (70%), although other organisms (such as, *Enterobacter, Klebsiella, Pseudomonas,* and *Proteus*) can cause infection. UTI secondary to group B streptococcus is more common in neonates. Several factors are believed to contribute to the etiology of UTIs. Most UTIs are thought to be ascending (i.e., the infection begins with colonization of the urethral area and ascends the urinary tract). If the infection progresses to the kidney, intrarenal reflux deep into the kidneys can lead to scarring. However, the most important risk factor for the development of pyelonephritis in children is VUR, which can be detected in 10% to 45% of young children who have symptomatic UTIs. Furthermore, reflux of infected urine from the bladder increases the risk of pyelonephritis. This damage to the kidney occurs in the compound papillae, which have wide and gaping

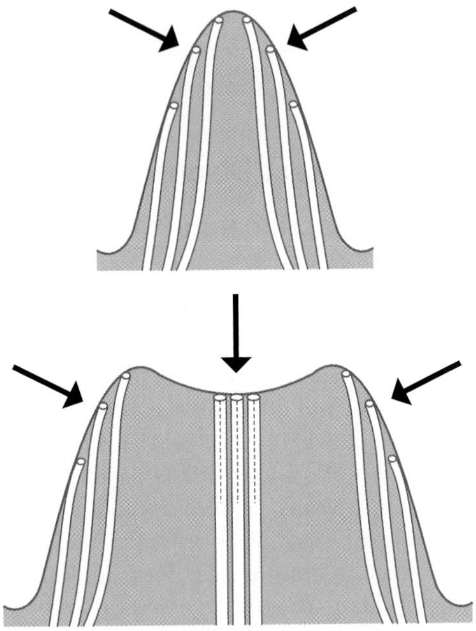

• **Figure 35-2** Most renal papillae are conical, with papillary ducts that open obliquely into the renal pelvis *(top)*. These do not allow intrarenal reflux. But some kidneys have compound papillae, formed by the fusion of conical papillae *(bottom)*. These have papillary ducts with gaping openings at right angles to urine flow and do permit intrarenal reflux. (From Ransley PG: Intrarenal reflux: anatomical, dynamic and radiological studies—part I, *Urol Res* 5[2]:61–69, 1977.)

openings allowing intrarenal reflux. The compound papillae are located in the upper and lower poles of the kidney, which is the usual site of scarring. Simple conical papillae have angled, slit-like openings that resist intrarenal reflux (Fig. 35-2).

Host resistance factors and bacterial virulence factors are also important in the etiology of UTIs. Host resistance factors include the presence of a structural abnormality or dysplasia (such as, VUR, obstruction, or any other anatomic defect) or the presence of functional abnormalities (such as, dysfunctional voiding or constipation). Other factors affecting resistance include female gender (having a short urethra), poor hygiene, irritation, sexual activity or sexual abuse, and pinworms.

Several bacterial factors are known, but the two most important ones are adherence and virulence of the bacteria. Bacteria that have fimbriae or pili are able to anchor or adhere to the surface of the bladder mucosa. This adherence allows the bacteria to resist the bladder's defensive cleansing flow of urine and causes tissue inflammation and cell damage. Adherence may also play a role in bacteria ascending the urinary tract. Virulence refers to the toxicity of substances released by bacteria. The greater the virulence, the greater the damage to the urinary tract. Both of these factors enhance colonization of the urinary tract and aid in the persistence and effect of the bacteria.

The risk of UTI in infants 2 to 24 months old is about 5%. The incidence in females is more than twice that of males (2.27%); uncircumcised boys have a rate 4 to 20 times greater than circumcised boys (AAP Subcommittee on Urinary Tract Infection, Steering Committee on Quality Improvement and Management, 2011). There is a greater frequency in premature and low-birth-weight infants. Females older than 12 months old have 2.1% prevalence; after the first year of life, it is also more common to find a UTI in females than in males with an overall incidence of 1% to 3% to in girls and 1% in boys (Elder, 2011d). The incidence of UTI is often increased in adolescent girls as they become sexually active. Recurrence is common, often within the first year after the initial infection.

Clinical Findings

History

The following information should be obtained:

- Family history of VUR, recurrent UTI, or other kidney problems
- Prenatally diagnosed renal abnormality
- Previous infection: Request records from the evaluation of past infections and diagnostic studies performed
- Circumcision
- Risk factors for infants 2 to 24 months old with no other source of infection (AAP Subcommittee on Urinary Tract Infection, Steering Committee on Quality Improvement and Management, 2011)
  - Female—white race, age younger than 12 months old, temperature 39° C or higher, fever for 2 days or more
  - Male—nonblack race, temperature 39° C or higher, fever for more than 24 hours
- Hygiene habits: Wiping front to back
- Voiding patterns: Frequency, abnormal stream, complete emptying, dribbling, and enuresis
- Constipation, perianal itching (pinworms)
- Irritants, such as nylon underwear or clothing (spandex, tight pants or shorts that rub); bubble bath or sitting in soapy bath water
- High BP
- Sexual activity, masturbation, or sexual abuse
- Other infection: Pinworms, diaper rash

Physical Examination

See Table 35-2 for age-related symptoms.

- General appearance (toxic appearing?)
- Vital signs: Temperature, BP
- Growth parameters: Growth may be decreased with chronic UTI or renal insufficiency, especially in infants
- Flank pain or tenderness in the costovertebral angle
- Abdominal examination: Suprapubic tenderness, bladder distention or a flank mass (obstructive signs), mass from fecal impaction
- Genitalia: Vaginal erythema, edema, irritation, or discharge; labial adhesions; uncircumcised male, urethral ballooning; weak, dribbling, threadlike stream
- Neurologic examination (if voiding is dysfunctional): Perineal sensation, lower extremity reflexes, sacral dimpling, or cutaneous abnormality

TABLE 35-2 Clinical Findings of Urinary Tract Infection in Children of Various Ages

Neonates	Infants	Toddlers and Preschoolers	School-Age Children and Adolescents
Jaundice	Malaise, irritability	Altered voiding pattern	"Classic dysuria" with frequency, urgency, and discomfort
Hypothermia	Difficulty feeding	Malodor	
Failure to thrive (FTT)	Poor weight gain	Abdominal/flank pain*	Malodor
Sepsis	Fever*	Enuresis	Enuresis
Vomiting or diarrhea	Vomiting or diarrhea	Vomiting or diarrhea*	Abdominal/flank pain*
Cyanosis	Malodor	Malaise	Fever/chills*
Abdominal distention	Dribbling	Fever*	Vomiting or diarrhea*
Lethargy	Abdominal pain/colic	Diaper rash	Malaise

*Findings increase likelihood of pyelonephritis.

Diagnostic Studies

The method used to collect urine has an effect on the interpretation of results. It is acceptable to collect urine for UA only from a non–toilet-trained child by using a sterile, adhesive bag carefully placed over well-cleaned genitals. If the bagged urine results in a positive leukocyte esterase or nitrite test, a child younger than 24 months old has risk factors, or the patient is symptomatic, additional urine should be collected by sterile catheterization or suprapubic aspiration. Older children, who can void on command, should be able to obtain a clean-catch void. Having the female child sit backward on the toilet separates the labia and decreases contamination. See the Diagnostic Studies section earlier in this chapter for other pertinent information.

- Urine culture by standard culture methods is essential to confirm the diagnosis. If the culture shows greater than 100,000 colonies of a single pathogen in a clean catch urine specimen, greater than 50,000 in a catheterized or suprapubic specimen, or if there are 10,000 colonies of a single pathogen and the child is symptomatic, the child is considered to have a UTI (Elder, 2011d; Shaw, 2015)
- UA should be used only to raise or lower suspicion. Suspicious findings include foul odor, cloudiness, nitrites, leukocytes, alkaline pH, proteinuria, hematuria, pyuria, and bacteriuria.
  - Nitrite chemical tests are reliable on urine specimens when gram-negative bacteria are present and when the urine has been in the bladder for 4 hours or longer. False-positive results are rare, whereas false-negative results are common.
  - Leukocyte esterase chemical tests detect pyuria, but pyuria may arise from causes other than UTI.
- Microscopic evaluation of uncentrifuged urine may be helpful if bacteria are seen.
- Gram stain may be helpful if bacteria are identified.
- Bacterial identification and determination of sensitivities are necessary in patients who appear toxic or could have pyelonephritis, have relapses or recurrent UTI, or are nonresponsive to medication.
- Complete blood count (CBC) (elevated WBC count), erythrocyte sedimentation rate (ESR), C-reactive protein (CRP), BUN, and creatinine should be done if the child is younger than 1 year old, appears ill, or if pyelonephritis is suspected.
- Serum procalcitonin level of more than 0.5 ng/mL is an accurate and reliable biologic marker for renal involvement during a febrile UTI, pyelonephritis, and with renal scarring, so it may be useful in the clinical diagnosis and treatment of UTIs (Leroy et al, 2011)
- Blood culture should be done if sepsis is suspected (see Chapter 24).

Differential Diagnosis

The differential diagnosis includes urethritis, vaginitis, viral cystitis, foreign body, sexual abuse, dysfunctional voiding, appendicitis, pelvic abscess, and pelvic inflammatory disease. Any child who has acute fever without a focus, FTT, chronic diarrhea, or recurrent abdominal pain should be evaluated for UTI.

Management

Goals of treatment are to quickly identify the extent and level of infection; to treat appropriately to eradicate infection; to provide symptomatic relief; to find and correct anatomic or functional abnormalities; and to prevent recurrence and new or progressive renal damage (AAP Subcommittee on Urinary Tract Infection, Steering Committee on Quality Improvement and Management, 2011). When deciding on a treatment plan, the child's age, gender, symptoms, the suspected location of the UTI and antibiotic

ALGORITHM

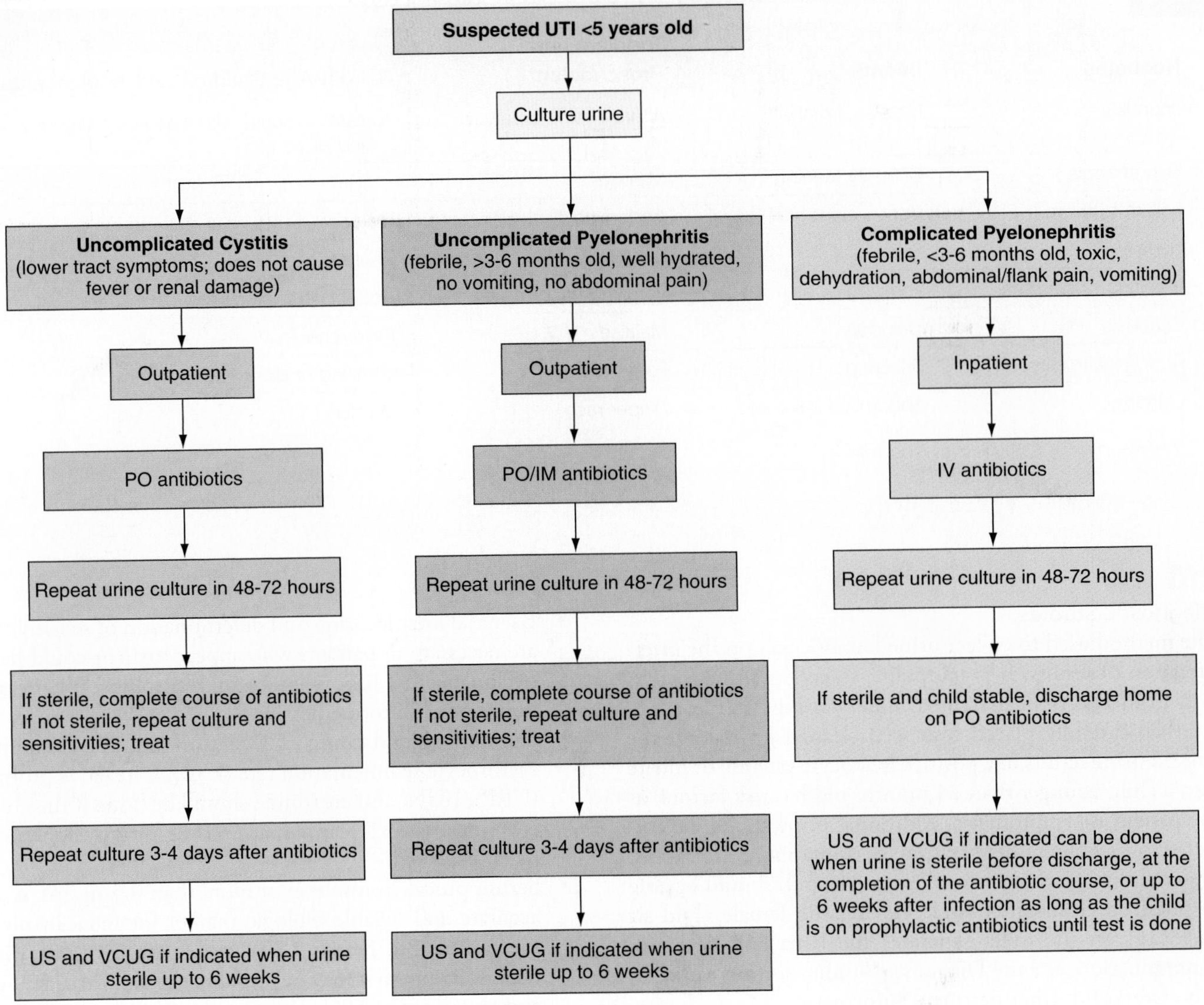

• **Figure 35-3** Suspected urinary tract infection *(UTI)* algorithm. *IM,* Intramuscular; *IV,* intravenous; *PO, per os* (by mouth, orally); *US,* ultrasound; *VCUG,* voiding cystourethrogram.

resistance patterns in the community must be considered. Figure 35-3 outlines treatment of UTI in the child.

Infants 2 to 24 Months Old

To diagnose UTI, the child should have both a UA suggesting infection (positive leukocyte and/or nitrite tests) and urine culture from a sterile catheterization or suprapubic aspiration (SPA) with at least 50,000 cfu/mL. Risk factors have been identified to help steer management. See the AAP Guideline (AAP Subcommittee on Urinary Tract Infection, Steering Committee on Quality Improvement and Management, 2011).

Asymptomatic Bacteriuria

If there is an absence of leukocytes on UA, no treatment is indicated.

Uncomplicated Cystitis

There is no agreement on the most effective antimicrobial agent or dosage for treating a UTI (Fitzgerald et al, 2012). Short-term antibiotics of 3 to 5 days may be as effective in treating non-febrile bladder infections as standard 7- to 10-day dosing with no increased risk of recurrence (Elder, 2011d). Children 2 to 24 months old and febrile children should have 7 to 14 days of antibiotics. Specific recommendations for the febrile child can be found in the AAP Guideline (AAP Subcommittee on Urinary Tract Infection, Steering Committee on Quality Improvement and Management, 2011). Choice of antibiotic should be made based on regional antibiotic resistance patterns and culture and sensitivity results. Recommended oral medications include the following (Elder, 2011d; Lee et al, 2015):

- Trimethoprim-sulfamethoxazole (TMP-SMX): More than 2 months old—8 to 12 mg/kg TMP component in two divided doses; adolescents, 160 mg TMP component every 12 hours.
- Amoxicillin: Younger than 3 months old—20 to 30 mg/kg/day in two divided doses every 12 hours; older than 3 months old—25 to 50 mg/kg/day in two divided doses; adolescents, 250 to 500 mg every 8 hours or 875 mg every 12 hours.
- Amoxicillin clavulanate (doses for amoxicillin component): Younger than 3 months old—30 mg/kg/day in two divided doses; older than 3 months old—20 to 45 mg/kg/day in two or three divided doses; adolescents—250 to 500 mg every 8 hours or 875 mg every 12 hours.
- Cephalexin: 50 to 100 mg/kg/day divided in four doses and given every 6 hours (maximum dose of 4 g/day).
- Cefixime: Older than 6 months old—16 mg/kg/day divided every 12 hours for first day, then 8 mg/kg/day divided every 12 hours to complete 13-day treatment; adolescents—400 mg every 12 to 24 hours.
- Cefpodoxime proxetil: 2 months to 12 years old—10 mg/kg/day divided every 12 hours (maximum dose of 400 mg/day); adolescents—200 to 800 mg/day divided every 12 hours (maximum dose of 800 mg/day).
- Ciprofloxacin extended release: Older than 18 years old—500 mg once a day for 3 days.
- Nitrofurantoin: Older than 1 month old—5 to 7 mg/kg/day divided every 6 hours (maximum 400 mg/24 hours); adolescents—50 to 100 mg/dose every 6 hours (macrocrystals) or 100 mg twice a day (dual release).
- Recurrent UTI: Further evaluation required (ultrasound, if not done previously and VCUG). Use of prophylactic antibiotics (Box 35-1) is controversial
- Acute pyelonephritis: Oral therapy is equally as effective in treating pyelonephritis and preventing kidney damage as parenteral antimicrobials (Engorn and Flerlage, 2015).
  - Hospitalization is required if severity of symptoms warrants—dehydrated, vomiting, or not drinking. Children 1 month old and younger should be admitted and provided a parenteral regimen.
  - Young children with uncomplicated pyelonephritis (well hydrated, no vomiting, no abdominal pain) can be effectively treated with cefixime, ceftibuten, or amoxicillin clavulanate.
  - Adolescents with uncomplicated pyelonephritis can be treated with either amoxicillin clavulanate (875/125 mg twice a day) or ciprofloxacin (500 mg twice a day or extended release 1000 mg once a day).
- Follow-up urine culture should be done 48 to 72 hours after initiating treatment if symptoms persist or organism resistance is found in the community.
  - If the culture is not sterile or if no clinical improvement is seen, antibiotic change should be based on sensitivity report received. Urine should be sent for bacterial identification and sensitivity studies now if not performed initially and an alternative broad-spectrum antibiotic should be used pending those results. Culture should again be repeated after 48 to 72 hours if response to therapy limited.
- Follow-up cultures are not routinely needed; however, when obtained for recurrent problems should be obtained 3 to 7 days after finishing antibiotic treatment.
- Repeat urine culture should be done with any fever, illness, dysuria, or frequency.

• BOX 35-1 Radiologic Workup and Prophylaxis for Urinary Tract Infections

Why Do a Radiologic Workup?

- To identify any structural or functional abnormality of the urinary tract
- To identify any renal scarring or damage

Who Requires a Workup?

- Order a renal and bladder ultrasound on children with the first positive urine culture and with fever and systemic illness. In children with one or more infections of the lower urinary tract (dysuria, urgency, frequency, suprapubic pain), renal and bladder ultrasound may be considered; however, assessment and treatment of bladder and bowel dysfunction is most important (Elder, 2011d).
- If the renal ultrasound is abnormal, a DMSA or VCUG is indicated.

What Test Should Be Done and When?

- Renal and bladder ultrasound
- VCUG if ultrasound is positive or concerning clinical picture
- Nuclear imaging scan (DMSA): Done to detect renal scars or parenchymal inflammation and ideally done 6 months after infection when the inflammatory changes in the kidney have resolved (Elder, 2011e; Feld and Mattoo, 2010)
- IVP: Done if further definition of structure or function of the kidney is needed but is rarely indicated

What about Prophylaxis?

- There is controversy about if and when prophylaxis should be used (AAP Subcommittee on Urinary Tract Infection, Steering Committee on Quality Improvement and Management, 2011; Feld and Mattoo, 2010). If a decision to use prophylaxis is made and depending on the source, between one quarter to one half of the treatment dose of antibiotic may be given at bedtime.
  - Nitrofurantoin: Older than 2 months old: 1 to 2 mg/kg as a single daily dose; expensive; liquid form poorly tolerated; consider sprinkling capsules over applesauce, yogurt, pudding
  - TMP-SMX: TMP 2 mg/kg as a single daily dose or 5 mg/kg twice per week (based on TMP component) if older than 1 month
  - Cephalexin: 10 mg/kg as a single daily dose
  - Amoxicillin: 10 mg/kg as a single daily dose; can be used for a newborn or premature infant; not used past the first 2 postnatal months; shelf life for liquid is 14 days

DMSA, Dimercaptosuccinic acid; *IVP,* intravenous pyelogram; *TMP-SMX,* trimethoprim-sulfamethoxazole; *VCUG,* voiding cystourethrogram.

TABLE 35-3 Radiologic Studies Done for Evaluation of Urinary Tract Conditions

Study	Cost	Advantages	Disadvantages	Use
Ultrasound	Least expensive	Shows structure, shape, and growth Detects structural abnormality, obstruction, pyelonephritis, large scars Painless, low risk, no radiation, noninvasive, available	Does not detect small scars of VUR Poor visualization of ureters Does not measure renal function or transient injury to kidney	Initial evaluation with first UTI and follow-up
Voiding urosonography (VUS)		Uses second-generation contrast agent that is safe, sensitive, and is radiation-free method for detection and grading of VUR Superior to VCUG	Requires intravesical administration of contrast	May be used if ultrasound evaluation abnormal
Voiding cystourethrogram (VCUG) (radiographic)	Least expensive	Detects and grades VUR if high or low pressure, high or low bladder volumes, during voiding, during early or late bladder filling Visualizes bladder and urethra (especially in males) and diverticula	Does not detect obstruction, pyelonephritis, scars Greater radiation than with scan Requires intravesical administration of contrast	Indicated in infants and children with abnormal ultrasound
VCUG (nuclear)	More expensive	Visualizes bladder and reflux Constantly monitors for transient reflux Less radiation	Discomfort of catheterization No urethral visualization Unable to grade reflux	Follow-up of VUR to evaluate siblings of child with VUR Follow-up of surgery
Dimercaptosuccinic acid (DMSA) renal scan (nuclear)	Most expensive	Detects acute inflammation, scars, and obstruction Earlier detection of parenchymal damage—large or small scars, permanent or focal—than with IVP (1 to 3 years old)	Does not detect VUR or measure renal function Does not evaluate calyces, ureters, bladder, or urethra	Follow-up for fever of unknown origin and negative ultrasound in neonates To diagnose acute pyelonephritis To detect renal scars
Computed tomography (CT) (contrast)	Expensive	Detects obstruction, pyelonephritis, large scars	Does not detect small scars or VUR Risk of allergic reaction, acute renal failure	Trauma

IVP, Intravenous pyelogram; *UTI,* urinary tract infection; *VUR,* vesicoureteral reflux.

- Phenazopyridine may be given at 12 mg/kg/day for 6- to 12-year-olds and 200 mg for those older than 12 years old, three times a day for dysuria.
- Radiologic workup (Table 35-3) is recommended to identify any structural or functional abnormality of the urinary tract and any renal scarring or damage.
  - Children younger than 2 years old with the first UTI should have a renal and bladder ultrasound as soon as the urine is sterile or when the prescribed antibiotic has been completed. Additionally, all children with fever or diagnosed with pyonephritis or with recurrent UTIs should have a renal and bladder ultrasound. VCUG does not need to be done routinely with first febrile UTI. However, if ultrasound reveals hydronephrosis, scarring, or other atypical or concerning findings, DMSA scan should be completed. If DMSA scan is unavailable, VCUG can be utilized (Elder, 2011d).
  - DMSA scan may be recommended for children with a febrile UTI or when a diagnosis of pyelonephritis is uncertain. If the DMSA scan is abnormal, then a VCUG is recommended (Elder, 2011d).

Patient and Family Education, Prevention, and Prognosis

The following should be discussed with parents and/or patients:

- Clear explanation of the cause, potential complications, and overall treatment plan, including both short- and long-term plans.

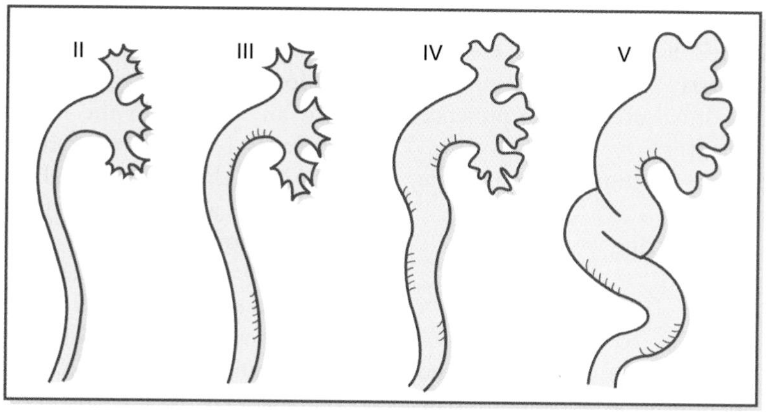

• **Figure 35-4** International reflux grading. Grade I (not shown): Ureter only. Grade II: Ureter, pelvis, and calyces; no dilation, normal calyceal fornices. Grade III: Mild or moderate dilation or tortuosity (or both) of ureter, and mild or moderate dilation of renal pelvis but no or slight blunting of the fornices. Grade IV: Moderate dilation or tortuosity (or both) of ureter and moderate dilation of renal pelvis and calyces. Complete obliteration of sharp angles of fornices but maintenance of papillary impressions in majority of calyces. Grade V: Gross dilation and tortuosity of ureter; gross dilation of renal pelvis and calyces; papillary impressions are no longer visible in majority of calyces. (From Lebowitz RL, Olbing H, Parkkulainen KV, et al: International system of radiographic grading of vesicoureteral reflux, International Reflux Study in Children, *Pediatr Radiol* 15[2]:105–109, 1985.)

- Frequent and complete voiding and increased quantities of fluids, especially water. Sometimes scheduled voiding times, voiding with knees spread apart, or double voiding (voiding and then immediately attempting to void again) can be helpful.
- Proper hygiene and avoiding irritants, such as bubble baths and perfumed soaps. Avoid wearing tight pants, especially spandex pants. Wear cotton underwear. Treat perineal inflammation to help prevent UTI.
- Treatment of constipation; pinworms.
- Sexually active females should be encouraged to drink water before intercourse and void immediately afterward.
- Decrease intake of bladder irritants, such as the "four Cs" (caffeine, carbonated beverages, chocolate, citrus), aspartame (NutraSweet), alcohol, and spicy foods.
- Importance of prompt medical attention with recurrence of fever and/or duration of fever for more than 48 hours, especially if younger than 24 months old.
- Cranberry juice is considered helpful in preventing the adherence of *E. coli* in the urethra but must be consumed in large quantities in order to be effective (see Chapter 43).

According to Fitzgerald and colleagues (2012), "The relationship between UTI, renal scarring, and VUR is unclear, as is the progression of uncomplicated UTI to pyelonephritis and subsequent damage to the kidneys." Major risk factors for renal damage include delay in treatment of pyelonephritis, younger than 1 year old, anatomic or neurogenic obstruction, severe reflux, dysplasia, and multiple infections. The same acute inflammatory process responsible for eradication of bacteria is also responsible for damage to renal tissue and subsequent scarring.

Vesicoureteral Reflux

VUR is regurgitation of urine from the bladder up into the ureters and potentially to the kidney. The major concern with VUR is the exposure of the kidney to infected urine and the potential to cause pyelonephritis. Primary VUR is the most common type and is typified by an abnormally short ureter and ineffective valve. Secondary VUR is due to bladder outlet obstruction and can be functional or structural. It is graded according to an international classification (Fig. 35-4). Grade I does not reach the renal pelvis; grade II extends up to the renal pelvis without dilation; grade III describes reflux to the renal pelvis with mild to moderate dilation of the ureter and the renal pelvis; grades IV and V (high grade) include definite distention of the ureters and renal pelvis and can include hydronephrosis or reflux into the intrarenal collecting system (Elder, 2011e).

VUR is the most common anatomic abnormality found in young infants and children with UTI. Approximately 30% to 40% of children with affected siblings have reflux, and 50% of children with affected mothers have reflux (Elder, 2011e). A meta-analysis identified that children who have UTIs more often and have associated bladder and bowel dysfunction are more at risk for renal scarring (Peters et al, 2010).

Clinical Findings

History

The history may be positive for a previous UTI, abnormal voiding pattern or dysfunction, unexplained febrile illness, chronic constipation, and/or UTI symptoms. History may be positive for VUR in related family members.

Diagnostic Studies

The following studies are ordered, as indicated, to identify obstructive uropathy and dysplasia:

- Ultrasonography (may be normal even in the presence of reflux)
- VCUG establishes the presence of reflux, determines the grade, and gives high detail
- DMSA scan to look for renal scarring

Management

The goal of treatment is the prevention of infection and subsequent scarring. Early identification and appropriate treatment of infection achieve this goal. Table 35-4 presents a summary of the American Urological Association (AUA) guideline on management of primary VUR (Peters et al, 2010). The guideline statements are labeled as standards, recommendations, and options based on the level of evidence and degree of flexibility in application.

- Most children outgrow their reflux, probably secondary to an increase in the intramural length of the ureter. Grades I and II reflux resolve spontaneously in up to 85% of children, grade III reflux resolves spontaneously in 50%, and grade IV reflux resolves spontaneously in 30%; however, grade V is unlikely to resolve spontaneously. VUR tends to resolve earlier in African American children. Older children who present with VUR and those with bilateral VUR tend to have lower rates of spontaneous resolution. Very few children with low-grade VUR require surgery (Elder, 2011e).
- Providers should treat underlying comorbidities, such as constipation and dysfunctional voiding.
- Prophylactic antibiotics may be used when a child has VUR to prevent UTI, pyelonephritis, renal injury, and

TABLE 35-4 Management of Primary Vesicoureteral Reflux in Children

	Standard*	Recommendation†	Option‡
Initial Evaluation of a Child with Vesicoureteral Reflux			
General evaluation	Thorough history and physical examination Measure weight, height, and BP Serum creatinine if bilateral renal cortical abnormalities are found	UA for proteinuria and bacteriuria; if UA indicates infection, obtain urine culture and sensitivities	Baseline serum creatinine may serve as an estimate of GFR
Imaging procedures	None	Renal ultrasound to assess upper urinary tract	DMSA renal imaging to assess the status of the kidneys for scarring and function
Assessment of voiding patterns	Information related to symptoms of BBD should be elicited, especially urinary frequency and urgency, prolonged voiding intervals, daytime wetting, perineal/penile pain, holding maneuvers to prevent wetting, and constipation or encopresis		
Family and patient education	Family and patient education should include a discussion of the rationale for treating VUR, the equivalency of certain treatment approaches, assessment of likely adherence to the treatment plan, determination of parental concerns, and accommodation of parental preferences when treatment options offer a similar risk-benefit balance		

TABLE 35-4 Management of Primary Vesicoureteral Reflux in Children—cont'd

Standard*	Recommendation†	Option‡
Initial Management of the Child with Vesicoureteral Reflux		
Child <1 year old with VUR	History of febrile UTI: Low-dose CAP is recommended because of the increased risk of morbidity from recurrent UTIs in this age group No history of febrile UTI: CAP is recommended with VUR grades III to V identified through screening	No history of febrile UTI: CAP may be offered for VUR grades I to II Circumcision may be considered: Goal of management of VUR is to prevent febrile UTI and renal injury and circumcised males have a decreased incidence of UTIs CAP may be considered in the absence of BBD Observation without CAP with prompt initiation of antibiotic therapy for UTI
Child >1 year old with UTI and VUR	If BBD is present, treatment of BBD is indicated before any surgical intervention Treatment options for BBD include behavioral therapy, biofeedback, anticholinergic medications, alpha-blockers, and treatment of constipation and encopresis Monitor effectiveness of BBD treatment CAP is recommended for the child with BBD and VUR due to the increased risk of UTI while BBD is present and being treated	Surgical intervention for VUR (both open and endoscopic methods) may be considered (even as initial therapy)
Follow-up management of the child with VUR	Ongoing monitoring of weight, height, BP; UA for proteinuria and bacteriuria (including culture and sensitivity if necessary) annually Ultrasound every 12 months to monitor renal growth and parenchymal scarring VCUG every 12 to 24 months with longer intervals in patients with lower rates of spontaneous resolution (grades III to V VUR) in order to limit the overall imaging studies performed DMSA imaging when renal ultrasound is abnormal, when there is a greater concern for scarring due to breakthrough UTI or grades III to V VUR, or if serum creatinine is elevated	Follow-up cystography may be an option: Grades I to II VUR because of high rate of spontaneous resolution A single normal VCUG can be used to establish resolution DMSA for follow-up of VUR to detect new renal scarring, especially after a febrile UTI

Continued

TABLE 35-4 Management of Primary Vesicoureteral Reflux in Children—cont'd

	Standard*	Recommendation†	Option‡
Interventions for the child with breakthrough UTI (BT-UTI)		Symptomatic BT-UTI (fever, dysuria, frequency, FTT, or poor feeding): A change in therapy is recommended; treat infection with appropriate antibiotic Child on CAP with BT-UTI: Consideration should be given for open surgical or endoscopic correction Child on CAP with a single BT-UTI without evidence of previous or new renal cortical abnormalities: Changing to an alternative antibiotic agent is an option before surgical correction Child not on CAP with BT-UTI: Initiation of CAP is recommended	Child not receiving CAP with afebrile UTI: Initiation of CAP is an option (not all pyelonephritis presents with fever) Surgical intervention for VUR may be used; studies have shown a reduction in the occurrence of febrile UTIs in patients who have had surgical correction compared with those on CAP
Follow-up management after resolution of VUR		Following spontaneous or surgical resolution of VUR: General evaluation, including monitoring weight, height, BP, and UA for protein and UTI, is recommended annually through adolescence if either kidney is found to be abnormal by ultrasound or DMSA scan With occurrence of febrile UTI following resolution of surgical treatment of VUR: Evaluation for BBD or recurrent VUR is recommended Long-term concerns of hypertension (especially during pregnancy), renal function loss, recurrent UTI, and familial VUR in the child's siblings and offspring should be discussed with family and child	Following spontaneous or surgical resolution of VUR if both kidneys are normal by ultrasound or DMSA scan: General evaluation, including monitoring weight, height, BP, and UA for protein and UTI, annually through adolescence is an option

Data from Peters CA, Skoog SJ, Arant BS Jr, et al: Summary of the American Urological Association guideline on management of primary vesicoureteral reflux in children, *J Urol* 184(3):1134–1144, 2010. The complete guideline is available at www.auanet.org/content/guidelines-and-quality-care/clinical-guidelines.cfm?sub=vur2010.

BBD, Bladder and bowel dysfunction; *BP,* blood pressure; *CAP,* continuous antibiotic prophylaxis; *DMSA,* dimercaptosuccinic acid; *FTT,* failure to thrive; *GFR,* glomerular filtration rate; *UA,* urinalysis; *UTI,* urinary tract infection; *VCUG,* voiding cystourethrogram; *VUR,* vesicoureteral reflux.

*Most rigid treatment policy.

†Less rigid; there is sufficient evidence, even if not highest quality, to advocate for a particular clinical approach.

‡Most flexible; evidence of relatively equal strength and quality supporting more than one approach; with any being acceptable or justifiable.

other sequelae. Prophylaxis for children younger than 1 year old and for grades II to IV in older children is recommended (AUA, 2010; Elder, 2011e), although a number of other studies have questioned the efficacy of prophylactic antibiotics for both VUR and recurrent UTI (Peters et al, 2010). Recommended medications used for prophylaxis should be given at bedtime and are listed in Box 35-1. The duration of prophylaxis depends on the age of the child, the severity of the VUR, patient compliance, presence of renal scarring, and recurrent infections on prophylaxis.

- Consideration of endoscopic surgery with the use of hyaluronic acid/dextranomer injected into the bladder at the ureter outlet is reporting good outcomes (Kaye et al, 2012) and may be considered at any stage of reflux from grades I to IV. Open surgery is reserved for higher grades of reflux and/or failed medical management.
- Interval urine cultures are performed with symptoms of unexplained illness.
- Repeat VCUG once 12 to 18 months after the diagnosis of reflux to monitor reflux and scarring. Routine follow-up studies are recommended every 1 to 2 years,

depending on the reflux grade, gender, and whether both or only one kidney is affected. BP and growth parameters should be checked at least yearly.
- Nephrology consultation is indicated in the presence of higher-grade reflux, notable scarring, a solitary or atrophic kidney, hypertension, elevated creatinine, or evidence of abnormal kidney function with any grade of reflux.

Patient and Family Education, Prevention, and Prognosis

- VUR does not cause scarring, infection does; but VUR is a risk factor for pyelonephritis and subsequent scarring. Prompt treatment of UTI should be instituted. Management, prevention of UTIs, and compliance must be understood by families. The necessity of urine culture with any suspicious symptoms should also be emphasized. The potential for untreated, chronic UTI leading to chronic renal disease must be explained. BP and growth should be monitored.
- Screen all siblings younger than 3 years old for VUR.
- Prophylactic medicines are best given at night because of urinary stasis while asleep.
- The guidelines discussed in the Patient and Family Education, Prevention, and Prognosis section of uncomplicated cystitis should be reviewed.

Preexisting renal damage may be present, and new renal scarring can occur. Children with grades I and II reflux usually have resolution of the reflux if infections are prevented or treated early. Reflux nephropathy is a common cause of hypertension; however, renal injury does not occur unless infection or high bladder pressures are present (Elder, 2011e).

Hematuria

Hematuria is defined as the presence of five or more RBCs per HPF in three consecutive fresh, centrifuged specimens obtained over several weeks (Pan and Avner, 2011b). The number of RBCs per HPF considered to be abnormal varies and ranges from any to more than 5 per HPF in unspun urine to more than 5 to 10 per HPF in spun urine. For management purposes, *hematuria* in this text is defined as more than two RBCs per HPF in unspun urine or five per HPF in spun urine. The term *gross hematuria* is related to the concentration of RBCs rather than to the location or significance of the disorder. Brownish, tea-colored urine with casts or protein is usually glomerular in origin. Clots and red-to-pink urine with isomorphic RBCs but no protein usually originates from the lower tract. Factors causing hematuria can arise anywhere in the urinary system, from the urinary meatus to the kidneys. Urine can be discolored and urine dipsticks can be positive for RBCs when there is myoglobinuria or hemoglobinuria, in which case no RBCs are seen on microscopic examination (Pan and Avner, 2011b), so dipstick hematuria should be confirmed via UA. Hematuria can be microscopic or macroscopic. Microscopic hematuria may be either persistent or transient.

The causes of macroscopic hematuria include hypercalciuria, immunoglobulin A (IgA) nephropathy, glomerulonephritis (GN), and idiopathic. UTI, hydronephrosis, tumor, cystitis cystica, polyps, or epididymitis are characterized by macrohematuria less than 1% of the time. However, 50% of children with gross hematuria have UTIs. The incidence of hematuria is 0.5% to 2% when confirmed with repeat UA (Pan and Avner, 2011b).

Clinical Findings

History

- Previous medical history of cystic kidney disease, sickle cell disease, systemic lupus erythematosus (SLE), malignancy
- Family or previous history of hematuria, nephrolithiasis, cystic kidney, hemoglobinopathy, sickle cell disease or trait, SLE, hypertension, congestive heart disease, malignancy, deafness, renal failure
- Preceding illness: Viral or streptococcal pharyngitis or impetigo
- Onset, duration, pattern, and timing of hematuria; color of urine
- Dysuria, urgency, frequency or enuresis
- Presence of pain (back, abdominal, or flank) with voiding
- Straining or squatting with urination (tumor)
- Strenuous exercise or trauma (including bladder catheterization)
- Trauma, foreign body
- Sexual activity or abuse
- Current menstruation
- Edema, rash, pallor, or arthralgias
- Certain drugs (sulfonamides, nitrofurantoin, salicylates, phenazopyridine, toxins [lead, benzenes]) and foods (food color, beets, blackberries, rhubarb, and paprika) can discolor the urine but will not result in RBCs in the urine (Pan and Avner, 2011b)
- Symptoms related to chronic renal disease (Box 35-2)

• BOX 35-2 Seven "Red Flags" for Chronic Renal Failure

1. FTT (poor growth, fatigue, anorexia, nausea, gastroesophageal reflux, vomiting)
2. Chronic anemia (normochromic, normocytic, nonresponsive to medication)
3. Complicated enuresis (daytime frequency, urgency, incontinence, chronic constipation, encopresis, infrequent voiding, straining to void, recurrent UTI)
4. Prolonged, unexplained vomiting or nausea (especially in the morning), anorexia, weight loss without diarrhea
5. Hypotension
6. Unusual bone disease (e.g., rickets, valgus deformity, fracture with minor trauma)
7. Poor school performance (e.g., headache, fatigue, inattention, withdrawal from activities)

FTT, Failure to thrive; *UTI,* urinary tract infection.

Physical Examination

- Growth parameters: FTT or falling growth curves (chronic renal insufficiency or long-standing acidosis)
- Vital signs, especially BP
- Malformed ears (congenital renal disease)
- Oliguria or anuria
- Edema, hypertension, and proteinuria, which are suggestive of glomerular disease
- Flank pain, which is suggestive of an upper tract disorder
- Abdominal or flank mass, which suggests an obstruction, such as Wilms tumor, cystic disease, or posterior valves
- External genitalia: Excoriation, bleeding, foreign body, abuse

Diagnostic Studies

- Urine dipstick analysis for pyuria, proteinuria, hematuria, and concentration
  - If greater than 1+ hematuria by dipstick (which equals three RBCs/HPF or 0.02 mg/dL hemoglobin), microscopic examination for RBCs is needed to differentiate RBCs from hemoglobinuria or myoglobinuria.
  - The most significant differentiating factor is the presence of proteinuria. If present, rapid evaluation and early referral to a nephrologist are essential. See section on Nephrotic Syndrome.
- Microscopic examination of the urine includes RBCs, size and shape of the cells, casts, crystals, and WBCs
  - Distorted, misshapen RBCs of different sizes suggest glomerular disease.
  - Crystalluria is most commonly caused by hypercalciuria.
- Urine culture
- 24-hour urine collection
- First morning UA on first-degree relatives
- Renal ultrasound if Wilms tumor or nephrolithiasis is suspected. Spiral helical computed tomography (CT) scan is the most sensitive modality for diagnosing nephrolithiasis, but there is a large radiation exposure (Pan and Avner, 2011b).
- If there are systemic symptoms (e.g., edema, hypertension, changes in urine output), consider further evaluation as described in the Nephritis and Glomerulonephritis section (Pan and Avner, 2011a)
- Renal biopsy is recommended for recurrent gross hematuria and coexisting nephritic syndrome, hypertension, renal insufficiency, systemic illness, and parent anxiety (Pan and Avner, 2011b)
- Cystoscopy, which is invasive and costly, is rarely used in children

Differential Diagnosis

Categories of hematuria to be considered in the diagnostic workup of hematuria are (Pan and Avner, 2011b):

- Gross hematuria
  - Urine color is red or tea-colored; microscopic examination shows RBCs.
  - Common causes are poststreptococcal glomerulonephritis (PSGN), renal disease, UTI, trauma, coagulopathy, crystalluria, and nephrolithiasis. Recurrent episodes of gross hematuria are rare.
  - Consider Henoch-Schönlein purpura (HSP) when there is gross hematuria in the presence of abdominal pain, with or without bloody stools, arthralgias, and purpuric rash (see Chapter 25).
  - Consider IgA nephropathy with gross hematuria in the presence of acute illness or strenuous exercise.
  - Sickle cell disease and trait can cause recurrent gross hematuria (mostly males, unilateral kidney).
  - Rhabdomyosarcoma causes gross hematuria and voiding dysfunction (Pan and Avner 2011b).
- Symptomatic microscopic hematuria
  - Greatest attention and methodic approach are required. History and physical examination guide the workup.
  - Renal disease is more likely if microscopic hematuria is accompanied by proteinuria on a first morning sample.
- Other nonspecific symptoms (fever, malaise, weight change), extrarenal symptoms (malar rash, purpura, arthritis, headache, dysuria, abdominal or flank pain, edema, oliguria) may be present.
- Asymptomatic microscopic hematuria rarely indicates significant renal disease.
  - Family history is important to assess for benign familial hematuria.
  - Hypercalciuria is commonly associated with asymptomatic microscopic hematuria, which leaves patients prone to symptomatic urolithiasis. The diagnosis is made by laboratory examination of urine. The spot calcium-creatinine ratio done on the first morning specimen is elevated to more than 0.2, or the 24-hour urinary calcium to more than 4 mg/kg/day. Hypercalciuria is also associated with immobilization, diuretics, vitamin D intoxication, hyperparathyroidism, and sarcoidosis (Pan and Avner, 2011b).
  - Regularly monitor for hypertension and proteinuria.
- Asymptomatic hematuria with proteinuria is worrisome for renal disease and further evaluation for renal problems is required.
- Consider evaluating for orthostatic proteinuria (see Proteinuria section). Persistent proteinuria is more indicative of a glomerular process.
- Other differential diagnoses to consider include:
  - Pseudohematuria occurs when a false-positive dipstick reading is noted, but no RBCs are found on the microscopic examination. The two most common causes are myoglobinuria and hemoglobinuria (see Table 35-1).
  - Extrarenal hematuria is common with systemic bleeding disorders and is evidenced by macroscopic and microscopic hematuria.
  - Although rare, renal stones (nephrolithiasis) or calcification (nephrocalcinosis) can occur. If suspected, a

renal ultrasonogram can be included as part of the workup.

- Hematuria caused by external irritation of the urinary meatus will resolve with healing and removal of the offending irritant (diaper rash, soaps, bubble bath, lotions) or avoidance of the offending behavior (e.g., scratching, masturbation, sexual activity).

Management

A progressive approach to evaluating hematuria should be undertaken with the goal of not overlooking serious, treatable, progressive conditions while at the same time avoiding unnecessary studies (Fig. 35-5). Referral is indicated if there is gross hematuria if the cause is unclear, symptomatic

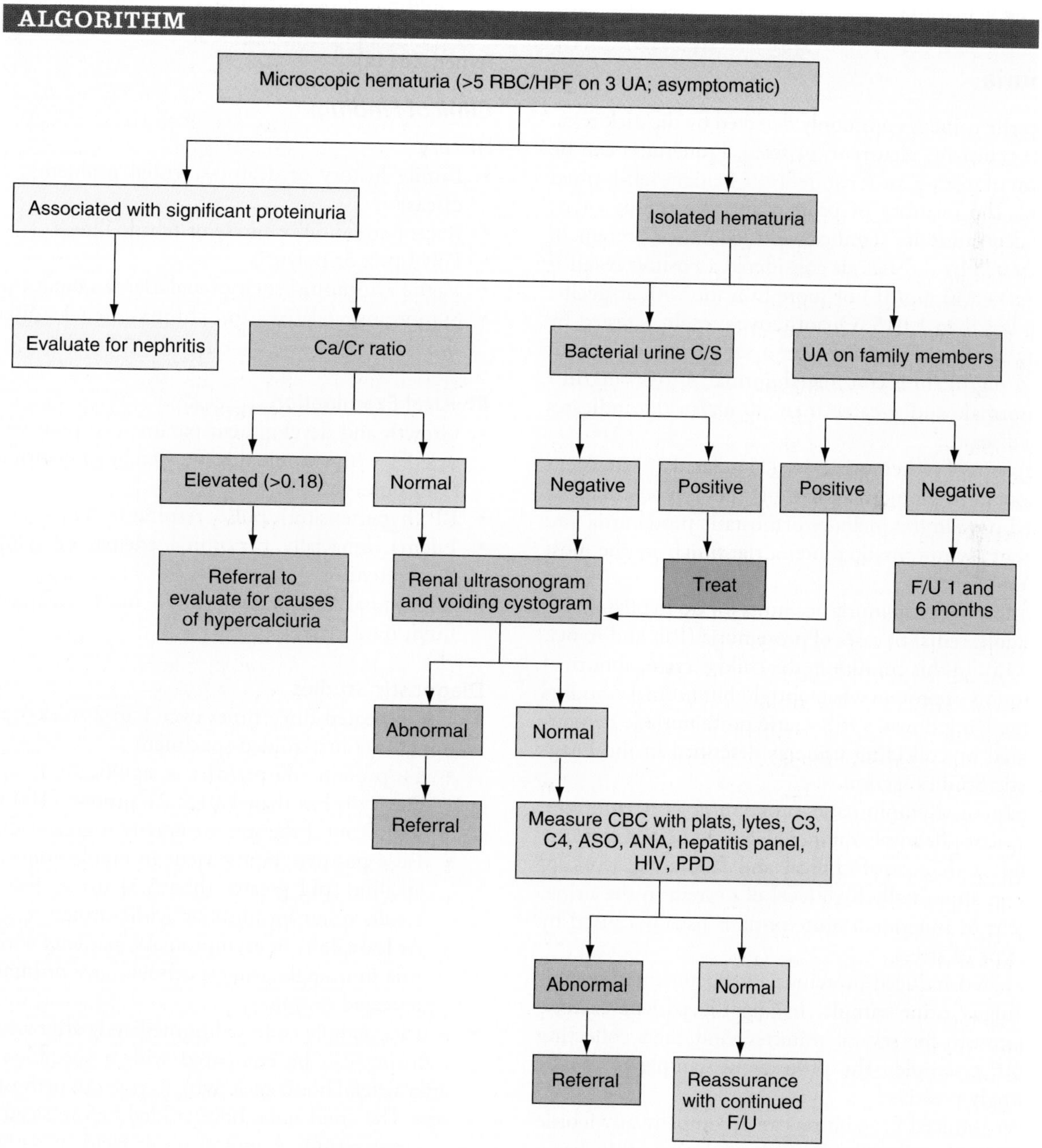

• **Figure 35-5** Management of asymptomatic microscopic hematuria algorithm. *ANA,* Antinuclear antibody; *ASO,* antistreptolysin O; *C3,* complement 3; *C4,* complement 4; *Ca/Cr,* calcium/creatinine ratio; *CBC,* complete blood count; *C/S,* culture/sensitivity; *F/U,* follow-up; *HIV,* human immunodeficiency virus; *lytes,* electrolytes; *plats,* platelets; *PPD,* purified protein derivative; *RBC/HPF,* red blood cells per high-power field; *UA,* urinalysis. (Adapted from Dershewitz RA, editor: *Ambulatory pediatric care*, ed 3, Philadelphia, 1999, Lippincott-Raven.)

microscopic hematuria, or persistent asymptomatic hematuria and proteinuria as renal biopsy may be indicated (Pan and Avner, 2011b). Asymptomatic hematuria requires periodic evaluation every 1 to 2 years to reevaluate for coexisting conditions or proteinuria and to revisit family history of hematuria or hearing deficits.

Patient and Family Education, Prevention, and Prognosis

Patient education should stress the importance of follow-up for evaluation of the hematuria. Prognosis depends on the cause of the hematuria.

Proteinuria

Protein in the urine is commonly detected by dipstick tests. It may be transient, recurrent, or fixed. Proteinuria can be a symptom of disease, or it can reflect a benign, self-limited condition. The quantity of protein and the timing of its presence determine its significance. Qualitative protein in urine, as tested by dipstick, is considered a positive result if it registers 1+ (30 mg/dL) or more in urine with a specific gravity of less than 1.015. Quantitative protein is tested by measuring a volume of urine over a set period. A level of less than 4 $mg/m^2/hr$ is considered normal, 4 to 40 $mg/m^2/hr$ is abnormal, and greater than 40 $mg/m^2/hr$ indicates nephritic disease.

Four groups of proteinuria exist: (1) isolated, (2) transient or functional, (3) glomerular, and (4) tubulointerstitial.

- Isolated proteinuria includes orthostatic proteinuria and persistent asymptomatic proteinuria, which are the most common.
  - Orthostatic proteinuria accounts for up to 60% (75% in adolescents) of cases of proteinuria (Pais and Avner, 2011a). In this condition, the child excretes abnormal amounts of protein when upright but normal amounts when lying down. Orthostatic proteinuria is demonstrated by collecting urine as described in the Diagnostic Studies section.
  - Persistent asymptomatic proteinuria is a common, transient phenomenon in which an otherwise healthy child, with normal clinical and laboratory workup, has an abnormally high level of protein in the urine.
- Transient or functional proteinuria is usually caused by some type of stress.
  - Exercised-induced proteinuria is documented by collecting a urine sample, having the patient exercise vigorously for several minutes, and then collecting another sample. The postexercise sample is usually strongly positive.
  - Fever-induced proteinuria can accompany any febrile state and usually subsides with resolution of the fever. Other stress-related causes include cold exposure, infection, congestive heart failure, and seizures. This type of proteinuria usually resolves in 1 to 2 weeks, and if resolution has been verified, no further workup is required.
- Glomerular proteinuria and tubulointerstitial proteinuria are the least common types and are characterized by high levels of proteinuria. Some authorities believe that children with persistent proteinuria, even at low levels, should be followed with a high index of suspicion for an underlying, progressive renal disorder.

Proteinuria originates from problems with glomerular filtration, tubular reabsorption or secretion, or both. The child is often asymptomatic. If proteinuria is significant enough to cause hypoproteinemia, edema is present. The incidence of proteinuria is cited at 30% to 55% in school-age children. It persists, however, in up to 6% of children when four consecutive urine specimens are tested (Pais and Avner, 2011a).

Clinical Findings

History

- Family history of deafness, visual problems, and renal disease
- Recent strenuous exercise or febrile illness
- Polydipsia or polyuria
- Vague symptoms, such as malaise, fatigue, or pallor
- Symptoms related to chronic renal disease (see Box 35-2)

Physical Examination

- Growth and development parameters (poor weight gain or FTT with chronic disease; weight gain with nephrotic syndrome)
- BP (hypertension), pulse, respiratory rate
- Edema, especially periorbital edema, or symptoms of fluid retention
- Abdominal examination for a mass, enlarged kidney, fluid, tenderness

Diagnostic Studies

- UA (repeated three times over 1 to 2 weeks), preferably done on a first-voided specimen:
  - 1+ protein (30 mg/dL) is significant if the specific gravity is less than 1.015; 2+ protein (100 mg/dL) is significant if the specific gravity is greater than 1.015.
  - False-positive results occur in highly concentrated or alkaline (pH greater than 5.5) urine. False-negative results occur in dilute or acidic urine.
  - At least 75% of asymptomatic patients with proteinuria in a single urine specimen have normal urine on repeated testing.
- A urine sample collected immediately after arising in the morning can be compared with a specimen collected after several hours of activity to rule out orthostatic etiology. The child must have voided before sleep to obtain accurate results. A typical result yields negative to trace amounts on the first-morning specimen, but 1+ or greater on the second specimen. If the result is equivocal, back-to-back urine samples (from arising to bedtime and bedtime to arising) can be evaluated for quantitative protein.

- Microscopic urine: RBCs or WBCs (or both), casts, bacteria, oval fat bodies, or other abnormalities are present in most pathologic conditions.
- A urine protein-to-creatinine ratio on a first morning voided sample. Normal values are less than 0.5 mg/dL in children younger than 2 years old and less than 0.2 mg/dL in children older than 2 years; greater than 2 mg/dL is considered nephritic (Pais and Avner, 2011a). An abnormal urine protein-to-creatinine ratio requires further testing.
- A 12- or 24-hour timed urine collection for creatinine (normal: 14 to 20 mg/kg/24 hr) and protein excretion (normal: less than 4 $mg/m^2/hr$) is elevated with proteinuria. A back-to-back sample collection (see earlier) is done to compare active or upright and resting levels.
- If protein in urine is greater than 4 $mg/m^2/hr$, check the CBC, electrolytes, BUN, creatinine, albumin/total protein, C3, C4, cholesterol, liver functions, and urine culture. Perform an ultrasonogram, VCUG, and radionuclide scans as indicated. Evaluate for systemic disease as indicated (e.g., antinuclear antibody [ANA], antistreptolysin O [ASO], streptozyme, hepatitis B, human immunodeficiency virus [HIV], tuberculosis).

Differential Diagnosis

Pseudoproteinuria can be caused by semisynthetic penicillins or anti-inflammatory agents.

Management

The persistence, quantity, and presence of other abnormalities (e.g., hematuria) are key in evaluating proteinuria (Fig. 35-6).

- If protein by dipstick is trace or 1+ and specific gravity is greater than 1.015, offer reassurance; do monthly recheck of urine for 4 to 6 months. If protein is persistent, refer the patient to a nephrologist.
- If protein by dipstick is greater than 1+, evaluate the child for orthostatic proteinuria (see Fig. 35-9)
- If first morning urine protein is 1+ or 2+, perform either a quantitative 12- to 24-hour urine protein excretion test or a random urine total protein-creatinine ratio and UA with microscope. Proceed as shown in Figure 35-6.
- If protein by dipstick is greater than 2+, evaluate for nephrotic syndrome (see later section).
- If hematuria is present, evaluate for nephritis (see later section).
- Follow-up is important to monitor for any change in status.
- Refer to a nephrologist if persistent unexplained nonorthostatic proteinuria, any hematuria or RBC or WBC casts, polyuria or oliguria, nephrotic levels of protein, elevated BUN or creatinine, elevated BP, systemic complaints (e.g., joint pain, rashes, or arthralgias), or a child with a family history of renal failure, GN, sensorineural hearing loss, or kidney transplantation.

Patient and Family Education, Prevention, and Prognosis

Patient education should stress the importance of follow-up to evaluate the cause of proteinuria. Children with mild asymptomatic proteinuria who have a normal first-morning specimen do not require extensive testing for kidney disease but should be monitored annually.

Nephrotic Syndrome

Nephrotic syndrome is due to excessive excretion of protein in urine as a result of alterations in the integrity of the glomerular filtration barrier. The main mechanism of the massive protein loss is increased glomerular permeability. The loss can be selective (albumin only) or nonselective (including most serum proteins), and such selectivity is an important distinction in diagnosis. The classic definition of nephrotic syndrome is massive proteinuria (3 to 4+ protein with UA, greater than 40 $mg/m^2/hr$ or a protein : creatinine ratio on a first morning void of greater than 2 to 3 : 1), hypoalbuminemia (less than 2.5 g/dL), edema, and hyperlipidemia. Edema formation results from a decrease in the plasma oncotic pressure due to a loss of serum albumin, which causes water to extravasate into the interstitial space. This then leads to decreased intravascular volume with decreased renal perfusion and activation of the renin-angiotensin system (Pais and Avner, 2011b). With protein loss, the liver increases its synthesis of protein and thereby causes concurrent hyperlipidemia and lipiduria. In addition, the reduced intravascular volume stimulates antidiuretic hormone, which enhances the reabsorption of water. Nephrotic syndrome can be congenital, idiopathic, or secondary.

- Congenital (early onset) can be associated with genetic mutation or congenital infection (Lennon et al, 2010). It can be associated with other syndromes and is generally not responsive to corticosteroids.
- Ninety percent of the children who have nephritic syndrome have idiopathic nephritic syndrome. There are five histologic types of idiopathic nephritic syndrome: (1) minimal change disease (minimal change nephrotic syndrome [MCNS]), (2) mesangial proliferation, (3) focal segmental glomerulosclerosis, (4) membranous nephropathy, and (5) membranoproliferative GN. MCNS is the most common type of nephritic syndrome and is found in 85% of the children younger than 6 years old. Focal segmental glomerulosclerosis accounts for 20% to 30% of the cases of nephrotic syndrome in adolescents (Pais and Avner, 2011b).
- Secondary nephrotic syndrome occurs in association with or secondary to systemic disorders (e.g., SLE, HSP), infectious processes (e.g., syphilis, hepatitis B, HIV, or malaria), drug toxicities (e.g., nonsteroidal anti-inflammatory drugs [NSAIDs], mephenytoin), allergens, or other renal disorders (e.g., IgA or congenital nephritis). Secondary nephritis should be suspected in children

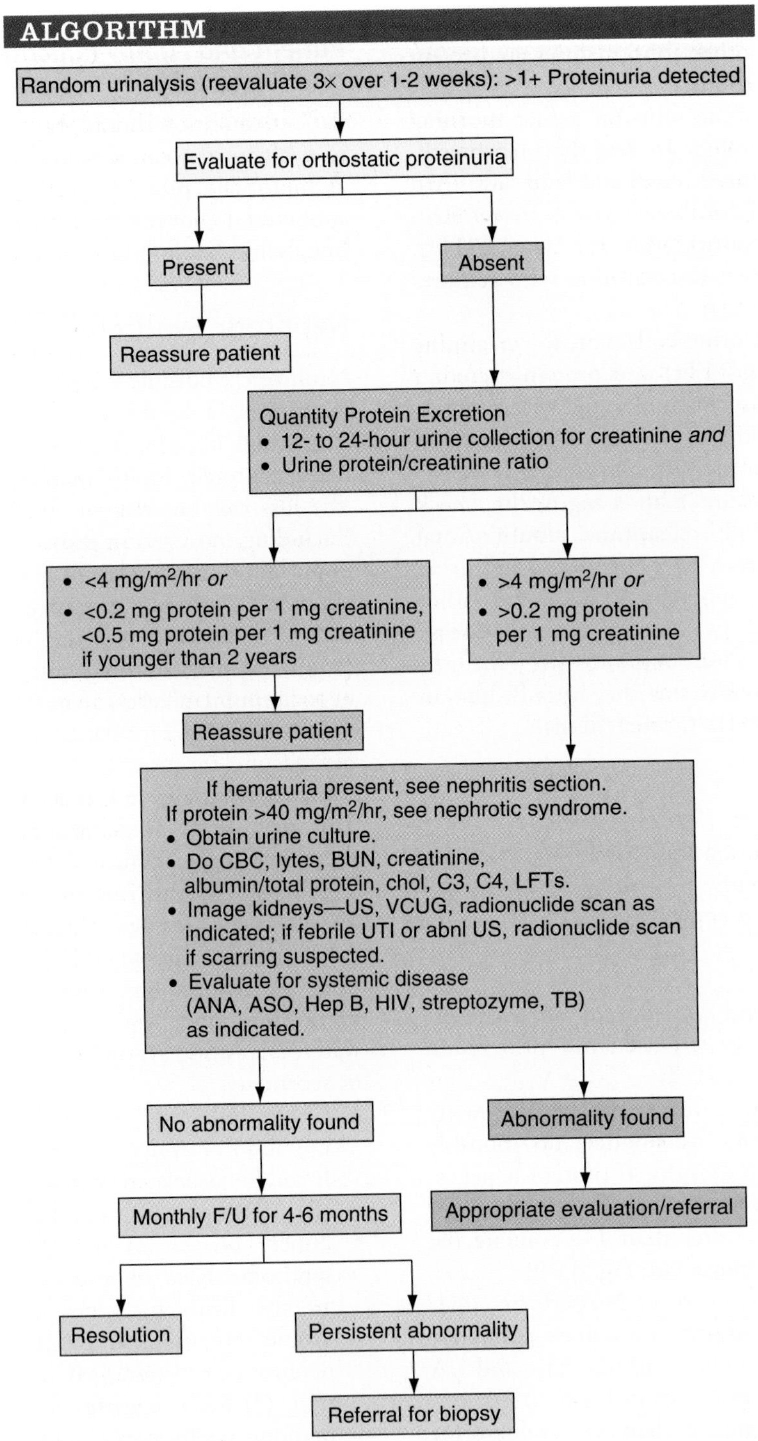

• **Figure 35-6** Evaluation of proteinuria algorithm. *abnl,* Abnormal; *ANA,* antinuclear antibody; *ASO,* antistreptolysin O; *BUN,* blood urea nitrogen; *C3,* complement 3; *C4,* complement 4; *CBC,* complete blood count; *chol,* cholesterol; *F/U,* follow-up; *Hep B,* hepatitis B; *HIV,* human immunodeficiency virus; *LFT,* liver function test; *lytes,* electrolytes; *TB,* tuberculosis; *US,* ultrasound; *UTI,* urinary tract infection; *VCUG,* voiding cystourethrogram. (Adapted from Dershewitz RA, editor: *Ambulatory pediatric care*, ed 3, Philadelphia, 1999, Lippincott-Raven.)

older than 8 years old who present with hypertension, hematuria, and other systemic symptoms of disease (Pais and Avner, 2011b).

Nephrotic syndrome is a chronic disease characterized by periods of remission (when both the urinary protein excretion and serum albumin normalize) and relapses (recurrence of proteinuria and hypoalbuminemia after complete remission). Ninety-five percent of the children with MCNS are "steroid responders," having remission with steroid treatment. Steroid responsiveness is the best prognostic indicator for nephrotic syndrome (Pais and Avner, 2011). Of the remaining children, most are steroid resistant and show no response to steroid treatment. A small number of cases are either partial responders with minimal response to steroids or are steroid dependent and require high doses of prednisone with frequent relapses.

Nephrotic syndrome occurs as a result of genetic, immune, systemic, nephrotoxic, allergic, infectious, malignant, vascular, or idiopathic processes. The actual mechanism of nephrotic syndrome has been extensively studied, and the understanding of its histopathology is better than the understanding of its pathogenesis. The primary mechanism is believed to be immunologic. The incidence of idiopathic nephrotic syndrome in the United States is 2 to 3 per 100,000 per year, with a 15 times greater incidence in children than in adults (Pais and Avner, 2011b). Thirty percent to 60% of children with nephrotic syndrome have a history of atopic disease, and 3% have a family history of a similar nephrotic syndrome (Lennon et al, 2010).

Clinical Findings

History

- History of allergy in up to 50% of children with MCNS
- Edema is the cardinal clinical feature, especially periorbital edema, dependent areas (tight shoes or underwear), and lax tissues (puffy eyes).
- Low urine production
- Gastrointestinal symptoms: Anorexia, paleness, listlessness, diarrhea, vomiting, abdominal pain (right upper quadrant)
- Respiratory difficulties secondary to ascites, effusion, pneumonia if advanced disease

Physical Examination

- Edema initially in tissues of low resistance and dependent: Periorbital, scrotal, and labial. If generalized, can become massive (anasarca)
- Anorexia, irritability, fatigue, abdominal discomfort, and diarrhea
- Muscle wasting, malnourishment, growth failure if prolonged
- If the disease is progressive, hydrothorax with respiratory difficulty
- Hypertension; normal BP if hypovolemic
- Chronically ill-appearing

Diagnostic Studies

- UA and microscopic examination (protein of 2+ or greater, hyaline and fine granular casts, microhematuria [in 33%], elevated specific gravity, fat bodies, and casts in urine).
- Quantitative urine protein excretion (24-hour collection or protein-creatinine ratio on a random first-morning urine).
- CBC; electrolytes, BUN, creatinine (normal); calcium; serum albumin (less than 2 g/dL), total protein; liver enzymes; triglycerides, lipoproteins, cholesterol (elevated); C3 and C4 (normal); ANA; varicella antibody test in case of exposure while on corticosteroids (Lennon et al, 2010).
- Consideration of Venereal Disease Research Laboratory (VDRL), hepatitis B surface antigen, HIV, malaria, purified protein derivative (PPD) as indicated by history.
- Neonatal or infant nephrotic syndrome requires a karyotype because male pseudohermaphroditism can be associated with Denys-Drash syndrome.
- Referral with possible kidney biopsy is recommended if criteria for MCNS are not met, systemic disease is present, hypertension and hematuria are present, hypocomplementemia or nonselective proteinemia is present, patient is older than 7 years or an adolescent, patient is nonresponsive to steroids, or if relapses are frequent.

Differential Diagnosis

Infants (newborn to 1 year old) usually have congenital renal problems, children 7 years old and older are likely to have focal glomerulosclerosis or mesangial proliferative GN, and teens have membranous nephropathy. The differential diagnosis includes hypoproteinemia from starvation, liver disease, and protein-losing enteropathy; none of these conditions has associated proteinuria. GN should also be considered in the differential diagnosis.

Management

Nephrotic syndrome is a complex, often chronic disorder that responds to careful management with a gratifying long-term positive outcome. The diagnosis is made with 95% certainty on clinical impressions. A major goal is to control edema while awaiting definitive remission.

- Consultation with and/or referral to a nephrologist should occur because of the constantly changing strategies for managing these children.
- Hospitalization may be necessary initially if disease is severe.
- Prednisone (2 mg/kg/day; maximum 60 mg) to induce remission, which can occur as early as 14 days as evidenced by diuresis. Steroids are continued for at least 4 to 6 weeks. A crushed or quartered pill is economical and often easier to give than liquid. Once remission occurs, steroid therapy is tapered and weaned over several months. There is less chance of relapse if corticosteroids are continued for several months after the first episode of nephrotic syndrome (Pais and Avner, 2011b). Relapses are treated with a short course of steroids and the patient is weaned as soon as the proteinuria resolves.
- Non-corticosteroid medications (cyclophosphamide and cyclosporine) are used by nephrologists if the child is steroid-dependent, steroid-resistant, or relapses frequently (Pais and Avner, 2011b).
- Activity and diet recommendations: No limitation is placed on activity. During active disease, salt may be restricted by nephrology. At other times, a diet appropriate for age is recommended.
- Diuretics and albumin replacement are sometimes used in the acute phase. Home BP monitoring may be recommended.
- Daily home proteinuria testing may be recommended to monitor the child and identify exacerbations as soon as

possible. Relapses are defined as persistent proteinuria greater than 2+ every day for 3 days.

- Routine immunizations should be given according to schedule but during remissions and when the child is on minimal immunosuppression. Live vaccines, including varicella, can be given after steroid therapy has been discontinued for 1 month (Pais and Avner, 2011b). Annual influenza vaccine is also recommended.
- Monitoring and prompt treatment of infection are essential as infection is a major complication of nephritic syndrome. Sepsis workup should be done with any fever and broad-spectrum antibiotics given until the organism is identified (Pais and Avner, 2011b). Immunosuppressed children who are exposed to varicella zoster must be given varicella-zoster immune globulin within 96 hours of exposure to prevent the disease.

Complications

Children with nephrotic syndrome are susceptible to pneumococcal, *E. coli, Pseudomonas,* and *Haemophilus influenzae* infection because of fluid stasis; such infection is seen as peritonitis, pneumonia, cellulitis, or septicemia. Hypertension or hypotension is a possibility. Because the child is in a hypercoagulable state, thromboembolism is possible. Protein losses and compromising edema are also potential complications.

Patient and Family Education, Prevention, and Prognosis

Patient education should stress the importance of continued, regular care to monitor renal function and the early treatment of the disease or concurrent infections. Families must know that relapses are the rule. An understanding of the disease process, side effects of steroids, recognition of infection, and the importance of monitoring proteinuria for relapses is crucial. If chronic steroid treatment is needed, the child and family must understand the side effects of the medication. The prognosis is good in steroid responders, with relapses that decrease in frequency as the child grows older, typically without any residual renal dysfunction.

Nephritis and Glomerulonephritis

Nephritis is a noninfectious, inflammatory response of the kidneys characterized by varied degrees of hypertension, edema, proteinuria, and hematuria that can be either microscopic or macroscopic with dysmorphic RBCs and casts. Nephritis is classified as acute, intermittent, or chronic. Primary GN occurs when the original and predominant structure impaired is the glomerulus. Secondary GN occurs when renal involvement is secondary to systemic disease (e.g., SLE, HSP, primary vasculitis, Goodpasture syndrome, or drug hypersensitivity reactions). Involvement can be in the glomerulus or the interstitium and either localized in one part of the kidney or generalized throughout. GN refers to inflammation primarily in the glomeruli; interstitial nephritis refers to inflammation in the interstitium primarily caused by drug reactions. PSGN is the classic form of GN.

Acute nephritis most commonly occurs as PSGN, which is characterized by a history of streptococcal infection within the prior 2 weeks and an acute onset of edema, oliguria, hypertension, and gross hematuria. Consider an alternative diagnosis if the following findings are present: nephrotic levels of protein, lack of evidence for a post-infection mechanism, rapidly deteriorating renal function, or clinical or laboratory findings suggesting other forms of GN (e.g., rash, positive ANA).

Intermittent gross hematuria and proteinuria syndromes include the following:

- IgA nephropathy, or Berger disease, is the most common chronic GN in children of European Asian descent and is uncommon in African Americans; it has a 2 : 1 male preponderance. It is an immunologic entity causing recurrent gross and microscopic hematuria and often proteinuria. It is present in about one third of persons biopsied for persistent microscopic hematuria. It is often precipitated by viral infections or strenuous exercise, and each episode lasts less than 72 hours. BP is normal, no edema is present, and C3 is normal. Definitive diagnosis is made by biopsy. The prognosis is good in the absence of elevated serum creatinine or nephrotic-range proteinuria, although progression to chronic renal insufficiency can occur.
- Hereditary or familial nephritis involves many disorders, but the best known is Alport syndrome. More common and severe in males, with onset before 15 years old in 75% of children, this condition is inherited as an X-linked dominant trait. The initial manifestation is isolated, persistent, microscopic hematuria with intermittent macrohematuria and variable proteinuria, occurring with an upper respiratory infection or exercise. Laboratory abnormalities are variable; biopsy verifies the diagnosis. Extrarenal abnormalities, including neurogenic deafness, ocular abnormalities, and macrothrombocytopenia, are often found. Vision and hearing screening are essential with referral for any abnormalities. Severe forms of the disease can lead to end-stage renal disease, which is often heralded by hypotension.
- Familial or benign recurrent nephritis, also known as *thin-basement-membrane disease,* is a disorder inherited as an autosomal dominant trait with unknown etiology. Episodes are characterized by macroscopic and microscopic hematuria and mild proteinuria, often precipitated by upper respiratory tract infection. Laboratory values other than UA are normal. The diagnosis is confirmed by biopsy, which may not be needed if the disease is mild and confirmed in relatives. In the absence of notable proteinuria, deafness, ocular defects, renal failure, and with normal biopsy findings, the prognosis is excellent.

Chronic nephritis is most commonly known as *membranoproliferative GN* and is distinguished by four types based on biopsy. Chronic nephritis can be found after acute nephritis or when investigating nonspecific complaints, such as anorexia, intermittent vomiting, and malaise. It is manifested by diminished renal function that ultimately has detrimental effects on other organ systems. Types I and II may respond to steroids, but the overall prognosis is guarded. Pyelonephritis, discussed earlier in the Pyelonephritis section, is inflammation of the renal parenchyma, calyces, and pelvis caused by bacteria.

The inflammatory response of the kidneys results from various causes, such as infection, an immunologic response, a drug or toxin, and vascular or systemic disorders. PSGN is an immune response by the host to a group A beta-hemolytic streptococcal infection, whereas acute postinfectious glomerulonephritis (APGN) can be caused by bacterial, fungal, viral, parasitic, or rickettsial agents.

PSGN is the most common form of nephritis in childhood, occurs most often between 5 and 12 years old, occurs more often in males (2:1), and is unusual in children younger than 3 years old. The incidence of APGN is difficult to determine because of the large number of patients with subclinical cases (Pan and Avner, 2011a).

Clinical Findings

History

- Streptococcal skin (more likely) or pharyngeal infection within the past 2 to 3 weeks (PSGN). Classically a latent period of 7 to 10 days elapses between infection and the onset of symptoms; if fewer than 5 days or more than 14 days, consider other causes.
- Abrupt onset of gross hematuria.
- Reduced urine output (with diuresis in 5 to 7 days).
- Lethargy, anorexia, nausea, vomiting, abdominal pain.
- Chills, fever, backache (pyelonephritis).
- Medication taken in the past few weeks.

Physical Examination

- Hypertension that is transient and resolves in 1 to 2 weeks
- Edema, especially periorbital edema, or abrupt onset with weight gain
- Circulatory congestion—dyspnea, cough, pallor, pulmonary edema if severe
- Ear malformations
- Flank or abdominal pain or a mass (in polycystic kidney or malignancy [e.g., Wilms tumor])
- Costovertebral angle tenderness (in pyelonephritis)
- Rashes or arthralgias (with SLE, HSP, or impetigo)
- Evidence of trauma or abuse

Diagnostic Studies

- UA with microscopic examination—tea color; elevated specific gravity; macrohematuria and microhematuria; proteinuria not exceeding the amount of hematuria; pyuria in PSGN; granular, hyaline, WBC, or RBC casts; and dysmorphic RBCs
- Serum C3 or C4 (low early in disease, returning to normal in 6 to 8 weeks), total protein and albumin (elevated)
- CBC, ESR, ASO titer (elevated), streptozyme test (positive), anti–deoxyribonucleic acid (DNA) antibody titer
- Electrolytes, BUN, creatinine, and cholesterol
- Fluorescent antinuclear antibody (SLE), hepatitis titers, sickle cell or hemoglobin electrophoresis, tuberculin PPD, and fluorescent treponemal antibody absorption (syphilis)

Differential Diagnosis

Acute nephritis also occurs as part of systemic illnesses, such as SLE, HSP, hemolytic-uremic syndrome, vasculitis, or as a reaction to drugs or irradiation.

Management

Consultation with a nephrologist is recommended in all cases (Fig. 35-7).

PSGN treatment is supportive because resolution occurs spontaneously 95% of the time. The course does not seem to be affected by corticosteroids, immunosuppression, or other treatment modalities. During the peak of oliguria and hypertension in the first few days of illness, hospitalization may be required with fluid and sodium limitation and diuretic, antihypertensive, and antibiotic treatment if cultures are positive. Resolution occurs once diuresis begins. Gross hematuria persists for 1 to 2 weeks, urine can be abnormal for 6 to 12 weeks, and microscopic hematuria can persist for up to 2 years. Complement levels return to normal in 6 to 8 weeks (Pan and Avner, 2011a).

- Acute nephritis—possible hospitalization with treatment, as described previously.
- IgA nephropathy—annual follow-up with BP, UA, and determination of renal function.
- Benign familial or hereditary nephritis—perform audiometry and review family medical history. Hereditary markers are being developed for this disease.
- Benign recurrent nephritis—monitor UA and renal function every 1 to 2 years.
- Chronic nephritis—a team approach is required to adequately provide care.

Complications

Prolonged oliguria and renal failure can occur if acute nephritis progresses. Hypertensive encephalopathy or congestive heart failure can occur secondary to PSGN. Irreversible parenchymal damage causes hypertension and renal insufficiency.

Patient and Family Education, Prevention, and Prognosis

Patients with PSGN may have macrohematuria or microhematuria for up to 6 to 12 months, but the long-range outcome is excellent. Thin-basement-membrane disease has a good outcome. IgA nephropathy with severe histologic findings has a poor outcome, especially if the child is African American. Patient education should stress the importance of continued, regular care to monitor renal function.

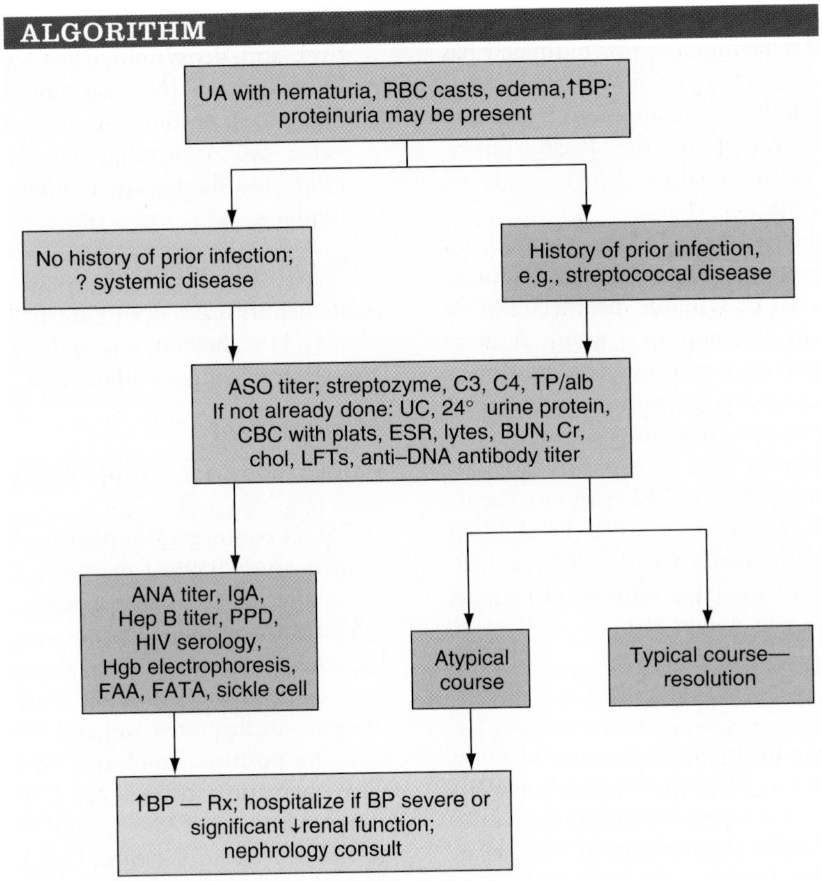

• **Figure 35-7** Evaluation of nephritis algorithm. *ANA,* Antinuclear antibody; *ASO,* antistreptolysin O; *BP,* blood pressure; *BUN,* blood urea nitrogen; *C3,* complement 3; *C4,* complement 4; *CBC,* complete blood count; *chol,* cholesterol; *Cr,* creatinine; *DNA,* deoxyribonucleic acid; *ESR,* erythrocyte sedimentation rate; *FAA,* fluorescent antinuclear antibody; *FATA,* fluorescent treponemal antibody absorption; *Hep B,* hepatitis B; *Hgb,* hemoglobin; *HIV,* human immunodeficiency virus; *IgA,* immunoglobulin A; *LFT,* liver function test; *plats,* platelets; *PPD,* purified protein derivative; *RBC,* red blood cell; *Rx,* prescribe; *TP/alb,* total protein/albumin; *UA,* urinalysis; *UC,* urine culture.

Renal Tubular Acidosis

Dysfunction of renal tubule transport capability results in a condition known as *renal tubular acidosis (RTA).* Several distinct types of RTA have been identified. Type I, classic or distal RTA (dRTA), occurs when the defect is in the distal tubule. When the defect occurs in the proximal tubules, it is known as *proximal RTA (pRTA), type II,* or *bicarbonate-wasting RTA.* Type III has been reclassified as a subtype of type I that occurs primarily in preterm infants. Type IV, also known as *hyperkalemic RTA,* occurs with problems in the functioning of aldosterone most commonly following relief of obstructive uropathy (Sreedharan and Avner, 2011).

The diagnosis depends on a combination of clinical features, laboratory values, and response to treatment.

- RTA is suggested by a serum carbon dioxide level less than 20, especially if the anion gap is normal (12 ± 4 mEq/L). Anion gap = $Na^+ - (Cl^- + HCO_3^-)$.
- dRTA (type I) is suggested by hypokalemia, hyperchloremia with a serum CO_2 less than 16, and urine pH greater than 5.5.
- pRTA (type II) is suggested by hypokalemia, hyperchloremia with a serum CO_2 less than 16, and urine pH less than 5.5.
- Type IV is suggested by hyperkalemia.

Fanconi syndrome is an uncommon and more complex form of pRTA (type II) with associated glycosuria, phosphaturia, aminoaciduria, and a defect in vitamin D metabolism manifested as nausea, anorexia, intermittent vomiting, and possibly rickets.

RTA is often an isolated and primary problem with unknown cause. It is seen most typically in children evaluated for growth failure and is often revealed when illness, dehydration, or starvation stresses a child. RTA is more common in males than females, with pRTA being the most common form seen in children.

Dysfunction in the transport capability of the renal tubules affects either the reabsorption of filtered bicarbonate, excretion of hydrogen ion, or both and results in a metabolic acidosis. The proximal tubule, which normally absorbs 85% of bicarbonate, is able to reabsorb only 60% of bicarbonate from filtered urine in patients with pRTA.

The distal tubule continues to function and reabsorbs approximately 15% of the bicarbonate, and the urine is acidified (pH less than 5.5). However, a large amount of bicarbonate is wasted. As the body adapts, a new threshold for serum bicarbonate is set, usually around 14 to 16 mEq/L (Sreedharan and Avner, 2011).

A defect in the ability of the distal renal tubule to excrete hydrogen is the cause of dRTA. This defect causes complete loss of reabsorption of the final 15% of bicarbonate and an inability to acidify urine (pH greater than 5.5). Type IV RTA is characterized by a deficiency in the production or responsiveness of aldosterone and impaired ammonia production. Type IV RTA is often associated with an obstructive uropathy or other transient phenomenon in infancy (Sreedharan and Avner, 2011).

Clinical Findings

History

- Failure to gain weight (especially) and height—the most common symptoms
- Polyuria and polydipsia
- Muscle weakness (caused by hypokalemia)
- Irritability before eating, satiation after eating, vomiting, diarrhea, or constipation in dRTA
- Preference for liquids over solid foods, poor appetite, or anorexia, especially with type IV

Physical Examination

- Arrested growth curve toward the end of the first year with prior consistent growth
- Normal physical examination and development

Diagnostic Studies

Studies include serum electrolytes, including CO_2 (hypokalemia, hyperchloremic metabolic acidosis), renal function tests (BUN, creatinine), calcium, phosphorus, alkaline phosphatase, and UA (first-morning void) to test for glucose and pH.

If any of the laboratory findings are abnormal, consider the following:

- A 24-hour creatinine clearance to establish the normal GFR, calcium (normal less than 4 mg/kg/24 hr), and calcium-creatinine ratio
- Renal ultrasonography to determine the anatomy and rule out nephrocalcinosis, nephrolithiasis, hydronephrosis, obstructive uropathy, and parenchymal damage

Differential Diagnosis

Primary RTA must be differentiated from secondary RTA, which can be due to many disease states or conditions, such as other causes of growth failure (e.g., FTT), hypothyroidism, and systemic acidosis.

Management

Goals of management include correcting the acidosis and maintaining normal bicarbonate (greater than 20 mEq/L), thereby restoring growth and minimizing complications.

- Oral alkalizing medications are given to achieve these goals. Dosing is determined by the type of RTA: dRTA requires low doses, often between 2 and 5 mEq/kg/day; pRTA requires high doses, often between 5 and 15 mEq/kg/day and sometimes as high as 20 mEq/kg/day. The dose must be titrated to the child's response as determined by weight and laboratory results (CO_2 and electrolytes). Initiate medication at 3 mEq/kg/day, and check laboratory results in a few days. Titrate the dose until a serum bicarbonate level of 20 to 22 mEq/L is achieved (Shaw, 2015). To maintain as normal a bicarbonate level as possible, doses should be given frequently throughout the day (with meals) and as late as possible at night (at bedtime).
  - Bicitra (sodium citrate and citric acid or Shohl solution), equals 1 mEq bicarbonate/mL and is relatively pleasant tasting.
  - Polycitra (sodium and potassium citrate and citric acid), equals 2 mEq bicarbonate/mL and is less palatable. Giving it in juice, water, or formula may ease its administration. Polycitra is especially useful if the child is hypokalemic or requires an excess quantity or if compliance is an issue.
  - $NaHCO_3$ tablets are available in 325-mg strength (4 mEq bicarbonate) and 650-mg strength (8 mEq bicarbonate).
  - 8 oz baking soda mixed with 2.65 L of distilled water equals 1 mEq/mL of bicarbonate.
- The response to medication helps confirm the diagnosis and type of RTA. dRTA has a rapid response to treatment, and normal bicarbonate levels are maintained with little difficulty. pRTA requires higher doses to normalize bicarbonate and is less easily maintained. Type IV RTA requires mineralocorticoid treatment if aldosterone is deficient.
- Maximizing caloric intake to enhance growth can be accomplished by emphasizing solid foods for all meals and snacks, and avoiding water and non-caloric foods. Providing nutritional supplements is also ideal.
- Meticulous follow-up is imperative. Weight and laboratory results should be monitored biweekly to monthly until weight gain is established and CO_2 is stabilized. Weighing should be done on the same scale.
- Pseudoephedrine should be avoided because it is minimally excreted in alkalinized urine and associated with a risk of intoxication.
- Referral to a pediatric nephrologist is necessary for any child who is not growing well despite treatment, or whose laboratory values are not normalizing with treatment, has unusual laboratory results, has type IV RTA, or has any complication of RTA.

Complications

It is rare to have complications with pRTA. Hypercalciuria can occur with dRTA, leading to nephrocalcinosis, nephrolithiasis, renal parenchymal destruction, and occasionally renal failure. Rickets are sometimes found in type IV RTA.

Patient and Family Education, Prevention, and Prognosis

Patient education should stress the importance of continued, regular care to monitor renal function and growth. Isolated pRTA responds quickly to treatment, with children showing catch-up growth and obtaining normal maximum height. pRTA resolves spontaneously without recurrence of symptoms, often within 1 to 2 years but at worst over the first decade of life (Sreedharan and Avner, 2011). dRTA usually lasts a lifetime; type IV resolves with correction of the underlying problem.

Nephrolithiasis and Urolithiasis

Urinary stones can be found anywhere in the urinary tract. In North America, most children have stones in the kidneys; bladder stones occur in less than 10% of the pediatric cases and are most often related to urologic abnormalities. Bladder stones are endemic to other parts of the world and are likely related to diet.

The prevalence of urinary stones varies by region, with a higher incidence in the Southeast United States and in Caucasians, with a slightly higher incidence in males than in females. Seventy-five percent of children who have nephrolithiasis have an identifiable predisposition to stone formation. Metabolic risk factors account for more than 50% of cases, structural abnormalities account for 32%, and infections account for 4%. Hypercalciuria is the most common metabolic cause (accounts for 30% to 60%) of urinary calculi and is a condition with many causes including renal tubular dysfunction, endocrine disturbances, bone metabolic disorders, UTI, familial idiopathic hypercalcemia, and medications (Elder, 2011c). Hyperoxaluria is found in up to 20% of children with nephrolithiasis. Hyperuricosuria has been documented in 2% to 10% of children with stone formation. Cystine stones account for less than 1% of urinary stones.

Clinical Findings

History

- Family history of nephrolithiasis, arthritis, gout, or renal disease
- Stones or fragments passed in urine
- Dietary history high in protein, sodium, calcium, and oxalate intake
- Colic in an infant
- History or symptoms suggestive of a UTI in a preschooler

Physical Examination

- Abdominal, flank, or pelvic pain (occurs at all ages, but present in 94% of adolescents)

Diagnostic Studies

- UA shows gross or microscopic hematuria (90%) and when cultured 20% of children also have UTI (Shaw, 2015)
- Hypercalciuria is diagnosed by a 24-hour urinary calcium excretion greater than 4 mg/kg. Screening may be performed on a random urine specimen by measuring the calcium : creatinine ratio (mg/dL : mg/dL) and greater than 0.2 suggests hypercalciuria in an older child; normal ratios may be as high as 0.8 in infants younger than 7 months old (Porter and Avner, 2011)
- Abdominal radiography, abdominal ultrasound, and/or CT scan
- Analyze stone composition to aid in the diagnosis of the metabolic abnormality, which present in up to 75% of children with a kidney stone (Shaw, 2015)

Differential Diagnosis

Other diagnoses causing flank pain should be considered (e.g., UTI, pyelonephritis or trauma). Just slightly more than half of preschool children with nephrolithiasis have flank pain, so other afebrile illnesses, including gastrointestinal viral syndromes and early appendicitis, chronic recurrent abdominal pain of no known cause, and emotional stress should be considered in the preschool child.

Management

Increased fluid intake is the first line of therapy for all stone types regardless of the cause. In adolescents, a goal of 2 L of urine output per day is helpful. Stone removal may be required if the stone is not passed and severe symptoms continue for a significant amount of time. Extracorporeal shockwave lithotripsy (ESWL) is safe in children; long-term kidney damage has not been validated in follow-up studies. Skin bruising and hematuria are almost universal side effects of ESWL. Stones may also be removed by using rigid or flexible endoscopes passed through the urethra into the bladder or ureter. Renal calculi may also be removed percutaneously, and open surgical lithotomy is still an option if other techniques fail.

Refer to a dietary expert for nutritional advice. Dietary restrictions control stone formation and renal injury in most metabolic disorders contributing to stone formation. Refer to urologist for a complete metabolic evaluation if stone or fragments are passed or seen in the urinary system on imaging studies.

Patient and Family Education, Prevention, and Prognosis

Recurrence rates are high if left untreated, and patients with hyperuricosuria may continue to have symptomatic or asymptomatic calculi. Despite an excellent response to therapy, children with nephrolithiasis require long-term follow-up with a nephrologist because of the potential for renal insufficiency and end-stage renal disease.

Wilms Tumor

Wilms tumor, the most common malignancy of the genitourinary tract, is typically recognized as a firm, smooth mass in the abdomen or flank. It is staged according to the Children's Oncology Group as follows:

- Stage I: The tumor is limited to the kidney and can be completely excised with the capsular surface intact.
- Stage II: The tumor extends beyond the kidney but can still be completely excised.
- Stage III: There is postsurgical residual nonhematogenous extension confined to the abdomen.
- Stage IV: There is hematogenous metastasis, most frequently to the lung.
- Stage V: There is bilateral kidney involvement.

This malignancy manifests as a solitary growth in any part of either or both kidneys. There are approximately eight cases of Wilms tumor per million children younger than 15 years old with 500 new cases every year. Most Wilms tumors occur in children between 2 and 5 years old. The peak incidence and median age at diagnosis is 3 years old. About 1% to 2% of children with Wilms tumor have a family history of Wilms, and the tumor is inherited in an autosomal dominant manner (Anderson et al, 2011). An important feature of Wilms tumor is the occurrence of associated congenital anomalies including renal abnormalities, such as cryptorchidism, hypospadias, duplication of the collecting system, ambiguous genitalia, hemihypertrophy, aniridia, cardiac abnormalities, and Beckwith-Wiedemann, Denys-Drash, and Perlman syndromes. Wilms tumor occurs with equal frequency in both sexes although males are diagnosed younger. There is a higher frequency in African Americans and a lower frequency in Asians.

Clinical Findings

History

- The most frequent finding is increasing abdominal size or an actual palpable mass.
- Pain is reported if the mass has undergone rapid growth or hemorrhage.
- Fever, dyspnea, diarrhea, vomiting, weight loss, or malaise may be reported.

Physical Examination

- A firm, smooth abdominal or flank mass that does not cross the midline may be noted.
- BP is elevated if renal ischemia is present (rare).
- A left varicocele is found in males if the spermatic vein is obstructed.
- A careful examination is needed to rule out congenital anomalies.

Diagnostic Studies

- Chest and abdominal radiography is performed to differentiate neuroblastoma, which is usually calcified.
- Abdominal ultrasonography is used to differentiate a solid from a cystic mass or hydronephrosis and multicystic kidney.
- UA demonstrates hematuria in 25% to 33% of children.
- A CBC, reticulocyte count, and liver and renal chemistry studies are performed.
- A CT scan of the chest, abdomen, and pelvis to stage the disease and bone marrow is done by the oncology team.

Differential Diagnosis

Neuroblastoma is the main differential diagnosis (the mass often crosses the midline). Multicystic kidney, hydronephrosis, renal cyst, or other renal malignancies are additional conditions to consider.

Management

Diagnostic workup is the initial urgent priority, with concurrent referral to a pediatric cancer center for treatment. Surgery is scheduled to remove the affected kidney and possibly the ureter and adrenal gland; combined chemotherapy and radiotherapy are instituted if the disease is advanced or histologic findings are unfavorable. Close follow-up after the initial treatment should be coordinated with the cancer team.

Complications

The lungs and liver are the most common sites of metastasis. High BP is possible because of renal ischemia and occasionally leads to cardiac failure. Scoliosis resulting from radiation therapy is uncommon because radiation exposure is carefully controlled.

Patient and Family Education, Prevention, and Prognosis

The prognosis is determined by the histology of the neoplasm, by the patient's age (the younger the better), the size of the tumor, positive nodes, and, most significantly, the extent or stage of the disease. The cure rate is about 80% to 90% for infants with stage 4S; children with high-risk neuroblastoma have survival rates between 25% to 35%; reoccurrence of the disease has a less than 50% response to alternative chemotherapeutic agents (Zage and Ater, 2011). A pediatric urologist should determine if a child should be allowed to participate in sports on an individual basis (American Academy of Family Physicians [AAFP] et al, 2010). Use of kidney protectors is highly recommended during sports. New information on the long-term sequelae for the treatment of Wilms tumors and the present trials and treatment recommendations can be accessed at the National Wilms Tumor Study.

Common Genitourinary Conditions in Males

Hypospadias

Hypospadias is a common congenital abnormality in which the urethral meatus is located anywhere from the proximal glans to the perineum on the ventral surface (underside) of the penis. Chordee, a ventral bowing of the penis, occurs when a tight band of fibrous tissue pulls on the penis. *Torsion* refers to rotation of the penis to the right or left.

The etiology of hypospadias is unknown. It is believed that the endocrine system probably has an important role, but what that role is remains unclear. The primitive gonad in the eighth week of embryonic development differentiates into male or female. As the genital tubercle enlarges, developmental arrest occurs along the line of urethral fusion and causes hypospadias.

Hypospadias occurs in 1 in 250 male infants with an increased risk if family members have hypospadias. Ten percent of boys with hypospadias also have undescended testicles, inguinal hernia, or hydrocele (Elder, 2011a).

Clinical Findings

History

- A family history of a male relative with genitourinary problems may be reported.
- The child sits to void or urinates on the floor in front of the toilet unless he holds his penis to direct the stream.

Physical Examination

In a newborn, the classic finding is a dorsally hooded foreskin. It is essential to visualize the urethral meatus. Pulling the ventral shaft skin in a downward and outward direction facilitates visualization. The deformity is described by location—glanular, coronal, subcoronal, mid-penile, penoscrotal, scrotal, or perineal and/or as distal (60%), mid-penile (25%), or proximal (15%).

Other findings include a urinary stream that aims downward rather than straight, inguinal hernia or undescended testicles (10%), and/or chordee (Elder, 2011a).

Differential Diagnosis

The differential diagnosis includes intersex abnormalities.

Management

The goal of surgical repair is to have a functional penis that appears normal. Circumcision must not be done because the foreskin may be used in the surgical repair. Referral should be made to a pediatric urologist at birth. Surgery to correct hypospadias is best done around 6 to 12 months old. Considerations in scheduling surgery include the risk of anesthesia at this age is similar to older toddlers, penile growth is slow over the next few years, the child does not remember the procedure, and the postoperative analgesia needs are less than in older children. Repair is usually accomplished in a one-stage outpatient procedure, unless it is a complex defect.

Complications

With unrepaired hypospadias, peer taunting of boys and problems with erections are possible complications. Intersex abnormalities are possible if associated with cryptorchidism.

Patient and Family Education, Prevention, and Prognosis

Education and reassurance regarding the etiology, repair, and outcome should be provided. Careful assessment of the newborn should be done when hypospadias is reported in a family member. Hypospadias is usually an isolated anomaly, but it does require further workup to assess the anatomy of the urinary system for other anomalies.

Cryptorchidism (Undescended Testes)

Cryptorchidism describes a testis that does not reside in and cannot be manipulated into the scrotum. A retractile testis is out of the scrotum, but can be brought into the scrotum and remains there. A gliding testis can be brought into the scrotum, but returns to a high position in the scrotum once released. An ectopic testis lies outside the normal path of descent. An ascended testis is one that has fully descended, but has spontaneously re-ascended and lies outside the scrotum. A trapped testis is one dislocated after herniorrhaphy. Any testis that is not in the scrotum is subject to progressive deterioration. Undescended testes is a common disorder that often causes great anxiety for parents.

Testes develop in the abdomen and descend in the seventh fetal month to the upper part of the groin, subsequently progressing through the inguinal canal into the scrotum. Failure of the testes to descend can be caused by mechanical lesions or can be secondary to hormonal, chromosomal, enzymatic, or anatomic disorders.

An undescended testis is the most common genitourinary disorder in boys, occurring in 3.4% in term newborns. Testicular descent occurs at 7 to 8 months gestation, so it is therefore more common in preterm (30%), low-birth-weight, and twin infants. A great majority of undescended testes descend spontaneously during the first 3 months of life but after 6 months old it is rare (0.8%) for them to descend. Cryptorchidism is bilateral in 10% of cases. Retractile testes are bilateral and most common in boys 5 to 6 years old (Elder, 2011b).

Clinical Findings

History

- Family history of undescended testes or testicular malignancy
- Testes not consistently descended during the infant's bath
- Risk factors include prematurity, hypospadias, congenital subluxation of the hip, low birth weight, Down syndrome, Klinefelter syndrome
- Other congenital, endocrine, chromosomal, or intersex disorders

Physical Examination

Having the child sit cross-legged or frog-legged, squat, or stand can facilitate testicle descent and palpation.

- Scrotal rugae less fully developed
- Bilateral or unilateral absence of a testicle
- Retractile testes, which move between the scrotum and external ring, but can be manipulated to the lower part of the scrotum and remain there; in children 3 months

to 7 years old, retraction is especially common with tactile stimulation of the area or cold
- Gliding testes that lie between the scrotum and external ring and can be manipulated to the lower part of the scrotum, but return to the high position
- Location:
  - Prescrotal (at the external inguinal ring)
  - Canalicular, high or low (between the external and internal rings), the most common type
  - Ectopic (superficial inguinal, femoral, or perineal)
  - Intraabdominal (above the internal inguinal ring), not palpable, occurring in less than 15% of males with undescended testes
  - Indirect inguinal hernia

Diagnostic Studies

None are indicated except in newborns with potential sex abnormalities, hypopituitarism, Down syndrome, or congenital adrenal hyperplasia. The risk of intersex abnormality is 27% if hypospadias and unilateral or bilateral cryptorchidism are present.

Differential Diagnosis

Anorchism and chromosomal abnormalities are the differential diagnoses.

Management

The goals of treating undescended testes are to improve fertility outcome, decrease malignancy potential, and minimize the psychological stress associated with an empty scrotum. Management is surgical intervention for the congenital undescended testes between 9 and 15 months old. Hormonal therapy has not demonstrated efficacy in stimulating testicular descent. Surgery at 6 months old is appropriate if orchiopexy is performed by a skilled pediatric urologist or surgeon with an attendant and skilled pediatric anesthesiologist. In a child younger than 1 year old, regular examination to assess the position of the testes should be performed at every well-child care visit. If the testes remain undescended, referral to a pediatric urologist or surgeon should occur by 6 months old. Referral should also occur if a retractile testis does not retain scrotal residence. If undescended testes are found after 1 year old, the child should be immediately referred to a pediatric urologist or surgeon for treatment.

Complications

Poor testicular development, infertility, malignancy, vulnerability to trauma, testicular torsion, and inguinal hernia are possible complications of undescended testicles.

Patient and Family Education, Prevention, and Prognosis

Histologic changes have been shown in an undescended testis as early as 6 months old, with irreversible changes shown by 2 years old that contribute to infertility and are associated with malignancy. Infertility as a complication of cryptorchidism has been reported in as many as 15% of men with unilateral undescended testes and 35% to 50% if bilateral (Elder, 2011b). Testicular malignancy in males with cryptorchidism is reported to have an incidence two to four times higher than the general population. Correction of undescended testes does not diminish the incidence of testicular cancer, although an increased incidence in testicular tumors has been observed if orchiopexy is done at later ages. Malignancy is more common with an intraabdominal testis. A testicular neoplasm in one child mandates examination of his male siblings (Elder, 2011b).

Testicular self-examination should be taught to all adolescents but especially to these young men (Fig. 35-8). The website for the Testicular Cancer Awareness Week has a patient handout sheet on testicular self-examination and provides the opportunity to sign up to receive monthly reminders to perform testicular self-examination.

Undescended testes do not resolve with puberty; retractile testes generally settle into the scrotum by puberty. Open discussion of the problem, management, and potential complications is essential initially, as well as over time. Participation in contact sports is discouraged because of the risk of losing the one viable testicle to trauma.

Hydrocele

A common cause of painless scrotal swelling is a hydrocele, a collection of serous fluid in the scrotal sac. A noncommunicating hydrocele has a collection of fluid only in the scrotum. If the processus vaginalis remains patent so that fluid moves from the abdomen to the scrotum, it is called a *communicating hydrocele* and is more likely to be associated with a hernia (Fig. 35-9).

Incomplete closure of the processus vaginalis through which the testes descend into the scrotum allows a hydrocele to develop. Incidence is 0.5% to 2% in neonates (Elder, 2011b).

Clinical Findings

Hydroceles that persist beyond 1 year old are assumed to be in conjunction with a hernia. In older children, they also occur after trauma, with an inflammatory illness, or neoplasm.

History

- Intermittent or constant bulge or lump in the scrotum, often more distally placed. Scrotal size increases with activity and decreases with rest.
- Overlying skin may be tense.
- No distress or vomiting.

Physical Examination

- Asymmetry or a scrotal mass present; if swelling is present in the inguinal area, a hernia is probable; swelling is usually unilateral (Table 35-5)
- Testes descended

In the realm of "if it ain't broke, don't fix it," there has been a substantial increase in information about prostate cancer. However, testicular cancer is the most common cancer in men 15 to 35 years old, an age when we do not want to admit the possibility of illness. If detected early, it is among the easiest to cure. For men in this age group, a once-a-month simple self-examination is suggested. This can help catch this cancer at an early stage.

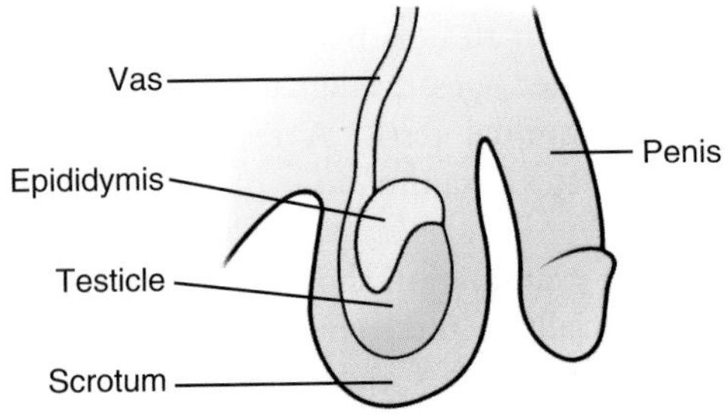

The most convenient time to examine yourself is while taking a shower or bath. The warm water causes the skin to relax, making the examination of the underlying tissues easier.

First:

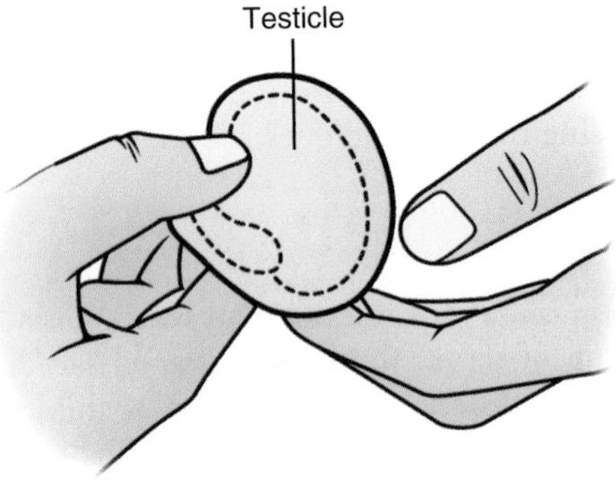

Examine your testicles. Slowly roll each testicle between thumb and forefingers. Try to find any hard, nonsensitive bumps.

Second:

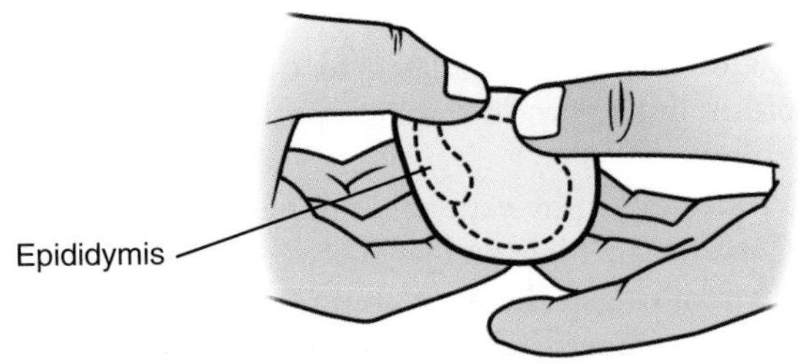

Examine the epididymis for lumps. This crescent-shaped cord is behind each testicle. This area is tender so do not be alarmed.

Third:

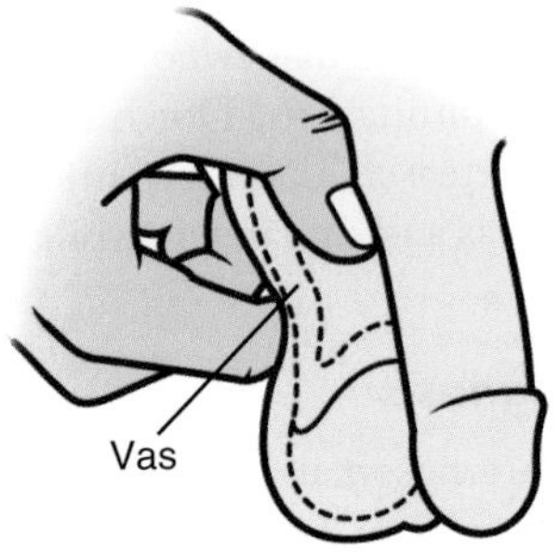

Examine the vas deferens, the sperm carrying tube that extends from the epididymis of each testicle.

Symptoms:

In early stages, testicular cancer may be symptomless. When symptoms do occur, they include:

* Lump on testicle, epididymis, or vas deferens
* Enlargement of a testicle
* Heavy sensation in groin area or testicles
* Dull ache in groin or abdomen area

If you find a lump or have any of the above symtoms, see your physician or NP immediately for an accurate diagnosis.

• **Figure 35-8** Self-examination for testicular cancer. *NP,* Nurse practitioner. (From The Testicular Cancer Resource Center: *The self exam, The Testicular Cancer Resource Center* (website), 2013, Available at http://tcrc.acor.org/. Accessed October 30, 2015; The American Cancer Society: *Testicular self-exam, American Cancer Society* (website), 2013, Available at www.cancer.org/cancer/testicularcancer/moreinformation/doihavetesticularcancer/do-i-have-testicular-cancer-self-exam. Accessed October 30, 2015.)

- Translucent on transillumination (pink or red glow)
- Noncommunicating hydrocele—scrotal sac tense, slightly blue tinged, fluctuant, and does not reduce; no swelling in the inguinal region
- Communicating hydrocele—fluid in the scrotal sac comes and goes (probably flat in the morning, swollen later in the day)

Differential Diagnosis

Hernia, undescended testicle, retractile testicle, and inguinal lymphadenopathy are the differential diagnoses.

Management

- Noncommunicating hydrocele: Fluid is generally absorbed spontaneously; no treatment is indicated unless the hydrocele is so large that it is uncomfortable or persists longer than 1 year.
- Communicating hydrocele: Many communicating hydroceles will resolve without surgery and deserve observation (Koski et al, 2010). If the hernia persists for more than 1 year, referral for surgical intervention is recommended.

For children over 12 months old, a diagnostic evaluation by the urologist is warranted if the congenital hydrocele has

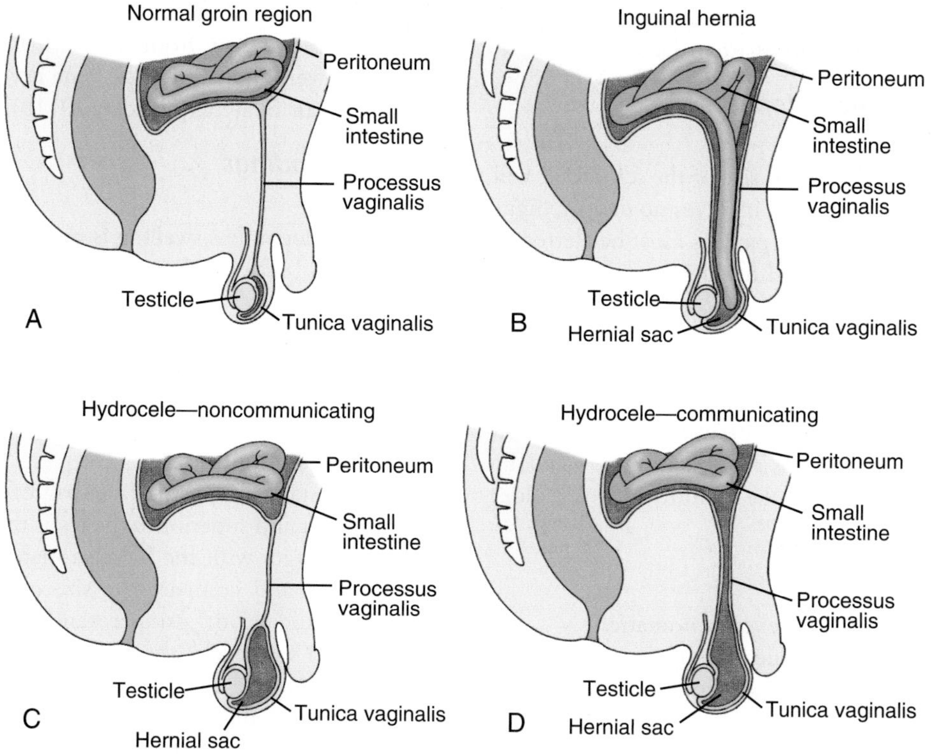

• **Figure 35-9** Hydroceles and hernias. **A,** Groin region of the normal male infant. **B,** An inguinal hernia is the protrusion of bowel into the groin region. **C,** A hydrocele is a collection of fluid within the processus vaginalis. In a noncommunicating hydrocele, the scrotal swelling does not change in size or shape because there is no connection with the abdominal cavity. **D,** In a communicating hydrocele, the processus vaginalis remains open from the scrotum to the abdominal cavity, and scrotal swelling may vary in size during the course of an infant's day. (From Betz CL, Hunsberger M, Wright S: *Family-centered nursing care of infants*, ed 2, Philadelphia, 1994, Saunders.)

TABLE 35-5 Physical Findings in Scrotal Swellings

Condition	Tender	Red	Blue	Cremasteric Reflex	Transillumination
Chronic					
Hydrocele	–	–	+	+	+
Tumor	–	–	–	+	–
Varicocele	–	–	–	+	–
Acute					
Torsion of newborn	–	–	+	–	–
Torsion of older child	+	+	–	–	–
Torsion of appendage	+	+	–	+	–
Epididymitis	+	+	–	+	–
Trauma	+	–	+	±	–

From Kaplan GN: Scrotal swelling in children, *Pediatr Rev* 21(9):312, 2000.

not resolve or with the initial onset of clinical findings. Surgery is usually done on an outpatient basis.

Patient and Family Education, Prevention, and Prognosis

Reassure parent that the increased size of the scrotal sac will resolve, usually by 1 year old, and involves no danger. Signs of hernia must be explained, and parents must be alerted to observe and report any abnormal findings.

Spermatocele

A benign, painless scrotal mass or cyst on the head of the epididymis or testicular adnexa containing sperm is called a *spermatocele.* A spermatocele is an uncommon, generally benign finding and occurs in the mature male or older adolescents.

Clinical Findings

- Scrotal swelling but otherwise asymptomatic
- Painless, mobile cystic nodule usually less than 1 cm in size, superior and posterior to the testicle that transilluminates
- No change in size with the Valsalva maneuver
- An ultrasound may be ordered if large and bothersome or painful

Differential Diagnosis

A varicocele and an epididymal cyst (identical in appearance, but not containing sperm) are the differential diagnoses.

Management

No treatment is required unless the cyst is large and bothersome or painful in which case referral to an urologist is recommended.

Patient and Family Education, Prevention, and Prognosis

Any pain or discomfort should be reported. Testicular self-examination assists in early detection of this disorder in later adolescence.

Varicocele

A varicocele is a benign enlargement or dilation of testicular veins causing a painless scrotal mass of varying size that may feel like a "bag of worms." It is usually found on the left side.

The etiology of varicoceles is probably multifactorial, with the physiologic changes associated with puberty playing some role. A varicocele is caused by valvular incompetence of the spermatic vein resulting in dilated or varicose veins. Varicoceles are rare before 10 years old and may be indicative of malignancy. They occur in 5% of adolescent males and 15% of adult males. Up to 85% to 95% arise on the left side because the left spermatic vein drains into the left renal vein and arterial compression of the renal vein obstructs blood flow from the vein. In contrast, the right spermatic vein drains into the vena cava. Only 2% of varicoceles occur bilaterally (Elder, 2011b).

Clinical Findings

History

- Usually a painless swelling is noted in the left side of the scrotum, occasionally a "dull ache" or "heavy" feeling if large.
- Scrotal swelling with prolonged standing causes pain; swelling and pain resolve on reclining. Pain can occur with strenuous physical activity.

Physical Examination

- In the standing position, a "bag of worms" can be felt posterior and superior to the testis that collapses on lying and enlarges with the Valsalva maneuver.
- Measure and compare the size of both testes (length, width, and depth) using a standard orchidometer.
- Grade 3 varicocele, the classic "bag of worms," is larger than 2 cm and easily visualized; grade 2 varicocele is 1 to 2 cm in diameter and is easily palpable when the adolescent is standing but not visualized; grade 1 varicocele is the most common, very small, and difficult to palpate (the Valsalva maneuver may help).

Diagnostic Studies

- Ultrasonography to rule out malignancy in children younger than 10 years old
- Serial ultrasonography to measure testicular size every 6 to 12 months of age

Differential Diagnosis

Varicoceles must be differentiated from other testicular masses, such as lipoma, hernia, hydrocele, spermatocele, and tumors.

Management

Asymptomatic grade 1 varicocele with normal testicular volumes usually does not require intervention in adolescence but is followed by ultrasonographic monitoring of testicular size every 6 months. Any change in comfort level should be reported. Referral to a surgeon or urologist should be made if the varicocele is grade 2 or 3, if the varicocele is painful, if the difference in testicular volume is marked (greater than 2 mm by ultrasound), if the varicocele is right sided or bilateral, or if testicular growth becomes retarded over a 6- to 12-month period (Elder, 2011b). Ligation is the usual procedure, completed on an outpatient basis with few complications.

Complications

Atrophy or testicular growth arrest, as noted by a discrepancy in testicular size, can occur. Lower fertility rates with decreased sperm concentration and motility have been noted and are factors in an aggressive surgical approach for the adolescent male with grade 2 or 3 varicocele. Hydrocele may be an insignificant, self-limiting complication following surgery.

Patient and Family Education, Prevention, and Prognosis

A varicocele is the most common cause of infertility. Because of this, early identification is essential. All patients should be counseled about the long-term risks to fertility. Correction of testicular atrophy and an improved sperm count and fertility have been noted in 80% to 90% of those undergoing surgery early in adolescence (Elder, 2011b). Testicular self-examination assists in early detection of this disorder.

Inguinal Hernia

A scrotal or inguinal swelling (or both) that includes abdominal contents is an inguinal hernia (see Fig. 35-9). In females, inguinal hernias cause swelling in the inguinal area and labia majora.

Incomplete closure of the processus vaginalis through which the testes descend into the scrotum allows the presence of abdominal contents in the inguinal canal or scrotum and thus the development of a hernia. Males who are obese or weight lifters or have a family history of undescended testes are at high risk for hernias. Having a sibling with an inguinal hernia increases one's risk, and 11.5% of patients have a family member with a history of inguinal hernia (Aiken and Oldham, 2011).

Inguinal hernias are much more common in males than in females (8 to 10 : 1), occurring in 1% to 5% of boys. Premature infants are at increased risk (7% to 30% of males, 2% of females). More than 50% of hernias are diagnosed during the first year of life, with the peak incidence in the first 3 months of life. Bilateral hernias are common (10% to 20%). Unilateral hernias are more likely to occur on the right side (50% to 60%) than the left (30%) (Aiken and Oldham, 2011). Indirect hernias are a congenital condition and are the most common type in children younger than 3 years old. Direct hernias increase in incidence after 3 years old and are usually acquired. Incarceration is more likely to occur within 2 weeks of initial diagnosis of the hernia. There does not seem to be any increased risk of incarceration based on age (Gholoum et al, 2010).

Clinical Findings

History

- Family or personal history of undescended testes
- Swelling in the inguinal area, scrotum, or both that comes and goes and increases with crying or straining
- Prematurity, weight lifting, or obesity

Physical Examination

- Swelling is found in the inguinal area, scrotal area (labia majora in females), or both.
- The hernia is reducible with pressure on the distal end.
- Transillumination does not occur unless the bowel is filled with fluid.
- Direct hernias push outward through the weakest point in the abdominal wall.
- Indirect hernias push downward at an angle into the inguinal canal.
- The child is fussy and has a distended abdomen if the hernia is incarcerated.
- Silk glove sign: A sensation of two surfaces rubbing against each other while one palpates the spermatic cord as it crosses the pubic tubercle.

Diagnostic Studies

An abdominal radiograph can be helpful if air is present below the inguinal ligament. Ultrasonography can differentiate a hernia from a hydrocele and is especially helpful if an incarcerated hernia is suspected.

Differential Diagnosis

Hydrocele, undescended testes, and inguinal lymphadenopathy are included in the differential diagnosis.

Management

If a child is seen with a hernia, an attempt should be made to reduce it, and the child should be referred to a surgeon or urologist for repair within 1 to 2 weeks. Even if no swelling is seen at the visit but is elicited by the history, the child should be referred to a surgeon or urologist. Inguinal hernias do not resolve spontaneously. Premature infants should have the hernia repaired prior to discharge. If the hernia is not easily reduced; if it is painful; or if a hard, tender, or red mass is present; refer immediately. If reduction has been difficult and ischemia is ongoing, hospitalization and surgical repair within 24 to 48 hours are indicated.

Complications

Incarceration and strangulation of a hernia cause pain, irritability, erythema, vomiting, and abdominal distention. The overall incidence of incarceration is 12% to 17%, and two thirds of incarcerated hernias occur during the first year of life (Aiken and Oldham, 2011). Both of these conditions should be treated as a surgical emergency. Bowel ischemia is of immediate concern, and testicular injury can occur from torsion as a result of the direct pressure of the incarcerated hernia or as a result of ischemia from cord compression. Because of the 40% to 60% contralateral occurrence of hernias in children, bilateral exploration is usually done at the time of surgery in infants younger than 1 year old.

Patient and Family Education, Prevention, and Prognosis

If surgery is deferred, parents must be aware of the signs and symptoms of incarceration (tenderness, redness, crying, nausea, vomiting, abdominal distention) and be cautioned to seek immediate evaluation by a health care provider should they occur.

Testicular Masses

A mass located on the testicle is most often a malignancy. Testicular tumors can occur at any age; 35% of prepubertal testicular tumors are malignant. Most of the tumors are yolk sac tumors; however, rhabdomyosarcoma and leukemia can appear in this age group; 98% of painless testicular tumors in adolescents are malignant (Elder, 2011b).

Clinical Findings

History

- Family history of testicular cancer
- Sensation of fullness or heaviness
- Possibly no complaints because testicular masses cause little or no pain and are often small
- Cryptorchidism, trauma, and atrophy

Physical Examination

- A hard, painless testicular mass that does not transilluminate.
- There may be an associated hydrocele.
- The abdomen and supraclavicular areas should be assessed for any palpable nodes.

Diagnostic Studies

- If a tumor is suspected, serum levels of alpha-fetoprotein, beta-human chorionic gonadotropin (β-hCG), and lactate dehydrogenase are indicated.
- Scrotal sonography is indicated to establish the exact location of the mass and differentiate a cystic from a solid mass.
- CT scan is indicated to evaluate for metastasis.

Differential Diagnosis

Intratesticular masses, which are almost always malignant, must be differentiated from extratesticular masses, such as hernia, varicocele, hydrocele, or spermatocele.

Management

Any child or adolescent with a testicular mass must be referred immediately for further evaluation. Treatment is dependent on the stage and type of tumor and can include orchiectomy, irradiation, and chemotherapy.

Patient and Family Education, Prevention, and Prognosis

Metastasis may occur before the initial tumor is noticed. Pay attention to complaints about back or abdominal pain, unexplained weight loss, dyspnea (pulmonary metastases), gynecomastia, supraclavicular adenopathy, urinary obstruction, or a "heavy" or "dragging" sensation. Early detection and therapeutic intervention can lead to a 90% survival rate; 90% of relapses occur in the first 12 months after treatment. Testicular examination must be routinely done during physical examinations and must also be taught to adolescent males (see Fig. 35-8).

Phimosis and Paraphimosis

Phimosis refers to a foreskin that is too tight to be retracted over the glans penis. Physiologic or primary phimosis occurs over the first 6 years of life when the glans has not completely separated from the epithelium. Pathologic or secondary phimosis occurs when the foreskin cannot be retracted after previously being retracted or after puberty. Paraphimosis is the opposite—a retracted foreskin that cannot be reduced to the normal position.

Phimosis can be congenital or acquired from infection and inflammation under the foreskin. Paraphimosis causes constriction of the penis and results in pain, edema of the glans, and possible necrosis. Paraphimosis is most common in adolescents and can follow masturbation, consensual sexual activity, sexual abuse, or forceful retraction.

Clinical Findings

History

- May be a history of infection or inflammation of the penis
- Retraction of the foreskin with an inability to reduce it (paraphimosis)
- Pain and dysuria
- Signs of urinary obstruction—ballooning of the foreskin with urination and/or abnormal intermittent urinary stream

Physical Examination

- Phimosis—a tight, pinpoint opening of the foreskin with minimal ability to retract the foreskin; foreskin flat and effaced
- Pathologic phimosis—thickened rolled foreskin
- Paraphimosis—edema and bluish discoloration of the glans and foreskin

Management

- Phimosis: Normal cleansing with gentle stretching of the foreskin until resistance is felt. Most foreskins are retractable by 5 or 6 years old. Never forcefully retract the foreskin. Circumcision is indicated if urinary obstruction or infection is present. Persistent phimosis can be treated with a corticosteroid cream three times per day for a month (Elder, 2011a). This frequently allows successful retraction of the foreskin and promotes awareness of improved hygiene.
- Paraphimosis: Reduction may be accomplished by lubricating the foreskin and glans and simultaneously compressing the glans and placing distal traction on the foreskin. If this technique is not successful, surgical release of the constricting band must be done to prevent necrosis of the glans. Paraphimosis is a

surgical emergency (Elder, 2011a). Investigation of events leading to the paraphimosis is needed to rule out sexual abuse.

Patient and Family Education, Prevention, and Prognosis

Infection, urinary obstruction, and reflux can occur with phimosis; however, a tight foreskin in uncircumcised males is normal and usually resolves by 6 years old. It is not an indication for circumcision. Necrosis of the penis is possible with paraphimosis. The foreskin of infants and children should never be forced back.

Balanitis and Balanoposthitis

Balanitis is an inflammation of the glans; *balanoposthitis* is an inflammation of the foreskin and glans penis occurring in males with phimosis or in uncircumcised males. Accumulation of debris under the foreskin, probably resulting from poor hygiene, irritates the foreskin and glans and leads to infection. If purulent discharge with fiery-red erythema and moist translucent exudates is present, streptococcal etiology should be considered. Normal skin flora is the usual cause of infection, but gram-negative bacteria can be involved. If a urethral discharge is present, a sexually transmitted infection (STI) must be considered. Occasionally trauma or allergy can be the cause.

Clinical Findings

- A fussy infant or pain and dysuria in an older child. Edema and inflammation are noted on the foreskin and glans.
- Cultures may be helpful in determining cause if infectious

Management

Antibiotics, both topically and orally, as directed by the cultures, along with warm soaks in the bathtub are prescribed. Depending on the swelling, topical steroids might also be prescribed.

Patient and Family Education, Prevention, and Prognosis

Paraphimosis can occur with severe infections; however, forcible retraction of the foreskin is to be avoided. A review of proper hygiene and the removal of irritants are needed. Occurrence is not an indication for circumcision.

Scrotal Trauma

Trauma to the scrotum most often occurs as a result of sports participation or play. Direct blows to the scrotum and straddle injuries are the most common causes of trauma. In a prepubertal child, the testicle is often spared damage because of the small size and mobility of the testes. Damage can occur when the testicle is forcibly compressed against the pubic bones. Significant symptoms (swelling, discoloration, and tenderness) from minor trauma suggest an underlying tumor.

Clinical Findings

- Pain after some type of injury; older children and adolescents usually report a specific mechanism of injury, time, and place.
- Swelling, discoloration, ecchymosis, and tenderness of the scrotum are common.
- Clear transillumination is compromised if a hematoma is present.
- Ultrasound is useful to differentiate the degree and type of injury and assess for testicular rupture.

Differential Diagnosis

Urethritis, epididymitis, orchitis, and prostatitis should all be included in the differential diagnosis. Degrees of injury include the following:

- Traumatic epididymitis: Inflammation, but no infection. Pain and tenderness with scrotal erythema and edema and a tender indurated epididymis develop within a few days after injury. UA and Doppler ultrasonographic findings are normal. The course is usually acute but short-lived.
- Intratesticular hematoma
- Hematocele with contusion and ecchymosis of the scrotal wall with severe scrotal injury
- Testicular torsion

Management

NSAIDs, cool compresses, scrotal support or elevation, and bed rest are modalities used to help relieve pain. An enlarging scrotum merits immediate surgical exploration, as does hematocele.

Patient and Family Education, Prevention, and Prognosis

On rare occasion, testicular rupture can occur and be manifested by massive swelling and ecchymosis. Prevention is the best approach to this disorder; an athletic cup should be worn when participating in any sport in which injury could occur. A testicular mass should be considered cancer until proved otherwise.

Testicular Torsion

Testicular torsion is the result of twisting of the spermatic cord, which subsequently compromises the blood supply to the testicle. Generally, there is a 6-hour window following a testicular torsion before significant ischemic damage and alteration in spermatic morphology and formation occurs (Elder, 2011b).

Normal fixation of the testis is absent, so the testis can rotate and block lymphatic and then blood flow. Torsion can occur after physical exertion, trauma, or on arising. Torsion can occur at any age but is most common in adolescence and is uncommon before 10 years old. The left side is twice as likely to be involved because of the longer spermatic cord.

Clinical Findings

History

- Sudden onset of unilateral scrotal pain, often associated with nausea and vomiting. The pain is unrelenting.
- History of bouts of intermittent testicular pain. Prior episodes of transient pain are reported in about half of patients.
- Minor trauma, physical exertion, or onset of acute pain on arising is possible.
- May be described as abdominal or inguinal pain by the embarrassed child.
- Fever is minimal or absent.

Physical Examination

- Ill-appearing and anxious male, resisting movement
- Gradual, progressive swelling of involved scrotum with redness, warmth, and tenderness
- The ipsilateral scrotum can be edematous, erythematous, and warm
- Testis swollen larger than opposite side, elevated, lying transversely, exquisitely painful
- Spermatic cord thickened, twisted, and tender
- Slight elevation of the testis increases pain (in epididymitis it relieves pain)
- Transillumination can reveal a solid mass
- The cremasteric reflex is absent on the side with torsion
- Neonate—hard, painless, non-transilluminating mass with edema or discolored scrotal skin

Diagnostic Studies

- UA is usually normal and pyuria and bacteriuria indicate UTI, epididymitis, or orchitis.
- Doppler ultrasound: Testicular flow scan considered if Doppler ultrasound within normal and time allows.

Differential Diagnosis

Torsion of the testicular or epididymal appendage, acute epididymitis (mild to moderate pain of gradual onset), orchitis, trauma (pain is better within an hour), hernia, hydrocele, and varicocele are included in the differential diagnosis.

Management

Testicular torsion is a surgical emergency, and identification with prompt surgical referral must occur immediately. Occasionally manual reduction can be performed, but surgery should follow within 6 to 12 hours to prevent retorsion, preserve fertility, and prevent abscess and atrophy. Contralateral orchiopexy may be done because of a 50% occurrence of torsion in nonfixed testes. Rest and scrotal support do not provide relief.

Patient and Family Education, Prevention, and Prognosis

Testicular atrophy, abscess, or decreased fertility and loss of the testis as a result of necrosis can occur if the torsion persists more than 24 hours.

Torsion of the Appendix Testis

Torsion of the appendix testis (appendix epididymis) is a common cause of acute scrotal pain and is often misdiagnosed. It most commonly occurs in the prepubertal age group and may be a response to hormonal stimulation. Recurrence is not uncommon, because there are a number of appendages. This condition is the most common cause of testicular pain in boys 2 to 10 years old (Elder, 2011b).

Clinical Findings

- Gradual onset of scrotal pain
- "Blue dot" sign, which is a subtle blue mass visible through the scrotal skin: Early in the process there may be a 3- to 5-mm tender indurated mass on the upper pole (Elder, 2011b).
- Doppler ultrasonography or testicular flow scan considered if Doppler ultrasound within normal and time allows.

Differential Diagnosis

Testicular torsion, acute epididymitis, orchitis, trauma, hernia, hydrocele, and varicocele are included in the differential diagnosis.

Management

Testicular torsion is a self-limited condition; inflammation resolves in 3 to 5 days. Management includes NSAIDs, limited activities or bed rest until pain is gone, and warm compresses to the scrotum. Surgery is rarely indicated but might be necessary if testicular torsion cannot be ruled out or if symptoms do not resolve spontaneously in a few days.

Epididymitis

Epididymitis is an inflammation of the epididymis that is painful and acute and commonly caused by *Neisseria gonorrhoeae* or *Chlamydia trachomatis* in the sexually active adolescent, with infection initially present in the urethra or bladder. However, it can also be caused by a viral, coliform bacterial, or tubercular infection; by chemical irritation; by anomalies of the genitourinary tract; or by dysfunctional voiding. It is rare before puberty, but it can occur in younger boys with the offending organism *E. coli*. It may occur in children younger than 2 years old with genitourinary tract abnormalities (Elder, 2011b).

Clinical Findings

History

- Trauma and sexual encounters within past 45 days
- Painful scrotal swelling, usually gradual but can be acute in onset
- Dysuria and frequency or obstructive voiding
- Fever, nausea, vomiting

Physical Examination

- Scrotal edema and erythema are noted.
- The epididymis is hard, indurated, enlarged, and tender; the spermatic cord is tender.
- The testis has normal position and consistency.
- The cremasteric reflex is normal (not present in older adolescents).
- Prehn sign can be elicited—elevation of testis relieves pain (in torsion it increases pain).
- Hydrocele may be present as a reaction to inflammation.
- Urethral discharge may be present, purulent in gonorrhea, and scant and watery in chlamydial infection.
- Rectal examination reveals prostate tenderness and can produce a urethral discharge.

Diagnostic Studies

- UA: Pyuria and occasional bacteria may be present
- CBC: Elevated WBC count
- Urethral culture and Gram stain: Urine nucleic acid amplification tests may be done for gonococci and chlamydia
- Testing for other STIs and HIV if there is a history of sexual activity
- Doppler ultrasonography or radionuclide imaging to differentiate torsion of the testis
- Follow-up VCUG, ultrasonography, or both in prepubertal children and in those who deny sexual activity, to identify urogenital problems

Differential Diagnosis

The differential diagnosis includes testicular torsion of the spermatic cord or appendix testis, hernia, hydrocele, varicocele, spermatocele, trauma, tumor, or concomitant urethritis. Testicular cancer has been confused with epididymitis.

Management

Management is directed toward symptom relief and treatment of a causative organism if found. Bed rest, scrotal support, and elevation are indicated. Apply ice packs as tolerated. Sitz baths and analgesics or NSAIDs are administered to relieve pain. Antibiotic treatment includes the following (Centers for Disease Control and Prevention [CDC], 2010):

- First line: Ceftriaxone (250 mg intramuscularly one time) plus doxycycline (100 mg twice a day for 10 days)
- Alternative treatments: Ofloxacin (300 mg twice a day for 10 days) or levofloxacin (500 mg once a day for 10 days)
- Referral to a urologist is indicated if a solitary testicle is involved, if a prompt response to treatment does not occur, or if a question about the diagnosis remains. Treatment of sexual partner(s) from the past 60 days is indicated if caused by an STI. Intercourse should be avoided until cured. Follow-up is needed within 3 days if no improvement is seen or if symptoms recur after treatment. Follow-up after antibiotics is recommended to ensure that no palpable mass remains.

Patient and Family Education, Prevention, and Prognosis

Infertility, abscess formation, testicular infarction, and late atrophy are possible but rare complications of epididymitis. Because epididymitis is usually caused by an STI, partners must be evaluated and treated. Patients must understand the sexually transmitted etiology of this disease. Pain and edema usually resolve within 1 week.

For a complete list of references, please visit http://evolve.elsevier.com/Burns/pediatric/.

36 Gynecologic Disorders

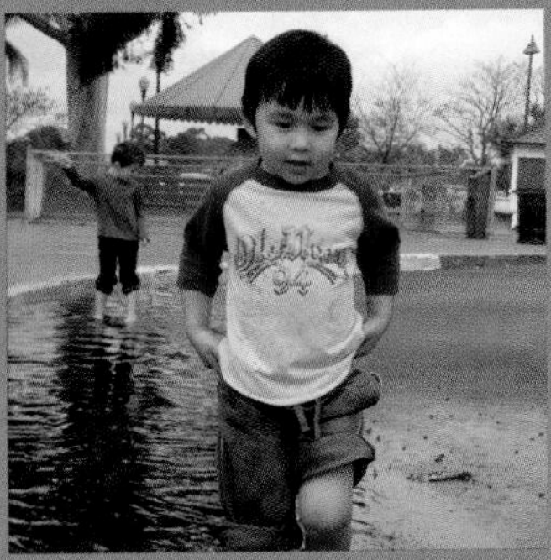

TERAL GERLT AND NANCY BARBER STARR

Pediatric gynecology can provide the primary care provider (PCP) with varied and interesting challenges. Knowledge, sensitivity, and comfort with gynecology aid the pediatric provider in working with the child or adolescent and the parent. Educating children and adolescents about their bodies as they mature is essential. Approaching issues that may be considered personal or embarrassing openly and directly allows more comprehensive care and an opportunity for anticipatory guidance. Establishing and maintaining a good relationship with parents and adolescents helps ease the transition during which adolescents take an increasingly larger role in determining their own care.

Gynecologic issues range from normal transitions that may be perceived as abnormal to serious systemic diseases or abnormalities. The provider should have an elevated index of suspicion in all cases so as to not overlook significant signs and symptoms. At the same time, most conditions are normal and can be easily addressed, reassuring the child, adolescent, and/or parent that all is well and that her body is developing normally.

Standards of Care

Healthy People 2020 (U.S. Department of Health and Human Services, 2013) has multiple objectives that are applicable to children and adolescents. Those that fall into pediatric gynecology are to promote responsible sexual behaviors and reduce teen pregnancies, sexually transmitted infections (STIs), and human immunodeficiency virus (HIV) infections in adolescents.

Bright Futures recommends as a routine part of annual health supervision that all adolescents be asked about sexual health behaviors that place them at risk for pregnancy, STIs, and HIV (Tanski and Garfunkel, 2010). Further, they should receive counseling about responsible sexual behavior, including abstinence and the use of contraception and condoms. All sexually active adolescents should be screened for STIs (gonorrhea, chlamydia, and syphilis if living in an endemic area) and HIV infection. The *Guide to Clinical Preventive Services* (U.S. Preventive Services Task Force, 2014) also recommends screening all sexually active women 24 years old and younger for chlamydia.

Anatomy and Physiology

For the first 6 to 7 weeks of gestation, male and female fetuses are sexually undifferentiated, both having two bipotential gonads and bilateral paramesonephric (müllerian) and mesonephric (wolffian) ducts. At this point testicular differentiation begins at the direction of the testes-determining factor on the Y chromosome. In the male gonad, the Sertoli cells produce antimüllerian hormone (AMH) that inhibits müllerian duct development, and the Leydig cells produce testosterone, which maintains wolffian duct development and causes them to differentiate into the epididymis, vas deferens, and the seminal vesicles.

Without the influence of the Y chromosome, the female gonads develop into ovaries by about 8 weeks' gestation, and by 20 weeks the fetal ovary reaches mature compartmentalization. The müllerian ducts become the uterus and fallopian tubes, and the wolffian ducts regress. By week 22 of gestation, canalization to create the uterine cavity, cervical canal, and the vagina is complete.

The external genitalia are neutral primordial and able to develop into either male or female structures. The presence of testosterone from the testes masculinizes the external genitalia, whereas the lack of androgens allows female genitalia to form.

In utero, maternal estrogen thickens and enlarges the female genital structures. After birth, maternal hormones are withdrawn resulting in the desquamation of the hypertrophic walls of the uterus. The mucus from the cervix results in the physiologic leukorrhea of the newborn period. As the hormonal influences continue to decrease, the endometrial shedding may be accompanied by bleeding.

Between 8 weeks and 7 years old, without maternal or endogenous estrogens, the labia majora are flat, the labia minora are thin, and neither offers protection to the genitalia. The absence of fat pads results in an open labia whenever the child is in the squatting position. In addition, this thin atrophic genital epithelium is readily traumatized.

The function of the reproductive system is controlled by the hypothalamic-pituitary-ovarian (HPO) axis. This complex process begins in the neurologic system (the hypothalamus), involves the endocrine system (the anterior pituitary), and completes its cycle with the gonads (ovaries). Initially this cycle causes sexual maturation, and once that is completed the ongoing release of hormones controls the menstrual cycle, pregnancy, and lactation.

Puberty

Puberty is the "coming together of multiple systems and influences, including genetic, metabolic, and hormonal factors" (Speroff and Fritz, 2005, p 178). It is a process usually starting with early breast development (thelarche), then growth of pubic and axillary hair (pubarche), and finally the first menses (menarche).

What sets this all in play is the reactivation of the HPO axis that has been suppressed since shortly after birth. The catalyst for this is unknown; however, there is a reduction of gonadotropin-releasing hormone (GnRH) suppression and decreased sensitivity of the negative feedback to estrogen, which leads to increasing GnRH pulsations to the anterior pituitary. This stimulates the anterior pituitary to release the gonadotropins, follicle-stimulating hormone (FSH), and luteinizing hormone (LH). These in turn stimulate the ovaries to synthesize estrogen (gonadarche). Increasing estrogen stimulates breast development, vaginal and uterine growth, skeletal growth, and female fat distribution. Independent of the HPO axis, increasing levels of adrenal androgens (adrenarche) lead to the growth of pubic and axillary hair. Finally, by midpuberty, there is enough estrogen to cause endometrial proliferation, and the first menses occurs (menarche). Because early cycles are anovulatory 50% to 80% of the time in the first 2 to 3 years after menarche, menstrual irregularities and 21- to 45-day cycle lengths are common. Anovulatory cycles may continue 10% to 20% of the time up to 5 years after menarche.

On average, it takes approximately 4½ years to traverse all the pubertal stages. The mean age of menarche in Caucasian girls is between 12 and 13 years and slightly earlier for African American girls in the United States. This age has remained unchanged for more than 50 years. If a girl has not started breast development by 13 years old or had menarche by 16 years old, she is experiencing delayed puberty and should be evaluated for medical or genetic conditions. Likewise, precocious puberty, the early development of secondary sex characteristics, needs further evaluation. However, the age at which a further workup is recommended varies by source. Traditionally the definition of precocious puberty is breast or pubic hair development in girls younger than 8 years old. In 1999, the Lawson Wilkins Pediatric Endocrine Society (LWPES) developed revised guidelines in response to research findings. Their recommendation, which remains unchanged since 1999, is to evaluate only if secondary sexual characteristics develop before 7 years old in Caucasian American girls and before 6 years old in African American girls (Kaplowitz and Oberfield, 1999). Mansfield and Neinstein (2008) recommend that girls with both breast development and pubic hair at age 7 to 8 should have a review of history and growth and bone age testing for height prediction. Other pediatric endocrinologists argue that lowering the age of workup will miss girls with significant pathology. In a review article, Sørensen and colleagues (2012) estimate that using the LWPES criteria could misdiagnose 5% to 10% of girls with central precocious puberty.

Menstrual Cycle

The menstrual cycle is controlled by the HPO axis. It is essential that PCP have an understanding of this complicated feedback system for the evaluation of menstrual disorders.

The average adult menstrual cycle is 28 days with a range of 21 to 34 days. Figure 36-1 illustrates the female reproductive cycle. The four phases of the cycle are:

- Menses—4 days plus or minus 2 days
- Follicular—10 to 14 days
- Ovulation—10 to 12 hours after LH surge
- Luteal—consistently close to 14 days plus or minus 3 days

The Follicular Phase

Initial follicular development occurs without hormonal influence. However, it is the stimulation by FSH that moves the follicles to the preantral stage. The antral follicle is the dominant follicle and is established during cycle days 5 to 7, leading to increased levels of estradiol by day 7 (Figs. 36-1 and 36-2). The increasing estradiol suppresses FSH and leads to LH secretion. Estrogen also modifies the gonadotropin molecule, increasing the quality and the quantity of FSH and LH midcycle. LH levels rise steadily during the late follicular phase, stimulating the theca in the production of androgen. The action of FSH in the granulosa permits the dominant follicle to use androgen to make estrogen, further increasing estrogen production. FSH also stimulates LH receptors to form on the granulosa cells.

It is not the gonadotropins alone acting on the follicle; growth factors and autocrine and paracrine peptides also influence the feedback loop. Inhibin B, which is secreted by the granulosa cells in response to FSH, suppresses pituitary FSH. Activin, from the pituitary and the granulosa, augments FSH secretion and action, and insulin-like growth factor (IGF) acts to enhance all actions of FSH and LH.

The *preovulatory follicle* occurs when the estrogen levels are sufficient to induce the LH surge; the increasing LH initiates luteinization and progesterone production in the granulosa. This rise in progesterone assists the positive feedback action of estrogen and may be needed to stimulate the

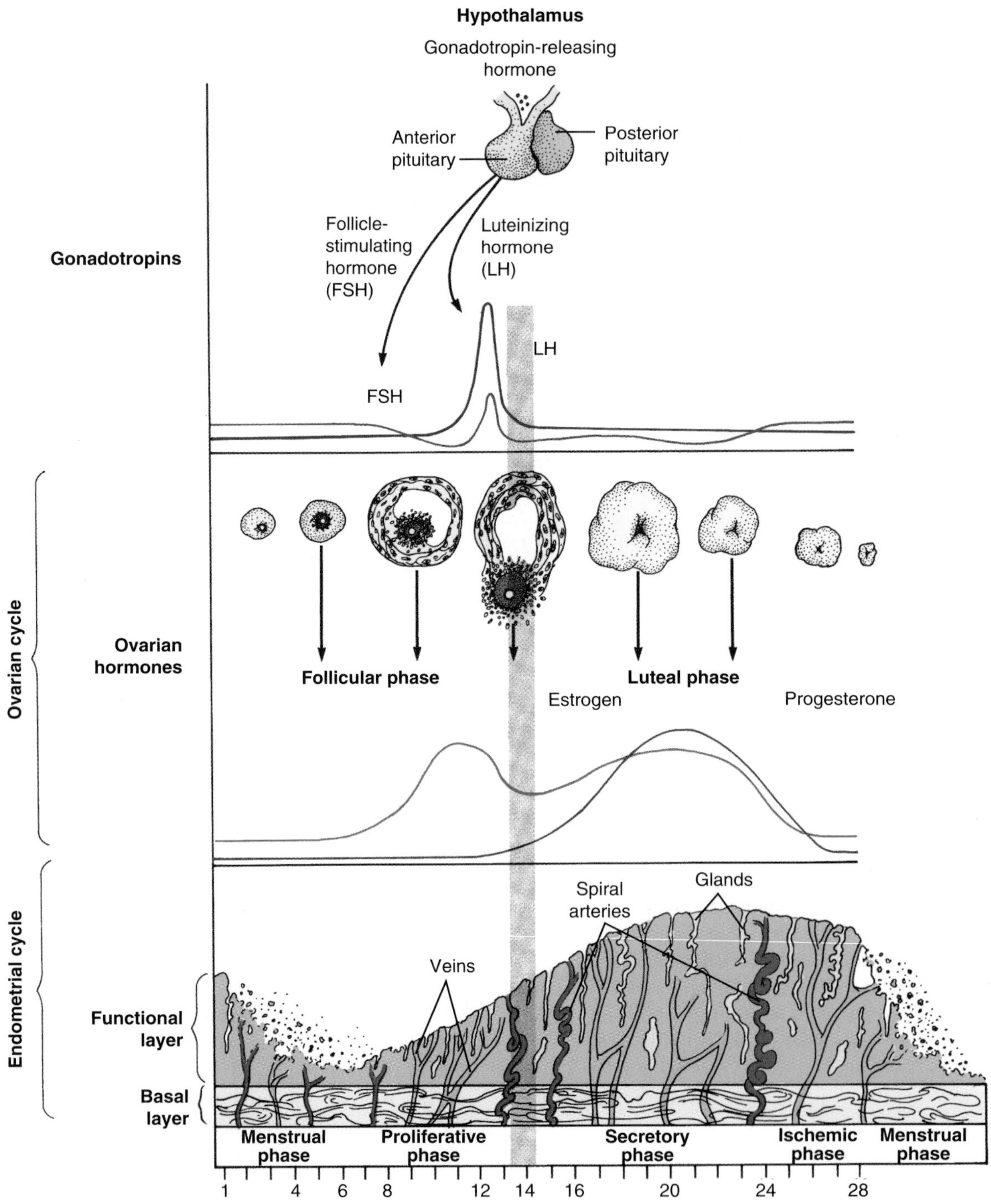

• **Figure 36-1** Female reproductive cycle showing changes in hormone secretion and in the ovary and the uterine endometrium. (From Gorrie T, McKinney E, Murray S: *Foundations of maternal newborn nursing*, ed 2, Philadelphia, 1998, Saunders.)

FSH peak midcycle. An increase in local peripheral androgens also occurs midcycle from the thecal tissue of lesser follicles (Fig. 36-3).

Ovulation

The LH surge stimulates continuation of miosis in the oocyte, luteinization of the granulosa, and production of progesterone and prostaglandins within the follicle. Progesterone augments the activity of the proteolytic enzymes that, together with prostaglandins, are responsible for the digestion and rupture of the follicular wall. The progesterone-influenced midcycle rise in FSH assists to free the oocyte from follicular attachments, to convert plasminogen to the proteolytic enzyme, plasmin, and to guarantee that adequate LH receptors are present to allow a normal luteal phase.

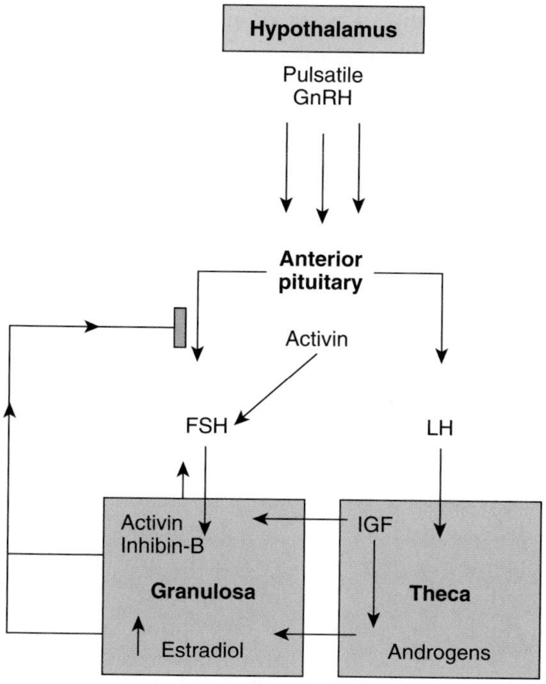

• **Figure 36-2** Early follicular to midfollicular phase. *FSH,* Follicle-stimulating hormone; *GnRH,* gonadotropin-releasing hormone; *IGF,* insulin-like growth factor; *LH,* luteinizing hormone; *orange box* represents negative feedback. (Data adapted from Fritz MA, Speroff L: *Clinical gynecologic endocrinology and infertility*, ed 8, Philadelphia, 2011, Wolters Kluwer Health/Lippincott Williams & Wilkins.)

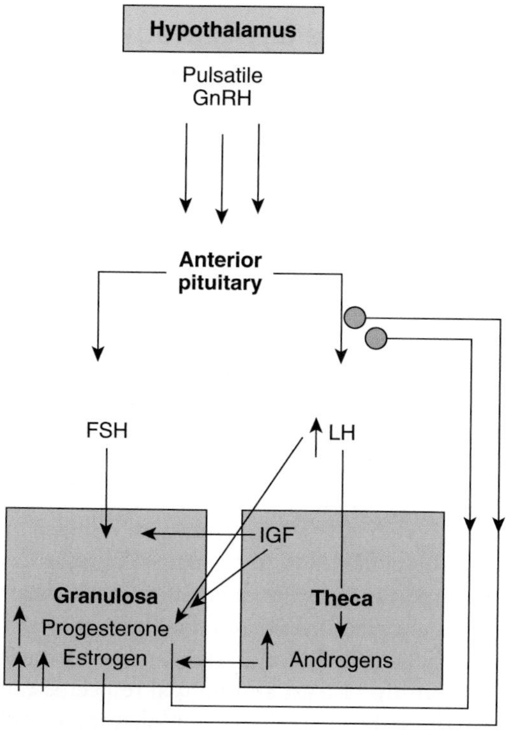

• **Figure 36-3** Late follicular phase to ovulation. *FSH,* Follicle-stimulating hormone; *GnRH,* gonadotropin-releasing hormone; *IGF,* insulin-like growth factor; *LH,* luteinizing hormone; *orange circle* represents positive feedback. (Data adapted from Fritz MA, Speroff L: *Clinical gynecologic endocrinology and infertility*, ed 8, Philadelphia, 2011, Wolters Kluwer Health/Lippincott Williams & Wilkins.)

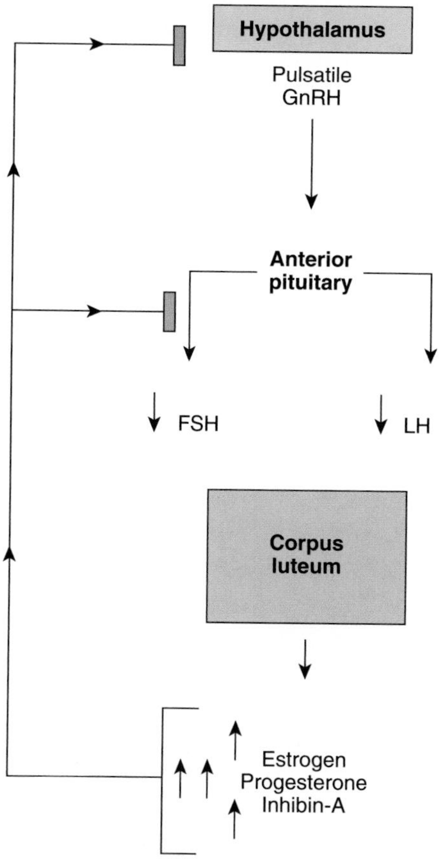

• **Figure 36-4** Early luteal to midluteal phase. *FSH,* Follicle-stimulating hormone; *GnRH,* gonadotropin-releasing hormone; *LH,* luteinizing hormone; *orange boxes* represent negative feedback. (Data adapted from Fritz MA, Speroff L: *Clinical gynecologic endocrinology and infertility*, ed 8, Philadelphia, 2011, Wolters Kluwer Health/Lippincott Williams & Wilkins.)

The Luteal Phase

A normal luteal phase requires both consummate preovulatory follicular development and the continued support of LH. Centrally, progesterone, estrogen, and inhibin A suppress new follicular growth. The regression of the corpus luteum may involve the luteolytic action of estrogen produced by the corpus luteum itself and is interceded by a modification in local prostaglandin and endothelin-1 concentrations (Fig. 36-4).

Luteal-Follicular Transition

The loss of the corpus luteum causes a fall in circulating levels of estradiol, progesterone, and inhibin A. The decreasing inhibin A eliminates the suppression of FSH secretion in the pituitary. The decrease in estradiol and progesterone permits a rapid increase in the frequency of GnRH pulsatile secretion and the elimination of negative feedback on the pituitary. The loss of inhibin-A and estradiol and the increasing GnRH pulsations join to permit greater secretion of FSH as compared with LH, which in turn increases in the frequency of episodic secretion of FSH. This increase in FSH is influential in rescuing an approximately 70-day-old

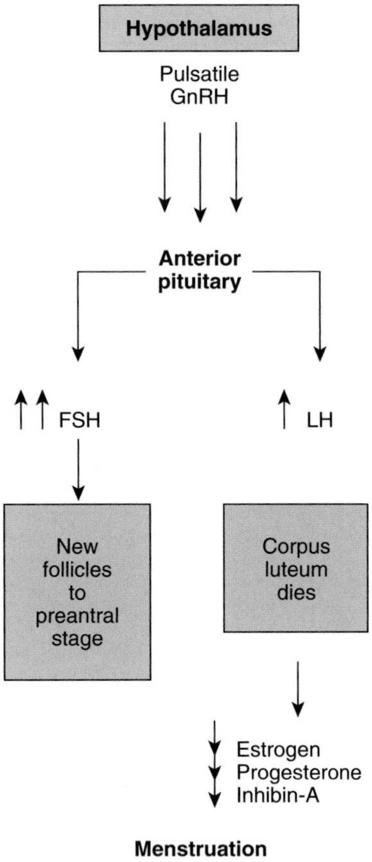

• **Figure 36-5** Luteal-follicular transition. *FSH,* Follicle-stimulating hormone; *GnRH,* gonadotropin-releasing hormone; *LH,* luteinizing hormone. (Data adapted from Fritz MA, Speroff L: *Clinical gynecologic endocrinology and infertility*, ed 8, Philadelphia, 2011, Wolters Kluwer Health/Lippincott Williams & Wilkins.)

group of follicles from atresia. This allows a dominant follicle to begin its emergence, and the cycle begins again (Fig. 36-5).

Pathophysiology and Defense Mechanisms of the Gynecologic System

The primary disorders of the gynecologic system can be classified as menstrual cycle disorders, inflammatory reactions, infection, and reproductive problems. Pubertal development is a complex but normal process. Adolescents may be seen with common menstrual problems, such as mittelschmerz or dysmenorrhea. Abnormal uterine bleeding (AUB), endometriosis, and amenorrhea are three less common menstrual cycle disorders that require the provider to differentiate normal growth and developmental variations from systemic disorders or disease (especially neurologic, endocrine, and reproductive problems). The female athlete is especially prone to exercise-related menstrual problems.

An inflammatory response can occur in either the external or internal genitalia. Local reactions involve the external genitalia and can be caused by dermatologic disorders or skin irritation from factors, such as normal leukorrhea, chemical or allergic reactions, or nonspecific causes. Internal inflammation caused by infection is not always as obvious.

The warm, moist environment of the reproductive tract provides an ideal place for infection. Viral pathogens, such as herpes simplex virus (HSV) and human papillomavirus (HPV), or fungal infection can manifest as vulvitis or a vaginal infection. *Trichomonas,* a protozoal infection, colonizes the vaginal vault. By contrast, bacterial infections caused by chlamydia and gonorrhea can ascend into the upper genital tract where pelvic inflammatory disease (PID) can cause tubal damage.

Reproductive problems occur as a result of structural, hormonal, or endocrine disorders or as sequelae of infection. Refer to a gynecologic or endocrine text for further information.

The gynecologic system has both anatomic and physiologic defense mechanisms. The labia majora and the pubic hair provide a barrier that serves as the first line of defense. The vagina, serving as an exit for mucosal secretion, menstrual fluids, and products of conception, also provides a means of defense with its natural downward and outward flow of secretions. Additionally, with increasing estrogen exposure, the vaginal epithelial tissue thickens and an acid pH develops, discouraging infection. The small external cervical os, a thick mucous plug, and the downward flow of cervical secretions provide barriers to entry to the uterus. A chemical barrier is also established by the cervical enzymes and antibodies.

Assessment of the Gynecologic System: Health Supervision Visits for Female Adolescents

The American Congress of Obstetricians and Gynecologists (ACOG) recommends that young female adolescents have an initial reproductive health visit between 13 and 15 years old to provide preventive care, anticipatory guidance, and screening (ACOG, 2014). This visit includes discussions of sexual development and reproductive issues rather than problem-focused care. Counseling and education about normal menses and patterns, pregnancy prevention, STIs, and HIV are essential; a pelvic examination is performed only if concerns arise that indicate this examination is warranted (discussed later).

This visit is the perfect opportunity to discuss confidentiality with the patient and her parents. All need to understand the importance of confidentiality in the health care provider–patient relationship and the limits to confidentiality imposed by state and local statutes and/or medical necessity. A relationship of trust and mutual respect is extremely important to establish so that the adolescent is willing to discuss intimate matters.

History

The history taken depends on the age of the child and chief complaint. Histories for specific conditions are included later in this chapter. An in-depth sexual history for the adolescent can be found in Chapter 15. The sexual history should be completed with the parent out of the room.

- Family history
- Maternal age at menarche and any problems encountered
- Dysmenorrhea, AUB, or endometriosis
- Diabetes mellitus or thyroid disease
- Bleeding or clotting disorders
- Cancer of the female reproductive system
- Genetic or pubertal development disorders
- Knowledge of pubertal development
- Age at breast and pubic hair development, age at menarche
- Length of cycles, longest and shortest interval between menses, duration of flow, estimated blood loss, last normal menstrual period (LNMP)
- Dysmenorrhea
- Sexual history and current sexual activity
- Knowledge about sexuality and discussions with parent or guardian (see Chapter 15)
- Age at first intercourse (voluntary or forced)
- Type of activity (oral, vaginal, anal)
- Partners of opposite sex, the same sex, or both
- Number of sexual partners in previous 60 days, 12 months, lifetime
- Previous vaginal infections or STIs, current exposures to STIs
- Papanicolaou (Pap) test date and results if history of previous Pap
- Contraceptive history
  - Current method—type, duration, frequency of use, problems and satisfaction
  - Past methods—type, duration, frequency of use, problems and satisfaction
- Obstetric history, as appropriate

Physical Examination

A girl's first gynecologic examination can influence her attitude toward future gynecologic care. When a gynecologic examination is performed, the child or adolescent should maintain a feeling of being in control by giving her as many choices as possible. Options include if she would like someone else in the room with her; the position of the table; use of a hand mirror to observe; and when possible, the timing of the examination. It is important that the provider take the time to establish rapport, preserve modesty, give choices, and obtain consent to examine. This requires flexibility and time from the care provider but demonstrates respect for the adolescent. It is also important that the parent understands what the examination entails and why it is necessary.

Prepubertal Child

There are a variety of positions in which to examine the vulva, vestibule, and lower vagina of a prepubescent girl. Lying on a table, supine, with feet together and knees out ("frog legged") is generally the most comfortable for patients and provides both ease of examination and obtaining of any necessary cultures by the PCP. Another alternative is sitting up in the parent's lap with feet and knees frog legged. Putting the parent on the examination table with feet in the stirrups and the child on his or her lap with feet to the outside of the parent's legs is another alternative. If examination of the entire vagina is necessary, putting the child in knee-chest position on the examination table is the best position for noninvasive, internal examination of the vulva and vagina.

Examine or note the following:

- Breasts, abdomen, and inguinal area
- Presence and distribution of pubic hair
- Presence and distribution of body hair—face, chest, back, abdomen, legs, arms
- Skin lesions
- State of hygiene
- Anus for cleanliness, excoriation, or erythema
- Sexual maturity rating (SMR) or Tanner staging (see Chapter 8 and Fig. 8-3)
- Genital examination with gentle traction on the labia majora
- Size of clitoris (approximately 3×3 mm prepubertal)
- Signs of estrogenization (prepubertal vaginal mucosa—moist, thin, and red; postpubertal vaginal mucosa—moist and dull pink)
- The hymen is normally smooth and continuous and is described as crescent shaped, annular, or redundant (Fig. 36-6). Also note:
  - Presence of notches or tags—normal variation
  - Presence of hymenal ridge—usually without sequela
  - Imperforate hymen
  - Periurethral bands

The significance of the diameter of the hymenal opening as a diagnostic finding is debated. Both transverse and anteroposterior diameters are dependent on age, relaxation, method of examination, and type of hymen. In general, the older and more relaxed the child, the larger the opening. It is also larger with retraction and in the knee-chest position. In the 3- to 6-year-old, a range of normal findings for the transverse diameter is 1 to 6 mm and for the anteroposterior diameter, 1 to 7 mm. Obesity in young children is associated with hymenal openings larger than average for age (e.g., a 2-year-old with a 4-mm opening when average is 2 mm).

Adolescent

- Inspect the skin for acne.
- Examine the breasts; note Tanner stage.
- Palpate the thyroid.
- Inspect hair distribution on face, chest, back, arms, legs, and abdomen.
- Inspect the external genitalia and determine the Tanner stage.
- Vaginal examination alone may be adequate to assess for irregular bleeding, severe dysmenorrhea, vaginal discharge, and amenorrhea. However, a speculum and a

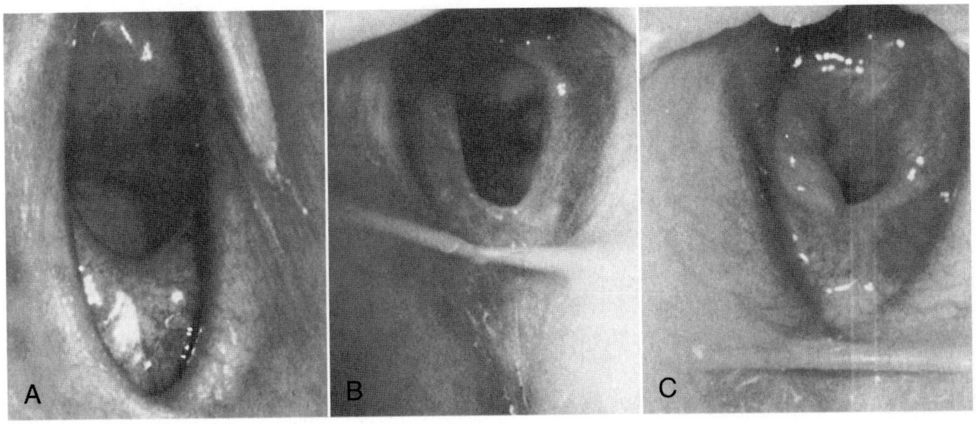

• **Figure 36-6** Types of hymens, photographed through a colposcope. **A,** Crescentic hymen. **B,** Annular hymen. **C,** Redundant hymen with crescent appearance after retraction. (From Emans SJ: Vulvovaginal problems in the prepubertal child. In Emans SJ, Laufer MR, Goldstein DP, editors: *Pediatric and adolescent gynecology*, ed 5, Philadelphia, 2005, Lippincott Williams & Wilkins.)

bimanual examination may be necessary based on symptoms and history.

Diagnostic Studies

The routine care of the child and adolescent without gynecologic complaints does not require diagnostic studies. When indicated, the following studies can be helpful as diagnostic tools. Specific studies and techniques are discussed with each diagnosis in subsequent sections in this chapter. Collection of specimens must be done with care. Techniques that are helpful include using a small amount of saline as a vaginal wash, using a soft plastic eyedropper or feeding tube, or using a moistened cotton swab. Tests may include:

- Wet mounts of vaginal secretions
- Saline for microscopic examination to look for white blood cells (WBCs), clue cells, trichomonads, and bacteria
- 10% potassium hydroxide (KOH) for whiff test and microscopic examination to look for yeast (branching hyphae and spores) (Fig. 36-7)
- pH of vaginal mucus (neutral in prepubescent; less than 4.5 once pubertal)
- Urine-based nucleic acid amplification test (NAAT), cultures, and/or serologic blood tests for STIs
- Other tests as indicated, including pregnancy test by urine or serum, BiGGY agar culture (suspected yeast infection), or ultrasound

Cervical Cancer Screening

The American Cancer Society (2014), ACOG (2012), and U.S. Preventive Services Task Force (2014) all recommend that cervical cancer screening with Pap testing should begin at 21 years old and occur every 3 years thereafter. The prior annual Pap testing policy has been abandoned due to over-diagnosis of cervical pathologic conditions and unnecessary interventions. This change is a result of understanding the natural history of HPV infections, which is the causative agent of most cervical cancer. There is evidence that the majority of low-grade HPV lesions regress spontaneously. The Centers for Disease Control and Prevention (CDC) (2012) reports the overall prevalence of high-risk HPV is 23%. For adolescents 14 to 19 years old, the rate is 35%; for women in their 20s, the rate decreases to 29%.

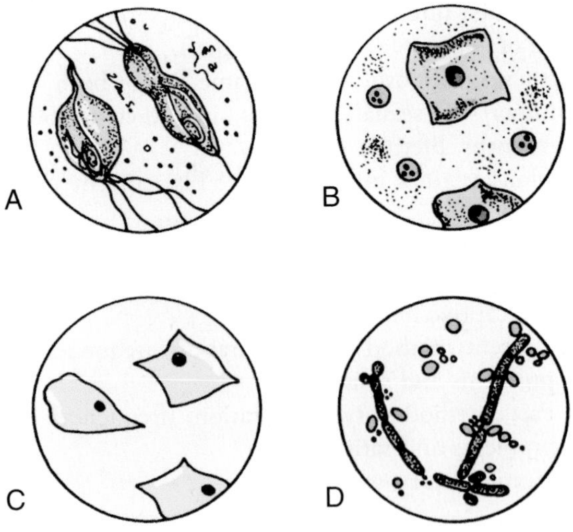

• **Figure 36-7** Drawings of vaginal smears. **A,** *Trichomonas.* **B,** Clue cells of bacterial vaginosis (BV). **C,** Leukorrhea. **D,** Candida. **A, B,** and **C** are saline preparations; **D** is a potassium hydroxide (KOH) preparation. (From Emans SJ: Vulvovaginal problems in the prepubertal child. In Emans SJ, Laufer MR, Goldstein DP, editors: *Pediatric and adolescent gynecology*, ed 5, Philadelphia, 2005, Lippincott Williams & Wilkins.)

Management Strategies

Anticipatory Guidance, Counseling, and Education

Anticipatory guidance related to gynecologic issues is important to both the child or adolescent and parents. Attention to appropriate genital hygiene can help prevent some potential childhood problems. The transition to puberty and establishment of menses is eased with appropriate education and counseling beforehand. With the advent of puberty and the increasing interest in sexuality, a great deal of guidance is needed to help the adolescent and her parents through these transitions. See Chapters 8 and 15 for further discussion of these topics.

Counseling and education related to normal gynecologic conditions and disorders of the gynecologic system need to be tailored to the child or adolescent and the parents. See Chapter 15 for more information on sexuality counseling. Confidentiality is a matter to be established with both the parents and the adolescent. Some states have specific laws that allow providers to treat adolescents for obstetric and family planning conditions without parental knowledge or consent.

Adolescent Pregnancy Prevention

There are several common goals in adolescent pregnancy prevention. These goals can be achieved by supporting a positive or protective environment, connecting the adolescent to an intervention program, and providing appropriate health care services. Prevention goals include the following:

- Maintain sexual health and promote sexual responsibility.
- Assist adolescents to make informed choices, recognizing educational, social, and economic effect of choices.
- Encourage abstinence and delay onset of intercourse.
- Provide contraceptive counseling and selection of a contraceptive method if sexually active or anticipating sexual activity, or for any adolescent who has recently experienced a spontaneous abortion, as part of third-trimester health teaching before delivery, or at the time of an elective termination of pregnancy.

Appropriate health care services are important in preventing adolescent pregnancy. This care should include confidentiality with minimal or no financial barriers; easy availability (e.g., timed for easy access, on site at school, or easy transportation to site); and a full range of contraceptive services for male and female adolescents (see Contraception for specific methods).

The CDC (2014b) addresses several core factors the evidence-based pregnancy prevention programs share, as listed in Box 36-1. The National Campaign to Prevent Teen and Unplanned Pregnancy (2008) has also outlined actions that parents can take to help protect against pregnancy (Box 36-2).

• BOX 36-1 Common Components of Evidence-based Teen Pregnancy Prevention Programs

- Knowledge of sexual issues, HIV, other STIs, and pregnancy (including methods of prevention)
- Perception of HIV risk
- Personal values about sex and abstinence
- Attitudes toward use of condoms (pro and con)
- Perception of peer norms and sexual behavior
- Individual ability to refuse sex and to use condoms
- Intent to abstain from sex or limit number of partners
- Communication with parents or other adults about sex, condoms, and contraception
- Individual ability to avoid HIV/STI risk and risk behaviors
- Avoidance of places and situations that might lead to sex
- Intent to use a condom

HIV, Human immunodeficiency virus; *STI*, sexually transmitted infection.

• BOX 36-2 What Parents Can Do to Protect Against Pregnancy

- Be clear about your sexual values and attitudes.
- Talk with your children early and often about sex, and be specific.
- Supervise and monitor your children and adolescents.
- Know their friends and families.
- Discourage early, frequent, and steady dating.
- Discourage dating of older persons.
- Encourage education and future goals.
- Know what your kids are watching, reading, and listening to.
- Build a strong, close relationship from an early age.

Contraception

Contraceptive Counseling and Education

Significant and specific knowledge is required for PCPs to offer reproductive health and contraceptive services to adolescents. An in-depth discussion is beyond the scope of this text; however, excellent management references are available. The authors recommend *Contraceptive Technology* by Hatcher and colleagues (2011) and *A Clinical Guide for Contraception* by Speroff and Darney (2011). Contraceptive counseling needs to be individualized and at the adolescent's developmental level. It is also important not to overwhelm the patient with too much information at one time. Ascertain what methods she knows about or is thinking about using. Frequently the provider needs to dispel misconceptions about risks related to various methods and educate on the menstrual and health benefits. It may take more than one visit to find a compatible contraceptive method. However, the adolescent should not leave the office without understanding the risk of pregnancy and STIs and HIV with unprotected sex. She should have education about and a prescription for emergency contraception (EC), know that condoms are a must for safer sex, and have practiced how to apply a condom correctly.

Factors identified as predictive of failure or success with contraception are listed in Box 36-3. Antecedent risk factors to unintentional pregnancy are listed in Box 36-4.

• BOX 36-3 Factors Predicting Success or Failure with Contraception

- Age: Adolescents 15 years old and younger are at highest risk for pregnancy because 40.9% report using no method of contraception at their first episode of intercourse. In comparison, only 9.9% of females 17 to 19 years old report using no method (Abma et al, 2010). Noncompliance with the first method chosen (previous method failure).
- Not acquiring a method of contraception at the first reproductive health visit.
- Frequency of family planning visits in the preceding 12 months: Increased compliance with clinic attendance appears to correlate with effective contraceptive use by client.
- Coital frequency: Adolescent females who have sexual intercourse more than six times per month are at greater risk of becoming pregnant.
- Length of time between first coitus and initiation of birth control use: The longer adolescents delay seeking services for contraception, the less likely they are to use a highly reliable method consistently and correctly.

• BOX 36-4 Risk Factors for Unintentional Pregnancy

- Early onset of sexual activity, especially before 15 years old
- Early onset of substance use, including cigarettes, alcohol, and illicit drugs
- Lesbian or bisexual; these females are as likely to have sex with males as heterosexuals, but their pregnancy rate is more than doubled (CDC, 2014c)
- Low educational expectation, poor academic achievement or dropout
- Low perception of life options; living in an environment where adolescent pregnancy is commonplace and accepted
- Poor grades and academic achievement
- Behavior problems, including truancy and delinquency
- Negative peer influence
- Poor contraceptive compliance or failure with a contraceptive device
- Nonintact families (those without both biologic mother and father present)
- Lack of family involvement; an intolerable home situation as defined by the teen
- Loss of parent by death, separation, divorce, or foster placement
- Depression or family history of mental illness
- Cultural values that favor adolescent pregnancy
- Prior history of sexual or physical abuse or neglect or violence at home (Cox, 2012)

Initial Screening to Assess for Appropriate Contraception

History

For the most part, adolescent girls are healthy with no contraindications for hormonal contraceptive methods. However, it is important to get a personal history related to cardiovascular and peripheral vascular disease, diabetes, headaches, liver and gallbladder disease, and current medications (including prescription, over-the-counter [OTC], herbal, and dietary supplements). The World Health Organization (WHO), using evidence-based methodology, has developed medical eligibility criteria for starting contraceptive methods (WHO, 2010). The authors recommend using the WHO website to access the most recent updates.

Physical Examination

- Height and weight; body mass index (BMI)
- Blood pressure
- Thyroid examination
- Breast examination, including Tanner staging
- Auscultation of heart and lungs
- Abdominal examination
- Pelvic examination (not a requirement to start oral contraceptive pills [OCPs])

Diagnostic Studies

- NAAT on urine, cervix or vaginal wall or cultures for gonorrhea and chlamydia as indicated
- Wet mounts when indicated by presence of abnormal vaginal discharge
- Complete blood count (CBC) or hemoglobin or hematocrit and rubella titer as indicated
- Syphilis serology with known STI, particularly condylomas or genital ulcers and if residing in endemic areas
- HIV

Hormonal Methods of Contraception (Coitus-Independent Methods)

Oral Contraceptive Pills

In addition to contraception, OCPs also offer cycle regulation, protection from endometrial and ovarian cancer, decreased iron deficiency anemia, and slowing the progression of endometriosis.

Types of Preparations. Two basic preparations are available: a combination oral contraction (COC) formulation that contains estrogen (less than 50 mcg) and progestin in a low dose, and a progestin-only minipill. Most women in the United States use the combination formulation, in either monophasic or triphasic formats. Progestin-only pills (POPs) are prescribed for women in whom estrogens are contraindicated (e.g., lactating women or women with medical contraindications to estrogen). Generally they are not the first choice for nonlactating adolescents because of irregular bleeding and higher failure rates. Mechanism of action, theoretic and use effectiveness, benefits, disadvantages, and side effects are listed in Table 36-1. The

TABLE 36-1 Hormonal Methods of Contraception: Mechanism of Action, Theoretic and Use Effectiveness, Benefits, Disadvantages, Side Effects, Failure, and Efficacy

Method	Mechanism of Action	Theoretic and Use Effectiveness	Benefits	Disadvantages	Side Effects, Failure, and Efficacy
Oral contraceptive pills (OCPs)	Suppression of ovulation (90% to 95% with COC and 50% with POP) Thickening of cervical mucus, blocking penetration of sperm Alteration of endometrial lining Alteration of tubal motility	Perfect use failure rate is 0.3% Typical first-year failure rate in all women is 8%	High rate of effectiveness Simple method to use Ease of discontinuing use Rapid reversal of effects after discontinuing medication Beneficial effects on the menstrual cycle Reduction of premenstrual symptoms Decreased dysmenorrhea Decreased flow Medical benefits: For women younger than 20 years old, the estimated death rate while on an OCP is 0.3 per 100,000 nonsmoking users (2.2 per 100,000 smoking users), as compared with that of childbirth, for which the estimated maternal death rate in the United States was 18.5 per 100,000 live births in 2013 (Kassebaum et al, 2014) Other health benefits: Reduction of anemia risks Decreased incidence of gonorrheal PID, resulting in less morbidity (chronic pelvic pain, decreased incidence of ectopic pregnancies, and less infertility) Protection against formation of ovarian cysts (COCs) Reduction of ovarian and endometrial cancer (COCs) Ortho Tri-Cyclen and Estrostep are approved by FDA for treatment of acne	No protection from STIs—need to use condoms Daily use difficult for some women Triphasic OCPs: Confusion about color of package Less flexibility of use by the prescriber (e.g., difficult to use for periods greater than 21 days or for management of ovarian cysts, endometrial bleeding, or AUB) Some adolescents find triphasic preparation confusing, especially if they forget to take a pill POPs: Irregular bleeding Effectiveness decreases dramatically if even one pill is missed; manufacturer recommends that POPs be taken at the same time every day and that a backup method of birth control be used if even one pill is missed or taken more than 3 hours late (Hatcher et al, 2011) May increase acne No protection from STIs—need to use condoms	Nausea and vomiting Breakthrough bleeding (spotting) Breast tenderness Headaches Mood changes OCP failure: Method failure or method ineffectiveness Patient failure/user effectiveness—68% still use OCPs 1 year after initiation; most discontinuance is for nonmedical reasons Concurrent drug interaction, such as with anticonvulsants, tetracycline, St. John's wort, and possibly oral antifungals OCPs can increase the action of diazepam, tricyclics, chlordiazepoxide, and theophylline

Continued

TABLE 36-1 Hormonal Methods of Contraception: Mechanism of Action, Theoretic and Use Effectiveness, Benefits, Disadvantages, Side Effects, Failure, and Efficacy—cont'd

Method	Mechanism of Action	Theoretic and Use Effectiveness	Benefits	Disadvantages	Side Effects, Failure, and Efficacy
Injectable contraception	Inhibits ovulation by inhibiting LH surge (normal ovulation occurs within 6 months after the last injection in approximately 50% of women; however, 25% will take up to 1 year to return to a normal menstrual pattern) (Speroff and Darney, 2011) Creates shallow, atrophic endometrium, unsuitable for implantation Increases thickening of cervical mucus, decreasing sperm penetration	The lowest expected pregnancy rate is 0.3 per 100 women with the typical failure rate of 3%	One-time dosing every 3 months Good method for adolescents who want to keep contraception private from family and friends Gynecologic benefits (e.g., decreases in PID, ectopic pregnancy, and endometriosis)	Menstrual irregularities (including amenorrhea or decreased menstrual flow) Weight gain Headache Breast tenderness Acne Hirsutism Psychological effects, such as moodiness, depression, change in libido Evidence of bone density loss in adolescents; osteopenia Intramuscular injection Need to use condoms to prevent STIs Increased risk for low birthweight in infants exposed in utero	
Postcoital hormonal contraception *or* emergency contraception (EC)	Inhibits ovulation May affect tubal transport				Nausea, vomiting, breast tenderness, headache, and dizziness The progestin-only methods have fewer side effects (Speroff and Darney, 2011) Plan B One Step has a 1% failure rate Yuzpe method has a 2% to 3% failure rate

AUB, Abnormal uterine bleeding; *COC,* combination oral contraceptive; *FDA,* U.S. Food and Drug Administration; *LH,* luteinizing hormone; *PID,* pelvic inflammatory disease; *POP,* progestin-only pill; *STI,* sexually transmitted infection.

initial use of an OCP requires special attention to dosing, preparation, timing, patient education, and follow-up.

Dosing. Initial dosing for a combination OCP should be at 30 to 35 mcg estrogen, with low progestin potency per tablet. Most providers have one or two OCPs that are favorites for first-time use in women without special conditions. There are 20-mcg combination OCPs available, should an ultra-low dose estrogen formulation be desired. The selection of an OCP can also be individualized based on menstrual characteristics or patient sensitivity. For example, a client with a history of cystic acne can be tried on an OCP in which the progestins are desogestrel or norgestrel, or on Ortho Tri-Cyclen or Estrostep, the only OCPs with U.S. Food and Drug Administration (FDA) approval for use in acne. For clients with hirsutism or polycystic ovary syndrome (PCOS), a low androgenic potency pill is used, such as Ortho-Cyclen, Desogen, or Ovcon-35. For clients who miss pills, using a monophasic 30- to 35-mcg pill provides more protection against escape ovulation than a 20-mcg estrogen, progestin only, or triphasic pill. Adolescents who demonstrate estrogen sensitivity can be tried on a more androgenic pill (such as, Lo/Ovral, Nordette, or Loestrin) or a 20-mcg preparation (such as, Alesse).

Preparation. Given the vast selection of products available to the health care provider, choose a few favorites that are on formulary and/or have a cheaper generic version. Box 36-5 has a list of questions to review in helping make a selection.

Timing. Ideally, OCPs should not be started until the adolescent has had three to six regular periods after menarche, but sexually active or other high-risk teens can be put on OCPs even before menarche. OCPs can be started 3 to 4 weeks postpartum (if breastfeeding, POPs) or after a first-trimester therapeutic abortion (Hatcher et al, 2011). Speroff and Darney (2011) add the caveat that to reduce the risk of postpartum venous thromboembolism only POPs should be used until after 6 weeks postpartum whether lactating or not.

• BOX 36-5 Steps in Choosing a Combined Oral Contraceptive with Low-Dose Estrogen

1. Does the adolescent have a contraindication to estrogen use?
2. If yes, consider the use of a progestin-only formulation.
3. If the client can use estrogen, the provider can select from among numerous products, considering the following:
   - The number of micrograms of estrogen in the preparation
   - Availability of the pill on formulary
   - Ease of understanding the packaging of the pill
   - Price of the pill to the adolescent and possibly the clinic
   - Previous adverse event or experience the adolescent may have had with a specific preparation
4. Consider other clinical factors, such as acne, nausea or vomiting, spotting or breakthrough bleeding, and absence of withdrawal bleeding.

There are several ways in which OCPs can be initiated:

- Quick start—same day start in certain circumstances
  - If within 72 hours of unprotected sex, use EC now and start OCPs the next day.
  - If pregnancy can be ruled out or there was no unprotected sex since the last menses, may start same day and use backup (condoms) for 7 days or until menses starts. This is a preferable method for adolescents because it is less complicated and has a higher rate of continuation.
- Start first day of menses
- Start within 5 days after menses and use backup (condoms) for 7 days
- First Sunday after menses started and use backup (condoms) for 7 days

Another timing issue is the pattern of COC use. The majority of pill packs come with 28-day cycling: 21 days of active tablets and 7 days of placebo tablets, with the woman having a monthly withdrawal bleed during the placebo week. For years, providers have recommended various patterns of monophasic COC use to prevent withdrawal bleeds. Women can skip the placebo week of their pill packs for one, two, or three cycles to decrease the number of withdrawal bleeds per year. This is particularly helpful in women with endometriosis, menorrhagia, severe dysmenorrhea, and menstrual migraines. Extended-cycle COCs are also available, packaged with 84 active pills and 7 inactive pills, giving women only four withdrawal bleeds per year.

Patient Education. Provide clear instructions on the correct way to start OCPs and need for consistent use. Include in the instructions:

- To take the pill every day in the order presented in the pill pack—no matter what your body is doing or what your friends say.
- How to make up missed or forgotten pills and the use of a backup method
  - One missed pill: Take as soon as possible (ASAP) and take next pill as usual.
  - Two missed pills: Take one pill ASAP and one pill in 12 hours. Then continue with the remainder of the pack and use backup for 7 days. Additionally, offer EC if pills are missed in first week of pack.
  - If more than two pills are missed, take EC and restart OCPs the next day and use backup for the next 7 days. If EC is declined, skip missed pills and continue the rest of the pack and use backup until next menses (Hatcher et al, 2011).
- Common side effects and the need to call if questions or concerns arise.

All adolescents should also use condoms along with any other method used for contraception for protection from STIs and HIV. Additionally, all adolescents should have a prescription for EC and understand how and when to use them.

Follow-up Management. Provide an emergency follow-up number and instruct the client on indications for calling. Schedule a return appointment. The return visit gives the

• BOX 36-6 The Mnemonic ACHES Used to Teach and Assess for Risks of Oral Contraceptive Pills

Abdominal pain: Have you experienced abdominal pain (severe)?
Chest pain: Have you noticed chest pain (severe), cough, or shortness of breath?
Headaches: Do you have headaches (severe), dizziness, weakness, or numbness?
Eye problems: Have you had a change in vision (loss or blurring) or other eye problems or speech problems?
Severe leg pain: Have you had any severe leg pain, especially in the calf or thigh?

health care provider an opportunity to assess the physiologic effects of the OCP and the adolescent's acceptance and use of this particular contraceptive method.

Adolescents tend to be acutely aware of and sensitive to body changes and processes. As a result, they may incorrectly interpret physical signs, exaggerate the effects of OCPs on their bodies, and discontinue the OCP use without consulting their health care provider. At the follow-up visit, the provider should reemphasize the noncontraceptive benefits of the OCP, have the client discuss concerns about the OCPs, discuss the lower risks of OCPs compared with those of pregnancy, and review and reclarify directions and side effects.

Interview the client for STI exposure, compliance, satisfaction with medication, and perceived side effects. The use of the mnemonic, ACHES (Box 36-6), can help guide assessment questions, and can be used carefully to help the teenager understand more clearly the risks of OCPs without unduly concerning her. Physical examination parameters during the return visit include weight and blood pressure measurements and any laboratory follow-up.

Other Methods of Hormonal Contraception

Hormonal contraception can also be delivered in other preparations (Box 36-7).

Postcoital Hormonal Contraception or Emergency Contraception

Preparations. EC is designed to be used after unprotected intercourse to prevent an unwanted pregnancy. Plan B One Step is one tablet of levonorgestrel that should be taken within 72 hours of unprotected intercourse for the highest efficacy. As of June 2013, it was made available in the United States OTC for all women without age restrictions. A generic version of levonorgestrel EC (AfterPill) is available online for half the price of Plan B One Step retail. Ulipristal acetate (Ella) is a formulation that can be taken up to 5 days after unprotected intercourse; it requires a prescription in all cases. Regular OCPs (combination) may also be used at recommended dosages; this regimen is referred to as the *Yuzpe method.* POPs are another alternative. See *Contraceptive Technology* (Hatcher et al, 2011) for specifics. There are no contraindications to EC for progestin-only formulations.

Clinical Management. All adolescents should have EC, in advance, for self-administration as needed. This is intended for such times as when a condom breaks or there has been a lapse in birth control method. An emergency contraceptive is more effective the earlier it is taken after unprotected intercourse. Studies have shown that when readily available, the use of EC does not increase unprotected sex (Speroff and Darney, 2011).

If a client has a need for EC and does not meet parameters for Plan B:

- Assess for pregnancy using a rapid high-sensitivity urine pregnancy test. If LNMP has been within 1 month, a pregnancy test is not necessary.
- Instruct patient to return for a pregnancy test if no menses occurs within 3 weeks.
- Instruct patient to abstain from intercourse until the start of her next cycle or use condoms 100% of the time.
- Discuss a long-term birth control method; review current method and effectiveness for client.
- Schedule return visit in 3 to 4 weeks.

Barrier Methods of Contraception (Coitus-Dependent Methods)

Mechanism of action, theoretic and use effectiveness, and benefits and disadvantages of barrier methods of contraception are listed in Table 36-2.

Condoms

Condoms are the most common barrier method of contraception. Used effectively they can prevent pregnancy and decrease STI transmission. In the CDC's 2013 Youth Risk Behavior Surveillance System data, 59.1% of high school students stated they used condoms for their last act of sexual intercourse (Kann et al, 2014).

More than 100 brands of condoms are available in an array of sizes (most are 170 × 50 mm), textures, lubricants, colors, and scents. Ninety-nine percent use latex condoms, and less than 1% use either natural skin or the newer polyurethane condoms. The polyurethane condoms are not subject to breakdown by petroleum-based lubricants, are latex-free, and have an improved taste over latex. However, they are less elastic, which increases slippage and breakage. They should be reserved for those with latex allergies. Protocol for use includes:

- *Use every time!*
- Apply correctly, allowing for 0.5-inch tip at end and removing any trapped air.
- Remove correctly after intercourse. Hold on to the condom while withdrawing the penis from the vagina to prevent the condom from coming off in the vagina. Replace if used for oral or anal sex before intravaginal intercourse.
- Avoid use of petroleum-based lubricants, such as petroleum jelly, shortening, and oil-based vaginal therapeutics, such as Monistat or Femstat.

• BOX 36-7 Other Methods of Hormonal Contraception

Contraceptive Patch

The contraceptive patch (Ortho Evra) is a 20-cm^2 transdermal adhesive patch consisting of progestin (17-deacetylnorgestimate) and ethinyl estradiol placed on the trunk, buttock, or arm once a week for 3 weeks and removed for 1 week to allow for a withdrawal bleed. The advantage of the patch is that it does not require the user to remember a daily oral contraceptive pill (OCP). Disadvantages include the visibility of the patch, which precludes privacy of method, and the need to remember to replace the patch when indicated. The patch also has decreased efficacy in women who weigh more than 198 pounds (90 kg). It costs about the same as OCPs (except for generic forms) and has the same precautions and side effects as OCPs. There is some evidence that the patch may have an increased risk of nonfatal venous thromboembolism (VTE) over OCPs in some women. Careful screening of VTE risk is recommended.

Vaginal Ring

The vaginal contraceptive ring (NuvaRing) is a self-administered contraceptive, consisting of a soft, flexible, 2-inch transparent plastic ring with a hole in the middle. It is 0.125-inch thick and is impregnated with estrogen and progestin. It is inserted vaginally once a month on or before the fifth day of menses, left in place for 3 weeks, removed for 1 week to allow for a withdrawal bleed, and then a new ring is inserted. Placement over the cervix is not necessary. As long as it is in contact with the vagina, it is working. The failure rate is the same as OCPs: typical use 8%, and perfect use 0.3%. Advantages include that it is coitus independent, does not involve the use of messy creams or gels, and is only dealt with once a month. It does not provide protection against sexually transmitted infections (STIs); there is some initial breakthrough bleeding, and the user must be comfortable inserting and removing the device and be able to adhere to the usage schedule.

Injectable Contraception: Medroxyprogesterone Acetate (Depo-Provera)

A single 150-mg intramuscular or 104-mg subcutaneous injection inhibits ovulation for 13 weeks. Dosage adjustment for body weight is not necessary. Always evaluate for pregnancy before giving the initial dose. It is preferable to deliver the initial injection before day 5 of the menstrual cycle to minimize pregnancy potential. Injections are usually given at 12-week intervals. If more than 13 weeks have transpired between injections, evaluate for pregnancy before giving the injection. Mechanism of action, theoretic and use effectiveness, benefits, and disadvantages are listed in Table 36-1. Medroxyprogesterone acetate is a contraceptive method of choice for patients with the following characteristics: seeking a long-term, reversible, highly reliable, private method of contraception; those for whom use of estrogen is contraindicated (e.g., patients with a previous thromboembolic episode, lupus, sickle cell anemia); those with seizure disorders—improves control (Speroff and Darney, 2011); those with poor compliance using other contraceptive methods; those with menstrual hygiene issues, such as individuals with an intellectual disability, because medroxyprogesterone acetate often causes amenorrhea after two injections.

Subdermal Implant Contraception

Implanon and Nexplanon are the only current implanted form of progestin-only contraception on the market in the United States. They are both a one-rod, 3-year subdermal implant that has a newer form of progestin (etonogestrel), however, Nexplanon (second generation) is radiopaque and is easier to insert than Implanon. The method of action is the same as other progestin-only methods. The advantage of an implant is that it provides long-acting contraception. Disadvantages include surgical insertion and removal procedures and side effects, such as irregular bleeding, weight gain, and acne. It is a more successful method for mature adolescents committed to long-term contraception.

Intrauterine Device

The levonorgestrel-releasing intrauterine system (LNG-IUS) is one of the two intrauterine devices (IUDs) available in the United States. The American Congress of Obstetricians and Gynecologists (ACOG) states that IUDs are safe to use in adolescents and do not increase the risk of infertility (AGOG, 2012a). As with any hormonal contraceptive method thorough counseling and education are required as is careful screening. Advantages include long-acting contraception that reduces blood loss during menses by 90% (Dayananda et al, 2012). Adverse or side effects are no different in adolescents than in adult women. See *Contraceptive Technology* (Hatcher et al, 2011) and *A Clinical Guide for Contraception* (Speroff and Darney, 2011) for detailed information.

- Check expiration date on the package, and make sure package is intact.
- Use only once and discard.
- Keep a prescription for an emergency contraceptive handy.

Diaphragm

Available for more than 100 years, there are three types of diaphragms in sizes from 50 to 105 mm, available by prescription only. For most adolescents, the 65- to 75-mm sizes of the coil spring or flat spring diaphragms are commonly prescribed. The diaphragm may be placed in the vagina over the cervix up to 1 hour before intercourse. It can be left in place for 24 hours, but it must be left a minimum of 6 to 8 hours. Reapplication of spermicide is required with subsequent intercourse. Protocol for use: *Use every time!*

Cervical Cap

The cervical cap, like the diaphragm, is available by prescription only. It may be left in place for 48 hours; however, subsequent intercourse within 6 hours or more requires additional intravaginal spermicide. The cervical cap should probably be reserved for those adolescents who are older, more motivated to comply with contraception, and able to place and remove the device. Protocol for use: *Use every time!*

TABLE 36-2 Barrier Methods of Contraception: Mechanism of Action, Theoretic and Use Effectiveness, Benefits, and Disadvantages

Method	Mechanism of Action	Theoretic and Use Effectiveness	Benefits	Disadvantages
Condoms	Prevent sperm from entering vagina	First-year failure rate among typical users is 15% First-year failure rate among perfect users is 2% Concomitant, perfect use of condoms with a spermicide has an estimated probability of contraceptive failure of 0.3%; this is equivalent to perfect-use failure rate with an OCP	Encourages male participation Appeals to those who have episodic intercourse and for sexual debuts (Lohr, 2008) Is inexpensive and accessible Use of lubricated condoms reduces mechanical friction and vaginal or penile irritation Decreases the risk of transmitting STIs Eliminates postcoital vaginal discharge Helps maintain erection for some men Has few contraindications	Condom breakage or slippage; approximately 2% to 6% of condoms fail as a result of breakage or slippage. Natural-skin condoms are contraindicated if there is a risk of infection by sexually transmitted viruses (e.g., hepatitis B virus, HPV, HSV, and HIV). Either partner may be allergic to latex. Male partner may fail to accept responsibility for use. Some men cannot maintain an erection when a condom is used.
Other barrier methods (diaphragm, cervical cap, female condom, contraceptive sponge)		Effectiveness of any of these methods is influenced by the patient's ability to use the method consistently and correctly, along with her own personal fertility characteristics Patients who are younger than 30 years old and have intercourse four or more times a week experience higher failure rates Diaphragm failure rate is 16% in typical users Cervical cap failure rate averages 16% to 32% Female condom pregnancy rates are reported to be 21% Sponge failure rate with typical use is 14% to18%	Diaphragms and female condoms help prevent transmission of STIs and decrease risk of PID, bacterial and viral infection, and cervical neoplasia Female condoms and the sponge are accessible OTC	Barrier methods are contraindicated if there is a history of toxic shock syndrome. Female condoms cost about $2 versus 50¢ to $1 for male condoms and have a visible outer ring. Sponges cost about $3 per sponge. Cervical caps are contraindicated if there has been a full-term delivery within the past 6 weeks, if there has been a recent spontaneous or induced abortion, or if there is vaginal bleeding from any cause, including menstrual flow. Allergic reaction may occur in those sensitive to rubber, latex, or polyurethane. Abnormalities in vaginal anatomy can interfere with satisfactory fit or placement of any of the devices. Diaphragm can cause recurrent urinary tract infections. For diaphragms and caps, trained personnel may not be available to fit device or lack the time to instruct patient adequately on use of method. Patient must be able to learn correct insertion and extraction techniques. Patient may not feel comfortable touching self or may find procedure messy and unpleasant.

TABLE 36-2 Barrier Methods of Contraception: Mechanism of Action, Theoretic and Use Effectiveness, Benefits, and Disadvantages—cont'd

Method	Mechanism of Action	Theoretic and Use Effectiveness	Benefits	Disadvantages
Spermicides	A combination of an inert base or carrier (foam, cream, jelly, suppository, or tablet) with active spermicidal agent nonoxynol-9 or octoxynol, which kills sperm by permeating the cell membrane	Estimated 15% failure rate among perfect first-year users Among typical users, failure rate is about 29%	Medically safe, with same efficacy as barrier methods or condoms Available OTC without a prescription; no need to access medical system No need for partner involvement with decision-making or implementation Used as backup option while waiting to start OCPs, for missed OCPs, or between relationships	Can cause allergic reaction in those sensitive to spermicidal agent or base Can be difficult for some people to learn correct insertion technique Abnormalities in vaginal anatomy can prevent correct placement or product retention (e.g., septum, prolapse, double cervix)

HIV, Human immunodeficiency virus; *HPV,* human papillomavirus; *HSV,* herpes simplex virus; *OCP,* oral contraceptive pill; *OTC,* over the counter; *PID,* pelvic inflammatory disease; *STI,* sexually transmitted infection.

Female Condom

The female condom is a device with an inner ring or dome that fits next to the cervix. An outer ring fits around the external opening to the vagina. The single-use condom acts as a barrier to prevent sperm from entering the vagina and may reduce the risk of STIs. Protocol for use: *Use every time!*

Contraceptive Sponge

The sponge is made of soft, disposable polyurethane foam and contains the spermicide nonoxynol-9. After it is moistened with water and inserted into the vagina, it becomes effective immediately and protects against pregnancy for the next 24 hours without the need to add spermicidal cream or jelly—even with repeated acts of intercourse. Protocol for use: *Use every time!*

Spermicides

Spermicides are marketed in various formats:

- Foams, creams, or jellies that can be used alone or in combination with a condom or diaphragm
- Spermicidal suppositories that are intended for use alone or with a condom; require a 10- to 15-minute wait before intercourse to allow the product to effervesce
- Vaginal contraceptive film that can be used alone or with a condom or diaphragm; film contains 72 mg of nonoxynol-9 in a thin sheet that is placed next to the cervix 15 minutes before intercourse

Protocol for use: *Use every time!* Keep adequate supply and store properly, be alert to timing of product placement before intercourse, place in vagina at appropriate time, and insert new application of product before every episode of repeated intercourse.

Less Useful Contraceptive Methods for Adolescents

Most methods may be considered for use in the mature and motivated adolescent. However, the following methods are usually not recommended for use with sexually active adolescents because of higher failure rates, the need for more maturity, and proven and committed use of contraceptives:

- Periodic abstinence
- Fertility awareness or rhythm method because of the more irregular cycles of adolescents
- POPs unless indicated

Specific Gynecologic Conditions of Children

Labial Adhesions

The fusion of tissue between the labia minora that appears to cover the vaginal opening is a common, benign condition in infants and prepubertal girls. It is also called *agglutination, synechia vulvae,* or *vulvar adhesion* if only the lower half of the labia minora is involved (Fig. 36-8).

Before puberty the vaginal tissues are in a hypoestrogenized state and are prone to inflammation and denudation. As the tissues heal, adhesion of the labia can occur. Mechanisms for the initial insult are irritation, infection, and trauma. The most common precipitant is an asymptomatic, nonspecific vulvovaginitis caused by poor hygiene. There is debate about whether lack of hygiene, masturbation, fondling, and subsequent irritation from sexual abuse are potential causes in older females. Labial adhesions occur primarily in girls 3 months to 6 years old, but can persist until puberty (Emans, 2012). They typically resolve spontaneously—50% within 6 months, 90% within 12 months, and 100% within 18 months (Nield, 2009).

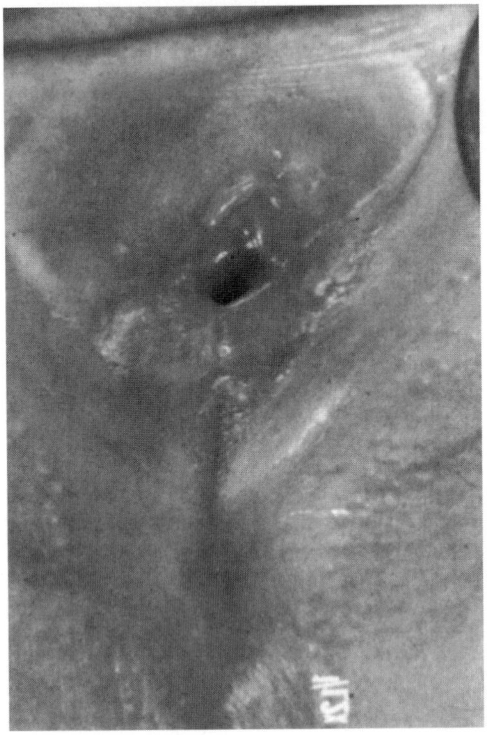

• **Figure 36-8** Labial adhesions that are thinned and almost translucent inferiorly following topical estrogen therapy.

Clinical Findings

History

The history may include concern about rash in genital area, parental concern about vaginal opening, and/or dysuria, difficulty voiding, or local discomfort.

Physical Examination

Physical examination reveals a thin, flat membrane of varying length from the posterior fourchette to the clitoris. The degree of opening near the clitoris varies. The vulva appears flat with a central line of fusion. The urethra may or may not be visualized, and there may be urinary dribbling.

Differential Diagnosis and Complications

Scarring, imperforate hymen, clitoral hypertrophy, and disorders of sex development (DSD) are the differential diagnoses. Urinary tract infections and re-adhesion following mechanical lysis can occur.

Management

The treatment of labial adhesions is somewhat controversial. Table 36-3 outlines steps that are generally accepted. In asymptomatic labial adhesions, observation is often the best treatment. The presence of symptoms of urinary tract infection, pain with activity, and change in behavior dictate treatment. Forceful separation is always contraindicated, because it may result in trauma to the child and recurrence of adhesions.

Patient and Family Education

Premarin cream can cause breast tenderness, transient breast enlargement, and vulvar pigmentation or erythema, which

TABLE 36-3 Treatment of Labial Adhesions

Degree of Involvement	Treatment	Prognosis
No urinary tract infection, no obstruction, no parental concern	No treatment. Reassure and observe.	Resolution with puberty and estrogenization of tissue.
Opening ensures urinary and vaginal drainage, but treatment desired	Apply ointment (e.g., A&D Ointment or petroleum jelly) nightly with cotton-tipped swab with gentle pressure. Following separation, maintain good hygiene and mild ointment (e.g., Vaseline) nightly for 6 to 12 months.	Separation within 8 weeks. If not, double check technique to ensure gentle pressure is being applied. If persists, see use of estrogen cream below.
Urinary and vaginal drainage impaired	Apply estrogen-containing 1% cream (e.g., Premarin) bid for 3 weeks with cotton-tipped swab then at bedtime for another 2 to 3 weeks. Use gentle pressure until separation occurs. Following separation, use petroleum jelly nightly as outlined above.	Separation occurs 50% of the time within 2 to 3 weeks. If not, check technique to ensure pressure is being applied and continue for another 3 weeks. If unresponsive, may anesthetize with 5% lidocaine ointment or EMLA cream, then gently tease the adhesions with a Calgiswab (Emans, 2012). Always avoid forceful separation.

bid, Bis in die (twice a day); *EMLA,* eutectic mixture of local anesthetics.

resolves after discontinuing the cream. The incidence of recurrence can be decreased with careful attention to perineal hygiene and the daily application of A&D Ointment until puberty.

Vulvovaginitis

Vulvovaginitis refers to inflammation, often with discharge, from infection or irritation. *Vulvitis* refers to inflammation of the vulva alone, whereas *vaginitis* refers to vaginal discharge, often with pruritus and irritation that may be secondary to the vulvitis.

Age is important in differentiating the etiology of vulvovaginitis. In prepubescent children several factors make vulvovaginitis a common problem. The lack of estrogen stimulation leaves the vulvar skin thin and the vaginal mucosa atrophic and contributes to minimal vaginal secretions with neutral pH. The lack of pubic hair and labial fat pads diminishes barrier protection, and the proximity of the vaginal opening to the anus predisposes prepubertal females to irritation and infection of the vulva and vagina. Poor hygiene, including wiping technique and lack of hand washing, and irritants (such as, bubble bath, harsh soaps, sand from playtime, or tight-fitting clothing) provide additional insults. Being overweight is also a risk factor.

Prepubescent vulvovaginitis most commonly is nonspecific (up to 75%). Other causes include foreign bodies (most often toilet paper), bacterial infection (often group A beta-hemolytic streptococci), or pinworms (Emans, 2012).

Clinical Findings

The clinical findings pertaining to vulvovaginitis are found in Table 36-4.

History

The history for the prepubertal child includes the following:

- Onset: Less than 1 month usually associated with specific diagnosis, whereas a longer period of time more likely nonspecific (Emans, 2012)
- Characteristics:
  - Genital irritation, itching, pain, inflammation
  - Vaginal discharge—note onset, quantity, color, type (bloody, mucoid), odor, consistency, and duration
  - Nighttime perianal itching
  - Urinary complaints, including dysuria and enuresis
- Recent medications, especially antibiotics
- Possible trauma, foreign body, pinworm infestation, or sexual abuse
- Previous occurrences and treatment used
- Underlying illnesses (e.g., streptococcus infection, dermatosis, diabetes, immunosuppression)
- Perineal hygiene
- Use of harsh soaps and bubble bath
- Tight-fitting or nylon underwear or clothing
- Superabsorbent diapers

Physical Examination

A good light and magnifying glass may aid in the physical examination. Prepubertal examination includes inspection, possible vaginal otoscopy in frog-leg or knee-chest position, and rectal examination.

Diagnostic Studies

- pH and wet mounts of vaginal secretions
- Microscopic examination for WBCs, clue cells, trichomonads, and bacteria
- 10% KOH for whiff test and microscopic examination to look for yeast (branching hyphae and spores) (see Fig. 36-7)
- Bacterial culture of vaginal secretions
- Slide with 20% KOH of skin scraping for yeast
- Pinworm eggs visualized on tape slide under microscope
- Cultures for gonorrhea and chlamydia if suspected sexual abuse

Differential Diagnosis

Atopic dermatitis, psoriasis, seborrhea, lichen sclerosus, or other dermatosis; labial adhesions; polyps or tumors; systemic diseases, such as Kawasaki or Crohn; STIs; and sexual abuse are included in the differential diagnosis.

Management

General treatment measures for any type of vulvovaginitis are listed in Box 36-8.

Prepubertal Nonspecific Etiology

Specific recommendations include the following (see also Table 36-4):

- If persistent, prescribe antibacterial cream at night (e.g., Bactroban, Sultrin, or clindamycin) for 2 weeks.
- If persistent after 3 weeks, prescribe a trial of amoxicillin, amoxicillin and clavulanate, or one of the cephalosporins.
- If symptoms still persist, use estrogen cream at bedtime for 2 to 3 weeks, then every other night at bedtime for 2 weeks to thicken vulvar epithelium.
- If recurrent vulvovaginitis, a 1- to 2-month course of low-dose cephalexin or trimethoprim-sulfamethoxazole (TMP-SMX) at bedtime should be tried.
- If a specific infection is found, treat as outlined here or refer to appropriate section.
- If therapy fails, refer to a pediatric gynecologist.
- If an STI is found in a child, a complete workup for sexual abuse is indicated.

Contact Dermatitis

Steroids and hormonal cream can be used to thicken vaginal skin and minimize irritation.

Foreign Body

- If foreign body remains after irrigation, refer to a pediatric gynecologist.

TABLE 36-4 Evaluation and Treatment of Vulvovaginitis

	Signs and Symptoms	Characteristics of Vaginal Discharge	Etiology	Laboratory Data	Treatment
Nonspecific vaginitis	Itching, burning; dysuria; varied vulvitis	Scant to copious; brown to green; mucoid; foul smelling, poor hygiene	Irritation from contact with various substances; normal UA	pH variable; no odor on whiff test; microscopic: leukocytes, bacteria, debris	Refractory cases may need topical estrogen or antibiotics
Physiologic leukorrhea	None or minimal itch or burn; minimal vulvitis; 6 to 12 months before menarche; possible mild erythema	Scant to moderate; clear to white; odorless; nonirritating	Endogenous hormones 6 to 12 months before menarche	pH <4.5; no odor on whiff test; microscopic: epithelial cells, lactobacilli; normal UA	No treatment needed; explain and reassure
Chemical or mechanical	Itch, erythema, vulvar inflammation, dysuria	Scant amount; yellow to white	Bubble bath, perfumed soap, lotion; tight-fitting clothes, sand or dirt from playground, overweight	pH <4.5; no odor on whiff test; microscopic: leukocytes, epithelial cells	Remove irritant; topical steroids
Foreign body	Dysuria, discomfort, bleeding, minimal vulvar excoriation; history of foreign body in other orifices	Purulent, persistent, dark brown, foul smelling (18%), bloody (82%)	Toilet paper (prepubescent); tampons (adolescent); condoms or object used for masturbation	pH >4.5; odd odor on whiff test; microscopic: WBCs, epithelial cells with bacteria and debris; UA normal	Remove foreign body with forceps or in prepubertal child, by irrigating with warm saline and small feeding tube at the hymenal opening with child in frog-leg (knee-chest position)
Bacterial	Acute respiratory, enteric, or skin infection	Green color, foul, copious with possible bleeding	*Streptococcus* (most common), *Escherichia coli, Enterococcus, Shigella, Staphylococcus,* or other bacteria	Strep test positive; culture positive	Penicillin, erythromycin, amoxicillin, broad-spectrum cephalosporin or other antibiotic as indicated
Candidiasis	Itching, burning, vulvar inflammation, external dysuria, dyspareunia	Thick, white, curdy cottage cheese–like, adherent, odorless; vulva red, edematous with satellite lesions	*Candida albicans;* recent antibiotic or steroid use; diabetes or immunodeficiency; pregnancy	pH <4.5; no odor on whiff test; microscopic: fungal hyphae and buds or spores; culture positive for *Candida* (see Fig. 36-2)	Azole cream topically or intravaginally; *or* fluconazole 150-mg oral tab—single dose
Pinworms	Recent exposure to pinworms; perineal itching, especially at night; anal excoriation, erythema, and lesions from scratching	No discharge	*Enterobius vermicularis* spread from anus	Normal UA; tape test reveals eggs	Albendazole 400 mg once; repeat in 2 weeks; treat family members Hand washing and daily change of underwear and clothes as well as sheets
Bacterial vaginosis (BV)	Foul odor, especially after menses or intercourse; often asymptomatic; no inflammation; abdominal pain or irregular prolonged bleeding	*Homogeneous, thin milky white discharge adherent to vaginal walls and pools in posterior fornix; increased amount	*Gardnerella vaginalis,* mycoplasmas, and anaerobic bacteria; caused by replacement of normal vaginal flora; may or may not be sexually transmitted	*pH >4.5; fishy odor on whiff test; microscopic: *clue cells, few lactobacilli, gram-negative rods, no WBCs	Treat if symptomatic with metronidazole 500 mg orally twice a day for 7 days *or* metronidazole gel 0.75% 5 g intravaginally at bedtime for 5 days *or* clindamycin cream 2% 5 g intravaginally at bedtime for 7 days

UA, Urinalysis; *WBC,* white blood cell.
*Three of these findings needed to diagnose bacterial vaginosis (BV).

• BOX 36-8 General Treatment Measures for Vulvovaginitis

1. Hygiene
   - Wash hands frequently.
   - Wipe front to back.
   - Change underwear every day.
   - Blow-dry perineal area with cool to warm air (especially if overweight).
2. Clothing
   - Wear absorbent white underwear, changing once or twice daily; do not wear underwear at night.
   - Wear loose clothing—no pantyhose or tight clothes.
   - Avoid spandex and sleeper pajamas.
   - Change out of swimsuit after swimming.
3. Comfort and healing measures
   - Take sitz bath with thorough drying.
   - Blow-dry for 10 to 15 minutes once or twice daily with cool to warm air or pat dry with towel.
   - Apply hydrocortisone cream 1% once or twice daily for itching.
   - Use oral diphenhydramine or hydroxyzine if itching is severe.
4. Protective measures
   - Avoid bubble baths and perfumed lotions or powder.
   - Use mild soap (e.g., Dove, Basis, Neutrogena).
   - Avoid shampoo in bath water.
   - Use protective ointment twice a day (e.g., petroleum jelly, A&D Ointment, Aquaphor).
   - Avoid bleach or fabric softener in wash, double rinse.
   - Urinate with knees spread apart to minimize urinary reflux.

- A broad-spectrum antibiotic, such as amoxicillin or a cephalosporin, may be indicated if infection is apparent.

Bacterial Infection

Obtain cultures and prescribe appropriate treatment; penicillin or erythromycin is usually used.

Candida Infection

- Topical antifungal creams are usually successful; treatment failure or recurrence may indicate a resistant organism.
- If appropriate, evaluate for STIs.
- Complicated candidal infections (severe local, recurrent in an immunocompromised host) require documentation by culture, workup for predisposing conditions, longer duration of treatment.

Pinworms

See Chapter 33 for discussion of rectal pinworms.

Gonorrhea, Chlamydia, or Trichomoniasis

A prepubescent child needs to be treated and evaluated for suspected child abuse (if any of these conditions are found). See the CDC guidelines for treatment of STIs in later section (CDC, 2014b).

Complications

Labial adhesions can occur.

Patient and Family Education, Prognosis, and Prevention

Follow up in 5 days if there is no improvement. Recurrence is common, especially with poor hygiene, in overweight girls, and during upper respiratory infection.

Normal Gynecologic Variations

Mittelschmerz

Pelvic pain that occurs at the time of ovulation, midway between menstrual periods, is referred to as *mittelschmerz* (middle pain). The etiology is unclear, but pain is probably caused by follicular rupture and the irritation of the peritoneum from the follicular fluid. The incidence is unknown, although some ultrasonographic studies have detected follicular fluid midcycle in 40% of women with normal cycles (Laufer, 2012).

Clinical Findings

History and Physical Examination

- Pain occurs midway between cycles, although not with irregular cycles
- Dull, achy pain in lower abdomen lasting a few minutes to several hours
- Recurrent discomfort at same time in each cycle
- Pain occasionally severe and crampy, persisting up to 3 days
- Pain with palpation on either or both sides of lower abdomen overlying the ovaries may be present

Differential Diagnosis

Included in the differential diagnosis is appendicitis, torsion or rupture of an ovarian cyst, and ectopic pregnancy.

Management

The etiology and benign nature of the pain should be explained to the adolescent and parent. A heating pad may provide some relief, and analgesics, especially prostaglandin inhibitors (ibuprofen, naproxen) may be used (see Box 36-9 for dosages). Rarely, OCPs may be prescribed to suppress ovulation. Provide reassurance and comfort measures. The adolescent should be encouraged to return if the pain worsens or changes or if she is concerned.

Dysmenorrhea

Painful menstruation with cramping in the lower abdomen or pelvis is the most common gynecologic problem seen in adolescence. Primary dysmenorrhea has no pelvic pathologic condition identified, whereas secondary dysmenorrhea is due to a pelvic pathologic condition.

• BOX 36-9 Common Prostaglandin Inhibitors Used to Treat Adolescent Menstrual Disorders

- *Ibuprofen:* 400 to 800 mg three times a day with a loading dose of 800 mg; maximum dose of 2400 mg/24 hours
- *Naproxen:* 500 mg at onset followed by 250 to 500 mg every 6 to 12 hours; maximum dose of 1250 mg/24 hours
- *Naproxen sodium:* 550 mg at onset followed by 275 mg every 6 to 12 hours; maximum dose of 1375 mg/24 hours
- *Mefenamic acid:* 500 mg at onset followed by 250 mg every 6 hours
- *Meclofenamate:* 100 mg initially; 50 to 100 mg every 6 hours

Primary dysmenorrhea is painful menses caused by an exaggerated production of prostaglandins, primarily prostaglandin $F_2\alpha$, in the secretory endometrium. This causes uterine contractions and vasoconstriction leading to ischemia and pain. The elevation of prostaglandins is brought about by falling progesterone levels during the luteal phase of ovulatory cycles.

Secondary dysmenorrhea may be prompted by endometriosis; complications of pregnancy; outflow obstruction; ovarian cysts, fibroids, or other uterine abnormalities; or infection. Dysmenorrhea is present in more than 50% of adolescents and has been reported in up to 93%. It is the leading cause (greater than 10%) of absenteeism from school or work, with increasing incidence in those who describe the pain as severe (Laufer, 2012).

Clinical Findings

History

For primary dysmenorrhea, ask about the following:

- Menstrual history
- Attitudes and beliefs about menstruation
- Onset—usually 6 to 24 months after menarche
- Location—lower midabdominal area radiating to back, thighs
- Duration and timing of pain—usually begins with menses and lasts less than 2 days
- Character—mild to severe cramping
- Associated symptoms—nausea, vomiting, diarrhea, headache, fatigue, nervousness, dizziness, urinary frequency, lower back or thigh pain
- Ameliorating or aggravating factors
- Treatments or medications tried, including complementary and alternative medicine (CAM)
- Sexual activity
- Number of days of school or activities missed
- Cigarette smoking
- Family history of dysmenorrhea

For secondary dysmenorrhea, the following history should be further explored:

- Onset (with menarche or 2 to 3 years postmenarche)
- Pelvic pain at times other than menstruation (worsens over time)
- Character of pelvic pain (dull and constant rather than crampy)
- History of infection, menorrhagia, intermenstrual bleeding, or abnormal vaginal discharge
- Dyspareunia
- History of sexual abuse
- Family history of endometriosis

Physical Examination

A complete physical examination is recommended and required for secondary dysmenorrhea. A speculum and bimanual examination may be deferred if the adolescent is not sexually active, if the dysmenorrhea is mild, if it does not interfere with daily activities, or if the dysmenorrhea is responding to treatment and without suspicion of pathologic condition. However, the external genitalia should be examined and a cotton swab inserted into the vagina to rule out hymenal abnormalities and/or a vaginal septum. A rectoabdominal examination also helps rule out adnexal tenderness and masses (Laufer, 2012).

Diagnostic Studies

The following are ordered only if indicated:

- NAATs or cervical cultures for gonorrhea and chlamydia
- CBC with sedimentation rate if PID is suspected
- Pregnancy test
- Pelvic ultrasound if abnormalities are suspected

Differential Diagnosis

Endometriosis, PID, chronic pelvic pain, obstructive malformations, and/or other pathologic conditions of the reproductive tract are included in the differential diagnosis. Nongynecologic causes of pelvic pain (such as, constipation, Crohn disease, and irritable bowel syndrome) should be considered.

Management

Primary Dysmenorrhea

- Prostaglandin synthetase inhibitors provide relief in 70% to 80% of patients (Laufer, 2012). They should be administered at onset of menses or, if cramping precedes menses, at onset of symptoms. Treat the patient for the duration of the pain, usually 1 to 2 days. The trial period should extend for three cycles; if no relief is experienced, an alternative prostaglandin inhibitor should be tried. See Box 36-9 for specific prostaglandin inhibitors. Nonsteroidal anti-inflammatory drugs (NSAIDs) are advantageous as first-line therapy, because they need to be taken for only 2 to 3 days. Ibuprofen and naproxen are widely used in clinical practice, but if ineffective, use one of the fenamates. Taking NSAIDs with food helps prevent abdominal complaints.
- OCPs are widely used for dysmenorrhea. Because they suppress ovulation, total progesterone-induced prostaglandin production is decreased in the endometrium. A 30- to 35-mcg estrogen-progestin combination pill may be used for a 3- to 6-month trial if

prostaglandin inhibitors are not successful (Laufer, 2012). The Cochrane Review Group (Wong et al, 2009) found OCPs may be more effective for dysmenorrhea than placebo; however, interpretation was limited due to the variable quality of the randomized controlled trials (RCTs) reviewed.
- CAM is likely to be beneficial per the Cochrane Review Group (Proctor and Farquhar, 2004) (see Chapter 43 for further CAM therapies).
  - Application of topical heat
  - Thiamine 100 mg/day
  - Toki-shakuyaku-san (herbal remedy) 2.5 g three times daily
  - High-frequency transcutaneous electrical nerve stimulation (TENS)
  - Vitamin E, 500 units/day
  - Magnesium
- Follow up by telephone or visit to adjust dose or change medication as needed; the adolescent should be seen again in 3 to 4 months. If failure to respond after 6 months of treatment or if pain worsens over time, a further workup is warranted.

Secondary Dysmenorrhea

Secondary dysmenorrhea requires a full diagnostic workup and often a referral for gynecologic care.

Patient and Family Education and Prevention

Exercise and stress reduction may help decrease pain. A well-balanced diet with ample amounts of fiber and water, in addition to decreasing caffeine, chocolate, and salt intake, may be useful to control dysmenorrhea.

Adolescent Pregnancy

Adolescent pregnancy occurs in girls or young women between 13 and 19 years old, although pregnancy is possible for any girl who has ovulatory cycles. Pregnancy has been seen in girls before their first menstrual cycle and in those as young as 10 or 11 years old. Except for a slight increase in 2006 and 2007, the rate of teen pregnancy has been declining annually with an overall decrease of 6% from 2011 to 2012 (CDC, 2014b). However, the rates for Hispanics and African American adolescents, though decreasing, are still twice as high as that of non-Hispanic whites (CDC, 2014b). The decline has been regarded as evidence of more effective contraceptive practices, delayed sexual debuts, and a decrease in sexual activity. Regional and social determinates have been found to play a role in teen pregnancy rates. Across the South and Southwest and in rural areas the pregnancy rates are higher regardless of ethnicity. Social determinates that correlate with adolescent pregnancy are poverty, low levels of education (teen and family), family dysfunction, history of sexual abuse, neighborhood segregation, and health inequities (CDC, 2014b). Other factors that have been associated with teen pregnancy include having a sibling who is a teen parent, decreased parental monitoring of the adolescent, academic underachievement, poor sense of personal efficacy, depression, and substance abuse (Cox, 2012).

Clinical Findings

History

Inquire about the following:
- Menstrual history; menarche; cycle regularity—normally how many days apart, how many days of flow; LNMP and/or last bleed
- Contraceptive use—method, consistency rate; if on a hormonal method, any missed pills, late patch or ring replacement, late medroxyprogesterone acetate injection, and so on.
- Sexual history (see Chapter 15)
- Associated symptoms: Breast sensitivity, nipple tenderness (1 to 2 weeks after conception), fatigue, nausea, urinary frequency (2 weeks after conception)
- Patients often have vague complaints (e.g., headache, abdominal discomfort, dizziness, and vaginal and urinary symptoms)

Physical Examination

There are three classic signs of pregnancy, each of which may be observed during the pelvic examination:
1. Hegar sign: Softening of the isthmus of the uterus (the area between the cervix and the uterine body). This may be observed before there is uterine enlargement.
2. Chadwick sign: Dark bluish or purplish discoloration of the vaginal and cervical epithelium, the result of increased blood supply to the pelvis. This is usually observed before uterine growth.
3. Uterine enlargement: Occurs at 5 to 6 weeks and initially is a result of changes in the uterine muscle rather than growing gestation. Uterine sizing is traditionally done by bimanual examination and recorded in weeks of estimated gestation.

Fetal heart tones may be auscultated by Doppler at 10 to 12 weeks' gestation.

Diagnostic Studies

Pregnancy testing is done in cases of suspected pregnancy. Urine testing is the chosen test for the ambulatory setting because results can be obtained rapidly, and the test is accurate and inexpensive. Current urine tests can detect human chorionic gonadotropin (hCG) in the urine down to 25 international units/L. Normal serum levels at the time of the first missed menses are between 50 and 100 international units/L.

Serum testing is of two types; a qualitative test can detect hCG down to 5 international units/L but will not measure the exact amount. A quantitative β-hCG can measure the exact amount of β-hCG in the serum and is indicated for serial measurements to evaluate for ectopic pregnancy, molar pregnancy, or to rule out gestational trophoblastic neoplasia (GTN) following a molar pregnancy.

If the pregnancy test result is positive, routine laboratory diagnostics include the following:

- Cervical cultures for gonorrhea and chlamydia
- Cervical cytology
- Vaginal pH with saline and KOH wet mounts
- Urinalysis and culture
- Routine prenatal blood work: Includes blood type and Rh, syphilis serology, rubella titer, CBC with differential, and screening for hepatitis B and HIV. Another test to consider is an abnormal hemoglobin screen in women of African American, Asian, or Mediterranean descent for sickle cell trait and thalassemias. Women of Ashkenazi Jewish and French-Canadian descent should be referred for testing for Tay-Sachs.
- Possibly vaginal and/or pelvic ultrasonography to determine gestation accurately

Differential Diagnosis

The differential diagnoses for pregnancy are amenorrhea from another etiology, nonviable intrauterine pregnancy, ectopic pregnancy, and molar pregnancy.

Management and Education

Prompt diagnosis assists with pregnancy planning, early onset of prenatal precautions (e.g., avoidance of OTC medications and herbal preparations without provider approval; the dangers of alcohol, smoking, and illicit drug use), and prenatal care. Early care also allows women considering an abortion ample time for counseling, decision-making, and obtaining an abortion in the first trimester, when the procedure is safest.

If the pregnancy test result is negative, the provider should talk with the adolescent about her situation. Is she in a steady relationship, was this date rape, were drugs and alcohol involved, was this forced or consensual sex, how old is the partner, and so on? The counseling should be tailored to her individual needs in addition to general education regarding the risk of unprotected intercourse, the potential for pregnancy and STIs and HIV, and reliable methods to protect her in the future.

If the pregnancy test result is positive, the visit should include the following:

- Dating parameters and pelvic examination to determine gestational age
- Counseling for pregnancy options, including continuing pregnancy and retaining custody of child, continuing pregnancy and placing child for adoption, or termination
- Assessment of the involvement of her social support system including family, partner, and any significant others: The provider should encourage parental involvement in the decision-making and may need to role-play and/or serve as mediator for the teenager in informing others. Some states have parental notification laws in place around the issue of abortion, and in most, health care providers are mandatory reporters of statutory rape. Providers must be aware of laws of the state in which they practice.

Initiation of referrals as appropriate for the decision made:

- If the choice is continuing the pregnancy and prenatal care is not part of the provider's practice, the adolescent should be referred to another provider or, if available in the community, a comprehensive adolescent pregnancy program to initiate medical, nutritional, psychosocial, and educational services.
- If adoption is the option of choice, refer to the appropriate legal or social service agency, or both. Look for agencies in the community that offer comprehensive preadoption and postadoption counseling.
- If the choice is terminating pregnancy, refer to an appropriate resource for abortion counseling and the procedure.
- Make additional referrals as indicated for Women, Infants, and Children (WIC) program, Medicaid coverage, and community health nurse involvement. Public health–based research indicates that there is a significant positive effect on pregnancy, parenting, and childrearing outcomes if home visits are made by community health nurses.

Complications

Young age in a pregnant woman is an inherent risk factor, even with good prenatal care. Adverse outcomes are common in pregnant teenagers and include the following: maternal anemia, preeclampsia, excessive weight gain or poor weight gain, puerperal complications, and potential social consequences (e.g., educational, economic, and occupational delay); fetal and neonatal low birth weight, intrauterine growth restriction, prematurity, and minor acute infections

Specific Gynecologic Problems of Adolescents

Breast Concerns: Mastalgia, Cysts, and Fibrocystic Changes

Breast tenderness or pain is fairly common in up to 40% of adolescents (DiVasta et al, 2012). Many teens have premenstrual discomfort, tenderness from hormonal contraception or early pregnancy. Severe pain is not a normal variation and needs further evaluation. Adolescents frequently have dense breast tissue which can make examination difficult. Fibrocystic changes can feel like thick cord-like areas with diffuse nodes and lumps without distinct masses. Cysts are palpable fluid-filled versus a solid mass.

Clinical Findings

History

- LNMP: discomfort noted in relationship to menstrual cycle?

- Lumps, masses, or specific points of pain?
- Erythema or heat over tender areas, fever
- Nipple discharge
- Medications, including hormonal contraceptives
- Sexually activity
- Stress, exercise
- Type of bra—underwire, poor support, sport bra, and so on
- Family history of benign breast disease or breast cancer

Physical Examination

- Vital signs
- Careful breast examination with gentle compression to evaluate for nipple discharge
- Note symmetry, masses, areas of fibrotic tissue, tenderness, erythema and/or heat

Diagnostic Studies

- Pregnancy test—regardless of sexual history
- CBC if indicated to rule out infection
- Ultrasound and/or referral—if indicated by findings, such as a cyst or lump

Differential Diagnosis

The differential includes mild mastalgia from typical non-concerning etiologies, infection, fibrocystic breast changes, breast cysts, fibroadenomas, mass of unknown etiology, and breast cancer.

Management

After the history and examination if the clinician is confident that the breast complaint is of a benign etiology, watch and wait is in order. Have the teen keep a diary of symptoms in relation to her menstrual cycle. Teach her how to do a self-breast examination as you do a clinical examination so that she can learn what is normal for her. Educate her on the probable diagnosis and prognosis of the condition. Cyclic mastalgia will usually improve over time, and she may use NSAIDs for discomfort. Most breast cysts will resolve spontaneously; however, if not, refer for further evaluation (DiVasta et al, 2012). Fibrocystic breast changes may improve as she ages and the breast density decreases. Counsel about the benign nature of this condition and that she is not at an increased risk of breast cancer.

Have her return for another examination the week after her next menses. The cyclic changes in the breast will be the least noticeable at that time. Review her diary for typical patterns. Continue education and reassurance. However, if on examination or ultrasound there is a suspicious mass, refer for further evaluation.

Amenorrhea

Amenorrhea is lack of menstruation and is described as either primary or secondary. *Primary amenorrhea* is defined as either absence of menarche by 16 years old with normal pubertal growth and development or absence of menarche by 14 years old in the absence of secondary sexual characteristics. *Secondary amenorrhea* is defined as the absence of menstruation for at least three cycles or more than 6 months in females who have an established menstrual pattern.

There are multiple etiologies for primary and secondary amenorrhea. When evaluating a young woman for amenorrhea, pregnancy should be ruled out first, regardless of sexual history. Amenorrhea is usually categorized by clinical findings and laboratory results into broad areas of causation. Speroff and colleagues (1973) devised a compartmental system to categorize amenorrhea that is still in use today (Fritz and Speroff, 2011). They distinguish between compartment 1, disorders of the outflow tract or uterine target organ; compartment 2, disorders of the ovary; compartment 3, disorders of the anterior pituitary; and compartment 4, disorders of the central nervous system (CNS; hypothalamic). Emans and DiVasta (2012) use the organs in the HPO axis to categorize etiology. Others, using the lab results from gonadotropins and prolactin, categorize etiology into hypogonadotropic, hypergonadotropic, normogonadotropic, hyperprolactinemic, and anatomic. Grouping in some manner assists the provider to delineate the origin of an individual adolescent's amenorrhea (Table 36-5).

Clinical Findings

History

- Maternal and sibling age of menarche
- Family history of menstrual irregularities, eating disorders, diabetes, thyroid disease, or genetic disorders
- Any prenatal exposure to hormones
- Detailed history of growth and pubertal development (sequence and tempo)
- Menstrual calendar (last menses, number and pattern of cycles, age at menarche)
- Chronic systemic disease or illness or previous surgery, radiation, or chemotherapy
- Nutrition, including eating habits, dieting, weight fluctuations
- Exercise patterns, including amount and intensity, level of participation, weigh-ins, or standards for weight that must be kept
- History of stress fractures
- Bowel patterns or abdominal pain
- Headache or visual change
- Galactorrhea, hirsutism, acne
- Medication use (contraceptives, phenothiazines, or antihypertensives)
- Sexual activity, contraceptive use
- Stress, recent change in environment, or depression
- Substance use (including anabolic-androgenic steroids)

Physical Examination

- Height, weight, BMI, nutritional status, blood pressure, pulse
- Sexual maturation rating

TABLE 36-5 Differential Diagnosis of Amenorrhea

	Primary	Secondary
Hypogonadotropic		
Compartment IV	Delayed puberty	Psychological disorder
Hypothalamic	Chronic illness Eating disorders Excessive exercise Kallmann syndrome	Depression Eating disorders Excessive exercise
Compartment III	Pituitary disease	Pituitary disease
Pituitary	Hyperprolactinemia	Hyperprolactinemia Sheehan syndrome
Thyroid		Hypothyroid
Hypergonadotropic		
Compartment II	Premature ovarian failure	Premature ovarian failure
Ovaries	Gonadal dysgenesis PCOS	PCOS
Adrenals	Adrenal hyperplasia	Adrenal hyperplasia
Anatomic	Müllerian agenesis	Asherman syndrome
Compartment I	Androgen insensitivity	
Outflow	Imperforate hymen Vaginal septum	
Hyperprolactinemia		
Compartment III	Medication/drugs	Medication/drugs
Pituitary	Macroadenoma Tumor	Macroadenoma Tumor Lactation

Data from Emans SJ, DiVasta AD: Amenorrhea in the adolescent. In Emans SJ, Laufer MR, editors: *Pediatric and adolescent gynecology*, ed 6, Philadelphia, 2012, Wolters Kluwer/Lippincott Williams & Wilkins; Speroff L, Fritz MA: *Clinical gynecologic endocrinology and infertility*, ed 7, Philadelphia, 2005, Lippincott Williams & Wilkins.
PCOS, Polycystic ovary syndrome.

- Complete neurologic examination, including cranial nerves, fundoscopic examination, and visual fields
- Midline facial defects or other congenital anomalies or stigmata of Turner syndrome
- Palpation of thyroid
- Breast examination with gentle compression to identify galactorrhea
- Palpation of abdomen and groin for masses, tenderness
- Examination of skin, hair distribution, and genitalia for signs of virilization
- External genital examination for estrogenization of vaginal mucosa (indicates ovarian function), vaginal and hymenal patency, and clitoromegaly (androgen excess)
- Digital vaginal examination and speculum examination if any abnormality is suspected
- Bimanual examination

Diagnostic Studies

Initial laboratory studies include pregnancy test regardless of sexual history, thyroid-stimulating hormone (TSH), FSH, and prolactin. Follow the algorithm (Fig. 36-9) for complete evaluation.

Differential Diagnosis

The differential diagnoses for primary amenorrhea and secondary amenorrhea have considerable overlap (see Table 36-5). The exceptions are a few genetic conditions that cause primary amenorrhea (e.g., Turner syndrome). The most common causation of amenorrhea in the adolescent falls within the hypogonadotropic-hypothalamic category. An important marker of hypogonadotropic hypogonadism is the female athlete triad of amenorrhea, eating disorder, and osteoporosis (Emans and DiVasta, 2012), especially common in gymnasts, figure skaters, ballet dancers, and long-distance runners at elite or highly competitive levels. The pressure for the ideal body for the sport and the intense exercise required may lead to this triad (see Chapter 13 for a discussion of this triad).

Management

The treatment of amenorrhea obviously depends on its cause. Restoration of ovulatory cycles leads to the best long-term prognosis, and this is often accomplished through estrogen-progestin therapy. The PCP may need to consult and/or refer to a pediatric gynecologist or endocrinologist depending on the etiology. Anxiety about amenorrhea is common, and frequent reassurance is necessary. Young women should be made aware of the long-term skeletal effects of amenorrhea and instructed on adequate diet, reasonable exercise, and calcium supplementation to prevent osteoporosis.

Abnormal Uterine Bleeding

AUB refers to uterine bleeding that is excessive, prolonged, or unpatterned. It can be described as follows:

- Polymenorrhea: Fewer than 21 days between menses
- Menorrhagia: Normal intervals with excessive flow or duration of menses
- Metrorrhagia: Irregular frequency of cycles with bleeding between cycles
- Menometrorrhagia: Excessive amount of bleeding with irregular frequency of cycles

AUB is a diagnosis of exclusion, so any other causes of pathologic conditions must first be ruled out. AUB can be classified as mild, moderate, or severe based on hemoglobin level, duration of cycle, and quantity of bleeding.

The mechanism of AUB appears to be a delay in the maturation of the negative feedback cycle and is not related to structural pathologic conditions or medical illness (Gray

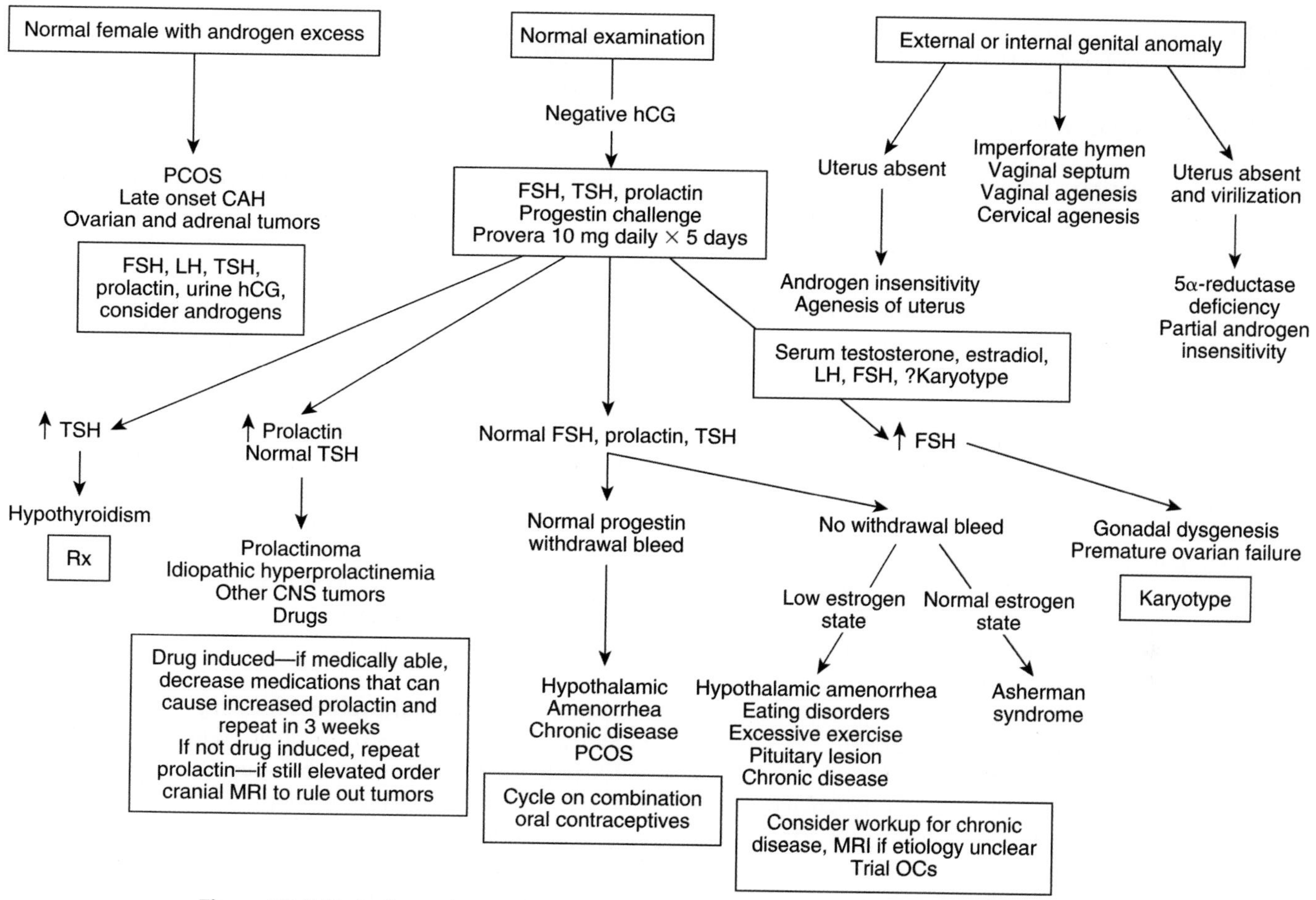

• **Figure 36-9** Evaluation and management of **amenorrhea**. *CAH,* Congenital adrenal hyperplasia; *CNS,* central nervous system; *FSH,* follicle-stimulating hormone; *hCG,* human chorionic gonadotropin; *LH,* luteinizing hormone; *MRI,* magnetic resonance imaging; *OC,* oral contraceptive; *PCOS,* polycystic ovary syndrome; *Rx,* medication; *TSH,* thyroid-stimulating hormone. (Adapted from Emans JS, DiVasta A: Amenorrhea in the adolescent. In Emans SJ, Laufer MR, editors: *Pediatric and adolescent gynecology,* ed 6, Philadelphia, 2012, Wolters Kluwer/Lippincott Williams & Wilkins.)

and Emans, 2012). Estrogen production continues without the balancing decrease in FSH, which would suppress estrogen. This results in abnormal endometrial thickening. The abnormal endometrium then sheds in a disorderly manner manifested by heavy, irregular, or prolonged bleeding. There is great variation in what is considered to be a normal menstrual cycle, especially in adolescents. Normal can range from 21 to 45 days between periods, with duration of flow from 3 to 7 days and 30 to 40 mL of blood loss (10 to 15 soaked tampons or pads) per cycle. Periods that last longer than 8 to 10 days with blood loss in excess of 80 mL are considered excessive (Gray and Emans, 2012).

AUB is frequently seen in adolescents (Gray and Emans, 2012). Anovulation is the most common cause of AUB in the adolescent; however, not all anovulatory cycles result in AUB. Adolescents with sustained anovulation (e.g., as a result of eating disorders, weight fluctuations, competitive athletics, chronic illness, or endocrine disease) have an increased incidence of AUB. Anovulation can also be due to stress or illness, thus appearing in adolescents after several years of regular cycles (Gray and Emans, 2012).

Clinical Findings

History

- Family history of bleeding disorders or dyscrasias, thyroid dysfunction, or diabetes mellitus
- Menstrual history: Onset, pattern, duration, quantity, and color; last menstrual period; breakthrough bleeding; dysmenorrhea; passing of clots, number of tampons or pads used; longest and shortest intervals between cycles
- Associated menstrual symptoms (e.g., premenstrual syndrome [PMS])
- Sexual activity and contraception used
- Postcoital bleeding
- Previous infection or STIs
- Vaginal discharge, pelvic pain
- Galactorrhea, hirsutism (endocrine disease), or other chronic disease
- Bleeding gums, nosebleeds, bruises, hemorrhage (bleeding disorders)
- Hair loss, sleep disorders, cold intolerance, constipation (thyroid symptoms)
- Recent stressors, medications, or substance use

- Exercise and eating patterns, weight, weight fluctuations, laxative use, body image
- Genital trauma, sexual abuse
- Effect of bleeding on lifestyle

Physical Examination

- Height, weight, BMI, body type, and fat distribution
- Vital signs (temperature, pulse, respiratory rate), orthostatic blood pressures
- Observation for acne, hirsutism, clitoromegaly (evidence of androgen excess)
- Breast examination for galactorrhea
- Thyroid palpation
- Observation for petechiae, bruising, pale color
- Abdominal examination for mass or tenderness
- Pelvic examination, including digital and speculum examination for foreign bodies, cervical lesions. In young, non–sexually active girls, the speculum examination may not be necessary per provider discretion.
- Tanner staging
- Bimanual and rectoabdominal examination

Diagnostic Studies

The following are ordered as indicated:

- Pregnancy test regardless of sexual history
- CBC with differential, platelet count, reticulocyte count
- Sedimentation rate or C-reactive protein (CRP) (if infection or inflammation is suspected)
- Coagulation studies: Prothrombin time, partial thromboplastin time, bleeding time (if bleeding disorder is suspected or there has been a significant drop in hemoglobin)
- Thyroid function test, blood sugar, prolactin level (if systemic disease is suspected), markers for PCOS (free and total testosterone, sex hormone-binding globulin and androstenedione)
- Wet preparations and cultures for gonorrhea and chlamydia if patient is sexually active
- Ultrasound of pelvis if mass is palpated, anomaly is suspected, bimanual examination cannot be completed, or condition is unresponsive to treatment

Differential Diagnosis

The differential diagnoses include pregnancy or pregnancy-related complications (postabortion, ectopic pregnancy); stress; excessive participation in athletics; eating disorders, including overweight; drug use; systemic diseases, such as blood dyscrasias (20% of patients with coagulation defects have excessive menstrual bleeding especially with first menses); infection (e.g., STIs); trauma, including forceful intercourse or rape; foreign bodies, including intrauterine device; tumors; anomalies; endometriosis; endocrine disorders (e.g., thyroid disorder, diabetes mellitus, prolactinoma); debilitating or chronic diseases (especially lupus, hepatic or renal diseases); reproductive tract disorders, including malignancy; and medications, including OCPs, progesterone implants, and injectables (Gray and Emans, 2012).

Management

The goals in managing AUB include controlling bleeding, preventing endometrial hyperplasia, preventing and treating anemia, restoring quality of life, and preventing recurrence. The following will enable the provider to manage AUB (Gray and Emans, 2012):

Mild Abnormal Uterine Bleeding

A shortened cycle or menses longer than normal with flow slightly to moderately increased or unpredictable; hemoglobin greater than 12 g/dL:

- Observe and reassure.
- Have patient start and maintain a menstrual calendar.
- Prescribe iron supplementation and dietary interventions to prevent anemia.
- Use prostaglandin inhibitors to reduce heavy bleeding (see Box 36-9).
- Consider OCPs for 3 to 4 months to decrease menorrhagia and stabilize menses.
- Reevaluate in 3 months.

Moderate Abnormal Uterine Bleeding

Shortened (1 to 3 weeks), irregular cycle with moderate to heavy bleeding, hemoglobin between 10 and 12 g/dL:

- Prescribe 30 to 35 mcg monophasic combination OCPs with a potent progestin (Gray and Emans, 2012).
  - If not currently bleeding, use same day start (see Contraception section).
  - If currently bleeding, start with one OCP twice daily for 3 to 4 days until bleeding stops. Then continue with one daily until finished with that pack, skip the placebo week, and start another pack without a withdrawal bleed. If bleeding resumes when OCPs are decreased to one per day, resume taking twice daily until first pack is completed and start a second pack, taking one OCP daily without a withdrawal bleed. Occasionally the twice daily dose will not stop the bleeding. Add one OCP every 3 to 4 days up to four OCPs per day. After the bleeding stops, decrease the dose by one pill every 3 to 4 days until down to one per day. Continue OCPs without a withdrawal bleed until the patient is completing a regular pill pack at one pill per day. If unable to control bleeding with four OCPs per day, consult and/or referral is necessary.
- Add antiemetic to control the nausea of higher doses of estrogen.
- Usual length of treatment with OCPs is 6 months.
- Alternatively, prescribe a progestin, such as medroxyprogesterone acetate (5 to 10 mg every day for 10 to 14 days started on the 14th day of cycle for 1 to 2 months). OCPs are more effective at stopping active bleeding.
- Have patient start and maintain a menstrual calendar.
- Prescribe iron supplementation plus 1 mg folic acid per day.
- Reevaluate at least monthly until condition is stable.
- Reassess after 6 months.

Severe Abnormal Uterine Bleeding

Irregular, prolonged, heavy bleeding; hemoglobin less than 10 g/dL:

- Refer to gynecologist and hospitalize if active bleeding is heavy and adolescent is hemodynamically symptomatic; treatment may include transfusion, intravenous hormonal therapy, and dilation and evacuation (D&E).
- Manage as moderate AUB if not actively bleeding.

Complications

Anemia, profuse bleeding, shock, and side effects of OCPs can occur. A long history of anovulation and AUB increases the risk of infertility and endometrial carcinoma.

Patient and Family Education and Prognosis

Encourage individual to keep a calendar of bleeding days and amounts. This includes keeping track of the number of pads or tampons used to increase accuracy. Educate the patient and her parents about the use of OCPs as a medication in the treatment of AUB. It is important that OCPs be taken as directed. Suddenly stopping it midcycle will result in resumed bleeding. Prognosis is excellent if AUB is due to anovulation and immaturity of the HPO axis; these adolescents respond well to treatment, and most will develop regular menstrual patterns within 4 years of menarche.

Endometriosis

Endometriosis is the proliferation of ectopic endometrial tissue outside the pelvic cavity. It is primarily manifested by dysmenorrhea that progressively worsens. Other symptoms include acyclic pelvic pain, gastrointestinal complaints, and dyspareunia. Adolescents usually experience pain, and as many as 62% of adolescents with endometriosis have both cyclic and acyclic pain.

The cause of endometriosis is unknown. A risk factor is early menarche. Several theories have been developed to explain the possible cause of endometriosis, including retrograde menstruation; embryonic müllerian remnants, coelomic metaplasia; lymphatic, vascular, and iatrogenic dissemination; genetic factors; immunologic or hormonal problems or defects: and environmental exposures (Laufer, 2012).

The incidence rate in adolescents is difficult to obtain because endometriosis is rarely studied in this age group. In a systemic review, Janssen and colleagues (2013) found that 70% to 75% of adolescents with untreatable dysmenorrhea or pelvic pain had a diagnosis of endometriosis on laparoscopy. In contrast, 49% of adolescents who had treatable pain reduction were diagnosed with endometriosis.

Clinical Findings

History

- First-degree relative with endometriosis
- Deep unilateral or bilateral pain described as sharp or dull
- Chronic pelvic pain that is cyclic and/or acyclic and mildly to severely disabling, disrupting routine and causing missed school days or emergency department visits without definitive diagnosis
- Bladder and bowel dysfunction; rectal pain
- Dyspareunia
- Cyclic leg pain

Physical Examination

- Tender, enlarged, or fixed ovaries
- Adnexal masses, thickening, or tenderness
- The pelvic examination is most often unremarkable, with mild to moderate pelvic tenderness on palpation

Diagnostic Studies

The following are ordered as indicated:

- CBC, urine testing, or cervical cultures for gonorrhea and chlamydia to rule out infectious cause
- Ultrasound (helpful to evaluate anatomic structures; however, nonspecific for diagnosing endometriosis)

Differential Diagnosis

Primary dysmenorrhea, PID, appendicitis, ovarian cysts, müllerian anomalies, eating disorders, lactose intolerance, irritable bowel syndrome, chronic constipation, and depression are included in the differential diagnosis.

Management

- Have adolescent keep pain diary.
- Proceed with trial of cyclic OCPs and NSAIDs.
- If unresponsive and the patient is younger than 18 years old, refer for a laparoscopic evaluation. If older than 18 years old, may try empiric trial of GnRH agonist. If pain improves, a diagnosis of endometriosis can be made (ACOG, 2005).
- Supportive phone follow-up for side effects of medications and painful flare-ups is essential.
- See at 1- to 3-month intervals to provide support and reevaluate.
- Diet and exercise are important aspects in coping with chronic pain.
- Stress reduction techniques and support groups may also be helpful.

Complications

Miscarriage and infertility can occur. Endometriomas are rare in the adolescent age group. Gastritis, which may be treated with histamine-2 blockers, is seen frequently.

Prognosis and Prevention

Endometriosis is a chronic disease, and remission and exacerbation are to be expected. Stressful events often cause exacerbation. The goals of treatment are to control pain and prevent infertility.

Vaginitis and Vaginal Discharge

Vaginitis refers to an inflammation or infection of the vulva and vaginal wall with or without discharge from the vagina.

At puberty, the pH changes from 7 to 4.5, vaginal mucosa thickens, acidogenic bacteria predominate, and lactobacillus stabilizes the environment; all these changes offer protection from infection. Adolescent vaginitis is most often due to a specific cause, often secondary to sexual contact. Normal physiologic leukorrhea occurs 6 to 12 months before puberty. Yeast, group A beta-hemolytic streptococci or other infections, foreign bodies (toilet paper fragments, tampon), and pinworms are possible causes. Bacterial vaginosis (BV), trichomoniasis, or other STIs (discussed later in this chapter) must also be considered. Up to one half of female gynecologic complaints are related to vaginitis. *Candida vaginitis,* BV, and *Trichomonas* are the most common infecting agents (Berlan et al, 2012).

Clinical Findings

History

- Onset: How long have the symptoms been present?
- Location—vulva, vagina, perineum, and/or anus
- Characteristics:
  - Genital irritation, itching, pain, and inflammation
  - Vaginal discharge—note onset, quantity, color, type (bloody, mucoid), odor, consistency, and duration
  - Urinary complaints, including dysuria
  - Pelvic pain and/or dyspareunia
  - Ameliorating or aggravating factors
- Treatments or medications tried including CAM
- Previous occurrences and treatment used
- Recent medications, especially antibiotics
- Use of contraception
- Possible trauma, foreign body, or sexual abuse
- History of sexual activity, menstrual irregularities, or STI or STI exposure
- Perineal hygiene and/or use of harsh or perfumed soaps and bubble bath
- Use of tampons or pads, with deodorant
- Douching, personal sprays, or any other hygiene measures
- Underlying illnesses (e.g., streptococcus infection, dermatosis, diabetes, immunosuppression)

Physical Examination

The examination of the adolescent should include the careful inspection of the perianal area and a speculum examination to visualize the cervix and vaginal walls. If the adolescent has not initiated vaginal intercourse, vaginal secretions can be collected with a saline-moistened cotton swab. See Table 36-4 for physical examination findings.

Diagnostic Studies

The following should be considered (and see Table 36-4):

- pH of vaginal secretions
- Wet mounts of vaginal secretions
- Saline for microscopic examination to look for WBCs, clue cells, trichomonads, and bacteria
- 10% KOH for whiff test and microscopic examination to look for yeast (branching hyphae and spores) (see Fig. 36-7)
- NAATs on urine, cervix, or vaginal wall, cultures for gonorrhea and chlamydia if indicated
- Urinalysis and culture if urinary tract infection (UTI) suspected

Differential Diagnosis

The differential diagnoses include normal physiologic discharge, yeast vaginitis, BV, trichomoniasis and other STIs, foreign body, and contact or allergic dermatitis.

Management

See Table 36-4 for treatment. Some CAM recommendations include:

- For yeast: Decrease foods high in simple carbohydrates; avoid foods with yeast or mold; increase fiber, garlic, ginger, cinnamon; live lactobacillus (1 to 2 billion live organisms per day) and acidophilus in diet
- For BV: Lactobacillus in the diet, and vaginal boric acid capsules

Complications

BV can contribute to PID, endometritis, postsurgical infection (abortion), and adverse pregnancy outcomes, such as preterm labor and birth, premature rupture of the membranes, and chorioamnionitis. Trichomoniasis has been linked with premature rupture of membranes and preterm delivery.

Patient and Family Education, Prognosis, and Prevention

Follow up in 5 days if there is no improvement. For the sexually active adolescent, recommend not using diaphragm or condom until 3 days after treatment with topical vaginal cream or tablet. Recommend frequent changes of tampons and use of a pad, especially at night, or ceasing the use of tampons.

Sexually Transmitted Infections

Multiple organisms are responsible for STIs in adolescents and children. Gonorrhea, chlamydia, syphilis, HSV, and HPV are the most common STIs affecting the lower female reproductive tract. *Trichomonas* (discussed in previous section), hepatitis B, and HIV also are recognized as STIs. See Chapter 24 for discussion of hepatitis B and HIV (systemic STIs). The term *sexually transmitted infection* is usually used instead of *sexually transmitted diseases (STDs).* Diagnosis can also be made in terms of the location of the infection (e.g., vaginitis, cervicitis, or urethritis) if causal organism is unknown.

STIs are a significant public health problem, placing a heavy financial health burden on society, having a tremendous effect on individuals' lives, and playing an important role in the transmission of HIV. Much progress has been made in treating STIs, with historic low incidence rates for gonorrhea and syphilis. However, the highest STI rates in the industrial world still occur in the United States (CDC, 2014a).

Considered an epidemic, STIs have the highest rates in adolescents. The CDC reports that of the 20 million new STIs per year almost half occur in adolescents and young adults 15 to 24 years old. Furthermore, one in four female adolescents have an STI, but young women between 15 and 19 years old have decreasing rates of *Chlamydia trachomatis* and *Neisseria gonorrhoeae* with the 20- to 24-year-old group increasing rates for both sexes (CDC, 2014a). Adolescents at highest risk for acquiring STIs include youth in detention facilities, male homosexuals, and injection drug users. Minorities, especially African Americans, are disproportionally affected.

Factors contributing to this epidemic are the increasingly early age and frequency of sexual activity, inconsistent use of contraceptive and protective devices, physiologic characteristics that predispose adolescents to infection, adolescents' lack of access to and use of health care, and societal influences (Box 36-10). Another factor that may contribute to higher reported numbers of STIs is the increased use and availability of accurate screening tests for diseases, especially chlamydia.

Most STIs must be reported, and the provider must be aware of each state's specific rules. All 50 states allow adolescents to be evaluated and to receive treatment for STIs confidentially. Management of children younger than 13 years old with STIs requires a coordinated effort between the PCP and child protective authorities.

Gonorrhea, caused by *N. gonorrhoeae,* a nonmotile, gram-negative diplococcus, is often found in carriage with chlamydia or other STIs. In 2009 the gonorrhea rate was the lowest it has been since data collection was started in 1941. However it has been increasing; and in 2014, the rate was 110.7 cases per 100,000, which reflects a 5.1% increase since 2013. Among 15- to 19- year-olds, the rate was 430.5 per 100,000, which relected a 5% decrease; among 20- to 24-year-olds, the rate was 533.7 per 100,00, reflecting a 2.8% increase (CDC, 2014a). The infection is often asymptomatic, and untreated gonorrhea can progress to PID.

C. trachomatis infection is the most frequently reported bacterial STI, with a rate of 456.1 cases per 100,000 reported in 2014 (CDC, 2014a). This rate is increasing 2.8% since 2013; however, some of the increase is thought to be a reflection of more effective screening. Young women have the highest percentage of these cases with a reported rate of 2941 per 100,000 in 15- to 19-year-olds, and 3651 per 100,000 in 20- to 24-year-olds. This reflects a 4.2% decrease among 15- to 19-year-olds, and a continued increase in 20- to 24-year-olds (CDC, 2014a). All sexually active young women in this age group should be screened at least annually, because chlamydia is frequently asymptomatic. Untreated chlamydia can progress to PID; as many as 20% to 40% of the women with untreated infections develop PID, and 20% of those may lose their fertility.

Syphilis, caused by *Treponema pallidum,* is a motile spirochete with a rate of 6.3 per 100,000 in 2014. Although the rate continues to increase (15.1% since 2013), the good news is that there has been no increase among young women. The rate for 15- to 19-year-olds is 2.5 per 100,000; and for 20- to 24-year-olds, the rate is 4.5 per 100,000 (CDC, 2014a). Congenital syphilis is 11.6 cases per 100,000 in 2014, a 27.5% increase since 2013, following the 2012 rate of 7.8%, which was the lowest it has been since 1988 (CDC, 2014a).

HSV has two identified serotypes: HSV-1 and HSV-2. Although either type may infect any part of the body, most recurrent genital herpes is a result of HSV-2. Asymptomatic HSV infections are responsible for the transmission of most cases of genital herpes. Type 2 in prepubescent children is reportable in some states.

HPV is a small deoxyribonucleic acid (DNA) virus. More than 30 types of HPV can infect the genital tract. Visible warts are usually caused by HPV types 6 or 11. A person may be infected with multiple types of HPV. Types 16, 18, 31, 33, and 35 have been strongly associated with cervical cancer and vulvar, penile, and anal squamous intraepithelial neoplasia (CDC, 2015). Markowitz and colleagues (2013) found the prevalence of HPV infection to be 26% in 14- to 19-year-old females.

• BOX 36-10 Risk Factors for Sexually Transmitted Infections

- Adolescent younger than 15 years old
- Sexually active adolescent, especially with two or more partners in 6 months, high frequency of intercourse, or high rate of new partners
- Use of drugs or alcohol or other high-risk behaviors
- Pregnancy or abortion
- Homosexuality
- Victim of abuse, rape, or incest
- Incarcerated, runaway, homeless, in group shelter or detention home
- Clients in sexually transmitted infection (STI) clinics or with any other STI or previous history of STI
- Lack of family availability; low level of parental support and monitoring
- Beliefs about normative behaviors among peers
- Inappropriate health care behaviors (e.g., not seeking medical care, not adhering to treatment regimen, failure to recognize symptoms, delay in notifying partners, nonuse of barrier contraceptive)

Data from Biro FM, Rosenthal SL: Adolescent STDs: diagnosis, developmental issues, and prevention, *J Pediatr Health Care* 9:256–262, 1995; Bonny AE, Biro FM: Recognizing and treating STDs in adolescent girls, *Contemp Pediatr* 15:199–143, 1998; Shrier LA: Bacterial sexually transmitted infections: gonorrhea, chlamydia, pelvic inflammatory disease, and syphilis. In Emans SJ, Laufer MR, Goldstein DP, editors: *Pediatric and adolescent gynecology*, ed 5, Philadelphia, 2005, Lippincott Williams & Wilkins.

Clinical Findings

History

Many patients are asymptomatic. The history should assess the following:

- Type of sexual activity (including oral, vaginal, anal sex/intercourse) and contraceptive use
- Number of sexual partners over 60 days, 12 months, and lifetime; heterosexual or homosexual (or both) activity

- Known exposure or previous STIs
- Use of drugs or alcohol
- Vaginal discharge (amount, color, odor), pruritus, irregular or painful bleeding, dysmenorrhea, dyspareunia
- Dysuria, urinary urgency or frequency
- Abdominal or pelvic pain
- Skin rashes or lesions, ulcers, warts
- Systemic symptoms, such as fever, malaise, headache

See Box 36-10 for risk factors for STIs and Box 36-11 for CDC's five P's mnemonic. Table 36-6 provides history specific to each STI, and Chapter 15 has further details on obtaining a thorough history.

Physical Examination

- General examination—skin rashes and lesions, lymphadenopathy
- Abdominal examination—hepatic or splenic enlargement or tenderness in right upper quadrant
- Pelvic examination—inspection of external genitalia and vaginal mucosa, vaginal pH and discharge, cervical erythema, friability and mucopus, bimanual examination for cervical motion tenderness, uterine size, adnexal tenderness
- Rectal examination

• BOX 36-11 Centers for Disease Control and Prevention's Five Ps

1. **P**artners
   - Do you have sex with men, women, or both?
   - In the past 2 months how many partners have you had sex with?
   - In the past 12 months how many partners have you had sex with?
2. **P**revention of pregnancy
   - Are you or your partner trying to get pregnant? If no, what are you doing to prevent pregnancy?
3. **P**rotection from STIs
   - What do you do to protect yourself from STIs and HIV?
4. **P**ractices
   - To understand your risks for STIs, I need to understand the kind of sex you have had recently.
   - Have you had vaginal sex, meaning "penis in vagina sex"?
     - If yes: Do you use condoms: never, sometimes, or always?
   - Have you had anal sex, meaning "penis in rectum/anus sex"?
     - If yes: Do you use condoms: never, sometimes, or always?
   - Have you had oral sex, meaning "mouth on penis/vagina"?

   For condom answers:
   - If "never": Why don't you use condoms?
   - If "sometimes": In what situations or with whom do you not use condoms?
5. **P**ast history of STIs
   - Have you ever had an STI?
   - Have any of your partners had an STI?

Additional questions to identify HIV and hepatitis risk:
- Have you or any of your partners ever injected drugs?
- Have any of your partners exchanged money or drugs for sex?
- Is there anything else about your sexual practices that I need to know?

From Centers for Disease Control and Prevention: *Sexually transmitted diseases treatment guidelines*, CDC (website), 2015, available at www.cdc.gov/std/tg2015/default.htm. Accessed on November 20, 2015.
HIV, Human immunodeficiency virus; *STI,* sexually transmitted infection.

Diagnostic Studies

In deciding which studies to order, the provider needs to know the difference in and accuracy of tests. Methods that are sufficiently accurate for adolescents (presumptive tests) are not adequate for children who are being evaluated for possible abuse (see Chapter 17).

- Gonorrhea: Culture on selective media with determination of penicillin resistance is the definitive test for gonorrhea in women. Nucleic acid hybridization tests (DNA probes) and NAATs are also available for gonorrhea testing. NAATs are more reliable when done by cervical swab testing than with urine testing. Gram stains of vaginal discharge or cervical secretions are not recommended (CDC, 2015).
- Chlamydia: Culture is the only acceptable method to diagnose possible sexual abuse cases; many family planning clinics use direct immunofluorescent smears; however, DNA probes and NAATs are acceptable in adolescents, especially in high-prevalence populations. NAATs can be done on a cervical swab of the vaginal wall or urine and are therefore preferable for adolescents.
- Syphilis: Direct visualization with darkfield microscopy or direct immunofluorescent antibody (DFA) test is definitive. Serologic nontreponemal tests (Venereal Disease Research Laboratory [VDRL], rapid plasma reagin [RPR], or automated reagin test) correlate with disease activity, decline after treatment, and are used to monitor disease progress. Treponemal tests (fluorescent treponemal antibody absorption [FTA-ABS] and microhemagglutination test for *T. pallidum* [MHA-TP]) are confirmatory, but once positive they usually remain so for years.
- Herpes: Culture of scraped vesicle or ulcer is the preferred method. Type specific serologic testing is available; however, testing is not recommended for the general population.
- HPV: Testing is not recommended in the adolescent.

Differential Diagnosis

Chancroid, lymphogranuloma venereum, cytomegalovirus, hepatitis, granuloma inguinale, and molluscum are included in the differential diagnosis.

Management

The guidelines identified in this section are those recommended by the CDC (2015) for uncomplicated, initial treatment of STIs. Other recommendations and options for children weighing less than 45 kg and for recurrent and

TABLE 36-6 **Sexually Transmitted Infection History, Physical Examination, and Initial Treatment**

	History	Physical Examination	Treatment
Gonorrhea *(Neisseria gonorrhoeae)*	Often asymptomatic (33%); dysuria; vaginal discharge or bleeding; dyspareunia	Profuse, thick, green discharge, urethritis, cervicitis; Skene or Bartholin gland abscess; exudative pharyngitis	Ceftriaxone 250 mg IM one time *plus* azithromycin 1 g PO in a single dose Report to state health department Follow-up cultures not needed if ceftriaxone used
Chlamydia *(Chlamydia trachomatis)*	Often asymptomatic (30% to 70%); spotting, vaginal discharge; dysuria, pyuria; mild abdominal pain or foreign body sensation in eyes possible	Clear to white or yellow discharge, mucopurulent cervicitis with edema, erythema, hypertrophy; Fitz-Hugh–Curtis syndrome (right upper quadrant pain); conjunctivitis	Azithromycin 1 g PO in a single dose *or* Doxycycline 100 mg PO bid for 7 days* Report to state health department Test of cure not recommended unless pregnant
Syphilis *(Treponema pallidum)*	Primary: Vaginal, anal, or oral chancre Secondary: Copper-penny rash especially on palms and soles, lymphadenopathy, mucocutaneous lesions	Single painless papule with serous discharge, smooth base, raised edges; painless regional lymphadenopathy	Benzathine penicillin G 2.4 million units IM in a single dose *or* If penicillin allergy and not pregnant, doxycycline 100 mg PO bid for 14 days* *or* Tetracycline 500 mg PO qid for 14 days* Test for gonorrhea, chlamydia, and HIV at time of infection and in 3 months Follow with RPR or VDRL titers at 6, 12, and 24 months; should have fourfold decline by 6 months Report to state health department
Herpes simplex virus (HSV)	Painful rash, blisters and ulcers; burning and irritation 24 hours before outbreak; dysuria; other systemic complaints	Clear to white to yellow discharge; vesicles on erythematous base that become ulcers in 1 to 3 days; extragenital lesions; lymphadenopathy	Primary: Acyclovir 400 mg tid for 7 to 10 days *or* 200 mg five times a day for 7 to 10 days Recurrent: Acyclovir 400 mg tid for 5 days *or* Acyclovir 800 mg bid for 5 days or tid for 2 days Comfort measures: Sitz bath, dry heat, lidocaine jelly 2%
Human papillomavirus (HPV)	Asymptomatic or subclinical unrecognized; can be painful	Warts, friable or pruritic (or both); moist, cauliflower-like anogenital and inguinal 4 to 6 weeks after exposure	Patient-applied treatment (see text). Provider-applied treatment (see text): Cryotherapy, podophyllin resin, TCA or BCA, or surgical removal

Alternate regimens and regimens for pregnancy, infants and children can be found on the CDC website.
Data from Centers for Disease Control and Prevention (CDC): *Sexually transmitted diseases: treatment guidelines*, CDC (website), 2015, available at www.cdc.gov/std/tg2015/default.htm Accessed November 20, 2015.
BCA, Bichloracetic acid; *bid,* bis in die (twice a day); *HIV,* human immunodeficiency virus; *IM,* intramuscular; *PO,* per os (by mouth, orally); *qid,* quater in die (four times a day); *RPR,* rapid plasma reagin; *TCA,* trichloroacetic acid; *tid,* ter in die (three times a day); *VDRL,* Venereal Disease Research Laboratory.
*Contraindicated if younger than 8 years old.

complex cases are found in that CDC resource and in adolescent gynecology or child abuse literature. The goals of treatment include making a prompt diagnosis, determining the mode of acquisition, instituting appropriate treatment, preventing complications, contacting appropriate authorities, ensuring appropriate follow-up, and educating the adolescent and partner about risk reduction. Adolescents in the United States can consent to confidential diagnosis and treatment of STIs, and the PCP must be aware of each state's regulations (see www.guttmacher.org/statecenter/spibs/spib_MACS.pdf).

Several options for pharmaceutical treatment are given for each disease (see Table 36-6). When determining appropriate treatment, consideration should be given to the site of infection, the resistance patterns in the community, concurrent infections, side effects of the medication, and cost. Box 36-12 has general treatment measures for STIs. Other management measures include:

1. Gonorrhea (uncomplicated, patient weighing more than 99 pounds [45 kg]): Evaluate and treat all partners exposed in the previous 30 to 60 days and treat last sexual partner if more than 60 days since last intercourse.
2. Chlamydia (uncomplicated genital infection):
   - Treat last partner and any partner exposed within the 60 days before the onset of symptoms.
   - Rescreen 3 to 4 months after positive test result because a high prevalence of *C. trachomatis* infection is found in women who had a chlamydial infection in the preceding several months. Reinfection is usually the cause of infection and elevates the risk for PID.
3. Syphilis (primary or secondary):
   - The same laboratory tests (RPR or VDRL) should be used for follow-up and should decrease fourfold by 6 months and become nonreactive 1 year after treatment in primary cases. If still reactive after 12 months, retreat and reevaluate for HIV.
   - Treat all partners exposed during symptomatic period and for the 3 months before onset of infection.
   - An acute febrile reaction (Jarisch-Herxheimer reaction) with myalgia, headache, and other symptoms can occur within 24 hours after treatment.
   - Refer if symptoms of secondary or tertiary syphilis is present.
4. Genital herpes: No treatment will eradicate the disease. Treatment or prevention of acute outbreaks is the goal of therapy:
   - Use daily suppressive treatment if episodes occur six times or more in a year. This reduces the frequency of episodes by more than 70% to 80%.
   - Test for other STIs as indicated.
   - Counsel to abstain from sexual activity when active lesions are present and inform sexual partners.
   - Inform that transmission of HSV can occur during asymptomatic periods.
   - Stress the risk of perinatal infection and follow pregnancies closely.
   - Educate regarding course of disease, self-inoculation, transmission, and asymptomatic viral shedding.
   - Suggest dietary modifications including increased intake of vitamin C, B-complex and B_6 vitamins, zinc, and calcium to boost the immune system. A diet high in lysine and low in arginine (e.g., eating fish, chicken, cheese, and most fruits and vegetables and avoiding chocolate, peanuts, and white and wheat flour) may be helpful.
5. HPV: No treatment will eradicate this disease. The goal should be to remove visible warts and reduce symptoms. The benefit of identification and treatment of subclinical infections has not been established. Patient preference and treatment availability should guide treatment course; spontaneous resolution occurs in most cases. Warts on moist surfaces respond better to topical treatment than do warts on drier surfaces.
   - Patient-applied treatment: Treat with podofilox 0.5% solution or gel, or imiquimod 5% cream. Wash treated area with mild soap and water 6 to 10 hours after application. Warts should clear after 8 to 10 weeks. Safety in pregnancy is not determined
   - Provider-applied treatment: Treat external visible warts with (1) cryotherapy with liquid nitrogen or cryoprobe every 1 to 2 weeks, (2) 10% to 25% podophyllin resin in benzoin washed off in 1 to 4 hours to decrease local irritation, repeated weekly (safety in pregnancy not established), (3) trichloroacetic acid (TCA) or bichloracetic acid (BCA) applied in small amounts, dried to frosting consistency, followed by baking powder or baking soda to remove unreacted acid, repeated weekly, or (4) surgical removal with scissors, shave, curette, or electrosurgery.

BOX 36-12 General Treatment Measures for Sexually Transmitted Infections

- Have patient abstain from sexual intercourse until patient and partner are cured (treatment complete and symptoms resolved). Consequences of untreated STIs should be explained.
- Test for other STIs, including hepatitis B, HIV, BV, and *Trichomonas.*
- Notify, examine, and treat all partners of patient for any STI identified or suspected.
- Report STIs to state health department. Reporting to appropriate authorities is important to identify those at risk, recognize new strains, and assess extent of infection in community and the effect of prevention efforts.
- Provide regular sex health assessment including vaginal examination and testing for STIs.
- Give hepatitis B, HPV vaccines if not done already.
- Discuss safer sex practices, including abstinence and use of condoms.
- Educate and counsel about complications and transmission of STIs and perinatal consequences.

BV, Bacterial vaginosis; *HIV,* human immunodeficiency virus; *HPV,* human papillomavirus; *STI,* sexually transmitted infection.

- Change treatment if there is no response after three patient-applied treatments or six provider-applied treatments.
- Use only one treatment modality at a time to prevent increased complications.
- Advise patient that an inflammatory reaction is common before resolution.
- After cryotherapy, pain, necrosis, and blistering are common.
- Refer patients with cervical warts, suspected abuse, or extensive lesions in difficult areas for gynecologic treatment. Intralesional interferon or laser surgery may be necessary in severe cases.
- No change in the schedule for Pap testing is necessary with clinical warts.
- Advise patient that recurrence is common, most often in the first 3 months following treatment.

Complications

In general, perinatal transmission, disseminated infection, and increased risk for chronic hepatitis are possible. PID, ectopic pregnancy, and infertility are possible sequelae to gonorrhea and chlamydia. Tertiary disease is a risk with syphilis. An increased risk of HIV transmission has been found with other STIs. HPV infection is linked with cervical dysplasia and cancer.

Patient Education and Family Education

Prevention occurs at a variety of levels and in a variety of ways. Primary prevention seeks to reduce the number of new cases of STIs. This best occurs before sexual debut by delaying initiation of sexual intercourse. If the adolescent currently is or plans to become sexually active, promoting the use of condoms and partner communication skills to avoid exposure to STIs is imperative. Address these topics specifically, using knowledge, attitudes, and behaviors to guide education, as well as considering developmental needs, cultural values, misperceptions, and social skills. Peer facilitators are useful. Hepatitis B, HPV, and possibly hepatitis A immunizations are recommended. Secondary prevention seeks to reduce the numbers of existing cases by early detection and treatment through well-woman care and STI screening (recommended every 6 months for those at risk). Access to health care for treatment and follow-up, monitoring for sequelae, partner notification, and evaluating risk behaviors are important aspects to successful secondary prevention. Tertiary prevention seeks to minimize the psychological and biologic sequelae of STIs including minimizing perinatal complications, infant morbidity and mortality rates, and reducing the frequency of PID and its complications. Identifying coping strategies and means of increasing self-esteem are also important aspects.

Treatment of any STI in a child should be coordinated with the laboratory, child protective services, and the state authorities. Important family factors that reduce risk behaviors include perceived parental support, degree of family closeness, communication among family members, parenting style, and parental supervision and monitoring.

Pelvic Inflammatory Disease

Considered an ascending infection, PID refers to infection and inflammation involving the upper genital tract (uterus, fallopian tubes, ovaries, or peritoneal tissue). PID is either acute (less than 3 weeks' duration) or chronic. The classic picture is acute salpingitis that causes lower abdominal pain, vaginal discharge, and fever with an onset after menses. However, PID is difficult to diagnose because symptoms are widely varied.

PID is often a polymicrobial infection, with gonorrhea and chlamydia being the two most common STIs causing PID. Vaginal flora, other aerobic and anaerobic organisms, group B streptococcus, genital mycoplasma, and gram-negative bacteria also are implicated. Approximately 33% of cases of PID are in adolescents. The two risk factors considered to be most significant among teenagers are multiple sexual partners and the high prevalence of STIs in this age group. Other risk factors include increased susceptibility of adolescents to infection, cervical ectopy and thinner cervical mucus, recent instrumentation or intrauterine device use, previous PID, history of lower genital tract infection (including gonorrhea, chlamydia, trichomoniasis, and BV), and nonuse of contraceptives of any type.

Clinical Findings

PID in adolescents is often subtle and can go undiagnosed, contributing to the inflammatory sequelae. Criteria for diagnosis of PID have been identified, including a set of minimal, low-threshold criteria prompting early intervention (Box 36-13).

History

- Sexual history, including number of partners and type of activity
- Last menstrual period, contraceptive use, and previous STI or PID
- Lower abdominal pain or tenderness (acute onset with gonorrhea, subtle with chlamydia)
- Intermenstrual bleeding
- Malaise, dysuria, nausea, vomiting, chills, dyspareunia

Physical Examination

The physical examination includes abdominal examination for bilateral lower quadrant tenderness (most common initial symptom) and possibly right upper quadrant pain (Fitz-Hugh–Curtis syndrome—inflammation of liver capsule) with occasional peritoneal signs; speculum examination, and bimanual examination (see Box 36-13).

Diagnostic Studies

- CBC (WBCs greater than 10,000), erythrocyte sedimentation rate (ESR), CRP
- Microscopic examination of cervical discharge, NAATs or culture for gonorrhea and chlamydia, serologic test (syphilis)
- Pregnancy test (ectopic)

BOX 36-13 Criteria for Diagnosing Pelvic Inflammatory Disease

Minimum criteria for treating PID in sexually active adolescents with pelvic or lower abdominal pain and no other cause for illness identified include one or more of the following pelvic examination findings:

- Cervical motion tenderness
- Uterine tenderness
- Adnexal tenderness

Additional lower-genital-tract inflammatory findings that support the diagnosis:

- Cervical friability
- Cervical exudates
- Predominance of leukocytes in the vaginal secretions

Additional criteria that support a diagnosis of PID:

- Oral temperature >101° F (>38.3° C)
- Abnormal mucopurulent cervical or vaginal discharge
- Presence of abundant WBCs in saline microscopy of vaginal secretions
- Elevated ESR
- Elevated CRP
- Laboratory documentation of cervical infection with gonorrhea or chlamydia

Most specific criteria for diagnosing PID, warranted in selected cases:

- Endometrial biopsy with histopathologic evidence of endometritis
- Transvaginal sonography or magnetic resonance imaging showing thickened fluid-filled tubes with or without free pelvic fluid or tubo-ovarian complex
- Laparoscopic abnormalities consistent with PID

Data from Centers for Disease Control and Prevention (CDC): Sexually transmitted diseases: treatment guidelines, *MMWR Morb Wkly Rep* 59(RR-12):63–64, 2010.
CRP, C-reactive protein; *ESR,* erythrocyte sedimentation rate; *PID,* pelvic inflammatory disease; *WBC,* white blood cell.

- Urinalysis and culture if symptoms of pyelonephritis or cystitis
- Pelvic ultrasound (if adnexal enlargement or tubo-ovarian abscess suspected)

Differential Diagnosis

Acute appendicitis, ectopic pregnancy, torsion of an ovarian cyst, ruptured corpus luteal cyst, salpingitis, tubo-ovarian abscess, endometritis, acute pyelonephritis, gastroenteritis, vaginitis, and functional pain are included in the differential diagnosis.

Management

Outpatient treatment regimens are delineated in Table 36-7. Goals of treatment include the relief of acute discomfort and prevention of infertility and other sequelae. More than one diagnosis is possible. Empiric treatment should be initiated in sexually active young women if the minimal criteria are met. Treatment should be initiated as soon as possible with broad-spectrum coverage to minimize long-term sequelae. Follow-up should occur within 72 hours. Patients should demonstrate clinical improvement as evidenced by defervescence, decreased abdominal tenderness, and decreased uterine, adnexal, and cervical motion tenderness. If no clinical improvement, the patient will need hospitalization.

TABLE 36-7 Outpatient Treatment Regimens for Pelvic Inflammatory Disease

Regimen A	Regimen B
Ceftriaxone 250 mg IM in a single dose	Cefoxitin 2 g IM in a single dose *and* Probenecid 1 g orally administered concurrently in a single dose
Plus	**Plus**
Doxycycline 100 mg orally bid for 14 days	Doxycycline 100 mg orally bid for 14 days
With or Without	**With or Without**
Metronidazole 500 mg twice daily for 14 days	Metronidazole 500 mg twice daily for 14 days

Data from Centers for Disease Control and Prevention (CDC): *Sexually transmitted diseases: treatment guidelines*, CDC (website), 2015, available at www.cdc.gov/std/tg2015/default.htm. Acessed November 20, 2015.
bid, Bis in die (twice a day); *IM,* intramuscular.

Hospitalization is also recommended in the following situations: a surgical emergency cannot be excluded; pregnancy; lack of response to oral antibiotics; inability to tolerate oral antibiotics; severe illness with nausea, vomiting, or high temperature; or tubo-ovarian abscess (CDC, 2015).

Other recommendations include:

- Treatment of any sexual partners exposed within 60 days of onset of symptoms. Abstinence from intercourse until partners have been treated.
- Additional follow up of patient 7 to 10 days after treatment.
- Rescreen for chlamydia and gonorrhea 3 to 6 months after treatment. HIV screening should be offered.
- PID is a reportable STI in some states.

Complications

Infertility (13% to 50% attributable to PID, a higher percentage with subsequent episodes); tubo-ovarian abscess; ectopic pregnancy (sixfold to tenfold increased risk); perihepatitis (Fitz-Hugh–Curtis syndrome); chronic pelvic pain; dyspareunia; and repeated PID can occur (Shrier, 2012).

Prevention

Decrease prevalence and transmission of STIs by promoting abstinence and barrier methods (condoms, diaphragms, cervical caps, and spermicidal foams). Screen sexually active adolescents for gonorrhea and chlamydia every 6 months.

For a complete list of references, please visit http://evolve.elsevier.com/Burns/pediatric/.

37 Dermatologic Disorders

LEAH G. FITCH AND LAUREN BELL GAYLORD

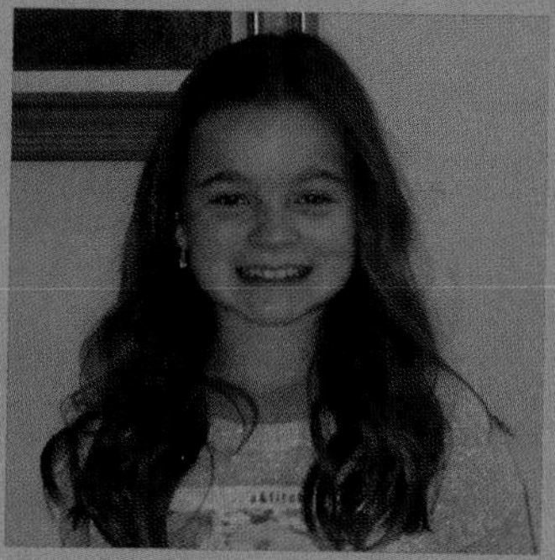

The skin is the body's largest organ and one of its most important. Skin conditions reflect physical and emotional health and often give clues to underlying conditions. Skin functions are multiple. Beauty is often defined by the appearance of the skin. Emotions are expressed by blushing and sweating. Skin conveys many impressions through its sensory functions, including reaction to touch, heat, cold, pressure, and pain. Additionally, the skin provides a protective physiologic covering, the first line of defense against injury from chemical, physical, and microorganic invaders. Homeostasis is maintained through fluid regulation and thermoregulation.

Disruptions in the skin account for a significant percentage of all pediatric office visits. The primary care provider plays an essential role in maintaining skin integrity, identifying and minimizing skin disruptions, maximizing healing, and educating parents and children about skin care.

Skin development is constant from embryogenesis throughout life. During the embryonic period (the first 2 months of gestation), the skin differentiates into several layers. The skin changes and develops throughout childhood and adolescence, achieving adult skin thickness and characteristics in the late teenage years. Melanin in the skin reaches adult levels by 1 year old. Vascularization is well developed by the end of the second year of life. Cutaneous nerves develop until puberty and beyond. Sebaceous glands cease production between 6 and 12 months old, but they become active again at around 7 years old. Eccrine sweat function begins between 2 and 18 days old, although full function is not in place until 2 or 3 years old. The apocrine glands become active at puberty. Hair grows approximately 1 cm per month. Nails are spoon shaped and thin from infancy until 2 to 3 years old.

Anatomy and Physiology

The skin is composed of three layers: the epidermis, the dermis, and the subcutaneous layer (Fig. 37-1). The epidermis and dermis together vary from 1.5 to 4 mm in thickness (Cohen, 2013).

The epidermis, a thinner outer layer, functions as a protective barrier between the body and the environment and is comprised of five layers of stratified squamous epithelium. Most epidermal cells are keratinocytes, and the replication and maturation of the keratinocytes is called *keratinization.* New keratinocytes of the basal layer mature and are shed approximately every 28 days. The outer horny layer is called the *stratum corneum* and is responsible for much of the barrier protection against microorganisms and irritating chemicals. It impedes the exchange of fluids and electrolytes with the environment and provides strength for the skin. Melanin protects deoxyribonucleic acid (DNA) from damage by ultraviolet (UV) light irradiation. It is produced in the basal layer of the epidermis and contributes to the color of the skin, eyes, and hair. Ambient moisture influences the epidermal barrier, with either excess or inadequate amounts contributing to microscopic and macroscopic breaks.

The dermis is the thicker middle layer that contributes strength, support, and elasticity to the skin. It is a tough, leathery mechanical barrier that also regulates heat loss, provides host defenses of the skin, and aids in nutrition and other regulatory functions. The dermis is primarily composed of fibrous connective tissue (made up of fibroblasts and collagen), with some elastic fibers and a mucopolysaccharide gel. It includes mast cells, inflammatory cells, blood and lymph vessels, and cutaneous nerves that elicit sensations. These specialized receptors are a defense mechanism to protect the skin surface from environmental trauma.

Underlying the dermis is subcutaneous tissue primarily composed of adipose tissue. It contains arteries and arterioles that assist in skin thermoregulation. The subcutaneous tissue insulates, cushions against trauma, provides energy, and metabolizes hormones.

Skin appendages include the hair, nails, sweat glands, and sebaceous glands. Hair follicles are found over the entire body except for the palms, soles, knuckles, distal and interdigital spaces, lips, glans and prepuce of the penis, and areolae and nipples of the breast. Two types of hair can be found on the body. Terminal hair is thick, visible, and found

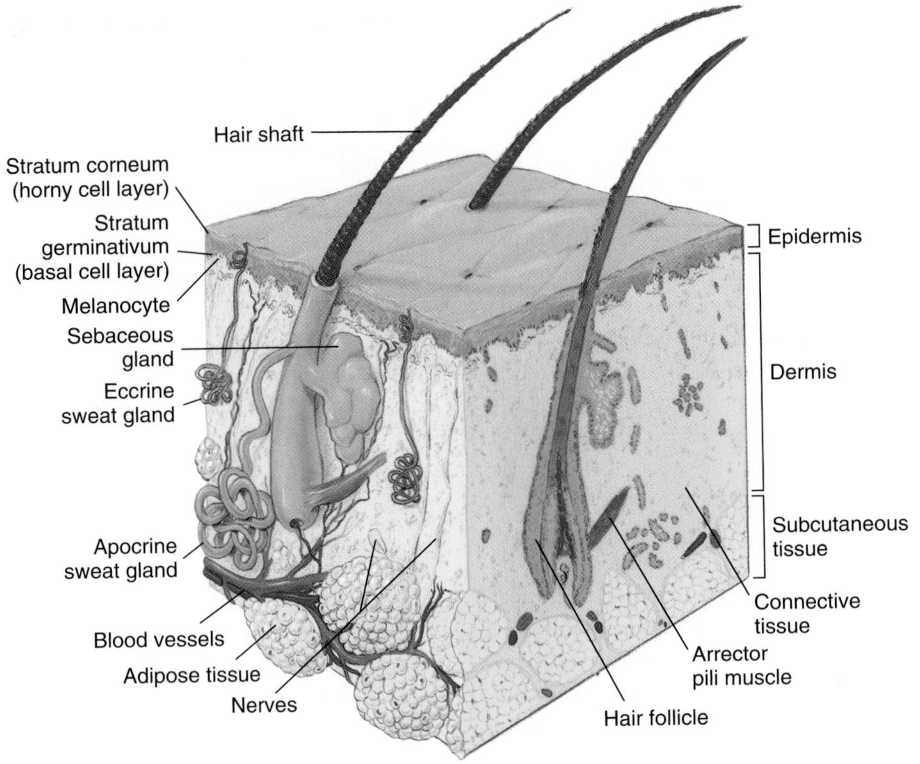

• **Figure 37-1** Structure of the skin. (From Jarvis C: *Physical examination and assessment*, ed 6, Philadelphia, 2012, Saunders/Elsevier.)

on the scalp, axillae, and pubis. Very fine vellus hair is found over the remainder of the body. The visible portion of the hair is the shaft. The hair root is embedded in the dermis as a pilosebaceous unit, consisting of a hair follicle and a sebaceous gland. The hair shaft may be straight, wavy, helical, or spiral. Following an acute febrile illness or stress, there may be hair thinning for several months.

Nails are epidermal cells converted to keratin that grow continually. The nailbed, underneath the nail plate, is composed of layers of epidermis and dermis, which serve as structural support. The nail root lies just under the epidermis.

There are three types of sweat glands: eccrine, ceruminous, and apocrine. *Eccrine glands* are distributed over the entire body. They help maintain fluid and electrolyte balance and body temperature and provide some excretory function. *Ceruminous glands* are located in the external ear canal and secrete a waxy pigmented substance called cerumen. *Apocrine glands* are located primarily in the axillary, genital, and periumbilical areas. They open into hair follicles, require androgens to stimulate their secretions, and are thought to be responsible for body odor.

Found in conjunction with hair follicles, sebaceous glands contribute to the epidermis protection and are distributed over the entire body except the soles, palms, and dorsa of the feet. These glands secrete sebum (oil) when stimulated by androgen and function to prevent excessive water evaporation, minimize heat loss, and lubricate the skin and hair.

Pathophysiology and Defense Mechanisms

Disruption of the skin and subcutaneous tissue occurs through a variety of assaults. These include:

- Bacterial, fungal, and viral infections
- Allergic and inflammatory reactions
- Infestations
- Vascular reactions
- Papulosquamous and bullous eruptions
- Congenital lesions
- Hair and nail disorders

There are three identified cutaneous reactions to trauma, infection, or inflammation: pigment lability, follicular response, and mesenchymal response. Pigment lability occurs as postinflammatory hypopigmentation or hyperpigmentation. If superficial, with changes in the epidermis only, normal pigmentation returns in about 6 months (e.g., in diaper rash, seborrhea, tinea, or pityriasis alba). If dermal changes happen, dermal tattooing may occur, causing long-term or permanent changes (e.g., excoriated acne, impetigo, varicella, and contact dermatitis). An exaggerated follicular response results in prominent papule and follicle formation, especially with atopic dermatitis, pityriasis rosea, syphilis, or tinea versicolor. A mesenchymal response, which often follows varicella, ear piercing, burns, or any surgical procedure, causes scars and keloids (scars that thicken and extend beyond the margins of the initial injury).

Special Dermatologic Considerations in Children with Dark Skin or from Diverse Cultural or Ethnic Groups

Knowledge of normal variations in children with different levels of skin pigmentation and/or from diverse ethnic or cultural groups is important for assessing and treating dermatologic conditions. Skin reactions to injury, inflammation, common skin conditions, and cultural practices are varied. A wise pediatric health care provider listens to parents, because they are often the first to detect subtle changes in color or texture of the skin. This section discusses some of the dermatologic differences of children with dark skin.

Preventive care for children with dark skin should be implemented in routine well-child care. The following are initial areas to include:

- Immunize against varicella to prevent scarring.
- Use insect repellents.
- Treat early signs and symptoms of pruritic or inflammatory conditions (e.g., acne, eczema) and infections.
- Advise against overuse of pomades and complications.
- Reduce causes of traction alopecia.
- Use moisturizing agents and eliminate soaps for dry, itchy skin.
- Use oral antipruritics for dry, itchy skin.
- Caution about the use of topical medications, especially high-potency steroids, benzoyl peroxide, and isotretinoin.
- Avoid trauma and any procedures that can induce keloids.

Cutaneous Reaction Patterns

Pigment lability is common and tends to be more obvious in dark-skinned individuals regardless of race. People of color are especially prone to the development of keloids and hypertrophic scars, sometimes from relatively minor skin trauma. Other exaggerated responses common in darker-skinned individuals include lichenification and vesicular or bullous reaction to bites or staphylococcal infection. African American children may have an exaggerated cutaneous response to common disorders of the skin.

Normal Variations and Common Problems

The following are normal variations or common problems in children with dark skin:

- Variation in color and texture of skin from one part of the body to another
- Pigmentation of gingiva, mucous membrane, sclerae, and nails correlates with degree of cutaneous pigmentation
- Increased areas of melanin in thicker-skinned areas (elbow, knee)
- The terms *Futcher line* or *Ito line* describe the vertical line that separates the hyperpigmented dorsal and extensor surfaces from less pigmented ventral surfaces; this line of differentiation follows Voigt lines and is most noticeable on the extremities
- Mongolian spots and increased numbers of café au lait spots (see later discussion)
- Normal exfoliation produces a fine layer of gray scales
- Color alterations (jaundice, anemia, cyanosis) are difficult to assess
- Erythema may appear as a purplish tinge and be difficult to detect
- Kinky, wooly, tightly curled hair with closely knit growth that tangles when dry and mats when wet
- Atopic dermatitis (see Chapter 25) with prominent follicular pattern with pityriasis alba and postinflammatory hypopigmentation

Cultural or Ethnic Practices with Skin Sequelae

Grooming, cosmetic, or healing practices of cultural or ethnic groups contribute to various conditions that may be seen. These include the following:

- Hair pomade—acne
- Bleaching creams—discoloration and erythematous nodules
- Chemical or thermal hair straighteners—alopecia, fragile hair shaft, scalp contact dermatitis
- Tightly braided, twisted, locked hair (dreadlocks), and tight ponytails—traction folliculitis followed by traction alopecia that can be permanent and cause scarring (Cafardi, 2012)
- Henna for superficial tattooing—orange discoloration of skin, increased bilirubin levels in infants
- Decorative practices—scars or tattoos
- Healing practices used during significant illness that produce burns—circular 1- to 2-cm scars on chest, periumbilicus, wrists, ankles, or back
- Coining—petechiae and ecchymoses, especially on chest and back
- Cupping—circular ecchymoses on neck, chest, back, and arms

Assessment of the Skin and Subcutaneous Tissue

History

The history should assess the following:

- History of present illness
  - Onset and duration of present or recent illness (e.g., respiratory or gastrointestinal)
  - Most common concerns (e.g., pruritus, scaling, alterations in cosmetic appearance)
  - Symptom analysis: Questions to ask about an eruption or lesions include:
    - What did the rash or lesion(s) originally look like?
    - How has it changed in appearance?

    - Is the way it looks today typical of its appearance?
    - Where did the eruption first begin?
    - Has the rash or lesion spread to other locations (pattern of spread)?
    - How long has the rash been present?
    - Does it come and go?
    - Has the lesion blistered, bled, or had discharge?
    - Does it itch?
    - What have you used to treat it and what was the effect?
  - Parts of the body not affected by the rash or lesions (e.g., face, soles, palms)
  - Associated systemic symptoms (e.g., fever, malaise, pain) associated with lesion or eruption
  - Factors that alleviate, trigger, or worsen skin symptoms
  - Exposure to things that could cause skin reactions (e.g., medication, foods, animals, plants, new substances, people with similar symptoms or illness, soaps, hair products, lotions, detergents)
  - Allergies to things that could cause skin reactions
  - Medication (prescription and over the counter) taken over the past few days, including creams, ointments, powders, or lotions (It is often helpful to have patients bring medications that they have used to the appointment.)
  - Prior incidents of a similar rash
  - Recent travel
  - How much is the problem affecting your life or feelings about yourself?
- Family review of systems
  - Similar symptoms
  - Skin disorders or history of atopy disorders (asthma, seasonal or drug allergies or atopic dermatitis)
  - Chronic illnesses with related dermatologic findings
- Client review of systems and past medical history
  - Usual state of health and recent illnesses
  - Skin, hair, and nails: Skin type (dry or oily), recent and long-term changes, previous incidence of skin disease
  - Eyes, ears, nose, and throat: Swelling, itching, crusting, discharge or circles around eyes, nasal mucus discharge, patency or irritation, dry mouth, lesions, or pain
  - Chest: Wheezing, coughing, or respiratory difficulty
  - Chronic illnesses with related dermatologic findings

Physical Examination

When seeing a child with a dermatologic condition, it is essential to assess whether the child is ill. This clinical impression helps the provider differentiate serious illnesses from the majority of dermatologic conditions. The entire body, not just exposed skin, needs to be examined. Attention should be given to the eyes, nose, mouth (mucous membranes, teeth), lymph nodes, and lungs because a skin disorder may be a cutaneous manifestation of other disease. The dermatologic examination includes a thorough look at the skin, scalp, hair, palms and soles, nails, and anogenital region.

Special techniques for examination of the skin may be required. Good light (daylight is best) is essential to a good examination. A source of direct light, such as a gooseneck lamp, is the best alternative. Other helpful tools include a magnifying glass, a ruler, a glass slide, and a Wood's lamp (UV light). A glass slide gently pressed on the skin (diascopy) allows viewing of the skin with and without capillary filling. A Wood's lamp is used to examine fluorescent-positive fungal infections and depigmenting skin disorders, such as vitiligo.

Identification of the type of lesion and correct use of terminology are essential to good dermatologic care. Essential documentation includes the following:

- Location and type of lesion
- Color, color changes, size, and shape
- Arrangement (e.g., isolated, grouped, linear, annular, zosteriform)
- Pattern (e.g., sun-exposed area, symmetry)
- Distribution of lesion (e.g., regional, generalized, crops)
- Border (e.g., indistinct, well-circumscribed)
- Consistency (e.g., firm, soft, mobile)

Primary skin lesions (Box 37-1) include changes that arise from previously normal skin. These descriptions should be memorized and used. *Secondary* skin lesions (Box 37-2) result from changes in primary lesions. *Vascular* skin lesions (Box 37-3) involve the blood supply. Other useful descriptive terms are listed in Box 37-4. Vesicles, pustules, scaling, and color changes should be noted when considering differential diagnoses.

• BOX 37-1 Primary Skin Changes to Lesions

Bulla: Vesicle larger than 1 cm
Comedo: Plugged, dilated pore; open (blackhead), closed (whitehead)
Cyst: Palpable lesion with definite borders filled with liquid or semisolid material
Macule: Flat, nonpalpable, discolored lesion, 1 cm or smaller
Nodule: Raised, firm, movable lesion with indistinct borders and deep palpable portion, 2 cm or smaller
Papule: Solid, raised lesion of varied color with distinct borders, 1 cm or smaller
Patch: Macule, larger than 1 cm
Plaque: Solid, raised, flat-topped lesion with distinct borders, larger than 1 cm
Pustule: Raised lesion filled with pus, often in hair follicle or sweat pore
Tumor: Large nodule, may be firm or soft
Vesicle: Blister filled with clear fluid
Wheal: Fleeting, irregularly shaped, elevated, itchy lesion of varied size, pale at center, slightly red at borders

• BOX 37-2 Secondary Skin Changes to Lesions

Atrophy: Thinning skin, may appear translucent
Crusts: Dried exudate or scab of varied color
Desquamation: Peeling sheets of scale
Erosion: Oozing or moist, depressed area with loss of superficial epidermis
Excoriation: Abrasion or removal of epidermis; scratch
Fissure: Linear, wedge-shaped cracks extending into dermis
Keloid: Healed lesion of hypertrophied connective tissue
Lichenification: Thickening of skin with deep visible furrows
Scales: Thin, flaking layers of epidermis
Scar: Healed lesion of connective tissue
Striae: Fine pink or silver lines in areas where skin has been stretched
Ulcer: Deeper than erosion; open lesion extending into dermis

• BOX 37-3 Vascular Skin Lesions

Angioma or hemangioma: Papule made of blood vessels
Ecchymosis: Bruise, purple to brown, macular or papular, varied in size
Hematoma: Collection of blood from ruptured blood vessel, larger than 1 cm
Petechiae: Pinpoint, pink to purple macular lesions that do not blanch, 1 to 3 mm
Purpura: Purple macular lesion, larger than 1 cm
Telangiectasia: Collection of macular or raised dilated capillaries

• BOX 37-4 Descriptive Terms for Dermatologic Lesions

Acral: Involving extremities (hands, feet, ears, and so on)
Annular: Ring-shaped
Arcuate: Arc-shaped
Circinate: Circular
Confluent: Running together
Contiguous: Touching or adjacent
Diffuse or generalized: Scattered, widely distributed
Discrete: Distinct and separate
Eczematous: Referring to vesicles with oozing crust
Grouped: Arranged in sets
Guttate: Small, droplike
Herpetiform: Referring to grouped vesicles resembling those of herpes
Iris: Arranged in concentric circles, one inside the other
Linear: Arranged in a line
Localized: In a limited area
Nummular: Coin-shaped
Pedunculated: Having a stalk
Polycyclic: Oval with more than one ring
Reticular: Netlike
Serpiginous: Snakelike, creeping
Symmetric: Balanced on both sides
Target lesion (iris or targetoid): Erythematous papule or plaque characterized by a red to violet dusky center surrounded by a raised, edematous pale ring and red periphery
Telangiectatic: Referring to dilated terminal vessels
Umbilicated: Depressed or shaped like a navel
Verrucous: Wartlike
Zosteriform: Resembling shingles, following a nerve root or dermatome

Diagnostic Studies

A few simple laboratory tests are helpful in identifying or excluding dermatologic disorders. Proper procurement of the sample is important. Lesions can be scraped with a No. 15 blade or a toothbrush and scales or debris placed on a glass microscope slide or in culture material. The No. 15 blade is also useful for exfoliating a blister. It is important to scrape under any scabs to get a sample of the organisms present. Moistening the lesion may facilitate this. Scrapings can be obtained from the edges of skin lesions, from plucked hair (getting the root is essential), from the nail plate, or from subungual debris. Laboratory tests that can be used include the following:

- Microscopic examination of skin scrapings:
  - Potassium hydroxide (KOH) can be used to examine for fungal disorders (hyphae or spores; Fig. 37-2). Scrape fine scales from the edge of the lesion onto a glass slide. Add a drop of KOH 20% to dissolve debris, and cover with a coverslip. Let sit for 20 to 30 minutes or heat gently (do not boil). Use ×10 magnification to examine.
  - Wright, Giemsa, or Wright-Giemsa stains are used to examine for bacteria, white cells, and multinucleated giant cells (or Tzanck cells found in viral lesions, such as herpes, varicella, or zoster) in scrapings of skin lesions, ulcers, or vesicles. Allow scrapings to air-dry, then stain with Wright or Giemsa stain, or both. Use ×40 magnification to examine for bacteria and multinucleated giant cells.

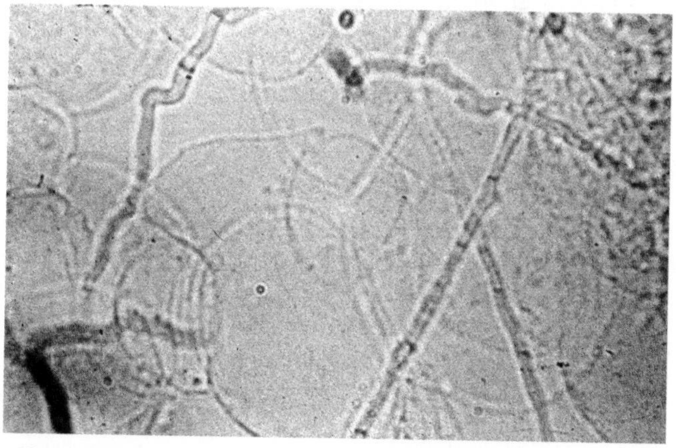

• Figure 37-2 Fungal elements (hyphae: long septae, branching rods) as seen on microscopic examination of a potassium hydroxide (KOH) preparation. (From Cohen B: *Pediatric dermatology*, ed 4, Philadelphia, 2013, Saunders/Elsevier.)

- Microbial culture of lesions for bacteria, viruses, or fungi. Simple, inexpensive culture methods for fungal organisms include the dermatophyte test medium (DTM) and InTray CCD (includes *Candida*). Skin or nail scrapings

or hairs, including the root, are applied so that they break the agar surface. A color change is noted in 1 to 5 days.
- Patch or skin testing for allergic or contact reactions is usually done by dermatologists or allergists.
- Skin biopsy following local anesthesia may be by punch or shave method for any tumor, palpable purpura, persistent dermatitis, or blister that is not otherwise definitively diagnosed. Such procedures often require referral to a dermatologist.
- Complete blood count (CBC) and erythrocyte sedimentation rate (ESR) may evaluate infection or inflammation.

Management Strategies

Hydration and Lubrication

Adequate skin hydration is essential to prevent and treat skin conditions. If the skin is overhydrated, the bonds between cells at the stratum corneum loosen and the barrier is broken. If the skin is too dry, it cracks, again breaking the barrier.

Bathing

Bathing is an efficient means of hydrating and lubricating the skin, especially with dry skin or in dry climates. Lukewarm, not hot, water should be used. The bath should last long enough for skin to become moisturized without becoming supersaturated or "pruned." Bubble-bath solutions are especially irritating and should be avoided. Soaping and shampooing should be done at the end of the bath followed by thorough rinsing. The skin should be patted dry and a lubricating agent applied immediately. Baths containing baking soda or colloidal oatmeal may help relieve pruritus. Bathing and other heat exposures can make a rash seem worse temporarily.

Environmental Considerations

Because water is essential to skin integrity, environmental humidity also plays a role. Excessive humidity (greater than 90%) or deficient humidity (less than 10%) can cause disruption of the skin. Macerated skin benefits from less humidity. Itching from excessively dry skin can be relieved by increasing ambient humidity (e.g., using a vaporizer or humidifier). In hot temperatures, itching can be alleviated by air conditioning. Water consumption also plays a role in maintaining proper skin hydration, and children should drink plenty of water.

Skin Care Agents

Soaps, Oils, and Colloids

Non-allergic, mild soaps are best or soap substitutes. Colloid oatmeal and bath oils are also helpful.

Moisturizers and Lubricants

Moisturizers and lubricants treat chronic dryness and inflammation of the skin by retaining water in the skin. Composed of petrolatum or a mixture of petrolatum and lanolin, moisturizers and lubricants are most effective when applied to damp skin.

Wet Dressings

For acute oozing, crusting, or itching skin, wet dressings help dry the skin, decrease itching, and remove crusts. Thin cloths, such as diapers, handkerchiefs, or strips of sheets, make the best wet dressings. Dressings should be moderately wet but not dripping, with lukewarm water and applied for 10 to 20 minutes two to four times daily over a period of 48 to 72 hours. During the treatment dressings must be kept wet either by removing and rewetting or by applying water directly to the dressing. Alternative solutions include saline (1 teaspoon salt with 1 pint of water) or Burow solution (1 Domeboro tablet [aluminum acetate; calcium acetate] with 1 pint of cool or tepid water). The medication in creams or ointments applied following wet dressings is absorbed more effectively. A slightly more intense technique involves applying a steroid ointment or cream to the skin; then covering the skin with a wet dressing and then a dry dressing (e.g., a sleeper, pajamas, or long johns are wetted, put on, and covered with a dry sleeper or long johns) (Cathcart and Theos, 2011). The dressing is changed every 6 hours for 24 to 72 hours or is used overnight for 5 to 10 nights. When using this technique, care must be taken to prevent excessive steroidal absorption by applying steroid only to areas needing it, especially in infants and young children.

Occlusive Dressings

Occlusive dressings decrease water evaporation from the skin and enhance hydration and absorption of topical medications. Plastic wrap is placed over the affected area after hydrating the skin and applying cream or ointment; these dressings should not be left on longer than 8 hours. Ointments, oils, urea compounds, and propylene glycol used alone are occlusive. Skinfolds serve as naturally occurring occlusive areas. Lichen simplex chronicus, dyshidrotic eczema, and psoriasis are skin conditions that benefit from occlusion.

Other Considerations

- Irritants and sensitizing agents, such as wool, sweat, and saliva, should be avoided.
- Allergens and foods that most commonly cause skin reactions include milk, eggs, wheat, tomatoes, citrus, chocolate, fish, and nuts.

Sunscreens and Sunblocks

Sunscreens and sunblocks protect the skin from UV light and are graded by their ability to provide sun protection. Daily application of a fragrance-free sunscreen with a sun protection factor (SPF) of 30 is recommended (American Academy of Dermatology [AAD], 2014). Children who are extremely photosensitive should use sunscreen with levels of SPF 30 or higher. Sunscreens that act by absorbing UV light in the B range include para-aminobenzoic acid (PABA) or

PABA esters, cinnamates, salicylates, benzophenones, and anthranilates. Only benzophenones protect from UV rays in the longer UVA range. Sunblocks including titanium dioxide, zinc oxide, and talc scatter light and act as protective barriers. They are especially useful on the nose, ears, and lips.

Chemical-containing sunscreens should be applied 30 minutes before exposure to the sun to allow binding of the agents to the stratum corneum. Sunblocks can be applied immediately before sun exposure. Reapply sunscreens after swimming, excessive periods of perspiration, or after washing or showering. Sunscreen is never a substitute for sensible sun protection, which includes limiting exposure to intense sun rays. Other protective strategies include wearing protective clothing, hats with visors, and sunglasses with UV protection.

Medications

General Considerations

Dermatologic conditions are most commonly treated with topical medications. Topical therapy restores hydration, alleviates symptoms, reduces inflammation, protects the skin, reduces scale and debris, cleanses, and eradicates causative organisms.

Thought must be given not only to the medication used in treating skin conditions but also its preparation (Box 37-5) and vehicle (Fig. 37-3), including stabilizers, preservatives, and perfumes. Occasionally an individual is sensitive to a medication vehicle or preparation, and symptoms are aggravated rather than relieved. Common agents that cause sensitization include ethylenediamine, lanolin, parabens, thimerosal, diphenhydramine, propylene glycol, "caines," and neomycin. The following guidelines for use of preparations may be helpful:

- Acute inflammation—wet dressings, powders, suspension lotions, alcohol- or water-based lotions, or aerosols
- Chronic inflammation—creams, oil-based lotions or gels, ointments
- Patient's tolerance for and willingness to use certain vehicles
- Patient's environment (dry or humid)

All topical medications except powders have enhanced absorption if applied to skin immediately after it has been saturated with water. Occlusion enhances absorption (see previous discussion). Application of the topical medication is best done in one direction, preferably along the hair follicles, without rubbing, applied with a single motion. Use an adequate but not excessive amount.

• BOX 37-5 Preparations of Topical Medications

Creams: Contain more water than oil and therefore are less occlusive; better used with less dry skin, in high-humidity areas, in summertime, and on parts of body that naturally cause occlusion (body folds); often accepted better by patient but must be applied every 2 to 3 hours

Gels: Alcohol based, provide good penetration of skin but can burn on application; primarily used for acne and in hairy areas

Lotions: Mixtures of powder and water, useful for drying, cooling, and soothing actions; *emulsion lotions* contain some oil, so are not as drying as lotions; lotions come in suspension or solution

Oils: Fluid fats that hold medication to the skin as barriers or occlusive agents

Ointments: Best used with dry skin; composed primarily of oil with little or no water; provide most potent concentration of medication because of their occlusive action on skin; generally need to be used only every 12 hours; tend to leave a greasy feeling and can cause heat retention from decreased evaporation

Pastes: Made of a combination of powder and oil, which makes them somewhat difficult to apply and remove, but effective in providing dryness and protection for skin

Powders: Absorb moisture and reduce friction, provide cooling, decrease itching, increase evaporation

Shampoos: Liquid soaps or detergents for cleaning the hair and skin (e.g., tar for psoriasis or seborrhea, antifungal shampoos for tinea versicolor or tinea corporis)

Antibacterial Agents

Soap, antibacterial soap, and topical antiseptics thoroughly cleanse the skin and reduce the number of bacteria on the skin. Topical antibiotics are applied to treat minor skin infections. Products containing neomycin should be avoided because of the high incidence of contact sensitization. Oral antibiotics may be necessary to treat more significant bacterial skin infections. If methicillin-resistant *Staphylococcus aureus* (MRSA) is suspected, obtain a culture and sensitivity of the drainage (see Chapter 24).

Antifungal Agents

Many topical antifungals are over-the-counter medications. Oral antifungals are used for hair and nail infections or refractory skin infections. Because of concerning side effects and minimal clinical experience in children, oral antifungals should be used with caution in children; many of these drugs are not U.S. Food and Drug Administration (FDA) approved for pediatric use (antifungal agents are listed in Table 37-4).

Antiviral Agents

Topical antivirals are used to control cutaneous herpes infections. Oral antivirals, such as acyclovir, can shorten the course of the infection and can be used in children with acute or recurrent herpetic skin infections.

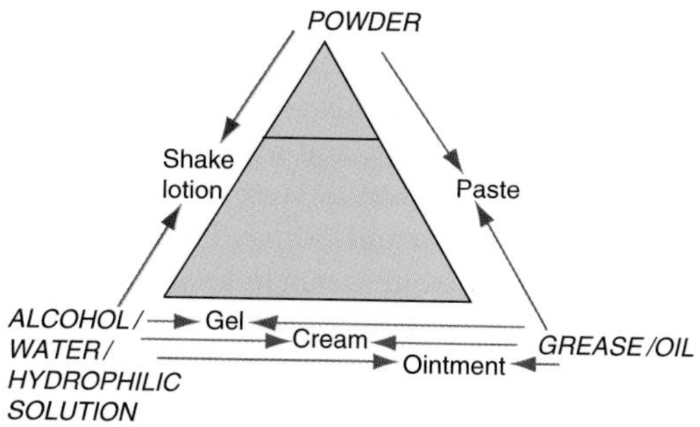

• Figure 37-3 Vehicles for dermatologic therapy. See Box 37-5 for description.

Wart therapy agents destroy keratinocytes. These include salicylic acid and lactic acid collodion, salicylic plaster, salicylic solution, liquid nitrogen, cantharidin, podophyllum, and trichloroacetic acid.

Antiacne Agents

Topical keratolytics are used in acne to relieve follicular obstruction by inhibiting bacterial growth and promoting peeling of the skin. The two most common keratolytics, benzoyl peroxide and retinoic acid, are the first line of treatment for mild acne and are used in combination with other agents for moderate or severe acne. The oral retinoid, isotretinoin, is effective in nodulocystic acne that is not responsive to other combination treatments. Patients taking isotretinoin should be monitored by a dermatologist, with tightly controlled follow-up and prescriptions. The use of isotretinoin is contraindicated in pregnancy because of teratogenic effects.

Topical antibiotics are most effective in maintaining control of acne. Clindamycin, erythromycin, and sulfacetamide have few side effects and are the most commonly used topical antibiotics. Systemic antibiotics (such as, tetracycline, doxycycline, minocycline, and erythromycin) are effective in treating inflammatory acne. Antibiotics work by decreasing the population of *Propionibacterium acnes*.

Some estrogen-containing oral contraceptives are being combined with antiandrogen for treating acne. Ortho Tri-Cyclen, Yaz/Loryna, and Estrostep are oral contraceptives approved for acne by the FDA (Bolognia et al, 2014). Photodynamic therapy is also an option.

Anti-Inflammatory Agents

Topical glucocorticoids are frequently used to reduce inflammation, decrease itching, and promote vasoconstriction without causing the widespread systemic effects of oral steroids. They are subdivided into three categories: high potency, moderate potency, and low potency (Table 37-1); and they are classified as fluorinated or nonfluorinated. Nonfluorinated steroids are less potent and have fewer side effects.

The key to using topical steroids is to be familiar with a few low-, medium-, and high-potency steroids and use them consistently. Brand-name preparations often have a more consistent base and potency. Ointments are more potent than creams, creams are more potent than lotions, and foams are more effective in hairy areas. Absorption is enhanced in areas that are traumatized or denuded.

Primary care providers should rarely use high-potency topical steroid preparations. Always use the lowest potency available, use them sparingly, and for the shortest length of time possible. Only low-potency steroids should be used on the face, buttocks, groin, and axillae. Potential side effects of prolonged topical steroid use include skin atrophy, striae, increased fragility of the skin, hypopigmentation, secondary infection, acneiform eruption, folliculitis, miliaria, hypertrichosis, telangiectasia, and purpura. Oral glucocorticoids (prednisone) are used only in acute situations and are limited to short courses. Intralesional steroid injections may be used by a dermatologist to control localized eczema, lichen planus, or psoriasis.

Antipruritic Agents

Antihistamines are used both for sedation and to relieve itching. The most commonly used antihistamines are hydroxyzine, cetirizine, fexofenadine, and diphenhydramine. Topical antihistamines, especially diphenhydramine HCl and "caine" medications, should be avoided because of the possibility of contact sensitization.

Topical Calcineurin Inhibitors

This class of immunosuppressive, nonsteroidal anti-inflammatory topical medication is used for short-term or intermittent long-term treatment of atopic dermatitis when conventional therapy is inadvisable, ineffective, or not tolerated. Immunomodulators are expensive and cannot be used in children younger than 2 years old (see Chapter 25).

Scabicides and Pediculicides

These agents are toxic to mites and lice. Crotamiton, permethrin, and pyrethrin plus piperonyl butoxide are used in children but should be used sparingly. Lindane is no longer recommended for use in children.

Hair and Scalp Preparations

Antimicrobial, tar, keratolytic, and detergent shampoos are used on the hair and scalp when needed for infection, psoriasis, dandruff, dermatitis, or general cleansing.

Patient and Family Education

It is essential to spend adequate time with the patient and parents to discuss the child's skin condition and the family's concerns and needs. Education regarding the disease, plan of treatment, and potential risks and benefits should be provided. Because disorders of the skin are so visible, time must be spent discussing the short- and long-term prognoses and potential plans to prevent complications, recurrence, and spread.

Bacterial Infections of the Skin and Subcutaneous Tissue

Diagnosis and treatment of common bacterial infections are listed in Table 37-2.

Impetigo

Impetigo is a common contagious bacterial infection of the superficial layers of the skin. It has two forms: nonbullous, with honey-colored crusts on the lesions, and bullous (Fig. 37-4). Impetigo is usually caused by group A *streptococcus (Streptococcus pyogenes), Staphylococcus aureus,* or MRSA. Often streptococcus and staphylococcus can be

TABLE 37-1 Topical Corticosteroids

Class	Generic Name	Trade Name	Potency
1	Betamethasone dipropionate, augmented 0.05% Clobetasol propionate 0.05% Diflorasone diacetate 0.05% Halobetasol propionate	Diprolene 0.05% Diprolene AF 0.05% Temovate 0.05% Dermovate 0.05% Psorcon 0.05% Ultravate 0.05%	High potency↑↑↑↑
2	Amcinonide Betamethasone dipropionate Diflorasone diacetate Halcinonide Fluocinonide Desoximetasone Mometasone furoate	Cyclocort ointment 0.1% Diprosone ointment 0.05% Florone ointment 0.05% Maxiflor ointment 0.05% Halog cream 0.1% Halciderm 0.1% Lidex cream 0.05% Metosyn 0.05% Lidex ointment 0.05% Topicort cream 0.25% Elocon ointment 0.1%	↑↑↑
3	Betamethasone dipropionate Betamethasone benzoate Betamethasone valerate Fluticasone propionate	Diprosone cream 0.05% Benisone gel 0.025% Valisone ointment 0.1% Betacap 0.1% Cutivate ointment 0.05%	↑↑
4	Triamcinolone acetonide Flurandrenolide Fluocinolone acetonide	Aristocort ointment 0.1% Kenalog ointment 0.1% Adocortyl 0.1% Cordran ointment 0.05% Synalar cream 0.025%	↑
5	Desonide Flurandrenolide Fluocinolone acetonide Clocortolone pivalate Betamethasone valerate Hydrocortisone valerate Hydrocortisone butyrate Prednicarbate 0.1%	Tridesilon ointment 0.05% Cordran SP cream 0.05% Fluonid cream 0.01% Synalar 0.025% Synalar cream 0.01% Cloderm cream 0.1% Valisone cream 0.1% Westcort cream 0.2% Locoid cream 0.1% Dermatop cream/ointment	Medium potency↓↑
6	Hydrocortisone 1%, urea 10% Desonide 0.05% Alclometasone dipropionate	Alphaderm cream 1% Locorten cream 0.03% Tridesilon cream 0.05% DesOwen cream Aclovate cream 0.05% Modrasone 0.05% Desonide 0.05%	↓↓
7	Hydrocortisone 1% Dexamethasone Methylprednisolone acetate Prednisolone	Hytone cream 1%; Cobadex 1%; Dioderm 0.1%; Mildison 1%; Hytone ointment 1% Hexadrol cream 0.04% Medrol ointment 0.25% Meti-Derm cream 0.5%	↓↓↓
8	Hydrocortisone 0.5%	Cortaid cream	Low potency

From Cohen BA: *Pediatric dermatology*, ed 3, Philadelphia, 2005, Mosby/Elsevier, p 11; Taketomo CK, Hodding JH, Kraus DM: *Pediatric dosage handbook*, ed 17, Hudson, OH, 2011, Lexi-Comp; Weston WL, Lane AT, Morelli JG: *Color textbook of pediatric dermatology*, ed 4, St. Louis, 2007, Mosby/Elsevier.

TABLE 37-2 Diagnosis and Treatment of Common Bacterial Infections

	Causative Organism	Presentation	Area of Involvement	Treatment	Prevention
Impetigo	*Staphylococcus aureus* or *Streptococcus pyogenes*	Honey-colored crust on erythematous base, or blisters that rupture, leaving varnish-like coat	Superficial layers of skin (epidermis)	Topical antibiotic if minor; oral antibiotics (amoxicillin/clavulanate, cephalexin, dicloxacillin, cloxacillin, or clindamycin) if more significant infection	Moisturize skin; thoroughly cleanse any break in skin
Cellulitis	Most commonly group A streptococcus (GAS) or *S. aureus*	Erythema, swelling, tenderness; irregular borders with significant induration resembling an orange peel is associated with GAS	Dermis and subcutaneous tissue	Oral antibiotic depending on likely organism; amoxicillin clavulanate (first-line) or cephalexin or dicloxacillin	Same as above
Folliculitis	*S. aureus*	Pruritus, erythematous papule or pustule at hair follicle	Hair follicle	Warm compresses, topical keratolytics, topical antibiotics, or antistaphylococcal antibiotic if severe	Same as above; good hygiene and antibacterial soap

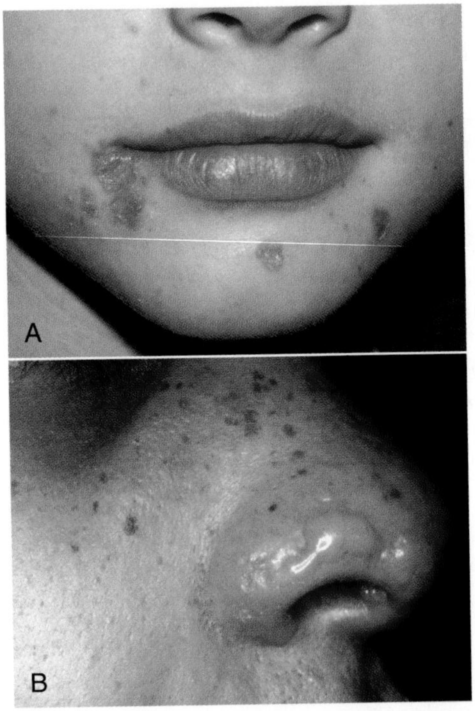

• **Figure 37-4 A,** Nonbullous impetigo. **B,** Bullous impetigo. (From Bologia J, Schaffer JV, Duncan KO, et al: *Dermatology essentials*, Philadelphia, 2014, Saunders/Elsevier.)

cultured from an impetigo lesion. Nonbullous impetigo accounts for more than 70% of cases, with *S. aureus* as the most common pathogen. Nonbullous impetigo usually follows some type of skin trauma (e.g., bites, abrasions, or varicella) or another skin disease, such as atopic dermatitis. Bullous impetigo occurs sporadically, develops on intact skin, and is more common in infants and young children. Certain epidermal types of *S. aureus* produce a toxin that causes bullous skin lesions.

Bacterial colonization of the skin occurs several days to months before lesions appear; the organism usually spreads from autoinoculation via hands, towels, clothing, nasal discharge, or droplets. Impetigo occurs more frequently with poor hygiene; during the summer months; in warm, humid climates; and in lower socioeconomic groups. Streptococci that cause pharyngitis rarely cause impetigo and vice versa. Secondary bacterial infections of underlying skin problems (dermatitis, varicella, psoriasis) are most commonly caused by staphylococci (Cohen, 2013).

Clinical Findings

History

- Pruritus, spread of the lesion to surrounding skin, and earlier skin disruption at the site
- Weakness, fever, and diarrhea may accompany bullous impetigo

Physical Examination

The following can be found:

- Nonbullous, classic, or common impetigo—begins as 1- to 2-mm erythematous papules or pustules that progress to vesicles or bullae, which rupture, leaving moist, honey-colored, crusty lesions on mildly erythematous, eroded skin; less than 2 cm in size; little pain but rapid spread
- Bullous impetigo—large, flaccid, thin-wall, superficial, annular, or oval pustular blisters or bullae that rupture, leaving thin varnish-like coating or scale

- Lesions are most common on face, hands, neck, extremities, or perineum; satellite lesions may be found near the primary site, although they can be anywhere on the body
- Regional lymphadenopathy

Diagnostic Studies

Gram stain and culture are ordered if identification of the organism is needed in recalcitrant or severe cases.

Differential Diagnosis

Herpes simplex, varicella, nummular eczema, contact dermatitis, tinea, kerion, and scabies are included in the differential diagnosis.

Management

Management involves the following:

- Topical antibiotics may be used if the impetigo is superficial, nonbullous, or localized to a limited area. Topical treatment alone provides clinical improvement but may prolong the carrier state (Weston and Morelli, 2013). In localized regions, topical antibiotics (such as, bacitracin, polymyxin B, and neomycin) may be used, but, given the increasing resistance to traditional topical antibiotics, mupirocin and retapamulin are considered better choices for topical treatment (Cohen, 2013; Weinberg and Tyring, 2010; Weston and Morelli, 2013). Oral antibiotics are recommended for multiple lesions or nonbullous impetigo with infection in multiple family members, child care groups, or athletes. Treat for *S. aureus* and *S. pyogenes* because coexistence is common (Cohen, 2013).
  - Cephalexin: 40 mg/kg/day for 7 to 10 days
  - Amoxicillin/clavulanate: 50 to 90 mg/kg/day for 7 to 10 days
  - Dicloxacillin: 15 to 50 mg/kg/day for 7 to 10 days
  - Cloxacillin: 50 to 100 mg/kg/day for 7 to 10 days
  - Clindamycin: 10 to 25 mg/kg/day for 7 to 10 days
- For widespread infection with constitutional symptoms and deeper skin involvement, use an oral antibiotic active against beta-lactamase–producing strains of *S. aureus*, such as amoxicillin/clavulanate, dicloxacillin, cloxacillin, or cephalexin.
- If an infant has bullous impetigo, use parenteral beta-lactamase–resistant antistaphylococcal penicillin, such as methicillin, oxacillin, or nafcillin.
- If there is no response in 7 days, swab beneath the crust, and do Gram stain, culture, and sensitivities. Community-acquired MRSA should be considered. This organism is more susceptible to clindamycin and trimethoprim-sulfamethoxazole (TMP-SMX) (see Chapter 24 for treatment of MRSA).
- Educate regarding cleanliness, hand washing, and spread of disease.
- Exclude from day care or school until treated for 24 hours.
- Schedule a follow-up appointment in 48 to 72 hours if not improved.

Complications

- Cellulitis may occur with nonbullous impetigo and present in the form of ecthyma (infection involving entire epidermis) or erysipelas (spreading cellulitis with induration).
- Lymphangitis, suppurative lymphadenitis, guttate psoriasis, erythema multiforme, scarlet fever, or glomerulonephritis may occur following infection with some strains of *Streptococcus*. Acute rheumatic fever is a rare complication of streptococcal skin infections.
- Staphylococcal scalded skin syndrome (SSSS) is a blistering disease that results from circulating epidermolytic toxin–producing *S. aureus*. SSSS is most common in neonates (Ritter disease), infants, and children younger than 5 years old. It manifests abruptly with fever, malaise, and tender erythroderma, especially in the neck folds and axillae, rapidly becoming crusty around the eyes, nose, and mouth. Nikolsky sign (peeling of skin with a light rub to reveal a moist red surface) is a key finding. Treatment may include hospitalization and parenteral antibiotics, especially for young children (Berk and Bayliss, 2010). Antibiotics of choice are intravenous (IV) or oral dicloxacillin, a penicillinase-resistant penicillin, first- or second-generation cephalosporins, or clindamycin. Quicker healing without scarring results if steroids are avoided, there is minimal handling of the skin, and ointments and topical mupirocin are used at the infection site (Berk and Bayliss, 2010; Patel and Patel, 2010). Severe cases may need treatment similar to extensive burn care.

Patient and Family Education

- Thorough cleansing of any breaks in the skin helps prevent impetigo.
- Postinflammatory pigment changes can last weeks to months.
- The patient should not return to school or day care until 24 hours of antibiotic treatment is completed.

Cellulitis

Cellulitis is a localized bacterial infection often involving the dermis and subcutaneous layers of the skin. It is commonly seen following a disruption of the skin surface from an insect or animal bite, trauma, or a penetrating wound. Cellulitis is more common in children with diabetes and immunosuppression. Periorbital cellulitis is discussed in Chapter 29.

In children, cellulitis is often periorbital, perivaginal, perianal, or buccal, or it involves a joint or an extremity. *Streptococcus pneumoniae* and *S. aureus* are the most common causes. Buccal cellulitis and infections over joints are most commonly caused by *Haemophilus influenzae* and occur in children 3 months to 3 years old, but the incidence has decreased since the introduction of the *H. influenza* vaccine (Bolognia et al, 2014; Hagiya and Otsuka, 2014). Periorbital and orbital cellulitis are most commonly caused by streptococcal species (*S. pneumoniae* and group A beta-hemolytic streptococci [GABHS]). Most cases of cellulitis of the extremities and perianal area are caused by streptococci or *S. aureus*. MRSA can also cause cellulitis with pus accumulation. Rarely, other aerobic, anaerobic, and fungal organisms can cause cellulitis in immunocompromised individuals.

Clinical Findings

History

- A previous skin disruption at the site or recent upper respiratory infection *(H. influenzae).* Note that edema that occurs within 24 hours of an insect bite is most likely to be inflammatory, whereas edema that occurs between 48 to 72 hours is more likely to be infectious.
- Fever, pain, malaise, irritability, anorexia, vomiting, and chills can be reported.
- Recent sore throat or upper respiratory infection.
- Anal pruritus, stool retention, constipation, and blood-streaked stools.

Physical Examination

- Erythematous, indurated, tender, swollen, warm areas of skin with poorly demarcated borders
- Blue to purple tinge to the cellulitis is often associated with *H. influenzae* (Daum, 2011)
- Regional lymphadenopathy
- Well-demarcated perianal erythema up to 2 cm around the anus; the erythema may extend to the vulva and vagina
- Erysipelas—a superficial variant of cellulitis—presents with rapidly advancing lesions that are tender, bright red, have sharp margins and an "orange peel" look and feel

Diagnostic Studies

Most cellulitis cases are treated empirically. CBC and blood culture are done if the child is febrile, appears ill or toxic, or is younger than 1 year old. Leukocytosis is common. Positive blood cultures are low, ranging from 1% to 18% of cases. Perform Gram stain and culture of the erythematous area if unusual organisms are suspected, pus is present (which is more typical of MRSA), or the child looks toxic. An aspirate at the point of maximum inflammation is more likely to yield a causative organism than one taken from the leading edge, although the bacterial counts tend to be low with either method. Gram stains and cultures lead to identification of the causative organism in less than 25% of cases (Gunderson, 2011).

Differential Diagnosis

Pressure erythema, giant urticaria, contact dermatitis, popsicle panniculitis (reaction to cold exposure), early erythema nodosum, subcutaneous fat necrosis, herpetic whitlow, and diaper dermatitis are included in the differential diagnosis.

Management

Immediate antibiotic therapy is required.

- Hospitalization is recommended if the child is a febrile neonate or infant, is acutely ill or toxic, or has periorbital cellulitis.
  - Neonates with cellulitis require a full septic workup and initiation of empiric therapy with methicillin or vancomycin and gentamicin or cefotaxime (Cohen, 2013).
- Antibiotic therapy
  - As noted earlier, prompt administration of antibiotics is essential.
  - If a streptococcal infection is suspected, penicillin is the drug of choice.
    - A hospitalized febrile acutely ill infant or child should have penicillin, up to 2 million units per day.
    - Benzathine penicillin: 600,000 to 1,200,000 units IM for one dose.
    - Penicillin V: 30 to 60 mg/kg/day orally for 10 days.
    - If allergic or concern for multiple organisms a third-generation cephalosporin, such as 50 to 75 mg/kg ceftriaxone intramuscularly (IM) once a day.
  - If suspected organism is staphylococcus:
    - An initial IM dose of ceftriaxone 50 to 75 mg/kg/dose, then dicloxacillin 50 to 75 mg/kg/day orally, divided four times a day for 10 days or cephalexin 50 to 100 mg/kg/day orally, divided three times a day for 10 days.
    - If MRSA suspected, clindamycin 10 to 30 mg/kg/day orally divided three times a day for 10 days.
  - If suspected organism is *H. influenzae:*
    - Amoxicillin clavulanate 50 to 90 mg/kg/day orally for 10 days.
    - Methicillin or a third-generation cephalosporin is also an option.
- Follow up in 24 hours to assess response and observe toxicity. Continue daily visits until child is recovering. Counsel parents to call the provider immediately or return for an urgent visit if the infection is not improving or is getting worse.

Complications

Recurrent perianal streptococcal infection, septicemia, necrotizing fasciitis (NF), and toxic shock syndrome (TSS) are possible complications and all require immediate referral for care and hospitalization.

- NF is a rare infection in children and has two subtypes. Type I is generally a polymicrobial infection that usually affects children who have an underlying disease. Type II, commonly referred to as *flesh-eating strep,* is an acute, rapidly progressing necrotic invasion of GABHS through the skin and subcutaneous tissue to the

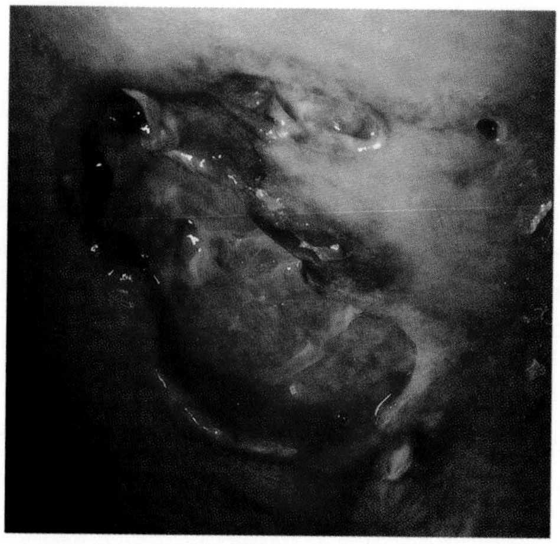

• **Figure 37-5** Necrotizing fasciitis (NF). (From Bologia J, Schaffer JV, Duncan KO, et al: *Dermatology essentials*, Philadelphia, 2014, Saunders/Elsevier.)

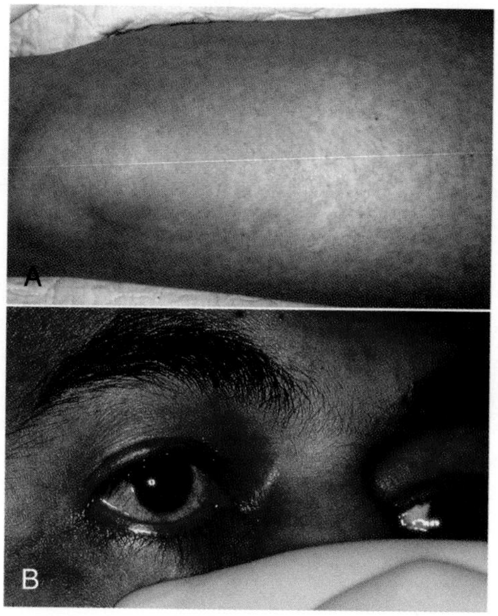

• **Figure 37-6** Toxic shock syndrome (TSS). (From Bologia J, Schaffer JV, Duncan KO, et al: *Dermatology essentials*, Philadelphia, 2014, Saunders/Elsevier.)

fascial compartments. It is more common in otherwise healthy children or children with varicella. NF is more common in boys younger than 5 years old and children with diabetes, skin injury, surgery, immunodeficiency, IV drug use, malnutrition, and obesity. NF begins as cellulitis (usually on the leg or abdomen in infants) with severe pain, edema, fever, and bullae on an erythematous surface. It quickly progresses to ulcer, eschar, and gangrene within 2 days. Prompt treatment (hospitalization, surgical debridement, and fluid management), prolonged antibiotic treatment (penicillin), and intravenous immunoglobulin (IVIG) may be lifesaving, because the overall mortality rate is high (Fig. 37-5).

- TSS is an acute febrile illness with rapid onset that causes significant fever, vomiting and diarrhea, engorged mucous membranes, hypotension, a diffuse macular or sunburn-like rash, conjunctival injection, and multiple organ system involvement. *S. aureus* or *S. pyogenes* (group A streptococci) are the causative agents associated with TSS, and incubation can be as little as 14 hours. Both organisms can be associated with invasive infection (e.g., pneumonia, osteomyelitis, bacteremia, or endocarditis) or focal tissue invasion that is rapidly progressive (Rodriguez-Nunez et al, 2011). Initially recognized in menstruating adolescents, TSS is also found in males and younger children. *S. aureus* is usually the causative agent in menstruating females. Nasal packing, surgical procedures, and postpartum condition are some factors linked to nonmenstrual TSS. Treatment is intensive, requires hospitalization, and consists of fluid management, antibiotics, and other supportive measures. Staphylococcal TSS has a mortality rate of 3%, whereas streptococcal TSS has a mortality rate of 30% to 60% (Berk and Bayliss, 2010). It is a reportable disease in most states (Fig. 37-6).

Patient and Family Education

- Thorough cleansing of any break in the skin helps prevent cellulitis.
- Keep bites, scrapes, and rashes clean and bandaged until healed to prevent them from being infected by staphylococcal bacteria.
- Frequent hand washing is essential.
- Immunize against *H. influenzae.*
- Perianal spread can occur through shared bath water.
- See Chapter 24 regarding treatment of children and families with MRSA infection.

Folliculitis and Furuncle

A superficial bacterial inflammation of the hair follicle is called *folliculitis;* a deeper infection with involvement of the base of the follicle and deep dermis is called a *furuncle* (boil) (Fig. 37-7).

Obstruction of the follicular orifice is the most important factor contributing to the development of folliculitis, but a moist environment, maceration, poor hygiene, occlusive emollients, and prolonged submersion in contaminated water are also factors. *S. aureus* is a common causative organism as is *Pseudomonas aeruginosa,* which causes hot-tub folliculitis. *Escherichia coli* is also implicated. These infections are more common in males than in females.

Clinical Findings

History

- Pruritus with folliculitis; tenderness with furuncle
- Hot-tub exposure

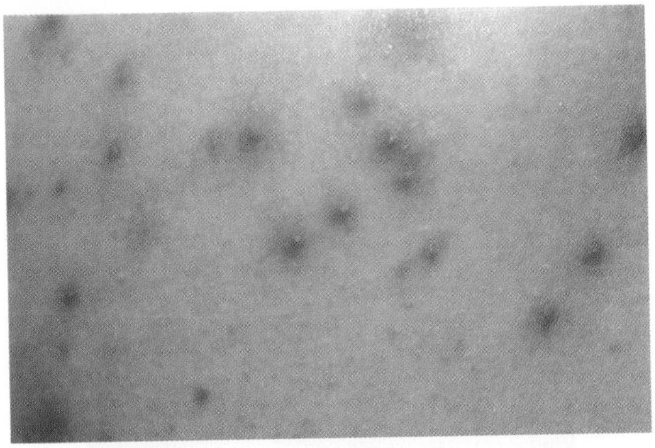

• **Figure 37-7** Staphylococcal superficial folliculitis. (From Weston WL, Lane AT, Morelli JG: *Color textbook of pediatric dermatology*, ed 4, St. Louis, 2007, Mosby/Elsevier, p 69.)

- Irritating surface agent
- Occasional fever, malaise, or lymphadenopathy

Physical Examination

The child often is asymptomatic, but the following can be seen:

- Discrete, erythematous 1- to 2-mm papules or pustules on an inflamed base centered around a hair follicle
- Involvement of face, scalp, extremities (typically thighs and upper arms), buttocks, and back
- Nodules with larger areas of erythema and tenderness (furuncle)
- Pruritic papules, pustules, or deep red to purple nodules, most dense in areas covered by swimsuit 8 to 48 hours after exposure (hot-tub folliculitis)

Diagnostic Studies

Gram stain and culture are occasionally ordered. In the case of persistent or difficult-to-treat folliculitis, consider the possibility of MRSA.

Differential Diagnosis

Cellulitis, *Candida* infection, tinea, acne pustules, and chemical folliculitis constitute the differential diagnosis.

Management

The following steps are taken:

- Warm compresses after washing with soap and water several times a day
- Topical keratolytics, such as benzoyl peroxide 5% to 10% twice a day for 5 days, especially if chronic or recurrent
- Topical antibiotic, such as erythromycin or clindamycin, in cream, gel, solution, or ointment twice a day for 10 to 14 days for superficial folliculitis
- Antistaphylococcal beta-lactamase–resistant antibiotics, such as dicloxacillin 15 to 50 mg/kg/day divided four times a day for 7 to 10 days, or cephalexin 40 to 50 mg/kg/day divided three times a day for 7 to 10 days in severe or widespread cases
- Review of good personal hygiene habits; avoid shaving until resolved
- Follow-up treatment in 1 week for folliculitis, in 1 day for furuncle or abscess, which may need incision and drainage
- Identify and eliminate predisposing factors
- If recurrent, look for nasal or skin carrier state

Complications

Deep abscess formation or carbuncles can occur. *Sycosis barbae* occurs on the chin, upper lip, and jaw, especially in adolescent African American males.

Patient and Family Education

Good personal hygiene and an antibacterial soap minimize spread to other household members. Hot-tub folliculitis resolves in 5 to 14 days but can recur up to 3 months after exposure.

Fungal Infections of the Skin

Diagnosis and treatment of common fungal infections are listed in Table 37-3.

Candidiasis (Moniliasis)

Candidiasis is a fungal infection of the skin or mucous membranes commonly called a *yeast infection* or *thrush*. See Chapter 36 for discussion of vaginal candidiasis.

Candida albicans, a yeastlike fungus, is commonly found on skin and oral, vaginal, and intestinal mucosal tissue. Although *Candida* is part of the normal flora, overgrowth and penetration of inflamed skin or mucous membranes can occur when there is a localized or systemic alteration in host defenses. Candidiasis is more common in infants, obese children, adolescents, and chronically ill or immunocompromised children. It also is often seen as a secondary infection in persistent diaper rashes or with antibiotic, oral steroid, or oral contraceptive use. Systemic infection with candidiasis is not discussed in this text (Figs. 37-8, 37-9, and 37-10).

Clinical Findings

History

The history often includes antibiotic or steroid use over the previous weeks and occurrence of a rash in a moist, warm area.

Physical Examination

- Mouth—friable, adherent white plaques on an erythematous base on the mucous membranes (thrush); cracked lips (cheilitis); fissured and inflamed corners of the mouth (angular cheilitis)
- Intertriginous areas (neck, axillae, or groin)—bright erythema in flexural folds

TABLE 37-3 Diagnosis and Treatment of Common Fungal Infections

Infection	Causative Organism	Clinical Findings	Management	Complications
Candidiasis	*Candida albicans*	Moist, bright-red diaper rash with sharp borders, satellite lesions; may have associated white spots in mouth, mucous membranes, or corner of mouth	Topical or oral antifungal, generally nystatin; diaper area hygiene	Paronychia or onychomycosis
Tinea corporis	*Trichophyton tonsurans, T. rubrum, Microsporum canis*	Pruritic, slightly erythematous circular lesion with a slightly raised border and central clearing; well demarcated	Topical antifungals; identify and treat source; exclude from day care until treated; use oral medications for resistant cases	Tinea incognita from steroid treatment
Tinea cruris	*Epidermophyton floccosum, T. rubrum, T. mentagrophytes*	Raised-border, scaly lesion on upper thighs and groin; penis and scrotum spared; symmetric	Same as for tinea corporis; loose clothes, absorbent medicated powder	Possible secondary infection
Tinea pedis	*T. rubrum, T. mentagrophytes*	Vesicles and erosions on instep; fissure between toes with scaling and erythema; diffuse scaling on weight-bearing surfaces with exaggerated scaling in creases; pruritus	Same as for tinea corporis; absorbent medicated powder; cotton socks; open-toed shoes; moisturize	Reinfection common
Tinea versicolor	*Malassezia furfur (Pityrosporum orbiculare, Pityrosporum ovale)*	Multiple scaly, discrete oval macules on neck, shoulders, upper back, and chest; hypopigmented to hyperpigmented areas; fail to tan in summer	Selenium shampoo; ketoconazole shampoo; topical imidazoles	50% recurrence rate

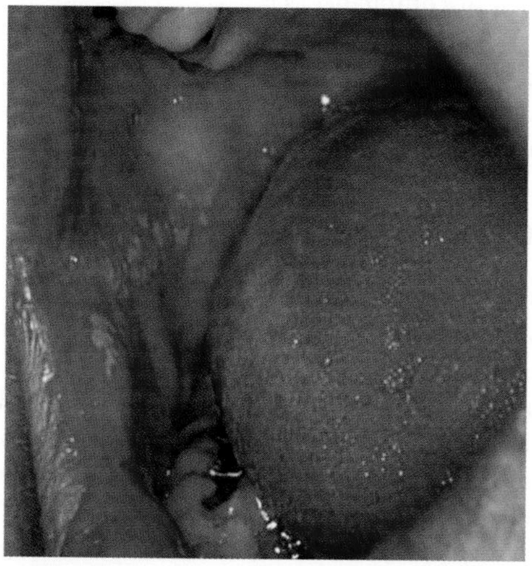

• **Figure 37-8** Thrush. (From Bologia J, Schaffer JV, Duncan KO, et al: *Dermatology essentials*, Philadelphia, 2014, Saunders/Elsevier.)

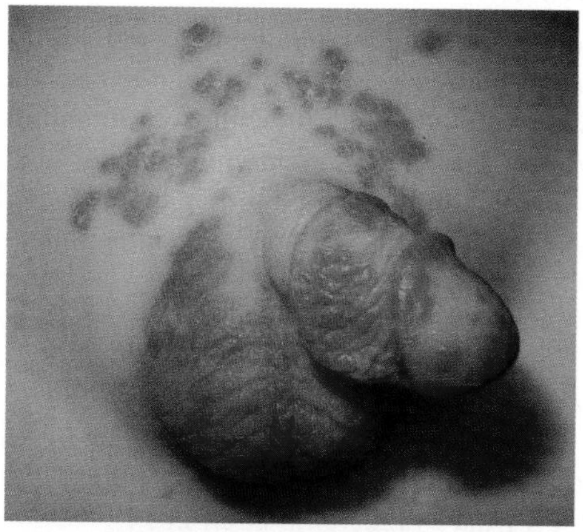

• **Figure 37-9** Candidiasis of the suprapubic area. (From Bologia J, Schaffer JV, Duncan KO, et al: *Dermatology essentials*, Philadelphia, 2014, Saunders/Elsevier.)

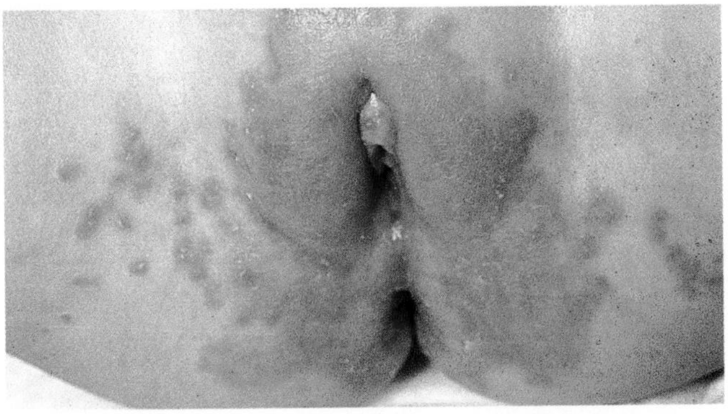

• **Figure 37-10** Diaper candidiasis. (From Cohen B: *Pediatric dermatology*, ed 4, Philadelphia, 2013, Saunders/Elsevier.)

- Diaper area—moist, beefy-red macules and papules with sharply marked borders and satellite lesions; erosions may also be present
- Vulvovaginal area—thick, cheesy, yellow discharge; erythema; edema; and itching
- Nail plates—transverse ridging of the nail plate, loss of cuticle, and mild proximal lateral periungual erythema (chronic paronychia)

Diagnostic Studies

If treatment failure or questionable diagnosis occurs, KOH-treated scrapings of satellite lesions or mucosa reveal yeast cells and pseudohyphae (see Fig. 37-2).

Differential Diagnosis

The differential diagnoses include erythema toxicum, miliaria, staphylococcal pustulosis, transient neonatal pustulosis, neonatal herpes simplex, and congenital syphilis.

Management

The following steps are taken (Table 37-4):

- Thrush: Oral nystatin suspension four times a day, or gentian violet 1% to 2% aqueous solution applied twice a day until 1 to 2 days after white adherent patches are gone. If breastfeeding, the mother should put the solution on her nipples to eliminate reinfection. A second course is sometimes needed to clear the infection.
- If resistant to treatment, oral fluconazole 6 mg/kg the first day in a single dose; then 3 mg/kg/dose daily for 14 days (Taketomo et al, 2011).
- Thrush (in older children), cheilitis and angular cheilitis: Clotrimazole troche 10 mg dissolved slowly five times a day for 14 days (Taketomo et al, 2011).
- Skin infection: Topical antifungals (such as, nystatin, miconazole, clotrimazole, ketoconazole, ciclopirox, or econazole) applied to skin at every diaper change until the rash is gone plus an additional 1 to 2 days (Weston and Morelli, 2013). Avoid antifungal/corticosteroid combination medications.
- If inflammation is severe, 1% hydrocortisone can be applied simultaneously to the diaper area for 1 or 2 days (Bolognia et al, 2014). Topical mupirocin applied four or five times a day may be effective (Cohen, 2013).
- Keep area dry and cool. Minimize skin irritation:
  - Frequent diaper changes.
  - Leave diaper area open to air as much as possible.
  - Blow-dry with warm air (low setting) for 3 to 5 minutes at diaper change (especially helpful in intertriginous areas in infants and obese children).
  - Avoid rubber pants.
  - Use mild soap and water; rinse well; avoid diaper wipes.
  - Avoid powders and other medications not prescribed, such as baby powder.
  - Discontinue oral antibiotics and steroids when possible.
  - Discard or sterilize pacifiers.
  - Educate about avoiding underlying predisposing factors (e.g., lip licking).
  - Add topical or oral antibiotic if secondary infection is suspected.
    - Nail involvement (chronic paronychia) can be treated with topical application of antifungal cream twice daily, but it will take several months for the nail plate to grow out normally; oral fluconazole may be needed for severe or resistant involvement.

Complications

Chronic mucocutaneous candidiasis resulting from immunologic deficit can occur and is heralded by widespread involvement (oral, skin, nails). Paronychia may occur with thumb sucking.

Patient and Family Education

Emphasize good hand washing. Treatment failure is usually due to lack of compliance.

Tinea Capitis

See later section on alopecia.

Tinea Corporis

Tinea corporis, commonly called *ringworm,* is a superficial fungal skin infection found on the non-hairy skin of the body. It is also identified by the part of the body affected (e.g., tinea manuum [hand], tinea barbae [beard], tinea faciei [face]) (Figs. 37-11 and 37-12). Tinea corporis is most commonly caused by the dermatophytes *Microsporum canis, Trichophyton, Microsporum,* and *Epidermophyton* species (Bolognia et al, 2014; Cohen, 2013). Transmission comes as the stratum corneum is invaded following direct contact with infected humans, animals, or fomites. The exact mechanism is unknown but is probably due to a toxin causing an inflammatory response. Infection is common in children. Contact sports (especially wrestling), hot and humid climates, crowded living conditions, and immunosuppression

TABLE 37-4 Antifungal Medications

Drug Generic Name	Strength and Formulation	Application	Mode of Action, Indications, Side Effects, and Comments
Topical Medications			
Imidazoles			
Clotrimazole	1% cream, lotion, solution and powder	Twice daily	Fungistatic; erythema, stinging, blistering, peeling, edema, pruritus, hives, burning
Econazole nitrate	1% cream	Daily or twice daily	Fungistatic; burning, pruritus, stinging, erythema; may have antibacterial effects
Ketoconazole	2% cream and shampoo	Daily or twice daily	Fungistatic; irritation, dry skin, pruritus, stinging
Miconazole nitrate	2% cream, powder, and lotion	Daily or twice daily	Fungistatic; irritation, maceration, urticaria, allergic contact dermatitis, pruritus; economical
Allylamines			
Naftifine HCl	1% cream and gel	Daily or twice daily	Fungicidal; burning, stinging, erythema, pruritus, irritation
Terbinafine HCl	1% cream and solution	Daily or twice daily	Fungicidal; pruritus, irritation, burning
Ethanolamine			
Ciclopirox olamine	1% cream, lotion, gel and nail lacquer (8% solution)	Twice daily; nail lacquer applied daily at bedtime	Fungicidal; irritation, erythema, burning
Others			
Gentian violet	1% to 2% solution	Twice daily	Topical antiseptic/germicide; staining, burning, vesicle formation
Nystatin	100,000 units/gram cream, powder, and ointment	Twice or four times a day	Fungistatic; rare adverse reactions; effective against yeast only
Selenium sulfide shampoo	1% and 2.25% shampoo, 2.5% lotion	Daily for lotion Twice weekly for shampoo for 2 weeks then once every 1 to 4 weeks as needed	Used for tinea capitis (reduces transmission), tinea versicolor, and seborrheic dermatitis (shampoo may be used as lotion); thought to block the enzymes involved in growth of epithelial tissues; discoloration of hair, alopecia
Tolnaftate	1% cream, powder, and solution; aerosol powder and solution also available	Two to three times daily	Fungistatic; rare adverse reactions; pruritus, stinging
Oral Medications			
Clotrimazole	10 mg troche	1 troche five times a day dissolved slowly in mouth	Treatment of oral candidiasis; gastrointestinal symptoms; hepatotoxicity
Fluconazole	10 mg/mL and 40 mg/mL; 50, 100, 150, and 200 mg tablets	3 to 6 mg/kg/day in single dose for 2 weeks for oropharyngeal candidiasis; day 1 dosage is 6 mg/kg (children) and 200 mg/dose (adults) followed by daily therapy of 3 mg/kg/dose (pediatric) and 100 mg/dose (adults)	Approved for pediatric use for oropharyngeal, esophageal, or disseminated candidiasis; possible drug interactions; caution with liver or kidney dysfunction and arrhythmias

Continued

TABLE 37-4 Antifungal Medications—cont'd

Drug Generic Name	Strength and Formulation	Application	Mode of Action, Indications, Side Effects, and Comments
Griseofulvin	Ultramicrosized: 250 mg ultramicrosized = 500 mg microsized Microsized: 125 mg/mL 500 mg tablets	>2 years old: 10 to 15 mg/kg in single or in two divided doses; maximum dose 750 mg/day 10 to 20 mg/kg/day given daily or two divided doses (consider 20 to 25 mg/kg/day for tinea capitis); maximum dose 1 g/day	Fungistatic; mainstay of therapy; excellent safety profile and extensive use Duration of treatment: Tinea corporis: 2 to 4 weeks; tinea capitis: 4 to 6 weeks or longer; tinea pedis: 4 to 8 weeks; tinea unguium: 4 to 6 months or longer Evaluate clinical status frequently, and consider CBC, LFTs, renal function after 8 weeks of therapy or with status change while on treatment; possible drug interactions
Ketoconazole	100 mg/mL suspension 200 mg tablets	Children >2 years old: 3.3 to 6.6 mg/kg/day in single dose Adolescents and adults: 200 to 400 mg/dose/day	Less effective than griseofulvin and higher risk of hepatotoxicity
Nystatin	100,000 units/mL	Infants: 2 mL four times a day after meals Children/adolescents: 400,000 to 600,000 units four times a day—swished about in mouth	Treatment of oral candidiasis
Terbinafine	125 mg/packet of granules 250 mg tablets	Granules: Tinea capitis in children >4 years old: <25 kg: 125 mg once daily for 6 weeks; 25 to 35 kg: 187.5 mg once daily for 6 weeks; >35 kg: 250 mg once daily for 6 weeks Onychomycosis dosage once daily for 6 weeks (fingernails) or 12 weeks (toenails) as follows: 10 to 20 kg: 62.5 mg; 20 to 40 kg: 125 mg; >40 kg: 250 mg	Treatment of tinea capitis in children >4 years old; costly; possible drug interactions

Data from Paller AS, Mancini AJ: *Hurwitz clinical dermatology: a textbook of skin disorders of childhood and adolescence*, ed 4, Philadelphia, 2011, Saunders; Taketomo DK, Hodding JH, Kraus DM: *Pediatric dosage handbook*, ed 17, Hudson, OH, 2011, Lexi-Comp; Weston WL, Lane AT, Morelli JG: *Color textbook of pediatric dermatology*, ed 4, St. Louis, 2007, Mosby.
CBC, Complete blood count; *LFT,* liver function test.

increase the risk of tinea corporis. Autoinoculation accounts for spreading lesions (Cohen, 2013).

Clinical Findings

History

Contact with a person or animal with ringworm is sometimes reported.

Physical Examination

- Classical appearance of lesions: Annular, oval, or circinate with one or more flat, scaling, mildly erythematous circular patches or plaques with red, scaly borders
- Lesions spread peripherally and clear centrally or may be inflammatory throughout with superficial pustules
- Often prominent over hair follicles
- Multiple secondary lesions may merge into a large area several centimeters in diameter

Diagnostic Studies

If treatment failure or questionable diagnosis occurs:

- KOH-treated scrapings of border of lesion reveal hyphae and spores (see Fig. 37-2)
- Fungal culture
- Wood's lamp does not fluoresce most tinea infections *(Trichophyton tonsurans)*
- Fungal culture of the lesion

Differential Diagnosis

Pityriasis rosea herald patch, nummular eczema, psoriasis, seborrhea, contact dermatitis, tinea versicolor, granuloma

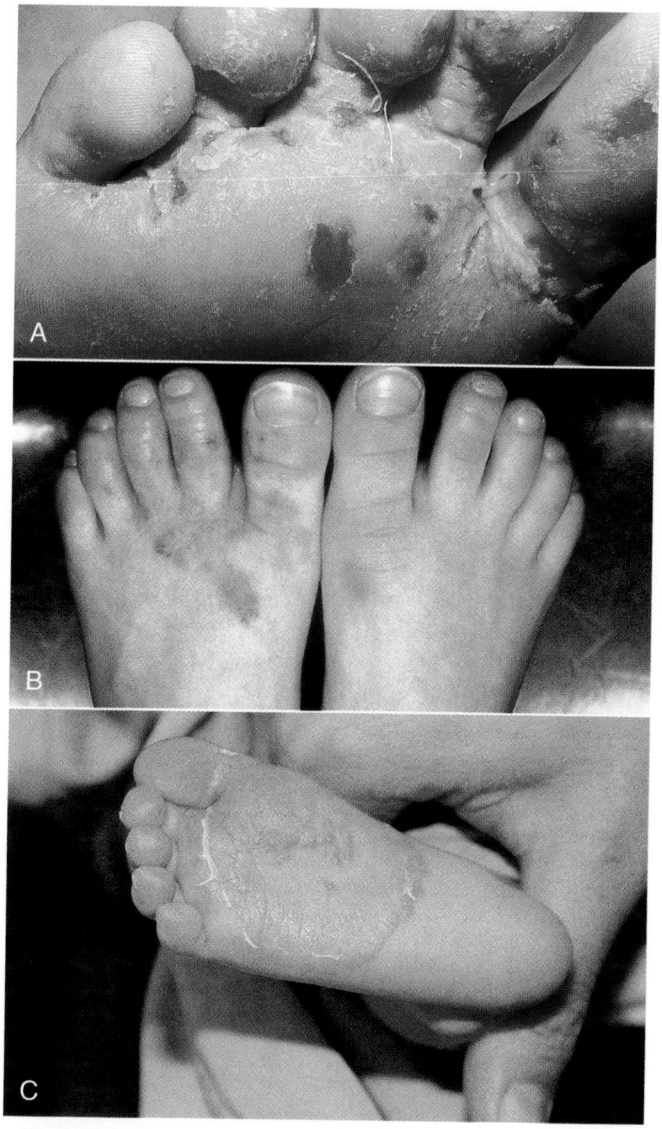

• **Figure 37-11** Tinea pedis. (From Cohen B: *Pediatric dermatology*, ed 4, Philadelphia, 2013, Saunders/Elsevier.)

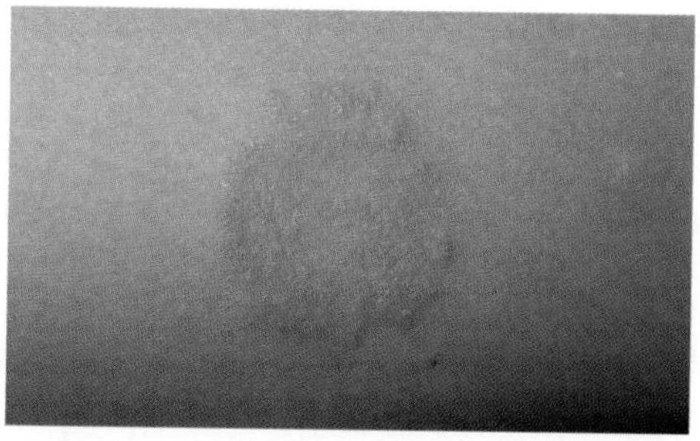

• **Figure 37-12** Tinea corporis, ringworm. (From Bologia J, Schaffer JV, Duncan KO, et al: *Dermatology essentials*, Philadelphia, 2014, Saunders/Elsevier.)

annulare, and Lyme disease are in the differential diagnosis.

Management

- For superficial or localized tinea corporis, topical antifungals (see Table 37-4) (such as miconazole or clotrimazole) are generally effective. Antifungal and steroid combinations should be avoided. Apply cream to the lesion, including a zone of normal skin, twice a day until clinical resolution, which can take 1 to 4 weeks. Prescription antifungals (e.g., econazole, ciclopirox) penetrate the skin more effectively but are more expensive.
- Tinea faciei (face), extensive infection, immunosuppression, coexisting tinea infections on scalp or nails, or infection that is unresponsive to topical treatment may require systemic treatment. Griseofulvin (see Table 37-4) is the systemic drug of choice for children older than 2 years old. Treatment typically lasts for 2 to 4 weeks, and the medications should be taken with fatty foods for better absorption. Because of the risk of hepatotoxicity, nephrotoxicity, and neutropenia, patients requiring extended therapy should have a CBC and liver and renal function 8 weeks after initiating therapy and every 8 weeks until treatment is stopped. Tinea corporis gladiatorum may require systemic therapy, because it is endemic among wrestling team members.
- Identify and treat contacts.
- Educate about communicability of lesions and length of treatment.
- Exclude from day care or school until 24 hours after treatment has begun.
- Follow up in 2 weeks or sooner if lesions are not responding. If unresponsive, diagnosis is incorrect or resistance is possible. Culture to confirm diagnosis and change class of antifungal used.

Complications

Tinea incognito is a dermatophyte infection that has been altered by the use of topical calcineurin inhibitors (e.g., tacrolimus and pimecrolimus) or steroid creams, either alone or in combination with a topical antifungal. The lesions improve but there is a rapid relapse when the creams are stopped and chronic infection persists. Occasionally a pruritic papulovesicular rash on the trunk, hands, or face that is caused by a hypersensitivity response to the fungus may occur and is known as an *id response* (Bolognia et al, 2014).

Patient and Family Education

Find the source of infection and treat or eliminate it to prevent recurrence. Keep skin dry following application of antifungal.

Tinea Cruris

Tinea cruris, commonly called *jock itch,* is a superficial fungal skin infection found on the groin, upper thighs, and intertriginous folds. Caused by the dermatophyte *Epidermophyton floccosum, Trichophyton rubrum,* or *Trichophyton mentagrophytes,* tinea cruris rarely occurs before adolescence and is more common in males, obese individuals, or those with hyperhidrosis or experiencing chafing from tight clothes or moisture. It is extremely common.

Clinical Findings

History

- Hot, humid weather, tight clothing, vigorous physical activity and chafing, or contact sport, such as wrestling
- Often associated with tinea pedis

Physical Examination

- Erythematous to slightly brown, sharply marginated plaques with a raised border of scaling, pustules or vesicles; central clearing may be present
- Usually bilateral and symmetric, but not always
- Occurs on inner thighs and inguinal creases; penis, scrotum, and labia majora generally spared
- Occasionally occurs in perianal region or on the buttocks and/or abdomen

Diagnostic Studies

If treatment failure or questionable diagnosis occurs:

- KOH-treated scraping reveals hyphae and spores
- Fungal culture

Differential Diagnosis

Psoriasis, candidiasis, contact dermatitis, seborrhea, intertrigo, and erythrasma are in the differential diagnosis.

Management

Management is the same as for tinea corporis. Duration of topical treatment is usually 4 to 6 weeks. Antifungal and steroid combinations are to be avoided. Do not use steroids because of risk of atrophy and striae. Advise the patient to wear cotton underwear and loose clothing and to use absorbent antifungal powder. If tinea pedis is suspected, advise the patient to put socks on before underwear to prevent the spread of the infection. Maintain good hygiene following a wrestling event (e.g., bathing as soon as possible, sole use of towel; dry thoroughly).

Tinea Pedis

Tinea pedis is a superficial fungal skin infection found on the feet, commonly called *athlete's foot.* There are three clinical forms: (1) vesicles and erosions on the instep of one or both feet; (2) an occasional fissure between the toes with surrounding scale and erythema; and (3) rare diffuse scaling on the weight-bearing surface of the foot with exaggerated scaling in creases (moccasin foot) often extending to lateral foot margins.

Caused by the dermatophytes *T. rubrum* or *T. mentagrophytes,* tinea pedis is uncommon in preadolescent children and is more common in males. It is acquired through direct contact with contaminated surfaces (e.g., warm moist environment of showers and locker room floors) and often occurs with tinea cruris (see Fig. 37-11).

Clinical Findings

History

- Sweaty feet
- Use of nylon socks or nonbreathable shoes
- Exposure in family or at school
- Itching, intense burning, stinging, foul odor
- Microtrauma to feet—cracks, abrasions, nicks, cuts
- Contact with damp areas (e.g., swimming pools, locker room, showers)

Physical Examination

- Red, scaly, cracked rash on soles or interdigital spaces and instep, especially between the third, fourth, and fifth toes
- Infection initially presents as white peeling lesions becoming erythematous, vesicular, macerated, fissured, and scaly
- Dorsum of foot remains clear
- Chronic infection manifested by a moccasin pattern with diffuse scaling (plantar hyperkeratosis) and mild erythema

Diagnostic Studies

Laboratory studies are the same as those for tinea corporis.

Differential Diagnosis

Contact dermatitis, atopic dermatitis, dyshidrotic eczema, psoriasis, pitted keratolysis, and juvenile plantar dermatosis (red, dry fissures of weight-bearing surface) are in the differential diagnosis.

Management

Management is the same as for tinea corporis. Antifungal medication should be applied 1 cm beyond the borders of the rash twice daily until 7 days after clearing. Usual treatment is 3 to 6 weeks. In rare cases, griseofulvin may be required, and treatment for 6 to 8 weeks is usually recommended. Additionally:

- Advise patient to keep feet dry, use absorbent antifungal powder or sprays, wear cotton socks, avoid scratching, and wear shoes that allow the feet to breathe or go barefoot when home. Thoroughly dry feet and between toes after using a commercial showering facility.
- Rinse feet with plain water or water and vinegar; dry carefully, especially between the toes. Moisturize and protect feet to prevent splitting and cracking.
- Aluminum chloride (Drysol, CertainDri, Xerac AC, or Arrid Extra Dry antiperspirant sprays) may be used for hyperhidrosis.
- Acute vesicular lesions can be treated with wet compresses two to four times daily for 10 to 15 minutes in addition to application of topical antifungals.

- Moccasin-type tinea pedis may need the addition of a keratolytic agent (lactic acid or urea) with the application of antifungals.
- Tennis shoes may be washed in the machine with soap and bleach.
- Physical education or sports may be continued.
- Follow up in 2 to 3 weeks or sooner if lesions are not responding.

Complications

A secondary bacterial infection, indicated by foul odor, can occur. An allergic reaction to fungus, called an *id response,* is manifested by a vesicular eruption on the palms and sides of fingers and occasionally on the trunk and extremities.

Tinea Versicolor

Tinea versicolor is a superficial fungal infection, also called *pityriasis versicolor,* that tends to be persistent and occurs predominantly on the trunk. The lesions do not tan in the summer and become relatively darker in winter months (Fig. 37-13).

This infection is caused by a yeastlike organism, *Malassezia furfur* (referred to as *Pityrosporum orbiculare* and *Pityrosporum ovale*) and occurs more commonly in adolescents than in younger children, in chronically ill and immunocompromised children, and in warmer seasons and humid climates. Breastfeeding infants can acquire the organism from their mother and exhibit facial lesions.

Clinical Findings

History

The infection is associated with warm, humid weather. Occasional mild itching may occur.

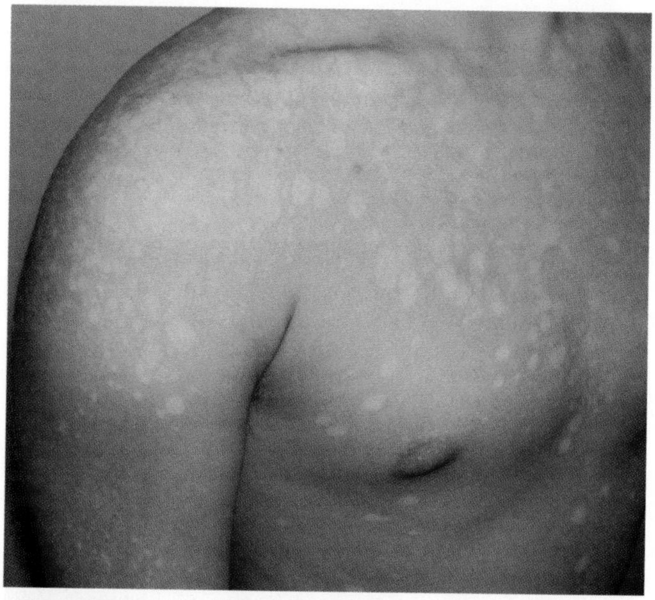

• Figure 37-13 Tinea versicolor. (From Marks JG, Miller JJ: *Lookingbill and Marks' principles of dermatology*, ed 4, Philadelphia, 2006, Saunders/Elsevier.)

Physical Examination

Multiple, annular, scaling, discrete macules or patches, ranging from hypopigmented in dark-skinned individuals to hyperpigmented (salmon-colored to brown) in light-skinned individuals, are seen on the neck, shoulders, upper back and arms, chest midline, and face (especially in children). They tend to have a guttate or raindrop pattern.

Diagnostic Studies

KOH scrapings, though not necessary, reveal short curved hyphae and circular spores ("spaghetti and meatballs"). Scrapings fluoresce yellow-orange under Wood's lamp if not cleansed recently.

Differential Diagnosis

Pityriasis alba, pityriasis rosea, vitiligo, postinflammatory hypopigmentation or hyperpigmentation, seborrhea, and secondary syphilis are included in the differential diagnosis.

Management

The following steps are taken (Bolognia et al, 2014):

- Selenium sulfide 2.5% lotion or 1% shampoo (over the counter) applied in a thin layer several hand-widths beyond lesions for 30 minutes twice a week for 2 to 4 weeks followed by monthly applications for 3 months to help prevent recurrences. Older adolescents can use ketoconazole 2% shampoo as directed earlier or for smaller areas of infection, topical imidazoles (e.g., clotrimazole, miconazole, ciclopirox, or terbinafine solution) or topical azoles (e.g., ketoconazole or oxiconazole) applied twice daily for 2 to 4 weeks.
- Resistant or severe cases in older adolescents sometimes require oral antifungal treatment with fluconazole 200 to 400 mg by mouth once weekly for two to three doses. Follow up in 1 month.

Patient and Family Education

- Sun exposure makes lesions appear hypopigmented as the surrounding skin tans.
- Repigmentation takes several months.
- If the patient is taking oral antifungal medication, encourage exercise to induce sweating, because this may enhance concentration of medication in the skin.
- Skin irritation occurs with overnight application.
- Absence of flaking when skin is scraped is a sign of effective treatment.

Viral Infections of the Skin

Herpes Simplex

In the active state, herpes simplex virus (HSV) causes contagious infections of the skin and mucous membranes ranging from mild to life threatening. HSV infection can be either primary or recurrent. Primary infection occurs in individuals without circulating antibodies after direct contact with secretions or mucocutaneous lesions of an infected individual. Incubation takes days to weeks and then manifests itself anywhere from subclinical to severe infection. The virus then becomes dormant in certain nerve cells until reactivated by triggering factors, such as stress, menses, illness, sunburn, windburn, and fatigue. Recurrent infection occurs in individuals previously infected who had either clinical or subclinical manifestations of infection.

HSV type 1 (HSV-1) usually affects the oral mucosa, pharynx, lips, and occasionally the eyes, causing a herpes labialis infection, commonly called *cold sores* or *fever blisters* (see Fig. 37-15). HSV-2 infection commonly occurs as a neonatal infection (see Chapter 40) or herpetic vulvovaginitis (see Chapter 36) or progenitalis. Type 1 can also be found in the genital area, and type 2 can be found on the lips and mouth. Herpetic keratoconjunctivitis is discussed in Chapter 29; other information may be found in Chapter 24.

Herpetic whitlow, occurring on a finger or thumb, is a swollen, painful lesion with an erythematous base and ulceration resembling a paronychia. It occurs on fingers of thumb-sucking children with gingivostomatitis or adolescents with genital HSV infection.

HSV is transmitted by close contact with skin, mucous membranes, and body fluids, often through a break in the skin or by autoinoculation. Lesions occur in children of all ages, are contagious as long as they are present, and have an incubation period of 2 to 12 days. Primary lesions usually occur before 5 years old, are more painful and extensive, and last longer.

Clinical Findings

History

In primary herpes, fever, malaise, sore throat, and decreased fluid intake can occur. Primary genital HSV presents with painful vesicles in genital areas. In recurrent HSV infection, there is often a painful prodrome of burning, tingling, paresthesia, and itching at the involved site. Recent acute febrile illness or sun exposure may also be reported.

Physical Examination

The following are seen on physical examination:

- HSV-1
  - Gingivostomatitis: Pharyngitis with grouped vesicles on an erythematous base that ulcerate and form white plaques on mucosa, gingiva, tongue, palate, lips, chin, and nasolabial folds; lymphadenopathy and halitosis are present (Fig. 37-14)
  - Herpes labialis: Cluster of small, clear, tense vesicles with an erythematous base that become weepy and ulcerated, progressing to crustiness, usually only on one side of the mouth and on the vermillion border—classic cold sore (Fig. 37-15)
  - Herpetic whitlow on hand or fingers: Deep-appearing vesicles (Fig. 37-16)

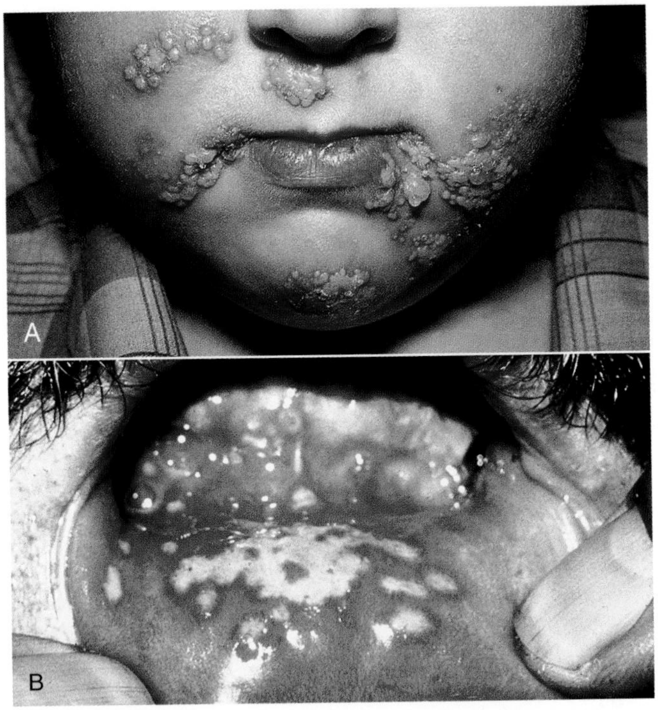

• **Figure 37-14** Herpetic stomatis. (From Cohen B: *Pediatric dermatology*, ed 4, Philadelphia, 2013, Saunders/Elsevier.)

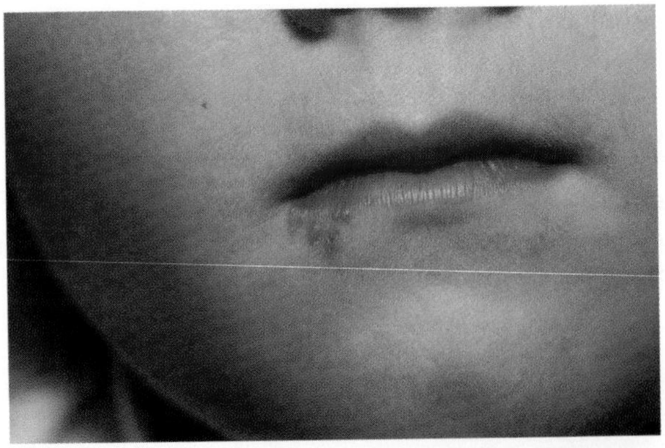

• **Figure 37-15** Herpes labialis. (From Weston WL, Lane AT, Morelli JG: *Color textbook of pediatric dermatology*, ed 4, St. Louis, 2007, Mosby/Elsevier, p 128.)

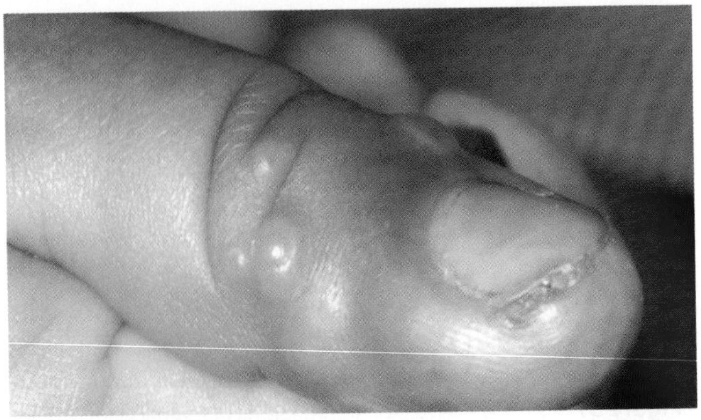

• **Figure 37-16** Herpetic whitlow. (From Cohen B: *Pediatric dermatology*, ed 4, Philadelphia, 2013, Saunders/Elsevier.)

- Common sites of involvement: Lips, hand, fingers, nose, cheek, forehead, and eyes; can also occur in the genital area
- HSV-2
  - Grouped vesicopustules and ulceration with edema
  - Primary lesions on vaginal mucosa, labia, or perineum in females and on the penile shaft or perineum in males; females may have cervical involvement; oral lesions are possible
  - Recurrent lesions on labia, vulva, clitoris, or cervix in females and on the prepuce, glans, or sulcus in males; generally less severe cutaneous lesions
  - Regional lymphadenopathy

Diagnostic Studies

A Tzanck smear can be done on fluid from the lesions to identify epidermal giant cells; however, it does not distinguish HSV-1 from HSV-2. Viral cultures are the gold standard for definitive diagnosis. Direct fluorescent antibody (DFA) tests, enzyme-linked immunosorbent assay (ELISA) serology, and polymerase chain reaction (PCR) tests are usually only used with severe forms of HSV infection.

Differential Diagnosis

The differential diagnosis includes aphthous stomatitis, hand-foot-and-mouth disease, varicella, impetigo, folliculitis, and erythema multiforme.

Management

Management can be guided by considering the host (e.g., age, area and extent of involvement, and immune status) and the drug needed (Table 37-5). Treatment includes:

1. Burow solution compresses three times a day to alleviate discomfort
2. Acyclovir 20 to 40 mg/kg/dose orally five times a day for 5 days, or 200 mg five times a day for 7 to 10 days (maximum pediatric dose 1000 mg/day) may be indicated to help shorten the course and alleviate symptoms for children older than 2 years old with the following conditions:
   - Any underlying skin disorder (e.g., eczema)
   - A severe case
   - An immunocompromised disease
   - Systemic symptoms with primary genital infection
   - Occasionally for initial severe gingivostomatitis

   Acyclovir is most effective if started within 3 days of disease onset. Famciclovir or valacyclovir are additional antiviral agents approved for use in adults.
3. Topical acyclovir ointment may help for initial genital herpes infections but is often not beneficial for recurrent infections.
4. Oral acyclovir 200 mg five times a day for 5 to 10 days may speed healing of herpetic whitlow (see Fig. 37-16).
5. Antibiotics for secondary bacterial (usually staphylococcal) infection:
   - Mupirocin: Topically three times a day for 5 days
   - Erythromycin: 40 mg/kg/day for 10 days
   - Dicloxacillin: 12.5 to 50 mg/kg/day for 10 days
6. Oral anesthetics for comfort; use with caution in children (the child needs to be able to rinse and spit):
   - Viscous lidocaine 2% topical
   - Liquid diphenhydramine alone or combined with aluminum hydroxide or magnesium hydroxide as a 1:1 rinse (maximum of 5 mg/kg/day diphenhydramine in case it is swallowed); it can also be applied to the lesions with cotton-tipped swabs
7. Newborn infant, immunosuppressed child, child with infected atopic dermatitis, or child with a lesion in the eye or on the eyelid margin; consult with or refer to an appropriate provider
8. Offer supportive care, such as antipyretics, analgesics, hydration, and good oral hygiene

TABLE 37-5 Diagnosis and Treatment of Herpes Simplex and Herpes Zoster

Presentation		Clinical Findings	Treatment	Education
Herpes simplex	Gingivostomatitis as primary infection; herpes labialis or herpes facialis as recurrent infection	Pharyngitis with erythematous vesicles, near, on, and/or in mouth; small, clear vesicles on erythematous base progressing to crusting	Burow solution; acyclovir in primary case or underlying disorder; antibiotics if secondary infection; oral anesthetics; supportive care	Degree and duration of contagion; triggers to infection
Herpes zoster	Reactivation of latent varicella virus, especially after mild cases or in infants younger than 1 year old or immunocompromised host	Two or three clustered groups of vesicles on erythematous base, especially over thoracic or lumbosacral dermatomes; pain (can be severe), itch, tingle is minimal in children	Burow solution; antihistamine; drying lotions; possible acyclovir; silver sulfadiazine; antibiotics if secondary infection	New vesicles occur for up to 1 week; takes 2 to 3 weeks to resolve; contagious until lesions stop erupting and are crusted over; varicella vaccine to prevent

9. Exclude from day care only during the initial course (gingivostomatitis) and if the child cannot control secretions
10. Recurrent, frequent, and severe HSV infection may be treated with acyclovir prophylaxis for 6 months

Complications

Eczema herpeticum or Kaposi varicelliform eruption is discussed in Chapter 24. HSV has also been implicated as a possible cause of erythema multiforme and Stevens-Johnson syndrome (SJS).

Patient and Family Education

Recurrence of infection, possible triggering factors, and avoidance measures should be discussed. Triggers can include physical and psychological stress, trauma, fever, exposure to UV light, illness, menses, and extreme weather. Contagiousness of lesions and oral secretions must be understood. Explanation of the course of primary disease, with fever lasting up to 4 days and lesions taking at least 2 weeks to heal, is important.

Herpes Zoster

Herpes zoster (HZ) is a recurrent varicella infection commonly called *shingles* (Fig. 37-17). Caused by reactivation of the latent varicella zoster infection from the sensory root ganglia, HZ occurs in 10% to 20% of all individuals, is rare in childhood, and occurs more frequently with increasing age (three times more common in adolescents than preschoolers). HZ is more common following mild cases of varicella infections before 1 year old (threefold to twentyfold increased risk) and in immunocompromised children.

Clinical Findings

History

Burning, stinging pain, tenderness to light touch, hyperesthesia, or tingling precedes eruption by about 1 week, although this is less common in children. The lesions can be extremely itchy and painful.

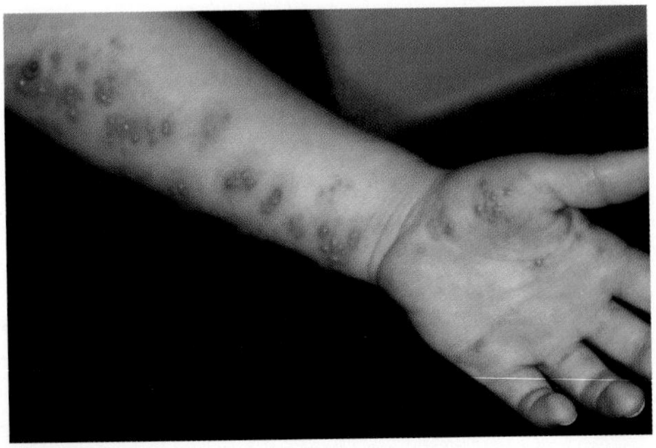

• **Figure 37-17** Herpes zoster (HZ). (From Weston WL, Lane AT, Morelli JG: *Color textbook of pediatric dermatology*, ed 4, St. Louis, 2007, Mosby/Elsevier, p 134.)

Physical Examination

- Two or three clustered groups of macules and papules progress to vesicles on an erythematous base. These vesicles become pustular, rupture, ulcerate, and crust.
- Lesions develop over 3 to 5 days and last 7 to 10 days. Lesions may develop for up to 1 week followed by crusting and healing during the next 2 weeks. In children, delayed chronic pain, known as *postherpetic neuralgia,* is rare.
- Lesions commonly follow the dermatomes of the second cervical to lumbar nerves and the fifth to seventh cranial nerves with scattered lesions outside these areas.
- Lesions do not cross midline (key to diagnosis); sharp demarcation at the midline with occasional contralateral involvement.
- Lymphadenopathy may occur.

Diagnostic Studies

The diagnosis is clinical. If needed, Tzanck smear or viral culture can distinguish HZ from HSV infection. Bacterial culture or Gram stain can be used to distinguish from impetigo. A DFA stain of vesicle base scrapings is beneficial in the difficult to diagnosis case and results are timely.

Differential Diagnosis

Local cutaneous HSV infection and impetigo are differential diagnoses.

Management

Management steps include the following:

1. Burow solution compresses three times a day to alleviate discomfort
2. Warm, soothing baths
3. Antihistamines for itching
4. Analgesics for discomfort; do not use salicylates
5. Ointment (such as, Aquaphor or Vaseline) to moisturize the lesions and decrease itching
6. Antiviral medications are not recommended for use in all children with HZ:
   - Acyclovir 30 mg/kg/day divided four times a day for 5 days may be useful for children who are immunosuppressed, have ocular herpes, or have Ramsay-Hunt syndrome (Weston and Morelli, 2013)
7. Antibiotics for secondary bacterial (usually staphylococcal) infection:
   - Mupirocin topically twice daily
   - Dicloxacillin 12.5 to 25 mg/kg/day for 7 to 10 days
8. Refer for immediate ophthalmologic examination if eyes, forehead, or nose is involved

Complications

Complications are rare except in immunocompromised children. Occasionally HZ is the initial finding in acquired immunodeficiency syndrome (AIDS), especially if more than one dermatome is involved. Eczema herpeticum may occur.

Patient and Family Education

- New vesicles appear for up to 1 week and take 2 to 3 weeks to resolve. Illness is usually mild.
- The child is contagious for varicella until lesions are crusted. If the lesions can be covered, the child does not need to be excluded from school or child care. If the lesions cannot be covered, the child should avoid contact with others until the lesions are crusted (Cohen, 2013).

Molluscum Contagiosum

A benign common childhood viral skin infection with little health risk, molluscum contagiosum often disappears on its own in a few weeks to months and is not easily treated (Fig. 37-18). This poxvirus replicates in host epithelial cells. It attacks skin and mucous membranes and is spread by direct contact, by fomites, or by autoinoculation (typically scratching). It is commonly found in children and adolescents. The incubation period is about 2 to 7 weeks but may be as long as 6 months (Weston and Morelli, 2013). Infectivity is low but the child is contagious as long as lesions are present.

Clinical Findings

History

- Itching at the site
- Possible exposure to molluscum contagiosum

Physical Examination

- Very small, firm, pink to flesh-colored discrete papules 1 to 6 mm in size (occasionally up to 15 mm)
- Papules progressing to become umbilicated (may not be evident) with a cheesy core; keratinous contents may extrude from the umbilication
- Surrounding dermatitis is common

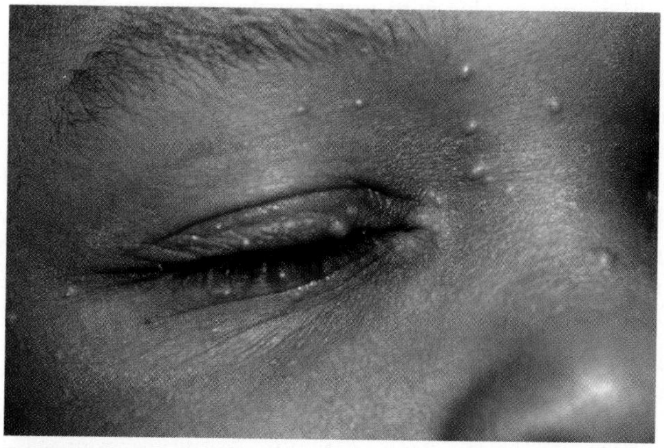

• **Figure 37-18** Molluscum contagiosum. (From Weston WL, Lane AT, Morelli JG: *Color textbook of pediatric dermatology*, ed 4, St. Louis, 2007, Mosby/Elsevier, p 144.)

- Face, axillae, antecubital area, trunk, popliteal fossae, crural area, and extremities are the most commonly involved areas; palms, soles, and scalp are spared
- Single papule to numerous papules; most often numerous clustered papules and linear configurations
- Sexually active or abused children can have genitally grouped lesions
- Children with eczema or immunosuppression can have severe cases; those with human immunodeficiency virus (HIV) infection or AIDS can have hundreds of lesions

Differential Diagnosis

Warts, closed comedones, small epidermal cysts, blisters, folliculitis, and condyloma acuminatum are included in the differential diagnosis.

Management

- Untreated lesions usually disappear within 6 months to 2 years but may take up to 4 years to completely go away. There is no consensus on the management of molluscum contagiosum and no evidence-based literature to show that any treatment is superior to placebo. Therapy may be necessary to alleviate discomfort, reduce itching, minimize autoinoculation, limit transmission, and for cosmetic reasons. Genital lesions may need to be treated to prevent spread to sexual partners.
- Mechanical removal of the central core is to prevent spread and autoinoculation. Using eutectic mixture of local anesthetics (EMLA) cream (lidocaine/prilocaine) 30 to 45 minutes before the procedure reduces discomfort. Curettage is done with a sharp blade to remove the papule. Piercing the papule and expressing the plug is an option but is painful.
- There are reports that irritants (such as, surgical tape, adhesive tape, or duct tape) applied each night can result in lesion resolution.
- Topical medications may prove beneficial. Recheck the patient in 1 to 2 weeks to determine need for retreatment.
  - Liquid nitrogen applied for 2 to 3 seconds (easiest but also painful).
  - Trichloroacetic acid 25% to 50% applied by dropper to the center of the lesion, followed by alcohol (use with caution). Surround the lesion first with petroleum jelly.
  - Cantharidin 0.7% in collodion applied by dropper to the center of the lesion, followed by alcohol. Salicylic or lactic acid or KOH or podophyllin can also be used.
  - Podofilox 0.5% topical solution or gel, or imiquimod 5% applied daily with a toothpick or cotton-tipped swab.
  - Tretinoin or tazarotene cream or gel applied to lesion each night.
  - Silver nitrate, iodine 7% to 9%, or phenol 1% applied for 2 to 3 seconds.

- Cimetidine 30 to 40 mg/kg/day in two divided doses orally for 6 weeks if topical treatment fails.
- Sexual abuse of children with genitally grouped lesions should be suspected and evaluated.
- Evaluate for HIV infection if hundreds of lesions are found.
- Wait and see approach—spontaneous clearing occurs over years.

Complications

Molluscum dermatitis, a scaly, erythematous, hypersensitive reaction, can occur and will respond to moisturizer; avoid hydrocortisone because it causes molluscum to flare. Impetiginized lesions, inflammation of the eyes or conjunctiva, and scarring can occur.

Patient and Family Education

Patients are contagious, but there is no need to exclude them from day care or school. Children with impaired immunity, atopic dermatitis, or traumatized skin are at greater risk for broader spread. Severe inflammation is possible several hours after application of cantharidin. Scarring is unusual.

Warts

Warts are common childhood skin tumors characterized by a proliferation of the epidermis and mucosa infected by the human papillomavirus (HPV). There are over 100 HPV types, and each one produces characteristic lesions in specific locations (e.g., verruca vulgaris, verruca plana, verruca plantaris, and condyloma acuminatum). Trauma promotes inoculation of the HPV (Koebner phenomenon); as a result, most warts are on the hands, fingers, elbows, and plantar surfaces of the feet.

The transmission of warts from person to person depends on viral and host factors, such as quantity of virus, location of warts, preexisting skin injury, and cell-mediated immunity. Transmission is from fomites or skin-to-skin contact, and autoinoculation is frequent. Incubation is from 1 to 6 months, possibly years.

Although a large percentage of all warts resolve spontaneously within 3 to 5 years, there is a high recurrence rate. Cutaneous warts are rarely a serious health concern but present cosmetic problems for children and their families (Cohen, 2013).

Clinical Findings

History

The history can include exposure to someone with warts. Though most common on the extremities, warts can occur anywhere on the body, including the face, scalp, and genitalia.

Physical Examination

- Common warts (verruca vulgaris) are usually elevated flesh-colored single papules with scaly, irregular surfaces and occasionally black pinpoints, which are thrombosed blood vessels. They are usually asymptomatic and multiple and are found anywhere on the body, although most commonly on the hands, nails, and feet. They may be dome shaped, filiform, or exophytic (Fig. 37-19). Filiform warts project from the skin on a narrow stalk and are usually seen on the face, lips, nose, eyelids, or neck. Periungual warts are common, occurring around the cuticles of the fingers or toes.

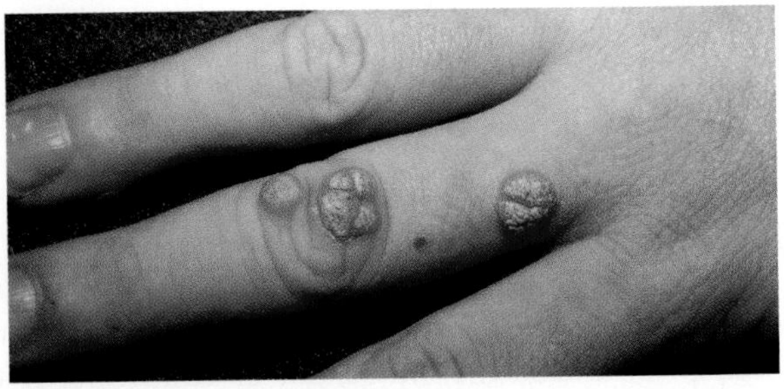

• **Figure 37-19** Multiple common warts (verruca vulgaris). (From Weston WL, Morelli JG: *Pediatric dermatology DDx deck*, Philadelphia, 2013, Elsevier/Saunders.)

- Plantar warts (verrucae plantaris or mosaic) are commonly found on weight-bearing surfaces of the feet. They grow inward and disrupt skin markings.
- Flat warts (verruca plana or juvenile warts) are seen commonly on the face, neck, and extremities. They are small, slightly elevated papules and number from few to several hundred.
- Condylomata acuminata on genital mucosa and adjacent skin are multiple, confluent warts with irregular surfaces, light color, and cauliflower-like appearance (Fig. 37-20).

Differential Diagnosis

The differential diagnosis includes calluses, corns, foreign bodies, moles, comedones, and squamous cell carcinoma.

Management

There is no single effective treatment for warts; watchful waiting is an option. The recurrence rate is high; they typically do not resolve with just a single treatment. No treatment is necessary if the warts are asymptomatic. The decision to treat should be based on location, number and size of lesions, discomfort, and whether they are cosmetically objectionable. Treatment should not be harmful, and scarring should be avoided. Genital warts found in young children or in adolescents who are not sexually active should create suspicion of sexual abuse. Specific treatment options are outlined in Box 37-6. Follow up in 2 to 3 weeks to evaluate response.

Complications

Scarring from removal can occur. A ring of satellite warts may develop at the edge of the blister following treatment with cantharidin. Immunocompromised hosts can have extensive involvement.

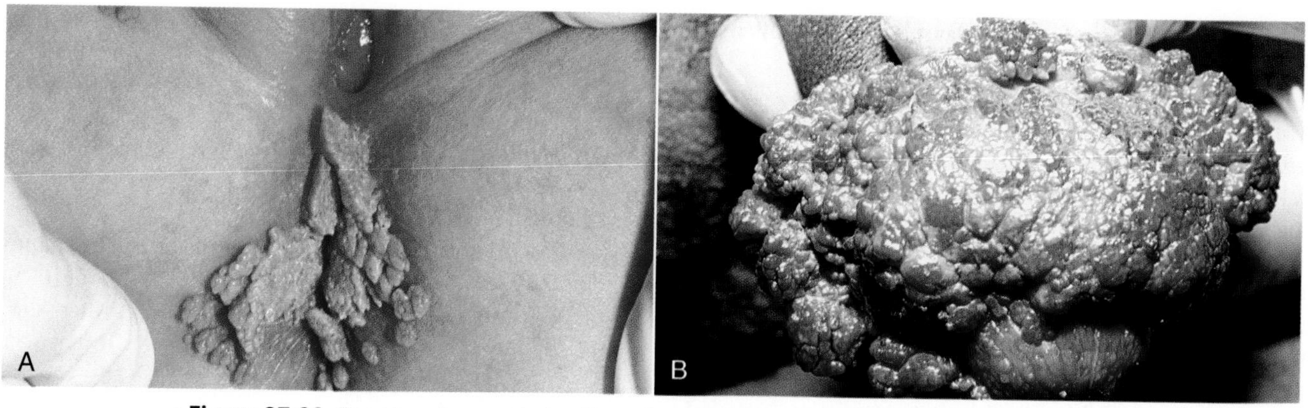

• **Figure 37-20** Condylomata acuminata. (From Cohen B: *Pediatric dermatology*, ed 4, Philadelphia, 2013, Saunders/Elsevier.)

• BOX 37-6 Treatment Options for Warts

- Keratolytics eliminate the wart by causing an inflammatory response and topical peeling. They are often available over the counter, cause little pain, and are low in cost and risk, but they are slow to work.
  - Salicylic acid paints with a concentration of greater than 20% are applied with a toothpick once or twice a day for 4 to 6 weeks. On thick skin, a combination of 16.7% salicylic acid and 16.7% collodion is more effective. This method is useful for common or periungual warts, but it is not effective with warts larger than 5 mm in diameter.
  - Salicylic acid plasters with 40% concentration are cut to size and taped in place for 3 to 5 days. After the plaster is taken off, the area should be soaked for 45 minutes and the dead epidermis removed. A new plaster is then applied. Treatment can last 3 to 6 weeks. This method is useful for plantar warts.
  - Retinoic acid gel 0.025% to 0.05% applied once or twice daily brings resolution in 4 to 6 weeks. This method is useful for flat warts, but it does not work for common, plantar, or periungual warts.
- Occlusion with duct tape: Place on for 12 hours a day for 6 days in a row, followed by soaking and scraping of epidermis; is easy, painless, and inexpensive.
- Destructive agents eliminate the wart by causing necrosis and blister formation. Most techniques are painful and require patient cooperation.
  - Cryotherapy: Liquid nitrogen is applied for 2 to 10 seconds until an area 1 to 3 mm beyond the wart turns white or patient complains of pain; goal is to induce blister formation above the dermal-epidermal junction. Take care not to freeze the wart too vigorously. Caution should be used when freezing warts over joints and the lateral aspects of digits. This method is uncomfortable and often not tolerated by children. Retreatment is often necessary. Cantharidin 0.7% is applied directly to the wart with a toothpick and covered with tape for 24 hours. This is a potent blistering agent that creates a blister in 2 to 3 days that is sloughed after 7 to 14 days. This method is useful for periungual and some plantar warts. Do not use on other body surfaces.
  - Podophyllum 25% solution in compound benzoin tincture is applied to the wart with a toothpick; it should be washed off in 4 hours; may be repeated in 1 week. Podofilox, available over the counter for home use, is applied twice a day for 3 days. After a 4-day rest period, the 3-day cycle may be repeated as necessary. This technique is useful for common or genital warts.
  - Surgical excision of warts can lead to scarring that can be more painful than the wart itself, but can be highly effective for large individual warts. Surgery by snipping with scissors, not scalpel, is useful for filiform warts.
  - Laser treatments are often as effective as cryosurgery, but can be painful and require several treatments for complete resolution.
- Immunotherapy modalities stimulate an immune response to HPV. These newer treatment modalities do not have controlled studies evaluating their effectiveness.
  - Oral cimetidine, a histamine 2–receptor-blocking agent, may improve immunity to HPV. It is used in conjunction with other modalities at a dose of 20 to 30 mg/kg divided twice a day for 3 to 4 months.
  - Imiquimod cream creates cell-mediated immunity in surrounding areas and is often effective as a home treatment. It is applied daily for 1 to 2 months.
  - Contact sensitization and interferon injection are methods used by dermatologists, usually in adult patients.

HPV, Human papillomavirus.

Patient and Family Education

A blister, sometimes hemorrhagic, may form 1 to 2 days after liquid nitrogen treatment. Redness and itching may herald regression of a wart. Parents and patients must be warned that multiple or prolonged treatment is often necessary.

Infestations of the Skin

Pediculosis

Pediculosis (lice infestation) can affect the scalp (most common), body (uncommon), or pubic area (considered a sexually transmitted disease). Infestation is defined by some as the presence of either nits (eggs) or lice and by others as presence of lice alone.

Lice infestation is caused by three subspecies, *Pediculus humanus capitis* and *corporis* (head and body) or by *Phthirus pubis* (pubic). The adult female louse, which survives by sucking human blood, deposits 6 to 10 eggs per day on a gluelike substance about 4 mm from the scalp on the hair shaft in a waterproof shell. Nits incubate for about 1 week, hatch and grow into adult lice over another 1 to 2 weeks, then begin laying eggs. Head lice live approximately 30 days on a host and lay up to 100 nits. Transmission is by direct or indirect contact, often by sharing hairbrushes, caps, clothing, or linen or through close living quarters, or sexual activity (pubic lice).

Pediculosis capitis is common in children. Head lice are not considered a health hazard, because they do not spread disease. All socioeconomic groups are affected, but lice are most common in school-age Caucasian females, with the peak season occurring from August to November. Lice are uncommon in African American children (Guenther, 2014).

Pediculosis corporis is uncommon in childhood. The louse is rarely seen on the body; rather it attaches to clothing and intermittently pierces the skin. It is the only louse that can carry human disease (e.g., epidemic typhus and trench fever).

Pubic lice may involve the scalp, eyebrows, or eyelashes but primarily are found in the pubic area. Clothing and bed linens are a source of residence. If pediculosis pubis is found in a child, sexual abuse must be considered.

Clinical Findings

History

- A history of infestation in a family, friend, or day care contact
- Dandruff-like substance in the hair
- Itching of the scalp, scratching, and irritability if infestation has been present for a few weeks
- Reports of a crawling sensation in the scalp

Physical Examination

- Head lice
  - Lice can be visualized; nits can be seen as small white oval cases attached tightly to a hair shaft. Nits are usually laid within 4 mm of the scalp; as the hair grows, the nits and empty shells are found farther from the scalp, indicating more long-term infestation.
  - Care must be taken to differentiate hair casts, epithelial cells, and other debris from nits.
  - Common sites are the back of the head, nape of the neck, and behind the ears; eyelashes can be involved. Scalp excoriations and occipital or cervical adenopathy can be present.
- Body lice
  - Excoriated macules or papules may be present (secondary bacterial infection of the skin may develop).
  - Belt line, collar, and underwear areas are common sites.
  - A hemorrhagic pinpoint macule is seen where the louse extracted blood.
  - Axillary, inguinal, or regional lymphadenopathy can be present.
- Pubic lice
  - Excoriation and small bluish macules and papules may be present.
  - Eyelashes can be involved; spread to other short-haired areas (thighs, trunk, axillae, beard) may occur.

Diagnostic Studies

- Microscopic examination of a hair shaft can more clearly identify nits.
- Test for other sexually transmitted diseases if pubic lice found; specifically gonorrhea and syphilis.

Differential Diagnosis

Scabies, dermatitis herpetiformis, and necrotic excoriations are in the differential diagnosis. Rule out sexual abuse if pubic lice are found.

Management

Correct diagnosis is imperative to effective management. Treatment is recommended when live lice and viable nits are observed, because nonviable nits (which do not necessarily indicate the presence of lice) can persist on the hair shaft for several months.

Treatment options are varied and controversial. Lice are growing resistant to available pharmacologic treatment options mainly in children who have been treated multiple times. Treatment failure is common, whether as a result of poor technique or actual medication resistance. This has led to the trial of many alternative treatments. Over-the-counter medications, prescription medications, and dangerous substitutes (e.g., kerosene) may be used by parents. It is recommended that providers follow local resistance patterns when determining treatment. Table 37-6 outlines recommended treatment.

Pediculicides are a first-line treatment option. They are toxic substances, however, and should be used only as directed and with care. Pregnant women and nursing mothers should not be exposed to pediculicides; they should not be used to treat lice in babies (National Pediculosis Association, 2009). The National Pediculosis Association also advises caution in children with allergies, asthma, epilepsy, other chronic illness, or open wounds; those undergoing chemotherapy, using other medications, or already overexposed to pediculicides.

Proper pediculicide application is key to success. Prior to use, do not use a shampoo that contains conditioner or cream rinse, or petrolatum products on the hair or scalp. Keep the pediculicide out of the eyes. If applying to damp hair, make sure the hair is damp, not wet (dilutes the pediculicide). Do not rewash the hair for 1 to 2 days following treatment. Reapply in 7 to 10 days.

TABLE 37-6 Diagnosis and Treatment of Pediculosis and Scabies

	Clinical Findings	Treatment
Pediculosis (head lice)	History of infestation; itchy scalp, scratches; postoccipital nodes; occasional visualization of lice or nits (small white oval cases), commonly on back of head, nape of neck, behind ears, possibly eyelashes	Key to treatment is proper technique! *First step:* Apply pediculicide: permethrin *or* pyrethrin plus piperonyl butoxide *Second step:* Remove nits: comb hair with fine-toothed comb in 1-inch sections with special attention to nape of neck and behind ears *Third step:* Cleanse the environment: check family, friends, day care/school contacts; clean sheets, towels, clothing, and headgear; store other items in plastic for 2 days; vacuum; soak brushes and combs; follow up in 2 weeks with daily recheck at home by parent May return to school after pediculicide treatment; "no nit" policies are not recommended
Scabies	Key finding: Itching, worse at night, and complaints are more significant than physical findings; fitful sleep, crankiness; curving burrows, especially in webs of fingers, sides of hands, folds of wrist, armpits, forearms, elbows, belt line, buttocks, proximal half of foot and heel; secondary excoriation; infants may have lesions on palms, soles, scalp, face, posterior auricle and axilla, folds, red-brown; may be <10 lesions total or may be dozens (typical of infants); lesions may occur in the form of firm nodules in infants	Treat with permethrin 5%, repeated in 1 week; use antihistamine, hydrocortisone, or nonsteroidal anti-inflammatory drugs (NSAIDs) for itching; simultaneously treat family members (even if asymptomatic), friends, and school/day care contacts Cleanse environment: Linens and clothing, vacuum, store anything else in plastic bags for 2 days; rash and itch persist for up to 3 weeks after treatment; return to school 24 hours after treatment

- Permethrin 1% cream rinse is the treatment of choice for head lice because of its safety (can be used in children older than 1 month old), efficacy, and 10-day residual. Hair should be shampooed and towel dried (damp), permethrin applied, left on for 10 minutes, and then rinsed. Hair should not be rewashed for at least 24 to 48 hours. Apply again in 7 to 10 days (Engorn and Flerlage, 2015).
- Spinosad was approved in 2011 for infestations in patients 4 years old and older. It is applied to dry hair and left on 10 minutes before rinsing.
- Benzyl alcohol, a prescription medication that is not ovicidal, is applied to dry hair and left on for 10 minutes before rinsing. Repeat the application in 7 days to kill newly hatched lice. Benzyl alcohol is contraindicated in children younger than 6 months old.
- Pyrethrin, a natural extract from the chrysanthemum plant, is effective as a pediculicide but not as an ovicide. A 10-minute shampoo is applied to dry hair, with a repeat application in 7 to 10 days. Pyrethrin is contraindicated in children with allergy to ragweed. Because pyrethrin does not kill both lice and eggs, treatment failures are more common than with permethrin.
- Topical ivermectin is a single-dose, 10-minute application to dry hair. It is approved for children 6 months old and older.
- Lindane is a prescription organochloride that effectively kills lice and nits. It is a neurotoxin, and there are safety concerns because of potential central nervous system effects on the child and long-term environmental contamination. Therefore, it is recommended for use only in patients who have failed to respond to adequate doses of other approved agents. For head lice, a 1% lindane shampoo is used, left on the hair for 4 minutes, then rinsed; for body lice, cream or lotion may be applied for 8 to 12 hours (overnight) and then rinsed off; for pubic lice, a 1% shampoo is applied for 10 minutes, then rinsed off. Retreatment is not recommended (Guenther, 2014).
- Malathion lotion 0.5% is an organophosphate with a pine-needle–oil base that is available only by prescription. It is a potent lice killer that binds to the hair shaft for 4 weeks and it is considered the most effective therapy for killing lice and nits. It is not recommended in children younger than 2 years old. The drug is flammable, and if ingested causes severe respiratory distress. Malathion 0.5% lotion should be applied to dry hair, be allowed to dry, and then carefully rinsed off 8 to 12 hours later. The treatment should be repeated in 7 to 10 days if live lice are still seen (Guenther, 2014).

The second step in treatment for lice is removal of nits, although this is may not be an absolutely necessary step. Proper technique is the key to success. A good light, a magnifying glass, and tweezers are useful. A wide-toothed comb may be used initially to straighten the hair, but a fine-toothed nit-removal comb is necessary to remove nits.

- Some products claim to dissolve the substance (cement) that attaches the nit to the hair to facilitate removal. A 1 : 1 vinegar-to-water solution applied to the scalp, then covered with a warm, moist towel for 30 minutes before beginning to comb may also help.
- Use a proper nit-removal comb with fine teeth (included in most pediculicide kits).
- Comb damp hair for a minimum of 20 to 30 minutes, working from the top of the scalp down in 1-inch sections. Pay special attention to the nape of the neck and behind the ears.
- If eyelashes are involved, coat with petroleum jelly two or three times a day for 8 to 14 days and manually remove nits.
- Comb-outs and inspection should be repeated every night for 2 to 3 weeks to ensure cure.

The third step in lice treatment is thorough cleansing of the environment.

- Examine family members, friends, school, and day care contacts. Do not treat family members if nothing is found because of the emergence of treatment-resistant lice and pediculicide toxicity.
- Launder sheets, towels, clothing, and headgear in hot water and machine dry on hot cycle for 20 minutes, iron, or dry clean.
- Any item that cannot be washed or dry-cleaned should be stored in a plastic bag for 2 weeks.
- Hot iron or vacuum play areas, floors, rugs, and furniture.
- Soak brushes, combs, and hair accessories in pediculicide, alcohol, or Lysol for 1 hour, followed by a hot-water rinse.
- Spraying or fumigating the house is not recommended.

Alternative treatments include herbal or essential oils, such as olive oil, pine oil, tea-tree oil, margarine, mayonnaise, dog shampoo, styling gels, and petroleum jelly, all of which suffocate and kill the lice. Further evidence-based studies are needed regarding these practices. Definitely avoid wrapping the hair in plastic and putting the child under a hair dryer or washing the hair with gasoline or kerosene.

Treatment failure is not unusual. Common mistakes that lead to recurrence of lice include dilution of pediculicide by applying to wet, not damp hair; use of a shampoo with conditioner or cream rinse before treatment; inadequate combing techniques; not cleansing personal care items; and not screening and treating family members and close contacts. However, with proper use of a pediculicide, if lice reappear, reinfection from contact with an untreated individual is a more likely cause.

There are neither formal recommendations, nor FDA approval for dealing with resistance. Some methods for treating resistant lice include the following:

- Use Nix (permethrin 1%) creme rinse for 4 to 8 hours instead of 10 minutes.
- Use Nix (permethrin 1%) creme rinse under a shower cap overnight.
- Use Elimite (permethrin 5%) cream overnight.

Body lice are treated by improving hygiene and cleaning clothes. Wash infested clothing and dry at hot temperatures on a weekly basis for several weeks. Pediculicides are not necessary (Guenther, 2014). Pubic lice are treated as pediculosis capitis.

Complications

Secondary bacterial infection can occur.

Patient and Family Education

Items for discussion include the following:

- Daily to weekly checks or combing for lice or nits should be carried out at home.
- Educate family members about the expected course, that lice infestation is not a social disease, and about the need to avoid excessive or unnecessary retreatment. Do not use extra amounts; do not treat more than three times with the same medication without being seen by a care provider; do not mix pediculicides.
- Children should not be excluded or sent home from school because of lice. Parents should be notified and informed that the child should be treated. The American Academy of Pediatrics (AAP) discourages "no-nit" policies in schools, because such policies have been ineffective in controlling head lice transmission and result in excessive lost school and workdays (Frankowski et al, 2010).

Scabies

Scabies is caused by the mite, *Sarcoptes scabiei,* which is an obligate human parasite that burrows into the epidermis and causes intense itching (Fig. 37-21). Scabies is a highly contagious infestation spread through close contact and shared clothing or linen. The female mite burrows into the skin, laying up to three eggs a day as she travels. The eggs hatch in about 3 to 4 days and mature into adult mites in 10 to 14 days. The female mite has a lifespan of 15 to 30 days. Sensitization, which causes intense itching, occurs

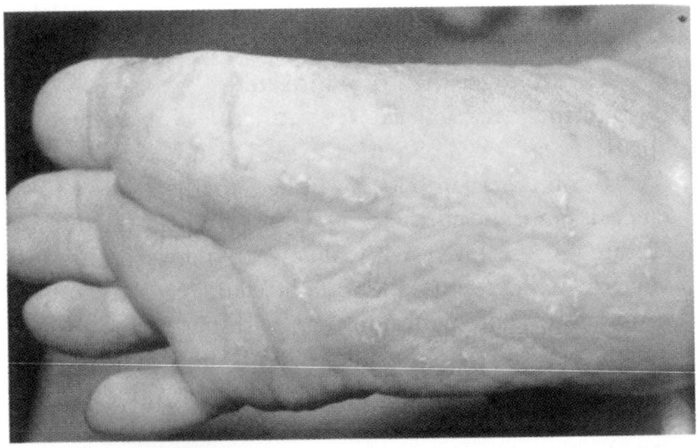

• Figure 37-21 Scabies. (From Aly R, Maibach H: *Atlas of infections of the skin*, Philadelphia, 1999, Saunders, p 176.)

approximately 3 weeks after infestation. Scabies occurs in all socioeconomic groups and in all age groups. However, infestation of African Americans is rare.

Clinical Findings

History

- Key finding: Itching, worse at night, initially mild but progressively more intense
- Fitful sleep, crankiness, or rubbing of hands and feet (infants)

Physical Examination

- Complaints are significantly greater than examination findings.
- Characteristic lesions include curving S-shaped burrows, especially on webs of fingers and sides of hands, folds of wrists and armpits, forearms, elbows, belt line, buttocks, genitalia, or proximal half of foot and heel.
- Vesiculopustular lesions tend to be found in infants and young children. They classically have vesicular lesions on palms, soles, scalp, face, posterior auriculae, and axillae, concentrated in the folds; head and neck lesions typically are red-brown vesicopustules or nodules. However, any child younger than 2 years old can have an unusual manifestation.
- Secondary lesions include itchy papules, red-brown nodules from inflammatory response, crusting, excoriation, and other signs of secondary infection.
- Infants classically have dozens of lesions; older children may have fewer than 10.

Diagnostic Studies

- Microscopic examination of scrapings from an unscratched burrow in saline or mineral oil can reveal an eight-legged mite, eggs, or feces. Do not use KOH because it dissolves the mites, eggs, and feces. Burrows and fresh papules are best for specimen collection.
- Burrow ink test: Apply a drop of ink or rub a washable felt-tipped pen across suspected burrow. Wipe off excess ink and examine with magnifying glass for an ink-stained burrow.

Differential Diagnosis

Papular urticaria; atopic, seborrheic or contact dermatitis; insect bites; folliculitis; lichen planus; and dermatitis herpetiformis are included in the differential diagnosis.

Management

Management involves the following:

1. Pharmacologic treatment begins with applying a thin layer of scabicide to the entire body, excluding the eyes. Areas of special importance are under the fingernails, the scalp, behind the ears, all folds and creases, and the feet and hands. In general, the scabicide should be reapplied in 7 days on all symptomatic patients.
2. Permethrin 5% cream remains the drug of choice for the treatment of scabies. Despite frequent use over the past two decades, there is no clear evidence of resistance to permethrin 5% cream for the treatment of classic scabies (Gunning et al, 2012). It is indicated for use in children as young as 2 months old (Cohen, 2013). Parents and patients should be educated on proper application of a thin layer of cream to the entire body from the neck down, and rinsing after 8 to 14 hours. Application may be repeated in 1 week (Gunning et al, 2012). Unlike adults and older children, infants generally present with lesions on the face, neck, scalp, and hands and feet; be sure to include these areas on application, avoiding the areas around the eyes and mouth (Bethel, 2014). The treatment of crusted or Norwegian scabies has proven to be more difficult due to common misdiagnosis. Ivermectin 200 mcg/kg is recommended orally on days 1, 2, 8, 9, and 15 of treatment, in conjunction with full body application of permethrin cream 5% for 7 days, then twice weekly until resolved (Gunning et al, 2012). Due to a lack of safety data, ivermectin is not recommended for children younger than 5 years old, or less than 15 kg (Cohen, 2013). Antihistamines (hydroxyzine or diphenhydramine) or topical 1% hydrocortisone can be helpful for itching, which can last for several weeks after successful treatment.
3. Simultaneous treatment of family members, friends, and school and day care contacts, even if asymptomatic, is essential.
4. At time of treatment, linens and any clothing worn during the past 48 hours should be washed with hot water, put into a hot dryer for 20 minutes, or dry-cleaned. The house should be vacuumed.
5. Store nonwashable items in sealed plastic bags for a minimum of 1 week.

Resistance to medication is not common and continued infestation is usually due to treatment failure rather than resistance. Reasons for treatment failure include an incorrect diagnosis, not applying medication to the whole body, or not treating all members of the household. The child may develop postscabetic eczema that can be misdiagnosed as treatment failure. Evaluate and treat with topical corticosteroids.

Complications

A secondary bacterial infection is possible and should be treated. Postscabetic syndrome is common, with visible lesions and pruritus persisting for days to weeks following treatment; nodular lesions can persist for weeks to months. Norwegian scabies is a nonpruritic, crusted, scaling infestation with thousands to millions of mites occurring in immunosuppressed or institutionalized patients.

Patient and Family Education

Educate the family about the course of disease. Rash and itching persist for up to 3 weeks following treatment. Avoid overbathing and further irritation of the skin. The child should not be infectious 24 hours after treatment and may return to school or day care.

Allergic and Inflammatory Reactions of the Skin

Acne Vulgaris

Acne is an inflammatory disorder of the pilosebaceous unit in which excess sebum, keratinous debris, and bacteria accumulate, producing microcomedones. The microcomedones may be noninflamed or inflamed lesions. Although rarely a serious disorder, acne may cause permanent scarring and decreased self-esteem, and occasionally heralds underlying disease. It is often of significant concern to the adolescent, having a serious effect on social development (Fig. 37-22).

Acne is the most common skin disorder and affects approximately 80% to 85% of individuals between 11 and 30 years old in the United States (Paller and Mancini, 2011). Four mechanisms contribute to this sebaceous follicle disorder:

- Sebaceous follicles become plugged with keratinous material.
- Colonies of anaerobic bacteria grow deep in the follicle, primarily *P. acnes,* but coagulase-negative staphylococci and *M. furfur* can be involved.
- Sebum is overproduced and androgen production increases, resulting in expansion of the follicle.
- Inflammation occurs and pustules form secondary to trapped *P. acnes* and sebum. The bacteria release chemotactic factors that attract neutrophils to ingest the bacteria and release hydrolytic enzymes.

Acne usually begins at the onset of puberty, occurring earlier in girls (12 to 13 years old) than boys (14 to 15 years old). It tends to improve in the summer and worsens with menses and stress. The pathogenesis of acne is multifactorial; gender, age, genetic factors, and environment are significant factors. Although not a serious physical disorder, acne has been associated with psychosocial morbidity and decreased emotional well-being. "Patients with even mild to moderate acne have demonstrated high scores on the Carrol Rating Scale for Depression and an increased prevalence of suicidal ideation" (Paller and Mancini, 2011, p 167).

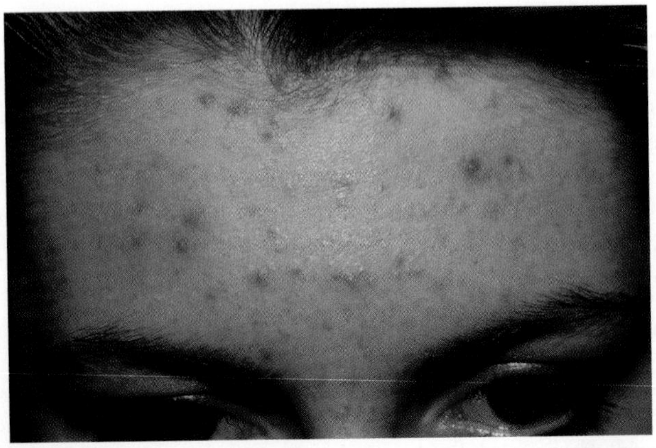

• **Figure 37-22** Acne vulgaris. (From Weston WL, Lane AT, Morelli JG: *Color textbook of pediatric dermatology*, ed 4, St. Louis, 2007, Mosby/Elsevier, p 27.)

Neonatal acne occurs in about 20% of normal newborns; infants are occasionally affected by acne. Neonatal acne is thought to be related to either stimulation of sebaceous glands by maternal androgens or transient adrenal and gonadal androgen production. Infantile acne may occasionally be associated with hyperandrogenism.

Clinical Findings

History

- Family history of acne
- Stage of pubertal development and menstrual history
- Facial and hair products used, especially occlusive products or pomades
- Oral and topical prescription medication, especially oral contraceptives, antibiotics, or steroids
- Current or previous acne treatment and results
- Sports participation, especially if wearing football pads, helmets, headbands, or other protective devices
- Jobs, such as cooking at a fast-food grill or working at a gas station
- Other medical conditions

Physical Examination

Lesions most commonly are found on the face, back, and chest.

- Noninflammatory lesions:
  - Microcomedone—a follicular plug as a result of obstruction of the pilosebaceous unit (hair follicle and sebaceous gland) typically localized on the face and trunk.
  - Open comedone (blackhead)—a noninflammatory lesion or papule, firm in consistency, caused by blockage at the mouth of the follicle and occurring on the face, upper back, shoulders, and chest. The black color is thought to come from oxidized keratinous material at the follicular opening. This is the main lesion in early adolescence.
  - Closed comedone (whitehead)—a noninflammatory lesion, semisoft in consistency, caused by blockage at the neck of the follicle. This is a precursor to inflammatory acne.
- Inflammatory lesions occur secondary to rupture of noninflamed lesions into the dermis and can include papules, pustules, excoriation, lesion crusting, nodules, cysts, scars, and sinus tracts (confluent nodules likely to scar).

The severity of acne is determined by the quantity, type, and spread of lesions. It is helpful to use a diagram of the face or a grading graph to identify the number and type of lesions to allow more precise patient follow-up. If only open and closed comedones are found, the disorder is called *comedonal acne.* Most adolescents have a combination of comedones, red papules, and pustules called *papulopustular acne,* which can be mild or severe. *Nodulocystic acne* is the most severe form and requires more intensive intervention. Specific types of acne include *frictional,* occurring from rubbing of bras, tight clothes, or headbands; *pomadal,* along the temple and forehead, as a result of pomades or oil-based cosmetics; *athletic,* on forehead, chin, or shoulders, caused by helmets and pads; and *hormonal,* with a beard distribution.

Differential Diagnosis

Cosmetic, mechanical, environmental, or drug-induced acne; rosacea; flat wart; milia; perioral dermatitis; and folliculitis are included in the differential diagnosis.

Management

The goals of acne management are to (1) reduce the excess production of sebum, (2) counteract the abnormal desquamation of epithelial cells, (3) decrease the proliferation of *P. acnes*, and (4) prevent or decrease scarring. Choice of treatment depends on the extent, severity, and duration of disease; type of lesions; and psychological effects the adolescent is experiencing (Table 37-7 and Box 37-7).

- Education is the first priority. The adolescent must have realistic expectations and understand the pathophysiology and the process of treatment, including the fact that the acne often worsens before improving. Reading

BOX 37-7 Medications Commonly Used in Treating Acne

Topical Keratolytic or Comedolytic Agents

Retinoids
- Tretinoin: 0.01% to 0.025% gel; 0.025% to 0.1% cream; 0.1% microgel
- Tretinoin/clindamycin (combination topical)
- Tazarotene: 0.05% to 0.1% cream; 0.05% to 0.1% gel
- Adapalene: 0.1% gel or cream; 0.3% gel

Benzoyl peroxide: 2.5% to 20% gel; 5% and 10% cream; 5% to 20% lotion or wash
Azelaic acid: 20% cream; 15% gel

Topical Antibiotics

Clindamycin: 1% solution, lotion, gel, pledget, foam
Erythromycin: 1% to 2% solution, 3% gel or swabs
Erythromycin: 3% with benzoyl peroxide 5% gel
Clindamycin: 1% with 5% benzoyl peroxide

Oral Antibiotics*

Tetracycline: 250 to 500 mg per dose twice a day
Erythromycin: 250 to 500 mg per dose twice a day
Minocycline: 50 to 100 mg per dose twice a day (associated with more side effects)
Doxycycline: 50 to 100 mg per dose twice a day

*From Paller AS, Mancini AJ: *Hurwitz clinical pediatric dermatology: a textbook of skin disorders of children and adolescence*, ed 4, Philadelphia, 2011, Elsevier.

TABLE 37-7 Treatment of Acne

Type of Acne	Lesions	Initial Treatment	If Not Improving
Comedonal	Open or closed comedones	Choose one: Benzoyl peroxide: 5% gel daily (if mild) Tretinoin: 0.025% cream daily (if moderate) Adapalene: 0.1% gel	Combine benzoyl peroxide with tretinoin or increase strength of tretinoin to 0.05%
Mild papulopustular	Red papules, few pustules	**Option 1**. Choose one: Benzoyl peroxide: 5% to 10% daily Adapalene: 0.1% gel Azelaic acid: Twice a day (if mild) *Plus* topical antibiotic twice a day **Option 2**. Choose one: Erythromycin: 3% with 5% benzoyl peroxide daily to twice a day (if moderate) Clindamycin: 1% with 5% benzoyl peroxide daily to twice a day	Increase benzoyl peroxide to twice a day *or* Combine benzoyl peroxide with tretinoin (for comedones) Substitute topical antibiotic twice a day (for inflammatory acne)
Moderate to severe papulopustular	Red papules, many pustules	Choose one: Benzoyl peroxide: 5% and tretinoin 0.025% Adapalene: 0.1% gel Azelaic acid (if comedonal) Topical antibiotic twice a day (if no comedones) *Plus* oral antibiotic twice a day	Increase strength of treatment *or* Refer to dermatologist
Nodulocystic, scarring, or unresponsive	Red papules, pustules, cysts, and nodules	Choose one: Oral antibiotics twice a day and tretinoin 0.05% daily Adapalene (0.1% gel) and benzoyl peroxide (10% gel) twice a day (if comedonal) Adapalene: 0.1% gel and topical antibiotic	Refer to dermatologist for oral isotretinoin

materials about acne and its treatment provide support for self-management efforts.

- Wash face twice a day with a mild soap, such as Dove, Neutrogena, or Aveeno Cleansing Bar. Avoid scrubbing, rubbing, picking, and squeezing. Medication should be applied lightly.
- Use of a comedone extractor can cause scarring and should be discouraged. Hot soaks applied to pustules may help their resolution.
- All products used on the face should be labeled as *noncomedogenic.*
- Identify and discontinue use of aggravating substances, such as oil-based cosmetics, pomades, hair spray, mousse, and face creams.
- Identify possible aggravating factors, such as stress; hot, humid weather; and jobs involving frying oil or grease.
- Reassure that no scientific evidence indicates that any particular foods adversely affect acne; however, a well-balanced diet is important to maintaining healthy skin.
- Discuss psychosocial concerns and provide support.
- Remind the adolescent that results take months and that adherence to treatment is essential to improvement.
- Sun exposure helps clear acne for some adolescents but may worsen it for others. Sunscreen use is recommended, and caution about sun exposure should be given if a medication that increases photosensitivity is being used.

- Medications used in treatment of acne vary by action, route of administration, and strength. They include topical and systemic preparations; keratolytic or comedolytic agents; those with antibacterial or antibiotic effects; hormonal agents; and preparations that have a combination of actions.
- Topical keratolytic or comedolytic agents, used to minimize follicular obstruction and break up microcomedones, are the first line of acne treatment. They may be dispensed in a combination form with a topical antibacterial agent. Many strengths and forms are available, the strongest being the gels, if tolerated; creams are the least drying. A general rule is to start low (in strength) and slowly (in frequency) and advance as tolerated or needed. A useful technique to decrease the incidence of irritation is to start therapy only for 3 nights a week and slowly increase to a nightly application over a few weeks. A minimum of 4 to 6 weeks of treatment is required before improvement is seen. There are three topical retinoids (tretinoin, adapalene, and tazarotene) and two agents that possess both antibacterial and keratolytic properties (benzoyl peroxide and azelaic acid). Each works by a different mechanism. They can be used together and interchangeably. Dryness, erythema, irritation, and scaling can occur with these products, and the strength and frequency of use must be adjusted for this.
  - Tretinoin is a keratolytic that causes sun sensitivity. A pea-sized application should be made 20 minutes after washing the face. Initially it is used every other night, advancing to every night. Sensitivity to tretinoin is worst in the first 2 weeks of use and decreases thereafter.
  - Adapalene seems to cause less irritation and less photosensitivity, and it has better efficacy.
  - Tazarotene is a keratolytic to be used once daily.
  - Azelaic acid is antibacterial and keratolytic. It is useful in individuals with sensitive or dark skin and is also effective in treating acne rosacea.
  - Benzoyl peroxide, the most frequently used topical preparation for acne, is used once or twice a day, depending on the severity of acne and dryness of skin. It is a powerful antimicrobial with comedolytic and anti-inflammatory effects. Use in combination with topical antibiotics causes less antibiotic resistance.
- Topical antibiotics are used to control the inflammatory process, usually most helpful in moderate inflammatory acne. They are used to maintain control after treatment with oral antibiotics, and are applied to the entire skin surface, not just to problem areas. They should not be applied within 30 minutes of shaving. Erythromycin can have up to a 51% resistance rate (Paller and Mancini, 2011).
  - Topical clindamycin, erythromycin, or sulfacetamide is used once or twice a day, either alone or in combination with other topical medications.
  - Topical erythromycin with benzoyl peroxide and clindamycin with benzoyl peroxide are combination products that are more effective than either drug alone and have less resistance from *P. acnes.* This combination is especially effective in mild to moderate inflammatory acne or as an adjunct to oral therapy (Paller and Mancini, 2011).
- Oral antibiotics are used in addition to topical agents to decrease the concentration of *P. acnes* and to decrease the degree of inflammation if there is no response to topical agents. Systemic antibiotics should be used for the shortest time possible, rarely longer than 6 months, and often require 3 to 4 weeks to see improvement. Once improvement is noted, the dose should be tapered to a daily dose, and then discontinued.
  - Tetracycline should be taken with 8 ounces of water 1 hour before or 2 hours after eating. Tetracycline should not be used by pregnant or breastfeeding females or in children younger than 9 years old. Photosensitivity reactions can occur. The usual dose is 250 to 500 mg twice daily.
  - Erythromycin can be taken with food, but gastrointestinal upset is common, and vulvovaginal candidiasis can be problematic. The usual dose is 250 to 500 mg twice daily.
  - Minocycline can be taken with food, although dairy products decrease absorption. Side effects include

blue-black discoloration in scars, photosensitivity, and hypersensitivity reactions. The usual dose is 50 to 100 mg twice daily.
    - Doxycycline can be taken with food (dairy products decrease absorption), but has the highest rate of photosensitivity reactions. The usual dose is 50 to 100 mg twice daily.
- Oral retinoids are used for severe, recalcitrant nodulocystic acne. Isotretinoin is contraindicated in pregnancy (pregnancy Category X drug known for its teratogenic effect) and requires evaluation by a dermatologist before use. Its association with depression and suicide is controversial. The usual course is 20 weeks; there are many side effects, and CBC, liver function tests (LFTs), human chorionic gonadotropin (hCG), and urinalysis for pregnancy must be monitored every month while the patient is taking the medication. The iPledge program creates a registry for all patients being treated with isotretinoin. The FDA requires health care providers, female patients, and pharmacists to access the iPledge website monthly after office visits and before filling their prescription for documentation regarding pregnancy, blood donation, and contraceptive counseling.
- Hormonal and other therapies: Hormonal therapies can be used in females to oppose effects of androgen on sebaceous glands, such as antiandrogens (e.g., spironolactone, flutamide) and androgen receptor blockers; oral contraceptive pills (OCPs) provide estrogen and a progestin, and some are FDA approved to treat acne vulgaris. Intralesional steroid therapy for large cysts or nodules is sometimes used; resurfacing lasers and dermabrasion are used for acne scarring.
- Noncomedogenic moisturizers can be used for dryness, which is common with treatment. Noncomedogenic makeup is also available and helpful in treating these patients.

Follow-up visits should occur at least every 4 to 6 weeks until control is established, defined as when lesions clear or only a few new lesions appear every 2 weeks. Refer to a dermatologist for nonresponsive or severe cases.

Mild cases of neonatal or infantile acne are best treated with a plan of watchful waiting and gentle daily cleansing with soap and water. In mild comedonal acne, sparing use of topical tretinoin is recommended. Use 2.5% benzoyl peroxide or topical antibiotics for mild inflammatory acne. Have the parents apply these agents every other night.

Complications

Failure can be due to lack of patient motivation, lack of education, inappropriate treatments, initial treatment that was too strong, or expectations of a quick fix. Psychological effects include decreased self-esteem and poor body image, problems with interpersonal relationships, self-consciousness, embarrassment, depression, and decreased athletic participation, especially in gymnastics, swimming, and wrestling. Resistance of *P. acnes* to tetracycline, erythromycin, and minocycline is increasing.

Atopic Dermatitis

See Chapter 25.

Contact Dermatitis

Contact dermatitis is an acute or chronic inflammation resulting from a hypersensitive reaction to a substance (either irritants or allergens). Common types of contact dermatitis include the following:

- Dry skin dermatitis caused by extremely low humidity (less than 30%), excess soap or cleansing cream use, or inadequate rinsing of soap products
- Nickel dermatitis from contact with jewelry, belts, snaps, or eyeglasses
- Lip-licker dermatitis caused by frequent lip licking, most often in dry, cold weather
- Phytophotodermatitis from sun exposure following contact with plants or juices, such as limes, lemons, carrots, celery, figs, parsnips, or dill; manifests as a blistered lesion on an erythematous base and may be confused with a burn
- Plant oleoresins, such as poison ivy, oak, or sumac; contact can be direct or indirect (exposure to burning plant material); oils may be inhaled, causing damage to lung tissue (Urushiol, the allergen in poison ivy, oak, and sumac can remain on contaminated items, such as clothing, animal hair, toys, and sports equipment resulting in sequential outbreaks due to reexposures.)
- Juvenile plantar dermatosis, manifested as dryness, cracking, and erythema of weight-bearing surfaces of the feet, initially the big toes; it mimics tinea pedis, often found in children with atopic dermatitis
- Latex dermatitis, associated with the use of products containing latex, such as protective gloves

Substances such as saliva, urine, and feces; baby wipes; bubble bath; agents that dry the skin; and adhesives often cause contact dermatitis. Diaper dermatitis is the most common form (see following section). Contact dermatitis can also be caused by allergens. Allergic reactions occur as an immunologic response to an antigen penetrating the skin. There are two phases: sensitization and elicitation. Allergic dermatitis is seen only after sensitization to an allergen has occurred and a subsequent type IV delayed hypersensitivity response has activated an immune cascade. Common causes are contact with shoes (components, such as rubber and potassium dichromate); nickel; clothes with woolen or rough textures; topical medications (e.g., neomycin and lanolin); perfumed soaps or cosmetics (including lanolin); preservatives; or poison ivy, oak, or sumac. Sometimes the cause is obvious; often no specific cause can be identified. Although it occurs at any age, contact dermatitis is extremely common in children (Tan et al, 2014).

Clinical Findings

History

- Contact with any new or unusual substances
- Repeated exposure to any substance or item
- Diarrhea or infrequently changed diapers
- Rash localized to specific area(s)

Physical Examination

The area of involvement offers clues to the causative agent. Often the rash is localized to one area and has sharp borders. Common examples include a linear-type rash secondary to wearing a necklace or bracelet, circular areas from snaps on clothing, or inflammation of the earlobes from jewelry or a reaction pattern on the toes and dorsum of the foot from shoes. The severity of the rash depends on the length of exposure and the concentration of the irritant. Minimal contact may produce only mild erythema, whereas prolonged or concentrated contact may produce significant erythema, edema, and blistering with possible crusting and secondary infection. Irritant reactions tend to be immediate, whereas allergic ones are delayed.

- A chafed appearance with shiny, mild to severely erythematous, peeling, or dry, fissured skin or red patches and plaques with secondary scales may be seen if the reaction is due to an irritant. For example, the dorsum of the hand may exhibit the above characteristic appearance with frequent hand washing with irritating soaps.
- Erythema, vesicles, and weeping may be present in the acute stage of allergic contact dermatitis. The lesions are pruritic.
- Hyperpigmentation and lichenification are seen in chronic conditions.
- A generalized idiosyncratic (id) reaction can develop to an allergen. An id reaction occurs as a secondary or "sympathy" rash distant from the primary site of exposure.

Differential Diagnosis

The differential diagnosis includes atopic dermatitis, impetigo, herpes simplex, psoriasis, and seborrhea.

Management

Appropriate skin care, recognizing and eliminating offending agents, and treating inflammation are key to managing contact dermatitis successfully. Identify and avoid the substance (irritant or allergen) causing the dermatitis. General treatment measures include:

- Burow solution soaks or oatmeal baths and cool compresses (1 teaspoon salt/pint water) applied for 20 minutes every 4 to 6 hours to soothe vesicular rashes.
- Water and either petrolatum-based or lanolin-and-petrolatum–based emollients applied to the skin to restore moisture to areas of dryness and chafing.
  - Petrolatum-based emollients include dimethicone, white petrolatum, and Vaseline Dermatology Formula.
  - Lanolin-and-petrolatum–based emollients should not be used if there is inflammation.
- Topical corticosteroids used two or three times daily give relief in 2 or 3 days, although it may take 2 or 3 weeks for complete healing. Occasionally oral corticosteroids are used for short periods if the area of allergic involvement exceeds 10% of the skin surface (10 to 14 days, tapered the last 7 days).
- Do not use flavored lip creams in cases of lip-licker dermatitis. Emollient lotions and petroleum-based emollients can moisturize the skin and discourage lip licking because of their bad taste.
- Oral antihistamines are helpful if itching and scratching are problems.

Resolution may take 2 to 3 weeks. Refer to a dermatologist or an allergist for patch testing if the dermatitis worsens, fails to respond, or recurs. Allergic contact dermatitis can develop into chronic dermatitis if left untreated. Psoralen and UVA treatment, narrow-band UVB treatment, systemic treatment with immunomodulators, and targeted biologic therapy may be considered if unresponsive to other measures (Tan et al, 2014).

Diaper Dermatitis

Diaper dermatitis is the most frequent contact dermatitis seen in children and one of the most common skin disorders of infants (Table 37-8; Fig. 37-23). The initial rash is termed *irritant contact diaper dermatitis.* A variation of this is called *tidewater* or *tidemark dermatitis* and is found at the diaper edges. *Jacquet dermatitis,* a severe form manifested by punched-out lesions or erosions primarily on the labia and buttocks, is especially prone to secondary infection.

Factors contributing to diaper dermatitis include the following:

- Improper hygiene and cleansing methods
- Chemical irritation caused by prolonged contact with skin products, urine, feces, or breakdown products. Feces and its breakdown products are the major factors
- Mechanical irritation from diapers or skinfolds
- Occlusion of skin with use of diapers and plastic or rubber pants
- Other skin dermatoses aggravated by wearing diapers (e.g., seborrhea, atopic dermatitis, or psoriasis)
- In the diaper area around the anus, the rash is often due to diarrhea; if the skin is affected but the folds are spared, urine is often responsible

Clinical Findings

History

- Type of diapers and diaper covering used; recent change in brand or laundering products
- Frequency of wet diapers and stools
- Frequency of diaper changes and methods of cleansing used
- Any new baby care products used

TABLE 37-8 **Diagnosis and Treatment of Diaper Dermatitis**

Type	Cause	Presentation and Location	Other Characteristics	Treatment
Irritant contact dermatitis	Related to wearing diapers; contact with urine and feces	Chapped, shiny, erythematous, parchment-like skin with possible erosions on convex surfaces; creases spared	Peaks at 9 to 12 months old; may progress to involve creases; skin may be dry	Frequent diaper changes, gentle cleansing; greasy lubricant; sitz bath, air-dry; 0.5% to 1% hydrocortisone for inflammation
Candidiasis	Related to wearing diapers; a superinfection with *Candida*	Shallow pustules, fiery-red scaly plaques on convex surfaces, inguinal folds, labia, and scrotum	Satellite lesions, oral thrush; recent antibiotic or diarrhea; occurs at any age	Antifungal cream plus same measures as for contact dermatitis
Miliaria or intertrigo	Related to wearing diapers; a result of heat and occlusion	Discrete vesicles or papules (miliaria); erythematous, scaly, maceration in skinfolds	Sweat retention or friction associated	Self-limited (miliaria); avoid precipitating factors; care as for contact dermatitis
Seborrhea	Exaggerated by wearing diapers; overgrowth of *Malassezia* yeast in areas of sebaceous gland activity	Greasy, erythematous scales, well circumscribed in creases of skin, groin; spared convex surfaces	Onset at 3 to 4 weeks old; also occurs on face or body; often superinfected with *Candida*	Ketoconazole and/or hydrocortisone is treatment of choice
Atopic dermatitis (AD)	Exaggerated by wearing diapers; exact cause unknown	Increased number of lines in skin; areas of excoriation in folds and convex surfaces and buttocks; less widespread	AD in other areas; usually begins in first year of life; scratches skin with diaper change; hyperlinear skinfolds with diffuse borders	Skin care as for contact dermatitis and as indicated for AD (see Chapter 25); antibiotics for bacterial infection
Psoriasis	Exaggerated by wearing diapers; psoriasis evolves in response to chronic trauma	Erythematous, well-defined sharp, scaly plaques on convex surfaces and inguinal folds; less widespread	Psoriasis affects other places; rare occurrence if found, usually at 6 to 18 months old	Treatment often required for weeks or until toilet trained; steroids; ketoconazole if *Candida* present
Bacterial dermatitis	Usually caused by staphylococcal or streptococcal infection	Red, denuded areas or fragile blisters; crusting and pustules in suprapubic area and periumbilicus	Usually in newborn, can occur anywhere	Nystatin if yeast is present as well; mupirocin if minimal; amoxicillin clavulanate or cephalexin

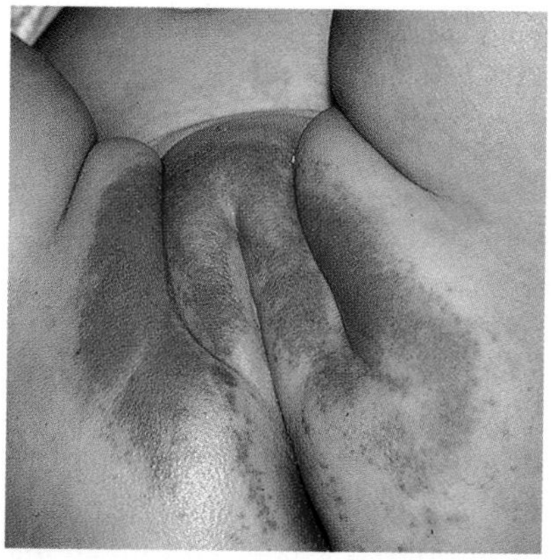

• **Figure 37-23** Diaper dermatitis. (Adapted from White G, Cox N: *Diseases of the skin*, ed 2, St. Louis, 2006, Mosby/Elsevier.)

- Medication taken (particularly antibiotics) or used on rash
- Present or recent use of antibiotics

Physical Examination

Erythema, edema, and vesiculation are typically the first characteristic changes observed. Chronic changes include scale, lichenification, and increased or decreased pigmentation. Other findings associated with specific causative factors can include the following:

- Chemical causes
  - Shiny, peeling, erythematous macular or papular rash confluent in the diaper area, sparing folds
  - Head of penis erythematous and dry
  - Erythema primarily on buttocks and around anus (fecal irritation)

- Mechanical causes
  - Erythematous, macerated (acute) or dry (chronic), hyperpigmented area prominent along edges of diaper or plastic or rubber pants
  - Erythematous, macerated folds caused by overlapping skin
- Hygiene problems
  - Any finding listed previously
  - Poor hygiene in general

Differential Diagnosis

Differential diagnoses include contact dermatitis; bacterial, viral, or monilial infection; atopic dermatitis; psoriasis; seborrhea; scabies; and congenital syphilis.

Management

The best treatment is prevention!

1. Keep diaper area dry, clean, and aerated.
   - Frequent diaper changes are essential; every 1 to 2 hours is recommended with one change at night and a minimum of eight changes in a 24-hour period for infants. Cleanse the area well with water at every diaper change and use mild soap, rinsing well following a stool. Avoid vigorous cleansing because this can worsen matters. Avoid using wipes.
   - Use a greasy lubricant if skin is dry.
   - Use a protective barrier ointment or cream, such as Desitin (cod liver oil with zinc oxide), A&D Ointment, Aquaphor, petrolatum, or zinc oxide at the first sign of irritation.
2. Proper use of diapers
   - In addition to frequent changes, use thick or absorbent diapers.
   - Avoid use of rubber or plastic pants.
   - Cloth diapers should be soaked, prerinsed, washed in a mild soap, double rinsed with ¼ cup of vinegar, and dried in the sun if possible.
   - Disposable diapers must be large enough not to bind and should never be worn with rubber pants.
3. Treatment of diaper rash
   - Sitz baths in warm water for 10 to 15 minutes four times a day.
   - Expose diaper area to air by leaving diaper off or by blow-drying with low heat three or four times a day.
   - Burow solution soaks or compresses four times a day if skin is weepy.
   - Diaper cream containing undecylenic acid or zinc oxide to decrease the friction and exposure to moisture.
   - Hydrocortisone 0.5% or 1% applied as a thin layer three times a day for no more than 5 days, especially if skin is dry, for moderate to severe diaper dermatitis. Do not use fluorinated steroids.
   - Increase intake of fluids to dilute urine. In older infants, 2 to 3 ounces of cranberry juice acidifies the urine.
   - If the rash has been present for more than 3 days or if there is no response to the aforementioned measures, add a topical antifungal cream, such as clotrimazole or miconazole. If there is still no response, a trial of oral antifungal is indicated (see Monilial Dermatitis section).
   - Any recalcitrant rash should be referred to a dermatologist.
   - Follow up by phone in 1 to 2 days. If not improved, reassess within 1 week.

Complications

Secondary infection with bacteria, viruses, or fungi can occur (see previous sections). Red flags that could indicate systemic disease or require consultation with a dermatologist include severe erosions or ulcers; bullae or pustules; large papules or nodules, purpura, or petechiae; and redness or scaliness over entire body.

Seborrheic Dermatitis

Seborrhea is a chronic inflammatory dermatitis commonly called *cradle cap* in infants or *dandruff* in adolescents. The condition is thought to be related to overproduction of sebum because it commonly occurs in areas with large numbers of sebaceous glands. It may be an overgrowth of *Malassezia ovalis* (formerly *P. ovale*), a saprophytic yeast, which is universally present on the human body. Seborrhea occurs most often in early infancy and adolescence, is associated with blepharitis, and is more common in spring and summer.

Clinical Findings

History

Note age of onset (infancy or adolescence).

Physical Examination

In infants, erythematous, flaky to thick crusts of yellow, greasy (waxy appearance) scales occur predominantly on the scalp, but also on the face, behind the ears, on the neck and trunk, and in the diaper area (Fig. 37-24). In adolescents there are mild flakes with some erythema and yellow, greasy scales on the scalp, forehead, nasal bridge, and eyebrows; behind the ears; on the face and flexural surfaces; and in intertriginous areas. The dermatitis is not pruritic and has no pustules.

Differential Diagnosis

Atopic dermatitis, psoriasis, *Candida* infection, contact dermatitis, tinea, scabies, and pityriasis rosea are included in the differential diagnoses.

Management

Three categories of agents may be helpful in the treatment of seborrheic dermatitis in both infants and adolescents. These include antifungal agents, anti-inflammatory agents, and keratolytic agents (Goldenberg, 2013):

- Antifungal: Azoles, selenium sulfide
- Anti-inflammatory: Topical steroids, topical calcineurin inhibitors

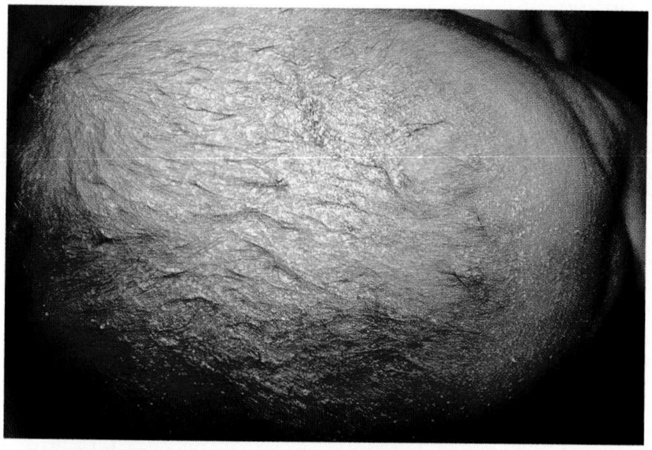

• **Figure 37-24** Seborrheic dermatitis. (From Cohen B: *Pediatric dermatology*, ed 4, Philadelphia, 2013, Saunders/Elsevier.)

- Keratolytic (remove excess scale): Topical salicylic acid, urea

Seborrhea in infants may be self-limited, typically resolving spontaneously in the first year of life (Cohen, 2013). There are no FDA-approved medical treatments for seborrheic dermatitis in children younger than 2 years old (Schmidt, 2011).

- Mineral oil may be applied to the scalp for 5 to 10 minutes before shampooing with a mild shampoo. Scales can be removed with a soft brush or toothbrush (Weston and Morelli, 2013). For thicker scales, the scalp may be soaked in warmed mineral oil overnight then washed with a mild shampoo (Schmidt, 2011).
- Treatment for adolescents with seborrheic dermatitis includes (Schmidt, 2011):
  - Facial dermatitis
    - Daily ketoconazole 2% topical preparations (cream, shampoo, gel, or foam)
    - Intermittent use of low-potency topical corticosteroids (0.05% desonide cream or lotion)
    - Calcineurin inhibitors are good for face and ears
  - Scalp dermatitis
    - Medicated shampoos (tar, salicylic acid, ketoconazole, or selenium sulfide) two or three times a week (one to four times per month for African Americans) alternated with prescription-strength shampoos (ketoconazole 2.5%, selenium sulfide 2.5%) (Schmidt, 2011). Shampoo should be left on the scalp for 5 to 10 minutes before scrubbing crusts and then rinsing.
    - Topical corticosteroids added weekly for recalcitrant dermatitis (leave-in foams or solutions work best)
- Body and skinfold seborrheic dermatitis: The same regimens mentioned previously can be used on the body.

Educate parents about the etiology, control measures, and the need to continue treatment for a few days after resolution, and arrange for follow-up in 1 to 2 weeks.

Complications

Secondary infection with bacteria or *Candida* can occur. Severe, generalized seborrhea is commonly found in persons infected with HIV.

Drug Eruptions

Drugs taken systemically can result in a variety of skin reactions. The two most common types of drug-related eruptions found in children are a morbilliform (measles-like) rash (also called an *exanthematous reaction* manifested by erythematous macules and/or papules) and urticaria typified by erythematous wheals (Table 37-9). Morbilliform rash is discussed here and urticaria is discussed later in the section on vascular reactions. Although not described in this chapter, other drug-related dermatologic reactions include acute generalized exanthematous pustulosis, drug hypersensitivity syndrome, serum sickness-like reaction, vasculitis, fixed drug eruption, acneiform eruptions, and SJS.

The morbilliform, or exanthematous, rash is the most common allergic skin reaction to a drug (Fig. 37-25). The rash may be an immunologic or nonimmunologic reaction to the drug. The most common drugs causing reactions are nonsteroidal anti-inflammatory drugs (NSAIDs), penicillins, cephalosporins, and sulfonamide antibiotics (including TMP-SMX combinations), anticonvulsants, and oral fluconazole or ketoconazole antifungal drugs (Weston and Morelli, 2013). The risk of this type of eruption is increased if the child also has a viral infection (e.g., the rash that appears after giving penicillin to a child with Epstein-Barr virus). Exanthematous rashes typically have their onset within 1 to 2 weeks of starting a new medication and can occur after the medication has been stopped. If there is a rechallenge of that medication, the reaction can occur within a few days (Paller and Mancini, 2011). Repeated exposure can progress to anaphylaxis.

Clinical Findings

History

- Medication taken within the past 3 weeks
- Varying degrees of itching—can be intense
- Rash worsens even after medicine is discontinued for up to 5 days
- Possible systemic symptoms—low-grade fever, arthralgia, arthritis, lymphadenopathy, edema

Physical Examination

Findings include the following:

- Condition often begins as a fairly symmetric, macular erythematous rash that becomes papular and confluent.
- Patches of normal skin are scattered throughout areas of involvement.
- Rash begins on the trunk, where it is a brighter red, more confluent, and extends distally to the extremities, including the palms and soles.
- Rash may turn brownish red and desquamate in 7 to 14 days.

TABLE 37-9 Differentiating Drug Eruptions, Urticaria, and Erythema Multiforme

	Drug Eruption	Urticaria	Erythema Multiforme
Etiology	Reaction to medication, especially penicillin, cephalexin, erythromycin, sulfa drugs, NSAIDs, barbiturates, isoniazid, carbamazepine, phenytoin	Hypersensitive reaction; immunologic antigen-antibody response to release of histamines; often unknown cause; possible reaction to food, drug, insect bite or sting, pollen; possible reaction to infection, especially streptococcal, sinus, mononucleosis, hepatitis	Immune-mediated hypersensitivity reaction often to infection, especially HSV; also to many other agents
Clinical findings	Symmetric, macular, erythematous to papular, confluent morbilliform rash; intense itching; patches of normal skin throughout; begins on trunk, extends distally, including palms and soles; face with confluent erythema	Key finding: Appears suddenly, fades in 20 minutes to 24 hours Family history of hives; possible atopy; intense itching; mild erythema, annular, raised wheals with pale centers; lesions scattered or coalesced; blanch with pressure; associated edema of eyelids, lips, tongue, hands, feet	Key finding: Target or iris lesions: Lesions fixed, symmetric, typical distribution on hands, feet, elbows, knees, also face, neck, trunk History of infection, especially herpes labialis; variety of lesions on skin and mucous membranes—macules, papules, vesicles, early lesions, such as, urticaria; possible oral mucous membrane involvement
Treatment	Stop drug and label as allergen to the child; give antihistamine, antipruritic, prednisone if severe; lubricate skin; rash can last 7 to 14 days; use medical alert bracelet	Quick resolution; identify and remove offending agent if possible and treat; stop antibiotic; give oral antihistamines; topical antipruritics; epinephrine or prednisone if anaphylactic, angioedema, or refractory; refer if >6 weeks' duration	Identify, treat, discontinue trigger if possible; treat infection; supportive measures for hydration, prevention of secondary infection, relief of pain; oral antihistamines, cool compresses; oral lesions—mouthwash, topical anesthetics; lesions last 5 to 7 days, recur in batches over 2 to 4 weeks, resolve without scarring or sequelae

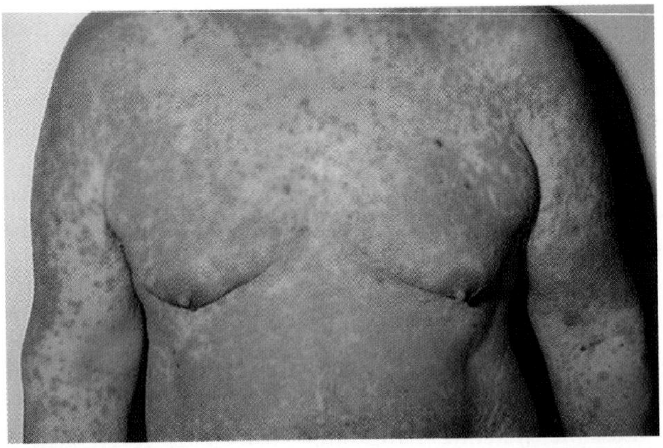

• **Figure 37-25** Allergic drug reaction. (From Lookingbill DP, Marks JG: *Principles of dermatology*, ed 2, Philadelphia, 1993, Saunders, p 218.)

- The face often has confluent areas of erythema.
- Mucous membranes are typically spared.

Diagnostic Studies

The following are ordered if necessary for differential diagnosis:

- CBC, monospot test, C-reactive protein (CRP), anti-nuclear antibodies, anti-streptolysin O (ASO), cold agglutinins
- Chest radiograph

Differential Diagnosis

Viral exanthem; measles; toxic erythema, such as in scarlet fever, staphylococcal scarlatina, or Kawasaki disease; TSS; roseola; and erythema infectiosum are included in the differential diagnosis.

Management

Decisions about whether a drug is to be implicated depend on the patient's previous history of taking the drug, the experience of the general population with the drug, the morphology and timing of the rash, and other possible explanations for the rash (e.g., viral illness). The following steps are taken:

1. Discontinue the suspected drug.
2. Label the patient's medical record with the potential allergen.
3. Prescribe antihistamines if itching is present; recommend a lubricant and antipruritics as adjuncts.

4. Systemic steroids are not usually indicated in a morbilliform drug eruption (Newell and Horii, 2010). If severe reaction, give prednisone 1 to 2 mg/kg/day for 5 to 7 days.
5. Schedule follow-up visit as determined by severity of reaction and other illness.

Refer to allergist for skin testing to confirm allergy if there are limited or no alternative medications, for desensitization, to clarify drug allergy, for severe parental anxiety, or if symptoms are severe and life threatening.

Complications

Body heat and water loss can occur if the rash is severe. Progression of the rash if medicine is continued can lead to toxic epidermal necrolysis (TEN) or SJS (see Erythema Multiforme, Stevens-Johnson Syndrome, Toxic Epidermal Necrolysis section) or allergic interstitial nephritis.

Patient and Family Education

- The rash can last 7 to 14 days with itching, and it may worsen before getting better.
- There is potential risk from further exposure to that drug or related ones; alternative therapies should be explained.
- Identification and communication of the child's allergy are imperative. If the child has a life-threatening allergy, wearing a medical alert bracelet or necklace is essential.

Vascular Reactions of the Skin

Urticaria and Angioedema

Urticaria and angioedema are hypersensitivity reactions (usually a type I reaction—immunoglobulin E [IgE] mediated) commonly called *hives* (Fig. 37-26). Urticaria involves the superficial dermis; in contrast, angioedema involves the deeper dermis and subcutaneous tissue.

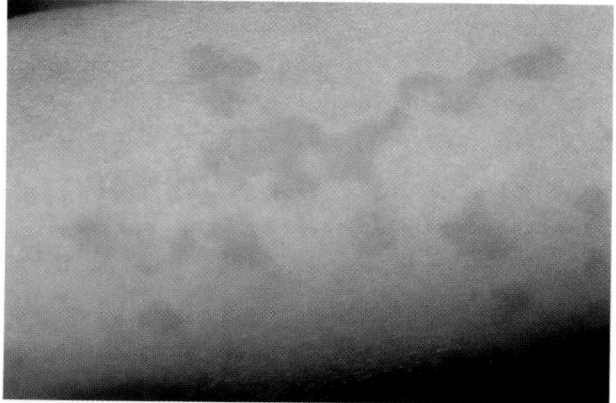

• **Figure 37-26** Urticaria. (From Weston WL, Lane AT, Morelli JG: *Color textbook of pediatric dermatology*, ed 4, St. Louis, 2007, Mosby/Elsevier, p 259.)

Urticaria and angioedema are the result of a complex interplay of immunologically mediated antigen-antibody responses to the release of histamine from mast cells and other vasoactive mediators, such as leukotrienes and prostaglandins. Vasodilation and increased vascular permeability cause erythema and the characteristic wheal of urticaria. Onset is usually rapid, and resolution occurs within a few days of onset. Possible causative factors include the following:

- Reactions to foods (e.g., nuts, eggs, shellfish, strawberries, tomatoes), stings (e.g., bees, wasps, scorpions, spiders, jellyfish), bites (e.g., mosquitoes, fleas, mites), parasites (scabies), or pollen
- Reaction to skin contact with antigens, such as chemicals, latex, fish, or caterpillars
- Response to bacterial, viral, or fungal infections, especially streptococcal or sinus infection, mononucleosis, hepatitis, adenoviruses, and enteroviruses
- Cholinergic response to physical stimuli (e.g., heat or cold, sun or water [aquagenic urticaria], tight clothing, vibrations) or stress
- Reaction to drugs (about 10% of urticaria, usually acute in nature; salicylates and penicillins are the two most common) (Paller and Mancini, 2011)
- Genetic origin
- Concurrent with inflammatory systemic diseases (e.g., collagen-vascular or inflammatory bowel disease)
- Immunologic (rare)
- Idiopathic or unknown

Portals of entry for the causative agent include infection (most common), ingestion, injection, or inhalation.

Urticaria and angioedema are more common in children than adults, and about 50% of patients with urticaria also have angioedema. Children who get both angioedema and urticaria tend to have more severe reactions.

Urticaria occurs sometime in the lives of about 15% of the population. Transient or acute urticaria lasts less than 6 weeks; chronic, recurrent, or persistent urticaria lasts more than 6 weeks.

Angioedema is an extension of the reaction into the subcutaneous tissue with indistinct borders, and tends to involve the face (especially the eyes), hands, and feet (Weston and Morelli, 2013). It is gradual in onset and often involves reactions to medication. Hereditary angioedema is a rare autosomal dominant disorder that results from either a deficiency or dysfunction of the first component of complement (C-esterase inhibitor). It is life threatening and usually manifests before 10 years old, typically with exacerbations in adolescence, often following trauma (e.g., dental work, surgery, or accident). It is manifested by repeated episodes of swelling of the extremities, face, and throat, accompanied by abdominal pain that becomes progressively more severe (Paller and Manicini, 2011). Severe airway edema, if untreated, is often the cause of death.

Clinical Findings

History

- Family or previous history of hives, angioedema, connective tissue disease, juvenile arthritis
- Possibility of atopy
- Intense itching and scratching
- Ingestion (within 4 hours) of nuts, shellfish, chocolate, berries, spices, egg white, milk, fish, sesame
- Ingestion or injection of medicines (e.g., penicillin, sulfa drugs, sedatives, diuretics, analgesics, acetylsalicylic acid), additives, or preservatives
- Injection of diagnostic agents, vaccine, insect venom, blood
- Infection with upper respiratory infectious agent, virus, streptococcus, mononucleosis; hepatitis; parasites
- Inhalation of animal dander, pollen, dust, smoke, or aerosols
- Flea or mite bites
- Cold, heat, exercise, sun, water, pressure, or vibration

Physical Examination

Location of lesions may help determine the cause (e.g., a lesion around the mouth or tongue is likely due to an ingested agent). Findings can include the following:

- Urticaria is seen as mildly erythematous, annular, raised wheals or welts with pale centers from 2 mm to several centimeters in diameter; however, they can be of various shapes. Such lesions typically:
  - Are scattered or coalesced but generalized
  - Appear suddenly as individual lesions and fade in anywhere from 20 minutes to less than 24 hours, reappearing in other areas later; if fixed more than 48 hours, it is not urticaria
  - Blanch with pressure
  - Seem to be intensified with heat
  - Appear as wheals after rubbing or stroking the skin (dermatographism)
  - Occur most commonly as papulovesicular lesions with central punctate lesion and wheals in toddlers (papular urticaria)
  - Can appear as large, blotchy, erythematous lesions with 1- to 3-mm central wheals (cholinergic urticaria)
- Angioedema is seen as asymmetric, localized, nondependent and transient edema.
  - Typically less pruritic than urticaria
  - May involve the upper airway and progress to life-threatening obstruction
  - Can cause associated edema of eyelids, lips, tongue, hands, feet, and genitalia

Diagnostic Studies

If urticaria with possible anaphylaxis from an insect bite is suspected, refer to an allergist for testing and hyposensitization. If fever is present, evaluate for underlying disease.

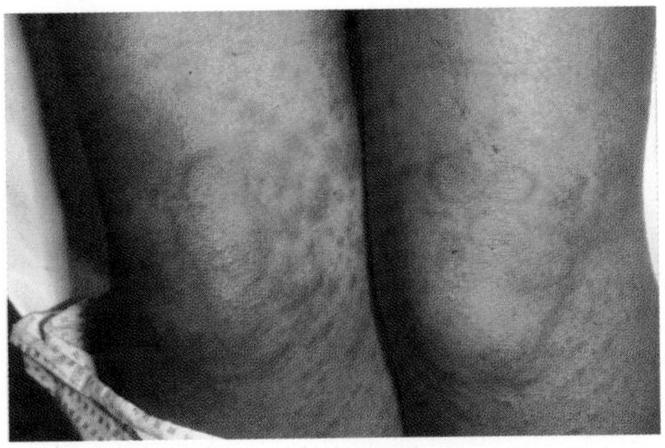

• **Figure 37-27** Erythema multiforme. (From Arndt KA, Wintroub BU, Robinson JK, et al: *Primary care dermatology*, Philadelphia, 1997, Saunders.)

Differential Diagnosis

Contact dermatitis, atopic dermatitis, scabies, erythema multiforme (lesions are fixed with dusky centers and appear within 72 hours; Fig. 37-27), mastocytosis, reactive erythemas, vasculitis, psoriasis, and juvenile arthritis are also included in the differential diagnosis (see Table 37-9).

Management

Control of symptoms is the main goal of treatment. The following steps are taken:

1. Identify and remove the offending substance if possible. Stop all antibiotics. Avoid any possible food or environmental trigger.
2. Test for dermatographism by stroking the skin, for cholinergic urticaria by applying heat or observing immediately after exercising, for cold urticaria by applying cold packs, for pressure urticaria by applying weighted bands for several minutes, and for water urticaria by applying wet compresses.
3. Administer medications as indicated.
   - Oral antihistamines, such as diphenhydramine 0.5 to 1 mg/kg/dose every 4 to 6 hours as needed (maximum 50 mg/dose and 300 mg/day) or hydroxyzine 0.6 mg/kg/dose every 6 hours as needed (400 mg/day maximum) until itching and urticaria are resolved. Nonsedating antihistamines are less effective, but if needed, astemizole, cetirizine, or loratadine are best. Urticaria is less likely to recur if the antihistamine is continued for 1 to 2 weeks after resolution.
   - Topical antipruritics may be helpful.
   - Aqueous epinephrine 1:1000 (subcutaneously 0.01 mL/kg up to 0.3 mL) may be needed if anaphylaxis or significant angioedema with swelling of the face, mucous membranes, and airway is present.
   - Prednisone: 1 to 2 mg/kg/day for 1 week with rapid taper only if refractory to other measures or if angioedema is present with swelling of lips and face.
4. Follow-up visit if not improved within 48 hours.

Chronic urticaria persisting longer than 6 weeks needs evaluation for infection or systemic causes or referral for further evaluation.

An emergency epinephrine kit (EpiPen Jr, 0.15 mg; or adult, 0.3 mg) should be prescribed for children after the first episode or with recurrent episodes of life-threatening urticaria or angioedema.

Complications

Angioedema or anaphylaxis occurs by the same mechanism as urticaria.

- Anaphylactic symptoms require emergency intervention.
- Serum sickness begins with hives, but has other systemic symptoms (e.g., fever, arthralgias, malaise, lymphadenopathy, or proteinuria).
- If urticaria is from a drug reaction, rechallenge with the drug is more likely to cause anaphylaxis.

Patient and Family Education

The following are needed:

- Explanation of causes (often unknown), course, and treatment. The entire episode usually resolves in 24 to 48 hours, rarely extending beyond 3 to 4 weeks. Further evaluation is needed only if urticaria lasts longer than 8 weeks.
- Papular urticaria hypersensitivity often declines within 6 to 12 months.
- Physical urticarias last 2 to 4 years in most cases, but occasionally persist into adulthood.
- Occasionally macular blue-brown lesions are found on resolution of urticaria.
- Avoid allergen if known; wear a medical alert bracelet in case severe reaction occurs. Refer for hyposensitization if life-threatening symptoms occur.
- Carry an epinephrine kit if indicated.

Erythema Multiforme, Stevens-Johnson Syndrome, Toxic Epidermal Necrolysis

In the past, erythema multiforme minor, Stevens-Johnson syndrome (SJS) (also known as *erythema multiforme major*), and toxic epidermal necrolysis (TEN) were thought to be related disorders. However, erythema multiforme minor is a distinct disorder that does not progress to SJS or TEN. Erythema multiforme is an acute, usually benign, self-limited eruption characterized by target lesions and minor mucosal involvement (papules and varying bullae); it is rarely associated with complications. SJS and TEN are considered to represent a distinct syndrome that occurs with variable expression along a continuum. SJS and TEN are associated with significant risk of morbidity and mortality.

Erythema multiforme usually follows an infection, with approximately 80% of cases of classic erythema multiforme attributed to HSV, in particular, herpes labialis or progenitalis lesion(s) (see Fig. 37-31). The herpetic lesion may have healed or had a subclinical presentation but led to an immune response in the body. Erythema multiforme tends to be recurrent as do herpes lesions. Erythema multiforme may also be associated with other viruses, such as EBV, cytomegalovirus (CMV), and other herpesviruses (Weston and Morelli, 2013).

Clinical Findings

History

- With erythema multiforme
  - Recent or current infection with herpes virus (herpes labialis or progenitalis)
  - Exposure to UV light or trauma to area
  - Low-grade fever, malaise, and myalgia
- With SJS or TEN
  - SJS is usually caused by medication or viral illness
  - SJS can have a prodrome of high fever, cough, sore throat, vomiting, diarrhea, chest pain, and arthralgia that usually lasts 1 to 3 days (but can last from 1 to 14 days) followed by the onset of lesions
  - TEN is nearly exclusively caused by medication (Treat, 2010)
  - TEN begins with a fever, sore throat, malaise, and generalized sunburn-like erythema

Physical Examination

It is important to differentiate the clinical findings of erythema multiforme from SJS and TEN.

- In erythema multiforme
  - Lesions vary from patient to patient, within a single episode, and with recurrence.
  - Lesions initially appear dusky, as red macules or edematous papules that evolve into target lesions with multiple, concentric rings of color change.
  - Lesions are fixed (another diagnostic clue), tend to be symmetric, and have a typical distribution predominantly on the face, extensor surface of the arms and legs, dorsum of the hands and feet, and the palms and soles.
  - The oral mucosa is commonly involved, and 50% of children will present with shallow oral lesions (Weston and Morelli, 2013).
- In SJS or TEN
  - SJS skin lesions typically are erythematous macules on the head and neck and can spread to the trunk and extremities with blister formation (within hours) that is often hemorrhagic, extensive, and confluent; mucosal involvement of eyes, nose, and mouth is widespread.
  - The TEN rash has rapidly coalescing target lesions and widespread bullae that become full-thickness epidermal peeling or sloughing within 24 hours; Nikolsky sign (peeling of skin with a light rub that reveals a moist red surface) is present. Conjunctivae, urethra, rectum, oral and nasal mucosa, larynx, and tracheobronchial mucosa may or may not be involved with TEN.

Diagnostic Studies

Studies are ordered as indicated by the clinical condition of the child.

Differential Diagnosis

Urticaria can be differentiated by lack of itching, lability of lesions, and shorter-lasting hives that are pale centrally, not target or iris lesions (see Table 37-9). Viral exanthems are more centrally located, confluent, and less erythematous. Purpura is present in vasculitis. In SSSS, the skin peels superficially (not full thickness) and is significantly red. Also included in the differential diagnosis are Kawasaki disease and lupus erythematosus.

Management

Care for erythema multiforme is generally supportive because the condition is self-limited.

- Symptomatic and supportive care: Maintain hydration, prevent secondary infection, and relieve pain.
  - Mild analgesics, cool compresses, and oral antihistamines, such as diphenhydramine
  - Soothing mouthwashes or topical anesthetics, such as Kaopectate or Maalox, mixed in equal parts with diphenhydramine
  - Topical intraoral anesthetics, such as dyclonine liquid or viscous lidocaine, are sometimes used with caution in older children and adolescents
  - Débridement of oral lesions with half-strength hydrogen peroxide
  - Wound care
  - IV fluids if oral hydration is not adequate
  - Systemic antihistamines, analgesics, and antimicrobials as needed
- Prevention of herpes simplex: Avoid sun exposure and use sunscreen and protective clothing.
- Prophylaxis for recurrent erythema multiforme treatment:
  - Oral acyclovir, for child weighing less than 40 kg, 20 mg/kg/day divided twice daily, or weighing more than 40 kg, 400 mg/day divided twice daily, for a 6- to 12-month trial with periodic stopping to reassess.
  - Acyclovir during an acute episode of erythema multiforme does not alter its course.

SJS and TEN are potentially life-threatening diseases. Children are typically admitted to the pediatric intensive care unit (PICU) or burn unit for wound care, management of hydration and electrolyte issues, nutritional support, and pain control. IVIG should be started as quickly as possible in order to reverse the blistering and sloughing. The use of systemic corticosteroids is contraindicated in the treatment of SJS and TEN because of the increased risk of sepsis (Treat, 2010).

Complications

SJS and TEN are associated with significant morbidity including pneumonitis, sepsis, gastrointestinal bleeding, renal disease, keratitis, and other ophthalmologic disorders.

Patient and Family Education

Erythema multiforme lesions can erupt in crops that last 1 to 3 weeks, but resolve without scarring or sequelae, except for transient desquamation, scaling, or hyperpigmentation. Recurrence of erythema multiforme is common.

Papulosquamous Eruptions of the Skin

Pityriasis Rosea

Pityriasis rosea, meaning rose-colored flaking, is a common, mild, self-limited papulosquamous disease (Fig. 37-28).

The etiology of pityriasis rosea has not been established. There is debate as to whether it is caused by human herpesvirus 6 or 7 (HHV-6 or HHV-7). It is minimally contagious and occurs most commonly in the fall, early winter, and spring in temperate climates. Fifty percent of all cases occur before 20 years old, most commonly in adolescence, with males and females equally affected. Approximately 98% of cases result in lifelong immunity (Paller and Mancini, 2011).

Clinical Findings

History

Although most are otherwise well, a small percentage (5%) of patients experience a prodrome of mild symptoms including malaise, pharyngitis, lymphadenopathy, and headache before onset of rash. Those that have prodromal symptoms tend to have a more florid rash.

Physical Examination

- Herald spot or patch (70% of presentations): a 2- to 5-cm solitary, ovoid, slightly erythematous lesion with a finely scaled slightly elevated border that enlarges quickly with central clearing); typical locations for the herald patch include the trunk, upper arm, neck, or thigh.
- Secondary generalized lesions appear that are symmetric, small macular to papular, thin and round to oval. The lesions have thin scales centrally with thicker scales peripherally ("collarette" scales surround the lesions). They are also pale pink; more common on trunk and proximal extremities from neck to knees; typically spare the face, scalp, and distal extremities; and usually occur 2 to 21 days after the appearance of the herald patch (key finding).
- Christmas tree pattern—rash, especially on back, follows dermatome skin lines with oval lesions running parallel and wrapping around the trunk horizontally.
- Itching occurs in about 25% of cases particularly with secondary lesions.
- Oral lesions have punctate hemorrhages, erosions or ulcerations, erythematous macules, or annular plaques; such lesions occur in about 16% of patients.
- An atypical presentation can occur with lesions involving areas that are usually spared (e.g., the face, axilla, and/or groin). The face and neck are frequent areas of involvement in young children, especially African American children (Paller and Mancini, 2011).

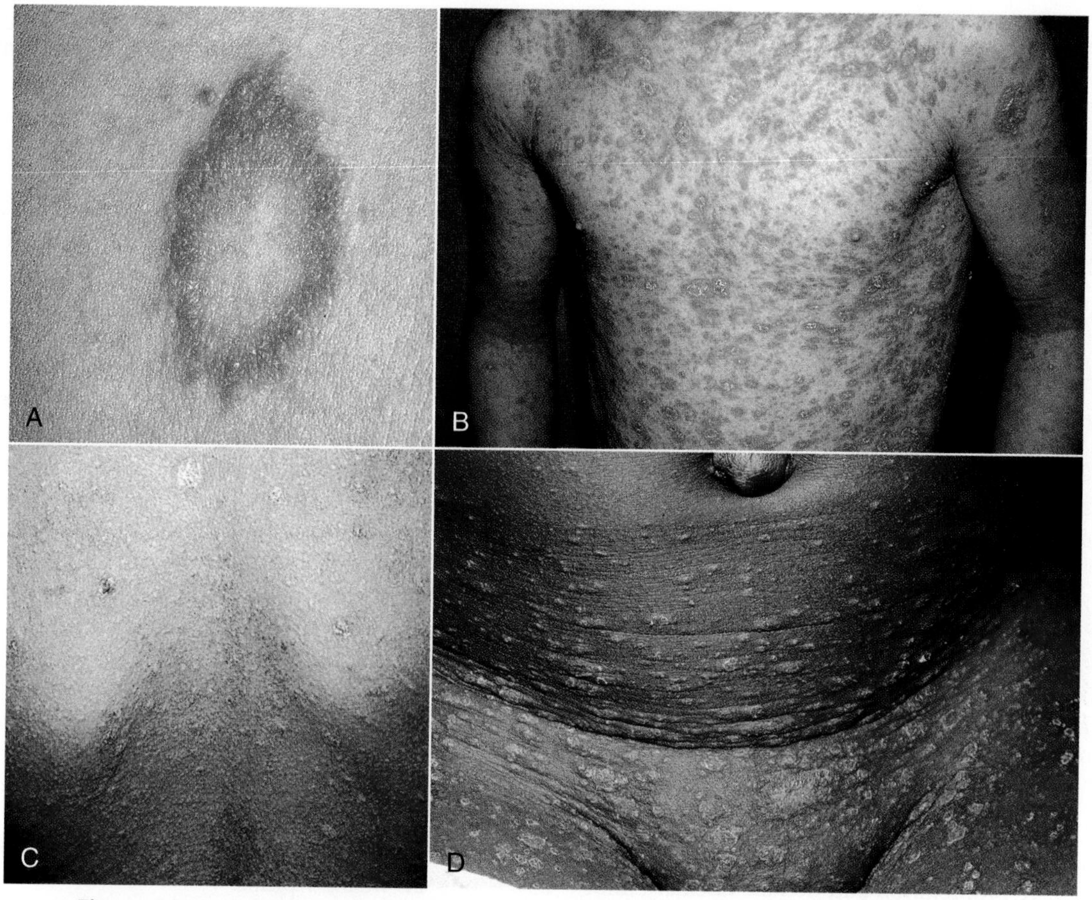

• **Figure 37-28** **A,** Herald patch. **B,** Numerous oval lesions on chest of white teenager. **C,** Christmas tree pattern on the back of a black adolescent. **D,** Small, papular lesions as well as larger scaly patches most prominent on abdomen and thighs of 5-year-old female. (From Cohen B: *Pediatric dermatology*, ed 4, Philadelphia, 2013, Saunders/Elsevier.)

Diagnostic Studies

If needed, a KOH preparation of a skin scraping is done to rule out tinea.

Differential Diagnosis

Include psoriasis, guttate psoriasis, nummular eczema, scabies, tinea (especially the herald patch), secondary syphilis, drug eruptions, or viral exanthems in the differential diagnosis.

Management

The following steps are taken:

- Application of calamine lotion (or other lotions containing menthol and/or camphor or pramoxine), tepid baths with Aveeno, antihistamines, and emollients as needed for itching.
- Topical steroids do not change the lesions or hasten recovery.
- Minimal sun exposure can help lesions resolve more quickly. Prevent sunburn.
- Oral erythromycin 250 mg four times a day for 2 weeks may hasten the resolution of the eruption (Weston and Morelli, 2013).

Patient and Family Education

Pityriasis rosea is a benign, self-limited, and noncontagious disease that has three cycles (emerging, persisting, and fading) with spontaneous resolution in 6 to 12 weeks. Transient pigmentary changes can occur, especially in African Americans. Recurrence is common.

Psoriasis

Psoriasis, a chronic papulosquamous skin disorder with spontaneous remissions and exacerbations, is characterized by thick silvery scales, varied distribution patterns, and an isomorphic (Koebner phenomenon) response (Fig. 37-29). Types of psoriasis include guttate psoriasis (following a streptococcal infection), psoriasis vulgaris, napkin psoriasis (occurring in the diaper area), inverse psoriasis (limited to areas that are normally spared), localized pustular psoriasis, generalized pustular or psoriatic erythroderma, and psoriatic arthritis.

Psoriasis is an immune-mediated disorder associated with genetic predisposition and environmental risk factors. Though the exact cause is unknown, chromosome 6p21.3 is linked to the development of psoriasis, and the

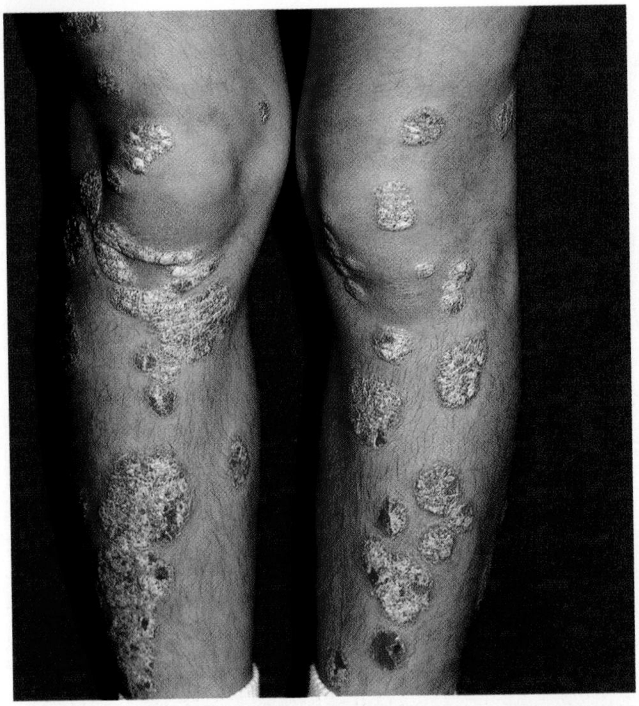

• **Figure 37-29** Psoriasis. (From Paller AS, Mancini AJ: *Hurwitz clinical pediatric dermatology: a textbook of skin disorders of childhood and adolescence*, ed 3, Philadelphia, 2006, Saunders/Elsevier, p 86.)

contributing gene is termed PSORSI. The disease results from keratinocyte proliferation and dermal vascular abnormalities. Trigger factors include infection, local trauma, stress (physical and psychological), and certain drugs (corticosteroids, lithium, beta-blockers, NSAIDs).

Psoriasis occurs at all ages; 30% of cases have onset in childhood (Lyon, 2011). Guttate psoriasis is often the first sign of psoriasis in children.

Clinical Findings

History

- The etiology of psoriasis includes both genetic and environmental factors; more than one third of patients have a family history of psoriasis (Cohen, 2013)
- Streptococcal infection of the oropharynx or perianal area before onset (guttate)
- Trauma before onset
- Itching (variable)

Physical Examination

- The scalp (encircling the hairline and external ears), elbows, knees, and buttocks (especially the diaper area in infants) are the most common sites of involvement. In children, the face may also be involved. Lesions are often found around areas of trauma (e.g., genitalia, palms, soles).
  - Plaque psoriasis: Discrete, initially erythematous, symmetric, well-marginated rash becoming papular with silver scales that may be trivial to widespread.
  - Guttate (teardrop) psoriasis: Widespread, symmetric, round, or oval 0.5- to 2-cm lesions occurring primarily on the trunk and proximal extremities, occasionally on the face, scalp, and ears and rarely on the palms or soles. There is less scaling than in psoriasis vulgaris.
  - Psoriasis vulgaris: Well-circumscribed, erythematous plaques with thick, silvery white scales concentrated on elbows, knees, scalp, and hairline, but also seen on eyebrows, around ears, and in intergluteal fold and genital area.
  - Koebner phenomenon (isomorphic response): Psoriatic lesions occur in areas of local injury, such as scratches, surgical scars, or sunburns.
  - Auspitz sign: Bleeding occurs when a scale is removed.
  - Nail signs: Nails have "ice pick" pits and ridges, are thick and discolored (yellowing), can have splinter hemorrhages or subungual hyperkeratosis, and can be separated from the nailbed (Lyon, 2011).
  - Napkin or diaper area psoriasis: Appears eczematous with sharply defined plaques, bright red coloration, shiny with large drier scales, affecting inguinal and gluteal folds.

Diagnostic Studies

- ASO if guttate pattern
- KOH-treated scrapings and culture to rule out fungal infection
- Venereal Disease Research Laboratory (VDRL) to rule out secondary syphilis

Differential Diagnosis

Pityriasis rosea, seborrhea, *Candida* infection, contact or irritant dermatitis, atopic dermatitis, tinea, dyshidrosis, secondary syphilis, and other nail-pitting conditions are included in the differential diagnosis.

Management

In children, treatment should be as conservative as possible. Medications and treatments should be rotated for best effectiveness. The following are treatment options:

- Sun exposure in moderate amounts alleviates lesions. Prevent sunburn.
- Emollient creams (such as, petrolatum, Eucerin, Aquaphor, or Cetaphil) for dry skin can minimize trauma and subsequent psoriasis and may improve psoriasis.
- Apply topical steroids two or three times a day for 2 to 3 weeks. They should be used intermittently but not discontinued spontaneously, because worsening can occur. Monitoring of the child during use is important. Small, localized lesions can be treated with topical fluorinated steroids. A moderate-potency steroid can be used on thick plaques and larger areas. Severe plaques on the elbows and knees may need a higher-potency steroid (see Table 37-1). Systemic steroids are not indicated and may worsen the condition, causing pustular flare.
- Tar or keratolytic shampoos (ketoconazole, anthralin, salicylic acid) can be used on the scalp.

- Mineral or olive oil and warm towels to soak and remove thick plaques.
- Follow up every 2 weeks until psoriasis is controlled and during exacerbations and then as needed.

A child with psoriasis necessitates a referral to the dermatologist and additional treatments that may be prescribed include:

- Keratolytic agents, such as sulfur 3% or salicylic acid 3% to 6%, to reduce thick, unresponsive plaques. Salicylic acid blocks UVB and should not be used in combination with phototherapy.
- Anthralin ointment for plaques that are resistant to steroids and tar. Apply ointment in high strengths (1% and higher) for 10 to 30 minutes once a day, then wash off. In lower strengths, leave on for 8 hours. Strength used is determined by tolerance. Anthralin stains skin and clothing and can irritate skin.
- Calcipotriol, a vitamin D analogue, is effective for mild to moderate plaque psoriasis in adults and children. Available in cream, ointment, and lotion, it is safe, effective, and well tolerated for short- and long-term treatment. Hypercalcemia is reported with application of excessive quantities over large areas.
- Tazarotene is a retinoid that may be effective in management of plaque psoriasis, but is often too irritating for use in childhood psoriasis (Paller and Mancini, 2011).
- Tacrolimus ointment, a calcineurin inhibitor, has demonstrated benefit when used for facial and intertriginous psoriasis in children (Paller and Mancini, 2011).
- UV light therapy may be used for disseminated, chronic, or recalcitrant disease. Narrowband UVB light therapy is preferred in children due to safety and efficacy (Cohen, 2013).
- Cyclosporine and methotrexate are systemic therapies used for recalcitrant and severe disease.
- Other treatment options include psoralens, intralesional steroids, retinoids, cyclosporine, biologic therapy, and immunotherapy.

Complications

The following complications are possible and require referral to a dermatologist:

- *Candida* infection: May be a secondary infection in the diaper area.
- Erythrodermic and pustular psoriasis: Unusual in childhood; characterized by generalized or local multiple 1- to 2-mm pustules with erythema and scaling also involving palms and soles; accompanied by malaise, fever, electrolyte and fluid imbalances, temperature instability, and leukocytosis; can be fatal.
- Exfoliative erythroderma: Rare manifestation, including desquamation and loss of hair and nails with previous history of psoriasis.
- Psoriatic arthritis: An inflammatory arthritis that is rare but increasing in frequency, most common in females 9 to 12 years old. Prognosis is good but should be referred to a rheumatologist.

Patient and Family Education

Emotional support and education are the most important aspects in dealing with psoriasis. Areas for discussion include the following:

- Psoriasis is chronic and involves spontaneous remissions and exacerbations. Control and relief are sought, but cure is not available. Treatment may require up to 1 month to determine effectiveness.
- Guttate psoriasis often resolves with antibiotic treatment for streptococcal infection. Psoriasis vulgaris may persist for months to years.
- Lifestyle changes help prevent recurrence. These include avoiding cutaneous injury, streptococcal infection, sunburn, stress, itching, bites, tight clothes and shoes, some medications (e.g., oral steroids, NSAIDs), and occlusive dressings. Good skin care, including regular use of emollients and avoiding irritating underarm deodorants and harsh soaps, may improve psoriasis and minimize recurrences. With nail involvement, avoid long fingernails or toenails and use of nail polish. Do not vigorously brush or comb hair if scalp area is affected.
- Psoriasis tends to improve during summer and with pregnancy.
- Psoriasis is considered stable if there are either no new plaques or if existing plaques are not enlarging.
- Refer patients to the National Psoriasis Foundation (see Additional Resources).

Lichen Striatus

Lichen striatus (LS) is peculiar to childhood, characterized by unilateral shiny papules along embryonic lines, or lines of Blaschko. Although the etiology is unknown, it is thought to be related to a cutaneous defect from an embryologic mutation of somatic cells. It is most common in school-age children and affects girls more than boys. LS is typically located on the extremities, upper back, or neck, but can be found on the palms, soles, nails, genitals, or face. Lesions spontaneously disappear after 3 to 12 months, but they may last up to 3 years. Short relapses occur on occasion.

Clinical Findings

History

Lesions appear spontaneously without prodrome.

Physical Examination

- Linear, shiny hypopigmented or flesh-colored, flat-topped papules with adherent scale
- Limited to one extremity, initially lesions coalesce in a linear distribution down an extremity
- Lesions involving a nailbed result in nail deformity
- Rarely are lesions noted on the face
- May be asymptomatic or may be intensely pruritic
- May resolve with hypopigmentation that lasts several months

Differential Diagnosis

The unilateral linear lesions are characteristic. However, differential diagnosis includes lichen planus, lichen nitidus, psoriasis, epidermal birthmarks, and linear Darier disease.

Management

Lesions generally resolve without treatment in 1 to 2 years. Lubricants and topical steroids may help to reduce scale and inflammation. Topical tacrolimus ointment has also been reported as a successful treatment option (Cohen, 2013).

Patient and Family Education

LS is a benign, self-limited, noncontagious disorder that results in complete resolution.

Keratosis Pilaris

Keratosis pilaris is a common finding on the extensor aspects of the extremities, buttocks, and occasionally the cheeks. The skin has a typical appearance of "chicken skin" with small bumps at the hair follicle. The etiology is unknown. It is not present at birth but is common from early childhood onward. Some believe it to be a disorder of abnormal keratinization; others believe it is a response to drying of the skin surface. Keratosis pilaris is more common in children with atopic disorders; in those living in cold, dry climates; and in winter months.

Clinical Findings

History

Keratosis pilaris appears spontaneously, without prodrome. It is usually asymptomatic, although most patients are bothered by the appearance and seek treatment.

Physical Examination

- Rough dry skin on the posterior upper arms, anterior thighs, buttocks, and cheeks
- Small papules with follicular plugs of stratum corneum
- Occasional diffuse eruption with small sterile pustules

Diagnostic Studies

Skin biopsy reveals inflammation outside the hair follicle; however, this is typically not needed because the diagnosis is easy to determine.

Differential Diagnosis

Microcomedones of acne, molluscum contagiosum, warts, milia, and folliculitis are often confused with keratosis pilaris.

Management

It is important to recognize keratosis pilaris as a benign disorder to avoid detrimental treatment. Management includes the following:

- In mild cases, lubricants and emollients to moisturize skin are sufficient for improvement.
- Topical keratolytics combined with lactic acid 12%, salicylic acid, urea creams, retinoids, and lubricants are applied several times daily.
- Antibiotics active against *S. aureus* are useful for folliculitis.

Patient and Family Education

The chronic but benign nature of keratosis pilaris should be stressed. Treatment takes weeks to months, and recurrence is common.

Congenital Lesions of the Skin

Vascular and Pigmented Nevi

Nevi are a common finding in children. The two most common types are vascular nevi (vascular malformations and hemangiomas) and pigmented nevi (e.g., mongolian spots, café au lait spots, acquired melanocytic nevi, atypical nevi, and lentigines).

Vascular nevi are caused by a structural abnormality (malformations) or by an overgrowth of blood vessels (hemangiomas) and are flat, raised, or cavernous. Flat lesions or vascular malformations include salmon patches (also called *macular stains*), an innocent malformation that is a light red macule appearing on the nape of the neck, upper eyelids, and glabella. Approximately 60% to 70% of newborns have a salmon patch on the back of the neck. Port-wine stains occur in 0.2% to 0.3% of newborns (Cohen, 2013). At 1 year old, 10% to 12% of Caucasian infants have a hemangioma—females three times more likely than males. There is also an increased incidence of hemangioma in premature neonates. Vascular malformations are always present at birth and do not resolve spontaneously. Precursor lesions of hemangiomas are present at birth 50% of the time. They undergo rapid growth (proliferative stage), stability (plateau phase), and regression (involution phase); 90% are completely resolved in children 9 to 10 years old (Paller and Mancini, 2011).

Pigmented nevi are caused by an overgrowth of pigment cells. Pigmented nevi most commonly seen are mongolian spots (found in up to 90% of African Americans, 62% to 86% of Asians, 70% of Hispanics, and less than 10% of Caucasians), café au lait spots (found in up to 33% of normal children and in 50% of patients with McCune-Albright syndrome), and acquired melanocytic nevi, the most common tumor of childhood. Atypical nevi, also called *dysplastic nevi,* are potential precursors for malignant melanoma. Dysplastic nevi are uncommon under 18 years old but have a higher incidence in melanoma-prone families (Paller and Mancini, 2011).

Clinical Findings

History

- Presence from birth, or age first noted
- Progression of lesion
- Familial tendencies for similar nevi, especially for history of melanoma

Physical Examination

Findings include the following (Box 37-8):

- Vascular malformations or flat vascular nevi are present at birth and grow commensurate with the child's growth.
- Hemangiomas are classified as superficial, deep (cavernous), or mixed. They may or may not be present at birth, but they usually emerge by 2 to 3 weeks of life. They may manifest initially as a pale macule, a telangiectatic lesion, or a bright red nodular papule. After appearing, hemangiomas go through a proliferative phase during which they grow rapidly and form nodular compressible masses, ranging in size from a few millimeters to several centimeters. Occasionally they may cover an entire limb, resulting in asymmetric limb growth. Rapidly growing lesions may ulcerate. The final phase of involution occurs slowly (10% per year) but spontaneously (30% by 3 years old, 50% by 5 years old, 70% by 7 years old, and 90% by 9 to 10 years old). Average involution begins between 12 and 24 months old, heralded by gray areas in the lesion followed by flattening from the center outward. Most hemangiomas appear as normal skin after involution, but others may have residual changes, such as telangiectasias, atrophy, fibrofatty residue, and scarring (Paller and Mancini, 2011).
- Pigmented nevi may be present at birth or acquired during childhood.
- Atypical nevi are larger than acquired nevi; have irregular, poorly defined borders; and have variable pigmentation.

• BOX 37-8 Common Vascular and Pigmented Lesions

I. Vascular malformations or flat vascular nevi
   A. Salmon patch or nevus flammeus: Light pink macule of varying size and configuration. Commonly seen on the glabella, back of neck, forehead, or upper eyelids.
   B. Port-wine stain: Purple-red macules that occur unilaterally and tend to be large. Usually occur on face, occiput, or neck, although they may be on extremities.

II. Hemangiomas
   A. Superficial (strawberry) hemangiomas are found in the upper dermis of the skin and account for the majority of hemangiomas.
   B. Deep cavernous hemangiomas are found in the subcutaneous and hypodermal layers of the skin; although similar to superficial hemangiomas, there is a blue tinge to their appearance. With pressure, there is blanching and a feeling of a soft, compressible tumor. Variable in size, they can occur in places other than skin.
   C. Mixed hemangiomas have attributes of both superficial and deep hemangiomas.

III. Pigmented nevi
   A. Mongolian spots: Blue or slate-gray, irregular, variably sized macules. Common in the presacral or lumbosacral area of dark-skinned infants; also on the upper back, shoulders, and extremities. The majority of the pigment fades as the child gets older and the skin darkens. Solitary or multiple, often covering a large area.
   B. Café au lait spots: Tan to light brown macules found anywhere on the skin; oval or irregular shape; increase in number with age.
   C. Acquired melanocytic nevi are benign, light brown to dark brown to black, flat, or slightly raised, occurring anywhere on the body, especially on sun-exposed areas above the waist.
      1. Junctional nevi represent the initial stage, with tiny, hairless, light brown to black macules.
      2. Compound nevi—a few junctional nevi progress to more elevated, warty, or smooth lesions with hair.
      3. Dermal nevi are the adult form, dome shaped with coarse hair.
      4. Atypical nevi usually appear at puberty, have irregular borders, variegated pigmentation, are larger than normal nevi (6 to 15 mm); usually found on trunk, feet, scalp, and buttocks.
      5. Halo nevi appear in late childhood with an area of depigmentation around a pigmented nevus, usually on trunk (see Fig. 37-34).
   D. Acanthosis nigricans is velvety brown rows of hyperpigmentation in irregular folds of skin, usually the neck and axilla; tags may also be present.
   E. Lentigines are small brown to black macules 1 to 2 mm in size appearing anywhere on the body in school-age children.
   F. Freckles: 1 to 5 mm light brown, pigmented macules in sun-exposed areas.

Differential Diagnosis

Hematomas or ecchymoses of child abuse are occasionally confused with some nevi. Non–insulin-dependent diabetes mellitus (NIDDM) often causes acanthosis nigricans.

Management

1. Flat vascular nevi
   - Salmon patches: Fade with time, usually by 5 or 6 years old; no treatment is needed.
   - Port-wine stains: A permanent defect that grows with the child, so cosmetic covering is often used. If forehead and eyelids are involved, there is potential for multiple syndromes, including Sturge-Weber, Klippel-Trenaunay-Weber, and Parkes Weber. Neurodevelopmental and ophthalmologic follow-up is needed. Referral to a dermatologist for possible laser treatment or cosmesis is required.
2. Hemangiomas
   - Reassure and educate the family about the nature and course of these nevi and that they are not related to anything the mother did during pregnancy.
   - Follow-up frequently, especially during the proliferation phase. Sequential photographs are helpful.
   - If the lesions are strategically placed (eye, lip, oral cavity, ear, airway, diaper area), ulcerating, multiple, very large, or grow very quickly, prompt referral to a dermatologist is indicated because early treatment is most effective. Steroids (intralesional and oral) are prescribed during the proliferation phase until growth is stabilized, then gradually tapered. Indications for steroid treatment are interference with physiologic functions (e.g., breathing, hearing, eating, and vision), recurrent bleeding or ulceration, high-output

congestive heart failure, Kasabach-Merritt syndrome, rapid growth that distorts facial features, or presence in the diaper area. Interferon-alpha may also be used. Treatment by surgery, cryotherapy, radiation, or injecting sclerosing agents often leads to scarring. Large, deep lesions can cause cardiovascular complications, disseminated intravascular coagulation, or compression of internal organs.
- Involution (without treatment) occurs at a rate of 10% per year. Scarring may be present if ulceration occurs; fibrofatty masses, atrophy, and telangiectasis can occur following involution. Laser therapy is effective management for residual telangiectasias (Paller and Mancini, 2011).

3. Pigmented nevi: Educate family about the nature of these lesions.
   - Mongolian spots: Document to distinguish from bruise; fade with time, usually no traces by adulthood.
   - Blue nevus: Heavily pigmented melanocytes in papule or nodule that can develop melanoma.
   - Café au lait spots: If six or more lesions larger than 5 mm in diameter are present in children younger than 15 years old and more than 1.5 cm in diameter for older individuals, or if axillary freckling (Crowe's sign), neurofibromas, or iris hamartomas is also present, refer child to rule out neurofibromatosis, McCune-Albright syndrome, tuberous sclerosis, LEOPARD* syndrome, epidermal nevus syndrome, Bloom syndrome, ataxia-telangiectasia, and Silver-Russell syndrome (Cohen, 2013).
4. Other disorders of hyperpigmentation that can appear in early childhood:
   - Acquired melanocytic nevi: Giant nevi (e.g., bathing trunk nevus). These children are at increased risk of developing melanoma and need referral to a dermatologist.
   - Atypical nevi appear most commonly in adolescents and require regular follow-up because of increased risk for melanoma. However, melanoma often manifests with new lesions rather than from transformation of current ones (see section on burns in Chapter 39 (Fig. 37-30).
   - Halo nevus: A depigmented ring around a pigmented nevus.
   - Spitz nevus: A smooth, pink to brown, dome-shaped papule often occurring on head and neck.
   - Nevus spilus: A light-brown speckled lentiginous nevus with darker papules within it can be congenital or acquired and has potential to develop into melanoma.
5. Guidelines for when a child with a nevus should be referred to a dermatologist are listed in Box 37-9.

*LEOPARD is an acroymn that stands for:
Lentigines (multiple)
Electrocardiographic conduction abnormalities
Ocular hypertelorism
Pulmonary stenosis
Abnormalities of genitalia
Retardation of growth
Deafness

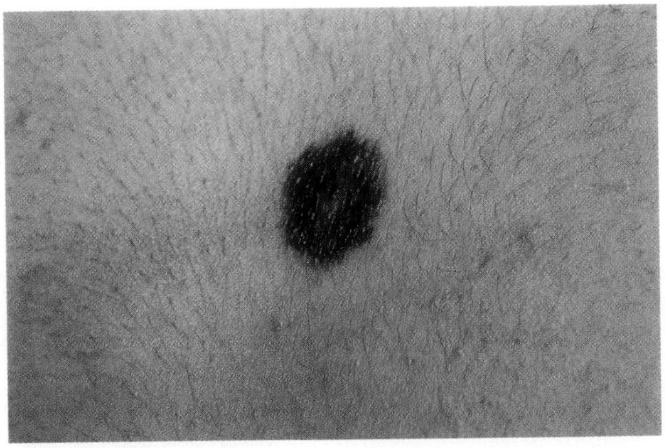

• **Figure 37-30** Atypical nevus with irregular borders and pink background. (Weston WL, Morelli JG: *Pediatric dermatology*, St. Louis, 2013, Elsevier, p 129.)

• BOX 37-9 When to Refer Nevi to a Dermatologist

- Suspicious appearing nevus (as identified by ABCDE signs—asymmetry, border, color, diameter, evolving)
- Rapidly growing or changing nevus
- More than 50 nevi
- One or more atypical nevi
- History of one or more first-degree relatives with melanoma
- Presence of a giant or large congenital nevus
- Signs of excessive sun exposure (increased nevi and freckles in exposed areas)
- History of immunosuppression and multiple nevi on examination

Complications

Ulceration, infection, platelet trapping, airway or visual obstruction, or cardiac decompensation can occur with large vascular nevi. Kasabach-Merritt syndrome occurs when thrombocytopenic hemorrhage occurs in a large, deep hemangioma. Melanoma in congenital nevi is possible. An autosomal dominant, familial, atypical mole and melanoma syndrome has been identified genetically. Children with multiple atypical nevi and family members with melanoma are at risk for childhood melanoma.

Patient and Family Education

Monitoring nevi that are at risk for developing melanoma is important as is teaching the family to watch nevi for any changes. Changes of particular concern are development of an off-center nodule or papule, color change, bleeding, persistent irritation, erosion, ulceration, and rapid growth. See Chapter 39 for more information.

Cutaneous Manifestations of Underlying Disease

Acanthosis Nigricans

Acanthosis nigricans is not a skin disease per se; rather it is typically a sign of an underlying problem. It may be related to:

- Heredity (autosomal dominant trait with no associated obesity): It may appear at birth or during childhood with proliferation during adolescence. Children of Native American, African American, Hispanic, Asian American, and Pacific Islander descent are at increased risk (Thoenes, 2012).
- Endocrine disorders (e.g., insulin resistance, hypothyroidism, hyperandrogenic states, Cushing syndrome)
- Obesity (more commonly seen in darker-pigmented individuals)
- Drug administration (e.g., oral contraceptives, stilbestrol use in young males, high levels of nicotinic acid)
- Malignancy (e.g., adenocarcinoma, Wilms tumor, and less commonly lymphoma)

All but the malignant form of acanthosis nigricans result in papillary hypertrophy, hyperkeratosis, and an increase in the number of melanocytes from keratocyte and dermal fibroblast changes. There is no gender predominance.

Clinical Findings

Acanthosis nigricans is characterized by symmetric, brown thickening of the skin. As time progresses the skin develops a velvety, leathery, warty, or papillomatous surface. The axillary areas (most commonly), neck, groin, belt line, dorsal surfaces of the fingers, in the mouth, around the areola of the breast, and umbilicus can be affected. In areas of maceration, odor or discomfort may be reported (Fig. 37-31).

Differential Diagnosis

Terra firma-forme dermatosis, a condition with lamellar hyperkeratosis, can occur anywhere on the body. Although it can look like dirt, terra firma-forme dermatosis is not related to hygiene and cannot be washed off with soap and water. Unlike acanthosis nigricans, however, the darkened skin of terra firma-forme dermatosis can be removed with vigorous rubbing with isopropyl alcohol. It is important to diagnose terra firma-forme dermatosis in order to avoid an extensive and expensive workup for an endocrine or metabolic disorder.

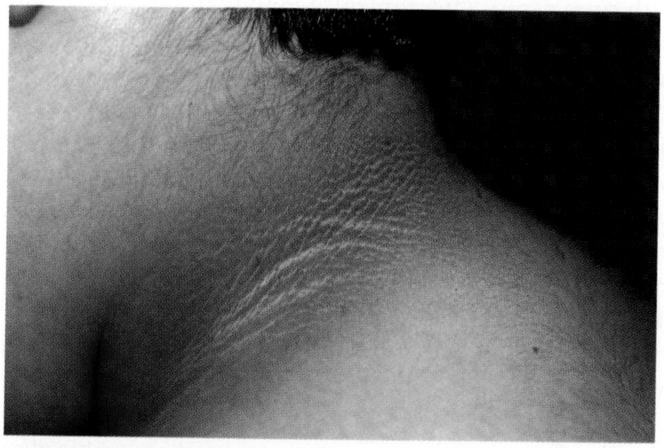

• **Figure 37-31** Acanthosis nigricans. (From Weston WL, Lane AT, Morelli JG: *Color textbook of pediatric dermatology*, ed 4, St. Louis, 2007, Mosby/Elsevier, p 331.)

Management

Treatment consists of addressing the underlying causes. This most commonly includes management of overweight (diet changes and weight loss) and correction of metabolic abnormality (hyperinsulinemia). In nonoverweight individuals, an underlying malignancy must be considered. The skin lesions themselves are benign, usually asymptomatic, and do not require intervention. Thicker lesions may cause discomfort and respond to topical retinoic acid cream or gel once daily. Dermabrasion and long-pulsed alexandrite laser therapy have also been used. Lac-Hydrin (12% lactic acid cream) can help soften lesions.

Patient and Family Education

It is important for patients to understand that acanthosis nigricans may be a cutaneous marker for an underlying condition such as insulin resistance and type 2 diabetes in obese individuals or for a malignancy. Associated tumors include gastric carcinoma, lymphoma, Hodgkin disease, and osteogenic sarcoma (Cohen, 2013). The condition may completely resolve with adequate treatment of the underlying disorder.

Lentigines

Lentigines are small, tan, dark brown or black, flat, oval or circular, sharply circumscribed lesions that appear in childhood and may increase in number until adulthood. They may also be seen on mucous membranes and may fade or disappear with time. Lentigines can be associated with various syndromes including LEOPARD syndrome and Peutz-Jeghers syndrome (Weston and Morelli, 2013).

Other Common Dermatologic Issues in Pediatrics

Vitiligo and Hypopigmentation Disorders

Lack of skin pigment, leaving white or light-colored areas, can be either hypopigmentation or vitiligo. It is congenital or acquired and appears in a diffuse or localized pattern. Vitiligo is presumed to be an immune disorder that has a genetic component. A patterned pigmentation loss with great variation in location, size, and shape of individual lesions, vitiligo occurs in 1% to 2% of the population worldwide, with 50% of cases appearing before 18 years old. Generalized vitiligo occurs most commonly in children, and it is generally associated with other autoimmune disorders, most commonly hypothyroidism (Weston and Morelli, 2013).

Hypopigmentation follows inflammation or injury to the melanocytes in the skin resulting from diseases (such as, atopic dermatitis, psoriasis, or pityriasis rosea), or from abrasions, burns, injury from liquid nitrogen, or severe sunburn.

Clinical Findings

History

- Family history of vitiligo, halo nevi, traumatic depigmentation of skin, or markedly premature graying of the hair (Paller and Mancini, 2011)
- Onset of depigmentation (birth or more recent)
- Presence of any systemic or skin diseases
- Any recent trauma to the skin; Koebner phenomenon is noted in about 15% of children with vitiligo

Physical Examination

- Vitiligo
  - Flat milk-white macules or papules with scalloped, distinct borders of varied size
  - Symmetric or asymmetric, possibly following a nerve segment
  - Few to multiple, seen most commonly on face and trunk
- Hypopigmentation
  - Macules and patches with irregular mottling and borders
  - Linear or patterned
  - May be associated hyperpigmented areas

Diagnostic Studies

For vitiligo, a skin biopsy and CBC, fasting glucose, thyroid function and antithyroid antibodies, early-morning serum cortisol, and VDRL are sometimes indicated. A Wood's light may be helpful in fair-skinned individuals to delineate a contrast between the normal and depigmented skin.

Differential Diagnosis

Pityriasis rosea, pityriasis alba, tinea versicolor, and albinism (which is seen at birth and affects eye color) are included in the differential diagnosis.

Management

The following steps are taken:

- Vitiligo
  - Broad-spectrum sunscreens are used to decrease the tanning of normal skin.
  - Cover-up agents, such as skin dyes and walnut oil, may be used.
  - Mild to moderate steroids may show success in some patients. Topical calcineurin inhibitors (e.g., tacrolimus ointment, pimecrolimus cream) eliminate atrophy, with 40% to 90% of pediatric patients showing a response to these treatments (Paller and Mancini, 2011).
  - Refer for treatment with psoralens, which may be used in combination with UVA radiation (best used in children younger than 9 years old). UVB may also be used.
  - Support groups help families because this can be a highly disfiguring condition, especially for those with dark complexions.
- Hypopigmentation
  - Reassure family that repigmentation will occur. Postinflammatory hypopigmentation is self-limited and lasts only a few months.

Complications

Vitiligo may be associated with other immune disorders or their symptoms, such as thyroid disease, diabetes mellitus, pernicious anemia, Addison disease, uveitis, and alopecia areata. Patients are at risk for severe sunburn.

Hair and Nail Disorders

Alopecia, hair loss from areas of skin that normally produce hair, can be limited to one area or scattered over the scalp and can be complete or leave residual hairs of differing lengths. The three main causes of hair loss are tinea capitis, traumatic alopecia, and alopecia areata (Table 37-10).

Tinea Capitis

Ringworm of the scalp and hair may be seen in four different manifestations: (1) diffuse fine scaling without obvious hair breaks and with subtle to significant hair loss; (2) discrete areas of hair loss with stubs of broken hairs (black-dot ringworm) (Fig. 37-32); (3) "classic" patchy hair loss and scaly lesions with raised borders; and (4) scaly, pustular lesions, or kerions. Tinea capitis occurs in a noninflammatory stage for 2 to 8 weeks and then becomes inflammatory.

The fungus invades the scalp and hair shaft, causing an inflammatory response and hair shaft fragility. *T. tonsurans* and *M. canis* are the most common organisms associated with tinea capitis (Weston and Morelli, 2013). Tinea capitis is transmitted by fomites when humans share hats, combs, and brushes, or by cats, dogs, or rodents. Tinea capitis is the most common dermatophyte infection of childhood, typically found in children 2 to 10 years old (Cohen, 2013; Michaels and Del Rosso, 2012). It is more common in boys and African American children.

Clinical Findings

History

Hair loss, itching, and contact with another person or pet with ringworm are sometimes reported.

Physical Examination

- Scaling, erythema, or crusting usually occurs.
- Bald patches or areas of broken hairs are noted.

TABLE 37-10 Diagnosis and Treatment of Alopecia

	Etiology	Clinical Findings	Treatment
Tinea capitis	*Trichophyton tonsurans* 90% to 95%; *Microsporum canis;* others	Fine diffuse scaling without obvious hair breaks and subtle to significant hair loss; hair loss discrete with stubs of broken hair; patchy hair loss with scaling and raised borders to lesions; scaly, pustular lesions or kerions	Griseofulvin taken with fatty food until 2 weeks after negative culture; prednisone if kerion present; culture family members; sporicidal shampoo; follow up in 2 weeks; launder sheets, clothes, vacuum house
Traumatic alopecia	Chemical, thermal, traction (hairstyling), friction (trichotillomania)	Traumatic: Incomplete hair loss with varying lengths Traction: Erythema and pustules, hair thins and breaks in certain areas, especially linear Trichotillomania: Circumscribed hair loss with irregular borders and broken hair of varied lengths, no erythema or scarring, especially frontal, parietal, or temporal	Traction: Avoid hairstyles that precipitate; use mild shampoo, gentle brushing; short course of antibiotics if pustules are present Trichotillomania: Discussion with parents, oil at night, counseling, behavioral modifications
Alopecia areata	Autoimmune mechanism	Family history; single or multiple round or oval patches of complete or near-complete hair loss; no erythema or scaling, scalp smooth with fine new hair growth, usually frontal or parietal; "exclamation hairs" present; nail ridging or pitting; occasional loss of body or pubic hair	Discussion and support; often self-limited course; if extensive, refer to dermatologist for alternative treatments; supportive care; prescription for wig; refer to National Alopecia Foundation

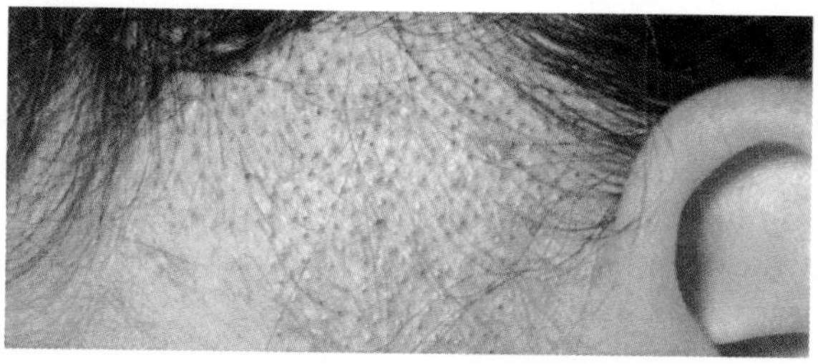

• Figure 37-32 Tinea capitis. (From Aly R, Maibach H: *Atlas of infections of the skin*, Philadelphia, 1999, Saunders, p 20.)

- *T. tonsurans* manifests as black-dot tinea, with tiny black dots that are the remainder of hair that has broken off at the shaft; no scalp scale is present (most common).
- *M. canis* leaves the hair broken and lusterless with a fine gray scale on the scalp.
- Occipital or posterior cervical adenopathy may be significant.
- A kerion is a boggy, inflamed mass filled with pustules. It results from a delayed inflammatory reaction. There may be regional lymphadenopathy, fever, and leukocytosis. The contents of the kerion are sterile.

Diagnostic Studies

Examine hair scrapings as follows:

- Wood's light fluoresces yellow-green (positive with *M. canis,* negative with *T. tonsurans*).
- KOH examination of scraped hair: Wait 20 to 40 minutes after application of KOH to examine. If Wood's light was positive, under microscopy the KOH-prepared outer surface of hair is coated with tiny mats of spores; if Wood's light was negative, hyphae and spores are present in hair shaft.
- Fungal culture of a completely plucked hair with its root (use a Kelly clamp) is most reliable.

Differential Diagnosis

Traumatic alopecia, alopecia areata, hypothyroid and hyperthyroid hair loss, seborrhea, atopic dermatitis, psoriasis, impetigo, and folliculitis are included in the differential diagnosis.

Management

Topical antifungals are ineffective. Antibiotic treatment is not indicated. The following steps are taken:

- Griseofulvin ultramicrosize at 10 to 15 mg/kg/day once daily or in two divided doses or griseofulvin microsize at 20 to 25 mg/kg/day once daily or in two divided doses for 6 to 8 weeks; taken with fatty food, such as ice cream, to enhance absorption. Treatment should be continued until clinical and mycologic cure (Taketomo et al, 2011).
- In addition to griseofulvin therapy, shampoo with selenium sulfide 2.5% or econazole or ketoconazole 2% (two or three times per week for 4 weeks) to decrease spore viability and keep other household members from being infected.
- If a long-standing kerion with severe inflammation is present, give prednisone 1 to 2 mg/kg/day for 5 to 14 days.

- Family members and pets should be checked for infection by fungal culture and treated if positive. Do not rely on lack of symptoms, as asymptomatic carriers are common.
- A follow-up visit should be scheduled after 2 weeks to evaluate response to treatment. Medication should be continued until 2 weeks after culture is negative. Follow-up should be continued every 2 to 4 weeks until new hair growth is evident.
- Monitoring of CBC, LFTs, and renal function is no longer required in children treated with oral griseofulvin due to its favorable safety profile; however, clinical monitoring is required with laboratory evaluation considered with a change in clinical status (Michaels and Del Rosso, 2012). In extended therapy with the medication, over 8 weeks, laboratory evaluation may be considered.
- If resistance to griseofulvin is encountered, oral itraconazole, terbinafine, fluconazole, and ketoconazole have been used, but are not all approved for use in children younger than 18 years old. Terbinafine is not FDA approved for this indication; however, some studies in children show it to be effective for resistant cases (see Table 37-4 for dosing).

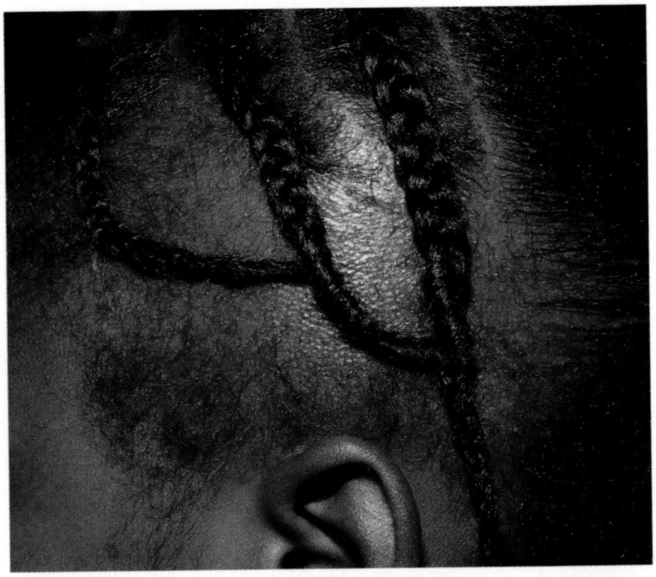

• **Figure 37-33** Traction alopecia. (From James WD, Berger TG, Elston DM: *Andrews' diseases of the skin: clinical dermatology*, ed 11, Philadelphia, 2011, Saunders/Elsevier.)

Complications

An id reaction to the fungus, not to the medication, can occur. It manifests either as a red, superficial edema or as scaly, red plaques and papules on the scalp and is treated with 1 to 2 weeks of topical or systemic steroids. Permanent hair loss and scarring can occur with an untreated kerion.

Patient and Family Education

- Sites and modes of transmission are identified (*M. canis,* animal source; *T. tonsurans,* human source) and treated.
- Side effects of medication should be explained and monitored; griseofulvin typically may result in gastrointestinal disturbances, photosensitivity, skin eruptions, and headache.
- Hair regrowth is slow (3 to 12 months) and, if a kerion was present, hair loss can be permanent.
- Laundering sheets and clothes in a hot water wash and hot dryer cycle and vacuuming may decrease spread in the family.
- Grooming practices (e.g., hair traction, greasy pomades, infrequent shampooing) may be predisposing factors.
- There is a high rate of asymptomatic carriers; culture is the only definitive means of identification.

Traumatic Alopecia

Traumatic hair loss, characterized by incomplete hair loss with hair of varying lengths, can be due to chemical exposure, thermal damage, traction, or friction. The most common forms are traction alopecia and trichotillomania. Traction alopecia, commonly seen in African American females, is due to hair styling. Common causes are cornrows, ponytails, or braids; tight curlers; or excessive brushing (Fig. 37-33).

Trichotillomania is a common disorder seen in children of all ages after infancy. Hair loss is varied and is caused by repeated pulling and/or excessive twisting of hair with fracturing of the longer hair shafts. Research indicates etiology is multifactorial, including genetic predisposition and environmental and behavioral variables. In preschoolers it is associated with habitual behaviors and situational stress. It can also be associated with obsessive-compulsive psychiatric disease in older children (Cohen, 2013). Trichotillomania after the preschool years is classified as an impulse control disorder.

Clinical Findings

History

- Various methods of hair styling with tight pull on hair
- Habits, such as nail biting, finger sucking, or hair twirling
- Any recent life changes or stressors
- Medications (e.g., anticonvulsants, antithyroid medications, beta-blockers, isotretinoin, lithium, oral contraceptives, vitamin A supplements, warfarin)
- Excess time spent lying supine

Physical Examination

The following findings are present:

- Possible erythema and pustules
- Thinning and breaking of hair in certain areas, tending to occur in a linear pattern related to hairstyle
- Circumscribed hair loss with irregular borders and broken hairs of varied length
- No erythema or scaling of the scalp
- Hair loss is commonly found on frontal eyelashes, parietal, and temporal areas with peripheral sparing, but also eyebrows

Differential Diagnosis

The differential diagnosis includes tinea capitis, alopecia areata, neonatal occipital alopecia, and child abuse (make sure no one but the child is pulling out the hair).

Management

The following steps are taken:
1. Traction alopecia
   - Avoid any hairstyle or device that causes traction on the hair, including cornrows, ponytails, braids, and curlers.
   - Use only mild shampoo, shampoo infrequently, use wide-toothed combs with rounded ends, and brush gently.
   - A short course of antibiotics is prescribed if pustules are present.
2. Trichotillomania
   - A straightforward discussion and ongoing support of the child and parents are essential. In very young children, trichotillomania is usually benign and resolves spontaneously. Older children and adolescents may require individual and family therapy. Attempt to relieve stress and cope with any traumatic events.
   - Applying oil to the hair at night makes it slippery and harder to pull.
   - Behavior modification programs may be needed for children with more severe trichotillomania. Cognitive-behavioral therapy and/or pharmacologic therapy may be indicated if behavior modification strategies prove unsuccessful (Labouliere and Storch, 2012).

Complications

Trichobezoars (hairballs) in the child with trichotillomania can cause gastrointestinal symptoms. Some children with trichotillomania have extensive psychopathologic conditions.

Patient and Family Education

The cause of the hair loss must be discussed and support offered to resolve issues. New hair growth can take 3 to 6 months.

Alopecia Areata

Alopecia areata is an asymptomatic, complete hair loss occurring primarily in frontal or parietal areas (Fig. 37-34). *Ophiasis* is a form of alopecia areata that begins in the frontal or occipital hairline and spreads along the hair margins.

The cause of alopecia areata is unknown, but it is thought to be an autoimmune mechanism. Twenty-seven percent to 60% of patients experience their first episode before 20 years old (Castelo-Soccio, 2014). Twenty-five percent of patients have a family history of alopecia areata (Weston and Morelli, 2013).

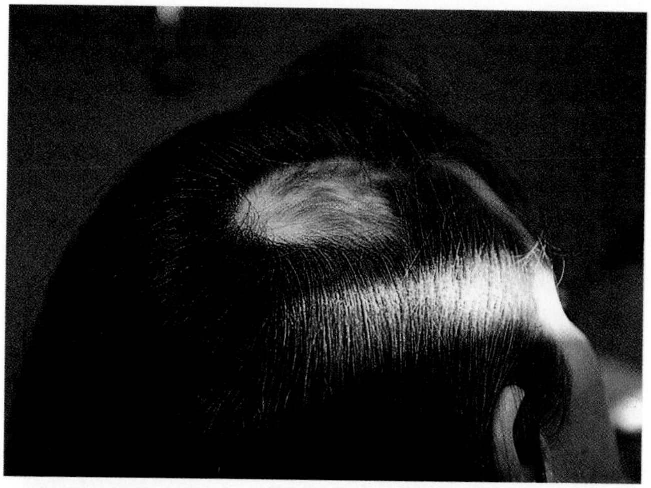

• **Figure 37-34** Alopecia areata. (From Thibodeau GA, Patton KT: *The human body in health & disease*, ed 5, St. Louis, 2010, Mosby/Elsevier.)

Clinical Findings

History

The history can include other family members with alopecia areata.

Physical Examination

- Single or multiple (up to three) round or oval patches of complete or nearly complete hair loss without erythema or scaling. Scalp is smooth with fine new hair growth.
- The frontal and parietal areas are involved 90% of the time.
- "Exclamation hairs" are narrower at the base, short, and broken off.
- Nail ridging or pitting (a helpful distinguishing factor).
- Occasional loss of body or pubic hair, or eyelashes or eyebrows.
- Possible atopic dermatitis or vitiligo.

Diagnostic Studies

The following are sometimes performed:
- KOH examination or fungal culture to rule out tinea
- Skin biopsy
- Thyroid screening, because it can be associated with autoimmune thyroiditis

Differential Diagnosis

Tinea capitis versus traumatic alopecia is the differential diagnosis.

Management

The following steps should be taken:
1. Open discussion and support of the child and parents. If only one or two patches are present, reassure that regrowth will occur.
2. If extensive involvement, refer to a dermatologist for treatment options. Treatment options include topical

corticosteroids, local irritants, topical minoxidil, topical sensitizers, and UV light therapy (Cohen, 2013).
3. Recommend wearing a wig, depending on the severity of involvement; prescribing the wig as a medical treatment helps defray the cost. Locks of Love is an organization that provides hairpieces to financially disadvantaged children younger than 21 years old and the National Alopecia Areata Foundation (see Additional Resources) is a national support group for affected children and families.

Complications

Self-esteem issues are common. *Alopecia totalis* is a loss of all the hair on the scalp. *Alopecia universalis* is a loss of all the hair on the body.

Patient and Family Education

All families should be put in touch with the National Alopecia Areata Foundation. The condition is self-limited in most school-age children and adolescents. Full recovery, often within 1 year, is more likely if three or fewer areas are involved and if onset is in late childhood. However, the greater the hair loss, the longer it takes for regrowth. Prognosis is guarded in infants and toddlers. Approximately one third of patients have a recurrence within months to years, with a worsening prognosis with each episode.

Onychomycosis

Onychomycosis is a fungal infection of the nail(s) typically with *T. rubrum* or *Candida* (Fig. 37-35). When the nail infection is due to a dermatophyte, it is often called *tinea unguium*. One or two nails are often involved. The infection may be superficial, hypertrophic (onychauxis), or cause separation of the nail plate from the tissue (onycholytic).

The infecting organism invades the nail, proliferates, and destroys the nail integrity, causing separation of the nail plate from the nailbed. The infection originates at the distal edge of the nail. It is uncommon during the first two decades of life, limited most commonly to adolescents and adults. When it occurs in children, there is often a concurrent tinea pedis or tinea manuum. There may be a relationship to the use of occlusive shoes. The causative organisms include *T. rubrum, T. mentagrophytes, E. floccosum*, and *C. albicans*. However, 50% of the time another condition is responsible for dystrophic nail.

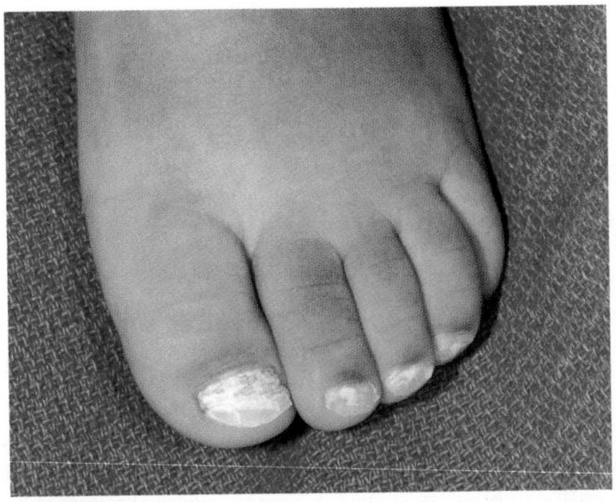

• **Figure 37-35** Onychomycosis. (From Paller AS, Mancini AJ: *Hurwitz clinical pediatric dermatology: a textbook of skin disorders of childhood and adolescence*, ed 3, Philadelphia, 2006, Saunders/Elsevier, p 461.)

Clinical Findings

History

The patient may report a thickened, discolored nail.

Physical Examination

- Opaque white or silvery nail that becomes thick, yellow, with subungual debris.
- Toenails are involved more often than fingernails with tinea.
- Fingernails are involved more often than toenails with *Candida.*
- Seldom symmetric; it may be one to three nails on one extremity.

Diagnostic Studies

KOH preparations and fungal cultures of the material under the nail are helpful in confirming the diagnosis.

Differential Diagnosis

Psoriasis (involves all nails and includes pitting), hereditary nail defects, dystrophy secondary to eczema or chronic paronychia, lichen planus, and trauma are the differential diagnoses.

Management

1. Successful treatment is difficult and requires oral medication. Griseofulvin can be used, but side effects, length of treatment, low cure rates, and high recurrence rates following treatment make successful management uncommon (Paller and Mancini, 2011).
2. Oral terbinafine, fluconazole, and itraconazole have a better short-term success rate than griseofulvin and a lower relapse rate. Treatment recommendations for onychomycosis are based on the site of infection (Taketomo et al, 2011):
   - Toenails
     - Itraconazole: 5 mg/kg/day for 12 weeks; or as pulse therapy, 5 mg/kg/day for 1 week each month for 3 months (Morelli, 2011)
     - Terbinafine: More than 40 kg, 250 mg tablet once daily for 12 weeks
     - Griseofulvin: 15 to 20 mg/kg/day (decrease dose if using ultramicronized form) for 6 to 18 months
     - Fluconazole: 6 mg/kg/week for 8 months
   - Fingernails
     - Itraconazole: 5 mg/kg/day for 6 weeks or 1 week each month for 2 months (Morelli, 2011)
     - Terbinafine: 4 to 6 mg/kg/day for 6 weeks
     - Fluconazole: 6 mg/kg/week for 4 months

3. Ciclopirox in nail lacquer used daily has high cure rates in adults, but it has not been studied in children. It has been used as monotherapy and adjunctive therapy (Paller and Mancini, 2011).
4. If triazoles are used, a careful history of current medications must be taken, because there are many interactions. Monitoring of CBC and hepatic function is recommended at onset of therapy and every 4 to 6 weeks.
5. *Candida* infection is treated with topical application of ketoconazole under occlusion (plastic glove covered by a cotton sock at bedtime) for 3 to 4 weeks.
6. Follow-up visits at 1-month intervals to monitor laboratory values are recommended; long-term follow-up every 6 months is suggested.

Patient and Family Education

The unfortunate truth to communicate is that cure is difficult to obtain and relapse is common.

Paronychia

Paronychia is a chronic or acute inflammation and infection around a fingernail or toenail. It is a common disorder in childhood and adolescence caused by bacteria (often *S. aureus,* occasionally *Streptococcus* or *Pseudomonas*), *Candida* (in infants with thrush or thumb sucking or when hands are frequently immersed in water), or herpes (Fig. 37-36). It is more common with tight shoes, or when nails are malaligned, or cut too short or with rounded edges.

Clinical Findings

History

Tenderness and drainage are reported and discomfort, especially with walking.

Physical Examination

- Proximal nailfold is erythematous, swollen, and tender; if chronic, may not be tender

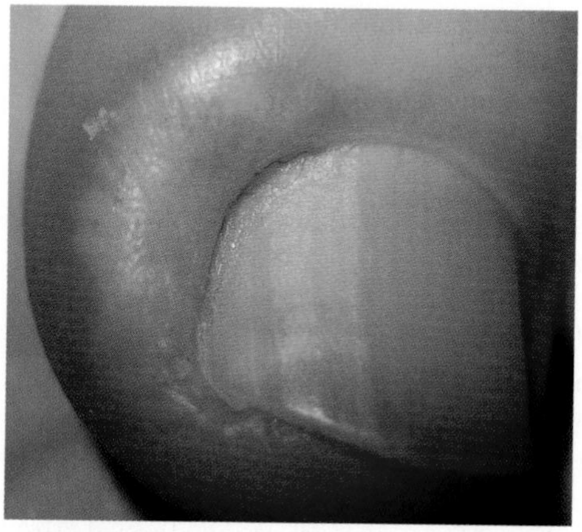

• **Figure 37-36** Paronychia. (From Bologia J, Schaffer JV, Duncan KO, et al: *Dermatology essentials*, ed 1, Philadelphia, 2014, Saunders/Elsevier.)

- Purulent exudate expressed
- Cuticle broken or absent
- Nontender erythema and edema with thickened, disrupted nail (*Candida* infection, often with secondary bacterial infection)

Diagnostic Studies

A culture of the exudate is occasionally done.

Differential Diagnosis

Herpetic whitlow (grouped vesicles on an erythematous base) and eczematous inflammation should be ruled out.

Management

Management includes the following:

- Systemic oral antibiotic if acute infection; coverage for staphylococcal infection may be required.
- If *Candida* is suspected, nystatin cream under occlusion (a plastic glove covered by a cotton stocking) every night for 3 to 4 weeks.
- If purulent area is full, loosen cuticle from nail with a No. 11 blade to allow exudate to escape.
- Frequent warm soaks, after which cotton pledgets are inserted beneath the nail to lift it.
- Instruction on proper trimming of nails and care of toenails:
  - Wear wide-toed shoes.
  - Trim nails straight across and not too short.
  - If condition is recurrent, refer for surgical removal of lateral portion of nail.
  - Do a follow-up visit in 1 month, as recurrent infection is possible.

Body Art

Tattoos and Body Piercing

A tattoo is an indelible mark fixed on the body by inserting pigment under the skin. Body piercing is the creation of a hole anywhere in the body (typically the ear, eyebrow, lip, naris, tongue, navel, nipple, or genitalia) to insert jewelry. Both are considered forms of *body art* that have been practiced throughout the ages in many cultures as rites of passage, as means of showing status or membership in a particular group, or as proof of virility.

Most tattoos or piercings are done in unregulated, unlicensed tattoo parlors, and some adolescents may tattoo or pierce themselves or their peers. Some states have legislation that prevents practitioners in tattoo parlors from tattooing minors or that requires parental consent before tattooing is done on a minor.

Adolescents obtain tattoos for many reasons, including making a personal statement, seeing it as a form of art or a fashion statement, or wishing to be daring. Piercing is considered less permanent than a tattoo. Adults and parents may see piercing or tattooing as a deviant behavior, a strange new trend, a fetish, a fad, or a fashion.

The incidence of tattooing and piercing has been increasing, especially in the adolescent population. In one study, 19% of boys and 17% of girls reported getting tattoos, but more girls (42%) than boys (16%) reported piercings (earlobes not included). Teens who participate in piercing and tattooing reported less interest in school, more deviant behavior, and substance abuse (Dukes and Stein, 2011).

Clinical Findings

History

Questions to discuss include the following:

- When and where was the body art obtained?
- Where is it located, and what care is being given?
- Were there any complications?

Physical Examination

Look for any symptoms of infection, erythema, crusting, or scabs.

Differential Diagnosis

Branding, the burning of the skin to create a permanent scar in a desired design via blowtorch or wire coat hanger in hot oil, is one differential diagnosis. *Self-mutilation,* a self-directed violence that ranges from altering physical appearance (e.g., ear piercing) to extreme forms (e.g., amputation), is another. Some forms are considered normal, but deviant forms are physically damaging, done in response to crisis, and demonstrate disconnectedness and alienation from others.

TABLE 37-11 Healing Time for Body Piercings

Type of Piercing	Time to Heal
Cheek, outer labia	2 to 4 months
Clitoris	1 to 2½ months
Ear cartilage, navel, nostril	2 months to 1 year
Earlobe, eyebrow	1½ to 2 months
Frenum (underneath tongue), nipple	2 to 6 months
Inner labia	1 to 2 months
Lip	2 to 3 months
Male genitalia	1 to 6 months
Nasal septum	6 to 8 months
Nasal bridge	2 to 2½ months
Tongue	1 to 1½ months

Data from Martel S, Anderson JE: Decorating the "human canvas": body art and your patient, *Contemp Pediatr* 19(8):86–102, 2002; Schnare SM: Tattooing, branding, and body piercing, *Women's Health Care* 1(4):21–28, 2002.

Management

1. Aftercare for tattoos:
   - Perform basic wound care, including not touching for 24 hours.
   - A moderate amount of oozing and local swelling is normal for 48 hours.
   - Scab should be left alone except for the application of antibiotic ointment.
   - Protect from rough surfaces that can traumatize; protect from sunburn.
   - Review signs and symptoms of infection.
2. Aftercare for body piercings
   - Wash hands before touching; cleanse area twice a day with antibacterial soap.
   - A moderate amount of oozing and swelling is normal; if crusts appear, remove with wet swab.
     - Tongue
       a. Use ice to minimize swelling.
       b. Rinse mouth 10 to 12 times a day with half-strength Listerine, twice a day with carbamide peroxide.
       c. No deep kissing for 48 hours; once healed, use dental dams for dental work, and avoid smoking.
     - Navel
       a. Slowest to heal, most likely area to reject jewelry.
       b. Cleanse twice a day with antibacterial soap.
       c. Avoid handling; avoid clothing that rubs for up to 1 year.
     - Nipples and genitalia
       a. Cleanse twice a day with antibacterial soap.
       b. Avoid manipulation and tight garments; cotton clothes are ideal.
       c. Use latex barriers with sexual activity.
3. Healing times are variable and should be considered. A tattoo may take 2 to 3 weeks to heal. Body piercing, depending on the site, can take from 4 to 8 weeks for ears to 6 to 12 months for navel and genital piercings (Table 37-11).
4. Infection can be treated with dicloxacillin 500 mg four times a day for 10 days. The decision to remove jewelry during an infection should be based on whether leaving it in place will provide a route for drainage, become an obstacle to healing, or be an ongoing source of infection.
5. Screen for high-risk behaviors.
6. Discuss the need to remove dangling ornaments during contact sports.

Complications

Common complications of tattooing or body piercing include infections, allergic reactions to the dyes or jewelry, and the transmission of blood-borne diseases, primarily hepatitis B and C, but potentially HIV. Other reported complications of tattoos include skin neoplasms, syphilis, leprosy, cutaneous tuberculosis, tetanus, hyperplasia, and granuloma annulare. Complications of piercings also in-

• BOX 37-10 Know the Facts about Getting a Tattoo or Body Piercing: Make an Informed Decision

- Unsterile tattooing and piercing equipment and needles can spread serious infections, hepatitis, or possibly even HIV.
- The law in many states prohibits the tattooing of minors.
- Asking a friend to apply a tattoo may ruin a friendship if the tattoo does not look like you thought it would.
- Tattoos and permanent makeup are not easily removed and in some cases may cause permanent discoloration.
- Tattoo removal is very expensive. A tattoo that costs $50 to apply may cost more than $1000 to remove.
- Blood donations cannot be made for 1 year after getting a tattoo, body piercing, or permanent makeup.

Before You Get a Tattoo or Body Piercing: Think Carefully

- First: Talk to your friends or others who have been tattooed or pierced. Ask them about their experience, the cost, pain, healing time, and so on. Ask them what they would do if they had a chance to do it over again.
- Second: Understand that you do not have to tattoo or pierce your body to belong. Remember that you are directly involved in decisions that affect your health and body. You can always change your mind or wait if you are not sure.
- Third: Because of potential complications, if you decide to get a tattoo or body piercing, never tattoo or pierce your own body or let a friend do it.

Health Risks to Consider Before You Act

- Both tattooing and piercing involve puncturing the skin to introduce a foreign material, jewelry, or ink, and the procedures carry similar risks. The primary health concern is introducing blood-borne germs or viruses into your body.
- Blood-borne illnesses, such as hepatitis B and C, tetanus, tuberculosis, and HIV infection, can lead to serious health problems or death.
- Make sure you have had the three series hepatitis B vaccination and a tetanus booster within the past 10 years.
- Localized infections, such as *Staphylococcus* or *Pseudomonas*, can lead to illness, deformity, and scarring.
- Tattoo troubles: *Tattoos are open wounds that may become infected*. Keep the new tattoo clean and moist with an ointment to prevent a scab from forming. If you are allergic to the inks in the tattoo, the site will not heal properly and scarring may occur.
- Piercing problems: Complications depend on the location of the piercing. Navel infections are the most common; it takes approximately 1 year for navel piercings to heal. Ear cartilage heals slowly. Tongue piercings may lead to tooth and enamel damage from biting on the jewelry and jewelry knocking against a tooth, partial paralysis if the jewelry pierces a nerve, and extreme inflammation during the first few days.

Selecting a Tattoo Artist or Piercer

- Visit several piercers or tattooists. The work area should be kept clean and have good lighting. If they refuse to discuss cleanliness and infection control with you, go somewhere else.
- Consent forms (which the customer must fill out) should be handled before tattooing. Reputable piercing and tattoo studios will not serve a minor without signed consent from parents. Check the laws in your state about tattooing of minors if you are younger than 18 years old.
- The tattooist or piercer should have an *autoclave*—a heat sterilization machine used to sterilize equipment between customers.
- Packaged, sterilized needles should be used only once and then disposed of in a biohazard container.
- Immediately before tattooing or piercing, the tattooist or piercer should wash and dry his or her hands and wear latex gloves. These gloves should be worn at all times while the tattoo or piercing is being done. If the tattoo artist or piercer leaves or touches other objects, such as the telephone, new gloves should be put on before the procedure continues.
- Only jewelry made of a noncorrosive metal, such as surgical stainless steel, niobium, or solid 14-karat gold, is safe for a new piercing.
- Leftover tattoo ink should be disposed of after each procedure. Ink should never be poured back into the bottle and reused.

HIV, Human immunodeficiency virus.

clude excessive bleeding, nerve damage, keloids, dental fracture, soft-tissue damage, and speech impediments.

Patient and Family Education

Provide information and encourage teenagers to thoroughly research and consider the idea of getting a tattoo or body piercing. Removing tattoos is expensive, not necessarily completely successful, and fraught with complication (e.g., scarring, rashes) (Box 37-10). Maintaining an open, nonjudgmental attitude when discussing the options and caring for adolescents who have body art is essential. Alternatives to discuss include temporary stick-on tattoos and use of henna or other body paints.

For a complete list of references, please visit http://evolve.elsevier.com/Burns/pediatric/.

38 Musculoskeletal Disorders

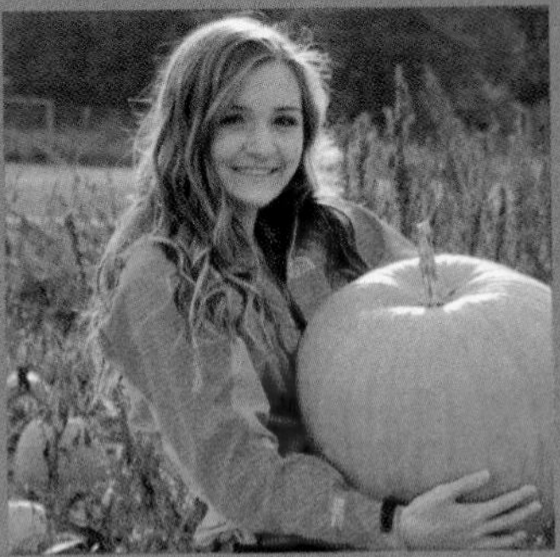

CYNTHIA MARIE CLAYTOR AND JAN BAZNER-CHANDLER

Musculoskeletal complaints are common in children and youth with one in eight seeking medical attention annually (Gunz et al, 2012). Common musculoskeletal disorders include athletic injuries, back pain, foot injuries, knee disorders, shin splints, and stress fractures. Congenital problems include spinal deformities, hip and foot anomalies, growth disorders and developmental delay, metabolic disorders, and neuromuscular disorders ranging from cerebral palsy to muscular dystrophy. A variety of other conditions can cause musculoskeletal findings, including intentional and unintentional injury, cancer, and juvenile idiopathic arthritis. Iatrogenic deformities that result from cultural practices, such as using a cradleboard, or from fetal position and intrauterine compression can also cause deformities. Disorders of the musculoskeletal system present unique problems because growth and development of this system contribute to the evolution of pathologic conditions over time. Limited mobility, pain, and deformity can interfere with the child's lifestyle. Children with functional disabilities may not be able to fully participate in all activities with peers and family or meet the physical requirements of various occupations. They may also face challenges related to self-esteem. Primary care providers must be vigilant and seek to help children and their families prevent these problems.

Primary care providers play a significant role in the early identification and management of children with orthopedic problems. They assess development of the musculoskeletal system, identify problems requiring early intervention, focus on lifestyle assessment and injury prevention, and monitor the long-term outcomes of orthopedic care. They are often the first to refer to specialists as needed for early diagnosis and treatment. When necessary, primary care providers help families integrate orthopedic care within the daily living activities at home and school and assist families to cope with the issues of disability, deformity, and long-term care.

Anatomy and Physiology

Limb formation occurs early in embryogenesis (4 to 8 weeks of gestation); primary ossification centers are present in all the long bones of the limbs by the 12th week of gestation. Development of the skeletal system begins around the 4th week of gestation, with ossification of the fetal skeleton beginning during the 5th month of gestation. The clavicles and skull bones are the first to ossify, followed by the long bones and spine. The epiphyses of the newborn's long bones are composed of hyaline cartilage. Soon after birth, the cartilage along the epiphyseal plate begins secondary ossification. The shape of the spine also changes from a C-shape at birth to an S-curve by late adolescence. As the child starts to walk, the lumbar curve develops. The sacrum starts out as five separate bones at birth—only to become fused as one large bone by 18 to 20 years old (Duderstadt and Schapiro, 2014).

Bone age, measured by radiographs of the left hand and wrist, can be used to quantitatively determine somatic maturation and serves as a mirror that reflects the tempo of growth. In adolescents, the skeletal growth spurt begins at about Tanner stage 2 in girls and Tanner stage 3 in boys. Growth peaks around stage 4 and then ends with stage 5. The growth spurt lasts longer in boys than in girls. The pelvis widens early in pubescent girls. In both sexes, the legs usually lengthen before the thighs broaden. Next the shoulders widen, and the trunk completes its linear growth. Bone growth ends when the epiphyses close.

Long bones have a growth plate, or physis, at each end that separates the epiphysis from the diaphysis or shaft. Openings through this plate allow blood vessels to penetrate from the epiphysis. In the growth plate, chondrocytes produce cartilage cells, dead cells are absorbed, and the calcified cartilage matrix is converted into bone. The entire growth plate area is weaker than the remaining bone, because it is less calcified. Because the blood supply to the growth plate comes primarily through the epiphysis, damage to epiphyseal circulation can jeopardize the survival of the chondrocytes. If chondrocytes stop producing, growth of the bone in that area stops (Fig. 38-1).

There are two ways that children's bones grow. Longitudinal growth occurs in the ossification centers; changes in bone width and strength take place via intramembranous ossification. The length of long bones comes from growth at the epiphyseal plates, whereas their diameter increases as

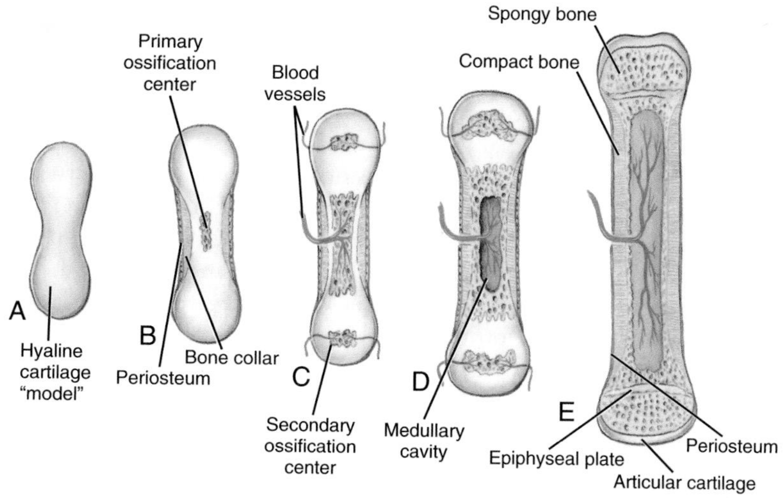

• **Figure 38-1** Growth plates and transition from cartilage to bone at the epiphyseal plate. **A,** Hyaline cartilage "model." **B,** Periosteum and bone collar form. **C,** Blood vessels and osteoblasts infiltrate primary ossification centers. **D,** Osteoclasts form the medullary cavity. **E,** Ossification is complete. Hyaline cartilage remains as articular cartilage and in the epiphyseal plate. (From Duderstadt KG, Schapiro NA: Musculoskeletal system. In Duderstadt KG, editor: *Pediatric physical examination: an illustrated handbook*, Philadelphia, 2014, Elsevier, p 260, Fig. 18-1.)

a result of deposition of new bone on the periosteal surface and resorption on the surface of the medullary cavity. Growth of the small bones, hip, and spine comes from one or more primary ossification centers in each bone. Apophyses are the sites for connection of tendons to bone. In children, these sites, which are similar to epiphyses, allow for growth and are weaker than bone. These sites can become inflamed with overuse, as occurs in Osgood-Schlatter disease.

The development of bones and muscles is influenced by use. Thus in infants and toddlers, the legs straighten and lengthen with the stimulus of weight bearing and independent walking. The infant is born with the full complement of muscle fibers. Growth in muscle length results from lengthening of the fibers, and growth in bulk comes from hypertrophy. Length of muscles is related to growth in length of the underlying bone. If a limb is not used, it grows minimally. Furthermore, if muscles and bones are not used in their intended normal manner, such as occurs with spastic diplegia, the forces for development tend to stimulate growth in abnormal patterns. Thus, scoliosis can develop or bowlegs may increase in severity. Muscle contractures occur if muscles are not used regularly and put through their full range of motion. The growth of fibrous tissue, tendons, and ligaments is also dependent on mechanical demands.

Nutritional, mechanical, and hormonal factors during the growth process influence the thickness of bones and the health of the marrow. Adequate protein, calcium, and vitamin D in the diet are key nutritional elements that affect the growth and development of a child's musculoskeletal system.

The muscle structures originate from the embryonic mesoderm and include tendons, ligaments, cartilage, and joints. Muscle fibers are developed by the 4th or 5th month of gestation and grow in tangent with their respective bones. The rate of muscle growth (muscle mass and cell sizes) speeds up dramatically around 2 years old, with girls exhibiting a greater rate of growth than boys until this gender trend is reversed at puberty (Duderstadt and Schapiro, 2014).

Pathophysiology and Defense Mechanisms

Pathophysiology

Muscles and bones can be affected by localized or systemic problems. Thus the initial orthopedic problem can be symptomatic of a larger problem (e.g., juvenile arthritis). Tendon and ligament injuries that result in sprains and strains or apophysitis are the result of traumatic injury or overuse.

Systemic Problems

Musculoskeletal presentation in children and adolescents can be a feature of potentially life-threatening conditions (such as, sepsis, malignancy, or nonaccidental injury) and chronic pediatric conditions (such as, inflammatory bowel disease, cystic fibrosis, and juvenile idiopathic arthritis, which is also known as juvenile arthritis).

Systemic problems can include chronic conditions, such as hemophilia, sickle cell disease, and arthritic diseases; neurologic problems, such as cerebral palsy; and various cancers, including osteosarcoma and leukemia. Children with metabolic problems, such as vitamin D–resistant rickets, have bony deformities. Acute systemic disorders can also affect the musculoskeletal system. For example, viruses and bacteria can infect joints and bones. In developing countries, tubercular infections of bones are common and devastating. Thus the pediatric provider must assess patients from a broad perspective, obtain a history to include other body systems, and order appropriate laboratory studies that might identify systemic problems.

Genetic Problems

Many genetic problems have an orthopedic component. Osteogenesis imperfecta (OI) is a genetic disorder characterized by decreased levels of collagen, the major protein of the body's connective tissue. Mutations in genes encoding type 1 collagen (COL1A1 or COL1A2 genes) account for approximately 80% of OI cases (Abdelgawad and Naga, 2014). Children with OI have bones that break easily, even from minor trauma. Down syndrome is a consequence of a trisomy 21 chromosome. The main orthopedic pathology is hypotonia and the possibility of loose joint capsules and ligaments. Children with Down syndrome have a higher incidence of scoliosis, dislocation of the hip, Legg-Calvé-Perthes disease (LCPD), instability of the patella, and pes planus (flat feet). Children with Marfan syndrome may have long spider-like fingers, low muscle tone, and lax joints that are prone to dislocate. Severe scoliosis may develop in children with neurofibromatosis, Turner syndrome, and Noonan syndrome. Girls with Turner syndrome may present with webbed neck, short stature, valgus deformity of the elbow, and short fourth metacarpal deformity. Children with Noonan syndrome can present with webbed neck, pectus carinatum or pectus excavatum, clumsiness, poor coordination, and motor delay. (See Chapter 41 for further discussion of various genetic conditions.)

Many orthopedic problems have a multifactorial inheritance pattern. Thus if one child in a family has a dislocated hip or scoliosis, the risk for these conditions increases for the other siblings. The pediatric provider needs to understand the genetic disorder to monitor related orthopedic problems, consider the genetic implications, and provide families with appropriate genetic information or refer them for genetic counseling.

Intrauterine Compression Deformations

The developing fetus moves its body parts frequently, and this movement influences musculoskeletal development. When the baby fills the uterine space, movements are restricted and body parts begin to assume the shape in which they are fixed. Because of in utero positioning, joint and muscle contractions can develop and are generally considered physiologic in nature. Fetal movement is required for proper development of the musculoskeletal system, and anything that restricts fetal movement can cause deformation from intrauterine molding. Two major intrinsic causes for deformations are neuromuscular disorders and maternal oligohydramnios. Extrinsic causes are related to fetal crowding that restricts fetal movement. Infants with deformations caused by extrinsic causes (e.g., breech position) have an excellent prognosis with corrections occurring spontaneously. Because much of the bony structure is cartilaginous, molding occurs with relative ease. Thus intrauterine positioning issues can result in tibial bowing and a 20- to 30-degree of hip flexion. Occasionally, a foot may be turned awkwardly, the legs might be fixed straight up with the feet near the ears, or the neck may be tipped to one side. Such positioning issues are outside the range of normal. The outcomes are deformities in various degrees. The longer the position is maintained, the more severe the problems are. In general, there is a tendency for bowing and late deformations to straighten; however, the effects related to in utero positioning may not fully abate until the child is 3 to 4 years old. More severe deformities (i.e., rigid metatarsus adductus [MA]) need to be referred to orthopedists for treatment as soon as they are found, because a softer skeleton is easier to realign in a positive direction.

Injuries

The unique differences in the pediatric skeletal system predispose children to injuries unlike those seen in adults. The important differences are the presence of periosseous cartilage, physes, and a thicker, stronger, more osteogenic periosteum that produces new bone called *callus* more rapidly and in great amounts. Sports- and recreation-related injuries account for a significant number of emergency department visits each year for children ranging in age from 5 to 14 years old. Physeal fractures in preadolescent children are the most common musculoskeletal injuries seen. Clavicular fractures are seen at all ages ranging from a newborn birth injury to trauma in adolescence. Injury to the clavicle is usually sustained by a fall on an outstretched hand or by direct force; approximately 80% of fractures occur in the middle third of the clavicle (Landry, 2011). Fractures of the wrist and forearm account for nearly half of all fractures in children. Tendinosis may occur in the young athlete in the rotator cuff from throwing motions and swimming, in the iliopsoas in dancers, and in the ankle of dancers, gymnasts, and figure skaters. Shoulder injuries can be acute or result from chronic overuse. Overuse injuries are common chronic injuries in children that are related to repetitive stress on the musculoskeletal system without sufficient time to recover. Apophysitis is an overuse injury unique to the skeletally immature active child or athlete and refers to the irritation, inflammation, and microtrauma that affect muscles, ligaments, tendons, bones, and growth plates (Wilson and Rodenberg, 2011).

The possibility of nonaccidental trauma should always be considered when orthopedic injuries, especially fractures, are present. Health care providers should have a high index of suspicion if an injury is unexplained, if the severity of injury is incompatible with the history, or if the injury is inconsistent with the child's developmental capabilities. Rib fractures and any unexplained fracture in a child younger than 3 years old, metaphyseal fractures, multiple fractures in various stages of healing, and complex skull fractures should be carefully evaluated (Flaherty et al, 2014). Management of traumatic injuries is discussed in Chapter 40. Assessment of nonaccidental trauma is also discussed in Chapter 17.

Defense Mechanisms

Fracture Healing

One of the major differences between the adult and the pediatric bone is that the periosteum in children is very thick. The major reason for increased healing speed of children's fractures is the periosteum, which contributes to the largest part of new bone formation around a fracture. Children have significantly greater osteoblastic activity in this area, because bone is already being formed beneath the periosteum as part of normal growth. This already active process is readily accelerated after a fracture. Periosteal callus bridges a fracture in children long before the underlying hematoma forms cartilage anlagen that go on to ossify. Once cellular organization from the hematoma has passed through the inflammatory process, repair of the bone begins in the area of the fracture. In most children, by 10 days to 2 weeks after a fracture, a rubber-like bone forms around the fracture and makes it difficult to manipulate. As part of the reparative phase, cartilage formed as the hematoma organizes is eventually replaced by bone through the process of endochondral bone formation. The more growth potential the child has, the more remodeling will occur. Furthermore, remodeling power is highest near the physis and across the coronal and sagittal planes (Abdelgawad and Naga, 2014).

Growth Plate Fractures

Fractures of the long bones can produce permanent deformities in children if the fracture occurs through the growth plate. The outcomes depend on the fracture location and type, the age of the child, the status of the blood supply to the physis, and the treatment. The Salter-Harris classification is based on the mechanism of injury, the relationship of the fracture line to the layers of physis, and the prognosis with respect to subsequent growth disturbance. There are five classifications (Fig. 38-2). Type I involves a fracture through the zone of hypertrophic cells of the physis with no fracture of the surrounding bone. Type II fractures, the most common type of growth plate fracture, are similar to type I except that a metaphyseal fragment is present on the compression side of the fracture. Growth disturbance in types I and II is rare.

Type III fracture involves physeal separation with fracture through the epiphysis into the joint. The fracture requires anatomic reduction, occasionally through an open approach. Type IV fracture involves the metaphysis, physis, and epiphysis. Type V fracture involves a compression or crushing injury to the physis. Type V fractures are rare and are difficult to diagnose initially due to the lack of radiologic signs. Types IV and V require anatomic reduction to prevent articular incongruity and osseous bridging across the physis. Certain growth plates are more prone to growth disturbances. Thus children should be reevaluated intermittently for 1 year after the healing to assess possible growth or functional disturbances.

Shaft Fractures

The mechanism of injury is an important part of the history in evaluating a child for a traumatic injury. Closed pediatric fractures are largely caused by low-energy activities and play; open fractures are generally caused by more force.

There are a variety of shaft fractures. In children between 9 months and 6 years old, torsion of the foot may produce an oblique fracture of the distal aspect of the tibial shaft without a fibula fracture. These fractures are usually the result of tripping while walking or running, stepping on a ball or toy, or falling from a modest height. The child is typically seen due to failure to bear weight, a limp, or pain when asked to stand on the involved extremity. Physical findings may be minimal, and radiographs may show the characteristic faint oblique fracture line crossing the distal tibial diaphysis and terminating medially. Treatment is immobilization. Fractures of the forearm in children most often result from a fall on an outstretched hand. This results in forceful axial loading with resultant bony failure in compression and bending. These forces generally cause torus or greenstick fractures. The rotational malalignment may not be identified and may be undertreated. During physical examination the provider should observe for soft tissue injury, subtle rotational deformities, and neurovascular involvement and compare with the contralateral limb.

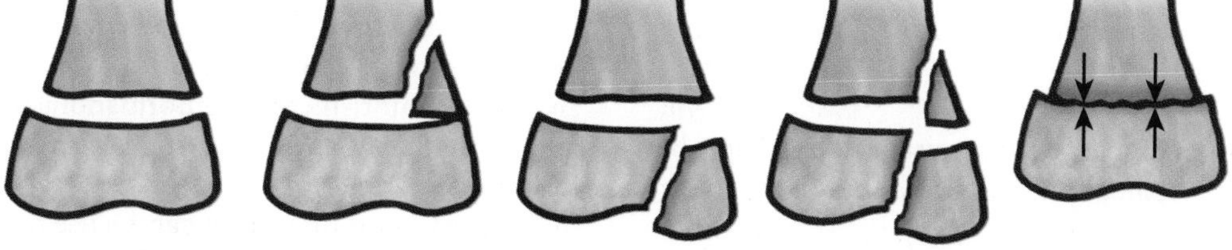

• **Figure 38-2** Salter-Harris classification of physeal fractures, types I to V. (From Wells L, Sehgal K, Dormans JP: Pediatric fracture patterns. In Kliegman RM, Stanton BF, St. Geme JW, et al, editors: *Nelson textbook of pediatrics*, ed 19, Philadelphia, 2011, Saunders/Elsevier, pp 2389–2391.)

Anteroposterior (AP), lateral radiographs, and oblique views of the wrist and forearm should be performed on all patients with a physical examination suggestive of fracture or dislocation. Furthermore, it is important to examine the entire arm and to consider radiographic views of the joints above and below suspected fractures. Failure to diagnose and treat rotational malalignment is the most common cause of loss of forearm rotation in children.

Assessment of the Orthopedic System

History

- History of present illness
  - Onset: Appearance of first symptoms; insidious or sudden; association with injury or strain; accompanied by any constitutional symptoms or signs (e.g., fever, malaise, swelling, ecchymosis)
  - Pain: Location and character, course of radiation, severity, extent of disability produced, effect of various activities including weight bearing, relief measures, changes from day to night or from day to day, child's refusing to move the painful part or assuming a pain-relieving position, effects of previous treatment, presence of pain or discomfort in other parts of the body
  - Deformity: Character (swelling, inflammation, contracture, joint stiffness, unusual positioning, appearance); first appearance and who noted it; association with injury or disease; rate of change; extent of disability; a cosmetic problem or a cause of embarrassment
  - Injury: How, when (time and date), why, and where; mechanism or manner in which injury was produced; involvement in organized or competitive sports
  - Altered function: Weakness, limp, decreased range of motion, loss or decrease sensation, loss of or alteration in perfusion that may be associated with circumferential swelling
  - Altered gait patterns: Toe walking, in-toeing or out-toeing, limping, shortened single-limb stance phase, Trendelenburg gait, steppage gait, or Gowers sign
  - Other factors or constraints: Type of shoe worn (e.g., platform shoes); use of backpack and amount of weight in backpack, amount of time spent at repetitive tasks or at computer station; sitting in TV squat or "W" position; aggravating factors: dominate hand; use of complimentary/alternative modalities
  - Medication use: Steroids, anti-inflammatories, analgesics
- Family history
  - Any family members with musculoskeletal problems; many orthopedic problems have a genetic component
- Medical history
  - Pregnancy history and birth history: Breech delivery, shoulder presentation, multiple births, oligohydramnios, asphyxia at birth; maternal alcohol or substance abuse
  - Development history: Milestones met at appropriate age, such as first walking and sitting; delays in achieving gross or fine motor developmental milestones
  - Illnesses, accidents, or surgeries: Trauma, meningitis, juvenile arthritis, chronic diseases; especially those affecting nutritional status (i.e., inflammatory bowel disease, sickle cell disease)
- Review of systems
  - Any infections, constitutional diseases, or congenital problems that might have an orthopedic component

Physical Examination

Special orthopedic examination techniques specific to children are described in the following sections and should be completed in addition to the normal orthopedic examination maneuvers.

Inspection and Palpation

Inspection of the skin noting the skin color, presence of swelling or atrophy, erythema, ecchymosis, scars, or unusual pigmentation is essential. The provider should observe the child's posture while sitting, standing, and walking, as well as assess and evaluate the proportion of the upper extremities to the lower extremities. In addition, the provider should palpate skin for differences or inconsistencies in temperature and perfusion and palpate bone and joints to ascertain tenderness, prominence, indentations, and crepitus. Evaluation of symmetry as well as range of motion, muscle size, strength, and tone should be a part of a musculoskeletal examination. Furthermore, when there is a concern regarding sensory or motor deficits, the provider should assess and evaluate the child's spinal nerves and deep tendon reflexes.

Range of Motion Examination

Range of motion is the normal range, flexion, extension, and rotation of a joint. Joint hypermobility is the ability of the joint to move beyond its normal range. Hypermobility of joints generally does not cause problems, although there is a slight increase in dislocation and sprain of the involved joint. The normal values of joint motion are age related and must be kept in mind (e.g., external hip rotation is greatest in early infancy). Passive range of motion, in which the examiner moves the joint, provides information about joint mobility and stability. It can also provide information about the limits of tendons and muscles that are contracted. Active range of motion, in which the child moves the joint, provides information about both muscle and bony structures working together for functional movement.

Limited range of motion can be the result of mechanical problems, swelling, muscle spasticity, pain, infection, injury, or arthritis. Note pain, stiffness, limitations or deviations, and rigidity.

Gait Examination

Ambulation typically begins between 8 and 16 months of age. The development of a normal gait is dependent on progressive neurologic maturation. Initially, a child's gait is characterized by a short stride length, a fast cadence, and slow velocity with a wide-based stance. The gait undergoes developmental changes. Walking velocity, step length, and duration of the single-limb stance increase with age, whereas the number of steps taken per minute decreases. A mature gait pattern is well established by 3 years old. Normal neurologic maturation results in efficiency and smoothness of gait; and by 7 years old, the gait characteristics are similar to those of an adult (Wells et al, 2011). A normal gait cycle consists of the stance phase, during which the foot is in contact with the ground, and the swing phase, during which the foot is in the air. The stance phase is further divided into three major periods: the initial double-limb support, followed by the single-limb stance, and then another period of double-limb support.

Observe the child walking without shoes and minimal covering. The stance and swing phases should be compared in both legs, and the range of motion of each joint should be evaluated. Inspect from the front, side, and back as the child walks normally, on his or her toes, and then on the heels. The gait should be smooth, rhythmic, and efficient. Ankle, knee, and hip movements should be symmetric and full with little side-to-side movement of the trunk.

Limping is a disturbance in normal pattern of gait. Abnormal gait can be antalgic or non-antalgic. An antalgic gait is characterized by a shortening of the single-limb stance phase to prevent pain in the affected leg. Painful or antalgic gaits serve to reduce stress or pain at the affected area. The trunk shifts to the opposite side to keep balance and reduce stress; the stance phase and stride length are shortened as compensatory mechanisms. Causes of a painful gait include infection, trauma, or acquired disorders. A non-antalgic gait may be caused by general weakness, spasticity, muscular disorders, or leg length discrepancies. For example, a Trendelenburg gait in which the trunk tips over the affected hip indicates hip disease and might or might not be painful because it also involves muscle weakness around the hip joint. Gait disturbances may become more apparent with fatigue.

Posture

To assess posture adequately, the child should be examined undressed to his or her underwear. The examiner needs to look at the child from the front, side, and back.

- Pelvis and hips should be level. Place hands on the iliac crest to test for a pelvic tilt caused by limb length discrepancy.
- Legs should be symmetric in shape and size. The patellae should be straight ahead.
- The feet should point straight ahead, with an imaginary line from the center of the heel through the second toe. There should be an arch (except in babies, in whom a fat pad obscures the arch) and straight heel cords.
- The spine should be straight, and the back should look symmetric, with shoulder and scapula heights and waist angles equal. There should be slight lordotic curves at the cervical and lumbar areas.

Special Examinations

Hip Examinations

Galeazzi Maneuver

The Galeazzi sign can signal conditions that cause leg length discrepancies. The Galeazzi maneuver includes flexing the hips and knees while the infant or child lies supine, placing the soles of the feet on the table near the buttocks, and then looking at the knee heights for equality (Fig. 38-3, *A*). The Galeazzi sign is positive if the knee heights are unequal. However, it is not reliable in children with dislocatable but not dislocated hips or in children with bilateral dislocation.

Barlow Maneuver

The Barlow maneuver dislocates an unstable or dislocatable hip posteriorly (Fig. 38-4, *A*). The infant is placed in the supine position with knees flexed. The hip is flexed, and the thigh is brought into an adducted position applying downward pressure. With hip instability, the femoral head slips/drops out of the acetabulum or can be gently pushed out of the socket; this is termed a *positive Barlow.* The dislocation should be palpable as this maneuver is performed. The maneuver needs to be done gently in a non-crying neonate/infant to keep from damaging the femoral head. The hips should be examined one at a time. The hip generally spontaneously relocates after release of the posterior force.

Ortolani Maneuver

The Ortolani maneuver can be done after the Barlow maneuver or separately (see Fig. 38-4, *B*). The Ortolani maneuver reduces a posteriorly dislocated hip. It is done to reduce a recently dislocated hip and is not done forcefully. The infant is in the supine position with both knees flexed. The thumb is placed near the lesser trochanter, and the pad of the second finger is positioned on the bony prominence of the greater trochanter. The leg is flexed at the hip and then abducted while pushing up with the fingers located over the trochanter posteriorly. The femoral head is lifted anteriorly into the acetabulum. A palpable *clunk* as the femoral head is relocated is considered a positive Ortolani sign. A mild *click* sound may be audible and is not considered a positive Ortolani sign. These clicks are common and normal sounds radiating from the knee or ankle (Duderstadt and Schapiro, 2014). Of note, a positive Ortolani may only be achieved during the first few months of life. Dislocations can occur later in infancy; therefore, the provider

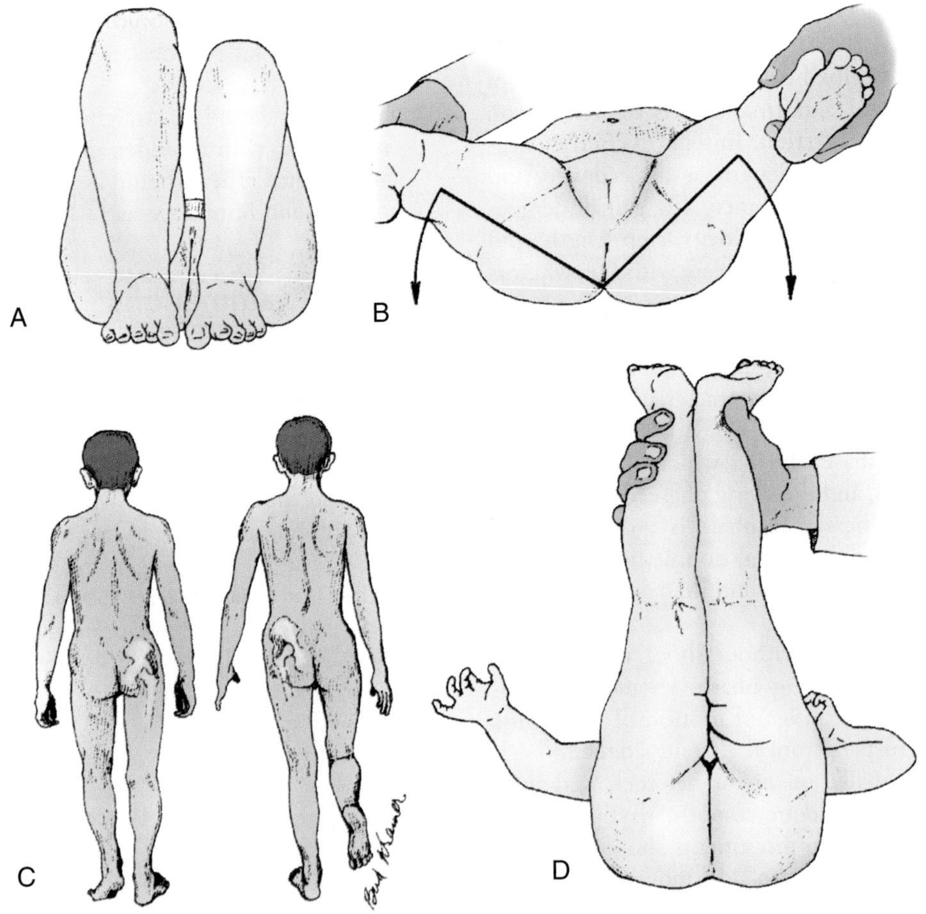

• **Figure 38-3** Physical findings in congenital hip dislocation. **A,** Leg length inequality is a sign of unilateral hip dislocation (Galeazzi sign). **B,** Limitation of hip abduction is often present in older infants with hip dislocation. Abduction of greater than 60 degrees is usually possible in infants. Restriction or asymmetry indicates the need for careful radiologic examination. **C,** Trendelenburg sign. In single-leg stance, the abductor muscles of the normal hip support the pelvis. Dislocation of the hip functionally shortens and weakens these muscles. When the child attempts to stand on the dislocated hip, the opposite side of the pelvis drops. **D,** Thigh-fold asymmetry is often present in infants with unilateral hip dislocation. An extra fold can be seen on the abnormal side. However, the finding is not diagnostic. It may be found in normal infants and may be absent in children with hip dislocation or dislocatability. (From Scoles P: *Pediatric orthopedics in clinical practice*, ed 2, St. Louis, 1988, Mosby.)

must test the hips using other strategies and note limited abduction in older infants until they are walking independently (Fig. 38-5).

Klisic Test

The Klisic test provides an observational sign of hip placement. The examiner places the tip of the third finger of one hand over the greater trochanter and the index finger of the same hand on the anterior superior iliac spine. An imaginary line is then drawn between the index and third fingers. Normally, the imaginary line points to the umbilicus. If the hip is dislocated, the imaginary line points halfway between the umbilicus and the pubis (i.e., the line points below the umbilicus). The Klisic sign is another physical assessment marker of hip dislocation (Sankar et al, 2011) (Fig. 38-6).

Trendelenburg Sign

The Trendelenburg test can be used to identify conditions that cause weakness in the hip abductors. The Trendelenburg sign is elicited by having the child stand and then raise one leg off the ground. If the pelvis (iliac crest) drops on the raised leg side, the sign is positive and indicates weak hip abductor muscles on the side that is bearing the weight. Normally the muscles around a stable hip are strong enough to maintain a level pelvis if one leg is raised (see Fig. 38-3, *C*). With bilaterally dislocated hips, a wide-based Trendelenburg limp is noted.

Medial (Internal) and Lateral (External) Rotations

The child is placed prone, and the knees are flexed 90 degrees. Medial rotation is measured as the legs are allowed

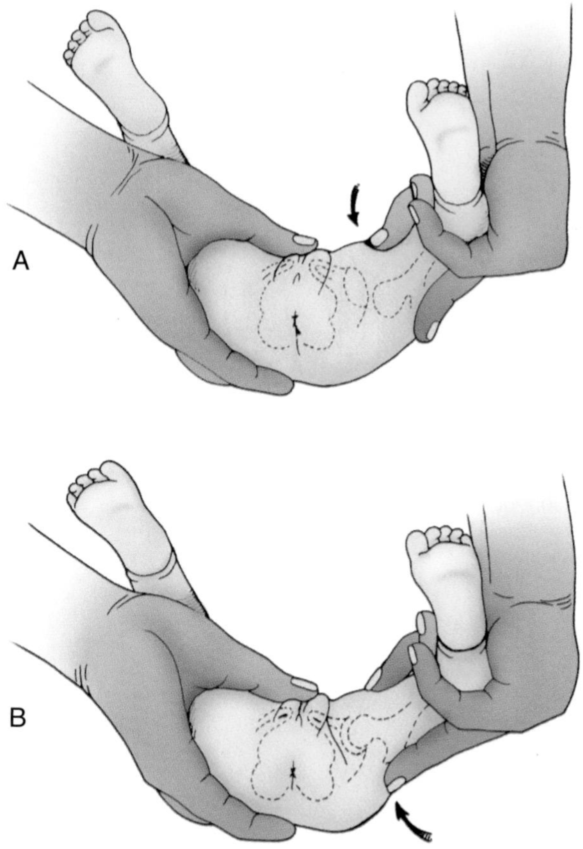

• **Figure 38-4** **A,** Barlow (dislocation) test. The "stabilizing hand" is positioned with the thumb on the symphysis and the fingers on the sacrum. The thumb of the abducting hand is placed on the inner aspect of the thigh and gives lateral pressure to the adductor region, while the hand (wrapped around the knee with the index finger on the lateral side of the thigh) provides gentle downward pressure. If there is hip instability, dislocation is palpable as the femoral head slips out of the acetabulum. Diagnosis is confirmed with the Ortolani test. **B,** Ortolani (reduction) test. With the infant relaxed on a firm surface, the hips and knees are flexed to 90 degrees. The hips are examined one at a time. Grasp the infant's thigh with the middle finger over the greater trochanter, and lift the thigh to bring the femoral head from its dislocated posterior position to opposite the acetabulum. Simultaneously the thigh is gently abducted, reducing the femoral head in the acetabulum. In a positive finding, the examiner senses reduction by a palpable, nearly audible "clunk." Test one hip at a time for both of these tests. (From Marcdante KJ, Kliegman RM, Jenson HB, et al, editors: *Nelson essentials of pediatrics*, ed 6, Philadelphia, 2011, Saunders/Elsevier.)

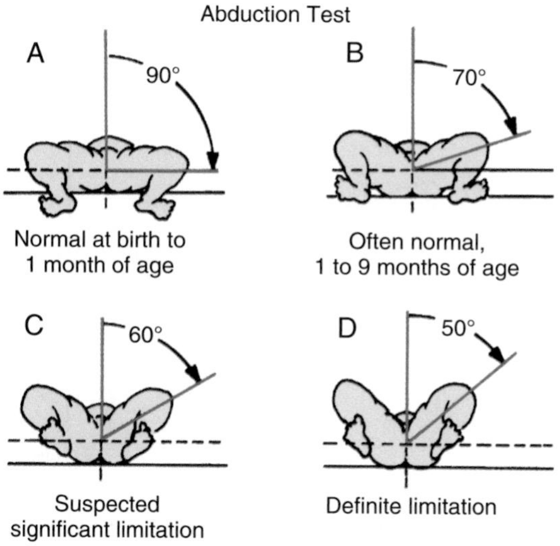

• **Figure 38-5** Hip abduction test. The child is placed supine, and the hips are flexed 90 degrees and fully abducted. Although the normal abduction range is quite broad (**A** and **B**), one can suspect hip disease in any patient who lacks more than 35 to 45 degrees of abduction (**C** suspicious and **D** abnormal). (From Chung SMK: *Hip disorders in infants and children*, Philadelphia, 1981, Lea & Febiger.)

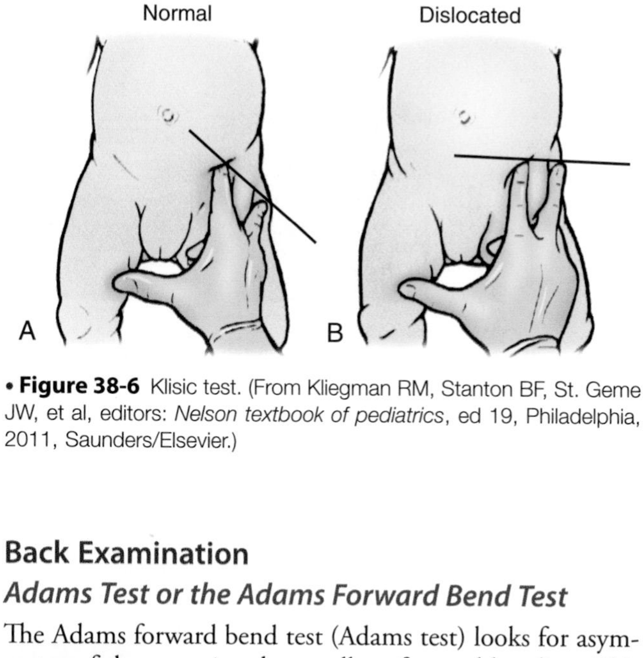

• **Figure 38-6** Klisic test. (From Kliegman RM, Stanton BF, St. Geme JW, et al, editors: *Nelson textbook of pediatrics*, ed 19, Philadelphia, 2011, Saunders/Elsevier.)

to fall apart as far as possible, using gravity alone or with light pressure. The angle between vertical (0 degree) and the leg position is the medial rotation. It is measured for each leg (Fig. 38-7, *A*). Asymmetric hip rotation is abnormal. Lateral rotation is measured by allowing the legs to cross while the child is still prone. The angle between vertical and the leg position is measured for each leg (see Fig. 38-7, *B*). Again, asymmetric hip rotation is abnormal. By 1 year old, a normal child has approximately 45 degrees of internal and external hip rotation.

Back Examination

Adams Test or the Adams Forward Bend Test

The Adams forward bend test (Adams test) looks for asymmetry of the posterior chest wall on forward bending. This position allows for evaluation of structural scoliosis. The child bends at the waist to a position of 90 degrees back flexion with straight legs, ankles together, and arms hanging freely or with palms together (in a diving position) but not touching the toes or floor (Fig. 38-8). The back is inspected for asymmetry of the height of the curves on the two sides or rib hump; the provider inspects the child's back by looking at it from the rear and side positions. The examiner should be seated in front of the child to best visually scan each level of the spine. If a rib hump is present, a scoliometer, if available, can be used to measure the angular tilt of the trunk. A spinal rotation greater than 5 to 7 degrees

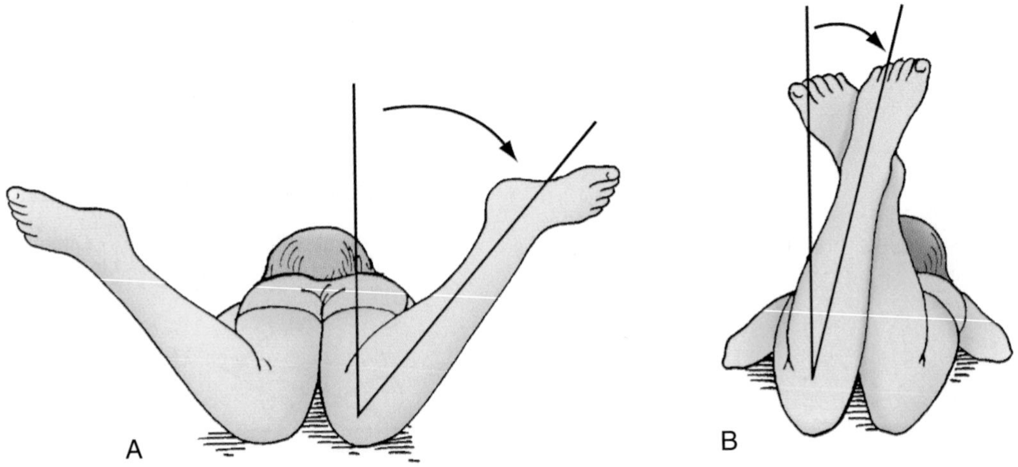

• **Figure 38-7** Hip rotation in extension. This is measured with the child in prone position and the knee flexed 90 degrees. The lower leg is vertically oriented. This is considered the neutral position. On outward rotation **(A),** the leg produces internal hip rotation, and on inward rotation **(B),** the leg produces external hip rotation. (From Thompson GH: Gait disturbances. In Kliegman RM, editor: *Practical strategies in pediatric diagnosis and therapy*, Philadelphia, 1996, Saunders.)

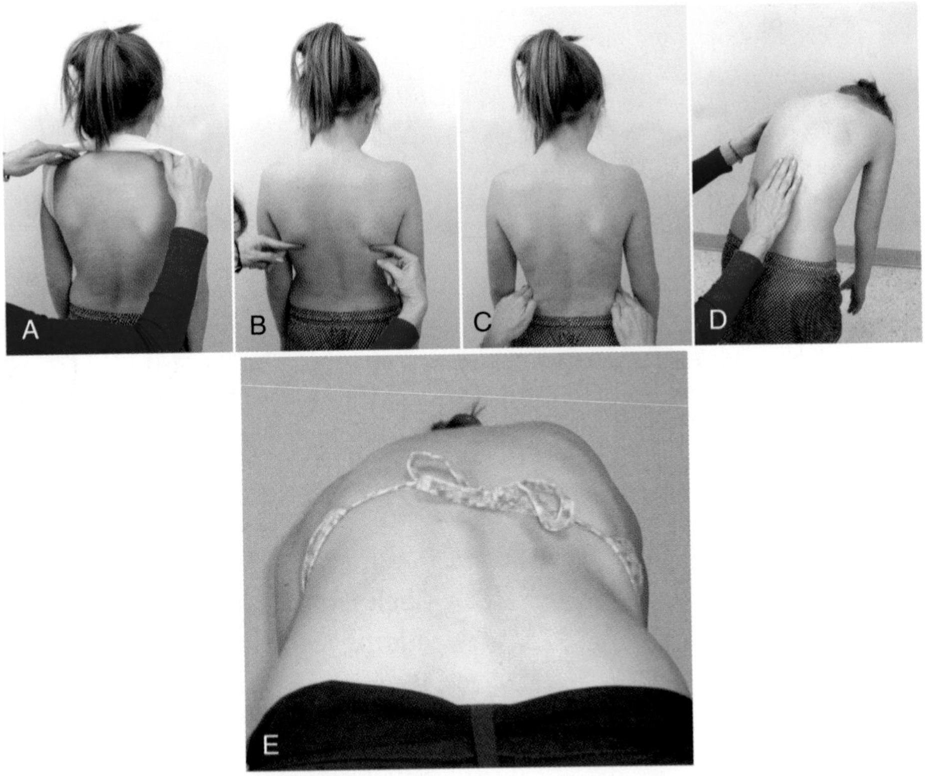

• **Figure 38-8** Asessment of the spine. **A**, Testing shoulder symmetry. **B**, Scapular symmetry. **C**, Iliac crest symmetry. **D,** Beginning Adams forward bend test. **E,** Positive rib hump. (From Skirven T, Osterman A, Dedorczk J, et al: Rehabilitation of the hand and upper extremity, ed 6, Philadelphia, 2012, Mosby; In Duderstadt KG, editor: *Pediatric physical examination: an illustrated handbook*, Philadelphia, 2014, Elsevier, p 277.)

measured by placing the scoliometer at the peak of the curvature indicates the need for further evaluation (Duderstadt and Schapiro, 2014).

Diagnostic Studies

Radiographs are an important diagnostic tool for the musculoskeletal system. Imaging should begin with standard radiographs of the area of concern. AP and lateral views of the affected area, bone, or joint are typically ordered to analyze the anatomic structures. Views of both extremities may be ordered so that comparisons can be made. Computed tomography (CT) scans augment radiographs to detail specific areas of the body, especially in identification of soft-tissue lesions. CT is useful in detailing the relationship of bones to their contiguous structures. Magnetic resonance imaging (MRI) gives excellent visualization of joints, soft tissues, cartilage, and medullary bone. It can distinguish among various physiologic changes that occur in bone marrow related to age and disease process. Ultrasonography can provide information about cartilaginous areas or tissues not visible on radiograph. The test is highly sensitive for detecting effusion of the hip joint. Bone scans (scintigraphy) are more sensitive than radiographs, demonstrate abnormal uptake earlier than conventional radiographs, and are useful in detecting causes of obscure skeletal pain. Although CT scanning and radiographs offer tremendous benefits in diagnosing and guiding care for children with musculoskeletal problems, providers must be mindful of the amount of radiation a child is exposed to and weigh the risks and benefits of their use.

Laboratory studies can help to identify systemic disease, infection, or inflammation. Erythrocyte sedimentation rate (ESR), C-reactive protein (CRP), complete blood count (CBC), blood cultures, rheumatoid factor, and antinuclear antibodies are hematologic tests that can assist in the diagnosis and management of bone disorders. Other laboratory tests also can provide an understanding of muscle metabolism (e.g., carnitine, lactic acid, leptin, pyruvates). Some bony lesions may need to be biopsied, and joint effusions and/or muscle tissue frequently needs to be sampled to determine specific disease pathologic conditions.

Management Strategies

Counseling

Counseling for orthopedic problems involves several components. The family should understand and have time to ask questions about all of the following issues:

- The pathologic condition, including possible etiologies
- The treatment plan
- The prognosis with and without treatment
- Any genetic implications of the diagnosis
- Long-term care issues

Counseling helps families cope with a poor, chronic, or challenging diagnosis and its short-term and long-term implications. Congenital problems are often identified prenatally, at birth, or shortly thereafter. Families need to be given the diagnosis truthfully, humanely, and as soon as possible. Issues of etiology need to be discussed to address parents' feelings of guilt for causing the problem and to discuss genetic implications, if any. A plan of care that is mutually agreed on by the family and the health care provider must be developed before the infant is discharged from the hospital or clinic.

Anticipatory Guidance: Musculoskeletal Development

Families are sometimes concerned about problems that providers believe are within normal limits and do not require an orthopedic referral. The provider should provide the child's family with a description of the child's predicted musculoskeletal development. Timelines and markers that parents can use to monitor their child's development are particularly helpful in allowing families to understand their child's pattern of growth. Misperceptions about the implications of minor variations need to be clarified, and the family should always be given the opportunity to return for further assessment or discussion if concerns remain. Examples of common concerns are flat feet in infants and toddlers, "bowed" legs in toddlers, and "knock-knees" in preschool children.

Shoes

The use of therapeutic shoes to correct orthopedic problems is controversial. Studies confirm that therapeutic shoes do little to correct deformities. Shoes for the average child should keep the feet warm and protected from injury. Shoes should be selected to fit properly and comfortably with room for growth. High-top shoes for toddlers may have the advantage of staying on little feet with fat pads better, but they do not provide additional support. Toddlers' feet do not need extra support. Features of a good shoe are as follows:

- Flexible sole—to allow as much free motion as possible; for young children, test to see if the shoe can be flexed in the parent's hand
- Flat—do not allow high heels
- Foot shaped—avoid pointed toes or other shapes that are not the normal configuration of the foot
- Fitted generously—better to be too large than too small
- Friction similar to skin—the soles should have the same friction as skin so that they are not slippery

Well-cushioned, shock-absorbing shoes are helpful in the child or adolescent athlete in order to decrease the chances of developing overuse syndrome. Shoe modifications may be needed in certain conditions. Shoe lifts are needed if limb length differences exceed 2.5 cm. Orthotics also can be used in certain orthopedic situations to more evenly distribute pressure on the sole of the foot and facilitate function.

Care of Children in Casts and Splints

Casts and splints serve various functions in the management of musculoskeletal injuries. They are applied in order to immobilize, promote healing, maintain bone alignment, diminish pain, protect the injury, and help compensate for surrounding muscular weakness. Splints are non-circumferential immobilizers that accommodate swelling. Splints are used in orthopedic conditions where swelling is anticipated: acute fractures or sprains and for initial stabilization of reduced, displaced, or unstable fractures before orthopedic intervention. Casts are circumferential immobilizers. They provide superior immobilization but are less forgiving and have a higher rate of complications. The use of casts and splints is generally limited to a short period of time. If prolonged immobilization is required, joint stiffness and muscle atrophy may occur and generally warrant physical or occupational therapy to regain function.

The child's cast should be kept cool, clean, and dry. Cover the cast with plastic wrap or a plastic bag when the child bathes or is in a situation in which the cast may get wet. If the cast becomes wet, a hair dryer set on cool setting can be used for drying small areas. If the cast becomes soiled, it can be cleaned with a slightly damp washcloth and cleanser.

The family should be taught how to do a circulatory inspection to check the function of nerves and blood vessels. Casts can be perceived by children to be itchy, and they may insert small toys or long thin objects that cannot be seen externally for relief. These objects or area swelling may impede the blood flow or neurologic innervation. The child's toes or fingers below the cast should be pink and warm to touch. The child should be able to feel all sides or his or her fingers or toes when touched and should be able to wiggle the fingers or toes. Skin care following cast and splint removal is imperative. For the first few days following splint and cast removal, the skin is delicate and sensitive. The skin may appear pale yellow and skin will be flaky. The family should be instructed to soak and gently cleanse the skin, pat dry, and avoid rubbing or peeling excess skin.

The family needs to know when to call the provider: if the toes or fingers are cold to touch and appear pale or blue, complaints of tingling or numbness, inability to move fingers or toes, and excessive swelling. Additional problems with casts (such as, foul smell, breakage, or loosening) should be reported. Furthermore, alteration in skin integrity following the removal of a cast or splint must be reported.

Physical and Occupational Therapy

Children with developmental delays, cerebral palsy, spine disorders, and torticollis may benefit from physical or occupational therapy. Treatments focus on improving gross and fine motor skills, balance and coordination, strength and endurance, as well as cognitive and sensory processing. Structured physical therapy post-orthopedic injury can be helpful.

Orthopedic Problems Specific to Children

Arm Problems

Annular Ligament Displacement

Annular ligament displacement, previously described as a subluxation of the radial head and frequently called *nursemaid's elbow,* is a frequent injury that occurs in children 6 months to 5 years old. The injury typically occurs when traction is applied to the arm of a young child, which is most often the result of pulling a child by the hand or grasping a child's hand to prevent a fall. This motion causes the annular ligament to slide over the head of the radius, where it becomes entrapped in the radial-humeral joint when the distal traction is released (Browner, 2013) (Fig. 38-9, *A*).

Clinical Findings

History. Often the history is nonspecific as to a report of an injury, and the parent may not have been aware of when the injury occurred. Alternatively, a caregiver will commonly report the child cried, complaining of arm pain after being pulled up by his or her arm, or swung by the arms. The caregiver typically reports that since the incident, the child has refused to bend or use the affected arm, crying out in pain if the arm is moved, particularly the elbow. The toddler with nursemaid's elbow may be comfortable and is reluctant to use the affected arm and hand.

The injury produces immediate pain and limited supination. The child typically shows no limitation of flexion or extension of the elbow, and swelling and ecchymosis are absent (Carrigan, 2011). The child will resist moving his or her arm and can be observed holding the affected arm against their body and slightly flexed.

Diagnostic Studies. Radiographs are not routinely recommended when the history and clinical presentation are classic. However, if obtained, radiography of the elbow is normal. If the history of the injury is not consistent with a mechanism expected to cause a nursemaid's elbow or if the physical examination lends to the possibility of additional injury, radiographs are indicated.

Differential Diagnosis

Subluxation has a classic history and presentation. If the child does not improve after the reduction procedure (see next section), a fracture of the elbow or clavicle should be considered. The clinical presentation of a fracture may be similar to that of a subluxation injury and therefore must be ruled out. Consider maltreatment if recurrent dislocations or other symptoms or signs are present.

Management

Two techniques can be used to reduce the radial head: supination and flexion or pronation. Do not attempt either procedure if epitrochlear tenderness is present, because this may be indicative of a more serious injury (e.g., fracture).

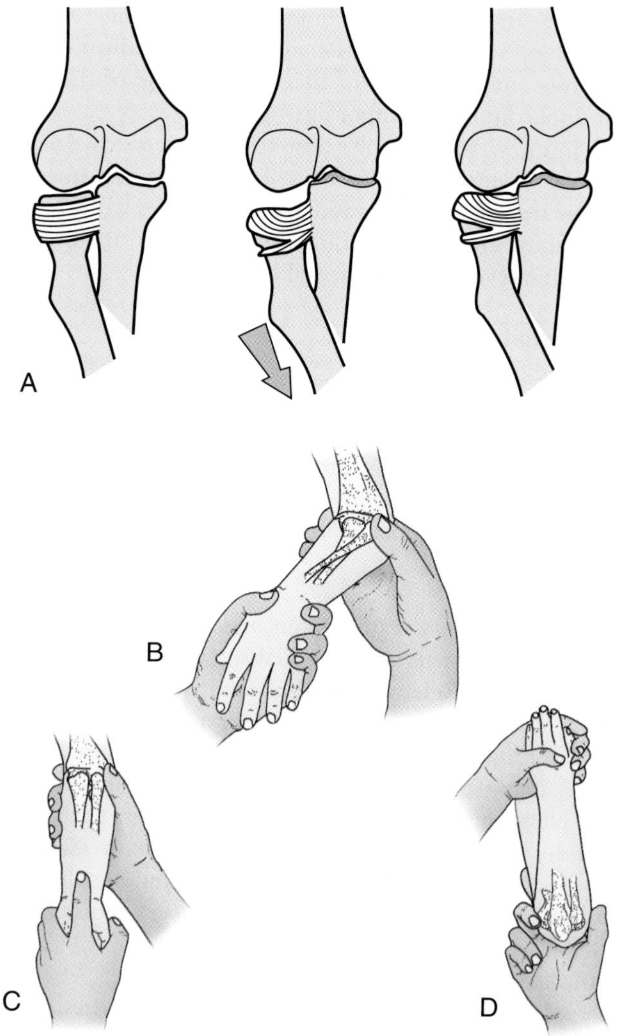

• **Figure 38-9** **A,** Annular ligament displacement, formerly known as *subluxation of the radial head.* The pathology of nursemaid's elbow, or pulled elbow. The anterior ligament is partially torn when the arm is pulled. The radial head moves distally, and when traction is discontinued, the ligament is carried into the joint. **B-D,** Reduction of radial head subluxation by supination and flexion technique. **B,** Grasp the palm of the child's hand as if to shake it. Axial traction is applied to the forearm with the wrist adducted to the ulnar side. Pressure is also applied directly over the radial head of the elbow. **C,** The forearm is supinated while axial traction and pressure are maintained over the forearm and radial head. **D,** Flex the elbow to the shoulder while supination and pressure are maintained over the radial head. (**A,** From Rang M: *Children's fractures*, ed 2, Philadelphia, 1983, JB Lippincott, p 193. Found in Kliegman RM, Stanton BF, St. Geme JW, et al, editors: *Nelson textbook of pediatrics*, ed 19, Philadelphia, 2011, Saunders/Elsevier. **B-D,** From Shah B: Reduction of radial head subluxation. In Finberg L, Kleinmn RE, editors: *Saunders manual of pediatric practice*, ed 2, Philadelphia, 2002, Saunders, p 1162.)

The steps to correct the subluxation involve the following:

- Approach the child in a slow, nonthreatening way and distract the child by talking or other diversionary tactics.
- Use either the supination and flexion technique as illustrated in Fig. 38-9, *B,* or the pronation technique. With the pronation technique, the provider gentle extends the elbow in order to fully pronate the child's forearm (palm down). Once full pronation and extension are achieved, the provider then releases the forearm and elbow and evaluates if the attempt at reduction was successful (Browner, 2013).
- A palpable or audible "pop" or "click" usually signals successful reduction. Typically the child begins reaching for objects again with the affected arm within 15 minutes of reduction. If reduction is successful, no further treatment is necessary.

Complications

Several attempts (up to three at reduction) may be necessary before the patient resumes normal use of the arm. If normal use does not follow reduction attempts, immobilization using a sling with prompt orthopedic follow-up is indicated. Recurrence of nursemaid's elbow occurs in approximately one third of patients. Therefore, education and anticipatory guidance should be provided to caregivers in an effort to prevent reinjury (Browner, 2013).

Patient and Parent Education

Key points to cover include the following:

- Instruct caregivers not to lift or pull the child by the hand or elbow.
- Instruct caregivers to lift the child from the axillae.

Brachial Plexus Injuries

The brachial plexus is a network of nerves in the shoulder arising from the spinal cord that enables movement and sensation in the shoulders, arms, and hands. Injury to the shoulder and brachial plexus during the birthing process is known as *obstetric brachial plexus palsy* or *neonatal brachial plexus palsy* and is the focus of this discussion. Brachial plexus injuries are typically classified using Narakas criteria, types I through IV (Table 38-1). Most injuries affect the upper brachial plexus (C5 and C6 nerve roots), resulting in weakness or paralysis of the shoulder and upper arm, and are known as *Erb-Duchenne (Erb) palsy.* More severe injuries involving the lower plexus (C7, C8, and T1 nerve roots) impair hand function and cause ipsilateral ptosis and miosis, known as *Dejerine-Klumpke (Klumpke) palsy* (Phua et al, 2012).

Risk factors for neonatal brachial plexus palsies may be divided into three categories: neonatal, maternal, and labor-related factors. Breech presentation and macrosomic infants are at increased risk for brachial plexus injuries. Maternal characteristics include diabetes, obesity, maternal age (more than 35 years), and maternal pelvic anatomy. Labor-related factors (such as, shoulder dystocia) account for approximately 45% of brachial plexus injuries. Vacuum extraction, direct compression of the fetal neck during delivery by forceps, or application of lateral traction on the head during delivery of the shoulder can cause stretching of the cervical nerve roots and eventually brachial plexus injury (Russman, 2015).

TABLE 38-1 Brachial Plexus Injury Using Narakas Classification

Name	Nerves and Muscles Involved	Prognosis
Narakas type I	C5 and C6; shoulder and biceps	Recovery usually complete
Narakas type II	C5 to C7; shoulder, biceps, and forearm extensors	Recovery usually complete
Narakas type III	C5 to T1	Variable with complete paralysis of limb; shoulder and biceps recovery is fair to poor with hand recovery variable
Narakas type IV	C5 to T1	Complete paralysis of the limb and Horner syndrome; shoulder and biceps recovery is fair to poor with hand recovery variable

Clinical Findings

History. History should include obstetric history, mode of delivery, and postnatal health of the infant.

Physical Examination. A thorough head-to-toe examination is required to identify any deformations or other injuries that may have occurred in utero or during delivery. Passive range of motion must be assessed, and newborn reflexes should be tested in order to identify neurologic deficits. Findings may include:

- Erb palsy, presenting with an adducted arm, which is internally rotated at the shoulder: The wrist is flexed, and the fingers are extended, resulting in a characteristic "waiter's tip" posture.
- Absent bicep reflex with asymmetric Moro and tonic neck reflex on the affected side
- Limp wrist and hand with absent grasp reflex (lower plexus involvement)
- Horner syndrome (ipsilateral ptosis, miosis, enophthalmos, anhidrosis) if the sympathetic fibers of the T1 nerve root are involved
- Occasionally hand paralysis with normal shoulder movement, which is a rare occurrence of an isolated C8 through T1 injury
- Ruptured intraabdominal structures, especially the liver and spleen, which require careful abdominal examination
- Limited neck movement due to damage to the sternocleidomastoid muscle; skull fracture
- Impaired respiratory effort as a result of diaphragmatic paralysis and flaccidity

Diagnostic Studies. Radiologic examination, electrophysiologic studies, and MRI are useful to confirm clinical diagnosis and the extent of the injury. X-rays of the chest and upper limbs are important because they reveal associated injuries, such as rib, transverse process, clavicle, or humeral fractures. Chest x-ray is necessary to rule out phrenic nerve injury. Electrodiagnostic studies with electromyography and nerve conduction velocities are used to determine severity of the neural lesion.

Differential Diagnosis

The differential diagnosis of upper extremity paralysis in a newborn includes epiphyseal separation of the humeral head, fracture of the clavicle or humerus, septic arthritis, acute osteomyelitis of the upper extremity, spinal cord injury, cervical cord lesions, and congenital malformations of the plexus and upper limb (Herring and Ho, 2014).

Management

A multidisciplinary team approach is ideal with referral to health professionals who specialize in treating brachial plexus injuries. Referral should be made in the first week of life. The initial goal of therapy is to maintain passive range of motion, supple joints, and muscle strength. Indications for surgical exploration and reconstruction of the brachial plexus include failure of recovery of elbow flexion and shoulder abduction from the third to the sixth month of life. The spectrum of nerve surgery includes neurolysis, neuroma resection, nerve grafting, and nerve transfers.

Complications

Late sequelae include internal rotation contractures, hypoplasia of the arm, altered sensibility, flexion contractures of the elbow, dislocations of the radial head, and psychological and social consequences.

Prognosis

Recovery can occur spontaneously and is highly dependent on the level and extent of nerve injury. In general, paralysis of the upper portion of the arm has a better prognosis than does paralysis of the lower part of the arm. If the paralysis is due to edema surrounding the nerve fibers (neurapraxia), spontaneous full recovery within a few weeks is likely; if it is due to disruption of the nerve fibers (axonotmesis), function generally returns in a few months. More severe injuries, total disruption of the nerves (neurotmesis) and root avulsion, require surgery with partial or complete recovery observed for several years. Fortunately, 50% of plexus injuries occur at the upper nerve roots (C5 to C6), involve neurapraxia and axonotmesis, and heal spontaneously (Russman, 2015).

Shoulder Problems

Clavicle Fracture

Clavicle fractures are seen in newborns, as a result of birth trauma, and in young children as a result of accidental and nonaccidental trauma. They can occur as a result of a direct hit or indirect trauma and are most commonly associated with a fall. Approximately 80% to 85% of these fractures occur in the middle third of the clavicle and 12% to 15% in the distal third. The clavicle is the first bone to ossify and the last physis in the body to close, usually not until 25 to 30 years old (Herring and Ho, 2014).

Clinical Findings

History. History varies depending on the age of the child.

In the neonate:

- Difficult delivery, high birth weight, midforceps delivery, and shoulder dystocia
- Irritability when infant is moved or lifted

In the older child:

- History of fall or trauma with focus on mechanism of injury

Physical Examination. In all children, look for the following:

- Pain with shoulder movement
- Decreased arm movement on affected side (asymmetric spontaneous arm movements) or absent Moro reflex
- Swelling, bony abnormality, discoloration, and/or crepitus elicited over fracture site
- Callus felt over fracture site within a few days
- Spasm of sternocleidomastoid muscle on affected side
- An associated Erb palsy

Diagnostic Studies. Imaging studies are recommended. Radiography with routine clavicle views is sufficient.

Differential Diagnosis

Brachial palsy, shoulder dislocation, or other bony problem should be considered.

Management

Management involves the following:

- Neonate
  - Incomplete fractures that do not cause pain need no treatment.
  - Immobilization of the shoulder is an option when movement results in a painful arm (usually with a complete fracture). Pin the sleeve of the infant's arm to the front of the shirt for 1 to 2 weeks.
- Older child
  - Sling immobilization for comfort to support the affected extremity is often sufficient. Generally sling immobilization can be discontinued at 3 to 4 weeks.
  - A figure-eight clavicle brace can be used if displacement results in a decreased shaft length. However, it is uncomfortable to wear, and its effectiveness is questionable.
  - Protection for 4 to 5 weeks is generally sufficient because union requires about 4 weeks of healing.
  - An older child may need analgesics or a nonsteroidal anti-inflammatory drug (NSAID) for pain.
  - The need for surgical intervention is uncommon with clavicle fractures. Surgery may be needed in open fractures, neurovascular compromise, multiple trauma, rib cage fractures, and those with greater than 100% displacement with severe skin tenting.

Prognosis

The prognosis is excellent. Often the injury in neonates is identified only at later primary care visits, when the callus lump is palpated, although the child may be irritable until the fracture is stable. The infant is usually asymptomatic within 7 to 10 days. Parents need information and emotional support. In older children, general healing time is 6 to 8 weeks with average return to noncontact sports in 4 to 6 weeks. Bony callus appears approximately 10 days post-injury as a painless, firm "lump."

Rib Problems

Costochondritis and Sternochondritis

Costochondritis is a common cause of chest pain in children and adolescents. The condition is characterized as an inflammatory process of one or more of the costochondral cartilages that causes localized tenderness and pain of the anterior chest wall. Most are idiopathic (Garry, 2015).

Trauma to the area and unaccustomed physical effort (lifting heavy objects or coughing) are factors known to cause costochondritis. Inflammation is the underlying problem.

Clinical Findings

History. Pain localized to the costosternal or costochondral junction is the major symptom. It often presents with tenderness over more than one rib as a result of referred pain. The primary rib that is inflamed and usually responsible for the symptoms is most often the one that exhibits the greatest sensitivity to palpation. Characteristics of the pain include the following:

- Acute or gradual onset; typically insidious occurring over several days or weeks
- Sharp, darting, or dull quality
- Radiation from chest to upper abdomen or back
- Occasional complaints of a feeling of tightness caused by muscle spasm
- Exacerbating factors may include coughing, sneezing, deep inspiration, movement of the upper torso and upper extremities

Physical Examination. Palpation reveals tenderness over the costochondral junction. The tenderness should be localized and is most common at the sternocostal cartilage of the second through the seventh ribs. The presence of pain, swelling (a unique bulbous enlargement of the joint commonly noted over a single upper costochondrial junction) with or without redness, and tenderness at the costal cartilage is referred to as *Tietze syndrome.* Ecchymosis may be seen in cases of trauma. Respiratory effort is normal. Auscultation of the lungs, heart, and abdomen is normal (Garry, 2015).

Diagnostic Studies. No diagnostic studies are needed, because history and physical findings are the key to the diagnosis. Chest radiography may exclude other possible causes but offers no diagnostic value. A CT scan can demonstrate swelling of the costal cartilage.

Differential Diagnosis

Rib fractures are the key differential diagnosis if pain is associated with an injury. Childhood rheumatic diseases also can have complaints similar to costochondritis but generally have other characteristic physical findings. Costochondritis is one of the differential diagnoses of pediatric chest pain (see Chapter 31).

Management

Treatment consists of using mild analgesia and NSAIDs to relieve discomfort and avoiding strenuous activity. Cough suppressants may be beneficial if cough is an aggravating factor. Stretching exercises and use of ice to the area can be useful. Parents and children need to be reassured that this is a benign self-limited condition and is not related to cardiac disease.

Back Problems

Back Pain

Children do not commonly complain of severe back pain. Most episodes of back pain in pediatric patients are brief with nonspecific findings and history. Back pain that warrants immediate attention includes children younger than 4 years old, persistent symptoms, self-imposed activity limitations, systemic symptoms, increasing discomfort, persistent nighttime pain, neurologic symptoms, history of tuberculosis or cancer, and back pain accompanied by unexplained weight loss (Kordi and Rostami, 2011). The older the child, the more likely the etiology of back pain is musculoskeletal in origin. Younger children who have such complaints should be carefully evaluated for occult pathologic conditions, and the provider's index of suspicion about underlying pathologic conditions should be raised. The young athlete is especially susceptible to back injury. Intense training can cause repetitive microtrauma. Back pain can result from sprains of the ligaments or muscles (or both) of the back caused by injury.

Clinical Findings

History. Onset, duration, location, frequency, and intensity of the pain are key questions to ask to form an initial impression. In addition, it is important that the provider differentiate between mechanical and inflammatory causes. Therefore, the history should include questions related to the timing of back pain, as well as aggravating or relieving factors. Specifically, the back pain reported with morning stiffness or prolonged rest is associated with inflammatory causes, whereas back pain reported with activity is associated with mechanical causes.

The following findings should alert the pediatric provider to possible pathologic conditions:

- Night pain
- Pain that prohibits play or activities
- Pain that persists or worsens
- History of trauma (vertebral fracture)
- Positive neurologic or musculoskeletal signs on examination
- Systemic signs, such as fever, chills, weight loss, and malaise
- Presence of any radicular symptoms, gait disturbances, muscle weakness, altered sensation, and changes in bowel and/or bladder function

In school-age children and adolescents, back pain can be associated with a history of the following:

- Muscle strain as a result of "overuse syndrome" from excessive muscular exertion, usually related to sports, commonly in sedentary children who recently increased their activity level
- Wearing high heels or platform shoes (females)
- Neck/shoulder, low back, and arm pain in relation to computer or video game use; excessive TV watching

Physical Examination. The examination should include a complete musculoskeletal and neurologic assessment with the child adequately exposed for the clinical examination. Inspect for any changes in alignment in the frontal or sagittal plane, and range of motion should be assessed in flexion, extension, and lateral bending. Younger children may be asked to pick up an object off the floor to assess spinal flexion. Palpation will reveal any areas of tenderness and/or muscle spasm. Palpate the top of the iliac wings while the child is standing to assess leg lengths. A careful neurologic examination should be performed.

Diagnostic Studies. A CBC with differential, ESR, and CRP are useful tests for infectious conditions; rheumatoid factor and antinuclear antibodies are useful tests for suspected rheumatologic disorders. Initially AP and lateral radiographs of the involved region of the spine are recommended. With lumbar back pain, right and left oblique views are recommended. MRI is most helpful when neurologic symptoms or findings are present. CT is superior to MRI for assessing bone involvement (Wells et al, 2011).

Differential Diagnosis

Occult pathologic conditions should be ruled out. Diskitis, vertebral osteomyelitis, vertebral fracture, or tumor can cause significant back pain in toddlers. Older children can experience these same problems in addition to intervertebral disk herniation, vertebral endplate fractures, low back stress fracture, and spondylosis. Back pain is a commonly reported symptom in somatizing children. Athletes with a history of low back pain lasting more than 1 month deserve careful evaluation. A low-back stress fracture or spondylosis needs to be included in the differential diagnoses.

Management

Treatment is determined by the findings on history and physical examination and can include referral for radiographs (AP and lateral views) and imaging studies or referral to a subspecialist physician or pediatrician. If the back pain is due to injury, pain management and physical therapy may be part of the treatment plan.

Scoliosis

Scoliosis is a three-dimensional deformity most commonly described as a lateral curvature of the spine in the frontal plane. There are two types of scoliosis: nonstructural and structural. Nonstructural, also known as *functional scoliosis,* involves a curve in the spine without rotation of the vertebrae. The curve is reversible, considering it is caused by conditions such as poor posture, muscle spasms, pain, or leg length discrepancy. Structural scoliosis involves a rotational element of the spine and has various classifications depending on the cause. The remaining discussion pertains to structural scoliosis.

The diagnosis is based on a curvature of more than 10 degrees using the Cobb method in which the angle between the superior and inferior end vertebrae (tilted into the curve) is measured by a radiologist (see Diagnostic Studies in the following text). In most pediatric cases, the etiology is unknown and is therefore termed and classified as idiopathic. Other classifications include congenital, in which vertebrae fail to form (e.g., hemivertebrae), and neuromuscular (e.g., cerebral palsy, neurofibromatosis, Marfan syndrome). Kyphosis, which results from disorders of sagittal alignment (such as, postural kyphosis and Scheuermann disease), is another classification of structural scoliosis. Kyphosis, commonly termed *round back,* is discussed following scoliosis.

- Idiopathic: Etiology is unknown and is likely multifactorial. It is the most common type of scoliosis. There are three types classified by age at onset:
  - Infantile (0 to 3 years old)
  - Juvenile (3 to 10 years old)
  - Adolescent (11 years old and older)
- Congenital: A structural anomaly present at birth (e.g., hemivertebrae) often associated with other congenital abnormalities, such as renal and cardiac anomalies; progression of curvature can worsen rapidly, particularly during periods of rapid growth (e.g., first 2 to 3 years of life and adolescence).
- Neuromuscular: Most common in non-ambulatory patients. Secondary to weakness/imbalance/spasticity of the muscles of the trunk caused by primary neuromuscular problems (e.g., cerebral palsy or muscular dystrophy). In contrast to idiopathic and congenital scoliosis, curves caused by neuromuscular disorders can continue to progress after skeletal maturity.

Idiopathic is the most common type of scoliosis. Its etiology is unknown, but it often has a familial or genetic pattern. The overall incidence of idiopathic scoliosis is approximately 2% to 3% with between 0.3% and 0.5% of children with scoliosis having curves greater than 20 degrees on radiography and less than 0.1% demonstrating curves greater than 40 degrees Cobb's angle.

Hormonal changes play a role in the disease process, and a rapid growth period is believed to be a significant factor in the progression of curvature associated with idiopathic scoliosis. In addition, the risk of curve progression depends on the amount of growth remaining, the magnitude of the curve, and gender. Although the incidence of idiopathic scoliosis is nearly equal in girls and boys, females have a much higher risk of developing curves more than 30 degrees (Spiegel and Dormans, 2011). The most common type of idiopathic scoliosis is found in adolescents and is the major focus of the remaining discussion.

Small to moderate scoliotic curves (10% to 30%) usually do not increase significantly after skeletal growth is complete but bear watching, particularly during periods of rapid growth velocity. Double S-curves and more severe curves are more likely to progress during the growth years. For a given child, however, the ability to predict progression is difficult, because even small curves (10% to 25%) can progress to severe deformity. Thus regular monitoring of any curve in a skeletally immature child is important (Table 38-2).

The female-to-male ratio increases with increasing curve magnitude. For curves less than 20 degrees, the risk for progression of the curve is low; these curves generally just need to be observed. However, for curves between 20 and 45 degrees, the risk for progression is high during growth, and early intervention is of paramount importance. In children with curves greater than 50 degrees, the spine loses its ability to compensate and progression is expected. Young premenarchal females with large curves are a vulnerable group, because their spines are skeletally immature with growth remaining. The majority of adolescents with idiopathic scoliosis have a right thoracic curve. Juvenile manifestation is uncommon, and infantile scoliosis is rare in the United States.

Clinical Findings

History. Scoliosis is generally painless, and insidious onset is typical. Generally there is no significant history. The provider should assess the following:

- Family history of scoliosis
- Age of menarche
- Etiologic factors related to the various causes of structural scoliosis

The presence of pain with a lateral curvature of the spine suggests an inflammatory or neoplastic lesion as the cause of the scoliosis. Some children with idiopathic scoliosis complain of mild pain that is activity related. Severe, constant, or night pain and point tenderness could be indicative of other pathologic conditions (e.g., metastatic tumor or stenosis) and warrants further investigation.

Physical Examination. Children of all ages should be evaluated in the standing position, from both the front and the side, to identify any asymmetry. Looking primarily at the straightness of the spine can be misleading, because scoliosis involves both rotation and misalignment of the vertebrae. The Adams forward bend position accentuates

TABLE 38-2 Scoliosis, Kyphosis, and Lordosis

	Curve	Etiology	Clinical Findings	Radiographs	Management
Scoliosis	Lateral	Classifications: Idiopathic (most common); neuromuscular; constitutional; secondary; congenital; miscellaneous; functional (leg length discrepancy—not scoliosis)	History: Positive family history; related to etiologies (classifications); painless curvature; typically have right thoracic curve	AP and lateral standing views to identify degree of curve; >10 degrees abnormal; may have one curve (C) or two curves (S); vertebrae show lateral deviation and rotation	Referral to orthopedic surgeon; brace or surgery; need to monitor progression of curve Most curves do not increase after growth complete; females with idiopathic scoliosis more likely to have curve progression and need close monitoring
Kyphosis	AP curve of thoracic spine	Familial (Scheuermann disease); secondary to tumor, trauma, and so on; congenital; postural, not true kyphosis	Postural round back	Narrow disk space and loss of normal anterior height of vertebrae	Postural: PT, dancing, and swimming can be helpful If structural, refer to an orthopedic surgeon for observation, bracing, or surgery
Lordosis	AP curve of lumbar spine	As a result of hip contractures; physiologic; family and racial groups; before puberty	Abdomen and buttock protuberant; if result of hip contractures, lordosis disappears when sitting	Standing lateral views	If lumbar spine flattens and lordosis disappears when child bends forward, it is physiologic and no treatment; if fixed, refer to an orthopedist

AP, Anteroposterior; *PT*, physical therapy.

the rotational deformity of scoliosis. Asymmetries to look for include:

- Unequal shoulder height
- Unequal scapula prominences and heights: Note that the muscle masses may be somewhat unequal, especially if the child uses one shoulder more than the other as in carrying books. Look for bony, not muscular, prominence.
- Unequal waist angles: The hip touches one arm, and the contralateral arm hangs free.
- Unequal rib prominences and chest asymmetry
- Asymmetry of the elbow to flank distance, and some deviation of the spine from a straight head-to-toe line
- Unequal rib heights when the child stands in the Adams forward bend position (see Fig. 38-8)

During the Adams test the examiner looks for asymmetry of the posterior chest wall on forward bending, the earliest abnormality seen. Rotation of the vertebral bodies toward the convexity results in outward rotation and prominence of the attached ribs posteriorly. The anterior chest wall may be flattened on the concavity due to inward rotation of the chest wall and ribs. Associated findings may include elevation of the shoulder, lateral shift of the trunk, and an apparent leg-length discrepancy.

Congenital scoliosis may be visible in the infant lying prone; it is sometimes more prominent if the infant is suspended prone. Inspect for skin abnormalities, sacral dimple, and hairy patches.

The physical examination should also include the following:

- Observation for equal leg lengths
- Examination of the skin for hairy patches, nevi, café au lait spots, lipomas, dimples
- Neurologic examination checking for weakness or sensory disturbance
- Cardiac examination with diagnosis of Marfan syndrome

Diagnostic Studies. Standing AP and lateral radiographs of the entire spine are recommended at the initial evaluation for patients with clinical findings suggestive of a spinal deformity. On the PA radiographs, the degree of curvature is determined by the Cobb method. An MRI is helpful when an underlying cause for the scoliosis is suspected based on age (infantile, juvenile curves), abnormal findings in the history and on physical examination, and atypical radiographic features. Atypical radiographic findings include uncommon curve patterns, such as the left thoracic curve, double thoracic curves, high thoracic curves, widening of the spinal canal, and erosive or dysplastic changes in the vertebral body or ribs. On the lateral radiograph, an increase in thoracic kyphosis or an absence of segmental lordosis may be suggestive of an underlying neurologic abnormality (Spiegel and Dormans, 2011).

Differential Diagnosis

Structural scoliosis must be differentiated from functional scoliosis. The latter disappears when the child is placed in the Adams forward bend position, whereas the former is enhanced in this position. Persistent functional scoliosis to one side in a child with a neuromotor problem can eventually become structural and must be managed with physical therapy or other means to prevent progression. Consider systemic problems, such as neurofibromatosis, cerebral palsy, multiple sclerosis, Rett syndrome, rickets, tuberculosis, and tumor.

Management

The primary aim of scoliosis management is to stop curvature progression and improve pulmonary function. Treatment options include observation, bracing, and surgical treatment. The management presented in this text addresses idiopathic scoliosis treatment. Of note, genetic testing is now available to provide a personalized treatment approach for selected patients diagnosed with adolescent idiopathic scoliosis. The ScoliScore is a genetic test that screens for more than 50 genetic markers (53 single nucleotide polymorphisms [SNPs]) linked to the progression of spinal curves and assigns a quantitative score to a patient's deoxyribonucleic acid (DNA) saliva sample. (See the SNP discussion in Chapter 41.) The score identifies the patient as having a low, medium, or high risk for curve progression (Bohl et al, 2014; Smith and Cruz, 2010). For children in the low-risk group, these prognostic data may lead to less frequent follow-up visits to specialists, avoiding or discontinuing bracing, and fewer radiologic tests. However, the test is only indicated for children with mild curves (10 to 25 degrees) with growth remaining (Ward et al, 2010). Combined with diagnostic information and clinical judgment, the results of the ScoliScore test serve as a guide for health care providers to optimize the treatment of scoliosis.

Idiopathic Scoliosis

Adolescent scoliosis can resolve, remain static, or increase. As a result treatment options vary considerably. Treatment decisions are based on the natural history of each curvature. Infantile scoliosis can resolve spontaneously; however, progressive curves require bracing and surgery in an attempt to slow the curve progression and prevent complications (e.g., thoracic insufficiency syndrome). Juvenile scoliosis is found more frequently in girls, and the curves are at high risk for progression and often require surgical intervention. The goal in treatment is to delay spinal fusion, allowing time for the pulmonary system and thoracic cage to have matured and maximum trunk height to be achieved. (See the various surgical procedures described in the following section.) The natural history includes the degree of skeletal maturity or growth remaining, the magnitude of the curve, and any associated diagnoses or medical conditions.

Observation is always indicated for curves less than 20 degrees. Bracing or surgery may be indicated for larger curves. Brace treatment may reduce the need for surgery, restore the sagittal profile, and change vertebral rotation. Indications for bracing are a curve more than 30 degrees. Additional indications for brace therapy include skeletally immature patients with curves of 20 to 25 degrees that have shown more than 5 degrees of progression. The efficacy of bracing for adolescent idiopathic scoliosis remains controversial. Some studies show brace treatment to be effective in preventing curvature progression; however, it has been found that the success of the treatment is proportional to the amount of time that the patient wears the brace. Various brace treatment protocols suggest wearing a brace as much as 23 hours per day; therefore, compliance is a significant factor for this treatment modality (Spiegel and Dormans, 2011).

Surgical treatment is indicated for children and adolescents who have progressive spinal deformity that do not respond to bracing and for those with curvature exceeding 45 to 50 degrees (Richards et al, 2014). There are various surgical procedures; all aim to control progressive curvatures. In the past, surgery was limited to arthrodesis (surgical fusion) of the spine.

In recent years, several procedures have been developed that are designed to postpone and, in some cases, eliminate the need for early spinal fusion and allow for growth. These include the vertical expandable prosthetic titanium rib (VEPTR). This procedure is indicated for children with restricted pulmonary function due to the curvature of their thoracic spine. The surgery involves implanting a prosthesis that serves to enlarge the constricted thorax. The prosthesis can be adjusted approximately every 4 to 6 months, thereby allowing for growth. The "growing rod" surgical procedure has shown success in patients with adolescent idiopathic scoliosis and involves inserting spinal rods that are used to exert distraction forces that are adjusted approximately every 6 months. The rods serve as an internal brace to control the curvature of the spine while allowing skeletal growth. A more recent procedure involves intervertebral spinal stapling or tethering. Unlike the VEPTR and growing rod procedures, intervertebral spinal stapling does not require repeat adjustments and, therefore, eliminates the need for repeat surgical procedures. Research on this technique is limited, and clinical indications have not been universally agreed upon. Further research is necessary and long-term results are yet to be determined.

Referral to an orthopedist or a center that specializes in working with infants and children with scoliosis is essential. Support must be given to the child and family through the diagnostic and treatment phases, considering school and peer factors. The primary care provider needs to assist the child with psychological adjustment issues that arise if bracing or surgery is recommended and instituted. Some specific concerns of the child can include self-esteem problems, managing hostility and anger, learning about the disease and its care, wondering about the long-term prognosis, and concerns about clothing and participation in sports and other activities.

Complications

Progressive scoliosis can result in a severe deformity of the spinal column. Severe deformities can result in impairment of respiratory and cardiovascular function and limitation of physical activities and decreased comfort. The psychological consequences of an untreated scoliosis deformity can be severe.

Prevention

Prevention is not possible; however, screening and early identification of children with scoliosis may help avoid more expensive, invasive care and prevent the long-term consequences of the disorder. Screening is effective, however, only if identified children are referred for care. Parents must be notified, a referral arranged, and follow-up ensured.

Kyphosis

The thoracic spine normally has between 20 and 45 degrees of posterior curvature, which is considered physiologic. *Kyphosis* is the term used to describe the condition when the normal posterior curvature of the thoracic spine becomes excessive or exaggerated and is outside the physiologic range of normal. With kyphosis, there is an AP forward curve of the thoracic spine with the apex posterior (i.e., the back is prominent). The most common clinical type of kyphosis is postural (postural round back). The curvature of the spinal column points backward and, when viewed from the side, gives the appearance of being humpbacked. In postural kyphosis, the Adams forward bend test demonstrates normalization of the lateral spine profile when viewed from the side (see Table 38-2), and the child can reverse the round-back appearance with active extension. Postural kyphosis is the most common type and is more common in girls than boys. It rarely causes pain, and the curvature is flexible.

Scheuermann kyphosis is an osteochondrosis that presents as an abnormality of the vertebral epiphyseal growth plates. Onset generally occurs in adolescence. The kyphosis is rigid, and the pain is located over the deformity and is worse at the end of the day. Scheuermann kyphosis is defined by vertebral wedging of 5 degrees or more on three adjacent vertebral bodies visualized on a standing lateral radiograph of the thoracic and lumbar spine. Associated radiographic findings include irregularities of the vertebral end plates, disk-space narrowing, and herniation of the intervertebral disk penetrating into the vertebral body (Spiegel and Dormans, 2011).

Management

Depending on cause and severity of the kyphosis, there are different treatment options. Postural kyphosis may be improved with an exercise and physical therapy program that strengthens the supporting muscles. Activities (such as, dancing or swimming) that require a full range of motion of the shoulders, back, and arms can be helpful. Adolescent kyphosis may be treated with a combination of a back brace, exercise, and physical therapy. Surgery may be required in children with structural problems that cause kyphosis and in adolescents with curvature of the back that exceeds 50 to 60 degrees. Kyphosis caused by infections or tumors may also require surgery.

Lumbar Lordosis

Lumbar lordosis, or hyperlordosis, is an AP curve of the lumbar area of the spine (i.e., the child stands with the abdomen and buttocks protuberant). It is the least common of the congenital spinal deformities and is often associated with kyphosis or scoliosis. Congenital lordosis deformity is usually progressive. Lordosis can be a secondary result of a hip problem in which full extension is limited by hip flexion contractures or from lumbosacral deformities.

Management

If the pediatric provider suspects lumbar lordosis, have the child bend forward. If the lumbar spine flattens and the lordosis disappears in the forward bending position, it indicates that the spine is flexible and the lordosis is only physiologic. This child should be seen for follow-up in 6 to 12 months, and the examination should be repeated to ensure continued physiologic findings. If the lordosis persists in the forward bending position, this indicates a fixed structural deformity and needs referral to an orthopedist. Lordosis resulting from hip flexion contractures is absent while sitting; it is commonly seen in children with cerebral palsy, spina bifida, and developmental dysplasia of the hip (see Table 38-2).

Hip Problems

Developmental Dysplasia of the Hip

Developmental dysplasia of the hip (DDH) represents a spectrum of anatomic abnormalities in which the femoral head and the acetabulum are in improper alignment and/or grow abnormally. This includes dysplastic, subluxated, dislocatable, and dislocated hips. Dysplasia is characterized by a shallow more vertical acetabular socket with an immature hip/acetabulum. In subluxation, the hip is unstable, and the head of the femur can slide in and out of the acetabulum. DDH occurs congenitally or develops in infancy or childhood. Dysplasia may be diagnosed many years after the newborn period.

Physiologic, mechanical, and genetic factors are implicated in DDH. Physiologic factors include the hormonal effect of maternal estrogen and relaxin that are released near delivery and produce a temporary laxity of the hip joint. Mechanical factors include constant compression in utero with restriction of movement late in gestation if the fetal pelvis becomes locked in the maternal pelvis. This is seen with first pregnancy, oligohydramnios, and breech presentation. The incidence of DDH is greater than normal in cultures that swaddle infants in extended position or place them on cradleboards because of such neonatal positioning.

In the unstable hip, the femoral head and the acetabulum may not have a normal tight, concentric anatomic relationship, which can lead to abnormal growth of the hip joint and result in permanent disability. In the newborn, the left hip is most often involved because this hip typically is the one in a forced adduction position against the mother's sacrum.

The hip can dislocate non-congenitally or in utero in children with certain muscular or neurologic disorders that affect the use of the lower extremities, such as cerebral palsy, arthrogryposis, or myelomeningocele. Dislocation results from the abnormal use of the extremity over time.

The incidence of DDH is estimated to range from 1.5 to 20 per 1000 live births in the United States. It is found more commonly with breech births and is four times more common in girls than boys. A positive family history (genetic risk factors) increases the risk for having a child with this problem. Other risk factors seen in infants that are associated with DDH include oligohydramnios, torticollis, and lower limb deformities, such as clubfoot, MA, and dislocated knee.

Clinical Findings

History. Risk factors for DDH include female gender, family history, high birth weight, breech positioning, and in utero postural deformities (Herring, 2014a).

Physical Examination. A hip examination should be performed on children as part of their well child supervision until they are 2 years old. Findings of DDH include the following:

- Screening tests are serial physical examinations of the hip and lower extremities. The Barlow and Ortolani tests are used to screen for DDH in neonates. Once an infant reaches the 2nd and 3rd months of life, the soft tissue surrounding the hips begins to tighten and the Barlow and Ortolani tests are less reliable. The Klisic and Galeazzi tests are used to screen older infants. Routine ultrasonography is not recommended; however, an ultrasound should be obtained if there is a high index of suspicion of dysplasia based on a positive clinical examination.
- Sixty percent to 80% of abnormal hips of newborns identified by physical examination resolve by 2 to 8 weeks.
- In the older infant, 6 to 18 months old:
  - Limited abduction of the affected hip and shortening of the thigh is a reliable sign (see Fig. 38-3, *B,* and Fig. 38-5).
  - Normal abduction with comfort is 70 to 80 degrees bilaterally. Limited abduction includes those cases with less than 60 degrees of abduction or unequal abduction from one side to the other (see Fig. 38-5).
  - Positive Galeazzi sign (see Fig. 38-3, *A*).
- Other findings include asymmetry of inguinal or gluteal folds (thigh-fold asymmetry is not related to the disorder [see Fig. 38-3, *D*]) and unequal leg lengths, shorter on the affected side.

In the ambulatory child who was not diagnosed earlier or was not corrected, the following might also be noted:

- Short leg with toe walking on the affected side
- Positive Trendelenburg sign (see Fig. 38-3, *C*)
- Marked lordosis or toe walking
- Painless limping or waddling gait with child leaning to the affected side

If the hips are dislocated bilaterally, asymmetries are not observed. Limited abduction is the primary indicator in this situation (see Fig. 38-5). Also in subluxation of the hip (not frankly dislocated), limited abduction again is the primary indicator. A waddling gait may also be noted.

Diagnostic Studies. Ultrasound is superior to radiographs for evaluating cartilaginous structures and is recommended for infants after 4 weeks of age. Use of ultrasonography prior to 4 weeks old has a high incidence of producing false-positive results. Ultrasound is used to assess the relationship of the femur to the acetabulum and provides dynamic information about acetabular development and stability of the hip. Radiologic evaluation of the newborn to detect and evaluate DDH is recommended once the proximal epiphysis ossifies, usually by 4 to 6 months (Sankar et al, 2011). Radiography prior to this is unreliable, because so much of the hip joint is cartilaginous in the young infant. AP and lateral Lauenstein (frog-leg) position radiographs of the pelvis are indicated.

Differential Diagnosis

The condition is relatively unique.

Management

The goal of management is to restore the articulation of the femur within the acetabulum. Many newborns with positive screening tests and abnormal hips resolve without intervention; however, prompt referral to an orthopedist is important. The orthopedist needs to reexamine the newborn to determine whether early treatment is necessary.

- The majority of neonatal hip instability cases resolve spontaneously by 6 to 8 weeks old. Close observation of these children is recommended.
- The treatment of choice for subluxation and reducible dislocations identified in the early phase is a Pavlik harness. The harness is applied with hips having greater than 90 degrees of flexion and with adduction of the hip limited to a neutral position. The success rate of Pavlik harness treatment is reported to be between 80% and 97%. Radiographic or ultrasound documentation can be used during treatment to verify the position of the hip. If the infant does not respond to treatment with the harness, surgical treatment may be needed.

- The earlier that treatment is started with the Pavlik harness, the better the prognosis for a successful outcome. The harness is worn 24 hours a day, except for bathing. The infant with a Pavlik harness should be seen weekly to ensure it fits properly, to identify complications associated with the use of the harness (e.g., avascular necrosis and femoral nerve palsy), and to ensure the femur is properly seated in the socket. Ultrasonography can be performed while the Pavlik harness is worn to assess hip reduction and acetabular development. The length of time the harness is worn depends on the age of the child, when it was applied, and whether or not reduction is successful. Generally the harness is worn full time for 3 to 6 weeks and then may be required only during waking hours for decreasing periods of time.
- For a child in a Pavlik harness or spica cast, cast care, skin care, and car safety when the child cannot easily be placed in a car seat are issues to be addressed. Furthermore, the child needs special attention to maintain developmental stimulation while immobilized. An orthopedist should be immediately consulted for any infant seen in a primary care setting who is in a Pavlik harness and exhibits excessive hip flexion (beyond 100 degrees) or abduction (beyond 60 degrees).
- The 6- to 18-month-old infant with a dislocated hip is likely to require either closed manipulation or open reduction. Preoperative traction, adductor tenotomy, and gentle reduction are especially helpful in preventing osteonecrosis of the femoral head. After the closed or open reduction, a hip spica cast is applied in order to maintain the hip in more than 90 degrees of flexion and avoid excessive internal or external rotation (Herring, 2014a). Triple diapering is not helpful, because the musculoskeletal forces far outweigh the force that can be exerted by the diaper material.
- Annual or biennial follow-up including radiographs to the point of skeletal maturity is recommended to evaluate for the possibility of late asymmetric epiphyseal closure (Herring, 2014a). Support the child and family through the treatment phases. Explain management goals clearly.

Complications

The Pavlik harness and other positional devices may cause skin irritation, and a difference in leg length may remain. There may be delay in walking if the child is put in a body cast. The long-term outcomes depend on the age at diagnosis, the severity of the joint deformity, and the effectiveness of therapy. Untreated cases may result in a permanent dislocation of the femoral head so that it lies just under the iliac crest posteriorly. Clinically, the child has limited mobility of this pseudo joint and related short leg. Forceful reduction can result in avascular necrosis of the femoral head with permanent hip deformity. Redislocation or persistent dysplasia can occur. Adult degenerative arthritis is associated with acetabular dysplasia.

Prevention

The condition cannot be prevented, but early identification resulting in early treatment significantly reduces the long-term consequences of the problem. Screening of all neonates and infants should include full hip abduction; examination for unequal inguinal and gluteal folds and unequal leg lengths; and Barlow, Ortolani, and Galeazzi maneuvers at every examination. The hip can dislocate at any point in early development, even up to the point of first ambulation. In older children, limited abduction, gait, and standing position, including the Trendelenburg position, add important information. Charting should always include notation about hip findings, because these can change at subsequent visits. The Ortolani test should only be used in the first 2 to 3 months of age.

Legg-Calvé-Perthes Disease

LCPD is a childhood hip disorder that results in infarction of the bony epiphysis of the femoral head. It presents as avascular necrosis of the femoral head. The basic underlying cause of LCPD is insufficient blood supply to the femoral head. There is an initial ischemic episode of unknown etiology that interrupts vascular circulation to the capital femoral epiphysis. The articular cartilage hypertrophies, and the epiphyseal marrow becomes necrotic. The area revascularizes, and the necrotic bone is replaced by new bone. This process can take 18 to 24 months. There is a critical point in these dual processes when the subchondral area becomes weak enough that fracture of the epiphysis occurs. At this time, the child becomes symptomatic. With fracturing, further reabsorption and replacement by fibrous bone occurs, and the shape of the femoral head is altered. Articulation of the head in the hip joint is interrupted. The bone re-ossifies with or without treatment; but without treatment, the femoral head flattens and enlarges, causing joint deformity. Lateral subluxation of the femoral head is associated with poor outcomes.

Etiology is unclear, but certain risk factors have been identified in children. These include gender, socioeconomic group, and the presence of an inguinal hernia and genitourinary tract anomalies. Boys are affected three to five times more often than girls; incidence increases in lower socioeconomic groups and in children with low birth weights. The disease is bilateral in 10% to 20% of children. It affects children 4 to 8 years old.

Clinical Findings

History. There can be an acute or chronic onset with or without a history of trauma to the hip, such as jumping from a high place.

- The most common presenting sign is an intermittent limp (abductor lurch), especially after exertion, with mild or intermittent pain.
- The most frequent complaint is persistent pain in the groin, anterior hip region, or laterally around the greater trochanter.

- Pain may be referred to the medial aspect of the ipsilateral knee or to the anterior thigh.
- Some children may report limited range of motion of the affected extremity.

Physical Examination. Findings may include the following:

- Antalgic gait with limited hip movement
- Trendelenburg gait resulting from pain in the gluteus medius muscle
- Muscle spasm
- Atrophy of gluteus, quadriceps, and hamstring muscles
- Decreased abduction, internal rotation, and extension of the hip
- Adduction flexion contracture
- Pain on rolling the leg internally

Diagnostic Studies. Routine AP pelvis and frog-leg lateral views are used to confirm the diagnosis, stage the disease, and follow disease progression and response to treatment. Radiographic findings can include smaller epiphysis, increased epiphyseal density, subchondral fracture line, lateralization of the femoral head, and other features. Changes in the epiphysis margin are discerned by the orthopedist and radiologist (Fig. 38-10). However, there may be no radiographic findings early in LCPD. Ultrasonography is useful in the preliminary diagnosis; capsular distention can be seen on sonographic images. Bone scans and MRI allow for precise localization of the bone involvement, but changes seen as bone marrow edema and joint effusions are nonspecific. CT is not typically used on a routine basis to evaluate patients with LCPD (Kim and Herring, 2014).

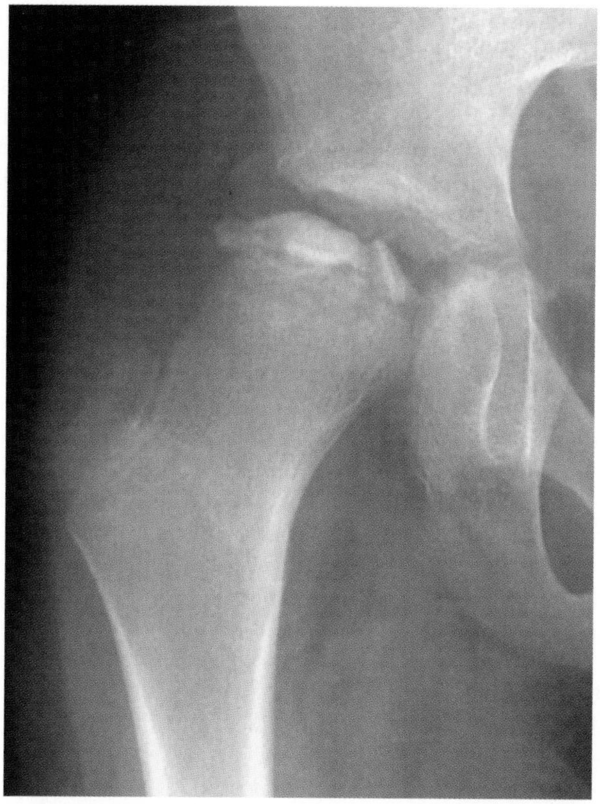

• **Figure 38-10** Anteroposterior (AP) radiograph of the right hip of an 8-year-old boy with Legg-Calvé-Perthes disease (LCPD). There is a collapsed, yet dense, capital femoral epiphysis with early fragmentation. The small medial triangle of the capital femoral epiphysis is uninvolved in the disease process. (From Behrman RE, Kliegman RM, Jenson HB, editors: *Nelson textbook of pediatrics*, ed 17, Philadelphia, 2004, Saunders.)

Differential Diagnosis

Acute and chronic infections, sickle cell disease, toxic synovitis, Gaucher disease, slipped capital femoral epiphysis (SCFE), osteomyelitis, juvenile rheumatoid arthritis, hemophilia, and neoplasm are included in the differential diagnosis.

Management

- Referral to an orthopedist is necessary. Because age of onset and the severity of LCPD can vary significantly from one child to another, there are various approaches to the management, and treatment remains controversial. Overall, the general approach is guided by the principle of containment of the femoral head within the acetabulum. To be successful, containment must be instituted while the femoral head is still moldable. Nonoperative containment can be achieved in a variety of ways and ranges from activity limitation, and protected weight-bearing, use of NSAID and physical therapy to maintain hip motion to bed rest with traction using casts to maintain hip abduction. Surgical approaches involve pelvic and femoral osteotomies of the proximal femur or pelvis.
- Support and monitor the child throughout treatment and recovery, including during interruption of school or other activities. Treatment and monitoring of LCPD can last months to years.

Complications

Osteoarthritis related to femoral head deformity and decreased use of the hip joint may occur, depending on the femoral head remodeling status. Older children have a poorer prognosis owing to the decreased opportunity for femoral head remodeling in the remaining growth period. Females with LCPD also have a poorer prognosis.

Prevention

The condition is not preventable, but early identification and treatment reduce the long-term complications of the disorder, such as premature degenerative arthritis in early adult life.

Slipped Capital Femoral Epiphysis

SCFE is a Salter-Harris type I fracture through the proximal femoral physis. Stress around the hip causes a shear force to be applied at the growth plate. Although trauma may play a role in the fracture, there is an intrinsic weakness in the physeal cartilage. The fracture occurs at the hypertrophic zone of the physeal cartilage. Stress on the hip causes the epiphysis to displace posteriorly and inferiorly to the metaphysis. Because the blood supply to the epiphysis crosses the weakened area, the epiphysis is at risk for avascular necrosis. The slippage is generally gradual, and the condition is categorized as stable or unstable based on the child's ability to bear weight (Jarrett et al, 2013).

SCFE typically occurs just after the onset of puberty, often in overweight and slightly skeletally immature boys. It is seen in children in whom puberty is delayed. African American children are affected slightly more than others. The incidence is slightly greater in boys than girls. In children younger than 10 years old, SCFE is associated with hypothyroidism, panhypopituitarism, hypogonadism, renal osteodystrophy, and growth hormone abnormalities. The mostly exclusive incidence of SCFE during the adolescent growth spurt indicates a hormonal role. Obesity, another risk factor, alters the level of circulating hormones and affects the mechanical load on the physis (Sankar et al, 2011).

Clinical Findings

Clinical presentation is often misleading and can result in delay of diagnosis and treatment.

History.

- A vague history of antecedent trauma
- Pain in affected hip, groin, thigh, or knee
- Some have complaints of limping or gait abnormalities

Physical Examination.

- Obesity: 60% of children diagnosed with SCFE have a weight in the 90th percentile or higher (Kienstra and Macias, 2015).
- Delayed puberty
- Pain in the groin or diffusely over the knee or anterior thigh
- Pain and decreased internal rotation
- Antalgic limp with short leg component (50% are up to 1 inch shorter on the affected side)
- As the epiphysis continues to slip, there may be a more pronounced limping and external rotation of the toes when walking
- External rotation of the thigh when the hip is flexed; lack of internal rotation of the hip with range of motion
- Mild atrophy of the thigh and gluteal muscles
- Limited abduction and extension
- With unstable SCFE, the child is unable to bear weight

Diagnostic Studies. Plain radiography is often the only image modality needed to diagnose and evaluate SCFE (Herring, 2014c). AP pelvis, frog-leg lateral, and true lateral views of the pelvis are obtained. Radiographic findings include flattening of the epiphyseal prominence, widening or irregularity of the growth plate, and narrowing of the area if the epiphysis has slipped posteriorly (Fig. 38-11). Radiographically, the slippage is measured using the Southwick method and can be classified as mild (less than 33% slippage of the epiphysis or less than a 30-degree slip angle), moderate (33% to 50% slippage of the epiphysis or 30- to 50-degree slip angle), or severe (greater than 50% slippage of the epiphysis or greater than 50-degree slip angle) (Kienstra and Macias, 2015).

Differential Diagnosis

LCPD, sepsis of the hip joint, and osteoarthritis should be considered.

Management

Treatment modalities aim to prevent further slippage by stabilizing the epiphysis and avoid complications, such as osteonecrosis and chondrolysis (Peck and Herrera-Soto, 2014).

- Refer immediately to an orthopedic surgeon.
- Place child on crutches or in a wheelchair. Non–weight bearing needs to be emphasized to prevent further slippage. Once the diagnosis is made, the child should be admitted to the hospital immediately and placed on bed rest.

Standard treatment for a stable SCFE involves percutaneous pinning and placement of a single cannulated screw through the femoral neck into the central aspect of the proximal femoral epiphysis. Recently, a new operative intervention for more severe and unstable SCFE (modified Dunn procedure) has emerged (Sankar et al, 2013). This procedure involves surgical dislocation of the hip and aims to restore the anatomical alignment of the proximal femur without disrupting the arterial blood supply to the femoral head, thereby decreasing the risk of avascular necrosis (Jarrett et al, 2013).

- There is a high incidence of contralateral SCFE within 6 to 12 months. The hip(s) need to be monitored until skeletal maturity is achieved.
- Support and monitor the child throughout the treatment phase, which includes interruption of school and activities during the recovery period. Contact sports are usually restricted by the orthopedist until growth is complete.

Complications

The two most severe complications of SCFE are avascular necrosis and chondrolysis. Avascular necrosis is loss of blood supply to the proximal femoral physis, resulting in death of a portion of the bone. It is the most serious complication and has a higher incidence of occurring if the slip is severe or unstable. Chondrolysis is acute cartilage necrosis and represents a loss of articular cartilage.

Prevention

SCFE is not a preventable condition. However, identification of the condition during the pre-slip period, when complaints of hip or referred knee pain, loss of motion, or weakness in the hip are present, allows early intervention. This can prevent deformity and long-term sequelae, such as premature degenerative arthritis in early adult life. If the child is overweight, advise about the need for weight reduction.

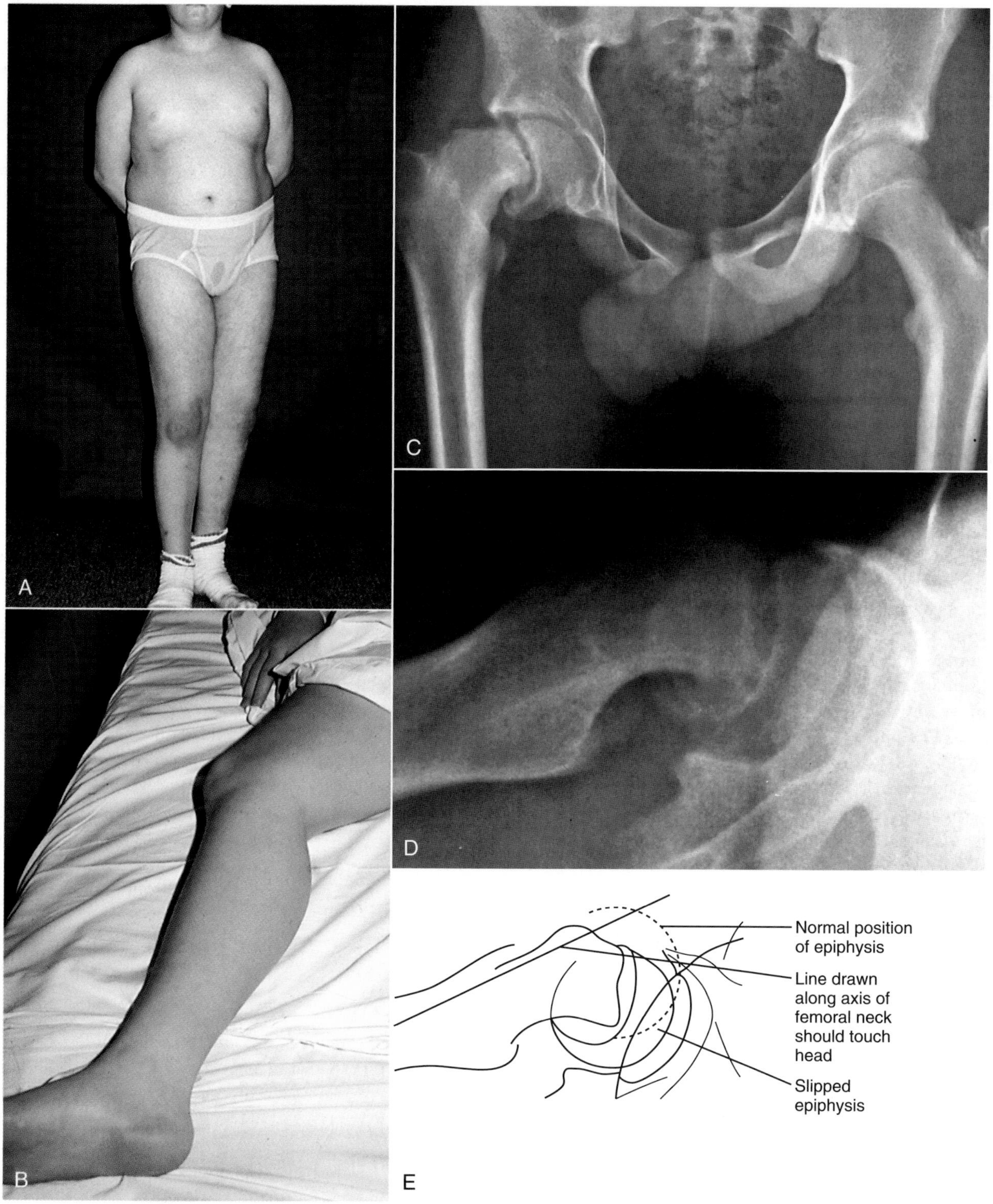

• **Figure 38-11** Slipped capital femoral epiphysis. **A,** Obese boy with a painful limp and reluctance to bear weight on right leg. **B,** In supine position, right leg is in external rotation to minimize discomfort. **C,** Anteroposterior radiograph shows right femoral head displaced medially to the femoral neck. **D,** Lateral view shows the femoral head displaced posteriorly to the femoral neck. **E,** A line drawn along the axis of the femoral neck normally touches the head. (From Basil Z, McIntire S: *Zitelli and Davis' atlas of pediatric physical diagnosis*, ed 6, Philadelphia, 2013, Saunders/Elsevier.)

Femoral Anteversion

Everyone has some degree of femoral anteversion. Femoral anteversion is a condition in which the head and neck of the femur are rotated at an increased angle anteriorly in relation to the femoral shaft and results in an in-toeing gait. Younger children have a somewhat wider angle. During infancy, the degree of anteversion is approximately 40 degrees and decreases with skeletal maturity (Herring, 2014b). An in-toeing gait is most noticeable in children 3 to 6 years old but is considered normal. By 10 to 12 years old, the normal angle (10 to 15 degrees) of anteversion is seen. Femoral anteversion is also called *internal femoral torsion,* the etiology of which is unknown and controversial. Some attribute a worsening of the condition to sitting in a "W" position, whereas others believe the anteversion is congenital and is not altered by position. A family history is often identified, and it occurs more commonly in girls than boys (2 : 1).

Clinical Findings

History.

- In-toeing gait, most noticeable with running
- Runs awkwardly (looks like an "eggbeater"); may actually trip as a result of crossing the feet while walking or running
- Possible family history
- History of "W" sitting

Physical Examination.

- In-toeing gait with patellae medial
- Internal (medial) rotation normally less than 70 degrees (mild deformity: 70 to 80 degrees; moderate: between 80 and 90 degrees; severe: greater than 90 degrees [see Fig. 38-7])
- External (lateral) rotation decreased (limited to 0 to 10 degrees)
- Knees medially rotated ("kissing patella") when standing

Diagnostic Studies. Radiographs are not merited unless surgery is contemplated.

Differential Diagnosis

Consider other rotational deformities, such as internal tibial torsion or MA. Cerebral palsy with a "scissoring gait" might be mistaken for severe femoral anteversion.

Management

The family should be informed that femoral anteversion is not harmful and there are no known serious consequences to the condition. Management includes observation of the child and referral to an orthopedist if medial rotations are significant (no external rotation of the hip in extension) or the child or family has significant concerns. Nonoperative management strategies (such as, shoe modifications, twister cables, and night splints) are ineffective. Operative correction is successful, but it carries the risk of complications. Osteotomy is rarely performed and is done only in the child older than 8 years old with significant cosmetic and functional deformity. The natural history of the condition is for the medial, or internal, rotation to decrease, providing some improvement.

Complications

Studies have shown that the condition does not cause flatfoot, bunions, knee problems, back difficulties, difficulties in running, or degenerative arthritis of the hip in adults. It is primarily a cosmetic problem unless it is severe enough to interfere with activities. Self-esteem can be affected.

Prevention

Excessive femoral anteversion cannot be prevented. Studies have shown that in-toeing is usually, but not always, self-correcting and is not prevented or improved with special shoes, braces, or exercises (Herring, 2014b).

Knee Problems

Genu Varum

Genu varum, or bowing of the legs, can be a physiologic or developmental variation of normal or a pathologic condition that involves a rotational deformity (Fig. 38-12). The term *bowlegs* is used to describe physiologic variations of the normal knee angle, resulting in bowing of the legs that is typically seen in children up to 2 years old, but it can be considered normal until 3 years old. The typical pattern of normal bowing seen in children is a symmetric lateral bowing of both tibias in the first year followed by bowlegs in the second year. Most bowing resolves spontaneously but

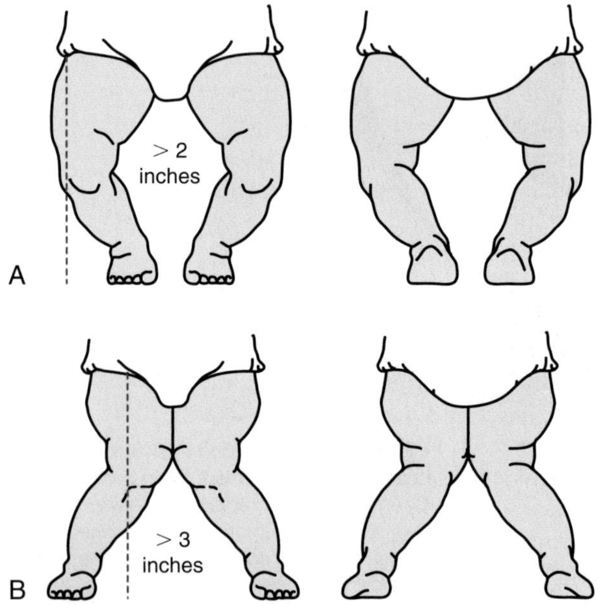

• **Figure 38-12** Genu varum and genu valgum. In genu varum **(A),** the knees are tilted away from the midline; measure the intercondylar (knee) distance with the ankles together. In genu valgum **(B),** the knees are tilted toward the midline; measure the intermalleolar distance with knees approximated.

can progress to persistent or pathologic varus. The angle between the tibia and femur is pronounced in varus (up to 15 degrees) in normal children before 1 year old. This is considered an in utero positioning effect. The angle approaches neutral by 18 months old and then proceeds to a valgus angle, with an average angle of 12 degrees from 2 to 3 years old. The angle then gradually decreases to 8 degrees in females and 7 degrees in males by adulthood. If the varus angle is greater than 15 degrees in infants, does not begin to decrease in the second year, is asymmetric, is associated with short stature, or is rapidly progressing, the condition is considered pathologic.

If the varus persists after 30 months of age or increases, it may represent Blount disease, rickets, tumor, neurologic problems, infection, or other conditions. A Salter fracture through the tibial growth plate can result in later genu varum as growth across the plate progresses unevenly.

With Blount disease (idiopathic tibia vara that affects the proximal tibia), there is an abnormal growth of the medial aspect of the proximal tibial epiphysis that results in progressive varus angulation of the tibia. Blount disease is rare, but it can occur in infancy (18 months to 3 years old), school years (4 to 10 years old), and during adolescence (11 years and older). It is seen more frequently in African American, Hispanic, and Scandinavian populations, is associated with obesity and early walkers, and commonly has a positive family history. Onset in infancy presents the highest risk for greatest deformity (Stevens, 2015).

Clinical Findings

History. Family history is important because certain heritable conditions—Marfan syndrome, OI, or vitamin D–resistant rickets—may predispose a child to this condition. Additional history may include progression since birth; increasing deformation is problematic.

Physical Examination.

- Tibial-femoral angle greater than 15 degrees
- Associated internal tibial torsion
- Lower extremity length discrepancy
- Intercondylar (knees) distance with the ankles together—measurement greater than 4 to 5 inches suggests the need for additional evaluation
- Joint laxity of the lateral collateral ligaments in older children

Diagnostic Studies. The standard radiograph for the older child is an AP of the lower extremities with the patellae facing forward and a lateral radiograph of the involved extremity. The length of each femur and tibia is measured, and diaphyseal deformities are noted. The mechanical axis is a line drawn from the center of the head of the femur to the center of the ankle; this line should bisect the knee (Stevens, 2015). In physiologic bowing, the deformity is gentle and symmetric, with a metaphyseal-diaphyseal angle less than 11 degrees, and normal appearance of the proximal tibial growth plate. In Blount disease, the bowing is asymmetric, abrupt, and with sharp angulation, and the metaphyseal-diaphyseal angle is greater than 11 degrees; there is medial sloping of the epiphysis and widening of the physis (Wells and Sehgal, 2011a).

Differential Diagnosis

Physiologic, persistent, and pathologic genu varum, metabolic (rickets), neurologic problems, Blount disease, infections, tumor, osteochondrodysplasias, and internal tibial torsion should be ruled out.

Management

- In physiologic genu varum (no increasing deformity):
  - No active treatment and resolves spontaneously. Corrective shoes and splinting are unnecessary.
  - Reassure parents; provide information about the natural progression of the problem.
  - Observe the child's condition over time (in 3 to 6 months) to be sure the problem is resolving, especially during the second year of life. Photographs of the legs for the chart can be helpful.
- In pathologic genu varum (increasing deformity):
  - Refer to an orthopedist. Blount disease may be treated with bracing in children younger than 3 years old. Bracing is effective and can prevent progression in 50% of these children. In children older than 4 years old, a proximal tibial valgus osteotomy and associated fibular diaphyseal osteotomy are the procedures of choice.
  - Monitor to be sure braces are used consistently with good fit.
  - Observe to be sure the problem is not worsening.

Complications

Knee degeneration and deformity result if pathologic genu varum is not treated.

Prevention

Early identification and referral reduce the complexity and expense of treatment and the residual deformities.

Genu Valgum

Genu valgum is commonly referred to as *knock-knees* (see Fig. 38-12). Females tend to have a somewhat higher degree of valgus knee posture than males, leveling off by 7 years old at 5 to 9 degrees compared with 4 to 7 degrees for boys. Physiologic genu valgum tends to peak at around 24 to 36 months old and lasts until about 7 to 8 years old. Normal valgus is achieved by 4 years old. Variation up to 15 degrees is possible until 6 years old. The condition can be considered developmental or physiologic. Pathologic conditions leading to valgus are metabolic bone disease (rickets, renal osteodystrophy), skeletal dysplasia, posttraumatic physeal arrest, tumors, and infection (Wells and Sehgal, 2011b).

Clinical Findings

History.

- Progression of the deformity
- Risk factors as listed previously

- Joint pains or stiff gait
- Older child may report knee pain due to the stretching of the medial aspect of the knee

Physical Examination.

- Bilateral tibial-femoral angle less than 15 degrees of valgus in the child up to 7 years old is considered normal; a valgus angle greater than 15 degrees is outside the range of normal
- Unilateral deformity
- Awkwardness of gait
- Subluxing patella
- Intermalleolar (ankles) distance with the knees together: Measurement greater than 4 to 5 inches suggests the need for additional evaluation (Wells and Sehgal, 2011b).
- Short stature: Genu valgum associated with short stature should be referred.

Diagnostic Studies. No radiographic studies are needed unless a pathologic condition is suspected. Long length AP radiographs of the leg in a weight-bearing stance are used for preoperative planning.

Differential Diagnosis

Rule out pathologic conditions of genu valgum.

Management

Deformities greater than 15 degrees and occurring after 6 years old are unlikely to correct with growth and require surgical management. In the skeletally immature, medial tibial epiphyseal hemi-epiphysiodesis is the surgical procedure. In the skeletally mature, osteotomy is necessary at the center of rotation of angulation.

Prevention

Preventive measures are the same as those for genu varum.

Osgood-Schlatter Disease

Osgood-Schlatter disease is caused by microtrauma in the deep fibers of the patellar tendon at its insertion on the tibial tuberosity. The diagnosis is usually based on history and physical examination. The quadriceps femoris muscle inserts on a relatively small area of the tibial tuberosity. Naturally high tension exists at the insertion site. In children, additional stress is placed on the cartilaginous site as a result of vigorous physical activity, leading to traumatic changes at insertion.

Osgood-Schlatter disease is often seen in the adolescent years after undergoing a rapid growth spurt the previous year. It occurs more frequently in boys than girls, with a male-to-female ratio of 3:1. This difference is probably related to a greater participation in specific risk activities by boys than by girls (Sullivani, 2015).

Clinical Findings

History.

- Recent physical activity (such as, running track, playing soccer or football, or surfboarding) commonly produces the condition.
- Pain increases during and immediately after the activity and decreases when the activity is stopped for a while.
- Running, jumping, kneeling, squatting, and ascending/descending stairs exacerbate the pain.
- The pain is bilateral in 20% to 50% of cases.
- Approximately 25% of patients give a history of precipitating trauma.

Physical Examination. Characteristic findings include the following (Sullivan, 2015):

- Pain may be reproduced by extending the knee against resistance, stressing the quadriceps, or squatting with the knee in full flexion
- Focal swelling, heat, and point tenderness at the tibial tuberosity
- Full range of motion of knee

Diagnostic Studies. The diagnosis is based on history and physical examination. Radiographs are not needed unless another pathologic condition is suspected.

Differential Diagnosis

Other knee derangements, tumors (osteosarcoma), and hip problems with referred pain should be considered. The referred pain of hip problems is diffuse across the distal femur without point tenderness at the tibial tubercle.

Management

Osgood-Schlatter disease is a self-limiting condition, with symptom management the key consideration. The following steps are taken:

- Avoid or modify activities that cause pain until the inflammation subsides.
- Ice or cold therapy to reduce pain and inflammation.
- Once the acute symptoms have subsided, quadriceps-stretching exercises, including hip extension for complete stretch of the extensor mechanism, may be performed to reduce tension on the tibial tubercle. Stretching of the hamstrings may also be useful.
- Use of NSAIDs is recommended by some but thought ineffective by others. Because this condition may last up to 2 years, their chronic use may be problematic.
- A neoprene sleeve over the knee may help stabilize the patella.
- A patella tendon strap that wraps around the joint just below the knee reduces the strain on the tibial tuberosity.
- Cylinder casting or bracing with limited weight bearing for 2 to 3 weeks may be used in severe cases.

Complications

In the postpubertal child, a residual ossicle in the tendon next to the bone may cause persistent pain. Surgical removal is indicated and will relieve the pain.

Prevention

The condition cannot be prevented, but earlier management may decrease the length of disability and the discomfort associated with it. Avoid overuse and encourage balanced training and adequate warm-up before exercise or sports participation. The use of kneepads may help protect the tibial tuberosity from direct injury for those who engage in sports that result in knee contact.

Tibial Torsion

Tibial torsion is a common problem in children that involves the twisting of the long bone along its long axis. *Tibial version* is the term used to describe the normal variation in tibial rotation. At birth, the tibias have a mean lateral rotation of 2.2 degrees and rotate laterally over time, with an adult mean lateral tibial rotation of about 23 degrees. Tibial torsion describes those rotations that are outside the range of normal. Medial tibial torsion (MTT), also known as *internal tibial torsion,* consists of abnormal medial rotation or twisting, resulting in in-toeing of the feet; lateral tibial torsion (LTT) consists of abnormal lateral rotation resulting in out-toeing (Wells and Sehgal, 2011a).

Tibial torsion may be congenital, developmental, or acquired. MTT is the most common cause of in-toeing during the second year of life and is often noted around 6 to 12 months old. In most cases, it is a physiologic condition that is the result of in utero positioning. In 90% of cases, internal tibial torsion gradually resolves on its own by the time the child reaches 8 years old. LTT is a cause of out-toeing in late childhood and is usually an acquired deformity. Contracture of the iliotibial band is the underlying problem.

Clinical Findings

Physical Examination. Observe the child's gait for in-toeing. The thigh-foot angle (TFA) is used to assess tibial rotation. With the child prone and the knees flexed 90 degrees, the foot and thigh are viewed from directly above (looking downward at the angle of the thigh and foot). The foot should be relaxed. MTT exists if the TFA is negative by more than 10 to 20 degrees (−10 to −20 degrees), bearing in mind the child's age. In-toeing is expressed in negative values (Fig. 38-13). The normal range at 13 years old is −5 to +30 degrees. Abnormal lateral torsion is associated with forward-pointing patellae and outward-pointing feet. A TFA measurement of greater than +30 degrees indicates abnormal LTT (Wells and Sehgal, 2011a).

Diagnostic Studies. Radiographs are usually not necessary.

Differential Diagnosis

Genu varum in which the problem originates at the knee with a tibial-femoral angle, femoral torsion (femoral anteversion), adducted great toe, and MA also produce in-toeing gaits. Adducted great toe (the searching toe) is a benign condition that resolves spontaneously. Lateral femoral torsion also causes an out-toeing gait. Screen for associated hip dysplasia and neuromuscular problems (cerebral palsy).

Management

- Treatment of tibial version (the normal variation in tibial rotation) is observation and monitoring.
- MTT should be referred to an orthopedist if the problem is significant (TFA greater than −20 by 3 years old). Stretching exercises or external rotational splints may be recommended. Surgical intervention may be needed for severe cases that persist into late childhood and cause significant functional problems.

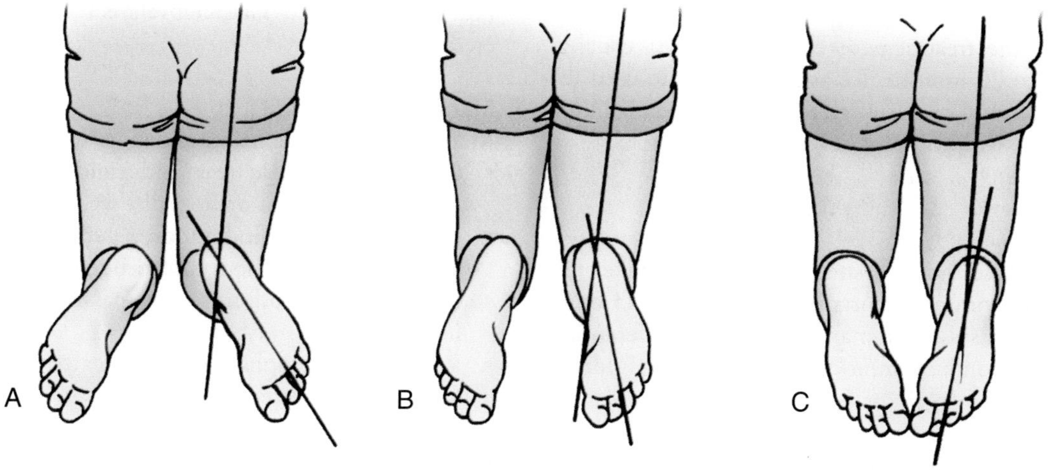

• **Figure 38-13** Thigh-foot angle (TFA). With the child in the prone position and the knees flexed and approximated, the long axis of the foot can be compared with the long axis of the thigh. The long axis of the foot bisects the heel and the second toe or lies between the second and third toes. **A,** External tibial torsion produces excessive outward rotation. **B,** Normal alignment is characterized by slight external rotation. **C,** Internal tibial torsion produces inward rotation of the foot and is a negative angle. (From Thompson GH: Gait disturbances. In Kliegman RM, Nieder ML, Super DM, editors: *Practical strategies in pediatric diagnosis and therapy*, Philadelphia, 1996, Saunders.)

- Special shoes are ineffective for the treatment of MTT. The avoidance of certain postures that are thought to exacerbate MTT is controversial (e.g., sleeping in the knee-chest position and sitting with the feet tucked under the buttocks).
- LTT with TFA greater than +30 degrees should be referred to an orthopedist, because it usually worsens with growth and does not correct spontaneously. Medial femoral torsion with pain also should be referred.

Complications

There are no complications with normal tibial version and no interference with activities. Tibial torsion (the TFA is outside the acceptable range of normal) can lead to significant functional problems in severe cases.

Popliteal Cysts

Popliteal cysts, or Baker cysts, result from egress of fluid through a normal communication of a bursa or may be caused by herniation of the synovial membrane through the joint capsule. Baker cysts appear much less frequently in children than adults.

Clinical Findings

The major findings are swelling behind the knee with or without discomfort. Cysts are generally located at or below the joint line.

Diagnostic Studies. Ultrasonography can distinguish between a fluid-filled cyst and solid tumor. Radiographs will show if there is soft calcification in the mass.

Differential Diagnosis

Rule out lipomas, xanthomas, vascular tumors, and fibrosarcomas.

Management

Observation is the treatment of choice. The cyst usually resolves in 10 to 20 months. Ice and NSAIDs are used to promote comfort and relieve pain. Surgical incision is indicated only when symptoms are severe and limiting.

Knee Injuries

Chapter 13 discusses issues related to the musculoskeletal examination and common sports injuries. Table 38-3 outlines the etiology, assessment, management, and differential diagnosis of common knee injuries that are seen in children and young adults.

Foot Problems

Pes Planus

Physiologic or flexible pes planus (flatfoot) is commonly seen in neonates and toddlers and is due to a fat pad in the arch that makes the appearance of the arch seem flat. This generally resolves by 2 to 3 years old but, in a small percentage of cases, can persist into adulthood. Flexible flatfoot is often familial, common, and benign. The arch is seen when the foot is suspended but flattens with weight bearing. Rigid flatfoot is pathologic.

There are three types of flatfeet: a flexible flatfoot, a flexible flatfoot with a tendo-Achilles contracture, and a rigid flatfoot. Flatfeet in neonates and toddlers are associated with physiologic ligamentous laxity. Flexible flatfeet persisting into adolescence are usually associated with familial ligamentous laxity, because there is often a familial tendency toward the problem. Flatfoot also is associated with certain syndromes (Marfan and Down syndromes), myelodysplasia, cerebral palsy, and obesity. Flatfeet may be secondary to muscle imbalance or weakness, a bony abnormality, or shortened heel cords.

History

Onset is noticed with weight bearing. The flexible flatfoot is painless and asymptomatic. Examine the shoes to see if there is abnormal wear on the inner side.

Physical Examination

Clinical manifestations include the following (Hosalkar et al, 2011):

- There is a normal longitudinal arch when examined in a non–weight-bearing position, but the arch disappears when standing.
- On standing, the hindfoot collapses into valgus, and the midfoot sag becomes evident.
- Generalized ligamentous laxity is commonly observed.
- Range of motion should be normal in flexible flatfoot.

Differential Diagnosis

Congenital vertical talus should be considered if the foot is rigid and no arch can be molded or if the foot has a rocker-bottom appearance. Calcaneovalgus foot might be considered also.

Management

Management involves the following:

- Only symptomatic feet and rigid flatfoot should be treated; refer to an orthopedist.
- For painful, flexible flatfoot, a removable, longitudinal arch support may be recommended by the orthopedist.
- If the Achilles tendon is tight, passive stretching may be helpful.
- Routine radiographs are not indicated unless pathologic flatfoot is suspected.

Complications

Flatfoot should be considered a variation of normal, unless there is pain or rigidity. Congenital vertical talus is difficult to treat and should not be missed. Some cases of flatfeet are symptomatic in adulthood; and in severe cases, the bones of the feet adapt to abnormal position with pronation and possible development of bunions.

TABLE 38-3 Characteristics of Various Types of Knee Injuries and Conditions

Condition	History, Mechanism of Injury	Clinical Findings	Management	Differential Diagnosis, Prognosis, and Comments
Quadriceps contusion	Typically a sports injury that results in bruising/contusion of the quadriceps muscle Injury can sometimes result from minor trauma or indirectly from tensile overload	Acute pain, swelling, and restriction of active and passive range of motion of hip and knee; tenderness over quadriceps	**RICE: R**est not to exceed 48 hours, **I**ce, **C**ompression wrap, and **E**levation Progressive leg and gravity-assisted ROM after rest Flexion of the knee is the last function to return to normal, so it is a good indicator for return to sport NSAID for pain relief	In teens, rule out rhabdomyosarcoma of the quadriceps, Ewing sarcoma, and osteosarcoma if there is swelling and pain in thigh without clear history of trauma
Meniscal tear (torn cartilage)	Associated with a significant injury in a youth; results from axial loading with rotation Tear of a normal meniscus is rarely seen in children <12 years old Congenital abnormal cartilage (discoid) can tear at any age	Pain, swelling, and limping Joint line tenderness and positive McMurray sign May report a sensation of a clicking or catching in the knee or a locking of the knee Can be isolated or occur in combination with ACL or MCL injuries	RICE initially MRI if suspected tear; arthrography with MRI to rule out nerve injury with a prior tear Pain management Surgical intervention: meniscectomy generally relieves symptoms	75% of patients develop degenerative articular changes on x-ray by 30 years old A small percentage of youths develop degenerative changes 3 to 5 years after injury Chondral fractures or injuries to articular cartilage have similar history and physical findings
Sprain of the anterior cruciate ligament (ACL)	Acute injury; typically there is a twisting or hyperextension while the foot is planted and knee extended Report of a "popping" feeling and knee shifting or pulling apart	Swelling/effusion and pain Instability with lateral movement Positive Lachman test	Following the injury, a knee brace or immobilizer is used until swelling and pain subside ACL reconstruction Pain management Neuromuscular training to prevent injury	Associated with MCL and meniscal tears
Sprains of the medial collateral ligament (MCL)	Most commonly injured ligament of the knee Valgus stress to an extended knee Reports tearing sensation with medial pain, swelling, stiffness	Instability with lateral movement and medial knee pain Tenderness over the MCL If tenderness extends along the distal femoral physis, suspect physeal fracture	RICE, splint, or hinged knee brace to protect against valgus stress Pain management Plain radiographs to look for physeal and epiphyseal fractures in skeletally immature children Surgical repair on an isolated collateral ligament is not beneficial; nonoperative treatment is the standard of care	Combined ACL and MCL injuries are common Physeal fractures are more common than MCL sprains in youths

Continued

TABLE 38-3 Characteristics of Various Types of Knee Injuries and Conditions—cont'd

Condition	History, Mechanism of Injury	Clinical Findings	Management	Differential Diagnosis, Prognosis, and Comments
Osteochondritis dissecans	Juvenile and adolescent types Common in 10- to 15-year-olds; boys more common than girls Isolation and sometimes sequestration of an osteochondral fragment without significant trauma May be caused by microtrauma, trauma, or may involve metabolic or genetic factors Pain increased with activity and diminished with rest plus intermittent effusions Locking and catching are unusual findings but may be present if bone fragments are detached	Activity-related pain and swelling Tenderness of the femoral condyle	Plain radiographs or MRI; 4 to 6 weeks of immobilization and non–weight bearing if <12 years old Youths >12 years old: Arthroscopic surgery Eliminate high-impact activities—non–weight bearing for several weeks until symptoms abate About 50% heal spontaneously with rest and protected weight bearing Surgical intervention if still symptomatic despite 6 to 12 months of conservative treatment, symptomatic loose body, or nonunion	Mimics symptoms of a torn meniscus Articular cartilage transplantation for selected patients
Dislocation of the patella	Associated with patellar malalignment Most cases involve lateral dislocation Pain and swelling Most occur in youths <20 years old Family history in 20% to 30% More frequently in girls than boys	Massive and tense effusion Tenderness at the medial border of the patella and medial retinaculum Guarding with gentle pressure on the medial patella with lateral displacement	Nonoperative management: 2 to 3 weeks of joint rest with splint or knee immobilizer (patella-stabilizing sleeve), then intensive rehabilitation Isometric exercises, especially of quadriceps 80% to 85% of cases are successfully managed with nonoperative treatment Surgical correction for recurrent dislocations or chronic instability	Outcomes with nonoperative therapy vs. acute surgery are similar Patellar dislocation tends to recur (recurrence is more frequent in younger child) but decreases over time Degenerative arthritis is common with or without surgery with recurrent dislocations

Data from Anderson SJ: Lower extremity injuries in youth sports, *Pediatr Clin North Am* 49:627–641, 2002; Hosalkar HS, Wells L: The knee. In Kliegman RM, Behrman RE, Jenson HB, et al, editors: *Nelson textbook of pediatrics*, ed 18, Philadelphia, 2007, Saunders/Elsevier; Landry GL: Management of musculoskeletal injury. In Kliegman RM, Behrman RE, Jenson HB, et al, editors: *Nelson textbook of pediatrics*, ed 18, Philadelphia, 2007, Saunders/Elsevier; McMahon P, editor: *Current diagnosis and treatment: sports medicine*, New York, 2007, Lange Medical Books/McGraw-Hill; Staheli LT, editor: *Pediatric orthopaedic secrets*, ed 2, Philadelphia, 2003, Hanley & Belfus.

ACL, Anterior cruciate ligament; *MCL,* medial collateral ligament; *MRI,* magnetic resonance imaging; *NSAID,* nonsteroidal anti-inflammatory drug; *ROM,* range of motion.

Patient Education

Parents need to understand that special shoes do not cure the problem, and arch supports do not help the foot to "grow" an arch.

Metatarsus Adductus

MA involves adduction of the forefoot relative to the hindfoot. When the forefoot is supinated and adducted, the deformity is termed *metatarsus varus*. The most common cause is intrauterine molding; the deformity is bilateral in 50% of cases (Hosalkar et al, 2011). A nonflexible foot, especially with heel valgus, or persistence may indicate a more serious problem.

Clinical Findings

History. There can be a family history.

Physical Examination.

- The forefoot is adducted, whereas the midfoot and hindfoot are normal.
- The lateral border of the foot has a convex shape with the base of the fifth metatarsal appearing prominent. Normally, this border should look straight. Sometimes spreading of the toes is noted with a wider space between the first and second toes.
- The foot should normally be straight. If one draws a line from the middle of the heel, it should pass through the second toe or between the second and third toes. In MA, the forefoot has an increased angle (greater than 15 degrees) or resists stretching (Fig. 38-14).
- To determine whether the foot is flexible or rigid, the heel is grasped with one hand while the forefoot is abducted with the other hand. In flexible MA, the forefoot can be abducted past midline.

Diagnostic Studies. Radiographs are not performed routinely. AP and lateral weight bearing are indicated in toddlers or older children with residual deformities. The AP radiographs demonstrate adduction of the metatarsals at the tarsometatarsal articulation and an increased intermetatarsal angle between the first and second metatarsals.

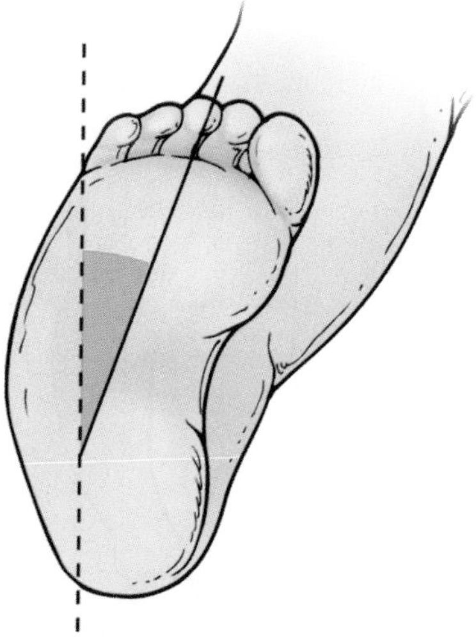

• **Figure 38-14** Metatarsus adductus (MA) angle. An angle (created by the intersecting lines) that is greater than 15 degrees indicates MA.

Differential Diagnosis

Consider congenital vertical talus, which will be rigid, or clubfoot, in which the foot is inverted and in the pointed-toe position. A careful hip examination should be performed to rule out DDH.

Management

Management is based on the rigidity of the deformity; most children respond to nonoperative treatment:

- For the flexible foot that can be brought past midline, the soft tissues can be stretched by the parents with each diaper change. Stretching is done as described under Physical Examination when the examiner determines whether the foot is flexible. Instruct the parents to hold the hindfoot in one hand and stretch the midfoot to overcorrect the deformity to the count of five and repeat five times. The soft tissues should blanch with each stretch. Be sure that the parent is not just pushing on the great toe. Feet that correct just to the neutral position may benefit from stretching exercises and retention in a slightly overcorrected position by a splint or reverse shoe. If there is no improvement in 4 to 6 weeks, serial plaster casts should be considered. Once flexibility and alignment are restored, orthoses or corrective shoes are generally recommended. Surgical treatment may be considered in the small subset of children with symptomatic residual deformities. Surgery is generally delayed until 4 to 6 years old (Hosalkar et al, 2011).
- For the nonflexible foot:
  - Refer to an orthopedist.
  - Educate the family that the treatment for infants may include serial short-leg casts or braces to stretch the foot (two or three casts for 2 weeks per cast) or other management if the bones of the foot are more severely affected. If the child is older than 2 to 3 years old, surgery may be needed to correct the problem.
  - Surgical treatment may be considered in patients with symptomatic residual deformities that have not responded to conservative treatment. Surgery is generally delayed until the child is 4 to 6 years old.

Complications

Early intervention can prevent more intensive therapeutic measures to correct the deformity.

Talipes Equinovarus

Talipes equinovarus (clubfoot) has three elements: the ankle is in equinus (the foot is in a pointed-toe position), the sole of the foot is inverted as a result of hindfoot varus or inversion deformity of the heel, and the forefoot has the convex shape of MA (forefoot adduction). The foot cannot be manually corrected to a neutral position with the heel down.

The etiology of clubfoot may be idiopathic (which tends to be hereditary), neurogenic (as seen with myelomeningocele), or associated with certain syndromes, such as arthrogryposis and Larsen syndrome. It varies in severity, with uterine positioning a factor in mild clubfoot. The incidence is 1:1000 live births, with approximately 50% of cases being bilateral. The etiology is thought to be multifactorial and likely involves the effects of environmental factors in a genetically susceptible host (Hosalkar et al, 2011). The problem is congenital and can be identified in neonates. It is more common in male infants.

Clinical Findings

History. Clubfoot is present at birth.

Physical Examination. The foot appears as described previously. A complete physical examination should be performed to rule out coexisting musculoskeletal and neuromuscular problems.

Diagnostic Studies. AP and lateral radiographs are recommended, often with the foot held in a maximally corrected position. Radiographic measurements can be made to describe malalignment between the tarsal bones. A common radiographic finding is "parallelism" between lines drawn through the axis of the talus and the calcaneus on the lateral radiograph, indicating hindfoot varus. Radiographs are not required as an infant to diagnosis the anomaly.

Management

The following steps are taken:

- Refer to an orthopedist as early as possible, ideally shortly after the infant is born, because the joints are most flexible in the first hours and days of life. Nonoperative treatment should be initiated as soon as possible after birth. The treatments include taping and strapping, manipulation, and serial casting. The Ponseti method of clubfoot treatment involves a specific technique for manipulation and serial casting. Weekly cast changes are performed; 5 to 10 casts are usually required. Up to 90% of children will need a percutaneous tenotomy of the heel cord as an outpatient followed by a long leg cast with the foot in maximal abduction and dorsiflexion. This is followed by a full-time bracing program for 3 months and then nightly bracing for 3 to 5 years. For older children with untreated clubfeet or for those who have residual deformity, osteotomies may be required in addition to the soft-tissue surgery (Hosalkar et al, 2011).
- Stiffness remains a concern at long-term follow-up. Although pain is uncommon in childhood and adolescence, symptoms may appear during adulthood.

Complications

With growth, the abnormality can become increasingly distorted, making correction more difficult. Calf hypoplasia and a shorter than normal foot can occur even with correction.

Overriding Toes

Overriding toes are generally identified at birth. Efforts to tape them into a correct position or otherwise modify their position are usually futile. Overriding of the second, third, and fourth toes generally resolves with time. Occasionally, if severe, they can be surgically improved. Shoe fit can be a problem.

In-Toeing and Out-Toeing Rotational Problems

When a child has an in-toeing or out-toeing gait, the degree of rotation and source of the rotational deformity must be assessed (Fig. 38-15). These include internal femoral torsion (femoral anteversion), internal tibial torsion, and MA. The causes of in-toeing usually are physiologic, are related to age, and resolve as the child grows (Table 38-4). In addition, in-toeing in children can vary with activities and from step to step.

Clinical Findings

History.

- Onset, progression, functional limitations, previous treatment, evidence of neuromuscular disorder, and significant family history

Physical Examination.

- Observe the gait. Note that the slightly older child may consciously or unconsciously improve or worsen the gait for the examiner. Asking the child to run may also be helpful.
- Lay the child prone on the examining table.
- Examine for femoral anteversion (medial and lateral rotations).
- Examine for internal or external tibial torsion (TFA).
- Examine for MA or other deformity.

The child may have a combination of any or all of the aforementioned problems.

Management

See the individual diagnoses for management strategies.

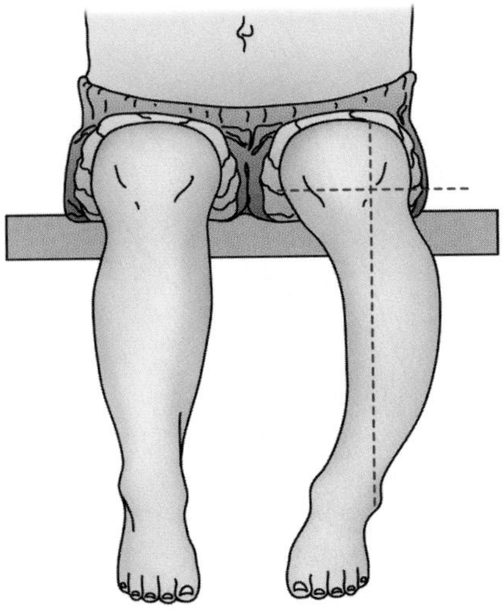

• **Figure 38-15** In-toeing from internal (medial) tibial torsion.

TABLE 38-4 Typical Cause of In-Toeing and Out-Toeing Rotational Problem

Cause	Possible Diagnoses	Typical Finding	Age at Manifestation
In-toeing	Equinovarus	Plantar foot flexion, forefoot adduction, and hindfoot varus	At birth
	Metatarsal adductus	Curved foot: Refer if not flexible	Birth to 6 months old
	Abducted great toe	Searching toe: Resolves spontaneously	Toddler period
	Medial tibial torsion (MTT)	Refer if thigh-foot angle (TFA) more than −10 to −20 degrees	12 to 18 months old
	Internal femoral torsion	Refer if >70 degrees medial and <10 degrees lateral hip rotation	2 to 5 years old
Out-toeing	Physiologic infantile out-toeing	Feet may turn out when infant is positioned upright: Resolves spontaneously	Early infancy
	Lateral tibial torsion (LTT)	Refer if TFA > +30 degrees	Late childhood
	Lateral femoral torsion	Refer if >2 standard deviations of the mean	Late childhood

Other Common Musculoskeletal System Findings Needing Attention

Toe Walking

Most young children walk on their toes until they establish the heel-toe pattern, usually within the first 6 months of walking. Consistent toe walking is frequently associated with neurologic problems, such as cerebral palsy. Autistic children or those with early muscular dystrophy may toe walk. Children with tight heel cords may toe walk. Unilateral toe walking can be associated with a short leg, as found with a dislocated hip. Toe walking also can be a habit, especially in children who used walkers or jumpers. In these children, toe walking generally resolves before 3 years old and is not associated with any musculoskeletal deformity. It is important to differentiate between the idiopathic toe walker and the child who toe walks because of a neuromusculoskeletal condition associated with tight heel cords and contractures.

Clinical Findings

History

The provider should assess:
- Onset
- Severity
- Neurologic history
- Use of a walker or jumper

Physical Examination

The examination should include:
- Looking at shoe wear to assess extent of toe walking. For example, is the heel worn?
- Assessing for tight heel cords. The foot should be brought beyond a 90-degree angle.
- Conducting a neurologic assessment.
- Measuring leg lengths and examining hips.

Management

Management depends on the etiology. Orthopedic management is needed for tight heel cords, unequal leg lengths, and hip problems.

Ganglions of the Hands

Ganglions are the most common benign lesions of soft tissue in children (see Popliteal Cysts). A ganglionic cyst is an acquired, mucinous, fluid-filled painless lesion that originates from the synovial-lined space. A ganglion grows out of a joint. It rises out of the connective tissues between bones and muscles.

Clinical Findings

Ganglions of the hand are hard, fixed masses commonly found on the wrist (commonly dorsal) and flexor aspects of the finger. The etiology of these cysts is unknown. Transillumination of the cyst with an otoscope or examination by ultrasonography plus findings on physical examination are keys to the diagnosis.

Management

Ganglionic cysts in children are rarely symptomatic and usually regress spontaneously. The likelihood of recurrence with any form of treatment is higher in children than the recurrence rate in adults with such lesions. Conservative care with rest and splinting can be tried. If conservative care fails to result in partial or complete resolution, refer for needle aspiration or surgical excision, which is the most reliable method to eliminate a ganglion because the tract that extends into the joint is removed. Steroid injections are not advised.

Leg Aches of Childhood

Extremity pain, often referred to as *growing pains* by the layperson, is a frequent clinical presentation. The pain is usually nonarticular; in two thirds of children, it is described as being located in the shins, calves, thighs, or popliteal fossa. It is almost always bilateral. The pain appears late in the day or is nocturnal, often awaking the child. The pain can last from minutes to hours. By morning, the child is almost always pain-free. Because it occurs late in the day and is often reported on days of increased activity, it may represent a local overuse syndrome, and it may be associated with decreased bone strength. Leg aches of childhood are generally not associated with serious organic disease, have a peak age incidence between 4 and 8 years old, and usually resolve by late childhood; 10% to 20% of school-age children experience intermittent leg aches (Anthony and Schanberg, 2011). However, it is important to differentiate these pains from more serious pathologic conditions; thus this is a diagnosis by exclusion. Restless legs syndrome (discussed in Chapter 14) is a more recently recognized common source of nocturnal leg pains in children.

Clinical Findings

History

Pain or leg aches are typically described as:

- Occurring characteristically in the evening or late in the day; may wake child up from sleep
- Pain gone in the morning with no limitation of activity
- Poorly localized and bilateral
- Occurring commonly in the front of the thighs, in the calves, and behind the knees
- Transient and occurring over a period of time as long as several years
- Not associated with a limp or disability
- No reported fevers or swelling
- No report of recent or remote trauma

Physical Examination

- Have the child stand on tiptoes and heels.
- Measure leg lengths.
- Evaluate range of motion. (Consider using the Pediatric Gait, Arms, Legs and Spine [pGALS] video as a visual guide on how best to examine the child's gait, arms, legs, and spine when doing the musculoskeletal examination; it is available on the Internet. See Additional Resources on the Evolve site.)
- Assess for swelling, erythema, and tenderness.
- Observe for limping.

Findings include normal physical examination with no joint pain or tenderness, guarding, swelling, erythema, or reduced range of motion.

Diagnostic Studies

There is no single diagnostic test. It is a diagnosis of exclusion.

Differential Diagnosis

Restless legs syndrome, neoplastic lesions, leukemia, sickle cell anemia, juvenile arthritis, and subacute osteomyelitis apophysitis must be ruled out (Duey-Holtz et al, 2012).

Management

Reassure the parents that these common complaints have a benign etiology and generally resolve spontaneously. Symptomatic treatment with heat and analgesic may be of benefit. Stress the need for parents to bring the child in for reevaluation if there is a change in symptoms or other signs emerge. Refer a child if the pain is localized to one region, is associated with swelling or other constitutional symptoms, is increasing in severity, or alters gait.

Limps

Deviations from normal age-appropriate gait pattern can be caused by a wide variety of conditions. A limp is usually mild and self-limited and caused by contusion, strain, or sprain. In some cases, the cause can be a sign of a serious inflammatory or infectious process. Age is an important factor in diagnosing the many causes of limping. Table 38-5 describes the various types of limps commonly seen in children.

Clinical Findings

History

A careful history is needed, including:

- Presence of pain
- History of trauma, past medical history
- Presence of fever, night sweats
- Weight loss or anorexia
- Type of limp (Table 38-6)
- Interference with activities
- Review of systems

Physical Examination

- Child should be unclothed during examination.
- Observe for areas of erythema, swelling, atrophy, and deformity.
- Observe each limb segment.
- Identify limp type: Have the child walk and run while distracted.
- Stance and swing phase should be compared in both legs.
- Range of motion of each joint should be evaluated, especially the hip.
- Complete a neurologic examination, including strength, reflexes, balance, and coordination.
- Assess Trendelenburg sign for hip stability.

Diagnostic Studies

A CBC with differential and measurement of ESR and CRP levels should be obtained to rule out infection, inflammatory arthritis, or malignancy. Imaging should include radiographs of the area of concern. When imaging the hip, frog-leg lateral views should be obtained. Ultrasound may be used to detect effusion of the hip joint. If radiographs and ultrasound are positive, a CT scan may be indicated.

TABLE 38-5 Types of Limp

Type of Limp	Cause	Characteristics	Examples
Antalgic	Pain: Typically due to infection, fracture, or trauma	Walking on a painful extremity results in an attempt to get weight quickly off affected side; gait has shortened stance phase*	Sore knee: Walks with fixed knee Sore toe: Tries not to roll off toe at toe-off phase of the stride Appendicitis causes slight slumping posture and shortened stride on the right side due to psoas muscle irritation
Trendelenburg gait/ abductor lurch	Hip problems: Typically developmental, congenital, or muscular disorders	Tilts over affected hip to decrease mechanical stresses; unaffected leg is off the ground during swing-through phase of gait	Hip dysplasia
Equinus/toe-to-heel gait	Neurologic incoordination	Unsteady, wide-based gait	Cerebral palsy: Toe-to-heel sequence to gait during stance phase due to heel-cord contractures
Circumduction	Functionally longer leg; knee or ankle stiffness	Longer leg progresses forward in swing motion	Leg length inequality/knee injury with hyperextension/ankle problems

*Stance phase: Represents 60% of the gait cycle; swing about 40%.

Differential Diagnosis

Fracture, DDH, LCPD, SCFE, tumor, infection, juvenile arthritis, and others should be considered (see Table 38-6).

Management

Refer the patient to an orthopedist immediately, unless the etiology is a mild strain or a local lesion that can be managed conservatively by the primary care provider.

Overuse Syndromes of Childhood and Adolescence

Overuse injuries, overtraining, and burnout among child and adolescent athletes are a growing problem. It is estimated that 30 to 45 million children and youth, ages 6 to 18 years old, participate is some form of sport activity (Lykissas et al, 2013). An overuse injury is microtraumatic damage to a bone, muscle, or tendon that has been subjected to repetitive stress without sufficient time to heal or undergo the natural reparative process. *Apophysitis* refers to the irritation, inflammation, and microtrauma of the apophysis. The risk of overuse injuries is more serious in the pediatric population, because the growing bones cannot handle as much stress as the mature adult bone. Typical overuse injuries of childhood are varus overload of the elbow ("Little League elbow"), Osgood-Schlatter disease, proximal humeral epiphysiolysis ("Little League shoulder"), patellofemoral pain syndrome, shin splints, and stress fractures (Table 38-7).

Clinical Findings

History

In-depth history about the sport played, activities performed (e.g., pitching, kicking, swinging), and hours played per week, including games and practice, needs to be determined. The provider must ask specific questions related to the child's pain. For example, what makes the pain better or worse? Further history and discussion with the child and adolescent should include questions related to the timing of the pain as it relates to the child's activity:

- Pain in the affected area after physical activity
- Pain during the activity without restricting performance
- Pain during the activity that restricts activity
- Chronic, unremitting pain even at rest

Physical Examination

The examination is dependent on the joint or limb involved. Check for deformity, warmth, swelling, range of motion, and ecchymosis. Observe for guarding of an extremity or limping.

Differential Diagnosis

Depending on the presenting symptoms, a plain film, CT, MRI, or bone scan may be indicated.

Management

Most of the injuries can be managed conservatively with proper and timely diagnosis. Treatment often involves resting and icing the extremity or joint, doing retraining and strengthening exercises, gradually reintroducing activities,

TABLE 38-6 Differential Diagnosis of Limping

Condition	Age	Pain (±)	Historical Findings	Clinical Findings	Causative Factors	Management
Developmental dysplasia of the hip (DDH)	Infant, toddler, child, adolescent	–	Breech delivery; MA; torticollis; poor treatment outcomes if not diagnosed at birth or shortly thereafter	Limited abduction; Trendelenburg; radiography at 2 to 3 months old; shortening of leg; acetabular dysplasia	Familial; joint laxity, positioning, maternal hormones	Newborn: No triple diapers; Pavlik harness to hold hips in flexion—see weekly; after 6 months old, traction or open reduction; after 18 months old, osteotomy
Leg length inequality	Toddler, child, adolescent	–	None	Circumduction gait; joint contracture; >1 cm discrepancy in leg lengths	Congenital; neurogenic; vascular; tumor; trauma; infection	Shoe lifts; epiphysiodesis (fusion of growth plate to arrest growth of the opposite side), if discrepancy 2 to 6 cm
Neuromuscular (NM) disease	Toddler, child, adolescent	–	Depends on cause	Depends on cause; equinus or abductor gait	Cerebral palsy, muscular dystrophy, and other NM diseases	Referral to appropriate specialists
Diskitis	Toddler, child, adolescent	+	Varied: fever, malaise, unwilling to walk, backache	Stiff back, ↑ ESR; positive x-ray within 2 to 3 weeks—narrow disk space, irregular vertebral body endplate; bone scan, CT, MRI show early findings early bone scan has typical findings	Bacterial infection in disk space *(Staphylococcus aureus)* or inflammatory response	Immobilization and antistaphylococcal antibiotic therapy
Septic arthritis	Toddler, child, adolescent	++	Moderate to high fever, malaise, arthralgias; irritability; progressive course	Redness, warmth, and swelling of joint—knee or hip; limited hip motion; ESR >25 mm/h	*S. aureus* likely organism	Appropriate antibiotic coverage (7 days, IV; 3 to 4 weeks total)
Acute hematogenous osteomyelitis	Toddler, child, adolescent	+	Varied: malaise, low-grade to high fever; may have severe constitutional symptoms; toxicity	Refusal to walk or move limb; point tenderness; limp; 7 to 10 days to see radiographic bony changes; 25% ↑ WBCs; ↑ CRP	*S. aureus* likely organism	Appropriate antibiotic coverage (generally 7 days, IV; 4 to 6 weeks total or until ESR normal)

TABLE 38-6 Differential Diagnosis of Limping—cont'd

Condition	Age	Pain (±)	Historical Findings	Clinical Findings	Causative Factors	Management
Neoplasm	Toddler, child, adolescent	+	Depends on type of neoplasm	Varied	Neoplasm—benign or malignant	Referral to oncologist
Trauma	Toddler, child, adolescent	+	Depends on type (fractures, strains, sprains)	Varied	Varied	Rule out physical abuse if discrepancy related to developmental capabilities, injury history, and type of injury
Occult trauma: toddler fracture	Toddler	+	Well child	Commonly radiograph (oblique view) shows spiral fracture of tibia; refusal to walk, mild soft tissue swelling	Trauma	See Trauma above
Transient synovitis	3 to 8 years old	+	Mild to moderate fever, mild irritability; resolves within 1 week	Limited hip motion; ESR <25 mm/h	Inflammatory reaction; unknown etiology; often URI (50%) prior	Rest
Juvenile arthritis (JA)	Childhood until 16 years old	+	Fever, rashes, ↑ WBCs; some iritis; joint stiffness and swelling; S&S >3 months	Mono-/polyarticular arthropathy; + ANA (25% to 88%); ↑ ESR in moderate/severe JA	Unknown; genetic (HLA) or environmental	Treat with NSAIDs initially; may need sulfasalazine, methotrexate; corticosteroids; joint replacements when older
Slipped capital femoral epiphysis (SCFE)	9 to 15 years old	+	>90th percentile weight; African American; male	Limited abduction and extension; external rotation of thigh if hip flexed	Multifactorial: mechanical; endocrine; trauma; familial	Needs immediate surgery; non–weight-bearing crutches until admitted; bilateral involvement does occur
Legg-Calvé-Perthes disease (LCPD)	4 to 8 years old	+	Acute or chronic onset; pain in hip, groin, knee; stiffness; male	+ Trendelenburg, shortening; ↓ abduction, internal rotation, hip extension; + radiographs but not early	Familial; breech birth; prior trauma (17%)	In female, tends to be more serious problem; bed rest, traction, then PT; bracing and surgery may be needed; bilateral involvement does occur

ANA, Antinuclear antibody; *CRP,* C-reactive protein; *CT,* computed tomography; *ESR,* erythrocyte sedimentation rate; *HLA,* human leukocyte antigen; *IV,* intravenous; *MA,* metatarsus adductus; *MRI,* magnetic resonance imaging; *NSAID,* nonsteroidal anti-inflammatory drug; *PT,* physical therapy; *S&S,* signs and symptoms; *URI,* upper respiratory infection; *WBC,* white blood cell.

TABLE 38-7 Overuse Injuries of Childhood: Characteristic Features and Their Treatment

Condition	Clinical Findings	Treatment	Comments
Osgood-Schlatter disease	Swelling and tenderness/ pain over tibial tubercle	NSAIDs, kneepad, knee immobilizer if severe pain for 1 to 2 weeks	Most resolve with time (12 to 18 months); x-ray only if pain persists (shows soft tissue swelling and possible residual ossicle); if pain persists, consider surgical incision of ossicle
Patellofemoral pain syndrome	Anterior knee pain	Rest, NSAIDs, retraining, and strengthening of quadriceps muscles	Arthroscopic surgery only if recurring problems
Proximal humeral epiphysiolysis ("Little League shoulder")	Shoulder pain—gradual onset; pain ↑ with throwing, especially curve ball	Modify activity; gradual restart, but limit intensity and frequency of throwing with retraining and muscle strengthening	Seen in skeletally immature children; radiographs show widening proximal humeral physis
Shin splints	Pain along medial border of tibia; child has a history of prolonged running	NSAIDs; ice after running; retraining and muscle strengthening after inflammation ↓; gradual return to running	Associated with poor running technique, hard running surface, muscle weakness; inadequate running shoes; sudden increase in running; is an inflammatory response; may need to consider exertional compartment syndrome
Stress fractures	Tenderness and swelling at site	Reduce or eliminate activity that caused injury for 10 to 14 days; may need to cast	Caused by microtrauma; most commonly seen in active teens, but can occur during childhood; proximal tibia most common site
Varus overload of the elbow ("Little League elbow")	Elbow pain with activity; locking and ↓ extension of elbow; medial humeral epicondyle tenderness	Rest; NSAIDs; ice; when pain-free, gradual return to activity with retraining; surgery if elbow instability	Leads to osteochondral lesions and stress fractures if severe; radiographs reveal widening proximal physis; also seen in gymnasts

NSAID, Nonsteroidal anti-inflammatory drug.

and using analgesics. NSAIDs help reduce the inflammatory component of the trauma. Patient and parent education is important to prevent further injury and disability and to allow the child to return to safe sport participation. If not managed properly and effectively, overuse injuries can affect normal physical growth and maturation. Health care providers can be instrumental in educating the active child, the parents, and the coaches in developing strategies to prevent overuse injuries. These include careful monitoring of training workload especially during growth spurts, providing time for pre-practice neuromuscular training to enhance strength and conditioning, and frequent evaluation of proper use and sizing of sporting equipment (DiFiori et al, 2014).

Muscle Diseases

The muscular dystrophies are a group of hereditary disorders of skeletal muscle that produces progressive degeneration of skeletal muscle leading to weakness. The muscular dystrophies are autosomal dominant, sex-linked, and can appear in several children in a family. The X-linked dystrophies are the most common with the most common dystrophy being Duchenne muscular dystrophy. The estimated incidence of Duchenne muscular dystrophy in the United States is 2 per 10,000 (Darras, 2015a).

Clinical Findings

History

- Disease becomes evident between 3 and 6 years old
- Family history of muscle disease
- Failure to achieve motor milestones, especially independent ambulation
- Toe walking
- Loss of motor skills, such as the ability to climb stairs easily
- Easy fatigue with physical activity

- A history of good days and bad days in relation to ability to accomplish physical activities
- Increasing difficulties with motor activities

Physical Examination

- Toe walking
- Large firm calf muscles
- Fibrotic or "doughy" feel to the muscles
- Widely based lordotic stance
- Waddling Trendelenburg gait
- Lower extremities show early weakness of gluteal muscle strength
- Positive Gowers' sign: Gowers' sign is obtained by asking the child to get up off the floor without help. The sign is positive if the child uses his or her arms to push off from the legs, gradually standing in a segmented fashion.

Management

Referral is necessary. These conditions may need to be handled by an interdisciplinary team with orthopedic, metabolic, and physical therapy, social service, and nursing care. Genetic counseling may be necessary, depending on the diagnosis.

The use of corticosteroids and deflazacort, which is not approved for use in children by the United States Food and Drug Administration and is not available in the United States, has been shown to preserve or improve strength, but each has significant side effects, including weight gain, osteopenia, and myopathy. Dexamethasone and triamcinolone should not be used, because they induce myopathy. Physical therapy is used to promote mobility and prevent contractures (Darras, 2015b). Surgery may be needed for severe contractures and scoliosis.

Patient and family support is needed. Muscle diseases are chronic, debilitating, and some are fatal conditions. Helping the child to lead as normal a life as possible while coping with his or her condition is a major task for parents and caregivers.

For a complete list of references, please visit http://evolve.elsevier.com/Burns/pediatric/.

39 Perinatal Disorders

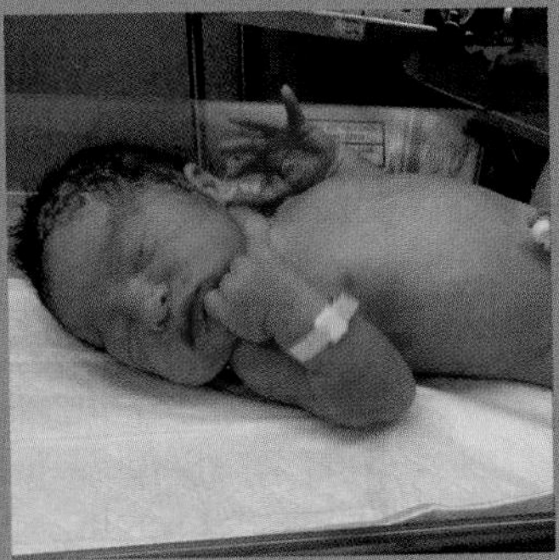

NAN M. GAYLORD AND ROBERT J. YETMAN

The neonatal period is remarkable for the vast array of physiologic changes that occur as the infant transitions from the intrauterine to extrauterine life. This period is a highly vulnerable time for the infant. In the United States, about two thirds of all deaths in the first year of life occur among infants less than 28 days old with the highest risk in the first 24 hours of life (MacDorman et al, 2013). Because serious health problems can arise for the infant in the hours after the initial transition to extrauterine life, the primary care provider must be prepared to manage these problems while providing psychosocial support and education for the families. An understanding of the physiology of fetal development, risk factors for potential problems, and pertinent physical findings is necessary to effectively assist the newborn's transition to extrauterine life.

Standards of Care

The overall goals of the Healthy People 2020 objectives related to maternal, infant, and child care are to improve maternal health and pregnancy outcomes and to reduce rates of disability in infants, thereby improving the health and well-being of women, infants, children, and families in the United States (U.S. Department of Health and Human Services, 2010). Since its inception in 1979, the Healthy People program suggests that the health of a population is reflected in the health of its most vulnerable members. A major focus of many public health efforts, therefore, is improving the health of pregnant women and their infants, including reductions in the rate of birth defects, risk factors for infant death, and death of infants and their mothers. Included among these goals are improvements in the rates of breastfeeding, ensuring that all newborns are screened for state-mandated diseases, reducing the proportion of children with a metabolic disorder who experience developmental delay requiring special education services, and increasing the percentage of healthy full-term infants who are placed to sleep on their backs.

The Guide to Clinical Preventive Services (U.S. Preventive Services Task Force, 2014) recommends the following preventive services for neonates:

- Prenatal screening for Rh(D) incompatibility; human immunodeficiency virus (HIV); hepatitis B; syphilis; chlamydia and gonorrhea
- Promotion of breastfeeding
- Neonatal screening for sickle hemoglobinopathies to identify infants who may benefit from antibiotic prophylaxis to prevent sepsis
- Screening for congenital hypothyroidism for all newborns the first 4 days of life
- Screening for phenylketonuria (PKU) for all newborns before discharge from the nursery: Infants who are tested before they are 24 hours old should receive a repeat screening test by 2 weeks old.
- Topical ocular prophylaxis of all newborn infants to prevent gonococcal ophthalmia neonatorum

Bright Futures: Guidelines for Health Supervision of Infants, Children, and Adolescents (Hagan et al, 2008) and the American Academy of Pediatrics (AAP) Committee on Practice and Ambulatory Medicine (AAP Task Force on Sudden Infant Death Syndrome, 2011) have detailed anticipatory guidelines for the newborn, first-week, and 1-month health supervision visits. *Guidelines for Perinatal Care* from the AAP and the American Congress of Obstetricians and Gynecologists (ACOG) is another thorough compendium of standards of caring for the newborn (Riley and Stark, 2012).

Anatomy and Physiology

The infant's intrauterine-to-extrauterine transition requires an extraordinary number of biochemical and physiologic changes. In utero, the placenta provides metabolic functions for the fetus. Oxygenated blood from the placenta arrives to the fetus through the umbilical vein. Because of high fetal pulmonary vascular pressure, this blood is shunted from the right to the left side of the fetus' heart through the foramen ovale or to the systemic circulation through the ductus arteriosus. At birth, the umbilical cord is severed. Simultaneously, the infant begins to breathe and the high pulmonary vascular pressure drops, allowing blood flow to the lungs for oxygenation. The foramen ovale and ductus arteriosus are no longer necessary and close after birth. The newborn becomes dependent on gastrointestinal tract function to absorb nutrients, renal function to excrete wastes and maintain chemical balance, liver function to metabolize and excrete toxins, and the functions of the immunologic system to protect against infection. Many newborn problems are related to poor transition to extrauterine life as a result of asphyxia, premature birth, congenital anomalies, or adverse effects of delivery.

A predictable series of changes or reactivities in vital signs and clinical appearance take place after the delivery of most normal infants (Fig. 39-1). The first period of reactivity includes sympathetic system changes, such as tachycardia, rapid respirations, transient rales, grunting, flaring and retractions, a falling body temperature, hypertonus, and alerting exploratory behavior. Parasympathetic system changes during the first period of reactivity include the initiation of bowel sounds and the production of oral mucus. After an interval of sleep, the infant enters the second period of reactivity. During this time, the oral mucus production again becomes evident, the heart rate becomes labile, the infant becomes more responsive to endogenous and exogenous stimuli, and meconium is often passed.

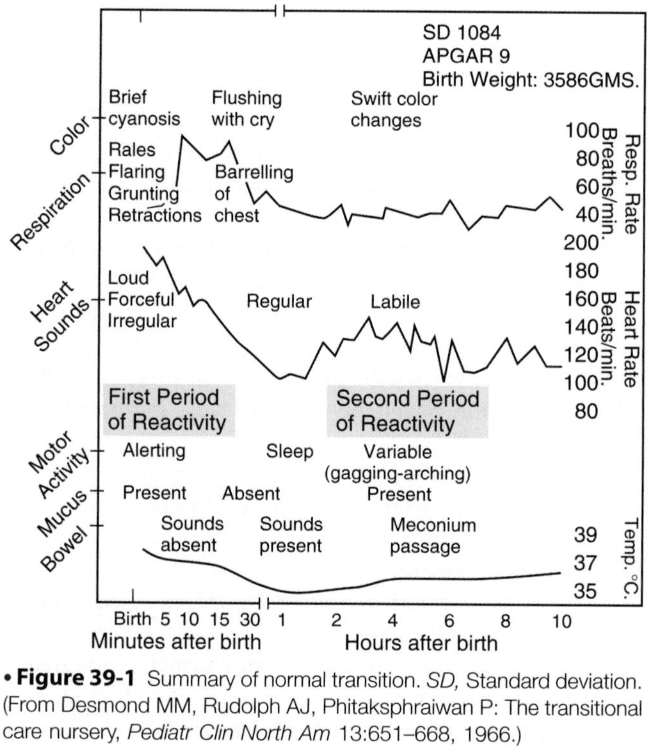

• **Figure 39-1** Summary of normal transition. *SD*, Standard deviation. (From Desmond MM, Rudolph AJ, Phitaksphraiwan P: The transitional care nursery, *Pediatr Clin North Am* 13:651–668, 1966.)

Pathophysiology

High-Risk Pregnancy

High-risk pregnancies are defined as those in which factors exist that increase the chances of abortion, fetal death, premature delivery, intrauterine growth retardation, fetal or neonatal disease, congenital malformations, intellectual disability, and other handicaps. Identification of a high-risk pregnancy is the first step toward prevention of neonatal problems (Box 39-1). Comprehensive and frequent prenatal visits for women with high-risk pregnancies are aimed at preventing complications in the newborn.

Acquired Health Problems

In utero exposure to poor nutrition, alcohol, drugs, viruses or bacteria, and maternal conditions, such as hypertension and diabetes, can result in prematurity and abnormalities at birth. The risk of neonatal problems increases with maternal age younger than 20 years old and older than 35 years old (see Box 39-1).

Genetic Problems

The presence of chromosomal abnormalities, congenital anomalies, inborn errors of metabolism, intellectual disability, and familial diseases increases the risk of the same condition in the infant. Because many conditions are not easily identifiable on physical examination, exploring family histories to identify newborns at risk for any inheritable diseases is important. Anticipation of various inherited conditions leads to their early identification and allows preparation for the management of potential problems.

Perinatal Complications and Injuries

Perinatal complications occur immediately before or during birth. Prolonged or dysfunctional labor increases the possibility of fetal distress. Prolonged rupture of the membranes and chorioamnionitis increase the risk of infant infection, and ruptured placenta previa increases the risk of infant blood loss. Cesarean deliveries, the use of forceps or vacuum extraction, and the type of maternal anesthesia used also pose threats. The term *birth injury* includes mechanical and anoxic trauma incurred by an infant during labor and delivery. Predisposing risk factors for birth injury include macrosomia, prematurity, cephalopelvic disproportion, dystocia, prolonged labor, and breech presentation. Birth injuries include caput succedaneum, cephalhematoma, subcutaneous fat necrosis on the buttocks or extremities, fractures of the skull, subconjunctival and retinal hemorrhages, intracranial hemorrhage, peripheral nerve palsies (brachial, phrenic, facial), fractured clavicle or humerus, ruptured liver or spleen, and hypoxic-ischemic insults. Proper steps to monitor and treat an infant with perinatal complications and injuries must be undertaken immediately after birth.

• BOX 39-1 Factors Associated with High-Risk Pregnancies

Demographic Social Factors

Maternal age <20 years old or >35 years old
African American race
Developmentally delayed mother or low educational status
Illicit drug, alcohol, cigarette use
Poverty, unemployed, homelessness
Unmarried or lack of support
Emotional or physical stress including depression and other mental health problems
Poor access to or use of prenatal care, underinsured or uninsured

Medical History

Diabetes mellitus
Hypertension, maternal hypercoagulable state, sickle cell disease, congenital heart disease
Asymptomatic bacteriuria
Autoimmune disease including rheumatologic illness (SLE)
Chronic medication
Sexually transmitted infections (colonization: herpes simplex, GBS, syphilis, HIV)

Prior Pregnancy

Intrauterine fetal demise or neonatal death
Previous infertility
Prematurity or low birth weight infant
Intrauterine growth retardation
Congenital malformation
Incompetent cervix
Blood group sensitization, neonatal jaundice
Neonatal thrombocytopenia
Hydrops
Inborn errors of metabolism

Present Pregnancy

Uterine bleeding (abruptio placentae, placenta previa)
Inception by reproductive technology
Poor weight gain or abnormal fetal growth
Multiple gestation, parity more than 5
Preeclampsia or eclampsia
Premature rupture of membranes
Short interpregnancy time
Polyhydramnios or oligohydramnios
High or low maternal serum alpha-fetoprotein

Labor and Delivery

Premature labor (<37 weeks) or prolonged labor
Postdates (>42 weeks) or prolonged gestation
Fetal distress
Immature L/S ratio: Absent phosphatidylglycerol
Breech presentation
Meconium-stained fluid
Nuchal cord
Forceps or cesarean delivery
Apgar score <4 at 1 minute

Neonate

Birth weight <2500 g or >4000 g
Birth before 37 or after 42 weeks of gestation
SGA or LGA
Hypoglycemia
Tachypnea, cyanosis
Congenital malformation
Pallor, plethora, petechiae

GBS, Group B streptococcus; *HIV*, human immunodeficiency virus; *LGA*, large for gestational age; *L/S*, lecithin-sphingomyelin ratio; *SGA*, small for gestational age; *SLE*, systemic lupus erythematosus.

The provider must be familiar with perinatal conditions that subject the newborn to a higher risk and be prepared to intervene quickly based on the available perinatal information.

Assessment of the Neonate

History

- Past maternal health history
- Past obstetric history
  - Number of previous pregnancies; number of infants born alive or stillborn
  - Number of elective or spontaneous abortions; number of preterm and term deliveries
  - Cesarean deliveries and indications for them
  - Health status of living children; if deceased, age and cause of death
- Family history
  - Genetically acquired conditions, birth defects, intellectual disability, or other diseases
  - Hypertension, hyperlipidemias, heart disease, or familial cancers
  - Age and health status of living relatives
  - Causes of death of family members
- Current obstetric history
  - Present health and medical history including depression or other mental health conditions
  - Age of mother
  - Prenatal care—duration of
  - Medications used during pregnancy including prescription, over-the-counter, and natural health products
  - Use of pregnancy-enhancing drugs or technology
  - Infections (including group B streptococcus [GBS] status and results of other screening tests) and illnesses during pregnancy
  - Alcohol, cigarettes, or other drugs used during pregnancy
  - Environmental exposures to heavy metals (mercury) or bacteria (listeria)
  - Hypertension or glucose intolerance

- Duration of labor, duration of ruptured membranes, analgesia, anesthesia, presentation and route of delivery, use of forceps
- Polyhydramnios (excessive fluid) or oligohydramnios (reduced fluid)
- Stained infant meconium or foul smelling amniotic fluid
- Fever
- Social history
  - Emotional stressors during pregnancy, including homelessness
  - Unplanned or unwanted pregnancy
  - Financial and emotional support
  - Dietary considerations (e.g., strict vegan diet)
  - Educational background of parents
  - Father's anticipated involvement in raising infant
  - Ages of other children in the home

Physical Examination

Immediately After Birth

Apgar Score

Immediate evaluation of the newborn infant at 1 and 5 minutes of age is a valuable routine procedure. An Apgar score is assigned to the baby based on the criteria in Table 39-1.

- Apgar score: 8 to 10
  - Vigorous, pink, and crying
  - Requires only warming, drying, gentle stimulation
  - Occasionally requires oxygen for a short period
- Apgar score: 5 to 7
  - Cyanotic
  - Slow, irregular respirations
  - Good muscle tone and reflexes
  - Responds to bag-and-mask ventilation
- Apgar score: 4 or less
  - Limp, pale, or blue
  - Apneic, slow heart rate
  - Maximal resuscitative efforts with bag and mask, chest compressions, intravenous (IV) volume expansion, and drug therapy

The 5-minute Apgar score is an indication of how well the resuscitation efforts have succeeded. Caution must be exercised when using the Apgar score to predict long-term outcomes of mortality and developmental delay. Only when combined with other factors, such as fetal status, umbilical cord or scalp blood pH, evidence of organ injury, or seizures, can the Apgar score be useful in determining long-term outcome (AAP, 2006). In actual practice, the decision to resuscitate an infant typically is based on a quick assessment of the heart rate, color, and respiratory rate, rather than the full 1-minute Apgar score (Fig. 39-2) unless resuscitative decisions have made prior to delivery when fetal anomalies are known.

Gestational Age

Maturational assessment of an infant's gestational age is based on the physical examination (Fig. 39-3). The assessment is done promptly after birth to confirm maternal estimated dates, and it is interpreted with information on the mother's menstrual history, obstetric milestones achieved during pregnancy, and prenatal ultrasonograms. An infant's length, weight, and fronto-occipital head circumference are measured and plotted on growth curves based on gestational age (Fig. 39-4). Infants whose weights fall above the 90th percentile for age are classified as large for gestational age (LGA); those whose measurements fall below the 10th percentile for age are classified as small for gestational age (SGA). Those whose measurements fall between the 10th and 90th percentiles are classified as appropriate for gestational age (AGA).

Temperature

Body surface area of the newborn infant relative to its weight is approximately three times that of the adult. Estimated rate of heat loss in the newborn is four times that of an adult (Carlo, 2011b). Body temperature falls precipitously in a cool environment unless adequate precautions are taken. Towel dry the infant after birth to prevent evaporative heat loss and place skin-to-skin with the mother if the infant is otherwise stable. Alternatively use a radiant

TABLE 39-1 Apgar Scores

Sign	Score 0	Score 1	Score 2
Heart rate (bpm)	Absent	Slow (<100)	>100
Respiratory effort	Absent	Weak cry; hypoventilation	Good; strong cry
Muscle tone	Limp	Some flexion of extremities	Well flexed
Reflex irritability (response of skin stimulation to feet)	No response	Some motion	Cry
Color	Blue; pale	Body pink; extremities blue	Completely pink

bpm, Beats per minute.

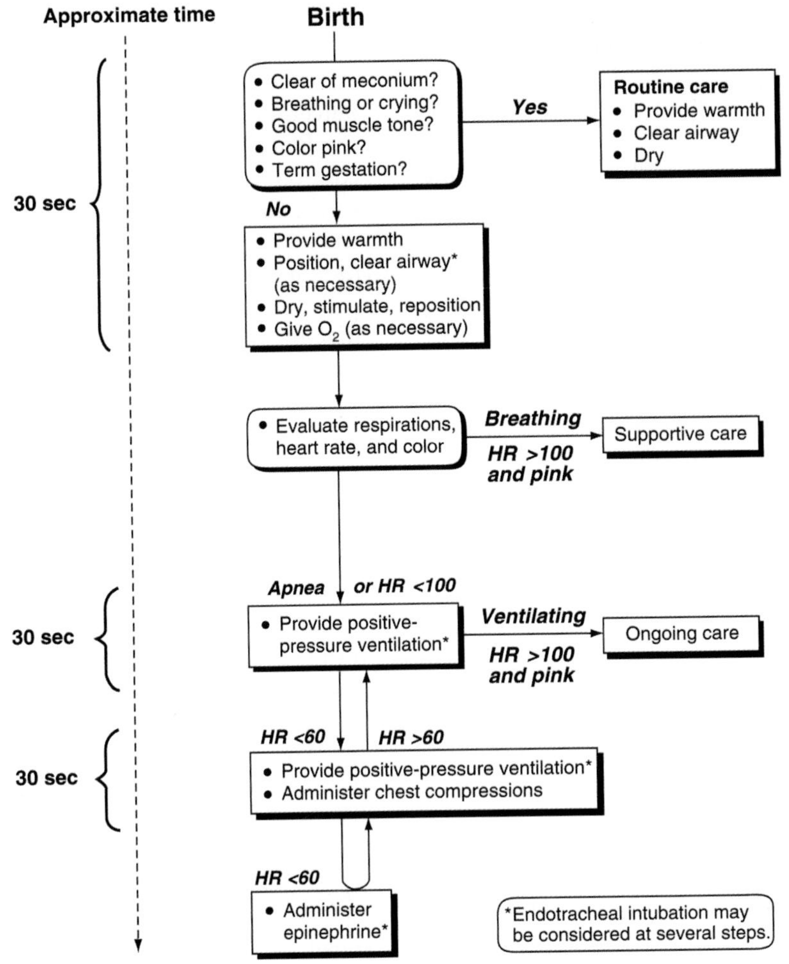

• **Figure 39-2** Resuscitation in the delivery room. *HR,* Heart rate. (From Niermeyer S, Kattwinkel J, Van Reempts P: International guidelines for neonatal resuscitation: an excerpt from the Guidelines 2000 for Cardiopulmonary Resuscitation and Emergency Cardiovascular Care: International Consensus on Science, *Pediatrics* 106(3):29, 2000.)

warmer, wrap infant in warm blankets, and cover the head to reduce heat loss when the baby will be held by parents.

Lungs

During a vaginal delivery, the squeezing action on an infant's chest as it passes through the pelvis and vagina assists in expulsion of amniotic fluid from the lungs. Further expulsion of amniotic fluid from the lungs and reversal of high pulmonary vascular resistance ensue with an infant's first large breaths. Careful bulb suctioning assists in clearing the amniotic fluid from the oropharynx. An infant born by cesarean delivery does not experience the squeezing action of a vaginal birth and is dependent on respiratory efforts and appropriate bulb suctioning to adequately clear the amniotic fluid. Auscultation of the newborn's lungs reveals bronchovesicular or bronchial breath sounds. Fine crackles can be present during the first few hours of life and is a variant of normal.

Umbilical Cord

The normal umbilical cord contains two thick-walled arteries and a single thin-walled vein. Vessel numbers other than this are abnormal and can be associated with congenital anomalies. The umbilical cord is clamped using sterile technique to prevent infection and bleeding.

After Stabilization

After a quick initial assessment in the delivery room to evaluate for obvious problems, a more complete physical examination is done (Table 39-2). When performing the physical examination, the infant's gestational age, age in hours, and stage of transition must be considered.

Diagnostic Studies

All states in the United States require screening of infants for a variety of congenital abnormalities, although the screening tests performed vary from state to state. Infants should be screened based on state law. Typically they are screened before they are discharged; if an initial screen was before 24 hours of life, rescreening should be done by 14 days old. Although most infants require no special screening tests, some are at risk for predictable complications in the

Text continued on p. 1092

MATURATIONAL ASSESSMENT OF GESTATIONAL AGE (New Ballard Score)

NAME ______________ SEX ______________

HOSPITAL NO. ______________ BIRTH WEIGHT ______________

RACE ______________ LENGTH ______________

DATE/TIME OF BIRTH ______________ HEAD CIRC. ______________

DATE/TIME OF EXAM ______________ EXAMINER ______________

AGE WHEN EXAMINED ______________

APGAR SCORE: 1 MINUTE ________ 5 MINUTES ________ 10 MINUTES ________

NEUROMUSCULAR MATURITY

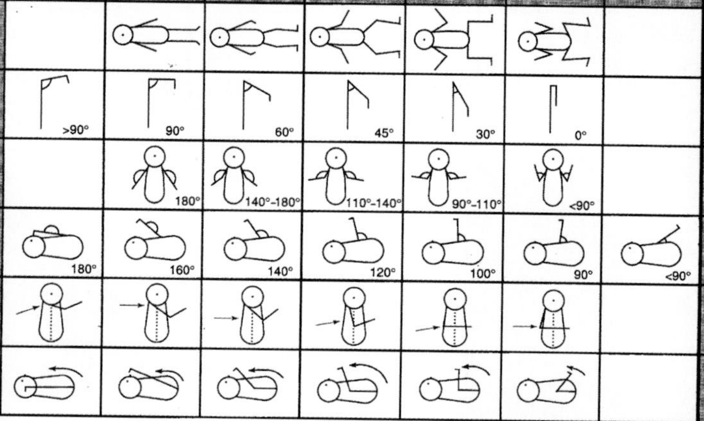

NEUROMUSCULAR MATURITY SIGN	SCORE -1	0	1	2	3	4	5	RECORD SCORE HERE
POSTURE								
SQUARE WINDOW (Wrist)	>90°	90°	60°	45°	30°	0°		
ARM RECOIL		180°	140°-180°	110°-140°	90°-110°	<90°		
POPLITEAL ANGLE	180°	160°	140°	120°	100°	90°	<90°	
SCARF SIGN								
HEEL TO EAR								

TOTAL NEUROMUSCULAR MATURITY SCORE

PHYSICAL MATURITY

PHYSICAL MATURITY SIGN	SCORE -1	0	1	2	3	4	5	RECORD SCORE HERE
SKIN	sticky friable transparent	gelatinous red translucent	smooth pink visible veins	superficial peeling &/or rash, few veins	cracking pale areas rare veins	parchment deep cracking no vessels	leathery cracked wrinkled	
LANUGO	none	sparse	abundant	thinning	bald areas	mostly bald		
PLANTAR SURFACE	heel-toe 40-50 mm:-1 <40 mm:-2	>50 mm no crease	faint red marks	anterior transverse crease only	creases ant. 2/3	creases over entire sole		
BREAST	imperceptible	barely perceptible	flat areola no bud	stippled areola 1-2 mm bud	raised areola 3-4 mm bud	full areola 5-10 mm bud		
EYE/EAR	lids fused loosely: -1 tightly: -2	lids open pinna flat stays folded	sl. curved pinna; soft; slow recoil	well-curved pinna; soft but ready recoil	formed & firm instant recoil	thick cartilage ear stiff		
GENITALS (Male)	scrotum flat, smooth	scrotum empty faint rugae	testes in upper canal rare rugae	testes descending few rugae	testes down good rugae	testes pendulous deep rugae		
GENITALS (Female)	clitoris prominent & labia flat	prominent clitoris & small labia minora	prominent clitoris & enlarging minora	majora & minora equally prominent	majora large minora small	majora cover clitoris & minora		

TOTAL PHYSICAL MATURITY SCORE

SCORE

Neuromuscular ______

Physical ______

Total ______

MATURITY RATING

score	weeks
-10	20
-5	22
0	24
5	26
10	28
15	30
20	32
25	34
30	36
35	38
40	40
45	42
50	44

GESTATIONAL AGE (weeks)

By dates ______

By ultrasound ______

By exam ______

Reference
Ballard JL, Khoury JC, Wedig K, et al: New Ballard Score, expanded to include extremely premature infants. *J Pediatr* 1991; 119:417-423. Reprinted by permission of Dr Ballard and Mosby-Year Book, Inc.

• **Figure 39-3** Classification of newborns by intrauterine growth and gestational age. (From Ballard JL, Khoury JC, Wedig K, et al: New Ballard score, expanded to include extremely premature infants, *J Pediatr* 119:417–423, 1991.)

CLASSIFICATION OF NEWBORNS (BOTH SEXES) BY INTRAUTERINE GROWTH AND GESTATIONAL AGE [1,2]

NAME ______________________ DATE OF EXAM ______________________ LENGTH ______________________

HOSPITAL NO. ______________________ SEX ______________________ HEAD CIRC. ______________________

RACE ______________________ BIRTH WEIGHT ______________________ GESTATIONAL AGE ______________________

DATE OF BIRTH ______________________

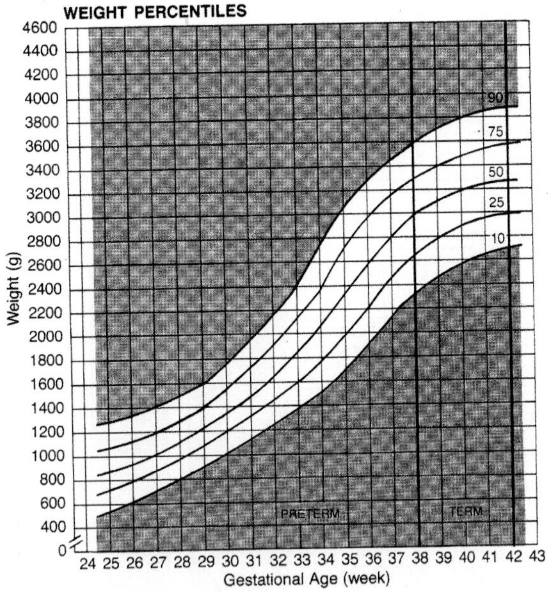

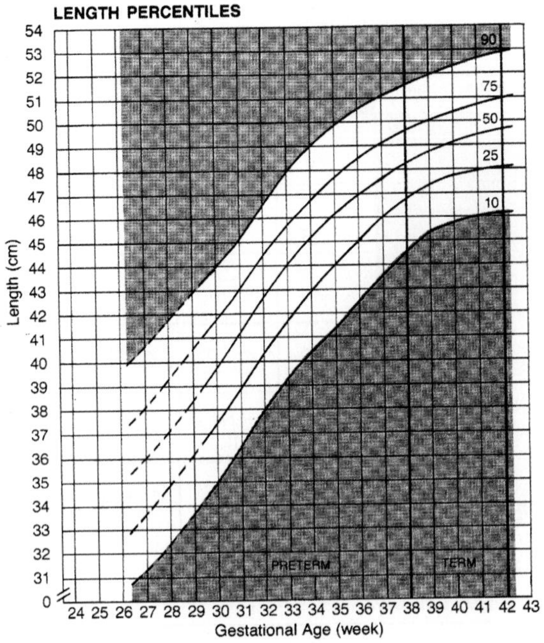

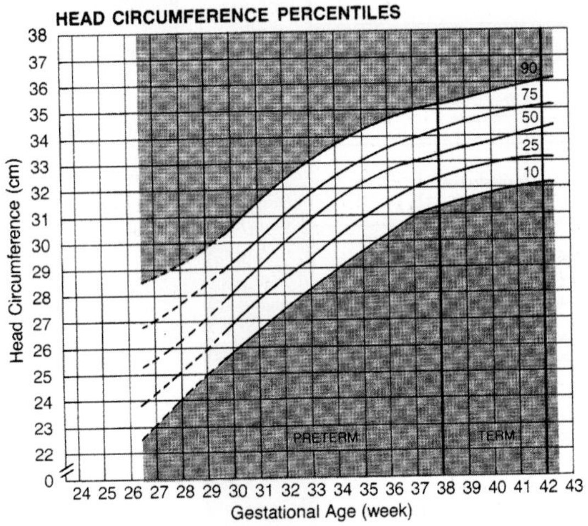

CLASSIFICATION OF INFANT*	Weight	Length	Head Circ.
Large for Gestational Age (LGA) (>90th percentile)			
Appropriate for Gestational Age (AGA) (10th to 90th percentile)			
Small for Gestational Age (SGA) (<10th percentile)			

*Place an "X" in the appropriate box (LGA, AGA or SGA) for weight, for length and for head circumference.

References
1. Battaglia FC, Lubchenco LO: A practical classification of newborn infants by weight and gestational age. *J Pediatr* 1967; 71:159-163.
2. Lubchenco LO, Hansman C, Boyd E: Intrauterine growth in length and head circumference as estimated from live births at gestational ages from 26 to 42 weeks. *Pediatrics* 1966; 37:403-408.

• **Figure 39-4** Newborn maturity rating and classification. (From Ross Hospital Formula System, Ross Products Division, Abbott Laboratories, Columbus, OH; adapted from Battaglia FC, Lubchenco LO: A practical classification of newborn infants by weight and gestational age, *J Pediatr* 71:159–163, 1967; Lubchenco LO, Hansman C, Boyd E: Intrauterine growth in length and head circumference as estimated from live births at gestational ages from 26 to 42 weeks, *Pediatrics* 37:403–408, 1966.)

TABLE 39-2 Physical Examination Findings

System	Findings
Vital signs and measurement	Check frequently in the first hours. Every 6 to 8 hours when stable. Evaluate temperature stability (97.7° to 99.3° F [36.5° to 37.4° C]) in open crib after transition to extrauterine environment. • Failure to maintain temperature suggests sepsis • Respirations = 30 and 60 breaths/min • Heart rate = 100 and 160 bpm • Significant molding of the head requires repeated measurements to verify size • Daily weight measurement with losses of up to 10% in the first 2 to 3 days are normal • *Weight loss of greater than 10%* often due to poor intake or excessive losses
Skin	Normal dermatologic findings: • Lanugo and vernix: Most common in premature infants • Dry and cracked skin: Most common in a postmature infant • Pallor: Causes include anemia, sepsis, cold stress, hypoglycemia, and seizures • Plethora: Causes include polycythemia or hyperthermia • Meconium staining: When the first stool passes in utero due to antenatal stress, staining of the infant's skin and fingernails results • Jaundice: Hematologic conditions
Head	• Sutures and molding: Vaginally delivered infants may demonstrate elongation of the anteroposterior diameter of the skull • Fontanelles: Anterior fontanelle = about 2 to 3 cm in diameter; the posterior fontanelle = about 1 cm in diameter (Fig. 39-5)
Face	Symmetric structures should be apparent, although unilateral facial edema as a result of delivery conditions may occur.
Eyes	Check symmetry, size, and slanting of palpebral fissures: • Uncoordinated eye movements: Intermittent uncoordinated eye movements (disconjugate gaze) during the first weeks after birth are common, improving by 2 to 4 months old and resolving by 6 months old. • Fixed disconjugate gaze is abnormal. • Conjunctivae: Reddening in the first 24 to 48 hours of life may be caused by the ocular prophylaxis agent. • Purulent discharge in the first days or weeks of life can be associated with gonococcus, chlamydia, or herpes. • Sclerae: Yellowing is associated with hyperbilirubinemia. Conjunctival hemorrhages secondary to delivery resolve spontaneously over the first weeks of life. Thinning of the sclera, common in African Americans, is manifested by dark blue or black patches. Blue sclerae are associated with osteogenesis imperfecta. • Red reflex: Absence of a red reflex may indicate the presence of lens opacities secondary to cataracts, congenital infection (rubella), or calcium metabolism abnormality. A white reflex can indicate retinoblastoma. Absence of the expected red reflex requires an immediate ophthalmologic evaluation.
Ears	Identify normalcy in the size, rotation, shape, position, and patency of the external auditory canal. Universal screening for detection of infants with hearing loss is recommended. Auditory brain response testing should be ordered for any infant in whom a question of hearing exists or are high risk (e.g., family history, in utero infection, craniofacial anomalies, syndromes associated with hearing loss) such as: • Low-set ears: Evaluate for dysmorphic features • Abnormalities in shape: Evaluate for genitourinary system abnormalities • Preauricular skin tags or significant pits: Can be a genetic red flag
Nose	Patency of the nasal passages can be tested by closing the mouth and one nostril at a time. If questionable, pass a small catheter into the nasopharynx to confirm patency. Nasal flaring is a sign of respiratory distress.
Mouth	Evaluate size and symmetry of the lips at rest and with movement: • Thin lips with a smooth philtrum are associated with fetal alcohol syndrome. • Cleft lip and palate can be associated with midline CNS abnormalities. Incomplete cleft palates are recognized by digital examination of the mouth for bony defects of the hard palate in the presence of normal palatal mucosa. • Excessive salivation can be related to reflux of gastric contents or esophageal atresia. • An excessively large tongue can be associated with genetic or metabolic abnormalities, such as hypothyroidism or Down syndrome.
Neck	Short neck indicates the possibility of Klippel-Feil syndrome or other vertebral problems. Webbing or redundant skin is seen in trisomy 21, Turner syndrome, and Noonan syndrome. Torticollis: Asymmetric shortening of the sternocleidomastoid muscle results in preferential turning of the head to one side.

Continued

TABLE 39-2 Physical Examination Findings—cont'd

System	Findings
Thorax	Evaluate for shape and symmetry. Normal = rounded appearance measuring about 2 cm less than the head circumference (approximately 33 cm): • Minimization of rounding occurs with RDS, atelectasis, and other diseases of decreased expansion of the chest. • Accentuation is seen in meconium aspiration. • Asymmetric movement occurs with unilateral pneumothorax. • Intercostal, subcostal, or supracostal retractions indicate respiratory distress Clavicles: • Vaginally delivered LGA babies are especially prone to fractures Nipples: • Fullness and sometimes secretion of a white milky substance are normal and are secondary to maternal hormonal stimulation. • Supernumerary and inverted nipples are common. • Redness surrounding the nipple, especially with purulent drainage, occurs in neonatal mastitis.
Lung	Coughing, retractions, and an intermittently increased respiratory rate occur immediately after birth, transitioning by about 12 hours of life to smooth and unlabored respirations at a rate of 30 to 60 breaths/minute. • Respiratory distress: Tachypnea, apnea (pauses in respiration >15 seconds), grunting (an infant's attempt to increase functional residual capacity, thereby improving gas exchange), interclavicular, subclavicular, or supraclavicular retractions, nasal flaring, and central cyanosis all indicate distress. Auscultation: • Rales or crackles are commonly heard immediately after birth as lung fluid is resorbed. Beyond the immediate postpartum period, rales can indicate pneumonia, delayed resorption of lung fluid, meconium aspiration, or pulmonary edema. • Unilateral absence of breath sounds occurs in pneumothorax, atelectasis, and pleural effusion. • Bowel sounds over the chest, especially with a scaphoid abdomen and significant respiratory distress, indicate a diaphragmatic hernia with displacement of abdominal contents into the chest.
Heart	Inspection: Observe neonate for adequacy of perfusion. Respiratory distress is common with cardiac abnormalities. Edema as a result of cardiac failure is rarely seen in the newborn. Palpation: • Point of maximal impulse is displaced from the fourth left intercostal space with pneumothorax, situs inversus, or dextrocardia. • Thrills or heaves are associated with murmurs and cardiac abnormalities. Auscultation: Heart rate is normally 100 to 160 bpm. Detection of skipped beats warrants electrocardiogram. Heart sounds may be muffled or displaced in the infant with a pneumothorax. Murmurs: Common in the newborn period, many murmurs disappear after a few hours or a few days. Significant murmurs should be investigated. Pulses: Brachial or radial pulses are compared with femoral or dorsalis pedis pulses for symmetry of impulse and strength. Delay or relative weakness of lower extremity pulses occurs in coarctation of the aorta. Blood pressure: By Doppler device using a 2.5- to 4-cm wide and 5- to 9-cm long cuff, compare with normal for age and gestation. Systolic blood pressures greater than 96 mm Hg are considered significant hypertension in the newborn, and systolic blood pressures exceeding 106 mm Hg are considered severe hypertension.
Abdomen	Normal abdomen is slightly protuberant, is soft, moves smoothly with respirations, and has fine bowel sounds scattered throughout. Absent bowel sounds can indicate ileus. • The liver is usually palpated 1 to 2 cm below the right costal margin; the spleen tip is sometimes felt at the left costal margin; kidneys, deep within lateral aspects of the abdomen measuring 3 to 4 cm in size, may be palpated. • Umbilicus: Midline outpouching from the sternum to the umbilicus is seen with weak abdominal musculature (diastasis recti); a large and protuberant umbilicus occurs with an umbilical hernia. The cord contains two arteries and a single vein. Absence of the second artery can be associated with congenital abnormalities. • Failure to pass stool in the first 24 to 48 hours of life or at all (meconium ileus) is associated with cystic fibrosis and Hirschsprung disease.

TABLE 39-2 Physical Examination Findings—cont'd

System	Findings
Genitalia	Male: • The urethral opening should be at the tip of the phallus with completely developed foreskin. Testes not located in the scrotal sac or inguinal canal but retrievable to the scrotum are normal. Testes not located in or relocated in the scrotal sac from the canal are considered to be undescended. • Hydrocele is identified by transilluminating fluid collection around the testis and is regarded as normal unless it is associated with inguinal hernia or it lasts more than 12 months. • Inguinal hernia with displacement of intestines into the scrotal sac is frequently non-transilluminating and is associated with scrotal bowel sounds. Inguinal hernias are sometimes apparent and reduced at other times. A surgical consultation is indicated. Female: • Labia majora are large and completely surround the labia minora. • Labia and vagina should be open, often with a white discharge. • Blood-tinged fluid in small amounts by day 2 to 3 is normal. Ambiguous genitalia: • Genitalia that do not appear to be completely masculinized or feminized. • Endocrine and genetic referrals are essential. Anus and rectum: • Patency of the rectum and placement of the anus should be noted.
Extremities, back, hip	• Intrauterine constraint and resultant molding cause mild curvatures of the feet and legs. • Fractures can occur anywhere as a result of the delivery process. • Dimples, hemangiomas, tufts of hair, or other lesions along the spine may be associated with spinal abnormalities, such as spina bifida occulta. • Perform Ortolani and Barlow maneuvers to assess for dislocated or dislocatable hips.
Neurologic examination	Observe tone, movement, and symmetry of the extremities while the infant is awake. Elicit the following reflexes: • Rooting • Sucking • Palmar grasp • Moro reflex • Ankle clonus (three or four beats is normal) • Stepping and placing response • Galant reflex • Asymmetric tonic neck reflex Cranial nerves: CN I (olfactory) is rarely tested. Vision (CN II) is tested by an infant's response to a bright light. CNs III, IV, and VI are tested by noting an infant's ability to gaze in all directions, although intermittent disconjugate gaze is normal through 6 months old. Adequate sucking and swallowing confirm presence of CNs V, IX, X, and XII. Symmetric movement of the face with crying confirms presence of CN VII. Hearing (CN VIII) is assessed by startle to loud noise and hearing screening.

bpm, Beats per minute; *CN,* cranial nerve; *CNS,* central nervous system; *LGA,* large for gestational age; *RDS,* respiratory distress syndrome.

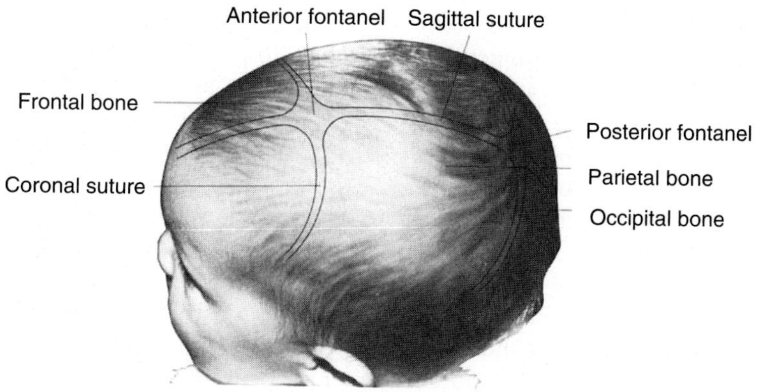

• Figure 39-5 Fontanelles and sutures. (From Betz CL, Hunsberger M, Wright S: *Family-centered nursing care of children,* ed 2, Philadelphia, 1994, Saunders, p 124.)

newborn period. Infants born to mothers with poorly controlled diabetes and LGA or SGA infants are at higher risk for hypoglycemia and usually require serum glucose level screening. Similarly, infants demonstrating Coombs test positivity because of maternal-child blood incompatibility are screened for evidence of hemolysis. Some nurseries screen both mothers and infants for syphilis; mothers should be screened for HIV and hepatitis B, unless it was done prenatally. Universal hearing screening is recommended by 1 month old (see Chapter 30), and special attention is paid to any newborn at higher risk for hearing loss as a result of low birth weight, rubella or other infection, malformation, trauma, asphyxia, prematurity, intensive care unit stay, or antibiotic use.

Management Strategies

Initial Care

Following birth, newborns require observation as they master the transition to the extrauterine environment. Components of care at this period include prophylaxis for eye infection with antibiotic ointment and vitamin K injection for hemorrhagic disease.

Establishing Feeding

Regardless of the route of feeding the family has chosen, the provider must ensure that the infant and parents have well-established feeding patterns before discharge. Follow-up care is scheduled in 2 or 3 days to ensure adequate ongoing nutrition. See Chapters 10 and 11 for more detailed information on breastfeeding and formulas.

Anticipatory Guidance Before Discharge

Physical Care

Umbilical Cord

Applying alcohol to the base of the cord traditionally has been recommended to aid in cord separation, although the utility of this practice has been questioned, especially in high income populations in industrialized areas; air-drying by tucking the diaper below the cord may be preferable (Suliman et al, 2010; Zupan et al, 2004). Some have recommended that bactericidal or antimicrobial agents may be used daily or a bactericidal agent with alcohol swabbing twice per day are effective in reducing colonization with *Staphylococcus aureus* around the healing umbilicus (Carlo, 2011d). After cord separation, which usually occurs at 10 to 14 days old, a slight bloody discharge can be seen for 1 to 2 days. Bellybands or coins to cover the navel are avoided, because these increase the chance of infection. If a foul-smelling discharge or erythema appears around the umbilicus, the infant should be evaluated immediately for sepsis. If a granuloma appears after the cord falls off, an application of silver nitrate helps to heal it.

Circumcision

Circumcision, the removal of the foreskin that normally covers the glans penis, is a controversial surgical procedure. The decision to circumcise is the parents' responsibility, although the provider can supply factual information on the risks and potential benefits of the procedure.

Proponents of circumcision claim that it keeps the glans penis cleaner; it lowers the chance for developing urinary tract infections (although the chance of urinary tract infections in uncircumcised males is only 1%); it reduces the incidence of penile cancer, phimosis, balanitis, adhesions, and occlusion of the urethral meatus; and it allows the boy to look more like his peers. The opponents of circumcision claim that it does not prevent sexually transmitted infection; that good hygiene prevents penile cancer; that circumcision leaves the glans open to the chance of cautery burns and meatal stenosis; and that because fewer boys are being circumcised, these boys will not be different from many of their peers. In 2012, the AAP issued a policy statement on circumcision stating that there is no evidence for routine circumcision, but that the benefits of the procedure are greater than its risks (AAP Task Force on Circumcision, 2012). Additionally, this statement advocates for circumcision access for all families desiring the procedure. In 2014, the Centers for Disease Control and Prevention (CDC) issued preliminary recommendations suggesting that uncircumcised at-risk heterosexual male patients and parents of newborn males should receive comprehensive counseling on the risks and benefits of circumcision (CDC, 2015). These recommendations note that the benefits of circumcision (especially the reduction in spread of HIV) outweigh the risks of the procedure.

Contraindications to circumcision include epispadias or hypospadias, ambiguous genitalia, exstrophy of the bladder, familial bleeding disorders, and illness. Complications of circumcision are rare but include infections, bleeding, gangrene, scarring, meatal stenosis, cautery burns, urethral fistula, amputation or trauma to the glans, and pain. For infants who undergo circumcision, procedural anesthesia is recommended. A variety of anesthesia techniques are available, including application of topical anesthetics (eutectic mixture of local anesthetics [EMLA] cream), dorsal penile nerve block, and subcutaneous ring block (Brady-Fryer et al, 2004). Postoperative pain relief measures in the form of sucrose on a pacifier, acetaminophen, soft music, and physiologic positioning of the infant in a padded environment are helpful.

Care of the uncircumcised baby includes gentle cleaning around the genital area. The skin normally adheres to the penis and is not retractable at birth, but loosens as the baby grows. The parents are counseled not to force the foreskin back. If the baby is circumcised, the penis should be cleansed daily with cotton balls dipped in tap water followed by the application of a small amount of petroleum jelly to the tip of the penis for the first 2 or 3 days after the procedure with each diaper change to prevent discharge from the penis sticking to the diaper.

Bathing, Oils, and Powders

Tradition favors that the infant not be immersed in a tub of water, but rather should be sponge bathed until the umbilical cord separates and the navel appears healed. Mild cleansing agents (such as, Dove, Caress, Neutrogena, and Basis) are gentle enough for infants' skin. Oils and greasy substances are not recommended because they tend to clog the skin's pores and can cause acne or rashes. Powders should be avoided because inhaling the talc could lead to respiratory problems. For dry skin, a lotion (such as, Keri, Eucerin, Aveeno, or Cetaphil) is recommended.

Diapers

Much controversy exists whether disposable or cloth diapers are the better choice for infants. The need for frequent changing and proper cleansing is the important message to deliver. Information on parenting is found in Chapter 5, information on sleep in Chapter 14, and information on injury prevention in Chapter 40.

Early Discharge and Follow-up

Newborns are often discharged after a relatively short period of hospital observation. Although "early discharge" is a common practice, infants can experience difficulty with breastfeeding, weight gain, jaundice, and dehydration, although outcome findings in mothers and newborns related to length of stay have been inconsistent and contradictory (Fink, 2011). The Newborns' and Mothers' Health Protection Act of 2008 prevents insurers from requiring hospital discharge before 48 hours for a vaginal delivery and 96 hours for a cesarean delivery (Department of the Treasury, Department of Labor, U.S. Department of Health and Human Services, 2008). Guidelines for early discharge of normal, healthy newborns are listed in Box 39-2. Plans for follow-up care within 48 to 72 hours and plans for ongoing health maintenance should be confirmed before discharge (Box 39-3). Even newborns who are hospitalized longer may need follow-up care within the first few days of life. All parents leaving the hospital with a newborn should have a confirmed time and place for follow-up, in addition to contacts in case of an emergency or questions.

Premature Infants and Newborns with Special Needs

Premature infants have special needs that must be addressed before discharge (Box 39-4). Newborns with special needs (e.g., anomalies, disease states, social situations) require early assessment, intervention, and referral before discharge to ensure that support, education, and follow-up are in place.

Common Neonatal Conditions

Skin Conditions

Table 39-3 lists newborn skin disorders.

• BOX 39-2 Guidelines for Early Discharge of Normal, Healthy Newborns

- No ongoing medical issues that require continued hospitalization
- Term (37 to 41 completed weeks) baby
- Stable vital signs for at least 12 hours before discharge:
  - Axillary temperature of 97.7° to 99.3° F (36.5° to 37.4° C) in open crib
  - Heart rate 100 to 160 bpm
  - Respiratory rate less than 60 breaths/minute
- Regular passage of urine and at least one stool
- Two successful feedings have been accomplished
- Normal physical examination
- No excessive bleeding at circumcision site
- The clinical significance of jaundice has been determined and appropriate follow-up plans made
- Evaluation and monitoring for sepsis based on maternal risk factors have been accomplished
- Infant laboratory data, including maternal syphilis, hepatitis B, and human immunodeficiency virus (HIV), and infant blood type and Coombs testing (as indicated) completed
- Appropriately timed neonatal metabolic and hearing screenings completed
- Initial hepatitis B administered
- Social support and continuing health care identified
- Social situation adequate: screen for drug abuse, previous child abuse, mental illness, lack of social support, lack of permanent home, history of domestic violence, communicable diseases in the household, teenage mother, inadequate transportation or communication abilities
- Appropriate medical home identified with early follow-up care achievable, preferably within 48 hours of discharge, but no later than 72 hours in most cases
- Mother knowledgeable in the care of the infant, including the following:
  - Feeding, with breastfeeding encouraged
  - Normal stool and urine frequency
  - Skin, genital, and cord care
  - Ability to identify illness (especially jaundice)
  - Proper safety (car seat, sleeping position, smoke-free environment, room sharing)
  - Smoke alarms in the home

Milia

Milia are multiple, firm, pearly, opalescent white papules scattered over the forehead, nose, and cheeks. Their intraoral counterparts are called *Epstein pearls*. Histologically, milia represent superficial epidermal inclusion cysts filled with keratinous material associated with the developing pilosebaceous follicle. No treatment is necessary because milia exfoliate spontaneously in most infants over the first few weeks of life (Fig. 39-6).

Sebaceous Hyperplasia

Sebaceous hyperplasia is characterized by prominent yellow-white papules at the opening of each pilosebaceous follicle, predominantly over the nose, forehead, upper lip, and cheeks. The overgrowth of sebaceous glands in response to the same androgenic stimulation that occurs in adolescence

• BOX 39-3 Guidelines for 48- to 72-Hour Follow-up Visit of the Normal, Healthy Newborn

- Review delivery and discharge summary for any identified follow-up needs (e.g., hearing screening, specialty referrals)
- Assess the infant's general health, weight, hydration, and jaundice; identify any new problems; review feeding, stooling, and urination
- Assess quality of bonding
- Reinforce maternal and family education
- Review outstanding laboratory data
- Perform neonatal screen or other tests (such as, bilirubin), if indicated
- Develop plan for health care maintenance, including emergency care, preventive care, immunizations, and periodic screenings
- Evaluate mother for post-partum depression
- Refer to Women, Infants, and Children (WIC) program eligibility screening as appropriate.

causes sebaceous hyperplasia. No treatment is required. These tiny papules diminish in size and disappear entirely within the first few weeks of life (Fig. 39-7).

Erythema Toxicum

Firm, yellow-white 1- to 2-mm papules or pustules with a surrounding erythematous flare characterize erythema toxicum. Lesions are clustered in several sites. These lesions usually develop at 24 to 48 hours old. The cause is unknown, although examination of a Wright-stained smear of the lesion reveals numerous eosinophils. Up to 50% of infants develop erythema toxicum, with a higher incidence in term than in premature infants. Pyoderma, candidiasis, herpes simplex, transient neonatal pustular melanosis, and miliaria should be considered (Table 39-4). No treatment is required; the course is brief and transient (Fig. 39-8).

Transient Neonatal Pustular Melanosis

Transient neonatal pustular melanosis is characterized by superficial vesicopustules that rupture easily and leave a halo

• BOX 39-4 Guidelines for Discharge and Follow-up of the High-Risk Neonate

Discharge Planning

- Demonstrate adequate weight gain, temperature control in open crib, adequate feeding without cardiorespiratory compromise, and mature and stable cardiorespiratory function.
- Ensure adequacy of immunizations based on infant's chronologic age and appropriate metabolic screenings.
- Screen for anemia and nutritional risks; begin therapy, if indicated.
- Conduct funduscopic evaluation if necessary.
- Ensure appropriate hearing screen has been completed.
- Identify all active medical or social problems through a review of the medical record and physical examination of infant; ensure home readiness has been evaluated, especially for the technologically dependent child.
- Complete car seat evaluation.
- Review with family member medications, feeding schedules, well child care, signs of illness, safety instruction, and appropriate response and follow-up for infants with active medical conditions.
- Identify family and community resources if infant is to be discharged on home oxygen therapy.
- Ensure adequate training of appropriate family members in cardiopulmonary resuscitation (CPR) and, if applicable, home apnea monitor or other equipment use.
- Consider need for visiting nurse, social service, respite care, support groups, early intervention services, or referral to the Women, Infants, and Children (WIC) program.
- Ensure that follow-up care is arranged to include a primary care provider and surgical or other subspecialty providers, if indicated.

Follow-up Planning

- Schedule follow-up hearing screen (if necessary) for infants with:
  - Craniofacial abnormalities
  - In utero infections
  - Birth weight less than 1500 g
  - Meningitis
  - Exchange transfusion for hyperbilirubinemia
  - Use of ototoxic medications
  - Apgar score of 0 to 4 at 1 minute or 0 to 6 at 5 minutes
  - Mechanical ventilation for 5 days or longer
  - Stigmata of syndrome associated with hearing loss
  - Failed initial screening
  - Family history of deafness
- Ensure that by about 4 to 6 weeks of chronologic age a dilated binocular indirect ophthalmoscopic examination has occurred for neonates with:
  - A birth weight of 1500 g or less or with a gestational age of <32 weeks
  - A birth weight between 1500 and 2000 g or gestational age of more than 32 weeks with an unstable clinical course including cardiorespiratory support, especially if infant is thought to be at high risk for retinopathy of prematurity (see Chapter 29)
- Additional examinations may be recommended based on the results of this first evaluation.
- Follow-up visits every 1 to 2 weeks, especially if infant is on oxygen therapy.
- Growth and development should be of prime interest at each routine outpatient visit with referral for formal developmental assessment if any concerns are identified.

TABLE 39-3 **Comparison of Newborn Skin Disorders**

Rash	Significant Maternal or Infant History	Rash Description	Diagnostics	Management/ Treatment
Milia	None	Firm, pearly, white papules over cheeks, nose, and forehead	None	Superficial inclusion cysts will spontaneously resolve
Sebaceous hyperplasia	None	Prominent, yellow-white papules over cheeks, nose, and forehead	None	Overgrowth of sebaceous glands will spontaneously resolve in first few weeks
Erythema toxicum	None Presents at 24 to 48 hours	Yellow-white papules with an erythematous base over cheeks, nose, and forehead	Wright stain demonstrates large number of eosinophils Cultures are sterile	Clears within 2 weeks, completely gone in 4 months
Transient neonatal pustular melanosis	None More common in darker skinned persons	Vesicopustules that rupture easily and leave a halo of white scales around a central macule of hyperpigmentation on trunk, limbs, palms, and soles	None	Spontaneous resolution in 2 to 3 days although hyperpigmentation can persist for up to 3 months
Sucking blisters	Results from vigorous sucking in utero on the affected part	Scattered superficial bullae on the upper arms and lips of infants at birth	None	Will resolve without additional intervention
Cutis marmorata	Accentuated physiologic response to cold	Lacy, reticulated, red or blue vascular pattern	None	Transient and will resolve with warming
Harlequin color change	None	Half of the baby's coloring is red and the other pale	None	Transient and will resolve
Nevus sebaceous	None	Yellow, hairless smooth plaque on head or neck	None	Total excision prior to adolescence; refer to dermatologist
Herpes simplex virus (HSV)	Mother may have active lesions or a history of disease	Grouped vesicles on erythematous base	DFA or ELISA detection of HSV antigens	Acyclovir

DFA, Direct fluorescent antibody; *ELISA,* enzyme-linked immunosorbent assay.

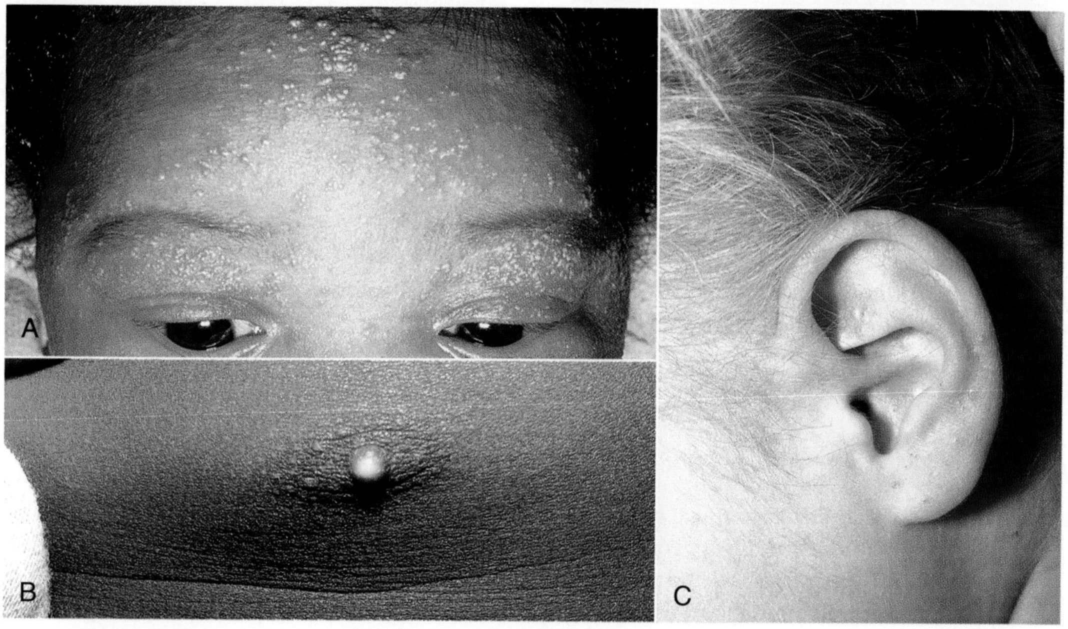

• **Figure 39-6** Milia. (From Cohen BA: *Pediatric dermatology,* ed 4, Philadelphia, 2013, Elsevier, Fig. 2-18A.)

TABLE 39-4 Comparison of Erythema Toxicum and Herpes Simplex Virus

Erythema Toxicum	Herpes Simplex Virus
Benign, self-limited	Pathologic, progressive
No specific maternal history	Frequently a history of maternal disease
Usually seen only in term infant	Can occur in infants of any gestational age
Begins on the second or third day of life, lasting as long as 1 week	Often begins late in the first week of life or early in the second week of life
Rash is evanescent, often involving the face, trunk, and extremities	Can be superficial and localized only to the presenting part (vertex or buttocks) or widespread and disseminated with or without cutaneous involvement
1- to 2-mm white papules or pustules on an erythematous base that occasionally may become somewhat vesicular	May manifest similar to sepsis without cutaneous findings or as grouped vesicles on an erythematous base on the presenting part about days 9 to 11 of life
Wright or Giemsa stain of lesion scraping demonstrates large numbers of eosinophils and no organisms; cultures are sterile	DFA staining or ELISA detection of HSV antigens of vesicle scrapings or growth of the organism from vesicle fluid is diagnostic
No specific therapy necessary	Acyclovir and other antiviral agents

DFA, Direct fluorescent antibody; *ELISA,* enzyme-linked immunosorbent assay; *HSV,* herpes simplex virus.

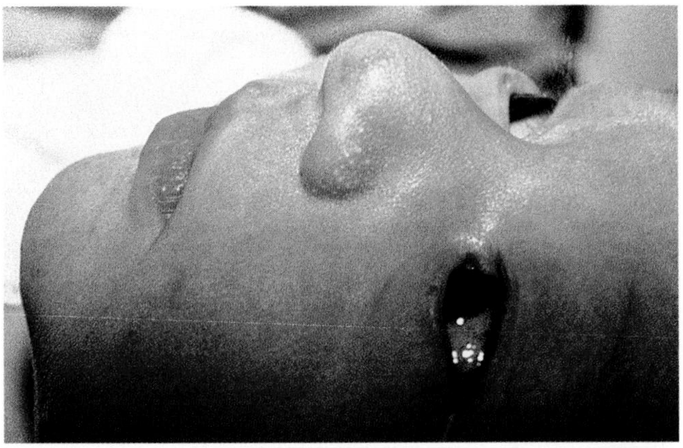

• **Figure 39-7** Sebaceous hyperplasia. (From Cohen BA: *Pediatric dermatology,* ed 4, Philadelphia, 2013, Elsevier, Fig. 2-15.)

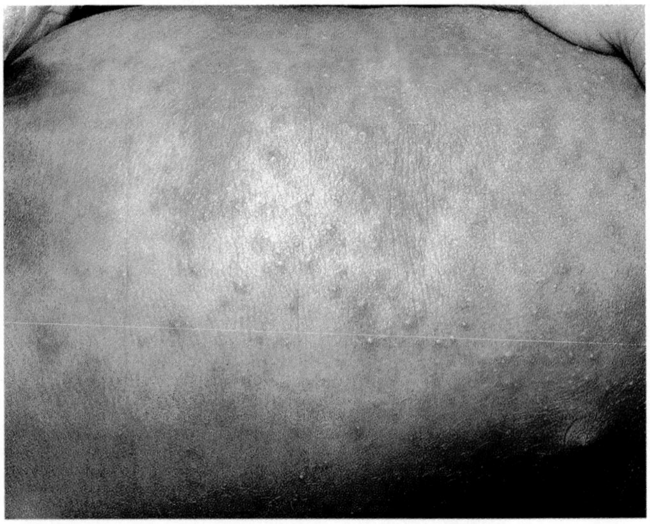

• **Figure 39-8** Erythma toxicum. (From Cohen BA: *Pediatric dermatology,* ed 4, Philadelphia, 2013, Elsevier, Fig. 2-11.)

of white scales around a central pinhead-sized macule of hyperpigmentation. Pustular melanosis is caused by increased melanization of the epidermal cells, with sites of predilection being the trunk, limbs, palms, and soles. It is more common in darker-skinned infants. Pyoderma and erythema toxicum are the differential diagnoses. No treatment is required. The pustular phase rarely lasts more than 2 to 3 days; hyperpigmented macules can persist for as long as 3 months (Fig. 39-9).

Sucking Blisters

Sucking blisters are solitary or scattered superficial bullae on the upper limbs and lips of infants at birth, commonly found on the radial aspect of the forearm, the thumb, and the index finger. These blisters result from vigorous sucking on the affected part in utero. No treatment is required. These bullae resolve rapidly without sequelae.

Cutis Marmorata

Cutis marmorata is a lacy, reticulated, red or blue cutaneous vascular pattern appearing over most of the body surface. The vascular change is a response to exposure to low environmental temperatures. It represents an accentuated physiologic vasomotor response that disappears with increasing age. Persistent and pronounced cutis marmorata occurs in Down and trisomy 18 syndromes. Cutis marmorata usually resolves upon warming the infant (Fig. 39-10).

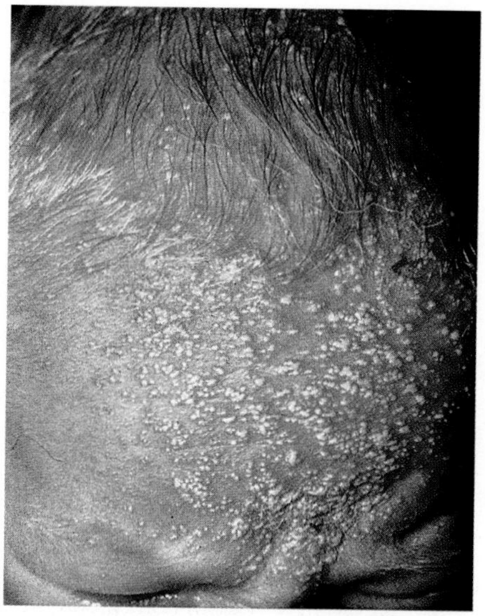

• **Figure 39-9** Transient neonatal pustular melanosis. (From Cohen BA: *Pediatric dermatology,* ed 4, Philadelphia, 2013, Elsevier, Fig. 2-12A.)

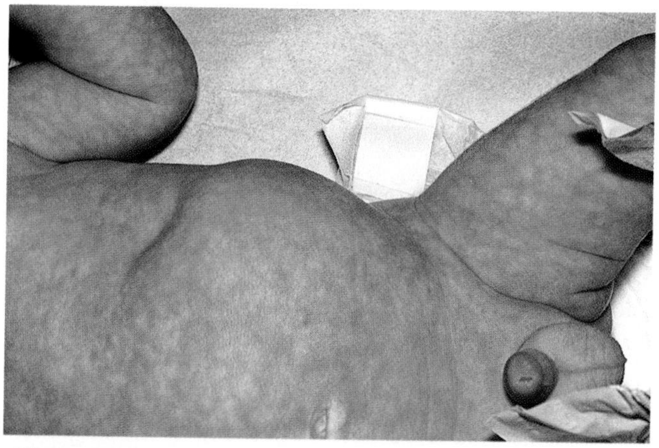

• **Figure 39-10** Cutis marmorata. (From Cohen BA: *Pediatric dermatology,* ed 4, Philadelphia, 2013, Elsevier, Fig. 2-8.)

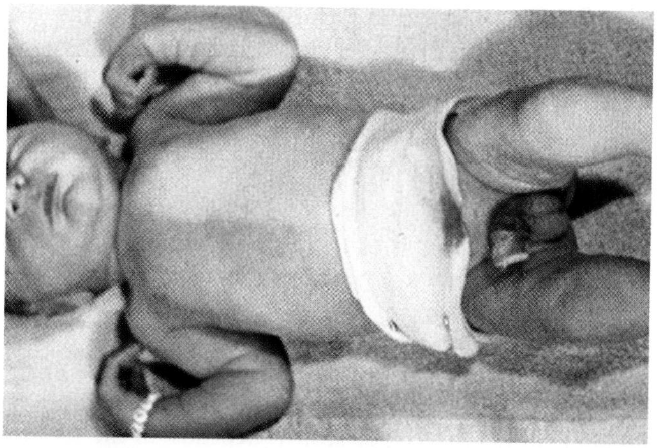

• **Figure 39-11** Harlequin color change. (From Cohen BA: *Pediatric dermatology,* ed 4, Philadelphia, 2013, Elsevier, Fig. 2-10.)

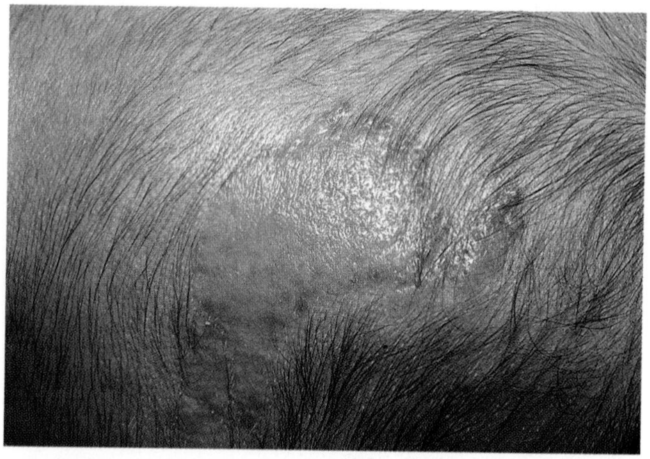

• **Figure 39-12** Nevus sebaceous. (From Cohen BA: *Pediatric dermatology,* ed 4, Philadelphia, 2013, Elsevier, Fig. 2-82A.)

Harlequin Color Change

Harlequin color change is a division of the body skin coloring from forehead to pubis into red and pale halves. The cause is unknown. No treatment is indicated with this transient and benign condition (Fig. 39-11).

Mongolian Spots, Café au Lait Spots, Salmon Patch (Nevus Simplex), and Port-Wine Stain (Nevus Flammeus, Port-Wine Nevus)

See Chapter 37 for a discussion of these skin conditions.

Nevus Sebaceous

Nevus sebaceous is a yellowish, hairless, sharply demarcated smooth plaque usually on the head and neck. Histologically these nevi contain an abundance of sebaceous glands. With maturity, usually during adolescence, the lesions become verrucous with large rubbery nodules. During adulthood, the lesions are complicated by secondary malignancies, most commonly basal cell carcinoma. Total excision before the onset of adolescence is recommended. Referral to a pediatric dermatologist prior to adolescence is warranted (Fig. 39-12).

Skin Dimpling

Deep skin dimples, in addition to pits and creases, can occur over bony prominences and in the sacral area. They occur in normal infants and in those with dysmorphologic syndromes, such as congenital rubella, deletion of the long arm of chromosome 18, and cerebrohepatorenal syndromes. No treatment is indicated if isolated and not associated with other findings.

Preauricular Sinus Tracts and Pits

Sinus tracts and pits occur anterior to the pinna and can be unilateral or bilateral. They result from imperfect fusion of the tubercles of the first and second branchial arches during gestational development, are familial, are more common in females and in African Americans, and occasionally are associated with other anomalies of the ears and face. Excision rarely is required for chronic infections and drainage. Confirmation of normal newborn hearing evaluation is warranted.

Amniotic Constriction Bands

In utero fibrous strands that encircle fetal parts can cause permanent depression of the underlying tissue, producing defects in the underlying structure. Found in otherwise normal infants, these bands are thought to result from intrauterine rupture of the amnion with formation of fibrous strands. Sometimes there are associated abnormalities, including craniofacial anomalies and thoracic or abdominal wall defects. Treatment depends on the severity of deformities produced. Constriction bands on the limbs are often managed in consultation with plastic surgery.

Supernumerary Nipples

Solitary or multiple accessory nipples and sometimes areolae occur in unilateral or bilateral distribution along a line from the midaxilla to the inguinal area. The cause is unknown. Urinary tract anomalies very rarely occur in conjunction with the finding. Usually no treatment is necessary.

Branchial Cleft and Thyroglossal Cysts and Sinuses

Cysts and sinuses in the neck can be unilateral or bilateral and can open onto the cutaneous surface or drain into the pharynx. Thyroglossal cysts and fistulas are defects located in or near the midline of the neck, extending to the base of the tongue. Thyroglossal cysts occasionally contain aberrant thyroid tissue and mucinous material. Thyroglossal cysts and sinuses form along the course of the first and second branchial clefts of the neck as a result of improper closure during embryonic life. These anomalies can be inherited as autosomal dominant traits. Antibiotic therapy is indicated for infections of the cysts or sinuses, which are rare in the neonatal period. Surgical excision is recommended for thyroglossal cysts.

Head, Face, and Eye Conditions

Caput Succedaneum

Caput succedaneum is a diffuse swelling of the soft tissue of the scalp with possible underlying bruising; the swelling usually crosses the suture lines (Fig. 39-13). Caput succedaneum originates from trauma as the baby descends through the birth canal.

Clinical Findings

- Primigravida and traumatic delivery
- Obvious swelling and bruising in the parietal regions of the scalp
- Swelling that crosses suture lines
- Frequently associated with molding

Differential Diagnosis

Cephalhematoma is the differential diagnosis.

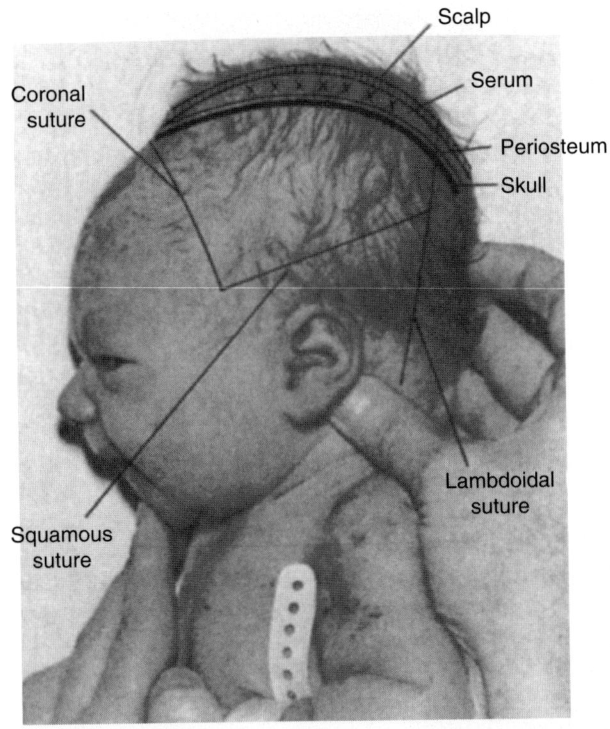

• **Figure 39-13** Caput succedaneum. (From Betz CL, Hunsberger M, Wright S: *Family-centered nursing care of children,* ed 2, Philadelphia, 1994, Saunders, p 124.)

Management

No treatment is necessary because swelling resolves spontaneously over a few days. If the lesion is large, observe the baby for the development of jaundice as the blood from bruising is reabsorbed.

Cephalhematoma

Cephalhematoma is a collection of blood in the subperiosteal area of the scalp that does not cross the suture lines. Frequently no noticeable bruising of the area is seen (Fig. 39-14). Cephalhematoma results from trauma occurring during a difficult delivery. The swelling appears hours to days after delivery.

Clinical Findings

- Primigravida and traumatic delivery may be part of the history
- Swelling in the parietal area that does not cross suture lines
- Rarely associated with a skull fracture, coagulopathy, or intracranial hemorrhage

Differential Diagnosis

Caput succedaneum and cranial meningocele should be considered as differential diagnoses.

Management

No treatment is indicated because the condition resolves in a few weeks to months. Calcification of the hematoma can

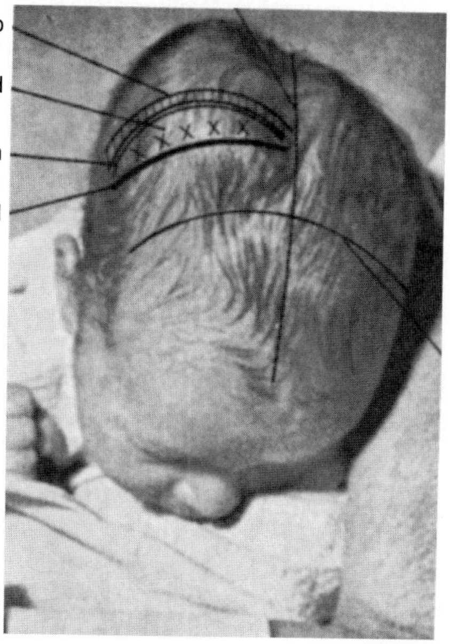

• **Figure 39-14** Cephalhematoma. (From Betz CL, Hunsberger M, Wright S: *Family-centered nursing care of children,* ed 2, Philadelphia, 1994, Saunders, p 124.)

occur, which is felt as bony prominences on the cranium. Observe for hyperbilirubinemia.

Craniotabes

Craniotabes is thinning of the bone of the scalp. This is a normal variation of the parietal bone, usually near the sagittal suture line.

Clinical Findings

- Prematurity
- A "ping-pong ball" effect when pressing on the parietal bone

Management

No treatment is necessary because craniotabes resolves spontaneously. If persistent, pathologic causes, such as rickets, should be investigated.

Cleft Lip and Palate

Cleft lip results from failure of embryonic structures surrounding the oral cavity to join. Cleft palate appears when the palatal shelves fail to fuse. Various degrees of clefts are seen. Genetic factors influence the development of cleft lip more than cleft palate; however, both occur sporadically. A combination of cleft lip and cleft palate is more common than one without the other. Cleft lip with or without cleft palate occurs in about 1 in 750 Caucasian births. Cleft palate alone occurs in 1 in 2500 Caucasian births (Tinanoff, 2011). Clefts are more common in males. In most cases, a genetics consultation is warranted.

Clinical Findings

- A varying degree of cleft, from a small notch to a complete separation
- Unilateral or bilateral cleft
- Involvement of the soft palate, hard palate, or both
- A bifid uvula, which may indicate a submucosal cleft palate

Management and Complications

Surgical repair is indicated, the timing of which is individualized. Special nipples and feeding techniques are used until surgery can be performed. Breastfeeding and bottle feeding may be successful, depending on the severity of the cleft. Speech evaluation and perhaps therapy are necessary in later years. Dental restoration is often needed. Team management is preferred. Middle ear, nasopharyngeal, and sinus infections, as well as associated hearing loss can occur.

Congenital Cataracts, Glaucoma, and Retinopathy of Prematurity

See Chapter 29.

Cardiac Conditions

See Chapter 31.

Respiratory Conditions

Respiratory Distress Syndrome

Respiratory distress syndrome (RDS), formerly known as *hyaline membrane disease,* occurs secondary to surfactant deficiency, resulting in alveolar atelectasis and decreased lung compliance. This is the most common pulmonary disease in the newborn (Table 39-5). The incidence rises rapidly at gestational ages less than 33 to 34 weeks, and the incidence increases with decreasing gestational age and/or weight. An estimated 50% of all neonatal deaths result from RDS or its complications (Carlo and Ambalavanan, 2011).

Clinical Findings

History.

- Diabetic mother (increased incidence at older gestational ages in infants of diabetic mothers)
- Preterm, precipitous, or cesarean delivery
- Multiple births and previously affected siblings
- Asphyxia and/or cold stress

Physical Examination.

- Tachypnea, grunting, intercostal retractions, nasal flaring, duskiness, and/or cyanosis
- Breath sounds may be normal but often are diminished with harsh tubular quality
- Fine rales on deep inspiration

Diagnostic Studies. A radiograph of the chest shows a fine reticular granularity of the parenchyma and air bronchograms. Blood gas results indicate hypoxemia, hypercarbia, and mixed metabolic/respiratory acidosis.

TABLE 39-5 Clinical Comparison of Transient Tachypnea of the Newborn and Respiratory Distress Syndrome

Transient Tachypnea of the Newborn	Respiratory Distress Syndrome
Seen only in infants delivered at or near term; often in infants born by cesarean section	Found almost always in premature infants, with the greatest incidence in infants weighing <1500 g
Increased respiratory rate is invariably present; grunting and intercostal retractions are not always present	Usually, respiratory rate is increased, infants grunt at expiration, nasal flaring is noted, and sternal and intercostal retractions are commonly seen
Cyanosis is not a prominent feature	Cyanosis in room air is a prominent feature
Air exchange is good; rales and rhonchi are usually absent	Auscultation reveals diminished air entry
Begins at birth, usually resolving in the first 24 to 48 hours of life	Progressive respiratory distress in the first hours of life
Chest radiograph shows central perihilar streaking with slightly enlarged heart with fluid in the fissure	Chest radiograph demonstrates reticulogranular, ground-glass appearance, and air bronchograms
Typical course involves gradual decrease in respiratory rate with resolution in about 72 hours	Course variable depending on infant's gestational weight and age; usually, RDS begins to improve after about 5 days of life
No specific therapy other than maintaining oxygenation is usually necessary	Artificial surfactant and antenatal administration of steroids to the mother can reduce the severity of this disease; mechanical ventilation is commonly needed

RDS, Respiratory distress syndrome.

Management, Prognosis, and Prevention

Supportive care and mechanical ventilation are used as indicated. Administration of synthetic corticosteroids to women expected to deliver prematurely is indicated to reduce the severity of the problem. After delivery, the immediate use of exogenous surfactant has been found to reduce mortality rates and improve short-term respiratory status in preterm infants. The overall prognosis depends on the severity of the disease and the birth weight of the infant. The only fully effective preventive measure is elimination of prematurity (Carlo and Ambalavanan, 2011).

Transient Tachypnea of the Newborn

Transient tachypnea of the newborn (TTN) is a respiratory condition that results from incomplete evacuation of fetal lung fluid in full-term infants. TTN results from decreased pulmonary compliance and tidal volume and increased dead space secondary to slow absorption of fetal lung fluid. It is more common in cesarean deliveries.

Clinical Findings

- Usually disappears within 24 to 48 hours
- Tachypnea, expiratory grunting, intercostal retractions
- Auscultation without findings
- Occasionally responds to minimal oxygen

Diagnostic Studies. A chest radiograph shows prominent pulmonary vascular markings, fluid lines along fissures, overaeration, flat diaphragms, and occasionally pleural fluid.

Differential Diagnosis

The differential diagnoses are RDS and pneumonia (see Table 39-5).

Management and Prognosis

If the infant is not in significant respiratory distress, close observation and transcutaneous oxygen saturation monitoring can be sufficient until the absorption of fetal lung fluid is complete and tachypnea resolves. The need for supplemental oxygen therapy should be based on close oxygen monitoring. The use of mechanical ventilation in TTN is rare. Infants usually recover rapidly within 24 to 48 hours without intervention.

Meconium Aspiration Syndrome

Meconium aspiration syndrome occurs in term or postterm infants. This syndrome is a serious pulmonary disorder characterized by small airway obstruction, chemical pneumonitis, and secondary respiratory distress. In utero fetal distress and anoxia increase intestinal peristalsis and relax the anal sphincter, resulting in release of meconium into the amniotic fluid. Thick meconium is aspirated either in utero or with the first breath. Approximately 10% to 15% of all newborns are meconium stained, but only 5% of these infants develop respiratory problems (Ambalavanan and Carlo, 2011).

Clinical Findings

- Meconium in the amniotic fluid and below the vocal cords on resuscitation

- Tachypnea, intercostal retractions, grunting, and cyanosis within hours of delivery

Diagnostic Studies. A chest radiograph shows patchy infiltrates, coarse streaking of both lung fields, and flattening of the diaphragm.

Management, Prognosis, and Prevention

An infant born with meconium in the amniotic fluid but who is vigorous (strong respiratory effort, good muscle tone, and a heart rate of higher than 100 beats per minute [bpm]) does not need intubation and suctioning as had been previously recommended. Rather, ongoing treatment of the vigorous infant includes supportive care and standard management of respiratory distress. Intubation and suctioning of meconium stained infants is recommended only when the infant is depressed, not breathing, and has a heart rate of less than 100 bpm (ACOG Committee on Obstetric Practice, 2007). Severe meconium aspiration cases may require extracorporeal membrane oxygenation (ECMO). The mortality rate is increased in infants born with meconium staining. Meconium aspiration syndrome accounts for a significant proportion of neonatal deaths. Residual lung problems are possible, and central nervous system (CNS) injury from asphyxia can occur.

Gastrointestinal and Abdominal Conditions

Esophageal Atresia and Tracheoesophageal Fistula

In esophageal atresia, a blind pouch occurs in the esophagus with or without an associated fistula. Most infants (87%) have a proximal pouch, with the associated fistula connecting the distal esophagus and the trachea (Fig. 39-15). This defect occurs in 1 in 4000 births. Approximately one third of affected infants are born prematurely and have the highest risk for mortality (Khan and Orenstein, 2011).

Clinical Findings

History. The history includes maternal polyhydramnios and inability to pass a nasogastric tube into the stomach during resuscitation at birth or afterward in the nursery, especially in a child with vomiting. The diagnosis may be suspected prenatally with polyhydramnios and when a small stomach sac and blind pouch is found on prenatal ultrasonography but is difficult to diagnose (Garabedian et al, 2014) and other evaluations may be warranted.

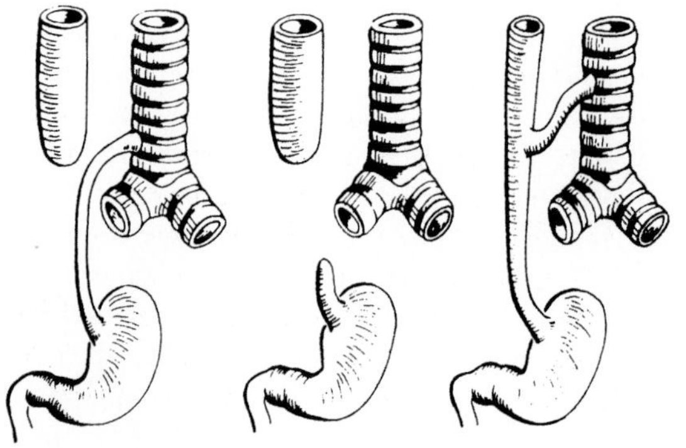

• Figure 39-15 The three most common types of esophageal atresia and tracheoesophageal fistula (TEF). (From Ein SH: Congenital malformations of the esophagus. In Wyllie R, Hyams JS, editors: *Pediatric gastrointestinal disease,* Philadelphia, 2006, Saunders/Elsevier.)

Physical Examination.

- Excessive oral secretions that require frequent suctioning
- Choking, coughing, and cyanosis, particularly during feedings
- Spitting or vomiting

Diagnostic Studies. Chest and abdominal radiographs show the nasogastric tube coiled in the pouch in the thoracic region. Carefully performed water-soluble x-ray evaluation of the upper esophagus demonstrates the exact location of the atresia and rules out tracheoesophageal fistula.

Differential Diagnosis

RDS, meconium aspiration, and congenital heart disease should be considered.

Management, Complications, and Prognosis

This is a surgical emergency requiring immediate intervention. A nasogastric tube can be inserted into the blind pouch to prevent aspiration until surgical repair can be accomplished. Preoperatively the infant should be placed in a prone position and suctioned frequently. Pneumonia, atelectasis, aspiration, postoperative strictures, and repeated surgery are possible complications. The survival rate postoperatively approaches 100% unless other congenital anomalies are present. Approximately 50% of affected infants have other congenital anomalies (Khan and Orenstein, 2011).

Duodenal Atresia

Duodenal atresia is a complete obstruction of the duodenum, ending blindly just distal to the ampulla of Vater. Duodenal atresia occurs in 1 in 10,000 to 30,000 births. It is associated with prematurity in 50% of cases, Down syndrome in 40% of cases, and other anomalies in up to 20% of cases (Bales and Liacourus, 2011).

Clinical Findings

History and Physical Examination. The history includes maternal polyhydramnios and is more common in prematurity and Down syndrome. The infant presents with bilious vomitus, abdominal distention, and jaundice.

Diagnostic Studies. Abdominal radiographs show a "double-bubble" pattern in the upright position secondary to air in the stomach and a distended duodenum.

Differential Diagnosis

Malrotation, duodenal obstruction, and annular pancreas should be considered.

Management, Complications, and Prognosis

Surgical intervention is indicated once the diagnosis of duodenal atresia has been made. Feedings should be discontinued and gastric suctioning applied. The prognosis depends on early identification and treatment and other associated anomalies. Aspiration of gastric contents can occur as a complication of this condition.

Volvulus

Volvulus is the twisting of a loop of bowel, causing intermittent or acute pain and obstruction, occurring in 1 in 6000 live births (Hunter & Liacourus, 2011a).

Clinical Findings

Physical findings include abdominal distention and bilious vomiting.

Diagnostic Studies. Intestinal obstruction is demonstrated on plain abdominal radiograph. Contrast studies demonstrate a "bird's-beak" obstruction in the proximal duodenum and a spiral (corkscrew) configuration of the duodenum.

Differential Diagnosis

Duodenal obstruction or atresia and annular pancreas are in the differential diagnosis.

Management, Complications, and Prognosis

Surgical repair and fluid replacement are indicated. The prognosis depends on identification of the volvulus and the urgency of surgery. Perforation, necrosis of the bowel, sepsis, and peritonitis are possible complications.

Pyloric Stenosis

Pyloric stenosis is characterized by hypertrophied pyloric muscle, causing a narrowing of the pyloric sphincter. Pyloric stenosis occurs in 3 per 1000 live births, with a fourfold increase in males compared with females (Hunter and Liacourus, 2011b). It tends to be familial and is seen more commonly in Caucasian first-born males.

Clinical Findings

History.

- Regurgitation and non-projectile vomiting during the first few weeks of life
- Projectile vomiting beginning at 2 to 3 weeks old
- Insatiable appetite with weight loss, dehydration, and constipation
- An association of pyloric stenosis with the administration of erythromycin in the first 2 weeks of life has been demonstrated

Physical Examination.

- Weight loss
- Nonbilious vomitus that can contain blood
- A distinct "olive" mass that is often palpated in the epigastrium to the right of midline
- Reverse peristalsis visualized across the abdomen

Diagnostic Studies. Ultrasound, with measurement of the pyloric muscle thickness, is used in most centers. An upper gastrointestinal series demonstrates a "string sign," indicating a fine, elongated pyloric canal may be required if ultrasound is unavailable or inconclusive.

Management and Prognosis

Surgical intervention (pyloromyotomy) is indicated after correction of fluid and electrolyte imbalance. Vomiting can continue for a few days after surgery, although it is not as significant as it was preoperatively; feedings should be introduced gradually. The prognosis is excellent.

Hirschsprung Disease (Congenital Aganglionic Megacolon)

Hirschsprung disease is an absence of ganglion cells in the bowel wall, most often in the rectosigmoid region, resulting in a portion of the colon having no motility. This disorder occurs in 1 in 5000 births. It is the most common cause of neonatal obstruction of the colon and accounts for approximately 33% of all neonatal obstructions. The disease is familial, affects males four times more commonly than females, and is common in children with trisomy 21. Additional anomalies are sometimes present (Hunter and Liacourus, 2011b).

Clinical Findings

- Failure to pass meconium within the first 48 hours of life
- Failure to thrive, poor feeding
- Chronic constipation, vomiting, abdominal obstruction
- Diarrhea, explosive bowel movements, or flatus
- Down syndrome

Diagnostic Studies. Radiographs indicate dilated loops of bowel (Fig. 39-16). A biopsy determines the absence of ganglion cells.

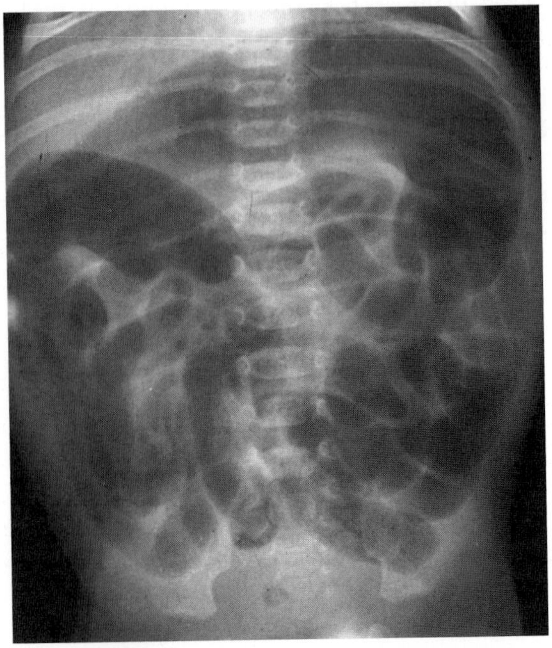

• **Figure 39-16** Dramatic dilation of bowel consistent with Hirschsprung disease. (Photo courtesy of Lawrence H. Robinson, professor of Radiology and Pediatrics, University of Texas Medical School, Houston, TX.)

Differential Diagnosis

The differential diagnosis includes acquired functional megacolon, colonic inertia, chronic idiopathic constipation, obstipation, small left colon syndrome, meconium plug syndrome, and ileal atresia with microcolon.

Management

Surgical resection of the affected bowel is indicated, with or without a colostomy.

Imperforate Anus

Imperforate anus is the lack of a rectal opening. This condition occurs in about 1 in 4000 births, about half associated with another anomaly (often the VACTERL syndrome consisting of **V**ertebral dysgenesis, **A**nal atresia [imperforate anus], **C**ardiac anomalies, **T**racheo**E**sophageal fistula, **R**enal anomalies, and **L**imb anomalies). Congenital heart disease, esophageal atresia, intestinal atresia, annular pancreas, intestinal malrotation or duplication, bilateral absence of the musculus rectus abdominis, trisomy 21, finger and hand anomalies, omphalocele, bladder exstrophy, and exstrophy of the ileocecal area are associated conditions (Stafford and Klein, 2011).

Clinical Findings

The history includes lack of passage of meconium. Findings include no obvious opening in the rectal area, although in girls stool passage may occur through a rectovaginal fistula. Endoscopic examination and ultrasound identify the degree of malformation.

Management

Immediate surgical repair with or without performing a colostomy is indicated. Long-term management related to bowel functioning may be needed because some children will have trouble with bowel emptying or incontinence.

Omphalocele and Gastroschisis

An omphalocele is a protrusion of the sac of intestines into the base of the umbilical cord. The intestines are covered by the peritoneum without overlying skin. Occurrence is 1 in 5000 to 10,000 births. Gastroschisis is similar in appearance with intestinal contents protruding through the abdomen with no protective peritoneal covering. Gastroschisis occurs in about 1 in 10,000 to 20,000 live births when there is failure to close the lateral ventral folds of the developing abdominal wall. With omphalocele, serious associated conditions occur in 50% of newborns including chromosomal abnormalities (trisomy 13 and 18), congenital diaphragmatic hernia, and a variety of cardiac problems. Concomitant hypoglycemia and macroglossia suggest Beckwith syndrome. Associated congenital anomalies are rare with gastroschisis (Carlo, 2011d).

Clinical Findings

Examination reveals a saclike protrusion covered by the peritoneum without overlying skin at the midabdomen.

Management and Complications

Maintain body temperature. Apply protective gauze and wrap abdomen with cellophane to prevent heat and fluid loss. When the infant is stable, surgical repair is indicated. Ileus is a common complication.

Necrotizing Enterocolitis

Necrotizing enterocolitis (NEC) is characterized by varying degrees of mucosal or transmural necrosis of the intestine. The usual onset is in the first 2 weeks of life, but it can be later in very low birth weight infants. The cause is unknown, but the condition is much less common in infants who are breastfed and have minimal feeds before bolus feeds are initiated. Infants that have immature colons that have become necrosed from trauma or injury are at especially high risk of developing this condition. NEC occurs in 3% to 5% of neonates in the neonatal intensive care unit (NICU), with the vast majority (90% to 93%) of these cases occurring in premature infants, especially those between 500 and 750 g (Sneedharan and Liacouras, 2011).

Clinical Findings

History.

- Prematurity, SGA, asphyxia, polycythemia
- Maternal hemorrhage, preeclampsia, cocaine exposure in utero
- Exchange transfusions, umbilical catheters

Physical Examination.

- Abdominal distention, vomiting, bloody stools (25%)
- Apnea, lethargy
- Evidence of disseminated intravascular coagulation (DIC), rapid progression of shock

Diagnostic Studies.

- Sepsis workup should be done.
- An abdominal radiograph shows pneumatosis intestinalis, a specific air pattern.

Differential Diagnosis

The differential diagnosis includes sepsis, intestinal obstruction, volvulus, Hirschsprung disease, anal fissures, and neonatal appendicitis.

Management, Complications, and Prognosis

- Prescribe systemic antibiotics following sepsis workup.
- Stop feedings, initiate gastric suctioning, maintain electrolyte balance, give oxygen as needed, and initiate surgical consultation.
- Obtain serial abdominal radiographs to follow course of disease.
- Delay oral feedings in very low birth weight infants for at least 1 week after definitive diagnosis; when feedings are begun, they typically are continuous slow drip before advancing to bolus.

The mortality rate is 10% to 50%, causing 1000 deaths per year. Ileus and perforation are early complications. Sequelae to NEC include feeding intolerance, stricture formation, and short-bowel syndrome, especially after intestinal resection (Sneedharan and Liacouras, 2011).

Meconium Ileus

Meconium ileus is an impaction of the bowel with meconium, causing intestinal obstruction. Meconium ileus is associated with cystic fibrosis and maternal polyhydramnios. About 80% to 90% of patients with meconium ileus have cystic fibrosis; about 10% to 20% of patients with cystic fibrosis have meconium ileus. Infants with meconium ileus may have associated intestinal disorders, including atresia, stenosis, volvulus, or perforations, and symptoms suggestive of cystic fibrosis (Sneedharan and Liacouras, 2011).

Clinical Findings

- History of failure to pass meconium within 48 hours of life.
- Clinical findings of abdominal distention and persistent vomiting.

Diagnostic Studies. A radiograph shows bowel loops of varying width, often with a grainy appearance at points of heaviest meconium concentration.

Management and Prognosis

Treatment is individualized; high enemas (with water-soluble contrast material) or laparotomy can be used. The survival rate is good. Identification of any underlying disorders should be undertaken, and referral to a gastrointestinal specialist may be necessary.

Diaphragmatic Hernia

In diaphragmatic hernia, abdominal contents herniate into the thoracic cavity. A diaphragmatic hernia is caused by failure of the pleuroperitoneal canal to close completely during embryologic development. It occurs on the left side 80% to 90% of the time with a frequency of about 1 in 2000 to 5000 live births; the condition is more common in females (Maheshwari and Carlo, 2011).

Clinical Findings

History. After birth, immediate respiratory failure occurs secondary to pulmonary hypertension or pulmonary hypoplasia. The degree of respiratory distress is related to the amount of functional lung capacity. Any newborn with respiratory distress should be evaluated for diaphragmatic hernia.

Physical Examination.

- Respiratory distress with tachypnea, cyanosis, absence of breath sounds
- Scaphoid abdomen, bowel sounds heard in the chest (rare)
- Heart tones best heard in the contralateral chest

Diagnostic Studies. A chest radiograph shows fluid and air-filled loops of intestine in the chest. The mediastinum is displaced toward the unaffected side, usually to the right.

Management and Prognosis

- As soon as the diagnosis is suspected, the infant should be positioned with the head and chest higher than the abdomen.
- Intensive respiratory support, which often includes ECMO
- Surgery, with intensive respiratory and metabolic support

The mortality rate is about 30%, depending on the degree of lung hypoplasia (Maheshwari and Carlo, 2011).

Hydrocele and Inguinal Hernia

See Chapter 35.

Umbilical Hernia

Umbilical hernia is a weakness or imperfect closure of the umbilical ring.

Clinical Findings

Findings include a soft swelling in the umbilical area that can be reduced, often associated with diastasis recti.

Management, Prognosis, and Education

Surgery is not required unless the hernia persists beyond about 5 years of age, strangulates, becomes nonreducible, or dramatically enlarges in size. Most umbilical hernias resolve spontaneously by 1 year old, but some can take up to 4 to 5 years to resolve. Lesions with fascial defects greater than 1.5 cm in diameter have a lower rate of spontaneous closure. Incarceration is extremely rare. Counsel parents to avoid taping coins or placing bellybands over the umbilicus, because these efforts do not help and can contribute to infection.

Renal Conditions

Acute Renal Failure

The newborn normally produces 1 to 3 mL/kg/hr of urine and urinates within the first 48 hours of life—most within the first 24 hours of life. A stressed neonate may develop decreased renal function. Urine output less than 0.5 mL/kg/hr can indicate acute renal failure and puts the infant at risk for disrupted body fluid homeostasis. Multiple causes of renal failure can be identified, including stress during the prenatal period, dehydration, sepsis, anoxia, shock, administration of nephrotoxic drugs, renal dysgenesis, obstructive uropathy, congenital heart disease, hemorrhage, and renal vein thrombosis.

Clinical Findings

- Neonatal history of decreased or no urinary output; maternal oligohydramnios
- Pallor, edema, lethargy, vomiting, seizures, coma
- High or low blood pressure
- Pulmonary edema, congestive heart failure, or arrhythmias
- Abdominal mass, myelomeningocele, or prune-belly syndrome

Diagnostic Studies. Order the following, as indicated:

- Bladder tap or catheterization to confirm adequacy of urinary output
- Urinalysis to identify hematuria or pyuria
- Urine osmolarity, sodium, and potassium values to measure kidney filtration
- Serum blood urea nitrogen, creatinine, sodium, and potassium values to measure kidney filtration (although in the first days of life these values may be more reflective of maternal renal function)
- Complete blood count (CBC) including differential and platelets for evidence of thrombocytopenia, sepsis, or renal vein thrombosis

Management and Prognosis

- Replace fluid loss (approximately 30 mL/kg every 24 hours), then restrict fluid and diet.
- Maintain strict intake, output, and fluid and electrolyte balance.
- Monitor blood pressure.
- Dialysis is sometimes indicated.
- The prognosis depends on the cause and the degree of renal failure.

Hydronephrosis

Hydronephrosis is a significant dilation of one or both kidneys possibly caused by an obstruction of the uretero-pelvic junction, posterior urethral valves, ectopic ureterocele, prune-belly syndrome, or ureteral or ureterovesical obstructions. Obstructive uropathy is slightly more common in males.

Clinical Findings

- Findings on prenatal ultrasonogram
- Asymptomatic in early stages
- Decreased urinary output or abdominal mass

Management and Prognosis

Surgical repair may be necessary depending on the cause of the hydronephrosis and if spontaneous resolution does not occur by 6 to 12 months old. The longer the obstruction lasts, the less likely renal function will return to normal.

Cystic Kidney Disease

The presence of multiple cysts of various sizes and shapes in the kidney can be either an autosomal dominant or autosomal recessive disease. The autosomal dominant form usually appears in the fourth or fifth decade of life and can be associated with hepatic cysts or cerebral aneurysms. In the autosomal recessive form, which also usually has hepatic cysts, the infant has abdominal masses at birth. The adult form (autosomal dominant) occurs in 1 per 500 to 1000 individuals; the juvenile form (autosomal recessive) occurs in 1 per 10,000 to 40,000 live births (Suchy, 2011). A renal ultrasonogram is done to document the disorder.

Clinical Findings

- Maternal oligohydramnios in the juvenile form
- Abdominal lobular mass
- Hematuria
- Hypertension

Differential Diagnosis

Multicystic dysplastic kidney, hydronephrosis, von Hippel-Lindau disease, tuberous sclerosis, Wilms tumor, and renal vein thrombosis are included in the differential diagnosis.

Management and Prognosis

Monitor kidney function, check with renal ultrasound for enlargement of cysts, and observe for signs and symptoms of infection. Hypertension may be difficult to control. Nephrectomy may be necessary if no regression in cyst size is seen or a significant complication develops. Dialysis or transplantation is sometimes considered for those infants with profound renal failure. With severe involvement, the neonate is at risk for death from pulmonary or renal insufficiency.

Renal Artery or Vein Thrombosis

Injury to the kidney occurs when there is decreased blood flow to the kidney due to thrombus formation in the vessel.

Clinical Findings

In the newborn, this condition is often associated with asphyxia, dehydration, shock, and sepsis. Maternal diabetes is a rare cause. Sudden onset of gross hematuria may be noted. Findings include a firm flank mass. Ultrasonography shows marked enlargement of the kidney. The hematocrit is low. The urine contains protein and often blood.

Differential Diagnosis

Other causes of hematuria (such as, hydronephrosis, cystic disease, Wilms tumor, hemolytic-uremic syndrome, and renal abscess) are included in the differential diagnosis.

Management

- Maintain fluid and electrolyte balance.
- Monitor blood pressure.
- Prophylactic anticoagulation therapy occasionally is given to prevent thrombosis in the contralateral kidney.
- Nephrectomy is not necessary unless chronic infection or uncontrollable hypertension occurs.

Neuroblastoma

A neuroblastoma is a solid tumor of unknown cause that originates from neural crest tissue along the craniospinal axis. The majority of neuroblastomas develop in the abdomen, usually in the adrenal gland. About 500 new cases of neuroblastoma are diagnosed each year; it is the most commonly diagnosed neoplasm in neonates (Zage and Ater, 2011).

Clinical Findings
- An unexplained fever, mass, and symptoms related to the site of the tumor
- Ascites and/or firm, irregular, nontender mass in abdomen
- Pallor, hypotension, irritability
- Possible external tumors in newborn, such as skin lesions similar to those of congenital rubella syndrome

Diagnostic Studies. The following help to assess and stage the disease:
- CBC, basic chemistry panel
- Renal radiographs to detect calcifications
- Ultrasound, computed tomography (CT) or magnetic resonance imaging (MRI) of abdomen
- Radiograph or CT scan of chest
- Skeletal survey or bone scan
- Urine catecholamines, homovanillic acid (HVA) and vanillylmandelic acid (VMA)
- Bone marrow aspirate and biopsy

Differential Diagnosis
Wilms tumor, hydronephrosis, renal vein thrombosis, and lymphoma are included in the differential diagnosis.

Management and Prognosis
Although some neuroblastomas regress without therapy (usually only those in children younger than 1 year old), treatment generally involves surgical removal followed by radiation therapy or chemotherapy. The prognosis depends on the age of the patient and the stage of the tumor.

Renal Agenesis
Renal agenesis is failure of the kidney to form normally. Bilateral agenesis is incompatible with life, and occurs in 1 in 3000 births (Elder, 2011).

Clinical Findings
History. Maternal oligohydramnios is noted in bilateral agenesis. Unilateral renal agenesis usually is detected on prenatal ultrasound or when the child is evaluated for other congenital anomalies or for urinary tract infection.

Physical Examination.
- Single umbilical artery associated with unilateral agenesis
- Associated anomalies involving the gastrointestinal or urinary tract and skeleton, especially with Potter syndrome (bilateral agenesis)
- Low-set ears, senile appearance, broad nose, and receding chin consistent with Potter syndrome

Management and Prognosis
Monitor for proteinuria and hypertension. Infants with bilateral disease die within a few months of life.

Endocrine Conditions
Congenital Hypothyroidism and Congenital Adrenal Hyperplasia
See Chapter 26.

Metabolic Conditions
Hypoglycemia
In the term infant, serum glucose levels rarely fall below 35 mg/dL in the first 3 hours of life, below 40 mg/dL between 3 and 24 hours of life, or below 45 mg/dL thereafter. Infants at higher risk of developing hypoglycemia include SGA infants and those with diabetic mothers, asphyxia at birth, sepsis, erythroblastosis fetalis, glycogen storage disease, or galactosemia (Table 39-6).

Clinical Findings
- Evidence of sepsis or asphyxia
- Infant of a diabetic mother (IDA), SGA
- Lethargy, poor feeding, and regurgitation
- Apnea, jitteriness, pallor, sweating, cool extremities
- Seizures

Management and Prognosis
See the Management column in Table 39-6. Infants with symptomatic hypoglycemia, particularly low birth weight infants and infants of diabetic mothers, are at risk for poor intellectual development as compared with asymptomatic infants. Prognosis for normal intellectual function is guarded in infants with prolonged and severe hypoglycemia.

Infant of a Diabetic Mother
An infant born to a mother whose pregnancy is complicated by poorly controlled gestational or insulin-dependent diabetes mellitus is referred to as an *infant of a diabetic mother (IDM)*. Maternal hyperglycemia causes fetal hyperglycemia and fetal hyperinsulinemia, leading to increased hepatic glucose uptake and glycogen synthesis, accelerated lipogenesis, and augmented protein synthesis (Carlo, 2011c) (see Table 39-6).

Clinical Findings
- History of a mother with diabetes, especially those who are poorly controlled
- Large and plump neonate with large viscera
- Puffy facies, plethora
- Hyperexcitability during the first 3 days of life, although hypotonia, lethargy, and poor sucking also occur

Management, Complications, and Prevention
See Table 39-6. Cardiomegaly is common (30%), and heart failure occurs in 5% to 10% of infants. Congenital anomalies are increased threefold; cardiac malformations (15 times greater) and lumbosacral agenesis are most common (Carlo, 2011c). A predisposition to obesity in childhood can extend into adult life. Symptomatic neonatal hypoglycemia, which can occur upon cutting of the umbilical cord, increases the risk of impaired intellectual development. Strict management of blood glucose levels in mothers with diabetes decreases the risk of severe problems in the infant.

TABLE 39-6 Identification and Management of Hypoglycemia, Infant of Diabetic Mother, and Polycythemia in the Newborn

Condition	Clinical Finding	Workup	Management
Hypoglycemia	Blood glucose <30 mg/dL; infant with history of SGA; poorly controlled diabetic mother (IDM); at risk for sepsis, asphyxia, erythroblastosis fetalis, lethargy, poor feeding, regurgitation, apnea, jitteriness, pallor, sweating, cool extremities, and seizures	Serum glucose—measure within 1 hour of birth, every 2 hours until 6 to 8 hours of life, then every 4 to 6 hours until 24 hours of life	Give normoglycemic high-risk infants oral or gavage feedings with breast milk or formula at 1 to 3 hours of life and continue every 2 to 3 hours for 24 to 48 hours; IV glucose at 8 mg/kg/min if serum glucose less than 30 to 35 mg/dL and oral feedings poorly tolerated.
Infant of diabetic mother (IDM)	IDM: Large, plump infant with large viscera; puffy facies; plethora; hyperactivity first 3 days; ± hypotonicity, lethargy, poor suck; ± cardiomegaly and murmur	Intensive observation and care Serum glucose—measure within 1 hour of birth, then frequently for the next 6 to 8 hours, especially for macrosomia or growth restriction	If clinically well and normoglycemic, initially give oral or gavage feedings with infant formula or breast milk started within 2 to 3 hours old and continued at 3-hour intervals. If infant is unable to tolerate oral feeding, discontinue feeding and give 10% glucose by peripheral IV infusion at a rate of 4 to 8 mg/kg/min with the appropriate dose for each patient individually adjusted. Treat hypoglycemia, even in asymptomatic infants, with IV infusions of glucose.
Polycythemia	Cyanosis, tachypnea, respiratory distress; hyperbilirubinemia; infant with history of diabetic mother; IUGR, postmaturity, SGA exposed to chronic hypoxia; recipient of twin-twin transfusion; delayed clamping of umbilical cord; plethora; and feeding disturbance	Hematocrit ≥65%	Phlebotomy and replacement with saline or albumin or partial exchange transfusion to reduce hematocrit to 50%

From Engorn B, Flerlage J: *The Harriet Lane handbook*, ed 20, Philadelphia, 2015, Elsevier.
IUGR, Intrauterine growth restriction; *IV,* intravenous; *SGA,* small for gestational age.

Orthopedic Conditions

Fractured Clavicle and Brachial Palsy

See Chapter 38.

Polydactyly and Syndactyly

Polydactyly is a condition that varies from a skin tag to a fully formed finger or toe with a nail; they most commonly extend from the postaxial side. Polydactyly occurs in 2 per 1000 births, more commonly in the African American population (Hosalkar et al, 2011). In contrast, syndactyly can be identified by finding fingers or toes fused by skin and sometimes bone. Syndactyly can be seen as part of a variety of syndromes.

Clinical Findings

A positive family history is found in 30% of cases (Carrigan, 2011; Hosalkar et al, 2011). In polydactyly, a floppy digit is seen on the foot or hand. It varies in degree of formation. Syndactyly is webbing of two digits, partially or to the tip of the digit.

Management

For polydactyly, surgical removal of the floppy extra digit is indicated. If the digit is stabilized by bone, surgical removal is deferred until the patient is older, when function can be assessed. Surgical separation of syndactyly is recommended until the child is at least 2 to 3 years old. Close physical examination for other congenital anomalies is undertaken.

Central Nervous System Conditions

Congenital Hydrocephalus

Congenital hydrocephalus is an overaccumulation of cerebrospinal fluid (CSF) in the brain's ventricles at birth, occurring in 1 of 1000 live births (Venkataramana and Mukundan, 2011). Malformations, infections, intraventricular hemorrhage (IVH), and disorders in brain development can lead to congenital hydrocephalus. The incidence varies depending on which of these conditions is causative. Cranial ultrasonography shows dilated ventricles. Often an MRI is obtained to further define anatomy.

Clinical Findings

- Head circumference enlarging or rapidly increasing in size
- Cranial sutures separated by large, tense fontanelles

Management

Medications that decrease CSF production (e.g., acetazolamide), a ventriculoperitoneal shunt, or both are used. Referral to a pediatric neurosurgeon should be prompt.

Intraventricular Hemorrhage

IVH occurs within the ventricles of the brain, usually within the first 72 hours of life. Risk factors include prematurity, RDS, hypoxic-ischemic or hypotensive injury, increased or decreased cerebral blood flow, hypertension, hypervolemia, and reduced vascular integrity. The incidence of IVH decreases with increasing gestational age. Infants weighing less than 1000 g are especially prone to severe IVH (Carlo, 2011a).

Clinical Findings

- Risk factors include SGA, prematurity, and others mentioned earlier
- Diminished or absent Moro reflex, apnea
- Poor muscle tone, lethargy, somnolence
- Periods of pallor or cyanosis
- Failure to suck well
- High-pitched, shrill cry; seizures
- Bulging fontanel or sudden increase in head circumference

Diagnostic Studies. Ultrasonography is used to classify IVH into grades I to IV based on the presence and quantity of blood in the ventricles or brain tissue. Screening cranial ultrasounds are routinely performed on all premature infants. Recommendations include screening infants between 1250 and 1500 g at 3 to 7 days and before discharge; on infants weighing between 1000 and 1250 g at 3 to 7 days, at 28 days, and before discharge; and on infants less than 1000 g at 3 to 7 days, at 10 to 14 days, at 28 days, and before discharge (Carlo, 2011a).

Management and Prognosis

Treatment may include the following:

- Glucocorticoid given antenatally to reduce the risk of severe RDS to prevent hypoxia
- Supportive management and minimal stimulation
- Indomethacin to reduce the severity of IVH
- Acetazolamide to decrease CSF production
- Repeated lumbar punctures
- Ventriculoperitoneal shunt or external ventriculostomy

Outcome is related to white matter involvement, with grade IV lesions being associated with the most adverse outcome.

Hypoxic-Ischemic Insults

Hypoxic-ischemic insult in the newborn is divided into three stages of injury (stages I, II, and III, or mild, moderate, and severe) (Table 39-7). Brain damage results from fetal hypoxia or ischemia over an extended period. The initial hypoxic or ischemic insult is followed by metabolic and respiratory acidosis. Compensatory mechanisms, such as shunting blood through the ductus to maintain perfusion of the brain, heart, adrenals, kidneys, liver, and intestines, ultimately fail if the insult is severe enough. Depending on the organ(s) most damaged, a variety of signs and symptoms can be seen; 15% to 20% of infants with hypoxic-ischemic encephalopathy die in the neonatal period, and up to 30% develop permanent neurodevelopmental disabilities. Causes of the initial hypoxic or ischemic insult include abruptio placentae, hemorrhage, cord compression, mechanical injury, severe maternal hypertension or diabetes, and inadequate resuscitation of the infant (Carlo, 2011a).

Clinical Findings

Infants can have apnea, pallor, cyanosis, and bradycardia unresponsiveness to stimulation.

Seizure activity can be a consequence of a hypoxic-ischemic event.

Management and Prognosis

The prognosis depends on the effectiveness of managing the underlying symptoms. Severe complications (hypoxia, hypoglycemia, shock) and encephalopathy characterized by flaccid coma, apnea, and seizures are associated with a poor prognosis (Carlo, 2011a). An infant who remains neurologically abnormal after the initial recovery phase (2 weeks) likely has suffered permanent neurologic impairment. A low Apgar score at 20 minutes, absence of spontaneous respirations, and persistence of abnormal neurologic signs at 2 weeks of age predict death or severe cognitive and motor deficits; Apgar scores done at 1 and 5 minutes are far less predictive of outcome (AAP, 2006).

Myelomeningocele

A myelomeningocele is the result of failure to close the posterior neural tube and the vertebral column. This is the most severe form of neural tube defect occurring in 1 per 4000 live births (Kinsman and Johnston, 2011). Genetic and environmental factors are believed to play a causative role (see Chapter 28 for more information).

Clinical Findings

- History of poor prenatal intake of folic acid and exposure to hyperthermia or valproic acid

TABLE 39-7 Hypoxic-Ischemic Encephalopathy in Term Infants

Signs	Stage 1	Stage 2	Stage 3
Level of consciousness	Hyperalert	Lethargic	Stuporous, coma
Muscle tone	Normal	Hypotonic	Flaccid
Posture	Normal	Flexion	Decerebrate
Tendon reflexes/clonus	Hyperactive	Hyperactive	Absent
Myoclonus	Present	Present	Absent
Moro reflex	Strong	Weak	Absent
Pupils	Mydriasis	Miosis	Unequal, poor light reflex
Seizures	None	Common	Decerebration
Electroencephalogram	Normal	Low-voltage changing to seizure activity	Burst suppression to isoelectric
Duration	<24 hours if progresses, otherwise may remain normal	24 hours to 24 days	Days to weeks
Outcome	Good	Variable	Death, severe deficits

Adapted from Sarnat H, Sarnat M: Neonatal encephalopathy following fetal distress: a clinical and electroencephalopathic study, *Arch Neurol* 33:696, 1976; cited in Kliegman RM, Stanton BF, St Geme JW, et al, editors: *Nelson textbook of pediatrics*, ed 19, Philadelphia, 2011, Saunders/Elsevier.

- Saclike cyst containing meninges and spinal fluid covered by thin layer of partially epithelialized skin; 75% found in the lumbosacral area
- Flaccid paralysis of lower extremities
- Absence of deep tendon reflexes
- Lack of response in lower extremities to touch and pain
- Constant urinary dribbling

Management, Prognosis, and Prevention

Surgical repair and multidisciplinary supportive management are indicated. The mortality rate is 10% to 15% in aggressively treated children with most deaths occurring before 4 years old. At least 70% have normal intelligence, but seizure disorders, hydrocephalus, learning disabilities, and neurogenic bowel and bladder are more common than in the general population (Kinsman and Johnston, 2011). Prenatal folic acid supplementation (400 mcg/day) with a daily multivitamin is helpful in preventing neural tube defects and should be taken by all females of childbearing age. Prenatal vitamins have at least 400 mcg of folic acid/vitamin; however, additional folic acid supplementation (4000 mcg) is recommended for those women who have had a child with a neural tube defect (AAP, 2014; CDC, 2014a).

Hematologic Conditions

Polycythemia

Polycythemia is characterized by a central hematocrit of 65% or higher. Polycythemia can occur in a variety of conditions, including IDM, cyanotic congenital heart disease, and infants with growth retardation who were exposed to chronic fetal hypoxia that stimulated erythropoietin production and increased red blood cell production. Polycythemia occurs in 1% to 2% of term AGA births, depending on the etiology (see Table 39-6).

Clinical Findings

- Diabetic mother and hypoglycemia in the infant as a result, feeding disturbances
- Recipient of a twin-twin transfusion, delayed clamping of umbilical cord although infants with polycythemia may be asymptomatic with hyperbilirubinemia
- Cyanosis (persistent fetal circulation), tachypnea, respiratory distress
- Postmature infant, SGA infant

Management and Prognosis

See Table 39-6. Long-term problems may include speech deficits, abnormal fine motor control, reduced intelligence quotient (IQ), and other neurologic abnormalities as a result of the decreased brain tissue perfusion both with and without intervention.

Hemorrhagic Disease in the Newborn

Severe transient deficiencies of vitamin K–dependent clotting factors lead to bleeding. Hemorrhagic disease is caused by a lack of free vitamin K in the mother and absence of bacterial intestinal flora normally responsible for synthesis of vitamin K in the infant. Vitamin K–dependent clotting factors (factors II, VII, IX, and X) are normal at birth, but decrease within 2 to 3 days, increasing the incidence of early-onset bleeding in all newborns. Breast milk is a poor source of vitamin K; late-onset bleeding (occurring 1 to 3 months after birth) is rare, but may be seen in exclusively breastfed infants. A particularly severe form of deficiency of vitamin K–dependent coagulation factors occurring in the first day of life has been reported in women receiving the anticonvulsants phenytoin and/or phenobarbital.

Clinical Findings

- Anticonvulsant (phenytoin or phenobarbital) use by the mother
- Prematurity
- Exclusive breastfeeding without vitamin K supplementation
- Failure to administer parenteral vitamin K at birth
- Neonatal hepatitis or biliary atresia
- Gastrointestinal, nasal, subgaleal, or intracranial bleeding or bleeding at the site of an injection or circumcision

Diagnostic Studies. Prothrombin time, blood coagulation time, and partial thromboplastin time are prolonged.

Differential Diagnosis

This disorder may be the result of DIC or congenital bleeding disorders unrelated to vitamin K.

Management, Prevention, and Prognosis

- In the child with evidence of hemorrhagic disease, IV infusion of 1 to 5 mg of vitamin K is needed. Improvement of coagulation defects and cessation of bleeding should occur within a few hours.
- If a newborn is delivered at home, confirm vitamin K was given.
- Prevention of early- and late-onset bleeding is achieved by routinely giving 1 mg of natural oil-soluble vitamin K intramuscularly within 1 hour of birth.
- Prognosis of a child sustaining a hemorrhagic event depends on the site and extent of bleeding.

Anemia

Anemia is characterized by less than the normal range of hemoglobin for birth weight and postnatal age. Anemia at birth occurs secondary to acute blood loss before or during delivery. Acute blood loss after delivery can be external (gastrointestinal, circumcision site, umbilical stump), internal (fracture site, cephalhematoma, pulmonary hemorrhage, injured internal organ), or secondary to hemolysis or congenital aplastic or hypoplastic anemia.

Clinical Findings

- Twin-twin transfusion
- Unexpected tearing or delayed clamping of umbilical cord resulting in neonatal blood loss
- Internal hemorrhage (fracture, cephalhematoma, internal organ trauma)
- Umbilical stump or circumcision bleeding
- Pallor, congestive heart failure, and shock possible

Management and Prognosis

Treatment depends on the cause and symptoms. An asymptomatic full-term infant with a hemoglobin level of 10 g/dL can be observed, whereas a symptomatic neonate born after abruptio placentae or with severe hemolytic disease of the newborn warrants transfusion. Treatment with blood should be balanced by concern about transfusion-acquired infection with cytomegalovirus (CMV), HIV, and hepatitis B and C viruses. Prognosis depends on the cause and severity of the anemia.

Blood in Vomitus or Stool

Bright red or dark red blood in the vomitus or stool can be seen without clinical evidence of blood loss. This problem often is caused by ingestion of maternal blood during delivery.

Clinical Findings

Bright red or dark red blood is seen in vomitus or stool.

Diagnostic Studies. Blood of maternal origin can be differentiated from infant blood by testing for fetal hemoglobin using the Apt test.

Differential Diagnosis

The differential diagnosis includes infant gastrointestinal bleeding caused by trauma, duplication of bowel, intussusception, volvulus, hemangioma or telangiectasia of bowel, rectal prolapse, vitamin K deficiency, or anal fissure.

Management

No treatment is necessary if blood is of maternal origin, although breakdown of maternal blood may exaggerate neonatal jaundice.

Jaundice

Jaundice, a clinically apparent accumulation of bilirubin in the skin, causes a yellowish orange or sometimes green hue to the skin. Jaundice becomes apparent when serum bilirubin levels exceed 5 to 7 mg/dL and usually advances in a pattern from the infant's head to the toes (Table 39-8). Physiologic jaundice is the most common type of jaundice in the newborn period with the infant showing no signs of illness. Classic physiologic jaundice is characterized by a rise in bilirubin from approximately 1.5 mg/dL in cord blood to 5 to 6 mg/dL on the third day of life, declining to a normal adult level (less than 1.3 to 1.5 mg/dL) by 10 to 12 days in Caucasian and African American infants. Asian infants reach 8 to 12 mg/dL on day 4 to 5 and decline more slowly; 2% of Asian newborns and 1% of Caucasians and African Americans have serum bilirubin greater than 20 mg/dL in the first week of life. Breast milk jaundice is often included in the category of physiologic jaundice and can be divided into early-onset and late-onset types. Early-onset breast milk jaundice develops within 2 to 4 days of birth and is believed to occur as a result of infrequent breastfeeding and insufficient intake leading to decreased intestinal motility. Late-onset breast milk jaundice develops 4 to 7 days after birth, peaks at 10 to 15 days of life, and frequently persists. See Chapter 11 on breastfeeding for more information.

Nonphysiologic (pathologic) jaundice appears at less than 24 hours of age and may last longer than 8 days. The

TABLE 39-8 Diagnostic Features of the Various Types of Neonatal Jaundice

Diagnosis	Nature of Van Den Bergh Reaction	Jaundice		Peak Bilirubin Concentration		Bilirubin Rate of Accumulation (mg/dL/day)	Remarks
		Appears	Disappears	mg/dL	Age (days)		
Physiologic jaundice							Usually relates to degree of maturity; infant shows no signs of illness
Full-term	Indirect	2 to 3 days	4 to 5 days	10 to 12	2 to 3	<5	
Premature	Indirect	3 to 4 days	7 to 9 days	15	6 to 8	<5	
Hyperbilirubinemia caused by metabolic factors							Metabolic factors: hypoxia, respiratory distress, lack of carbohydrates
Full-term	Indirect	2 to 3 days	Variable	>12	First week	<5	Hormonal influences: cretinism
Premature	Indirect	3 to 4 days	Variable	>15	First week	<5	Genetic factors: Crigler-Najjar syndrome, transient familial hyperbilirubinemia Drugs: Vitamin K, novobiocin
Hemolytic states and hematoma	Indirect	May appear in first 24 hours	Variable	Unlimited	Variable	Usually >5	Erythroblastosis: Rh or ABO incompatibility Congenital hemolytic states: Spherocytic, nonspherocytic Infantile pyknocytosis Drugs: Vitamin K; enclosed hemorrhage—hematoma
Mixed hemolytic and hepatotoxic factors	Indirect and direct	May appear in first 24 hours	Variable	Unlimited	Variable	Usually >5	Infection: Bacterial sepsis, pyelonephritis, hepatitis, toxoplasmosis, cytomegalic inclusion disease, rubella Drugs: Vitamin K
Hepatocellular damage	Indirect and direct	Usually 2 to 3 days	Variable	Unlimited	Variable	Variable; can be >5	Biliary atresia; galactosemia; hepatitis, infection

From Brown AK: Diagnostic features of the various types of neonatal jaundice, *Pediatr Clin North Am* 9:589, 1962; as cited in Kliegman RM, Stanton BF, St Geme JW, et al, editors: *Nelson textbook of pediatrics*, ed 19, Philadelphia, 2011, Saunders/Elsevier.

rate of increase in total bilirubin is rapid at more than 0.5 mg/dL/hr. Total bilirubin levels are frequently more than 12.5 mg/dL before 48 hours old, or the direct bilirubin exceeds 1.5 to 2 mg/dL. Kernicterus or bilirubin encephalopathy involves toxicity of the nervous system resulting from very high levels of bilirubin. The estimated minimal level of risk for kernicterus and thus considering exchange transfusion is probably at 25 to 30 mg/dL in healthy term infants (AAP, 2004).

Jaundice is observed during the first week of life in approximately 60% of term infants (Sneedharan and Liacouras, 2011). Causes include the following:

- Increased rate of hemolysis: ABO incompatibility, Rh incompatibility, abnormal red blood cell shapes (spherocytosis, elliptocytosis, pyknocytosis, and stomatocytosis), red blood cell enzyme abnormalities (glucose-6-phosphate dehydrogenase deficiency, pyruvate kinase deficiency)
- Decreased rate of conjugation: Immaturity of bilirubin conjugation (physiologic jaundice), congenital familial nonhemolytic jaundice (inborn errors of metabolism affecting glucuronyl transferase system and bilirubin transport), breast milk jaundice
- Abnormalities of excretion or absorption: Sepsis, hepatitis (viral, parasitic, bacterial, toxic), metabolic abnormalities (galactosemia, glycogen storage disease, IDM, cystic fibrosis), biliary atresia, choledochal cyst, obstruction of ampulla of Vater (annular pancreas), drugs

Clinical Findings

The following are risk factors for the development of significant hyperbilirubinemia:

- Hemolytic disease, anemia
- Inborn errors of metabolism
- Early or severe jaundice
- Ethnic or geographic origin associated with hemolytic anemia
- Hepatobiliary disease
- Previous sibling required phototherapy
- ABO or Rh incompatibilities in previous pregnancies
- Sepsis risk for the infant, such as prolonged rupture of maternal membranes
- Macrosomic IDA

Physical Examination.

- Jaundice at birth or at any time during the neonatal period, depending on the underlying condition, with face affected first, followed by the shoulders, chest, and abdomen. Jaundice from deposition of indirect bilirubin in the skin tends to appear bright yellow or orange; jaundice of the obstructive type (direct bilirubin) appears greenish or muddy yellow, with the difference apparent only in severe jaundice.
- The accuracy of estimating an infant's true bilirubin level based on skin color alone is poor. However, a crude estimate of the level of jaundice can be based on the dermal zone in which the jaundice is noticed. This estimate should not be used to determine bilirubin levels or management, but it might help determine whether acquiring a total serum bilirubin (TSB) or a transcutaneous bilirubin (TcB) is warranted.
  - Head and neck—a mean bilirubin of 6 mg/dL
  - Trunk and umbilicus—a mean bilirubin of 9 mg/dL
  - Groin including the upper thighs—a mean bilirubin of 12 mg/dL
  - Knees and elbows (including the ankles and wrists) or to the feet and hands (including the palms and soles)—a mean bilirubin of 15 mg/dL
- Petechiae, bruising, hepatosplenomegaly, or signs of infection
- Lethargy, hypotonia, poor feeding, and loss of the Moro reflex are common initial signs of bilirubin toxicity to the brain (kernicterus). These symptoms are subtle and indistinguishable from those of sepsis, asphyxia, hypoglycemia, intracranial hemorrhage, and other acute illnesses in the neonate.
- Diminished tendon reflexes, respiratory distress, failure to suck, opisthotonos, bulging fontanelle, twitching of face or limbs, seizures, and a shrill, high-pitched cry are later signs of kernicterus.

Diagnostic Studies.

- TcB
- TSB level (indirect and direct) for infants who have a TcB more than 15, for darker skinned infants, or for infants under phototherapy
- If the provider suspects that the total bilirubin is significantly elevated for the age of the infant, additional blood can be drawn and held for further testing, eliminating a return visit, stick, and/or unnecessary expense if all of the tests are not later indicated. Tests that may be indicated include:
  - ABO, Rh, blood type, isoimmune antibodies of mother (should be available at prenatal and delivering hospital), Coombs test on infant (many times this is done at delivery and held in the hospital's laboratory)
  - Hemoglobin, hematocrit, reticulocyte count

Elevated indirect (unconjugated) serum bilirubin with a normal reticulocyte count and negative Coombs test indicates conditions such as physiologic jaundice, breast milk jaundice, or congenital familial nonhemolytic jaundice. Elevated indirect serum bilirubin with an increased reticulocyte count indicates increased hemolysis secondary to conditions, such as isoimmunization (positive Coombs test, such as caused by ABO or Rh incompatibility), abnormal red blood cell shape, or red blood cell enzyme abnormalities. Elevated indirect and direct serum bilirubin with a negative Coombs test and a normal reticulocyte count indicates hepatitis, metabolic abnormalities, biliary atresia, choledochal cyst (in the bile duct), gastrointestinal or pancreatic obstruction, sepsis, or drugs.

Pathologic jaundice requires a more in-depth workup for the cause. Risk factors include:

- Appearance of jaundice in first 24 hours of life
- Rise of bilirubin greater than 0.5 mg/dL/hr
- Conjugated bilirubin greater than 2 mg/dL

Management and Prevention

Prevention of severe hyperbilirubinemia and bilirubin encephalopathy in infants requires the promotion and support of successful breastfeeding, systematic assessment of the newborn for the risk of hyperbilirubinemia, early and focused follow-up based on the risk assessment, and treatment when indicated.

- Promote breastfeeding by advising mothers to put the baby to the breast 8 to 12 times per day for the first several days and discourage the use of routine supplementation of water or dextrose water.
- In the healthy full-term (greater than 35 weeks) infant, physical findings, bilirubin level according to age, and designation of risk are helpful in determining the course of treatment (Figs. 39-17, 39-18, and 39-19).
- Phototherapy is used to treat elevated indirect hyperbilirubinemia. Home phototherapy can be used for those infants without risk factors and with TSB levels 2 to

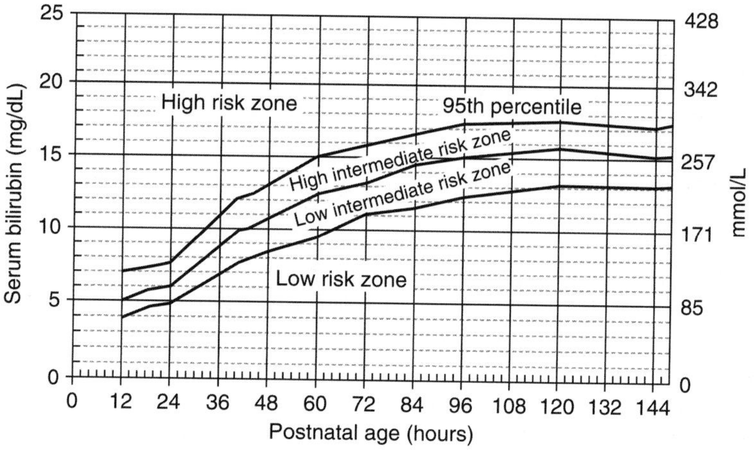

• **Figure 39-17** Nomogram for designation of risk in 2840 well newborns at 36 or more weeks' gestational age with birth weight of 2000 g or more or 35 or more weeks' gestational age and birth weight of 2500 g or more based on the hour-specific serum bilirubin values. (From the Academy of Pediatrics Subcommittee on Hyperbilirubinemia: Clinical practice guideline: management of hyperbilirubinemia in the newborn infant 35 or more weeks of gestation, *Pediatrics* 114:297–316, 2004.)

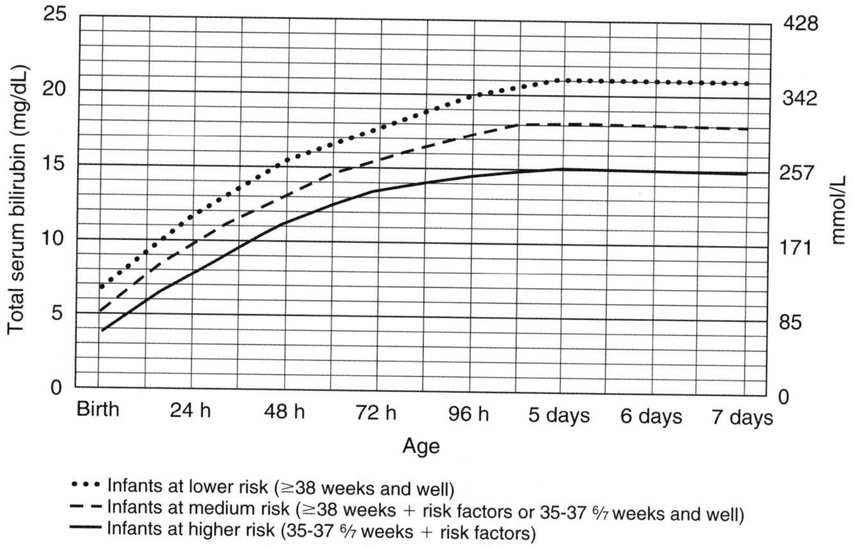

• **Figure 39-18** Guidelines for phototherapy in hospitalized infants of 35 or more weeks of gestation. (1) Use total bilirubin. Do not subtract direct-reacting or conjugated bilirubin. (2) The risk factors are isoimmune hemolytic disease, glucose-6-phosphate dehydrogenase (G6PD) deficiency, asphyxia, significant lethargy, temperature instability, sepsis, acidosis, or albumin <3 g/dL (if measured). (3) For well infants 35 to 37 6/7 weeks, total serum bilirubin (TSB) levels can be adjusted for intervention around the medium risk line. It is an option to intervene at lower TSB levels for infants closer to 35 weeks and at higher TSB levels for those closer to 37 6/7 weeks. (4) It is an option to provide conventional phototherapy in hospital or at home at TSB levels 2 to 3 mg/dL (35 to 50 mmol/L) below those shown but home phototherapy should not be used in any infant with risk factors. (From the Academy of Pediatrics Subcommittee on Hyperbilirubinemia: clinical practice guideline: management of hyperbilirubinemia in the newborn infant 35 or more weeks of gestation, *Pediatrics* 114:297–316, 2004.)

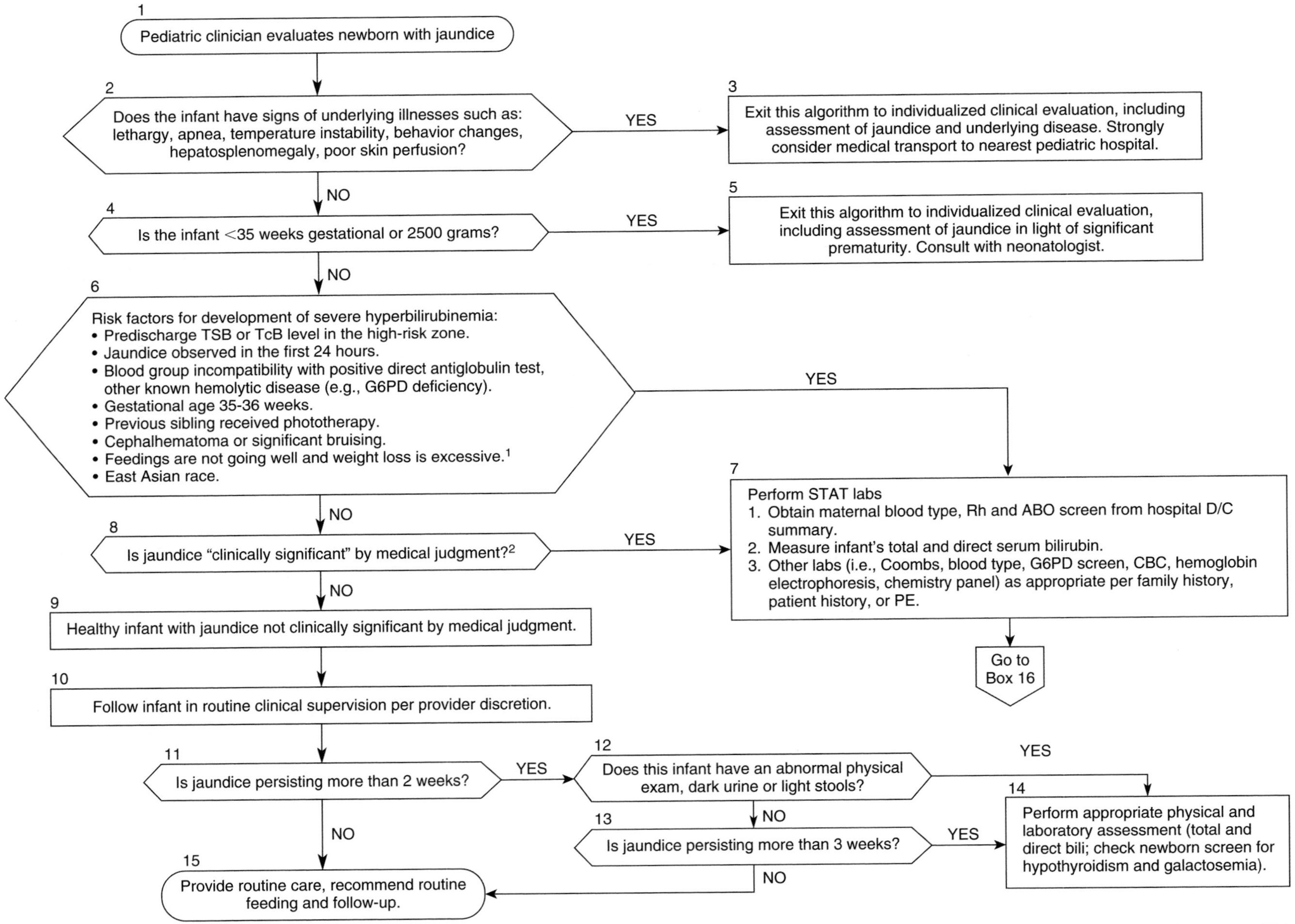
1
Pediatric clinician evaluates newborn with jaundice
2
Does the infant have signs of underlying illnesses such as: lethargy, apnea, temperature instability, behavior changes, hepatosplenomegaly, poor skin perfusion?
YES
3
Exit this algorithm to individualized clinical evaluation, including assessment of jaundice and underlying disease. Strongly consider medical transport to nearest pediatric hospital.
NO
4
Is the infant <35 weeks gestational or 2500 grams?
YES
5
Exit this algorithm to individualized clinical evaluation, including assessment of jaundice in light of significant prematurity. Consult with neonatologist.
NO
6
Risk factors for development of severe hyperbilirubinemia:
• Predischarge TSB or TcB level in the high-risk zone.
• Jaundice observed in the first 24 hours.
• Blood group incompatibility with positive direct antiglobulin test, other known hemolytic disease (e.g., G6PD deficiency).
• Gestational age 35-36 weeks.
• Previous sibling received phototherapy.
• Cephalhematoma or significant bruising.
• Feedings are not going well and weight loss is excessive.1
• East Asian race.
YES
7
Perform STAT labs
1. Obtain maternal blood type, Rh and ABO screen from hospital D/C summary.
2. Measure infant's total and direct serum bilirubin.
3. Other labs (i.e., Coombs, blood type, G6PD screen, CBC, hemoglobin electrophoresis, chemistry panel) as appropriate per family history, patient history, or PE.
Go to Box 16
NO
8
Is jaundice "clinically significant" by medical judgment?2
YES
NO
9
Healthy infant with jaundice not clinically significant by medical judgment.
10
Follow infant in routine clinical supervision per provider discretion.
11
Is jaundice persisting more than 2 weeks?
YES
12
Does this infant have an abnormal physical exam, dark urine or light stools?
YES
14
Perform appropriate physical and laboratory assessment (total and direct bili; check newborn screen for hypothyroidism and galactosemia).
NO
13
Is jaundice persisting more than 3 weeks?
YES
NO
NO
15
Provide routine care, recommend routine feeding and follow-up.

• **Figure 39-19** Algorithm for the management of neonatal hyperbilirubinemia in the outpatient setting. *CBC,* Complete blood count; *D/C,* discharge; *ED,* emergency department; *F/U,* follow-up; *G6PD,* glucose-6-phosphate dehydrogenase; *PE,* physical examination; *Rh,* rhesus; *T. bili.,* total bilirubin; *TcB,* transcutaneous bilirubin; *TSB,* total serum bilirubin. (Modified and used with permission of the Multnomah County Health Department, Primary Care Division, Portland, OR.)

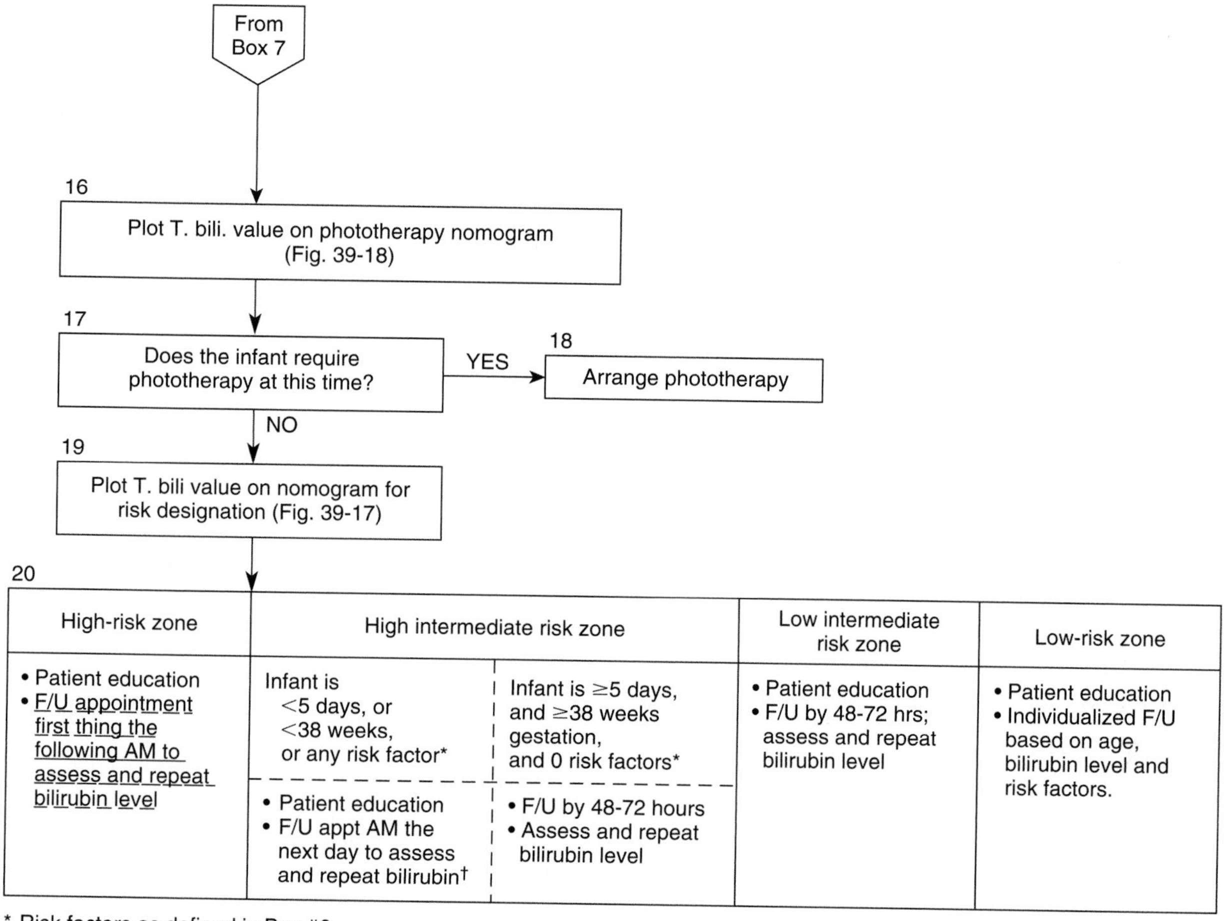

* Risk factors as defined in Box #6
† If infant's bilirubin levels have stabilized at the high intermediate risk zone or below, follow up can be slightly later than the above recommendations

[1] Weight loss of >10% of birth weight is excessive at 72-96 hrs, or >12% after 96 hrs. Breastfed babies usually reach their maximum weight loss on day three. To additionally assess adequacy of intake in breastfed infants consider normal 4-6 wet diapers/24 hours; 3-4 stools/day by day four. Change from meconium to yellow soft breast stool by day four.

[2] Severely jaundiced infants should be referred immediately to the ED for assessment in order to expedite medical intervention.

• Figure 39-19, cont'd

3 mg/dL less than those shown in Fig. 39-18. Phototherapy is contraindicated with elevated direct bilirubin. The infant should be dressed only in a diaper and should be wearing eye shields. Three types of phototherapy are used:
- Banks of overhead lights placed close to the infant requires eyepatch with removal at regular intervals, taking care to prevent corneal abrasions; monitoring of temperature; increased fluid intake in response to evaporative water losses; and avoidance of oral drugs because of decreased absorption
- Biliblanket (fiberoptic pad) allows ongoing interaction between mother and infant
- Bilibed

- If the breastfeeding infant requires phototherapy, breastfeeding should be continued. It is also an option in some situations to interrupt temporarily breastfeeding (have the mother pump to maintain her supply) and substitute formula for 24 hours. In breastfed infants receiving phototherapy, supplementation with expressed breast milk or milk-based formula is appropriate if the infant's intake is inadequate, weight loss is excessive (greater than 10% of birth weight), or the infant seems dehydrated.
- Rebound bilirubin testing (measurement of bilirubin after phototherapy is discontinued) is not required in full-term newborns with physiologic jaundice.
- Guidelines for exchange transfusion levels are available in the AAP practice parameter on the management of hyperbilirubinemia (AAP, 2004).

Infections of the Newborn

Three mechanisms for acquiring neonatal infections exist:
- Transplacental, when the mother acquires an organism that invades her bloodstream and passes through the placenta

- Vertical, when organisms in the vagina invade the amniotic fluid within the uterus
- Horizontal, when the newborn is exposed to environmental agents after birth

Syphilis is transplacentally acquired; herpes, gonorrhea, GBS, *Listeria, Escherichia coli,* and *Chlamydia trachomatis* are typically vertically acquired (Martin and Fanaroff, 2015). Staphylococcal infection is the most common horizontal infection. The most common means for horizontal transmission is unwashed hands.

Risk factors for sepsis (systemic infection) in the newborn include early rupture of amniotic membranes followed by preterm labor, prolonged rupture of membranes, maternal fever, maternal diagnosis of chorioamnionitis, maternal tachycardia, fetal tachycardia, and malodorous amniotic fluid. The neonate with sepsis can be asymptomatic or, due to delayed immune response to local infection, have nonspecific symptoms of infection, such as poor feeding or temperature instability (Martin and Fanaroff, 2015). Organisms quickly invade the systemic circulation, and significant deterioration occurs before it can be clinically recognized. Because of the serious nature of neonatal sepsis, a newborn with significant risk factors or a clinically unstable neonate without perinatal risk factors warrants investigation and initiation of appropriate antibiotics (Box 39-5).

• BOX 39-5 Neonatal Sepsis

History

"Not doing well"
Temperature instability (often hypothermia)
Jitteriness
Poor feeding, vomiting
Irritability or lethargy
Apnea or respiratory distress
Seizures

Physical Examination

Jaundice
Pallor
Petechiae or purpura
Rash
Hepatosplenomegaly
Poor tone and perfusion
Tachycardia or bradycardia
Tachypnea
Cyanosis, grunting, flaring, retractions

Laboratory Evaluation

Blood for CBC with differential, platelet count, and culture (evaluating for anemia; increase or decrease in WBC count with left shift; thrombocytopenia); serum ammonia for urea cycle defects
Urine for analysis and culture typically not done in the first 72 hours of life because of low yield
CSF often obtained for protein, glucose, cell count, and culture (evaluating for elevated protein and WBC count; depressed glucose)

Management

Combination broad-spectrum antibiotic coverage for gram-positive cocci, gram-negative bacilli, and *Listeria* is recommended. Consider adding coverage for herpes infection when suspected. *Listeria* is treated with ampicillin; *GBS* can be treated with the penicillins and the cephalosporins; gram-negative organisms are well covered by aminoglycosides and some cephalosporins.

CBC, Complete blood count; *CSF*, cerebrospinal fluid; *GBS*, group B streptococcus; *WBC*, white blood cell.

Toxoplasmosis

Toxoplasmosis is an infection caused by *Toxoplasma gondii,* an obligate intracellular protozoan. *T. gondii* infects most species of warm-blooded animals, particularly cats. Cats excrete oocysts in their stools; intermediate hosts include cattle, pigs, and sheep. Humans become infected by consumption of poorly cooked meat or by accidental ingestion of oocysts from soil or in contaminated food. Depending on the timing of the infection, 17% to 65% of untreated women who acquire toxoplasmosis during gestation transmit the parasite to their fetuses (McLeod, 2011).

Clinical Findings

- Prematurity and low Apgar scores
- Infants with congenital infection are asymptomatic at birth in 70% to 90% of cases (AAP, 2012)
- Jaundice, anemia, hepatosplenomegaly
- Chorioretinitis, microcephaly

Diagnostic Studies. CT of the brain shows calcifications or hydrocephalus. The CSF shows high protein, low glucose, and evidence of *T. gondii.* Serum immunoglobulin G (IgG), IgM, IgA, and IgE antibodies against toxoplasmosis are seen. The organism can be isolated by inoculation into mice or tissue culture of blood from the placenta, the umbilical cord, or the infant.

Differential Diagnosis

Sepsis, syphilis, and hemolytic disease are considered in the differential diagnosis.

Management, Prognosis, and Prevention

Pyrimethamine plus sulfadiazine (with folic acid supplementation) for up to 1 year is often recommended. Treatment usually eliminates the manifestations of toxoplasmosis, such as active chorioretinitis, meningitis, encephalitis, hepatitis, splenomegaly, and thrombocytopenia. However, infants with extensive involvement at birth often have mild to severe impairment of vision, hearing, cognitive function, and other neurologic functions. No protective vaccine is available. Pregnant women should be informed not to handle raw meat or contaminated cat litter, to wash fruits and vegetables before consumption, to cook meat and eggs well, and to drink pasteurized milk.

Congenital Rubella

Rubella is a ribonucleic acid (RNA) virus. Rubella is transmitted by person-to-person contact; the virus infects the placenta and is transmitted to the fetus. It occurs more frequently in the winter and spring.

Clinical Findings

History.

- Maternal infection before 16 weeks of gestation
- Negative rubella titers in mother at beginning of pregnancy
- As many as 50% of infected women are asymptomatic (AAP, 2012)

Physical Examination.

- May be asymptomatic in the newborn period
- Cataract or glaucoma and microphthalmia, hearing loss
- "Blueberry muffin" skin lesions, congenital heart disease
- Intellectual disability

Diagnostic Studies. The rubella virus can be isolated from nasopharyngeal secretions, conjunctiva, urine, stool, and CSF. Alternatively, measurement of serum immunoglobulins may be helpful.

Management and Prevention

No specific drug therapy is available. Monitoring and intervention for developmental, auditory, visual, and medical needs improve the quality of life for these children. Congenital rubella is now a rare occurrence because of widespread administration of an effective vaccine (AAP, 2012). All women of childbearing age should have rubella serology titers, and vaccine should be given to IgG-seronegative women who are not pregnant.

Cytomegalovirus

CMV, a member of the herpesvirus family, is transmitted via intimate and household contact with virus-containing secretions and blood products. When CMV is introduced into a household, it is likely that all members will acquire the infection. CMV is transmitted to the infant via the placenta. Infections are distributed worldwide, and most humans have become infected by the time they reach adulthood. CMV causes congenital infection in 1% to 2% of all live births in the United States. When pregnant women acquire the virus, a 30% to 40% transmission rate to the fetus is seen (AAP, 2012; Martin and Fanaroff, 2015).

Clinical Findings

- Maternal infection (although many women are asymptomatic)
- As many as 90% of infected newborns are asymptomatic
- SGA and/or intrauterine growth retardation
- Jaundice, hepatosplenomegaly
- Petechial rash, chorioretinitis
- Cerebral calcifications, microcephaly

Diagnostic Studies. CMV is isolated in cell cultures from urine, saliva, or other body fluids. Techniques for detection of viral deoxyribonucleic acid (DNA) by polymerase chain reaction (PCR) are available from selected reference laboratories. Proof of congenital infection requires obtaining specimens within 3 weeks of birth. Viral isolation or a strongly positive test for serum IgM anti-CMV antibody is considered diagnostic.

Management, Prognosis, and Prevention

Limited data in infants suggest that ganciclovir may be helpful in decreasing progression of hearing impairment; consultation with an expert is recommended (AAP, 2012). Monitor urine for CMV for 18 to 24 months. The outcome of symptomatic congenital CMV infection is poor; a 20% to 30% mortality rate and a 90% to 95% morbidity rate, characterized by psychomotor retardation, microcephaly, hearing loss, seizures, chorioretinitis, optic atrophy, intellectual disability, and learning disabilities, are seen. At greatest risk for acquiring the infection are susceptible pregnant women exposed to the urine and saliva of CMV-infected children who attend day care centers (AAP, 2012). Hand washing and simple hygienic measures should be reinforced in this population.

Group B Streptococcus

GBS, a gram-positive diplococcus, is the leading cause of sepsis in infants from birth to 3 months old, resulting in significant perinatal morbidity and mortality rates. Early-onset disease usually occurs at birth or within the first 24 hours of life; late-onset disease occurs during the second week of life.

The organism forms colonies in the maternal genitourinary and gastrointestinal tracts. Pregnant women are usually asymptomatic, but they can manifest chorioamnionitis, endometritis, or urinary tract infection. Infants born of women who are highly colonized are more likely to become colonized. GBS is acquired by newborns following vertical transmission (e.g., ascending infection through ruptured amniotic membranes or contamination following passage through the colonized birth canal). As many as 50% of infants with early-onset disease are symptomatic at birth, indicating an intrauterine infection. The highest attack rate of early-onset GBS is in high-risk deliveries, premature SGA infants, very low birth weight infants, or those with prolonged ruptured membranes; full-term infants account for 50% of cases. Colonization of pregnant women and newborns ranges from 15% to 40%. Incidence of early-onset GBS disease has been reduced from about 1 to 4 cases per 1000 live births to about 0.3 cases per 1000 live births owing to widespread chemoprophylaxis (AAP, 2012).

Clinical Findings

History.

- Infants who are younger than 37 weeks of gestation
- Rupture of membranes 18 hours or more
- Maternal fever during labor more than 100.4° F (40° C) oral
- Previous delivery of a sibling with invasive GBS disease

- Maternal chorioamnionitis to include rupture of membranes and maternal fever with at least two of the following:
  - Maternal tachycardia (heart rate greater than 90 bpm)
  - Fetal tachycardia (heart rate greater than 170 bpm)
  - Maternal leukocytosis (white blood cell count greater than 15,000/mm^3)
  - Uterine tenderness
  - Foul-smelling amniotic fluid

Physical Examination.

- Poor feeding, temperature instability
- Cyanosis, apnea, tachypnea, grunting, flaring, and retracting
- Seizures, lethargy, bulging fontanelle
- Rapid onset and deterioration

Diagnostic Studies. Cultures of blood, CSF, or both are definitive; antigen identification tests are available but have poor specificity.

Differential Diagnosis

RDS, amniotic fluid aspiration syndrome, persistent fetal circulation, infection or sepsis from other organisms, and metabolic problems are included in the differential diagnosis.

Management, Prognosis, and Prevention

Initiate antibiotic therapy with a penicillin (usually ampicillin) and an aminoglycoside, often gentamicin, until GBS has been differentiated from *E. coli* or *Listeria* sepsis or other organisms (AAP, 2012).

- Ampicillin IV:
  - Infant younger than 7 days old: Give 200 to 300 mg/kg/day in three divided doses.
  - Infant older than 7 days old: Give 300 mg/kg/day in four divided doses.
- Gentamicin doses are found in Table 39-9.

TABLE 39-9 Gentamicin Doses

Gestational Age (Weeks)	Age (Days)	Dosage
≤29 or asphyxia, decreased renal function	0-7	5 mg/kg every 48 hours
	8-28	4 mg/kg every 36 hours
	>28	4 mg/kg every 24 hours
30 to 33	0 to 7	4.5 mg/kg every 36 hours
	>7	4 mg/kg every 24 hours
≥34	0 to 7	4 mg/kg every 24 hours
	>7	4 mg/kg every 12 to 18 hours

Adapted from Engorn B, Flerlage J: *The Harriet Lane handbook*, ed 20, Philadelphia, 2015, Elsevier.

- IV penicillin G is the treatment of choice for documented GBS infection.
  - Infant younger than 7 days old: Give 250,000 to 400,000 units/kg/day in three divided doses.
  - Infant older than 7 days old: Give 450,000 to 500,000 units/kg/day in four divided doses.
  - Duration of therapy is 10 (bacteremia without focus) to 14 days (uncomplicated meningitis).
- Consultation with pediatric infectious disease specialists is recommended.

Screening of all pregnant women for GBS at 35 to 37 weeks of gestation is recommended. Antepartum treatment of asymptomatic mothers carrying GBS is not recommended. The mortality rate of early-onset disease ranges from 10% to 40%; mortality rate is highest in very low birth weight infants and in those with low neutrophil count (less than 1500/mm^3), low Apgar scores, hypotension, apnea, and a delay in initiation of antimicrobial therapy. Chemoprophylaxis of high-risk, colonized, pregnant women is an effective method of preventing early-onset GBS infection. Consensus guidelines are developed by both the CDC (2010) and AAP (2012). The guidelines outline steps for a screening-based and risk-factor strategy to prevent GBS. Treatment consists of IV penicillin or ampicillin given to high-risk women at the onset of labor, repeated every 4 hours until the infant is born.

Listeriosis

Listeria monocytogenes is a small gram-positive rod isolated from soil, streams, sewage, certain foods, silage, dust, and slaughterhouses. The food-borne transmission of disease is related to soft-ripened cheese, whole and 2% milk, uncooked hot dogs, undercooked chicken, raw vegetables, and shellfish. The newborn infant acquires the organism transplacentally or by aspiration or ingestion at the time of delivery.

Clinical Findings

- Brown-stained amniotic fluid
- Generalized symptoms of sepsis
- Whitish posterior pharyngeal and cutaneous granulomas
- Disseminated erythematous papules on skin

Diagnostic Studies. Blood, CSF, meconium, and urine are cultured. The CSF shows elevated protein, depressed glucose, and a high leukocyte count. Cultures of the placenta and amniotic fluid also may be helpful.

Management and Prognosis

- Administer IV ampicillin and an aminoglycoside (gentamicin) as initial therapy for severe infections.
- After clinical response occurs or for less severe infections in normal hosts, administer ampicillin alone.
- The duration of therapy is 10 to 14 days for infections without meningitis and 14 to 21 days for infections with meningitis (AAP, 2012).

Transplacentally acquired listeriosis often results in spontaneous abortion. The death rate of premature infants with *Listeria* pneumonia noted within 12 hours of birth approaches 100%. Mortality rate varies from 20% to 50% if disease develops between 5 and 30 days of birth, and it is especially high in premature infants. Intellectual disability, paralysis, and hydrocephalus have been noted in survivors of *Listeria* meningitis (Martin and Fanaroff, 2015).

Congenital Varicella

Varicella-zoster virus (VZV) is a herpesvirus. Humans are the only source of infection for this highly contagious virus. The infectivity rate for congenital varicella syndrome in infants born to mothers with chickenpox is 2% when infection occurs between 7 and 20 weeks of gestation (LaRussa and Marin, 2011).

Clinical Findings

- History of maternal chickenpox infection
- Limb atrophy
- Scarring of the skin
- Eye manifestations

Diagnostic Studies. Diagnosis of VZV is made by immunofluorescent staining of vesicular scrapings.

Management, Prognosis, and Prevention

Some experts recommend acyclovir for pregnant women with varicella, especially in the second or third trimester (AAP, 2012). Varicella-zoster immune globulin (VariZIG) is recommended for the term newborn infant whose mother had an onset of chickenpox within 5 days before delivery or within 48 hours after delivery. All exposed premature infants younger than 28 weeks of gestation or 1000 g or less birth weight should receive VariZIG; exposed premature infants 28 weeks of gestation and older whose mothers lack serologic evidence of disease or a reliable history of disease also require VariZIG (AAP, 2012). Despite having received VariZIG, about 50% of infants may still develop a mild varicella infection. If VariZIG is not available, then immunoglobulin intravenous (IGIV) is recommended. VariZIG is not indicated if the mother has varicella-zoster (shingles) only. Airborne and contact precautions are recommended for neonates born to mothers with varicella. If the infant is still hospitalized, such precautions are continued for 21 days from last exposure or 28 days if they received VariZIG.

Prevention efforts are targeted to potential mothers. Varicella vaccination is recommended for nonpregnant women of childbearing age who have no history of varicella infection (AAP, 2012) (see Chapter 24).

Sexually Transmitted Infections

Gonorrhea

Neisseria gonorrhoeae is a gram-negative diplococcus that occurs only in humans. The organism lives in exudate and secretions of infected mucous membranes. The organism is transmitted primarily through sexual contact and parturition. Gonococcal infections in the newborn are acquired primarily during delivery.

Clinical Findings

There is a history of maternal gonococcal infection. Findings include conjunctivitis, and rarely as septicemia, pneumonia, or joint infection.

Diagnostic Studies. Culture of eye exudate is positive for *N. gonorrhoeae*.

Management and Prevention

Administer a single dose of intramuscular ceftriaxone 25 to 50 mg/kg (not to exceed 125 mg) for prophylaxis of infants born to mothers with active gonorrhea. Because gonorrheal conjunctivitis can rapidly lead to blindness, all infants are given eye prophylaxis at birth with erythromycin 0.5% ophthalmic ointment (AAP, 2012).

Chlamydia

Chlamydial infection is caused by an obligate intracellular parasite, *Chlamydia trachomatis,* and is the most common sexually transmitted infection in the United States. Acquisition occurs in approximately 50% of infants born vaginally to infected mothers and in some infants delivered by cesarean section with intact membranes. The risk of developing conjunctivitis is 25% to 50% in infants who have acquired *C. trachomatis;* the risk with pneumonia is 5% to 20% (AAP, 2012).

Clinical Findings

- History of maternal chlamydial infection
- Conjunctivitis a few days to several weeks after birth
- Infant commonly afebrile with normal activity level
- Pneumonia 2 to 19 weeks after birth

Diagnostic Studies.

- Tests for detection of *C. trachomatis* without cell culture include DNA probe, direct fluorescent antibody (DFA) staining, enzyme immunoassay (EIA), and nucleic acid amplification (PCR, ligase chain reaction [LCR]).
- Routine bacterial cultures are not helpful.
- Gram stain and culture of discharge from the eye (must include epithelial cells from the palpebral conjunctival sac because chlamydia is an obligate parasite) are necessary for diagnosis.

Management and Prevention

Oral erythromycin suspension (50 mg/kg/day in four divided doses for 10 to 14 days) is given for both conjunctivitis and pneumonia (AAP, 2012; Workowski et al, 2015). Appropriate treatment of the pregnant woman before delivery prevents disease in the newborn. Prophylaxis with oral erythromycin of the asymptomatic infant born to an untreated but *Chlamydia*-positive woman generally is contraindicated because of the increased risk of developing hypertrophic pyloric stenosis in the infant exposed to erythromycin.

Syphilis

Syphilis is caused by the spirochete *Treponema pallidum,* which crosses the placenta in an infected mother. Routine maternal serologic testing is legally required during prenatal care in all states.

Clinical Findings

- Maternal infection and positive serologic testing
- The majority of neonates are asymptomatic at birth
- Failure to thrive, restlessness, fever, persistent rhinorrhea
- Maculopapular or bullous dermal lesions, hepatosplenomegaly

Diagnostic Studies. Evaluation needs to be individualized depending on the adequacy of maternal treatment and follow-up for syphilis. Consultation with infectious disease may be indicated. CSF evaluation shows high protein, low glucose, high white blood cell count, and positivity on Venereal Disease Research Laboratory (VDRL) test. Serum liver enzymes are elevated with liver involvement, and serum rapid plasma reagin (RPR) test is positive.

Management and Prognosis

For proven or highly probable congenital syphilis, the CDC recommends 10 consecutive days of crystalline penicillin G 100,000 to 150,000 units/kg/day, given as 50,000 units/kg/dose IV every 12 hours during the first 7 days of life and every 8 hours thereafter (Workowski et al, 2010). Procaine penicillin G 50,000 units/kg IM/dose daily in a single dose for 10 days is the only acceptable treatment regimen for congenital syphilis and for all infants born to seropositive mothers without a documented history of adequate treatment. If more than 1 day is missed, the entire course must be restarted. For infants with less certain evidence of syphilis, alternative regimens are available; referral to the latest CDC guidelines is recommended (Workowski et al, 2010). Untreated congenital syphilis can lead to severe multiorgan involvement. Infants who are appropriately treated have a good prognosis.

Herpes Simplex Virus

Three clinically distinguishable categories of herpes simplex virus (HSV) (Fig. 39-20) infection exist: (1) disseminated disease, (2) CNS disease, and (3) disease restricted to the skin, eyes, and mouth (AAP, 2012) (see Table 39-3). HSV is transmitted by direct contact with infected maternal genitalia during the birth process. Transplacental transmission occurs but has been reported in only a few cases. The risk of neonatal infection is highest with primary genital infection (see Chapter 24 for further discussion).

Clinical Findings

The mother may have active lesions and deliver vaginally. Vesicles in the skin, eye, and mouth are found. Signs or symptoms of encephalitis, pneumonia, or sepsis can also be present.

Diagnostic Studies. The virus is isolated in tissue cultures obtained from vesicles, nasopharyngeal or conjunctival swabs, urine, stool, and tracheal secretions; alternatively, vesicle scrapings can be evaluated for antigens with rapid diagnostic tests.

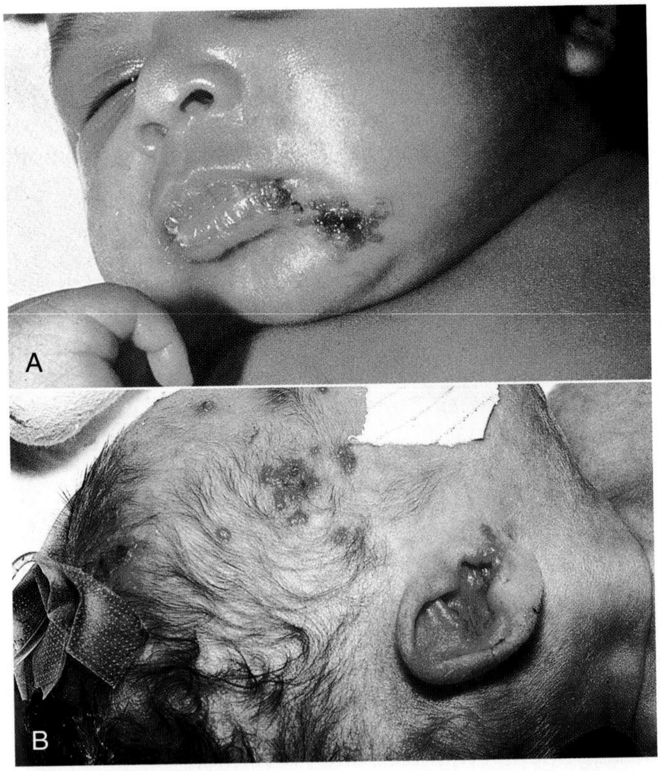

• **Figure 39-20** Herpes simplex virus (HSV). (From Cohen, BA: *Pediatric dermatology,* ed 4, Philadelphia, 2013, Elsevier, Fig. 2-45 A and B.)

Management, Prognosis, and Prevention

Acyclovir 60 mg/kg/day IV given every 8 hours for 14 days (skin, eyes, and mouth infection) or 21 days (disseminated or involving the CNS) (AAP, 2012). Additionally, treatment with ophthalmic drugs (1% trifluridine, 0.1% iododeoxyuridine, or 3% vidarabine) is used for infants with ocular involvement (AAP, 2012). Despite effective antiviral therapy, disseminated neonatal HSV infections and localized encephalitis are associated with considerable morbidity and mortality. Some obstetricians provide antiviral therapy in the final weeks of life for women with a history of HSV. The risk of acquiring this serious infection is lowered by performing cesarean delivery before rupture of membranes in any pregnancy in which signs or symptoms of HSV infection occur.

Human Immunodeficiency Virus

HIV, a retrovirus, is transmitted to the newborn via the placenta or at birth secondary to exposure to maternal blood (see Chapter 24 for further discussion).

Neonatal Abstinence Syndrome

The medical issues surrounding newborns whose mothers abuse substances during their pregnancy are serious concerns. Although the incidence varies by location, 3.39 per 1000 births are affected by maternal drug abuse (Association of State and Territorial Health Officials, 2014). In one

TABLE 39-10 Neonatal Drug-Withdrawal Scoring System

Signs	Score			
	0	1	2	3
Tremors (muscle activity of limbs)	Normal	Minimally increased when hungry or disturbed	Moderate or marked increase when undisturbed; subside when fed or held snugly	Marked increase or continuous even when undisturbed, going on to seizure-like movements
Irritability (excessive crying)	None	Slightly increased	Moderate to severe when disturbed or hungry	Marked even when undisturbed
Reflexes	Normal	Increased	Markedly increased	
Stools	Normal	Explosive, but normal frequency	Explosive, more than 8 days	
Muscle tone	Normal	Increased	Rigidity	
Skin abrasions	No	Redness of knees and elbows	Breaking of the skin	
Respiratory rate/minute	<55	55 to 75	76 to 95	
Repetitive sneezing	No	Yes		
Repetitive yawning	No	Yes		
Vomiting	No	Yes		
Fever	No	Yes		

Reprinted with permission from Lipsitz PJ: A proposed narcotic withdrawal score for use with newborn infants: a pragmatic evaluation of its efficacy, *Clin Pediatr* 14(6):592–594, 1975.

study, mothers who stated they had used cocaine or had a positive drug screen had a significantly higher risk of infections, including syphilis, gonorrhea, hepatitis, and HIV; psychiatric, nervous, and emotional disorders; and abruptio placentae. The prevalence of serious and life-threatening medical outcomes is low in drug-abusing pregnant women. However, the disadvantaged social and environmental conditions that are often characteristic of the lifestyle of these women may compound the risk for infection and poor neurodevelopmental outcome. Elimination of in utero exposure to drugs of abuse can occur only if identification of a potential problem is identified in a high-risk mother and referral to a substance abuse prevention program is accomplished.

Use of both "street drugs" and prescription medications place the infant at risk for poor neurologic outcomes and withdrawal symptoms at birth. Multidrug intake is common; however, the classes of drugs of abuse generally can be divided into opioids, CNS stimulants, CNS depressants, and hallucinogens. The onset of neonatal symptoms can begin at birth or up to about 14 days after birth; symptoms may last from a few days to about 18 months. Symptomatic neonates need both pharmacologic and non-pharmacologic intervention for withdrawal symptoms; asymptomatic neonates need non-pharmacologic interventions as identified later (Hudak and Tan, 2012). Use of an objective scoring tool helps guide therapy. The Neonatal Drug-Withdrawal Scoring System (Lipsitz, 1975) can be found in Table 39-10. The Lipsitz tool offers the advantages of a relatively simple numeric system and a reported 77% sensitivity using a value of 4 as an indication of significant withdrawal signs. A more comprehensive scoring system (21 symptoms and different assigned score for each) is the Modified Finnegan's Neonatal Abstinence Scoring Tool, which can be found at www.lkpz.nl/docs/lkpz_pdf_1310485469.pdf.

Cocaine (Crack) Exposure

Cocaine is a local anesthetic and CNS stimulant that some believe to be a teratogen that crosses the placenta.

Clinical Findings

Maternal exposure to cocaine or crack and positive maternal and/or infant urine drug screen for cocaine are found. Premature labor, abruptio placentae, intrauterine growth restriction, and fetal asphyxia with meconium staining are possible. Many infants will show no adverse effects from maternal use of cocaine and no clinically documented neonatal withdrawal syndrome for cocaine has been identified (Carlo, 2011c).

Management, Complications, and Prevention

- Do not breastfeed because cocaine is detectable in breast milk.
- Close neurodevelopmental follow-up and testing are necessary through the first several years of age.

- Involvement of the Department of Child and Family Services is essential.

Heroin and Methadone Exposure

Heroin and methadone are narcotics that cross the placenta.

Clinical Findings

History.

- Maternal exposure to heroin or methadone
- Urine drug screen positive for opiates in mother and/or infant
- Increased incidence of stillbirths and SGA infants, but probably not congenital anomalies

Physical Examination.

- Tremors and hyperirritability often more coarse than those with hypoglycemia
- Limbs rigid and hyperreflexic, fist sucking
- Skin abrasions secondary to hyperactivity
- Tachypnea, poor feeding, high-pitched cry
- Vomiting, diarrhea
- Low birth weight or SGA in 50% (Carlo, 2011c)

Symptoms of heroin withdrawal occur in up to 75% of infants, usually beginning in the first 48 hours of life, depending on the daily maternal dose, duration of addiction, and most recent maternal dose. Symptoms of methadone withdrawal occur in up to 90% of infants. A higher incidence of symptomatology is seen if the last dose was taken within 24 hours of birth. Overall the withdrawal syndrome is more severe and more prolonged with methadone than with heroin (Carlo, 2011c).

Differential Diagnosis

The differential diagnosis includes hypoglycemia and hypocalcemia.

Management and Prevention

Supportive management, such as swaddling, frequent feedings, and protection from external stimuli is needed. Education regarding sudden infant death syndrome (SIDS) is imperative, because these infants are at increased risk. The Department of Child and Family Services must be involved before discharge. Medications (such as, phenobarbital, tincture of opium, and methadone) can be used if symptoms such as severe irritability, vomiting and diarrhea, seizures, temperature instability, or severe tachypnea are noted. Pregnant women who are addicted to heroin should be encouraged to enter a treatment program.

Fetal Alcohol Syndrome

See Chapter 42.

Sudden Infant Death Syndrome and Apparent Life-Threatening Events

The accepted definition of SIDS is the sudden death of an infant younger than 1 year old that remains unexplained after a complete case investigation, including performance of a complete autopsy, examination of the death scene, and review of the clinical history (Hunt and Hauck, 2011). SIDS rarely occurs in the first month of life, with 90% of deaths occurring between 1 and 6 months old, peaking at 12 weeks old (85% occur between 2 and 4 months old). SIDS is the most common cause of death in infants between 1 and 6 months old, accounting for 5000 deaths per year. African American infants are at twice the risk, and a higher frequency of SIDS is seen in male infants and in the winter months, although the seasonal difference in rates is decreasing (AAP Task Force on Sudden Infant Death Syndrome, 2011; Hunt and Hauck, 2011). An apparent life-threatening event (ALTE) is defined as an episode that is frightening to the observer and that is characterized by some combination of apnea (central or occasionally obstructive), color change, marked change in muscle tone, choking, or gagging. In some cases, the observer fears that the infant has died.

The diagnosis of SIDS is one of exclusion, because the specific cause remains unknown. It cannot be predicted or prevented, although placing the infant in a supine position has been shown to decrease the incidence of SIDS and is the recommended sleep position for infants. The National Institutes of Health has monitored sleep position since 1992, and prone sleeping has decreased from 70% to less than 15%. At the same time, the SIDS death rate has fallen by about 53% in the United States (AAP Task Force on Sudden Infant Death Syndrome, 2011).

Three main pathophysiologic mechanisms are considered to contribute to SIDS: decreased arousal, asphyxia and rebreathing, and thermal stress. Experts have considered as possible causes respiratory obstruction, restrictive clothing, and hyperthermia. Factors associated with SIDS include ALTE, poverty, lack of prenatal care, low birth weight, SGA, preterm birth, young maternal age, high parity, maternal smoking and drug use, and co-sleeping.

Clinical Findings

History

- Maternal: Cigarette smoking, drug or alcohol use; no or poor prenatal care; bottle feeding; poor education; unmarried; multiparity; maternal age younger than 20 years old; short intervals between pregnancies; anemia
- Infant: Prematurity (less than 37 weeks); low birth weight (less than 2500 g) or SGA; twins or other multiple births; Apgar score less than 6 at 5 minutes; apnea; poor weight gain; anemia; intensive care unit stay; neonatal respiratory abnormality, bronchopulmonary dysplasia, previous ALTE; previously healthy infant with or without recent upper respiratory infection (URI) symptoms
- Socioeconomic, other: Low-income family; crowded living conditions; poor housing conditions; prior SIDS in family; prone sleeping position, soft bedding, overheating; co-sleeping, especially with smoke, alcohol, or mind-altering drug use; race, ethnicity, culture (higher rates in African American and American Indian and Alaska Native children)

Physical Examination

- No sign of injury (nonaccidental trauma must be ruled out)
- Frothy blood-tinged secretions in mouth and nares
- Intrathoracic petechiae on autopsy
- Retention of peri adrenal brown fat on autopsy

Diagnostic Studies

Autopsy and death scene evaluation must be done. A skeletal bone survey may be done if a concern about abuse exists.

Differential Diagnosis

Aspiration; suffocation; infant botulism or poisoning; cardiac or respiratory disease; hypoxemia; infection; metabolic disorders; child abuse, Munchausen syndrome, or shaken baby syndrome; and CNS abnormalities should be ruled out. Bed sharing, especially if the parent is large, appears to be associated with an increased likelihood of some SIDS-like deaths (AAP Task Force on Sudden Infant Death Syndrome, 2011).

Management and Prevention

Management is aimed at assisting the family to cope with the loss of the child. The first response of the family is disbelief and shock.

- Obtain a thorough history from the caretaker within a short period of time after the death. Do not accuse the family of any wrongdoing. Focus the questioning on the cause of death to better understand the circumstances.
- Reassure caretaker and family that it was not their fault and the death could not have been prevented.
- Offer support and counsel to families as soon as possible after death.
- Supply names of different support groups to help the family overcome grief.
- Provide follow-up for at least 1 year.
- Assist surviving siblings. Observe their reaction to the death and refer for counseling if necessary. Help them understand that it was not their fault and alleviate their feelings of guilt. Allow children to verbalize their feelings. Assist parents to deal with their other children; suggest that parents give extra love, attention, and reassurance to their other children.

• BOX 39-6 Measures that Aid in Preventing Sudden Infant Death Syndrome

- Breastfeeding is recommended.
- Infants should be immunized (reduces risk by 50%).
- Place infants on their backs to sleep until at least 6 months old. The National Institutes of Health has a "Safe to Sleep" program with parent information, stickers, and video.
- Use a firm mattress. Do not use bumper pads or soft bedding or have stuffed animals in bed. Infants should not sleep on a sofa or chair, or on a waterbed or in bed with an adult.
- Avoid overheating and overbundling; room temperature should be 68° to 72° F (20° to 22.2° C).
- Avoid alcohol and drugs (including smoking) while pregnant and breastfeeding, and while in bed.
- Do not allow cigarette smoking within the house or car.
- Avoid bed sharing and co-sleeping.
- Separate but proximate caregiver sleeping environments are recommended.
- Consider pacifier use at naptime and bedtime (but not in breastfed infants until after the first month of life when feedings are established).
- A variety of products to maintain an infant's sleep position are commercially available; their efficacy and safety have not been thoroughly investigated and cannot be recommended.
- For at-risk infants, educate parents and caregivers regarding pros and cons of apnea monitor use. Cardiopulmonary resuscitation instruction is recommended.

- Evaluate need for home monitoring. Because the rate of SIDS in succeeding children is low (less than 2%) and because monitoring a child cannot prevent a SIDS episode from occurring, controversy remains about whether to monitor succeeding children (AAP Task Force on Sudden Infant Death Syndrome, 2011). Monitors are recommended by some in the following instances: when more than one child in a family has died from SIDS; in infants with ALTEs; in infants with tracheostomy or other airway problems; in infants with neurologic problems affecting respiratory control; and in infants with chronic lung disease.

Box 39-6 lists measures that aid in the prevention of SIDS.

For a complete list of references, please visit http://evolve.elsevier.com/Burns/pediatric/.

40 Common Injuries

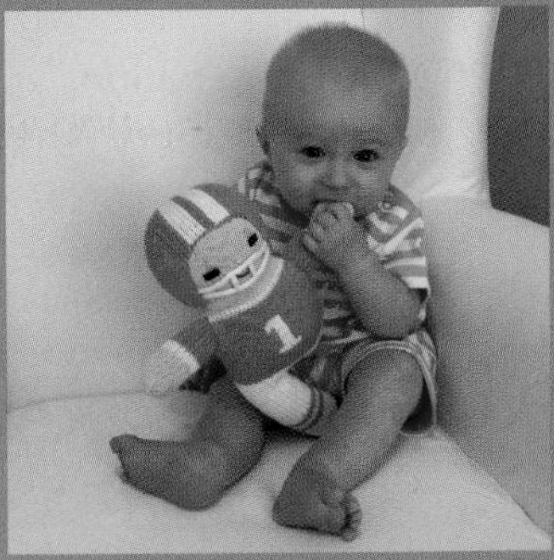

SARA D. DEGOLIER, DAWN LEE GARZON

Unintentional injuries are the leading cause of death and account for over 9 million nonfatal injuries, almost 8,500 deaths, and 8.7 million emergency department (ED) visits each year among children aged 1 to 19 (Centers for Disease Control and Prevention [CDC], 2012a). Injury prevention is as important as appropriate management strategies for this important public health concern. Injured children may be cared for with (1) a simple home treatment by the parent, caregiver, or supervising adult; (2) intervention by the provider in the primary care setting; (3) referral to a medical specialist or inpatient facility; or (4) a combination of these. Modifying the potential for injury before it occurs is a key factor of injury management. Health care professionals have a responsibility to educate families to prevent injuries from occurring.

Unintentional injury prevention involves anticipatory guidance to help parents provide a safe environment and developmentally appropriate supervision. Effective injury prevention strategies in children and adolescents focus on understanding and modifying risk factors, developing community-wide programs, and promoting health policy that focuses on injury prevention. When implementing prevention strategies, it is important to consider that injury occurrence and severity vary, depending on several factors including age, race, gender, residence, and socioeconomic status.

Principles of Injury Control

The most effective injury prevention education focuses on specific, usable information to decrease injury risk rather than broad, nonspecific recommendations. For example, teaching children and parents how to purchase and size a bicycle helmet is more effective than telling children to "always use a bike helmet." Anticipatory guidance provided by health providers at well-child visits should be geared to the developmental stage of the child. Written materials, audiovisual presentations, peer counseling, and one-to-one interaction with a health professional are all effective teaching and learning strategies. However, safety information should be provided in moderate doses, with reinforcement or repetition at subsequent visits. This strategy helps ensure that the prevention education points are well received and used by caregivers, patients, and their families. Passive injury prevention is the most effective strategy for reducing injury and involves the implementation of safety measures that do not require caregivers to change their behavior to make the environment safer for their children. This prevention strategy includes modification of everyday items in the child's environment. Examples include the use of child-resistant caps on medicines and cleaning products, and safety design in toys.

Another safety approach includes environmental modification, such as the use of smoke and carbon monoxide detectors, safe roadway design to reduce traffic volume and speed in residential neighborhoods, window locks, and firearm safety locks. Providers can advocate for local and national prevention strategies and support programs, such as the Safe Kids USA campaign (see Additional Resources). They can also play a key role by supporting injury prevention legislation or initiatives. Public and consumer awareness is crucial for successful prevention programs.

Although most children with serious injuries are seen first in EDs, primary care providers have a professional obligation to remain current in basic life support techniques. Competence in performing emergency cardiopulmonary resuscitation and emergency intervention for choking (whether it be for infants, children, or adults) is critical for all licensed health professionals in clinical practice settings. Likewise, all parents and caregivers should be encouraged to enroll in a basic pediatric life support program, especially parents and caregivers of infants and children at risk for cardiopulmonary arrest.

Approach to Trauma

Three main components essential to the management of an injured child include obtaining an appropriate history, identifying the mechanism of the injury, and performing a thorough physical examination. If the injury is life threatening or there has been any deterioration in the child's condition, a trauma severity assessment must immediately be

TABLE 40-1 Classification and Disposition of Trauma by Severity

Category	History	Vital Signs	Local Findings	Physical Examination: Laboratory/ Radiologic Studies	Physical Examination: Probable Disposition
Mild	Minimal force	Normal	Superficial only	Few	Discharge
Moderate	Significant force	Normal	Suspicious for internal injury	Intermediate	Evaluate
Severe	Critical force	Abnormal	Indicative of internal injury	Many	Immediate therapy; admit

From Lee LK, Fleischer GR: An approach to the injured child. In Fleischer GR, Ludwig S, et al, editors: *Textbook of pediatric emergency medicine,* ed 6, Philadelphia, 2010, Lippincott Williams & Wilkins, p 1234.

performed. Primary assessment of the injured child should occur within the first 5 minutes of initial contact and includes assessment of:

- Respiratory status and airway
- Circulation
- Vital signs
- A brief history (allergies, medications, past medical history, and events surrounding the injury)
- Rapid assessment of essential organ status; cardiopulmonary resuscitation must be initiated if indicated

Once the patient is stabilized, a secondary assessment should include:

- A complete physical examination
- Laboratory and radiographic studies as indicated

Assessment of the patient's vital signs, physical examination, and laboratory tests should be repeated as indicated based on the injury and initial diagnostic study results. The definitive care phase includes stabilization of local injuries and preparation of the patient and family for transport to the ED if necessary (Table 40-1).

The practitioner should always consider nonaccidental trauma (physical abuse) when a child presents with an injury and the caregiver explanation for the injury is not consistent with the injury itself. According to Chiesa and Sirotnak (2014), red flags in the injury history provided by the caregiver can include an absent history, a history that changes each time the caregiver gives the history, or a history with significant detail lapses. Improbable or illogical explanations of the injury from the caregiver is also concerning.

Common Pediatric Injuries

The abnormal transfer of energy either by mechanical, thermal electric, chemical, or radiation between a moving or stationary object to a target is now recognized at the etiology of most injuries. Mechanical energy transfer, for example when a rough or hard surfaced object lacerates or scrapes the skin, is the most common type of injury (Baker and Li, 2012).

Trauma to the Skin and Soft Tissue

Abrasions

Description and Epidemiology

Abrasions are superficial skin injuries, often the result of falls or friction that involve epidermal trauma. The depth of skin tissue involvement varies depending on the amount of force and friction that the skin encounters at the time of injury. The most serious form of abrasion is an avulsion, a trauma that results in loss of the epidermal, dermal, and subcutaneous layers.

Assessment

History. Seek information about the cause and type of injury, the possibility for foreign objects in the wound, and the presence of dirt at the accident scene.

Physical Examination. Determine the extent of the abrasion and the presence of dirt, grime, or other foreign body (e.g., tar). Findings include an area of skin that appears scraped off and may include oozing of serous fluid and blood. Increasing pain, swelling, warmth, redness, and red streaking of the injured area might indicate secondary infection. Assess the surrounding tissue and extremity (if the injury is located on an extremity) for circulation, sensation, motion, and function.

Differential Diagnosis

The injury history and physical findings are the keys to diagnosis. Any other skin condition that can cause loss of epidermis, such as a burn, is included in the differential diagnosis.

Management

Appropriate first-aid care is important to prevent infection. Most abrasions of the skin can be managed at home unless the abrasion is deep, involves a large area, is associated with severe pain, or has a significant amount of dirt, grime, tar, or a foreign body in the wound. Because of the increased risk of infection, parents of a child who is immunocompromised should contact the child's provider either by phone and/or office visit. Abrasion management includes:

- Thoroughly cleansing the wound. The area can be scrubbed with soap or an antibacterial cleanser using a wet gauze or soft surgical nailbrush. Gentle irrigation with copious amounts of water or normal saline (300 to 1000 mL depending on the surface area of the wound) is the preferred method to thoroughly cleanse a wound and prevent infection. The larger the surface area, the more irrigation solution is needed to ensure proper cleansing. Povidone-iodine, alcohol, and peroxide should not be used on open wounds. If dirt or dark-colored matter is not adequately removed, new skin may grow over the particles, resulting in a permanent tattoo. A secondary infection may occur as well if all debris is not removed. Remove pieces of loose skin with sterile scissors and remove foreign particles with tweezers. If tar particles are present, rub the wound area with petrolatum, and then repeat normal saline or water irrigation.
- Small abrasions can be left open to the air or may require a small bandage.
- Cover larger abrasions with a sterile nonadherent dressing. Antibiotic ointment such as bacitracin/polymyxin B may be applied, especially to abrasions of the elbows or knees to prevent cracking or reopening of the wound because of constant movement and stretching of the joints.
- Protect abrasions of the hands, feet, or areas overlying joints from friction and dirt until a protective dry scab is formed.
- Instruct the caregiver to wash the abrasion at least every 24 hours and reapply the dressing and antibiotic ointments until a protective dry scab is formed. Instructions regarding the signs and symptoms of infection should also be provided.
- Tetanus prophylaxis should be administered if the wound is significant or if the child has not received a tetanus immunization within the previous 5 years. The use of Tdap is the preferred vaccination for children 10 to 11 years old and older (see Chapter 24).

Puncture Wounds

Description and Epidemiology

Puncture wounds result from penetration of varying levels of skin and underlying tissue. These wounds are typically classified as superficial or deep. Glass, wood splinters, toothpicks, needles, nails, metal, staples, thumbtacks, and bites are common sources of injury. Although the majority of puncture wounds heal without problems, a sizable minority of these injuries are complicated by infections that can lead to cellulitis, fasciitis, septic arthritis, or soft-tissue abscesses.

Staphylococcus aureus and beta-hemolytic streptococci are normal flora of the skin and are common causes of secondary infections in puncture wounds. *Pseudomonas aeruginosa* colonizes on the rubber soles of tennis shoes and is a common pathogen for plantar puncture wounds when the puncture occurs through the sole of a tennis shoe and into the foot. Osteomyelitis can occur if the puncture wound penetrates a bone or joint and is most commonly caused by *P. aeruginosa* in nondiabetic patients and is most commonly caused by *S. aureus* in diabetic patients (Baddour, 2013). Cat and dog bites can cause wound infection from *Pasteurella multocida.*

When considering risk for infection, the location and depth of the wound and the presence of a foreign object are important components. For example, deep penetrating injuries to the forefoot with a dirty object, especially if they involve the plantar fascia, have a higher risk of infection than wounds to the arch or heel area. The forefoot has less overlying soft tissue than other plantar surfaces and is the major weight-bearing area of the foot; therefore, cartilage and bone can be involved. The metatarsophalangeal joint region is also at high risk for infection for the same reasons. Puncture wounds through the soles of tennis shoes can transfer bacteria into the tissue while simultaneously impairing wound drainage, placing the child at higher risk for a secondary infection.

Assessment

The assessment of a child with a minor wound begins by excluding more serious and sometimes occult injuries.

History. Important information to elicit after a report or suspicion of a puncture wound includes the following:

- Date and time of injury and history of wound care provided at time of injury and thereafter.
- Identification of the penetrating object and the type and estimated depth of penetration. If it is not known what object penetrated the skin, the likelihood of an imbedded foreign body is high.
- Location and condition of the penetrating object. Was the object clean or rusty, jagged or smooth?
- Whether all or part of the foreign object was removed.
- Type and condition of footwear that was being worn (pertinent to injuries to the foot) or if the child was barefoot.
- Immunization status for tetanus coverage (see Chapter 24).
- Presence of any medical condition that increases the risk for infectious complications.

Physical Examination. A good light source is necessary to assess and treat a puncture wound. Note circulation, movement, and sensation of the area next to the injury. Determine the amount of involvement of underlying tissue or bone structures. For plantar puncture wounds, have the patient lie prone with the feet positioned at the head of the examining table and the knees slightly flexed (Buttaravoli and Leffler, 2012). Assess the wound for length and depth, presence of debris or penetrating object, and signs of infection.

Examination findings consistent with *cellulitis* include:

- Localized pain or tenderness, swelling, and erythema at the puncture site (may be more obvious at dorsum of the foot for plantar puncture wounds)

- Possible fever
- Pain with flexion or extension of the extremity involved
- Decreased ability to bear weight
- For plantar puncture wounds, pain along the plantar aspect of the foot during extension or flexion of the toes may indicate deep tissue injury, thus a higher risk of infection

Examination findings consistent with *osteomyelitis-osteochondritis* include:

- Extension of pain and swelling around the puncture wound and to the adjacent bony structures
- Exquisite point tenderness over the bone
- Fever
- Increasing erythema
- Decreased use of the affected extremity

Examination findings consistent with *pyarthrosis* (septic arthritis) include:

- Pain, swelling, warmth, and erythema over the affected joint
- Decreased range of motion and weight bearing of the affected joint
- Fever

Diagnostic Studies. Plain film radiograph should be ordered if any of the following occur:

- A suspicion of a retained foreign object.
- There is a tremendous amount of pain at the site of the wound, localized tenderness is noted over the wound, there is discoloration underneath the skin surface, or there is a palpable mass noted at or near the wound entry site (Baddour, 2013).
- There was penetration of a joint space, bone or growth cartilage, or the plantar fascia of the foot.
- The puncture site has signs of infection and is from a nail injury.
  - Most metal and glass foreign bodies can be seen on a plain radiograph. However, if the foreign object is not radiopaque or if the x-ray is negative despite suspicion of foreign object in the wound, computed tomography (CT), ultrasound, and magnetic resonance imaging (MRI) are useful diagnostic tools (Buttaravoli and Leffler, 2012).
  - Bone scans are sensitive but not specific for osteomyelitis. Radiographs are specific, but findings for osteomyelitis are noted late. Clinical examination and laboratory studies and imaging should be considered early in the diagnosis of osteomyelitis (Erickson and Caprio, 2014).
  - A complete blood count (CBC) and blood culture may be needed. An elevation in the white blood cell count might indicate infection.
  - An erythrocyte sedimentation rate (ESR) and C-reactive protein (CRP) are nonspecific inflammatory markers and are helpful in the diagnosis and management of bony inflammation and infection.
  - A wound culture is indicated prior to starting antibiotics if the wound appears infected.

Differential Diagnosis

The history and physical examination provide the diagnosis.

Management

The circumstance surrounding the penetrating injury and the presenting symptoms are the best indicators of whether the injury is superficial and will heal uneventfully or if it will result in infectious complications. Buttaravoli and Leffler (2012) suggest the following practical and straightforward approach to the management of puncture wounds:

- For the majority of superficial or simple puncture wounds, débridement with an antiseptic solution after scrubbing the wound surface is sufficient. Consider the use of wound irrigation. Ensure that there are no foreign bodies present.
- A No. 10 scalpel may be used to gently shave off the cornified epithelium surrounding the puncture wound to aid in the removal of debris that collected around the point of entry.
- For wounds where debris is noted, gently slide the plastic sheath of an over-the-needle catheter down the wound track and move the catheter sheath in and out while irrigating with copious amounts of normal saline until debris no longer flows from the wound. A local anesthetic agent may be necessary for débridement and irrigation procedures.
- Obtain imaging studies as indicated. If imaging studies demonstrate that the foreign object has invaded bone, growth cartilage, or a joint space, refer the child immediately to an orthopedic surgeon. Always suspect a retained foreign object if the puncture wound is infected, the infection is not responding to antibiotic therapy, or if pain or aching of the injured site is still present weeks after the injury. In order to prevent a catastrophic outcome, wounds that are deep or highly contaminated should be referred to an orthopedic surgeon so that débridement can take place in an operating room (Buttaravoli and Leffler, 2012).
- Following careful wound cleansing, the wound can be covered with a simple bandage. Deeper wounds that require more extensive exploration should have a small sterile wick of iodoform gauze placed in the wound track in order to keep the edges open, thus aiding in granulation tissue growth and wound healing. Remove the gauze 2 to 3 days after placement (Selbst and Attia, 2010).
- Children with simple, uncomplicated puncture wounds do not need antibiotics; however, if there are signs of infection, the puncture is the result of a cat bite, or if the wound is deep or contained debris, antibiotics should be part of the treatment plan. Appropriate antibiotics for puncture wounds include amoxicillin clavulanate or cephalexin. Clindamycin should be used when children are allergic to penicillins. Plantar puncture wounds require ciprofloxacin. If methicillin-resistant *Staphylococcus aureus* (MRSA) is cultured from the wound or pus is present at the puncture site, then trimethoprim-sulfamethoxazole (TMP-SMX)

or clindamycin is recommended until sensitivities are known. All antibiotics should be prescribed for 7 to 14 days depending on severity of infection (Baddour, 2013). A recheck appointment should be scheduled 48 hours from the start of antibiotics for the patient receiving outpatient therapy.

- Surgical débridement for removal of a foreign body and/or abscess drainage should be considered with an infected puncture wound (Baddour, 2013).
- Treatment for severe infections secondary to puncture wounds, such as septic arthritis and osteomyelitis, includes surgical débridement and parenteral antibiotics (Hosalkar et al, 2011).
- Tetanus prophylaxis is indicated if it has been more than 5 years since the last tetanus vaccine or if the date of the last tetanus vaccine is unknown. Consider passive immunization with tetanus immune globulin (TIG) or initiation/continuation of a primary tetanus series (DTaP, Tdap, or Td as appropriate) for children who have never been immunized or are behind in their vaccinations (see Chapter 24).

Patient and Parent Education

Home care management for a puncture wound includes:

- Cleanse the wound two times a day and when soiling of the wound occurs. Use warm water and soap, and then apply bacitracin or triple antibiotic ointment to the wound.
- Cover the wound with a dressing, such as an adhesive bandage.
- Observe closely for signs and symptoms of infection and if infection is suspected, notify the provider immediately; rapid reevaluation is necessary. Further evaluation is required if a puncture wound continues to cause localized or spreading pain or discomfort.

Ingrown Toenail and Nail Hematoma

Description and Epidemiology

Onychocryptosis (ingrown toenail) and nail hematomas are common occurrences in pediatrics. Ingrown toenails are caused by several factors, including abnormal position of the toenail on the nailbed, tight and improperly fitting shoes, trauma to the nail, and improper toenail trimming. The great toe is the most commonly affected. An ingrown toenail occurs when the lateral edge of the toenail pierces the lateral nail fold of the skin, entering the dermis layer (Goldstein and Goldstein, 2014). Subungual hematomas are blood accumulations under an intact nail. Subungual hematomas may be accompanied by lacerations or fractures of the distal phalanx (Tuft fractures). Tuft fractures are commonly associated with fingertip crush injuries.

Management

- Ingrown toenail
  - Pack cotton under the nail edge to elevate the nail, and educate the patient to repack the cotton daily to prevent infection.
  - Soak the affected foot in warm water mixed with Epsom salts for 20 minutes, three times a day. Keep the foot or affected toenail clean and dry.
  - Encourage frequent elevation of the affected toe as well as minimal activity to aid in healing.
  - Educate about the importance of clipping nails straight across with extension of toenail just over the edge of the nailbed. Properly fitting shoes are also important.
  - Systemic antibiotics are rarely needed and should be reserved for severe cases.
  - For persistent ingrown toenails with or without infection, consider a referral to a podiatrist.
- Subungual hematoma
  - Determine whether a digital or regional nerve block is needed (proper training is required).
  - Attempt to lift the nail to examine for the presence of significant nailbed injuries.
  - Irrigate nail surface with saline solution, then clean with chlorhexidine or isopropyl alcohol.
  - Uncomplicated nail hematomas can be drained (nail trephination) by primary care providers. Make one or more holes in the area of the nail hematoma with either a portable heat cautery device or the end of an untwisted heated-to-red paperclip (heated to melt the nail). Ensure the holes are large enough to drain the hematoma. Remove the cautery device immediately after creating a hole to ensure that the underlying tissue is not cauterized, subsequently blocking the drainage of fluid.
  - Antibiotics generally are not needed. For open Tuft fractures, an oral antibiotic (typically a first-generation cephalosporin) is used to prevent infection, such as cellulitis or osteomyelitis.
  - Tuft fractures are often able to be managed in the primary care setting with orthopedic consult if needed. An aluminum splint can be used to immobilize a Tuft fracture for 2 to 3 weeks.
  - Nail injuries that involve lacerations or a crushing fracture of the distal phalanx should be referred to an orthopedist.
  - Home care includes educating patient and parent to monitor for signs of infection (increased redness, swelling, pain, or purulent drainage) and to return for further care if infection is suspected. Instruct soaking of affected nailbed three times per day with antibacterial soap until the drainage has stopped and the underlying skin has healed.

Lacerations

Description and Epidemiology

Lacerations are deep cuts to the skin caused by a wide variety of mechanisms and are most common on the face, scalp, and hands. Lacerations are one of the leading causes of ED visits (Hollander and Weinberger Conlon, 2014). Facial lacerations account for a significant proportion of lacerations seen in the pediatric population and occur more often in males than females (Hwang et al, 2013). Lacerations often require more complicated treatment than other minor wounds, because they can be associated with occult injuries to the deeper tissues and require careful exploration.

Shear, tension, and compression injuries are the three most common lacerations, result from varying mechanisms and have the potential to vary the treatment plan. Shear injuries are caused by sharp objects and tend to cause minimal, if any, damage to the tissues surrounding the injury. Shear injuries heal quickly and have the lowest potential for wound infection. The greatest danger of shear injuries is the potential for damage to nerve, tendon, and vascular structures that may require more complicated repair that should only be attempted in the ED or operating room by a skilled surgeon.

Tension lacerations are caused from stresses on the skin, usually secondary to the force of a blunt object at less than a 90-degree angle. The skin tears due to the stress and causes an irregularly shaped edge to the injury. These types of lacerations are accompanied by damage to surrounding tissues. A classic example is when a child falls and bumps his or her head on the dull edge of a piece of furniture, causing the skin to break open.

Compression lacerations are caused by a crush injury, usually involving blunt force of an object at a 90-degree angle. This type of laceration usually has irregular, often stellate wound edges. Compression injuries can cause significant injury to adjacent tissues and have the highest incidence of wound infections.

Assessment

History. Key questions to ask when assessing a laceration include:

- How did the injury happen? Determining the mechanism of injury is essential in identifying the potential extent of tissue damage, the presence of contaminants, and the possible presence of a foreign body, such as dirt, debris, glass, and splinters.
- How long ago (number of hours) did the injury occur? Length of time since injury can influence the treatment plan for the patient.
- Does the child have allergies to antibiotics or anesthetics?
- What is the child's tetanus immunization status? Is there a need for further immunization?

Physical Examination. Key points in the examination of a laceration include:

- Perform a neurovascular examination, including evaluation of pulses, motor function, and sensation distal to the laceration.
- Evaluate the range of motion, especially with wounds involving the distal forearm, wrist, and hand due to the high potential for tendon injury.
- Determine whether the wound edges approximate and note the degree of tension at the wound site.

Differential Diagnosis

The history and physical examination provide the diagnosis.

Management

Providers may repair the wound using sutures, staples, glue, or tape, as indicated. Minor lacerations to the scalp, arms, and legs are commonly managed by primary care providers. Significant wounds to the face, hands, or genital areas should be referred to a specialist, such as an orthopedic surgeon who specializes in hand repair, or a plastic surgeon for plastic and reconstructive surgery (particularly for the face).

The steps in wound management are summarized as follows (Selbst and Attia, 2010):

1. *Decision to close the wound:* Children are less likely than adults to get wound infections. In fact, the infection rate from sutured lacerations in children is 2%. Most wounds may be closed using a primary wound closure (i.e., bringing the edges of the skin together, known as "approximation") as soon after the injury as possible to speed healing, prevent infection, and improve the cosmetic result. Delayed closure increases the risk of infection. Some researchers suggest a "golden period" for wound closure of 6 hours. However, wounds considered low risk for infection, such as a clean knife wound to an extremity, can be closed even 12 to 24 hours after the injury. Other guidelines to consider in wound closure include the following:
   - Most facial wounds may be closed up to 24 hours after initial injury in order to provide the child with the most optimal cosmetic outcomes. Depending on the severity of the laceration or potential for infection (such as, a dog bite), repair and management may be best performed in the operating room.
   - Risk of infection is inversely related to the blood flow to the body part where the laceration occurs. The lower the blood flow, the higher the infection risk. For example, a hand or foot laceration is far more likely to become infected than a scalp laceration, because the extremities of the body have lower blood perfusion than the head and scalp.
   - Contaminated wounds, crush wounds, and lacerations in children who are immunocompromised are at high risk for infection and should be closed within 6 hours of injury.
   - Animal, human, or barnyard animal bites should be left open for healing by secondary intention, which is a process of healing by granulation and re-epithelialization. The potential of scar formation increases with this method, but the benefits of improved healing and decreased infection outweigh the cosmetic negative.
   - Delayed primary closure consists of closing of a wound 3 to 5 days after initial injury when the risk of infection decreases. This type of closure is

recommended for selected heavily contaminated wounds and those associated with extensive damage, such as high-velocity missile injuries, crush injuries, and explosion injuries. Initial management of such injuries should include wound cleansing, débridement, and a sterile dressing. Close follow-up is recommended in order to check for infection and for wound closure (Selbst and Attia, 2010).

2. *Anesthesia:* Appropriate use of local anesthetic and conscious sedation is essential for successful repair of lacerations in children. Proper wound care includes wound exploration and careful cleansing—both painful procedures made worse by fear and anxiety. Infiltration of the wound with local anesthetic, such as 1% lidocaine with or without epinephrine (depending on location of laceration), can also help control bleeding. LET (lidocaine, epinephrine, tetracaine), LAT (lidocaine, adrenaline, tetracaine), and TAC (tetracaine, adrenaline, cocaine) are topical solutions placed on minor wounds 20 to 30 minutes prior to cleansing or repair procedures to help with pain management and to control bleeding. Topical solutions such as these cannot be used on eyes, ears, nose, fingers, genitals, or toes. Textbooks are available that address procedures in primary care that include excellent information on local anesthetic and wound closure. It is also helpful for clinicians to attend workshops that focus on wound management.
3. *Hair:* Hair near the wound usually creates minimal difficulty during repair and generally does not need to be removed. In any case, hair should not be shaved because to do so can damage hair follicles and increase the risk of infection. Instead, the hair should be clipped with scissors when necessary. Alternatively, petroleum jelly can be used to keep unwanted scalp hair away from the wound while suturing. Eyebrow hair should not be removed because this may lead to abnormal or slow regrowth.
4. *Wound cleansing:* The preferred method of wound cleansing is *irrigation* to reduce bacterial contamination and prevent subsequent infection. Normal saline or safe tap water may be used for wound irrigation (Fernandez and Griffiths, 2012). A general rule for the volume needed for saline irrigation is to use 50 to 100 mL of normal saline per centimeter of the wound or laceration. More solution may be needed if the wound is unusually large or contaminated. Use a large irrigating syringe (20 to 50 mL) to provide enough force to cleanse the wound. A splash guard attached to the syringe is recommended to reduce splatter during irrigation. *Scrubbing* the wound should be reserved only for particularly "dirty" wounds when irrigation does not remove contaminants completely. Forceps may also be required to remove foreign debris from the wound when saline irrigation is unsuccessful. It is important to remove all foreign debris to decrease infection risk and prevent tattooing of the skin. Chlorhexidine or povidone-iodine surgical scrub preparations may be used to clean the skin *surrounding* the wound but are not recommended for use in the wound itself. Hydrogen peroxide and alcohol are also not recommended for wound cleansing. These agents may be irritating to tissues, causing slow healing times, and may increase infection by damaging white blood cells.
5. *Wound exploration:* The wound must be explored for presence of foreign bodies, deep tissue layer damage, injury to nerve or blood vessel, or joint involvement. It is imperative that the wound depth be determined. Wound probing is done with a cotton-tipped swab, a hemostat, or a needle holder. Deep lacerations should be referred to an ED for layered closure. If tendon injury is suspected or if bone is exposed, referral to an orthopedist is the standard of care.
6. *Wound débridement:* Gentle removal of unattached loose tissues may be done with sterile instruments. Débridement is advantageous because it helps to remove contaminant from the wound and creates more approximated wound edges. The approximation of wound edges allows for easier wound repair and cosmetic acceptability for the patient after the wound heals. Although it is helpful to excise necrotic skin, excessive trimming of irregular lacerations should not be attempted. Excessive removal of tissue can create a defect that is difficult to close or that may increase tension at the wound margin, making scarring more likely.
7. *Wound closure:* Several methods are available for wound closure.
   - *Traditional stitches* (or sutures) are often used to close lacerations. This involves "sewing" the skin together with a needle and surgical thread. This procedure usually requires an injection and/or topical use of an anesthetic and bandaging the wound afterward. Simple, uncomplicated lacerations to the scalp, trunk, arms, or legs may be closed with sutures (called *primary closure*). Choice of suture material and type of stitch used is dependent on the wound itself. In general, an absorbable suture material is used for closure of structures deeper than the epidermis, and nonabsorbable sutures are used to close the outermost layer of a laceration. Deep sutures promote more efficient healing of the wound by relieving skin tension and decreasing dead space. The wound type determines the size of the suture material. Wounds on the face require a smaller size, such as a 6.0 tensile strength; wounds over joints, the trunk, and extremities require a stronger tensile strength size, such as a 3.0, 4.0, or 5.0.
   - *Staples* can be used for the scalp, trunk, and extremities (not including the hands and feet) and provide a more rapid closure time than with sutures. Laceration repair with staples is associated with a lower infection rate but can be more painful to remove and also may not result in as cosmetically appealing

a closure after the wound has healed. Staples should not be used if MRI or CT is going to be necessary.
- *Surgical tape,* such as Steri-Strips, is used for small superficial wounds. Surgical tape cannot be used on wounds in moist areas or in areas of tension, such as flexor or extensor surfaces. Surgical tape should also be avoided in wounds on small children, who will most likely remove the tape prematurely.
- *Topical skin adhesive,* also known as *skin glue,* is used for simple lacerations with clean edges. The adhesive is applied on top of the skin while the edges of the wound are held together. Usually two or three applications of the adhesive are applied to ensure adequate closure. Adhesive in the wound or between wound margins should be avoided. Skin glue takes less time to apply than stitches and forms a strong, flexible bond over the top of the wound. Topical skin adhesive should not be used on areas of skin where there is tension, such as over a joint, due to the high probability of the wound reopening and thus requiring healing by secondary closure, causing increased risk of scarring. A bandage is not required for cover after tissue repair with skin glue. The topical skin adhesive sloughs off the wound as it heals, usually in 7 to 10 days, and does not require a return visit for suture removal. Infection risk is minimal due to antimicrobial properties of the adhesive. Minimal scarring is associated with this method of laceration repair.

8. *Dressing:* A simple repaired laceration may be covered with an adhesive bandage. For more complex repaired injuries, dress the wound with nonadherent gauze for the first layer followed by a second layer of plain gauze if needed and secured in place with adhesive tape or elasticized gauze (tubular net bandage).
9. *Immunization:* Give tetanus booster or tetanus immunoglobulin as indicated.
10. *Antibiotic controversy:* Antibiotic prophylaxis of clean wounds is not indicated. Its use in contaminated wounds may be helpful, but careful wound cleaning with extensive irrigation followed by prompt wound closure (when indicated) are the most effective safeguards in preventing infection. See the Bites and Stings section in this chapter for specific antibiotic coverage indicated for lacerations.
11. *Suture and staple removal:* The timing for removal of staples and sutures depends on their location (Table 40-2).

Patient and Parent Education

Instructions for wound care at home are best given in writing and should include the following information:

- Patient can briefly shower 48 hours after sutures are in place without worrying about the risk of possible infection. However, dry the area well and keep it dry at all times after showering.

TABLE 40-2 Suture and Staple Removal Guide

Location of Sutures	Length of Time Before Removal
Facial	3-5 days
Scalp	7-10 days
Upper extremity	7-10 days
Trunk	10 days
Lower extremity	8-10 days
Over a joint	10-14 days

- Note signs and symptoms of infection that warrant an early recheck (redness, swelling, discharge, increased pain).
- Give instructions about cleansing and bandaging the wound; instructions vary based on severity of the wound. For surgical tape and topical skin adhesive, do not use topical antibiotic ointment or lotions because they will remove the adhesive.
- List any restrictions on activities.
- Identify a date for a return appointment.

Burns

Description and Epidemiology

According to the CDC, every day more than 300 children from birth to 19 years old are treated in emergency rooms for burn-related injuries and two children die from burns or burn complications in the United States (CDC, 2012b). Intentionally inflicting burns to a child is, unfortunately, a common form of abuse, and every burn injury in a child should be evaluated for a potential etiology of abuse or neglect. Intentionally inflicted burn injuries often leave a characteristic pattern.

Common causes of burn injuries include grills, hot soups, hot water, curling irons, house fires, and appliances, such as hot stoves or coffee pots. Serious injury or death frequently occurs among children who are injured in residential fires (Joffe, 2013). Younger children tend to sustain more scald injuries from steam or hot liquid, and older children tend to incur burns more often from flame and direct contact with fire (CDC, 2012b). Scald burns have the potential to cause deeper injuries, depending on how long the skin is in contact with the substance. The longer the contact, the deeper the scald burn is. Thermal burns in children are deeper, involving more layers of the skin than the same burn in adults due to children having thinner skin than adults.

A burn injury to one or more layers of the skin and underlying tissues causes varying degrees of damage. Burns are classified by depth of injury, percentage of body surface area (BSA) involved, location of the burn, and association with other injuries. The classification system for burns has changed from first, second, and third degree to superficial,

superficial (partial or deep), and full thicknesses in order to better identify the need for surgical intervention. The term *fourth-degree burn* has not been changed and is designated to identify burns that extend into the muscle, fascia, and/or bone and are potentially life-threatening (Rice and Orgill, n.d.).

- Superficial burns involve only the epidermis. The skin is erythematous, inflamed, and painful, but there are no blisters. Superficial burns typically heal in 3 to 7 days, have little risk of scarring, and require only symptomatic treatment. Sunburn is a common example of a superficial burn.
- Partial-thickness burns involve the epidermis and the dermis to a variable degree. The dermal appendages are always preserved and provide a source for regeneration.
  - Superficial partial-thickness burns are red, very painful, mottled, moist, and blistered. These burns usually heal in 7 to 14 days, and scarring may occur.
  - Deep partial-thickness burns appear pale and yellow. These burns are less painful and weepy than superficial partial-thickness burns. Deep partial-thickness burns take longer to heal (3 weeks), and scarring is more likely to occur.
- Full-thickness burns are major thermal injuries in which the epidermis and dermis are completely destroyed. The skin appears whitish (a waxy white appearance) or leathery. The surface is dry and nontender to palpation. Fluid losses can be profound with this degree of burn. Full-thickness burns usually require skin grafting, are associated with permanent scarring, and take several weeks to heal.
- Full-thickness burns with extension into deep tissues, also known as *fourth-degree burns,* involve destruction and/or extensive injury of muscle, fascia, nerves, tendons, vessels, and bone. They typically require surgical intervention and skin grafting.

Burns involving large surfaces of the body generally vary as to their degree of depth. Burn wounds are dynamic, and the effect of dermal ischemia (affected by infection, exposure, and dehydration) may not be readily apparent at first. Their depth can change from day to day. The percentage of BSA and the part(s) of the body affected are also key factors to determine treatment, disposition, and prognosis (Table 40-3). Multiple methods have been devised to estimate the BSA affected. For example, the area covered by a child's palm (from wrist crease to finger crease), also called the "rule of the palm," is considered to represent 1% of total BSA (TBSA) and may be used for estimating the extent of small burns covering less than 10% of BSA (Antoon and Donovan, 2011). Free software to calculate BSA in pediatric burn victims is available at www.sagediagram.com/.

Assessment

History. The following information should be obtained:

- Description of how the burn occurred, including agent of injury and length of time agent was in contact with the skin, circumstances surrounding the injury, when it occurred, and likelihood of other injuries, such as trauma or smoke inhalation
- Initial and subsequent treatment of the burn
- Previous history of burn injuries
- Other current medical problems, medications, allergies, and tetanus status
- Suspicion of child abuse if the injury does not match the history and mechanism described (see Chapter 17)

Physical Examination. The physical examination should begin by conducting a primary assessment of the airway. The most common cause of death during the first hour after a burn injury is respiratory impairment. Inhalation injury produces upper airway edema that can proceed with alarming speed to complete airway obstruction. Children with any sign of airway compromise should immediately be placed on 100% oxygen via a nonrebreather mask and transported to the hospital via ambulance and emergency medical services (EMS) for further care and management. Airway complications should be suspected if there is loss of consciousness, death of another victim, presence of facial or neck burns, burns or soot over the nasal passages or oral cavity, or presence of cough, wheezes, or crackles on auscultation (Mandel and Hales, n.d.). Once the patient is stable, a thorough physical examination requires the following determinations:

- Percentage of BSA affected (see Table 40-3)
- Type of burn and associated injuries
- Distribution and pattern of the burn with particular concern for circumferential burns to the thorax that may cause poor chest expansion and declining oxygen saturation
- Burn depth—classified as superficial, partial thickness, or full thickness
- Assessment of the vascular status of extremities
- Presence of any complicating medical condition

Diagnostic Studies

- A CBC is indicated to establish baseline levels. The hematocrit is often elevated secondary to fluid loss. Initial elevation of the white blood cell count is most always secondary to an acute phase reaction, but later may be an indicator of infection.
- A basic metabolic panel may reveal elevated potassium due to cell breakdown. Blood urea nitrogen (BUN) and creatine kinase are used to assess renal function, rhabdomyolysis, and tissue perfusion.
- A urinalysis, particularly the specific gravity, helps determine hydration status, and presence of myoglobin may suggest acute tubular necrosis secondary to muscle tissue destruction and breakdown.
- Baseline clotting studies and typing and crossmatching may be indicated if there is associated trauma or if surgical intervention, such as grafting, is considered.
- Pulse oximetry, arterial blood gases, carboxyhemoglobin (for inhalation or suspected inhalation injury), and chest radiographs are indicated if there is airway involvement or vascular instability.

TABLE 40-3 Estimation of Surface Area Burned Based on Age*

Area	Age (Years) Birth to 1	1 to 4	5 to 9	10 to 14	15	Adult
Head	19	17	13	11	9	7
Neck	2	2	2	2	2	2
Anterior trunk	13	13	13	13	13	13
Posterior trunk	13	13	13	13	13	13
Right buttock	2.5	2.5	2.5	2.5	2.5	2.5
Left buttock	2.5	2.5	2.5	2.5	2.5	2.5
Genitalia	1	1	1	1	1	1
Right upper arm	4	4	4	4	4	4
Left upper arm	4	4	4	4	4	4
Right lower arm	3	3	3	3	3	3
Left lower arm	3	3	3	3	3	3
Right hand	2.5	2.5	2.5	2.5	2.5	2.5
Left hand	2.5	2.5	2.5	2.5	2.5	2.5
Right thigh	5.5	6.5	8	8.5	9	9.5
Left thigh	5.5	6.5	8	8.5	9	9.5
Right leg	5	5	5.5	6	6.5	7
Left leg	5	5	5.5	6	6.5	7
Right foot	3.5	3.5	3.5	3.5	3.5	3.5
Left foot	3.5	3.5	3.5	3.5	3.5	3.5

From Joffe MD: Burns. In Fleisher GR, Ludwig S, Henretig FM, et al, editors: *Textbook of pediatric emergency medicine,* ed 6, Philadelphia, 2010, Lippincott Williams & Wilkins, p 1285.

*This modification by O'Neill of the Brooke Army Burn Center Diagram shows the change in surface area of the head from 19% in an infant to 7% in an adult. Proper use of this chart provides an accurate basis for subsequent management of the burned child.

- Cardiac monitoring may be needed for electrical burn injury and as otherwise indicated.
- Culturing of critical burn wounds may need to be done weekly or more frequently if infection develops.

Differential Diagnosis

Chapter 17 discusses intentional burn injuries resulting from child abuse. Scalded skin syndrome caused by staphylococcal infection can cause skin exfoliation, but the clinical presentation clearly differentiates it from an accidental burn injury. Management is similar to that used for burn management.

Management

Determining the need for admission to a hospital or burn center involves many factors, including burn depth, percentage of BSA injured, and mechanism of the burn injury. Other factors that influence hospital or burn center admission include risk of infection, pain control, functional and cosmetic outcomes, and social considerations. Children with burn injuries who meet the following criteria should be admitted to the hospital or burn center for further management (Krennerich, 2015; Mandt and Grubenhoff, 2014):

- Burns involving more than 20% TBSA
- Partial-thickness burns involving more than 10% TBSA
- Full-thickness burns involving more than 2% TBSA
- Circumferential burns
- Burns involving critical areas, such as the hands and feet, genitalia, and perineum; and burns overlying joints
- Full-thickness burns
- Chemical burns, electrical burns (including lightning injury), inhalation injury
- Suspicion of child abuse or unsafe home environment
- Presence of an underlying chronic illness

The outpatient treatment of minor burns is an option only for superficial burns (first degree) and partial-thickness burns (second degree) to less than 10% of BSA. Referral and consultation with a burn specialist should be made depending on the severity and location of the burn. Box 40-1 outlines the primary care management of superficial and partial-thickness burns.

• BOX 40-1 Management of Superficial and Partial-Thickness Burns in the Primary Care Setting

1. Maintain proper nutrition and hydration to enhance healing.
2. Management of superficial burns (Morgan and Miser, n.d.):
   - Cleanse the burn and surrounding skin with lukewarm water and soap.
   - Burns with an intact epidermis, such as superficial or superficial partial thickness wounds, do not require a topical antimicrobial agent.
   - A nonadherent dressing, such as Adaptic, followed by a gauze dressing may be applied for larger more severe superficial burns and changed twice a day or when soiled if risk of infection is present, such as on a hand. Otherwise leave the superficial burn open to air.
   - Aloe vera has some antibacterial properties and may be used to help with healing and soothing the skin. Lanolin may cause itching and is best not to use.
   - Administer analgesics, such as acetaminophen or ibuprofen, as indicated for pain relief.
3. Management of superficial partial-thickness burns (Morgan and Miser, n.d.):
   - Administer adequate analgesic medication. Narcotics may be needed before wound care is performed and during the day. Switch to over-the-counter acetaminophen or ibuprofen as the pain subsides.
   - Cleanse the wound with mild soap and tap water.
   - Monitor the burn daily for the first few days to ensure proper healing, and assess for infection. Dressing changes and wound cleansing with débridement should be performed twice a day or as needed for soaked or soiled dressings until the burn has healed.
   - If bullae or blisters are present and intact, leave them intact. They act as a natural bandage to keep bacteria out. Most bullae or blisters open eventually on their own, but while left intact, they protect the underlying skin from infection and allow time for internal healing.
   - Gently débride open blisters to remove devitalized tissue and residue from prior dressing changes.
   - Superficial partial thickness burns with an intact epidermis do not require a topical antimicrobial agent.
   - For any nonsuperficial burn to prevent infection, apply bacitracin or 1% silver sulfadiazine cream to the clean débrided area followed by the application of sterile petrolatum gauze. Next apply a dry gauze outer dressing. Do not apply a circumferential gauze wrap because of the risk of impaired circulation if swelling occurs. Instead, tubular stretch gauze netting may be used to hold the dressing in place.
   - Do not use 1% silver sulfadiazine if the patient has a sulfa allergy or if the burn is on the face. This product is an antimicrobial and soothing agent but has the potential to stain skin, which is why its use should be avoided on facial burns.
   - Biologic and or synthetic dressings may be more beneficial depending on the burn. Consult with a burn specialist if considering use.
   - Itching occurs commonly during the healing process triggered oftentimes by activity, heat, and stress. Use mittens for young children to prevent scratching if itching occurs. If needed, administer an antihistamine, such as diphenhydramine.
   - If a partial-thickness burn involves an extremity, keep it elevated to reduce edema and compromise of blood flow to the burned area. Individuals with circumferential burns of an extremity may need to be admitted to the hospital for observation so that compartment syndrome does not develop.
   - Another option for partial thickness burn management is the use of Aquacel Ag dressing (ConvaTec). Aquacel Ag is a dressing that is impregnated with silver ion, which helps prevent infection. Apply the Aquacel Ag after cleansing and débridement of the burn is complete. Cover the burned area with sterile gauze and leave in place for 7 days, with close wound monitoring (Tenenhaus and Rennekampff, 2014).

Patient and Parent Education

The following points are important components of patient and parent education:

- Emphasize use of sunscreen protection to prevent sunburn. This is very important for skin that is recovering from a burn because the skin is prone to hyperpigmentation from sunlight for up to a year following the burn injury. All skin that has been burned should be protected from sun for at least 12 months. Encourage parents to protect their child from excessive sun exposure, to avoid exposure as much as possible between 10 AM and 3 PM when the risk of sunburn is higher, and to use a sunscreen with a sun protection factor (SPF) of 25 (or higher) if sun exposure is unavoidable.
- Discuss home and environmental safety issues related to burn prevention at health maintenance visits. Key points to discuss with families include (CDC, 2012b):
  - Install and maintain smoke alarms in the home on every floor and near rooms where people sleep.
  - Keep the hot water heater thermostat at 120° F or lower.
  - Never leave cooking food on the stove or hot food unattended.
  - Create and practice a family fire escape plan for the home.
- Reinforce safety issues after a burn injury has occurred (e.g., scald prevention, safekeeping of matches and cigarette lighters, safe use of electric cords and outlets).
- Teach first-aid measures for burns (e.g., submerge minor burned area in tepid water; do not use butter, margarine, and oil-based creams and lotions; rinse chemical burns in cold water, and flush skin thoroughly for at least 20 minutes).
- Inform parents of serious or long-term consequences of burns: frequent and significant sunburns during early childhood can predispose to skin cancers in later life; electric burns cause thermal injury to skin (contact burn); if an arc is created and there is passage of electrical

current through the body, there is a potential for cardiac dysrhythmias and neurologic impairment following the burn.
- Inform parents that the extent of scarring is difficult to predict with certainty; that scarring depends on depth of the burn, length of time needed for healing, whether grafting was done, and the child's age and skin color; and that scars remain immature for the first 12 to 18 months and go through color and texture changes as the child grows. Most minor scald injuries from hot liquids heal quickly with little or no scarring.

Contusions and Hematomas

Description and Epidemiology

A contusion, or bruise, is an injury in which the skin is not broken but trauma has caused effusion into muscle and subcutaneous tissue with injury to the vessels and possibly the nerves. In children, contusions can occur anywhere on the body but are most often seen on the extremities.

Contusions are common in children and are caused by blunt trauma, most often as a result of falling or bumping into objects during play. Participation in contact sports puts children at increased risk for contusions. Bruises to the trunk, face, or head should raise a red flag for possible child abuse. A careful history must be taken to determine whether the explanation of the injury is consistent with the child's condition and his or her independent report of what happened.

Hematomas are localized collections of extravasated blood that are relatively or completely confined within a space or potential space. In essence, a hematoma is a raised, palpable ecchymosis or bruise. Hematomas can be associated with most types of minor and major wounds; they must be observed closely for signs of infection and, in some instances, drained.

Assessment

History. The following should be assessed:
- Cause of bruise
- Treatment given
- History of easy bleeding or bruising, or slow healing

Physical Examination. The following should be determined:
- Circulatory status and discoloration
- Motor and sensory function: sensation, mobility, and range of motion
- Involvement of underlying structures
- Presence of swelling
- Pain or point tenderness

If there is any evidence of circulatory compromise, such as lack of pulse, it is important to seek care in the ED immediately.

Differential Diagnosis

Hemophilia, von Willebrand disease, and purpura should be considered. Myositis ossificans, a complication of contusions rarely seen in children, can be confused with osteogenic sarcoma.

Management

For contusions involving extremities:
1. Acute treatment of contusions (Buttaravoli and Leffler, 2012):
   - Prescribe rest, ice, compression, and elevation (RICE):
     - Rest and restrict movement of the affected part utilizing an Ace wrap or splint as needed to maximize immobilization.
     - Ice (a bag of ice wrapped in a towel) should be applied to the injury for 10 to 20 minutes every 1 to 3 hours for the first 24 hours. Never apply ice directly to the skin.
     - Compression: Apply a pressure bandage, such as an Ace wrap, to help prevent swelling. Ensure the bandage or wrap is not too tight to ensure proper circulation.
     - Elevate the affected body part (ideally, above the level of the heart) to prevent swelling.
   - Provide appropriate analgesia. Acetaminophen with or without hydrocodone, or a nonsteroidal anti-inflammatory drug (NSAID), such as ibuprofen, is a good choice. NSAID use should be limited to the first 2 to 3 days after the injury.
2. From 24 to 48 hours after the acute phase of tenderness and swelling:
   - Warm compress use has limited benefit and should not be recommended for treatment (Buttaravoli and Leffler, 2012).
   - Do range-of-motion and strengthening exercises.
3. For 5 to 7 days, avoid exercise that involves the contused area.
4. Key management points to remember:
   - Reserve radiographs for suspected foreign bodies or bone fracture.
   - Refer severe injuries for orthopedic management.

Complications

Most contusions heal quickly without sequelae, but severe trauma to the quadriceps muscle can lead to myositis ossificans if not treated properly or, with large hemorrhage, to compartment syndrome.

Patient and Parent Education

Explain to parents the expected color changes of ecchymosis from purple discoloration to greenish and that the ecchymosis may also migrate to other surrounding tissues. Arrange for follow-up if discomfort continues or increases. Encourage parents to provide their children with a physical environment that minimizes risk of injury. Return to activities is determined by the degree of injury and resolution of subjective symptoms. Physical or occupational therapy may be needed for larger muscle contusions to assist in return to full function (Buttaravoli and Leffler, 2012). Table 40-4 provides a list of prevention strategies for

TABLE 40-4 Common Injuries and Prevention Strategies

Medical Condition	Prevention Strategies	Comments
Lacerations/ contusions/ abrasions	• Protective equipment is essential.	These injuries are mostly related to baseball (contusion/ abrasion), soccer, cycling, and ice hockey (lacerations).
Blisters	• Wear socks. • Wear properly fitted shoes. • Use powder, petroleum jelly, or a product, such as Second Skin, on reddened or at-risk areas.	

contusions, as well as other minor injuries that can occur among children.

Bites and Stings

Animal and Child Bites

Description and Epidemiology

Children can be bitten by pets, stray animals, or humans, especially other children. Most animal bites are to the head and neck in infants and very young children and to the upper extremities in older children. In contrast, most bites caused by other young children occur on the upper extremities.

Each year, an estimated 1% of ED visits during the summer months are due to animal or human bite wounds (AAP, 2014). About 80% to 90% of bites are dog bites (both provoked and unprovoked) (Ginsburg, 2011). Boys are attacked more often than girls. Dog and cat bites are often caused by animals known to the child. The risk of infection from a dog bite is between 2% and 15%. The risk of infection from a cat bite (despite early medical attention) is at least 50%. Cat bites cause puncture wounds and tend to be deeper than dog bites. Dog bites can cause abrasions, puncture wounds, and lacerations, with or without an associated avulsion of tissue. Limited data define the incidence of human bite injuries, but it is suspected that human bites are the leading cause of injury in child care centers. All human bite wounds, regardless of mechanism of injury, should be considered at high risk for infection. Other animal bites, such as rat bites, are not reportable, so there is a paucity of information about their epidemiology (Ginsburg, 2011). Clenched-fist bites are the most serious of human bites and typically are the result of fighting. In this type of injury, the closed fist hits the teeth of another resulting in laceration(s) of the skin typically over the third and fourth metacarpals. These human bite injuries are high risk for infection and joint compromise.

Assessment

History. Ask about the circumstances surrounding the bite including the type of animal, domesticated or feral animal, provoked or unprovoked attack, and location of the attack. History of drug allergies and immunization status of the child also should be ascertained.

Physical Examination. The wound should be assessed for the type, size, and depth of injury. Explore for the presence of foreign material and the status of underlying structures. If the bite is on an extremity, assess its range of motion and sensory intactness. Likewise, assess functioning of the facial nerve with deep facial bite injuries. At minimum, a diagram of the injury should be recorded in the child's chart (Ginsburg, 2011). If possible, it is best to photograph the injury for documentation.

Diagnostic Studies. Aerobic and anaerobic cultures should be obtained from wounds exhibiting signs of infection (Buttaravoli and Leffler, 2012). A radiograph of the affected part should be obtained if it is likely that a bone or joint could have been penetrated or fractured or if retained foreign material may be present.

Differential Diagnosis

The differential diagnosis includes lacerations or puncture wounds from other causes.

Management

Management involves both physical and psychological care of the child and includes the following (Mandt and Grubenhoff, 2014):

- Administer tetanus booster and rabies prophylaxis if indicated (consult with local animal control or public health department).
- Provide/administer appropriate analgesia or anesthesia.
- Débride avulsed or devitalized tissue and remove foreign matter.
- Using normal saline, irrigate the wounds using high pressure (greater than 4 pounds per square inch) and high volume (greater than 1 L).
  - Isolated puncture wounds should not be irrigated, instead soak the wound in a diluted solution of tap water and povidone-iodine for 15 minutes.
- Prescribe a 3- to 5-day course of prophylactic antibiotics for all human and cat bites, and for the following types of bite or wound characteristics: hand, puncture, overlying bone fracture, substantial crushing tissue injuries or if requiring débridement, or those involving tendons, muscles, or joint spaces. In addition, antibiotic coverage is needed for wounds in children who are immunosuppressed. For outpatients, prescribe a broad-spectrum antibiotic, such as amoxicillin clavulanate (first choice). Penicillin-allergic individuals should be treated with an extended spectrum cephalosporin or trimethoprim-sulfamethoxazole plus clindamycin (Hodge, 2010).

- Rabies exposure prophylaxis also should be considered if there is any question about possible exposure. The CDC provides guidelines on prophylaxis for possible rabies (see Additional Resources). The local health department is also a good resource for guidance on postexposure prophylaxis for rabies.
- Some controversy exists over whether bite wounds should be closed primarily with delayed closure (3 to 5 days after injury) or allowed to heal by secondary intention (leaving the wound open). Factors to consider are the type, size, and depth of the wound; the anatomic location; presence of infection; the time interval since the injury; and the potential for cosmetic disfigurement. Surgical consultation should be obtained for all deep or extensive wounds and those involving the bones, joints, or hands. Because of the excellent blood supply to the face, facial lacerations are at less risk for infection. Many plastic surgeons advocate primary closure of facial bite wounds that have been brought to medical attention within 5 to 6 hours and have been thoroughly irrigated and débrided. Because of concern about scarring, the provider may refer facial wounds for plastic surgery repair.
  - There is consensus that bites involving the hand or foot should not be sutured but allowed to drain. Hand and foot bites less than 1.5 cm are best left to heal by secondary intention; bites greater than 1.5 cm should have delayed primary closure.
  - Bite wounds more than 8 to 12 hours old should not be sutured except for facial wounds that can be sutured up to 24 hours, maximum.
  - A single layer of nonabsorbable sutures is best (avoid multiple closure layers).
    - Refer children with severe bites. Obtain a surgical consult if there is evidence of or concern about nerve, tendon, and/or ligament injury or if a joint space was involved. Hospitalization, reconstructive surgery, and long-term follow-up may be indicated.
    - Discuss the child's fears and management of any behavioral problems that may result (see Chapter 19).
    - Report dog and wild animal bites to animal control.

Complications

Secondary infection is the most common complication of mammalian bites and can lead to cellulitis and lymphangitis, requiring hospitalization. *Streptococcus* and *Staphylococcus* are common organisms associated with infected animal and human bites; anaerobic infection is also possible. Species of gram-negative bacteria (such as, *P. multocida* from dog and cat bites and *Eikenella corrodens* from human bites) can also cause infections (Krennerich, 2015). The potential for rabies, human immunodeficiency virus (HIV), and hepatitis B and C exposure must also be considered.

Patient and Parent Education

Preventive education and actions should include the following:

- Teach children to avoid stray animals, be cautious around domesticated animals, and not tease or provoke any animal.
- Emphasize the importance of parental supervision of children as they play with pets.
- Do not keep typically wild animals as pets in families with very young children.
- Do not allow pets to roam freely.
- Never leave infants or young children alone with dogs or cats; animals with histories of aggression are inappropriate in households with children.
- Report stray animals promptly to animal control officials.

Hymenoptera

Description and Epidemiology

Bees, hornets, yellow jackets, fire and harvester ants, and wasps belong to the Hymenoptera order of insects and have common antigens in their venom. Among the Hymenoptera order, the Vespidae (hornets, wasps and yellow jackets), Apidae (honeybees and bumblebees), and Formicidae (fire ants) generally can cause allergic reaction from their sting. Cross-reactivity of the allergens present within family venoms occurs for all except the Apidae family (Casale and Burks, 2014). Immunoglobulin E–dependent hypersensitivity is the underlying cause of reactions. Histamines, leukotrienes, prostaglandins, and other inflammatory factors are released, causing local or systemic symptoms.

Bees and wasps ordinarily do not sting unless frightened, bothered, or hurt. Yellow jackets are aggressive. Fire ants may cause multiple, painful stings. Reactions to stings by these insects can vary from mild, local responses to life-threatening anaphylaxis with wheezing and urticaria. Most children experience only a local reaction, but some children suffer severe systemic reactions, which can progress to medical emergencies unless prompt intervention is initiated.

Assessment

History. The child usually reports being bitten or stung. There may be a past history of a local or systemic reaction following an insect bite.

Physical Examination. Findings include the following:

- Mild reaction consists of local redness, pruritus, pain, edema, and possibly generalized urticaria.
- Severe reactions, including anaphylaxis, are characterized by local signs, plus any of the following:
  - Watery eyes
  - Hives
  - Difficulty in breathing, wheezing
  - Difficulty swallowing
  - Hoarseness, thickened speech
  - Gastrointestinal disturbances, abdominal pain
  - Dizziness, weakness, confusion
  - Collapse, unconsciousness, even death

    - Fire ant bites are characterized by vesicles that develop into sterile pustules

Diagnostic Studies. Diagnosis of a Hymenoptera order of insect sting acutely is usually based on history and physical examination alone. For systemic reactions, refer to an immune-allergist for venom-specific immunoglobulin E testing and identification after resolution of the reaction.

Differential Diagnosis

Other insect bites or dermatologic eruptions that produce similar symptoms are included in the differential diagnosis.

Management

The following steps are taken:

- For *mild local* reactions:
    - If the stinger is visible, flick it off with the edge of a sharp object (e.g., knife blade or credit card), taking care to not squeeze the attached venom sac.
    - Apply cool compresses locally or cool baths.
    - Administer an antihistamine, such as diphenhydramine at 1 to 2 mg/kg per dose every 4 to 6 hours (37.5 mg/day maximum under 5 years old; 150 mg/day 6 to 11 years old; 300 mg/day maximum for over 12 years old), or hydroxyzine 2 mg/kg/day, in divided doses every 6 to 8 hours daily (50 mg/day maximum under 6 years old; 50 to 100 mg/day maximum over 6 years old), for treatment of pruritus.
    - Topical glucocorticoid creams or ointments may help to reduce itching.
- For *moderate* to *severe* reactions:
    - Moderate reactions may need to be treated with oral antihistamines, corticosteroids, and inhaled bronchodilators (if wheezing).
    - Institute emergency measures for treatment of anaphylactic reactions and transport to the ED as quickly as possible.
    - Hospitalize for anaphylactic shock.
- Epinephrine: 0.01 mg/kg (0.01 mL/kg/dose of 1:1000 aqueous epinephrine per dose intramuscularly in the mid-anterolateral aspect of the thigh; maximum dose of 0.5 mg in adults and 0.3 mg in children). Dose may be repeated every 5 to 15 minutes if the patient has recurrent or refractory symptoms. Usually the patient will respond after one or two doses (Casale and Burks, 2014; Simons et al, 2012).
- Antihistamines should be given immediately following epinephrine (and repeated every 6 hours for up to 3 days) but not as a substitute for epinephrine; give both histamine type 1 (H_1) and type 2 (H_2) blockers. Administration of both H_1 and H_2 blockers together has been shown to help alleviate histamine-mediated symptoms better than when H_1 blockers have been used alone (Shahzad Mustafa, n.d.). Give diphenhydramine 1 to 2 mg/kg; up to 50 mg intravenous (IV) for the H_1 blocker and ranitidine 1 mg/kg up to 50 mg IV for the H_2 blocker (Covar et al, 2014).
- Glucocorticoids are not helpful in treating acute reactions but may help to prevent a potential late phase reaction also known as *biphasic anaphylaxis* (Covar et al, 2014; Shahzad Mustafa, n.d.).
- Give IV methylprednisolone (1 mg/kg every 4 to 6 hours to a maximum of 50 mg for a child, 50 to 100 mg for adults), or for less severe reactions oral prednisolone (1 mg/kg; 50 mg maximum) (Covar et al, 2014).
- Nebulized albuterol (2.5 to 5 mg/dose) should be given either with a metered dose inhaler (MDI) or a nebulizer in patients with a history of asthma and/or those who present with bronchospasm or wheezing (Cheng, 2011).
- IV fluids should be administered if the child is hypotensive as a result of anaphylactic shock.
- Administer high-flow oxygen (warm humidified) by non-rebreather mask.
- Tracheostomy should be performed if laryngeal edema is life threatening.

Referral to an allergist is indicated for any child who has life-threatening respiratory symptoms (e.g., stridor or wheezing) or hypotension. Venom immunotherapy desensitization is highly effective (98% protective) in preventing further systemic reactions. Children younger than 16 years old who have only urticaria or angioedema do not require venom immunotherapy, because only 10% of these children will have systemic reactions with subsequent stings.

Patient and Parent Education

Key issues to discuss with moderate to severe reactions include the following:

- Importance of wearing a medical alert tag or bracelet
- Proper use of an insect sting kit that includes two self-injectable epinephrine pens and the need to have a kit always readily available for emergency use
- Prevention of stings by avoiding areas likely to be infested with these insects, not wearing bright-colored clothing, and not using perfumed products

Mosquitoes, Fleas, and Chiggers (Red Bug or Harvest Mites)

Description and Epidemiology

Mosquito bites are the most common insect bites for infants and children. Mosquitoes are the vectors of many important diseases in humans and cause irritating local skin reactions when they bite. Similarly, flea and chigger (also known as *red bug* or *harvest mite*) bites produce local skin eruptions.

Fleas that commonly attack humans in the United States include the human flea, cat flea, and dog flea. The six-legged larvae of harvest mites are responsible for the skin eruption characteristic of chigger bites. Harvest mites live on grain stems, shrubs, grass, and vines. As humans or animals pass by, the larvae attach themselves to the skin and inject an irritating secretion. The harvest mites then drop to the ground or are scratched off within 1 to 2 days. There is a seasonal pattern to mosquito, flea, and chigger bites.

Assessment

History. The following may be reported:

- Mosquito or flea bites
  - Known mosquito or flea bite or seasonal time
  - Presence of cat, dog or furry animal in child's environment
  - Complaints of a brief stinging sensation followed by itching
- Chigger bites
  - Complaints of itching followed by dermatitis
  - History of playing or walking in grassy areas, parks, or other harvest mite habitat near woods and water

Physical Examination. Mosquito bites are characterized by the following:

- Local irritation in unsensitized children
- Urticarial wheals that itch and last several hours to days in sensitized children or firm papules or nodules that last a long time
- Central punctum (sometimes noted)
- Secondary impetigo from scratching of skin lesions

Flea bites are characterized by the following:

- Urticarial wheal or papule surrounded by redness in a sensitized person
- Often, central hemorrhagic puncta
- Progression of wheals into bullae in highly sensitized individuals, especially young children
- Grouping of multiple lesions, commonly found on arms, ankles, legs, feet, thighs, waist, buttocks, and lower abdomen
- Bites are commonly in a classic linear configuration, which is referred to as the "breakfast, lunch, and dinner" sign

Chigger bites are characterized by the following:

- Discrete, bright-red papules 1 to 2 mm in diameter that often have hemorrhagic puncta
- Lesions mainly seen on legs (sock area) and belt line but can be widespread
- Wheals, papules, or papulovesicles in sensitized individuals
- Blisters if a secondary hypersensitivity reaction; purpuric lesions or bullae
- Intense pruritus reaching a peak on the second day and decreasing over the next 5 to 6 days, but can persist for months
- Possible secondary impetigo from scratching lesions
- May see the embedded chiggers

Diagnostic Studies. The presence of fleas or harvest mites is diagnostic; otherwise, no studies are done.

Differential Diagnosis

The diagnosis is often obvious, but the differential diagnosis can include insect bites that produce similar papular, vesicular lesions, or other skin conditions.

Management

Management consists of controlling pruritus and can include measures such as the following:

- Cool compresses
- Topical corticosteroids (e.g., 1% hydrocortisone cream)
- Topical antipruritic agents, such as calamine lotion (Riemann and High, n.d.); avoid topical diphenhydramine
- Oral antihistamines (e.g., diphenhydramine) if topical corticosteroids do not provide relief
- Removal of embedded chiggers (can be withdrawn by covering the insect with alcohol, mineral oil, nail polish, or ointment)
- Colloidal oatmeal baths (clean tub thoroughly after bath to avoid fall risk from oil residue left behind)
- Treatment of secondary skin lesions as indicated
- Elimination of fleas by treating animals and cleaning carpets, bedding, upholstered furniture; avoid areas that are potentially infested with mosquitoes, fleas, or chiggers
- Insecticides should be used with caution

Patient and Parent Education

Prevention of insect bites is a key component in education. Bites can be prevented by eliminating mosquitoes, fleas, and chiggers from the environment or by preventing their contact with the skin.

- Use insect repellents (generally effective against mosquitoes and harvest mites).
- Wear protective clothing to cover the body and tuck pants into shoes or socks.
- Wear neutral-colored clothes (white, green, tan, and khaki do not attract mosquitoes).
- Avoid scented hair sprays, powders, soaps, lotions, creams, and perfumes, because they can attract all forms of stinging insects.
- Mosquitoes are attracted to bright clothing and sweaty skin and are drawn to humans by scent.
- Treat suspected animal carrier for fleas, and spray carpets and other infested areas; spray yards and grassy places for fleas in those environments that the child frequents.
- Vacuum carpets daily if fleas are seen on household pets.
- Avoid playing in areas of harvest mite habitat.

Ticks

Description and Epidemiology

Ticks are blood-sucking arachnids classified into three families: Ixodidae (hard ticks), Argasidae (soft ticks), and Nuttalliellidae (soft ticks). They are vectors of significant diseases, such as rickettsial infection (e.g., Rocky Mountain spotted fever and Q fever), Colorado tick fever, ehrlichiosis, tularemia, and Lyme disease.

Ticks are found in grass, shrubs, vines, and brush and attach themselves to various animals and humans. The female tick sucks blood from the skin and can inject a toxin while sucking blood. Lyme disease transmission in the United States is primarily by the *Ixodes scapularis* (deer) tick. However, *I. ricinus* is the vector of Lyme disease in northern California and Oregon. Transmission of Lyme disease requires at least a 24-hour tick attachment. Tick bites are most common from early spring to early fall and are associated with both acute and chronic dermatoses. Rocky Mountain spotted fever occurs throughout the United States but is most common in the southeastern and central regions. Ehrlichiosis, also called *human monocytic ehrlichiosis (HME)* caused by *Ehrlichia chaffeensis,* is endemic to the south central, southeastern, and middle Atlantic states within the United States (Sexton, 2014).

Another tick-borne illness, similar to HME, is human granulocytic anaplasmosis (HGA) caused by *Anaplasma phagocytophilum* and *Ehrlichia ewingii.* HGA is quickly becoming more common than HME and is prevalent in the northeast, upper Midwest, south central, and southeastern parts of the United States (Sexton, 2014).

Assessment

History. Assess for a report of known tick bite and exposure to a tick habitat. However, many individuals may have no recall of tick bites. Less than 50% of patients with Lyme disease remember being bit by a tick due to the small size of the tick at the time of the bite (Buttaravoli and Leffler, 2012).

Physical Examination. Findings include the following:

- The initial bite is painless and innocuous; thus the tick is frequently undetected or detected only after several days of attachment.
- Hypersensitivity reactions are common and can include papules, nodules, bullae, ulceration, and necrosis.
- In Lyme disease, an infiltrated lesion with a distinct surrounding erythematous halo develops and can last for 1 to 2 weeks.
- Rickettsial infections most often present with fever, severe headache, myalgia, and pulmonary symptoms (Levin and Weinberg, 2014).
- A small pruritic nodule, lasting for months or years, can result if the tick's mouthparts are left in the skin.
- Tick-borne relapsing fever has an incubation period of 7 days on average and is characterized by sudden onset of high fever, chills, headaches, malaise, myalgia, and arthralgias. Treatment of tick-borne relapsing fever is with either tetracycline or erythromycin (Buttaravoli and Leffler, 2012).
- Tick paralysis can occur 4 to 6 days after tick attachment (usually to the scalp or neck) and is characterized by acute ascending paralysis. The paralysis is caused by a neurotoxin released from the tick during skin attachment. The treatment is tick removal, and symptoms usually resolve after tick removal in 24 hours for patients in the United States, but in Australia, tick paralysis symptoms have been known to worsen briefly before resolution of symptoms occurs (Buttaravoli and Leffler, 2012).
- Other signs depend on the tick-related illness that can develop; erythema chronicum migrans can develop around the bite in 2 to 3 weeks and progress to a disseminated rash and Lyme disease.

Diagnostic Studies. Identification of the tick is diagnostic. Diagnostic studies are ordered depending on the disease for which the tick is the vector.

Differential Diagnosis

The differential diagnosis of local reactions to simple tick bites includes other insect bites. Many different diseases result from tick bites and their sequelae. The presentation of tick-related diseases is variable and depends on the illness for which the tick is the vector.

Management

The most effective means of managing tick-borne infection is through prevention (see the following Patient and Parent Education section). Prompt removal of any ticks is also important in helping to prevent tick-borne illnesses. Complete removal of the tick is essential. If fragments of mouthparts or the proboscis are left in the skin, local symptoms can continue. To remove ticks, wear gloves and firmly grasp the tick with forceps, tweezers, or gloved fingers as close to the skin as possible (try to grasp its head and not crush the tick). Avoid placing pressure on the tick's abdomen. Gently pull straight upward with steady, even pressure. Wash the area with soap and water and save the tick for identification. If any part remains, a skin punch biopsy will remove the rest.

Although medical intervention varies with the specific disease, illnesses resulting from tick bites are best managed with prompt use of antibiotics, such as amoxicillin or doxycycline. Antibiotic prophylaxis for asymptomatic tick bites is generally not recommended especially if the tick has been attached for less than 24 hours.

Patient and Parent Education

The following key points should be made:

- Avoid areas known to be infested with ticks (especially brush and overgrown areas).
- Avoid sitting on logs or leaning against trees.
- Wear protective clothing—preferably light colored to see ticks better (e.g., long-sleeved shirts tucked into long pants and pants tucked into socks).
- Use DEET-containing insect repellents. Spray onto clothes and hats or directly onto the skin, but do not apply to the face or non-intact skin. Also inform parents that repellents occasionally cause allergic or toxic effects. Skedaddle 7.25% and OFF 10% are effective agents and have a good safety profile. Use a higher SPF of sunscreen if applying insect repellents because the SPF may be decreased.
- Inspect children for ticks after exposure or walking in areas likely to be infested; check for ticks every 2 to 3 hours during a hike. Carefully check the scalp, hairline, neck, behind the ears, armpits, legs, back of knees, and groin, because these areas are favorite hiding places of ticks.
- Take a brisk shower after a hike to help remove ticks that are not firmly attached. Wash off tick repellents with soap.

Spiders and Scorpions

Description and Epidemiology

Most spider bites are innocuous and do not cause reactions. If reactions occur, they are generally a minor, localized response that can be mistaken for a flea, bedbug, or some other insect bite. Most spiders cannot bite humans because of their short and fragile fangs, and almost all spiders avoid humans unless provoked. There are two main spiders common in the North American continent that can cause serious complications: the black widow *(Latrodectus mactans)* and the brown recluse *(Loxosceles reclusa).*

The black widow spider has a globular body about 1 cm across that is shiny black with a red or orange hourglass marking on its underside. It is found throughout the United States. The black widow spider prefers to live in cool, dark, dry places in buildings and little-used structures, such as woodpiles, garages, basements, and tool sheds or less frequented outbuildings. This particular type of spider often spins its web on outdoor furniture, which explains why many black widow spider bites are received around the genital and buttock areas. The black widow has neurotoxic venom.

The brown recluse, one of the most dangerous spiders in the United States, has an oval light fawn to dark chocolate-brown body; it is approximately 1 cm long (adults range from 1 to 5 cm in total length) with a dark brown violin-shaped band extending from its eyes partially down its back. The brown recluse is endemic in south Midwest and southeastern states. Although it can be transported anywhere in the United States and there is some evidence that global warming may be contributing to expansion of its range to northern Midwest states, colonization has not occurred outside its endemic range (Saupe et al, 2011). The brown recluse spider typically lives in dark, dry places (attics, basements, boxes) and storage closets among clothes; when living outdoors it resides in grasses, rocky bluffs, and barns. The brown recluse bites only in self-defense. The venom of the brown recluse can be hemolytic and necrotizing with extension caused by a spreading factor.

Only about 30 of the 1400 reported scorpion species in the world can produce fatal stings (LoVecchio, 2013). Scorpions have a stinging apparatus in their tail. They are nocturnal and found in the southwestern and southern United States. Scorpions commonly live in cool, dark places during the day and are known to crawl into sleeping bags, shoes, and discarded clothing. Scorpions prefer to avoid stinging unless they are provoked or attacked (Mayo Clinic Staff, 2014). Human stings by scorpions are usually accidental and most commonly occur when a person unintentionally steps on a scorpion or reaches under wood or rocks (LoVecchio, 2013).

Assessment

History. Assess the known history of a spider bite or activities in, or travel to, an environment that is frequented by these spiders. The characteristic appearance of the spider helps in its identification. Children are more vulnerable to spider and scorpion bites than adults.

Physical Examination. The characteristic features are identified for each type of spider bite:

- Black widow spider bites (Swanson et al, 2013):
  - Initially most bites are asymptomatic or mild pain is noted at the bite site.
  - The bite wound most often has a center punctum with a blanched circular patch and a surrounding erythematous perimeter.
  - Thirty to 120 minutes after the bite, symptoms may start to occur, including tremors, weakness, shaking of the effected extremity, local paresthesias, diaphoresis, headaches, nausea, and/or vomiting.
  - Muscle pain is the most common symptom and usually occurs in the back, extremity muscles, or abdomen. Severe abdominal pain is characteristic with abdominal wall rigidity that can be confused for a surgical abdomen, such as appendicitis or cholecystitis. Muscle pain is self-limited and resolves within 24 to 72 hours without treatment.
  - Muscle rigidity and tenderness may also be noted adjacent to the bite site and/or myoclonus of the affected limb may occur.
  - In children, facial swelling and generalized erythema are common occurrences—typically, young infants and children will also present as distressed, inconsolable, and refusing to eat, along with a history of using a crib that was just taken from storage.
  - Vital signs are normal in 70% of patients, but tachycardia, tachypnea, and hypertension have been noted secondary to anxiety, venom effects, or pain.
  - Rare findings include pulmonary edema, cardiovascular collapse, cardiomyopathy, priapism, rhabdomyolysis, hematuria, Horner syndrome, compartment syndrome, toxic epidermal necrolysis, and death.
- Brown recluse spider bites (Vetter and Swanson, 2014a):
  - Brown recluse bites typically occur on the inner thigh, upper arm, or thorax and look like 2 small punctum marks with surrounding erythema. Central pallor eventually is noted around the punctum marks but is not usually seen soon after the bite.
  - Usually the initial bite is painless, but on occasion, a burning sensation or pain has been noted.
  - Pain then may develop over the following 2 to 8 hours after the initial bite and increases in severity with resolution within 1 week of onset.
  - The wound may develop a dark, depressed center over 24 to 48 hours, resulting in a dry eschar that ulcerates. The ulcerative wound may then evolve into a necrotic region several days following the initial bite. The necrotic and ulcerative regions usually are noted with bites over buttocks and thighs, where fatty tissue is located. The necrotic lesion may expand for up to 10 days after the initial bite, and then it heals, usually over several weeks, without needing surgical repair and without scarring.

- Some patients develop itching or a morbilliform rash.
- Systemically, malaise, nausea, vomiting, fever, or myalgias may occur.
- Rarely, complications of acute hemolytic anemia, disseminated intravascular coagulopathy, coma, renal failure, myonecrosis, rhabdomyolysis, and/or death occur.

- Scorpion bites (LoVecchio, 2013):
  - Most scorpion bites in the United States and Mexico cause local or no pain with minimal if any swelling, and the puncture site is not very visible.
  - Bites from *Centruroides exilicauda* and *C. suffusus* are the most dangerous within the United States and Mexico and can cause:
    - Paresthesias, remote pain, and unexplained agitation with uncontrollable crying in children
    - Systemic reactions include abnormal eye movements, blurred vision, restlessness, fasciculations, shaking, jerking movements of the limbs and body, stridor, wheezing, respiratory failure, hyperthermia, hypersalivation, rhabdomyolysis, multiple organ failure, pancreatitis, sterile cerebrospinal fluid pleocytosis, metabolic acidosis, and death
    - Children are at much higher risk for severe symptoms and death secondary to a scorpion bite than adults

Differential Diagnosis

Other spider bites and conditions that result in similar cutaneous manifestations or systemic findings, or both, are included in the differential diagnosis.

Management

In cases in which venomous spider bites are suspected or confirmed, refer to the appropriate medical specialist or toxicologist. Treatment for black widow spider bites includes cleansing the wound with soap and water and administering pain medication, antiemetics, and muscle relaxants (such as, benzodiazepines) as needed and tetanus prophylaxis as indicated (Vetter et al, 2014b). For severe symptoms, consider use of an antivenin (Vetter et al, 2014b). Most brown recluse bites tend to heal without incident. Bites with necrotic centers generally require tetanus prophylaxis, pain medication, application of ice or cold compresses, and elevation of the extremity. Surgical excision and skin grafts may be needed if extensive necrosis occurs. Scorpion stings may be managed immediately with application of cold compresses to the affected area, raising the stung limb above the heart, staying calm, administering acetaminophen or ibuprofen for pain control, and antivenin administration when available. Intensive care is needed in severe cases for sedation and management of cardiorespiratory and neurologic complications.

Patient and Parent Education

The focus of patient and parent education is prevention. Careful monitoring of environments in which these spiders tend to live and prompt treatment, if bitten, are important. Use caution when near woodpiles and attics, and always shake out shoes and sleeping bags before using them.

Snakebites

Description and Epidemiology

Worldwide, there are 600 different species of venomous snakes causing an average of at least 100,000 to 125,000 deaths per year (White and Cheng, 2014). Approximately 5,000 snakebites are reported to the American Association of Poison Control Centers annually, and most of the snakebite victims are males (Cheng and Seifert, 2014). Venomous snakes include indigenous pit vipers (Crotalinae) (such as, rattlesnakes, cottonmouths, water moccasins, and copperheads) and the Elapidae (coral snake).

Southern and western states, including Texas, Florida, California, Arizona, Louisiana, Georgia and North Carolina, account for the highest rate of venomous snakebite occurrences due to the warmer climate zones that snakes favor (Cheng and Seifert, 2014). The snake injects venom that contains a variety of toxins into the soft tissue; the venom can be carried throughout the body via the blood and lymph systems. Snake venom reactions can be divided into three types: cytotoxic, hemotoxic, and neurotoxic. Cytotoxic envenomation presents with localized pain, swelling, and ecchymosis; compartment syndrome may develop in severe cases. Hematologic effects include hemolysis, fibrinogen activation, and thrombocytopenia. Neurologic toxicity can include taste abnormalities, local paresthesias, seizures, altered mental status, and fasciculations. Children bitten by snakes suffer more severe effects than adults. Rattlesnake and cottonmouth snakebites typically produce more severe clinical effects, such as swelling, pain, bruising, nausea, vomiting, tachycardia, tachypnea, and hypotension (Cheng and Seifert, 2014).

Assessment

History. Assess for report of a snakebite. It is helpful to determine the type of snake. Pit vipers have a large triangular head and vertically oriented elliptical pupils, unlike the round pupils of nonvenomous snakes. Copperheads and rattlesnakes have diamond-shaped patterns of varying colors. Coral snakes have black heads, followed by yellow and red bands that are followed by black bands.

Physical Examination. Characteristic features indicating the presence of venom include the following:

- Severe local reaction soon after the bite with intense pain, burning, discoloration, edema, and hemorrhagic effects
- Proximal extension of ecchymosis and swelling during the first few hours after the bite with later fluid-filled or hemorrhagic bullae and necrosis
- Peripheral and central neurologic symptoms, including worsening weakness, numbness or tingling of the face and/or extremities, diplopia, and lethargy
- Increased salivation, metallic taste in the mouth, sweating, nausea, and vomiting
- Evidence of hematologic coagulopathy, such as hematemesis, melena, and hemoptysis
- Respiratory distress and shock that can lead to death

Diagnostic Studies. Coagulation studies and other laboratory tests are ordered as indicated by the child's condition.

Management

For nonvenomous bites, simply clean the wound, give tetanus prophylaxis if necessary, and administer appropriate pain medication. Give oral antibiotic therapy for 5 days with amoxicillin/clavulanic acid if there is presence of a secondary infection. If there is any uncertainty about the identity of the snake, contact poison control and observe for venomous symptoms for at least 3 to 4 hours.

If a venomous snakebite is suspected, the effects (including possible death) depend on the size of the child, site of the bite, type of snake, and degree of envenomation, plus the effectiveness of treatment. Up to 25% of venomous snakebites are "dry" bites and are therefore asymptomatic. In the case of a rattlesnake bite, there is a period of 6 to 8 hours between the bite and death in which effective treatment can be instituted to reverse the effects of the venom. Treatment of all snakebites includes rapid transportation to a medical center, referral to appropriate medical specialists, antivenin therapy, and treatment for shock and respiratory difficulties.

Patient and Parent Education

Prevention of snakebite is important. Parents and patients who live or vacation in areas where pit vipers are found should be familiar with emergency first-aid treatment of snakebites. First-aid measures include the following (Cheng and Seifert, 2014):

- Remove the patient from the area where the snakebite occurred.
- Splint the affected extremity and minimize the patient's movements.
- Remove any jewelry, watches, or constrictive clothing from the affected extremity.
- Do not elevate the affected extremity; lay or sit the person down with the bite at the level of the heart.
- Do not give the person alcohol or a caffeinated beverage to drink.
- Do not give drugs, such as narcotics, that could impair clinical evaluation.
- Cleanse the wound with soap and water.
- Do not use a tourniquet, compression dressing, or ice packs.
- Do not cut the bite area and attempt to suction out the venom.
- Transport immediately to a medical facility.

Heat and Cold Injuries

Frostbite

Description and Epidemiology

Frostbite occurs when ice crystals form within the soft tissues as a consequence of exposure to cold. The freezing of tissue impairs circulation to the affected area and results in constriction and vaso-occlusion. This causes microvascular changes, leading to cellular destruction and the release of inflammatory mediators that also cause damage. Frostbite most commonly involves distal, relatively poorly perfused regions of the body, such as fingertips, toes, earlobes, and the nose. In children, areas that have poor heat-generating ability and insulation, including the cheeks and chin, are also at high risk for frostbite. However, any area of skin that is exposed to prolonged cold can be affected.

Exposure to temperatures ranging from 28.4° to 14° F (−2° to −10° C) can cause frostbite. Factors such as duration of exposure, increased wind velocity, dependency of the extremity (limb in a dependent, not elevated position), application of emollients, fatigue, injury, high altitude, immobility, and general health can potentiate the effects of cold. Exposure to very cold chemicals (e.g., liquid nitrogen or oxygen) also produces instant frostbite.

Assessment

History. The provider should assess the following:

- Exposure to cold temperatures
- Sensory changes (initial pain, then numbness if deeply frostbitten)
- Complaints of throbbing pain after thawing

Physical Examination. Typical initial findings include the following:

- Frozen area is cold.
- Skin is red at first, then appears pale or waxy white or slightly yellow or may have a bluish tint if deeply frostbitten.
- In early stages, tissue blanches; in later stages, it feels doughy or rock hard.

On rewarming, the extent of tissue damage becomes apparent. Deep frostbite occurs when tissues are icy hard and without deep tissue resilience. With deep frostbite the following signs and symptoms appear with rewarming:

- Cyanosis or mottling
- Erythema and swelling
- Numbness that evolves into complaints of burning pain
- Vesicles and bullae that appear within 24 to 48 hours
- Gangrene in severe frostbite

Table 40-5 describes the four levels of frostbite.

Differential Diagnosis

The differential diagnosis includes other conditions that produce similar cutaneous manifestations and injury; a history of exposure to extreme temperatures is the key to the diagnosis.

Management

Severe frostbite should be managed by medical specialists. Treatment includes rapid rewarming procedures, pain management, medical and surgical management of tissue necrosis, prevention of infection, and amputation if needed. Damaged skin should never be massaged or rubbed with snow or ice. Early treatment of mild frostbite includes the following:

- Cover affected area with other body surfaces and warm clothing.
- Avoid pressure or any rubbing of the affected area.

TABLE 40-5 The Four Categories of Frostbite

Category by Degree	Description	Complication
First (frostnip)	Redness, edema, transient discomfort; reversible within a few hours	Normal skin appearance within a few hours; may have mild desquamation
Second	Notable redness and swelling; numbness becomes burning pain in 12 to 24 hours; bullae and vesicles form	Sensory neuropathy and cold sensitivity are residuals after healing
Third	Hemorrhagic bullae or waxy, mummified skin	Extensive tissue loss
Fourth	Involvement of full-thickness skin, muscle, tendon, bone	Amputation is likely

- Pain control as needed.
- Topical aloe and oral ibuprofen orally inhibit prostaglandins and thromboxane, thus limiting inflammation (Zafren and Crawford Mechem, n.d.).
- *Do not use local dry heat*; this practice is dangerous and can cause tissue damage.

Patient and Parent Education

Education of children and parents about the prevention and initial management of frostbite is important. Essential points include the following:

- Use of appropriate clothing when exposed to extreme cold temperatures
- Survival skills for travelers, hikers, or winter sports participants who are exposed to cold temperatures or who could become lost
- Immediate rewarming of skin that is white by covering with warm clothing or another body surface
- Danger of rubbing affected area with snow or ice or massaging; these practices are contraindicated because they lead to mechanical trauma

Hypothermia

Description and Epidemiology

Hypothermia is the condition in which body core temperature falls below 95° F (35° C). At less than 95° F (35° C), the human body loses its ability to generate sufficient heat to maintain bodily functions. Hypothermia can be the result of environmental exposure. Body heat is lost by radiation of heat to nearby objects, evaporation of moisture from the skin and respiratory system, convection of heat from the skin's surface into cooler air, or conduction of heat to objects in direct contact with the body. The effect of cool ambient temperatures is exacerbated by wind, moisture, and lack of appropriate clothing or shelter. Predisposing factors include malnutrition, underlying medical illness, adrenal insufficiency, sepsis, central nervous system injury, hypoglycemia, major trauma, burns, hypothyroidism, and drug overdose or child abuse/maltreatment (Corneli and Bolte, 2013a). Although most cases of accidental exposure are seen in winter, hypothermia can occur in other seasons during wet, windy weather. It can also occur quickly with cold-water emersion.

Children are at increased risk of hypothermia because of their relatively larger BSA, proportionately larger head, smaller body fluid volume, less developed temperature-regulating mechanisms, and decreased amount of protective body fat. Children are also less able to escape on their own from a cold environment and are more likely to wander off from adult supervision. Newborns, particularly low-birth weight or premature infants, very young children, and children who are ill, fatigued, poorly nourished, or have experienced trauma are at high risk.

Hypothermia results in cutaneous vasoconstriction and increased heat production by shivering and thyroxine releases. Hypothermia that is not associated with environmental exposure may be a sign of other life-threatening illnesses or injuries. Secondary hypothermia is not discussed here.

Assessment

History. The following are assessed:

- Exposure to low ambient temperatures
- Risk factors (e.g., age, physical condition)

Physical Examination. Signs of hypothermia progress from early to late stages and include the following:

- Decreasing body temperature
- Shivering that disappears in moderate hypothermia
- Pallor or blue lips and skin
- Disorientation, listlessness, sleepiness
- Decreased pulse and respiration
- Decreasing neurologic status and eventually coma and death

Diagnostic Studies. No studies are done if hypothermia is mild and responds to basic treatment measures.

Differential Diagnosis

Shock is the differential diagnosis.

Management

For mild hypothermia (greater than 89.6° F [32° C] body temperature) in early stages of cooling, remove the child from the cold environment, replace wet clothing, and provide warm liquids if the patient is conscious and able to drink. Placing the child in a warm water bath can be effective. As the body cools further, it can no longer generate adequate heat itself, so external sources of heat must be provided. Provide heat with warm blankets, heat lamps, hot-water bottles, or, if none of these is available, use the classic technique of placing the child skin-to-skin with a warm person of normal temperature in a sleeping bag or blanket. Administration of warmed IV normal saline should be considered for treatment of mild hypothermia and is a necessity for treatment of moderate to severe hypothermia.

Children with severe hypothermia (less than 82° F [28° C] body temperature) require active internal and external rewarming. Heated saline lavage of the pleural space, bladder, stomach, and/or peritoneum should be used for internal warming. Forced-air external rewarming (e.g., Bair Hugger heated blanket) and warmed, humidified 100% oxygen via non-rebreather mask are also important therapies implemented in combination with active internal rewarming (Corneli and Bolte, 2013b). Children who require forced-air external and/or active internal rewarming should be transferred to an ED because of the risk of cardiovascular instability and death.

Patient and Parent Education

Instruct parents about the risks of hypothermia in young children. Emphasize the need to monitor children's activities in cold weather and to provide adequate supervision and protection from exposure. The higher metabolic rate of normal, healthy children keeps them warm, and they may not feel the effects of short-term exposure to the cold. Thus they may not want a jacket, sweater, hat, or mittens when their parents believe they need them. Having a survival kit along with families or teens on camping trips or traveling in uninhabited areas may save a life.

Hyperthermia: Common Heat-Related Illness

Description and Epidemiology

Hyperthermia is a life-threatening increase in body core temperature. Heat cramps, heat exhaustion, and heat stroke are types of hyperthermia. Heat cramps are painful muscle cramps that are probably caused by electrolyte depletion associated with insufficient blood supply to an exercising muscle. Heat exhaustion is caused by excessive sweating associated with inadequate intake of water and salt in a hot environment. Heat stroke is defined as a core temperature of more than 104° F (40° C) combined with central nervous system dysfunction secondary to environmental heat exposure (Ishimine, 2012). Heat cramps and heat exhaustion often occur during sports activities (see Chapter 13). Heat stroke is a life-threatening condition. This section more specifically discusses heat stroke.

Heat-related illness results from an ineffective response of the body's thermoregulatory mechanisms to environmental conditions. The body's normal response to overheating is cutaneous vasodilation, sweating, and decreased heat production through inhibiting shivering. Evaporation through sweating is the body's primary cooling mechanism. Air temperature higher than body temperature, high humidity, and dehydration negatively affect the body's cooling mechanisms and compromise the process of evaporation. Internal body temperature then increases. All children are at risk for hyperthermia or heat stroke when exposed to high air temperature, especially if the heat is combined with high humidity and if steps are not taken to keep the child cool. Age, exertion, illness, obesity, and poor nutrition also exacerbate the hyperthermia risk. Compared with adults, children sweat less, begin to sweat at a higher internal temperature (or set-point), have a higher metabolic rate thus producing more body heat and lower cardiac output, and are more susceptible to dehydration because of proportionately larger BSA. Children with some genetic myopathies have malignant hyperthermia, which is a pathologic reaction to anesthetic.

Assessment

History. Assess the following:

- Exposure
- Excessive exercise
- Overdressing for the climate
- Inadequate fluid intake or the use of water or other low-sodium fluids during prolonged and strenuous exercise
- Previous episode of heat stroke
- Heat cramps: Complaints of intermittent muscle cramping (no rigidity)
- Heat exhaustion: Complaints of thirst, weakness, headache, fatigue, dizziness, malaise, myalgias and muscle cramps, nausea, and vomiting; core temperature is normal or slightly elevated and the patient still sweats
- Heat stroke: Delirium, stupor, or coma—central nervous system dysfunction

Physical Examination. Signs of heat exhaustion include the following:

- Appears anxious and diaphoretic
- Tachycardia with normal blood pressure
- Temperature 104° F (40° C) or lower
- Headache, fatigue, weakness, dizziness, mild confusion

Signs of heat stroke include all the symptoms of heat exhaustion listed earlier, are progressive, and include the following:

- Body temperature 104° F (40° C) or higher
- Hot, dry, red skin
- Presence or absence of the ability to sweat
- Initially a rapid, strong pulse that becomes progressively weaker
- Initially constricted pupils, progressively dilated
- Initially a deep, rapid "snore like" breathing that becomes progressively weaker
- Tremors, increasing dizziness, and weakness
- Confusion, irritability, anxiety (central nervous system dysfunction)
- Headache
- Loss of appetite, nausea, vomiting, diarrhea
- Decreasing blood pressure, tachyarrhythmia
- Seizures, hallucinations, collapse
- Renal insufficiency, disseminated intravascular coagulation (DIC), liver failure, cardiogenic shock, coma, and death

Diagnostic Studies. CBC and urinalysis, along with electrolyte monitoring may be necessary for significant heat cramps and heat exhaustion. Heat stroke requires extensive laboratory studies and monitoring of physiologic parameters.

Differential Diagnosis

Fever differs from hyperthermia in that it is an alteration of the body's hypothalamic set point in response to a pathologic illness or condition.

Management

The management of heat-related illness includes the following:

- Heat cramps—usually mild
  - Cooling measures
  - Rest
  - Oral sodium replacement with electrolyte fluids or liberally salted foods
- Heat exhaustion
  - Rest in a cool or well-ventilated environment
  - Oral sodium replacement with electrolyte fluids or liberally salted foods
  - If weak or impaired level of consciousness, administer IV replacement of electrolytes (initial bolus of 10 to 20 mL/kg normal saline)
- Heat stroke—focuses on cardiovascular support and normalizing body temperatures
  - All individuals with heat stroke will die without treatment and require intensive or emergency care. Heat stroke patients should be transported to a medical facility as quickly as possible. Cooling therapies should be stopped once the core temperature reaches 100.4° F (38° C) to prevent overshooting and thus creating a state of hypothermia (Ishimine, 2012).
  - First-aid management includes the following steps:
    - Remove the child from the heat source.
    - Apply cold packs, wet sheets, or towels, or spray the body with lukewarm water. The body responds quickly to cooling of the neck, head, abdomen, and inner thighs.
    - Use a fan to cool and circulate air over the child and to facilitate evaporation.
    - Be alert for vomiting; prevent aspiration.
    - Administer IV benzodiazepines (e.g., midazolam) to prevent shivering, which generates heat (Ishimine, 2012).
    - When the body temperature is lowered to the desired level, stop cold packs, monitor, and be prepared to reapply cold packs if temperature increases.
    - Alcohol baths are contraindicated due to the potential for alcohol poisoning.
    - Acetaminophen and ibuprofen have no role in the treatment of heat stroke.
    - All children with heat stroke should be admitted to a pediatric intensive care unit (ICU) to monitor and to manage any potential complications such as DIC, rhabdomyolysis, or end organ failure (Ishimine, 2012).

Patient and Parent Education

Instruct parents on the risks of hyperthermia (e.g., never leave an infant or a child in a closed car or continuously exposed to direct sunlight) and that children who suffer heat stroke are at a higher risk for subsequent heat-related illnesses. Teach ways to prevent hyperthermia:

- Keep children well hydrated. Offer water often during active play and athletic events or practices. Water is the primary replacement fluid; electrolyte-based sports drinks are also acceptable for intense sweating or prolonged exercise.
- Make sure children are well rested and have good nutritional intake.
- Provide appropriate clothing (e.g., sunshades, hats, and light-reflective shirts that allow ventilation).
- Regulate children's activity levels to environmental conditions (e.g., limit active play if it is very hot or humid).
- Acclimatize child gradually to changes in environment.

Motor Vehicle Trauma

Description and Epidemiology

Motor vehicle trauma continues to be the leading cause of death among children in the United States, with significant mortality and morbidity rates in all age groups. In 2012, 1,139 children from birth to 14 years old died in motor vehicle crashes, and approximately 179,000 were injured. Overall, there has been a 45% decrease in fatalities in children from this age group since 2003; however, there was a slight increase of 3% from 2011 to 2012. Alcohol impairment was a factor in 239 (20%) of these pediatric fatalities, with 124 of the deaths occurring in a car with a driver whose blood alcohol concentration was 0.08 or higher (National Highway Traffic Safety Administration [NHTSA], n.d.a).

Positioning young children in rear seats and correctly using child restraint systems (CRSs) can prevent fatalities from motor vehicle trauma and can reduce the number and severity of injuries to children. NHTSA noted that child safety seats used correctly reduced the risk of fatal pediatric injuries in passenger vehicles by 71% in infants younger than 12 months and by 54% in the 1- to 4-year-old group (NHTSA, 2014a). Nonetheless, many children ride unrestrained or incorrectly restrained. Forty percent of the children who died in motor vehicle accidents in 2012 were unrestrained (NHTSA, 2014a). Serious injury or death caused by airbags is also more likely if a child is not properly restrained or if a child in a rear-facing child safety seat is incorrectly placed in the front seat (NHTSA, 2014a). Seat belt usage is significantly higher in states with primary seat belt enforcement laws (i.e., drivers can be stopped and cited by law enforcement officials for failure to wear a seat belt) versus those with secondary enforcement laws (i.e., drivers can be cited if they are stopped for another traffic violation and are not wearing a seat belt).

In addition to not using restraints, a number of common errors have been found in the way CRSs are used (Box 40-2). The most common errors are loose vehicle safety straps attached to the CRS and loose harness straps

• BOX 40-2 Common Errors in the Use of Child Restraint Systems

- Seat belt is not tight enough.
- Rear-facing seat is not positioned at a 45-degree angle.
- Harness straps are not snug (infant may be wrapped in a "cocoon" of blankets).
- Harness straps in infant, rear-facing seat is not at or below shoulders of infant.
- Harness straps in child, forward-facing seat is not at or above shoulders of child.
- Retainer clip in child, forward-facing seat is not at armpit level.
- Seat belt is not in locked mode.
- Infants and toddlers younger than 2 years old are placed in forward-facing position.

securing the child to the CRS. Providers should assess the parents' use of CRSs and correct errors. This may mean accompanying parents to the parking lot to observe how children are placed in the restraint. CRS use should be reviewed at each well-child visit, and children should be involved in the discussion from a very early age. Both parents and children should receive positive reinforcement for proper use of CRSs. Information from NHTSA on which restraint system is appropriate for the size, age, and condition of the child should be shared with parents (see Additional Resources).

The 2011 NHTSA guidelines are based on emerging evidence and research related to child restraint technologies and include recommendations that take both the child's age and size into consideration (NHTSA, 2014c). Parents should be advised to register their child's car seat online with the manufacturer to receive notification in the event of a safety recall. There are child car seat inspection stations where a certified technician can inspect the safety seat and demonstrate how it should be correctly installed and used. NHTSA's website provides an inspection station locator for parents seeking information about the closest station to their home.

Pedestrian injuries or injuries involving bicycles, skateboards, and automobiles are common among children. Providers should discuss this issue with parents at each well-child visit, ask children about their pedestrian safety habits during the well-child visit, and support educational efforts to instruct children on pedestrian safety and age-appropriate safe use of bicycles or skateboards. Children of all ages need adult supervision related to motor vehicles. Adult supervision is especially important for younger children who are unaware of the dangers.

Adolescents, especially new drivers, are often involved in motor vehicle accidents because of their inexperience, immature judgment, or tendency to take risks. Legislation has been passed in all but one state to restrict adolescent driving. Enactment of "graduated driver" licensing (learner, intermediate, and fully licensed stages) laws began in the 1990s. Since the adolescent driving laws changed, there has been a significant decrease of fatalities in young drivers 15 to 20 years old. From 2003 to 2012, fatalities involving young drivers decreased by 49% (NHTSA, 2014b). Successful implementation of the law depends on parents acting as advocates for safety and supporting their adolescents' compliance with the regulations. Providers also can reinforce the message to teenagers that driving is a privilege that requires skill and maturity.

Graduated driver licensing legislation may require some or all of the following:

- Teens must complete driver education classes.
- Teens with learner permits may drive only with a fully licensed adult.
- Driving is restricted to certain times of day and/or without other teenagers in the car.

Another important education point for parents and health care providers to discuss with adolescent drivers is the danger involved in use of electronic equipment (e.g., cell phones, smartphones, texting) while driving. Motor vehicle accidents resulting in injury or death secondary to texting while driving are on the rise, and several states have implemented "no texting while driving" laws to address this issue. Providers should educate and remind parents and adolescent drivers of these laws. Parents should also be role models and not text or use handheld cell phones while driving.

For a complete list of references, please visit http://evolve.elsevier.com/Burns/pediatric/.

41 Genetic Disorders

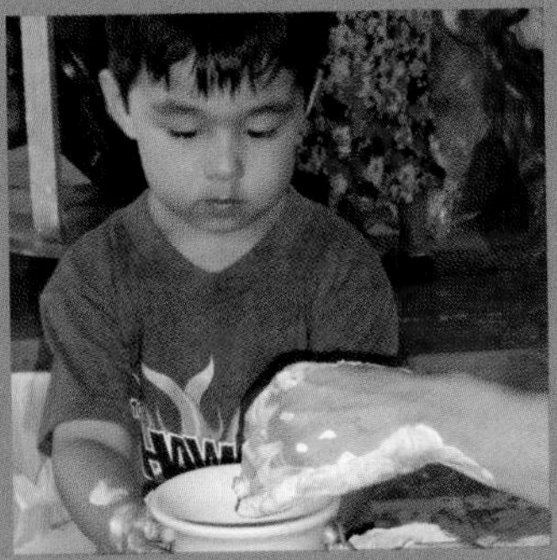

MARTHA DRIESSNACK AND SANDRA DAACK-HIRSCH

The future is not in front of us, but inside us.

JOANNA MACY

Our understanding of the human genome continues to evolve, transforming not only the field of genetics, but also our understanding of human embryology, physiology, and disease processes. In short, it is changing the way we diagnose, treat, and prevent human diseases. Genome-based science has now expanded beyond the study of single genes to include the interaction of genes across the genome, as well as how these interactions are influenced by the environment, random events, and epigenetic factors. Very few diseases are entirely genetic and inherited, and health care providers should no longer characterize disorders as genetic or non-genetic. Rather, all diseases, and, for that matter, individual response to treatment, have a genetic/genomic component.

At the same time, with the current emphasis on patient-centered care and patient engagement, children and families are becoming active participants in both their care and health care decisions. Of equal importance are the impact of the Internet and its delivery of all forms of information as they are learned, with instant commentary and interpretation by anyone willing to weigh in. Together, along with the sheer volume of daily information and emergent technologies, health care is being transformed for providers and consumers. Today's children are right in the mix, growing up at the intersection of the genome era and information age (Driessnack, 2009). An understanding of genetics will help primary care providers (PCPs) provide better care. The medical home model of care identifies PCPs as holding a crucial role in the management of patients who have the potential for or have been diagnosed with a genetic disorder (Genetics in Primary Care Institute [GPCI], 2014a). Core competencies in genetics for nurses at all levels of practice have already been established, communicated in *The Essentials of Baccalaureate Education for Professional Nursing Practice* (American Association of Colleges of Nursing [AACN], 2008), *The Essentials of Doctoral Education for Advanced Nursing Practice* (AACN, 2006), and the *Core Competencies in Genetics for Health Professionals* (National Coalition for Health Professional Education in Genetics [NCHPEG], 2007). In addition, there are specific resources available for PCPs through the Genetics in Primary Care Institute (GPCI), whose main mission is to work with providers to better understand and integrate genetics into their primary care practice (see Additional Resources).

This chapter provides a brief review of basic genetic concepts and terminology, genetic's contribution to disorders, and patterns of inheritance, along with insights into obtaining a family history and conducting a pediatric assessment using a genetics lens. The concept of epigenetics, emerging technologies, and some of the ethical challenges that can arise are introduced. Most importantly, key resources that maintain up-to-date, easily accessed information for busy providers are highlighted. Common genetic disorders found in children are discussed.

Basic Principles of Genetics

Each human is a unique being, established by the joining of one egg and one sperm, each of which provided a unique deoxyribonucleic acid (DNA) package. An individual's total DNA package is called a *genome.* Within each cell, genetic information flows from DNA to ribonucleic acid (RNA) to protein, with each gene coding for up to 20 different proteins. In other words, the information carried within the DNA dictates the end product (protein) that will be synthesized. Our genomes and their products, in turn, interact with the individual's internal and external environment in very complex ways.

Deoxyribonucleic Acid

DNA is a molecule that contains genetic instructions for the structure and function of all living organisms. DNA is made up of a string of nucleotides and each nucleotide consists of deoxyribose, a phosphate group, and one of four bases, called *adenine (A), cytosine (C), guanine (G),* and *thymine (T).* The two backbones of the DNA helix are formed by the deoxyribose and phosphate groups, whereas the rungs that hold them together are formed by complementary pairing (A-T and C-G) of the bases. The DNA helix is coiled, similar to a telephone cord, tightly encircling

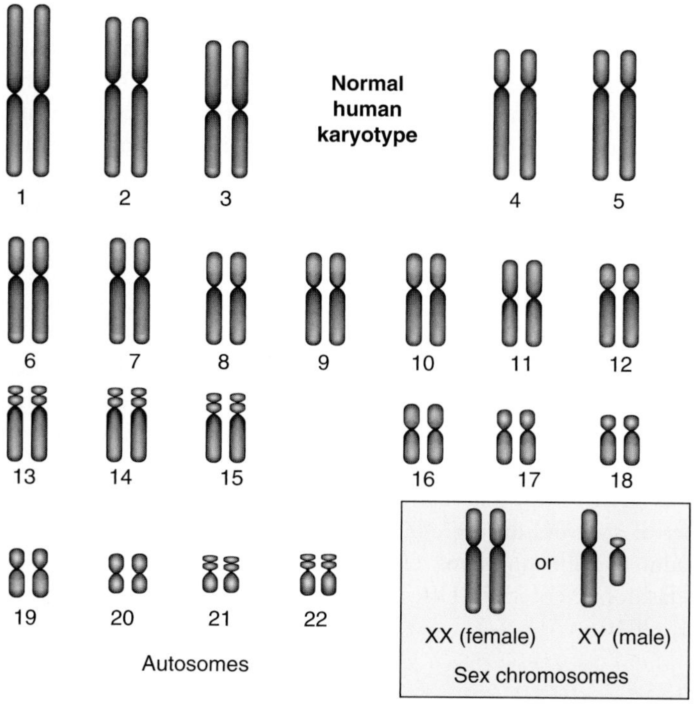

• **Figure 41-1** Normal human karyotype. (From Genetics Home Reference: Normal human karyotype, Genetics Home Reference (website), 2014, Available at http://ghr.nlm.nih.gov/handbook/illustrations/normalkaryotype. Accessed November 16, 2015.)

histone proteins. Uncoiled, each DNA strand is approximately 6 feet long. Although each person has a unique DNA package that reflects one in several million possible combinations from the four grandparents' genetic material, the base sequences of any two human genomes are thought to be 99.9% identical. In short, people are more alike than different, and the differences arise from only 0.1% of DNA. Yet, the slightest alteration in an individual's DNA sequence can have devastating health consequences. For example, sickle cell anemia is one of many diseases caused by the smallest of genetic changes—an alteration of a single nucleotide (one A, T, C, or G). On the other hand, some DNA alterations have no known effect on an individual, while still others appear to provide a benefit or protective action. For example, the same single nucleotide alteration that is responsible for sickle cell anemia can confer a survival advantage to unaffected carriers challenged with the malaria pathogen (Clancy, 2008; Thom et al, 2013). This is why sickle cell alterations, including both the trait and disease, persist in populations where malaria is endemic.

Chromosomes

Cytogenetics is the study of genetics at the chromosome level, where most of our genetic information is located. Each chromosome is a strand of DNA. In the nucleus of all normal human cells, with the exception of gametes, are 46 chromosomes arranged in 23 pairs. Twenty-two of the pairs are called *autosomes;* they look the same in females and males. The remaining pair, the sex chromosomes, differs between females and males, with two X chromosomes for females (XX) and one X and one Y chromosome (XY) for males. The 22 autosomes are numbered by size—from largest (1) to smallest (22). The picture of human chromosomes lined up in pairs is called a *karyotype* (Fig. 41-1).

Human somatic cells are *diploid,* containing 23 paired chromosomes. Diploid cells are replicated through the process of *mitosis,* which creates two identical daughter cells. In contrast, gametes, or germline cells (egg and sperm), are *haploid* cells, each containing only 23 chromosomes. Gametes are produced in the ovary or testicle during *meiosis,* where there is an exchange of genetic material, through crossing over and recombination, resulting in a random assortment of maternally and paternally derived genetic material in the daughter cells. Fusion at fertilization restores the 46-chromosome (23-pair) complement, with one of each chromosome pair from each gamete, creating a unique human being.

A chromosome has a long arm (q) and a short arm (p). Geneticists often use a diagram, or *ideogram,* which shows a chromosome's size and banding pattern. The bands are used to further describe the location of genes on each chromosome. For example, the cytogenic location of the *CFTR* gene (cystic fibrosis) is 7q31.2, which means the *CFTR* gene is located on the long arm (q) of chromosome 7, band 3, sub-band 1, and sub-sub-band 2. Other common symbols include *del,* for deletion, *dup,* for duplication, and + indicating an increased or − indicating a decrease in number. For example, 47, XY+21 indicates a male with three copies of chromosome 21 (Down syndrome), whereas

46, XX,8q– denotes a female with a deletion on the long arm of chromosome 8 (Tsai et al, 2011).

At the ends of each chromosome are protective caps, or *telomeres.* Telomeres, specific repetitive sequences of non-coding DNA, contain and protect the genetic information on the chromosome. The telomeres shorten each time a cell divides, losing their protective function over time until cells can no longer replicate and divide, and therefore die. This shortening process is the focus of ongoing research related to aging and cancer. Emerging research now suggests that growing up in a stressful environment can also leave lasting marks on young chromosomes. In particular, children from poor and/or unstable homes have been shown to have shorter telomeres than their unaffected peers (Madhusoodanan, 2014). This line of research parallels the work of the adverse childhood experiences (ACE) study whose findings suggest that as the number of stressors during childhood increase, the risk for adult health problems also increases in a strong and graded fashion (Centers for Disease Control and Prevention [CDC], 2010).

Genes

A gene is a specific *coding* sequence of DNA organized in small blocks of three letters (e.g., GGC, ATG) known as a *codon.* There are 64 different codons or words in the genetic code. To early geneticists, a gene was an abstract entity whose existence was only known through its reflected *phenotype,* or physical expression transmitted between generations (Gerstein et al, 2007). Later, genes on chromosomes were thought to be like beads on a string, each coding for one protein. However, we now know that one gene codes for an average of three proteins (National Human Genome Research Institute [NHGRI], 2014a). Today, genes are increasingly viewed through informational science and computational biology lenses, resulting in the infusion of information processing and systems language, including upstream regulation, exons, and introns. *Genotype* refers to an individual's collection of genes. The *phenotype* is the manifestation of the individual's genotype, because gene expression is both regulated by molecular mechanisms and modified by environmental factors. Phenotype includes an individual's physical features, organ structure, and biochemical and physiologic nature.

Each human inherits two copies of each gene, one copy, or *allele,* from each parent. Alleles are forms of the same gene with differences in their DNA sequence. These differences contribute to each person's unique features. If the two alleles at any given location (locus) are similar, the individual is *homozygous* for that gene; if the alleles are different, the individual is *heterozygous.* For example, a child with cystic fibrosis may have identical gene sequences (e.g., mutation F508del) in both alleles, and as such would be called *homozygous* for that mutation, whereas this child's parents most likely were heterozygous, each with only one copy of the gene mutation and one copy of a normal allele.

In humans, genes can vary in size from 200 to more than 2 million DNA bases. Humans are thought to have between 20,000 and 25,000 different genes. Although every human cell contains every gene, not all genes are active at once; certain mechanisms activate them, turning them on or off at various developmental points or at various locations within the body. Each gene also has coding sequences (exons), separated by non-coding sequences (introns), and occupies a specific location (locus) on a chromosome. Additionally, a small number of genes are situated in the mitochondria.

It was previously believed that differences in non-coding DNA sequences did not have relevance to human health and development. As such, the term *allele* was typically used to describe differences in DNA sequences; however, it now also refers to variations among non-coding DNA sequences, some of which are associated with increased risk for common diseases, such as diabetes, heart disease, and cancer (Genetics Home Reference, 2014).

Mutations

An allele is typically regarded as a *mutation* when its genetic variation is found in less than 1% of the population or a *polymorphism* when it is found in greater than 1% of a population; however, the cutoff of at least 1% prevalence is somewhat arbitrary (Clancy, 2008). The term *mutation* is typically used to mean a disease-causing variation, whereas a *polymorphism* is used to refer to a normal variation, or one that does not *directly* cause disease. But really the key difference between the classification of mutation and polymorphism is the frequency that each occurs.

One type of polymorphism is known as *single nucleotide polymorphisms,* or *SNP* (pronounced "snip"). SNPs are used to study the genetic contribution to multifactorial disorders, such as cleft lip and cleft palate, diabetes, heart disease, and cancer, as well as individual response to drugs (pharmacogenetics). A SNP is a single base pair alteration that is common in a given population. On average, SNPs are found every 300 to 2,000 nucleotides in the human genome, and scientists participating in the International HapMap Consortium have mapped millions of these small alterations (International Human Genome Sequencing Consortium, 2001) (see The International HapMap Project in Additional Resources). Typically, SNPs are not directly disease-causing mutations; however, they are biologically relevant because they help to identify individuals at increased risk for multifactorial disease and/or individuals at increased risk for adverse response to medications.

Mutations directly cause disorders and are further subclassified as *point mutations, nucleotide repeat expansions, copy number variants,* or *chromosome mutations.* It is important to remember that although these types of mutations can have a large effect on individual human health and development, human evolutionary changes are more likely to result from the accumulation over time of many mutations with small effects.

Point Mutations

Point mutations are single base pair changes, occurring at the level of the nucleotide, yet capable of changing the function of a gene or gene product. They are responsible for many single-gene genetic disorders, including sickle cell anemia and cystic fibrosis. Point mutations should not be confused with SNPs. Although both are single nucleotide differences in a DNA sequence, a SNP, by definition is present in at least 1% of the general population. There is no known disease-causing mutation that is that common.

Nucleotide Repeat Expansions

Nucleotide repeat expansions occur beyond single point changes. A repeat expansion is a mutation that increases the number of times the short DNA sequence is normally repeated. When the number of repeats increases beyond the normally tolerated limit, the mutation (i.e., repeat expansion) results in a genetic disorder. For example, almost all cases of fragile X syndrome are caused by an expansion of a trinucleotide (three-base-pair) repeat sequence (CGG) in the *FMR1* gene (Xq27.3) from a normal 5 to 40 times to over 200 times. The expansion makes the gene unstable, resulting in little or no protein output with an outcome of signs and symptoms of fragile X syndrome.

Copy Number Variations

A copy number variation (CNV) involves larger areas of chromosomes, beyond point mutations and repeat expansions. During egg and sperm production, unequal crossover events occur throughout the genome. When this happens, children may have lost or gained additional copies of genetic information that were present in either of their parents' chromosomes. Unlike other types of mutations that have been inherited for countless generations, geneticists now recognize that CNVs (which have a more recent origin) provide the genetic basis for common psycho-behavioral diseases, such as mental retardation, autism, and schizophrenia (Beckmann et al, 2007). The Autism Genome Project (AGP) found that some children with autism have an inherited duplication on chromosome 9q21.13, encompassing the four last exons of the *ANXA1* gene (Correia et al, 2014; Marshall and Scherer, 2012). This understanding has the potential to facilitate diagnosis and guide the development of treatments.

Chromosome Mutations

Chromosome mutations occur when even larger segments of a chromosome (involving many bands) are deleted, duplicated, rearranged, or translocated in such a way that there is a resulting alteration of the DNA sequence, a modification of the gene dosage, or a complete absence of a gene or several genes. For example, cri-du-chat syndrome (5p–) is caused by the deletion of the entire end of the short (p) arm of chromosome, whereas Down syndrome is caused by the addition of an entire chromosome. Chromosome mutations usually result in multi-organ, large effects, such as in Down syndrome in which the individual can have neurologic, eye, ear, orthopedic, cardiac, and other abnormalities.

Genetic Disorders

A genetic disorder is a disease caused in whole, or in part, by a change in DNA away from the normal sequence. Nearly all diseases are now thought to have a genetic component. Some diseases are caused by inherited mutations; other diseases are caused by spontaneous mutations that occur during the development of the gametes or in early human development, whereas still others are caused by acquired mutations in a gene or group of genes that occur during a person's life. Such mutations are not inherited from a parent but occur either randomly or due to a random event or environmental exposure (e.g., most forms of cancer). The majority of genetic disorders can be grouped under one of three categories: (1) monogenetic, or single-gene disorders, (2) chromosome disorders, or (3) multifactorial disorders. Mitochondrial disorders also occur but are less common.

Monogenetic Disorders

Monogenetic disorders occur when the mutation affects a single gene. The mutation may be present on one or both chromosomes and is most often classified as dominant, recessive, or X-linked. Dominant disorders are caused by the presence of the gene mutation on just one of the two inherited parental alleles; recessive diseases require the presence of the gene mutation on both of the inherited alleles; X-linked diseases are monogenic disorders confined to the X chromosome. They can be dominant or recessive. Some examples of monogenic disorders that should be familiar to PCPs are sickle cell disease, thalassemia, neurofibromatosis, hemophilia, Duchene muscular dystrophy, cystic fibrosis, fragile X syndrome, polycystic kidney disease, Marfan syndrome, and Tay-Sachs disease.

Chromosome Disorders

Chromosome disorders occur with changes in the number or structure of an entire chromosome, or large segments of it. For example, Down syndrome (trisomy 21) is caused by an extra copy of chromosome 21, Prader-Willi syndrome is caused by the absence of a group of genes on chromosome 15, and chronic myeloid leukemia (CML) results from a translocation in which portions of chromosomes 9 and 22 are exchanged resulting in a new, abnormal gene (NHGRI, 2014). Other examples of chromosomal disorders that should be familiar to providers in primary care are cri-du-chat syndrome (5p–), Williams syndrome, and DiGeorge syndrome, also referred to as *velocardiofacial* or *22q11 deletion syndrome.*

Chromosome disorders can also involve sex chromosomes, such as Klinefelter syndrome (XXY), which is caused by an extra X chromosome, and Turner syndrome (XO), which is caused by the absence of an X chromosome.

Another type of chromosomal disorder is called *mosaicism,* which occurs when an altered chromosomal arrangement occurs in some cells but not in others within the same individual. The clinical symptoms are usually milder and the prognosis improves with the fewer numbers of cells involved.

When taking a family history, PCPs should remember there is a high frequency of chromosomal disorders in spontaneous abortions and stillbirths. Further, the prevalence of chromosomal disorders due to nondisjunction increases with advancing maternal age.

Multifactorial Disorders

Multifactorial disorders result from a combination of genetic and environmental factors. Recurrence risks are based on empirical statistics—observations based on data collected from thousands of family histories transformed into probabilities. Although these disorders tend to cluster in families, the exact recurrence risk is difficult to predict because the individuals' or couples' precise genetic and environmental risks are usually not known. Therefore, a population-based recurrence risk rather than a personal recurrence risk is given. One example of a multifactorial disorder includes neural tube defects (NTD), such as spina bifida or anencephaly. We know that NTDs appear in females more often than males and once a child is born with a NTD, the chances for those parents to have another child with a NTD in a future pregnancy increase (Online Mendelian Inheritance in Man [OMIM], 2013). The rate of NTDs decreases with sufficient maternal folic acid supplementation, as long as that supplementation starts at least 3 months prior to conception and continues for the first month of pregnancy (Tsai et al, 2011). In contrast, the rate of NTDs increases when mothers have uncontrolled diabetes or take certain medications (e.g., valproic acid) (U.S. Food and Drug Administration [FDA], 2013). The specific combination of genetic factors or how they interact with each other or other environmental factors is unknown. Other examples of multifactorial disorders that should be familiar to PCPs are congenital heart defect, club foot, cleft lip/palate, pyloric stenosis, Hirschsprung disease, hip dysplasia, and asthma.

Teratogens

A *teratogen* is any agent that results in, or increases the incidence of, a congenital malformation. Although teratogens have traditionally been considered as environmental toxins altering critical embryonic and fetal development events, it appears that genomic factors can have significant modifying effects to the teratogen. The same teratogenic exposure can induce a severe malformation in one embryo, while failing to do so in another, even though the timing and dose of the exposure were similar (Wlodarczyk et al, 2011). A teratogen may also affect the embryo at one developmental point but not at a different one. The Organization of Teratology Information Specialists (OTIS) provides both health care providers and the public with evidence-based information about exposures during pregnancy and while breastfeeding (see MotherToBaby in Additional Resources). The world's most notorious teratogen is probably thalidomide; however, clinicians today are probably more familiar with fetal alcohol spectrum disorder (FASD), which results from prenatal exposure to alcohol. However, exposures can also include viruses, including rubella, cytomegalovirus, and toxoplasmosis, and medications, such as warfarin, lithium, tetracycline, and phenytoin.

Mitochondrial Disorders

Although the majority of an individual's DNA is found in chromosomes within the nucleus of a cell, a small amount of genetic material is found in the mitochondria located in the cytoplasm, outside the nucleus. This genetic material is known as *mitochondrial DNA (mtDNA)* and contains only 37 genes. Each cell contains hundreds to thousands of mitochondria, which also means there are more opportunities for mutations. Mitochondrial disorders are caused by mutations in mtDNA (i.e., non-chromosomal DNA) and are typically progressive disorders affecting the brain and muscles. Mitochondrial disorders are characterized by exclusively maternal (matrilinear) transmission. When many normal mitochondria are present, the effects from the aberrant mtDNA may be minimal. Some examples of mitochondrial disorders that should be familiar to PCPs are Leber hereditary optic neuropathy (LHON), Leigh syndrome, non-syndromic deafness mitochondrial encephalomyopathy, lactic acidosis, and stroke-like episodes (MELAS). Of note, mtDNA also provides individuals with genealogic information about their female ancestral line.

Patterns of Inheritance

Terminology

One of the important outcomes of taking a family history is the ability to recognize basic inheritance patterns; however, it is important to understand that there can be variable phenotypes, making some patterns of inheritance harder to detect. There are a few terms that clinicians need to understand, including penetrance, expressivity, pleiotropy, variable age of onset, and anticipation (Table 41-1).

Mendelian Inheritance Patterns

Genetic disorders caused by mutations in a single gene are usually inherited in one of several patterns, commonly referred to as *Mendelian* (after Gregor Mendel, known as the father of genetics) patterns of inheritance. They include autosomal dominant (AD), autosomal recessive (AR), X-linked dominant, and X-linked recessive, as well as maternal or mitochondrial inheritance. In contrast, most

TABLE 41-1 Definitions of Gene Expression Variables

Term	Definition	Examples
Penetrance—complete or incomplete	Proportion (%) of individuals with a specific genotype that exhibit the corresponding disease phenotype. Complete: Everyone with a specific disease genotype (100%) manifests the corresponding phenotype Incomplete: Some (varying %) of the affected individuals manifest the phenotype	Complete: Huntington disease Incomplete: Breast cancer from BRCA1 or BRCA2 mutation
Expressivity (variable expressivity)	Degree to which a phenotype is expressed. Can vary by compilation and/or severity, even within families.	Van der Woude syndrome: Children can have a cleft lip, cleft palate, or both. Children can have pits near the center of the lower lip; mounds, and/or missing teeth.
Pleiotropy	One genotype results in multiple, seemingly unrelated phenotypes	Marfan syndrome: From joint hypermobility and limb elongation to aortic and heart disease, vision problems, caused by a dislocated lens in either one or both eyes, as well as varying severity, timing of onset, and rate of progression
Variable age of onset	Phenotypic expression does not emerge until later in life	Alzheimer or Parkinson disease
Anticipation	Some phenotypes become more severe and/or appear at an earlier age as a genetic disorder is passed from one generation to the next	Myotonic dystrophy, fragile X syndrome, Huntington disease

chromosomal disorders are not passed from one generation to the next.

Autosomal Dominant

This type of single genetic disorder is characterized by the inheritance of a single copy of a mutated gene located on one of the autosomal chromosomes (chromosome 1-22). The gene mutation is passed on from only one parent but results in a genetic disorder. The paired gene from the other parent is normal. The parent passing on the gene mutation typically has the disorder. For the offspring, the risk of inheriting the mutation from an affected parent is 50%, regardless of sex and independent of having an affected sibling (Fig. 41-2). Children without the abnormal gene will neither develop the disorder nor pass it on. Examples of genetic disorders with an AD inheritance pattern include Huntington disease, Noonan syndrome, and neurofibromatosis type 1.

The clinician reviewing a child's family history should consider AD inheritance when a specific phenotype does not skip generations, both sexes appear equally affected, and male-to-male transmission occurs. However, penetrance, expressivity, pleiotropy, variable age of onset, and anticipation can interfere with one's ability to recognize AD inheritance. Further, some AD disorders, such as achondroplasia, have a high rate of *de novo* (new) mutations, making it highly likely that a pedigree will not reveal additionally affected relatives.

Autosomal Recessive

This type of single gene disorder requires inheritance of two copies of a mutated gene (one from each parent) located on one of the autosomal chromosomes (chromosome 1-22). Offspring who inherit only one abnormal gene in the pair are considered *carriers;* they can pass that gene to their children but are typically unaffected. For offspring of parents who both carry an AR mutation, there is a 25% chance of inheriting the mutation from both parents, thus developing the associated disorder, a 50% chance of inheriting one copy and becoming a carrier, and a 25% chance of not inheriting either mutation (Fig. 41-3). Examples of AR genetic disorders include cystic fibrosis, albinism, phenylketonuria, thalassemia, and sickle cell anemia.

The clinician reviewing a child's family history should consider AR inheritance when a specific phenotype affects multiple siblings, both sexes are affected, and/or the disorder appears to skip generations. A family's geographic ancestry and ethnic background, as well as consanguinity, can influence the likelihood of AR genetic disorders. For example, the gene mutations associated with cystic fibrosis occur most frequently in populations of European descent, and gene mutations associated with sickle cell anemia occur more frequently throughout sub-Saharan Africa, the Middle East, and the Indian subcontinent (Williams and Weatherall, 2012).

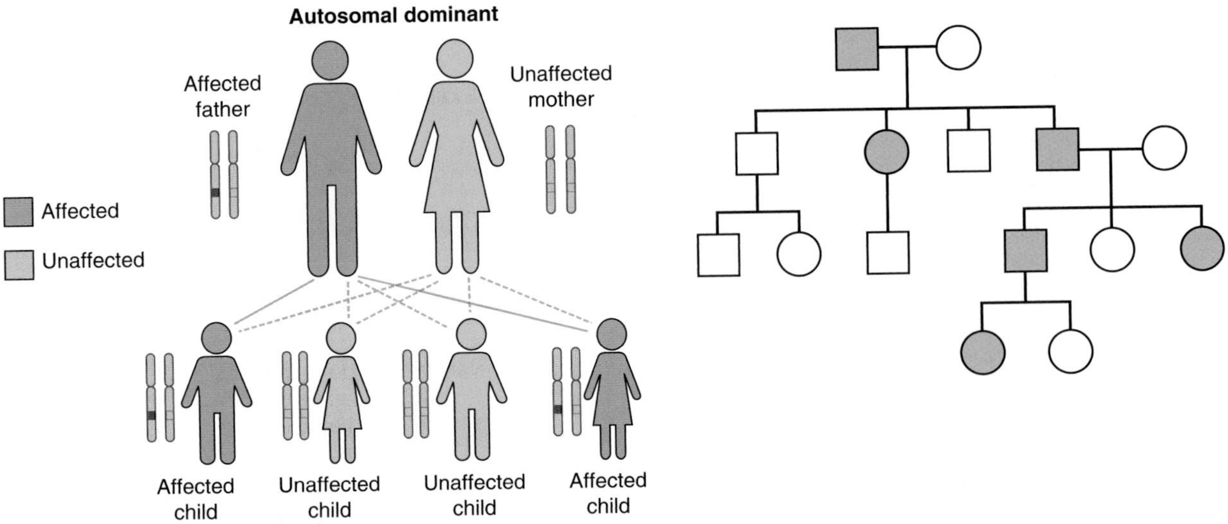

• **Figure 41-2** Autosomal dominant (AD) inheritance. (From Genetics Home Reference: Autosomal dominant, Genetics Home Reference (website), 2014, Available at http://ghr.nlm.nih.gov/handbook/illustrations/autodominant. Accessed November 16, 2015.)

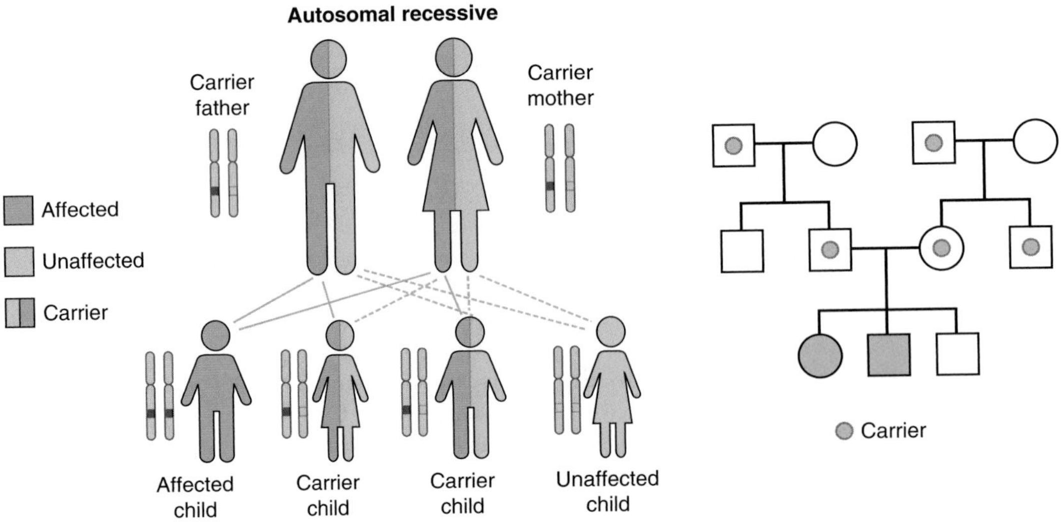

• **Figure 41-3** Autosomal recessive (AR) inheritance. (From Genetics Home Reference: Autosomal recessive, Genetics Home Reference (website), 2014, Available at http://ghr.nlm.nih.gov/handbook/illustrations/patterns?show=autorecessive. Accessed November 16, 2015.)

X-Linked Inheritance

Although X-linked inheritance patterns have traditionally been separated into subcategories of X-linked dominant or recessive, there is a move toward collapsing these categories, considering X-linked inheritance patterns across a spectrum. However, for the purposes of this chapter, they will be presented separately.

X-Linked Dominant

When a genetic disorder is classified as *X-linked dominant,* it means that a single abnormal gene on the X chromosome gives rise to the disease (Fig. 41-4). If the father is affected (abnormal X) and the mother is not, all of his female offspring will inherit the disease but none of his sons, because daughters always inherit their father's X-chromosome, whereas sons inherit their father's Y-chromosome. If the mother is affected (one abnormal X) and the father is not, there is only a 50% chance that each daughter or son will inherit the disorder, because mothers have two X chromosomes to pass on.

The clinician reviewing a child's family history should consider X-linked dominant inheritance when a specific phenotype affects both sexes in each generation, with slightly more females, and the absence of male-to-male transmission. Examples of genetic disorders with X-linked dominant inheritance include Rett syndrome and vitamin D-resistant rickets.

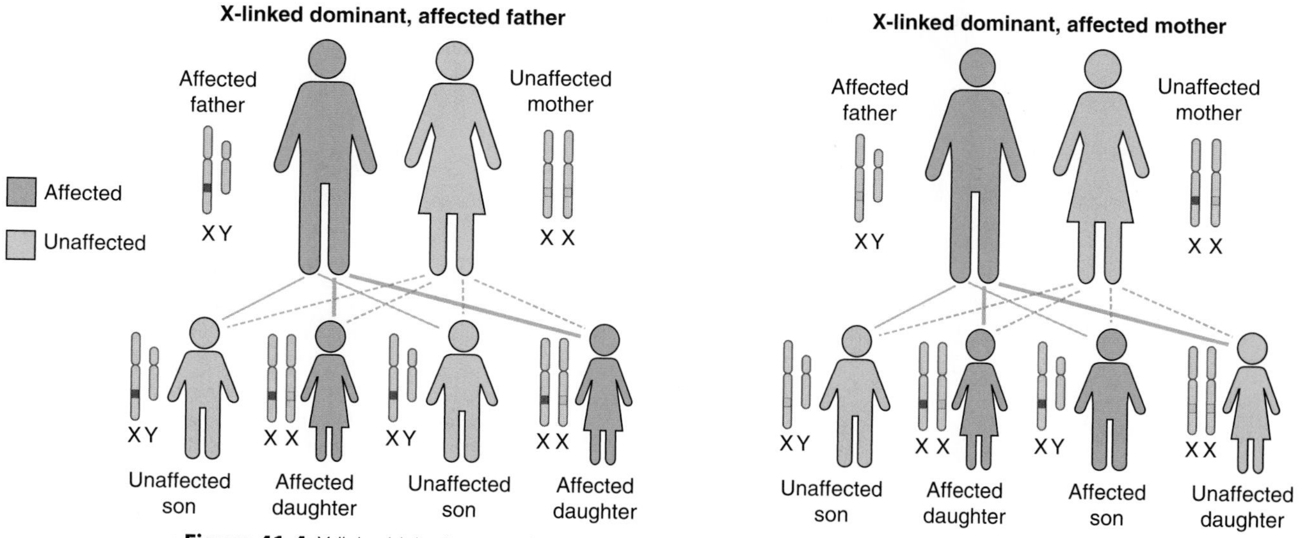

• **Figure 41-4** X-linked inheritance—dominant. (From Genetics Home Reference: Inheritance patterns, Genetics Home Reference (website), 2014, Available at http://ghr.nlm.nih.gov/handbook/illustrations/patterns?show=xlinkdominantfather. Accessed November 16, 2015; and Genetics Home Reference: Inheritance patterns, Genetics Home Reference (website), 2014, Available at http://ghr.nlm.nih.gov/handbook/illustrations/patterns?show=xlinkdominantmother. Accessed November 16, 2015.)

X-Linked Recessive

When a genetic disorder is classified as *X-linked recessive,* it usually occurs in males (Fig. 41-5). This pattern is seen because males have only one X chromosome, so a single recessive gene on that X chromosome will cause the disease. The Y chromosome does not contain most of the genes of the X chromosome and therefore cannot protect the male. When the father is affected (abnormal X), none of his sons will be affected, and all of his daughters will be *carriers.* If the mother is a carrier (one abnormal X), there is a 50% chance that each son will be affected. Daughters have a 50% chance of being a carrier like their mothers. Although females can have an X-linked recessive disorder, it is rare.

When reviewing a child's family history, one should consider X-linked recessive inheritance when a specific phenotype is noted in males more often or more severely than females. Examples of X-linked recessive disorders include Fabry disease, hemophilia A and B, G6PD deficiency, and Duchene muscular dystrophy. As with AD inheritance, some disorders (e.g., Duchene muscular dystrophy) have high rates of *de novo* (new) mutations, thus rendering the past family history negative.

Nontraditional Inheritance Patterns

Mitochondrial Inheritance

Another inheritance pattern arises from the mtDNA, which accordingly is called *mitochondrial inheritance* (Fig. 41-6). Mothers alone pass on mitochondrial mutations (i.e., matrilinear or maternal inheritance) because only egg cells contribute mitochondria to the developing embryo. Disorders that arise from mutations in mtDNA can appear in every generation, affecting both sexes. Although on average, males are more severely affected compared with females. Affected fathers do not pass this on, however. Examples of genetic disorders with maternal (mitochondrial) inheritance include LHON, myoclonic epilepsy with ragged red fibers (MERRF), and MELAS.

Codominant Inheritance

A gene disorder is categorized as having a *codominant inheritance* when two different alleles for a gene can be expressed and different combinations result in slightly different proteins (Fig. 41-7). There are a few genes with established codominant inheritance patterns; however some genetic disorders do not follow established patterns and are considered multifactorial in origin. Sometimes the specific gene(s) remain partially or fully unidentified. The best example of this type of inheritance is reflected in blood type (ABO blood group) determination.

Genomic Imprinting

Children typically inherit two copies of genes, one from their mother and one from their father, and both copies are active (i.e., turned on) in the cells together; however, in some cases only one copy needs to be expressed, and therefore the other copy is turned off or silenced during embryogenesis. The decision as to which gene remains working and which is silenced depends on the parent of origin. Only a small number of genes go through genomic imprinting, which occurs when the origin of the gene (maternal vs. paternal) is marked (imprinted) on the gene during the formation of egg or sperm cells through methylation. Imprinted genes tend to cluster together in the same regions of certain chromosomes (Genetics Home Reference, 2014). Improper imprinting can result in a child having two active copies or two inactive copies. Two major clusters of imprinted genes have been identified in humans, on chromosomes 11 and 15. Prader-Willi syndrome occurs when

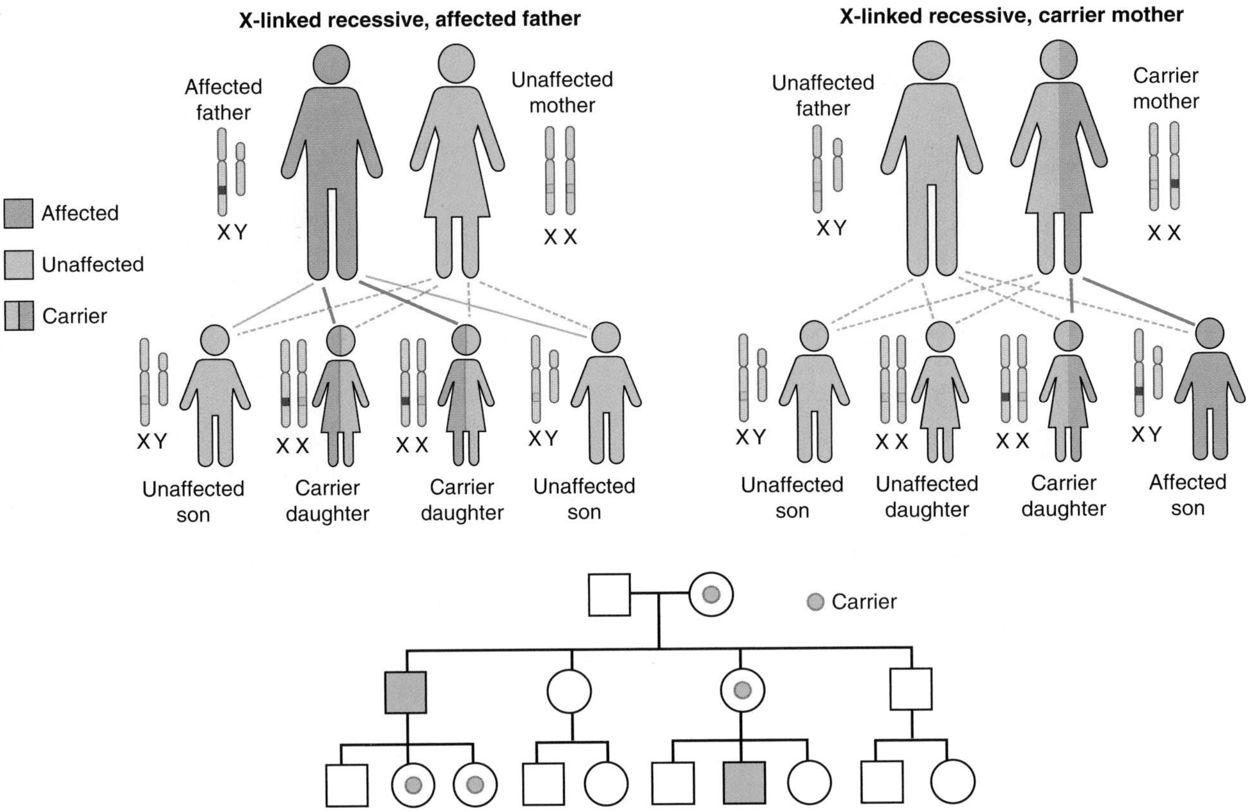

• **Figure 41-5** X-linked inheritance—recessive. (From Genetics Home Reference: Inheritance patterns, Genetics Home Reference (website), 2014, Available at http://ghr.nlm.nih.gov/handbook/illustrations/patterns?show=xlinkrecessivefather. Accessed November 16, 2015; and Genetics Home Reference: Inheritance patterns, Genetics Home Reference (website), 2014, Available at http://ghr.nlm.nih.gov/handbook/illustrations/patterns?show=xlinkrecessivemother. Accessed November 16, 2015.)

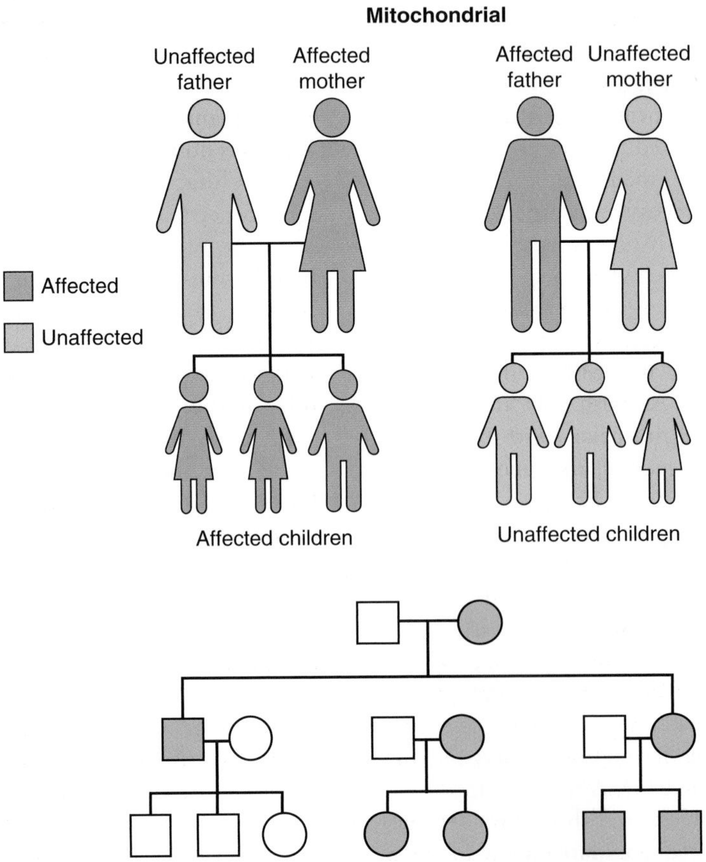

• **Figure 41-6** Mitochondrial inheritance. (From Genetics Home Reference: Inheritance patterns, Genetics Home Reference (website), 2014, Available at http://ghr.nlm.nih.gov/handbook/illustrations/patterns?show=mitochondrial. Accessed November 16, 2015.)

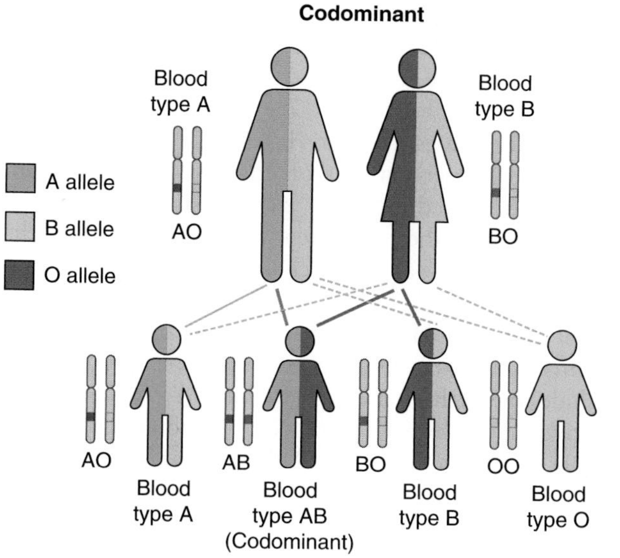

• **Figure 41-7** Codominant inheritance. (From Genetics Home Reference: Inheritance patterns, Genetics Home Reference (website), 2014, Available at http://ghr.nlm.nih.gov/handbook/illustrations/patterns?show=codominant. Accessed November 16, 2015.)

the paternally derived genes located in a specific chromosome 15 region are either improperly imprinted or deleted, whereas Angelman syndrome occurs when the maternally derived genes in the same area are either improperly imprinted or deleted. Thus, the developing embryo does not detect a paternal or maternal copy of chromosome 15, producing one syndrome or the other. Beckwith-Wiedemann and Russell-Silver syndromes are other examples of disorders influenced by genomic imprinting.

Uniparental Disomy

When a child receives two copies of one chromosome, or a part of a chromosome, from one parent and none from the other parent, it results in uniparental disomy (UPD). The child will be homozygous for every gene located on that chromosome, which increases the possibility of inheriting an AR disorder. UPD can occur as a random event during the formation of egg or sperm cells or may happen in early fetal development.

In many cases, UPD has no effect on a child's health or development, because most genes are not imprinted. Thus, it does not matter if a child inherits both copies from one parent or one copy from each parent. However, in some cases, maternal or paternal inheritance of a specific gene is important. Examples of genetic disorders that can arise from UPD include Prader-Willi and Angelman syndromes, which were also noted under genomic imprinting. Prader-Willi syndrome (caused by UPD) happens when the fetus inherits two maternal chromosome 15 (she or he is missing a paternally derived chromosome 15). Angelman syndrome (caused by UPD) happens when the fetus inherits two paternal chromosome 15 (she or he is missing a maternally derived chromosome 15).

Epigenetics

Epigenetics is the study of changes in gene function that occur without a change in DNA sequence (NHGRI, 2014b). Epigenetics regulates which genes get turned on and off. Its study is increasingly important in the identification and treatment of childhood diseases and developmental disorders. Unlike the genome, the epigenome is modifiable. Different experiences or exposures may influence the epigenetic profile of each cell through DNA methylation, histone modifications, and/or microRNA. Examples of factors that affect epigenetic changes include chemical exposures, diet, endocrine disruptive compounds, hypoxia, maternal physical state and age, placenta size, smoking, stress, and trauma. Many common adult disorders are now believed to be caused by epigenetic changes that occurred during that individual's childhood, including heart disease, hypertension, and obesity (see Let's Get Healthy: Epigenetics Game in Additional Resources).

Genetic Implications for Pediatric Primary Care

For pediatric PCPs, the integration of genetics, epigenetics, and accompanying technologies into their practice may seem overwhelming. The GPCI has developed *A Toolkit to Improve Care for Pediatric Patients with Genetic Conditions in Primary Care* (2014a) that guides providers through the process of identifying and caring for pediatric patients with genetic conditions, from collecting family health history, recognizing clinical red flags, and ordering genetic tests, to coordinating care with genetics' specialists and others (see Additional Resources).

Assessment

Family health history and the recognition of genetic red flags provide the foundation from which care evolves. Emphasis is on understanding genetic screening, working with children and families to understand the implications of a genetic workup and diagnosis, and coordinating care with genetic specialists. A complete head-to-toe physical and developmental assessment, combined with a comprehensive family health history, is important in identifying genetic disorders.

Family Health History and Pedigree

In primary care practice, taking the time to collect a child's family health history and pedigree can be just as important as information from a laboratory test, yet it is often underused (Tsai et al, 2011; Pyeritz, 2012). Individual and family involvement in family health history got a boost in 2004, when the U.S. Surgeon General declared Thanksgiving as the ideal day to investigate and/or update one's family health history. An individual's family history should be updated annually.

A Toolkit to Improve Care for Pediatric Patients with Genetic Conditions in Primary Care (GPCI, 2014a) provides step-by-step instructions, a downloadable pediatric genetic screening questionnaire, case examples with which to practice both collection and interpretation, and documentation of family history in electronic health records. Also helpful are the suggestions of wording and phrases to use throughout the family health history, as well as when asking about sensitive topics, such as adoption, consanguinity, death, or estranged family members. For example, the *Toolkit* (p. 29) suggests beginning with a purposeful explanatory statement, such as "I would like to ask you some questions about your health and about the health of your family members. Having this information will help to provide the best care for your child." Some suggestions for direct questions (p. 31) include: "Is there anyone with facial features that look different from other family members?" or "Are all your children with the same partner?" An example of an indirect question (p. 29) is: "Do you have any concerns about a condition that may be genetic that runs in your family?"

Table 41-2 suggests specific questions to use when conducting a comprehensive family health history.

Three-Generation Pedigree

The pedigree is a valuable visual record of genetic links and health-related information. It should include at least three generations and is much more helpful in visual, rather than in lists or narrative formats. It is important to remember that most disorders have some genetic component and the strength or pattern of traits or diseases may become apparent, based on the number or pattern of individuals in a family who are affected.

Refer to Figures 41-2 to 41-7 for the generic pedigrees highlighted under patterns of inheritance. Insights about families are gained, not only because families share genes, but also because they also often share environments, behaviors, and culture—all of which contribute to shared health problems.

All PCPs should be able to obtain, record, and interpret a three-generation pedigree, which is a construct that includes the health status of first-, second-, and third-degree relatives across three generations of the individual's or child's family (Brock et al, 2010). Although the aim for clinical practice is a three-generation pedigree, asking about only two generations, or in some cases asking about four generations, may be more appropriate, depending on the trait or disorder and family size (see Table 41-3 for proportion of genetic material shared by family relationships).

There is a set of standardized pedigree symbols that have been adopted internationally (Bennett et al, 2008). An overview of the symbols, as well as how to connect them to illustrate various family relationships, is provided in Figures 41-8 and 41-9. There are also multiple Internet resources to assist children, families, and providers in obtaining and documenting family health histories, including Genetic Alliance's "Does It Run in the Family" Toolkit (see Genetic

TABLE 41-2 General Screening for Genetic Conditions: The History

Question	Rationale/Comments
Does/Has anyone in the family have/had a birth defect?	To identify conditions that affect others in the family. If answer is yes, try to get more information about the nature of the defect.
Has anyone in the family had a stillborn baby? A baby who died early? A baby who died unexpectedly?	To identify unrecognized genetic disorders. Babies who died very early may have inheritable metabolic disorders. Distinguish from sudden infant death syndrome (SIDS).
Is there any chance that you and your partner are blood-related? Is this pregnancy a product of incest? Is there any history of consanguinity/incest in your extended family?	Consanguinity of partners closer than first cousins is a risk factor for autosomal recessive (AR) disorders. If yes, recommend genetics consultation.
What conditions/diseases/traits run in your family? Are there any conditions anyone in your family routinely sees a health care provider for?	Significant if early onset, two or more close relatives affected. Remember to ask about hearing/vision, growth disorders. Genetic heart disease and genetic cancer risks are important. If yes, recommend genetic consultation and monitoring.
Have you or your partner, or any of your/your partners' parents/siblings had three or more miscarriages? How about infertility issues?	May indicate a chromosome translocation. If yes, order a karyotype of the mother or father (or both). Difficulties becoming/maintaining a pregnancy may indicate a genetic syndrome.
Does anyone in the family have learning problems, mental retardation/behavioral disorders, developmental delays?	Look for multiple members affected and associated with dysmorphic features. If yes, recommend genetic consultation.
What is your ethnic/geographic heritage background? Your partner's?	Discovering where an individual's ancestors come from can help identify certain ethnic and/or population risk factors.

Alliance in Additional Resources) or NCHPEG's Family History Collection Tool (see National Coalition for Health Professional Education in Genetics [NCHPEG] in Additional Resources).

The process of constructing a family pedigree should begin with the core family, followed by added aunts and uncles, cousins, and grandparents. For all persons included in the pedigree, it is important to record their date of birth or age, relevant symptoms, traits, or disorders, as well as the ages of diagnosis, and the ages and causes of death. It is also important to record miscarriages, stillbirths, infertility, and any children relinquished for adoption (Tsai et al, 2011). An additional query should be made about the presence or possibility of consanguinity or incest. When pieces of family history are missing, it is important to note the information as missing, because the absence of information does not mean the child has not acquired genetic risk.

Genetic Red Flags from the History

Genetic red flags indicate the potential for genetic risk. For some providers, it is easiest to remember the Rule of Too/Two (GPCI, 2014b). Other providers find it helpful to use the SCREEN mnemonic to remember the important components to look for or ask about when obtaining a family health history. Another frequently cited mnemonic that organizes several principles is the F-GENES mnemonic (see Table 41-4).

In general, providers should pay attention if one or more of these genetic red flags emerge when taking a family health history: (1) multiple affected members with the same related disorder, (2) earlier age at onset than expected for the disorder, (3) a condition or disorder seen in the less-often affected sex, (4) the appearance of a disease in the absence of any known risk factors, (5) ethnicity or ancestral background, (6) unusual close relationships, such as consanguinity, by blood or through a common ancestor, (7) multifocal or bilateral occurrence in paired organs, and (8) intellectual impairment with or without major or minor malformations (Scott and Trotter, 2013).

TABLE 41-3 Degree of Relationship between Individual Family Members and Shared Genetic Material

Relationship	Amount of Shared Genetic Material	Example
First-degree relatives	25%	Children, full siblings, biologic parents
Second-degree relatives	50%	Grandparents, half siblings, aunts/uncles, nieces/nephews
Third-degree relatives	12.5%	Cousins

Physical Findings Indicating Genetic Disorders

It is important not only to identify red flags in the history but also to identify physical findings that can point to the presence of a particular genetic condition(s). Findings that are particularly notable include physical abnormalities (e.g., multiple café au lait spots, growth problems, and congenital anomalies) and neurologic abnormalities (including hearing loss, vision loss, developmental delay, mental retardation, hypotonia, progressive muscle weakness, and hard to control

TABLE 41-4 Mnemonics for Gathering and Interpreting the Genetic Health Data

Mnemonic	Meaning
Rule of Two/Too	***Too*** many of something: individual is *too* tall, *too* short, *too* early, *too* young, *too* different, and so on *or* ***Two*** birth defects, *two* cancers, *two* in a family, or *two* generations involved
SCREEN	**S**ome **C**oncerns about traits or diseases that run in the family **R**eproductive problems a history of **E**arly disease, death, or disability **E**thnicity of the patient **N**on-genetic risk factors or conditions that run in the family
F-GENES	**F**amily history: Multiple affected siblings in the same or individuals in multiple generations **G**roups (two or more) of congenital anomalies or anatomic variations **E**xtreme or exceptional presentation of a common condition(s), including early onset, recurrent miscarriage, bilateral disease **N**eurodevelopmental delay or degeneration (regression) **E**xtreme or exceptional pathology **S**urprising laboratory values

Adapted from Genetics in Primary Care Institute (GPCI): Genetic red flags, Available at https://geneticsinprimarycare.aap.org/YourPractice/Family-Health-History/Pages/Genetic%20Red%20Flags.aspx. Accessed November 20, 2015.

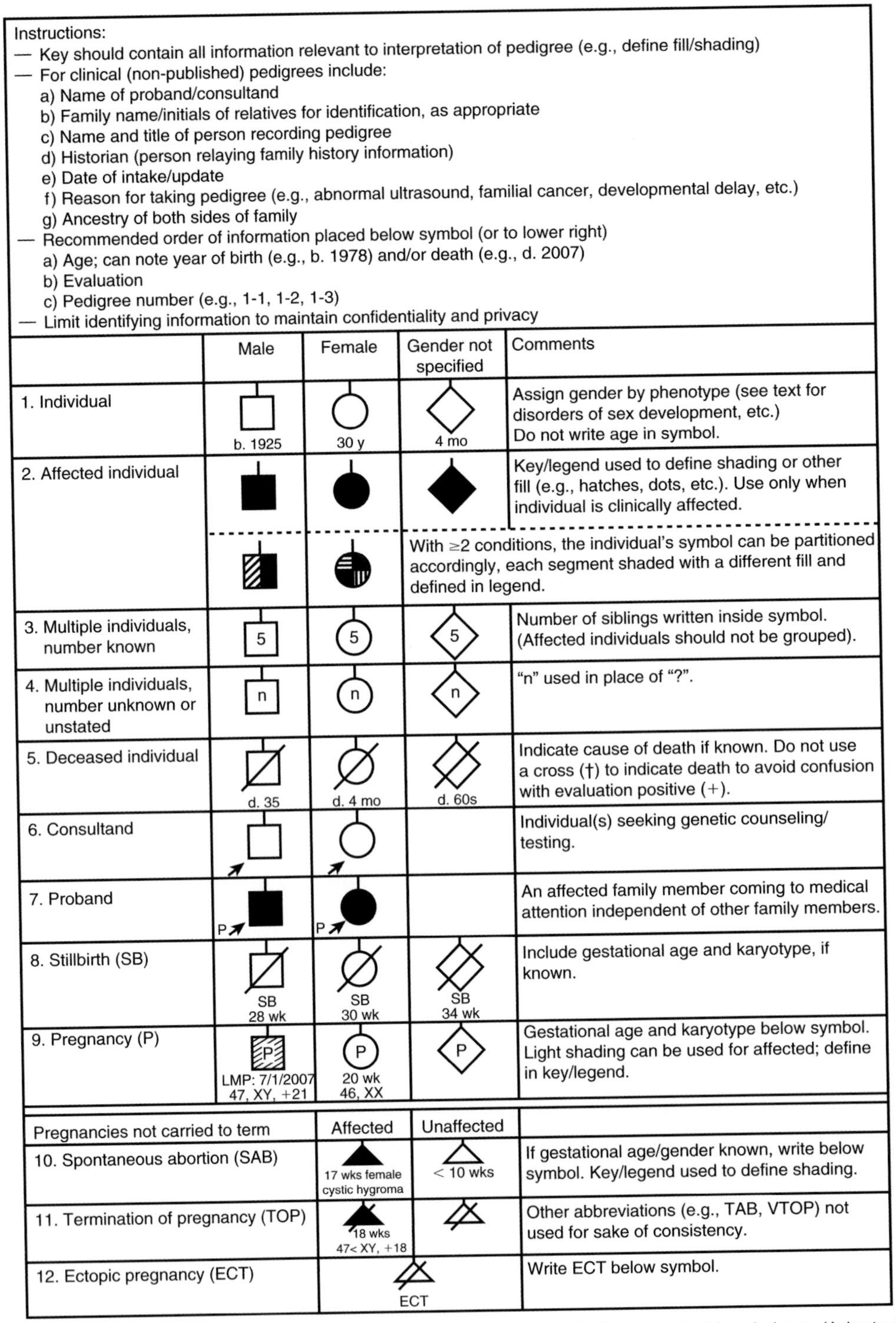
Instructions:
— Key should contain all information relevant to interpretation of pedigree (e.g., define fill/shading)
— For clinical (non-published) pedigrees include:
a) Name of proband/consultand
b) Family name/initials of relatives for identification, as appropriate
c) Name and title of person recording pedigree
d) Historian (person relaying family history information)
e) Date of intake/update
f) Reason for taking pedigree (e.g., abnormal ultrasound, familial cancer, developmental delay, etc.)
g) Ancestry of both sides of family
— Recommended order of information placed below symbol (or to lower right)
a) Age; can note year of birth (e.g., b. 1978) and/or death (e.g., d. 2007)
b) Evaluation
c) Pedigree number (e.g., 1-1, 1-2, 1-3)
— Limit identifying information to maintain confidentiality and privacy
Male
Female
Gender not specified
Comments
1. Individual
b. 1925
30 y
4 mo
Assign gender by phenotype (see text for disorders of sex development, etc.)
Do not write age in symbol.
2. Affected individual
Key/legend used to define shading or other fill (e.g., hatches, dots, etc.). Use only when individual is clinically affected.
With ≥2 conditions, the individual's symbol can be partitioned accordingly, each segment shaded with a different fill and defined in legend.
3. Multiple individuals, number known
5
5
5
Number of siblings written inside symbol. (Affected individuals should not be grouped).
4. Multiple individuals, number unknown or unstated
n
n
n
"n" used in place of "?".
5. Deceased individual
d. 35
d. 4 mo
d. 60s
Indicate cause of death if known. Do not use a cross (†) to indicate death to avoid confusion with evaluation positive (+).
6. Consultand
Individual(s) seeking genetic counseling/testing.
7. Proband
P
P
An affected family member coming to medical attention independent of other family members.
8. Stillbirth (SB)
SB 28 wk
SB 30 wk
SB 34 wk
Include gestational age and karyotype, if known.
9. Pregnancy (P)
P
LMP: 7/1/2007 47, XY, +21
P
20 wk 46, XX
P
Gestational age and karyotype below symbol. Light shading can be used for affected; define in key/legend.
Pregnancies not carried to term
Affected
Unaffected
10. Spontaneous abortion (SAB)
17 wks female cystic hygroma
< 10 wks
If gestational age/gender known, write below symbol. Key/legend used to define shading.
11. Termination of pregnancy (TOP)
18 wks 47< XY, +18
Other abbreviations (e.g., TAB, VTOP) not used for sake of consistency.
12. Ectopic pregnancy (ECT)
ECT
Write ECT below symbol.

• **Figure 41-8** Pedigree model. Common pedigree symbols, definitions, and abbreviations. (Adapted from Bennett RL, French KS, Resta RG, et al: Standardized human pedigree nomenclature: update and assessment of the recommendations of the National Society of Genetic Counselors, *J Genet Couns* 17[5]:424–433, 2008.)

seizure disorders). PCPs can hone their abilities by familiarizing themselves with advanced anthropomorphic measurement skills and by reviewing detailed descriptions and photographs of children and adults with various disorders (see Resources to Hone Physical Assessment Skills in Additional Resources).

Minor and Major Anomalies

Classification of features can appear somewhat arbitrary. A congenital anomaly or birth defect is an abnormality of structure or function that is present at birth. A physical finding is referred to as a *major anomaly* if it impairs normal body function (e.g., congenital heart disease, cleft palate),

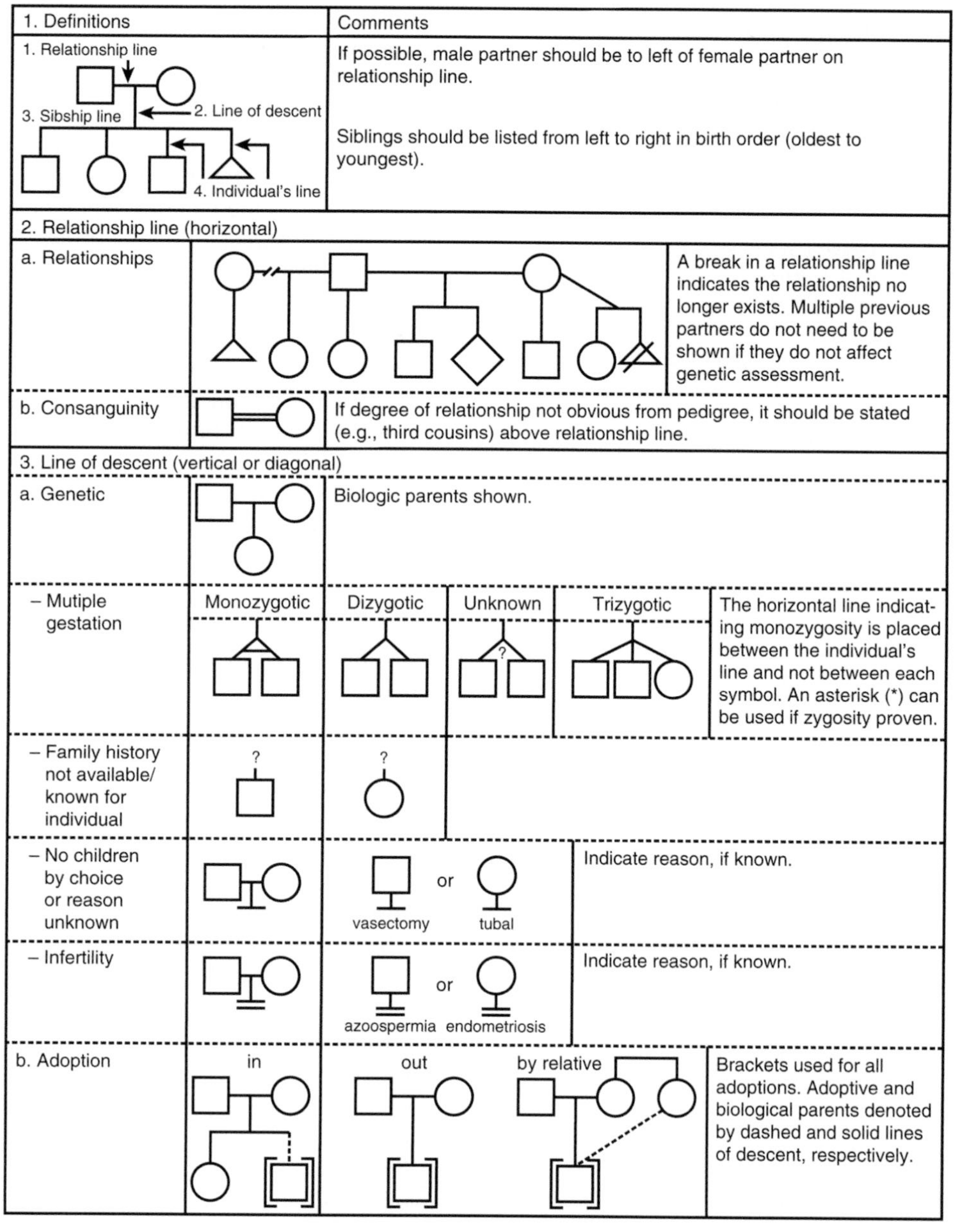

• **Figure 41-9** Pedigree line definitions. (Adapted from Bennett RL, French KS, Resta RG, et al: Standardized human pedigree nomenclature: update and assessment of the recommendations of the National Society of Genetic Counselors, *J Genet Couns* 17[5]:424–433, 2008.)

whereas a minor anomaly is more of a cosmetic variation, without impairing function (e.g., clinodactyly, small ear). This distinction is made because a genetic etiology is often considered when an individual has one major or more than two minor anomalies. Minor anomalies in the head, neck, and hand account for the majority of all minor anomalies (Table 41-5).

Malformations are birth defects that result from an intrinsic process, such as altered genetic or developmental processes. They typically result in a basic alteration in structure and occur early in gestation (e.g., cleft palate, anencephaly, limb agenesis). *Deformities* and *disruptions* are defects that result from an external process, resulting in an abnormal shape or positioning of a body part or organ. A deformity results from a distortion by a physical force, such as oligohydramnios or twins, on an otherwise normal structure (e.g., club foot), whereas a disruption refers to destruction of a tissue or structure that was previously normal (e.g., amniotic bands). In contrast, *dysplasia* is used to reflect abnormal cellular organization within tissues that results in a structural change (e.g., achondroplasia). When there is a set, recurrent pattern of features or malformations that often have a known genetic component, it is called a *syndrome.* An *association,* on the other hand, is a group of anomalies that occur more frequently than would be expected by chance alone. Associations do not have a predictable pattern or a unified etiology (e.g., VACTERL association—V = vertebral, A = anal anomalies, C = cardiac,

TABLE 41-5 Minor Malformations and/or Variations of Normal

General	Short/tall stature Body/limb disproportion Failure to thrive (FTT) or obesity
Craniofacial features	Unusual head shape/circumference/ fontanels Synophrys (fused eyebrows) Long eyelashes Hyper/hypotelorism Epicanthal folds Up/down slanting and/or short palpebral fissures Heterochromia, ptosis, cataract, glaucoma Low nasal bridge Abnormal ear position/shape/tags/ pits Short, long, or flattened philtrum Malar flattening Prominent metopic ridge Bifid uvula, high arched/cleft palate Natal teeth/central incisor Micrognathia
Hands/feet	Abnormal creases Short/long digit(s) Prominent digital pads Clinodactyly (incurved fingers) Syndactyly (fused digits) Polydactyly Camptodactyly (bent/flexed) Dysplastic nails
Hair/skin	Abnormal hair line or color Increased numbers or anterior location of hair whorl Hirsutism Hypopigmented/hyperpigmented patches Pigmented nevi
Neck	Short, webbing
Chest	Widely spaced or supernumerary nipples Abnormal chest shape
Abdomen/genitalia	Redundant umbilicus Shawl scrotum

TE = trachea-esophageal fistula, R = radial and/or renal anomalies, L = limb anomalies). The numbers of malformation syndromes described are increasing on a daily basis. The clinician needs to think in terms of phenotypic analysis, which begins with a complete physical and developmental assessment (Table 41-6).

Diagnostic Studies

No single genetic test can identify all genetic disorders. Equally important, findings from genetic testing completed for one individual can impact other family members. The increased availability and use of genetic screening and testing in children led the American Academy of Pediatrics (AAP) and the American College of Medical Genetics and Genomics (ACMG) to update their policy statements on newborn screening, diagnostic genetic testing, carrier testing, predictive genetic testing in children, and the disclosure of genetic test results (Hamid, 2013). In addition, they added a statement about direct-to-consumer genetic testing, strongly discouraging the use of this type of genetic testing in children. As highlighted in their policy statement, decisions about whether to offer genetic screening and/or testing should be informed by the best interest of the child (AAP Committee on Bioethics, Committee on Genetics and ACMG Social, Ethical, and Legal Issues Committee, 2013). One peer-reviewed resource for health care providers, called *GeneTests* (see Additional Resources), provides current information about available genetic tests and where they can be done.

Screening

Screening is used in asymptomatic populations to identify individuals who need further evaluation and/or testing. Pediatric providers need to be familiar with newborn and prenatal screening. The family health history and specific tests that screen for disorders increasingly thought to have a genetic basis, such as autism, are also important screening tools.

Newborn Screening

Newborn screening, which is used just after birth, is used to identify genetic disorders that can benefit from early diagnosis and treatment. This screening began over 50 years ago with the testing for phenylketonuria (PKU) and is considered the first genetic population-based screening program (Saul, 2013). Today, effective newborn screening involves a sophisticated network of coordinated efforts among public health agencies, PCPs, and specialists. It involves individual and family education, mass screening for a select subset of congenital or inherited conditions, and short- and long-term follow-up plans for newborns who screen positive. Each state determines the conditions included on their newborn screening panel; however, there is a national Recommended Universal Screening Panel (RUSP), which currently lists 31 core conditions and 26 secondary conditions, for which every baby should be screened. The RUSP is not a law, serving only as a guide for states. Clinicians should check the National Newborn Screening and Genetics Resource Center and/or Baby's First Test (see Additional Resources), where the latest information on the conditions included in each state's newborn screening is continually updated.

Following up a positive newborn screen is stressful for both the clinician and the family. Being well prepared will make the initial contact with the family more effective. The ACMG developed actions (ACT) sheets that provide clinicians with the steps to be taken after an initial positive screening result with an accompanying algorithm. Their

TABLE 41-6 Selected Syndromes, Associated Findings/Developmental Cues

Syndrome	Clinical Findings	Developmental Cues
Down (trisomy 21)	• Short stature • Brachycephaly • Midface hypoplasia with flat nasal bridge • Brushfield spots • Epicanthal folds with palpebral fissures that slant down to midline • Small mouth with protruding tongue • Myopia • Small ears • Lax joints (atlantoaxial instability) • Short broad hands and feet and digits • Single palmar crease • Clinodactyly • Exaggerated space between great and second toes • Congenital heart disease • At risk for leukemia, Alzheimer disease, hypothyroidism	• Intellectual disability/developmental delays • Hearing loss • Hypotonia as infant
Turner (X0) (Fig. 41-10)	• Short stature for family • Short neck with webbing and low posterior hair line • Posteriorly rotated ears • Ptosis • Short fourth and fifth metacarpals • Short legs • Hyper-convex nails • Cardiac disease, bicuspid aortic valve, coarctation of the aorta • Hip dysplasia, scoliosis, and/or kyphosis • Horseshoe kidney • Chronic OM, with conductive hearing loss • Delayed puberty/infertility	• Nonverbal learning disabilities • Hearing loss • Strabismus
Klinefelter (XXY) (Fig. 41-11)	• Tall, with long arm span • Dental decay • Small penis, cryptorchidism or small testes • Gynecomastia • Skin striae • Delayed puberty • Autoimmune disorders • Scoliosis • Malignancies, including male breast cancer	• Delayed expressive language • Shy, withdrawn • Immature for age • ADHD
Fragile X (Fig. 41-12)	• Facial features: Long narrow face, high-arched palate/dental crowding, prominent ears develops in second decade • Poor growth, GER, feeding problems, diarrhea • Strabismus, ocular disorders • Recurrent OM/sinus infections • Seizures • Macroorchidism (puberty) • Joint hyperlaxity • Sleep problems, obstructive sleep apnea • Elevated risk for obesity • Short stature • Increased risk for congenital malformations • Possible in girls (Kidd et al, 2014)	• Intellectual disability • Language delays • Autism spectrum disorder • Behavioral problems (e.g., anxiety, attention, aggression) • Stereopathies, such as hand-flapping
Prader-Willi	• Decreased fetal movement/position • Failure to thrive • Short stature • Central obesity • Hypothalamic insufficiency • Strabismus • Myopia/hyperopia • Sleep apnea • Enamel hypoplasia • Scoliosis	• Motor delays • Poor coordination • Language delays • Mild intellectual disability • Compulsive hyperphagia • Behavioral phenotype: Tantrums, stubborn, rigidity, skin picking, high pain tolerance, ADHD, compulsiveness

Continued

TABLE 41-6 Selected Syndromes, Associated Findings/Developmental Cues—cont'd

Syndrome	Clinical Findings	Developmental Cues
Angelman	• Seizures • Global developmental delays • Abnormal gait, arms held high/flexed elbows • Hypotonic trunk with hypertonic limbs (commando crawl) • Feeding/growth problems • Acquired microcephaly	• Speech delay, but adequate receptive language • Intellectual disability • Spontaneous (persistent) social smile/fits of laughter • Hand flapping • Loves water • Abnormal sleep
Beckwith-Weidemann	• Omphalocele or umbilical hernia • Macroglossia • Facial nevus flammeus • Facial features: Nevus flammeus, helical pits, prominent eyes, anterior ear lobe creases • Large placenta/long umbilical cord • Hypoglycemia • Cardiomegaly • Dental malocclusion with maxillary underdevelopment	• Normal • Articulation issues
DiGeorge (also known as velocardiofacial or 22q11 deletion syndrome)	• Congenital heart defect • Palate abnormalities • Facial features: Long tubular nose, crumpled ears, hypertelorism, malar hypoplasia • Hypotonia • Early feeding problems • Constipation • Chronic otitis media/sinusitis • Polydactyly • Vertebral anomalies • Strabismus	• Developmental disability • Communication disorders, including delayed speech and hypernasality • Psychiatric disorders
Marfan (Fig. 41-13)	• Tall, long limbs • Aortic root dilatation, mitral valve prolapse/regurgitation • Ectopia lentis, myopia, retinal detachment, exotropia/strabismus • Spontaneous pneumothorax • Connective tissue problems, including pectus deformities, joint hyperextensibility	• Normal
Fetal alcohol spectrum disorder (FASD; Fig. 41-14)	• Poor prenatal and postnatal growth • Hypotonia, poor coordination • Cardiac defects (e.g., VSD, ASD) • Narrow eyes, microphthalmia, large epicanthal folds, microcephaly, small upper jaw, smooth groove in upper lip, thin upper lip • Simian creases common	• Delayed development in three or more areas: cognitive, speech, motor, psychosocial

Adapted from Stephan MJ, Geneman B: The baker's dozen: 13 can't miss syndromes, 2011, available at www.aap.org/en-us/about-the-aap/Committees-Councils-Sections/Section-on-Uniformed-Services/Documents/The_Bakers_Dozen-Stephan.pdf#search=health%20supervision%20genetics. Accessed September 14, 2014; Kidd SA, Lachewicz A, Barbouth D, et al: Fragile X syndrome: a review of associated medical problems, *Pediatrics* 134(5):995–1005, 2014.
ADHD, Attention-deficit/hyperactivity disorder; *ASD*, atrial septal defect; *GER*, gastroesophageal reflux; *OM*, otitis media; *VSD*, ventricular septal defect.

website (www.ncbi.nlm.nih.gov/books/NBK55827/) contains the latest versions of the ACT sheets, which are regularly revised based on new tests and information.

Prenatal Screening

Prenatal screening is used during pregnancy to detect a genetic and congenital disorder before birth. Both screening and diagnostic tests may occur prenatally. Prenatal screening tests are typically offered to all women to screen for common genetic disorders (such as, Down syndrome) and congenital anomalies (such as, NTDs), or to select women who might be at higher risk based on age, ancestral, or ethnic background, or a specific family history of the genetic disorder. All forms of genetic testing for the specific purpose of diagnosing a fetus can be performed directly on the fetus by collecting fetal cells through a chorionic villus sample (CVS) or amniocentesis. In contrast, pre-implantation testing is used to detect genetic changes in embryos created through

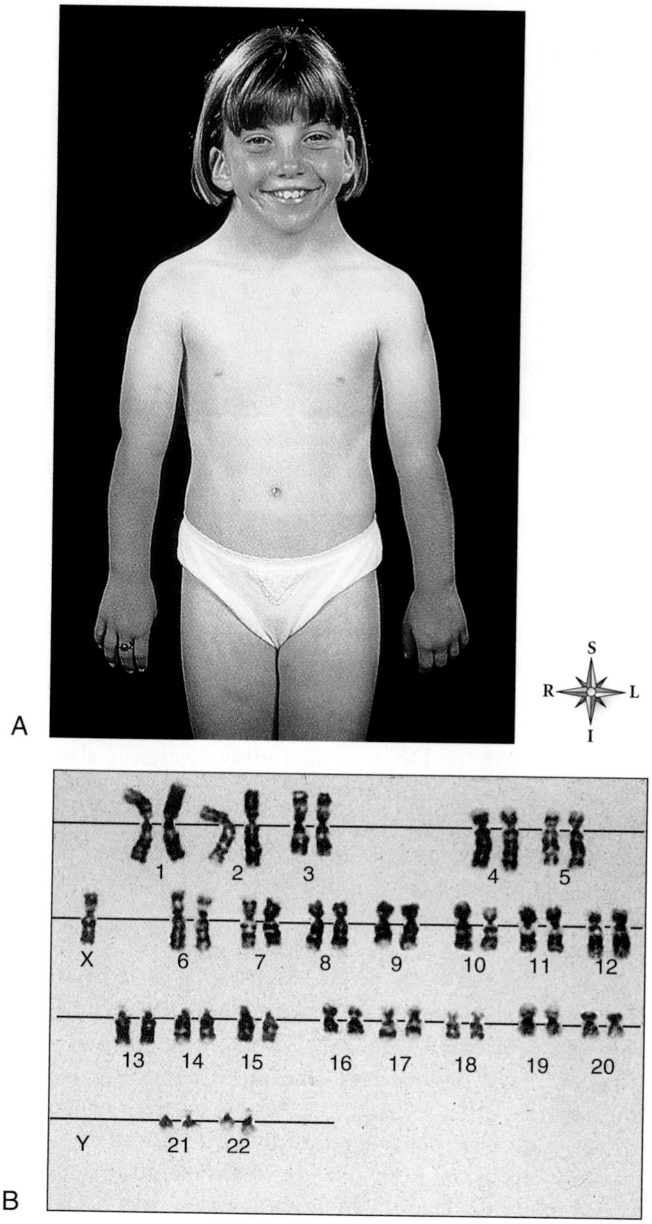

• **Figure 41-10** Turner syndrome. (From Patton KT, Thibodeau GA: *The human body in health & disease,* ed 6, St Louis, 2014, Mosby/Elsevier.)

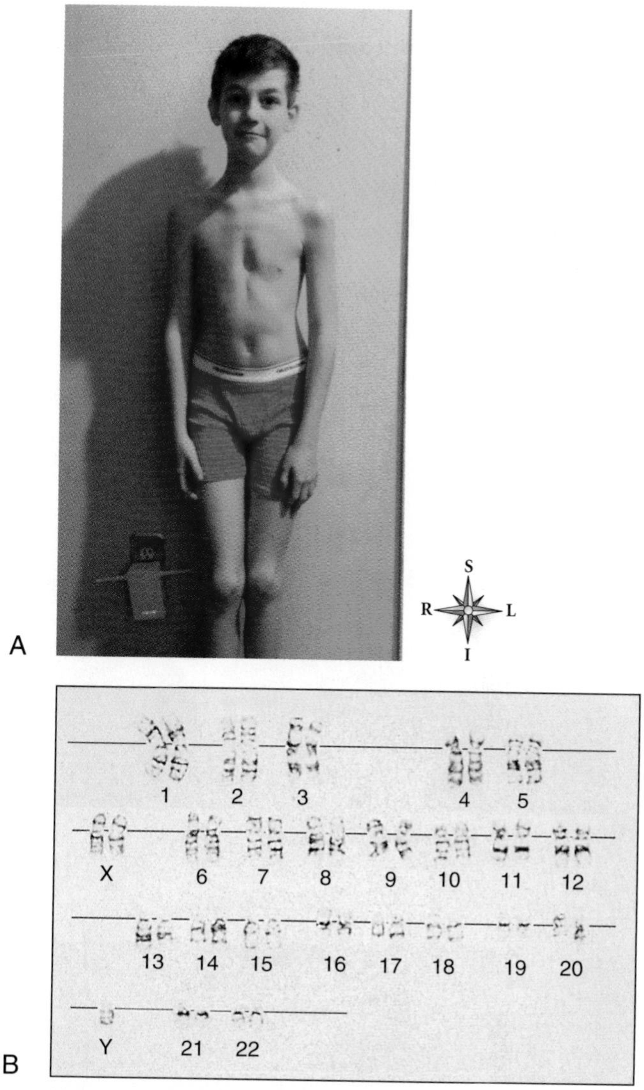

• **Figure 41-11** Klinefelter syndrome. (From Patton KT, Thibodeau GA: *The human body in health & disease,* ed 6, St Louis, 2014, Mosby/Elsevier.)

assisted reproductive techniques before they are implanted to initiate the pregnancy in the woman.

Diagnostic Genetic Testing

Diagnostic testing is used to confirm a diagnosis and is used in a symptomatic individual or in response to a positive screening test. Such tests are selected depending on the type or specific disease one is trying to confirm. Specific practice guidelines can help providers choose which test to order. For example, a chromosomal test would be used to confirm Down syndrome (trisomy 21) in a newborn. For a male preschooler who is unable to hop despite what appears to be muscular calves leading to a suspicion of Duchenne muscular dystrophy, a specific DNA test that confirms more than 95% of cases would be ordered. The test has been designed to identify missing or duplicated sections in the dystrophin (DMD) gene [Xp21.2] (National Institute of Neurological Disorders and Stroke [NINDS], 2014).

The main types of diagnostic genetic testing include karyotype, fluorescence in situ hybridization (FISH), biochemical testing, chromosomal microarray, molecular testing, and next generation sequencing. *Karyotype* is used to identify and evaluate the size, shape, and number of chromosomes. *FISH* is used to locate and detect a specific area of a particular chromosome, including subtle missing, additional, or rearranged chromosomal material by labeling a known chromosome sequence with fluorescent tags to see the location of genetic material. Unlike most other techniques used to study chromosomes, FISH does not have to be performed on cells that are actively dividing, making it more versatile. *Biochemical testing* is used to study the amount, activity level, or structure of proteins and enzymes

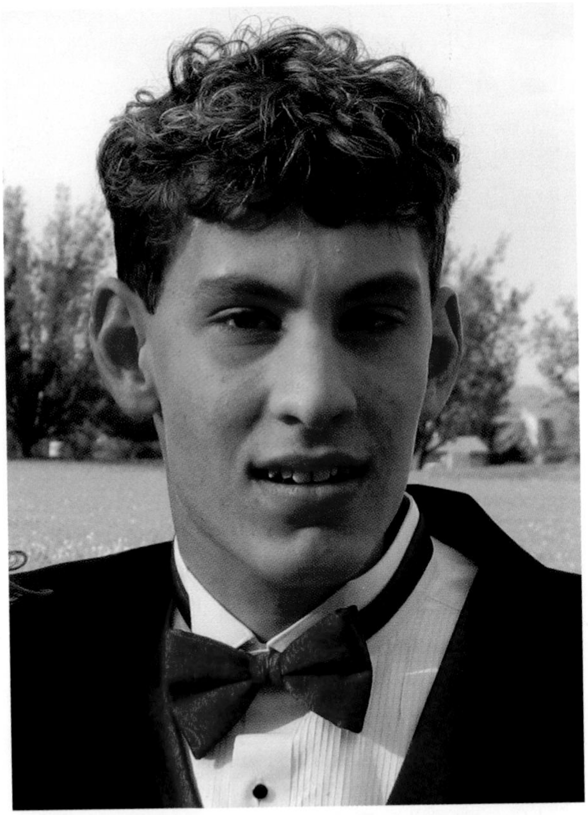

• **Figure 41-12** Fragile X syndrome.

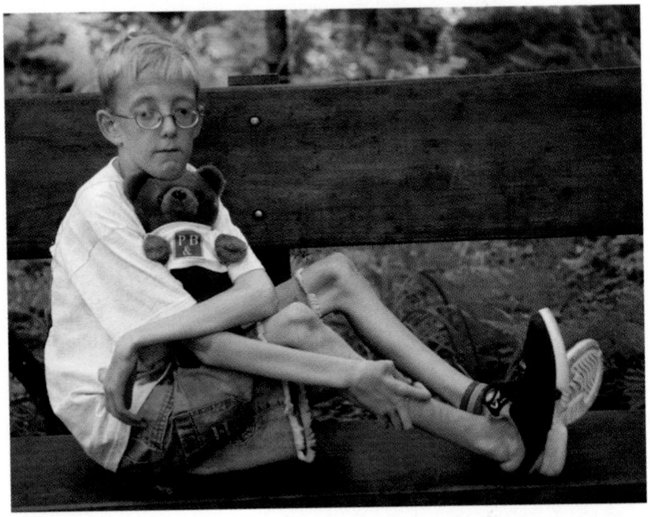

• **Figure 41-13** Marfan syndrome. Courtesy The Marfan Foundation.

that result from gene mutations. Many metabolic syndromes are screened for and diagnosed using biochemical testing. *Chromosomal microarray* is used to detect microdeletions or duplications (such as, CNVs) in any of the chromosomes but not specific gene mutations. Microarray testing is noted to have a superior diagnostic yield over karyotyping for similar clinical features, including developmental disabilities (Ellison et al, 2012). *Molecular testing* is

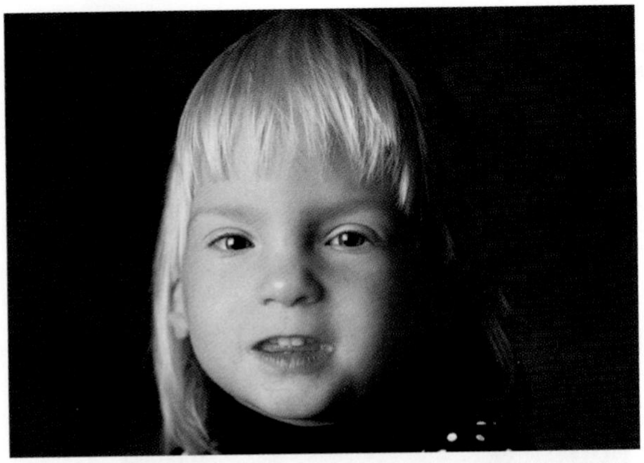

• **Figure 41-14** Fetal alcohol spectrum disorder (FASD). (In McKinney E, et al: *Maternal-child nursing,* ed 4, Philadelphia, 2013, Saunders/Elsevier. From Fortinash KM, Holoday Worret PA: *Psychiatric mental health nursing,* ed 5, St Louis, 2012, Mosby/Elsevier.)

used to detect specific single gene mutations (e.g., deletions, insertions, and single base pair changes) known to cause single gene disorders. Molecular techniques are used to directly detect aberrant sequences changes in a targeted gene or short length of DNA or to indirectly detect aberrant changes in DNA structure by identifying size variations in fragments of DNA from the targeted locus or gene. *Next generation sequencing* is used to detect a single mutation among many genes and can detect several sequence changes with one test (Table 41-7).

Carrier Testing

Carrier testing is used to identify individuals who have one copy of a gene mutation that causes a known disorder when two copies are present (AR conditions). Individuals with one copy are often referred to as having the trait or being a carrier, rather than having the disease. Carrier testing is typically offered to individuals who are planning a family, focusing on information about the couple's risk of having a child with the genetic disorder. Parents can be tested to see if they are carriers of one of the mutations leading to cystic fibrosis or if they have sickle cell or thalassemia trait. Carrier testing is also done to identify non-manifesting females of X-linked diseases. These women are referred to as "carriers" of X-linked diseases, such as Duchenne muscular dystrophy and hemophilia.

Other Testing

Predictive and presymptomatic tests are used when asymptomatic individuals are interested in learning if they have a gene mutation associated with a disorder and are typically offered when there is a family history of a genetic disorder. *Predictive testing* identifies mutations that increase an individual's *risk* of developing a genetic disorder (such as, breast or colon cancer), whereas *presymptomatic testing* identifies mutations that predict whether an individual will develop disorders (such as, Huntington disease or hemochromocytosis). The results of both types of tests help individuals

TABLE 41-7 **Diagnostic Genetic Testing**

	Karyotype	Fluorescence In Situ Hybridization	Microarray	Molecular Testing*
Detects *large* deletions or duplications	X	X	X	
Detects deletions or duplication in *part* of a chromosome		X	X	
Detects *small* deletions or duplications			X	
Detects translocations	X			
Detects *very small* structure and sequence changes and single gene mutations				X

*Including DNA sequencing.

and their providers make decisions about health care and reproductive planning. Generally these tests are not done in children. It is considered more ethical for children to make the decision about receiving this information when they are older and able to make such decisions as adults.

Pharmacologic testing is used to learn ahead of time what the best drug or best dose of a drug will be for a person. The goal of this testing is to guide the provider in tailoring drugs to an individual's genetic makeup. *Forensic testing* is most often used in pediatric practice to establish biologic relationships between individuals, such as establishing paternity. Forensic testing can also be used to identify catastrophic victims and/or crime victims/suspects.

Primary Care Management of Children with Genetic Disorders

Genetics Referral

Providers should consider a genetics consultation and/or referral when a child's family history is positive for a genetic condition for which the child is at risk, as well as for children with developmental, growth, and/or structural disorders, or inborn errors of metabolism. PCPs should include these specialists in their referral networks not only to provide guidance in terms of appropriate tests but also to have a trusted source of information to navigate this constantly evolving field. Their expertise in diagnosis, understanding inheritance patterns and recurrence risk, genetic testing, the nuanced mechanisms of genetic disorders, and evolution of clinical manifestations across the lifespan makes them invaluable resources for pediatric PCPs.

Genetics counseling is one specific aspect of the genetics referral. Families often need genetics information in order to make decisions that will affect their lives, especially reproductive plans. Genetic counseling should help families understand the diagnosis of concern, its course, and management. It should also help the family to understand the way that heredity influences the disorder, including risks of recurrence and carrier status. Strategies to reduce risk of recurrence and choosing a plan of action are part of genetics counseling. Finally, coping with a genetic diagnosis, its prognosis, and the risks of recurrence should be discussed in counseling.

Genetics specialists can also help the PCP develop emergency plans when clinical management is needed (e.g., myotonic dystrophy, porphyria, mitochondrial and glycogen storage diseases). Further, they can also offer guidance with difficult end-of-life conversations that may include post-mortem investigations, as well as providing continuity as children with genetic disorders transition out of pediatric practice to adult care.

The PCP's role is to help the family find a genetics specialist or counselor; initiate referrals with screening pedigrees, medical records, and other information; and evaluate the family's understanding of genetic counseling information provided to them. It is very important to prepare the child and family for the consultation and/or referral so that they understand the role of the specialist in the child's overall care. In particular, the clinician can anticipate for the family the need to obtain family health history and records, as well as requested neurodevelopmental testing, imaging studies, and child/family photographs.

The provider needs to decide which patients to test, when to test, which family members to test, how to interpret results, and when to refer for medical genetics consultation. In some cases, genetic retesting may be appropriate given the tremendous progress in this field over the recent past. Managing this care in a cost-effective, efficient way is challenging. Shared decision-making with the family and the child is essential (Scott and Trotter, 2013).

Primary Care for Children with Genetic Disorders

Children diagnosed with genetic disorders still need to be assigned to medical homes where care is accessible, continuous, comprehensive, patient- and family-centered, coordinated, compassionate, and culturally effective. In other words, these children have pediatric primary needs, too.

All primary care clinicians should follow age-appropriate health supervision guidelines as much as possible, knowing there may be some exceptions. Specific health supervision guidelines, developed by the AAP Committee on Genetics, are available for children with achondroplasia, Down syndrome, fragile X, Marfan syndrome, neurofibromatosis, Prader-Willi syndrome, sickle cell disease, Turner syndrome, and Williams syndrome. Each of these guidelines is available, updated regularly, and provide resources, specific assessment needs, cautions, available growth charts, current and emerging research, and syndrome-specific management guidelines. These guidelines, along with specific genetic counselling and management needs, are outlined in their publication *Medical Genetics in Pediatric Practice* (Saul, 2013). See Table 41-8 for some important highlights; however, the published guidelines should be the primary source(s) for managing primary health care.

Ethical Issues

From the inception of the Human Genome Project, the National Human Genome Research Institute (NHGRI) had

TABLE 41-8 Some Monitoring Suggestions for Children with Common Genetic Disorders

Genetic Disorder	Primary Care—Heads up!
Achondroplasia	• Monitor growth using specialized growth chart • Monitor for developmental (motor) delays • Annual hearing evaluation • Monitor for obstructive sleep apnea • Caution—hydrocephalus, spinal cord compression
Angelman syndrome	• Monitor for speech impairment • Monitor for scoliosis • Monitor for behavior problems (frequent laughing, fascination with water) • Monitor for feeding disorders/GER • Monitor for scoliosis • Increased sensitivity to heat
Beckwith-Wiedemann syndrome	• Anticipate hypoglycemia (newborn) • Monitor growth/hemihyperplasia (limb length discrepancies) • Monitor for feeding problems secondary to macroglossia • Caution—embryonal tumor risk • Caution—cardiac/renal anomalies
Down syndrome	• Monitor growth using specialized growth chart • Monitor for obstructive sleep apnea • Annual vision/hearing evaluation • Annual thyroid screen • Caution—increased risk for leukemia, duodenal atresia • Caution—cardiac anomalies
Fragile X syndrome	• Monitor for developmental/behavior problems • Monitor otitis media/sinus • Monitor sleep problems/obstructive sleep apnea • Monitor for obesity • Monitor vision • Caution—autism • Caution—hypertension, mitral valve prolapsed
Klinefelter syndrome	• Monitor growth and development, especially speech • Monitor for scoliosis • Annual thyroid screen • Caution—delayed puberty/gynecomastia/low testosterone • Caution—increased risk for autoimmune disorders, breast cancer
Marfan syndrome	• Monitor growth using specialized growth chart • Monitor for orthopedic problems, including protrusion acetabuli, pectus abnormalities, scoliosis, pes planus • Monitor BP (hypertension) • Annual ophthalmology screen (ectopia lentis) • Avoid contact sports • Caution—spontaneous pneumothorax • Caution—aortic root dilatation, mitral valve prolapse

TABLE 41-8 Some Monitoring Suggestions for Children with Common Genetic Disorders—cont'd

Genetic Disorder	Primary Care—Heads up!
Neurofibromatosis—type 1	• Monitor growth using specialized growth chart • Monitor for learning disabilities • Annual ophthalmology screen (Lisch nodules, optic gliomas) • Monitor BP • Monitor for scoliosis • Caution—tibial dysplasia
Noonan syndrome	• Monitor growth using specialized growth chart • Annual vision/hearing screen • Monitor for developmental delays • Caution—cardiac anomalies (hypertrophic cardiomyopathy) • Caution—coagulopathies • Caution—renal anomalies
Prader-Willi syndrome	• Monitor growth using specialized growth chart • Monitor for developmental delay/intellectual disability • Monitor for speech problems (articulation) • Monitor for behavioral problems • Annual vision/hearing screen • Caution—hyperphagia and obesity
Turner syndrome	• Monitor growth using specialized growth chart • Monitor for nonverbal learning disabilities • Annual vision/hearing screen • Monitor BP (hypertension) • Annual thyroid screen • Monitor for scoliosis • Caution—cardiac/renal anomalies • Estrogen supplementation with puberty
Sickle cell disease	• Annual trans-Doppler evaluations from ages 2 to 16 years old and long-term transfusion therapy to prevent stroke in patients with abnormal results (Yawn et al, 2014)

Yawn BP, Buchanan GR, Afenyi-Annan A, et al: Management of sickle cell disease summary of the 2014 evidence-based report by expert panel members, *JAMA* 312(10):1033–1048, 2014; Hersh JH, Saul RA, Committee on Genetics: Health supervision for children with fragile X syndrome (review), *Pediatrics* 127(5):994–1006, 2011.

BP, Blood pressure; *GER*, gastroesophageal reflux.

the foresight to anticipate the string of ethical, legal, and social issues that were to arise as part of advancing the science of genomic research. Housed within NHGRI is the Ethical, Legal, and Social Implications (ELSI) program. A few of the ethical issues include the rights to privacy and confidentiality, the rights to know, not know, the duty to warn, disclosure of incidental findings, and genetic discrimination.

The Genetic Information Nondiscrimination Act (GINA) was passed in 2008 with all aspects of the law in effect in November 2009. The intent of the legislation was to protect individuals from the misuse of genetic information in health insurance and employment and remove barriers to the use of genetic services. GINA does not affect health care. However, under GINA, *health insurers* cannot use an individual's genetic information to set eligibility requirements, establish insurance premiums, or request certain genetic tests. Further, *employers* cannot request, require, or purchase genetic information about an employee or family member, and they cannot use an individual's genetic information in decisions about job hiring, firing, assignments, or promotions (GPCI, 2014a). Unfortunately, GINA does not provide protection when a condition is already diagnosed or manifest, even if that condition is genetic. Further, GINA does not apply to life, disability, or long-term insurers. The types of genetic information protected under GINA include family health history, carrier testing, prenatal genetic testing, predictive testing, and other assessments of genes, mutations, or chromosomal changes. There are a few groups exempt from GINA, which include members of the military, veterans receiving care through the Veteran's Administration, those using the Indian Health Service, and federal employees enrolled in the Federal Employees Health Benefits program. However, the military, veterans, and federal employees have other protections that mirror GINA.

For a complete list of references, please visit http://evolve.elsevier.com/Burns/pediatric/.

42 Environmental Health Issues

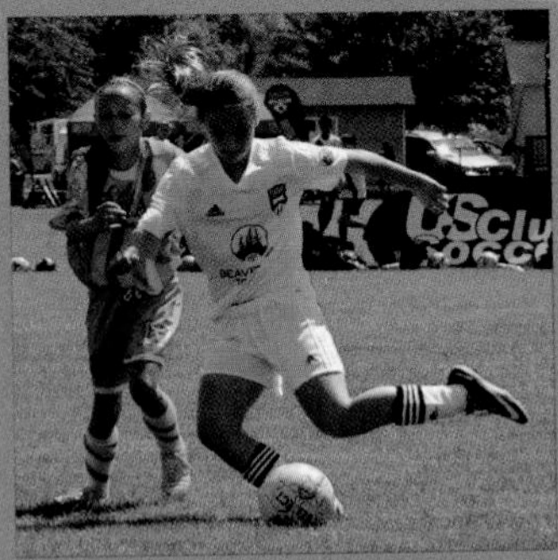

ARDYS M. DUNN, JENNIFER BEVACQUA, AND CATHERINE E. BURNS

All things are connected. Whatever befalls the earth befalls the children of the earth.

CHIEF SEATTLE, THE SOUL OF AN INDIAN

The environment is a basic determinant of human health and illness. About one third of the global burden of disease can be attributed to three major categories of environmental risk factors: (1) water, sanitation, and hygiene; (2) indoor air quality; and (3) outdoor air quality. Children are particularly vulnerable to environmental factors. Worldwide, nearly 3 million children younger than 5 years old die each year as a result of environment-related diseases, including diarrhea and respiratory infections (World Health Organization [WHO], 2014). Environmental factors are estimated to contribute to 100% of lead poisoning, 30% of asthma, 5% of cancers, and about 10% of neurobehavioral disorders. The *annual* cost of environment-related illness in children in the United States in 2008 has been calculated at $76.6 billion (Trasande and Liu, 2011).

Chemicals, natural and synthetic, constitute a large part of the environmental risk to health, contaminating water, soil, and air. There is sufficient scientific evidence of a causal link between prenatal or childhood exposure to methyl mercury, polychlorinated biphenyls (PCBs), polychlorinated dibenzofurans, active maternal smoking (during pregnancy), environmental tobacco smoke (ETS) (during childhood), and 2, 3, 7, 8-tetrachlorodibenzo-p-dioxin and adverse health outcomes in children and adults (Röösli, 2011).

In the United States, 1 in 33 children is born with defects, and there may be an association with the father's environmental exposure as well the mother's (Carter et al, 2011; National Birth Defects Prevention Study [NBDPS], 2014). Chemical exposure of the father or mother prior to conception, at the time of conception, and (for the mother and fetus) during pregnancy results in a gene-environment interaction that accounts for most adverse developmental outcomes of pregnancy (Mattison, 2010). Concern has been raised that human exposure to genetically modified organisms (GMOs) and to hormones fed to animals may contribute to cancers, hepatorenal toxicity, and long-term reproductive problems (Bawa and Anilakumar, 2013). In 2014, the U.S. Department of Health and Human Services (HHS) and the Centers for Disease Control and Prevention (CDC) updated the 2009 Fourth National Report on Human Exposures to Environmental Chemicals, confirming that almost all subjects studied had measurable levels of many industrial toxins in their blood and urine (CDC, 2014c). Yet despite the known effects of many environmental agents and despite the presence of toxins in almost all humans, a great deal of uncertainty about the relationship between the environment and disease and illness remains. This uncertainty is related specifically to the fact that (1) the extent of exposure may be unclear; (2) there can be a long latency period between exposure and appearance of illness; (3) an individual may have exposure to multiple confounding agents; (4) exposure may need to occur during a "window of vulnerability" (e.g., during the period when a particular body system is forming prenatally) for the agent to have an effect; (5) some individuals may have a genetic susceptibility to an exposure, whereas others do not; (6) some agents can cause several problems; (7) some problems can be related to several agents; and (8) much research in environmental health has been short term, or conducted on animals, so results may not translate to human development. Providers often feel inadequate to the task of managing environmental health concerns. To date, nursing and medical schools do not devote sufficient time to teaching about environmental health, and continuing education may be limited (Gehle et al, 2011).

To complicate matters, this uncertainty on the part of providers and in the field of pediatric environmental health occurs in a social and economic context where profit, not concern for health, drives corporate behavior. In the United

States, for example, the Toxic Substances Control Act of 1976 (TSCA) authorizes the U.S. Environmental Protection Agency (EPA) to require testing and reporting of some chemicals and to restrict mixing of some toxic substances. However, of the approximately 84,000 chemicals registered for use in the United States, only about 200 have been tested by the EPA and only five have been banned (Jackson, 2010). Safety testing of a chemical is often done by the company producing it, and the results may not need to be made public. About 20% of chemicals used (almost 17,000) are not reported to the EPA because companies claim that they represent "confidential business information" and disclosure of any information about them would jeopardize the company's "competitiveness" in the marketplace (EPA, 2010; Wilson, 2012). In addition, the cost of testing and regulating chemicals to ensure safety is balanced against the health problems that those chemicals might cause; and, to date, United States industry has successfully argued that it can be "too costly" to control pollution and restrict exposure for many chemicals. Finally, many chemicals used in cosmetics, foods, drugs, and pesticides are exempt from disclosure laws (Davis, 2014). Although corporations state that they do not intend to cause health problems with their products, examples of environmental contamination, advertising to vulnerable groups (e.g., cigarettes to adolescents), cover-ups of harmful findings, regulatory violations, and conflict of interest in research occur frequently (Shrader-Frechette, 2011).

Given this corporate-driven environment, and because it can be difficult to establish direct cause and effect between chemicals and health, it would be prudent to adopt a precautionary approach to environmental toxins. The *precautionary principle,* which operates in many European nations (Romano et al, 2011), stipulates that chemicals should not be introduced into the environment until they have been proven to be safe. In the United States, unfortunately, the opposite is true; regulatory agencies (e.g., the EPA) must demonstrate that a chemical in question represents an "unreasonable risk" to human health in order to ban its use. Health care providers across the United States must advocate for use of the precautionary principle to control exposure to environmental toxins nationally and internationally (American Academy of Pediatrics [AAP] Council on Environmental Health, 2011).

The current situation is grim, but it is important to note that health care providers are increasingly aware of the problem, and many efforts are being made to address environmental health in pediatric practices. A network of regional pediatric environmental health specialty units (PEHSUs) has been created to provide information, clinical consultation, and support for pediatric providers (see Additional Resources on Evolve website). In 2011, the American Academy of Pediatrics (AAP) updated its pediatric environmental health manual for providers (Etzel and Balk, 2012) and has a Council on Environmental Health to develop policy and guide research and practice. Educators are developing curricula and preparing materials for students in health disciplines (Beitz and de Castro, 2010; Jamil et al, 2010), and tools for assessment and management of environmental variables continue to be written (Judson et al, 2012). The American Board of Preventive Medicine certifies physicians in the subspecialty of medical toxicology, and a medical specialty in environmental medicine has been proposed (le Moal and Reis, 2011).

The human genome project has introduced the concept of exposomes, "the measure of all the exposures of an individual in a lifetime and how those exposures relate to health" (CDC, 2014b) and the new field of exposomics is leading the study of this relationship. In Europe, the Human Early Life Exposome (HELIX) project proposes to clarify the relationship between early life exposure to environmental factors and child health, using innovative assessment tools and biomarkers (Vrijheid et al, 2014). New technology allows for more sophisticated assessment of how chemicals affect the human body, and intricacies of the environment-health relationship are better understood. Use of systematic review methods (e.g., the Navigation Systematic Review Methodology) to synthesize research and more efficiently evaluate the relationship between environment and health is being advocated in an effort to link the science of environmental studies to evidence-based health practice (Woodruff and Sutton, 2014). In the United States, Congress authorized the National Children's Study in 2000 to investigate the root causes of many childhood and adult diseases. One hundred thousand children were to be followed from before conception until 21 years old, examining environmental influences on health, including diet, ambient air, and home and school environments, as well as interactions with various genetic traits. A vanguard study was done, and a tentative start date of 2015 was set for beginning the main study (National Research Council and Institute of Medicine, 2014), but the project, though considered worthwhile, was determined to be unfeasible and was terminated in 2014 due to budget constraints and project design (Altman et al, 2014; Collins, 2014).

Health care providers need to be able to give their clients the most accurate environmental health information available. Parents may suspect that an illness is associated with environmental conditions, or they may express concern about the risk of exposure to untested substances. The provider who is knowledgeable about the potential hazards of environmental exposure will be able to explain the possible connections, collect clear assessment data, and work closely with families to make appropriate treatment choices, including appropriate referral and consultation. If not personally knowledgeable, the provider should know where to get information. The National Organization of Nurse Practitioner Faculties (NONPF) in conjunction with the American Association of Colleges of Nursing (AACN) has identified the core competencies that nurse practitioners should recognize "environmental health problems affecting patients and provide health protection interventions that promote healthy environments for individuals, families, and communities" (HHS, 2002). This chapter is designed to help prepare providers to meet these competencies. In addition to direct patient care and education, primary health care providers can collaborate with other health care providers, conduct research to identify environmental problems, and advocate in the public arena (e.g., industry, policy, funding, and regulation) for more responsible management of environmental agents that affect health.

Principles for Understanding Children's Environmental Health

Children's Increased Risk for Environment-Related Illness

Children are particularly susceptible to environmental threats (Table 42-1). Prenatally and during childhood, children go through critical developmental periods or *windows of vulnerability,* during which exposure to toxins or other harmful substances affects growth or damages organs or body systems. For example, during the 26th day of gestation, a 50-mg dose of thalidomide will likely result in major malformations to an embryo but that same dose taken at the 10th week of gestation will have no effect (Brent, 2004). With some conditions, children are more likely to suffer health problems than adults exposed to the same substance. For instance, toxicants that cross the placenta (e.g., drugs, carbon monoxide [CO], mercury, lead, and cotinine [from ETS]) can contribute to low birth weight, spontaneous abortion, intrauterine growth retardation, birth defects, poor cognitive and behavioral development, and increased risk of cancer.

Children's rapidly growing tissues more readily absorb environmental toxins; the lungs, skin, and gastrointestinal (GI) tract of newborns are highly permeable, and a high gastric pH facilitates absorption. At the same time, newborns' immature organ systems more slowly metabolize drugs, making it more difficult for infants to detoxify and excrete harmful substances. Per pound of body weight, children consume more fresh fruit, water, milk, and juice and breathe more pollutants than adults, increasing exposure to pesticides or other chemicals. Children engage in more outdoor activities and are physically closer to many potentially harmful substances than adults. Crawling on floors, chewing on objects, and running and rolling in grass are behaviors that can result in lead poisoning, pesticide

TABLE 42-1 Environmental Risk Factors for Children at Different Stages of Development

Developmental Stage	Developmental Characteristics	Exposure Pathways (Physical Environment)	Biologic Vulnerabilities	Appropriate Responses in the Social Environment
Preconception	Maternal and paternal health status	Maternal/paternal reproductive organs may be compromised Maternal stores of toxicants in bones and fatty tissue can be mobilized during pregnancy	Problems with fertilization, implantation of ovum Damage to ovum or sperm	Research and education regarding long-term effects of environmental contaminants on reproductive system and subsequent offspring
Prenatal	Fetal development dependent on maternal health status and environmental exposure	Maternal blood supply via placenta Radiation Noise Heat	Tissue differentiation Rapid cell division and growth Organ development Metabolic pathways incomplete	Prenatal education, programs, and regulations regarding: • Alcohol • Cigarettes • Drugs • Metals
Newborn (0 to 2 months old)	Non-ambulatory Restricted environment High calorie, water intake High air intake Highly permeable skin Alkaline gastric secretions (low gastric acidity to about 3 years old)	Food: Breast milk, infant formula Dyes in clothing Soaps and shampoos Indoor air Tap/well water in home	Brain: Cell migration, neuron myelination, creation of neural synapses Lungs: Developing alveoli, rapid air exchange, narrow airways Bones: Rapid growth and hardening Other organs: Rapid growth Poor enzyme detoxification	Newborn-sensitive programs and regulations regarding PCBs Lead in drinking water and dust particles ETS Educate parents and policy makers concerning environmental hazards

TABLE 42-1 Environmental Risk Factors for Children at Different Stages of Development—cont'd

Developmental Stage	Developmental Characteristics	Exposure Pathways (Physical Environment)	Biologic Vulnerabilities	Appropriate Responses in the Social Environment
Infant/toddler (2 months to 2 years old)	Beginning to walk Oral exploration (mouthing) Restricted environment and near floors Increased time away from parents Minimal variation in diet: High intake of fruits, vegetables, and milk products per body weight	Food: Baby food, food additives, milk and milk products Air indoor layer effects: Air near floor contains more toxicants Tap/well water in home and day care Surfaces: Rugs, floors, lawns, playgrounds	Brain: Creation of synapses Lungs: Developing alveoli, rapid air exchange, narrow airways	Child-sensitive programs and regulations regarding: • Radon in the home • Residential pesticide use • Lead abatement • ETS Educate parents and policy makers concerning environmental hazards
School-age child (6 to 12 years old)	Beginning school Playground activities Increased involvement in group activities	Food at home and school Air: School, outdoor Water: School water fountains, tap/well water, swimming areas Playgrounds: Wood preservatives, pesticides, and fertilizers Other: Arts and crafts supplies, personal electronic equipment	Brain: Specific synapse formation, dendritic trimming Lung: Volume expansion Metabolic enzymes more active than in younger child	Child-sensitive programs and regulations regarding: • Asbestos abatement • Lead in school drinking water • Hazards in arts and crafts materials • ETS Educate parents and policy makers concerning environmental hazards
Adolescent (12 to 18 years old)	Development of abstract thinking Puberty Growth spurt Increased adherence to peer norms	Food Air Water Personal electronic equipment Other occupation Self-determination: Smoking, inhalations	Brain: Continued synapse formation Lung: Volume expansion Gonad maturation: Ova and sperm maturation Breast development Bone growth and calcification Muscle growth	Adolescent-sensitive programs and regulations regarding child labor and other issues, especially ETS Educate parents and policy makers concerning environmental hazards

Adapted from Gitterman BA, Bearer CF: A developmental approach to pediatric environmental health, *Pediatr Clin North Am* 48(5):1071–1083, 2001.
ETS, Environmental tobacco smoke; *PCB*, polychlorinated biphenyl.

poisoning, and respiratory problems, including asthma exacerbation. Adolescents are at increased risk if occupational hazards are present. All children living in poorer communities are at higher risk than others due to deteriorating housing and poor nutrition, high levels of environmental lead, toxic waste deposits, and limited access to health screening and treatment. In addition to the immediate risk during childhood, children have a longer time span for exposure to environmental toxins.

The Dynamics of Environmental Health Hazards

As noted, a direct cause-effect relationship between health and the environment may be impossible to determine. Using principles of epidemiologic relationships and toxicology, however, providers can better understand and explain to their patients the relationship between the two.

Epidemiologic Model: Assessment of Risk

A first step using an epidemiologic approach (Fig. 42-1) identifies the interactive factors in the environment, including *receptors* (i.e., hosts or living things that are susceptible or exposed to environmental agents); *toxins,* or harmful substances that might cause damage (i.e., the agent); and the environmental *medium,* or route by which exposure could occur (e.g., air, water, or food).

A second step of risk assessment using an epidemiologic model determines the possibility that harm could occur. A number of questions are asked when making this determination:

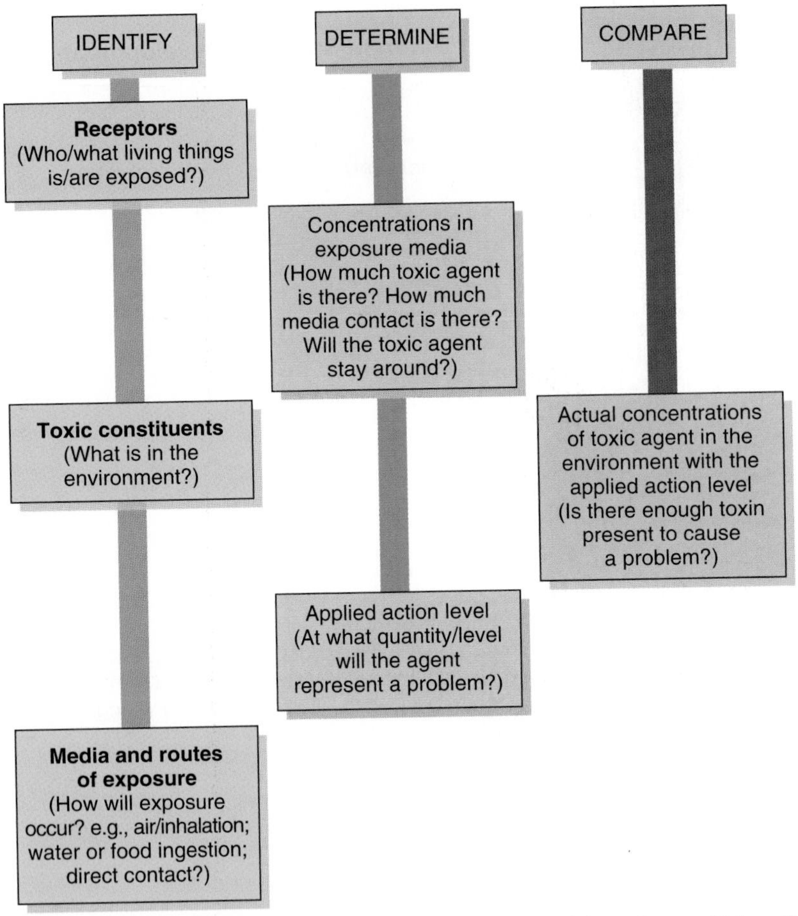

• **Figure 42-1** Risk assessment of environmental hazards. (Adapted from Oregon Poison Center and Health Division, Oregon Department of Human Resources: *Environmental hazards in perspective: seminar syllabus and environmental health resource notebook*, Portland, 1994, Oregon Department of Human Resources.)

- How *susceptible* is the receptor to the agent (e.g., age, gender, genetics, diet, and general health)?
- At what quantity (i.e., dose) will the agent present a problem or cause a response in this receptor? This amount is called the *applied action* or dose-response level. For some agents, like lead, *any* exposure represents a risk.
- What is the concentration of the toxic agent? How much is there? How strong is it? How long will it stay around? What is the extent of contact of the toxic agent with the receptor?

A final step in this process compares the actual environmental condition with the applied action level, asking the following question: With the amount of exposure present, is the individual at risk for health problems?

Toxicologic Principles

Toxicologic principles are those that the primary care provider has learned related to pharmacologic therapy: exposure, absorption, distribution, metabolism, tissue sensitivity, and effects—therapeutic or toxic. In fact, Paracelsus (1493-1541), considered the "father of toxicology," is reputed to have said, "All substances are poisons; there is none that is not a poison. The right dose differentiates a poison from a remedy."

Exposure

Contact of a biologic, chemical, or physical agent with the outer boundary of an organism (e.g., skin, lungs, and GI tract) constitutes exposure. The extent to which exposure creates a problem is an epidemiologic issue and depends on factors such as frequency and duration of exposure, concentration of the agent at the point of contact, and the susceptibility of the organism (e.g., an infant's skin burns much more easily than an adult's).

Absorption

Absorption is the process by which an agent is taken into the organism. It occurs in the skin, mucous membranes, lungs, or GI tract. Absorption involves active or passive transport (e.g., lipid-soluble chemicals, such as PCBs, are passively absorbed through the gut and stored in fat; lead is taken up through active transport in the GI tract and respiratory system and stored in bone or other tissues).

Distribution

Toxic agents are distributed throughout the organism via the blood and lymph systems. The ability of an agent to cross the blood-brain barrier (e.g., lead), the amount of blood flow to an organ, and the affinity of tissues to take up a particular agent (e.g., lipid-soluble chemicals are found in fatty tissues) all influence the degree to which a toxicant will be distributed throughout the body.

Metabolism

Metabolic enzymes in the body interact with toxic agents in several ways: (1) oxidation, reduction, and hydrolysis of the agent—the agent can be detoxified, but chemicals can also be activated and made more toxic during these processes; and (2) conjugation and breakdown to promote elimination, usually through the kidney. Metabolism is influenced by the individual's age, gender, nutritional status, genetic makeup, presence of other drugs, and disease or illness.

Tissue Sensitivity

Susceptibility and reaction of tissue to a particular agent can vary. The thalidomide example illustrates increased tissue susceptibility during a critical point of gestation.

Toxic Effects

Toxic effects include a wide range of pathologic conditions. Prenatal exposures can result in sterility, infertility, miscarriage, stillbirth, congenital malformations, fetal growth retardation, prematurity, and chronic illnesses. Paradoxically, for some environmental toxins (such as endocrine disruptors) small doses may have deleterious effects, whereas large doses do not; the larger doses simply kill the exposed cells rather than being used by the cells in an abnormal fashion.

• BOX 42-1 Screening Environmental History

The questions below are most often asked about the child's primary residence. One should always consider all places where the child spends time, such as day care centers, schools, and relatives' homes.

- Where does your child live and spend most of his/her time?
- What are the age, condition, and location of your home?
- Have you recently renovated or repaired your home, or do you have plans to do so?
- Does anyone in the family smoke?
- Do you have furry indoor pets?
- Do you have smoke detectors?
- Do you have a carbon monoxide (CO) detector?
- Have you had your home tested for radon?
- What type of heating/air system does your home have?
- Is your heating/air system regularly inspected and maintained?
- What is the source of your drinking water?
  Well water   City water   Bottled water
- What are the occupations of all adults in the household?
- Is your child protected from excessive exposure to the sun?
- Is your child exposed to any toxic chemicals of which you are aware?
- Does your child eat paint chips or chew on windowsills or other painted surfaces?
- Do you have any other questions or concerns about your child's home environment or symptoms that may be a result of his or her environment?

Data adapted from Agency for Toxic Substances and Disease Registry (ATSDR): *ATSDR case studies in environmental medicine. Taking a pediatric exposure history*, Atlanta, GA, 2013, Centers for Disease Control and Prevention; Etzel RA, Balk SJ: *Pediatric environmental health*, ed 3, Elk Grove Village, IL, 2011, American Academy of Pediatrics.

Primary Care Approach to Children's Environmental Health

Clinical Findings

History

Assessment of environmental health hazards should be integrated into health visits of both well and ill children. Boxes 42-1 and 42-2 and Figure 42-2 list essential questions to ask for an environmental history, including questions related to asthma.

Physical Examination

The physical examination should cover all body systems thoroughly. Evaluate agent-specific findings (e.g., burns caused by chemicals and neurotoxicity caused by mercury), but also look for subtle, nonspecific signs and symptoms (e.g., skin rashes and headaches). The effects of toxicants on the body can be subclinical or readily noted. Moreover, effects can occur immediately or a period of time after the exposure. These factors may contribute to a provider missing physical manifestations of toxicant exposure if one does not have an index of suspicion.

Diagnostic Studies

Laboratory studies can be performed on patients as indicated, based on signs and symptoms. Agent-specific laboratory studies, if available and reliable, can be helpful in determining treatment plans (Box 42-3). However, few tests are appropriate for use in primary care settings because of the following limitations:

- For the majority of toxins, valid and reliable tests have not been developed.
- For those toxins that do have tests, only select laboratories may be equipped to process them.
- Normal reference ranges may vary widely and may not clearly be evidence based to reflect levels at which toxicity (subclinical or clinical) appears.
- Turn-around time on specialized testing may not produce results in a clinically relevant time frame.
- Correlation between current toxicant level and harm may be poor. Levels may have returned to normal, despite damage done to the body; or a one-time sample can reflect recent active exposure but not measure the total body burden of the contaminant.

• BOX 42-2 Supplemental Environmental History

If a positive response is given to one or more of the questions in the Screening Environmental History, the primary care provider can ask the following questions:

General Housing Characteristics

- Do you own or rent your home?
- Was your home built before 1978? Before 1950?
- Has your child been tested for lead? If yes, what were the results?
- Is there a family member or playmate with an elevated blood lead level (BLL)?
- Does your child spend significant time in a location other than your home?

Indoor Home Environment*

- If a family member smokes, do they want to quit?
- Is your child exposed to smoke at school, day care, or a babysitter or relative's home?
- Do regular visitors to your home smoke?
- Does your home have carpet?
- Is the room where your child sleeps carpeted?
- Do you use a wood stove or fireplace?
- Have you had water damage, leaks, or a flood in your home?
- Do you see cockroaches in your home?
- Do you see rats and/or mice in your home?

Outdoor Environment/Air Pollution*

- Is your home near an industrial site, hazardous waste site, or landfill?
- Is your home near major highways or other high traffic roads?
- Are you aware of Air Quality Alerts in your community?
- Do you change your child's activity when an Air Quality Alert is issued?
- Do you live on or near a farm where pesticides are used regularly?

Food and Water Contamination

- If you use well water, has it been tested? When? With what results?
- Have you tested your water for lead?
- Do you mix infant formula with tap water?
- What types of seafood do you and your child normally eat?
- How many times a week do you and your child eat: shark, swordfish, tilefish, king mackerel, albacore tuna, other?
- How often do you and your child eat organically grown fruits and vegetables?
- How often do you wash fruits and vegetables before giving them to your child?

Toxic Chemical Exposures

Consider this set of questions for patients with seizures, frequent headaches, or other unusual or chronic symptoms.

- How often are pesticides applied inside your home?
- How often are pesticides applied outside your home?
- Where do you store chemicals/pesticides?
- How often do you use solvents or other cleaning or disinfectant chemicals?
- Do you have a deck or play structure built of pressure-treated wood?
- Have you applied a sealant to that wood in the past year?
- What do you use to prevent mosquito bites to your children?
- How often do you apply that product?

Occupations and Hobbies

- What type of work does your child/teenager do?
- Do any adults who live with the child work around toxic chemicals?
- If so, do they shower and change clothes before returning to the home?
- Does the child or any family member have arts, crafts, ceramics, stained glass work, or similar hobbies?

Health-Related Questions

- Have you ever relocated due to concerns about an environmental exposure?
- Do symptoms seem to occur at the same time of day?
- Do symptoms seem to occur after being at the same place every day?
- Do symptoms seem to occur during a certain season?
- Are family members/neighbors/coworkers experiencing similar symptoms?
- Are there environmental concerns in your neighborhood, child's school, or day care?
- Has any family member had a diagnosis of any of the following: asthma, autism, cancer, and/or learning disability?
- Does your child suffer from any of the following recurrent symptoms: Cough, headaches, fatigue, and/or unexplained pain (describe)?

Data adapted from Agency for Toxic Substances and Disease Registry (ATSDR): *ATSDR case studies in environmental medicine: taking a pediatric exposure history*, Atlanta, GA, 2013, Centers for Disease Control and Prevention; Etzel RA, Balk SJ: *Pediatric environmental health*, ed 3, Elk Grove Village, IL, 2011, American Academy of Pediatrics.

*For asthma, see Fig. 42-2.

Management of Environmental Conditions

Management of health and illness related to environmental factors uses a public health model of primary, secondary, and tertiary prevention (Table 42-2). A multidisciplinary approach that includes epidemiology, pediatrics, toxicology, public health, and health economics is necessary to achieve these levels of prevention. The "unknowns" of the relationship between health and environment can be frustrating for both providers and parents. In instances where providers may not have proof of a connection between a toxicant and symptom(s), yet the patient or family raises questions, the provider must listen to and validate the patient's concerns, conveying his or her own concern and willingness to work with patients to best manage the situation. In addition to caring for acute exposures, providers should inform patients and families about the nature of environmental contaminants and proven or suspected health risks. Providers should advocate for healthy environments via public policy, and work with other professionals to report, monitor, and

Specify that questions related to the child's home also apply to other indoor environments where the child spends time, including school, daycare, car, school bus, work, and recreational facilities.

		Follow up/ Notes
Is your child's asthma worse at night?	❑ Yes ❑ No ❑ Not sure	
Is your child's asthma worse at specific locations? If so, where? ______________________	❑ Yes ❑ No ❑ Not sure	
Is your child's asthma worse during a particular season? If so, which one? ____________	❑ Yes ❑ No ❑ Not sure	
Is your child's asthma worse with a particular change in climate? If so, which?________	❑ Yes ❑ No ❑ Not sure	
Can you identify any specific trigger(s) that makes your child's asthma worse? If so, what? ______________________	❑ Yes ❑ No ❑ Not sure	
Have you noticed whether dust exposure makes your child's asthma worse?	❑ Yes ❑ No ❑ Not sure	
Does your child sleep with stuffed animals?	❑ Yes ❑ No ❑ Not sure	
Is there wall-to-wall carpet in your child's bedroom?	❑ Yes ❑ No ❑ Not sure	
Have you used any means for dust mite control? If so, which ones? ______________________	❑ Yes ❑ No ❑ Not sure	
Do you have any furry pets?	❑ Yes ❑ No ❑ Not sure	
Do you see evidence of rats or mice in your home weekly?	❑ Yes ❑ No ❑ Not sure	
Do you see cockroaches in your home daily?	❑ Yes ❑ No ❑ Not sure	
Do any family members, caregivers or friends smoke?	❑ Yes ❑ No ❑ Not sure	
Does this person(s) have an interest or desire to quit?	❑ Yes ❑ No ❑ Not sure	
Does your child/teenager smoke?	❑ Yes ❑ No ❑ Not sure	
Do you see or smell mold/mildew in your home?	❑ Yes ❑ No ❑ Not sure	
Is there evidence of water damage in your home?	❑ Yes ❑ No ❑ Not sure	
Do you use a humidifier or swamp cooler?	❑ Yes ❑ No ❑ Not sure	
Have you had new carpets, paint, floor refinishing, or other changes at your house in the past year?	❑ Yes ❑ No ❑ Not sure	
Does your child or another family member have a hobby that uses materials that are toxic or give off fumes?	❑ Yes ❑ No ❑ Not sure	
Has outdoor air pollution ever made your child's asthma worse?	❑ Yes ❑ No ❑ Not sure	
Does your child limit outdoor activities during a Code Orange or Code Red air quality alert for ozone or particle pollution?	❑ Yes ❑ No ❑ Not sure	
Do you use a wood burning fireplace or stove?	❑ Yes ❑ No ❑ Not sure	
Do you use unvented appliances such as a gas stove for heating your home?	❑ Yes ❑ No ❑ Not sure	
Does your child have contact with other irritants (e.g., perfumes, cleaning agents, or sprays)?	❑ Yes ❑ No ❑ Not sure	

What other concerns do you have regarding your child's asthma that have not yet been discussed?

• **Figure 42-2** Environmental history form for pediatric asthma patient. (Used with permission of the National Environmental Education Foundation, Washington, DC. Available at www.neefusa.org/resource/asthma-environmental-history-form. Accessed December 2, 2015.)

control exposures. The regional PEHSUs and many online sources provide information and support for clinical, toxicologic, educational, and policy work (see Additional Resources).

Minorities and low-income populations are at higher risk for ill effects from environmental toxins and toxicants. Low-income communities, for example, are more likely than high-income communities to have air polluting and waste treatment facilities within their neighborhoods. Children from low-income families are disproportionately afflicted with high lead levels probably secondary to exposure to lead-based paint, which is a hazard in older homes. The environmental justice movement was begun in an effort to rectify these inequities, and it includes the Office of Environmental Justice (OEJ), housed within the EPA (EPA, 2014b), as well as numerous other nongovernmental organizations. Providers should be attuned to the reality of current inequities and environmental justice issues.

• BOX 42-3 Laboratory Tests Available to Test for Environmental Toxins

- Plasma lead levels
- Gas-liquid chromatography (for PCBs)
- Atomic absorption spectrometry (for mercury)
- Carboxyhemoglobin (for CO poisoning)
- 24-hour urine (for heavy metals)
- Plasma cholinesterase (ChE) levels (for pesticide metabolites, organophosphates)
- Urinary cotinine assays (for tobacco metabolites)

CO, Carbon monoxide; *PCB,* polychlorinated biphenyl.

Common Environmental Agents and Adverse Effects

This section presents a brief discussion of general pediatric poisoning and some common environmental agents that are particularly hazardous to children.

TABLE 42-2 Primary, Secondary, and Tertiary Prevention of Environmental Health Problems

Level of Prevention	Goals	Approaches	Examples
Primary	Prevent problems from occurring Maintain wellness	Education	Identify hazards: Explain problems that specific elements can cause (e.g., mercury in fish) Prevent exposure: Discuss steps that can be taken (e.g., using non-toxic cleaning materials in the home; keeping toxic compounds locked, out of reach)
		Assessment	Inspect school playgrounds Monitor environmental hazards (e.g., CO, lead and radon in homes and schools)
		Public policy	Conduct scientific research to develop biologic markers in children Enact and enforce regulations and restrictions that support healthy environments (e.g., air and water quality standards; ban of hydrofluorocarbons) Support 1997 Declaration of the Environment Leaders of the Eight on Children's Environmental Health (CPCHE, 1997)
Secondary	Detect problems early, provide for early treatment, and referral for identified cases	Testing	Test children for BLLs
		Reporting	"Reportable" conditions and diseases reported to public health departments; report, monitor and control environmental hazards
		Treatment	Refer identified cases for early treatment
Tertiary	Rehabilitation and restoration of health	Treatment	Evaluate any child with known exposure; conduct long-term evaluation given that effects may appear years later Treat clinically for specific conditions, acute, chronic, short and long term
		Abatement	Decontaminate environment (e.g., removal of asbestos or lead; clean up of Superfund and brownfields sites)
		Restoration	Restore healthy environment (e.g., wetlands and clean water sources)

From Canadian Partnership for Children's Health and Environment (CPCHE): 1997 declaration of environment leaders of the eight on children's environmental health, CPCHE (website), 1997, available at www.healthyenvironmentforkids.ca/resources/1997-declaration-environment-leaders-eight-childrens-environmental-health. Accessed September 14, 2014.

BLL, Blood lead level; *CO,* carbon monoxide.

General Pediatric Poisoning

Poisoning is the process in which a substance that interferes with the body's normal function is taken in by ingestion, inhalation, absorption, or injection. Poisoning is a major cause of pediatric injury. In the United States, more than 2.3 million poisonings occurred in 2011. Forty-nine percent occurred in children 5 years old or younger, underscoring the risk in young children. A total of 62% of all poisonings were in individuals younger than 19 years old; 70 fatalities due to poisoning occurred in this group (Bronstein et al, 2012).

Medications, plants, and chemicals are common causes of poisoning in children. The mouthing behavior of infants and normal curiosity of toddlers and preschoolers puts them at risk for accidental ingestion of toxic materials. Also, the storage practices of caregivers are often implicated as root causes of exposure in this age group. In 2011, the top five exposures in children 5 years old or younger were cosmetics and personal care products, analgesics, household cleaning substances, foreign bodies/toys/miscellaneous, and topical preparations. Children can also be exposed through breast milk and as a result of iatrogenic errors (e.g., prescribing errors, dispensing errors). Adolescents are more likely to intentionally abuse over-the-counter (OTC) and prescribed medications or chemicals for recreation. Moreover, adolescents are at higher risk to attempt or complete suicide using poisons or OTC or prescription medications (Bronstein et al, 2012).

Clinical Findings

History

The following are assessed:

- Type of substance taken in (e.g., product name and list of ingredients)
- Amount of intake
- Exact time of intake or exposure
- Route or method of intake
- Signs and symptoms and their progression over time
- Emergency care given
- Child's health status before poisoning (e.g., Any significant chronic illness? Is child taking prescription medication?)
- Contact information including phone and address if the assessment is via phone

Physical Examination

Findings vary greatly depending on the type and amount of poisonous substance, time since exposure, and susceptibility of the child. Reactions can be local, systemic, or both. Consult early with a Poison Control Center for guidance on how to proceed with the physical examination.

Questions to consider while conducting the physical examination include the following:

- Which body system or systems does the poison affect?
- What are specific signs of the poison's effect?
- When did the ingestion occur?
- How quickly does the poison have an effect?
- How susceptible is the child?
- What is the child's age and weight?

Diagnostic Studies

Analysis of specimens (e.g., emesis) can be helpful in determining the type of poison, if unknown. Serum or urine levels of some agents can be assessed (e.g., acetaminophen, opioids). In general, however, toxicology screens are not necessary, and diagnosis is made on the basis of history and in consultation with a poison control or pediatric environmental health center.

Differential Diagnosis

A history of exposure distinguishes suspected or known poisoning from acute-onset illness. Because there is not always an obvious episode of exposure, the provider should be suspicious of poisoning in otherwise well children who experience sudden seizures, GI distress, or cardiorespiratory collapse.

Management

Management approaches for ingested poisons vary with the type of poison, amount of exposure, time lapse since exposure, and susceptibility of the child. Observation alone may be sufficient (e.g., with warfarin); hospitalization and life-support may be necessary. Consultation with a Poison Control Center is strongly recommended. The goals of treatment are to:

- Maintain vital functions, airway, breathing, and circulation (ABCs).
- Counteract or neutralize effects of the poison:
  - Administer antidotes.
  - Decontaminate to reduce poison in the system (Box 42-4). Weigh risks of decontamination against positive effects.
  - Administer life-support measures to allow body to detoxify itself.
- Monitor child's condition. If managed at home, talk with caregiver approximately 30 minutes, 1, and 3 hours after ingestion.
- Alter treatment to respond to changes in the child's condition (e.g., continued monitoring, hospitalization).

Timing is critical when using decontamination procedures; and because decontamination procedures also contain risks, one must consider whether the technique chosen is likely to be of sufficient value to merit its use. Prompt cleansing action to remove a toxin from the skin (e.g., insecticide exposure) or from the eye may prevent major absorption. With ingested toxins, most liquid products are absorbed completely within 30 minutes and solids within 1 to 2 hours. Use of activated charcoal, an adsorbent agent, has been demonstrated to have good efficacy for many, but not all, toxins. With this agent, the toxins adhere to the GI surface, rather than being absorbed by its mucosa, and the toxins are excreted through the stool. There is no good evidence to support use of cathartics with activated

• BOX 42-4 Basic Decontamination Protocol

- Determine the need for decontamination by calling the Poison Control Center in your area.
- If clothing has been contaminated, strip the patient and double-bag clothing, then flush the entire body with plain water for 2 to 5 minutes. If contaminated with dust, keep clothing dry; remove carefully to minimize dust becoming airborne; if possible, apply dust mask or respirator to patient before removing clothing (brush dust from face first).
- Chemical contamination:
  - Scrub or irrigate open wounds for 5 to 10 minutes or longer using lukewarm water.
  - Irrigate eyes with sterile saline, balanced salt solution, or Ringer's lactate for at least 15 to 30 minutes.
  - Irrigate face, nose, and ear canals with normal saline using frequent suction.
  - Wash appendages (if that is only body part contaminated) without wetting the whole body, if possible.
  - Clean under nails with scrub brush and nail cleaner.
- Oily or greasy contamination:
  - Cleanse with soap or shampoo, followed by water flushing.

charcoal. A recent update of the position paper by the American Academy of Clinical Toxicology (AACT) and the European Association of Poison Centres and Clinical Toxicologists (EAPCCT) reaffirms that syrup of ipecac should not be used to treat poisoning (Höjer et al, 2013). Gastric lavage is not commonly recommended because it removes a small portion of gastric contents and may cause more harm than benefit. Whole-bowel irrigation with a polyethylene glycol (PEG) electrolyte into the stomach to cleanse the entire GI tract has been shown to be somewhat successful for substances that are absorbed slowly, such as iron or sustained-release medications (O'Donnell and Ewald, 2011). Other decontamination strategies that can be used in the hospital setting include diuresis, dialysis, and therapies for acute kidney injury (e.g., continuous renal replacement therapy [CRRT]). Occasionally, drug-induced liver injury (DILI) or hepatotoxicity caused by other agents (e.g., acetaminophen overdose with late presentation for care) leads to acute liver failure (ALF). ALF can ultimately result in the need for liver transplantation.

Patient and Family Education

Prevention is the best management for poisonings. Teach parents how to "poison-proof" their home, pointing out connections between the developmental stages of children and sources of poisoning. If a child is exposed to a toxic or potentially toxic substance, instruct parents to call the Poison Control Center *before* beginning treatment.

Heavy Metals

Several heavy metals, including lead, mercury, and arsenic, can cause severe toxic effects in children. Intoxication affects multiple organs in a variety of ways through widespread disruption of cellular functioning. Lead and mercury are particularly well known for their neurodevelopmental effects.

Lead

Lead poisoning is the presence of blood lead levels (BLLs) that cause toxic effects on multiple organ systems. A BLL of 5 mcg/dL or more is considered high, and the CDC recommends public health action be taken at this point. Despite this CDC "reference level," any amount of lead in the system has a toxic effect. There is no acceptable minimum threshold, and most neurocognitive damage (e.g., intelligence quotients [IQs] in children) occurs at levels less than 10 mcg/dL (Jakubowski, 2011). Therefore, primary prevention to eliminate environmental exposure is absolutely essential.

Exposure to lead is linked with many conditions, especially those related to the neurologic system, including lower IQs, attention-deficit/hyperactivity disorder (ADHD), reading problems, school failure, and delinquent and criminal behavior. Lead easily crosses the placenta, and prenatal lead exposure may be associated with schizophrenia (Opler et al, 2008) and autism (von Ehrenstein et al, 2014). GI, renal, musculoskeletal, reproductive, thyroid, and cardiovascular diseases can also occur. The effects of lead toxicity can be permanent, especially in children. Boys may be more susceptible than girls to the effects of prenatal exposure to low levels of lead (Jedrychowski et al, 2009).

Lead is absorbed through the GI system and lungs (lead dust). Absorption depends on the route of exposure and age and nutritional status of the individual. For example, 100% of lead inhaled into the lower lungs is absorbed. In children, up to 70% of lead in the GI tract can be absorbed, in contrast to about 20% in adults. Poorly nourished individuals, especially those with iron or calcium deficiencies, absorb lead more easily. Once ingested, lead circulates through the body attached to erythrocytes. It affects heme production, competes with calcium in any calcium-mediated process, alters certain enzyme functions (e.g., ferrochelatase in bone marrow), and damages the nervous system, both through direct nerve cell damage and interference with nerve conduction. Brain development is affected because lead inhibits the normal pruning process that eliminates multiple intercellular connections (Markowitz, 2011).

Children are exposed to lead primarily in their housing (i.e., dust and chips from deteriorating paint on interior surfaces, exposure to lead-based paints during renovation, and/or lead leached into water from lead pipes and solder). Some immigrant children enter the United States with high BLLs; others, including non-immigrant children, may be exposed to toys, candies, pottery, or home remedies that contain lead. Soil near old highways, deteriorating homes, mines, lead-using industries, and smelters can have high lead levels, and root vegetables can absorb lead from the soil. Cosmetics and dyes, insecticides, some dietary supplements, ammunition, fishing weights, and some vinyls contain lead. Artificial turf can represent a lead hazard, especially as it ages and deteriorates (Kim et al, 2012). Lead is not readily transferred in breast milk.

Although environmental lead sources and the incidence of elevated BLLs have decreased in the United States, lead poisoning continues to be a serious environmental health problem for young children. It is estimated that in 2010 over half a million American children 1 to 5 years old had BLLs of 5 mcg/dL or more (Wheeler and Brown, 2013), with a higher percentage of children living in poverty or low-income families having high BLLs (Vivier et al, 2011).

Clinical Findings

History. Every infant and child seen by a primary care provider should have a history taken to determine risk for lead exposure. Criteria that put the child at risk are:

- Living in a ZIP code with 27% or more of the houses built before 1950
- Receiving benefits from Medicaid or Woman, Infants, and Children (WIC) program
- Having a parent or guardian who answered "yes" or "don't know" to at least one question on the basic personal-risk questionnaire (see Box 42-2)

Every child who meets *any* of these three criteria should be screened for BLLs.

In addition to questions found in the basic environmental assessment tools, assessment for lead risk should include questions such as:

- What is the general condition of the child's residence?
- Is there evidence of peeling paint?
- Have there been recent renovations or repairs of the house?
- Are there outdoor areas where the child plays that could be contaminated?
- How does the family control dust and dirt that might be contaminated?
- Does the child exhibit pica?
- Does the child live near a lead smelter, battery recycling plant, or other industry likely to release lead?
- Does a family member or caregiver work with lead-based materials?
- In what hobbies do household members engage (e.g., ceramics, stained glass)?
- Are painted or unusual materials burned in wood stoves or fireplaces?
- Does the home contain vinyl mini-blinds made overseas and purchased before 1997?
- Does the child have access to imported foods or cosmetics?
- Does the family use complementary, herbal, or folk remedies?
- Is food prepared or stored in imported pottery or metal containers?
- Does the child have a retained lead bullet?

Physical Examination. Clinical signs of lead toxicity may not accurately reflect the amount of lead in the body, especially because most lead retained by the body is stored in the bones and is not measured by BLLs. One child can have high BLLs (e.g., 45 mcg/dL) with no obvious clinical signs. Another child may complain of severe GI problems with a lower lead level (e.g., 15 to 20 mcg/dL). Many children have subclinical effects that are difficult to identify but have serious health ramifications (e.g., neurocognitive damage with BLLs of 5 mcg/dL or less) or have symptoms that are easily confused with other conditions (e.g., anemia, constipation, abdominal pain, impaired hearing, learning disabilities, delayed growth, and/or hyperactivity). Many children do not demonstrate signs of acute toxicity until late in the disease. At higher levels, lead affects vitamin D metabolism, nerve conduction velocities, and hemoglobin synthesis that can lead to myocardial excitability, increased intracranial pressure, seizures, coma, and death.

Diagnostic Studies.

Screening. Providers should use state and local recommendations or policies, based on CDC guidelines, to guide their practice (CDC, 1997). All children at risk should be tested at 1 and 2 years old or 3 and 6 years old (if they have not been previously tested). Also, children who have any sign of lead toxicity should be screened. All children who have recently emigrated from other countries should be screened on arrival to the United States.

In 2006, the U.S. Food and Drug Administration (FDA) approved a rapid screening test that uses capillary blood and gives results in as little as 3 minutes. This test is exempt from Clinical Laboratory and Improvement Amendments of 1988 (CLIA) requirements; therefore, it can be administered in non-laboratory settings by individuals who are not laboratory technicians (FDA, 2014). If the preliminary screening result is 10 mcg/dL or greater, a venous sample should be drawn immediately for confirmation by laboratory testing (Advisory Committee on Childhood Lead Poisoning Prevention of the CDC, 2013). If there is doubt about the accuracy of the rapid test, 8 mcg/dL should be the standard for additional assessment and management.

Assessment of free erythrocyte protoporphyrin (FEP) and zinc protoporphyrin (ZPP) can be helpful because these are elevated in the presence of lead. Evaluate iron deficiency, including serum ferritin.

Differential Diagnosis

GI infections, other causes of anemia, growth retardation, behavior disorders, ADHD, and central nervous system (CNS) infections are included in the differential diagnosis.

Management

Management involves preventing the child's exposure to lead in the environment, treating the child for toxicity, monitoring BLLs, correcting dietary deficiencies (if any), and removing lead from the environment (i.e., lead abatement). Other children in the same household or environment where exposure could have occurred should be tested and treated as appropriate. Chelation is indicated to treat acute, severe, and life-threatening poisoning (Table 42-3), but there is controversy about its use for long-term exposure

TABLE 42-3 Management Recommendations for Lead Poisoning

Child has risk factors from screening criteria and/or there are no local or state guidelines on when to screen for lead levels.*
Yes: Draw blood sample and complete laboratory assessment.
No: Routine screening not recommended; provide caregiver dietary and environmental education.

Screening Sample: Blood Lead Levels	Action to be Taken†	Follow-Up Blood Lead Levels Monitoring
<5 mcg/dL	Not considered lead poisoning: • Provide caregiver/parent dietary and environmental education • Refer to social services as appropriate • Conduct environmental assessment to determine if child is exposed to a lead source (e.g., pre-1978 housing)	If high risk, retest in 6 months If low risk, no further testing necessary; ongoing monitoring for changes in environment
≥5 to 9 mcg/dL	Reference value requiring intervention: • Confirmatory venous blood test within 1 to 3 months	Early follow-up (two to four tests) by 3 months Later follow-up (after BLLs decline) at 6 to 9 months
10 to 44 mcg/dL • 10 to 19 mcg/dL	Confirmatory venous blood test within 1 week to 1 month‡	• Early follow-up 1 to 3 months§ Later follow-up at 3 to 6 months
• 20 to 24 mcg/dL		• Early follow-up 1 to 3 months§ Later follow-up at 1 to 3 months
• 25 to 44 mcg/dL		• Early follow-up 2 weeks to 1 month Later follow-up at 1 month Retest every month until results <15 mcg/dL for at least 6 months, then retest every 3 months until child is 36 months old
45 to 59 mcg/dL	Confirmatory venous blood test within 48 hours Complete history and physical examination Complete neurologic examination Lab work: Hgb or Hct and iron status (FEP or ZPP) Abdominal x-ray with bowel decontamination if indicated Chelation therapy, may be oral in ambulatory setting	Early follow-up as soon as possible Retest every month until results <15 mcg/dL for at least 6 months, then retest every 3 months until child is 36 months old
60 to 69 mcg/dL	Confirmatory venous blood test within 24 hours Complete history and physical examination Complete neurologic examination Lab work: Hgb or Hct and iron status (TIBC or SF) Abdominal x-ray with bowel decontamination if indicated Chelation therapy, may be oral in ambulatory setting	Early follow-up as soon as possible Retest every month until results <15 mcg/dL for at least 6 months, then retest every 3 months until child is 36 months old
≥70 mcg/dL	Medical emergency: Retest immediately as an emergency lab test with venous blood sample Hospitalize for IV chelation Proceed according to action for 45 to 69 mcg/dL	Early follow-up as soon as possible Retest every month until results <15 mcg/dL for at least 6 months, then retest every 3 months until child is 36 months old

Data adapted from Centers for Disease Control and Prevention (CDC): *Screening young children for lead poisoning: guidance for state and local public health officials*, Atlanta, 1997, CDC; Advisory Committee on Childhood Lead Poisoning Prevention of the Centers for Disease Control and Prevention (CDC): *Low level lead exposure harms children: a renewed call for primary prevention*, Atlanta, 2012, CDC.

BLL, Blood lead level; *FEP*, free erythrocyte protoporphyrin; *Hct*, hematocrit; *Hgb*, hemoglobin; *SF*, serum ferritin; *TIBC*, total iron-binding capacity; *ZPP*, zinc protoporphyrin.

*Universal screening is recommended, regardless of risk factors, if there are no state or local screening guidelines.

†In all cases of lead toxicity (≥5 mcg/dL):

- Inform caregiver of level of toxicity.
- Provide caregiver dietary and environmental education.
- Remove child from source of lead if known.
- Report to public health department.
- Initiate environmental investigation.
- Initiate lead hazard control/abatement.
- Refer to social services.

‡The higher the BLL, the sooner confirmatory testing should be done.

§May do at 1 month to ensure BLL are not rising rapidly.

or chronic intoxication because the therapy itself may be harmful and may outweigh the benefits of clearing the metal (Kosnett, 2010). Chelation therapy for levels higher than 20 mcg/dL and lower than 45 mcg/dL has not been shown to offer therapeutic benefits (CDC, 1997); and there is no evidence that chelation reverses cognitive impairments, so prevention is critical (AAP Committee on Environmental Health, 2005). It is also critical that providers do follow-up testing for children with positive lead screens. Lack of follow-up testing is an error of omission that can lead to permanent damage in the child.

Patient and Family Education

Prevention of lead poisoning is a public health responsibility. Use of Geographic Information Systems (GIS) allows public health officials to identify high-risk areas. Based on this information, focused, population-based screening programs (e.g., in Head Start classrooms) can be implemented, and the prevalence of lead toxicity in children can be discovered. Primary care providers also play a critical role in the process of preventing lead toxicity in children. The provider *must* take a lead exposure history and, using GIS information from public health sources, identify those children who need to be screened and tested, and institute appropriate treatment.

Parents need to be informed that lead abatement is absolutely essential; treatments such as chelation therapy and dietary changes (e.g., promoting iron-rich nutritional intake) are ineffective unless the child is returned to a clean house. Professional assessment of the level of contamination should be done, and professional abatement may be necessary. The provider can work with parents to identify ways to control lead dust and paint chips in older homes. Conventional vacuums can be used to help control lead dust and high-efficiency particulate air (HEPA) filtering vacuum cleaners can temporarily reduce lead loads, but levels soon rise if the source of lead remains (Yiin et al, 2002). Other strategies parents can use include the following:

- Block access to areas of the room where large peeling paint areas are found.
- Cover smaller peeling areas with sticky-backed paper.
- Damp-mop and damp-dust with household cleaners or lead-specific cleaning products (e.g., Ledizolv) twice weekly to decrease lead dust in the air; do not dry mop or sweep.
- Pick up and dispose of paint chips with a disposable rag or paper towel soaked in phosphate cleaner.
- Run water until temperature changes to flush pipes of lead sediment.
- Do not store or cook food in lead crystal or pottery that contains lead.
- Remove work clothes and wash hands before returning home if job is lead-related.

Inform parents that chelation therapy leads to a rapid fall in BLL but most children have a rebound increase within days or weeks of treatment; and repeated treatment may be necessary.

Mercury

Mercury is the second most common cause of heavy metal poisoning. Mercury exists in elemental forms (liquid or vapor), inorganic mercury salts, and organic forms such as methyl mercury, which is the most toxic to humans. Routes of exposure are most commonly through inhalation, ingestion, and skin absorption. Elemental mercury is poorly absorbed in its solid form, although the aerosolized form is absorbed easily by the lungs. Organic mercury (e.g., methyl mercury, ethyl mercury) is readily absorbed from the GI tract and through the skin.

Mercury has been labeled a "developmental neurotoxicant," and CNS tissue is the main target organ for mercury in humans. Once absorbed into the brain, mercury metabolizes to its inorganic form and cannot cross the blood-brain barrier to exit the brain. It causes permanent damage to the developing brain. Different effects (or degrees of effects) depend on the susceptibilities of the affected child at a given time. For the fetus, there is a dose-response relationship between maternal mercury levels and IQ (Etzel and Balk, 2012). Data from the National Health and Nutrition Examination Survey (NHANES) conducted by the CDC reveal that for the years 2009 to 2010, 2.3% of women of childbearing age had blood mercury levels greater than 5.8 mcg/L, which is the maximum acceptable daily exposure (i.e., reference dose) that the EPA has set as "not likely to be harmful." Based on birth rates, therefore, more than 75,000 newborns each year are at risk of in utero methyl mercury poisoning in the United States (EPA, 2014c). Inorganic mercury can be especially damaging to the kidney, causing tubular necrosis. Of note, ethyl mercury is a metabolite of thimerosal, a vaccine preservative, which is no longer used in the United States except in the multi-dose vial of influenza vaccine. In the 2000s, claims were made that thimerosal exposure was causally linked to an increased incidence of autism. Extensive prospective and retrospective research subsequent to these claims determined this link to be unfounded; no causal connection between thimerosal exposure and autism exists (CDC, 2014f). An information handout for parents can be accessed through the Immunization Action Coalition (see Additional Resources).

The presence of mercury in humans appears to be increasing. When tested in 1999 to 2000, 2% of the subjects in the 1999 to 2002 NHANES population had detectable inorganic mercury in their bodies; in a follow-up study done in 2005 to 2006, 30% of the same subjects had detectable inorganic mercury (Laks, 2009). In the United States, the concentration of methyl mercury in the body is greatest among older Asian men (Mortensen et al, 2014). Mercury is pervasive in the environment. Common sources are listed in Box 42-5; exposure and contamination varies for each type of mercury. It is emitted into the atmosphere largely by human activities (e.g., coal-fired industry, manufacturing) and occasionally by natural sources (e.g., volcanoes). From the atmosphere, mercury accumulates in clouds, falls as precipitation, and returns to soil, sediment, or bodies of

• BOX 42-5 Sources of Mercury Exposure

Finfish and shellfish with the highest levels of mercury:

- Mackerel, king
- Shark
- Swordfish
- Tilefish

Predator marine mammals (e.g., seals, whales) pose specific concern for children in Arctic regions.

Prenatal Exposure

- Exposure reflective of mother's mercury burden and ongoing exposures (e.g., dental amalgams, occupational hazards)

Infant Exposure

- Breast milk*
- Teething powders, soaps, organomercurial medicinals

Childhood Exposure

Exposure primarily through the home, school, and other places where child may spend time.

- Diet (fish, rice)
- Medicinal preparations (traditional medicines, nutraceuticals, homeopathic preparations, Ayurvedic medicines)
- Cosmetic goods (e.g., some soaps, creams)
- Dental amalgams
- Mercury-containing paints
- Broken or compromised oral or rectal thermometers
- Broken or compromised switches and pressure gauges (including sphygmomanometers†)
- Broken or compromised fluorescent light bulbs, thermometers
- Industrial sources (e.g., factories emitting aerosolized waste, parent tracking mercury home on shoes from workplace)
- School chemistry classes
- Batteries
- Antiques in the home
- Electronics
- In the developing world, child laborers in gold mining camps and waste scavenging sites

Adapted from World Health Organization (WHO): Children's exposure to mercury compounds, 2010, available at http://whqlibdoc.who.int/publications/2010/9789241500456_eng.pdf. Accessed November 17, 2014.
*Breast milk continues to be highly recommended as the exclusive food for the infant through 6 months and continuing thereafter nonexclusively. Formula does not have the full complement of nutrients and immune benefits of breast milk and is not completely free of pollutants.
†WHO recommends phasing out mercury-containing health care equipment.

water, where it is absorbed by plants and animals. In oceans, lakes, and streams, fish consume plants and smaller fish, leading to a process called *bioaccumulation.* Thus, larger and predatory fish (e.g., shark, swordfish, and tilefish) will have the highest levels of mercury and are the least safe to consume.

Clinical Findings

History. The signs and symptoms of mercury poisoning may be easily attributed to other processes. A careful history is essential to identify any possible exposures. Questions should focus on potential exposure (e.g., industrial exposure, mercury spills, consumer goods, and diet) and whether others in the household are experiencing similar symptoms.

Physical Examination. In the case of known or suspected mercury exposure, complete a full examination with special attention to the following systems:

- Respiratory system: Elemental mercury vapor produces chemical pneumonitis or necrotizing bronchitis, potentially progressing to acute respiratory distress syndrome (qualifying as respiratory failure).
- Neurologic system: Subacute exposures may include insomnia, forgetfulness, loss of appetite, tremor, peripheral neuropathy, visual impairments, and behavioral changes (e.g., emotional lability). Fetal exposure may result in Minamata disease: low birth weight, profound developmental delays, cerebral palsy, deafness, blindness, and seizures.
- Skin/musculoskeletal: Acrodynia ("pink disease") is the term for the constellation of findings in children (not adults) poisoned by mercury. This hypersensitivity reaction prominently affects the extremities, causing swelling, pain, weakness (particularly of pelvic area), and an erythematous maculopapular rash. Additionally, children with acrodynia may exhibit other organ system involvement listed here.
- GI system: Gingivostomatitis may result from chronic exposure. Acute exposure (e.g., ingestion of button batteries) may cause corrosive gastroenteritis, hematemesis, and pain with cardiovascular collapse or renal failure.
- Nephrologic system: Renal tubular dysfunction and hypertension may develop.

Diagnostic Studies. Blood mercury levels can be used to determine acute mercury exposure; however, due to the kinetics (e.g., half-life) of mercury, the result may not accurately reflect the level of toxicity. A blood level of less than 2 mcg/L is considered normal, but a normal level may not exclude mercury poisoning. A 24-hour urine sample can also be collected (less than 10 mcg/L is the reference range of "normal"). Hair analysis provides a more comprehensive look at mercury exposure but needs to be done in a controlled laboratory specializing in this test. The specific type of suspected or known exposure (elemental, inorganic or organic mercury; acute or chronic) will determine the best test, and its timing, in a specific circumstance. Poison Control Center personnel can assist with these determinations.

Differential Diagnosis

The differential diagnosis includes other poisonings, CNS, and/or psychiatric conditions. Rashes can be particularly confounding; therefore, a high level of suspicion and querying of environmental exposures is important when evaluating any rash. A patient with neurologic symptoms, along with rash, should always be evaluated for mercury and other poisonings.

Management

The initial measure is to remove the mercury source from the child's environment. This could include involving the local health department and, depending on the volume, a hazardous materials team or EPA-certified contractor for abatement. Other children in the environment should be evaluated for possible mercury poisoning.

The patient's case would best be managed by a pediatric toxicologist. The regional Poison Control Center or regional PEHSU, can provide a toxicologist to review the case and guide management.

Patient and Family Education

Education should focus on increasing awareness of sources of mercury and ways to prevent or limit exposure. Old thermometers, health care supplies, antiques, fluorescent light bulbs, and other common household items contain mercury. Elemental mercury, for example, can spill as a thick, bright silver liquid, very attractive to children. The EPA has specific instructions on how to clean up small mercury spills, including what *not* to do, such as vacuum or sweep up the spill (EPA, 2015). Fluorescent bulbs and other items that contain mercury should be recycled in accordance with local recommendations for hazardous materials. Alternatives to dental amalgams should be explored for dental caries.

As with all environmental toxicants, nurse practitioners and community members should maintain awareness of local environmental issues (e.g., mercury emissions from industrial plants) and actively participate in legislation and regulatory efforts to decrease pollution and, thus, improve the health of children. The EPA and FDA have released advice on fish consumption, in hopes of *increasing* fish consumption in women of childbearing age and in children while continuing to limit exposure to mercury (Box 42-6).

• BOX 42-6 Recommendations for Fish Consumption by Women of Childbearing Age and Children

- Eat 8 to 12 ounces of fish per week for women
- Eat two to three servings of appropriate proportions per week for children
- Choose fish lower in mercury (avoid predatory fish: shark, swordfish, king mackerel, tilefish)
- Eat no more than 6 ounces of albacore tuna per week
- When eating fish that have been caught from local streams, rivers, and lakes, pay attention to fish advisories on those bodies of water
- When adding more fish to your diet, stay within your calorie needs

From U.S. Environmental Protection Agency (EPA), U.S. Food and Drug Administration (FDA): FDA and EPA issue updated draft advice for fish consumption: advice encourages pregnant women and breastfeeding mothers to eat more fish that are lower in mercury, EPA (website), 2014, available at http://yosemite.epa.gov/opa/admpress.nsf/596e17d7cac720848525781f0043629e/b8edc480d8cfe29b85257cf20065f826!OpenDocument and www.fda.gov/Food/FoodborneIllnessContaminants/Metals/ucm393070.htm. Accessed December 2, 2015.

Arsenic

Arsenic is a highly poisonous chemical element, a heavy metal that occurs naturally in the environment in organic and inorganic forms. Arsenic is found in many different compound forms and salts, such as arsenic acid, arsenic trioxide, and arsenate; some compounds (e.g., arsine) are gaseous, colorless, nonirritating substances with an odor of garlic. Arsenic may act upon cardiovascular, dermal, neurologic and GI systems. Cancers of the genitourinary, pulmonary, or dermal systems may result depending on the route of exposure (Agency for Toxic Substances and Disease Registry [ATSDR], 2011a). Acute poisoning usually causes neurologic GI symptoms. Infant mortality is higher in mothers who are exposed to arsenic (Rahman et al, 2010).

Incidence of arsenic exposure is unknown. In addition to its natural occurrence, arsenic is used commercially in pesticides, herbicides, rodenticides, and wood preservatives. Arsenic trioxide is also used in glassmaking and some pigments. Drinking water and foods can be contaminated with arsenic (e.g., apple juice, rice). Children can also be exposed through contact with treated wood used to construct play structures. Chromated copper arsenate (CCA), which was used extensively before 2004 as a wood treatment to prevent decay and insect damage, can leach into soil and sand surrounding play structures. Currently, most residential building materials do not contain CCA, but the EPA has not banned its use nor required removal of structures built before 2004, so children are still at risk. Burning treated wood releases arsenic into the air, where it can be inhaled. Industrial processes can also release arsenic into the environment.

Clinical Findings

History and Physical Examination. An exposure history is essential in determining whether arsenic poisoning has occurred. Physical signs and symptoms depend on the dose, route, and duration of exposure. A partial list includes the following (ATSDR, 2010):

- Cardiovascular: Hypotension, shock, arrhythmias, edema
- Respiratory: Respiratory tract irritation, pulmonary edema, bronchitis, pneumonia
- Neurologic: Sensorimotor peripheral axonal neuropathy, neuritis, muscle cramps, headache, weakness, lethargy, delirium, encephalopathy, hyperpyrexia, tremor, seizure, coma
- GI and hepatic: Garlic odor of breath, abdominal pain, nausea, vomiting, thirst, anorexia, gastroesophageal reflux, diarrhea, dysphagia, transaminitis, liver necrosis, cholangitis
- Renal: Hematuria, oliguria, proteinuria, uremia, tubular necrosis
- Hematologic: Hemolysis, anemia, leukopenia, thrombocytopenia, disseminated intravascular coagulation (DIC)

- Dermal: Mees lines (transverse white lines in nail beds developing weeks to months after exposure), dermatitis, melanosis or pigment changes, hyperkeratosis
- Other: Rhabdomyolysis, conjunctivitis

Diagnostic Studies. A 24-hour urine sample is the preferred specimen; serum levels can also be measured but are less accurate because the half-life is very short. A laboratory reference value of less than 35 mcg/L in a 24-hour urine is considered within normal limits for all age groups. Concentrations higher than 100 mcg/L indicate acute arsenic intoxication (ATSDR, 2011a), although intervention may be needed for lower levels. Consult with a toxicologist to determine if exposure warrants laboratory evaluation and treatment.

Management

Minimizing exposure by identifying and removing the arsenic source is of utmost importance. For severe exposures, acute stabilization with gut decontamination (e.g., activated charcoal, gastric lavage) and/or chelation may be necessary. Monitor renal and hematologic function acutely and with follow-up. Treatment should be done in consultation with a pediatric toxicologist.

Parents and providers can work with schools and communities to assess for and manage arsenic contamination of play structures. Test water supplies that are suspected to be contaminated. Bottled water, distilled water, or home treatment units that remove arsenic should be used if drinking water is contaminated. Health care providers should support regulatory standards for production and use of arsenic-containing products to ensure protection of children's health.

Ambient Air Pollution: Indoor and Outdoor

Air quality is an important environmental factor in childhood illness, especially respiratory conditions such as asthma. Since the 1970s, outdoor air quality has improved in many areas as a result of local, state, and federal regulations, but air pollution continues to contribute significantly to adverse health effects. Gaseous pollutants include CO, sulfur oxides, hydrocarbons, ozone, and nitrogen oxides. Human activity that results in burning of fossil fuels is the chief source of these gases. Coarse, fine, or ultrafine particulate matter (from dust, dirt, soot, smoke, and liquid drops) is inhaled and can cause respiratory irritation. Patients and caregivers can check online at www.airnow.gov for daily updates on local outdoor air quality (AirNow, 2014).

Indoor air quality is affected by many factors, including ETS, construction materials and practices (e.g., air-tight, energy-efficient buildings with decreased ventilation have increased concentration of pollutants), cleaning products, furniture, and more. Because up to 90% of an individual's time is spent indoors in our current culture, exposure to airborne toxicants is a significant concern. As with outdoor air pollution, indoor air pollution can exacerbate asthma or other ailments. Source control and proper ventilation are essential components of management. For patients with asthma, utilize the screening questionnaire in Figure 42-2 to assess possible triggers.

As mentioned earlier, children are especially susceptible to air quality problems because they are experiencing rapid lung development; have smaller, narrower airways; breathe more rapidly; are more physically active than adults; and spend more time on the floor. Very young children spend notably more time indoors. This section discusses several of the more common indoor and outdoor airborne toxicants that influence children's health status: ETS, CO, radon, particulate matter, asbestos, and molds.

Environmental Tobacco Smoke

ETS, the presence of tobacco smoke in the air, is the single largest preventable cause of death and disease in the United States. Tobacco smoke contains more than 7,000 chemicals, about 70 of which are carcinogens. These include formaldehyde, benzene, polonium, vinyl chloride, chromium, arsenic, lead, cadmium, CO, hydrogen cyanide, ammonia, butane, and toluene (CDC, 2011).

ETS has been associated with a wide range of health problems during pregnancy and among infants and children. It is estimated that it causes an annual excess of 6,000 deaths among children 5 years old and younger. A major surgeon general's report highlights these problems. Effects can be grouped into several categories (Samet and Sockrider, 2014; USDHHS, 2014):

- Quality of life and costs
- Prematurity and prenatal mortality: Spontaneous abortion is higher among women who smoke.
- Fetal growth and development: Newborns of smoking mothers are more likely to have low birth weight and cleft lip and palate. The respiratory and growth outcomes are related to smoking in the second and third trimesters (Prabhu et al, 2010).
- Childhood growth and development: Prenatal ETS decreases the IQ of the offspring (Minnes et al, 2011). ETS affects physical growth and is associated with cognitive and behavioral problems in children. Effects include hypertonicity and irritability in newborns and behavioral problems in older children, including oppositional defiant disorder, conduct disorder, delinquency, and ADHD.
- Sudden infant death syndrome (SIDS)
- Respiratory symptoms and illness—especially lower respiratory illness including bronchitis, bronchiolitis, pneumonia, asthma, overall impaired lung function: Prenatal ETS exposure affects the respiratory health of children after birth. In children 2 years old and younger, prenatal or postnatal passive smoke exposure is associated with a 30% to 70% increased risk of wheezing and a 21% to 85% increase in the incidence of asthma (Burke et al, 2012).
- Atherosclerosis: Pubertal children with a history of long-term exposure to passive cigarette smoke, especially Caucasian males, are at increased risk of premature coronary artery disease.

- Middle ear disease: Children who live with ETS have more recurrent otitis media and middle ear effusions.
- Childhood cancer
- Infant gastroenteritis
- Impaired immune system function

A number of reasons for increased respiratory problems among children exposed to ETS have been proposed including:

- Changes to airway tissue development
- Suppression of phagocytic activity in pulmonary tissues
- Alteration in neural control of the airway
- Alteration in immune system function that can slow the body's response to infection (Wilson et al, 2012)

In addition, ETS may have an epigenetic effect on the fetus, causing adverse changes in the developing organism. More than 241 genes ($p < 0.05$) tested from the placentas of smoking and nonsmoking mothers showed a change in genetic expression in those mothers who smoked (Bruchova et al, 2010). In some conditions, tobacco may be a complicating rather than causal factor, and other variables such as socioeconomic status and diet must also be considered.

Children are exposed to tobacco smoke primarily through cigarettes, cigars, or pipes used by parents, other family members, visitors in the home, day care providers, teachers, or others smoking around them. Although smoking has decreased in the United States, nearly 50% of children between 3 and 18 years old are exposed to cigarette smoke regularly, either at home, in the family car, or in places where smoking is still allowed (HHS, 2014). Eleven percent of women report smoking during pregnancy and 16% of women report smoking after pregnancy (CDC, 2014a). Even if smokers smoke outside, open windows, or use fans, the child is still exposed to ETS and is at risk for its effects. Also third-hand smoke, smoke contamination that remains after a cigarette has been extinguished, is found on a smoker's clothes and body and on materials and surfaces in areas where smokers have been. It appears that health risks from third-hand smoke may last for years as tobacco chemicals linger and combine with other compounds in the environment (Ferrante et al, 2013; Sleiman et al, 2010).

Smoking is generally initiated and established during adolescence. Ninety percent of adult smokers tried their first cigarette before 21 years old. It is encouraging that trends over the past few decades indicate fewer and fewer children are beginning to smoke or continue to smoke after they try tobacco. Although 22.4% of students state they currently use some form of tobacco, that is a decrease from 43.4% in 1997; and the Youth Risk Behavior Survey (2013 data) revealed that only 15.7% of high school students across the United States smoked at least once in the past 30 days and 5.6% smoked on more than 20 of the past 30 days (Kann et al, 2014). Older, Caucasian students tend to smoke more than younger students and those from other ethnic groups. Boys tend to be heavier smokers, with 28% of 12th-grade males smoking currently. Less than 9% of students reported using smokeless tobacco at least once in the 30 days before the survey, and 12.6% reported smoking cigars. Data from these studies indicate that it is easy for children to purchase cigarettes. About 18% of students who currently smoke purchased cigarettes as underage consumers from stores or gas stations (Kann et al, 2014).

In addition to typical tobacco smoke exposures (e.g., cigarettes), there are somewhat novel ways for children, adolescents, and adults to use tobacco and similar products: *hookahs* (a water pipe), electronic cigarettes (e-cigarettes), *snus* (similar to, but different from, chewing tobacco), *kreteks* (tobacco mixed with cloves and other ingredients), *bidis* (Southeast Asian hand-rolled cigarettes), and dissolvable tobacco. The increasing use of hookahs and e-cigarettes is particularly concerning. Smoke from hookahs appears to contribute to significantly more particulate matter than cigarettes (Kumar et al, 2015), as much as a 73-fold increase in nicotine in the blood and significant exposure to carcinogens (St Helen et al, 2014). E-cigarettes, battery-powered devices that provide nicotine and additives (carcinogens, irritants) in aerosol form, present health risks similar to regular cigarettes. They may be flavored (e.g., menthol, cherry, chocolate, or vanilla). From 2011 to 2012, use of e-cigarettes doubled among middle and high school students (CDC, 2013).

Clinical Findings

A thorough and accurate history is required to assess the extent to which ETS affects a child's health. The physical problems for which children are treated vary, and the pediatric health care provider should suspect tobacco smoke as a factor in children who have recurrent respiratory and ear infections.

History. Collect data about the following:

- Three screening questions have proven effective for identifying which children are at greatest risk of exposure to ETS:
  1. "Does the mother smoke?"
  2. "Do other family or household members, caregivers, or others who frequently visit smoke?"
  3. "Do these people smoke inside the house?"
- How often and for how many hours per day is the child exposed to ETS?
- Is the child ever in a car while someone is smoking?
- Has the child experienced health problems that may be associated with ETS (e.g., cough, colds, or ear infections)?

Physical Examination and Diagnostic Studies. These will be specific to the physical signs and symptoms of the child (Table 42-4).

Management

The best treatment for adverse effects of ETS is prevention; every effort should be made to ensure that the child's environment begins and stays smoke-free. Pregnant women should be strongly advised not to smoke at any time during their pregnancy. Children and adolescents should be discouraged from starting to smoke. All children should be

TABLE 42-4 Air Pollutants and Relationship to Disease

Substance	Source	Health Effects/ Systems Affected	Signs and Symptoms	Prevention Strategies
Environmental tobacco smoke (ETS)	First-, second-, or third-hand smoke from cigarettes, cigars, pipes Novel sources include e-cigarettes, snus, kreteks, bidis, hookahs, and dissolvable tobacco	Respiratory Cardiac Growth Neurologic	Bronchitis Bronchiolitis Pneumonia Asthma Otitis media Premature coronary artery disease Low birth weight SIDS Cognitive delays	Adults and siblings in child's environment stop smoking or limit exposures as much as possible Enroll child in day care that is smoke-free Prevent child from starting smoking Recommend smoking cessation programs Health care provider recommendation of and support for decision to stop smoking
Radon	Air Water Generally concentrated in basements and underground	Respiratory	Lung cancer	Test air in basements and first floor of home for radon levels Avoid having children play in basements of homes with radon Consult mitigation company to reduce high levels Provide good ventilation Stop smoking
Particulate matter	Outdoor: • Industrial pollution • Gasoline and diesel exhaust • Pollens • Natural phenomena (e.g., forest fires, volcanic activity) Indoor: • Wood stoves • Dust mites • Animal dander • Cockroach particles • Molds and more	Respiratory Cardiovascular	Bronchitis Pneumonia Wheezing Chronic cough Decreased lung function Asthma Lung cancer Cardiovascular conditions	When outdoor air pollution is high, keep children indoors, decrease outdoor playtime Use HEPA filters for heating/air conditioning, vacuuming Check heating system to ensure it is clean Cover mattresses, wash bedding frequently Launder or discard stuffed animals
Molds	Damp areas (leaking roofs/walls/floors, wet basements, backed-up sewers) Humidifiers Steam from shower, bath, or cooking Wet clothes House plants Dry leaves	Respiratory Dermatologic CNS	Cough Wheezing, dyspnea Sinus congestion Watery, itchy, light-sensitive eyes Sore throat Skin rash Headaches, memory loss, mood changes Myalgias, pain Fever	Maintain dry, clean environment Affected areas can be cleaned with hot water and detergent; may require deep scrubbing Bleach solutions are not routinely recommended; exceptional circumstances (i.e., the environment of immunocompromised patient) may require bleach solution to remove mold If unable to thoroughly clean, discard moldy materials to prevent spores from being released when materials dry Use dehumidifiers and air conditioners as necessary Fix leaks and seepage promptly Use exhaust fans in kitchens and bathrooms Ensure carpets do not get moist (do not place carpets in areas likely to be moist, such as bathrooms)

TABLE 42-4 Air Pollutants and Relationship to Disease—cont'd

Substance	Source	Health Effects/ Systems Affected	Signs and Symptoms	Prevention Strategies
Asbestos	Construction materials: • Insulation • Ceiling and floor tiles • Shingles	Respiratory	Lung irritation Lung disease later in life with repeated exposure	Prevent exposure to asbestos products: If buildings that contain asbestos are in good repair, leave asbestos in place; if there is a question of possible exposure, contact a certified asbestos professional to check it Use asbestos abatement measures as appropriate when renovating If parents' workplace is a source of asbestos exposure, remove clothing and bathe before coming in contact with children

CNS, Central nervous system; *HEPA,* high-efficiency particulate air; *SIDS,* sudden infant death syndrome.

informed about the dangers associated with smoking, and nonsmoking youth should be praised for their decision to not smoke. Family-based smoking prevention programs can be effective; parents can become nonsmoking role models. Parental and caregiver monitoring is useful. School-based smoking prevention programs could be implemented, using school nurses or school-based health clinics.

Providers should assist those youth who do smoke to quit. Smoking cessation is a difficult process for youth, just as it is for adults, and it depends on a number of biologic, behavioral, and psychosocial factors. A complicating factor is the developmental level of most adolescents; they do not have the cognitive, emotional, and social skills of adults who themselves find quitting challenging. Also, young people vastly underestimate the addictive qualities of tobacco. Nonetheless, many young people try to stop smoking. Forty-eight percent of the students questioned in the Youth Risk Behavior Survey had tried to quit in the year before the study (Kann et al, 2014). Evidence-based recommendations for tobacco cessation that relate to children and adolescents are found in Box 42-7. Pediatric providers can use the "five As" discussed in Chapter 9 to structure their smoking cessation counseling. These include:

- Assess: Systematically identify tobacco users, assess and document their status and willingness to quit.
- Advise to quit: Strongly urge all smokers to quit.
- Agree on a plan to quit: Use a motivational interviewing strategy (see Chapter 9) to develop a mutual plan of action to quit smoking.
- Assist in quit attempt: Aid the patient in quitting by supporting a plan and providing education; assist with nicotine replacement therapy as needed, or refer to a smoking cessation program in the community.
- Arrange follow-up: Schedule follow-up contact. Follow through with continuing support and assessment.

The pediatric provider should also strongly encourage parents to stop smoking. In instances where the parent, caregiver, or household member is unable or unwilling to quit, the environment should be altered as much as possible. The parent should take measures to limit exposure: smoking outside the home, using a "smoking jacket" that stays outside, washing hands after smoking, ensuring adequate ventilation, and not smoking in cars or other enclosed spaces. Alternative day care arrangements should be explored if there is smoking at the child's day care center.

BOX 42-7 Tobacco Use Prevention: Clinical Practice Recommendations for Children and Adolescents

Recommendation 1

Clinicians should ask pediatric and adolescent patients about tobacco use and provide a strong message regarding the importance of totally abstaining from tobacco use. (Strength of evidence = C)

Recommendation 2

Counseling has been shown to be effective in treatment of adolescent smokers. Therefore, adolescent smokers should be provided with counseling interventions to aid them in quitting smoking. (Strength of evidence = B)

Recommendation 3

Second-hand smoke is harmful to children. Cessation counseling delivered in pediatric settings has been shown to be effective in increasing abstinence among parents who smoke. Therefore, to protect children from second-hand smoke, clinicians should ask parents about tobacco use and offer them cessation advice and assistance. (Strength of evidence = B)

From the Agency for Healthcare Research and Quality (AHRQ): Treating tobacco use and dependence: 2008 update, (website), available at www.ahrq.gov/professionals/clinicians-providers/guidelines-recommendations/tobacco/index.html. Accessed December 2, 2015.

Carbon Monoxide

CO is a colorless, odorless, tasteless, nonirritating poisonous gas. It is formed by incomplete combustion of any fossil fuel. Improperly vented indoor heating systems, kerosene space heaters, charcoal grills, hibachis, and Sterno stoves emit CO, as do wood stoves, gas stoves, pool heaters, and gas-powered engines (e.g., car exhaust fumes). Methylene chloride, an industrial solvent and paint-stripping agent, is metabolized in the liver to CO.

Because of its characteristics, CO is not readily detected in the environment. In the body, it binds to hemoglobin 240 times more easily than oxygen does, forming carboxyhemoglobin, and diminishing oxygen-carrying capacity. It may also affect the body through more complex mechanisms. It crosses the placenta and has a particular affinity for fetal hemoglobin so that the fetus of a pregnant woman exposed to CO will be affected more than the mother. Smokers have higher carboxyhemoglobin levels than nonsmokers. In all cases, the net result is tissue hypoxia. CO exposure is responsible for thousands of emergency department visits and an average of 430 deaths annually in the United States (CDC, 2014e).

Clinical Findings

Assessment should include the following:

- History of exposure or risk of exposure
- Evidence of similar symptoms in more than one person in a specific setting, with no other known cause; because of their higher oxygen use and higher minute ventilation, however, children may experience symptoms sooner than do adults around them.
- Clinical signs and symptoms:
  - Children exposed to CO have nonspecific neurologic and GI symptoms, including headache (the most common presenting symptom), drowsiness, confusion, nausea, vomiting, alterations in vision, or syncope. Severe CO poisoning may present with cardiac effects (arrhythmias, pulmonary edema, myocardial ischemia, chest pain) and more profound neurologic effects (seizure, coma).
  - Infants and toddlers will more likely exhibit more subtle, nonspecific findings of irritability or difficulty feeding.
- Some long-term, low-level exposure symptoms that have been reported include chronic headaches, learning difficulties, and behavioral problems. Rarely patients may experience *delayed neuropsychiatric syndrome,* consisting of variable degrees of cognitive deficits occurring 3 to 240 days after the exposure; in approximately 90% of cases of this syndrome, there has been a loss of consciousness due to CO (Shprecher and Mehta, 2010). Women exposed to increased CO pollution from automobile traffic have been found to experience more preterm births (Stieb et al, 2012).
- It is of utmost importance to recognize that standard pulse oximetry does *not* differentiate between oxyhemoglobin (what it usually measures) and carboxyhemoglobin. The provider should not rely on standard pulse oximetry when there is suspicion of CO poisoning. A CO oximeter can be used, if available, or the provider can test serum levels. Arterial or venous blood gas should be obtained to measure serum carboxyhemoglobin levels and assess for acidosis. Management should *not* be delayed while waiting for lab results.

Management

Acute CO poisoning is treated by removing the source and providing 100% (high flow) oxygen to compete with the CO. High flow oxygen shortens the half-life of carboxyhemoglobin from 5 to 6 hours to 40 to 60 minutes. Hyperbaric oxygen therapy is also used for severe cases. Consult with a toxicologist. Long-term neurologic sequelae may occur, so follow-up of development is essential.

Patient and Family Education

CO detectors are available for installation in homes and are the best assurance against CO exposure. Some states require CO detectors for all new homes. Family and community education should include warnings against using space heaters, barbeques, gas stoves, or engines in unventilated areas. Determining the CO source should be paramount for all exposures in order to prevent risk to others.

Radon

Radon is a colorless, odorless, gas produced by the decay of naturally occurring uranium in soil, rock, and water. As radon decays, some of its products change to an isotope of polonium, a radioactive element that, when inhaled, can cause lung damage leading to cancer. In the atmosphere, radon is diluted and has no health effect. When concentrated in an enclosed area, it represents a risk. Radon enters homes through basement floors, cracks in concrete foundations, sumps, or drains. Radon is more prevalent in certain geographic areas although levels can vary widely from house to house due to differences in ventilation, construction, and design. Therefore, all homes should be tested, even if in a "low risk" zone (EPA, 2014a).

Radon is the second leading cause of lung cancer in Americans, responsible for approximately 21,000 deaths annually (EPA, 2013b). Tobacco smoke provides a vehicle for radon to enter the lungs, adding to the risk of radon-induced cancer for smokers and individuals exposed to ETS. Well water, by nature, is filtered through the soil and may be contaminated with radon. Radon in water has been associated with a slightly increased incidence of gastric cancer and leukemia.

Clinical Findings

Exposure to radon has no acute or subacute health effects, so clinical findings are absent in children. Environmental screening is performed in hopes of avoiding long-term or chronic health problems later in life. All homes, except residences above the second floor in multilevel buildings, should be tested for radon. Radon detector kits can be purchased in hardware, home improvement, or department stores and are available from the National Safety Council (see Additional Resources). These tests are easy and relatively inexpensive. Short-term (2 to 90 days) or long-term (3 to 12 months) testing can be done. The long-term testing gives a more accurate measure of the average radon exposure, because levels fluctuate over time and with changes in seasons; however, if testing needs to be done quickly, short-term testing is used.

Management

Radon mitigation involves decreasing the amount of radon entering the home and removing radon that is present (see Table 42-4). Although the EPA does not yet have standards for safe radon levels in water, it recommends that homes with a radon level of 4 picocuries per liter (pCi/L) or higher in indoor air be repaired immediately. Mitigation companies may be certified by the National Environmental Health Association (NEHA) or the National Radon Safety Board (NRSB). Children and families should not spend significant amounts of time in high-risk areas of the home (e.g., basements). Parents need education to understand the risks because radon is not a widely known contaminant.

Particulate Matter

Particulate matter is air pollution consisting of extremely small particles and liquid droplets. These can have adverse effects on respiratory and cardiovascular function. Particulate matter is a pervasive by-product of industrial production, gasoline and diesel engines, wood-burning stoves, and natural phenomena (e.g., volcanic activity, grass and forest fires, and blowing dust) sometimes occurring obviously as smog or soot. Most school buses use diesel fuel and are a source of particulate matter exposure for children.

The Clean Air Act is a U.S. federal law designed to control air pollution on a national level; it is managed and enforced by the EPA and was last amended in 1990. Particulate matter is just one element that the Clean Air Act targets. The diameter of particulate matter is measured in micrometers, and the EPA has set standards for coarse and fine concentrations. Coarse particulate matter (2.5 to 10 micrometers in diameter) can be filtered by the nasal mucosa or trachea and removed by coughing or sneezing. Fine particulate matter (2.5 micrometers in diameter or smaller) is of concern, because it can be inhaled and carried deep into lung tissue. Ultrafine particles also represent a serious health problem. These particles are so small (less than 100 nanometers) that they can penetrate cells, carrying toxic compounds into the individual's DNA and other critical areas. To date, they are not regulated. In 2012, the EPA updated its national air quality standard for fine particulate matter to an annual health standard of 12 micrograms (mcg) per cubic meter. The EPA estimates that this action will save the United States $4 to $9 billion *annually* by decreasing mortality rates and the incidence of heart attacks, strokes, and childhood asthma (EPA, 2012b).

Residents of urban and industrial areas can be exposed to high levels of particulate matter, and concentrations increase in summer months and when there is more combustion present (e.g., rush-hour traffic). Agricultural areas can also have significant levels of particulate matter. The amount of indoor particulate matter, including dust mites, cockroach particles, and animal dander, varies among households, but there is concern that low-income residences may have disproportionately high levels of dust, mouse, and cockroach residue.

Clinical Findings

Parents can keep a diary of their child's illness episodes and the circumstances surrounding them, to help determine if increased air pollution, dust, insects, or pets in the home are associated with illness. An environmental history can also help in this determination. The provider should conduct a complete respiratory and cardiovascular examination. Pulmonary function tests could be considered.

Management

The goal of management is to decrease the amount of particulate matter in the environment and limit the child's contact with particulate matter (see Table 42-4 for suggested strategies).

Ammonia

Ammonia is a colorless gas found naturally in the environment. Liquid ammonia is an artificial product made for household and industrial uses. Ammonia is a frequent ingredient in household cleaning products. At levels found naturally in the environment, ammonia has no untoward health effects. However, exposure to liquid ammonia can irritate and burn skin, eyes, throat, and lungs. Ingestion can result in corrosive damage to the mouth, throat, and stomach. Caregivers should be advised to choose safe cleaning agents or ensure that children cannot access more toxic agents. Ingestion or exposure that is concerning should be reviewed with the regional Poison Control Center prior to treatment.

Volatile Organic Compounds

Volatile organic compounds (VOCs), as the name implies, are a class of compounds that are volatile (evaporate easily) and are organic (contain carbon); this does not, however, mean they are naturally occurring. Commonly recognized VOCs include acetone, formaldehyde, and automotive gasoline. Formaldehyde is the only regulated VOC (EPA, 2012a). VOCs are used in thousands of household and industrial products. Levels are frequently higher indoors than outdoors (due to lack of ventilation). Certain activities, such as paint stripping, can raise levels to 1000 times more than background outdoor levels. Some VOCs are known carcinogens. Acute symptoms in direct relation to VOC exposure should be managed in coordination with a Poison Control Center. See Table 42-4 for health effects and exposure prevention strategies.

Molds

Molds are a diverse group of species belonging to the kingdom *Fungi*. Some molds reproduce by aerosolizing spores. Molds thrive in damp spaces, but spores can be found in dry environments, dust, dry leaves, and storage areas. Common sources of mold exposure for children are listed in Table 42-4. Aspergillus (black mold), Alternaria, Penicillium, Streptomyces, Epicoccum, and Cladosporium are the most common household molds. Their natural purpose in the environment is biodegradation of natural materials (e.g., plant matter), a process essential to provide balance in nature. Molds also have been used to create medicines (e.g., penicillin, cyclosporine) and food products (e.g., tempeh, certain cheeses).

Human exposure to molds is through inhalation or contact. Most people have no reaction to mold exposure but those with increased sensitivity or compromised immune systems are vulnerable and disease may occur (see Box 42-8 for a list of infections with respiratory or neurologic presentations; fungal infections of the skin are discussed in Chapter 37).

In the United States, there appears to be an increasing prevalence in children with sensitivity (e.g., allergies, atopy) to molds, pollens, and other natural environmental elements. The "hygiene" or "biodiversity hypothesis" may partly explain this phenomenon. This hypothesis proposes that when people (children, in this instance) have reduced contact with nature, including environmental microbiota, their immunoregulatory circuits are inadequately stimulated. As a result, via complex mechanisms, their immune system may not mature enough to be able to prevent or terminate inappropriate inflammatory responses (Hanski et al, 2012). According to this hypothesis, molds themselves, particularly outdoors, should not be strictly avoided in early childhood. Unless there are obvious untoward effects that require treatment, caregivers should be careful not to over-sterilize their children's environment.

Clinical Findings

Children have an increased risk of asthma, dyspnea, wheeze, cough, respiratory infections, allergic rhinitis, bronchitis, and eczema when exposed to molds. Assessment questions clarify the nature of symptoms, usually a spectrum of allergic reactions (see Table 42-4), and identify the cause of the symptoms:

- Is there a pattern to the symptoms (daily or seasonally)?
- Are symptoms aggravated by any particular environment?
- Has the child recently travelled to other areas (e.g., the fungus *Coccidioides,* which is the cause of valley fever, is more common in dry, dusty areas of Southwestern United States, Mexico, and Central America)?
- Is there obvious mold in the home, school, or where the child spends time?
- Are symptoms relieved when the child changes environments?
- What has the family done to remediate the environment?

Laboratory tests can be used to measure antigens, antibodies, or to conduct immunoassays but may not reliably indicate exposure or establish causal relationships between mold and illness.

Differential Diagnosis

The differential diagnosis includes other causes of allergic reactions, upper respiratory infections, or asthma exacerbations. Reaction to molds can be confused with pesticide poisoning.

Management

Treatment of acute conditions includes antifungal medication, supportive care, and control of allergic symptoms (e.g., use antihistamines to control itching or sneezing; see Chapters 25 and 37 for discussion of allergies and their management). Moisture in the environment must be controlled (less than 50% humidity is recommended) and mold must be removed. Children's sleeping areas, in particular, should be clean and dry. Dehumidifiers can be used. Contaminated carpets and ceiling tiles can be removed. Walls, showers, and baths should be cleaned with detergent and water. Routine use of a bleach solution to clean mold is *not* recommended because it can cause adverse respiratory problems and it does not remove dead mold spores, which can cause problems in some people. Professional remediation may be required in homes or buildings with severe mold infestations. Parents and caregivers should be advised to research remediation techniques and choose a company that does not use dangerous chemicals in the cleanup process.

• BOX 42-8 Fungal Infections Secondary to Mold Exposure

- Aspergillosis
- Blastomycosis
- Coccidioidomycosis
- *Cryptococcus neoformans* infection
- *Cryptococcus gattii* infection
- Histoplasmosis
- Mucormycosis (rare)
- Pneumocystis

Asbestos

Asbestos is the name given to a group of incombustible fibrous magnesium silicate minerals used most often in construction materials. Chrysotile is the only asbestos product still on the market; other forms are found in older buildings. Contamination by asbestos is measured in fibers per cubic centimeter of air. The Occupational Safety and Health Administration (OSHA) has mandated federal standards for asbestos, and some states have created their own standards and enforcement policies (OSHA, 2014).

Asbestosis is considered an occupational problem of adults, and smokers are at higher risk of asbestos-induced lung disease than nonsmokers. Any exposure to asbestos fibers is a risk, but repeated inhalation of the fibers is associated with significant lung disease later in life. Childhood exposure to asbestos may contribute to serious illness as an adult. There may be a latency period of 10 to 40 years or more before conditions such as pleural effusion, lung fibrosis, lung cancer, and mesothelioma in the pleura or peritoneum appear. Children can be exposed through direct contact with air in a contaminated building or with material or clothing parents bring home from their worksite. Levels in schools are generally low; and although asbestos is found in many buildings (e.g., tiles, pipes, and insulation), it is considered a hazard only if the material is disrupted through deterioration or renovation and fibers become airborne.

Clinical Findings

Assessment of disease is based on a history of exposure and signs and symptoms of respiratory distress. Exposure to asbestos does not typically produce acute symptoms, although high concentrations of asbestos dust can cause lung irritation, including cough, dyspnea, fatigue, and chest pain in both children and adults. The earliest symptom is usually breathlessness with exertion.

Management

There is no treatment for asbestosis. Preventing unnecessary exposure to asbestos fibers reduces the risk of inhalation and subsequent disease (see Table 42-4). If asbestos is present in the workplace, OSHA standards (not always enforced) require employers to provide workers with full-body suits and shoe covers that are left at the worksite; parents should be encouraged to work with their employers to minimize the possibility of bringing fibers into the home. Parents who work with asbestos should shower and change clothes before returning home. Parents should be informed of the adverse effects of asbestos exposure and reassured that their children are at low risk unless they spend significant amounts of time in older buildings that are in poor repair or undergoing renovation.

Hypochlorites, Pesticides, Endocrine Disruptors, and Noise

Sodium and Calcium Hypochlorite: Laundry Detergent

Sodium and calcium hypochlorite are main ingredients in bleach and other cleaning solutions and as disinfectants for drinking water and swimming pools. Hypochlorite is corrosive (especially undiluted) and can be irritating to the respiratory tract, GI tract, skin, and eyes (ATSDR, 2011b). Notably, the esophageal irritation or burns that result after bleach ingestion can lead to long-term complications, such as esophageal stricture. Because bleach is a common household item, it can be easy for children to access and use inappropriately. Curious toddlers or young children may inadvertently ingest bleach, whereas older children or adolescents may ingest bleach with suicidal intent. In either case, consult a toxicologist at the regional Poison Control Center to determine management.

An emerging public health concern includes laundry pod ingestions. A laundry pod is a single-load capsule (often brightly and attractively colored) that contains concentrated liquid detergent inside a water-soluble membrane that dissolves when in contact with moisture. These pods may resemble pieces of candy or toys to young children. Poison Control Centers in the United States are receiving increasing numbers of calls for laundry pod ingestions, with over 480 calls in a 1-month period in 2012. Common symptoms include vomiting, coughing or choking, irritant conjunctivitis or eye pain, and lethargy. Coma, seizures, long-term morbidity (e.g., swallowing dysfunction), and mortality have been reported (CDC, 2012). Significant symptoms should prompt contact with the regional Poison Control Center.

Pesticides

Pesticides are substances used to control, repel, or kill unwanted pests. Pests are defined as living organisms that are a health hazard or nuisance to humans, generally because they cause damage to crops, humans, animals, or belongings. Pests may include, but are not limited to, insects, rodents, weeds, fungi, algae, microorganisms, and prions.

Pesticides are classified as "general-use" or "restricted-use," depending on their level of toxicity to humans or the environment. Restricted-use pesticides require special handling by certified applicators. Labeling of pesticides varies by toxicity, with a skull and crossbones and the statement "DANGER-POISON" on the most toxic; "WARNING" on less toxic; and "CAUTION" on the labels of the least toxic. All pesticides are hazardous because they are intentionally designed to harm living organisms; and although they have arguably improved contemporary life (e.g., contributed to larger crop yields; limited infectious diseases such as West Nile virus, Lyme disease, and rabies; decreased incidence of asthma [e.g., by controlling cockroaches]), they also carry significant health risks.

In 2007, approximately 1 billion pounds of pesticides were used in the United States, costing about $12.5 billion (EPA, 2011a). The EPA is responsible for regulating pesticides, and pesticide products are subject to periodic reregistration with the EPA as a way to ensure safety review (EPA, 2013a). Prominent environmental groups, however, report there are flaws in this process that allow for major loopholes (Sass and Wu, 2013).

Herbicides are the most widely used pesticide, and pesticide-laced food products (generally sold at grocery stores) are a major source of exposure. Because of children's small size and large fruit and vegetable intake per unit of body weight, they ingest pesticides in foods at a disproportionately higher rate than adults. Farm workers and children who live on or near farms are exposed to agricultural pesticides. Garden and lawn use increases risks to children playing outdoors; pesticide can also be tracked indoors on shoes and clothing. Pesticide routes of exposure are mainly oral, inhalation, and dermal. Incidental exposure via residues is most common among children. The CDC's biomonitoring surveys of the population show widespread pesticide exposure in humans (CDC, 2014c).

Pesticides are increasingly implicated in problems with fetal development and childhood illness, although causal links are difficult to establish given the multiple combinations of ingredients and varied effects possible. Polyneuropathy, CNS dysfunction (neurologic and neurodevelopmental problems), hormonal disruption, cancer, dermatological problems, and pulmonary fibrosis have all been linked to various pesticides. Meta-analyses of studies show a link between childhood leukemia and prenatal maternal occupational exposure to pesticides (Van Maele-Fabry et al, 2010). Maternal pesticide exposure and Wilms tumor are also linked (Chu et al, 2010). Organophosphates and organochlorines are associated with neurologic and neurodevelopmental effects, including ADHD, psychomotor delays, and autism (Bouchard et al, 2010). Common home and garden pesticides may be linked to childhood brain tumor development (Greenop et al, 2013). Some pesticides have been identified as endocrine disruptors, contributing to precocious puberty, thyroid dysfunction, hormone-mediated congenital defects (e.g., hypospadias), and other endocrinopathies. Agricultural pesticides may contribute to asthma and similar respiratory problems (Etzel and Balk, 2012).

Chemicals labeled as "inert" are also raising concerns in the United States. One would interpret "inert" to mean "harmless," but many hazardous inert ingredients (e.g., coal tar, dibutyl phthalate, hydrochloric acid, kerosene, naphthalene, and nitric acid) have been shown to present risks of injury to humans. The EPA is considering changes to require industry to disclose more of the ingredients in products, but industry officials worry that having their secret formulations disclosed will affect their market share (Weingold, 2010).

Clinical Findings

Adverse effects of pesticide exposure can be acute or chronic, and all body systems can be affected, depending on the nature of the toxin and the extent of exposure. In acute exposure, assessment is the same as with general poisoning. Acute poisoning with organophosphates or carbamates results in clinical signs of cholinergic excess (i.e., bradycardia, tearing, salivation, bronchospasm, urination, emesis, diarrhea, and diaphoresis). Neurologic disorders may occur 24 to 96 hours after exposure and delayed neurotoxicity may occur 1 to 3 weeks after exposure. Acute kidney injury has also been reported (Bird, 2014). Chronic and/or low-level exposure may cause health problems not yet elucidated. Also, most data are based on adult studies. Children, with their differences in growth, metabolism, and physiology may fare differently from their adult counterparts.

Management

Pesticide exposure should be prevented. Specifics of management after exposure depend on the type and amount of pesticide taken in and the route of absorption. Information on treatment is available on product labels. When treating an individual who may have been exposed to pesticides, health care providers, by law, are entitled to access information about the implicated pesticides (see Additional Resources, National Pesticide Information Center). The EPA's Worker Protection Standard (WPS) also mandates that providers be able to access information on general- and restricted-use pesticides. Under the WPS, this information can be obtained from employers or manufacturers. Patients may be able to provide the clinician with the pesticide label. Treatment focuses on basic life support (as necessary) and the following:

- Decontamination (e.g., remove patient's clothes; wash skin; gastric decontamination as indicated). Note that pesticides may penetrate standard health care personnel gloves; special protective gear may be required.
- Consult with a Poison Control Center (acute) and/or PEHSU (acute or chronic).
- Seizure control.
- Report pesticide exposure to the local and state health department.

Patient and Family Education

The risks pesticides present to children are immense. Pesticide exposure may occur in unanticipated ways. Because exposures are additive, patterns of multiple contaminations must be recognized and a plan to regulate overall exposure developed. Education and awareness are key to preventing pesticide poisoning in children. Steps can be taken to reduce pesticide use, which in turn reduces exposure. Integrated pest management combines physical, cultural, biologic, and other means of pest control with minimal use of pesticides. For example, farmers might encourage use of cats to catch mice rather than using rodenticides, or school cafeterias personnel might use bait traps for cockroaches rather than chemical spray. Herbicides on athletic fields could be applied as spot treatments rather than broadcast widely. Individuals can take steps to avoid or limit exposure. For example, use of insect repellents can be reduced or eliminated; families can choose foods that are local, in season, and organically grown as much as possible. Not all foods labeled as organic are the same; check USDA labels, which include "100% organic," "organic" (i.e., at least 95% organic content), "made with organic" (i.e., 70% organic content for up to three ingredients), and "organic components" (i.e., products with less than 70% organic content). Organic foods are often more expensive than conventional foods, thus income disparities and environmental justice issues come into play. Regulation of pesticide use, on foods particularly, should be considered in order to provide all children with safe foods, not just those families that "can afford it." A list of hazardous and safer fruits and vegetables is found in Table 42-5.

Endocrine Disruptors

Endocrine disruptors are chemicals that are likely to have the most long-term ill effects upon living organisms on our

TABLE 42-5 Pesticide Content of Common Fruits and Vegetables*

"Dirty Dozen" (Buy These Organic)	"Clean 15" (Lowest in Pesticides)
Apples (worst)	Avocados (best)
Strawberries	Sweet corn
Grapes	Pineapple
Celery	Cabbage
Peaches	Sweet peas (frozen)
Spinach	Onions
Sweet bell peppers	Asparagus
Imported nectarines	Mango
Cucumbers	Papaya
Cherry tomatoes	Kiwi
Imported snap peas	Eggplant
Potatoes	Grapefruit
	Cantaloupe
	Cauliflower
Leafy greens (kale and collards) and hot peppers are not in "dirty dozen" but are of concern because the *toxicity* (not amount) of pesticides on them is greater than most.	Sweet potatoes

Adapted from Environmental Working Group: EWG's 2014 shopper's guide to pesticides in produce, EWG (website), 2014, available at www.ewg.org/foodnews/. Accessed September 14, 2014.
*Fifty-one items were ranked from those having greatest concentration of pesticides to those having the least.

planet. The book, *Our Stolen Future,* by Colborn and colleagues (1996), brought their existence to the forefront. Endocrine disruption by chemicals was first noted in wildlife studies and has subsequently been identified in humans.

Hormones regulate all human biologic processes. Endocrine disruptors alter the function of endocrine hormones through a variety of mechanisms, including binding to hormone receptors to mimic natural hormones, blocking hormone receptors, or altering the production or metabolism of endogenous hormones. Endocrine disruptors can interfere with gene expression, changing developing tissues in permanent ways. It is hypothesized that a U-shape effect occurs: Extremely low doses and extremely high doses have significant effects, thus traditional toxicologic concepts (such as, "dose-response") may not always apply. Concentrations as low as one tenth of a trillion of a gram can alter the womb environment.

Endocrine disruptors are found extensively in the environment including in food, water, soil, air, plastics, cosmetics, and drugs. They are primarily ingested, but exposure can also occur topically, transplacentally, or perhaps in other as yet unknown ways. The incidence of endocrine disruption is difficult, if not impossible, to quantify given the spectrum of disease incurred. It is likely that much endocrine disruption does not result in acute illness for which the patient or caregiver would seek care. Specific health problems associated with chemical-related endocrine disruption include decreased sperm counts, infertility, testicular cancer, cryptorchidism, hypospadias, decreased penis size, decreased rate of male births, overweight, thyroid abnormalities, decreased duration of lactation, decreased height, altered cholesterol metabolism, early menarche, and hypotonia (possibly related to thyroid abnormalities) (Etzel and Balk, 2012). Cancer caused by diethylstilbestrol (DES) is a classic example of a severe endocrine disruptor. In the 1970s, millions of pregnant women were prescribed DES to prevent miscarriage (an indication later proven false) but their offspring had an unusually high incidence of genitourinary malformations, and female offspring had a high incidence of vaginal cancers as adolescents or adults. In addition, endocrine disruptors negatively affect neural and immune system development (Kajta and Wójtowicz, 2013; Rogers et al, 2013).

A listing of some common endocrine disruptors, their sources, effects, and alternatives for use are found in Table 42-6. PCBs, bisphenol A (BPA), and phthalates are discussed in the following sections. Pesticides are discussed earlier and their endocrine effects are presented in Table 42-6.

Polychlorinated Biphenyls

PCBs are not very water-soluble and, as a result, are not generally found in high concentrations in drinking water. They dissolve readily in oils and accumulate in the fatty tissues of fish, birds, and mammals. Human exposure comes primarily through ingestion of contaminated foods and breathing indoor air contaminated by electrical devices that contain PCBs. For children, fetal and neonatal exposures are ubiquitous, usually via maternal ingestion of contaminated food. School children can be exposed through deteriorating building materials. In the United States, the workplace is a major source of exposure to PCBs. Although the health effects of PCBs, like many toxicants, are difficult to evaluate, known effects include rashes, upper airway irritation, GI discomfort, endocrine mimicry, and liver injury (ATSDR, 2011c).

Clinical Findings.

History.

- History of maternal ingestion of contaminated food
- Skin disorders, including hyperpigmentation, nail changes, and chloracne
- Hepatic dysfunction
- Low birth weight and developmental delays
- Behavioral symptoms
- Frequent respiratory infections

Physical Examination. Clinical effects are listed in Table 42-6.

Diagnostic Studies. Increased liver enzymes with severe exposure, although these findings are nonspecific.

TABLE 42-6 Endocrine Disruptors: Industrial Agents

Chemical Group	Sources	Known Toxic Effects	Alternatives
Bisphenol A (BPA)	Kitchen appliances, water bottles, baby bottles, compact disks, water coolers, aluminum food and drink cans, paints, dental sealants, water main filters, and more	Rodent studies: Neurodevelopmental abnormalities, hormonal aberrations (diabetes, obesity, precocious puberty), breast cancer, uterine cancer, prostate gland abnormalities	Breastfeed instead of bottle feed when possible If using bottles, use BPA-free bottles Discard scratched infant feeding items Do not put boiling water in plastics Do not heat liquids in plastics Make sure to use "dishwasher safe" and "microwave safe" containers Reduce use of canned foods (in favor of fresh or dried) Use glass, ceramic, porcelain, or stainless steel containers as alternatives to plastics Avoid use of plastics with #7 stamped on the bottom (NIEHS, 2014)
Polychlorinated biphenyls (PCBs)	Electrical capacitors, transformers, carbonless copy paper, caulking	Upper airway irritation Rashes, other dermatologic changes GI discomfort Endocrine disruption (growth, thyroid, breast tissue changes) Liver injury	Manufacture of PCBs now banned, but they persist in the environment Limit exposure to known sources PCBs bioaccumulate in food chain; monitor local fish advisories accordingly
Phthalates	Soft plastics: Toothbrushes, cosmetics/personal care products, plastic toys, food packaging, vinyl shower curtains, car seats, wallpaper, floor coverings, medical tubing, and more	Animal studies: Low birth weight, skeletal abnormalities, CNS abnormalities, reproductive aberrations, liver toxicity	Avoid plastic food containers (alternatives include glass, aluminum, and ceramic), plastic toys, plastic wrap and PVC Avoid plastics with #3 stamped on the bottom Select cosmetics and personal care products free of phthalates
Pesticides	Food Water Direct or indirect contact with plants, grass, and other areas treated with pesticides, insecticides, herbicides, or fungicides Direct or indirect contact with pesticide through dust, mists, sprays	Endocrine disruption: Precocious puberty, thyroid dysfunction, hormone-mediated congenital defects (e.g., hypospadias), and more Note that pesticides also have many other untoward, non-endocrine, effects (discussed in text)	Decrease need for pesticide use (e.g., discuss strategic gardening techniques with nursery personnel; use proper food storage indoors to reduce pest attraction) Consider tolerating low levels of non-harmful pests (e.g., ants, weeds) Use non-chemical methods (e.g., caulking cracks in walls, vacuuming, keep a clean kitchen, boiling water and vinegar to kill weeds in sidewalks) Use only amount recommended for purpose stated Protect skin from exposure when using; wash thoroughly after use Do not inhale or use on windy day Keep children and pets from treated areas Clean up any spills Keep pesticides from food/dishes Store pesticides safely out of children's reach, in original container and dispose at a registered pesticide disposal site Do not mix pesticides Decrease exposure in foods: Vary kinds of fruits and vegetables children eat Buy or grow organically grown foods when possible Wash and peel fruits and vegetables (many pesticides are in the product itself; washing and peeling will not remove them) Try to use in-season fruits and vegetables to avoid those sprayed for transport and preservation

CNS, Central nervous system; *GI*, gastrointestinal; *PVC*, polyvinyl chloride.

Differential Diagnosis. The differential diagnosis includes acne vulgaris, other causes of developmental delay, lead poisoning, and hypothyroidism.

Management. Avoid contact with PCB-contaminated food and environmental sources, especially prenatally. Benefits of breastfeeding outweigh risks; therefore breastfeeding should not be stopped unless directed by a toxicologist. Acute toxicities should be managed in coordination with the regional Poison Control Center.

Phthalates

Phthalates are colorless liquid industrial compounds used in the production of soft plastics, often referred to as *plasticizers.* The chemicals can readily leach from the plastic into the environment. Di(2-ethylhexyl) phthalate (DEHP) is the most frequently used compound. Phthalates are commonly found in cosmetics and fragrances of personal care products (ATSDR, 2011d; Engle et al, 2010). They are also found in plastic toys, toothbrushes, food packaging, vinyl shower curtains, car seats, wallpaper, floor coverings, medical tubing, and many other products. Metabolites are commonly found in the urine of the general United States population. Potential health effects of high exposure (to date, based on animal studies, because a direct causal relationship in humans is elusive) include low birth weight and skeletal and CNS abnormalities (in offspring of mothers who were exposed prenatally), reproductive abnormalities (males, in particular), liver toxicity, gastric irritation, and endocrine disruption (ATSDR, 2011d).

Management. Use glass, aluminum, or other alternatives instead of plastic food containers; avoid plastic toys, plastic wrap, and polyvinyl chloride (PVC). The recycling label #3 indicates the item contains PVC. Avoid personal care products with phthalates, although this chemical may sometimes be described as part of the "fragrance," so the general label may be misleading. Some hospitals have taken steps to phase out DEHP-containing products. This includes intravenous (IV) tubing, IV bags, umbilical catheters, and other soft plastic materials.

Bisphenol A

BPA is a chemical used in production of polycarbonate plastics and epoxy resins. Polycarbonates are rigid plastics used in kitchen appliances, reusable water bottles, baby bottles, compact disks, and water coolers. Epoxy resins are strong adhesives used as coatings (e.g., liners for food and beverage cans), in paints, dental sealants, and water main filters among other products.

There is concern that, at typical human exposure levels, BPA causes adverse effects on neurodevelopment and hormonal abnormalities (e.g., diabetes, obesity, precocious puberty, breast cancer, uterine cancer, and prostate gland abnormalities) in fetuses, infants, and children; there may possibly be transgenerational effects (National Institute of Environmental Health Sciences [NIEHS], 2015). An association between BPA and metabolic syndrome in adults has been established (independent of physical activity and other standard risk factors for metabolic syndrome) leading to concern that BPA may cause similar hormonal problems in children that have not yet been elucidated (Teppala et al, 2012).

In a recent NHANES survey, BPA was found in over 90% of the participants, underscoring the widespread exposure in the United States. Children of low-income families (receiving emergency food assistance) had statistically significant higher levels compared to children of families that did not receive emergency food assistance (Nelson et al, 2012).

Management. In response to public concerns, some companies are now beginning to voluntarily eliminate BPA from their products. The FDA amended its regulations in 2012 and 2013 to no longer provide for the use of BPA-based resins in baby bottles, "sippy cups," and infant formula packaging, respectively. Alternative actions to decrease BPA exposure in children are listed in Table 42-6.

Noise

Noise is defined as any sound, but is usually considered loud, harsh, unpleasant, or unwanted. Noise pollution is the presence of irritating, distracting, or physically dangerous noise. Sound has qualities of frequency or pitch (measured in cycles per minute and stated in hertz [Hz]), intensity or loudness (measured in decibel [dB] sound pressure levels [SPL]), periodicity, and duration (either continuous, short-term, or episodic). The human voice is approximately 50 to 60 dB SPL. The National Institute for Occupational Safety and Health (NIOSH) defines hazardous noise as 85 dB for an average of 8 hours of sound exposure (CDC, 2014d). "White noise" or very low-level background noise may also be unwanted, although it does not necessarily cause hearing loss; in fact, it appears to have a positive effect on some children with attention disorders, improving their cognitive performance (Söderlund et al, 2010). See Chapter 20 for further discussion of children with hearing loss. Chapter 30 also discusses ear disorders, and Table 42-7 lists decibels for common sounds.

The impact of noise on human health is varied. Noise-induced hearing loss (NIHL) and tinnitus are the most obvious effects. Hearing loss is a growing problem in the pediatric population, especially among adolescents. NHANES data from 2005 to 2006 indicate that 19.5% of children 12 to 19 years old have demonstrable hearing loss, mostly at higher frequencies, and often unilateral. This is a significant increase from the 1988 to 1994 NHANES finding that 14.9% of the same age cohort had hearing loss. Children from families below the federal poverty level are more likely to suffer hearing loss (Shargorodsky et al, 2010).

Humans are subject to NIHL from exposure to continuous noise or to sudden acoustic trauma that causes damage to the hair cells of the cochlea due to excessive vibration; extreme noise can rupture the tympanic membrane. Noise of more than 85 dB but less than 140 dB leads to temporary hearing loss—most often in the 4000 Hz range. Permanent hearing loss can result from one exposure to a sudden,

TABLE 42-7 Noise in the Environment

Noise Source	Decibels
Quiet library	30 dB
Moderate rainfall	50 dB
Typical conversation	60 dB
Blow-dryer, food processor	80 to 90 dB
Subway	90 dB
Chain saw	110 dB
Jackhammer	130 dB

Data from The American Speech-Language-Hearing Association (ASHA): Noise, ASHA (website), 2014, available at www.asha.org/public/hearing/noise/. Accessed August 7, 2014.

extreme noise (greater than 120 dB in children) of short duration, or from ongoing lower levels of noise. Permanent loss is often in the 3000 to 6000 Hz range. Music listened to with headphones, ear buds, and at concerts; firecrackers; electrical tools; and airport noise can cause hearing loss. Chronic, everyday noise causes sleep disturbance, distraction, impairment of cognitive function (e.g., poor reading comprehension, decreased memory), and an increased stress response (e.g., increased heart rate, blood pressure, adrenaline, and cortisol production); these in turn result in irritability, poor coping, lower achievement, and possibly other yet to be determined effects in children. Newborn infants are a particularly vulnerable group. It is important to recognize that excessive noise in nurseries and intensive care units may disrupt growth and development. Noise and hearing loss are often associated with tinnitus (Mazurek et al, 2010). Tinnitus in adolescents contributes to mental health stress, increased alcohol and illicit drug consumption, and school problems (Brunnberg et al, 2008).

Clinical Findings

History. A careful history looks at the following:

- Type of noise in child's environment
- Exposure to chronic noise
- Episodic acoustic trauma
- History of ear disease
- History of prematurity or exposure to ototoxic drugs

Physical Examination. The CDC recommends universal screening of all newborns for congenital or birth-related hearing loss. Automated auditory brainstem response (AABR) or otoacoustic emissions (OAEs) testing are commonly used. This testing establishes a baseline. Newborns with hearing loss should be seen by a specialist no later than 3 months of age. If the screening is normal, all children should be assessed for hearing using a pure-tone audiometer at the 4-, 5-, 6-, 8-, and 10-year-old well-child examinations. Visual examination of the tympanic membrane with insufflation should be done at every well-child visit. Tympanography can help rule out chronic middle ear effusion.

Management

NIHL is virtually 100% preventable. The goals of management are to:

- Increase awareness of the health hazard noise represents. Parents and children need to understand the relationship between noise and the auditory system. Every well-child visit should include questions related to the child's noise environment, and both children and parents should be given information on the dangers of excessive noise and how to avoid them. Primary care providers can work with parents and schools to offer a hearing loss management curriculum.
- Decrease noise in the environment. Parents and children should be encouraged to minimize noise in their environment, including efforts to:
    - Reduce volume on television and radios; turn off "background" TVs and radios.
    - Use ear buds and headphones cautiously, keeping the volume low enough to hear normal conversation.
    - Avoid loud music, firecrackers, and other sources of episodic, extreme noise.
    - Avoid loud noises; for example, do not vacuum or use appliances (e.g., blender) with infants nearby.
    - Create a "quiet" place in the home.
- Mitigate exposure to noise. Wear earplugs and earmuffs to protect against "unavoidable" noise. Commercial-quality ear protectors are available for use in the home (e.g., when electrical saws or other loud tools are used). Earplugs can be purchased at any drugstore.
- Implement standards to regulate noise. The Federal Noise Control Act of 1972 provides the mechanism to set standards, rules, and regulations for occupational, industrial, and residential noise (e.g., automobiles and construction). States and municipalities have also established standards for noise control. Pediatric providers can be a resource to policy makers by providing information about the health effects of excessive and chronic noise.

In summary, environmental hazards and toxins are pervasive and have significant impact upon the health of children around the world, beginning with fetal life and persisting into adulthood. Although many of the health outcomes are as yet unknown, and most are difficult to manage, prevention is possible by reducing hazards in the environment. The provider must take a public health perspective on this issue, recognizing that the patient at hand is not likely to be the only person in the family or community who has been exposed to or affected by a given hazard. When faced with patient health problems as a consequence of environmental exposure, the local clinician can enlist the help of experts in the field—the local or state health department, the EPA, a regional PESHU, or other sources. Through advocacy and policy development, the hazards can be reduced or eliminated from our air, water, food, and soil, creating a healthier environment for future generations than exists today.

For a complete list of references, please visit http://evolve.elsevier.com/Burns/pediatric/.

43

Complementary Health Therapies in Pediatric Primary Care: An Integrative Approach

CATHERINE G. BLOSSER

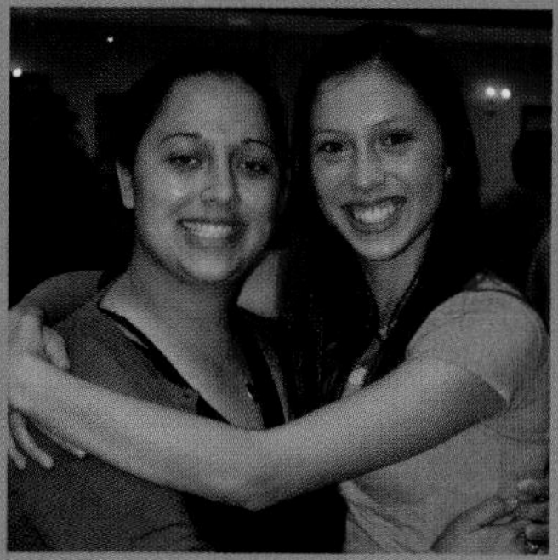

Traditional and complementary medicine is used in almost every country in the world and demand for its use is growing (World Health Organization [WHO], 2013). These forms of medical care are used in conjunction with or are the mainstay of primary health care. In Europe, up to 86% of some populations studied have used complementary and alternative medicine (CAM) (Fischer et al, 2014). In the United States, an estimated 4 in 10 adults and 1 in 9 children and youth between birth and 18 years old use CAM (Barnes et al, 2008).

Subsequently, the underlying clinical, academic, and philosophical foundations that drive conventional Western medicine have been undergoing a paradigm shift. Boundaries for health care and health delivery systems that were once rigid and exclusionary have been challenged. This has resulted in therapies that were once regarded as unconventional becoming an established part of the mainstream education and practices of nursing and medicine (e.g., the use of acupuncture to treat pain). At the same time, health delivery has been restructured to emphasize a "medical home" model based strongly on relationship-centered care between provider and patient. This personalized approach is at the core of integrative medicine and also addresses 21st-century pediatric health care concerns and needs (Vohra et al, 2012).

In discussing the paradigm shift, many conventional practitioners, including Dr. Snyderman who is quoted here, have noted that "[t]he integrative approach flips the system on its head and puts the patient at the center, addressing not just symptoms, but the real causes of illness. It is care that is preventive, predictive and personalized" (Bravewell Collaborative, n.d.). In an integrative model, the health care provider is required to fully consider the complex interplay between biology, culture, psychosocial, environment, and lifestyle choices. The focus becomes less on "curing diseases" and more on promoting health, healing, and preventing future disease. The integrative model utilizes the most efficacious treatments from both allopathic and CAM therapies, mindful of the scientific evidence behind both. Chronic health conditions are often more effectively addressed with this integration of therapies (Guarneri et al, 2010). Medical care also becomes less fractured, and costs decrease with an integrative approach. This can lead to fewer outside referrals for CAM treatments and/or provide more continuity of care when a child is using a CAM practitioner (Rakel and Weil, 2012).

Various phrases have been used to describe health practices that are not fully embraced by conventional Western medicine practices. These terms include *alternative, complementary, contemporary, holistic, integrative, folk, irregular, mind-body medicine, natural, New Age, new medicine, nonconventional, nontraditional, quackery,* and *vernacular medicine*. Many of these terms are erroneously viewed as implying "second rate" practices, and their use serves to restrict application of and regard for effective complementary therapies (Rakel and Weil, 2012). Currently, representatives of both the dominant and nondominant medical practices more routinely use the terms *integrative* and *complementary* rather than *alternative*. The National Institutes of Health's (NIH's) recent name change from the "National Center for Complementary and Alternative Medicine" (NCCAM) to the "National Center for Complementary and Integrative Health" (NCCIH) reflects the growing acknowledgment and acceptance of complementary (vs. alternative) therapies and encourages their integration into mainstream health care delivery (NCCIH, 2014a).

Much of the discussion regarding the use of CAM in the pediatric population centers around who the appropriate decision-makers are and the obligations of health care providers. The limitations of medical research in children make the decision-making more complex for providers, parents, and children/adolescents when weighing the benefits and safety of conventional *or* nonconventional treatments (Gilmour et al, 2011a).

Many pediatric health care providers may be asked about CAM therapies; providers may be curious, may suggest therapies, or may even be working collaboratively with CAM practitioners. In addition, they may not know whether or how their patients are using CAM. This chapter explores these topics so that the provider may have a better understanding of the multiple and complex issues and better meet the needs of children and families who seek a more integrated approach to their primary health care.

Standards and Guidelines

The National Patient Safety Goals (The Joint Commission, 2015) address medication reconciliation and require that complementary therapeutics (e.g., herbs, botanicals, and supplements) be included in the list of medications that a child or adolescent may be taking. The name, dosage, frequency, and purpose of the complementary product need to be noted in the medical record so that the provider can ascertain if there are any contraindications to using the product at the same time as other medications. This helps avoid any negative outcomes and ensures access to this information for other health care providers.

The American Association of Colleges of Nursing (AACN) Quality Safety Education for Nurses graduate competencies include the need for the health care provider to support patient-centered care based on the individual's values, culture, ethnicity, spiritual, and social preferences because these elements are often given as reasons individuals choose complementary health practices (Ventola, 2010). Additionally, providers need to know their own boundaries in order to avoid adverse risk when recommending a complementary practice; enhance a more positive organizational approach to complementary health practices so that individuals can feel free to discuss their use; utilize teamwork between conventional and complementary health practitioners; research complementary health approaches; and monitor outcomes (AACN, 2012).

The American Academy of Pediatrics (AAP) recognizes that the "best interest of the child" is always the guiding standard for providers, whether recommending a conventional or CAM approach. Disclosure regarding efficacy and safety is a universal principle; families should also be informed if there is a lack of information regarding a specific therapy. Providers are encouraged to keep an open mind, be nonjudgmental, be aware of cultural and ethnic practices of their patients, and educate patients about risks and benefits. The AAP offers the following standard (Adams et al, 2002):

> *If evidence supports both safety and efficacy, the physician should recommend the therapy but continue to monitor the patient conventionally. If evidence supports safety but is inconclusive about efficacy, the treatment should be cautiously tolerated and monitored for effectiveness. If evidence supports efficacy but is inconclusive about safety, the therapy still could be tolerated and monitored closely for safety. Finally, therapies for which evidence indicates either serious risk or inefficacy obviously should be avoided and patients actively discouraged from pursuing such a course of treatment.*

In addition, any treatment must be viewed as hazardous if its use delays the provision of proven conventional care for a serious medical condition.

The NCCIH has strategies that emphasize safe and efficacious use of CAM. These include better understanding the use of CAM by the pediatric population and within demographic subpopulations (e.g., cultural groups); better understanding the decision-making processes of patients choosing to use or providers who recommend CAM; studying the safety and risks of CAM for the pediatric population; and developing and conducting research into specific CAM interventions, practices, or disciplines that support healthy lifestyle behaviors (NCCIH, 2011).

The World Health Organization (WHO) recently issued the *WHO Traditional Medicine Strategy 2014-2023* to guide health care leaders of WHO Member States. This guide encourages Member States to formulate polices that recognize the potential contribution of traditional and complementary medicine (T&CM) to the overall health status and well-being of their populations; to promote safe, respectful, cost-efficient, and effective T&CM use by regulating and supervising products, practices, and providers of care; and to promote universal health coverage using integrative models into national health systems (WHO, 2013).

Complementary Therapies Used in Infants, Children, and Adolescents

The 2012 U.S. National Health Interview Survey (NHIS) CAM supplement provided information regarding CAM use by children 4 to 17 years old within the prior 12 months. Results revealed that approximately 20% of children used CAM (excluding multi-vitamins and multiminerals) or approximately 55% if specific vitamins and minerals are included. Thirty percent of those using CAM reported having emotional, mental, or behavior issues. About 20% of children reported having a chronic health condition, and of those with two or more chronic conditions, rates of CAM use doubled if pain was part of the chronic condition. Chiropractic/osteopathic manipulation was the most commonly used therapy that required a CAM practitioner (Child and Adolescent Health Measurement Initiative [CAHMI], 2012). A large pediatric CAM utilization study in Canada revealed usage rates exceeding 75%, depending upon the definition of CAM. Concurrent use of CAM and conventional medications was common (Adams et al, 2013). Cultures using nontraditional medicine that regard CAM practices as mainstream rather than "alternative" may be using CAM at higher rates.

Barnes and colleagues' (2008) extensive analysis of the 2007 NHIS CAM data (birth to 18 years old) sheds further light on the nuances of CAM use in children. Their analysis showed that the most commonly used therapies were *natural products* (e.g., *Echinacea,* fish oil/omega-3, combination herb pills, or flaxseed oil/pills), chiropractic practices, deep breathing, yoga, homeopathic treatment, traditional healers, massage, meditation, diet-based therapies, and progressive relaxation. CAM therapies were used predominantly for back and neck pain, head or chest colds, anxiety and stress, other musculoskeletal conditions, attention-deficit/hyperactivity disorder (ADHD), and insomnia. *Mind-body therapies* were most commonly used for anxiety and stress, insomnia, and nausea and vomiting; *biologically based therapies* were used for symptoms of fever, insomnia, reflux, and sinusitis; and *manipulation/bodywork* was used for abdominal pain, musculoskeletal conditions, and nausea and vomiting. Additional medical conditions or symptoms for which CAM was used included allergies, asthma, dermatologic conditions, developmental disorders, gastrointestinal (GI) conditions, headaches, insomnia, learning disabilities, overweight, and psychological conditions. These treatment modalities were not broken down by age group.

The 2007 NHIS also provided more information on the youth population utilizing CAM therapies. Use was higher among adolescents, non-Hispanic Caucasians, and those living in households earning more than $65,000, who had a college-educated parent, and who lived in states other than the South. Use was higher in those who also took prescription medicines in the past 3 months. The chosen therapies were used to both treat and prevent illnesses. CAM use in children was often predicated on difficulties accessing medical care; also, children experienced higher school absenteeism because of illness. There was little difference between CAM use and gender or race except for a preference for biologically based and manipulation/bodywork therapies by Caucasians as compared to non-Hispanic blacks and Hispanics. Nearly five times as many children used CAM if a parent also reported using CAM (Birdee et al, 2010). Approximately 30% of adolescents who suffered from chronic headaches used CAM. This rose to 41% for those who also reported having comorbid conditions that involved emotions, concentration, behavior, school attendance, or daily activities (Bethell et al, 2013). Youth with mental health issues reported using mind-body and biologically based therapies for either ADHD, anxiety, or depression (Kemper, 2012). Both the 2007 and 2012 surveys showed that CAM use was higher in those with private medical insurance and increased when clinical visits to a conventional provider also increased.

Little has been known about the use of homeopathic product (HP) remedies in children. Notable was a study that was administered to the same cohort of children at seven different times from their birth to 8½ years of age. Slightly less than 12% used HPs, with the most common age for administration around 7 years old. Parents were self-treating children with HPs 46% of the time versus having the remedy prescribed by a general practitioner (10%). Chamomile for teething and colic and arnica for soft-tissue bruising or cuts were the most commonly used products (Thompson et al, 2010).

Specific subsets of children in the United States use CAM therapies. A literature review by Kemper and colleagues (2008) found that of those who used CAM 50% were children with chronic, recurrent, and incurable conditions and up to 70% were homeless adolescents. Up to 64% had special needs, as defined by the Maternal and Child Health Bureau of the U.S. Department of Health and Human Services (Sanders et al, 2003).

Why Parents Seek Complementary Therapies for Their Children

Reasons cited by parents for choosing an array of CAM therapies for their children include (CAHMI, 2012; Ventola, 2010; WHO, 2013):

- Cost of conventional treatment
- Maintenance of health and prevention of diseases; treats the cause not just the symptoms of illnesses
- Dissatisfaction with impersonal nature of conventional care; CAM providers focus more on the whole person
- Ready access to CAM practitioners and effective marketing and promotion of CAM products (notably supplements)
- Only source of health care available or limited access to conventional care providers
- Failure of conventional medicine to have an effect on a specific condition or on chronic conditions. (Six or more concurrent health conditions were associated with higher CAM use according to the 2007 NHIS.)
- Awareness of complications and side effects produced by pharmaceuticals
- Discomfort associated with invasive procedures or diagnostics
- Ethnic and cultural beliefs consistent with spiritual beliefs or world view; historical influences
- Belief that CAM practices are more natural, less harmful, and more effective
- Parents are CAM users
- Belief that by combining conventional and nonconventional treatment a more effective approach to health care is achieved than either practice alone
- Awareness of the mind-body connection to affect the immune system response
- Desire for more parental, active participation in their child's treatment

Patient Disclosure about Use of Complementary and Alternative Medicine

In 1990, approximately 40% of patients told their conventional providers about using nonconventional treatments

(Eisenberg et al, 1993). Further studies of disclosure rates (including that by parents of pediatric patients) continue to vary from 40% to 60% (CAHMI, 2012; Erlichman et al, 2010; Shorofi and Arbon, 2010). A large Canadian study reported that the disclosure rate in a pediatric outpatient population was as low as 23% (Adams et al, 2013). The willingness to divulge the use of these products can depend largely on the relationship the individual or family has with their provider (Adams et al, 2013).

Moving toward an Integrated Health Care Model in Pediatrics

Increasing Acceptance of Integrative Health Care

One reason to integrate nonconventional therapies into pediatric primary care is that, in some cases, they work when conventional treatments do not. As an example, up to 30% of children with ADHD do not respond to pharmaceutical management or have side effects that limit use of medications. Efficacious CAM treatments (e.g., neurofeedback, omega-3s, or zinc supplements, which studies show may be beneficial [see Table 43-4 later in this chapter]) may complement established treatments (Searight et al, 2012). Also, the increase in chronic and stress-related conditions in children (along with parental demand) has led to efforts to increase providers' treatment options (e.g., the establishment of the pediatric integrative medicine [PIM] residency program at the University of Arizona). Although there are a number of reasons behind its growth, PIM is regarded as one of pediatrics' newest subspecialties and is a growing field in North America (Vohra et al, 2012).

Over the past 20 years, there has been growth in the number of medical schools teaching integrative strategies, in evidence-based research studies, and in numbers of patients seeking an integrative approach to their care. A survey of 29 U.S. academic medical centers and programs with integrative models of care that were affiliated with a hospital or health care system found that 62% treated pediatric patients, all provided care to adults, and 86% conducted research (Horrigan et al, 2012). A combination of mind-body, dietary/biologic, movement/energy, and manual interventions were the most frequently employed therapies; the most frequently prescribed interventions (in descending order) consisted of food/nutrition, supplements, yoga, meditation, acupuncture, massage, and pharmaceuticals. The integrative model was found most helpful for (in descending order) chronic pain, GI conditions, depression, stress, and cancer.

Scientific Observation and Complementary Medicine

Critics and advocates agree that whether the treatment is "mainstream" or "alternative," both conventional and nonconventional therapies need to be held to standards of the scientific method. CAM therapies are increasingly being subjected to the rigorous scientific study that meets Western criteria. This is of particular interest, because a landmark analysis found between a third and a half of the most-acclaimed scientific medical research findings (across medical disciplines) were false or exaggerated based upon the evidence being later refuted (Ioannidis, 2005). Subsequently, guidelines for all researchers to improve the credibility and efficiency of their studies have been recommended (Ioannidis, 2014).

Randomized controlled trials (RCTs) have been the cornerstone of measuring the effects of therapeutic interventions in conventional evidence-based medicine. However, RCTs may not reflect the complexity of symptom states or clinical responses most relevant to patients using CAM therapies. As an example, mind and body treatments affect a number of health domains and symptoms—all of which would need to be measured in a clinical trial (NCCIH, 2011). The effectiveness of a CAM treatment may also be influenced by the contextual or nonspecific effects of the relationship between the practitioner and the patient, a variable that is difficult to quantify. A PubMed search in 2011 showed that of 111 research articles about CAM therapies used in children, 31% used RCTs, 14% used meta-analyses or systematic reviews, and 21% used case-controlled or cohort/cross-sectional studies. The other methodologies offered less "empirical evidence" (Snyder and Brown, 2012).

Research in integrative medicine requires a shift from examining conventional research variables to looking at "the moderating variables that focus on the characteristics of individual people and the context in which they live" (Bravewell Collaborative, 2010). Advancements in technologies such as genomics, proteomics (study of proteins), metabolomics (study of chemical processes within living organisms), systems biology, and the analytic capacities of microprocessing and nanoprocessing will enable new scientifically based insight into an individual's expression of health and illness. This insight may lead to a greater appreciation of how "multiple variables interact in dynamic ways" and may further "the understanding about how the connections can be harnessed to produce" personalized health and healing treatments (Bravewell Collaborative, 2010, p 25). Conventional therapy research is more likely to be funded by pharmaceutical or large companies that are interested in developing and marketing drugs (Mayo Clinic, 2014); CAM research is limited by fewer numbers of researchers and CAM research institutions (Institute of Medicine [U.S.] Committee on the Use of Complementary and Alternative Medicine by the American Public, 2005). Additionally, conventional institutions doing CAM research may not have adequate peer review resources or may face difficulties obtaining institutional review board approval for pediatric CAM studies (Kemper et al, 2008).

The NCCAM (now NCCIH) was established in response to the need for scientific studies into CAM therapies. More than 2,500 research projects have been funded nationally and internationally; more than 3,300 scientific articles have been published in peer-reviewed journals (NCCIH, 2011). NCCIH does not include the pediatric population specifically among its priority groups for federally funded research. However, the AAP Section on Integrative Medicine (SOIM) is making an effort to address this deficit by (1) working with the Pediatric Research of Office Setting (PROS) Network and NCCIH to do more targeted CAM research in infants, children, and adolescents; (2) working with the U.S. Division on Health Care Finance and Practice Improvement to develop priorities, goals, and strategies for enhancing reimbursement for effective, appropriate CAM therapies; and (3) highlighting effective pediatric integrative clinical care models for interested pediatricians.

Examples of some NCCIH-related research projects applicable to pediatrics involve supplements to support the immune system; use of yoga, massage, and meditation for anxiety and stress; the effect of nutrition on inflammation; and the use of qigong massage therapy to calm autistic children. (Many of the results of these studies are referenced in Table 43-4.)

In addition to NCCIH, the NCI and the Office of Cancer Complementary and Alternative Medicine (OCCAM) sponsor a number of clinical research trials and studies at medical centers to evaluate CAM therapies for cancer. The Patient-Centered Outcomes Research Institute (PCORI), a nonprofit, nongovernmental organization authorized by Congress in the Patient Protection and Affordable Care Act of 2010, funds clinical trials comparing the benefits and safety of at least two approaches known to be effective for a particular clinical disorder. These trials can include drugs, medical technologies, CAM, behavioral interventions, and delivery systems (Selby, 2013). CAM research studies are readily available in the literature and increasingly found in well-regarded Internet reference sites: PubMed, NCCIH, National Library of Medicine, and Cochrane Collaboration, to name a few.

The Pediatric Complementary and Alternative Medicine Research and Education Network (PedCAM) endeavors to develop a pediatric CAM research agenda through an international consensus-driven priority building process. PedCAM disseminates a wide range of CAM information and is building collaborative relationships among researchers, educators, clinicians, and policymakers, both nationally and internationally (see Additional Resources).

Despite the difficulties CAM researchers face, some findings are clearly considered reliable and valid. Aetna Insurance Company, for example, recognizes that there is adequate evidence for the safety and effectiveness of CAM treatments for certain disorders. Therapies covered by this company include acupuncture, biofeedback, chiropractics, and electrical stimulation for pain (Aetna, 2014).

Media Marketing of Complementary Medicine

Families may seek treatment advice about a childhood illness from commercial retailers who sell CAM botanicals, particularly supplements. There is also much exposure to popular media and the Internet that promote botanicals (e.g., dietary supplements or St. John's wort for depression). Both primary care providers and pharmacists are in an excellent position to identify potential adverse drug interactions and counsel patients regarding supplements (Ventola, 2010).

Integrating Complementary Medicine into a Primary Care Practice

Common Principles of Integrative Care

When providers decide to bring a more integrative approach into their practice, they should begin by understanding the basic principles common to nonconventional treatment modalities. These include:

- A focus on wellness, that, in turn, prevents illness
- A belief in the body's ability to self-heal. (External interventions that stimulate the body's internal healing processes are a focus of care.)
- The understanding that health is a result of balanced energy forces (bioenergy) in the body
- An emphasis on using nutrition, plants, and other natural products to maintain or return to health
- Recognition and use of the individual's unique constitution, inner resources, and so forth to achieve health; each individual has strengths that facilitate healing

Health care providers who do not choose to integrate CAM therapies into their own practices can be effective by having sufficient knowledge, sensitivity, and willingness to support and help children and parents make informed decisions about their use. Table 43-1 lists many of the complementary therapies currently in use.

Talking with Patients about the Use of Complementary and Alternative Medicine

The topic of CAM use must be broached nonjudgmentally to help the family clarify the safety issues and explore how these products or services might fit into their child's management plan. The provider-patient relationship and the trust that builds when they explore mutual goals form the foundation for ongoing dialogue. Such relationship-centered care is particularly important when dealing with children and adolescents with chronic illnesses that are not easily treated (Rakel and Weil, 2012). Providers should not profess broad prohibitions and warnings about CAM use (Gilmour et al, 2011b). The child's health history should be expanded to include the following:

- CAM *products* that the child may be taking, including "alternative," "herbal," "natural products," and homeopathic and nutritional supplements
- CAM *therapies* that are being used (e.g., acupuncture, chiropractics, massage)
- Other practitioners the child may be seeing
- Other kinds of activities engaged in to address a particular problem
- The perception of any benefit gained from the complementary treatment
- The child's/family philosophy and self-care approach(es) to wellness and illness

TABLE 43-1 Complementary Therapies and Their Applications

Nonconventional Therapy	Theory Behind Use	Treatment Applications*
Whole Medical Systems (Diagnose and Treat Whole Body Systems)		
Acupuncture	Hair-thin sterilized, disposable needles inserted at specific anatomical points mobilize a limbic-paralimbic-neocortical network and its anticorrelated sensorimotor/paralimbic network at multiple levels of the brain to stimulate body to produce pain-relieving and mood-lifting chemicals or anti-inflammatory substances	Morning sickness of pregnancy, postoperative dental pain, chronic pain, asthma, allergies, nausea and vomiting, menstrual cramps, low back pain, addictions (e.g., smoking), MS pain
Ayurvedic medicine	A traditional form of medicine practiced in Indian cultures that treats imbalances or "doshas" within body that cause illness by using diet changes, herbal remedies, breath work, physical exercise, hatha yoga, meditation, and rejuvenation or detoxification programs	For primary health care disorders involving systems of GI, GYN, ENT, MS, circulation (including cardiovascular), psychological (including addictions)
Folk medicine (e.g., curanderismo, Native American healing, shamanism)	Form of healing embedded in many cultures; administered by folk healers Practices may involve prayer, healing touch, charms, herbal teas, tinctures, and magic rituals	Maladies treated run the gamut of those seen in primary health care; many symptoms are culturally based or have culturally based interpretation of disease
Homeopathy	Stimulates a healing response based on the "law of similars" by introducing a substance that is either the same as or similar to the disease (Infinitesimal doses of plants, minerals, and animal matter are used)	Used for wide range of primary care illnesses
Naturopathy	Uses many natural remedies to help restore health and balance in the body (e.g., diet, herbal medicine, hydrotherapy, acupuncture, homeopathy, and therapeutic massage) Practitioners often use similar diagnostic and testing procedures as Western medicine practitioners	Used for most primary health care issues (see Table 43-4 for specific conditions treated by naturopathy)
Traditional Oriental (Chinese) medicine	Combines practices and beliefs of acupuncture, acupressure, herbal remedies, massage, dietary changes, and bodywork, such as tai chi, breathing, and meditation, to stimulate vital body energy to rebalance life force	Used by one fourth of world's population for primary health care disorders
Mind-Body Therapies		
Acupressure	Similar principle as acupuncture but uses fingertips instead of needles to apply pressure Also incorporates breathing techniques to aid healing by balancing mind-body-spirit	Muscle tension, targeting a specific organ or glandular systems; usually more acceptable to children than acupuncture
Aromatherapy	Uses pure, essential, volatile oils containing oxygenated molecules to transport nutrients to cells of the body; believed to promote immunity and create a cellular environment in which disease-causing bacteria, fungi, and viruses cannot live Aromas of essential oils are either inhaled or absorbed through the skin	Stress, anxiety, depression, agitation, fatigue, immune disorders, acute and chronic pain, insomnia, intrapartum (to strengthen contractions)
Biofeedback	Empowers the mind to take control of conscious and autonomic processes; relaxation is focused on one muscle or function rather than on the whole body	HTN, insomnia, tension and migraine headaches, PTSD and depression, torticollis; chronic pain, JRA, RAP, functional voice disorders, urinary and fecal incontinence, postural training for scoliosis, ADHD
Deep breathing	Helps quiet the mind	Stress and/or tension, anxiety, insomnia, HTN, headaches

TABLE 43-1 Complementary Therapies and Their Applications—cont'd

Nonconventional Therapy	Theory Behind Use	Treatment Applications*
Guided imagery	Involves relaxation followed by visualization of calming images; technique practiced 20 to 30 minutes, several times a week	Chronic conditions including headaches, stress, HTN, anxiety; adjunct to cancer treatment
Hippotherapy	Uses the unique movements of a horse to achieve therapeutic benefits	Balance, fear, anxiety, lack of confidence, motor and social delays in children; mental health illnesses
Hypnosis	Uses an altered state of consciousness to access various levels of the mind to effect changes	Weight loss, drug addictions, smoking cessation, insomnia, pain and stress reduction, phobias
Meditation	A deep relaxation technique that can take many forms, from repeating a mantra to Sufi dancing	Stress-induced maladies; chronic illnesses
Music therapy	Music used to provide rhythmic cues to stimulate brain's motor systems to help build and strengthen connections among nerve cells in the cerebral cortex; used to boost immune function in children	Physical rehabilitation of cerebral palsy, ADHD, learning disabilities, Down syndrome, depression and anxiety, HTN, pain, weight gain for premature infants
Pet therapy	Therapy uses animals to help those with psychological issues	Anxiety, social isolation, poor sense of well-being, antipathy
Prayer	Uses the strongly held belief of the connection between the self and a higher power	All forms of health, illness, disease, and disability
Progressive relaxation	Successive tensing and relaxing each of the 15 major muscle groups, often used with deep breathing	Stress, tension, insomnia, anxiety, pain, HTN
Yoga	Works on breathing, body alignment, and posture to improve health; preventive	MS ailments; stress-related maladies; improves body flexibility, fitness, stamina, mental health; asthma, HTN
Energy Therapies		
Chromotherapy (color or light therapy)	Uses human sensitivity to seven colors to identify energy imbalances and evoke healing energies	Stress, depression, fatigue
Magnets, electromagnetic therapy (contraindications: acute injuries to bone and muscles, first-trimester pregnancy) (Not to be confused with magnetic pads, shoe inserts, jewelry.)	Uses the magnetic field or biofields to produce vasodilation, which increases blood flow and directs it more quickly to stressed or injured areas, aiding the healing process; may interfere with electric impulses triggering pain or stimulate release of endorphins	MS pain, headaches, nausea, osteoarthritis, fracture therapy, soft tissue injury
Qigong†	Ancient Chinese practice combining gentle physical movements, mental focus, and deep breathing to integrate mind, body, spirit, and stimulate movement of vital life energy (qi)	Asthma, arthritis, stress, lower back pain, allergies, diabetes, headaches, CVD, HTN, chronic pain, autism
Reflexology† (use with caution in pregnancy, avoid renal reflexes in those with suspected renal calculi	Massage technique based on the principle that proprioceptive nerve receptors in hands and feet correspond to all parts of the body, including organs and glands, Use thumb and fingers to massage reflex areas to detect diseases and to rebalances vital energy	Stress and anxiety, promote circulation, colic, irritability and reflux in infants, headaches; low back pain, some allergic and dermatology conditions, GI disorders, menstrual problems, arthritis
Reiki† (a.k.a. energy healing therapy)	A bodywork technique to stimulate healing energy within body	MS maladies, low hemoglobin levels, pain, stress/grief
Tai chi†	Stimulates and balances flow of chi or vital energy along acupuncture meridians	Improves body flexibility, fitness, stamina and energy, stress

Continued

TABLE 43-1 Complementary Therapies and Their Applications—cont'd

Nonconventional Therapy	Theory Behind Use	Treatment Applications*
Touch, therapeutic or healing	Affects ANS using subtle energy and vibration fields, spirit or vital source. Similar to qigong and Reiki	To reduce anxiety, insomnia, asthma, fatigue, pain
Biologically Based/Nutritionals/Orthomolecular Systems		
Balneotherapy	Therapy focuses on the beneficial effects of medicinal waters and involves bathing in water of various types	Low back pain, muscle spasm, stress, promotion of healing
Chelation	Involves IV injections of binding (chelating) agents that attach to toxic metals and wastes in the body that are then excreted in the urine	Arteriosclerosis, autism (experimental), lead poisoning (conventional use)
Diet (e.g., vegetarian, macrobiotic, Atkins, Ornish, Pritikin, Zone)	Desired effects achieved by eliminating calories, increasing fiber, decreasing fat, restricting fluids, and/or altering body's metabolism	Weight loss; prevention of heart disease and arteriosclerosis, HTN, diabetes; to enhance athletic performance
Herbalism (many phytomedicinals are not recommended for use in children; see Box 43-1)	Natural herbs are used over pharmaceutical derivatives; used extensively by naturopathic, homeopathic, and holistic practitioners The dried or extract form of the plant may be used as a tea, capsule, or topically	Used in place of many pharmaceuticals to treat a myriad of primary health care entities (see Table 43-4)
Megavitamin or high-dose vitamins (can produce adverse and/or toxic effects)	A form of "orthomolecular medicine" used to treat and prevent diseases; dosages beyond the RDA	Prevention and treatment of myriad illnesses
Nutrition	Places emphasis on a healthy, balanced diet to affect diet-related health issues; uses the MyPlate guidelines	Weight loss, food allergies, chronic diseases, vitamin and mineral deficiencies, nonpathological GI conditions (e.g., constipation)
Manipulative-Body Based Systems		
Chiropractic (contraindications: malignancies, bone or joint infections, acute fractures, arthropathies)	Regards the spinal column as the center of body's well-being; uses manipulation and massage of spinal vertebrae to restore proper flow of nerve impulses	MS pain, including low back pain, headaches, whiplash; torticollis
Craniosacral mobilization	Manipulates craniosacral mechanisms to free the flow of cerebrospinal fluid pathways that surround brain and spinal cord	TMJ, headaches, colic, vomiting, hypertonicity, tremor, irritability in infancy for infants after obstetrically complicated delivery; ADHD
Massage therapy (contraindications: clotting tendencies or communicable skin condition)	Hands-on bodywork techniques that knead and manipulate muscles, soft tissues, and connective tissues of the body; used to promote healing and relaxation, relieve sore and injured muscles, and improve sense of well-being and health	In infants: Prematurity and low birthweight, cocaine- and HIV-exposed, colic, disturbed sleep Diabetic children: To help normalize glucose levels Asthma, arthritis, autism, fatigue, stress, pain, digestive and circulatory problems, MS injuries, headaches
Osteopathy	Remobilization of joints and tissues to restore them to normal, structural positions and mobility	MS pain, torticollis
Pilates	Works on mind-body connection with exercise techniques to aid body flexibility and fitness	Restricted body flexibility

ADHD, Attention-deficit/hyperactivity disorder; *ANS,* autonomic nervous system; *CP,* cerebral palsy; *CVD,* cardiovascular disease; *ENT,* ears, nose, and throat; *GI,* gastrointestinal; *GYN,* gynecology; *HIV,* human immunodeficiency virus; *HTN,* hypertension; *IV,* intravenous; *JRA,* juvenile rheumatoid arthritis; *MS,* musculoskeletal; *MVA,* motor vehicle accident; *PMS,* premenstrual syndrome; *PTSD,* posttraumatic stress disorder; *RAP,* recurrent abdominal pain; *RDA,* recommended dietary allowance (established by the National Academy of Science); *TMJ,* temporomandibular joint.

*These applications may or may not be supported by scientific research; the listing of these therapies does not imply endorsement of proven efficacy.

†Also incorporates elements of manipulative body-based practices.

Some data from Snyder J, Brown P: Complementary and alternative medicine in children: an analysis of the recent literature, *Curr Opin Pediatr* 24:539–546, 2012.

• BOX 43-1 Herbals, Botanicals, and Diet Supplements: Precautions about Use in Children

Do Not Use

- Aristolochic acid–containing products (e.g., "Liqiang Xiao Ke Ling Thirst Quenching Efficacious" [a.k.a. birthwort, snakeroot, snake weed, sangree root, sangrel, serpentary, wild ginger])
- Arrow Brand Medicated Oil and Embrocation (also known as *Aceite Medicinal La Flecha* [Spanish])
- Glyburide-containing supplements ("Liqiang 4")
- Tiratricol- or fenfluramine-containing products (often marketed for weight loss)
- "Better than Formula Ultra Infant Immune Booster 17"
- Flu or avian flu preventive or treatment-promoting dietary supplements
- Body-building diet supplements (gamma hydroxybutyrate [GHB], gamma butyrolactone [GBL], 1,4-butanediol [BD]); many may also contain other harmful ingredients.
- Dieter's teas containing senna, aloe, cascara, castor oil, rhubarb root, buckthorn, or other plant-derived stimulant laxative
- Dietary weight loss supplements
- Ephedra (ma huang)
- Comfrey *(Symphytum officinale)*
- Crotalaria species (rattle pods) in herbal teas
- Borage *(Borago officinalis)*
- Coltsfoot *(Tussilago farfara)* in herbal teas
- Chaparral *(Larrea divaricata)*
- Foxglove *(Digitalis purpurea)*
- Germander *(Teucrium chamaedrys)*
- Ginkgo seeds (are toxic)
- Heliotropes
- Jin bu huan *(Lycopodium serratum)*
- Kava kava *(Piper methysticum)*
- Monkshood/wolfsbane/aconite *(Aconitum napellus, A. columbianum)*
- Rattlebox (*Crotalaria* spp.)
- Sassafras
- Senecio (ragwort, groundsel, golden ragwort) in herbal teas
- St. Ignatius bean (contains strychnine and brucine)
- Strychnos Nux Vomica tree seeds (contain strychnine)
- Pennyroyal oil (*Mentha pulegium, Hedeoma* spp.)
- *Prunus* spp. (amygdalin, laetrile)
- Lobelia
- Organ or glandular extracts

Use with Restrictions

Goldenseal/roots: Not for use in infants younger than 1 month old
Tea tree oil: Do not prescribe for internal use
Echinacea: Do not use in children younger than 2 years old
Pennyroyal: Do not prescribe for internal use

From Fetrow CW, Avila JR: *Professional's handbook of complementary and alternative medicines*, ed 3, Philadelphia, 2004, Lippincott Williams & Wilkins; Kuhn MA, Winston D: Part II: herb monographs. In Kuhn MA, Winston D, editors: *Kuhn & Winston's herbal therapy and supplements: a scientific and traditional approach*, Philadelphia, 2008, Lippincott Williams & Wilkins; Loo M: *Integrative medicine for children*, St. Louis, 2009, Elsevier, Chapter 7; U.S. Food and Drug Administration (FDA): FDA warning: consumers advised not to use Arrow Brand Medicated Oil &—Embrocation, Aceite Medicinal La Flecha, FDA (website), 2010: http://www.fda.gov/NewsEvents/Newsroom/PressAnnouncements/ucm213596.htm. Accessed December 15, 2014; U.S. Food and Drug Administration (FDA): FDA warns consumers not to feed infants "Better than Formula Ultra Infant Immune Booster 117," 2004, FDA (website): http://www.fda.gov/NewsEvents/Newsroom/PressAnnouncements/2004/ucm108229.htm. Accessed December 15, 2014.

Guidance is offered for clinicians counseling families about CAM in order to minimize legal risks of malpractice and/or professional discipline (AAP, 2001; Kemper et al, 2008). Suggested approaches in practice include:

- Determine whether the parents intend to abandon accepted and effective conventional treatments if the child's illness is life threatening or serious.
- Maintain knowledge about popular complementary practices, being prepared to discuss treatment options with children/families, including the benefits, possible limited evidence of efficacy, and side effects of the CAM therapy; be respectful of the child's/family values. The American Society of Health-System Pharmacists offers a good patient handout, *Using Alternative Medicines Safely,* on their website (see Resources on the Evolve site).
- Identify risks or possible deleterious effects, including diverting the child from an imminently necessary conventional treatment.
- Educate families about evaluating information regarding CAM treatments.
- Avoid communication of a negative bias or defensiveness about CAM therapies.
- Offer to assist in monitoring and evaluating CAM therapies chosen by the family.
- Evaluate the risk-benefit ratio of the CAM therapy as if you were another equally qualified clinician considering the same therapy; base your judgment on support from medical literature.
- Understand the local and state statutes and regulations governing licensure of CAM providers and specific therapeutic modalities.
- Understand state abuse and neglect laws because knowledge of CAM that is used as a substitute for conventional medical treatment of children with life-threatening illnesses may be reportable.
- Be familiar with the diagnostic tests practitioners of CAM use (Table 43-2).

The health care provider is not necessarily under any professional "duty of disclosure" to provide information about CAM therapies that are outside the range of conventional treatments or are of unproven efficacy. However, as evidence for a particular therapy increases, failure to disclose information may become a liability issue (Gilmour et al, 2011c). Some complementary practitioner advice may be contrary to conventional medicine recommendations or studies (e.g., the importance of food allergies in diagnosis and management of ADHD). This will put the primary care provider in an awkward position regarding appropriate

TABLE 43-2 Laboratory Tests in Integrative Medicine

Test	Explanation
Digestion/Nutrition	
Stool culture and analysis	Assesses digestion, absorption, metabolism, pancreatic function, inflammation, and fecal flora
Intestinal permeability: Double-sugar (lactulose and mannitol) challenge test	Measures the variable absorption of lactulose and mannitol
Small bowel bacterial overgrowth: Lactulose challenge test	Measures gas production (hydrogen and methane) over 2 hours to determine the level of bacterial fermentation in the distal small intestine
Lactose intolerance: Challenge test	Measures gas production to determine whether lactose is digested properly
Micronutrient testing	Assesses the level and function of specific nutrients in blood
Essential Fatty Acids	
Plasma fatty acids	Reflects nutritional intake and intestinal absorption of EFAs Rapid turnover is an indication of current fatty acid intake; allows assessment of triene-to-tetraene ratio
Red blood cell membrane fatty acids	Assesses fatty acid intake over past 2 to 4 months Correlated with cardiovascular disease risk
Environmental Testing	
Drinking water	Evaluates water for heavy metals, fluoride, and pH
Environmental pollutants: 24-hour urine	Tests urine for levels of common environmental pollutants, such as xylene, styrene, paraben, and phthalates
Heavy Metals	
Hair	Although of unknown value, hair tests for heavy metals have been used for the past 25 years by the U.S. Environmental Protection Agency to monitor environmental changes in toxic metals
Urine • Random and timed urine tests • Post provocation urine test	Used as a baseline evaluation before a chelating agent is given A chelating agent, such as EDTA (to bind lead) and DMSA or sodium DMPS (to bind mercury), is given before a timed urine test. The amount of heavy metal excreted in the urine is an indication of total body burden before chelation Test is useful to monitor treatment in an individual, but post provocation reference ranges are not available
Hormones	
Salivary/adrenal: Hormone levels of DHEA and cortisol	Measure free hormone availability and correspond with adrenal function
Salivary/female: Hormone levels of progesterone, testosterone, and estradiol	Correlate with free hormone availability Changes in salivary levels with hormone therapy make its use as a tool for monitoring treatment levels unclear
Serum: Hormone metabolites	2-hydroxyestrone/16-hydroxyestrone ratio in blood predicts recurrence of breast cancer
Urine: Hormone metabolites	2-hydroxyestrone/16-hydroxyestrone ratio in urine correlates with risk of breast cancer (low) and osteoporosis (high)
Immunology	
Immune function: Flow cytometry	Assesses natural killer cell (a type of lymphocyte) function, as well as presence and activity of immune cells and cytokines
Food allergies: Serum immunoglobulins—IgE and IgG	Measures immunoglobulin activation in the presence of various food antigens IgE, true allergic reaction to the food; IgG, intolerance
Nutrigenomics	Broad-based term to represent genomic testing that highlights individual biochemical needs for particular macro- and micronutrients Purely experimental at this point; no outcome studies have demonstrated clinical validity
Oxidative Stress Markers	
Lipid peroxides, isoprostane, 8-hydroxydeoxyguanosine	Markers of oxidative end tissue damage to fats, proteins, and DNA
Glutathione, TAC/TRAP superoxide dismutase	Markers of capacity to deal with oxidative stress

DHEA, Dehydroepiandrosterone; *DMPS,* dimercaptopropane sulfonate; *DMSA,* dimercaptosuccinic acid; *DNA,* deoxyribonucleic acid; *EDTA,* ethylenediamine-tetraacetic acid; *EFA,* essential fatty acid; *TAC,* total antioxidant capacity; *TRAP,* total reactive antioxidant potential.

Adapted from Rakel D: Appendix: laboratory testing resources in integrative medicine. In Rakel D, editor: *Integrative medicine*, ed 3, Philadelphia, 2012, Elsevier, pp 1004–1005.

advice at times. Blending the two approaches requires some thought and consideration.

For providers who are incorporating CAM therapies into their practices, it is recommended that informed consent be obtained and reference made to any conventional treatments that may be discussed and refused. An example of a comprehensive patient intake form can be accessed from the University of Arizona: Arizona Center for Integrative Medicine website (see Resources on the Evolve site). One should not refer children to a CAM practitioner without first having done a complete diagnostic evaluation, including:

- Determining the severity and acuteness of the illness and assessment of curability, effective treatment, and adverse effects from using conventional medicine.
- Studying the literature about the degree of invasiveness, safety, and efficacy of the chosen CAM treatment for the particular malady.
- Assessing the child's knowledge of and willingness to accept the risks and benefits of therapy.
- Reviewing any prescribed medications and drug interactions with CAM botanicals.

After the diagnostic evaluation of the child's complaint, the following steps should be taken to refer and/or assist those who wish to try CAM therapy:

- Establish a "short list" of CAM practitioners for referral purposes; be aware of the education, training, professional affiliations, and licensure status of any recommended CAM practitioner, if possible.
- Establish a collaborative relationship with CAM practitioners on the "short list."
- Provide the child/family with questions to ask the CAM practitioner during the first visit, including issues of safety, efficacy of any treatment, and reasonable expectations of measurable improvement.
- Review the recommended treatment plan with the child/family; encourage the child/family to keep a symptom diary.
- Monitor the child's response to treatment at monthly intervals.
- Note concurrent use of any prescribed medications.
- Document all interactions with the child/family.

Role of Diet in a Complementary Practitioner's Approach

Complementary practitioners may be more likely to identify allergies to foods and food additives as the etiology for many common childhood conditions including otitis media; upper respiratory infections; GI, urinary, and immunologic conditions; dermatitis; asthma; headaches; attention deficit hyperactivity; and autistic spectrum disorders. Genetics, the early introduction of solids, early weaning, genetic reengineering of food components, limited consumption of a variety of foods, hidden foods, additives and colorings, and impaired digestion may be offered as possible reasons for an increase in food sensitivities. An elimination diet may be utilized as both a diagnostic and a management strategy. An elimination diet handout is available on the University of Wisconsin Integrative Medicine Department website (see Resources on the Evolve site). See Table 43-2 for a listing and explanation of laboratory tests that are more commonly ordered by CAM practitioners.

Safety and Regulatory Issues

It is particularly important to ascertain the safety of certain treatment modalities by learning about any alternative product that the patient may be using, including its side effects, possible interactions with other medications, and mechanism of action. Mind-body techniques (e.g., prayer, guided imagery, spiritual healing, and relaxation) and acupuncture are not likely to interact with conventional medications. Providers should be aware of the possible harmful effect of products that are taken at high doses, such as herbal or phytomedicinal products, megadose combination nutritional supplements, colonics, or products taken in unconventional ways. Homeopathic remedies are highly diluted (the basis for most of the criticism) and are generally safe for infants, children, and pregnant and lactating women; there are few adverse side effects (Bergquist, 2012).

Safety and Efficacy of Dietary Supplements

A "dietary supplement" as defined in the Dietary Supplement Health and Education Act (DSHEA) of 1994 is a product taken by mouth that contains a "dietary ingredient" intended to supplement the diet (U.S. Food and Drug Administration [FDA], 2014). Supplements may include vitamins, minerals, herbs or other botanicals, amino acids, and substances such as enzymes, organ tissues, glandulars, and metabolites. Many supplements and/or their ingredients are imported (e.g., almost all vitamin C is from China). Even though the FDA is charged with monitoring manufacturers supplying pharmaceutical drugs to the United States, oversight remains a large concern. (An estimated 80% of pharmaceuticals sold in the United States are imported from China or India; the FDA has been adding international inspectors due to concerns about quality and safety.) However, the FDA has no authority to approve or monitor dietary supplements until there is a consumer complaint. Safety data, effectiveness, serving size, amount of nutrients, and other information are held by the manufacturers, and they are under no legal obligation to disclose the information to the consumer or the FDA. The FDA publishes comprehensive regulations for Current Good Manufacturing Practices that address the identity, purity, quality, strength, and composition of these supplements.

The majority of Member States of the WHO regulate herbal products, although they face the same difficulties with products being made in countries other than those in which they are sold. There is an ongoing effort for further regional and international collaboration on regulating such products (WHO, 2013). The European Union (EU) is adopting uniform legislation to regulate herbal products that can be prescribed or recommended.

Contamination and potency are of concern when patients use herbal (notably Ayurvedic herbal medicines) or folk remedies. Some traditional folk remedies or herbal preparations manufactured in third world countries (notably South Asia) contain heavy metals (lead, zinc, mercury, arsenic, aluminum, and tin), pesticides, and microorganisms. Other problems include content substitutions, adulterations or incorrect preparations, misleading advertising, improper labeling of contents, and failure to provide adequate amounts of the substance noted on the label (Gardiner and Low Dog, 2012). Prior, nonproblematic use of a product by an individual may not be a predictor of a future drug reaction because of potency inconsistency; lack of standardization regarding which parts of a plant are used; variations in plant ripeness, storage, and regional growth conditions; and the unknown influence of fertilizers, pesticides, and herbicides used during cultivation.

Most herbal/natural health products (NHPs) consumed in the United States have been historically safe; there have been few reports of adverse reactions (Gardiner and Low Dog, 2012). Such use has seldom led to litigation (Gilmour et al, 2011b; Kemper et al, 2008). In children, the most dangerous elements are the pyrrolizidine alkaloids, which can cause liver complications or death. These compounds occur in comfrey, borage, coltsfoot, and species of *Crotalaria* and *Senecio.* These plants are often found in herbal teas, particularly from Jamaica, Africa, and South and Central America. Chaparral, germander, and a Chinese medicine called *jin bu huan* can also cause liver toxicity. See Box 43-2 for a summary list of these herbs. Since 1993, the FDA has had a voluntary system in place, called *MedWatch,* for reporting adverse reactions to nutritionals and botanicals (see FDA under Resources on the Evolve site).

With 250,000 flowering plant species, the burden of knowing what is safe to use or not use becomes cumbersome. Although many herbs are harmless even in large amounts, others should be prescribed only by a knowledgeable herbalist or botanical professional. More than 1600 possible interactions have been identified between NHPs and conventional drugs (Natural Medicines Comprehensive Database, 2014). Although some of these drug interactions are insignificant, others can be serious. The appropriate herb in the appropriate quantity—like pharmaceutical medicines—is necessary to obtain the intended benefits. The medicinal effect of any one herb is thought to be the result of dozens of pharmacologically distinct actions. The herb may be causing physiologic changes in numerous subtle ways, none of which alone would produce the desired response. This mechanism contrasts with conventional medicines, which generally act by one of a few mechanisms of action and use "physiologically more significant pharmacologic" dosing.

Standardized extracts are more likely to ensure that a specific amount of an active compound is present. Western herbalists often use *simples* (the compound is made from one herb), whereas Chinese and Indian (Ayurvedic) medicines often blend together more than one herb. See Table 43-3 for a list of drug categories and NHP interactions, and see Box 43-2 for herbs contraindicated in pregnancy and lactation.

Some useful guidelines that clinicians can use when either advocating or advising about herbal and dietary supplements include:

- Use only single-herb supplements instead of combinations to prevent side effect confusion.
- Emphasize that "natural" does not mean "safe."
- Stop some herbal supplements minimally one week before any scheduled surgical procedure to prevent any alterations in coagulation, blood pressure, or interactions with anesthesia; communicate cessation to the surgeon. Botanicals to stop include, but are not limited to, angelica, anise, arnica, borage seed, celery, chamomile, clove, Danshen, Dong quai, ephedra, *Echinacea,* fenugreek, feverfew, fish oil, garlic, ginger, ginkgo, ginseng, goldenseal, hawthorn, horse chestnut, kava, licorice root, onion, papain, parsley, red clover, St. John's wort, sweet clover turmeric, and willow bark.
- Exercise caution when purchasing herbal products over the Internet.
- Avoid the use of herbs starting with the letter "G"—ginkgo, ginseng, garlic, ginger, or green tea if the patient is taking a drug that that is metabolized using the hepatic cytochrome P450 enzyme system (e.g., warfarin). The "G" herbs can either potentiate or inhibit the system, therefore altering the therapeutic effect or causing adverse effects.
- Research the NHP as thoroughly as possible, and look for these labels:
  - United States Pharmacopeia (USP) Dietary Supplement Verified seal: Product meets certain standards for contamination, adulteration, manufacturing processes, and pharmacologic properties.
  - National Sanitation Foundation (NSF) International: Sets standards, tests, and certifies products and systems, including Good Manufacturing Practices (GMP) for cleanliness, maintenance, and documented quality checks.
  - Natural Products Association (NPA; formerly National Nutritional Food Association TruLabel program: Includes a GMP process and a Natural Seal certification process that ensures ingredient quality and purity.
  - Consumer Lab (CL): Tests dietary supplements for composition, potency, purity, bioavailability, consistency of products.
  - Generally Recognized As Safe (GRAS) in the United States: Recognized as generally safe for its intended purpose as part of the Federal Food, Drug, and Cosmetic Act.
  - Herbal and NHPs manufactured and imported from Europe are generally regarded as safe because they have to comply with standards set by Commission E

BOX 43-2 Herbs in Pregnancy and Lactation: Precautions About Use*

Avoid in Pregnancy†

Aloe
Autumn crocus
Barberry root
Black cohosh root
Blessed thistle
Blue cohosh
Buckthorn bark and berry
Burdock
Chamomile (German and Roman)
Calendula
Cascara sagrada bark
Chasteberry
Cinchona bark
Cinnamon bark
Coltsfoot leaf
Comfrey herb, leaf, and root
Dong quai
Echinacea purpurea herb, injectable form
Ephedra (Ma Huang)
Evening primrose
Fennel oil and seed
Feverfew
Ginkgo biloba
Ginseng (American and Korean)
Goldenseal
Hops
Indian snakeroot
Juniper root
Kava kava
Licorice root (>100 mg glycyrrhizin)
Mayapple root and resin
Motherwort
Parsley herb and root
Passion flower
Pau d'arco
Pennyroyal
Peppermint oil or leaf
Petasites (butterbur) root
Red raspberry leaf
Rhubarb root
Rosemary
Sage leaf
Saw palmetto
Senna leaf
Shepard's purse
Slippery elm
St. John's wort
Tea tree oil
Thuga
Thyme
Uva ursi leaf
Vervain
White horehound
Wormwood
Yarrow
Yohimbe

Avoid During Lactation‡

Alfalfa
Aloe
Black cohosh
Bladderwrack
Blue cohosh
Borage
Buckthorn bark
Buckthorn berry
Bugleweed
Caraway oil
Cascara sagrada bark
Chasteberry
Comfrey
Coltsfoot leaf
Elecampane
Ephedra
Fennel
Fenugreek§
Garlic
Ginkgo biloba
Ginseng
Goat's rue
Indian snakeroot
Joe-pye
Kava kava
Licorice
Mayapple root
Male fern
Peppermint oil
Petasites (butterbur) root
Rhubarb root
Rue
Senna leaf
Stillingia
St. John's wort
Uva ursi
Valerian
Wormwood
Yarrow
Petasites (butterbur) root
Rhubarb root
Rue
Senna leaf
Stillingia
St. John's wort
Uva ursi
Valerian
Wormwood
Yarrow

Data from Fetrow CW, Avila JR: *Professional's handbook of complementary and alternative medicines*, Philadelphia, 2004, Lippincott Williams & Wilkins; Gardner Z, McGuffin M, editors: *American Herbal Products Association's botanical safety handbook*, ed 2, New York, 2013, CRC Press; Kuhn MA, Winston D: Appendix A: herbs contraindicated during pregnancy and breast-feeding. In Kuhn MA, Winston D, editors: *Kuhn & Winston's herbal therapy and supplements: a scientific and traditional approach*, Philadelphia, 2008, Lippincott Williams & Wilkins; Natural Medicines Comprehensive Database: Natural medicines used during pregnancy and lactation (website), 2014. http://naturaldatabase.therapeuticresearch.com/ce/ceCourse.aspx?s=ND&cs=&pc=11-102&cec=1&pm=5. Accessed December 12, 2014; Petrie K: Section I: complementary and alternative medicine in maternity care. In Ratcliffe SD, Baxley EG, Cline MK, et al, editors: *Family medicine obstetrics*, ed 3, Philadelphia, 2008, Mosby.

*This table is not a complete list of all herbs that should be avoided during pregnancy; Chinese herbs with potent effects to regulate qi, move blood, or drain downward are contraindicated.

†As single herb or as an ingredient in a combination product; product is deemed unsafe, has insufficient evidence of safety, or is likely unsafe.

‡Product is unsafe, has insufficient evidence of safety, or is likely unsafe.

§Used widely in some communities to increase production of milk in lactating mothers.

(Europe's equivalent of the FDA) (e.g., a label noting "original German formula" would be a good choice).

- In England, an herbal product is licensed and meets standards of safety and quality if it has a Marketing Authorization (MA) or Traditional Herbal Registration (THR) Scheme number on the label.

- Use websites, such as the American Botanical Council HerbClip Database, to determine if the product has been tested or reviewed. The Natural Medicine Comprehensive Database offers evidence-based information on safety, efficacy, interactions, and side effects for brand name conventional and NHPs, although there is a subscription fee to access this information. The NCCIH provides a list of herbal products that have been studied for specific conditions by that organization. The American Herbal Products Association (AHPA) has evaluated herbal safety for all botanical ingredients sold in North America. Each herb has been placed in one of three safety and interactions classes (see Resources on the Evolve site for websites for these groups).

Professional Oversight

Many states have licensing boards and professional organizations that set standards for nonconventional practitioners, including a requirement to carry malpractice insurance. The Federation of State Medical Boards has established policy and model guidelines for the use of CAM therapies when a physician recommends the therapy or when co-managing the patient with a CAM provider. Licensing requirements are subject to change, and families should be encouraged to review the credentials of any practitioner whom they are considering using. Currently there is no national licensure for CAM practitioners. State licensure requirements vary widely (NCCIH, 2013). Nurse practitioners (NPs) are advised to check the advanced Nurse Practice Act of their

TABLE 43-3 Potential Interactions between Some Pharmaceuticals and Herbal Products*

Drug Category	Herbs	Effect of Herb on the Drug's Action
Acetaminophen	Ginkgo Green tea Black cohosh	May cause intracranial bleeding Potentiates side effects Potentiates side effects
Anesthetics	Kava, valerian	Prolonged sedation—an additive effect
Antibiotics (ampicillin, ciprofloxacin, erythromycin)	Dandelion, fennel, khat; black cohosh with erythromycin	Decreased drug availability; increased side effects of erythromycin with black cohosh
Anticonvulsants, general	Cis-gamma-linolenic acid–rich herbs (evening primrose oil) Thujone-containing herbs (cedar, tansy, sage) Ginkgo Salicylate-rich herbs (e.g., cramp bark, willow, wintergreen)	Decreased therapeutic effect—may decrease seizure threshold; mechanism of action unknown Prevents conversion of vitamin B_6 into a form that promotes GABA Potential for decreased therapeutic effect Increased therapeutic effect with transient effects, per case reports; mechanism of action unknown
Anticonvulsants (ethosuximide, fosphenytoin sodium, phenytoin, carbamazepine, and others)	Shankhpushpi (an Ayurvedic product with many herbs) Gingko St. John's wort	Decreased effectiveness of phenytoin; decreases blood levels; lowered anticonvulsant action
Antidepressants—general Bupropion hydrochloride	Evening primrose oil, ginkgo, kava, ginseng Cis-gamma-linolenic acid–rich herbs (evening primrose oil)	May make a person more vulnerable to seizures by decreasing seizure threshold May cause mania
Tricyclics	Ma huang, St. John's wort, ginkgo, yohimbe, black cohosh	May enhance drug effects, causing restlessness; may increase blood pressure
SSRIs	St. John's wort, ma huang, black cohosh	Increased serotonergic effects and likelihood of adverse reactions (e.g., serotonin syndrome), restlessness
Barbiturates	Valerian, St. John's wort, kava	Increased side effects of drug, causing sleepiness, lethargy
Benzodiazepines	St. John's wort Kava, valerian	Decreased drug effect; may increase side effects and sedation; herb binds to GABA receptor sites, per animal and pharmacology studies Increased drug effects of sleepiness, lethargy
Mood stabilizers	Psyllium, ginseng	Psyllium, decreased drug concentration; ginseng may cause mania
MAOIs	St. John's wort Yohimbe Ma huang Panax ginseng, bioactive amines, licorice	May decrease effect of MAOIs Increases toxic effect of MAOIs Potentiates action of MAOIs, possibly causing life-threatening high blood pressure, high fever, coma Increased side effects that may lead to toxicity; licorice is a very strong MAOI
Corticosteroids	Laxative herbs (e.g., aloe, cascara, senna, yellow dock), Diuretic herbs (e.g., celery seed, corn silk, horsetail, juniper) Licorice Panax ginseng	Increased side effects; increased potassium loss per theoretical evidence Possible increased plasma levels as a result of increase in bioavailability CNS stimulation and insomnia, per case reports
Cyclosporine, tacrolimus	St. John's wort	Reduced blood levels; risk of transplant rejection
Diabetes medications, type 2 diabetes	Fenugreek, ginseng, karela or bitter melon *Echinacea,* green tea	May decrease blood sugar Can alter metabolic control
General medications	High-fiber herbs (e.g., flax, psyllium, acacia, slippery elm, marshmallow) "Hot" remedies (e.g., ginger, garlic, black pepper, red pepper)	Decreased absorption of drugs, per pharmacologic studies Increased absorption by causing vasodilation of intestinal wall

TABLE 43-3 Potential Interactions between Some Pharmaceuticals and Herbal Products—cont'd

Drug Category	Herbs	Effect of Herb on the Drug's Action
Iron	Tannin-rich herbs (e.g., caffeine-containing herbs, cat's claw, tea, uva ursi)	Decreased drug effect (may be due to tannin binding with iron to decrease absorption)
Laxative, stimulant (e.g., bisacodyl)	Aloe, cascara sagrada, senna, yellow dock	May increase laxative effect
Minerals	Fiber-containing herbs (flax, psyllium, acacia, slippery elm, marshmallow)	Decreased bioavailability, especially of Ca, Mg, Cu, Zn with psyllium
NSAIDs	Gastric irritant herbs (e.g., caffeine, rue, uva ursi) Nettles	Increased side effects and may increase gastric erosion and bleeding Increased therapeutic effect—increased effect of anti-inflammatory activity
Oral contraceptives, combination	Licorice, St. John's wort	Both may increase blood pressure; St. John's wort may increase clearance and cause breakthrough bleeding
Salicylates (e.g., aspirin)	Herbs that alkalinize urine (e.g., uva ursi) Tamarind Ginkgo, garlic	Decreased plasma levels caused by increased urine secretion Increased blood level of aspirin May cause prolonged bleeding by decreased platelet aggregation; eye hemorrhage
Theophylline	St. John's wort	May inhibit drug's effectiveness
Thyroid hormone	Horseradish Kelp	Decreased therapeutic effect by decreased thyroid function Increased therapeutic effect because kelp contains iodine, which may lead to hyperthyroidism

Ca, Calcium; *CNS*, central nervous system; *Cu*, copper; *GABA*, gamma-aminobutyric acid; *Mg*, magnesium, *SSRI*, selective serotonin reuptake inhibitor; *MAOI*, monoamine oxidase inhibitor; *NSAID*, non-steroidal anti-inflammatory drug; *Zn*, zinc.
Additional data from Danloff TA: Anesthesia and herbal supplements, *ASA Refresher Courses in Anesthesiology* 40(1):7–17, 2012; Laird J: Interactions between supplements and drugs: deciphering the evidence, *JAAPA* 24(12):44–46, 48–49, 2011.
*This is not a complete list of potential drug-herb interactions; a comprehensive drug-herbal interaction checker (e.g., Natural Medicines Comprehensive Database website) should be utilized.

state, the policies of their employer, and the relevant standards of practice before expanding their practice to incorporate some CAM modalities. NPs may have to pursue a broader interpretation and additional training or certification to ensure compliance with the terms of their state's Nurse Practice Act.

Continuing Education Opportunities

Over 60 academic medical centers or affiliated institutions in the United States and Canada now belong to the Academic Consortium for Integrative Medicine and Health. They offer clinical programs for medical students, residents, and other allied health professionals in integrative health care, clinical services, research, and/or education (Academic Consortium for Integrative Medicine & Health, n.d.). In Europe, CAM training and education for medical doctors is mostly provided through nonprofit associations and privately run schools and courses. Most European Union (EU) Member States include courses on CAM modalities in medical undergraduate curricula; some universities offer postgraduate training courses. There is an effort to institute state-recognized training courses and accreditation in the EU for CAM practitioners.

The NCCIH, American Medical Association, American Academy of Family Practice, American Nurses Association, American Nurse's Holistic Association, American Board of Integrative and Holistic Medicine, and other institutions (including hospitals) provide professional education in nonconventional treatment options. Many courses about CAM and herbal products are available online, and certifications of completion are offered. Integrative medicine conferences occur yearly in the United States; some conferences are specific to pediatrics.

Specific Complementary Therapies for Children and Adolescents

Table 43-4 lists some complementary treatments in use that address or augment pharmaceutical management of some health conditions present in children and/or adolescents. The complementary therapeutics in this table are based on evidence-based research as judged by the referenced authors

Text continued on p. 1237

TABLE 43-4 Complementary Treatments* for Some Health Conditions in Children and Adolescents

System/Field/ Diagnosis	Treatment Approach	Dosage	Benefit	Possible Side Effects	Research Citations Regarding Use
Cardiovascular					
Hypertension	**Herbal/Nutritional**				
	Garlic	350 mg twice daily or ½ to 2 cloves daily	↓ BP	Anticoagulant effect; GI irritation; garlic breath	Plotnikoff and Dusek, 2012; Xiong et al, 2015
	Omega-3 fatty acids (fish oil)	(See Omega-3 fatty acid diet at end of this table)	↓ BP, triglycerides, improves insulin sensitivity	Rare; GI irritation	Plotnikoff and Dusek, 2012; Miller et al, 2014
	Fish oil suppl	≥2 g/d			
	Cacao/dark chocolate (70% cocoa)	¼ of a standard-sized dark chocolate bar	↓ BP	None; no changes in weight, glucose, lipids	Plotnikoff and Dusek, 2012
	Coenzyme Q10	75 to 350 mg a day, taken with a meal containing some fat	↓ BP	Infrequent (GI discomfort, rash, headache; antiplatelet effect)	Plotnikoff and Dusek, 2012
	Mind-Body/Others				
	Biofeedback, device-guided breathing, transcendental meditation		↓ BP	None	Brook et al, 2013
	Tai chi, yoga, qigong	Use caution in those with low back pain	↓ BP	None	Plotnikoff and Dusek, 2012
Dental/Oral Health					
Aphthous stomatitis	**Herbal**				
	Deglycyrrhizinated licorice (DGL) (lozenges available as H-B12 Melts by OraCoat with 30 mg glycyrrhiza extract)	Lozenges: 1 (30 mg) lozenge melted in mouth in proximity of lesions every 6 hr; mouthwash of DGL (½ tsp with ¼ cup warm water) swished qid	Accelerates healing; under investigation as antiviral and immunomodulator	Rare allergic reactions if taken internally—do not swallow mouthwash; rare skin eruptions	Messier et al, 2012
	Tea tree oil	Apply topically bid; **not for ingestion**	Antifungal, antibacterial, anti-inflammatory	Rare allergic reaction	Pazyar et al, 2013 cite anti-inflammatory effect on gingival tissue
	Nutritional				
	Lactobacillus acidophilus	<12 yr: 2 tablets daily up to tid >12 yr: 4 tablets daily up to tid	Antifungal, antibacterial	None	Subiksha, 2014; home remedy
	Vitamins B_1, B_2, B_6, B_{12}, folic acid, iron	Multivitamin with minerals for age	Deficiencies in B vitamins occur more frequently in those with canker sores	None	Rakel, 2012

• Prevention	Vitamin B_{12}	≥18 yr: 1000 mcg, sublingually daily for 6 months	Prevention in those prone to canker sores	None; bright yellow coloration in urine	Rakel, 2012
Dental caries	**Xylitol**				
	Use a product that contains at least 50% of xylitol	4-6 g daily; 1 piece of gum chewed for 5 min qid (or 2 mints sucked)	Encourages remineralization; inhibits plaque; bacteria cannot colonize	None; diarrhea if recommended dose exceeded	American Academy of Pediatric Dentistry (AAPD), 2010; Nayak et al, 2014
Herpes simplex labialis	**Herbal**				
	70:1 lemon balm extract cream	Apply fairly thickly (1 mm) to help prevent outbreak; bid to qid at onset and 2-3 days after healing	Antiviral compounds; may prevent recurrences if used for initial infection; speeds healing	Safe; use with caution if taking thyroid medication; ↑ effects of barbiturates	Grassmann and Wissink, 2012; Schnitzler and Reichling, 2011
	Aloe vera (0.5% aloe extract cream)	Use topically several times daily at onset, for 2 wk	Speeds healing; anti-inflammatory	Contact dermatitis	Grassmann and Wissink, 2012
	Nutritional				
	L-Lycine	≥18 years: 1 g tid	Helps to prevent outbreak; has antiviral activity that blocks HSV replication	Diarrhea and abdominal pain if product used in excess (>10 g/day); may ↑ LDLs slightly	Grassmann and Wissink, 2012
Teething, infant	**Herbal**				
	Clove oil, topical	Dilute 1 gtt oil with 1-2 Tbsp of safflower oil; massage into gums bid/tid	Analgesic effect, antiviral, and antibacterial	Do not use >48 hr	Home remedy
Toothache, temporary relief	**Mind-Body**				
	Acupressure	Rub ice cube in the "anatomical saltbox" (Hoku point) for 5-7 min	Dulls pain	None	Shedletsky et al, 1984
	Acupuncture	For pre-dental pain management	↓ pain	None	Grillo et al, 2014
Dermatology					
Acne	**Herbal**				
	Goldenseal, extract or tincture (not for ingestion)	Teens: Use to wash face or apply on acne lesions	Antibacterial properties	Nontoxic at recommended dose	National Medicine Comprehensive Database, 2015 (anecdotal)
	Tea tree oil	Teens: 5% to 15% topical gel once daily or bid	Antiseptic and antifungal properties; comparable to 5% benzoyl peroxide with ↓ skin intolerance	Usually well tolerated; contact dermatitis in some; topical use unproven as male hormone disruptor (Carson, 2014)	National Center for Complementary and Integrative Health (NCCIH), 2012a; Zager, 2012

Continued

TABLE 43-4 Complementary Treatments* for Some Health Conditions in Children and Adolescents—cont'd

System/Field/ Diagnosis	Treatment Approach	Dosage	Benefit	Possible Side Effects	Research Citations Regarding Use
	Salicylic acid (OTC concentrations up to 2%)	Teens: Topically bid (start with 0.5% until tolerated and ↑ to 2%)	Breaks apart sebum plugs	Redness, irritation with higher concentration	Kemper, 2002; Zager, 2012
	Nutritional				
	Diet	↑ Low glycemic foods; eat organic dairy and meats; ↑ omega-3 foods (see Omega-3 diet at end of this table)	↓ immune-suppression; non-organic milk/meat may contain hormones	None	Kemper, 2002; Zager, 2012
	Zinc (picolinate, acetate, or monomethionine)	30 mg daily			Kemper, 2002; Zager, 2012
	Brewer's yeast	2 g tid			Zager, 2012
Atopic dermatitis/ skin irritations	**Herbal**				
	Aloe vera	All ages: Pure gel form or broken aloe leaf, applied TID	Antibacterial; anti-inflammatory	Contact dermatitis	Kuhn and Winston, 2008; Hajheydari et al, 2014
	Evening primrose oil	3 g PO daily; requires up to 16 wk for benefit	↓ scaling, inflammation, itching, severity	Rare, mild GI effects, headache	Bamford et al, 2013 (mixed results); Woolf et al, 2009a
	Atopiclair cream	≥6 mo old: apply tid	Anti-inflammatory	Safe for mild-moderate dermatitis dermatitis	Boguniewicz et al, 2008
• Severe, refractory atopic dermatitis	**Chinese Herbal**				
	Xiao Feng San	Taken orally; dosage dependent upon practitioner	Anti-inflammatory	None reported	Cheng et al, 2011
	Nutritional				
	Elimination diet†	Ensure adequate calcium, nutrients	Improvement in symptoms	Challenging; gives control to parents	Kaufman, 2012
	Combination probiotics inc. *Lactobacillus rhamnosus*	Infants/children: 5-10 billion CFU/d Teens: 20 billion CFU/d	Counteracts inflammatory response	None	Kaufman, 2012
	Omega-3 fatty acids (see Omega-3 fatty acid diet at end of this table)	Children: Fish oil suppl 1000 mg daily	↓ inflammation	Rare; platelet inhibition (stop 1 week prior to surgery)	Weydert, 2009a
• Diaper dermatitis, infant	**Nutritional**				
	Yogurt or probiotics containing live *L. acidophilus* bacteria or *Bifidobacterium bifidum*	Infants ≥6 mo: Give as yogurt; ½ to 1 cup daily PO <6 mo: Apply directly to diaper area	Thought to help replace the yeast on the skin	None noted	Kemper, 2002

Burns—minor	**Herbal**				
	Aloe vera (70% aloe vera gel or from fresh leaves)	Apply topically several times daily	Anti-inflammatory, anti-bacterial, aids wound healing	Contact dermatitis	Kemper, 2002; NCCIH, 2012b
	Calendula	Available in skin creams	Some anti-inflammatory properties; soothing	Rare rash	Kemper, 2002; Levatin, 2009a
	Mind-Body				
	Hypnosis		↓ pain and anxiety; ↑ coping skills	None	Culbert and Richtsmeier Cyr, 2009a
	Massage (of nonburned areas during healing; burned areas after healing)		For comfort, relaxation, ↓ pain and stress; ↓ itching, tightness; ↑ circulation, flexibility	None	McLellan, 2009a
Head lice	Bug Buster kit	Children: Combing regimen	Elimination of lice	None	WebMD staff, 2012
	Margarine; mayonnaise; petroleum jelly; Dr. Weil's mixture‡	Children: Apply heavy coating to hair and scalp; cover with shower cap overnight; wash out; comb repeatedly with nit comb		None; messy	Popular home remedy
Jock itch (fungal infection)	**Herbal**				
	Listerine mouthwash	Teens: Apply to groin area	Antifungal activity	Stings if placed in more delicate areas	Graedon, 2006
Molluscum contagiosum	**Herbal**				
	Combination: Tea tree oil and organically bound iodine	Children: 50:50 solution, applied bid to lesions	Antiviral, antibacterial; ↓ lesions by 30 days	Allergic dermatitis in sensitive patients; topical use not proven to be a male hormone disruptor (Carson, 2014)	Markum and Baillie, 2012
Onychomycosis	**Herbal**				
	Tea tree oil	Apply topically to affected nails bid for 3 mo	Antifungal, antibacterial, ↓ growth	Allergic dermatitis in sensitive people; topical use not proven to be a male hormone disruptor (Carson, 2014)	Flores et al, 2013

Continued

TABLE 43-4 Complementary Treatments* for Some Health Conditions in Children and Adolescents—cont'd

System/Field/ Diagnosis	Treatment Approach	Dosage	Benefit	Possible Side Effects	Research Citations Regarding Use
	Vicks VapoRub	>18 yr: Apply daily for up to 48 wk	Antifungal	None	Derby et al, 2011
	50:50 soln white vinegar/ amber Listerine mouthwash	Soak nails in soln 30 min/d for several months	Antifungal	Allergic dermatitis in sensitive people	Graedon, 2013
Warts, common	Duct tape (occlusive therapy)	Children/teens: Cover wart(s) with duct tape for 6 days (if falls off, replace); remove tape; soak wart in warm water and file with emery board; replace tape the next day and repeat regimen for 2 mo or until wart disappears	Most warts resolve within 1 month	None unless develops allergic reaction to tape	Iannelli, 2014
Ear/Nose/Throat					
Otitis media (OM)	**Nutritional**				
• Prevention of recurrent infection	Elimination diet†		Eliminates allergens that may impede immune system	None reported	Baral, 2009a
• Prevention	Xylitol gum	Older children: Chew two pieces five times daily	Anti-adhesive effects on oral micro-organisms; ↓ incidence OM	None; child must be able to chew gum safely; also may prevent caries	Kemper, 2002; Vernacchio et al, 2014
	Herbal				
Endocrine/Metabolic					
Diabetes, type 1 or 2, metabolic syndrome (not to be used at the exclusion of necessary pharmaceuticals)	**Nutritional**				
	Mediterranean diet (especially include onions) modified by ↓ high glycemic fruits/ grains; add chia grain; exclude eggs and other animal protein; ↑ fiber	As desired	Improved glycemic control; ↑ risk with meat/eggs; ↓ glucose with onions; 52% ↓ incidence of type 2 diabetes; ↑ quality of life	None	Linkner and Humphreys, 2012; McCarty et al, 2010; Nahas, 2012
Hypercholesteremia	**Nutritional**				
	Oat beta-glucan soluble dietary fiber	At least 3 g/d (about ½ cup cooked steel-cut oats = 4 g; 1 cup cooked rolled oats = 4 g; one instant package oats = 3 g)	Reduces plasma total and low-density lipoprotein cholesterol	None	Othman et al, 2011

PMS	**Herbal**				
• Breast tenderness	Evening primrose oil	Teens: 1.5 g bid (continuous)	May help ↓ tenderness	Possible minor GI symptoms	Gardiner and Kemper, 2000; Low Dog, 2012
• Insomnia	Valerian root	Teens: 2-3 g crude herb or std extract at hs	Mild sedative, sleep-promoting, anxiolytic	**Do not take if pregnant or lactating**	Low Dog, 2012
• Depression/ irritability	St. John's wort	Teens: 300 mg to 600 mg std to 3% to 5% hyperforin or 0.3% hypericin tid (continuous)	↓ depression	**Avoid** if taking an antidepressant, protease inhibitors, cyclosporine, any drug metabolized by cytochrome P-450 CYP3A4 system or P-glycoprotein	Low Dog, 2012
• Anxiety, moodiness	Black cohosh *(Cimicifuga racemosa)*	Teens: 20 to 40 mg bid std extract (triterpene glycoside)	↓ anxiety, tension, depression by binding 5-HT7 receptors	**Do not use if pregnant or lactating**	Low Dog, 2012
• Breast tenderness, anxiety, moodiness	Chasteberry *(Vitex agnus-castus)*	Teens: 250 to 500 mg/d dried fruit or 20-40 mg/d liquid extract	↓ secretion of prolactin; ↑ progesterone; binds opiate receptors	**Do not use if pregnant or lactating;** occasional minor skin irritations	Low Dog, 2012
	Nutritional				
• Mood swings	Calcium	Teens: 500-600 mg bid, as calcium carbonate or citrate	Improves mood; ↓ cramping, backache, nervousness	Avoid taking at same time: Iron supplements, tetracycline, steroids, pharmaceutical thyroid medications	Low Dog, 2012
• Cramps	Magnesium	Teens: 200 to 600 mg/d as chelate, citrate, or glycinate or as dietary sources (green leafy vegetables, tofu, legumes, nuts, seeds, whole grains)	Relieves dysmenorrhea, likely by inhibition of prostaglandin $F_{2\alpha}$	GI symptoms; cause in people with renal problems	Low Dog, 2012
• Depression	Vitamin B_6 (pyridoxine) or in active form as pyridoxal-5-phosphate or as part of multi-vitamin	Teens: 50-100 mg/d	May ↑ synthesis of serotonin, dopamine, norepinephrine, histamine, taurine	Reports of nerve damage with prolonged ingestion of 150 mg/day	Low Dog, 2012
	Diet	Eat diet high in fiber and low in saturated fat; avoid salt, processed foods, junk/fast foods, caffeine, sugar, and dairy	↓ serum estrogen; ↑ magnesium absorption; ↓ bloating; aid in glucose metabolism		Low Dog, 2012
	Mind-Body/Others				
	Relaxation, yoga, qigong		May be useful for certain individuals		

Continued

TABLE 43-4 Complementary Treatments* for Some Health Conditions in Children and Adolescents—cont'd

System/Field/ Diagnosis	Treatment Approach	Dosage	Benefit	Possible Side Effects	Research Citations Regarding Use
Gastrointestinal					
Abdominal pain, recurrent/ IBS	**Manipulative**				
	Hand acupuncture	Children: Use with essential oils—peppermint, roman chamomile, sweet fennel, ginger, rosemary, lavender, frankincense, mandarin	Causes relaxation of the proximal stomach	None; topical lavender not proven to be a male hormone disruptor (Carson, 2014)	Culbert and Richtsmeier Cyr, 2009b; Fitzgerald, 2009a
	Mind-Body/Energy				
	Therapeutic touch, CBT, biofeedback, hypnosis, meditation, yoga, Reiki		↑ self-regulation skills; improve sleep; restore energy flow		Weydert, 2012
	Herbal				
	Peppermint oil, enteric-coated only stated explicitly for enteric use	60-100 lb: 180-200 mg capsule tid >100 lb: 2 capsules tid	↓ pain by relaxing stomach muscles and supporting peristalsis	Possible heartburn, rectal discomfort/burning	Nightingale and Talley, 2013
	Chamomile: Extracts of 1 g/1 mL (1:1) or 1 g/4 mL (1:4) dilutions	Give three to five times daily: 35 lb: 1:1—4-8 gtts; 1:4—1/2 tsp 75 lb: 1:1—8-15 gtts; 1:4—1 tsp 150 lb: 1:1—15-30 gtts; 1:4—2 tsp	Anti-inflammatory effects; relaxation smooth muscle; anxiolytic	Safe, unless allergic to ragweed, asters, chrysanthemums, daisies	Nightingale and Talley, 2013
	Ginger (¼-inch slice fresh ginger root is about 10 g, (equivalent to dry powdered root in capsule of 1-2 g)	Fresh root can be brewed as tea, chopped and added to foods, soups, and salads ≥35 lb: 0.25-0.5 g dry powdered ginger root per day (2.5 g fresh) ≥75 lb: 0.5-1 g dry powdered root daily (5 g fresh) ≥150 lb: 1-2 g dry powdered root daily (10 g fresh)	Improves gastric motility; antispasmodic on visceral smooth muscle	Higher doses can cause GI upset; has antiplatelet effects	Nightingale and Talley, 2013
	Nutritional				
	Added fiber	↑ fruits, legumes, vegetables, whole grains	↓ constipation	None	Weydert, 2012
	Elimination diet		To detect/eliminate foods causing sensitivities		Weydert, 2012

	Use sucrose only; eliminate lactose, fructose, sorbitol		↓ clinical symptoms		Weydert, 2012
	Probiotics				
	LGG or combination *B. bifidum, L. acidophilus* or *Lactobacillus reuteri*	Children: 10 to 100 billion CFUs	↓ frequency and pain	None; **do not use** if immunocompromised or if has a central line	Weydert, 2012
Colic	**Nutritional**				
	12% sucrose solution	Infants: 5½ tsp sugar in 8 oz water: give 2 mL over 30-60 sec for 1-2 days during inconsolable crying	Analgesic—stimulates secretion of endogenous endorphins	None	Arikan et al, 2008
	Probiotics				
• Acute or preventive	*L. reuteri* (DSM 17938 strain used in studies of efficacy)	10^8 CFU/d (5 drops) for 90 days	↑ gut motility and function to ↓ gas, reflux, abdominal pain, cramping	None	Chumpitazi and Shulman, 2014; Savino et al, 2010
	Herbal				
	Tea with German chamomile, mint, fennel, licorice, or vervain; other herbs used by different cultures (anise, catnip, peppermint leaf, fennel, caraway seed, ginger root, dill)	Infants: Give in weak tea form (mix ½ to 1 tsp of herb in boiling water; steep 5 min): give ½ to 4 oz tid German chamomile tea: ½ cup or 150 mL; no more than tid at times of colic episode Mothers: drink same teas	Calming, sedating effects (antispasmodic on smooth muscles of digestive tract)	Rare allergic reaction (dermatitis, asthma, dyspnea, anaphylaxis) in people with hypersensitivity to daisy family	Kemper, 2002; Gardiner, 2007
	Chiropractic				
	Cranial sacral technique	Average of three treatments	Corrects rotational forces due to in utero positioning or from difficult labor or delivery	None reported	Spicer, 2009a (cites studies showing up to 94% resolution)
	Nutritional				
• Breastfed infants	Eliminate certain foods in mother's diet	For 1 wk no dairy, wheat, eggs, spicy food, caffeinated drinks, or foods causing gas in mother	Colic symptoms improved	None; counsel mother on alternative foods	Baral, 2009b

Continued

TABLE 43-4 Complementary Treatments* for Some Health Conditions in Children and Adolescents—cont'd

System/Field/ Diagnosis	Treatment Approach	Dosage	Benefit	Possible Side Effects	Research Citations Regarding Use
	Mind-Body/Others				
	Aromatherapy with essential oils of bergamot, Roman chamomile, ginger, mandarin	Place oil in a vaporizer/diffuser in infant's room			Fitzgerald, 2009a
	Acupressure	Gently squeeze the acupressure point between infant's thumb and finger (on the webbing)	Calms fussy infant		University of Maryland Medical Center, 2012a
	Massage (use lavender oil as massage vehicle)	Massage tummy lightly with baby on side, head somewhat down and bottom elevated; give 20-30 min after a meal; can extend massage to include entire body	Calming, relaxes	None if done gently; not proven to be a male hormone disruptor (Carson, 2014)	McLellan, 2009b (study involved massage three times daily)
	Motion	Gentle rocking or rolling in rhythmic and relaxed manner; can use front or backpack	Calming, relaxes	None	McLellan, 2009b
Crohn disease/IBD	**Nutritional**				
• Management of symptoms only; non-curative	Coconut (a medium-chain triglyceride [MCT]; anecdotal information of efficacy)	Eat 2 to 3 coconut macaroon cookies daily; add flaked coconut to cereal (1-2 tsp); use coconut milk in smoothies; oil in salads or for cooking; use as much as needed for control	Possible antibacterial effect from lauric acid in coconut fat decreases inflammation	None	Crohn's and Colitis Foundation of America, 2013; Graedon, 2012; Mañé et al, 2009
	Specific Carbohydrate Diet or other low refined sugar/carbohydrate diets	Diet available (see Gottschall in References)	Avoids carbohydrate overload and over fermentation in the intestines	Diet very restrictive	Suskind et al, 2014 (possible therapeutic option for pediatric Crohn disease)
	Dietary supplements	Take all these daily: Omega-3 (fish oil): 1000 mg Folate: 1 mg Calcium: 1000-1500 mg Vitamin D: 1000-2000 IU Vitamin B_{12}: 400 mcg Zinc: 15-20 mg (take with 2-4 mg/d copper) Iron: 30 mg (take with source of vitamin C) Magnesium: 500-1000 mg (in form of magnesium citrate, orotate, or aspartate for better absorption)	Reduces clinical symptoms and disease activity; replaces lost nutrients from inflammation and malabsorption; helps avoid other clinical symptoms (e.g., osteopenia, growth delay, skin disorders)		Weydert, 2009b

	Probiotics				
• Ulcerative colitis/IBD	LGG, *L. reuteri, bifidobacteria, Escherichia coli* Nissle, *Saccharomyces boulardii,* VSL#3	<26 lb: 10 billion CFU/day >26 lb: 20 billion CFU/day Use on trial basis for 2-3 mo; capsules can be opened and placed in liquids/soft foods	Remission	Well tolerated; **do not use** in preemies, those immunocompromised, or with central venous catheters	Floch, 2014; Greenfield, 2009a
Gastroenteritis/ diarrhea	**Herbal**				
	Berberine-containing plants (goldenseal, barberry, Oregon grape, or Chinese remedy—huanglian coptis chinensis) **Only use Chinese herbal preparations prepared by a licensed herbalist** Avoid agrimony, cocklebur, alder, or leaves and tops of betony—these contain high levels of cancer-causing tannins	Goldenseal: Toddlers and older children: ¼ - ½ tsp tincture or ⅛ tsp fluid extract tid/qid can be mixed with water or juice Berberine: Children: 5 mg/kg; adults: 25-50 mg tid or daily dosage up to 150 mg *Giardia:* Children, 5 mg/kg/day for 6 days; **stop vitamin C**	Demonstrated benefits of ↑ antimicrobial activity against bacteria (includes *E. coli, Shigella, Salmonella, Klebsiella, E. aerogenes*), fungi, protozoa, including *Giardia* When used with any indicated antibiotics, ↓ length of illness	Hypotension or hypertension, nausea, vomiting, diarrhea **Not recommended for infants younger than 1 month old or in those with jaundice**	Baral, 2009c; Kemper, 2002
	Nutritional				
• Prevention and treatment acute gastroenteritis	*LGG, L. reuteri, B. bifudum,* and/or *S. boulardii*	<26 lb: 10 billion CFU/day >26 lb: 20 billion CFU/day If using yogurt, make sure it contains these bacteria	↓ incidence and treatment of diarrhea in infants/ children; reinforces mucosal wall barrier	Flatulence, constipation **Do not use in those with impaired immune systems**	Ciccarelli et al, 2013; Floch, 2014; Greenfield, 2009b; Guarino et al, 2014
• Antibiotic-associated diarrhea with *Clostridium difficile*	*S. boulardii,* LGG, in combinations	Same as above for 3-4 weeks	Prevention *C. difficile* infection; fecal microbial transplantation effective as a cure	None	Floch, 2014; Greenfield, 2009b
• Preventive when taking antibiotic	LGG, *L. reuteri, B. bifidum*	Take along with antibiotic and continue for at least a week after antibiotic stopped	Prevention diarrhea	None; **do not use if immunocompromised**	Greenfield, 2009b
	5% carob pod powder (*Ceratonia siliqua*)	Infants to 1 yr: 1.5 g/kg/day in formula or in ORS or Pedialyte Children >1 yr: 1-15 g/kg/d in ORS or milk; stop 24 hr after first formed stool	Possibly tannins inhibit growth of bacteria and bind bacterial toxins	None; do not rely solely on this product	Kemper, 2002; University of Maryland Medical Center, 2012b
	Garlic (enteric-coated tablets/capsules, dried or powdered garlic, standardized for allicin content)	>1 yr: ½-1 clove (or 2-4 g/day) chewed, chopped, bruised, or crushed; do not use more than 2 cloves of raw garlic daily, as toxic in high doses	Treats *Entamoeba histolytica;* is antimicrobial; may interfere with microbial structures and functions	Garlic breath; has anti-clotting effect; burning mouth, rash, sweating, GI upset, lightheadedness	Baral, 2009c

Continued

TABLE 43-4 Complementary Treatments* for Some Health Conditions in Children and Adolescents—cont'd

System/Field/Diagnosis	Treatment Approach	Dosage	Benefit	Possible Side Effects	Research Citations Regarding Use
• Acute diarrhea	Acupuncture		Focuses on strengthening qi meridians	None	University of Maryland Medical Center, 2012b
IBS	**Herbal**				
	Peppermint oil, enteric-coated that states explicitly for enteric use only	60-100 lb: 180-200 mg capsule up to tid >100 lb: 2 capsules tid	↓ Pain by relaxing stomach muscles and supporting peristalsis	Heartburn, rectal burning	Grundmann and Yoon, 2014; Weydert, 2012
	Iberogast (combination of nine herbal extracts) (OTC)	Take tid and PO: Infants <3 mo: 6 gtts 3 mo-3 yr: 8 gtts 3-6 yr: 10 gtts 6-12 yr: 15 gtts ≥12 yr: 20 gtts	Reduces GI spasms and improves function and motility; relaxes stomach muscles; anti-inflammatory and anti-bacterial; regulates stomach acid; ↓ gas, and bloating	**Avoid if allergic to ragweed** (contains chamomile) or have sensitivity to licorice root (headaches, fatigue, ↑ BP)	Grundmann and Yoon, 2014
	Probiotics				
	L. acidophilus, L. plantarum, L. rhamnosus, B. breve, B. lactis, B. longum, B. infantis B5624, Streptococcus thermophilus have all been used	Once or twice daily	Relief of IBS symptoms	None; **do not use in the immunocompromised or with central lines**	Guandalini et al, 2014; Kennedy et al, 2014
	Mind-Body/Other				
	Hypnotherapy, CBT, yoga acupuncture	Use along with conventional treatments	Improved treatment outcomes	None	Guandalini et al, 2014; Kennedy et al, 2014
Nausea and vomiting	**Herbal**				
	Combination tea with chamomile, lemon balm, peppermint	Children: Small, frequent sips	Soothing	**Do not take if allergic to ragweed or daisy family of plants**	Kemper, 2002
	Goldenseal or barberry	Children: Tincture: 2-3 gtt in 4 oz water, sipped slowly over 1 hr	Helpful if child has vomiting and diarrhea	None reported at therapeutic levels	Kemper, 2002
	Basil tea	Older children: ½ oz dry basil and 1 cup boiling water; steep 5 min; strain		**Not recommended for infants or toddlers**	Kemper, 2002

	Ginger root: ¼-inch slice fresh ginger root (about 10 g is equivalent to dry powdered root in capsules of 1-2 g)	Powdered ginger: <3 yr: 0.25 g qid 3-6 yr: 0.50-0.75 g qid 6-12 yr: 1.25 g qid >13 yr: 2.50 g qid Ginger tea: 1 cup water to 1 tsp grated fresh ginger (simmer 5 min) or ¼ tsp fresh grated ginger in juice, applesauce, or cereal; or, ginger soda (with real ginger)	Helps to reduce nausea by promoting elimination of intestinal gas and reducing GI spasms	**Not for long-term use;** Use recommended doses as large doses can cause cardiac dysrhythmias, depress CNS, anti-coagulant effect	Kemper 2002; Saberi et al, 2014; Weydert, 2012
	Mind-Body/Energy				
	Hypnosis, Reiki, therapeutic touch	Age dependent	↓ recurrent nausea and vomiting	None reported	Kemper, 2002
	Acupressure or Acupuncture	Apply pressure 1 inch up from wrist crease, between the two tendons leading to the palm; repeat every 2 hr as needed to control nausea (can use travelers Nei-Kuan Point elastic wrist bands sold widely)	Delays onset of motion sickness; used in pregnancy; acupuncture controls post-op and chemotherapy-induced N/V	None reported	Hunt and Ernst, 2011
Genitourinary					
Nocturnal enuresis	**Mind-Body**				
• Nocturnal enuresis with other dysfunction	Biofeedback	For use in children ≥5 yr of age	↓ incontinence, dysuria, urgency	None	Culbert and Richtsmeier Cyr, 2009c; Ebiloglu et al, 2014
	Hypnosis	Trial of three to four visits to see if helps		Discontinue if no improvement	Culbert and Richtsmeier Cyr, 2009c; Huang et al, 2011
	Acupuncture	Several weeks of treatments		None	Huang et al, 2011
UTI prevention	**Herbal**				
	Cranberry juice, extract caps, or pure liquid extract mixed with OJ to ↓ tangy taste	Children/teens: Juice 150-600 mL/day Teens: 400 mg capsule once or bid	↓ adhesion of gram-negative and gram-positive bacteria to bladder wall cells	Safe; can ↑ urinary oxalate levels; use cautiously if has sugar sensitivity	Pettit, 2002; Williams et al, 2013
	Nutritional				
	Vitamin A Vitamin E Probiotics		Vitamins A and E support immune system, protect epithelial mucosal barrier; ↑ microflora balance	None	Sobouti et al, 2013; Williams and Craig, 2009

Continued

TABLE 43-4 Complementary Treatments* for Some Health Conditions in Children and Adolescents—cont'd

System/Field/ Diagnosis	Treatment Approach	Dosage	Benefit	Possible Side Effects	Research Citations Regarding Use
Neurology					
Attention-deficit disorder (ADD) or attention-deficit/ hyperactivity disorder (ADHD)	Homeopathy	Dosage dependent on practitioner; remedies may include *Stramonium, Cina, Hyoscyamus niger*		Considered safe alone or when combined with other CAM or allopathic medicine	Levatin, 2000b; University of Maryland Medical Center, 2013
	Herbal				
	Chamomile, hops, lemon balm, passionflower, or valerian	Children: For nighttime sleep hygiene	Promote calm, ↓ agitation; promote sleep	None; avoid kava	Kemper, 2012
	Ningdong (Chinese herb) (alternative to methylphenidate)	5 mg/kg/day (study dose)	↓ ADHD symptoms by helping regulate dopamine metabolism	Safe; fewer side-effects than methylphenidate	Li et al, 2011
	Nutritional				
	Dietary changes	See specific diet exclusions at end of this table. Diet changes preferable over giving listed supplements that follow; best to purchase organic foods to avoid pesticides; ensure adequate hydration	Results mixed; certain foods and additives may be causing neurotransmitter imbalances and fatty acid, vitamin, and mineral deficiencies, gut dysbiosis, or heavy metal toxicities	An elimination diet can put strain on family; best done in consultation with nutritionist None reported with suggested foods	Kemper, 2012; University of Maryland Medical Center, 2013
	Magnesium	200 mg daily	Regulates muscles and nerve function, helps with irritability, attention span, mental confusion	Diarrhea, drowsiness, weakness, lethargy if overdose; drug interaction with antibiotics and antihypertensives	University of Maryland Medical Center, 2013
	Zinc	35 mg/day	Regulates activity of brain chemicals, fatty acids, melatonin	Higher doses can be dangerous	University of Maryland Medical Center, 2013
	Fish oil supplements (omega-3 [EPA] and omega-6 [DHA]) plus diet changes noted at end of this table	500-2000 mg/daily combined EPA and DHA Ratio of omega-6 to omega-3 should be 4:1 Dietary omega-6: seeds, soy, canola oil, safflower oil, borage, red meats	Improves visual processing and motor coordination in those with dyslexia and dyspraxia—may help with ADHD	Safe to try; ↑ omega-3 has anticoagulant effect	Kemper, 2012

	Mind-Body/Energy				
	Yoga, tai chi, qigong (especially good for those with ADHD)	Twice weekly	↑ relaxation; ↓ anxiety, hyperactivity, inappropriate emotions; improves conduct	None reported	Culbert et al, 2009; Kemper, 2012
	Exercise	Minimum 30 min daily; martial arts particularly good	↑ brain-derived neurotrophic factor levels to enhance attention and memory; promote discipline	None	Kemper, 2012
	Music therapy (Hemi-Sync has music albums geared for ADHD)	Children listen to calm, low-pitched, slow-tempo music	↑ performance, ↓ tension and activity; calming effect on ANS; individual differences noted	High-pitched, fast, stimulating music can create tension, anxiety, activity, poor focus	Pelham et al, 2011; Rickson, 2006
	Neurofeedback	Takes 20-40 sessions over several weeks to learn techniques; age dependent	↑ attention and executive function	None	Steiner et al, 2014 (significant results over control)
	Musiko with Pepe (a behavioral therapy-oriented group training for children)	School age; combines music and physical activity	↑ concentration, impulse control; ↑ memory, social and emotional competence	None	Rothmann et al, 2014
	Meditation	Young children: A few minutes daily School age: 10 minutes bid Teens: 40-60 minutes daily	↑ attention, cognition, creativity; ↓ stress reactivity, absenteeism, behavioral problems, distractibility	None	Kemper, 2012
Autism	Qigong sensory training (QST)	A 15-minute massage protocol for parents taught by QST trainers; best if initiated pre-kindergarten	Opens sensory pathways for receiving coherent data from senses to improve sensory and regulatory responses, digestion, sleep	None	Silva et al, 2009, 2011
	Nutritional				
	Gluten-free/casein-free diet		Addresses abnormal intestinal permeability; ↑ buildup of opioid-like peptides; food allergies		Weydert, 2009c
	Omega-3 fatty acids (EFAs)	1000 mg EFA daily (combination of EPA, DHA, GLA)			Weydert, 2009c

Continued

TABLE 43-4 Complementary Treatments* for Some Health Conditions in Children and Adolescents—cont'd

System/Field/ Diagnosis	Treatment Approach	Dosage	Benefit	Possible Side Effects	Research Citations Regarding Use
	Probiotics				
	Lactobacillus GG, L. plantarum, L. paracasei, L. reuteri, L. acidophilus, Bifidobacterium infantis studied	Trial of 2-4 mo <12 kg: 10 billion CFU/day >12 kg: 20 billion CFU/day	Some autistic children have GI symptoms with ↑ irritability, anxiety, social withdrawal; ↓ GI symptoms with probiotics	None	Borre et al, 2014; Critchfield et al, 2011; Greenfield, 2009c
Cerebral palsy	Therapeutic (subthreshold) electrical stimulation (also known as neuromuscular electrical stimulation [NMES])		Pulses electricity into motor nerves; ↑ range of motion, strength and function		Wright et al, 2012
Headaches	**Herbal**				
	Feverfew *(Tanacetum parthenium)*	>12 yr: 125 mg up to tid; try for several months; sudden cessation may result in rebound headaches	↓ frequency; anti-inflammatory; if NSAIDs do not work, neither will feverfew (similar actions)	Mouth sores, abdominal pain; **do not use in pregnancy or if any clotting issues**	Mann and Coeytaux, 2012; NCCIH, 2012c
	Mind-Body/Other				
• Tension and migraine headaches	Biofeedback (including thermal biofeedback and bifrontal surface electromyography [EMG] biofeedback)	≥6 yr: As needed to master techniques (4 to 12 sessions over 6-10 wk); daily home practice results in greater improvement in pain	Child learns to dilate blood vessels to affect blood flow to the head and relax muscles; ↓ pain frequency/intensity	None; technique very popular with children familiar with computer age technology	Culbert and Richtsmeier Cyr, 2009d; Jones, 2014; Kemper, 2002
	Massage (to face, head, neck, shoulders) (alternative foot massage using reflexology points or cranial sacral)	Lotion: Mix 1-2 gtt lavender, peppermint, or eucalyptus oil with 1 tsp vegetable oil	Muscle relaxation; oil may help decrease pain sensitivity	None reported	Fitzgerald, 2009b; NCCIH, 2012c
	Self-hypnosis		Evidence of suppression in mast cell activation; ↓ frequency	None	Culbert and Richtsmeier Cyr, 2009d
	Progressive relaxation				Culbert and Richtsmeier Cyr, 2009d
	Chiropractic or cranial sacral therapy	All ages: Manipulation of cervical, skull, spinal vertebrae	Pain reduction, ↓ tissue restrictions	None to rare with cervical manipulation	NCCIH, 2012c; Spicer, 2009b
	Acupuncture (adjunct to allopathic care)	Age: As tolerant; non-needle techniques available	↓ frequency, days with migraine	None reported	NCCIH, 2012c; Wang et al, 2011

	Nutritional				
	Diet changes	Eliminate foods that typically cause headaches (see specific diet exclusions at end of this table); can try formal elimination diet[†]; ensure adequate hydration	Benefits children with frequent headaches; vitamin A excess ↑ intracranial pressure; vitamin D and zinc can cause HAs	None reported	Weydert, 2009d
	Riboflavin (B_2)	>12 years: 200 mg bid		None reported	American Headache Society, 2013; Mann and Coeytaux, 2012; NCCIH, 2012c
	Magnesium suppl (or increase magnesium-rich foods [nuts, legumes, dark leafy green vegetables, whole grain cereals and breads, seafood] and include ginger and hot peppers, garlic, onion, vegetable oils, fish oils)	Children: Targeted intake: 30-400 mg daily Teens: 400-500 mg/d	Lessens sensitivity to pain; low magnesium levels often found in patients with all types of headaches, including menstrual-related	Diarrhea, gastric irritation; pregnancy category A at 400 mg daily	Mann and Coeytaux, 2012; NCCIH, 2012c
	CQ10	Teens: 150-300 mg/d; 3 mo trial	↓ frequency	Rare GI symptoms	Mann and Coeytaux, 2012; NCCIH, 2012c
Insomnia, onset	**Herbal**				
	Melatonin	Take 1-2 hours prior to bedtime: <40 kg: 0.3-3 mg >40 kg: 6-10 mg	Advances circadian rhythms; ↑ sleep time	Regarded as safe	Kemper, 2010; Mann and Coeytaux, 2012
	Valerian root, crude herb or standardized extract of 0.8%	Trial 2-4 weeks; take at hs Children: 100-300 mg Adolescents: 300-900 mg	Mild anxiolytic effects; promotes sleep	Rare GI irritation	Kemper, 2010; Mann and Coeytaux, 2012
	Mind-Body				
	Music therapy (can pair with muscle relaxation)	All ages: Slow, soft music (music for sleep available commercially)	↑ sleep quality	None	Kotsirilos et al, 2011; Street et al, 2014
Pain	**Mind-Body/Others**				
• Postsurgical or procedural	Music therapy, deep breathing, guided imagery, distraction (videos, video games, stories, blowing bubbles), relaxation, hypnosis, massage; transcutaneous electrical nerve stimulation		↓ anxiety and pain by stimulating endogenous opioid and nonopioid systems		Bellieni et al, 2013; Cotton et al, 2014; Dobson and Bryne, 2014; Kemper and Danhauer, 2005

Continued

TABLE 43-4 Complementary Treatments* for Some Health Conditions in Children and Adolescents—cont'd

System/Field/Diagnosis	Treatment Approach	Dosage	Benefit	Possible Side Effects	Research Citations Regarding Use
• Postsurgical	Acupuncture	Can be used across age ranges, as tolerated	Useful as adjunct for pain control	None reported	Wu et al, 2009
	Nutritional				
• Neonates: Preoperative or painful procedures	Breastfeeding, breast milk supplementation; non-nutritive sucking	Give during procedure	↓ in pain scores vs. when infants swaddled or held		Shah et al, 2012
	12% glucose solution	Mix 5½ tsp sugar in 8 oz water; give 2 mL over 30-60 sec	↓ pain	None	Messerer et al, 2014
	Acupuncture		↓ neonatal infant pain scale scores and crying	None reported	Ecevit et al, 2011
• Chronic	Combination of acupuncture and hypnosis	10-15 min tid	Significant ↓ in pain, per studies	None	Zeltzer et al, 2002
	Mind-Body				
	Music therapy		↓ tension; calming effect on ANS		Kemper and Danhauer, 2005
	Yoga, especially Iyengar		↓ functional disability and lower back pain		Evans et al, 2013; Williams et al, 2009
• For acute or chronic pain	Acupuncture		Analgesic	None reported	NCCIH, 2014b
	Mind-Body				
	Deep breathing, biofeedback, meditation, hypnosis		Alter states of arousal; facilitate sense of control; ↓ anticipatory anxiety	None reported	Culbert and Richtsmeier Cyr, 2009e; Cunningham and Kashikar-Zuck, 2013
	Manipulatory				
	Massage		↓ distress, pain, tension, discomfort; improved mood	None	McLellan, 2009c; Suresh et al, 2008
	Nutritional				
	Omega-3 fatty acids (see Omega-3 diet at end of this table)	Omega-3 fatty acid suppl 1000 mg/d or in diet	Anti-inflammatory	Mild GI distress	Wagner et al, 2014; Wall, 2010

	Herbal				
	Boswellia serrata, standardized not enriched	>120 lbs.: 250-500 mg up to tid	Anti-inflammatory and analgesic effect	None to mild GI upset; platelet inhibition	Cameron and Chrubasik, 2014; Selfridge and Muller, 2012
	Tumeric	Topically, orally, or in diet as curcumin	Anti-inflammatory	Regarded as safe	Woolf et al, 2009b
• Leg cramps	**Nutritional**				
	Mustard, yellow	1 tsp as needed	Fast relief	None	Anecdotal report
Premature infants/ low birth weight infants	**Massage**				
	Moderate pressure	At least tid	Facilitates weight gain; ↓ medical complications; ↑ GI motility, brain development; shorter hospital stays and costs	None	Fallah et al, 2013; Rangey et al, 2014
	Music therapy		↑ weight gain	None	Lubetzky et al, 2010
Sedation	Music therapy (before sleep deprived EEG)	1-5 yr: Soothing music of voice, guitar, and/or soft percussion; culturally appropriate	Produces sleep for procedures	None	Loewy et al, 2005 (97% of music therapy vs 50% chloral hydrate subjects able to complete EEG)
Psychology					
Anxiety	**Mind-Body/Others**				
	Aromatherapy: Use bergamot, chamomile, lavender, rosemary, peppermint, lemon, sweet orange essential oils	2 or 3 gtt of the essential oil in a vaporizer	↓ irritability; anxiety; ↑ relaxation	None to rare allergic skin or respiratory reactions if sensitive to ragweed, aster, chrysanthemums (daisy family of plants)	Fitzgerald, 2009c; Jafarzadeh et al, 2013
	Belly breathing	Place child's hand over his or her belly button and picture it as a balloon; have child breathe in through nose slowly, counting to 3-4, and blowing up "belly balloon"; breathe out through mouth slowly to a count of 6-8, deflating "balloon"; do for 1-2 min, working up to 10-20 min	↓ stress, anxiety, pain, panic, and heart rate	None	Ditchek and Greenfield, 2002
	Music therapy		↑ quality of life (emotional, social, physical well-being); ↓ anxiety	None	Bufalini, 2009; Cincinnati Children's Hospital Medical Center, 2012; Lin et al, 2011

Continued

TABLE 43-4 Complementary Treatments* for Some Health Conditions in Children and Adolescents—cont'd

System/Field/ Diagnosis	Treatment Approach	Dosage	Benefit	Possible Side Effects	Research Citations Regarding Use
	Massage		Improved behavior; ↓ cortisol levels, BP	Rare reactions to pressure; allergy to oil	Cotton et al, 2014; Sherman et al, 2010
	Meditation		Calms via neuro pathways		Simkin and Black, 2014
	Therapeutic touch		↑ relaxation; ↓ pain and anxiety	None	Kemper et al, 2009
	Exercise	Determined by level of fitness; work up to 30-60 min/d		Consider existing health conditions	Lee, 2012
	Yoga		↑ coping; ↓ stress	None if healthy	Re et al, 2014
	Herbal				
	Valerian (*Valeriana officinalis*—1% std valerenic acid)	Trial 6 weeks: Teens: 150-300 mg in morning; 300-600 mg evening	↓ anxiety	Rare GI symptoms, headaches	Lee, 2012
Mood disorders (depression, bipolar disorder) • Mild to moderate depression	**Herbal**				
	Phototherapy				
	Bright, white (full-spectrum, 10,000 Lux light from special bulbs, lamps, light boxes)	All ages: 30-60 minutes daily—light needs to fall on eyes	↓ seasonal affective disorder	None	Schneider and Lovett, 2012
	Nutritional				
	Omega-3 fatty acids, vitamins B and C, tryptophan (in turkey, nuts, soybeans, cooked beans and peas), tyrosine (eggs, aged cheese, tofu, seafood)	Mediterranean-style diet and low-processed foods. Eliminate caffeine and simple sugars *or* supplement with omega-3 fatty oil 1000 mg/d; vitamin B complex; folate	Omega-3 and fatty acid intake boosts mood and vagal tone, modulates inflammatory responses to stressors	Omega-3: Rare interaction with anticoagulants	Kiecolt-Glaser, 2010; Rey et al, 2008; Weydert, 2009e
	Mind-Body/Others				
	Exercise; use as adjunct therapy)	All ages: At least 5 days out of 7 for 30-60 minutes	Improves energy, mood, appetite, sleep, self-esteem	Avoid if anorexic with compulsive over-exercising	Cooney et al, 2014; Toseeb et al, 2014

	Yoga, meditation, hypnosis, imagery, tai chi, mindfulness-based CBT, music therapy	Appropriate ages	Enhance efficacy of other treatments	None	Schneider and Lovett, 2012
	Acupuncture	Depends on age	Alters neurotransmitter levels	Rare	Schneider and Lovett, 2012
• Suicidal ideation	Mindful meditation	Mentored 3-12 minute silent meditation daily	↓ risk suicidal/self-harm thoughts	None	Britton et al, 2014 (small study)
Respiratory					
Asthma	**Nutritional**				
	Diet exclusions (see in footnotes at end of table)	Use onions, garlic liberally plus foods high in omega-3 fatty acids *or* suppl (teens: 500 mg cap bid/tid)	↑ allergic threshold and prevent acute attacks; onions and garlic inhibit release of inflammatory chemicals; omega-3 fatty acids improve airway responsiveness	Requires diet compliance; asthmatics that regularly eat fresh, fatty fish have significantly better lung function and decrease risk of asthma; can alter platelet function; caution in diabetics	Mark, 2012; Weydert, 2009f; D'Auria et al, 2014; Mark, 2012
	Vitamin B_6 (effects seen after 1 mo)	<50 lb: 8-15 mg bid 50-100 lb: 12-25 mg bid >100 lb: 25-50 mg bid	Improved peak flow rates; ↓ wheezing		Kemper, 2002; Mark, 2012; Weydert, 2009f
	Vitamin C	10-30 mg/kg/day in divided doses (max 250 to 500 mg once or twice daily)	Inhibits histamine release, promotes vasodilation; may ↓ EIB	None	Kemper, 2002; Mark, 2012
	Vitamin D_3	<4 yr: 400 IU/day ≥4 yr: 600 IU/day	↓ frequency asthma attacks	None	Mark, 2012
	Vitamin E	>100 lb: 200-400 IU daily	↓ oxidative damage to lungs; ↑ control	Do not exceed 400 IU/day	Mark, 2012; Weydert, 2009f
	Magnesium	<50 lb: 60-125 mg tid 50-100 lb: 100-200 mg tid >100 lb: 200-400 mg tid	Adequate levels necessary for lung function; affects asthma severity		Gontijo-Amaral et al, 2007; Mark, 2012
	Zinc (tablets or liquid)	1-10 yr of age: 15 mg/day >10 yr: 30-60 mg daily	Levels found to be lower in asthmatics	Take with food to avoid upset stomach	Baral, 2009d
	Selenium	1 yr to adolescence: 50-100 mcg daily Adolescents: 100-200 mcg daily	Levels found to be lower in asthmatics	GI distress; toxicity over 400 mcg daily	Baral, 2009d; Mark, 2012
	Probiotics				
	LGG, L. plantarum, L paracasei, L. reuteri, or *L. acidophilus, Bifidobacterium animalis*	<12 kg: 10 billion CFU/day >12 kg: 20 billion CFU/day Can mix with drinks or soft foods; try for 2-3 mo; if helps, continue	Possible ↑ interferon levels; ↓ inflammatory response	Well tolerated. **Do not use if immunocompromised, has a central line, or in preemies**	Greenfield, 2009d; Versalovic, 2013 (studies ongoing)

Continued

TABLE 43-4 Complementary Treatments* for Some Health Conditions in Children and Adolescents—cont'd

System/Field/Diagnosis	Treatment Approach	Dosage	Benefit	Possible Side Effects	Research Citations Regarding Use
	Mind-Body/Others				
	Acupuncture	Practitioner dependent; several treatments required	Study results mixed; some show effect	Rare	Mark, 2012; Pfab et al, 2014
	Hypnosis, guided imagery, belly breathing, biofeedback, yoga, Buteyko breathing technique (BBT)	Children can be good candidates	↓ symptoms and pharmaceutical medication use; ↑ effect in those with emotional component to illness	None	Mark, 2012
	Massage	Daily, up to 20 minutes	Improves peak airflow, ↓ asthma attacks	None reported	Fattah and Hamdy, 2011; Mark, 2012
	Physiotherapy (breathing exercises and massage of thoracic muscles [Lotorp method])		↓ respiratory symptoms during rest and exercise; ↑ chest expansion	None	Löwhagen and Bergqvist, 2014
	Qigong	Regular, self-conducted exercises practiced up to bid for <30 min (depending on response)	↑ peak air flow, ↓ asthma; ↓ costs, ED visits, pharmaceutical medication use	None	Chow and Choy, 2009
Upper respiratory infection/flu	**Herbal**				
	Echinacea purpurea (do not use prophylactically)	Teens: 1-2 mL extract in juice or water sublingually; or 150-300 mg powdered extract; or 1-5 mL tincture (1:5 in ethanol) tid/qid at onset of symptoms for 3-4 days	May boost immunity	Allergy to aster family; not recommended for use in younger children	Barrett, 2012; Karsch-Völk, 2014 (mixed results for prevention or treatment of the common cold)
	Astragalus root	2-6 yr: 4-8 gtt liquid standardized extract or tincture every 12 hr 6-12 yr: 8-15 gtt every 12 hr (caps: 250-500 mg every 12 hr) Teens: 4-7 g (up to maximum 28 g daily)	Stimulates immune system, and may have interferon-like effects	None **Do not use in those with progressive infections (e.g., tuberculosis, HIV) or autoimmune diseases);** can interfere with immunosuppressants	Barrett, 2012; Kemper, 2002
	Tea made from ginger, cinnamon, cloves, allspice, cardamom	Put ⅛ tsp of each into 2 cups of water to make a tea; or cut up 1-2 inches of ginger root, boil pieces in a quart of water for 10-20 min; strain; cool; may sweeten	Helps fight chills and fatigue; ginger combats one of the common cold viruses	None	Kemper, 2002

Nutritional				
Vitamin C	Children: 250 mg qid or four to five glasses of OJ daily at onset of cold; ↑ other citrus fruit, kiwi, berries, melon, bell pepper, broccoli Teens: 500-1000 mg tid for 3 to 4 days after URI onset; 1 g/d prevention	↓ symptoms and length of illness by activating neutrophils to oxidize inflammatory mediators and ↑ extracellular vitamin C	Regarded as safe; GI upset, diarrhea in high doses **Do not exceed 10 g daily**	Hemilä, 2013 (study done on cold-induced asthma); Barrett, 2012; Nahas and Balla, 2011
Vitamin D_3	School age: Up to 1200 IU daily	↑ immune function; may ↓ incidence of influenza	None in prescribed doses	Borella et al, 2014
Chicken soup; peppers (including cayenne), mustard, horseradish, salsa, other spicy foods; use organic chicken	Sip soup slowly throughout the day	Thins nasal secretions, increases nasal and sinus mucous mobility	None reported	Barrett, 2012
Garlic	Raw clove minced in mashed potatoes (1 medium clove = 100,000 units penicillin); do not exceed 2 cloves a day Kyolic liquid garlic: 1-5 yr: ½ tsp; 6+ yr: 1 tsp in grape juice bid	May kill cold viruses; supports immune function; ↓ incidence URI	Safe, occasional GI upset, odor, rash	Kemper, 2002; Lissiman et al, 2014
Zinc lozenges (teens or older only) **Do not use intranasal zinc**	>18 yr: 15-25 mg lozenge sucked every 2 hr *for 7 days only;* administer within 24 hours of onset of symptoms	May ↓ severity and length of illness by binding rhinoviral docking sites with somatic cells, inhibiting infectivity	Mouth irritation, GI upset; can suppress immunity if taken >7 days; smell and/or taste changes with nasal or lozenges (can be permanent with intranasal products)	Sego, 2009; Singh and Das, 2013
Probiotics				
L. rhamnosus, LGG, *L. acidophilus, Bifidobacterium animalis*	<12 kg: 10 billion CFU/day >12 kg: 20 billion CFU/day May mix into drinks or soft foods	May prevent/ lessen URI symptoms	None	Mark, 2012
Mind-Body/Others				
Aromatherapy: Oils of thyme, rosemary, peppermint, ravensara, tea tree, eucalyptus, or bergamot	Inhaled by vaporizer or steam	Helps relieve congestion; heats nasal passages to inhibits viral replication	None reported	Fitzgerald, 2009d

Continued

TABLE 43-4 Complementary Treatments* for Some Health Conditions in Children and Adolescents—cont'd

System/Field/ Diagnosis	Treatment Approach	Dosage	Benefit	Possible Side Effects	Research Citations Regarding Use
	Massage: May use oil of menthol, camphor, eucalyptus	Cradle infant/child on one's shoulder or chest; massage face, head, back, shoulders, anterior chest wall, lymph glands with emphasis on intercostals, scalenes, serratus, pectorals, trapezius; downward motion; mentholated ointment rubbed on soles of feet then covered with socks can decrease coughing and improve breathing	Relieves musculoskeletal pain from coughing; calms; oil may cool the nose, causing perception of decreased nasal congestion	Safe, but do not apply directly under nose in order to avoid aspiration	Fitzgerald, 2009d; McLellan, 2009d
	Acupuncture		Aids blocked sinuses; ↑ speed of mucociliary transport; ↑ immune function	Included in WHO list of recognized therapies	Loo, 2009

5-HT, 5-hydroxytryptamine; *ADHD*, attention-deficit/hyperactivity disorder; *ANS*, autonomic nervous system; *ASA*, acetylsalicylic acid (aspirin); *bid*, *bis in die* (twice a day); *BP*, blood pressure; *CAM*, complementary and alternative medicine; *cap*, capsules; *CBT*, cognitive behavioral therapy; *CFU*, colony-forming units; *CNS*, central nervous system; *d*, day; *DHA*, docosahexaenoic acid; *ED*, emergency department; *EEG*, electroencephalogram; *EFA*, essential fatty acids; *EIB*, exercise-induced bronchospasms; *EPA*, eicosapentaenoic acid; *GABA*, gamma-aminobutyric acid; *GI*, gastrointestinal; *GLA*, gamma-linolenic acid; *gtt*, *gutta* (drop); *HAs*, headaches; *HIV*, human immunodeficiency virus; *hs*, hora somni (at bedtime); *HSV*, herpes simplex virus; *HTN*, hypertension; *IBD*, irritable bowel disease; *IBS*, irritable bowel syndrome; *inc*, including; *IU*, international units; K^+, potassium; *LDL*, low-density lipoproteins; *LGG*, *Lactobacillus rhamnosus* GG; *min*, minutes; *mo*, month; *MSG*, monosodium glutamate; *N/V*, nausea and vomiting; *NSAID*, nonsteroidal anti-inflammatory drug; *OJ*, orange juice; *ORS*, oral rehydration solution; *OTC*, over the counter; *PMS*, premenstrual syndrome; *PO*, *per os* (by mouth, orally); *post-op*, postoperative; *qid*, *quarter in die* (four times a day); *RCT*, randomized-controlled trial; *soln*, solution; *SSRI*, selective serotonin reuptake inhibitor; *std*, standardized; *suppl*, supplement; *tid*, *ter in die* (three times a day); *URI*, upper respiratory infection; *UTI*, urinary tract infection; *WHO*, World Health Organization; ↑, increase(d); ↓, decrease(d).

*Inclusion of a complementary treatment in this table does not imply endorsement or efficacy by this textbook's authors; for reference only.

†See Resources on the Evolve site for University of Wisconsin Integrative Medicine Department Elimination Diet guidelines.

‡**DR. ANDREW WEIL'S MIXTURE FOR HEAD LICE:** Mix together: 2 oz olive or coconut oil; 20 gtts tea tree oil, 10 gtts either rosemary, lavender, or lemon essential oil. Rub into scalp and hair; cover with towel or shower cap for 1 hr only; wash thoroughly and comb repeatedly with nit comb (Weil, 1998).

OMEGA-3 FATTY ACID DIET includes: wild salmon, herring, mackerel, cod, sardines; fish oil; flax and hemp seeds; walnuts; algae.

SPECIFIC DIET EXCLUSIONS (also See Resources on the Evolve site for University of Wisconsin Integrative Medicine Department Elimination Diet guidelines):

Asthma: Eliminate dairy products, eggs, soy, wheat, peanuts, fish, yeast (breads, cheeses, and mushrooms); sulfites (dried fruits); pesticide residues (best to buy organic); food additives (e.g., tartrazine or yellow dye no. 5); citric acid; benzoates; aspartame.

Attention-Deficit Disorder or Attention-Deficit Hyperactivity Disorder: Eliminate artificial colors (blue 1,2; green 3; orange 8, red 3, 40; yellow 5, 6), flavors, and preservatives (butylated hydroxyanisole [BHA], butylated hydroxytoluene [BHT—often in packaged cereals], tertiary butyl hydroquinone [TBHQ]), sweeteners (Truvia, Neotame, Alitame); naturally-occurring salicylates (found in many fruits and vegetables); decrease refined foods and sugars; increase foods high in protein and complex carbohydrates; specific foods causing allergic reactions; buy organic foods; increase garlic, onions, eggs; increase foods high in calcium, magnesium, zinc, cold-water fish, walnuts, flax (omega-3). Can also try eliminating apples, oranges, benzoates (chewing gum, margarine, pickles, prunes, tea, raspberries, cinnamon, anise, and nutmeg), caffeine, corn, dairy, nitrates, propyl gallate, sulfites (dried fruits, mushrooms, potatoes, baked goods, canned fish, and relishes), peanuts, and tomatoes.

Headache: Avoid known dietary triggers (may need to try elimination diet). Avoid aged cheeses, some nuts, onions, chocolate, aspartame, processed meats with nitrates (e.g., hot dogs/pepperoni), monosodium glutamate (MSG), refined sugar, processed carbohydrates; limit caffeine, avoid foods high in omega-6 fatty acids; ensure adequate hydration.

as being clinically reasonable or holding clues to promising areas needing further research. Physician authors engaged in research were used as much as possible to compile this table. It is noted in the table if a treatment is a commonly used home remedy or if use is based on anecdotal evidence. *Inclusion of a complementary treatment in this table does not imply adequacy of evidence nor endorsement by this textbook's editors and authors.* Clinicians are strongly encouraged to consult references that cite research and safety precautions (see Resources on the Evolve site for some suggestions) before utilizing any CAM treatment modality and seek further formal education regarding aspects of CAM they wish to utilize. When referencing Table 43-4, knowledge of the following terms is useful:

- *Standardized:* An herbal product that contains a *specified concentration of one ingredient* of the plant; it may contain other nonstandardized ingredients from the same plant.
- *Essential oils:* Also known as *volatile* or *aromatic oils* that are found in many plants. These oils are highly concentrated and potent and are not to be taken internally.
- *Infusion:* Preparation similar to tea. The dried herb is steeped in boiling water for 5 to 10 minutes and strained; the preparation can be sweetened to make it more palatable; drink warm or cold.
- *Tincture:* A concentrated extract of an herb made with a mixture of cold water and alcohol. The tincture usually is diluted four or five times with water or juice for children; tinctures should not be given internally to children younger than 2 years old.

For a complete list of references, please visit http://evolve.elsevier.com/Burns/pediatric/.

Index

Note: Page numbers followed by "*f*" refer to illustrations; page numbers followed by "*t*" refer to tables; page numbers followed by "*b*" refer to boxes.

B

D

H

I

J

K

L

M

U

W

X

Y

Z